D0916987

The 5-Minute Clinical Consult 2012

20TH EDITION

The 5-Minute Clinical Consult 2012

20TH EDITION

Editor-in-Chief

Frank J. Domino, MD
Professor
Clerkship Director
Department of Family Medicine and Community Health
The University of Massachusetts Medical School
Worcester, Massachusetts

Associate Editors

Robert A. Baldor, MD
Professor
Department of Family Medicine and Community Health
The University of Massachusetts Medical School;
Vice-Chairman
Department of Family Medicine and Community Health
UMass Memorial Health Care
Worcester, Massachusetts

Jeremy Golding, MD
Professor of Family Medicine and of Obstetrics and Gynecology
The University of Massachusetts Medical School
Quality Officer - Department of Family Medicine and Community Health
UMass Memorial Health Care - Hahnemann Family Health Center
Worcester, Massachusetts

Jill A. Grimes, MD
Clinical Instructor
Department of Family Medicine
University of Massachusetts Medical School
Worcester, Massachusetts;
Private Practice
West Lake Family Practice
Austin, Texas

Julie Scott Taylor, MD, MSc
Associate Professor of Family Medicine
Director of Clinical Curriculum
Alpert Medical School of Brown University
Providence, Rhode Island

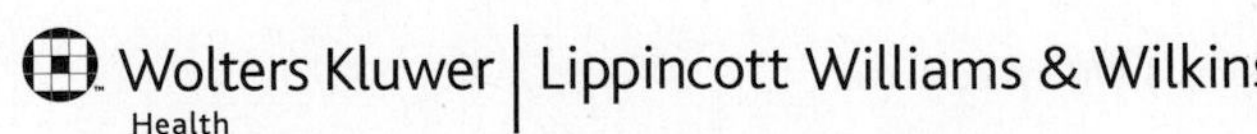

Philadelphia • Baltimore • New York • London
Buenos Aires • Hong Kong • Sydney • Tokyo

Acquisitions Editor: Avé McCracken
Product Manager: Michelle LaPlante
Vendor Manager: Bridgett Dougherty
Senior Manufacturing Manager: Benjamin Rivera
Marketing Manager: Kimberly Schonberger
Design Coordinator: Teresa Mallon
Production Service: Aptara, Inc.

Two Commerce Square
2001 Market Street
Philadelphia, Pa. 19103 USA
LWW.com

Printed in China

Library of Congress Cataloging-in-Publication Data

ISBN 13: 978-1-4511-3745-3
ISBN:10: 1-451-1374-51

To purchase additional copies of this book, call our customer service department at (800) 638-3030 or fax orders to (301) 223-2320. International customers should call (301) 223-2300.

Visit Lippincott Williams & Wilkins on the Internet: at LWW.com. Lippincott Williams & Wilkins customer service representatives are available from 8:30 am to 6 pm, EST.

10 9 8 7 6 5 4 3 2 1

CCS0311

"I'm just a tugboat, putting the big ships out to sea."
This is how my father viewed his role as a college professor and administrator. His greatest pride came not from his own accomplishments, but from seeing his students excel both in the academic realm and (more importantly) out in the real world. I believe my Dad embodied the spirit of all great teachers, regardless of their discipline, as he challenged his pupils to think critically, creatively and ethically, and then to act judiciously on those decisions.

I'd like to dedicate this edition to my father, Dr. William Litzinger, and all the wonderful teachers who continue to inspire their students. I am privileged that our editorial team is not only made up of such leaders, but led by my wonderful mentor, dear friend, and Professor of Medicine, Dr. Frank Domino. His generous offer to allow his associate editors a chance to dedicate our book is vintage Dr. Domino, as he continues to lift up those around him. To Frank—a sincere thank you.

Many of our authors are professors at medical schools spanning across our country and beyond, and I challenge all of our authors to recognize their topic is an extension of medical education, bringing current, evidence-based diagnostic and treatment guidelines outside the classroom and into our "real world" practices. Each author has the opportunity to be that effective teacher who directly impacts patient care across the globe. Again, I dedicate this book to each of you.

Finally, perhaps my greatest teachers in life are my husband, Drew, and our beautiful daughters, Brittany and Nicole. I am delighted my husband joins our team of authors this year, sharing his extensive clinical experience and medical wisdom from an anesthesia perspective. Every day I learn something new from each member of our family. Your love, support, patience and encouragement allow me to continue to dedicate my time and energy to this wonderful mission.

–Jill A. Grimes, MD

PREFACE

I don't know what your destiny will be, but one thing I know: the only ones among you who will be really happy are those who will have sought and found how to serve.

—Albert Schweitzer

All who participate in healthcare delivery, serve. If you are holding this book or looking at a screen, as a clinician, administrator or policy maker, you do so to help someone live a little better. This resource provides knowledge, but it is just one instrument in the toolbox of service. Adding skill, insight, and intuition makes you a master in your service.

I am honored to welcome you to the 2012 edition of the ***5-Minute Clinical Consult.*** Our editorial team has again collaborated with hundreds of authors to bring you this comprehensive and current resource whose mission is to assist in your service to your patients.

Using your feedback, we present this highly organized content and newly added features in print and online:

- Better and faster search functionality providing you with answers in **30 seconds or less**
- Current evidence-based designations highlighted in each topic's text
- A revised and updated Health Maintenance section
- More than 900 topics
- 200+ diagnostic and treatment algorithms linked to topics for quick diagnosis and treatment planning
- Video library for procedures and treatment
- Drug database from Facts & Comparisons including monographs, images, monthly updates and more
- More than 1,350 patient handouts in English and Spanish from The American Academy of Family Physicians linked directly from content
- Full-color images
- Updates that include new topics, videos, images, etc.
- Mobile version for quick reference on your Smartphone
- And more

Evidence based health care is the integration of the best medical information with the values of the patient ***and your*** skill as a clinician. We have improved our content and visibility of the best evidence, so you can focus on how to apply it.

The Health Maintenance recommendations included here have been updated through December 2010, based on the U.S. Preventive Services Task Force, and has been organized by age into *1-page* summaries.

Please check out the online and mobile versions at www.5minuteconsult.com. Your access is included in your purchase, allowing you to quickly reference the 5-Minute wherever needed. Included are over **900 topics** on the web via an easy-to-use interface. This new feature includes easy maneuverability between topics, algorithms, images, video procedures, and more as well as extra topics not in the book (including a pediatric section).

The algorithms section in the front of the book has been again expanded and includes both **diagnostic *and treatment* algorithms.** Our goal here is to provide you with a graphic method to evaluate an abnormal finding and how to prioritize treatment. I urge you to look through this section and recognize its utility.

Welcome to the 2012 edition of Lippincott Williams & Wilkins' 5-Minute Clinical Consult. The editorial team and I greatly value your observations and thoughts, so please drop me an email and share your thoughts, suggestions, and constructive criticism at 5MinConsultFeedback@lww.com.

Frank J. Domino, MD
Professor
University of Massachusetts Medical School
Worcester, Massachusetts
January 9, 2011

EVIDENCE-BASED MEDICINE

WHAT IS EVIDENCE BASED MEDICINE AND WHY IS THIS NEW?

Remember when we used to treat every otitis media with antibiotics? These recommendations came about because we applied logical reasoning to observational studies. If bacteria cause an acute otitis media, then antibiotics should help it resolve sooner, with less morbidity. Yet, when rigorously studied (via a systematic review), we found little benefit to this intervention.

The underlying premise of evidence-based medicine (EBM) is the evaluation of medical interventions, and the literature that supports those interventions, in a systematic fashion. EBM hopes to encourage treatments proven to be effective and safe. And when insufficient data exists, it hopes to inform you, on how to safely proceed.

EBM uses as endpoints of real patient outcomes; morbidity, mortality and risk. It focuses less on intermediate outcomes (bone density), and more on patient conditions (hip fractures).

Implementing EBM *requires* 3 components: the best medical evidence, the skill and experience of the provider, and the values of the patients. Should this patient be screened for prostate cancer? It depends on what is known about the test, on what you know of its benefits and harms, your ability to communicate that information, and that patient's informed choice.

"All this in 15 minutes" you ask? This is not an easy task. My goal is to provide you with the tools to assist in this process.

This book hopes to address the first EBM component; providing you access the best information in a quick format. While not every test or treatment has this level of detail, many of the included interventions here use systematic review literature support.

The language of medical statistics is useful to interpreting the concepts of EBM. Below is a list of these terms, with examples to help take the confusion and mystery out of their use.

POPULATION INFORMATION

These terms are designed to help you and epidemiologists look at the "community" as a whole, and determine how frequently disease occurs:

Prevalence: *Proportion of people* in a population who have a disease

"In the US, "0.3% (3 in 1,000) people over the age 50 have colon cancer"

Incidence: How many *new cases of a disease* occur in a population during an interval of time; for example, "the estimated incidence of colon cancer in the US is 104,000 in 2005"

TESTING INFORMATION

We often hear the words *Sensitivity* and *Specificity* and cringe. They are, at a minimum, very confusing. These terms are characteristics of a test, but they tell us little about the lab result we are holding in our hands. Rather, it is the *Predicative Value* that helps us interpret test results.

ML is a 53-year-old woman who you saw for a Health Maintenance visit; you ordered a *screening* mammogram and the report demonstrates an irregular area of microcalcifications. She is waiting in your office to receive her test results; what can you tell her?

Sensitivity (Sn): percent of People with Disease who test positive; for mammography, the Sensitivity is 71–96%.

Specificity (Sp): percent of People without Disease who test negative; for mammography, the Specificity is 94–97%.

Does this help in your discussion with ML? No, because these tests refer to characteristics of people who are known to have disease (sensitivity) or those that are known not to have (specificity) disease. What you have is an abnormal test result. To better explain this result to ML, you need to know the Positive Predictive Value.

Positive Predictive Value (PPV): Percent of **Positive** Test Results that are truly positive; the PPV for a woman 50–59 ~22%. Only 22% of abnormal screening mammograms in this group truly identified cancer. The other 78% are false positives.

Negative Predictive Value (NPV): Percent of negative test results that are truly negative.

You can tell ML only 1 out of 5 abnormal mammograms correctly identify cancer; the 4 are false positives, but the only way to know which mammogram is correct is to do further testing.

You may both find some comfort knowing the chance she has cancer is so low.

The PPV and NPV tests are population dependent, while the Sensitivity and Specificity are characteristics of the test, and have little to do with the patient in front of you. So when you receive an abnormal lab result, especially a screening test like mammography or PSA value, understand their limits based upon their PPV and NPV.

TREATMENT INFORMATION

In discerning the statistics of randomized, controlled trials of interventions, first consider an example. The Scandinavian Simvastatin Survival Study (4S): (*Lancet.* 1994;344(8934):1383–1389) found using simvastatin in patients at high risk for heart disease for 5 years resulted in deaths in 8% of patients vs. 12% of those on placebo; this results in a Relative Risk of 0.70, a Relative Risk Reduction of 33%, and a Number Needed to Treat of 25.

There are two ways of considering the benefits of an intervention with respect to a given outcome. The Absolute Risk Reduction (ARR) is the difference in the percent of people with the condition before and after the intervention. Thus, if the incidence of MI was 12% for the placebo group and 8% for the simvastatin group, the ARR is 4% (12–8% = 4%).

The Relative Risk Reduction (RRR) reflects the improvement in the outcome as a percentage of the original rate and is commonly used to exaggerate the benefit of an intervention. Thus if the risk of MI were reduced by simvastatin from 12% to 8% then the RRR would be 33% (4%/12% = 33%). 33% may appear better than 4%, the 4% that reflects the true outcome.

ARR is usually a better measure of *clinical* significance of an intervention. For instance, in one study, the treatment of mild hypertension was been shown to have a RRR of 40% over 5 years (40% fewer strokes in the treated group). However, the ARR was only 1.3%. Because mild hypertension is not strongly associated with strokes, aggressive treatment of mild hypertension yields only a small clinical benefit. Don't confuse Relative Risk Reduction with Relative Risk.

Absolute (or Attributable) Risk (AR): The percent of people in the placebo or intervention group who reach an end point; in the simvastatin study, the absolute risk of death was 8%

Relative Risk (RR): The risk of disease of those treated or exposed to some intervention (i.e., simvastatin) divided by those in the placebo group or who were untreated.

—If RR <1.0, it reduces risk—the smaller the number, the greater the risk reduction.

—If RR >1.0, it increases the risk—the greater the number, the greater the risk increase.

Relative Risk Reduction (RRR): The relative decrease in risk of an end point compared to the percent of that endpoint in the placebo group.

If you are still confused, just remember the RRR is an over estimation of the actual effect.

Number Needed to Treat (NNT): This is the number of people who need to be treated by an intervention to prevent one adverse outcome. A "good" NNT can be a large number (>100) if risk of serious outcome is great. If the risk of an outcome is not that dangerous, then lower (<25) NNTs are preferred.

The NNT should be compared to a similar statistic, the Number Needed to Harm (NNH). This is the number of people who have to be given treatment before one excess side effect or harm occurs. When the NNT is compared to the NNH, you and the patient can judge whether the benefit of the intervention is great enough to outweigh the risk of harm.

REFERENCES

To help you interpret diagnostic and treatment recommendations within the *5-Minute Clinical Consult*, we have graded the best information within the text, and highlighted this content.

An "A" grade means the reference is from the highest-quality resource, like a systematic review. A *systematic review* is a summary of the medical literature on a given topic that uses strict, explicit methods to perform a thorough search of the literature and then provides a critical appraisal of individual studies, concluding in a recommendation. The most prestigious collection of systematic reviews is from the Cochrane Collaboration (www.cochrane.org).

A "B" grade means the data referenced comes from high-quality randomized controlled trials performed to minimize bias in their outcome. Bias is anything that interferes with the truth; in the medical literature, it is often unintentional, but is much more common than we appreciate. In short, always assume some degree of bias exists in any research endeavor.

A "C" grade implies the reference used does not meet the A or B requirements; they are often treatments recommended by consensus groups (like the American Cancer Society). In some cases, they may be the standards of care. But implicit in a group's recommendation is the bias of the author or the group that supports the reference. For example, the American Urological Society's recommendation around screening for prostate cancer may be motivated by their need for funding rather than patient outcomes. Compare this to the highly valid recommendations of the U.S. Preventive Services Task Force (www.ahrq.gov), the organization that determines which health maintenance interventions are reasonable, and does so with the least bias.

BIAS

Bias is anything interferes with the truth. There are many types of bias that should be considered by the publishers of medical information. Below describes a number of bias types which often affects our care without us knowing it is present.

Publication bias occurs when research is not published; this is often when a study finds data that does *not* support an intervention. The motivation to publish information that "didn't work" is low. It is estimated that up to 40% of all medical research never gets published. So when you read of an intervention that "works," wonder if other studies were done that didn't show benefit and went unpublished.

Comparator bias occurs when research compares an intervention to placebo, when placebo isn't the standard of care. Knowing a new antibiotic is more effective than placebo for treating acute otitis media is not helpful if you typically use amoxicillin.

Why not release research comparing the new drug to the standard of care? Often, the research has been done, and the new drug proved no better. If this study does not get published, you have an example of Publication Bias.

Selection bias involves either using a tool that doesn't discriminate between populations selected or just reporting a just subset of study participants from a study. Either will result in the data being skewed because it can only be applied to small subset of people.

Attrition bias and the concept of intention to treat. Attrition bias is when researchers do not fully acknowledge and address how a study deals with participants who do not adhere to the research protocol or drop out completely. Intention to Treat Analysis hopes to diminish Attrition Bias by statistically considering the non-adhering or dropped out patients as unsuccessfully benefiting from the intervention.

Commercial (funder) bias involves who paid for the research being done, and do they have a vested interest in the outcome. Despite its size and scope, the recent *Jupiter* trial on treating low risk adults with a statin has been called into question as the company who funded the study makes the brand name drug used in the study and the lead author is part owner of the unique test employed in the trial. The data may be accurate, but until this is studied by less vested interests, some feel its outcome cannot be clinically applied.

I hope this brief introduction to EBM has been informative, clear, and helpful. If any of the information above seems unclear, or if you have a question, please drop me an email at 5MinConsultFeedback@lww.com

ACKNOWLEDGMENTS

This 20th edition of the *5-Minute Clinical Consult*, powered by its content, and supported by its ever-updated and improved interfaces, continues to be the most clinically useful tool in your health care box. From the diagnostic and treatment algorithms, through the knowledge components of each topic, and including the appendices like the Health Maintenance section, one cannot find a better collect of clinically useful content.

A book and Web site of this magnitude requires an equally broad effort from its supporting team. I wish to thank the dedication and tireless efforts of the team: Point-of-Care Editor, Ave McCracken; Senior Managing Editor, Michelle LaPlante; Kim Schonberger, Marketing Manager; Lisa McAllister, Director, Electronic Product Strategy; and Jennifer Gibson, Content Technology. They have given of themselves far beyond their call of duty, and I am deeply indebted to their effort. For the vision of making the 5-Minute the leading resource in health care around the world, my sincerest thanks to Diane Harnish, who brought us together. Lastly, my sincerest thanks for the gifts of Arlene and Marion.

This 2012 edition is the direct result of the dedication and insights of our Associate Editors. I wish to thank Drs. Robert Baldor, Jeremy Golding, Jill Grimes, and Julie Scott Taylor for their insights, hard work, and overwhelming commitment to the *5-Minute Clinical Consult.*

I wish to especially thank my wife, Sylvia, and my daughter, Molly, who have given greatly for this book.

The challenge of completing a book covering this broad a spectrum of medicine requires insights and skills far beyond my own. Many thanks to my mentors Bob Baldor and Mark Quirk who are an enormous support—always there to encourage, reassure, and impart wisdom.

Many in the academic and health care worlds are due thanks for support, insight, and friendship: Daniel Lasser, Alan Chuman, Michele Pugnaire, Karen Rayla, Isabel Feliciano, Phil Fournier, Erik Garcia, Jeff Stovall, Jim Comes, Len Levin, Judy Norberg, J. Herb Stevenson, Mick Godkin, Zainab Nawab, Sanjiv Chopra, Susan Gauquier, Vasilios (Bill) Chrisostomidis, James (Jay) Broadhurst, Danuta Antkowiak, Atreyi Chakrabarti, Kerry Morse, Mark Powicki, Steve Messineo, and the faculty and students of the University of Massachusetts Medical School.

Medicine is a challenge I have fortunately not had to meet alone. Thanks to my parents, Frank and Angela (Jean); my brother John and his family, Marylou, Cate, and Jane; Frank, Mary Anne, Diane, and David Christian; the Diana and Hymie Lipschitz family; and the Bob and Ruth Pabreza family; they are responsible for who I am and my success in life.

I am blessed with the best of friends; without them, I would not be a physician. Thanks to Bob Bacic, Ron Jautz, Richard Onorato, John Horcher, Auguste Turnier, Bob Smith, Paul Saivetz, Antoinette and (Gary) Francis, Bob and Nancy Gallinaro, Drew and Jill Grimes, Louay Toma, Laurie, Alan, Daniel, Jenny and Matt Bugos, Alan Ehrlich, Teri and Andy Jennings, Mark Steenbergen, John and Kathleen Polanowicz, Phil Pettine, Mark Shelton, Steve Bennett, Vicki Triolo, Michael Bernatchez, and Milo.

–Frank J. Domino, MD

CONTRIBUTING AUTHORS

Jose Abad, MD
University of California, Davis
Sacramento, California

Dawn Abbott, MD
Department of Internal Medicine
Rhode Island Hospital
Providence, Rhode Island

Cheryl Abel, PharmD
Assistant Professor of Pharmacy Practice
Massachusetts College of Pharmacy and Health Sciences
Manchester, New Hampshire

George Abraham, MD, MPH
Associate Professor
Department of Medicine
University of Massachusetts Medical School;
Associate Program Director
Department of Internal Medicine
Saint Vincent Hospital
Worcester, Massachusetts

Luis K. Abrishamian, MD
Department of Emergency Medicine
University of Southern California Medical Center
Los Angeles, California

Abdulrazak Abyad, MD, PhD, MBA, MPH, AGSF, AFCHSE
Director, Abyad Medical Center & Middle East Longevity Institute
Tripoli, Lebanon

Amos O. Adelowo, MD, MPH
Department of Obstetrics and Gynecology
University of Massachusetts Memorial Hospital
Worcester, Massachusetts

Ronald Adler, MD
Assistant Professor
Department of Family and Community Health
University of Massachusetts Medical School
Worcester, Massachusetts

Nitin Aggarwal, MD
Warren Alpert Medical School of Brown University
Providence, Rhode Island

Maria I. Aguilar, MD
Assistant Professor of Neurology
Department of Neurology
Mayo Clinic College of Medicine;
Consultant, Department of Neurology
Mayo Clinic Hospital
Phoenix, Arizona

Augusto Aguirre, MD
Department of Pathology
Corpath, Inc.
Columbus, Ohio

Francisco Aguirre, MD
Department of Pathology
Corpath, Inc.
Columbus, Ohio

Jaspal S. Ahluwalia, MD, MPH
Preventive Medicine
Walter Reed Army Institute of Research
Silver Spring, Maryland

Mazen J. AlBeldawi, MD
Department of Internal Medicine
Cleveland Clinic Foundation
Cleveland, Ohio

Antoin M. Alexander, MD
Associate Program Director
Staff Family Physician
Department of Family Medicine
David Grant Medical Center
Travis AFB, California

Fozia A. Ali, MD
Department of Family Medicine
University of Texas Health Science Center, San Antonio
University Hospital
San Antonio, Texas

Satya Allaparthi, MD
Fellow, Robotic Laparoscopic Urology
University of Massachusetts Medical School
Worcester, Massachusetts

Andrew Allegretti, MD
Department of Internal Medicine
Harvard Medical School
Massachusetts General Hospital
Boston, Massachusetts

Richard W. Allinson, MD
Associate Professor
Department of Ophthalmology
The Texas A&M University System, Health Sciences Center
College Station, Texas;
Senior Staff Physician
Department of Ophthalmology
Scott & White Clinic
Waco, Texas

Ginger Allister, MD
University of Massachusetts Medical School
Worcester, Massachusetts

Brian Alverson, MD
Assistant Professor
Department of Pediatrics
Warren Alpert School of Medicine
Brown University;
Head of Pediatric Hospitalist Section
Department of Pediatrics
Rhode Island Hospital
Providence, Rhode Island

James G. Anderson, MD
University of Massachusetts Medical School
Worcester, Massachusetts

Jeffrey Scott Anderson, MD
Department of Psychiatry
Vanderbilt University
Nashville, Tennessee

Nadeem Anwar, MD
Assistant Professor of Medicine
University of Massachusetts Medical School
Worcester, Massachusetts

Armin Arasheben, MD
Department of Family Medicine
State University of New York Upstate Medical Center;
Department of Medical Education
St. Joseph's Hospital
Syracuse, New York

Steffani Araya, MD
University of Massachusetts Medical School
Worcester, Massachusetts

Ivan A. Arenas, MD, PhD
Department of Internal Medicine
Framingham Union Hospital
MetroWest Medical Center
Framingham, Massachusetts

Paul Arguin, MD
Medical Epidemiologist
Centers for Disease Control and Prevention
Atlanta, Georgia

James J. Arnold, DO
Faculty
Department of Family Medicine
David Grant (USAF) Medical Center
Travis Air Force Base, California

Patricia K. Aronson, MD
Assistant Professor
Generalist Division
Department of Obstetrics and Gynecology
University of Massachusetts Memorial Medical Center
Worcester, Massachusetts

Elias Arous, MD
Associate Chief Medical Officer
Chief, Surgery
UMass Memorial Medical Center;
Professor of Surgery
University of Massachusetts Medical School
Worcester, Massachusetts

Melissa E. Arthur, LCSW, MA
Assistant Professor
Department of Family Medicine
SUNY Upstate Medical University;
Director, Behavioral Science
Family Medicine Residency
St. Joseph's Hospital
Syracuse, New York

Swati B. Avashia, MD
Clinical Assistant Professor
Department of Family Medicine
University of Texas Southwestern
Austin, Texas

Mouhanad Ayach, MD
University of Massachusetts
Fitchburg Family Medicine
Fitchburg, Massachusetts

Jennifer L. Ayres, PhD
Clinical Psychologist
University of Texas Southwestern Medical Center Austin
Austin, Texas

Stephen J. Bacak, DO, MPH

Elisabeth L. Backer, MD
Clinical Associate Professor
Department of Family Medicine
University of Nebraska Medical Center
Omaha, Nebraska

Yolanda Backus, MD
Family Practice
Rockville, Maryland

Elizabeth Bade, MD
Clinical Assistant Professor
Department of Family Medicine
University of Wisconsin School of Medicine and Public Health
Madison, Wisconsin;
Chief
Department of Family Medicine
Aurora Sinai Medical Center
Milwaukee, Wisconsin

Faisal Badri, MD
Consultant and Head of General Surgery Unit
Department of Surgery
Rashid Hospital and RH Trauma Center
Dubai, United Arab Emirates

Justin M. Bailey, MD
Assistant Professor
Department of Family Medicine
Uniformed Services University of Health Sciences
Bethesda, Maryland;
Faculty
Department of Medicine Residency
David Grant Medical Center
Travis Air Force Base, California

Sangeetha Balasubramanian, MD
Fellow
Department of Rheumatology
University of Massachusetts Medical School
Worcester, Massachusetts

Robert A. Baldor, MD
Professor
Family Medicine and Community Health
University of Massachusetts Medical School;
Vice-Chairman
Family Medicine and Community Health
University of Massachusetts Memorial Health Care
Worcester, Massachusetts

Jerry Balikian, MD
Professor
Departments of Medicine and Radiology
University of Massachusetts Medical School
Worcester, Massachusetts

Brent J. Barber, MD
Assistant Professor of Clinical Pediatrics (Cardiology)
Director, UMC Pediatric Cardiac Services
University of Arizona College of Medicine
Tucson, Arizona

David M. Barclay, III, MD, MPH, FAAFP
Associate Professor
Associate Chair
Undergraduate Education Department of Family and Community Medicine
Temple University School of Medicine
Philadelphia, Pennsylvania

Daniel J. Barker, MD
University of Massachusetts Medical School
Worcester, Massachusetts

Katharine Barnard, MD
Assistant Professor
Department of Family Medicine
University of Massachusetts Medical School;
Plumley Village Health Services
University of Massachusetts Memorial Medical Center
Worcester, Massachusetts

Timothy J. Barreiro, DO
Associate Professor of Medicine
Department of Internal Medicine
Ohio University College of Osteopathic Medicine;
Section Chief, Critical Care Medicine
Section of Pulmonary and Critical Care
Humility of Mary Health System, St. Elizabeth Hospital
Youngstown, Ohio

Michael C. Barros, PharmD, BCPS
Ambulatory Care Pharmacy Resident
Department of Pharmacy
Providence Veterans Affairs Medical Center
Providence, Rhode Island

Adam Barta, MD
Assistant Professor
Department of Family Medicine
University of Texas Southwestern, Austin
Austin, Texas

Kay A. Bauman, MD, MPH
Clinical Professor
Department of Family Medicine and Community Health
John A. Burns School of Medicine
University of Hawaii at Manoa
Honolulu, Hawaii

Francesca L. Beaudoin, MS, MD
Assistant Professor
Department of Emergency Medicine
Warren Alpert Medical School of Brown University;
Attending Physician
Department of Emergency Medicine
Rhode Island Hospital
Providence, Rhode Island

Armando Bedoya, MD
Warren Alpert Medical School at Brown University
Providence, Rhode Island

Petra Belady, MD
Department of Obstetrics and Gynecology
University of Massachusetts Medical School
Worcester, Massachusetts

Paul Belliveau, PharmD, RPh
Associate Professor of Pharmacy Practice
Massachusetts College of Pharmacy and Health Sciences
Worcester, Massachusetts;
Clinical Pharmacist
Pharmacy
Concord Hospital
Concord, New Hampshire

Daniel E. Belz, MD
Department of Family Medicine
University of Nebraska Medical Center
Omaha, Nebraska

Elise R. Bender, MD
University of Massachusetts Medical School
Worcester, Massachusetts

Sheldon Benjamin, MD
Director, Psychiatry Residency Training
Director, Neuropsychiatry
University of Massachusetts Medical School
Worcester Massachusetts

Andrew Bentley, MS
Clinical Herbalist
Private Practice
Lexington Complementary and Integrative Therapies
Lexington, Kentucky

Jamie Berkes, MD
Instructor, Hepatology
Department of Medicine
University of Illinois at Chicago Medical Center
Chicago, Illinois

Robert E. Berry, Jr., MD
Associate Professor Obstetrics and Gynecology
Obstetrics and Gynecology Residency Program Director
University of Massachusetts Medical School
UMass Memorial Medical Center
Worcester, Massachusetts

Bryan Beutel, MD
The Warren Alpert Medical School of Brown University
Providence, Rhode Island

Jacob L. Bidwell, MD
Assistant Professor of Family Medicine
University of Wisconsin Medical School
Milwaukee, Wisconsin

Dale E. Bieber, MD
Associate Professor
Department of Medicine
University of Iowa
Iowa City, Iowa

Garreth C Biegun, MD
House Staff Officer in Emergency Medicine
Warren Alpert Medical School
Brown University;
Resident Physician
Department of Emergency Medicine
Rhode Island Hospital, Lifespan Health System
Providence, Rhode Island

Kenneth M. Bielak, MD
Sports Medicine Fellowship
University Tennessee-Knoxville
Knoxville, Tennessee

Jhilam Biswas, MD
University of Massachusetts Medical School
Worcester, Massachusetts

Melissa Phillips Black, MD
Instructor of Clinical Medicine
Internal Medicine, Geriatrics Division
Emory University School of Medicine
Atlanta, Georgia

Robert M. Black, MD
Clinical Professor of Medicine
Department of Renal Medicine
UMass Medical School;
Chief, Division of Renal Medicine
St. Vincent Hospital & Fallon Clinic
Worcester, Massachusetts

Timothy L. Black, MD
Pediatric Surgeon
Department of Pediatric Surgery
Cook Children's Medical Center
Fort Worth, Texas

Joseph Blazuk, MD
University of Massachusetts Medical School
Worcester, Massachusetts

Kimberly Bombaci, MD
University of Massachusetts Medical School
Worcester, Massachusetts

Naomi F. Botkin, MD
Assistant Professor
Division of Cardiovascular Medicine
University of Massachusetts Medical School and Memorial Center
Worcester, Massachusetts

Jaclyn Boulais, MD
University of Massachusetts Medical School
Worcester, Massachusetts

Katherine Boyle, MD
University of Massachusetts School of Medicine
Worcester, Massachusetts

Doreen Brettler, MD
Department of Hematology/Oncology
University of Massachusetts Medical School
Worcester, Massachusetts

Ivan J. Briones, MD
University of Massachusetts School of Medicine
Worcester, Massachusetts

Juan-Pablo Brito-Campana, MD
Department of Endocrinology
Mayo Clinic
Rochester, Minnesota

Ekaterina Brodski-Quigley, MD
UMass Memorial Medical Center
Worcester, Massachusetts

Theodore R. Brown, DO, MPH
Preventive Medicine Officer
Headquarters, U.S. Central Command
Departments of Family, Preventive, and Occupational and Environmental Medicine
MacDill Air Force Base, Florida

Patricia Bruno, DO
Assistant Professor
Director of Inpatient Services;
Department of Family Medicine
University of Connecticut School of Medicine
Saint Francis Hospital and Medical Center
Hartford, Connecticut

Karen Bryant, MD
Hospitalist Program
Concord Hospital
Concord, New Hampshire

Kathleen Bryant, MS, APRN, BC
Family Nurse Practitioner
Montpelier Health Center
Central Vermont Medical Center
Montpelier, Vermont

Rebecca Burch, MD
UMass Memorial Medical Group
Worcester, Massachusetts

K. John Burhan, MD
Instructor
Department of Family Medicine
Creighton University School of Medicine
Omaha, Nebraska

John R. Burk, MD
Adjunct Professor
Integrative Physiology
University of North Texas Health Science Center;
Owner/Partner
Texas Pulmonary & Critical Care Consultants, PA
Fort Worth, Texas

Kristin Burke, MD
University of Massachusetts Medical School
Worcester, Massachusetts

Leah A. Burnett, MD
Department of General Surgery
University of Pittsburgh Medical Center / Mercy Hospital
Pittsburgh, Pennsylvania

Harold J. Bursztajn, MD
Associate Clinical Professor
Department of Psychiatry
Harvard Medical School;
Associate Clinical Professor
Department of Psychiatry
Beth Israel Deaconess Medical Center
Boston, Massachusetts

David E. Burtner, MD
Vice Chairman and Professor
Department of Family and Community Medicine
Mercer University School of Medicine
Macon, Georgia

Nancy Byatt, DO, MBA
Associate Professor
Department of Psychiatry
University of Massachusetts Medical School;
Attending Psychiatrist
Psychosomatic Medicine and Emergency Mental Health
Department of Psychiatry
University of Massachusetts Medical Center
Worcester, Massachusetts

Adriana Cabrera, PharmD
Assistant Professor of Pharmacy Practice
Massachusetts College of Pharmacy and Health Science;
Consulting Pharmacist
Department of Family Medicine
Family Health Center of Worcester
Worcester, Massachusetts

David Cachia, MD
Department of Neurology
University of Massachusetts Medical School
Worcester, Massachusetts

Marie Ellen Caggiano, MD, MPH
Assistant Professor
Department of Family Medicine and Community Health
University of Massachusetts Medical School;
Physician
Hahnemann Family Health Center
Worcester, Massachusetts

Mitchell A. Cahan, MD
Assistant Professor
Department of Surgery
University of Massachusetts Medical School;
Director of Acute Care Surgery
Department of Surgery
UMass Memorial Medical Center
Worcester, Massachusetts

Kristy M. Cahill, MD
University of Massachusetts Medical School
Worcester, Massachusetts

Katherine M. Callaghan, MD
Department of Obstetrics and Gynecology
University of Massachusetts Medical School
Worcester, Massachusetts

Jennifer A. Caragol, MD
Assistant Professor
Department of Family and Community Medicine
University of Kentucky
Lexington, Kentucky

Paloma F. Cariello, MD
Department of Infectious Diseases
University of Massachusetts Medical School
Worcester, Massachusetts

Stephanie Carinci, MD
Central Florida Neurologic Consultants
Deland, Florida

David Carne, MD
Department of General Surgery
Northeast Ohio University College of Medicine
Rootstown, Ohio;
Department of General Surgery
Akron General Medical Center
Akron, Ohio

Stephanie Carreiro, MD
Department of Emergency Medicine
Brown University;
Rhode Island Hospital
Providence, Rhode Island

Laurie A. Carrier, MD
Clinical Instructor
Department of Family and Community Medicine
Northwestern University Feinberg School of Medicine
Family Physician and Psychiatrist
Heartland International Health Center
Chicago, Illinois

Mary Cataletto, MD
Associate Professor of Clinical Pediatrics
Department of Pediatrics
SUNY Stony Brook
Stony Brook, New York;
Associate Director
Pediatric Pulmonology
Winthrop University Hospital
Mineola, New York

Jan Cerny, MD, PhD
Assistant Professor of Medicine
Department of Medicine
Division of Hematology and Oncology
University of Massachusetts Medical School;
UMass Memorial Medical Center
Worcester, Massachusetts

Olga M. Céron, MD
Retina/Vitreous Specialist
Staff Physician
Massachusetts Eye Research and Surgery Institution (MERSI)
Cambridge, Massachusetts

Teresa V. Chan, MD
Assistant Professor
Department of Otolaryngology—Head and Neck Surgery
University of Texas—Southwestern Medical Center
Dallas, Texas

Allen Chang, MD
University of Massachusetts Medical School
Worcester, Massachusetts

Felix B. Chang, MD
Assistant Professor
Department of Family Medicine and Community Health
University of Massachusetts School of Medicine;
Inpatient Service Director
UMass Fitchburg Family Medicine Residency Program
UMass Memorial Health Alliance Hospital
Leominster, Massachusetts

Phillip Chang, MBBS
Visiting Medical Officer
Department of Otolaryngology
St. Vincent's Hospital
Sydney, Australia

Denisse Tafur Chang, MD
Universidad de Especialidades Espiritu Santo
Guayaquil, Ecuador

Jason Chao, MD, MS
Professor
Department of Family Medicine
Case Western Reserve University;
Department of Family Medicine
University Hospitals Case Medical Center
Cleveland, Ohio

Arabinda Chatterjee, MD, FRCS, MS, D. Urology
Assistant Professor
Department of Family and Community Medicine
University of Massachusetts Medical Center
Worcester, Massachusetts;
Family Physician
Department of Family Medicine
Day Kimball Hospital
Putnum, Connecticut
William Backus Hospital
Norwich, Connecticut

Arka Chatterjee, MD
Department of Internal Medicine
University of Louisville School of Medicine
Louisville, Kentucky

Shaila V. Chauhan, MD
Assistant Professor of Obstetrics and Gynecology
Division of Reproductive Endocrinology
University of Massachusetts Medical School
Worcester, Massachusetts

Michael K. Chen, MD
Department of Family Medicine
University Hospitals Case Medical Center
Cleveland, Ohio

Stephanie Yu-hsuan Chen, MD
University of Massachusetts Medical School
Worcester, Massachusetts

Josue Chery, MD
University of Massachusetts School of Medicine
Worcester, Massachusetts

Vasilios Chrisostomidis, DO
Assistant Professor
Department of Family Medicine
University of Massachusetts Medical School
Worcester, Massachusetts

Atul R. Chugh, MD
Chief Fellow
Division of Cardiovascular Medicine
University of Louisville
Louisville, Kentucky

S. Lindsey Clarke, MD
Associate Professor
Department of Family Medicine
Medical University of South Carolina
Area Health Education Consortium
Charleston, South Carolina;
Director of Predoctoral Education
Montgomery Center for Family Medicine
Self Regional Healthcare
Greenwood, South Carolina

Deborah S. Clements, MD
Associate Program Director
Associate Professor
Department of Family Medicine
University of Kansas Medical Center
Kansas City, Kansas

Lisa Clemons, MD
Assistant Professor
Department of Family Medicine
University of Texas Southwestern—Austin;
Brackenridge Hospital
Austin, Texas

Kara M. Coassolo, MD
Attending Physician, Maternal Fetal Medicine
Department of Obstetrics and Gynecology
Lehigh Valley Health Network
Allentown, Pennsylvania

Cameron J. Codd, DO
Department of Obstetrics and Gynecology
Akron General Medical Center
Akron, Ohio

Naida Cole, MD
Alpert Medical School of Brown University
Providence, Rhode Island

Irene C. Coletsos, MD
University of Massachusetts Medical School
Worcester, Massachusetts

Dana M. Collaguazo, MD
Assistant Professor
Department of Emergency Medicine
The University of Iowa
Iowa City, Iowa

Jason Conforti, MD
University of Massachusetts Medical School
Worcester, Massachusetts

Nathan T. Connell, MD
House Staff Officer in Medicine
Department of Medicine
Brown University;
Rhode Island and The Miriam Hospitals
Providence, Rhode Island

Caitlin M. Connolly, MD
University of Massachusetts Medical School
Worcester, Massachusetts

Brynna Connor, MD
Department of Family Practice
University of Texas Southwestern-Austin
Austin, Texas

Kyle V. Contini, MD
Department of Family Medicine
Creighton University School of Medicine
Omaha, Nebraska

Maryann Cooper, PharmD
Assistant Professor of Pharmacy Practice
Hematology/Oncology
Massachusetts College of Pharmacy and Health Sciences
Manchester, New Hampshire
Worcester, Massachusetts

Michael Cooper, MD
University of Massachusetts Medical School
Worcester, Massachusetts

Macario C. Corpuz, Jr., MD
Assistant Professor
Department of Family Medicine and Community Health
University of Massachusetts Medical School;
Medical Staff
Department of Family Medicine
University of Massachusetts Memorial Hospital
Worcester, Massachusetts

Alan J. Cropp, MD
Professor of Medicine
Department of Internal Medicine
Northeastern Ohio Universities College of Medicine and Pharmacy
Rootstown, Ohio;
Medical Staff
Department of Internal Medicine
St. Elizabeth Hospital Health Center
Youngstown, Ohio

Katie Crowder, MD

Sandra Cuellar, PharmD, BCOP
Clinical Assistant Professor
Department of Pharmacy Practice
University of Illinois at Chicago College of Pharmacy;
Clinical Oncology Pharmacist
Department of Pharmacy Practice
University of Illinois at Chicago Medical Center
Chicago, Illinois

Hongyi Cui, MD, PhD
Assistant Professor of Surgery
Department of General and Laparoscopic Surgery
University of Massachusetts Medical School;
Associate Director, Acute Care Surgery
Department of Surgery
University of Massachusetts Memorial Medical Center
Worcester, Massachusetts

Paul T. Cullen, MD
Clinical Associate Professor
Department of Family Medicine
University of Pittsburgh
Pittsburgh, Pennsylvania;
Residency Program Director
Department of Family Medicine
Washington Hospital
Washington, Pennsylvania

James F. Cunagin, MD
Senior Clinical Instructor and Director of Behavioral Science, Department of Family Medicine
Senior Clinical Instructor, Department of Psychiatry
University Hospitals Case Medical Center
Case Western Reserve University School of Medicine
Cleveland, Ohio

Carol Curtin, MSW, LICSW
Research Assistant Professor
Department of Family Medicine and Community Health
E.K. Shriver Center
University of Massachusetts Medical School
Waltham, Massachusetts

Jennifer S. Daly, MD
Professor
Department of Medicine
University of Massachusetts Medical School;
Clinical Chief
Division of Infectious Diseases and Immunology
University of Massachusetts Memorial Health Center
Worcester, Massachusetts

Gaurav Dang, MD
Department of Family Practice
Summa Barberton Hospital
Barberton, Ohio

Akhil Das, MD
Assistant Professor of Urology
Department of Urology
Thomas Jefferson University;
Attending Physician
Department of Urology
Thomas Jefferson University Hospital
Philadelphia, Pennsylvania

Janice E. Daugherty, MD
Associate Professor
Department of Family Medicine
The Brody School of Medicine at East Carolina University;
Patient Care Privileges
PIH County Memorial Hospital
Greenville, North Carolina

Raul Davaro, MD
Associate Professor
Department of Medicine
University of Massachusetts
Worcester, Massachusetts

Autumn Davidson, MD
University of Massachusetts Medical School
Worcester, Massachusetts

Jessica Davidson, MD
University of Massachusetts Medical School
Worcester, Massachusetts

Marin Dawson-Caswell, DO
Assistant Professor
Department of Family Medicine
Louisiana State University Health Sciences Center
New Orleans, Louisiana

Lauren Michal de Leon, MD
Warren Alpert Medical School at Brown University
Providence, Rhode Island

Robert De Marco, MD
Professor and Immediate Past Chairman
Department of Internal Medicine
Northeastern Ohio Universities College of Medicine;
St. Elizabeth Health Center
Rootstown, Ohio

Peerawut Deeprasertkul, MD
Department of Internal Medicine
Metrowest Medical Center
Framingham, Massachusetts

Meaghan Delaney, MD
University of Massachusetts Medical School
Worcester, Massachusetts

Sophia L. Delano, MD
University of Massachusetts Medical School
Worcester, Massachusetts

Konstantinos E. Deligiannidis, MD, MPH
Assistant Clinical Professor
Department of Family Medicine and Community Health
University of Massachusetts Medical School;
UMass Memorial Health Care
Worcester, Massachusetts

Deborah DeMarco, MD
Associate Dean, GME
Professor of Medicine
Division of Rheumatology
University of Massachusetts Medical School
Worcester, Massachusetts

Penelope Dennehy, MD
Director, Division of Pediatric Infectious Diseases
Professor of Pediatrics
Hasbro Children's Hospital
The Pediatric Division of Rhode Island Hospital
Providence, Rhode Island

Amar Deshpande, MD
University of Miami Miller School of Medicine
Miami, Florida

Alicia R. Desilets, PharmD
Assistant Professor of Pharmacy Practice
Department of Pharmacy Practice
Massachusetts College of Pharmacy and Health Sciences
Manchester, New Hampshire

Richard F. DeSouza, MD
Department of Medicine
Brown University - Rhode Island Hospital
Providence, Rhode Island

Adam W. DeTora, MD
Department of Pediatrics
University of Massachusetts Medical School
Worcester, Massachusetts

Mathew J. Devine, DO
Senior Instructor
Department of Family Medicine
University of Rochester;
Associate Medical Director
Department of Family Medicine
Highland Family Medicine
Rochester, New York

Suneel Dhand, MD
Attending Physician
Department of Medicine
Fallon Clinic/Saint Vincent Hospital
Worcester, Massachusetts

David Dildine, MD
University Massachusetts Medical School
Worcester, Massachusetts

Rino H. Dizon, MD
Department of Family Medicine
David Grant Medical Center
Travis Air Force Base, California

Frank J. Domino, MD
Professor
Clerkship Director
Department of Family Medicine and Community Health
University of Massachusetts Medical School
Worcester, Massachusetts

David J. Donahue, MD
Medical Director
Department of Pediatric Neurosurgery
Cook Children's Medical Center;
Surgical Director
Pediatric Epilepsy Program
Cook Children's Medical Center
Fort Worth, Texas

Ryan Dono, MD
University of Massachusetts School of Medicine
Worcester, Massachusetts

Susan E. Donohue, MD
Assistant Professor
Department of Medicine
University of Massachusetts Medical School
Commonwealth Hematology and Oncology, PC
Worcester, Massachusetts

Anna Doubeni, MD
Assistant Professor
Family Medicine and Community Health
University of Massachusetts Medical School
Worcester, Massachusetts

Cary D. Douglass, MD
President
West Lake Family Practice, P.A.
West Lake Hills, Texas

Abigail Drucker, MD
Department of Obstetrics and Gynecology
Creighton University Medical Center
Omaha, Nebraska

Kaelen C. Dunican, PharmD, RPh
Assistant Professor
Department of Pharmacy Practice
Massachusetts College of Pharmacy and Health Sciences
Worcester, Massachusetts

Nedim Durakovic, MD
Alpert Medical School of Brown University
Providence, Rhode Island

Cheryl Durand, PharmD, RPh
Assistant Professor of Pharmacy Practice
Massachusetts College of Pharmacy and Health Sciences
Manchester, New Hampshire

William J. Durbin, MD
Professor, Residency Director
Department of Pediatric Infectious Disease
University of Massachusetts Medical School;
Chair, Department of Pediatric Infectious Disease
UMass Memorial Healthcare
Worcester, Massachusetts

Matthew J. Dykhuizen, MD
University of Massachusetts Medical School
Worcester, Massachusetts

Gerry Edwards, MD
Assistant Professor
Department of Family Medicine
State University of New York—Upstate Medical University;
Faculty Family Medicine Residency
St. Joseph's Hospital Health Center
Syracuse, New York

Shannon Ehleringer, DO
Department of Family Medicine
David Grant Medical Center
Travis Air Force Base, California

Alan M. Ehrlich, MD
Assistant Clinical Professor
Department of Family Practice
University of Massachusetts Medical School
Worcester, Massachusetts

William G. Elder, Jr., PhD
Associate Professor
Department of Family and Community Medicine
University of Kentucky College of Medicine;
University of Kentucky Chandler Medical Center
Lexington, Kentucky

Amy Ellingson-Itzin, MD
Department of Obstetrics and Gynecology
University of Massachusetts Medical School;
UMass Memorial Medical Center
Worcester, Massachusetts

Pamela I. Ellsworth, MD
Associate Professor of Urology/Surgery
Department of Surgery
The Warren Alpert School of Medicine at Brown University;
Pediatric Urologist
Department of Surgery
Hasbro Children's Hospital
Providence, Rhode Island

Kevin Engelhardt, MD
Department of Pediatrics
University of Arizona College of Medicine
Tucson, Arizona

Michael Engels, MD
University of Massachusetts School of Medicine
Worcester, Massachusetts

Joseph K. Erbe, MD
Staff Physician
Department of Family Medicine
David Grant Medical Center
Travis Air Force Base
Fairfield, California

Rasai L. Ernst, MD
Department of Family Medicine
University Hospitals Case Medical Center
Cleveland, Ohio

Martin A. Espinosa Ginic, MD
House Staff
Department of Graduate Medical Education
University of Louisville
University of Louisville Hospital
Louisville, Kentucky

Janelle M. Evans, MD
Department of Obstetrics and Gynecology
University of Massachusetts Medical School
Worcester, Massachusetts

Kristyn Fagerberg, MD
West Lake Family Practice
Austin, Texas

Ashley Falk, MD
Family Practice
Offutt Air Force Base, Nebraska

Nathan P. Falk, MD
Physician
Department of Family Medicine
University of Nebraska Medical Center
Omaha, Nebraska

Pang-Yen Fan, MD
Associate Professor of Medicine
Division of Renal Medicine
University of Massachusetts Medical School
Worcester, Massachusetts

Rhonda A. Faulkner, PhD
Director, Behavioral Medicine
Department of Family Medicine
University of Illinois College of Medicine at Saint Joseph Hospital
Chicago, Illinois

Neil J. Feldman, DPM
Central Massachusetts Podiatry, PC
Worcester, Massachusetts

Edward Feller, MD
Clinical Professor of Medicine
Adjust Professor of Community Health
Department of Gastroenterology, Public Health
Warren Alpert Medical School of Brown University
Providence, Rhode Island

Warren J. Ferguson, MD
Associate Professor
Department of Family Medicine and Community Health
University of Massachusetts Medical School;
Vice Chair
Department of Family Medicine and Community Health
UMass Memorial Medical Center
Worcester, Massachusetts

Lauren Ferrara, MD
New York Medical College
Valhalla, New York

Shawn M. Ferullo, MD
Assistant Professor
Department of Family Medicine
Boston University;
Assistant Director, Sports Medicine
Department of Family Medicine
Boston Medical Center
Boston, Massachusetts

Jo Ellen Feugate, MD, PhD
Department of Medicine
Arizona Arthritis Center
University of Arizona
Tucson, Arizona

Scott A. Fields, MD
Professor and Vice Chair
Department of Family Medicine
Oregon Health and Science University
Portland, Oregon

Stanley Fineman, MD
Associate Clinical Professor
Department of Pediatrics
Emory University School of Medicine
Atlanta, Georgia

Jonathon M. Firnhaber, MD
Clinical Assistant Professor
Department of Family Medicine
East Carolina University
Greenville, North Carolina

David Fish, MD
University of Massachusetts Medical School
Worcester, Massachusetts

Timothy P. Fitzgibbons, MD
Fellow
Department of Cardiology
University of Massachusetts Medical School
Worcester, Massachusetts

Jonathan M. Flacker, MD
Assistant Professor
Department of Medicine
Emory University;
Medical Director, Emory Clinic at Wesley Woods
Geriatrics
Wesley Woods Health Center
Atlanta, Georgia

Michael P. Flaherty, MD, PhD
Assistant Professor
Division of Cardiovascular Medicine
University of Louisville
Louisville, Kentucky

Sarah B. Fleisig, MD
Warren Alpert Medical School
Brown University
Providence, Rhode Island

Joseph A. Florence, MD
Professor/Director, Division of Programs
Department of Family Medicine
East Tennessee State University Quillen College
Johnson City, Tennessee

Terence R. Flotte, MD
Dean of the Medical School
Department of Pediatrics
University of Massachusetts Medical School;
Professor
Department of Pediatrics
University of Massachusetts Memorial Health Center
Worcester, Massachusetts

Mary K. Flynn, MD
Department of Family Medicine and Community Health
University of Massachusetts Medical School
Worcester, Massachusetts

Jay Gar-Yee Fong, MD
Assistant Professor
Department of Pediatric Gastroenterology
University of Massachusetts School of Medicine and Medical Center
Worcester, Massachusetts

Tiffany M. Forti, MD, MPH
Department of Obstetrics and Gynecology
University of Massachusetts Medical School;
UMass Memorial Healthcare
Worcester, Massachusetts

Grant C. Fowler, MD
Professor and Vice Chair
Department of Family and Community Medicine
University of Texas Medical School at Houston;
Assistant Chief
Department of Family Medicine
Memorial Hermann Hospital
Houston, Texas

Robert L. Frachtman, MD
Austin Gastroenterology, PA
Austin, Texas

Jennifer E. Frank, MD
Assistant Professor
Department of Family Medicine
University of Wisconsin
Madison, Wisconsin

Samuel Frank, MD
Assistant Professor of Neurology
Boston University School of Medicine
Boston, Massachusetts

Nancy J. Freeman, MD
Clinical Associate Professor of Medicine
Warren Alpert School of Medicine at Brown University;
Chief, Hematology/Oncology
Providence VA Medical Center
Providence, Rhode Island

Rebecca A. Frye, DO
Faculty
Department of Family Medicine
David Grant Medical Center
Travis Air Force Base, California

Matthew J. Furman, MD
Department of Surgery
University of Massachusetts Medical Center
Worcester, Massachusetts

Richard Gacek, MD
Director, Otology/Neurotology
UMass Memorial Medical Center;
Professor of Otolaryngology, University of Massachusetts Medical School
Worcester, Massachusetts

Heidi L. Gaddey, MD
Department of Family Medicine
David Grant Medical Center
Travis Air Force Base, California

J. Scott Gaertner, MD
West Lake Family Practice
Austin, Texas

Tyeese Gaines Reid, DO, MA
Emergency Medicine Resident
Yale-New Haven Hospital
New Haven, Connecticut

Stephanie Galica, MD
University of Massachusetts Medical School
Worcester, Massachusetts

Eric P. Gall, MD
Professor of Clinical Medicine (Rheumatology)
Interim Director of the Arthritis Center of Excellence
University of Arizona

Sumanth Gandra, MD, MPH
Infectious Disease Fellow
University of Massachusetts Medical School
Worcester, Massachusetts

Jennifer Gao, MD
Department of Internal Medicine
Alpert Medical School, Brown University
Providence, Rhode Island

Andrew Gara, MD
University of Massachusetts Medical School
Worcester, Massachusetts

Erik J. Garcia, MD
Assistant Professor
Department of Family and Community Medicine
UMass Memorial Medical Center
Worcester, Massachusetts

Juan Antonio Garcia, MD
Assistant Professor
Department of Family Medicine
University of Calgary
University of Calgary Medical Centre Sunridge
Calgary, Alberta
Canada

Luis T. Garcia, MD
Clinical Instructor
Department of Family Medicine
University of Illinois—Chicago campus;
Chairman and Program Director
Department of Family Medicine
Saint Joseph Hospital
Chicago, Illinois

Amit Garg, MD
Director, Residency Program
Department of Dermatology
Boston University School of Medicine;
Assistant Professor
Department of Dermatology
Boston Medical Center
Boston, Massachusetts

Christopher Garofalo, MD
Active Staff
Department of Family Practice
Sturdy Memorial Hospital
Attleboro, Massachusetts

William T. Garrison, PhD
Professor
Department of Pediatrics
University of Massachusetts Medical School;
Division Director
Developmental and Behavioral Pediatrics
UMass Memorial Healthcare
Worcester, Massachusetts

Gail Gazelle, MD
Assistant Clinical Professor of Medicine
Department of Medicine
Harvard Medical School;
Position Member
Division of General Medicine
Brigham and Women's Hospital
Boston, Massachusetts

Renata Gazzi, MD
Clinical Faculty
Department of Family Medicine
University of Illinois at Chicago;
Clinical Faculty/Attending Physician
Department of Family Medicine
Saint Joseph Hospital
Chicago, Illinois

Gerald Gehr, MD
Assistant Professor of Medicine
Dartmouth Medical School
Hanover, New Hampshire;
Hematology/Oncology Program
Dartmouth-Hitchcock Manchester
Norris Cotton Cancer Center Manchester
Manchester, New Hampshire

John J. Gentile, DMD
Department of Dental Medicine
University of Massachusetts Medical School
Worcester, Massachusetts

Thomas Germano, MD
Assistant Clinical Professor
Department of Emergency Medicine
Warren Alpert Medical School at Brown University;
Attending Physician
Rhode Island Hospital
Providence, Rhode Island

Jeff Ray Gibson, Jr., MD
Assistant Professor
Department of Anesthesiology
The Texas A&M University Health Sciences Center College of Medicine;
Senior Staff Anesthesiologist
Department of Anesthesiology
Scott & White Memorial Hospital
Temple, Texas

Timothy Gibson, MD
Assistant Professor
Department of Pediatrics
University of Massachusetts Medical School;
Chief
Hanshaw Hospitalist Service
Department of Pediatrics
UMass Memorial Children's Medical Center
Worcester, Massachusetts

Javed M. Gilani, MD
Clinical Professor
Department of Internal Medicine
Drexel University
Philadelphia, Pennsylvania;
Christiana Care Health System
Wilmington, Delaware

David B. Gilchrist, MD
Assistant Professor
Department of Family Medicine
University of Massachusetts Medical School
University of Massachusetts Memorial Hospital
Worcester, Massachusetts

Neil A. Gilchrist, PharmD
Adjunct Assistant Professor
Department of Pharmacy Practice
Massachusetts College of Pharmacy and Health Sciences;
Clinical Pharmacy Specialist
Department of Pharmacy
UMass Memorial Medical Center
Worcester, Massachusetts

Cheryl L. Gilmartin, PharmD
Clinical Assistant Professor
Department of Pharmacy Practice
College of Pharmacy
University of Illinois;
Clinical Pharmacist
Section of Nephrology
University of Illinois
Chicago, Illinois

John W. Gittinger, Jr., MD
Professor of Ophthalmology and Neurology
Department of Ophthalmology
Boston University School of Medicine;
Residency Program Director
Division of Ophthalmology
Boston Medical Center
Boston, Massachusetts

Alfred Chege Gitu, MD
Faculty Physician
Department of Family Medicine
Greenwood Family Medicine Residency Program;
Self Regional Healthcare
Greenwood, South Carolina

Richard H. Glew, MD
Professor Medicine, Molecular Genetics, and Microbiology
Department of Medicine
University of Massachusetts Medical School
Infectious Disease Consultant
Department of Medicine
University of Massachusetts Medical Center
Worcester, Massachusetts

Luke Godwin, MD
The Warren Alpert Medical School of Brown University
Providence, Rhode Island

Jeremy Golding, MD
Professor of Family Medicine and of Obstetrics and Gynecology
The University of Massachusetts Medical School
Quality Officer—Department of Family Medicine and Community Health
UMass Memorial Health Care—Hahnemann Family Health Center
Worcester, Massachusetts

Michael Golding, MD
Senior Attending
New Hanover Hospital
Medical Director, Psych Support Inc.
Raleigh, North Carolina

Walter K. Goljan, MD
Department of Internal Medicine
UMass Memorial Medical Center
Worcester, Massachusetts

Leonard G. Gomella, MD
The Bernard W. Godwin Professor of Prostate Cancer Chairman
Associate Director of Clinical Affairs
Department of Urology
Jefferson Medical College
Philadelphia, Pennsylvania

Christian D. Gonzalez, MD
Assistant Professor
Department of Anesthesiology
University of Massachusetts Medical School;
Director, Pain Medicine
Department of Anesthesiology
Worcester, Massachusetts

Herbert P. Goodheart, MD
Assistant Clinical Professor
Department of Dermatology
Mount Sinai College of Medicine
New York, New York

Jeffrey L. Goodie, PhD
Assistant Professor
Department of Family Medicine
Uniformed Services University of the Health Sciences
Bethesda, Maryland

Mark D. Goodman, MD
Associate Professor and Interim Chairman
Department of Family Medicine
Creighton University School of Medicine
Omaha, Nebraska

Ilya Gorbachinsky, MD
Wake Forest University Baptist Medical Center
Winston-Salem, North Carolina

Paul R. Gordon, MD, MPH
Associate Professor
Department of Family and Community Medicine
University of Arizona—College of Medicine
Tucson, Arizona

Yelena Gorfinkel, MD
Boston Medical Center
Boston, Massachusetts

Parag Goyal, MD
New York Presbyterian Hospital-Weill Cornell Medical Center
New York, New York

Heath A. Grames, PhD
Assistant Professor and Program Director for the Family Therapy Program
Department of Child and Family Studies
The University of Southern Mississippi
Hattiesburg, Mississippi

Chris Graves, MD
House Staff, Orthopaedics
University of Iowa Carver College of Medicine
Iowa City, Iowa

Caron J. Gray, MD
Associate Professor
Department of Obstetrics and Gynecology
Creighton University School of Medicine;
Chief of the Medical Staff
Creighton University Medical Center
Omaha, Nebraska

Michael Gray, MD
University of Massachusetts Medical School
Worcester, Massachusetts

Darius Greenbacher, MD
Assistant Professor of Emergency Medicine
Tufts University School of Medicine
Boston, Massachusetts

Ellen Greenblatt, BSC, MDCM
Associate Professor
Department of Obstetrics and Gynecology
University of Toronto;
Medical Director
Centre for Fertility and Reproductive Health
Mount Sinai Hospital
Toronto, Ontario
Canada

Jennifer J. Greene Welch, MD
Assistant Professor
Department of Pediatrics
Alpert Medical School Brown University;
Attending Physician
Division of Pediatric Hematology/Oncology
Department of Pediatrics
Hasbro Children's Hospital
Providence, Rhode Island

Ronald A. Greenfield, MD
Professor of Medicine and Chief
Infectious Diseases Section
Department of Medicine
University of Oklahoma Health Sciences Center;
VA Medical Center
Oklahoma City, Oklahoma

Pamela Lynn Grimaldi, DO
Assistant Professor
Department of Family Medicine and Community Health
University of Massachusetts Medical School;
Staff, Physician
Department of Family Medicine
University of Massachusetts Memorial Hospital
Worcester, Massachusetts

Drew Grimes, MD
Capital Anesthesiology Associates
Austin, Texas

Jill A. Grimes, MD
Clinical Instructor
Department of Family Medicine
University of Massachusetts Medical School
Worcester, Massachusetts;
Private Practice
West Lake Family Practice
Austin, Texas

Daria I. Grisanzio, PharmD, RPh
Adjunct Instructor
Department of Pharmacy Practice
Massachusetts College of Pharmacy and Health Sciences;
Clinical Research Fellow
Clinical Pharmacology Study Group
Worcester, Massachusetts

Joseph Grisanzio, MD
Consultant
Department of Medicine
Morton Hospital and Medical Center
Taunton, Massachusetts

Shanin Gross, DO
Assistant Professor, Attending Physician
Department of Family and Community Medicine
Penn State College of Medicine
Hershey Medical Center
Hershey, Pennsylvania

Marc Grossman, MD

Neil Grossman, MD
Department of Pediatrics
University of Massachusetts Medical School
Worcester, Massachusetts

Christopher Gudas, MD
University of Massachusetts Medical School
Worcester, Massachusetts

John A. Guisto, MD
Clinical Professor
Department of Emergency Medicine
University of Arizona College of Medicine;
Medical Director
Department of Emergency Medicine
University Medical Center
Tucson, Arizona

Adarsh K. Gupta, DO, MS
Assistant Professor
Department of Family Medicine
University of Medicine and Dentistry New Jersey-School of Osteopathic Medicine;
Attending Physician
Department of Family Medicine
Kennedy Memorial Hospital
Stratford, New Jersey

Gregory D. Gutke, MD, MPH
Physician Epidemiologist
Clinical Informatics Branch
Air Force Medical Support Agency
Brooks City-Base, Texas;
Physician Provider
Department of Occupational Health
Brooke Army Medical Center
Fort Sam Houston, Texas

Michael S. Guy, MD
Department of Obstetrics and Gynecology
Akron General Medical Center
Akron, Ohio

Krista Hachey, MD
The Warren Alpert Medical School of Brown University
Providence, Rhode Island

Mazen Hadid, MD

Laura Hagopian, MD
University of Massachusetts Medical School
Worcester, Massachusetts

Jessica Hahn, MD
University of Massachusetts Medical School
Worcester, Massachusetts

Diane M. Haleem, PhD, RN
Chair and Associate Professor of Nursing and Public Administration
Marywood University
Scranton, Pennsylvania

Jessica E. Haley, MD
Department of Pediatrics
University of Arizona;
University Medical Center
Tucson, Arizona

Thomas J. Hansen, MD
Associate Dean for Medical Education
Assistant Professor
Department of Family Medicine
Creighton University
Omaha, Nebraska

Allison Hargreaves, MD
University of Massachusetts Medical School
Worcester, Massachusetts

Natasha Harrison, MD
Department of Family Medicine
University of Pennsylvania School of Medicine
Philadelphia, Pennsylvania

Linda H. Hatch, MD

Fern R. Hauck, MD, MS
Associate Professor
Departments of Family Medicine and Public Health Sciences
University of Virginia School of Medicine
Charlottesville, Virginia

Beverly N. Hay, MD
Assistant Professor of Pediatrics
Department of Pediatrics
University of Massachusetts Medical School;
Chief, Division of Genetics
Department of Pediatrics
University of Massachusetts Memorial Health Care
Worcester, Massachusetts

Rajneesh S. Hazarika, MD, MS
Assistant Professor
Department of Family Medicine and Community Health
University of Massachusetts Medical School
Worcester, Massachusetts;
Physician
Department of Family Medicine
Health Alliance Hospital
Leominster, Massachusetts

Daithi S. Heffernan, MD
Department of Surgery
Division of Trauma and Surgical Critical Care
Alpert Medical School of Brown University;
Rhode Island Hospital
Providence, Rhode Island

Russell C. Hendershot, DO, MS
Associate Professor of Family Medicine
Chair of Family Medicine
Edward Via Virginia College of Osteopathic Medicine
Blacksburg, Virginia

Scott T. Henderson, MD
Assistant Director
Student Health Center
University of Missouri
Columbia, Missouri

Kerry Hensley, MD
University of Massachusetts Medical School
Worcester, Massachusetts

Benjamin Hilliker, MD
University of Massachusetts Medical School
Worcester, Massachusetts

Nadine T. Himelfarb, MD
Department of Emergency Medicine
The Warren Alpert Medical School of Brown University;
Rhode Island Hospital
Providence, Rhode Island

W. Jeff Hinton, PhD
Associate Professor
Director of Clinical Training for the Family Therapy Program
Department of Child and Family Studies
The University of Southern Mississippi
Hattiesburg, Mississippi

Vu Ho, MD
Boston Medical Center
Boston, Massachusetts

N. Wilson Holland, MD
Assistant Professor
Department of Medicine
Emory University School of Medicine;
Fellowship Program Director
Division of Geriatric Medicine
Staff Physician, Geriatrics and Extended Care
VA Medical Center
Atlanta, Georgia

David M. Holmes, MD
Clinical Associate Professor
Department of Family Medicine
State University of New York at Buffalo
Buffalo, New York

Michael P. Hopkins, MD, MEd
Professor and Chair
Northeastern Ohio University College of Medicine
Department of Obstetrics and Gynecology
Rootstown, Ohio;
Director
Department of Obstetrics and Gynecology
Aultman Health Foundation
Canton, Ohio

Mark C. Horattas, MD
Professor of Surgery
Department of Surgery
Northeastern Ohio Universities College of Medicine
Rootstown, Ohio;
Chief of Endocrine Surgery
Department of Surgery
Akron General Medical Center
Akron, Ohio

Evan R. Horton, PharmD
Assistant Professor of Pharmacy Practice
Massachusetts College of Pharmacy and Health Sciences
Worcester, Massachusetts;
Clinical Specialist
Department of Pharmacy (Pediatrics)
Baystate Medical Center
Springfield, Massachusetts

Kim House, MD
Medical Director
Atlanta Eagle's Nest—A Community Living Center
Decatur, Georgia

Elizabeth E. Houser, MD
Staff Urologist
Department of Urology
Seton Family of Hospitals
St. David's Family of Hospitals
Westlake Hospital
Austin, Texas

Jay U. Howington, MD
Associate Clinical Professor
Department of Surgery and Radiology
Mercer University School of Medicine;
Medical Director, Stroke Program
Memorial Health University Medical Center
Savannah, Georgia

Dennis E. Hughes, DO
Staff Attending Physician
Department of Emergency Medicine
Skaggs Regional Medical Center
Branson, Missouri

Karen A. Hulbert, MD
Assistant Professor
Department of Family and Community Medicine
Medical College of Wisconsin
Milwaukee, Wisconsin

Kam Hunter, MD
Clinical Educator, Family Medicine
Banner Health
Phoenix, Arizona

Caitlin Hurley, MD
University of Massachusetts Medical School
Worcester, Massachusetts

John C. Huscher, MD
Assistant Professor
Department of Family Medicine
University of Nebraska Medical Center
Omaha, Nebraska;
Staff Physician
Hospitalist
Faith Regional Health Services
Norfolk, Nebraska

Lawrence M. Hwang, MD
Assistant Clinical Professor
Department of Family Medicine
University of California Los Angeles
Los Angeles, California;
University of California Los Angeles Santa Monica and Orthopedic Hospital
Santa Monica, California

Robert J. Hyde, MD
Clinical Faculty
Department of Emergency Medicine
Christiana Care Health System
Newark, Delaware

Luis Idrovo Freire, MD
Neurologist
Hospital Ntra Sra del Rosario
Neurosonology Lab—Neurology Dept
Madrid Spain

Sabrina A. Indyk, MD
Department of Family Medicine
Resurrection Medical Center
Chicago, Illinois

Pablo I. Hernandez Itriago, MD
Medical Director
South End Community Health Center (SECHC)
Boston, Massachusetts

Mark Iverson, MD

Christine K. Jacobs, MD
Associate Professor
Department of Family and Community Medicine
St. Louis University School of Medicine
St. Louis, Missouri

Deepa Jagadeesh, MD, MPH
Hematology/Oncology Fellow
Department of Medicine—Hematology/Oncology
University of Massachusetts Medical School
Worcester, Massachusetts

Catherine Janes, MD
Assistant Professor
Attending Physician
Department of Pediatrics, Division of Pediatric Emergency Medicine
University of Massachusetts School of Medicine
University of Massachusetts Memorial Medical Center
Worcester, Massachusetts

Courtney I. Jarvis, PharmD
Associate Professor
Department of Pharmacy Practice
Massachusetts College of Pharmacy and Health Sciences
Worcester, Massachusetts;
Clinical Pharmacy Pharmacist
Department of Family Medicine
UMass Memorial Medical Center
Barre, Massachusetts

Joselyn Jedick, DO
Department of Family Medicine
Banner Good Samaritan Hospital
Phoenix, Arizona

Nathaniel J. Jellinek, MD
Clinical Assistant Professor
Department of Dermatology
Warren Alpert Medical School at Brown University
Providence, Rhode Island;
Dermatology Professionals, Inc.
East Greenwich, Rhode Island

Eric L. Jenison, MD
Professor
Department of Obstetrics and Gynecology
Northeastern Ohio Universities College of Medicine and Pharmacy
Rootstown, Ohio;
Chairman and Program Director
Department of Obstetrics and Gynecology
Akron General Medical Center
Akron, Ohio

John Jenkins, MD

Myrlene Jeudy, MD
University of Massachusetts Medical School
Worcester, Massachusetts

Adeliza S. Jimenez, MD
Department of Family and Community Medicine
University of Texas Health Science Center at San Antonio
San Antonio, Texas

Stacy Jones, MD

Maurice F. Joyce, III, MD
Department of General Surgery
Lahey Clinic
Burlington, Massachusetts

Patrick W. Joyner, MD
Department of Orthopaedic Surgery
Duke University Medical Center
Durham, North Carolina

Marc Jeffrey Kahn, MD
Professor of Medicine
Department of Medicine
Tulane University School of Medicine
New Orleans, Louisiana

Monica Kaitz, MD
Warren Alpert Medical School of Brown University
Providence, Rhode Island

Bharati Kalasapudi, MD
Warren Alpert Medical School of Brown University
Providence, Rhode Island

Abir O. Kanaan, PharmD, RPh
Assistant Professor
Department of Pharmacy Practice
Massachusetts College of Pharmacy and Health Sciences—Worcester/Manchester;
Clinical Specialist, Worcester Medical Center
Coronary Intensive Care Unit
Co-Director, Pharmacy Medication Safety Fellowship—Saint Vincent Hospital
Pharmacy Department
Worcester, Massachusetts

Packrisamy Kannan, MD
Senior Lecturer in Surgery
Department of Surgery
Dubai Medical College for Girls;
Senior Specialist Surgeon
Department of Surgery
Rashid Hospital & RH Trauma Center
Dubai, United Arab Emirates

Mark Kaplan, MD
Clinical Associate Professor of Orthopedics and Physical Rehabilitation
University of Massachusetts Medical School
Worcester, Massachusetts

Paul E. Kaplan, MD
President
Capitol Clinical Neuroscience
Folsom, California

Margo L. Kaplan-Gill, MD
Associate Professor
Department of Family Medicine
UMass Memorial Medical Center;
Family Health Center of Worcester
Worcester, Massachusetts

Rahul Kapur, MD, CAQSM
Assistant Director, Primary Care Sports Medicine Fellowship
Assistant Professor, Family Medicine and Sports Medicine
Department of Family Medicine and Community Health &
University of Pennsylvania Sports Medicine Center
University of Pennsylvania Health System
Philadelphia, Pennsylvania

Ioannis Karakis, MD
Department of Neurology
Boston University Medical Center
Boston, Massachusetts

Kristy Kedian Brown, DO
Associate Professor
Family Medicine
University of Massachusetts Medical School;
Faculty
Family of Medicine
University of Massachusetts Memorial Hospital
Worcester, Massachusetts

Molly P. Keegan, MD
Department of Emergency Medicine
University of Southern California Medical Center
Los Angeles, California

Rick Kellerman, MD
Professor and Chair
Department of Family and Community Medicine
University of Kansas School of Medicine—Wichita
Wichita, Kansas

Brandi Kelly, PharmD
MedTrak Services
Overland Park, Kansas

John J. Kelly, MD
Associate Professor
Department of Surgery
University of Massachusetts Medical School;
Chief
Department of Surgery
University of Massachusetts Memorial Medical Center
Worcester, Massachusetts

Kristen Kelly, MD
Department of Obstetrics and Gynecology
University of Massachusetts Medical School
Worcester, Massachusetts

Bevin Kenney, MD
Instructor in Medicine
Department of Internal Medicine
Harvard Medical School;
Brigham & Women's Hospital
Boston, Massachusetts

Robert M. Kershner, MD, MS
Eye Physician and Surgeon, Refractive and Cataract Surgery
Professor III, Microbiology, Anatomy and Physiology
Palm Beach State College
Palm Beach Gardens, Florida;
Clinical Professor of Ophthalmology
University of Utah School of Medicine
John A. Moran Eye Center
Salt Lake City, Utah;
Adjunct Professor Health Administration
Kaplan University
Ft. Lauderdale, Florida;
Ik Ho Visiting Professor of Ophthalmology
Chinese University of Hong Kong
Founder and Director Emeritus of Cataract and Refractive Surgery and Anterior Segment Fellowship Program
Eye Laser Center
Tucson, Arizona

Martin Kerzer, MD
Clinical Assistant Professor
Department of Family Medicine
Brown Alpert Medical School
Providence, Rhode Island;
Associates in Primary Care Medicine
Warwick, Rhode Island

Kerri Keslow, MD
Department of Family Medicine
Santa Monica-UCLA Medical Center and Orthopaedic Hospital
Santa Monica, California

Farah Y. Khan, MD
Department of Family Medicine
University of Texas Southwestern Medical School
Austin, Texas

Omar A. Khan, MD, MHS
Clinical Assistant Professor
Departments of Family Medicine and Public Health
University of Pennsylvania
Drexel University
Philadelphia;
Clinical Assistant Professor
University of Vermont
Burlington, Vermont

Saira Khan, MD
UT Health Science Center at San Antonio
Department of Family and Community Medicine
San Antonio, Texas

Salwa Khan, MD, MHS
Pediatric Hospitalist
Department of Pediatrics
Children's Hospital of Philadelphia
Philadelphia, Pennsylvania

Birgit N. Khandalavala, MD
Assistant Professor, Family Medicine
Creighton University
Omaha, Nebraska

Shefali B. Khandwala, DO
Assistant Clinical Professor
Department of Family Medicine
University of California at Irvine Medical Center
Orange, California

Morteza Khodaee, MD, MPH
Assistant Professor
Department of Family Medicine
University of Colorado Denver School of Medicine
Denver, Colorado

George E. Kikano, MD
Chair and Dorothy Jones Weatherhead Professor
Department of Family Medicine
Case Western Reserve University
University Hospitals of Cleveland
Cleveland, Ohio

Sam Seung Yeol Kim, MBBS, Mmed
Associate Clinical Lecturer
Department of Medicine
University of Sydney;
Surgical Resident
Department of Surgery
Westmead Hospital
Westmead, Sydney, Australia

Walter M. Kim, MD, PhD
University of Massachusetts Medical School
Worcester, Massachusetts

Scott E. Kinkade, MD, MSPH
Assistant Professor
Department of Family and Community Medicine
University of Texas Southwestern Medical Center at Dallas Southwestern Medical School;
Dallas, Texas

Rebecca G. Kinney, MD
Department of Family Medicine
Family Medicine Residency of Idaho
Boise, Idaho

George P. Kinzfogl, III, MD
Clinical Instructor
Department of Cardiology
Harvard Medical School
Boston, Massachusetts;
Heart Center of MetroWest
Framingham, Massachusetts

Jeffery T. Kirchner, DO
Clinical Associate Professor
Department of Family and Community Medicine
Temple University School of Medicine
Philadelphia, Pennsylvania;
Associate Director, Family Medicine Residency Program
Department of Family and Community Medicine
Lancaster General Hospital
Lancaster, Pennsylvania

Jason Kittler, MD, PhD, JD
Berkshire Medical Group
Pittsfield, Massachusetts

Michael Klein, MD
Warren Alpert Medical School
Brown University
Providence, Rhode Island

Michael S. Kleinman, DO
Department of Neurology
Boston University
Boston, Massachusetts

Dagmar Klinger, MD
Assistant Professor
Department of Medicine
University of Massachusetts Medical School;
Nephrologist
Department of Medicine
UMass Medical Center
Worcester, Massachusetts

Joshua T. Kluetz, DO
Family Medicine Residency
Resurrection Medical Center
Chicago, Illinois

William J. Knaus, II, MD
Department of Surgery
University of Texas Southwestern;
Department of Surgery
Parkland Hospital
Dallas, Texas

Teresa Knight, MD
Women's Health Specialists of St. Louis
Creve Coeur, Missouri

Ajar Kochar, MD
The Warren Alpert Medical School at Brown University
Providence, Rhode Island

Benjamin Kohnen, MD
David Grant Medical Center
Travis Air Force Base, California

Anjali Koka, MD
Department of Anesthesia, Critical Care and Pain Management
Massachusetts General Hospital
Boston, Massachusetts

Scott Kopec, MD
Department of Pulmonary Medicine
University of Massachusetts Medical Center
Worcester, Massachusetts

Galina Korsunsky, MD
MetroWest Medical Center
Framingham, Massachusetts

Anya S. Koutras, MD
Associate Professor
Department of Family Medicine
University of Vermont College of Medicine;
Faculty Attending
Department of Family Medicine
Fletcher Allen Health Care
University of Vermont
Burlington, Vermont

Michael S. Krathen, MD
Department of Dermatology
Boston University School of Medicine;
Department of Dermatology
Boston Medical Center
Boston, Massachusetts

Allison Kreiner, MD
Resident
Department of Obstetrics and Gynecology
Akron General Medical Center
Akron, Ohio

David W. Kruse, MD
Assistant Clinical Professor
Department of Orthopaedic Surgery
University of California, Irvine
Irvine, California

Rebecca Kruse-Jarres, MD, MPH
Assistant Professor
Department of Medicine
Tulane University
New Orleans, Louisiana

Eric J. Kujawski, DO
Sports Medicine Fellow
Department of Family Medicine
University of Tennessee
Knoxville, Tennessee

Santosh Kumar, MBBS
Department of Family Medicine
Freighton University Medical Center
Omaha, Nebraska

Tara N. Kumaraswami, MD
Department of Obstetrics and Gynecology
University of Massachusetts Medical School
Worcester, Massachusetts

Alphonsus K. Kung, MD
Department of Family Medicine and Community Health
University of Massachusetts Medical School
Worcester, Massachusetts

Jason M. Kurland, MD
Fellow, Department of Nephrology
Rhode Island Hospital/Brown University
Providence, Rhode Island

Daniel B. Kurtz, PhD
Assistant Professor
Department of Biology
Utica College
Utica, New York

Dylan C. Kwait, MD
Department of Radiology
Maimonides Medical Center
Brooklyn, New York

Chris G. Kyriakedes, DO
Professor, Emergency Medicine
Northeast Ohio Universities College of Medicine and Pharmacy
Rootstown, Ohio;
Attending Physician
Department of Emergency Medicine
Akron General Medical Center
Akron, Ohio

Mildred LaFontaine, MD
Department of Neurology
Concord Hospital
Concord, New Hampshire

Amara Lai, MD
Department of Family Medicine
Banner Good Samaritan
Phoenix, Arizona

Katherine Lang, MD
University of Massachusetts School of Medicine
Worcester, Massachusetts

Eduardo Lara-Torre, MD
Associate Professor
Department of Obstetrics and Gynecology
Virginia Tech-Cariolion School of Medicine;
Associate Residency Program Director
Department of Obstetrics and Gynecology
Carilion Clinic
Roanoke, Virginia

Lars C. Larsen, MD
Professor
Associate Dean for Academic and Faculty Development
Department of Family Medicine
The Brody School of Medicine at East Carolina University
Greenville, North Carolina

Austin Larson, MD
Department of Pediatrics
The Children's Hospital
Aurrora, Colorado

Richard A. Larson, MD
Professor
Department of Medicine, Section of Hematology/Oncology
The University of Chicago
Chicago, Illinois

Bonnie W. Lau, MD, PhD
The Warren Alpert Medical School of Brown University
Providence, Rhode Island

Margo Lauterbach, MD
Staff Psychiatrist
Neuropsychiatry Program
Sheppard Pratt Health System
Baltimore, Maryland

Ann Lavers, MD

Justin P. Lavin, Jr., MD
Professor
Department of Obstetrics and Gynecology
Northeastern Ohio College of Medicine
Rootstown, Ohio;
Vice Chairman, Chief of Maternal Fetal Medicine
Department of Obstetrics and Gynecology
Akron General Medical Center
Akron, Ohio

Alexis Lawrence, MD
University of Massachusetts Medical School
Worcester, Massachusetts

Jay Lawrence, MD
University of Massachusetts Medical School
Worcester, Massachusetts

Antonella M. Leary, MD
Assistant Professor
Department of Obstetrics and Gynecology
UMass Memorial Medical Center
Worcester, Massachusetts

Daniel J. Lee, MD
Assistant Professor
Department of Otology and Laryngology
Harvard Medical School;
Division of Otology and Neurotology
Department of Otolaryngology
Massachusetts Eye and Ear Infirmary
Boston, Massachusetts

Daniel T. Lee, MD
Associate Clinical Professor
Department of Family Medicine
David Geffen School of Medicine at UCLA
Los Angeles, California;
Staff Attending
Department of Family Practice
Santa Monica—UCLA Medical Center and Orthopaedic Hospital
Santa Monica, California

Justin A. Lee, MD
Department of Family Medicine
University of Colorado Health Sciences Center
Denver, Colorado

Juyong Lee, MD, PhD
Physician
Department of Internal Medicine
MetroWest Medical Center
Framingham, Massachusetts

Paul J. Lee, MD
Assistant Professor
Pediatrics
SUNY Stony Brook School of Medicine
Stony Brook, New York;
Attending Pediatrician
Pediatric Infectious Diseases
Winthrop-University Hospital
Mineola, New York

Matthew R. Leibowitz, MD
Assistant Clinical Professor
Department of Medicine
David Geffen School of Medicine at UCLA;
Attending Physician
Department of Infectious Diseases
UCLA Medical Center
Los Angeles, California

Meg Lekander, MD
Assistant Instructor in Family Medicine
Warren Alpert School of Medicine of Brown University
Providence, Rhode Island

Sergio A. Leon, MD
Rheumatology Fellow
Division of Rheumatology
University of Massachusetts Medical School
Worcester, Massachusetts

Andrew Leone, MD
Department of Urology
Brown Alpert Medical School;
Rhode Island Hospital
Providence, Rhode Island

Maya Leventer-Roberts, MD, MPH
Department of Pediatrics
Mount Sinai School of Medicine
Mount Sinai Kravis Children's Hospital
New York, New York

John M. Levey, MD
Clinical Chief, GI Division
Department of Digestive Disease
University of Massachusetts Medical School
Worcester, Massachusetts

Nikki Levin, MD, PhD
Associate Professor of Medicine
Division of Dermatology
University of Massachusetts Medical School
UMass Memorial Medical Center
Worcester, Massachusetts

Gary I. Levine, MD
Associate Professor
Department of Family Medicine
Brody School of Medicine
East Carolina University
Greenville, North Carolina

James H. Lewis, MD
Professor of Medicine
Division of Gastroenterology
Georgetown University Medical Center
Washington, District of Columbia

Desiree Lie, MD
Health Sciences Clinical Professor
Director, Research and Faculty Development
University of California, Irvine
Irvine, California

Brian K. Linn, MD
Medical Staff
Department of Family Medicine
North Arkansas Regional Medical Center
Harrison, Arkansas

Vasileios-Arsenios Lioutas, MD
Department of Neurology
Boston University Medical Center
Boston, Massachusetts

Janice A. Litza, MD
Assistant Professor
Department of Family Medicine
University of Wisconsin School of Medicine and Public Health
Madison, Wisconsin;
Aurora University of Wisconsin Medical Group
Aurora Healthcare
Milwaukee, Wisconsin

Kimberly E. Liu, MD, FRCSC
Assistant Professor
Department of Obstetrics and Gynecology
University of Toronto;
Staff Physician
Mount Sinai Hospital
Toronto, Ontario
Canada

Nancy Y. Liu, MD
Associate Professor of Clinical Medicine
Department of Medicine
University of Massachusetts Medical School
Worcester, Massachusetts

Samantha R. Llanos, PharmD, RPh
Adjunct Assistant Professor
Massachusetts College of Pharmacy
Worcester, Massachusetts

John Paul Lock, MD
Assistant Professor
Department of Medicine
University of Massachusetts School of Medicine
Worcester, Massachusetts

Madaiah Lokeshwari, MD
Hospitalist
Department of Medicine
Heywood Hospital
Gardner, Massachusetts

Rich Londo, MD
Assistant Professor of Clinical Family Medicine
Department of Family and Community Medicine
University of Illinois College of Medicine-Rockford
Rockford, Illinois

David Longstroth, MD
Contra Costa Health Services
Martinez, California

Claudia M. Lora, MD
Visiting Instructor
Department of Medicine
University of Illinois at Chicago;
Faculty
Department of Medicine
University of Illinois Medical Center
Chicago, Illinois

Claudine Lott, MD
University of Massachusetts Medical School
Worcester, Massachusetts

Jane K. Louie, MD
Attending Physician
Neurological Services, PC
MetroWest Medical Center
Framingham, Massachusetts

Zhen Lu, MD
Attending Physician
South Bay Family Medical Group;
Attending Physician
Torrance Memorial Medical Center
Torrance, California

Brock D. Lutz, MD
Partner
East Texas Infectious Disease Consultants
Tyler, Texas

Ann M. Lynch, PharmD, RPh
Assistant Professor
Department of Pharmacy Practice
University of Massachusetts College of Pharmacy Health Science
Worcester, Massachusetts

Paul E. Lyons, MD
Professor and Associate Chair
Department of Family and Community Medicine
Temple University School of Medicine
Philadelphia, Pennsylvania

Jonathan MacClements, MD
Director of Medical Education/DIO
Associate Professor and Chair/Program Director of the Family Medicine Department
Certificate of Knowledge American Society of Travelers' Health and Tropical Medicine
University of Texas Health Center at Tyler
Tyler, Texas

David C. Mackenzie, MD
Clinical Instructor
Department of Emergency Medicine
Brown University;
Rhode Island Hospital
Providence, Rhode Island

Heather Mackey-Fowler, MD
Assistant Professor
Department of Family Medicine and Community Health
University of Massachusetts Medical School;
Primary Care Physician
Department of Family Medicine
St. Vincent Medical Group
Worcester, Massachusetts

Theodore G. MacKinney, MD, MPH
Assistant Professor
Department of General Internal Medicine
Medical College of Wisconsin;
Staff Physician
Department of Internal Medicine
Froedtert Memorial Lutheran Hospital
Milwaukee, Wisconsin

Douglas W. MacPherson, MD, MSc(CTM)
Associate Professor
Department of Pathology and Molecular Medicine
McMaster University
Hamilton, Ontario, Canada;
President, Migration Health Consultants, Inc.
Cheltenham, Ontario, Canada

Tracy Madsen, MD
Department of Emergency Medicine
Brown University
Rhode Island Hospital
Providence, Rhode Island

Katherine M. Mahon, MD
Department of Family Medicine and Community Health
University of Pennsylvania Health System Presbyterian Medical Center
Philadelphia, Pennsylvania

Anne M. Mahoney, MD
Boston University School of Medicine
Boston, Massachusetts

Patrick Mailloux, DO
Assistant Professor of Medicine
Tufts University School of Medicine;
Associate Program Director
Critical Care Medicine Fellowship
Baystate Medical Center
Springfield, Massachusetts

Barbara A. Majeroni, MD
Clinical Professor
Department of Family Medicine
University of Buffalo, SUNY;
Attending Physician
Department of Family Medicine
Erie County Medical Center
Buffalo, New York

M. Keenan Mak, MD
Creighton University School of Medicine
Omaha, Nebraska

Dominique Malacarne, MD
The Warren Alpert Medical School
Brown University
Providence, Rhode Island

Maricarmen Malagon-Rogers, MD
Associate Professor
Department of Family Medicine
University of Tennessee Graduate School of Medicine;
Director, Pediatric Nephrology
Department of Pediatrics
University of Tennessee Medical Center, Knoxville
Knoxville, Tennessee

Melanie J.S. Malec, MD
Fellow
Department of Family Medicine
Case Western Reserve University;
University Hospitals Case Medical Center
Cleveland, Ohio

Samir Malkani, MD
Associate Professor of Clinical Medicine
Division of Diabetes
University of Massachusetts Medical School
Worcester, Massachusetts

Ronald L. Malm, DO
Assistant Professor
University of Wyoming;
Family Practice Residency Program
Cheyenne, Wyoming

Michael A. Malone, MD
Assistant Professor
Department of Family Medicine
Pennsylvania State College of Medicine;
Staff
Department of Family Medicine
Pennsylvania State Milton S. Hershey Medical Center
Hershey, Pennsylvania

Joshua M.V. Mammen, MD, PhD
Assistant Professor
Department of Surgery
University of Kansas
Kansas City, Kansas

Lee A. Mancini, MD, CSCS, CSN
Assistant Professor
Department of Family Medicine and Community Health
University of Massachusetts Medical School;
Sports Medicine Physician
Department of Family Medicine and Community Health
University of Massachusetts Medical Center
Worcester, Massachusetts

Daniel Mandell, MD
University of Massachusetts Medical School
Worcester, Massachusetts

Jeffrey Manning, MD

Mark J. Manning, DO, Med
Assistant Professor
Department of Obstetrics and Gynecology
University of Massachusetts Medical School;
UMass Memorial Medical Center
Worcester, Massachusetts

Mariann Manno, MD
Associate Professor
Departments of Pediatrics and Emergency Medicine
University of Massachusetts Memorial Medical Center;
Division Director
Department of Pediatrics
University of Massachusetts Memorial Children's Medical Center
Worcester, Massachusetts

Katherine A. Mansalis, MD
Department of Family Medicine
David Grant Medical Center
Travis Air Force Base, California

Aaron S. Mansfield, MD
Clinician-Investigator/Fellow
Department of Medicine/Division of Hematology
Department of Oncology
Mayo Clinic
Rochester, Minnesota

Eric Mao, MD
Warren Alpert Medical School at Brown University
Providence, Rhode Island

Murat Mardirossian, MD
Department of Family Medicine
University of California, Irvine
UC Irvine Douglas Hospital
Orange, California

Geoffrey M. Margo, MD, PhD
Clinical Associate Professor
Department of Psychiatry
University of Pennsylvania Health System;
Director, Consultation/Liaison Psychiatry
Department of Psychiatry
Pennsylvania Hospital
Philadelphia, Pennsylvania

Katherine L. Margo, MD
Assistant Professor
Department of Family Medicine and Community Health
University of Pennsylvania School of Medicine;
Faculty
Department of Family Medicine and Community Health
Presbyterian Hospital
Philadelphia, Pennsylvania

Kathy Mariani, MD
Assistant Professor
Center for Health & Well Being
The University of Vermont
Burlington, Vermont

Robert A. Marlow, MD, MA
Professor of Clinical Family Medicine
Department of Family and Community Medicine
University of Arizona College of Medicine
Tucson and Phoenix, Arizona;
Associate Director/Director of Research
Family Medicine Residency Program
Scottsdale Healthcare
Scottsdale, Arizona

William L. Marshall, MD
Associate Professor
Department of Medicine
University of Massachusetts Medical School;
Attending Physician
Department of Medicine
University of Massachusetts/Memorial Medical Center
Worcester, Massachusetts

Michelle T. Martin, PharmD
Clinical Assistant Professor
Department of Pharmacy Practice
University of Illinois at Chicago;
Clinical Pharmacist
Ambulatory Care Pharmacy
University of Illinois Medical Center at Chicago
Chicago, Illinois

Stephen A. Martin, MD, EdM
Instructor
Department of Family Medicine and Community Health
University of Massachusetts Medical School
Worcester, Massachusetts

A. Raquel Mateo-Bibeau, MD
Infectious Disease Specialist
Department of Medicine
John F. Kennedy Medicine Center
St. Mary's Medical Center
Atlantis, Florida

Donnah Mathews, MD
Assistant Professor
Department of Medicine
Alpert School of Brown University;
Attending Physician
Department of General Internal Medicine
Rhode Island Hospital
Providence, Rhode Island

Michele L. Matthews, PharmD
Assistant Professor
Department of Pharmacy Practice
Massachusetts College of Pharmacy Health Sciences
Boston, Massachusetts;
Clinical Pharmacy Specialist
Pain Management Center
Brigham & Women's Hospital
Chestnut Hill, Massachusetts

Jason Matuszak, MD
Department of Family Medicine
University of Buffalo;
Chief of Sports Medicine
Department of Sports Medicine
Excelsior Orthopaedics
Amherst, New York

Karen L. Maughan, MD
Associate Professor
Attending Faculty
Department of Family Medicine
University of Virginia
Charlottesville, Virginia

George Maxted, MD
Assistant Clinical Professor
Department of Family Medicine and Community Health
UMass Memorial Health Care
Worcester, Massachusetts

Aimee Mayo Nilsen, PharmD
Assistant Adjunct Faculty
Massachusetts College of Pharmacy and Health Sciences
Genzyme Corporation
Worcester, Massachusetts

Beth Mazyck, MD
Clinical Associate Professor
Department of Family Medicine and Community Health
University of Massachusetts Medical School
Worcester, Massachusetts;
Vice President of Medical Services
Community Health Connections, Inc.
Family Health Center
Fitchburg, Massachusetts

Elizabeth McAninch, MD
Physician
Department of Internal Medicine
University of Miami;
Jackson Memorial Hospital
Miami, Florida

Frank J. McCabe, MD
Clinical Instructor
Department of Ophthalmology
Tufts Medical Center
Boston, Massachusetts

Margaret McCormick, MS, RN
Clinical Assistant Professor
Department of Nursing
Towson University
Towson, Maryland

Timothy R. McCurry, MD
Clinical Assistant Professor
Department of Family Medicine
Stritch School of Medicine
Loyola University
Maywood, Illinois;
Program Director
Family Medicine Residency
Resurrection Medical Center
Chicago, Illinois

Elizabeth Colman McKeen, MD
Department of Pediatrics
Harvard University;
Massachusetts General Hospital for Children
Boston, Massachusetts

Patricia McQuilkin, MD
Assistant Professor
Department of Pediatrics
University of Massachusetts Medical School
Worcester, Massachusetts

Gary Mark McWilliams, MD
Executive VP Chief Ambulatory Services Officer
Ambulatory Operations
University Health System
San Antonio, Texas

Colleen F. Medeiros, PharmD, BCPS
Department of Internal Medicine
Boston Medical Center
Boston, Massachusetts

Eva Medvedova, MD
Fellow, Hematology and Oncology Fellow
Department of Medicine
University of Massachusetts Medical School
Worcester, Massachusetts

Erika Mello, MD
University of Massachusetts Medical School
Worcester, Massachusetts

Hannah Melnitsky, MD
University of Massachusetts Medical School
Worcester, Massachusetts

Timothy Menz, MD
University of Massachusetts Medical School
Worcester, Massachusetts

Tracy O. Middleton, DO
Chair, Family Medicine
Midwestern University
Arizona College of Osteopathic Medicine
Glendale, Arizona

James P. Miller, MD
Medical Director
Department of Pediatric Surgery
Cook Children's Medical Center
Fort Worth, Texas

Nathan Miller, MD, CAPT, MC
Department of Family Medicine
David Grant (USAF) Medical Center
Travis Air Force Base, California

Sandra Miller, MD
Assistant Director
Family Medicine Residency
Banner Good Samaritan Medical Center
Phoenix, Arizona

Jonathan Min, MD
University of Massachusetts Medical School
Worcester, Massachusetts

Jeffrey F. Minteer, MD
Clinical Associate Professor
Department of Family Medicine
University of Pittsburgh
Pittsburgh, Pennsylvania;
Program Director, Family Medicine Residency
Washington Hospital
Washington, Pennsylvania

Mark H. Mirabelli, MD
Assistant Professor
Department of Orthopaedics and Family Medicine
University of Rochester
Rochester, New York

Anna Mirk, MD
Instructor
Department of Geriatrics, Extended Care and Rehabilitation
Atlanta VA Medical Center
Decatur, Georgia

Ann Mitchell, MD
Associate Professor of Clinical Neurology
Department of Neurology
University of Massachusetts Memorial Medical Center
Worcester, Massachusetts

Jack H. Mitstifer, MD
Assistant Professor of Clinical Emergency Medicine
Department of Emergency Medicine
Northeastern Ohio Universities College of Medicine and Pharmacy
Rootstown, Ohio;
Chairman
Department of Emergency Medicine
Akron General Medical Center
Akron, Ohio

Vinod P. Mitta, MD
University of Southern California Keck School of Medicine
Los Angeles, California

Bryan K. Moffett, MD
Assistant Professor
Department of Internal Medicine
University of Louisville School of Medicine;
Hospitalist, Internal Medicine
University of Louisville
Louisville, Kentucky

Aaron Moore, DO
University of Massachusetts Medical School
Worcester, Massachusetts

Tiffany A. Moore Simas, MD, MPH, Med
Assistant Professor
Department of Obstetrics and Gynecology
University of Massachusetts Medical School;
Full-Time Generalist Obstetrician-Gynecologist
Department of Obstetrics and Gynecology
University of Massachusetts Medical Center—Memorial Campus
Worcester, Massachusetts

Wayne Morgan, MD
Combined Child/Adult Psychiatry
Department of Psychiatry
University of Massachusetts Medical School
Worcester, Massachusetts

Richard A. Moriarty, MD
Professor of Clinical Pediatrics
Department of Pediatrics
UMass Medical School;
Pediatric Infectious Disease Consultant
Department of Pediatrics
UMass Memorial Health Care
Worcester, Massachusetts

Anna K. Morin, PharmD
Associate Professor
Department of Pharmacy Practice
Massachusetts College of Pharmacy and Health Sciences;
Clinical Pharmacist
Department of Pharmacy Services
Worcester State Hospital
Worcester, Massachusetts

Peter Morse, MD
University of Massachusetts School of Medicine
Worcester, Massachusetts

Mohammad Ansar Mughal, MD
Eastern New Mexico Family Medicine
Roswell, New Mexico

Christian Müller, PhD
Assistant Professor
Department of Pediatrics
University of Massachusetts Medical School
Worchester, Massachusetts

Herbert L. Muncie, Jr., MD
Professor
Director of Student Education
Department of Family Medicine
Louisiana State University School of Medicine
New Orleans, Louisiana

Mallika Mundkur, MD
University of Massachusetts Medical School
Worcester, Massachusetts

Amanda Murchison, MD
Assistant Professor
Department of Obstetrics and Gynecology
Virginia Tech-Carilion School of Medicine;
Assistant Residency Program Director
Department of Obstetrics and Gynecology
Carilion Clinic
Roanoke, Virginia

Lawrence Murphy, MD
University of Massachusetts Medical School
Worcester, Massachusetts

Eleftherios Mylonakis, MD
Associate Professor of Medicine
Division of Infectious Diseases
Harvard Medical School
Massachusetts General Hospital
Boston, Massachusetts

Shashidhara Nanjundaswamy, MD, MBBS, MRCP, DM
Assistant Professor
Department of Neurology
University of Massachusetts Medical School;
Neurologist
Neurology
University of Massachusetts Memorial Health Care
Worcester, Massachusetts

Johra Nasreen, MD
Department of Family Medicine
University Hospital
University of Texas Health Science Center
San Antonio, Texas

David M. Navel, MD
Department of Family Medicine
David Grant Medical Center
Travis Air Force Base, California

Beverly L. Nazarian, MD
Clinical Associate Professor of Pediatrics
Department of Pediatrics
University of Massachusetts Medical School;
Pediatrician
Pediatric Primary Care
University of Massachusetts Medical Center
Worcester, Massachusetts

James G. Nee, MD
Clinical Faculty
Department of Family Medicine
University of Illinois—Chicago;
Clinical Faculty—Attending
Department of Family Medicine
Resurrection Healthcare—St. Joseph Hospital
Chicago, Illinois

Donald A.F. Nelson, MD
Director of Medical Informatics
Cedar Rapids Medical Education Foundation;
Active Medical Staff
Department of Family Medicine
St. Luke's Hospital
Cedar Rapids, Iowa

Elizabeth Ann Nelson, MD
Senior Associate Dean, Medicine-General Medicine
Baylor College of Medicine
Houston, Texas

Carla M. Nester, MD
Assistant Professor
Department of Medicine and Pediatrics
Division of Adult and Pediatric Nephrology
The University of Iowa Hospitals and Clinics
Iowa City, Iowa

Kristyn Newhall, MD
University of Massachusetts School of Medicine
Worcester, Massachusetts

Constance Nichols, MD
Clinical Associate Professor of Emergency Medicine
Director of Medical Informatics
University of Massachusetts Medical School
Worcester, Massachusetts

David L. Nickerson, PharmD
Department of Community Pharmacy Practice
Massachusetts College of Pharmacy and Health Sciences
Worcester, Massachusetts

Prachaya Nitichaikulvatana, MD
Fellow, Department of Rheumatology
University of Massachusetts Medical School
Worcester, Massachusetts

Laura L. Novak, MD
Associate Director
Barberton Family Practice Residency
Summa Barberton Hospital
Barberton, Ohio

Sean P. O'Reilly, MD
Assistant Professor of Medicine
Pulmonary, Allergy and Critical Care Medicine
University of Massachusetts Medical School;
UMass Memorial Healthcare
Worcester, Massachusetts

Kelly O'Callahan, MD
Instructor
Department of Medicine
University of Massachusetts Medical School;
Physician
Department of Gastroenterology
St. Vincent's Hospital
Worcester, Massachusetts

Jacqueline L. Olin, MS, PharmD, BCPS, CPP
Associate Professor of Pharmacy
Wingate University School of Pharmacy
Wingate, North Carolina

Ken S. Ota, DO
Department of Family Medicine
Banner Good Samaritan Medical Center
Phoenix, Arizona

Balakumar Pandian, MD
Assistant Professor
Internal Medicine & Pediatrics
University of Texas Southwestern;
Hospitalist
Department of Internal Medicine
Brackenridge Hospital
Austin, Texas

Kathleen Pangia, MD
University of Pennsylvania
Philadelphia, Pennsylvania

Debra Papa, MD
Assistant Professor of Obstetrics and Gynecology
UMass Memorial Health Care
University of Massachusetts Medical School
Worcester, Massachusetts

Jon S. Parham, DO, MPH
Associate Professor
Department of Family Medicine
University of Tennessee, Graduate School of Medicine;
Active Staff
Department of Family Medicine
University of Tennessee Medical Center
Knoxville, Tennessee

Douglas S. Parks, MD
Associate Professor
Family Practice Residency
University of Wyoming;
Chair
Department of Family Practice
Cheyenne Regional Medical Center
Cheyenne, Wyoming

Aleema Patel, MD
The Warren Alpert Medical School
Brown University
Providence, Rhode Island

Birju B. Patel, MD
Assistant Professor of Medicine
Emory University School of Medicine
Division of Geriatrics and Gerontology;
Department of Medicine
Atlanta VA Medical Center
Decatur, Georgia

Krunal Patel, MD
University of Massachusetts Medical School
Worcester, Massachusetts

Neepa Patel, MD
Department of Neurology
Boston Medical Center
Boston, Massachusetts

Nihal Patel, MD
University of Massachusetts Medical School
Worcester, Massachusetts

Nilay Patel, MD
Warren Alpert Medical School of Brown University
Providence, Rhode Island

Payal S. Patel, DO
Pediatric Hospitalist
Department of Pediatrics
Edward Hospital
Naperville, Illinois

Sagar C. Patel, MD
Warren Alpert Medical School of Brown University
Providence, Rhode Island

Elizabeth W. Patton, MD
Department of Obstetrics and Gynecology
Northwestern University
Prentice Women's Hospital
Chicago, Illinois

Rashmi V. Patwardhan, MD
Clinical Professor
Department of Medicine
University of Massachusetts Medical School;
Director Outpatient Clinic, Gastroenterology Division
Department of Medicine
University of Massachusetts Memorial Medical Center
Worcester, Massachusetts

Vilas Patwardhan, MD
Department of Internal Medicine
Massachusetts General Hospital
Boston, Massachusetts

Laura Paulin, MD, MHS
Montefiore Medical Center of the Albert Einstein College of Medicine
Bronx, New York

Ernest Pedapati, MD
Cincinnati Children's Hospital
Cincinnati, Ohio

Rade N. Pejic, MD
Assistant Professor of Family Medicine
Tulane University;
Lead Physician of Multi-Specialty Clinic
Department of Family Medicine
Tulane Medical Center
New Orleans, Louisiana

Elizabeth B. Pelkofski, MD
Department of Obstetrics and Gynecology
University of Massachusetts
Worcester, Massachusetts

Amy Pelletier, DO
Department of Pediatrics
Baystate Medical Center
Springfield, Massachusetts

Randall S. Pellish, MD
Assistant Professor of Medicine
Division of Gastroenterology
University of Massachusetts Medical School
University of Massachusetts Memorial Medical Center
Worcester, Massachusetts

Lisa Pelunis-Messier, PharmD
Adjunct Faculty Member
Department of Pharmacy
Clinical Pharmacy Research Services
Massachusetts College of Pharmacy
Worcester, Massachusetts

Douglas A. Pepple, MD
Department of Family Medicine
University of Illinois at Chicago;
University of Illinois at Chicago Medical Center
Chicago, Illinois

Ruben Peralta, MD
Director of Trauma and Critical Care Fellowship Program
Department of Surgery
Hamad Medical Corporation
Department of Medical Education;
Senior Consultant, Surgery, Trauma and Care
Department of Surgery
Hamad General Hospital
Doha, Qatar
United Arab Emirates

Adam B. Pesaturo, PharmD, BCPS
Critical Care Pharmacist
Department of Pharmacy Services
Baystate Medical Center
Springfield, Massachusetts

Kimberly A. Pesaturo, PharmD
Assistant Professor
Department of Pharmacy Practice
Massachusetts College of Pharmacy and Health Sciences;
Clinical Specialist-Pediatrics
Department of Pharmacy
University of Massachusetts Memorial Medical Center
Worcester, Massachusetts

Bobby X. Peters, MD
Assistant Professor
Department of Emergency Medicine
University of Iowa
Iowa City, Iowa

Nicole D. Pilevsky, MD
Private Practice
Obstetrics and Gynecology
Howard County General Hospital
Columbia, Maryland

Jochebed A. Pink, MD
University of Massachusetts Medical School
Worcester, Massachusetts

Barbara R. Pober, MD
Geneticist
Children's Hospital Boston
Boston, Massachusetts

Gregory A. Poland, MD
Mary Lowell Leary Professor of Medicine
Department of General Internal Medicine
College of Medicine, Mayo Clinic;
Director
Mayo Vaccine Research Group
Mayo Clinic
Rochester, Minnesota

Phyllis Pollak, MD
Associate Clinical Professor
Department of Pediatrics
University of Massachusetts Medical School;
Consultant
Department of Pediatrics
University of Massachusetts Medical Center
Worcester, Massachusetts

David A. Pope, MD
Private Practice
Mayo Health System
Janesville, Minnesota

Stacy E. Potts, MD
Assistant Clinical Professor
Department of Family Medicine and Community Health
University of Massachusetts;
Family Physician
Department of Family Medicine and Community Health
University of Massachusetts Memorial Health Care
Worcester, Massachusetts

Thomas Price, MD
Assistant Professor
Division of Geriatric Medicine and Gerontology
Emory University;
Chief, Department of Medicine
Wesley Woods Geriatric Hospital
Atlanta, Georgia

William A. Primack, MD
Professor of Medicine and Pediatrics
University of North Carolina Kidney Center
University of North Carolina School of Medicine
Chapel Hill, North Carolina

Kimberly Pringle, MD
Department of Emergency Medicine
Rhode Island Hospital and
Hasbro Children's Hospital
Providence, Rhode Island

Barbara Provo, MSN, APNP, CWOCN, FNP-BC
Coordinator
Wound and Ostomy Program
Froedtert Hospital
Milwaukee, Wisconsin

George Gunter A. Pujalte, MD
Clinical Lecturer
Department of Family Medicine
University of Michigan
University of Michigan Medical Center
Ann Arbor, Michigan

Elise H. Pyun, MD
Clinical Associate Professor
Department of Medicine
University of Massachusetts Medical School;
Rheumatology Attending
Department of Medicine
University of Massachusetts Medical Center
Worcester, Massachusetts

Juan Qiu, MD, PhD
Assistant Professor
Department of Family and Community Medicine
Pennsylvania State University College of Medicine;
Attending Physician
Department of Family Medicine
Mount Nittany Medical Center
State College, Pennsylvania

Jonna M. Quinn, DO
Aultman Hospital
Canton, Ohio

Naureen B. Rafiq, MBBS, MD
Instructor, Family Medicine
Creighton University Medical Center
Omaha, Nebraska

Mhd Basheer Rahmoun, MD
Assistant Professor, Adjunct
Department of Pharmacy Practice
Massachusetts College of Pharmacy and Health Sciences;
Clinical Research Fellow
Clinical Pharmacology Study Group
Worcester, Massachusetts

Jyoti Ramakrishna, MD
Assistant Professor
Department of Pediatrics
University of Massachusetts Medical School
University of Massachusetts Memorial Healthcare
Worcester, Massachusetts

Manju Ramchandani, MD
Private Practice
Mt. Vernon Family Health Center
Mt. Vernon, Illinois

Neha Raukar, MD
Assistant Professor of Emergency Medicine
Department of Bio-Med Emergency Medicine
Brown Alpert Medical School at Brown University
Providence, Rhode Island

Tejesh S. Reddy, MBBS
Department of Family Medicine
Creighton University
Omaha, Nebraska

Derek M. Richardson, Capt USAF AMC 60 MDOS/SGOF
Department of Family Practice
David Grant Medical Center
Travis Air Force Base, California

Tara J. Rizvi, MD
Assistant Professor
Department of Allergy, Immunology and Rheumatology
Baylor College of Medicine;
Attending Physician
Department of Rheumatology
Ben Taub General Hospital
Houston, Texas

Teresa M. Robb, MD
Clinical Instructor
Department of Obstetrics & Gynecology
Jefferson Medical College of Thomas Jefferson University;
Attending Physician
Department of Obstetrics & Gynecology
Albert Einstein Medical Center
Philadelphia, Pennsylvania

Michele Roberts, MD, PhD
Diplomate American Board of Pathology (AP/CP)
Diplomate American Board of Medical Genetics
Paxton, Massachusetts

Leslie Robinson-Bostom, MD
Associate Professor of Dermatology
Warren Alpert Medical School of Brown University
Providence, Rhode Island

Ann M. Rodden, DO, MS
Assistant Professor
Department of Family Medicine
Medical University of South Carolina
Charleston, South Carolina

Karla M. Rodriguez, MD
Department of Psychiatry
UMass Medical Center
Worcester, Massachusetts

Jennifer L. Rogers, MD
Aultman Hospital
Canton, Ohio

Lewis C. Rose, MD
Associate Professor
Department of Family and Community Medicine
University of Texas Health Sciences Center at San Antonio;
Active Medical Staff
Department of Family Medicine
University Hospital
San Antonio, Texas

Montiel T. Rosenthal, MD
Assistant Clinical Professor
Director of Maternity Services
Department of Family Medicine
University of Cincinnati;
Director of Prenatal Clinic
Department of Family Medicine
The Christ Hospital
Cincinnati, Ohio

Steven E. Roskos, MD
Associate Professor
Department of Family Medicine
Michigan State University
College of Human Medicine
East Lansing, Michigan

Julie L. Roth, MD
Assistant Professor
Department of Neurology
The Warren Alpert Medical School of Brown University
Providence, Rhode Island

Michael Rousse, MD, MPH
Hospitalist Director
Department of Medicine
Northeastern Vermont Regional Hospital
St. Johnsbury, Vermont

Paul G. Rubinstein, MD
Hematology/Oncology Fellow
Department of Medicine: Section of Hematology/Oncology
University of Illinois at Chicago Medical Center
Chicago, Illinois

Stephanie Ruest, MD
University of Massachusetts Medical School
Worcester, Massachusetts

Beth Ryder, MD
Assistant Professor of Surgery
Warren Alpert Medical School at Brown University
Providence, Rhode Island

Roland Saavedra, MD
Department of Family Medicine and Community Health
University of Massachusetts School of Medicine
Worcester, Massachusetts;

Aman D. Sabharwal, MD
Clinical Assistant Professor
Department of Medicine
Florida International University
College of Medicine;
Chief Utilization Officer
Jackson Health System
Miami, Florida

Anup Kumar Sabharwal, MD
Assistant Professor in Clinical Medicine
Endocrinology, Diabetes, and Metabolism
University of Miami
Miller School of Medicine
Miami, Florida

Stanley Sagov, MD
Assistant Professor
Department of Family Medicine
University of Massachusetts
Worcester, Massachusetts;
Chief of Family Medicine
Department of Medicine
Mount Auburn Hospital
Cambridge, Massachusetts

Karen I. Salomon-Escoto, MD
Assistant Professor
Department of Medicine
University of Massachusetts Medical School
Worcester, Massachusetts

Ricardo A. Samson, MD
Professor
Department of Pediatrics
The University of Arizona;
Chief
Section of Pediatric Cardiology
University Medical Center
Tucson, Arizona

Arthur B. Sanders, MD, MHA
Professor
Department of Emergency Medicine
University of Arizona;
Attending Physician
University Medical Center
Tucson, Arizona

Darshak Sanghavi, MD
Departments of Pediatrics and Cardiology
University of Massachusetts Medical School
Worcester, Massachusetts

Ann Saunders, MD
University of Massachusetts Medical School
Worcester, Massachusetts

Jennifer L. Savitski, MD
Clinical Instructor
Department of Obstetrics and Gynecology
Northeastern Ohio University College of Medicine
Rootstown, Ohio;
Assistant Residency Program Director
Department of Obstetrics and Gynecology
Akron General Medical Center
Akron, Ohio

Shailendra K. Saxena, MD
Assistant Professor, Family Medicine
Creighton University School of Medicine
Omaha, Nebraska

Dalia Sbat, PharmD
Adjunct Faculty
Department of Pharmaceutical Science
Massachusetts College of Pharmacy and Health Sciences
Worcester, Massachusetts;
Pharmacist
Walgreens Pharmacy
Shrewsbury, Massachusetts

Stephanie Scandale, MD
Assistant Clinical Professor
Department of Family Medicine
University of California, Los Angeles;
University of California, Los Angeles Santa Monica Hospital
Santa Monica, California

Fred Schiffman, MD
Vice Chairman, Department of Medicine
Sigal Family Professor of Humanistic Medicine
Clinical Director, Comprehensive Cancer Center
Professor of Medicine
Alpert Medical School of Brown University
The Miriam Hospital
Providence, Rhode Island

Eric Schmidt, MD
Clinical Associate Professor of Emergency Medicine
Co-Director, Undergraduate Medical Education
Department of Emergency Medicine
University of Massachusetts Medical School
Worcester, Massachusetts

Lisa M. Schroeder, MD
Assistant Director
Family Practice Residency Program
Summa Barberton Hospital
Barberton, Ohio

Alexandra Schultes, MD
Associate Professor
Department of Family Practice
University of Massachusetts
Worcester, Massachusetts

Bradford Schwartz, MD
University of Massachusetts Medical School
Worcester, Massachusetts

Deanna M. Scinto, PharmD
Adjunct Assistant Professor
Department of Pharmacy Practice
Massachusetts College of Pharmacy—Worcester
Worcester, Massachusetts

Christopher J. Scola, MD
Departments of Medicine and Rheumatology
Hartford Hospital
Hartford, Connecticut

Stephen M. Scott, MD, MPH
Assistant Professor
Department of Family and Community Medicine
Baylor College of Medicine
Houston, Texas

Gail Scully, MD, MPH
Assistant Professor
Department of Medicine
Division of Infectious Disease and Immunology
University of Massachusetts Medical School
Worcester, Massachusetts

David P. Sealy, MD
Clinical Professor
Department of Family Medicine
Director, Sports Medicine Fellowship
Department of Sports Medicine
Medical University South Carolina
Greenwood, South Carolina

Jose Oscar Seda, MD
Department of Family Medicine
University of Texas Health Science Center
San Antonio, Texas

Sheila M. Seed, PharmD, MPH
Associate Professor
Department of Pharmacy Practice
Massachusetts College of Pharmacy and Health Sciences
Worcester, Massachusetts

Patricia Seymour, MD
Department of Family Medicine and Community Health
University of Massachusetts Medical School
Worcester, Massachusetts

Amy Shah, MD
Department of Psychiatry
University of Cincinnati;
The University Hospital
Cincinnati, Ohio

Binay K. Shah, MD
Department of Hematology
St. Joseph Regional Medical Center
SJRMC Cancer Center
Lewiston, Idaho

Dhvani Shah, MD
Alpert Medical School
Brown University
Providence, Rhode Island

Archit Sharma, MD
Department of Family Medicine
Creighton University Medical Center
Omaha, Nebraska

Mohammed Shahsabebi, MD
Department of Community and Family Medicine
Duke University Medical Center
Durham, North Carolina

Sanjeev K. Sharma, MD
Associate Professor, Family Medicine
Creighton University School of Medicine
Omaha, Nebraska

Sujata Sharma, MD
Department of Family Medicine
Resurrection Medical Center
Chicago, Illinois

Douglas Shemin, MD
Associate Professor
Department of Medicine
Brown University School of Medicine;
Interim Director
Division of Kidney Diseases
Rhode Island Hospital
Providence, Rhode Island

David S. Shepro, MD
Assistant Professor
Department of Medicine
University of Massachusetts Medical School
Commonwealth Hematology and Oncology, PC
Worcester, Massachusetts

Awais Siddiki, MD
Department of Internal Medicine
University of Massachusetts Medical School
Worcester, Massachusetts

Aamir Siddiqi, MD
Associate Director
St. Luke's Family Medicine Residency
Aurora Health Care;
Vice President Medical Staff
Aurora Sinai Medical Center
Milwaukee, Wisconsin

Najmul H. Siddiqui, MBBS, MD
Department of Family Practice
Creighton University Medical Center
Omaha, Nebraska

Hugh J. Silk, MD
Assistant Professor
Department of Family Medicine and Community Health
University of Massachusetts Medical School;
Staff
Department of Family Medicine and Community Health
University of Massachusetts Memorial Medical Center
Worcester, Massachusetts

Matthew A. Silva, PharmD, RPh, BCPS
Assistant Professor
Pharmacy Practice
Massachusetts College of Pharmacy and Health Sciences;
Clinical Pharmacist
Department of Family Medicine/Pharmacy
Family Health Center of Worcester
Worcester, Massachusetts

B. Brent Simmons, MD
Assistant Professor
Department of Family Medicine
Drexel University-College of Medicine
Philadelphia, Pennsylvania

Linda Sinclair, MD
University of Massachusetts Medical School
Worcester, Massachusetts

Jaspreet Singh, DO

Manoj Singh, MD
Assistant Professor
Department of Family Medicine
University of Cincinnati;
Attending Physician
Department of Family Medicine
The Christ Hospital
Cincinnati, Ohio

Patrick Smallwood, MD
Assistant Professor of Psychiatry
Department of Psychiatry
University of Massachusetts Medical School;
Attending Psychiatrist/Medical Director of Psychosomatic Medicine and Emergency Mental Health
Department of Psychiatry
University of Massachusetts Medical Center
Worcester, Massachusetts

Robert A. Smith, DO
Colonel, Medical Corps
Deputy Commander for Clinical Service
U.S. Army Medical Department Activity
Heidelberg Germany

Stanley G. Smith, MA, MB, FCFP
Professor Emeritus
Department of Family Medicine
University of Western Ontario
London, Ontario, Canada

John C. Smulian, MD, MPH
Vice Chair and Chief of Maternal Fetal Medicine
Department of Obstetrics and Gynecology
Lehigh Valley Health Network
Allentown, Pennsylvania

Nancy J. Snapp, MD, MPH
Physician
Department of Family Medicine
International Community Health Services
Seattle, Washington

Michael Snyder, MD
Professor
Department of Medicine–Hematology/Oncology, Pathology
University of Massachusetts Medical School
Worcester, Massachusetts

Augustine J. Sohn, MD, MPH
Assistant Professor
Department of Clinical Family Medicine
Department of Family Medicine
University of Illinois at Chicago;
Attending Physician
Department of Family Medicine
University of Illinois Hospital
Chicago, Illinois

Weily Soong, MD
Clinical Associate Professor
Department of Pediatric Allergy and Immunology
University of Alabama School of Medicine;
Managing Partner
Alabama Allergy and Asthma Center
Birmingham, Alabama

Mia D. Sorcinelli, MD
Attending Physician
Department of Family Medicine
Lawrence General Hospital
Lawrence, Massachusetts

John Spangler, MD, MPH
Associate Professor
Department of Family and Community Medicine
Wake Forest University School of Medicine
Winston-Salem, North Carolina

Mikayla Spangler, PharmD, BCPS
Assistant Professor
Creighton University School of Pharmacy and Health Professions
Clinical Pharmacist, Creighton Family Healthcare
Omaha, Nebraska

Joshua J. Spooner, PharmD, MS
Director of Clinical and Outcomes Services
Advanced Concepts Institute
University of the Sciences in Philadelphia
Philadelphia, Pennsylvania

Kellie A. Sprague, MD
Assistant Professor
Division of Hematology-Oncology
Tufts University School of Medicine;
Assistant Director
Bone Marrow Transplant Program
Division of Hematology-Oncology
Tufts Medical Center
Boston, Massachusetts

Dana Sprute, MD, MPH
Assistant Professor
University of Texas Southwestern Medical Center;
Assistant Clinical Professor
University of Texas Medical Branch
Austin, Texas

Michelle St. Fleur, MD
University of Massachusetts Medical School
Worcester, Massachusetts

Joan M. Stachnik, PharmD, BCPS
Clinical Assistant Professor
Drug Information Group
Department of Pharmacy Practice
College of Pharmacy
University of Illinois Medical Center at Chicago
Chicago, Illinois

Michael S. Stalvey, MD
Assistant Professor, Pediatric Endocrinology
University of Massachusetts Medical School
Department of Pediatrics
Gene Therapy Center
Worcester, Massachusetts

Oscar Starobin, MD
Department of Cardiology
University of Massachusetts Medical Center
Worcester, Massachusetts

Mark Steenbergen, DO
Private Practice, Family Practice
Poughkeepsie, New York

Gillian S. Stephens, MD, MSc
Assistant Professor
Department of Family and Community Medicine
Saint Louis University
Saint Louis, Missouri

Debora B. Sternaman, PharmD
Regional Medical Scientist
Department of Medical Affairs
Boehringer Ingelheim
Georgetown, Texas

Edward C. Sternaman, II, MD
Hospitalist
Department of Internal Medicine
Seton Williamson
Round Rock, Texas

J. Herbert Stevenson, MD
Director, Sports Medicine Fellowship
Department of Family and Community Medicine
University of Massachusetts Medical School;
Director, Sports Medicine
Department of Family and Community Medicine
University of Massachusetts Memorial Medical Center
Worcester, Massachusetts

Sheila O. Stille, DMD, MAGD
Assistant Professor
Department of Family Medicine and Community Health
University of Massachusetts Medical School;
Program Director, General Practice Residency in Dentistry
Department of Family Medicine and Community Health
University of Massachusetts Memorial
Worcester, Massachusetts

Jeffrey G. Stovall, MD
Associate Professor
Department of Psychiatry
Vanderbilt University School of Medicine;
Residency Training Director, Adult Psychiatry
Vanderbilt Psychiatric Hospital
Nashville, Tennessee

Charles Strom, MD
University of Massachusetts School of Medicine
Worcester, Massachusetts

Ryung Suh, MD, MPP, MBA, MPH
Assistant Professor
Health Systems Administration
Georgetown University
Washington, District of Columbia;
Command Surgeon and Occupational Health Division Chief
Defense Threat Reduction Agency
Fort Belvoir, Virginia

James J. Sullivan, Jr., MD, USN
Emergency Medicine Department
University of Massachusetts Medical School
Worcester, Massachusetts

Karyn M. Sullivan, PharmD, MPH
Associate Professor
Department of Pharmacy Practice
Massachusetts College of Pharmacy and Health Sciences;
Clinical Pharmacist
Department of Pharmacy
St. Vincent Hospital
Worcester, Massachusetts

Laura Sullivan Eurich, MD
University of Massachusetts School of Medicine
Worcester, Massachusetts

Anna Svircev, DO, MPH
Department of Family Medicine
University of Colorado
Denver, Colorado

Sheela Swaminatha, MD
Department of Neurology
Georgetown University;
Department of Neurology
Georgetown University/DC Veterans Administration
Washington, DC

Sana Syed, MD
Department of Neurology
Boston Medical Center
Boston, Massachusetts

Vassiliki P. Syriopoulou, MD
Professor of Pediatrics
First Department of Pediatrics
Athens University;
Chief of Infectious Diseases
First Department of Pediatrics
Aghia Sophia Children's Hospital
Athens, Greece

Alfonso J. Tafur, MD
Assistant Professor of Medicine
Department of Cardiovascular—Vascular Medicine
Mayo Clinic
Rochester, Minnesota

Chris Tang, MD
Occupational Medicine
Care on Site
Long Beach, California

Nikki D.Y. Tang, MD
Warren Alpert School of Medicine at Brown University
Providence, Rhode Island

Dawn S. Tasillo, MD
Associate Clerkship Director
Department of Obstetrics and Gynecology
University of Massachusetts Medical School;
Assistant Professor
UMass Memorial Medical Center
Worcester, Massachusetts

Erica Tavares, PharmD, RPh
Clinical Pharmacist
Department of Pharmacy
UMass Memorial Medical Center
Worcester, Massachusetts

Julie Scott Taylor, MD, MSc
Associate Professor of Family Medicine
Director of Clinical Curriculum
Alpert Medical School of Brown University
Providence, Rhode Island

Peter Than, MD
Alpert Medical School, Brown University
Providence, Rhode Island

Richard J. Thomas, MD, MPH
Associate Professor
Department of Preventive Medicine and Biometrics
Uniformed Services University of the Health Sciences;
Acting Department Head
Department of Occupational Medicine
National Naval Medical Center
Bethesda, Maryland

Margaret E. Thompson, MD
Associate Professor
Department of Family Practice
Michigan State University College of Human Medicine
Grand Rapids, Michigan

Michelle A. Tinitigan, MD
Clinical Assistant Professor
Department of Family and Community Medicine
University of California-San Francisco
San Francisco, California

Rochelle J. Tinitigan, MD
Department of Family and Community Medicine
University of Texas Health Science Center at San Antonio
San Antonio, Texas

Moshe S. Torem, MD, DLFAPA
Professor of Psychiatry
Department of Psychiatry
Northeastern Ohio Universities College of Medicine
Rootstown, Ohio;
Chief of Integrative Medicine
Department of Medicine
Akron General Medical Center
Akron, Ohio

William A. Tosches, MD
Associate Clinical Professor of Neurology and Medicine
Department of Neurology
University of Massachusetts Medical School
Worcester, Massachusetts;
Chief of Neurology Service
Milford Regional Medical Center
Milford, Massachusetts

Alyssa H. Tran, DO
Department of Family and Community Medicine
University of Texas Health Science Center
University Hospital
San Antonio, Texas

Natasha A. Travis, MD
Assistant Professor of Medicine
Department of General Internal Medicine
Medical College of Wisconsin
Froedtert Hospital
Milwaukee, Wisconsin

Michelle Trivedi, MD
University of Massachusetts Medical School
Worcester, Massachusetts

Zoltan Trizna, MD, PhD
Private Practice, Dermatology
Austin, Texas

Katherine Tromp, PharmD
Assistant Professor
Department of Pharmacy Practice
Lake Erie College of Osteopathic Medicine
LECOM-Bradenton School of Pharmacy
Bradenton, Florida

Richard E. Trowbridge, MD
David Grant Medical Center
Travis AFB, California

Caroline Tschibelu, MD
Department of Emergency Medicine
Alpert Medical School at Brown University
Providence, Rhode Island

Kristin A. Tuiskula, PharmD
Assistant Professor
Pharmacy Practice
Massachusetts College of Pharmacy and Health Sciences
Worcester, Massachusetts

Katharine Tumilty, MD
University of Massachusetts Medical School
Worcester, Massachusetts

Auguste Turnier, MD
Internist/Gastroenterologist, Private Practice
Haddonfield, New Jersey

Lawrence E. Udom, MD, MPH
Department of Psychiatry/Family Medicine
University of Cincinnati, University Hospital
Cincinnati, Ohio

Katherine Upchurch, MD
Clinical Professor
Department of Medicine
University of Massachusetts Medical School;
Clinical Chief
Division of Rheumatology
UMass Memorial Medical Center
Worcester, Massachusetts

Eric Ursprung, MD
University of Massachusetts Medical School
Worcester, Massachusetts

Richard P. Usatine, MD
Professor
Department of Family and Community Medicine
University of Texas Health Science Center at San Antonio
San Antonio, Texas

Santiago O. Valdes, MD
Assistant Professor
Department of Pediatrics
University of Arizona
Tucson, Arizona

Anthony Valdini, MD
Director of Research
Director of the Faculty Development Fellowship
Director of Faculty Development
Greater Lawrence Family Health Center
Lawrence, Massachusetts

Ron Van Ness-Otunnu, MD
House Staff Officer
Department of Emergency Medicine
Warren Alpert Medical School of Brown University;
Rhode Island Hospital
Providence, Rhode Island

Adam Vasconcellos, MD
Alpert Medical School, Brown University
Providence, Rhode Island

Jake D. Veigel, MD
University of Massachusetts Primary Care Sports Medicine Fellowship
University of Massachusetts Medical School
Fitchburg, Massachusetts

Colleen Veloski, MD
Associate Professor
Department of Endocrinology
Temple University School of Medicine
Philadelphia, Pennsylvania

Richard Viken, MD
Professor
Department of Family Medicine
University of Texas Health Science Center at Tyler
Tyler, Texas

Siva Vithananthan, MD
University Surgical Associates Inc.
Providence, Rhode Island

Rishi Vohora, DO
Dept of Cardiology
University of Massachusetts Medical Center
Worcester, Massachusetts

Kenton I. Voorhees, MD
Associate Professor and Vice Chair, Education
Department of Family Medicine
University of Colorado Denver School of Medicine
Aurora, Colorado

Yongkasem Vorasettakarnkij, MD, MSc
Instructor, Department of Medicine
Faculty of Medicine
Chulalongkorn University
Bangkok, Thailand;
Program in Cardiovascular MR
Martinos Center for Biomedical Imaging
Massachusetts General Hospital
Charlestown, Massachusetts

Kimberle Vore, MD
Clinical Assistant Professor of Family Medicine
Department of Family Medicine
Penn State College of Medicine
Hershey, Pennsylvania;
Clinical Instructor
Department of Family Medicine
The Washington Hospital
Washington, Pennsylvania

John B. Waits, MD
Associate Professor/Program Director-Tuscaloosa Family Medicine Residency
Department of Family Medicine/Obstetrics and Gynecology
University of Alabama School of Medicine;
Physician
Department of Family Medicine/Obstetrics
DCH Regional Medical Center
Tuscaloosa, Alabama

Noah S. Walman, MD
Department of Family Medicine
University of Illinois at Chicago College of Medicine
Chicago, Illinois

Anne M. Walsh, PA-C, MMSc
Clinical Instructor
Department of Family Medicine
Keck School of Medicine
University of Southern California
Los Angeles, California

William V. Walsh, MD
Assistant Professor of Medicine
Division of Hematology Oncology
University of Massachusetts Medical School;
UMass Memorial Medical Center
Worcester, Massachusetts

Erik E. Wang, MD
Department of Emergency Medicine
Brown University;
Rhode Island Hospital
Providence, Rhode Island

Otis Warren, MD
Department of Emergency Medicine
Warren Alpert School of Medicine
Brown University
Providence, Rhode Island

Donald E. Watenpaugh, PhD
Adjunct Professor
Department of Integrative Physiology
University of North Texas Health Science Center
Fort Worth, Texas

Ramothea L. Webster, MD, PhD
Department of Family Medicine
SUNY Downstate Medical Center
Lutheran Medical Center
Brooklyn, New York

Kathryn W. Weibrecht, MD
Clinical Instructor
Department of Emergency Medicine
UMass Memorial Health Center
Worcester, Massachusetts

Patrice Weiss, MD
Professor
Department of Obstetrics and Gynecology
Virginia Tech-Carilion School of Medicine;
Residency Program Director and Vice-Chair
Department of Obstetrics and Gynecology
Carilion Clinic
Roanoke, Virginia

Nathan Weldon, MD
Department of Family Medicine
University of California, Irvine
Irvine, California

Andrew J. Westwood, MD
Department of Neurology
Boston Medical Center
Boston, Massachusetts

Chris Wheelock, MD
Faculty Southwest Washington Family Medicine
Clinical Instructor of Family Medicine University of Washington
Vancouver, Washington

Brett White, MD
Assistant Professor
Department of Family Medicine
Oregon Health and Science University
Portland, Oregon

Christopher C. White, MD, JD
Assistant Professor
Department of Psychiatry and Family Medicine
University of Cincinnati College of Medicine;
Medical Director, Psychiatric Consultation
Department of Psychiatry & Behavioral Neuroscience
University Hospital
Cincinnati, Ohio

Susan White, MD
Assistant Professor
Program Director, School of PA Studies
Manchester/Worcester Massachusetts College of Pharmacy & Health Sciences
Manchester New Hampshire

Michelle Whitehurst-Cook, MD
Associate Professor of Family Medicine
Associate Dean for Admissions
VCU School of Medicine
Richmond, Virginia

Kristine Willett, PharmD
Assistant Professor
Pharmacy Practice
Massachusetts College of Pharmacy and Health Sciences
Manchester, New Hampshire

Alan L. Williams, MD
Adjunct Professor of Family Medicine
Department of Family Medicine
Uniformed Services University of the Health Sciences
Bethesda, Maryland

Faren H. Williams, MD
Chief Physical Medicine and Rehabilitation
Clinical Professor
University of Massachusetts School of Medicine
Worcester, Massachusetts

Pamela M. Williams, MD, Lt Col, USAF, MC
Assistant Professor
Department of Family Medicine
Uniformed Services University of the Health Sciences
Bethesda, Maryland

Alan Williamson, MD
Department of Family Medicine/Sports Medicine
David Grant USAF Medical Center
Travis Air Force Base, California

Jessica Lenore Wilson, MD
University of Illinois at Chicago College of Medicine
Chicago, Illinois

Robyn D. Wing, MD
Department of Pediatrics
University of Massachusetts Medical School
Worcester, Massachusetts

Christopher M. Wise, MD
W. Robert Irby Professor of Medicine
Department of Internal Medicine
Division of Rheumatology
Virginia Commonwealth University Medical College of Virginia
Richmond, Virginia

Jeffrey D. Wolfrey, MD
Clinical Professor
Department of Family and Community Medicine
University of Arizona College of Medicine
Tucson, Arizona;
Residency Director
Department of Family Medicine
Banner Good Samaritan Medical Center
Phoenix, Arizona

Zerlina Wong, MD
The Warren Alpert Medical School of Brown University
Providence, Rhode Island

Kyle D. Wood, MD
Department of Urology
Wake Forest University Baptist Medical Center
Winston Salem, North Carolina

Fae G. Wooding, PharmD
Assistant Professor of Pharmacy Practice
Massachusetts College of Pharmacy and Health Sciences
Worcester, Massachusetts

Frances Y. Wu, MD
Clinical Assistant Professor
Department of Family Medicine
UMDNJ-New Jersey Medical School
Newark, New Jersey;
Assistant Director
Department of Family Practice
Somerset Medical Center
Somerville, New Jersey

Frederick Wu, MD
Assistant Professor
Department of Veterans Affairs, Atlanta Medical Center
Emory University School of Medicine
Decatur, Georgia

Congjun Yao, MD
Department of Family Medicine
University of Texas Health Science Center at San Antonio
San Antonio, Texas

Julie Yeh, MD, MPH
Assistant Professor
Department of Family, Community, & Preventive Medicine
Drexel University College of Medicine;
Medical Staff
Department of Family, Community, and Preventive Medicine
Hahnemann University Hospital
Philadelphia, Pennsylvania

Gary Yen, MD
Clinical Lecturer
Department of Family Medicine
University of Michigan
Ann Arbor, Michigan

Robert A. Yood, MD
Clinical Professor of Medicine
Department of Medicine
University of Massachusetts Medical School;
Chief
Division of Rheumatology
Fallon Clinic
Worcester, Massachusetts

James L. Young, MD, PhD
Program in Molecular Medicine
University of Massachusetts Medical School
Worcester, Massachusetts

Edward L. Yourtee, MD
Southern New Hampshire Internal Medicine Associates
Derry, New Hampshire

Leanne Zakrzewski, MD
Department of Family Medicine
University of California, Los Angeles, David Geffen School of Medicine
Los Angeles, California

Ali Zarrabi, MD
The Warren Alpert Medical School of Brown University
Providence, Rhode Island

John K. Zawacki, MD
Professor of Medicine
Department of Medicine
Division of Gastroenterology
University of Massachusetts Medical School;
UMass Memorial Health Care
Worcester, Massachusetts

William Zawatski, MD
University of Massachusetts Medical School
Worcester, Massachusetts

Katrina Darlene Zedan, MSPAS, PA-C
Department of Acute Care/Family Medicine
University of Texas Health Science Center–San Antonio
San Antonio, Texas

Liang Zhao, MD
University of Massachusetts Medical School
Worcester, Massachusetts

Peter J. Ziemkowski, MD
Assistant Professor
Department of Family Medicine
Michigan State University
East Lansing, Michigan;
Clerkship Director
Family Medicine Residency Program
MSU/Kalamazoo Center for Medical Studies
Kalamazoo, Michigan

Susan Ziglar, MD
Assistant Professor
School of Pharmacy
Wingate University
Wingate, North Carolina

Richard Kent Zimmerman, MD, MPH
Professor
Department of Family Medicine
University of Pittsburgh
Pittsburgh, Pennsylvania

Jill N. Zink, MD
Department of Surgery
Akron General Medical Center
Akron, Ohio

Gennine M. Zinner, RNCS, ANP
Clinical Instructor
Department of Nursing
MGH Institute of Health Professions
Boston, Massachusetts

Anthony M. Zizza, III, MD
University of Massachusetts Medical School
Worcester, Massachusetts

Deborah E. Zuckerman, MD
Clinical Instructor
Department of Ophthalmology
Tufts University School of Medicine
Boston, Massachusetts;
Active Staff Physician
Department of Ophthalmology
Winchester Hospital
Winchester, Massachusetts

Susan L. Zweizig, MD
Associate Professor
Division of Gynecologic Oncology
Department of Obstetrics and Gynecology
University of Massachusetts Medical Center
Worcester, Massachusetts

CONTENTS

Topics

U.S. Preventive Services Task Force Recommendations

This section is designed to be a quick reference to the best screening and prevention recommendations from the least biased sources. They are the United States Preventive Services Task Force (USPSTF), the U.S. Centers for Disease Control (CDC), the American Academy of Pediatrics, and the American Academy of Family Physicians. Each intervention receives an evidence-based grading set by the USPSTF. They are:

2005 TASK FORCE RATINGS

Strength of Recommendations

The U.S. Preventive Services Task Force (USPSTF) grades its recommendations according to one of five classifications (A, B, C, D, I) reflecting the strength of evidence and magnitude of *net benefit* (benefits minus harms).

A. The USPSTF strongly recommends clinicians provide [the service] to eligible patients. The USPSTF found good evidence that [the service] improves important health outcomes and concludes that benefits substantially outweigh harms.

B. The USPSTF recommends clinicians provide [this service] to eligible patients. The USPSTF found at least fair evidence that [the service] improves important health outcomes and concludes that benefits outweigh harms.

C. The USPSTF makes no recommendation for or against routine provision of [the service]. The USPSTF found at least fair evidence [the service] can improve health outcomes but concludes the balance of benefits and harms is too close to justify a general recommendation.

D. The USPSTF recommends against routinely providing [the service] to asymptomatic patients. The USPSTF found at least fair evidence that [the service] is ineffective or that harms outweigh benefits.

I. The USPSTF concludes the evidence is insufficient to recommend for or against routinely providing [the service]. Evidence the [service] is effective is lacking, of poor quality, or conflicting and the net benefit cannot be determined.

In 2008, the USPSTF updated their rating system for *all new recommendations*; they are:

GRADE DEFINITIONS AFTER MAY 2007

What the Grades Mean and Suggestions for Practice

The U.S. Preventive Services Task Force (USPSTF) has updated its definitions of the grades it assigns to recommendations and now includes "suggestions for practice" associated with each grade. The USPSTF has also defined levels of certainty regarding net benefit. These definitions apply to USPSTF recommendations voted on after May 2007.

Grade	Definition	Suggestions for Practice
A	The USPSTF recommends the service. There is high certainty that the net benefit is substantial.	Offer or provide this service.
B	The USPSTF recommends the service. There is high certainty that the net benefit is moderate or there is moderate certainty that the net benefit is moderate to substantial.	Offer or provide this service.
C	The USPSTF recommends against routinely providing the service. There may be considerations that support providing the service in an individual patient. There is at least moderate certainty that the net benefit is small.	Offer or provide this service only if other considerations support the offering or providing the service in an individual patient.
D	The USPSTF recommends against the service. There is moderate or high certainty that the service has no net benefit or that the harms outweigh the benefits.	Discourage the use of this service.
I Statement	The USPSTF concludes that the current evidence is insufficient to assess the balance of benefits and harms of the service. Evidence is lacking, of poor quality, or conflicting, and the balance of benefits and harms cannot be determined.	Read the clinical considerations section of USPSTF Recommendation Statement. If the service is offered, patients should understand the uncertainty about the balance of benefits and harms.

Levels of Certainty Regarding Net Benefit

Level of Certainty*	Description
High	The available evidence usually includes consistent results from well-designed, well-conducted studies in representative primary care populations. These studies assess the effects of the preventive service on health outcomes. This conclusion is therefore unlikely to be strongly affected by the results of future studies.
Moderate	The available evidence is sufficient to determine the effects of the preventive service on health outcomes, but confidence in the estimate is constrained by such factors as: • The number, size, or quality of individual studies. • Inconsistency of findings across individual studies. • Limited generalizability of findings to routine primary care practice. • Lack of coherence in the chain of evidence. As more information becomes available, the magnitude or direction of the observed effect could change, and this change may be large enough to alter the conclusion.
Low	The available evidence is insufficient to assess effects on health outcomes. Evidence is insufficient because of: • The limited number or size of studies. • Important flaws in study design or methods. • Inconsistency of findings across individual studies. • Gaps in the chain of evidence. • Findings not generalizable to routine primary care practice. • Lack of information on important health outcomes. More information may allow estimation of effects on health outcomes.

*The USPSTF defines certainty as "likelihood that the USPSTF assessment of the net benefit of a preventive service is correct." The net benefit is defined as benefit minus harm of the preventive service as implemented in a general, primary care population. The USPSTF assigns a certainty level based on the nature of the overall evidence available to assess the net benefit of a preventive service.
Current as of May 2008

These recommendations should be tailored to patients' preferences. For example, screening for carcinoma of the prostate receives an "I" recommendation, yet many providers (and their patients) are concerned. Use of a detailed *Informed Consent* discussion for prostate cancer screening empowers the patient and the clinician to use these recommendations in a patient-centered manner.

Absent are in these recommendations "vested interests." Many disease specific groups (American Cancer Society, the American Heart Association, National Osteoporosis Foundation, etc.) suggest interventions that serve *their* goals, but do not always have a strong evidence base (i.e. PSA testing for Prostate Cancer, Bone Mineral Density before age 65, etc.). The USPSTF provides the least biased evaluations.

—Frank J. Domino, MD
Editor-in-Chief

HEALTH MAINTENANCE: BIRTH TO 10 YEARS

(http://www.ahrq.gov/clinic/cps3dix.htm)

Leading causes of death:

- Perinatal infections
- Congenital anomalies
- Sudden infant death syndrome (SIDS)
- Accidents (drowning, abuse)
- Motor vehicle accidents

Recommended counseling, testing or interventions:

Height, weight, growth chart	
Immunizations (*http://www.cdc.gov/nip/ or www.immunizationed.org*)	(DPaT, IPV, Hib, hepatitis A, hepatitis B, MMR, pneumococcal, rotavirus, varicella, influenza 6 mo–18 years)
Counseling:	Injury prevention: –Car seats –Seat belts –Bicycle helmets –Smoke & carbon monoxide detector –Window/stair guards –Firearm storage
Breast fed infants	400 IU vitamin D started before 2 months
Congenital hypothyroidism	At birth
Dental caries in preschool children	Oral fluoride supplementation for children older than 6 months whose primary water source is deficient in fluoride –6 months–3 years 0.25 mg, –3–6 years 0.5 mg, –6–16 years 1.0 mg/day
Diet	Low Saturated Fat diet & Physical Exercise
Hearing screening	At birth
Lead screening	High risk: Minority, urban residency, low SES, house built before 1950, recent immigration
Obesity	Screen children >/= 6 years for obesity and offer/refer to comprehensive, intensive behavioral interventions to promote improvement in weight status
Substance abuse prevention	Tobacco, alcohol counseling
Tuberculosis screening	High risk: Urban residency, Low SES, recent immigration or exposure to recent immigrant
Vision screening: strabismus, amblyopia, visual acuity	For first 5 years of life

Insufficient to recommend for or against:

Dysplasia of the hip	By physical examination

HEALTH MAINTENANCE 11–24 YEARS

(http://www.ahrq.gov/clinic/uspstf/uspstopics.htm)

Leading causes of death:

- Motor vehicle accidents
- Unintentional injuries
- Homicide
- Suicide
- Malignant neoplasms

Immunizations: (*http://www.cdc.gov/vaccines/ or www.immunizationed.org*)	Tetanus-diphtheria-pertussis (Tdap), meningococcal (MCV4), human papilloma virus (females), varicella (2 total for those without immunity), influenza
Disease	**Recommended intervention (A or B grade)**
General	Height, weight, BMI, blood pressure, injury prevention (seat belts, firearms), low saturated fat diet, physical exercise
Alcohol & substance abuse screening	*
Breast & ovarian cancer by BRCA mutation	If high risk: Ashkenazi, or two 1° relatives with breast or ovarian cancer at <50 years of age
Cervical cancer screening	3 years after first intercourse or age 21
Chlamydia, gonorrhea and syphilis screening	If high risk: Sexually active, pregnancy, IV drug use
Depression	In clinical practices that have systems in place to assure accurate diagnosis, effective treatment, and followup.
Diabetes mellitus (non fasting glucose)	if BP >135/80
Domestic/family violence	If sexually active
HIV screening	If high risk: Sexually active, pregnancy, IV drug use
Hepatitis B	If high risk: Sexually active, pregnancy, IV drug use
Lipid disorders	20 to 35 if they are at increased risk for coronary heart disease (family history of premature CHD, diabetes, etc.)
Tuberculosis screening	If high risk: Travel, immigrant, alcohol abuse, IV drug use
Obesity (counseling for obese patients)	Screen children >/= 6 years for obesity and offer/refer to comprehensive, intensive behavioral interventions to promote improvement in weight status.
Folic acid for women	all women planning or capable of pregnancy take a daily supplement of 0.4 to 0.8 mg (400 to 800 μg) of folic acid
Tobacco cessation	Ask all adults about tobacco use and provide tobacco cessation interventions for those who use tobacco
Suicide screening	Depression*

*Additional screening

Alcohol abuse	"Risky"/"hazardous" alcohol use: >7 drinks per week or more than 3 drinks on any on occasion for women, and >14 drinks per week or more than 4 drinks on any one occasion for men. OR Screen: "on any occasion during the last 3 months, have had more than 5 alcohol drinks" or CAGE: Tried to CUT down, been ANGERED by questions about your drinking, felt GUILTY about your drinking, had an EYE OPENER (drink in the morning)
Domestic violence	Screen all at risk patients (all women, especially when pregnant) "Do you feel safe in your present relationship?" "Have you been hit, kicked, punched or otherwise hurt in the last year?"
Substance abuse	Question about drug use and related problems should be considered in all adolescent and adult.
Suicide	Risk factors include history of mood or other mental disorder, substance abuse, history of "deliberate self-harm"

Against (D grade)

Coronary heart disease via ECG, ETT, etc.
Hemochromatosis
Scoliosis screening
Testicular cancer

HEALTH MAINTENANCE 25–45 YEARS

(http://www.ahrq.gov/clinic/cps3dix.htm)

Leading causes of death

Accidental overdose (narcotics, etc.)
Motor vehicle accidents
Cardiovascular disease
Malignant neoplasm
HIV

Immunizations (*http://www.cdc.gov/nip/* or *http://www.immunizationed.org/*)

Tetanus	Tdap every 10 years or just at age 50 (if completed primary series)
Influenza	All adults

Disease	**Recommended intervention (A or B grade)**
General	Height, weight, BMI, blood pressure, injury prevention (seat belts, firearms), low saturated fat diet, physical exercise
Alcohol and substance abuse	*
Breast and ovarian cancer by genetic testing	Refer for genetic counseling if: Ashkenazi heritage, or two 1st degree relatives with breast or ovarian cancer at <50 years of age
Breast cancer screening by Mammography	Mammography starting at age >/= 40; repeat every 1–2 years
Cervical cancer screening	Begin 3 years after first intercourse
Coronary heart disease	Evidence is insufficient to recommend using nontraditional risk factors (high-sensitivity C-reactive protein (hs-CRP), ankle-brachial index (ABI), leukocyte count, fasting blood glucose level, periodontal disease, carotid intima-media thickness (carotid IMT), coronary artery calcification (CAC) score on electron-beam computed tomography (EBCT), homocysteine level, and lipoprotein(a) level) to screen asymptomatic men and women with no history of CHD to prevent CHD events
Depression	In clinical practices that have systems in place to assure accurate diagnosis, effective treatment, and follow up.
Diabetes mellitus, type II (if BP >135/80)	Random serum glucose if sustained blood pressure (either treated or untreated) greater than 135/80 mm Hg
Domestic/family violence	If sexually active
Diet/obesity	Intensive behavioral dietary counseling for patients with known risk factors for cardiovascular and diet-related chronic disease
Chlamydia, gonorrhea, syphilis testing	All adults who are at increased risk (sexually active, IV drug use, etc.)
HIV screening	All adults who are at increased risk (sexually active, IV drug use, etc.)
Hepatitis B	All pregnant women and those with multiple sexual partners, IV drug use, etc.
Lipid disorders	Men: 35 and older for lipid disorders & 20 to 35 if they are at increased risk for coronary heart disease (family history of premature CHD, diabetes, etc.) Women: 45 and older for lipid disorders & 20 to 35 if they are at increased risk for coronary heart disease (family history of premature CHD, diabetes, etc.)
Suicide screening	If depressed*
Tobacco abuse	Ask all adults about tobacco use and provide tobacco cessation interventions for those who use tobacco
Tuberculosis screening	If high risk: Travel, immigrant, alcohol abuse, IV drug use

*Additional screening

Alcohol abuse	"Risky"/"hazardous" alcohol use: >7 drinks per week or more than 3 drinks on any on occasion for women, and >14 drinks per week or more than 4 drinks on any one occasion for men. OR Screen: "on any occasion during the last 3 months, have had more than 5 alcohol drinks" or CAGE: tried to CUT down, been ANGERED by questions about your drinking, felt GUILTY about your drinking, had an EYE OPENER (drink in the morning)
Domestic violence	Screen all at risk patients (all women, especially when pregnant) "Do you feel safe in your present relationship?" "Have you been hit, kicked, punched or otherwise hurt in the last year?"
Substance abuse	Questioning about drug use and related problems should be considered in all adolescent and adult.
Suicide	Risk factors include history of mood or other mental disorder, substance abuse, history of "deliberate self-harm"

Recommends against

Aspirin	The USPSTF recommends against the use of aspirin for stroke prevention in women younger than 55 years and for myocardial infarction prevention in men younger than 45 years.

HEALTH MAINTENANCE 45–65 YEARS

(http://www.ahrq.gov/clinic/cps3dix.htm)

Leading Causes of Death

Cardiovascular Disease
Malignant Neoplasm
Accidents
Cirrhosis

Immunizations *(http://www.cdc.gov/nip/ or http://www.immunizationed.org/)*

Tetanus	Tdap every 10 years or just at age 50 (if completed primary series)
Influenza	All adults

Disease	**Recommended intervention (A or B grade)**
General	Height, weight, BMI, blood pressure, injury prevention (seat belts, firearms), low saturated fat diet, physical exercise
Alcohol and substance abuse	*Insufficient for population; screen at risk
Aspirin	Recommends use of aspirin for men age 45 to 79 and women age 55 to 79 years when potential benefit due to a reduction in myocardial infarctions outweighs the potential harm due to an increase in gastrointestinal hemorrhage.
Breast and ovarian cancer by genetic testing	Refer for genetic counseling if: Ashkenazi heritage, or two 1st degree relatives with breast or ovarian cancer at <50 years of age
Breast cancer screening by mammography	Mammography starting at Age >/= 50; repeat every 1–2 years
Cervical cancer screening	Begin 3 years after first intercourse
Chlamydia, gonorrhea, syphilis testing	All adults who are at increased risk (sexually active, IV drug use, etc.)
Colon cancer	Start at age 50–75 by fecal occult blood testing, sigmoidoscopy, or colonoscopy
Coronary heart disease	Evidence is insufficient to recommend using nontraditional risk factors (high-sensitivity C-reactive protein (hs-CRP), ankle-brachial index (ABI), leukocyte count, fasting blood glucose level, periodontal disease, carotid intima-media thickness (carotid IMT), coronary artery calcification (CAC) score on electron-beam computed tomography (EBCT), homocysteine level, and lipoprotein(a) level) to screen asymptomatic men and women with no history of CHD to prevent CHD events
Depression	In clinical practices that have systems in place to assure accurate diagnosis, effective treatment, and follow up.
Diabetes mellitus, type II if BP >135/80	Random serum glucose if sustained blood pressure (either treated or untreated) greater than 135/80 mm Hg
Domestic/family violence	*If sexually active
Diet/obesity	Intensive behavioral dietary counseling for patients with known risk factors for cardiovascular and diet-related chronic disease
HIV screening	All adults who are at increased risk (sexually active, IV drug use, etc.)
Hepatitis B	All pregnant women and those with multiple sexual partners, IV drug use, etc.
Lipid disorders	All Adults over 45 should be screened
Suicide screening	If depressed*
Tobacco abuse	Ask all adults about tobacco use and provide tobacco cessation interventions for those who use tobacco
Tuberculosis screening	If high risk: Travel, immigrant, alcohol abuse, IV drug use

*Additional screening

Alcohol abuse	"Risky"/"hazardous" alcohol use: >7 drinks per week or more than 3 drinks on any on occasion for women, and >14 drinks per week or more than 4 drinks on any one occasion for men. OR Screen: "on any occasion during the last 3 months, have had more than 5 alcohol drinks" or CAGE: Tried to CUT down, been ANGERED by questions about your drinking, felt GUILTY about your drinking, had an EYE OPENER (drink in the morning)
Domestic violence	Screen all at risk patients (all women, especially when pregnant) "Do you feel safe in your present relationship?" "Have you been hit, kicked, punched or otherwise hurt in the last year?"
Substance abuse	Questioning about drug use and related problems should be considered in all adolescent and adult.
Suicide	Risk factors include history of mood or other mental disorder, substance abuse, history of "deliberate self-harm"

HEALTH MAINTENANCE 65 YEARS AND ABOVE

(http://www.ahrq.gov/clinic/cps3dix.htm)

Leading causes of death

Cardiovascular disease
Malignant neoplasm
Stoke
COPD
Dementia

Immunizations *(http://www.cdc.gov/nip/ or http://www.immunizationed.org/)*

Tetanus	Tdap every 10 years or just at age 50 (if completed primary series)
Influenza	All adults

Disease	**Recommended Intervention (A or B Grade)**
General	Height, weight, BMI, blood pressure, injury prevention (seat belts, firearms), low saturated fat diet, physical exercise
Alcohol and substance abuse	*Insufficient for population; screen at risk
Aspirin	Recommends use of aspirin for men age 45 to 79 and women age 55 to 79 years when potential benefit due to a reduction in myocardial infarctions outweighs the potential harm due to an increase in gastrointestinal hemorrhage.
Breast and ovarian cancer by genetic testing	Refer for genetic counseling if: Ashkenazi heritage, or two 1st degree relatives with breast or ovarian cancer at <50 years of age
Breast cancer screening by mammography	Mammography through Age 75; repeat every 1–2 years; after age 75, at discretion
Cervical cancer screening	May cease to screen if had adequate recent screening and are not at high risk
Chlamydia, gonorrhea, syphilis testing	All adults who are at increased risk (sexually active, IV drug use, etc.)
Colon cancer	Start at age 50–75 by fecal occult blood testing, sigmoidoscopy, or colonoscopy
Coronary Heart Disease	Evidence is insufficient to recommend using nontraditional risk factors (high-sensitivity C-reactive protein (hs-CRP), ankle-brachial index (ABI), leukocyte count, fasting blood glucose level, periodontal disease, carotid intima-media thickness (carotid IMT), coronary artery calcification (CAC) score on electron-beam computed tomography (EBCT), homocysteine level, and lipoprotein(a) level) to screen asymptomatic men and women with no history of CHD to prevent CHD events
Depression	In clinical practices that have systems in place to assure accurate diagnosis, effective treatment, and follow up.
Diabetes mellitus, type II if BP > 135/80	Random serum glucose if sustained blood pressure (either treated or untreated) greater than 135/80 mm Hg
Domestic/family violence	*If sexually active
Diet/obesity	Intensive behavioral dietary counseling for patients with known risk factors for cardiovascular and diet-related chronic disease
HIV screening	All adults who are at increased risk (sexually active, IV drug use, etc.)
Hepatitis B	All pregnant women and those with multiple sexual partners, IV drug use, etc.
Lipid disorders	All adults over 45 should be screened
Suicide screening	If depressed*
Tobacco abuse	Ask all adults about tobacco use and provide tobacco cessation interventions for those who use tobacco
Tuberculosis screening	If high risk: Travel, immigrant, alcohol abuse, IV drug use

***Additional screening**

Alcohol abuse	"Risky"/"hazardous" alcohol use: >7 drinks per week or more than 3 drinks on any on occasion for women, and >14 drinks per week or more than 4 drinks on any one occasion for men. OR Screen: "on any occasion during the last 3 months, have had more than 5 alcohol drinks" or CAGE: tried to CUT down, been ANGERED by questions about your drinking, felt GUILTY about your drinking, had an EYE OPENER (drink in the morning)
Domestic violence	Screen all at risk patients (all women, especially when pregnant) "Do you feel safe in your present relationship?" "Have you been hit, kicked, punched or otherwise hurt in the last year?"
Substance abuse	Questioning about drug use and related problems should be considered in all adolescent and adult.
Suicide	Risk factors include history of mood or other mental disorder, substance abuse, history of "deliberate self-harm"

Diagnosis and Treatment: An Algorithmic Approach

This section contains flowcharts (or algorithms) to help the reader in the diagnosis of clinical signs and symptoms, and treatment of a variety of clinical problems. They are organized by the presenting sign, symptom or diagnosis.

These algorithms were designed to be used as a quick reference and adjunct to the reader's clinical knowledge and impression. They are not an exhaustive review of the management of a problem, nor are they meant to be a complete list of diseases.

ABDOMINAL PAIN, CHRONIC

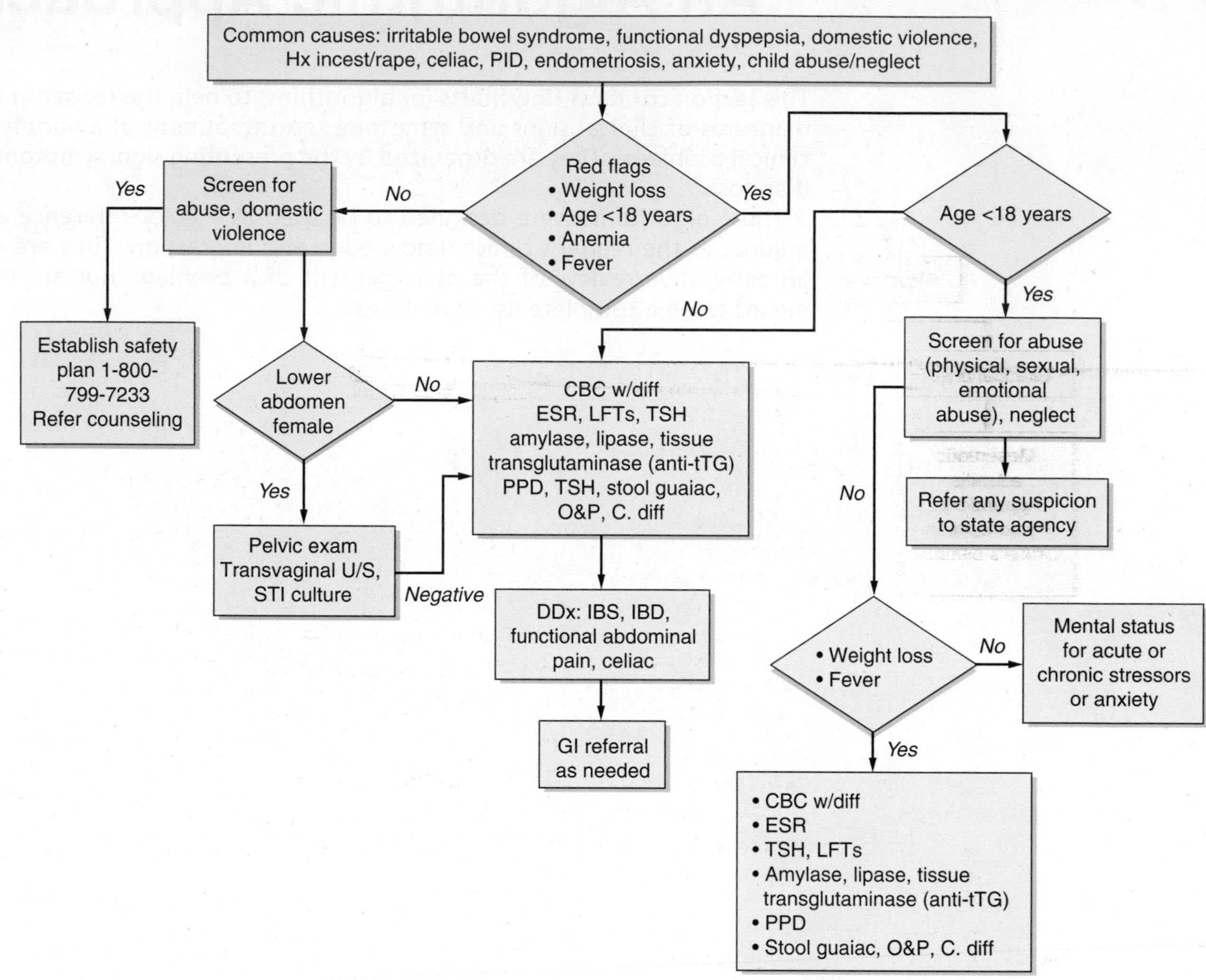

Common causes: irritable bowel syndrome, functional dyspepsia, domestic violence, Hx incest/rape, celiac, PID, endometriosis, anxiety, child abuse/neglect
Red flags
• Weight loss
• Age <18 years
• Anemia
• Fever
No
Yes
Screen for abuse, domestic violence
Yes
Establish safety plan 1-800-799-7233
Refer counseling
Lower abdomen female
No
Yes
Pelvic exam
Transvaginal U/S,
STI culture
Negative
CBC w/diff
ESR, LFTs, TSH
amylase, lipase, tissue transglutaminase (anti-tTG)
PPD, TSH, stool guaiac, O&P, C. diff
DDx: IBS, IBD, functional abdominal pain, celiac
GI referral as needed
Age <18 years
No
Yes
Screen for abuse (physical, sexual, emotional abuse), neglect
Refer any suspicion to state agency
No
• Weight loss
• Fever
No
Mental status for acute or chronic stressors or anxiety
Yes
• CBC w/diff
• ESR
• TSH, LFTs
• Amylase, lipase, tissue transglutaminase (anti-tTG)
• PPD
• Stool guaiac, O&P, C. diff

Josue Chery, MD

ABDOMINAL PAIN, LOWER

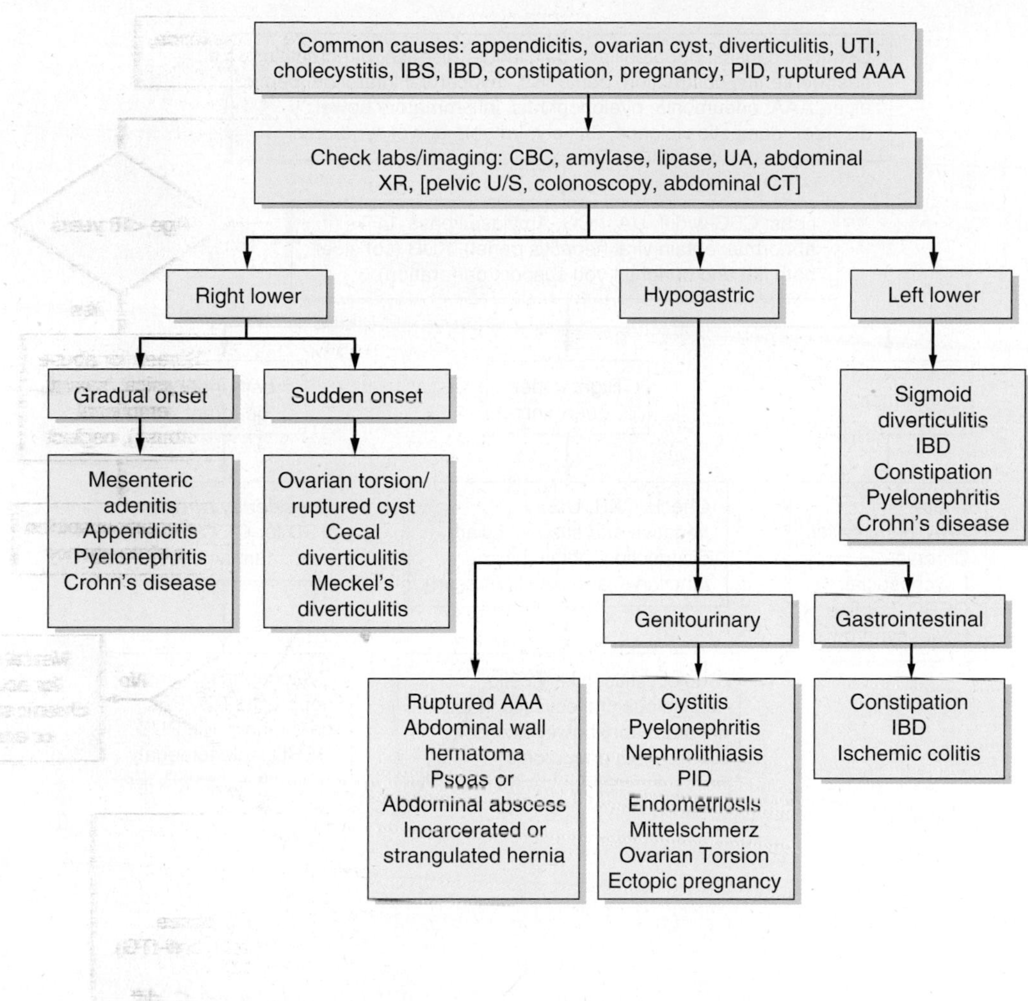

Nilay Patel, MD and Siva Vithananthan, MD

Scand J Gastroenterol. 1999;231(Suppl):3–8.

ABDOMINAL PAIN, UPPER

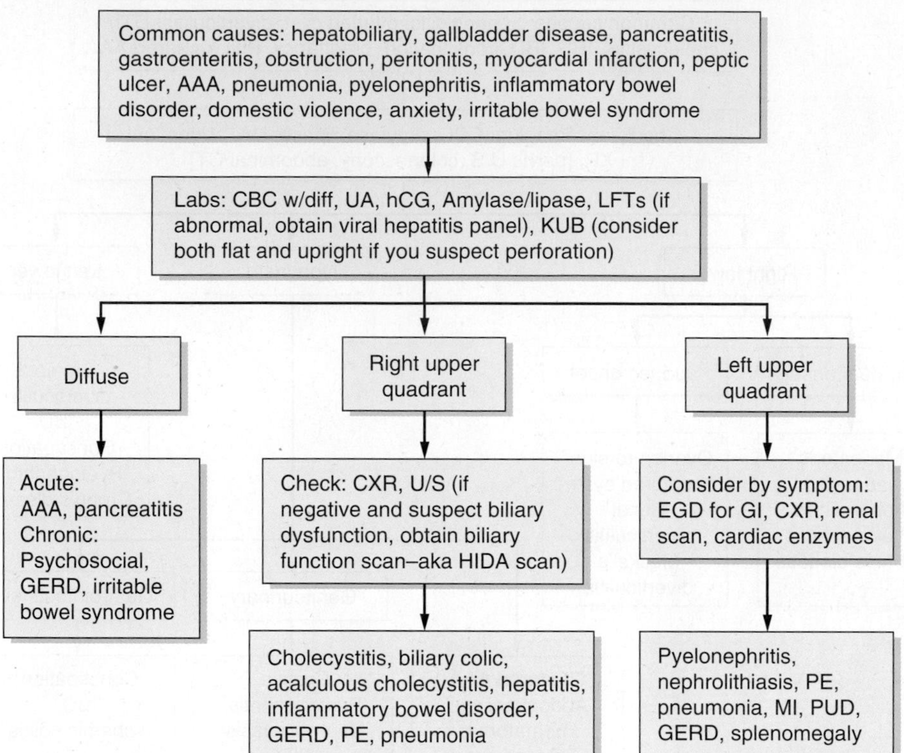
Common causes: hepatobiliary, gallbladder disease, pancreatitis, gastroenteritis, obstruction, peritonitis, myocardial infarction, peptic ulcer, AAA, pneumonia, pyelonephritis, inflammatory bowel disorder, domestic violence, anxiety, irritable bowel syndrome
Labs: CBC w/diff, UA, hCG, Amylase/lipase, LFTs (if abnormal, obtain viral hepatitis panel), KUB (consider both flat and upright if you suspect perforation)
Diffuse
Right upper quadrant
Left upper quadrant
Acute: AAA, pancreatitis Chronic: Psychosocial, GERD, irritable bowel syndrome
Check: CXR, U/S (if negative and suspect biliary dysfunction, obtain biliary function scan–aka HIDA scan)
Consider by symptom: EGD for GI, CXR, renal scan, cardiac enzymes
Cholecystitis, biliary colic, acalculous cholecystitis, hepatitis, inflammatory bowel disorder, GERD, PE, pneumonia
Pyelonephritis, nephrolithiasis, PE, pneumonia, MI, PUD, GERD, splenomegaly

Nilay Patel, MD and Siva Vithananthan, MD

Scand J Gastroenterol. 1999;231(Suppl):3–8.

ABDOMINAL RIGIDITY

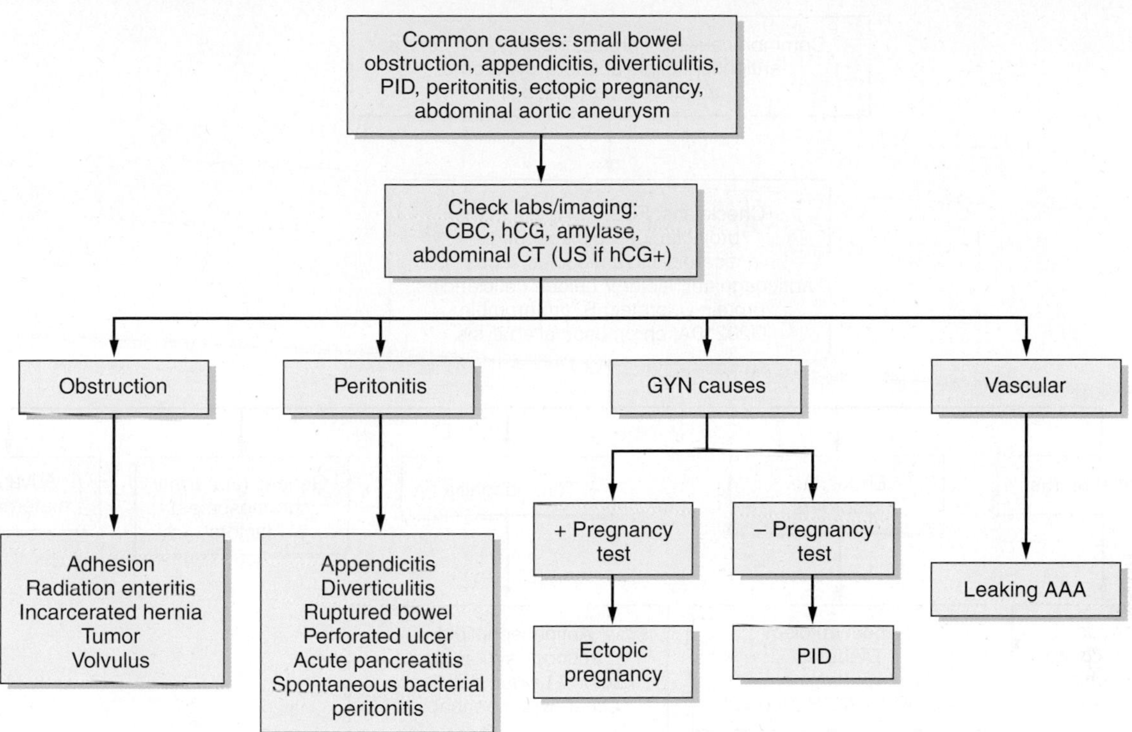

Robert A. Baldor, MD and Alan M. Ehrlich, MD

Med Clin North Am. 2008;92(3):599–625, viii–ix.

ABORTION, RECURRENT

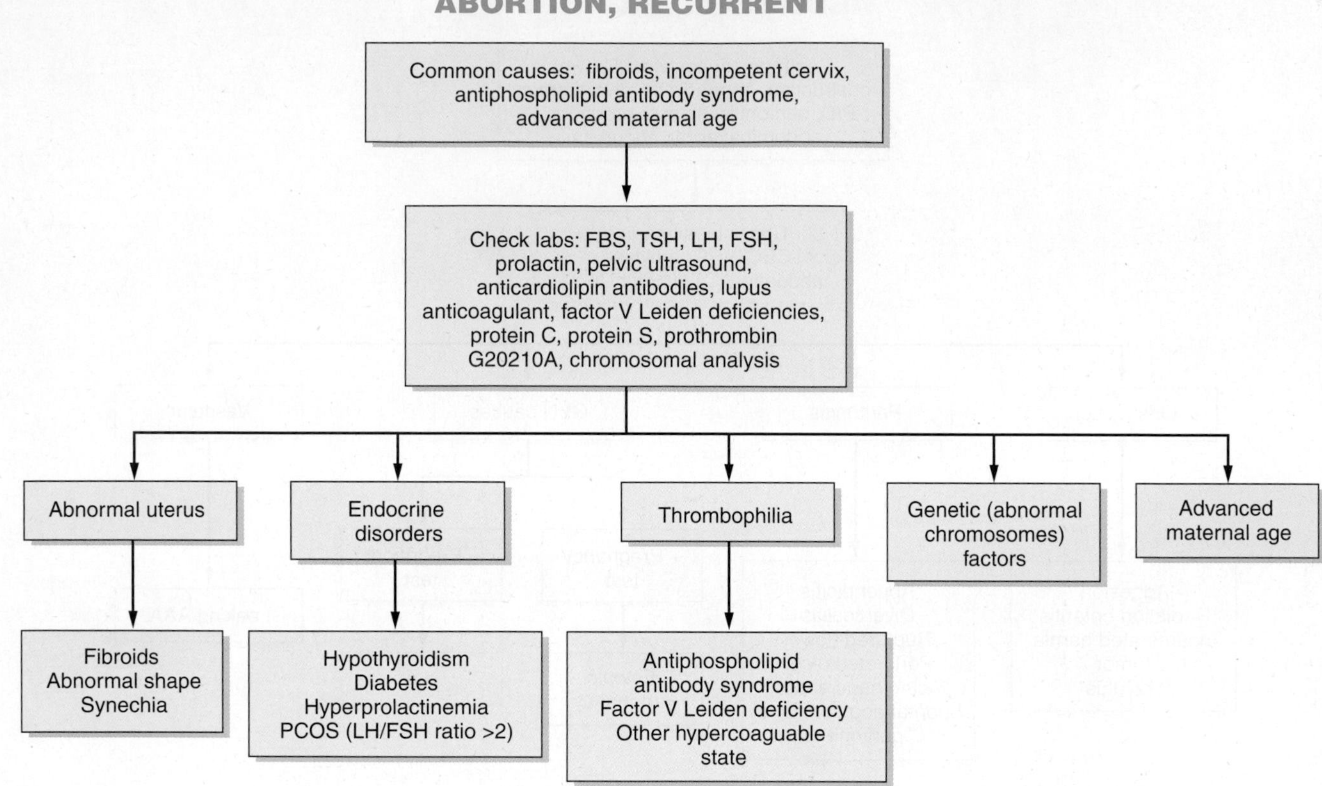

Robert A. Baldor, MD and Alan M. Ehrlich, MD

J Obstet Gynaecol Res. 2009;35(4):609–22.

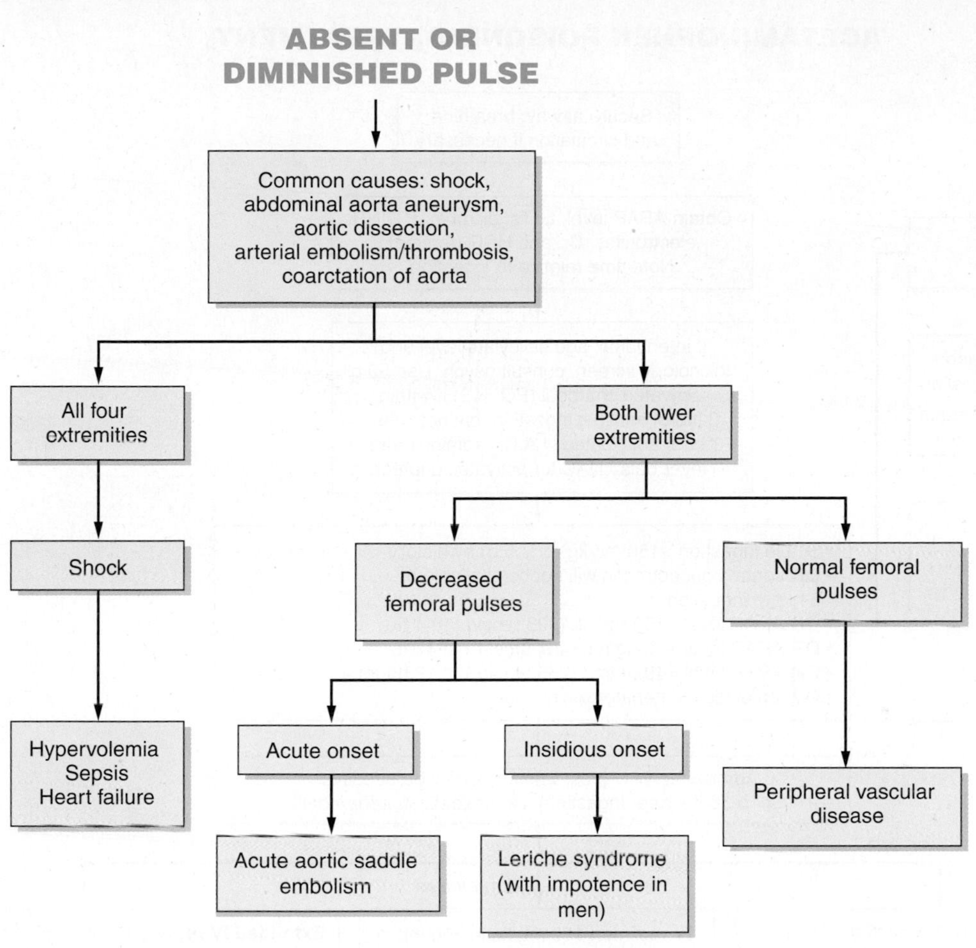

Robert A. Baldor, MD and Alan M. Ehrlich, MD

Semin Vasc Surg. 2009;22(1):10–6.

ACETAMINOPHEN POISONING, TREATMENT

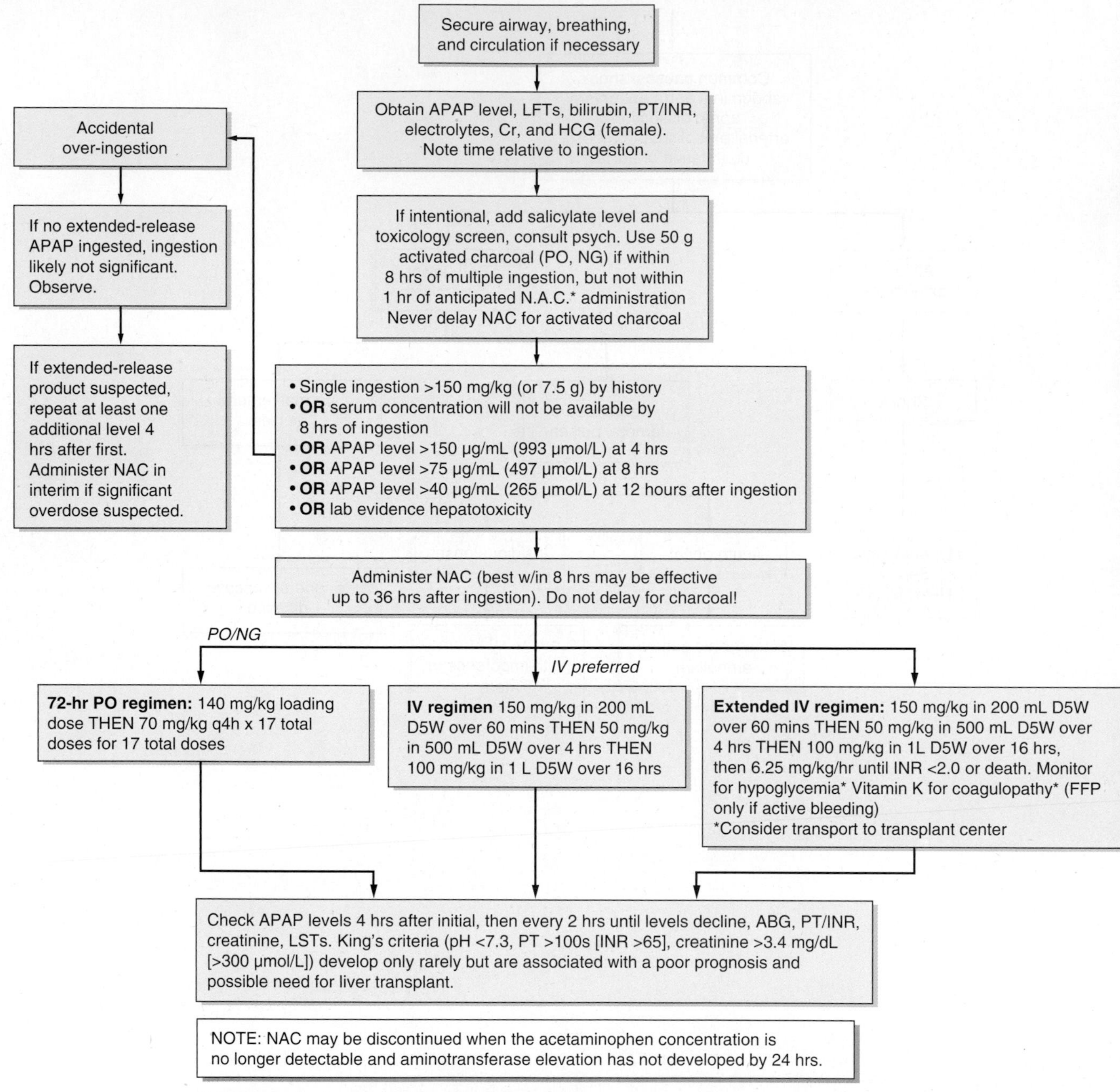

Secure airway, breathing, and circulation if necessary
Obtain APAP level, LFTs, bilirubin, PT/INR, electrolytes, Cr, and HCG (female). Note time relative to ingestion.
If intentional, add salicylate level and toxicology screen, consult psych. Use 50 g activated charcoal (PO, NG) if within 8 hrs of multiple ingestion, but not within 1 hr of anticipated N.A.C.* administration Never delay NAC for activated charcoal
• Single ingestion >150 mg/kg (or 7.5 g) by history
• **OR** serum concentration will not be available by 8 hrs of ingestion
• **OR** APAP level >150 μg/mL (993 μmol/L) at 4 hrs
• **OR** APAP level >75 μg/mL (497 μmol/L) at 8 hrs
• **OR** APAP level >40 μg/mL (265 μmol/L) at 12 hours after ingestion
• **OR** lab evidence hepatotoxicity
Accidental over-ingestion
If no extended-release APAP ingested, ingestion likely not significant. Observe.
If extended-release product suspected, repeat at least one additional level 4 hrs after first. Administer NAC in interim if significant overdose suspected.
Administer NAC (best w/in 8 hrs may be effective up to 36 hrs after ingestion). Do not delay for charcoal!
PO/NG
IV preferred
72-hr PO regimen: 140 mg/kg loading dose THEN 70 mg/kg q4h x 17 total doses for 17 total doses
IV regimen 150 mg/kg in 200 mL D5W over 60 mins THEN 50 mg/kg in 500 mL D5W over 4 hrs THEN 100 mg/kg in 1 L D5W over 16 hrs
Extended IV regimen: 150 mg/kg in 200 mL D5W over 60 mins THEN 50 mg/kg in 500 mL D5W over 4 hrs THEN 100 mg/kg in 1L D5W over 16 hrs, then 6.25 mg/kg/hr until INR <2.0 or death. Monitor for hypoglycemia* Vitamin K for coagulopathy* (FFP only if active bleeding)
*Consider transport to transplant center
Check APAP levels 4 hrs after initial, then every 2 hrs until levels decline, ABG, PT/INR, creatinine, LSTs. King's criteria (pH <7.3, PT >100s [INR >65], creatinine >3.4 mg/dL [>300 μmol/L]) develop only rarely but are associated with a poor prognosis and possible need for liver transplant.
NOTE: NAC may be discontinued when the acetaminophen concentration is no longer detectable and aminotransferase elevation has not developed by 24 hrs.

*APAP = Acetaminophen NAC = N-acetylcysteine

John Jenkins, MD

Med J Aust. 2008;188(5):296–301.

ACID PHOSPHATASE ELEVATION

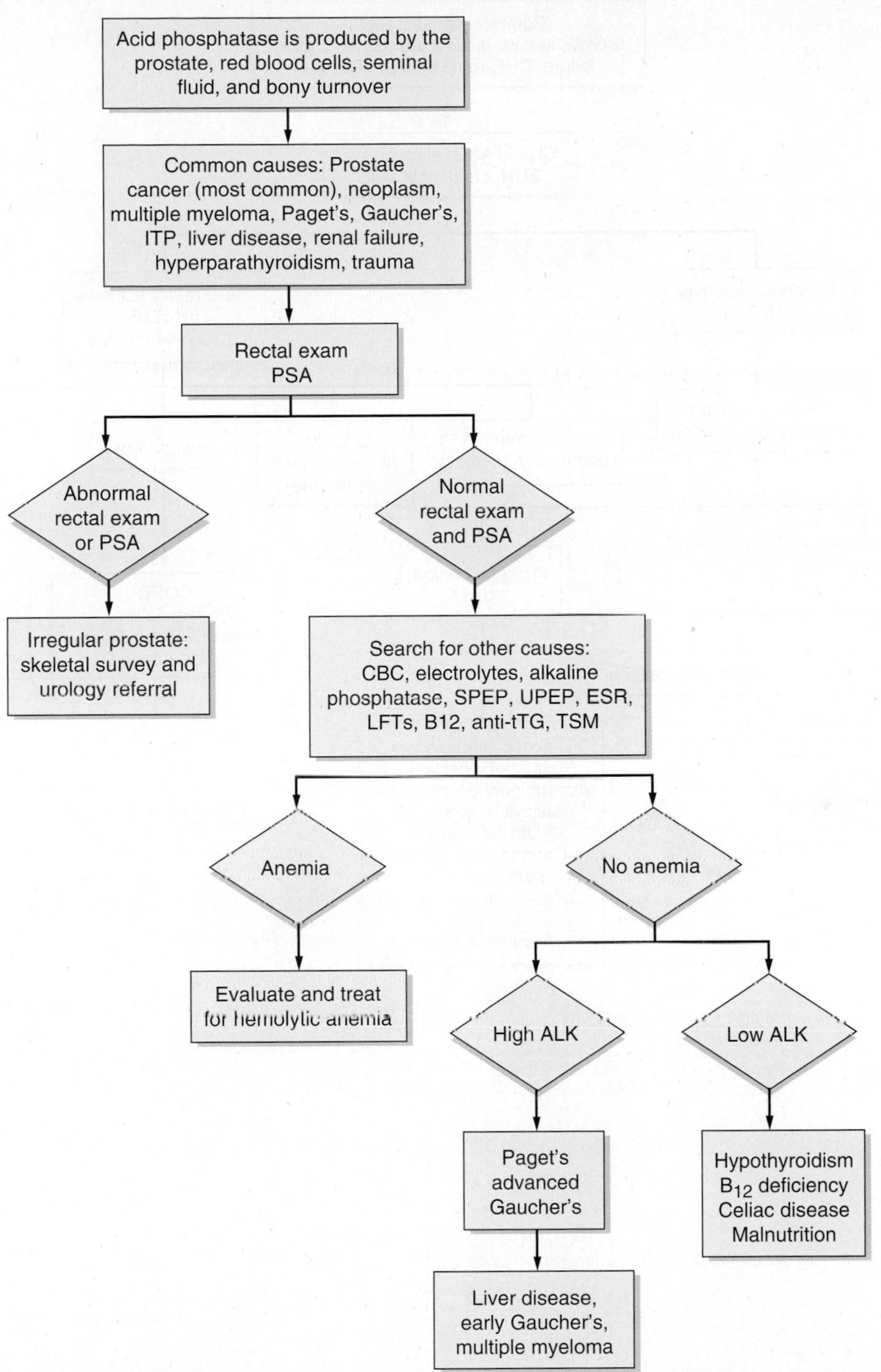

Laura Hagopian, MD and Michael Snyder, MD

ACIDOSIS

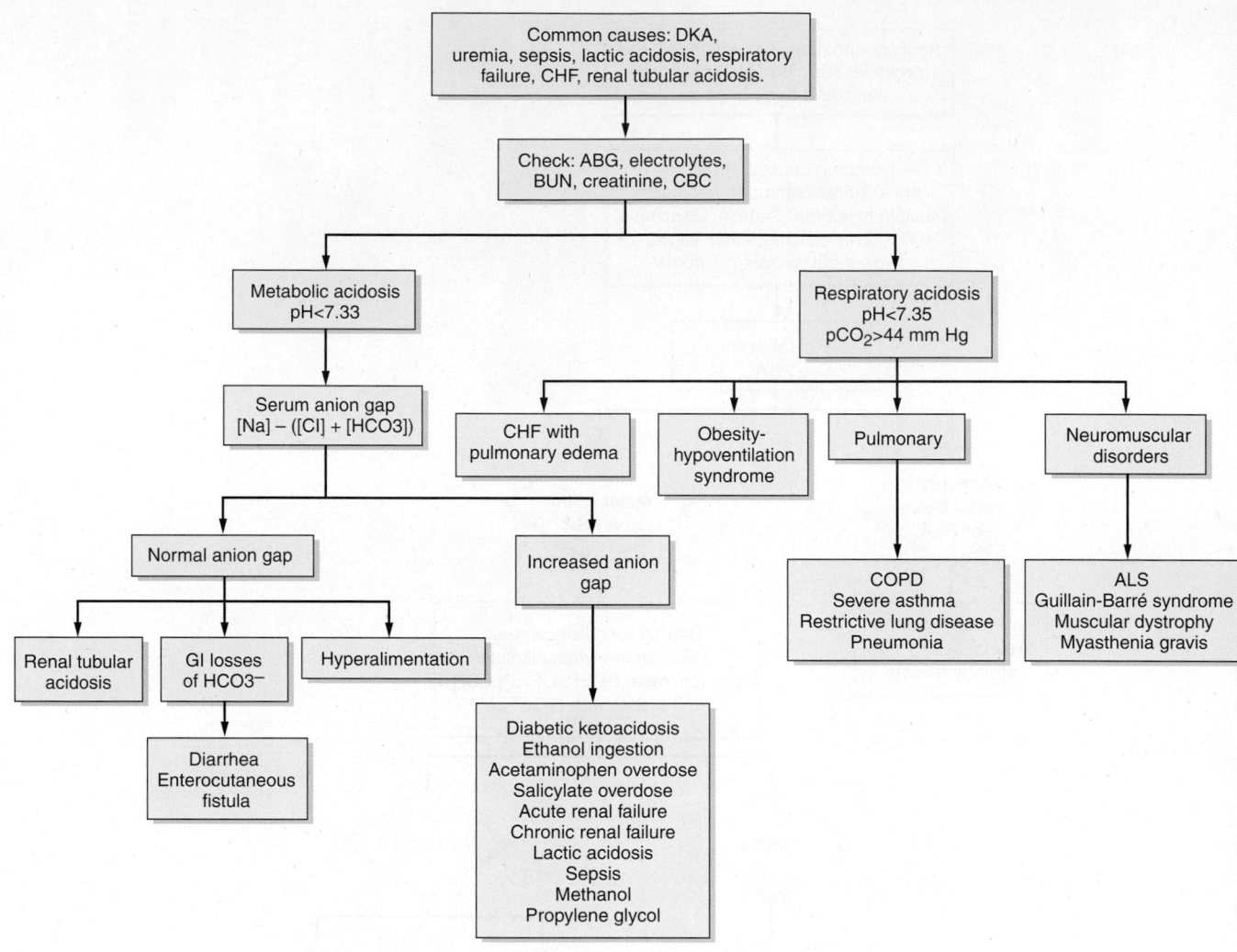

Common causes: DKA, uremia, sepsis, lactic acidosis, respiratory failure, CHF, renal tubular acidosis.

→ Check: ABG, electrolytes, BUN, creatinine, CBC

- Metabolic acidosis pH<7.33
  - Serum anion gap [Na] – ([Cl] + [HCO3])
    - Normal anion gap
      - Renal tubular acidosis
      - GI losses of $HCO3^-$
        - Diarrhea
        - Enterocutaneous fistula
      - Hyperalimentation
    - Increased anion gap
      - Diabetic ketoacidosis
      - Ethanol ingestion
      - Acetaminophen overdose
      - Salicylate overdose
      - Acute renal failure
      - Chronic renal failure
      - Lactic acidosis
      - Sepsis
      - Methanol
      - Propylene glycol
- Respiratory acidosis pH<7.35 pCO_2>44 mm Hg
  - CHF with pulmonary edema
  - Obesity-hypoventilation syndrome
  - Pulmonary
    - COPD
    - Severe asthma
    - Restrictive lung disease
    - Pneumonia
  - Neuromuscular disorders
    - ALS
    - Guillain-Barré syndrome
    - Muscular dystrophy
    - Myasthenia gravis

Robert A. Baldor, MD and Alan M. Ehrlich, MD

Diabetes Care. 2009;32(7):1335–43.

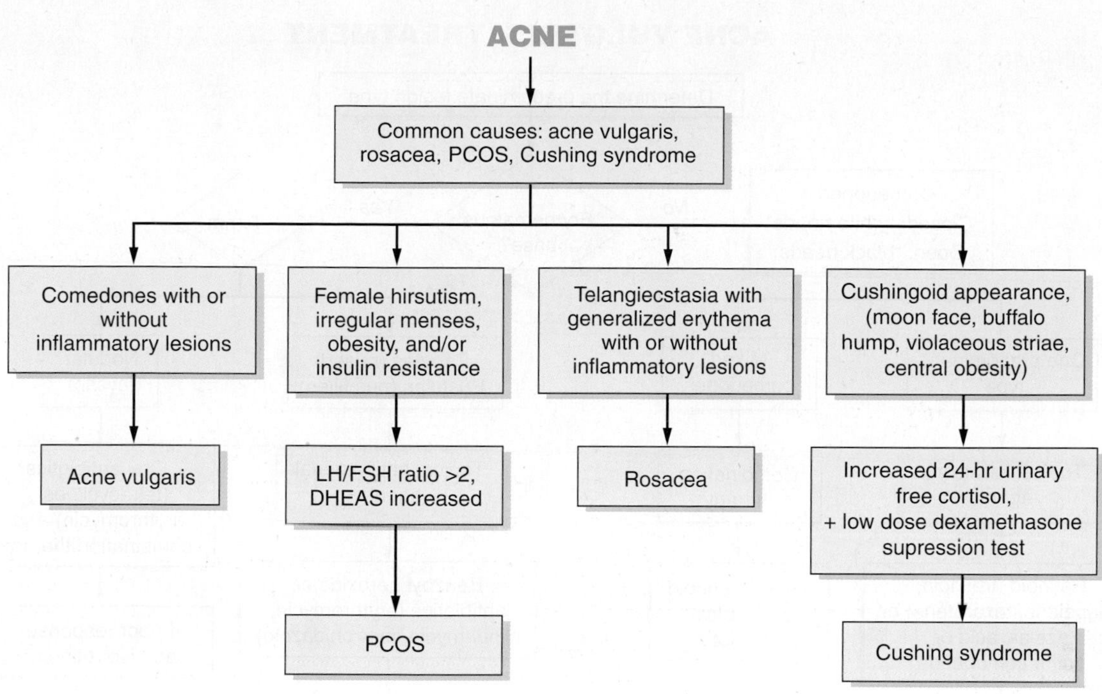

Robert A. Baldor, MD and Alan M. Ehrlich, MD

Dermatol Clin. 2009;27(4):459–71, vi.

ACNE VULGARIS, TREATMENT

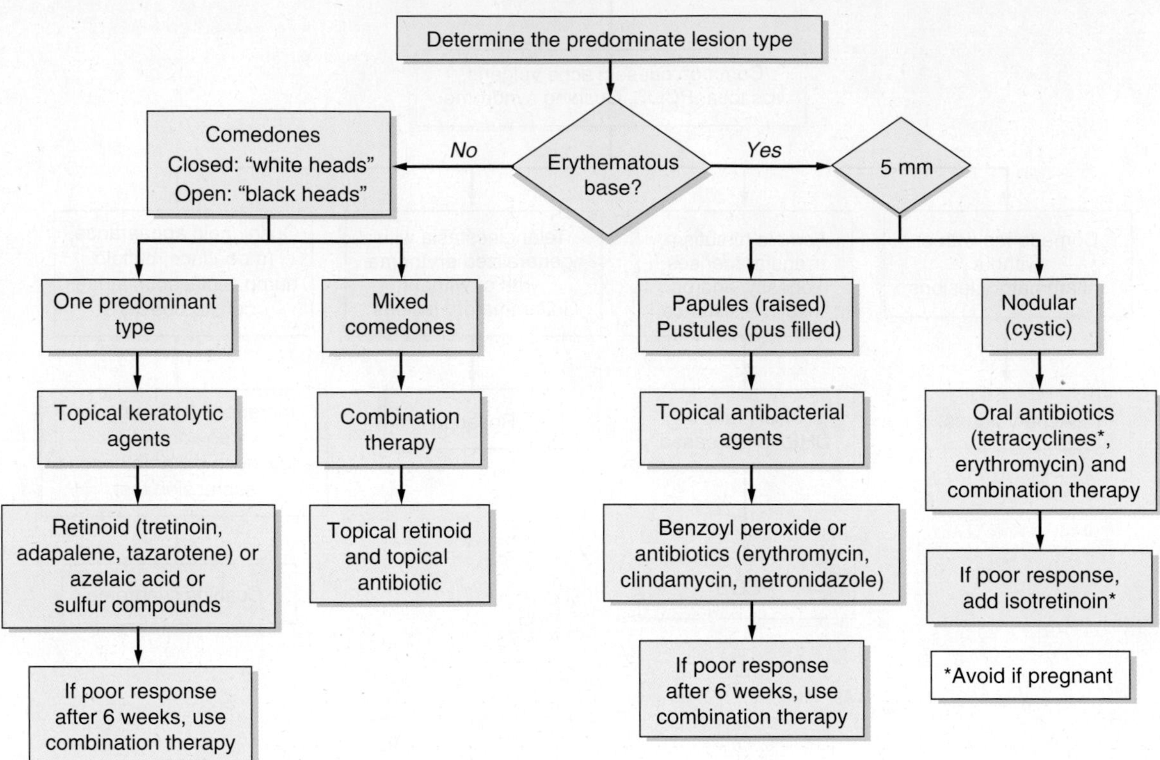
Determine the predominate lesion type
Erythematous base?
No
Yes
Comedones
Closed: "white heads"
Open: "black heads"
5 mm
One predominant type
Mixed comedones
Papules (raised)
Pustules (pus filled)
Nodular (cystic)
Topical keratolytic agents
Combination therapy
Topical antibacterial agents
Oral antibiotics (tetracyclines*, erythromycin) and combination therapy
Retinoid (tretinoin, adapalene, tazarotene) or azelaic acid or sulfur compounds
Topical retinoid and topical antibiotic
Benzoyl peroxide or antibiotics (erythromycin, clindamycin, metronidazole)
If poor response, add isotretinoin*
If poor response after 6 weeks, use combination therapy
If poor response after 6 weeks, use combination therapy
*Avoid if pregnant

Robert A. Baldor

Treat Guidel Med Lett. 2008;6(75):75–82.

ADRENOCORTICAL INSUFFICIENCY

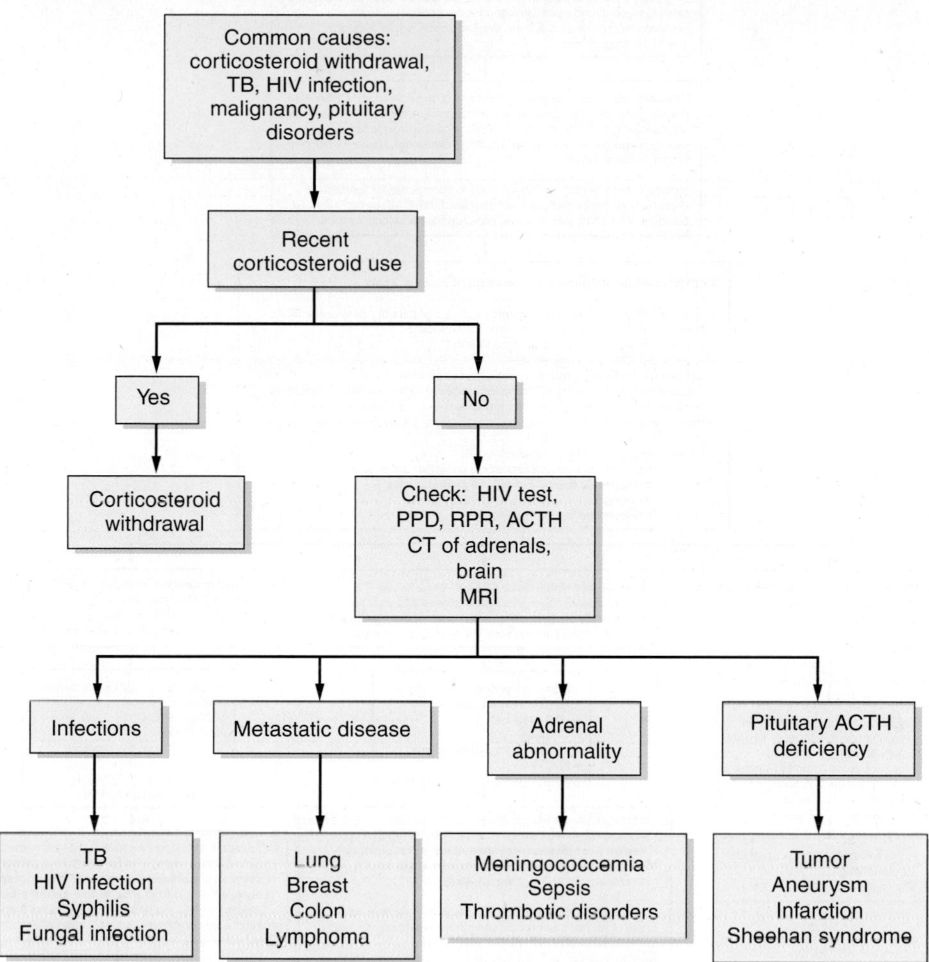

Robert A. Baldor, MD and Alan M. Ehrlich, MD

Ann Intern Med. 2003;139(3):194–204.

ALCOHOL WITHDRAWAL, TREATMENT

History: Duration and quantity of alcohol intake, time since last drink, previous episodes of alcohol withdrawal, concurrent substance use, pre-existing medical and psychiatric conditions, prior detoxification admissions, prior seizure activity, living situation, social supports, stressors, triggers, etc.

↓

Physical: VS (fever, tachycardia, tachypnea, hypertension), **CIWA** (see below), MSE (arousal, orientation, hallucinations), HEENT (diaphoresis, scleral icterus), CV (arrythmias, M/R/G), eval s/sx liver failure (ascites, varices, caput madusae, asterixis, palmar erythema), neuro (nystagmus, tremor, seizure activity)

Include assessment of conditions likely to *complicate*, *exacerbate* or *precipitate* alcohol withdrawal: arrhythmias, CHF, CAD, dehydration, GI bleeding, infections, liver disease, pancreatitis, neurologic deficits

↓

Clinical Institute Withdrawal Assessment of Alcohol Scale

- Nausea and vomiting 0–7; (7 constant nausea, frequent dry heaves/vomiting)
- Tremor 0–7; (7-severe, even with arms not extended)
- Paroxysmal sweats 0–7; (7-drenching sweats)
- Anxiety 0–7; (7-acute panic state)
- Agitation 0–7; (7-constantly thrashing about or pacing)
- Tactile disturbances 0–7; (4–7 for hallucinations, 1–3 for pruritus or paresthesias)
- Auditory disturbances 0–7; (4–7 for hallucinations, 1–3 for increased sensitivity)
- Visual disturbances 0–7; (4–7 for hallucinations, 1–3 for increased sensitivity)
- Headache, fullness in head 0–7
- Orientation and clouding of sensorium 0–4:
  - o cannot do serial additions or is uncertain about date
  - o disoriented to date but within 2 calendar days
  - o disoriented to date by > 2 days
  - o disoriented to place or person

↓

Mild withdrawal; CIWA 0–7 (onset 5–8 hours after cessation or significant decrease in consumption): Anxiety, restlessness, agitation, mild nausea, decreased appetite, sleep disturbance, facial sweating, mild tremulousness, fluctuating tachycardia and hypertension, possible mild cognitive impairment

↓

May be monitored as outpatient, *unless* pregnant, history of seizure d/o or withdrawal seizures, chronic or acute comorbid illness requiring inpatient observation, lack of ability to follow-up

↓

- Admit to inpatient detox program for monitoring
- Vital signs q4h; CIWA q1–3h

Moderate withdrawal; CIWA 8–14 (onset 24–72 hours after cessation): marked restlessness and agitation, moderate tremulousness with constant eye movement, diaphoresis, nausea, vomiting, anorexia, diarrhea

↓

- Admit to inpatient detox program
- Private room if possible
- Vital signs q4h
- CIWA q1–3h
- Institute seizure precautions
- IVF

↓

Diazepam 20 mg PO q1–2h until CIWA<8, **OR**
Diazepam 2–5 mg IV/min-maximum 10–20 mg q1h
If severe liver disease, severe asthma or respiratory failure, elderly, debilitated, or low serum albumin:
Lorazepam SL, PO 1–2 mg q2–4h PRN

Long-acting benzodiazepines (diazepam) have rapid onset of action, and provide smooth treatment course with fewer breakthrough symptoms.
Short-acting (lorazepam) may have lower risk when there is concern about prolonged sedation, e.g., elderly patients or those with severe hepatic insufficiency.

Severe withdrawal/delirium tremens; CIWA >15 (onset 72–96 hours after alcohol cessation): Marked tremulousness, fever, drenching sweats, severe hypertension and tachycardia, delirium

↓

- Admit to ICU for inpatient detox
- VS q30
- CIWA q1h
- NPO, IVF
- Lateral decubitus position, restrain if necessary
- Glucose, Na, K, PO4, Mg replacement as needed

↓

Diazepam 5–20 mg IV q10 min until calm, then q1hr to maintain light somnolence for duration of delirium
If severe liver disease, severe asthma or respiratory failure, elderly, debilitated, or low serum albumin:
Lorazepam 1–4 mg IV q10 min until calm, then q1h to maintain light somnolence for duration of delirium

(→ to Thiamine/adjunctive therapy box)

↓ (from moderate withdrawal)

Labs: Tox screen/BAL to assess need for and timing of withdrawal regimen; electrolytes, phos, Mg with severe withdrawal [B12 and folate repleted regardless of levels], amylase/lipase if sx pancreatitis, PT, PTT if suspect liver failure; CBC if suspect infection
Imaging: Head CT if history of trauma or mental status changes out of range expected for degree of withdrawal. Seizure workup if no history of withdrawal siezures. Head CT and EEG if focal neurologic signs or prolonged post-ictal state

↓

- **Thiamine** 100 mg IM/IV/PO q24h x 5 days; up to 1000 mg/day if oculogyric crisis

- Sympatholytic adjunctive therapy: Atenolol 50–100 mg q24
Beta blockers and clonidine may be used only in conjunction with benzodiazepines since *may mask symptoms of alcohol withdrawal and articially lower CIWA score*, reduce peripheral signs and symptoms of alcohol withdrawal but have not been shown to prevent or treat delirium or seizures

- Phenothiazines for hallucinosis: Haloperidol 2–5 mg IM/PO q1–4h max 5 mg/day
used only in conjunction with benzodinzepines. May lower seizure threshold, use with extreme caution.

↓

Discharge Planning:
- CIWA scores<8–10 for 24 hours
- Begin 1:1 or group therapy
- Discharge to treatment center, day program, home
- Facilitate entry into Alcoholics Anonymous
- Do not discharge with benzodiazepine rx
- Nutrition consult
- Social work consult

Alexis Lawrence, MD and Warren J. Ferguson, MD

N Engl J Med. 2003;348:1786.

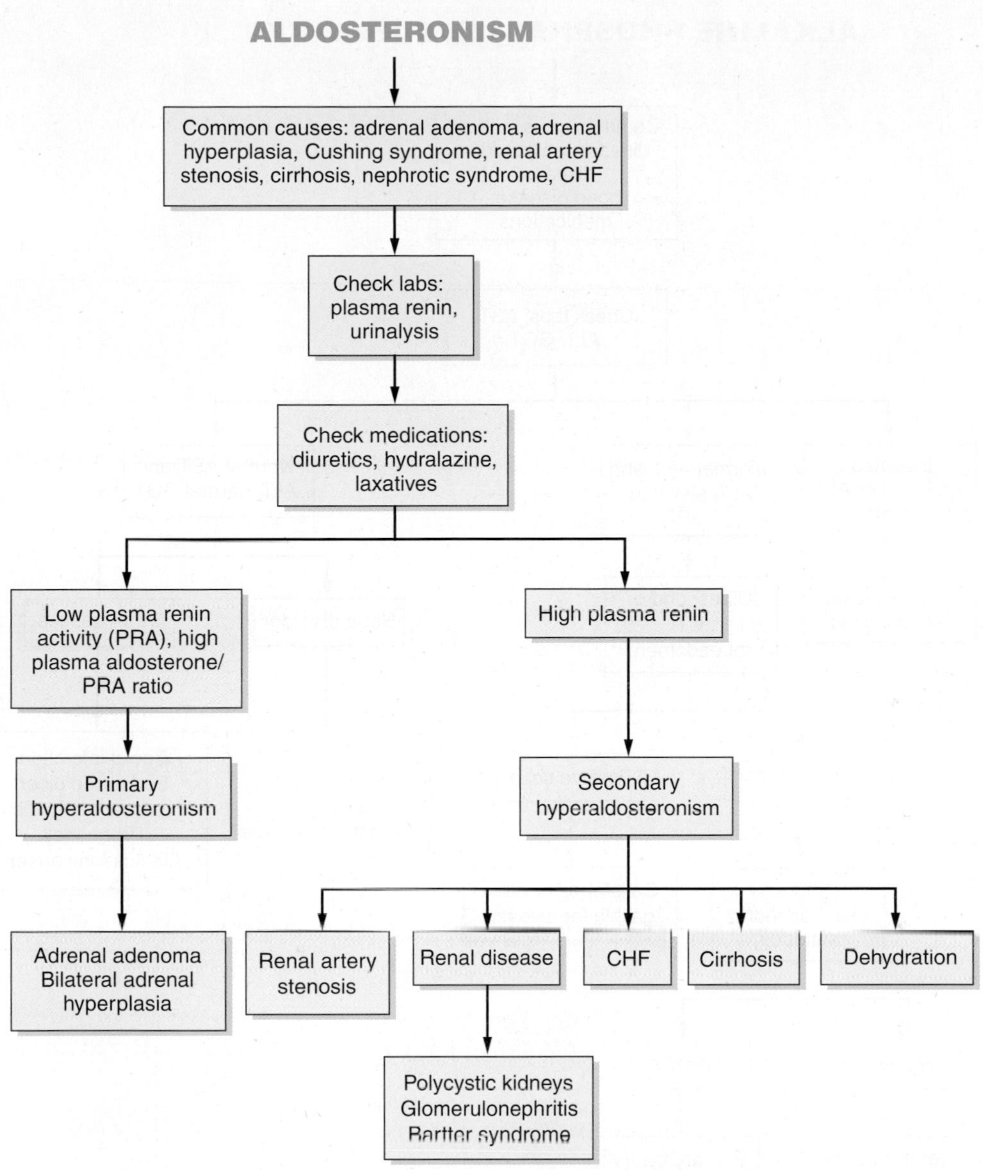

Robert A. Baldor, MD and Alan M. Ehrlich, MD

Cardiology. 1985;72(Suppl. 1):57–63.

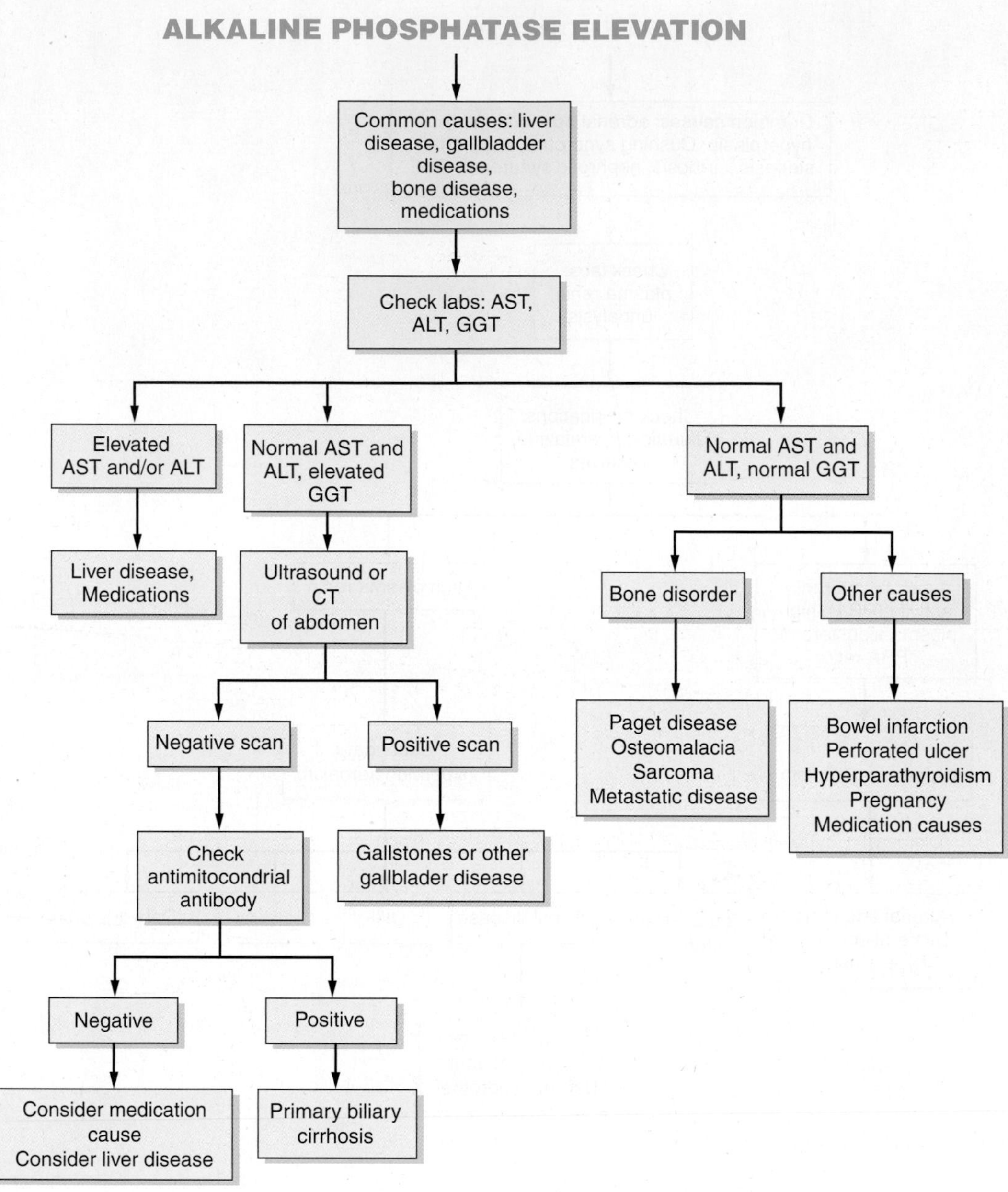
ALKALINE PHOSPHATASE ELEVATION
Common causes: liver disease, gallbladder disease, bone disease, medications
Check labs: AST, ALT, GGT
Elevated AST and/or ALT
Normal AST and ALT, elevated GGT
Normal AST and ALT, normal GGT
Liver disease, Medications
Ultrasound or CT of abdomen
Bone disorder
Other causes
Negative scan
Positive scan
Paget disease
Osteomalacia
Sarcoma
Metastatic disease
Bowel infarction
Perforated ulcer
Hyperparathyroidism
Pregnancy
Medication causes
Check antimitocondrial antibody
Gallstones or other gallblader disease
Negative
Positive
Consider medication cause
Consider liver disease
Primary biliary cirrhosis

Robert A. Baldor, MD and Alan M. Ehrlich, MD

J Fam Pract. 2001;50(6).

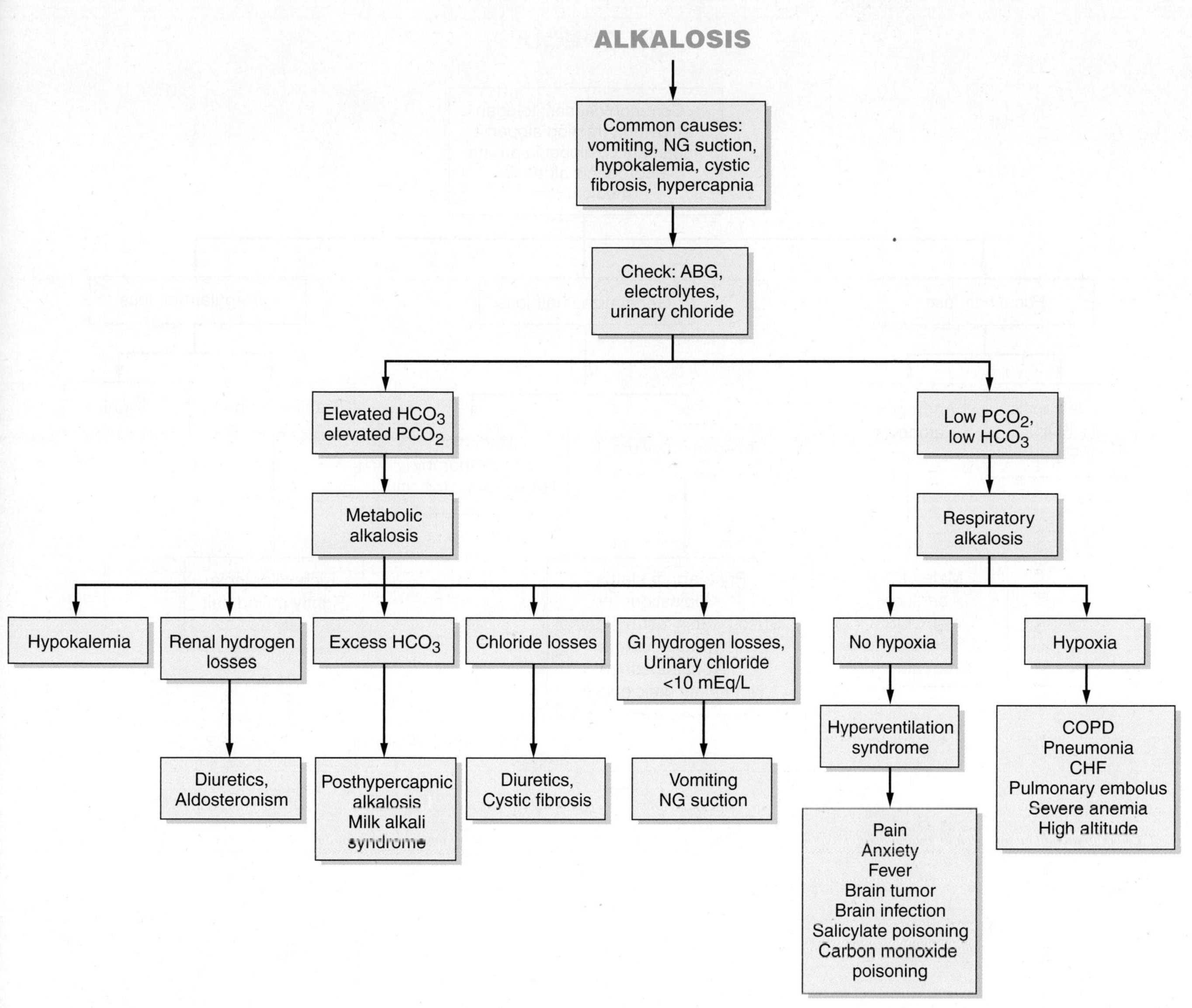
ALKALOSIS
Common causes: vomiting, NG suction, hypokalemia, cystic fibrosis, hypercapnia
Check: ABG, electrolytes, urinary chloride
Elevated HCO_3 elevated PCO_2
Low PCO_2, low HCO_3
Metabolic alkalosis
Respiratory alkalosis
Hypokalemia
Renal hydrogen losses
Excess HCO_3
Chloride losses
GI hydrogen losses, Urinary chloride <10 mEq/L
No hypoxia
Hypoxia
Diuretics, Aldosteronism
Posthypercapnic alkalosis Milk alkali syndrome
Diuretics, Cystic fibrosis
Vomiting NG suction
Hyperventilation syndrome
COPD Pneumonia CHF Pulmonary embolus Severe anemia High altitude
Pain Anxiety Fever Brain tumor Brain infection Salicylate poisoning Carbon monoxide poisoning

Robert A. Baldor, MD and Alan M. Ehrlich, MD

Nutr Clin Pract. 2008;23(2):122–7.

ALOPECIA

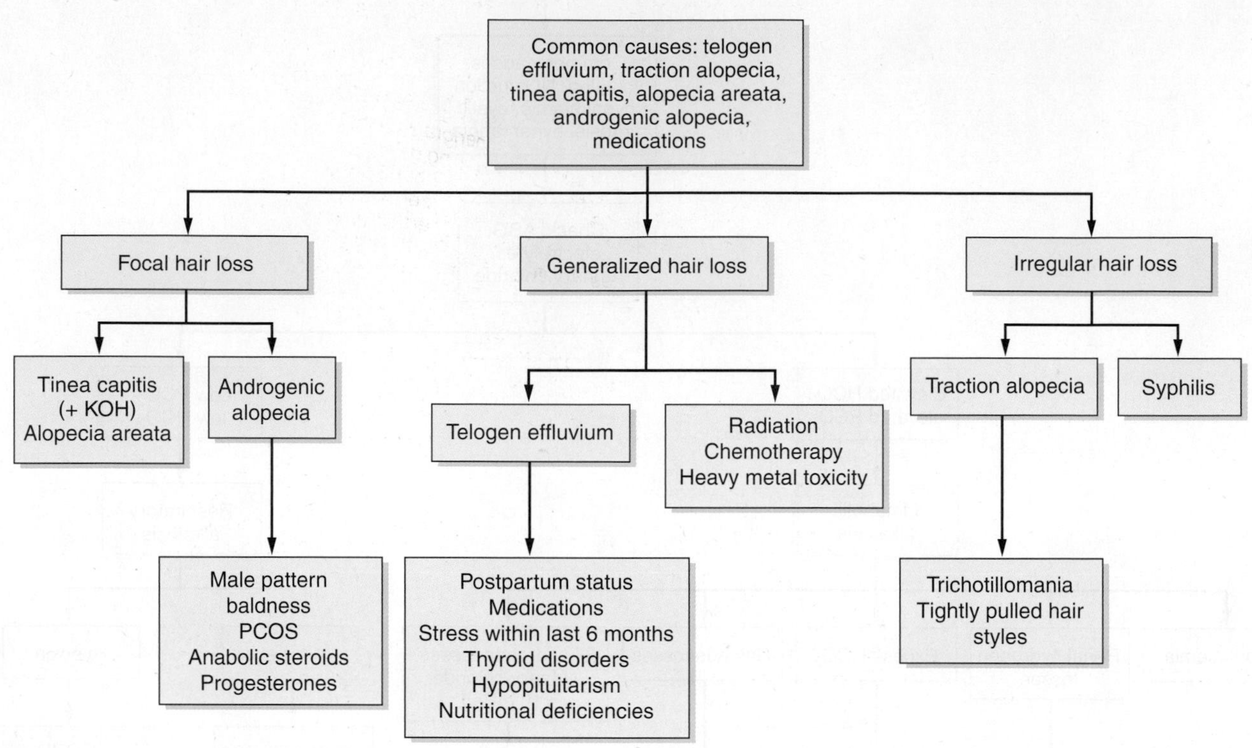

Robert A. Baldor, MD and Alan M. Ehrlich, MD

Am Fam Physician. 2009;80(4):356–62.

AMENORRHEA, PRIMARY (ABSENCE OF MENARCHE BY AGE 16)

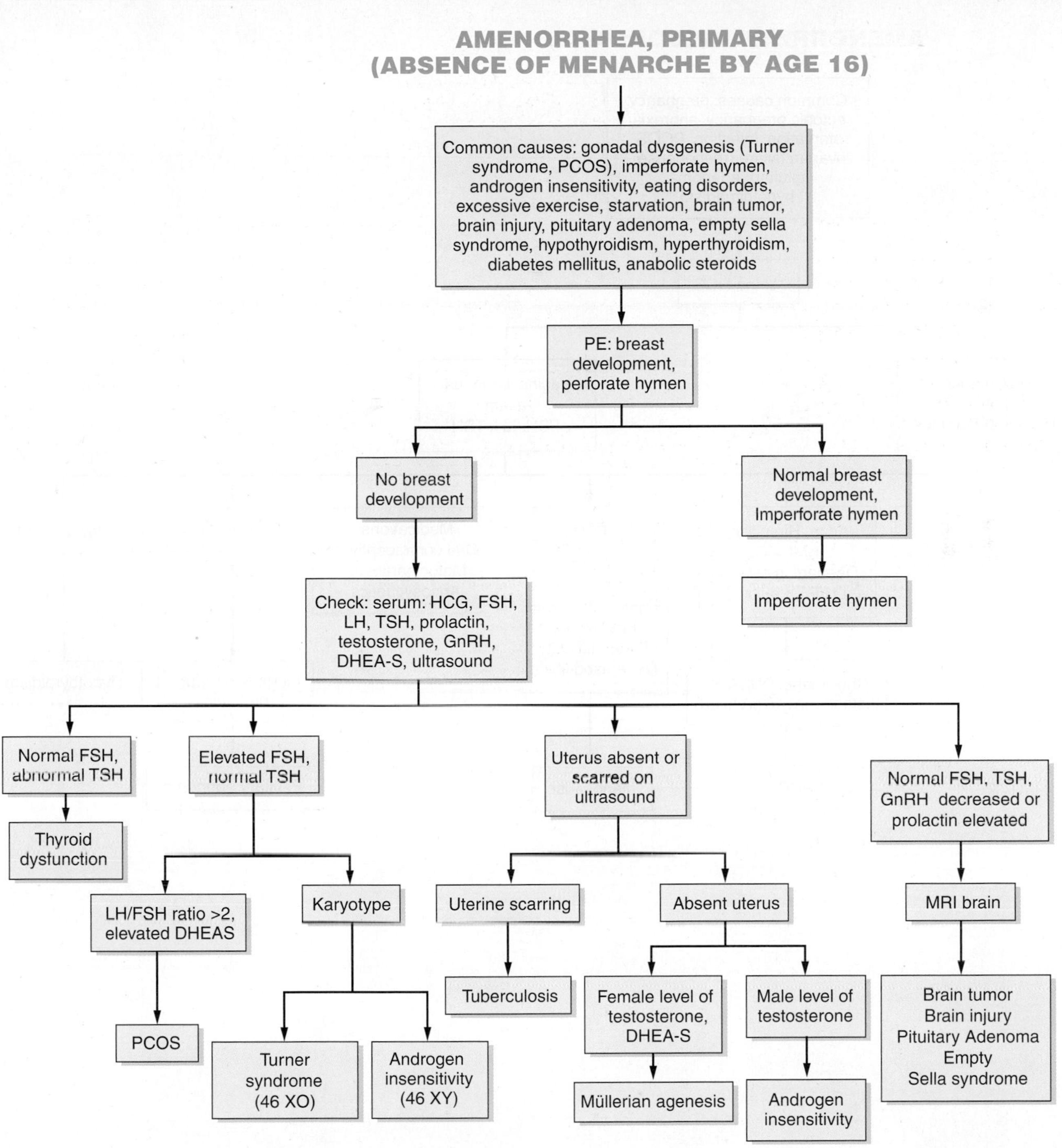

Robert A. Baldor, MD and Alan M. Ehrlich, MD

Am Fam Physician. 2006;73:1374–82.

AMENORRHEA, SECONDARY

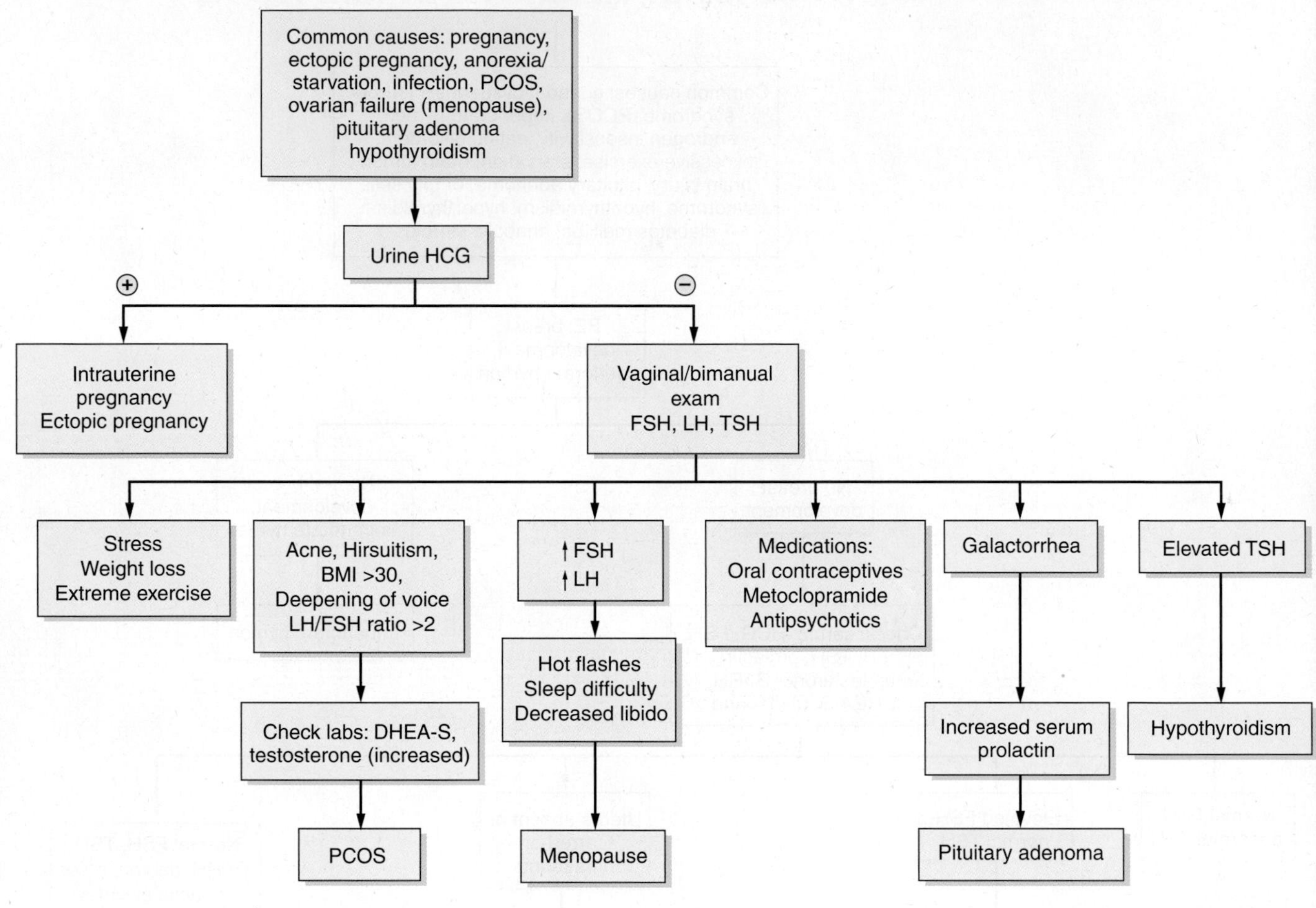

Robert A. Baldor, MD and Alan M. Ehrlich, MD

Am Fam Physician. 2006;73:1374–82.

AMNESIA

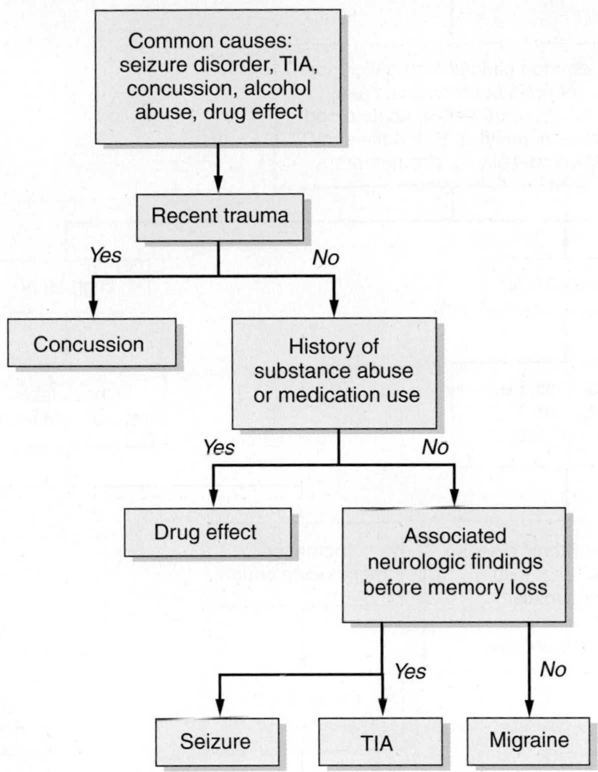

Robert A. Baldor, MD and Alan M. Ehrlich, MD

Ann Intern Med. 2007;146(6):397–405.

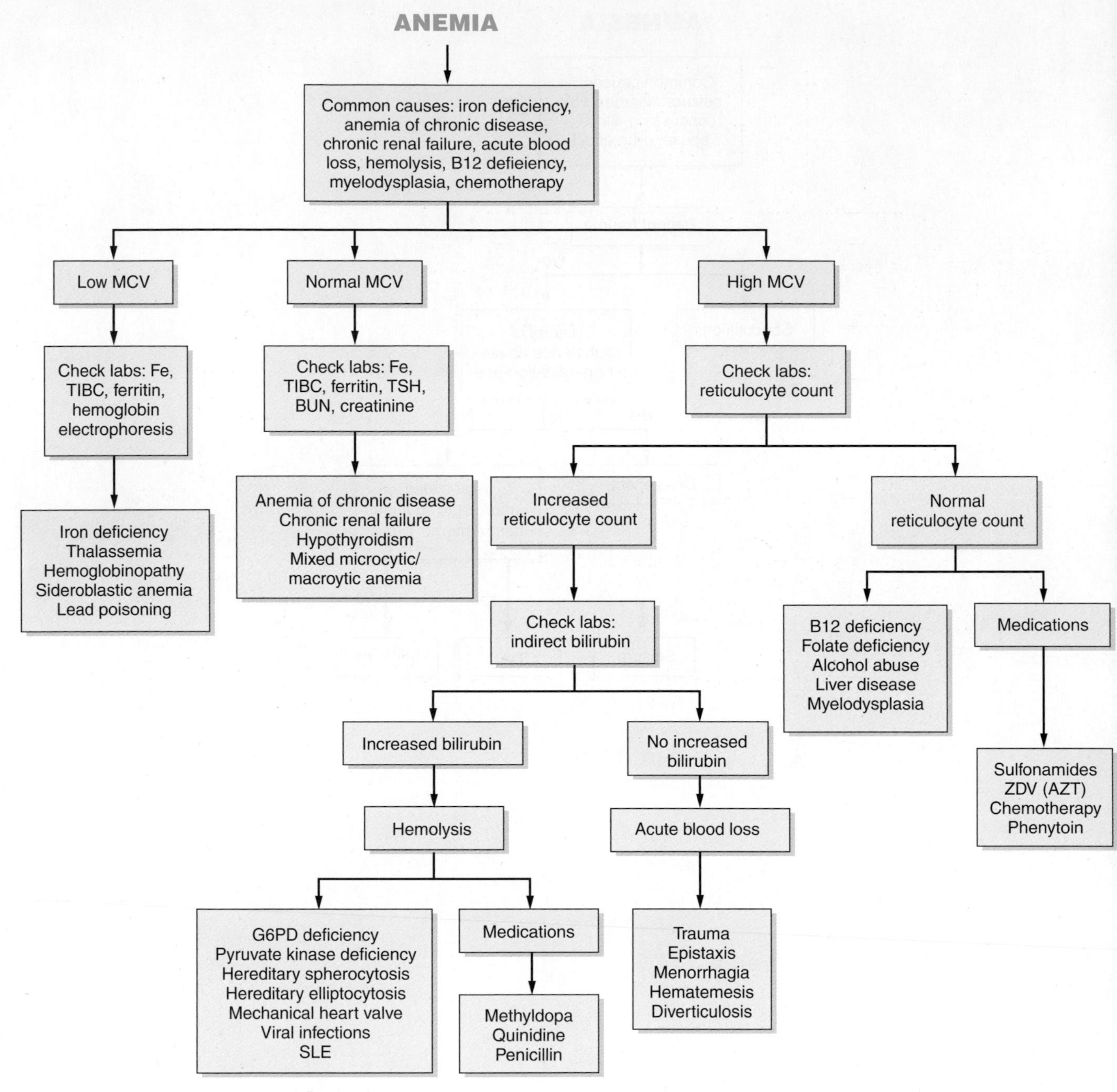
ANEMIA
Common causes: iron deficiency, anemia of chronic disease, chronic renal failure, acute blood loss, hemolysis, B12 defieiency, myelodysplasia, chemotherapy
Low MCV
Normal MCV
High MCV
Check labs: Fe, TIBC, ferritin, hemoglobin electrophoresis
Check labs: Fe, TIBC, ferritin, TSH, BUN, creatinine
Check labs: reticulocyte count
Iron deficiency
Thalassemia
Hemoglobinopathy
Sideroblastic anemia
Lead poisoning
Anemia of chronic disease
Chronic renal failure
Hypothyroidism
Mixed microcytic/ macroytic anemia
Increased reticulocyte count
Normal reticulocyte count
Check labs: indirect bilirubin
B12 deficiency
Folate deficiency
Alcohol abuse
Liver disease
Myelodysplasia
Medications
Increased bilirubin
No increased bilirubin
Sulfonamides
ZDV (AZT)
Chemotherapy
Phenytoin
Hemolysis
Acute blood loss
G6PD deficiency
Pyruvate kinase deficiency
Hereditary spherocytosis
Hereditary elliptocytosis
Mechanical heart valve
Viral infections
SLE
Medications
Methyldopa
Quinidine
Penicillin
Trauma
Epistaxis
Menorrhagia
Hematemesis
Diverticulosis

Robert A. Baldor, MD and Alan M. Ehrlich, MD

Am Fam Physician. 2000;62:1565–72.

ANOREXIA

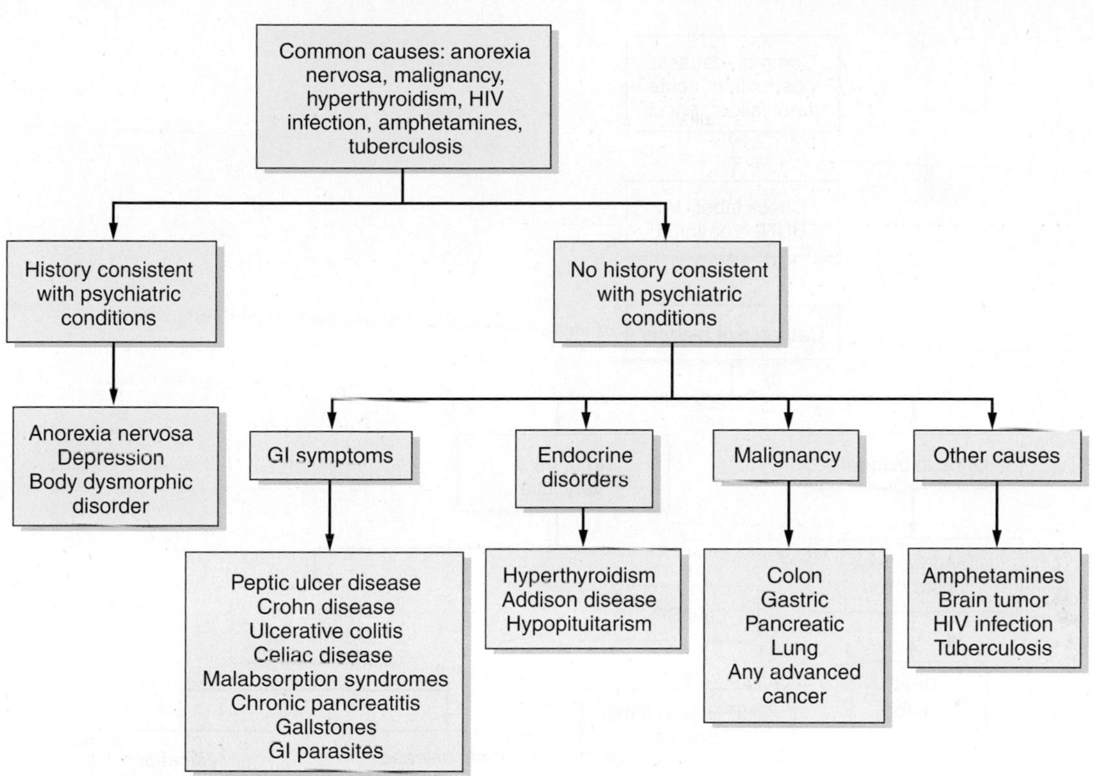

Robert A. Baldor, MD and Alan M. Ehrlich, MD

Am Fam Physician. 2003;67:297–304, 311–2.

ANURIA OR OLIGOURIA

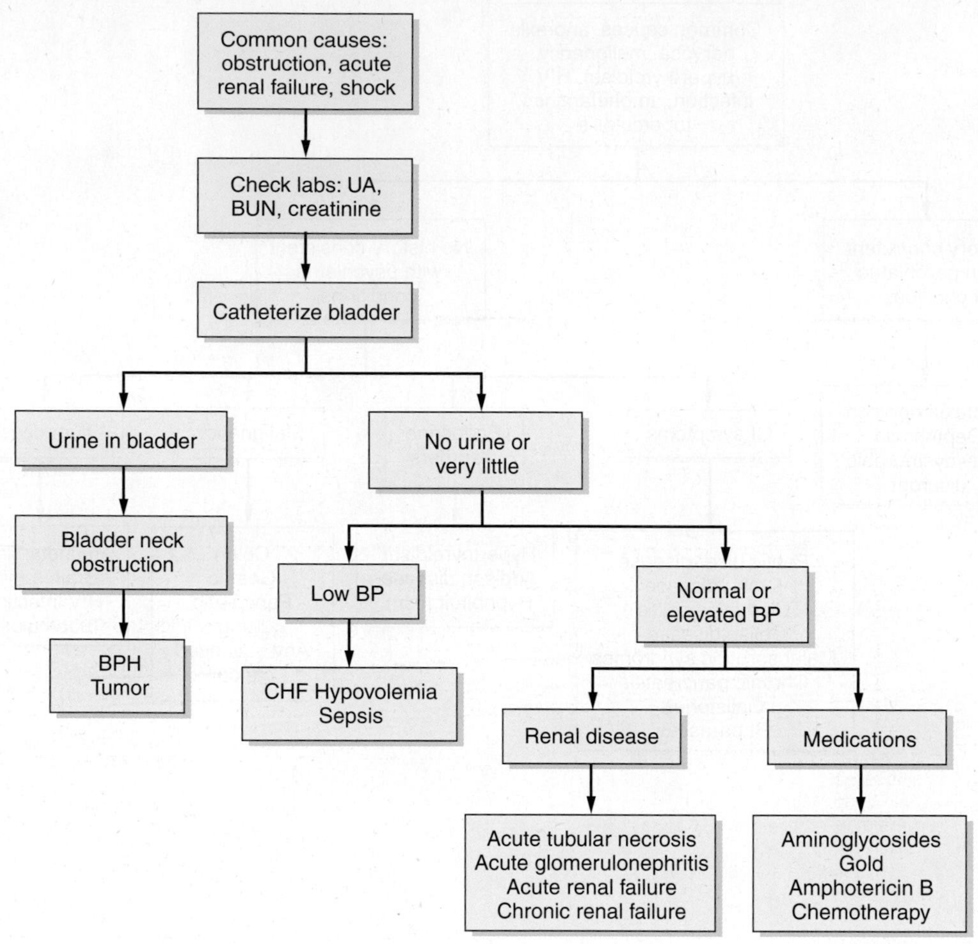

Robert A. Baldor, MD and Alan M. Ehrlich, MD

Am Fam Physician. 2000;61:2077–88.

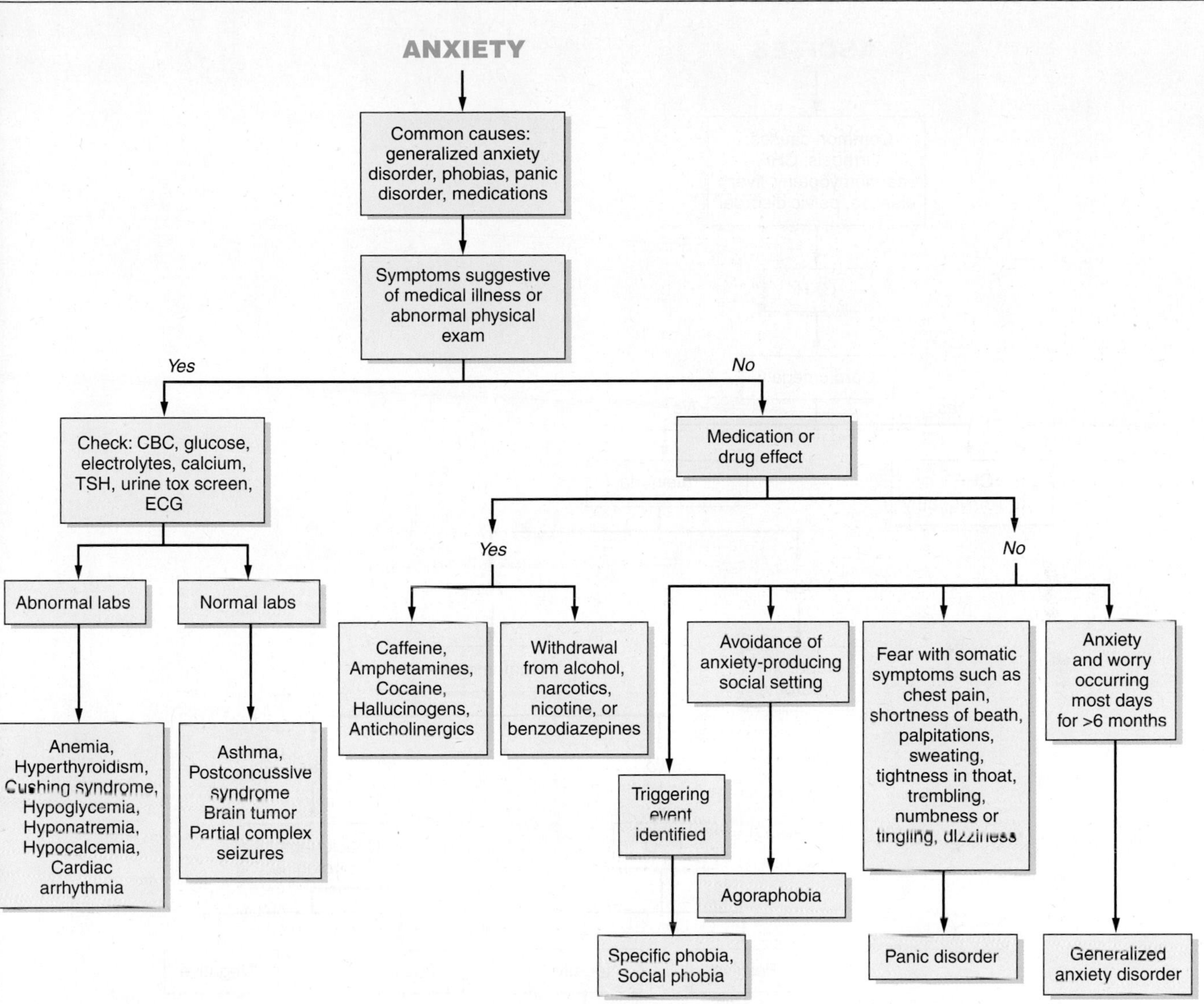
ANXIETY
Common causes: generalized anxiety disorder, phobias, panic disorder, medications
Symptoms suggestive of medical illness or abnormal physical exam
Yes
No
Check: CBC, glucose, electrolytes, calcium, TSH, urine tox screen, ECG
Medication or drug effect
Abnormal labs
Normal labs
Yes
No
Anemia, Hyperthyroidism, Cushing syndrome, Hypoglycemia, Hyponatremia, Hypocalcemia, Cardiac arrhythmia
Asthma, Postconcussive syndrome Brain tumor Partial complex seizures
Caffeine, Amphetamines, Cocaine, Hallucinogens, Anticholinergics
Withdrawal from alcohol, narcotics, nicotine, or benzodiazepines
Avoidance of anxiety-producing social setting
Fear with somatic symptoms such as chest pain, shortness of beath, palpitations, sweating, tightness in thoat, trembling, numbness or tingling, dizziness
Anxiety and worry occurring most days for >6 months
Triggering event identified
Agoraphobia
Specific phobia, Social phobia
Panic disorder
Generalized anxiety disorder

Robert A. Baldor, MD and Alan M. Ehrlich, MD

Am J Psychiatry. 1999;156:1677–85.

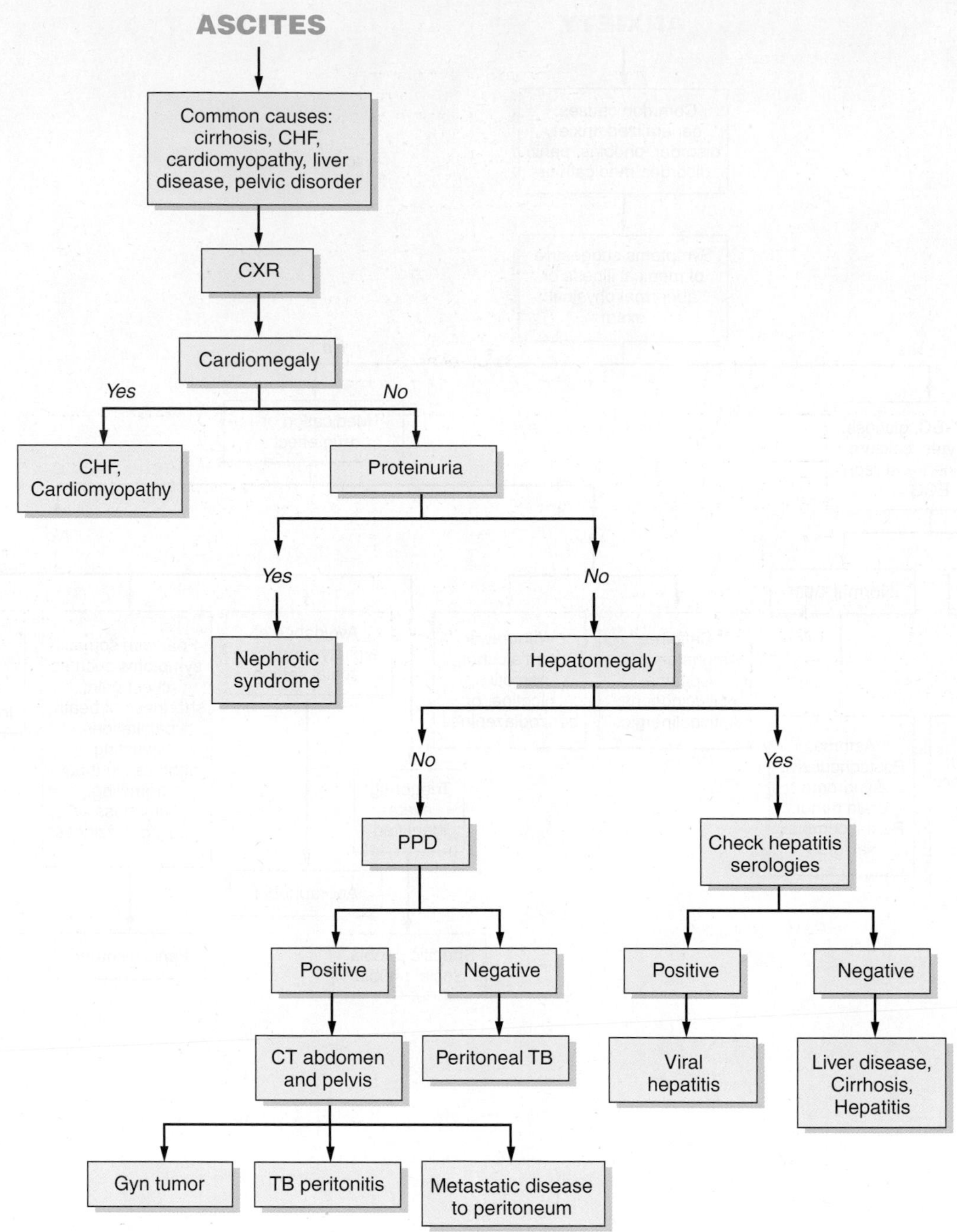

Robert A. Baldor, MD and Alan M. Ehrlich, MD

Am Fam Physician. 2006;74:767–76.

AST ELEVATION

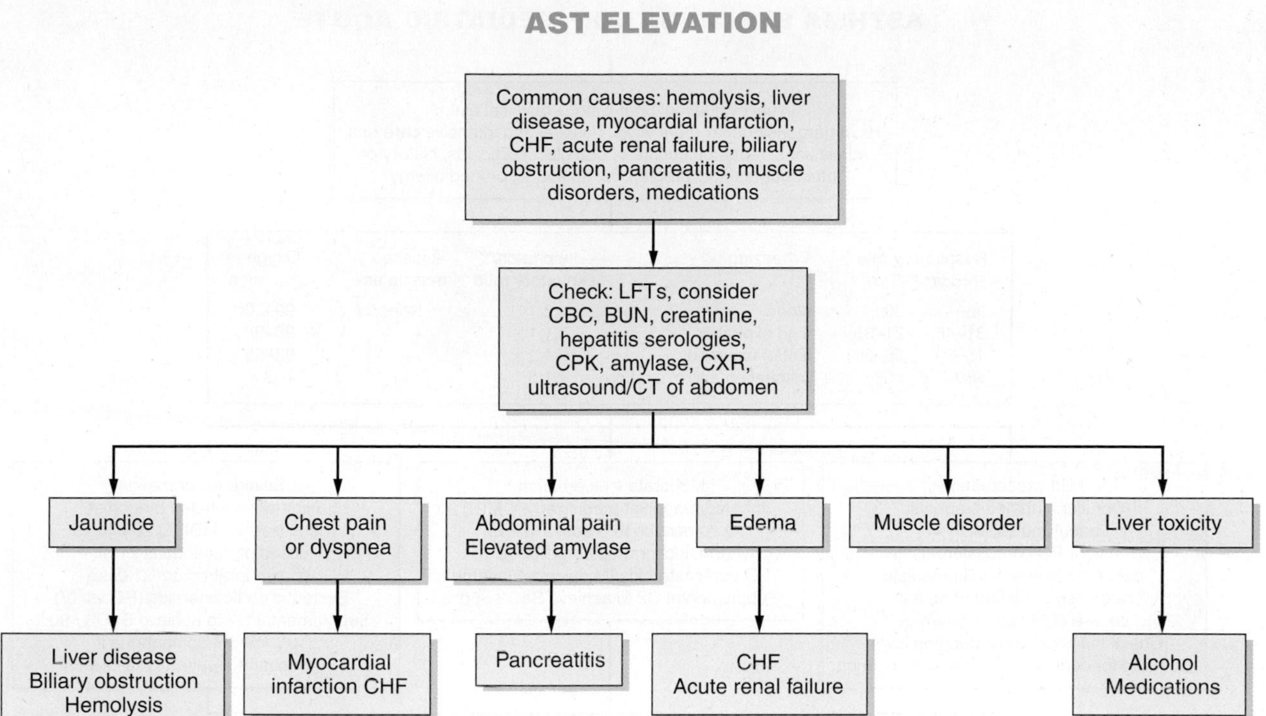

Robert A. Baldor, MD and Alan M. Ehrlich, MD

Am Fam Physician. 2005;71:1105–10.

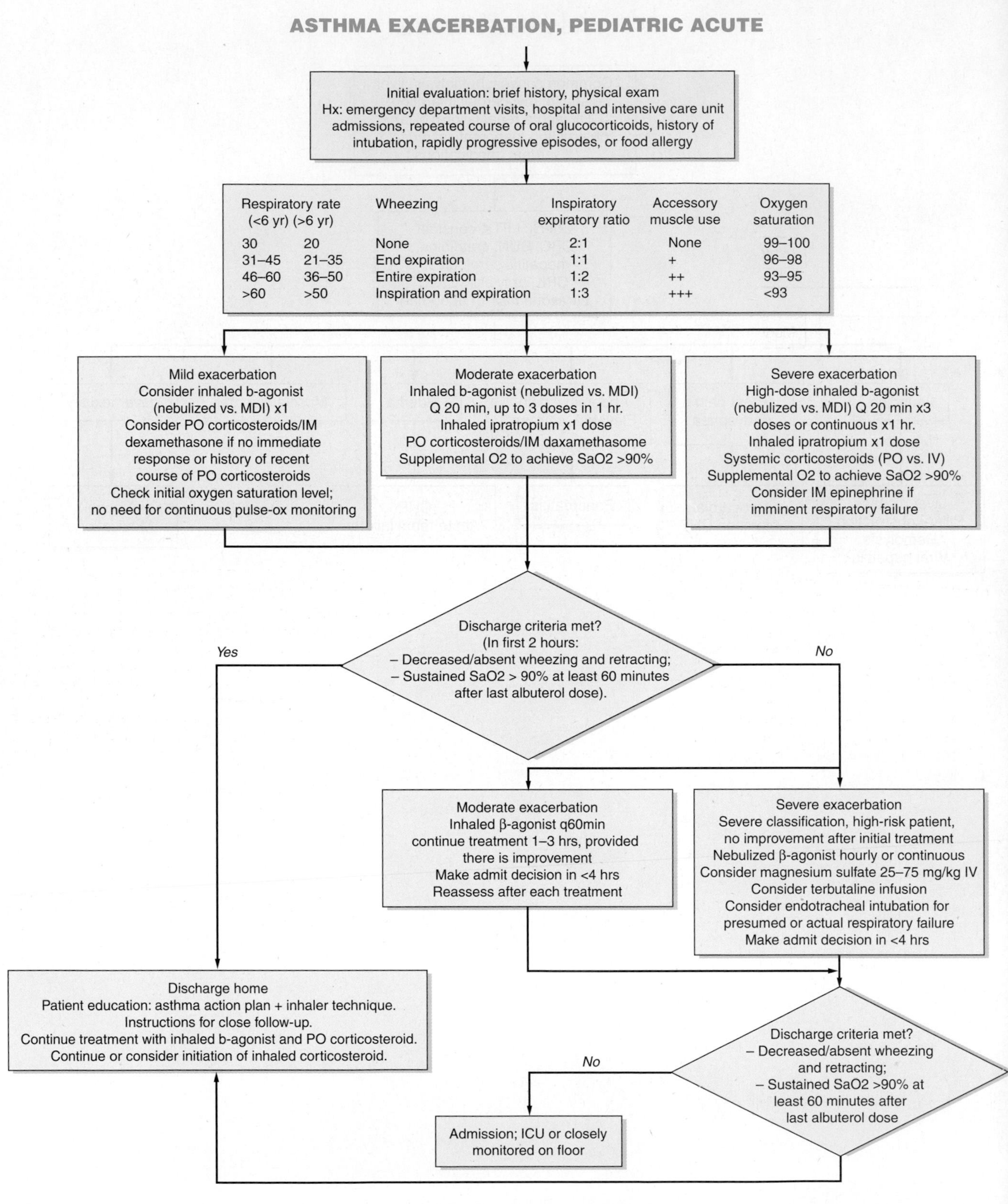

ASTHMA EXACERBATION, PEDIATRIC ACUTE
Initial evaluation: brief history, physical exam
Hx: emergency department visits, hospital and intensive care unit admissions, repeated course of oral glucocorticoids, history of intubation, rapidly progressive episodes, or food allergy
Respiratory rate (<6 yr) (>6 yr) | Wheezing | Inspiratory expiratory ratio | Accessory muscle use | Oxygen saturation
30 20 | None | 2:1 | None | 99–100
31–45 21–35 | End expiration | 1:1 | + | 96–98
46–60 36–50 | Entire expiration | 1:2 | ++ | 93–95
>60 >50 | Inspiration and expiration | 1:3 | +++ | <93
Mild exacerbation
Consider inhaled b-agonist (nebulized vs. MDI) x1
Consider PO corticosteroids/IM dexamethasone if no immediate response or history of recent course of PO corticosteroids
Check initial oxygen saturation level; no need for continuous pulse-ox monitoring
Moderate exacerbation
Inhaled b-agonist (nebulized vs. MDI) Q 20 min, up to 3 doses in 1 hr.
Inhaled ipratropium x1 dose
PO corticosteroids/IM daxamethasome
Supplemental O2 to achieve SaO2 >90%
Severe exacerbation
High-dose inhaled b-agonist (nebulized vs. MDI) Q 20 min x3 doses or continuous x1 hr.
Inhaled ipratropium x1 dose
Systemic corticosteroids (PO vs. IV)
Supplemental O2 to achieve SaO2 >90%
Consider IM epinephrine if imminent respiratory failure
Discharge criteria met? (In first 2 hours: – Decreased/absent wheezing and retracting; – Sustained SaO2 > 90% at least 60 minutes after last albuterol dose).
Yes
No
Moderate exacerbation
Inhaled β-agonist q60min
continue treatment 1–3 hrs, provided there is improvement
Make admit decision in <4 hrs
Reassess after each treatment
Severe exacerbation
Severe classification, high-risk patient, no improvement after initial treatment
Nebulized β-agonist hourly or continuous
Consider magnesium sulfate 25–75 mg/kg IV
Consider terbutaline infusion
Consider endotracheal intubation for presumed or actual respiratory failure
Make admit decision in <4 hrs
Discharge home
Patient education: asthma action plan + inhaler technique.
Instructions for close follow-up.
Continue treatment with inhaled b-agonist and PO corticosteroid.
Continue or consider initiation of inhaled corticosteroid.
Discharge criteria met? – Decreased/absent wheezing and retracting; – Sustained SaO2 >90% at least 60 minutes after last albuterol dose
No
Admission; ICU or closely monitored on floor

Catherine Janes, MD

Am Fam Physician. 2005;71:1959–68.

ATAXIA

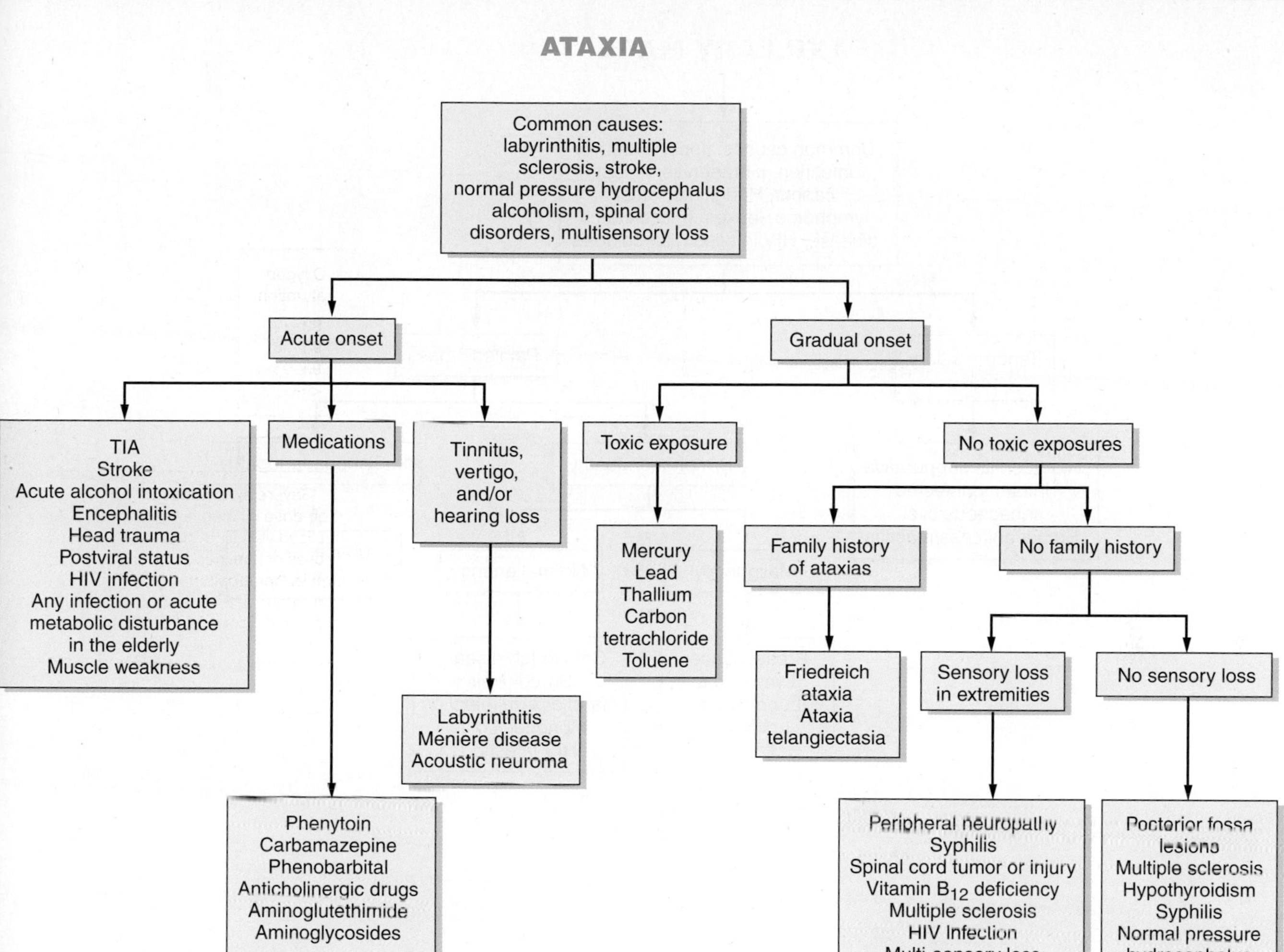

Robert A. Baldor, MD and Alan M. Ehrlich, MD

Arch Neurol. 2008;65(10):1296–303.

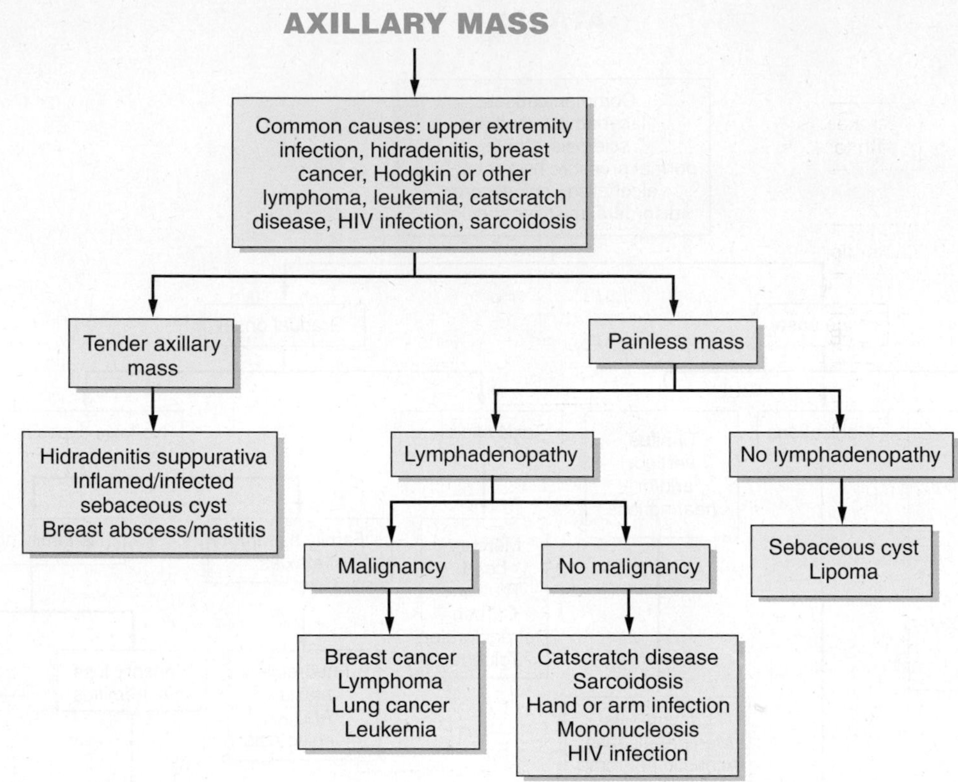

Robert A. Baldor, MD and Alan M. Ehrlich, MD

Ann Surg Oncol. 2000;7:411–5.

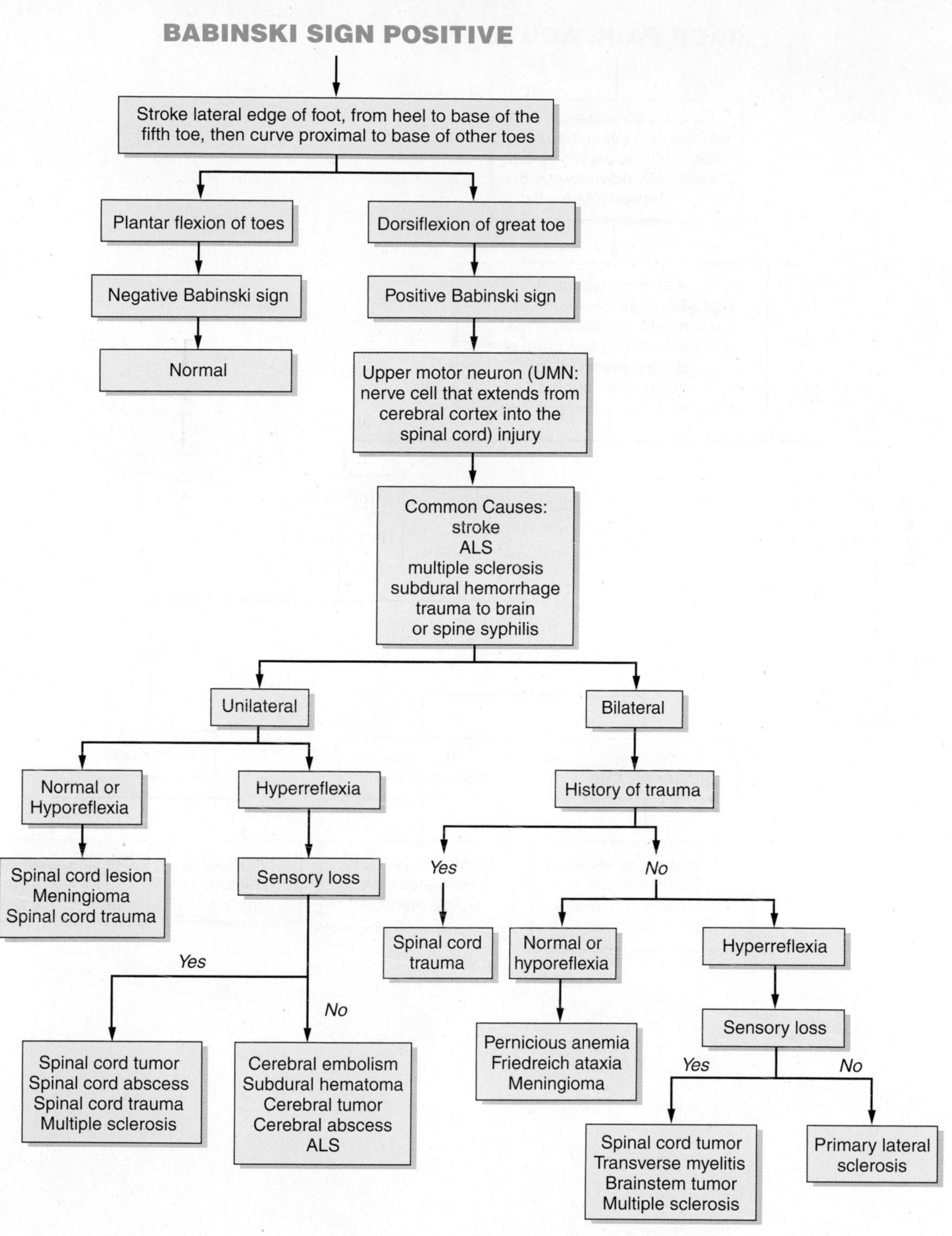
BABINSKI SIGN POSITIVE
Stroke lateral edge of foot, from heel to base of the fifth toe, then curve proximal to base of other toes
Plantar flexion of toes
Dorsiflexion of great toe
Negative Babinski sign
Positive Babinski sign
Normal
Upper motor neuron (UMN: nerve cell that extends from cerebral cortex into the spinal cord) injury
Common Causes: stroke ALS multiple sclerosis subdural hemorrhage trauma to brain or spine syphilis
Unilateral
Bilateral
Normal or Hyporeflexia
Hyperreflexia
History of trauma
Spinal cord lesion Meningioma Spinal cord trauma
Sensory loss
Yes
No
Spinal cord trauma
Normal or hyporeflexia
Hyperreflexia
Yes
No
Pernicious anemia Friedreich ataxia Meningioma
Sensory loss
Yes
No
Spinal cord tumor Spinal cord abscess Spinal cord trauma Multiple sclerosis
Cerebral embolism Subdural hematoma Cerebral tumor Cerebral abscess ALS
Spinal cord tumor Transverse myelitis Brainstem tumor Multiple sclerosis
Primary lateral sclerosis

Robert A. Baldor, MD and Alan M. Ehrlich, MD

J Neurol Neurosurg Psychiatry. 2002;73(4):360–2.

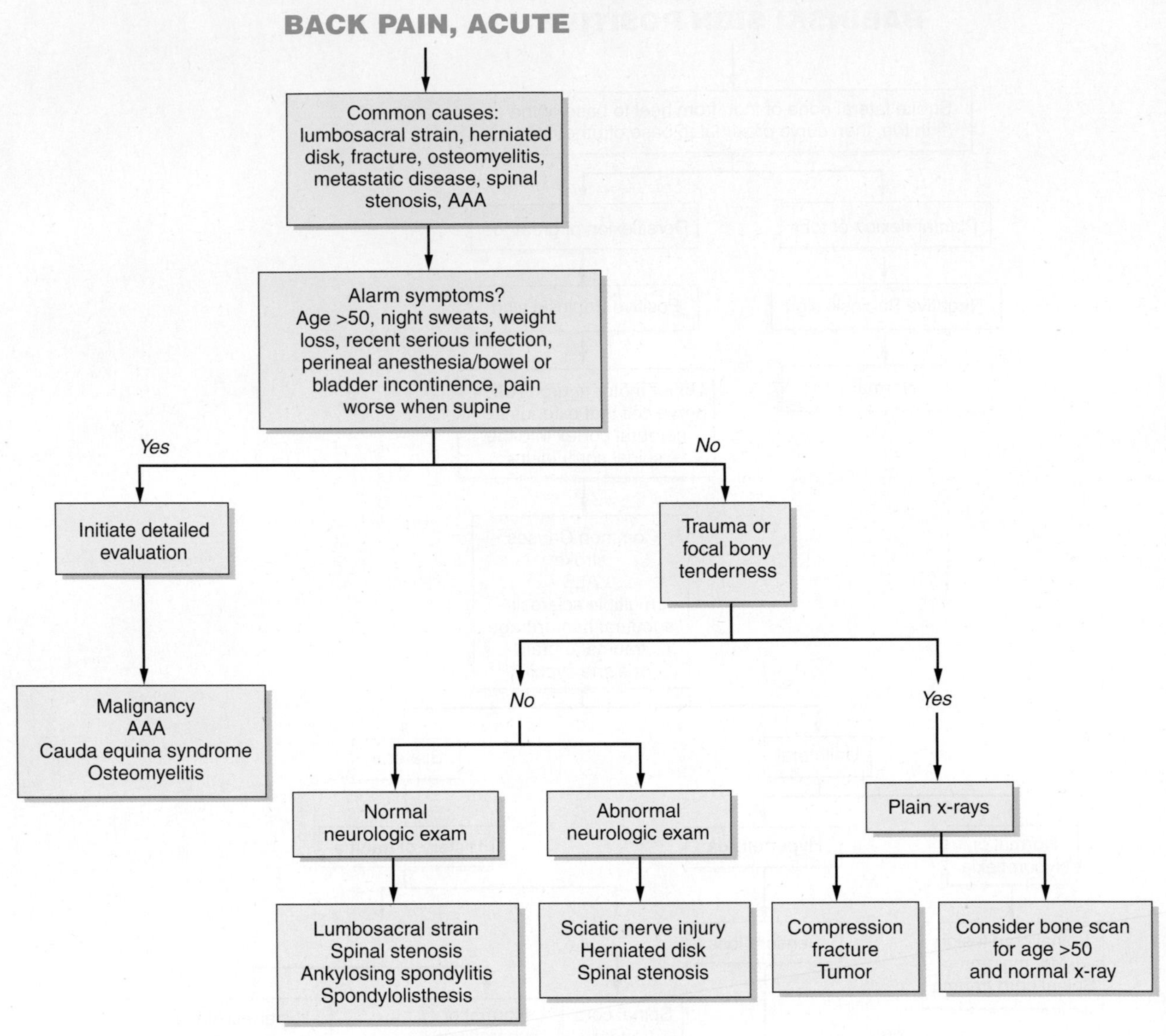
BACK PAIN, ACUTE
Common causes: lumbosacral strain, herniated disk, fracture, osteomyelitis, metastatic disease, spinal stenosis, AAA
Alarm symptoms? Age >50, night sweats, weight loss, recent serious infection, perineal anesthesia/bowel or bladder incontinence, pain worse when supine
Yes
No
Initiate detailed evaluation
Malignancy
AAA
Cauda equina syndrome
Osteomyelitis
Trauma or focal bony tenderness
No
Yes
Normal neurologic exam
Abnormal neurologic exam
Plain x-rays
Lumbosacral strain
Spinal stenosis
Ankylosing spondylitis
Spondylolisthesis
Sciatic nerve injury
Herniated disk
Spinal stenosis
Compression fracture
Tumor
Consider bone scan for age >50 and normal x-ray

Robert A. Baldor, MD and Alan M. Ehrlich, MD

Am Fam Physician. 2007;75:1181–8.

BLEEDING GUMS

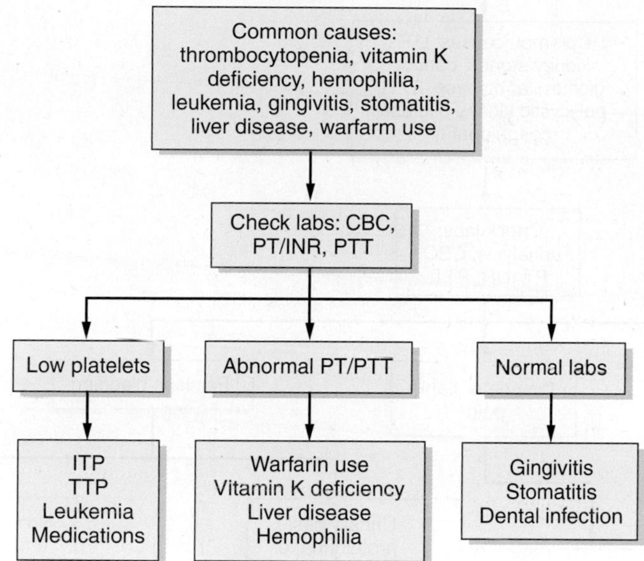

Robert A. Baldor, MD and Alan M. Ehrlich, MD

Compend Contin Educ Dent. 1999;20(10):936–40.

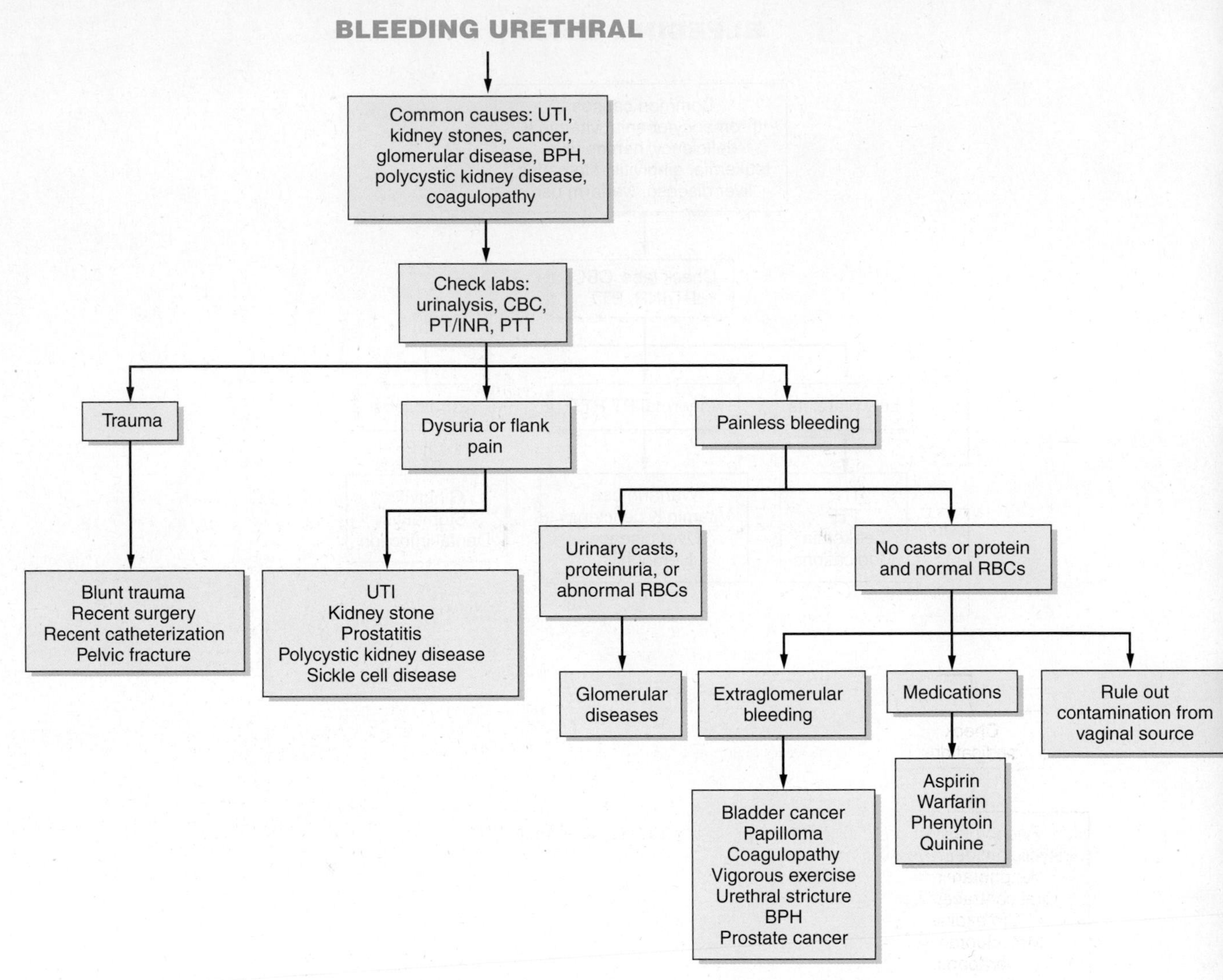
BLEEDING URETHRAL
Common causes: UTI, kidney stones, cancer, glomerular disease, BPH, polycystic kidney disease, coagulopathy
Check labs: urinalysis, CBC, PT/INR, PTT
Trauma
Dysuria or flank pain
Painless bleeding
Urinary casts, proteinuria, or abnormal RBCs
No casts or protein and normal RBCs
Blunt trauma
Recent surgery
Recent catheterization
Pelvic fracture
UTI
Kidney stone
Prostatitis
Polycystic kidney disease
Sickle cell disease
Glomerular diseases
Extraglomerular bleeding
Medications
Rule out contamination from vaginal source
Aspirin
Warfarin
Phenytoin
Quinine
Bladder cancer
Papilloma
Coagulopathy
Vigorous exercise
Urethral stricture
BPH
Prostate cancer

Robert A. Baldor, MD and Alan M. Ehrlich, MD

Am Fam Physician. 2001;63:1145–54.

BREAST DISCHARGE

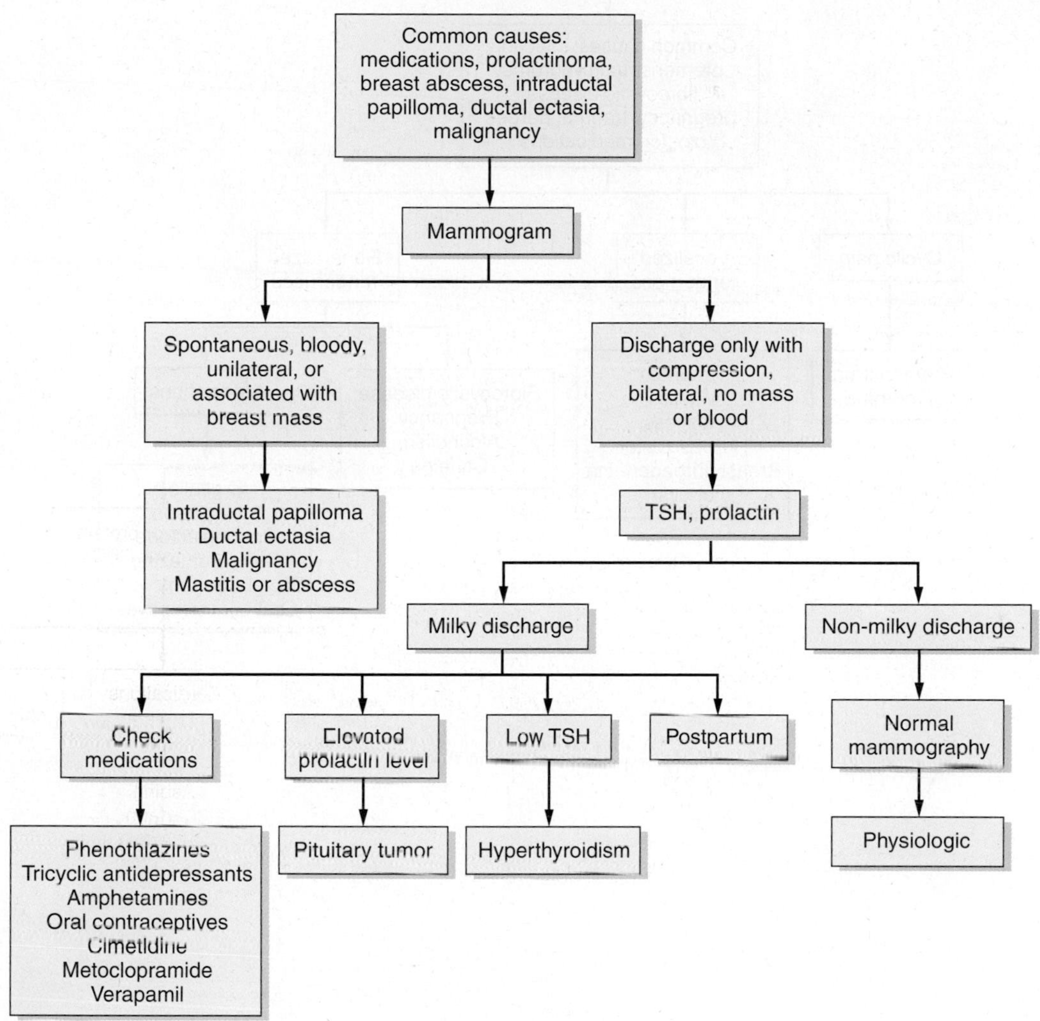

Robert A. Baldor, MD and Alan M. Ehrlich, MD

Breast J. 2009;15(3):230–5.

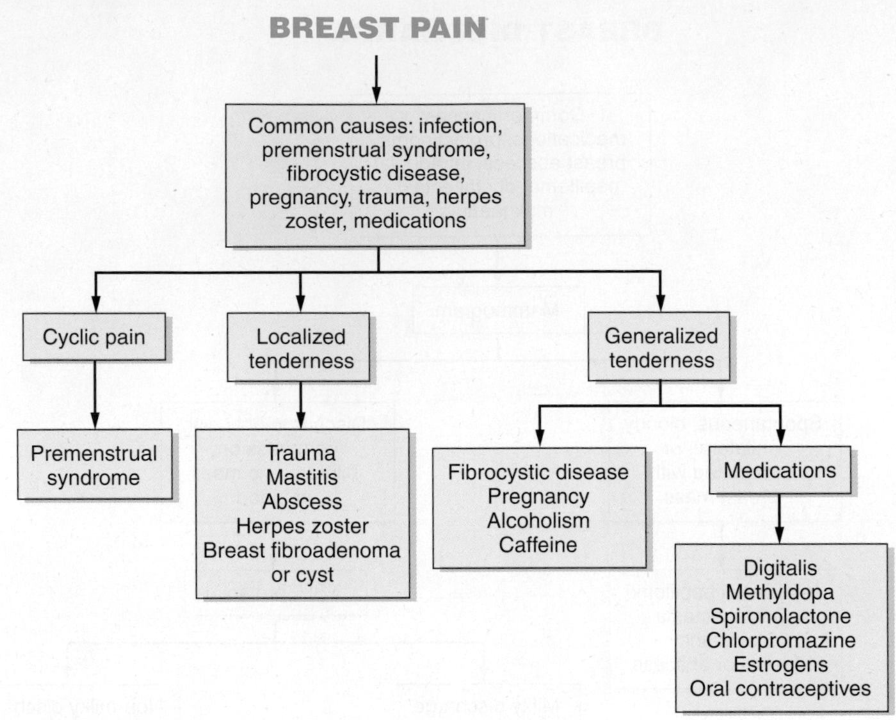

Robert A. Baldor, MD and Alan M. Ehrlich, MD

Obstet Gynecol Clin North Am. 2008;35(2):285–303.

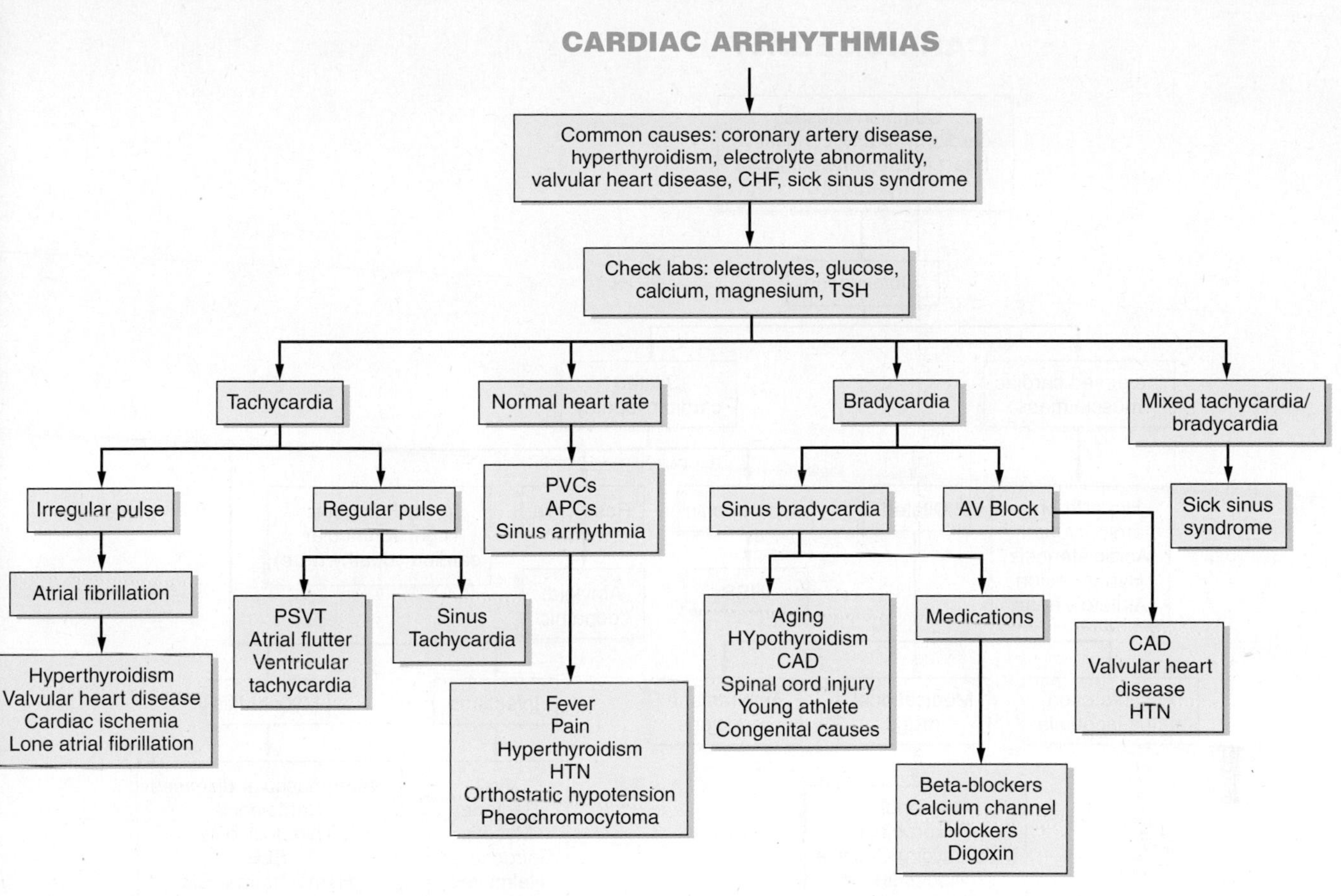

Robert A. Baldor, MD and Alan M. Ehrlich, MD

Am Fam Physician. 2005;743–50, 755–9.

CARDIOMEGALY

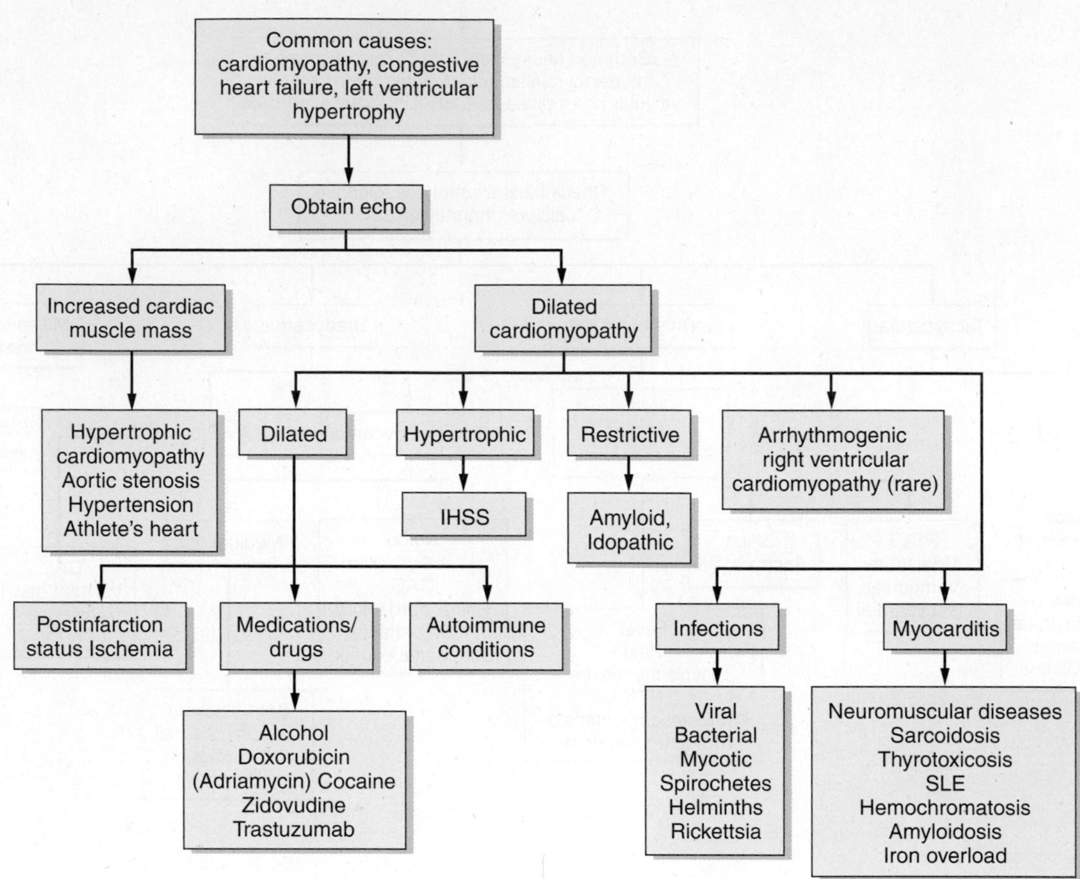

Robert A. Baldor, MD and Alan M. Ehrlich, MD

Eur J Echocardiogr. 2009;10(8):iii15–21.

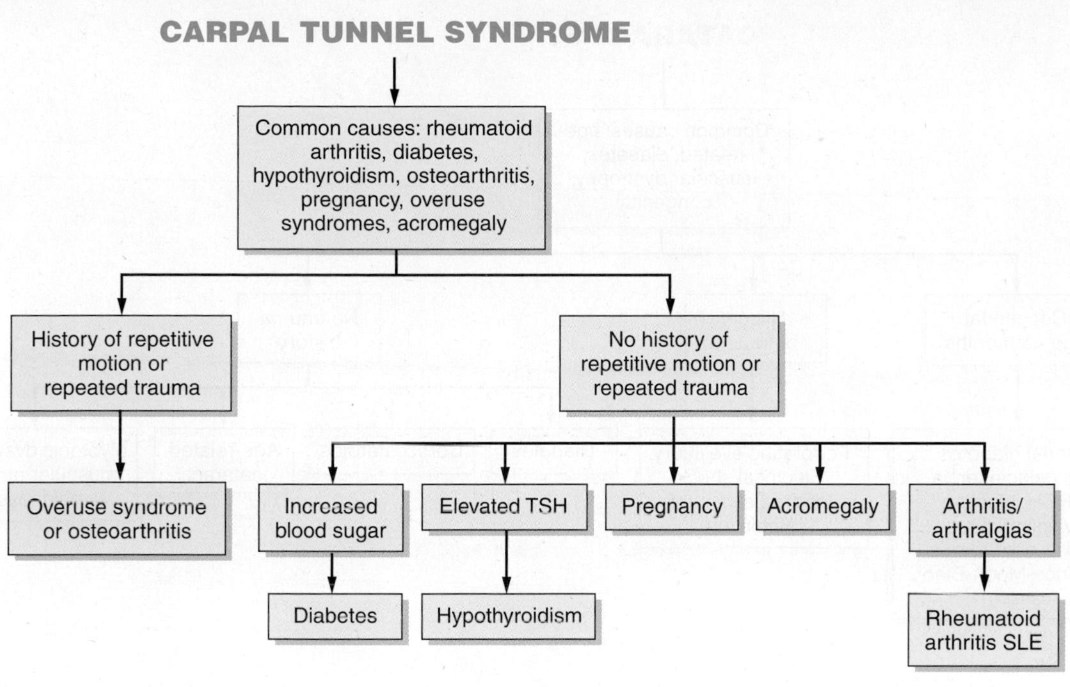

Robert A. Baldor, MD and Alan M. Ehrlich, MD

BMJ. 2007;335(7615):343–6.

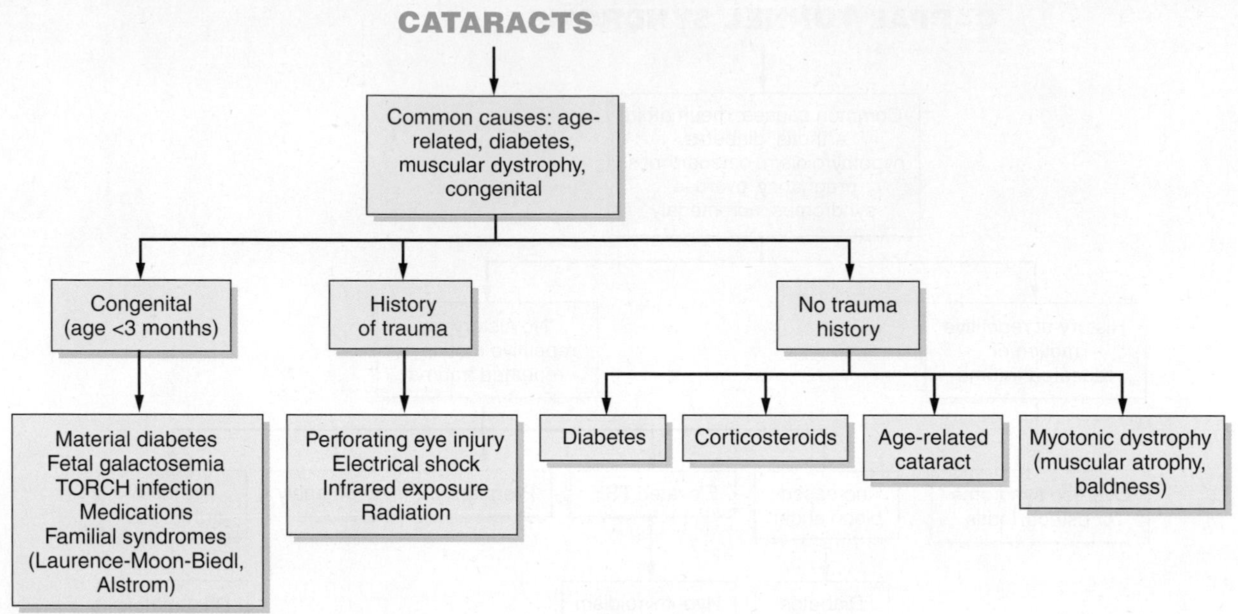

Robert A. Baldor, MD and Alan M. Ehrlich, MD

Ophth. 2010;117(8):1471–8.

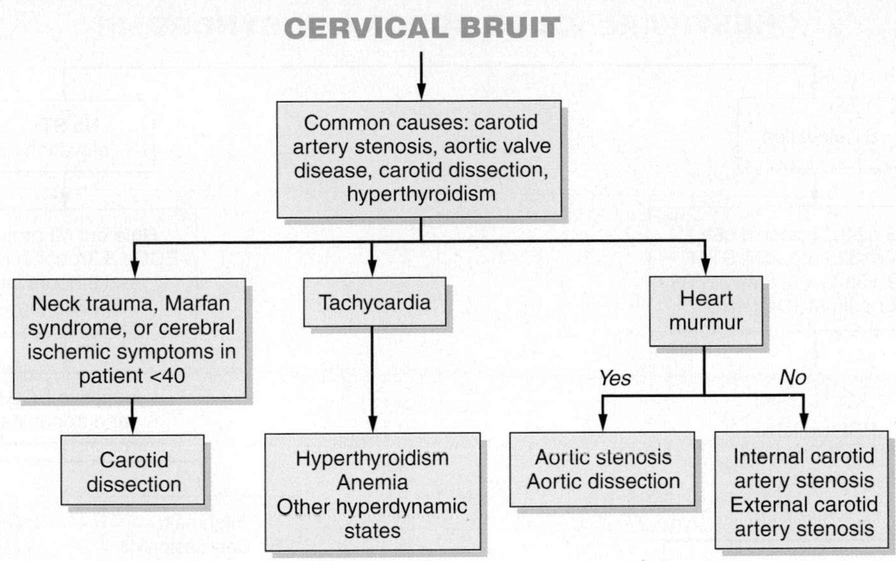

Robert A. Baldor, MD and Alan M. Ehrlich, MD

http://www.ncbi.nlm.nih.gov/bookshelf/br.fcgi?book=cm&part=A593

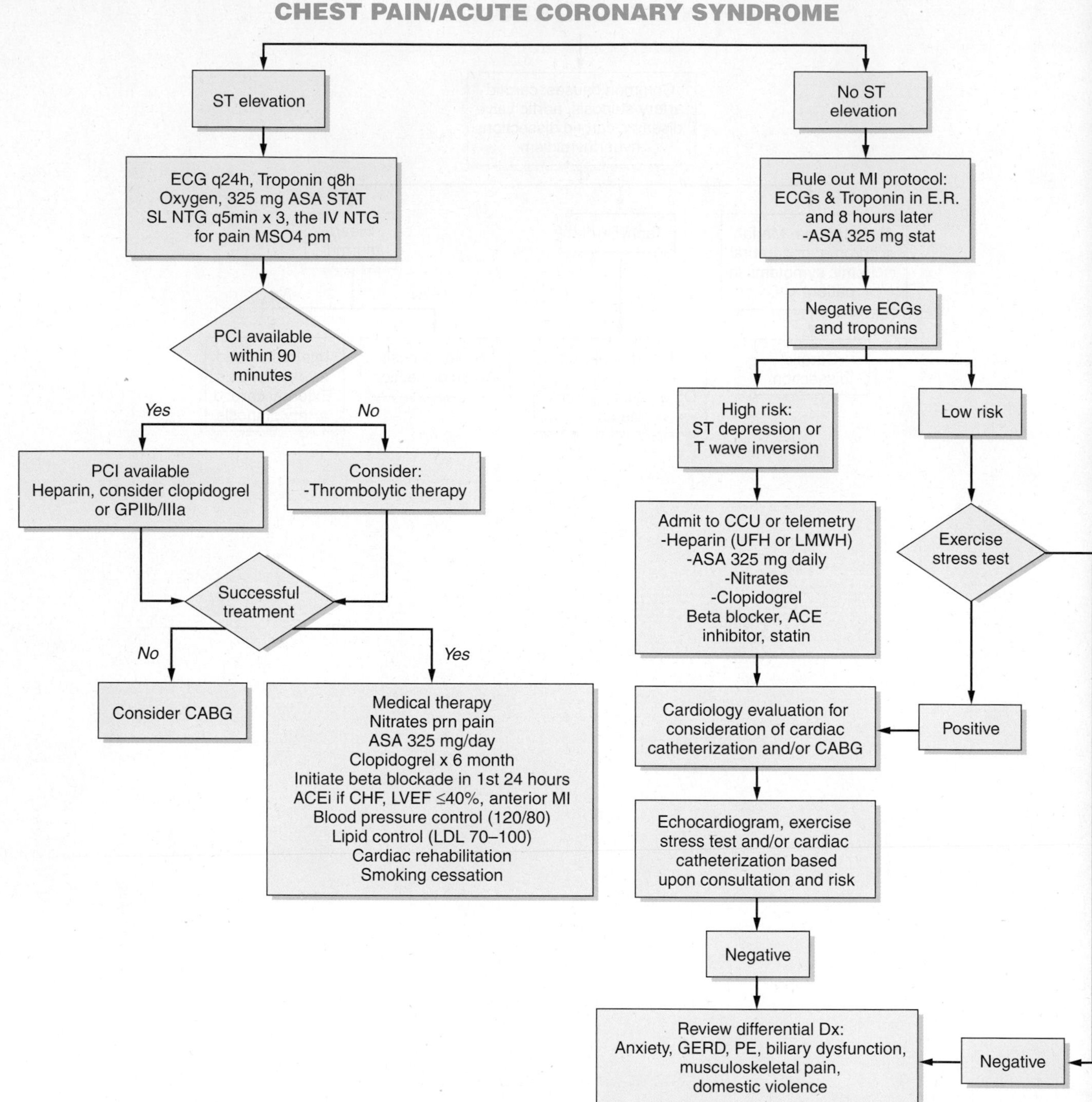

Allen Chang, MD and Naomi F. Botkin, MD

Circulation. 2005;112(22 Suppl):III55–72.

CHRONIC OBSTRUCTIVE PULMONARY DISEASE (COPD), DIAGNOSIS AND TREATMENT

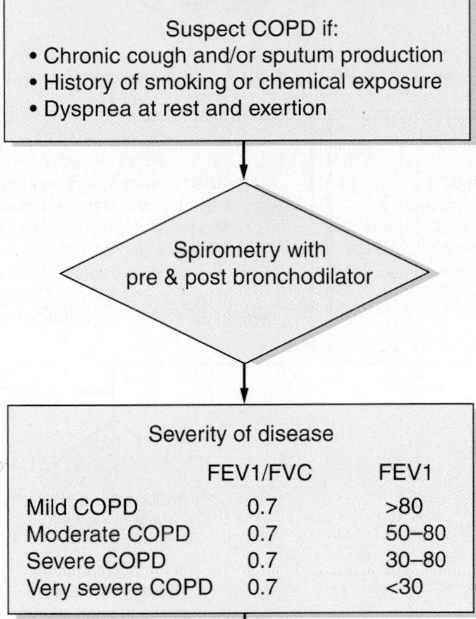

Suspect COPD if:
• Chronic cough and/or sputum production
• History of smoking or chemical exposure
• Dyspnea at rest and exertion
Spirometry with
pre & post bronchodilator
Severity of disease
FEV1/FVC FEV1
Mild COPD 0.7 >80
Moderate COPD 0.7 50–80
Severe COPD 0.7 30–80
Very severe COPD 0.7 <30

Functional dyspnea scale

0 Not troubled with breathlessness except with strenuous exercise.
1 Troubled by shortness of breath when hurrying or walking up a slight hill.
2 Walks slower than people of same age due to breathlessness or has to stop for breath when walking at own pace on the level.
3 Stops for breath after walking ~100 m or after a few minutes on the level.
4 Too breathless to leave the house or breathless when dressing or undressing.

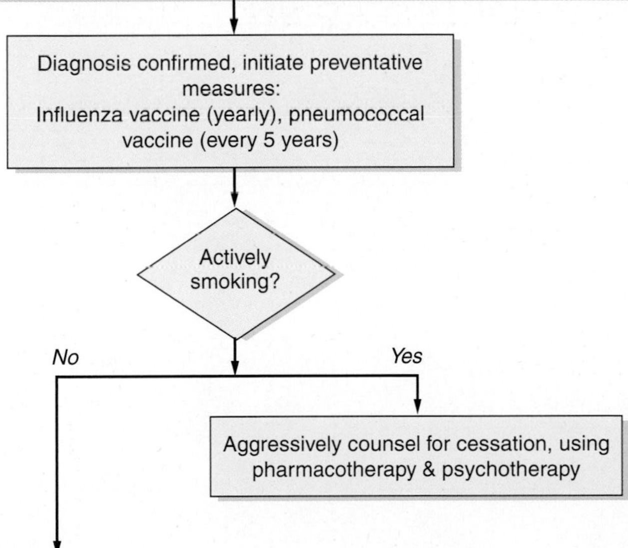

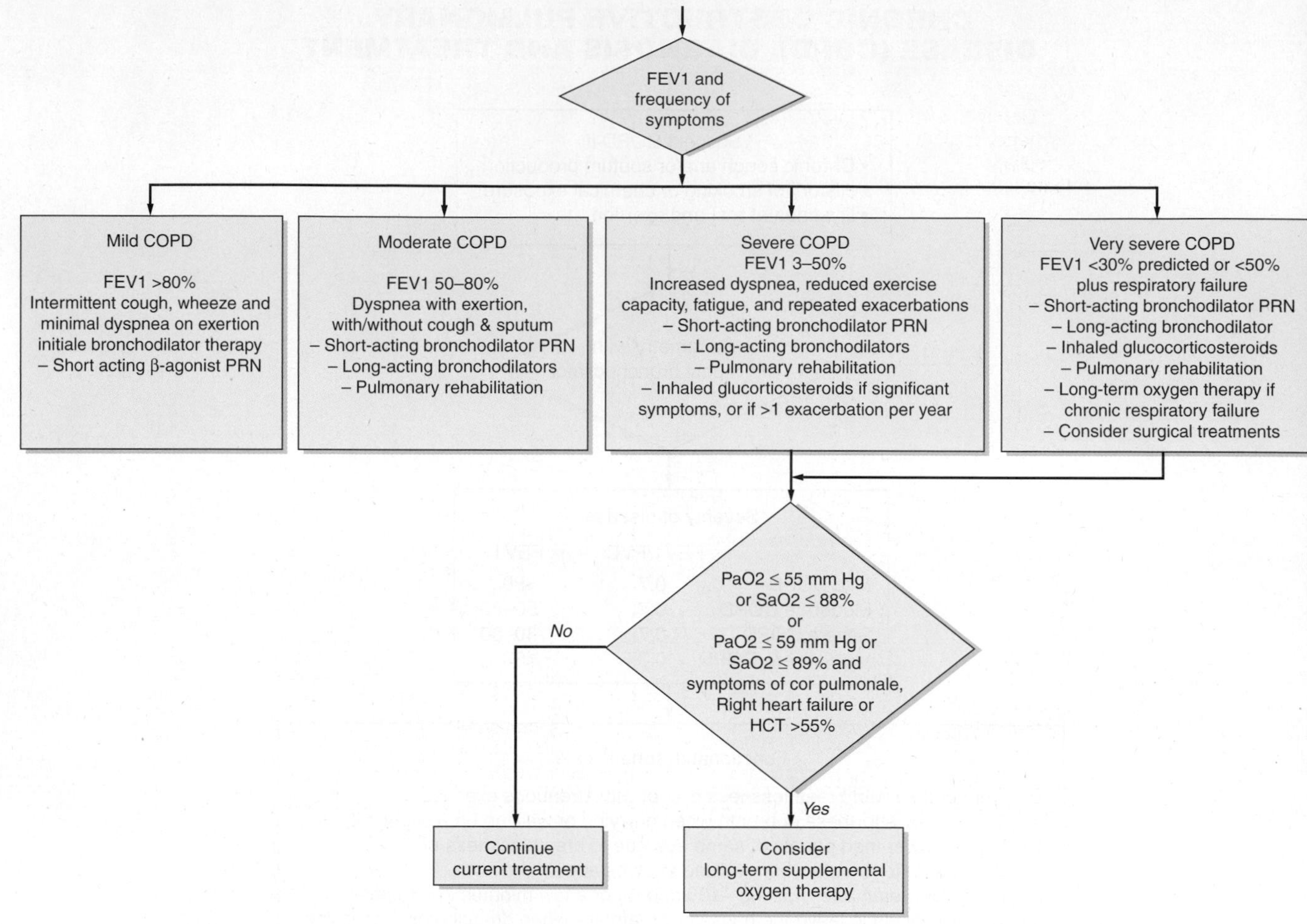

Laura Paulin, MD, MHS and Scott Kopec, MD

National Guidelines Clearinghouse. Global Initiative for Chronic Obstructive Lung Disease (GOLD); 2008.

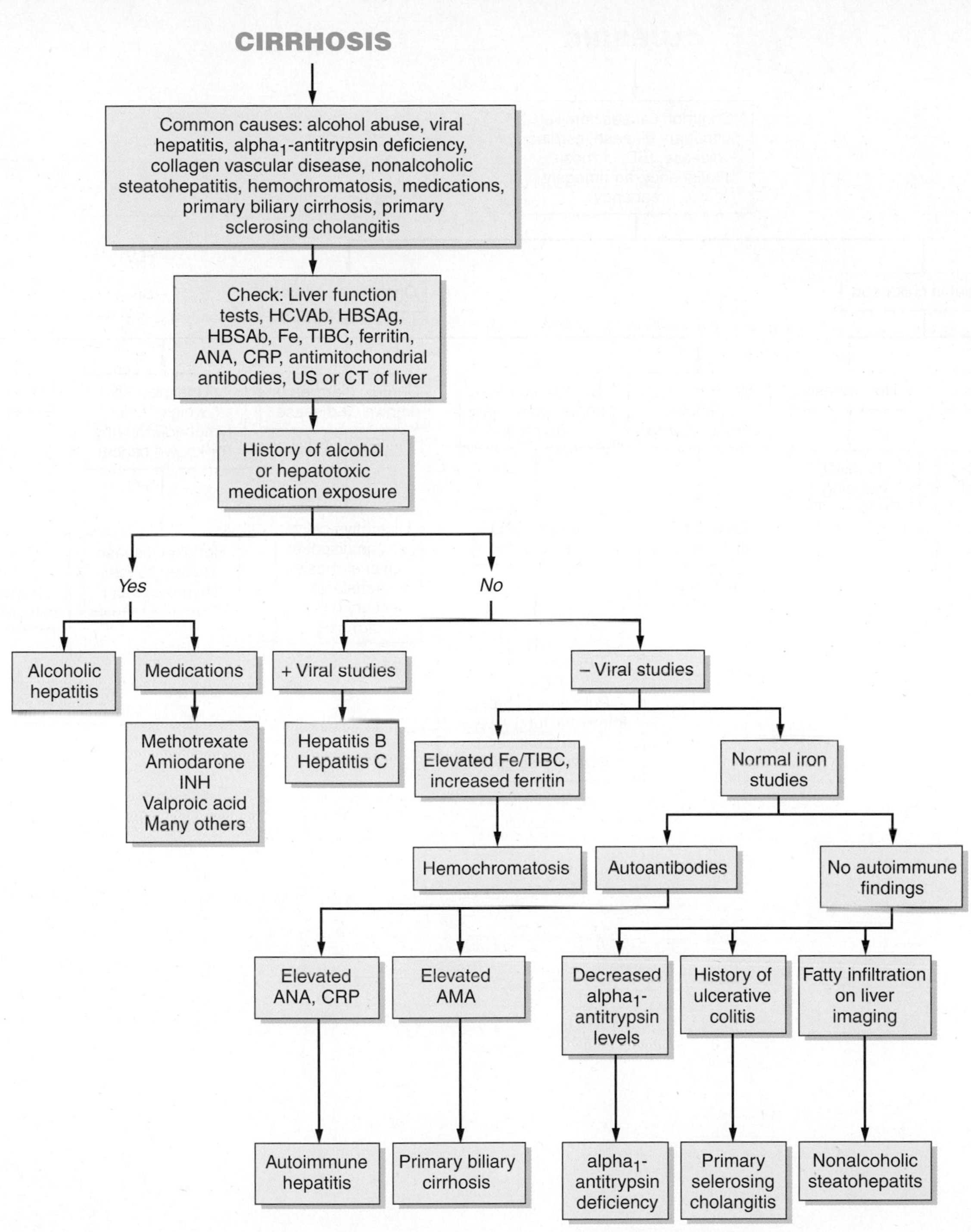
CIRRHOSIS
Common causes: alcohol abuse, viral hepatitis, alpha$_1$-antitrypsin deficiency, collagen vascular disease, nonalcoholic steatohepatitis, hemochromatosis, medications, primary biliary cirrhosis, primary sclerosing cholangitis
Check: Liver function tests, HCVAb, HBSAg, HBSAb, Fe, TIBC, ferritin, ANA, CRP, antimitochondrial antibodies, US or CT of liver
History of alcohol or hepatotoxic medication exposure
Yes
No
Alcoholic hepatitis
Medications
+ Viral studies
– Viral studies
Methotrexate
Amiodarone
INH
Valproic acid
Many others
Hepatitis B
Hepatitis C
Elevated Fe/TIBC, increased ferritin
Normal iron studies
Hemochromatosis
Autoantibodies
No autoimmune findings
Elevated ANA, CRP
Elevated AMA
Decreased alpha$_1$-antitrypsin levels
History of ulcerative colitis
Fatty infiltration on liver imaging
Autoimmune hepatitis
Primary biliary cirrhosis
alpha$_1$-antitrypsin deficiency
Primary selerosing cholangitis
Nonalcoholic steatohepatits

Robert A. Baldor, MD and Alan M. Ehrlich, MD

Med Clin North Am. 2009;93(4).

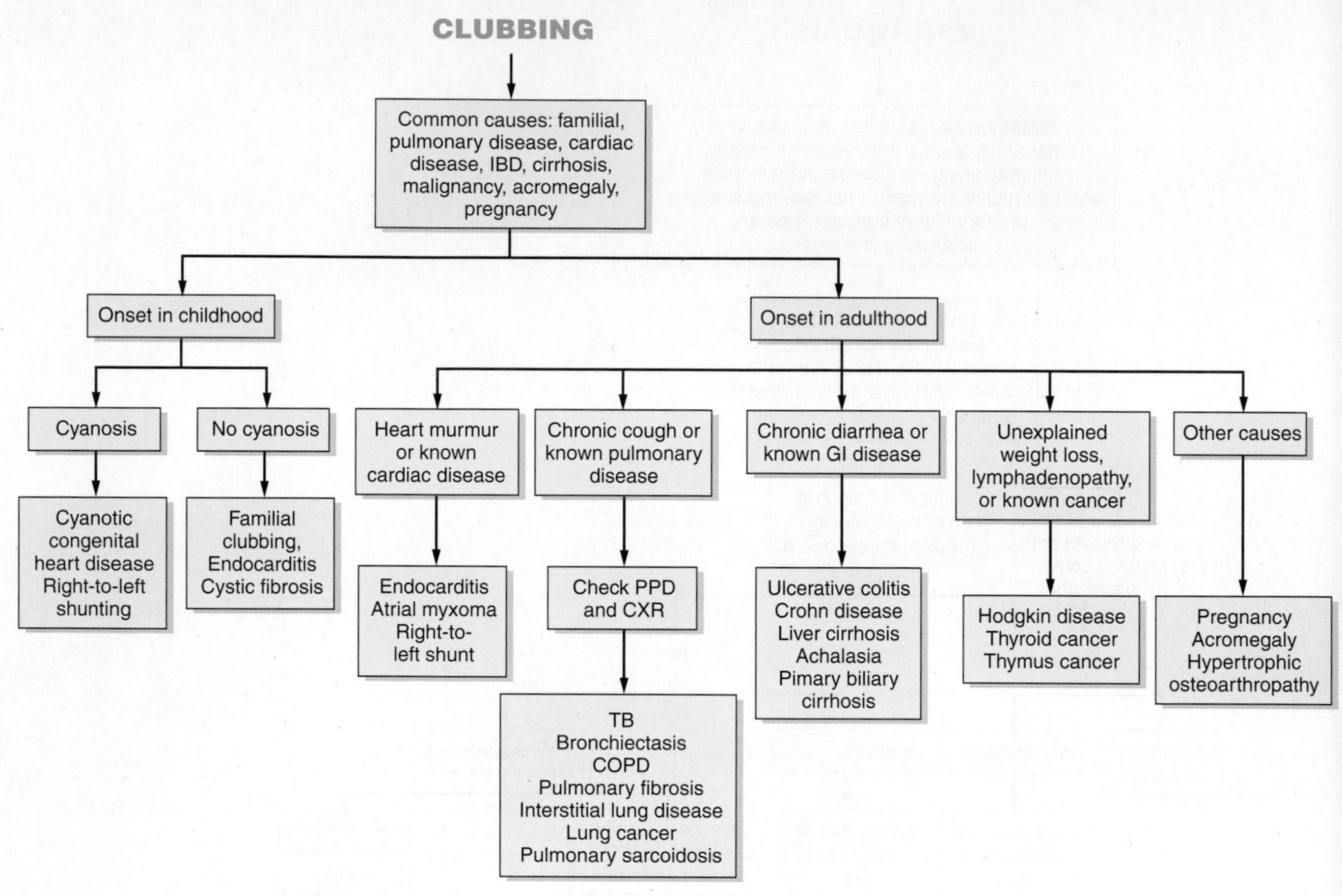

Robert A. Baldor, MD and Alan M. Ehrlich, MD

Clin Dermatol. 2008;26(3):296–305.

COMA

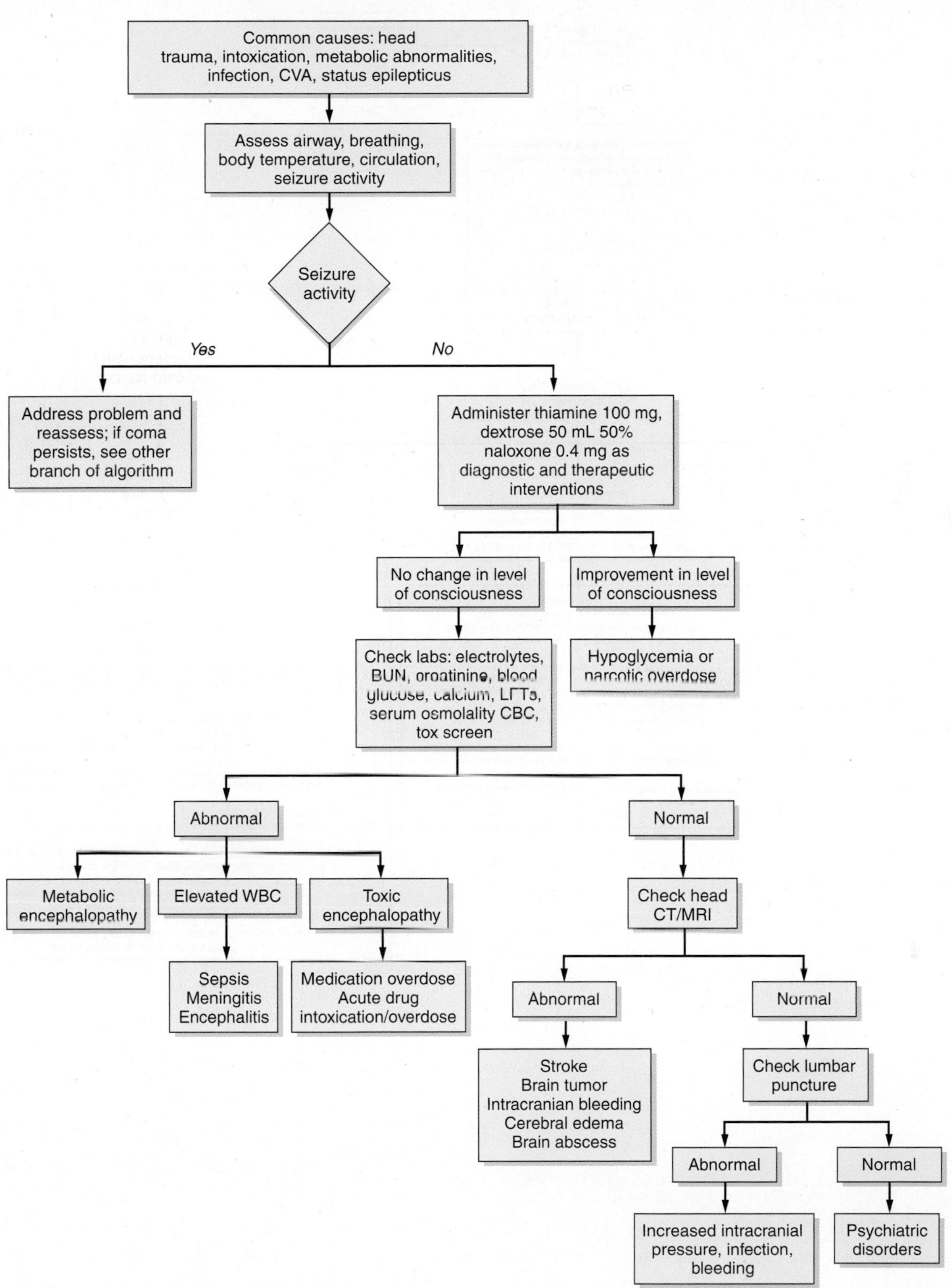

Robert A. Baldor, MD and Alan M. Ehrlich, MD

Neurol Clin. 2008;26(2).

CONCUSSION, SIMPLE EVALUATION AND MANAGEMENT (SPORTS)

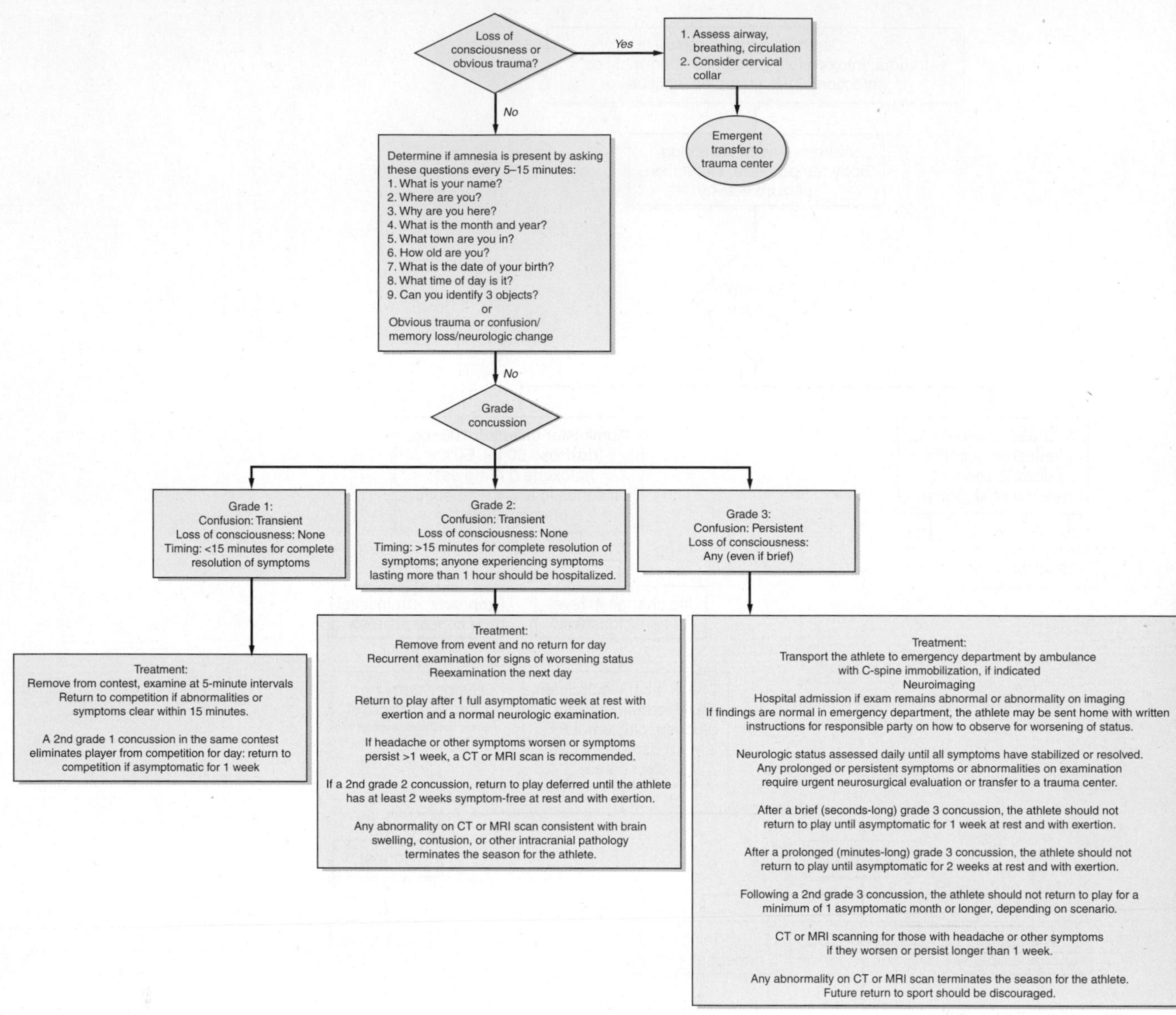

Armin Arasheben, MD and Jason Matuszak, MD

Br J Sports Med. 2005;39:691.

CONGESTIVE HEART FAILURE: DIAGNOSIS AND TREATMENT

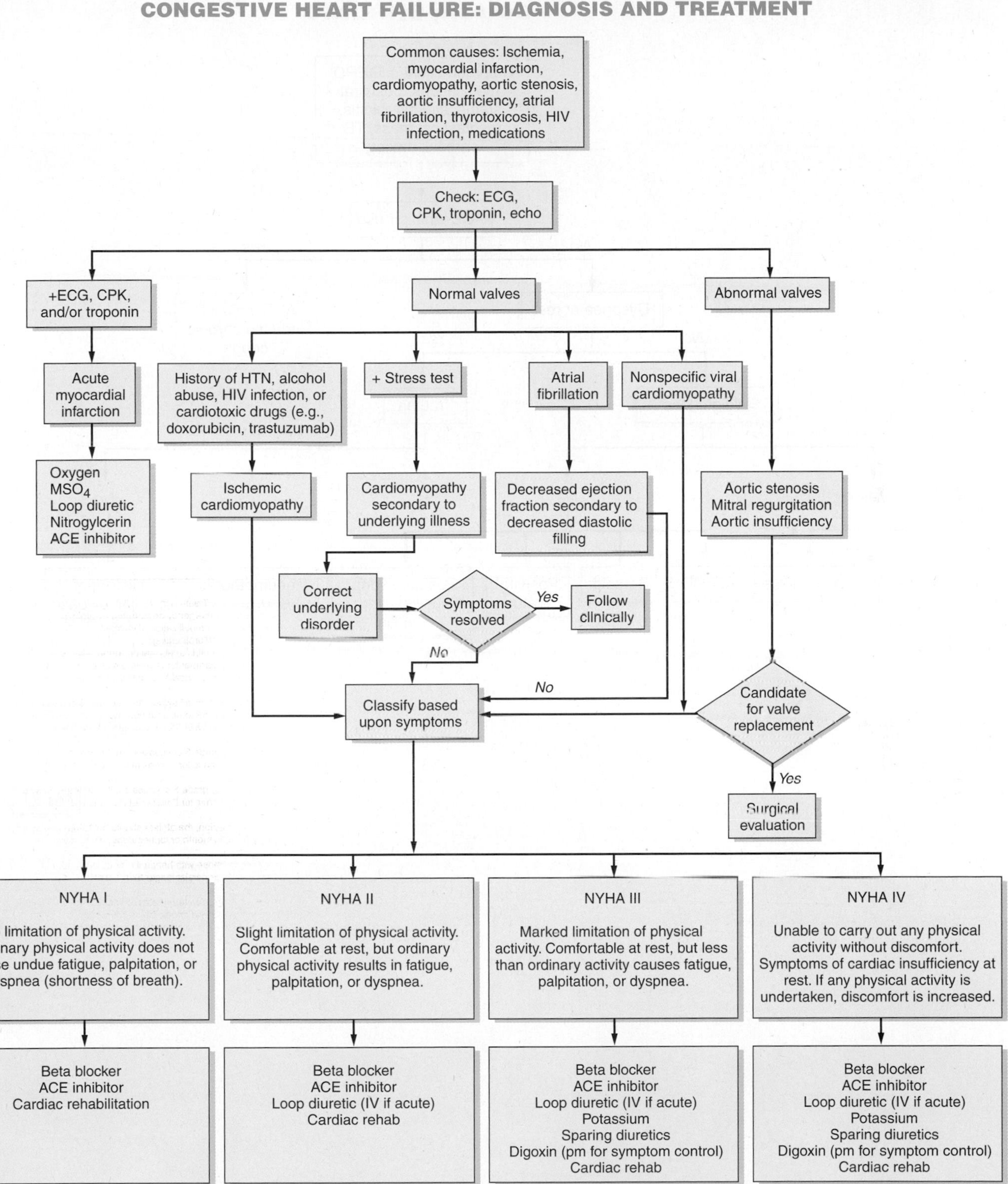

AICD, automated implanted cardiac defribrillator; NYHA, New York Heart Association classification

Robert A. Baldor, MD and Alan M. Ehrlich, MD

Joint ACC/AHA Guideline for Diagnosis and Management of Chronic Heart Failure in the Adult at guidelines.gov.

COUGH, CHRONIC

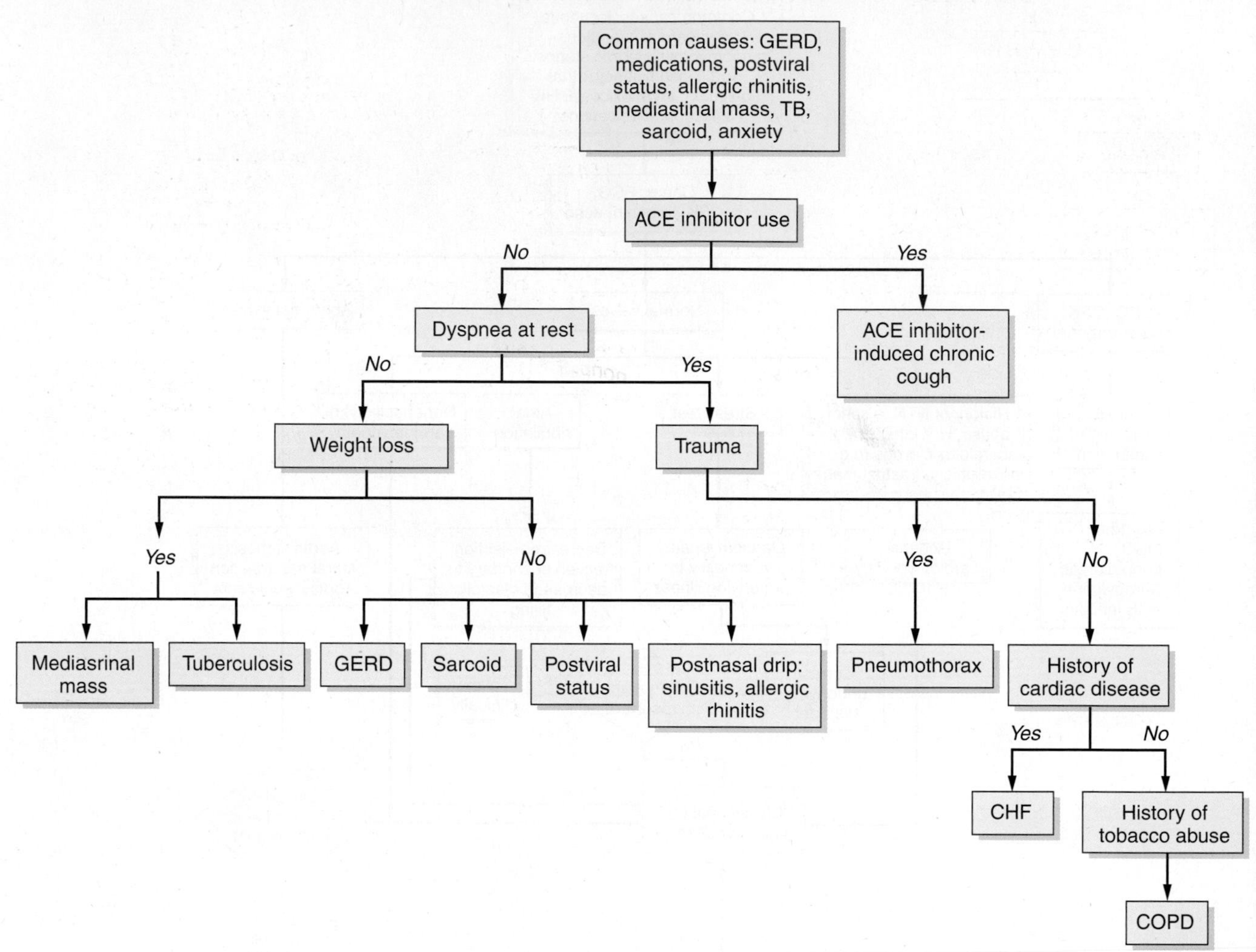

Robert A. Baldor, MD and Alan M. Ehrlich, MD

ACCP Guideline Chronic Cough Chest. 2006;129(1 Suppl):220S–1S.

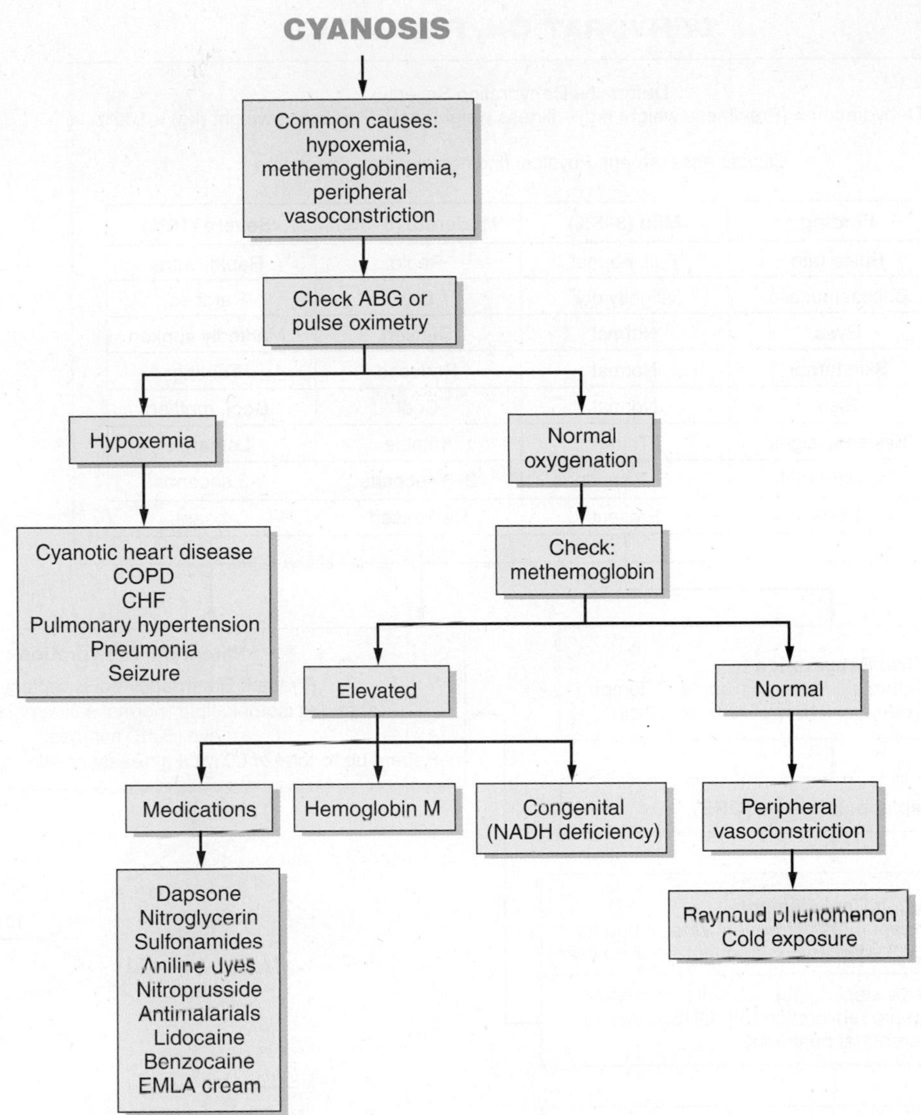

Robert A. Baldor, MD and Alan M. Ehrlich, MD

Am J Roent. 2005;189:241–7.

DEHYDRATION, PEDIATRIC

Determine Dehydration Severity:
% Dehydration = [Pre-illness weight (kg) – illness weight (kg)]/ Pre-illness weight (kg) x 100%
or
Clinical Assessment: Physical findings of volume depletion

Finding	Mild (3–5%)	Moderate (6–9%)	Severe (10%)
Pulse rate	Full, normal	Rapid	Rapid, weak
Buccal mucosa	Slightly dry	Dry	Parched
Eyes	Normal	Sunken	Markedly sunken
Skin turgor	Normal	Reduced	Tenting
Skin	Normal	Cool	Cool, mottled
Systemic signs	↑ Thirst	Irritable	Lethargic
Capillary refill	>1.5–2 seconds	2–3 seconds	>3 seconds
Tears	Present	Decreased	Absent

Oral Rehydration
(contraindications: Intractable vomiting, acute abdomen, severe gastric distention, >10 mL/kg/hr stool loss)

Oral Replace Solutions (ORS)

Deficit Replacement
Mild: 50 mL/kg ORS over 4 hrs in frequent small amounts
Moderate: 100 mL/kg ORS over 4 hrs in frequent small amounts

If continued, excessive stool output or severe, persistent vomiting and inadequate rehydration with ORS, consider parenteral treatment

Maintenance

ORS by age	ORS by weight per hour
Infants: 1 oz/hr	<10 kg: 4 mL/kg ORS
Toddlers: 2 oz/hr	11–20 kg: 40 mL + 2 mL/kg (per kg 11–20)
Older child: 3 oz/hr	>20 kg: 60 mL + 1 mL/kg (per kg >20)

Ongoing Losses

For every loose stool: 10 mL/kg ORS

For every emesis episode: 2 mL/kg ORS

Parenteral Rehydration
Phase I: Emergency bolus replacement
–20 mL/kg isotonic fluid (normal saline or lactated ringer) over 5–10 minutes
–Repeat up to total of 60 mL/kg; reassess etiology if no improvement

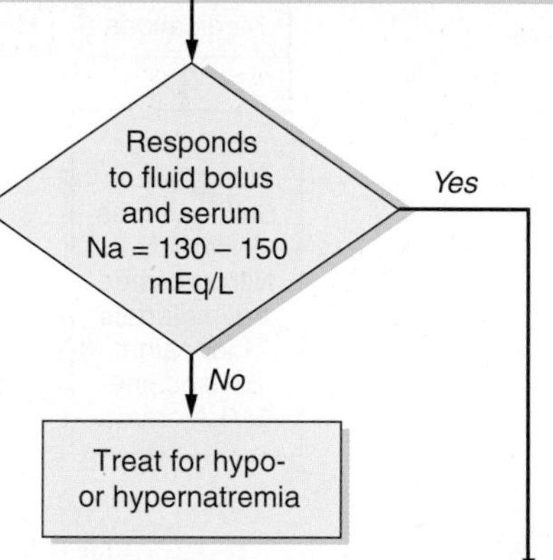

Phase II: Maintenance

a) 100 mL/kg for 1st 10 kg, then
50 mL/kg for next 10 kg, then
25 mL/kg for each kg >20 kg.
b) Give 1st half over 8 hours, 2nd half over next 16 hours.

Stephanie Galica, MD

Am Fam Physician. 2009;80(7):692–6.

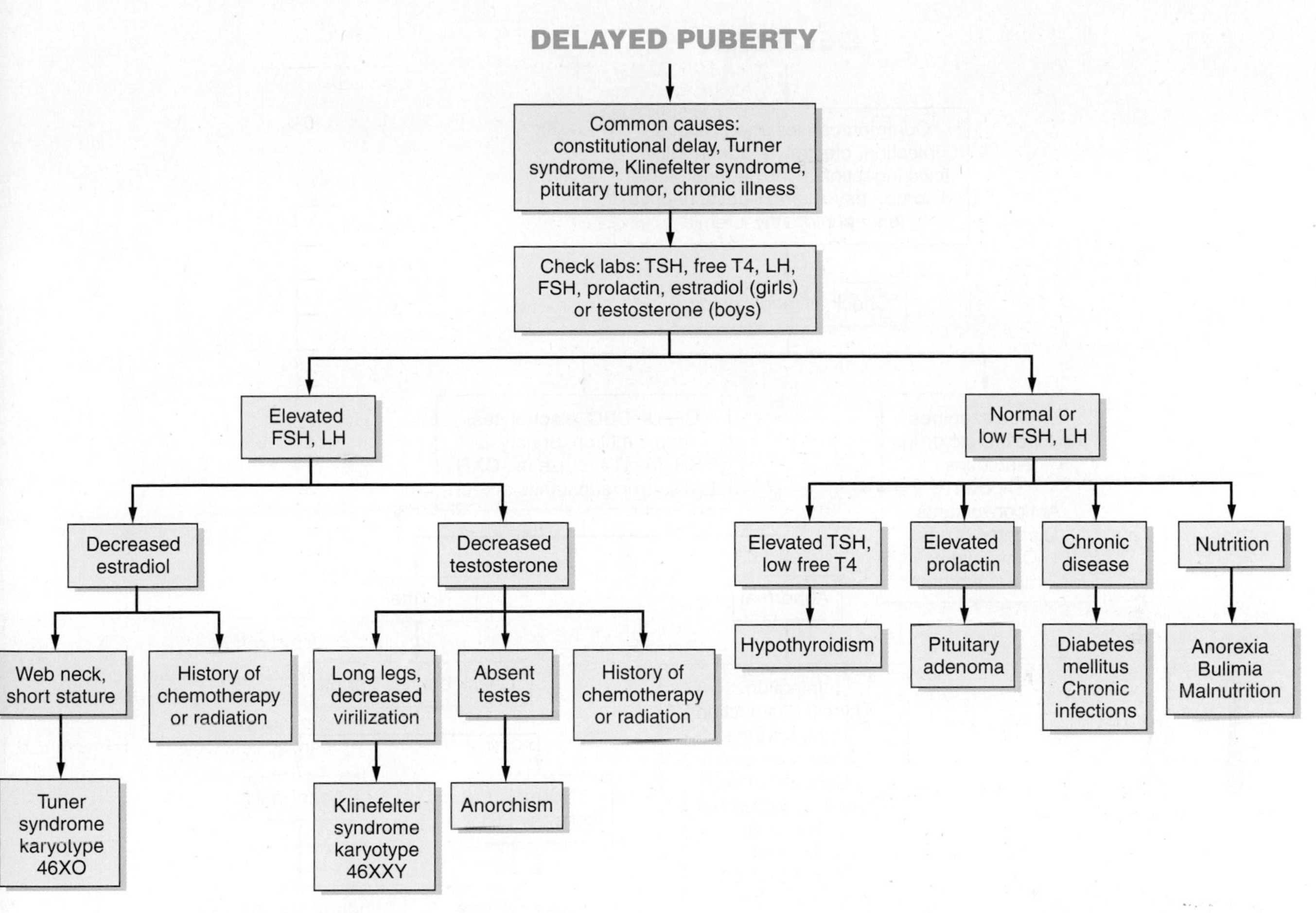
DELAYED PUBERTY
Common causes: constitutional delay, Turner syndrome, Klinefelter syndrome, pituitary tumor, chronic illness
Check labs: TSH, free T4, LH, FSH, prolactin, estradiol (girls) or testosterone (boys)
Elevated FSH, LH
Normal or low FSH, LH
Decreased estradiol
Decreased testosterone
Elevated TSH, low free T4
Elevated prolactin
Chronic disease
Nutrition
Web neck, short stature
History of chemotherapy or radiation
Long legs, decreased virilization
Absent testes
History of chemotherapy or radiation
Hypothyroidism
Pituitary adenoma
Diabetes mellitus Chronic infections
Anorexia Bulimia Malnutrition
Tuner syndrome karyotype 46XO
Klinefelter syndrome karyotype 46XXY
Anorchism

Robert A. Baldor, MD and Alan M. Ehrlich, MD

Am Fam Physician. 1999;60:209–24.

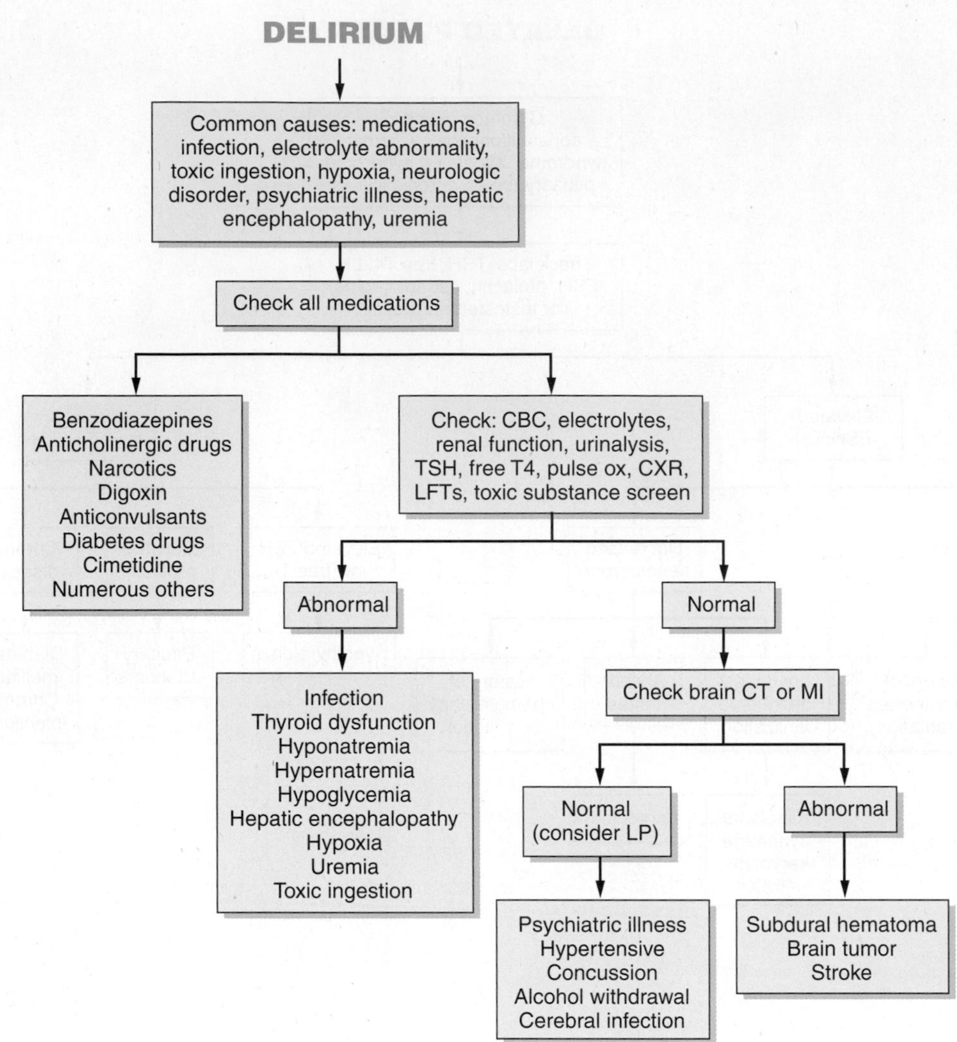
DELIRIUM
Common causes: medications, infection, electrolyte abnormality, toxic ingestion, hypoxia, neurologic disorder, psychiatric illness, hepatic encephalopathy, uremia
Check all medications
Benzodiazepines
Anticholinergic drugs
Narcotics
Digoxin
Anticonvulsants
Diabetes drugs
Cimetidine
Numerous others
Check: CBC, electrolytes, renal function, urinalysis, TSH, free T4, pulse ox, CXR, LFTs, toxic substance screen
Abnormal
Infection
Thyroid dysfunction
Hyponatremia
Hypernatremia
Hypoglycemia
Hepatic encephalopathy
Hypoxia
Uremia
Toxic ingestion
Normal
Check brain CT or MI
Normal (consider LP)
Psychiatric illness
Hypertensive
Concussion
Alcohol withdrawal
Cerebral infection
Abnormal
Subdural hematoma
Brain tumor
Stroke

Robert A. Baldor, MD and Alan M. Ehrlich, MD

Am Fam Physician. 2003;67:1027–34.

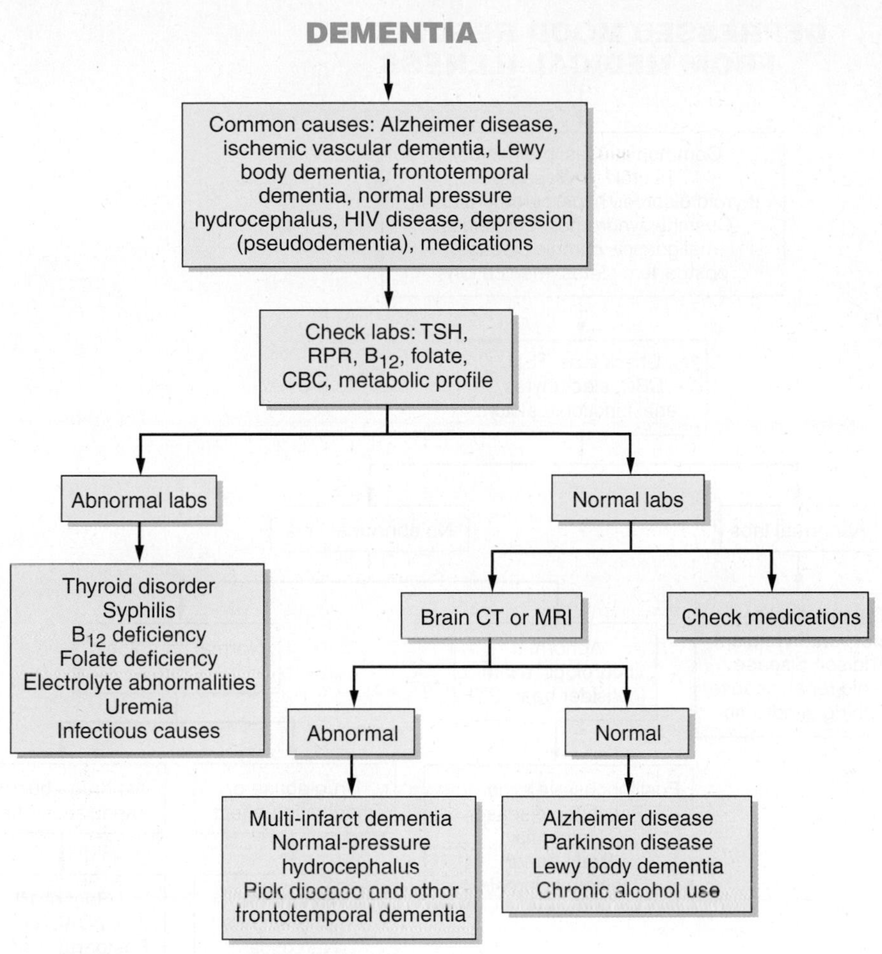

Robert A. Baldor, MD and Alan M. Ehrlich, MD

Neurology. 2001;56(9):1143–53.

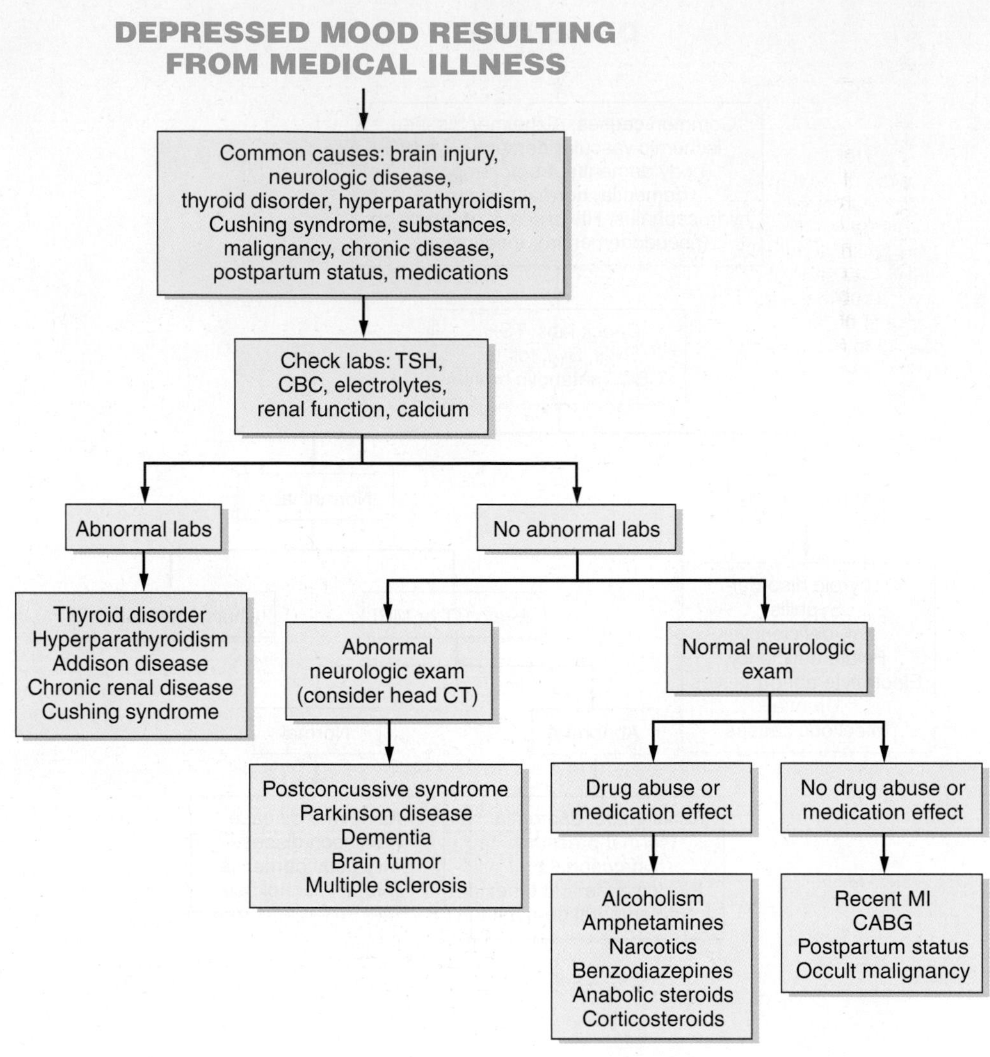
DEPRESSED MOOD RESULTING FROM MEDICAL ILLNESS
Common causes: brain injury, neurologic disease, thyroid disorder, hyperparathyroidism, Cushing syndrome, substances, malignancy, chronic disease, postpartum status, medications
Check labs: TSH, CBC, electrolytes, renal function, calcium
Abnormal labs
No abnormal labs
Thyroid disorder
Hyperparathyroidism
Addison disease
Chronic renal disease
Cushing syndrome
Abnormal neurologic exam (consider head CT)
Normal neurologic exam
Postconcussive syndrome
Parkinson disease
Dementia
Brain tumor
Multiple sclerosis
Drug abuse or medication effect
No drug abuse or medication effect
Alcoholism
Amphetamines
Narcotics
Benzodiazepines
Anabolic steroids
Corticosteroids
Recent MI
CABG
Postpartum status
Occult malignancy

Robert A. Baldor, MD and Alan M. Ehrlich, MD

Phys Sportsmed. 2009;37(2):141–5.

DEPRESSIVE EPISODE, MAJOR

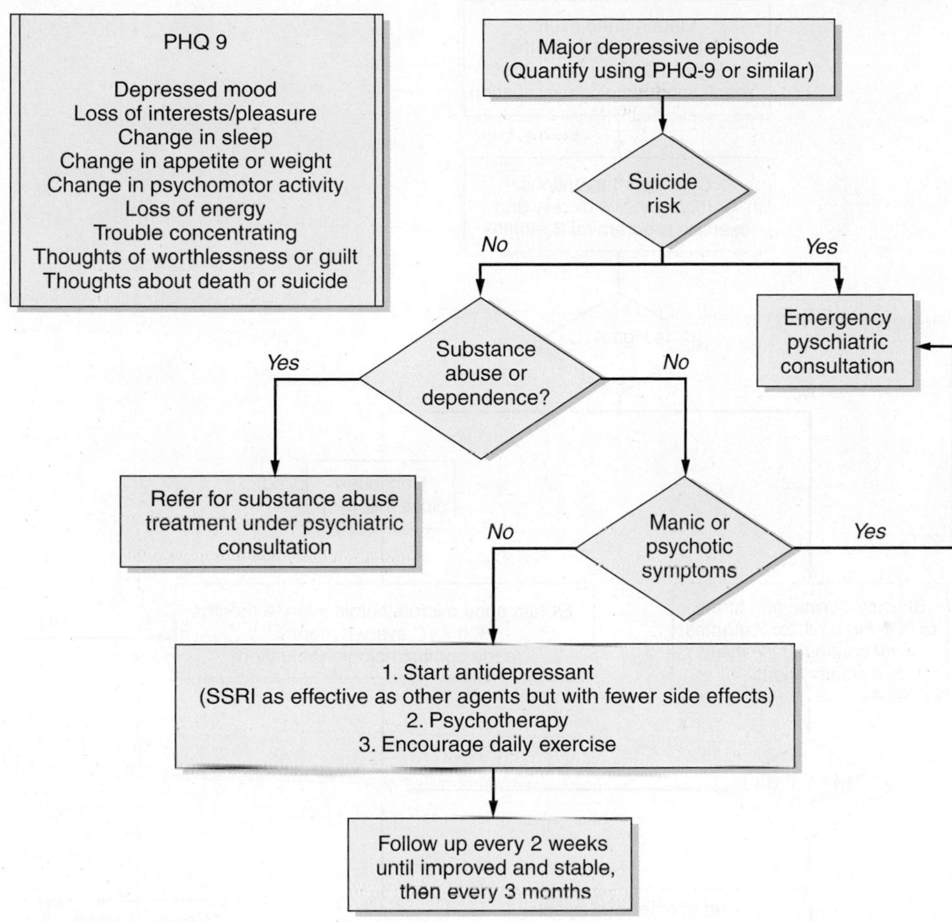

James F. Cunagin, MD

Depression. University of Michigan Health System; 2005 Oct. 20 at National Guidelines Clearinghouse.

DIABETES MELLITUS, TYPE 2

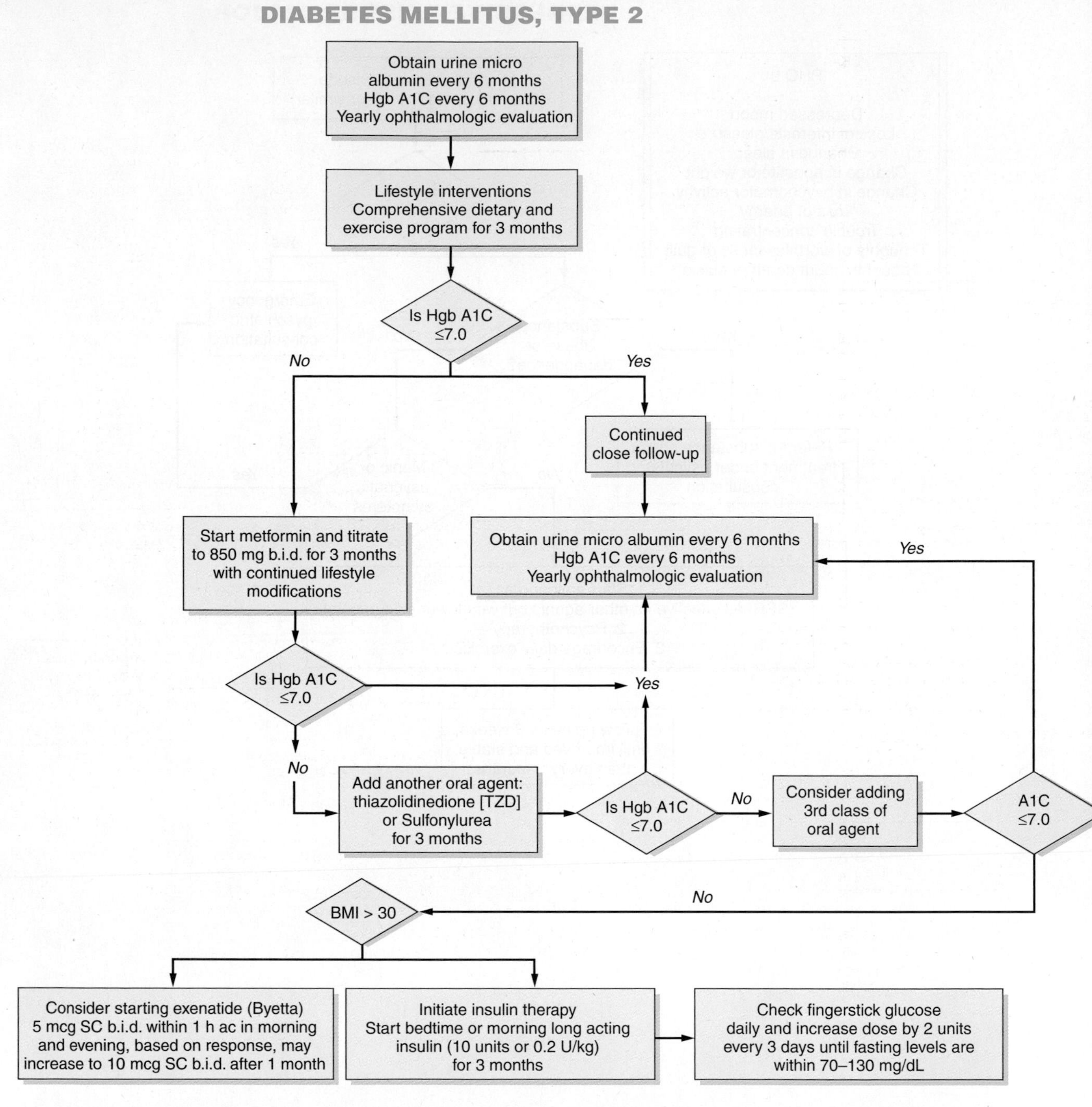
Obtain urine micro albumin every 6 months
Hgb A1C every 6 months
Yearly ophthalmologic evaluation
Lifestyle interventions
Comprehensive dietary and exercise program for 3 months
Is Hgb A1C ≤7.0
No
Yes
Continued close follow-up
Start metformin and titrate to 850 mg b.i.d. for 3 months with continued lifestyle modifications
Obtain urine micro albumin every 6 months
Hgb A1C every 6 months
Yearly ophthalmologic evaluation
Yes
Is Hgb A1C ≤7.0
Yes
No
Add another oral agent: thiazolidinedione [TZD] or Sulfonylurea for 3 months
Is Hgb A1C ≤7.0
No
Consider adding 3rd class of oral agent
A1C ≤7.0
No
BMI > 30
Consider starting exenatide (Byetta) 5 mcg SC b.i.d. within 1 h ac in morning and evening, based on response, may increase to 10 mcg SC b.i.d. after 1 month
Initiate insulin therapy
Start bedtime or morning long acting insulin (10 units or 0.2 U/kg) for 3 months
Check fingerstick glucose daily and increase dose by 2 units every 3 days until fasting levels are within 70–130 mg/dL

Frank J. Domino, MD

Am Fam Physician. 2003;67(5).

DIABETIC KETOACIDOSIS (DKA), TREATMENT

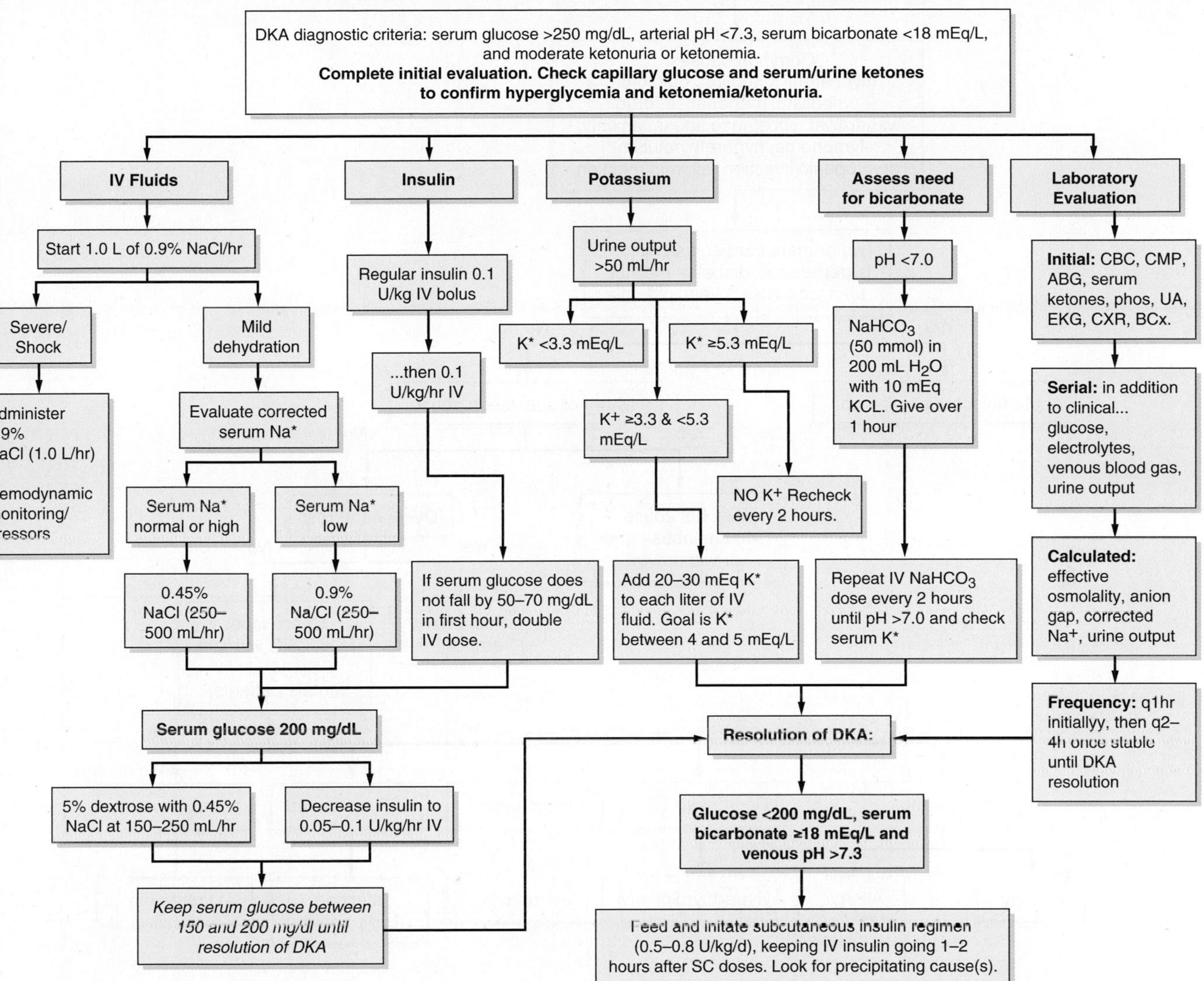

Kitabchi AE, Wall BM. Management of diabetic ketoacidosis. *Am Fam Physician*. 1999;60(2):455–64.
Kitabchi AE, Umpierrez GE, Miles JM, Fisher JN. Hyperglycemic crises in adult patients with diabetes. *Diabetes Care*. 2009;32(7):1335–43.
Trachetenbarg DE. Diabetic ketoacidosis. *Am Fam Physician*. 2005;71(9):1705–14.

John B. Waits, MD

LMAJ. 2003;168(7):859–6.

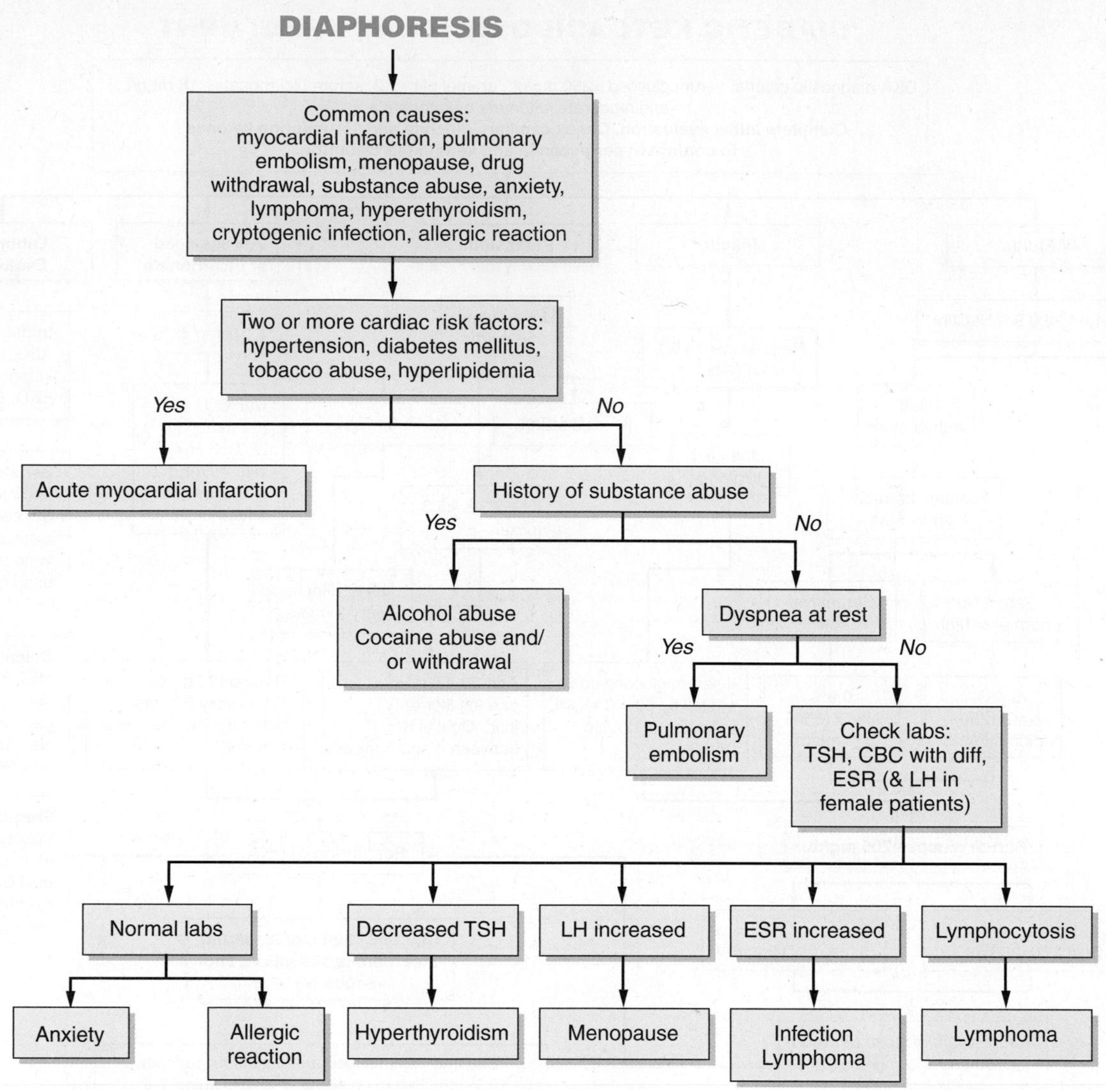

Robert A. Baldor, MD and Alan M. Ehrlich, MD

Depression University of Michigan Health System; 2005 Oct. 20 at National Guidelines Clearinghouse.

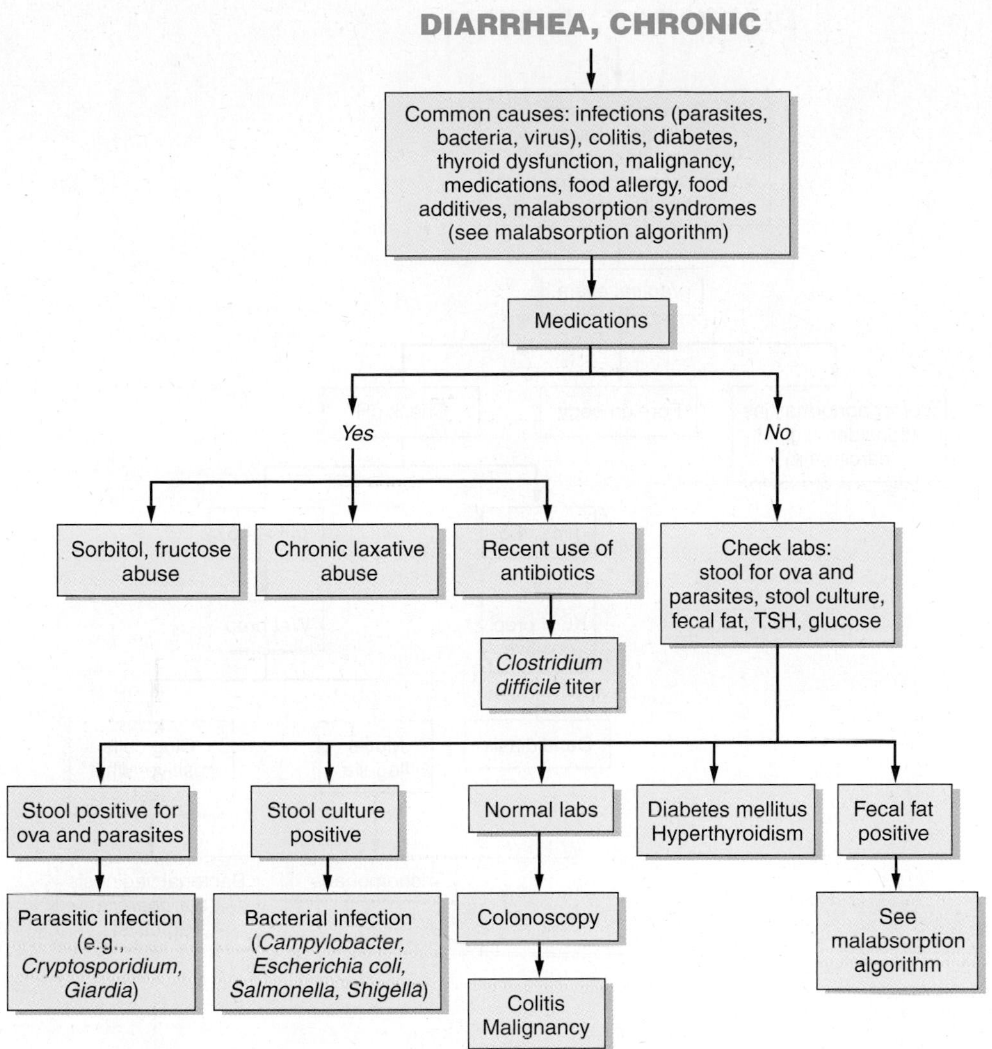

Robert A. Baldor, MD and Alan M. Ehrlich, MD

Institute for Clinical Systems Improvement (ICSI); 2009 May. 114 p. at National Guidelines Clearinghouse.

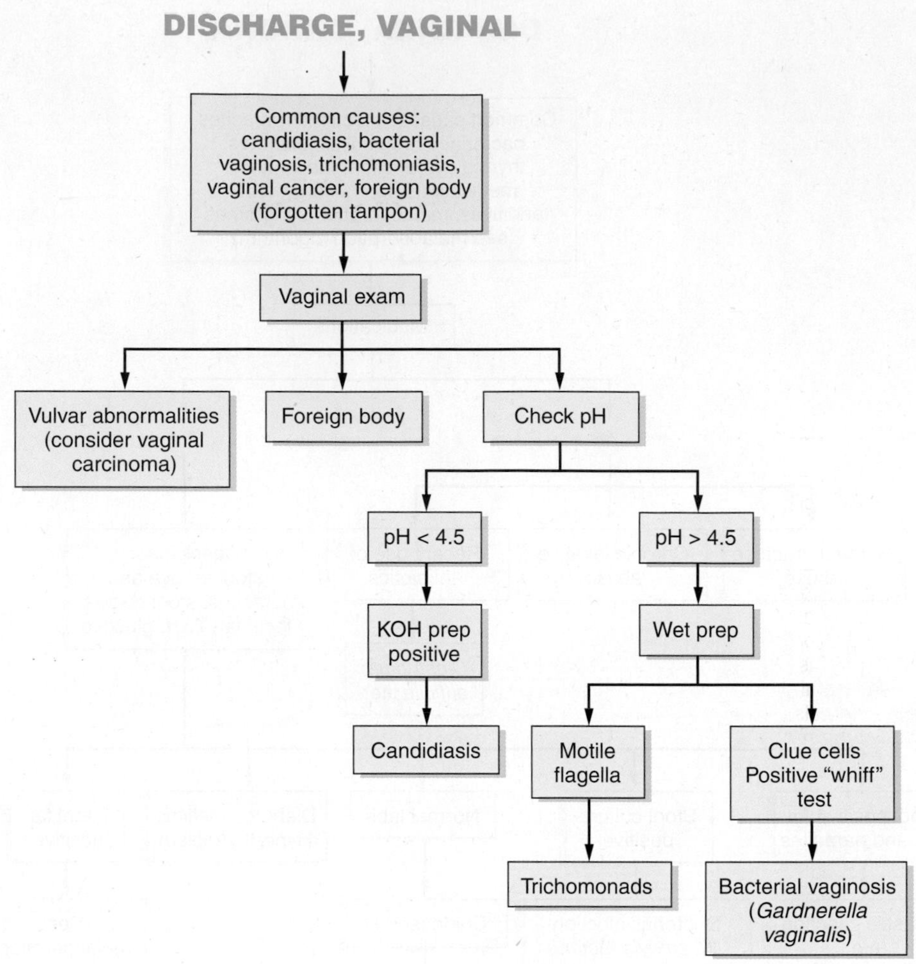

Robert A. Baldor, MD and Alan M. Ehrlich, MD

Primary Care Clin Office Pract. 2009;36(1).

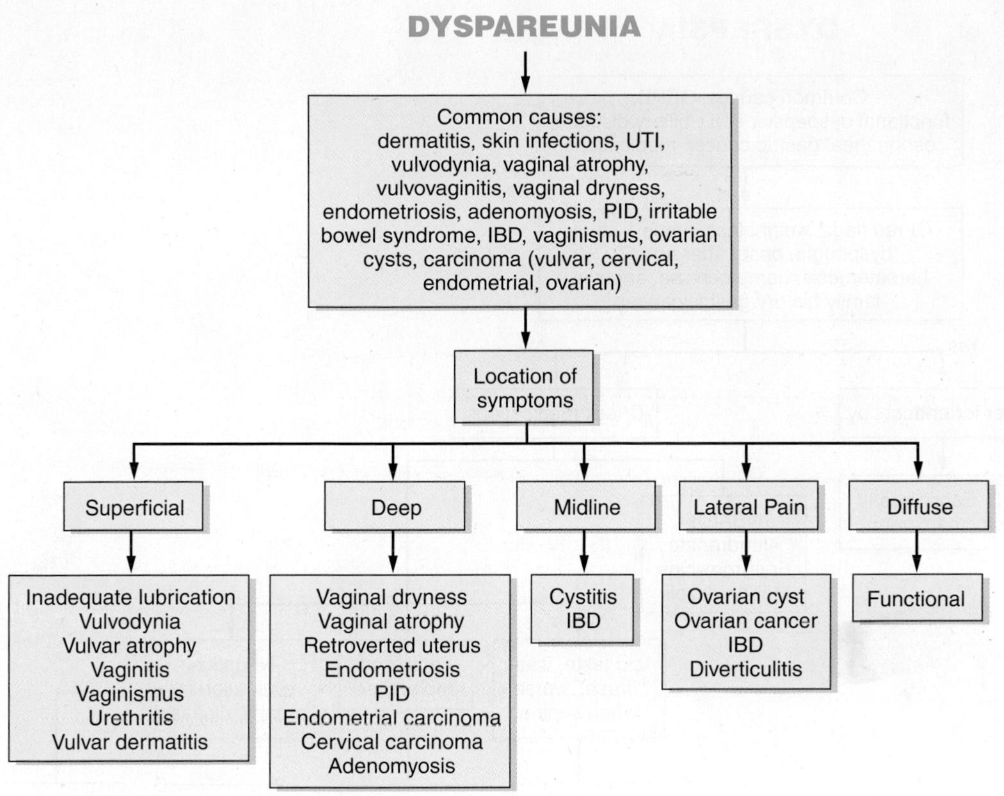
DYSPAREUNIA
Common causes: dermatitis, skin infections, UTI, vulvodynia, vaginal atrophy, vulvovaginitis, vaginal dryness, endometriosis, adenomyosis, PID, irritable bowel syndrome, IBD, vaginismus, ovarian cysts, carcinoma (vulvar, cervical, endometrial, ovarian)
Location of symptoms
Superficial
Deep
Midline
Lateral Pain
Diffuse
Inadequate lubrication
Vulvodynia
Vulvar atrophy
Vaginitis
Vaginismus
Urethritis
Vulvar dermatitis
Vaginal dryness
Vaginal atrophy
Retroverted uterus
Endometriosis
PID
Endometrial carcinoma
Cervical carcinoma
Adenomyosis
Cystitis
IBD
Ovarian cyst
Ovarian cancer
IBD
Diverticulitis
Functional

Robert A. Baldor, MD and Alan M. Ehrlich, MD

Obstet Gynecol Clin. 2006;33(4).

DYSPEPSIA

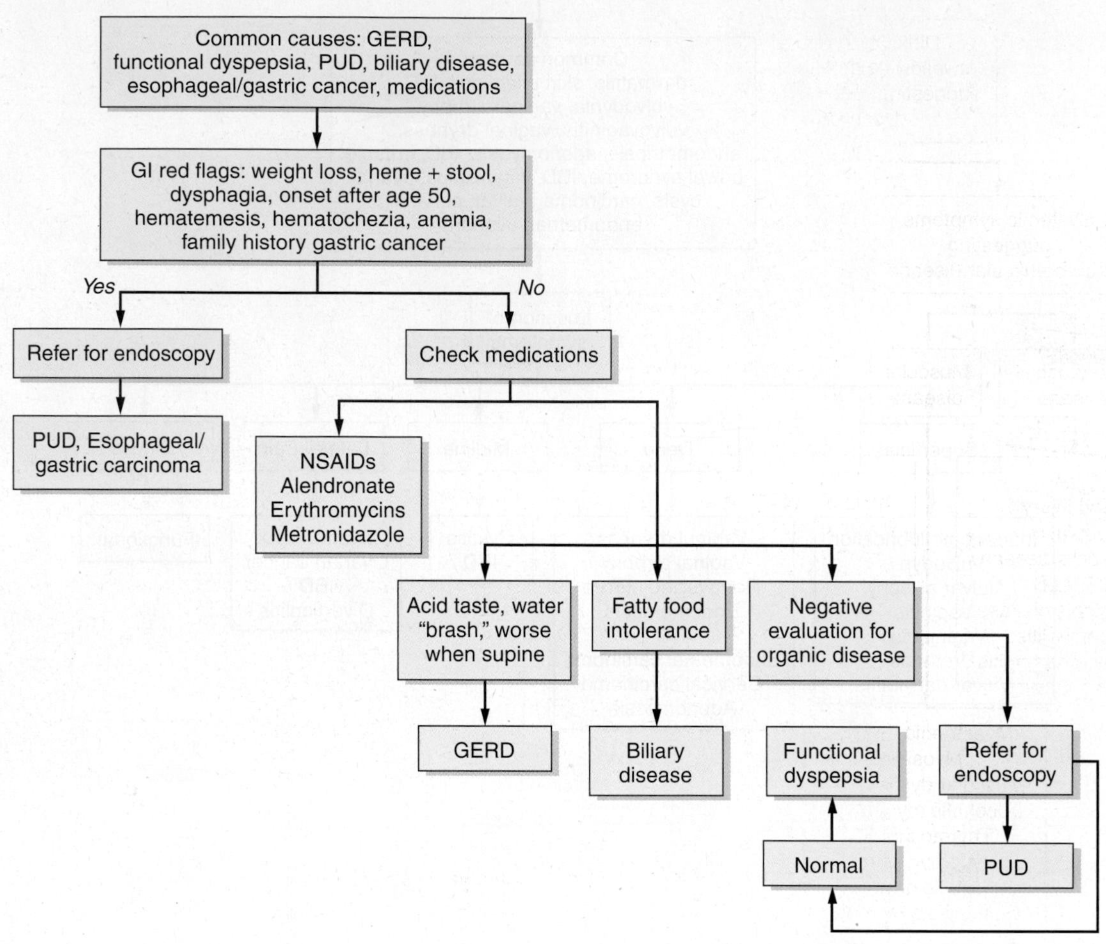

Robert A. Baldor, MD and Alan M. Ehrlich, MD

J Fam Pract. 2009;58(7 Suppl Short):S1–1.

DYSPHAGIA

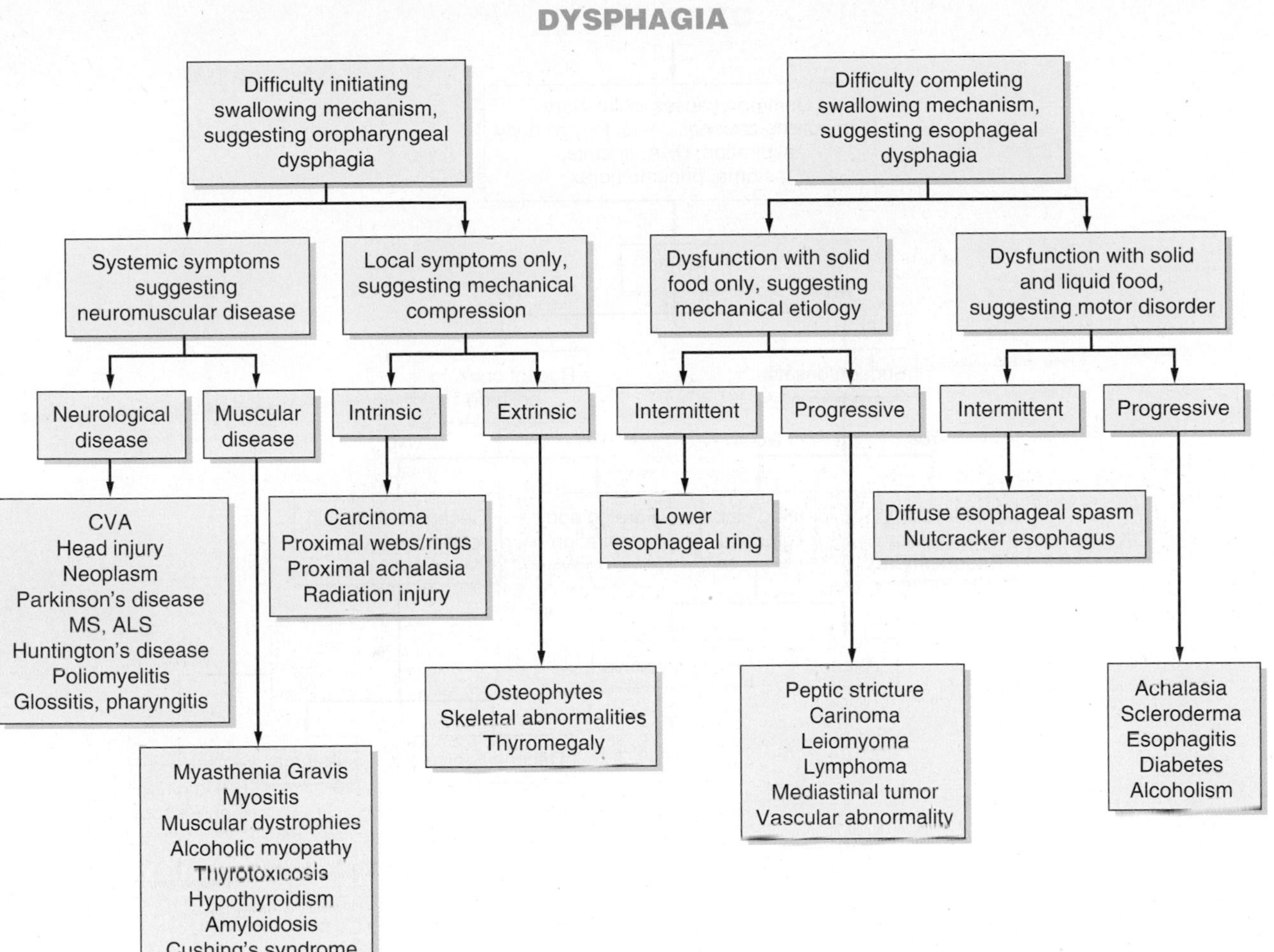

Parag Goyal, MD

Gastroenterol Clin North Am. 2003;32(2):553–75.

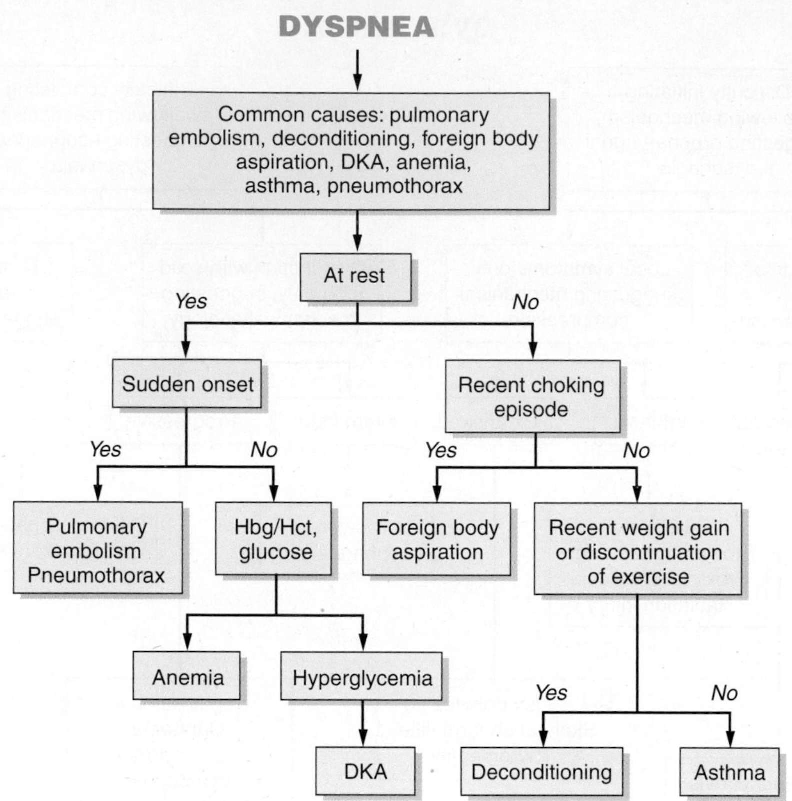

Robert A. Baldor, MD and Alan M. Ehrlich, MD

Diagnostic evaluation of dyspnea. *Am Fam Physician.* Feb 15, 1998.

DYSURIA

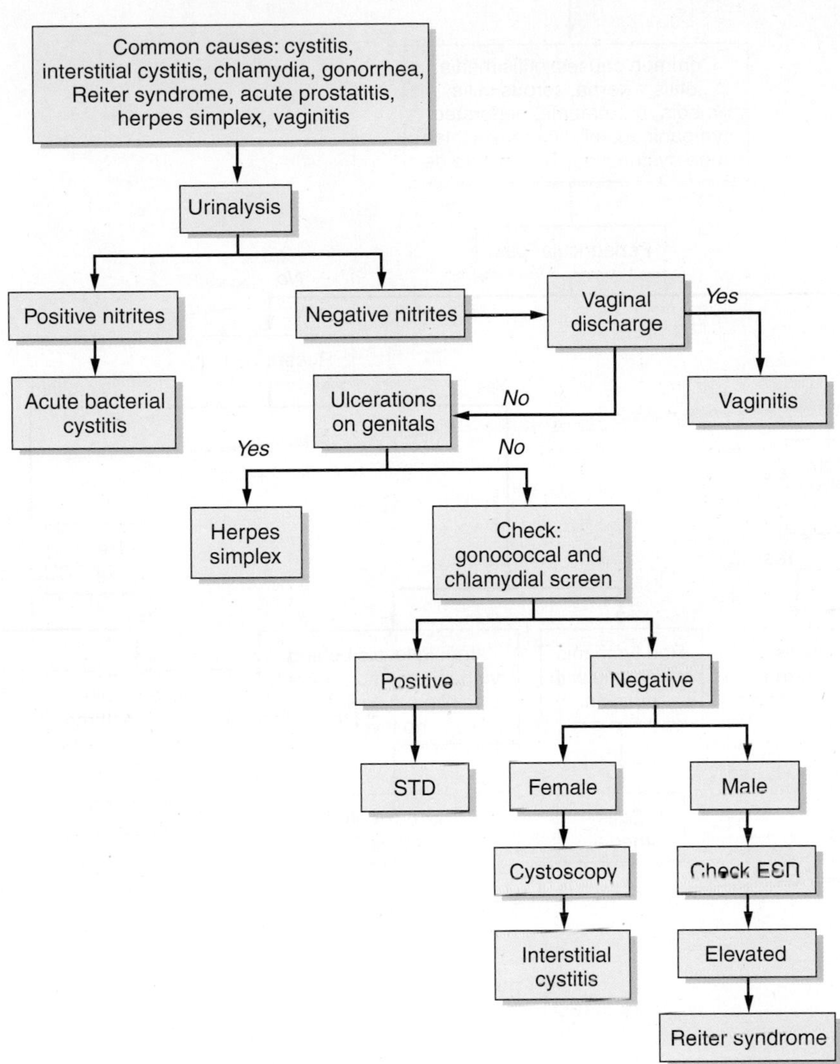

Robert A. Baldor, MD and Alan M. Ehrlich, MD

Am Fam Physician. 2002;65:1589–97.

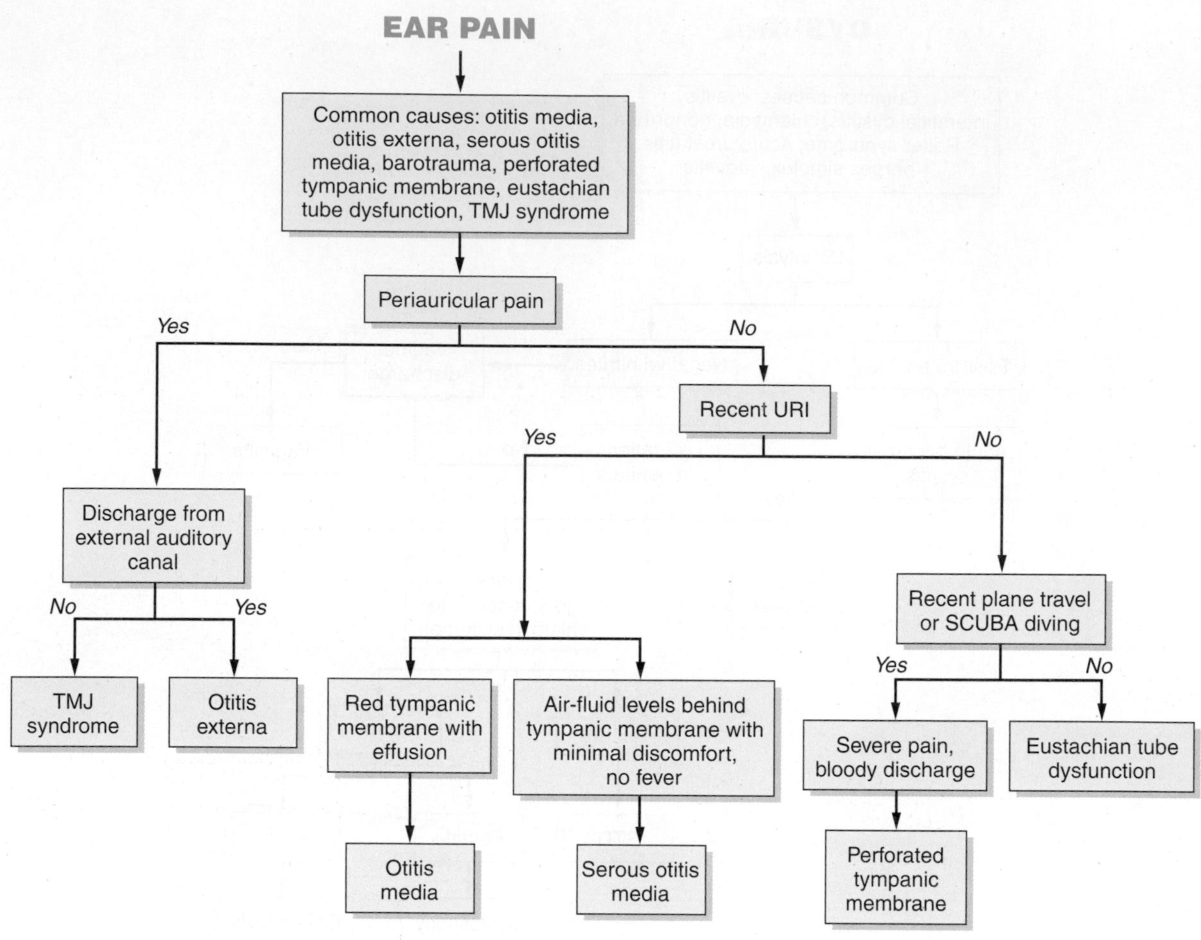

Robert A. Baldor, MD and Alan M. Ehrlich, MD

Am Fam Physician. 2008;77(5).

ECCHYMOSIS

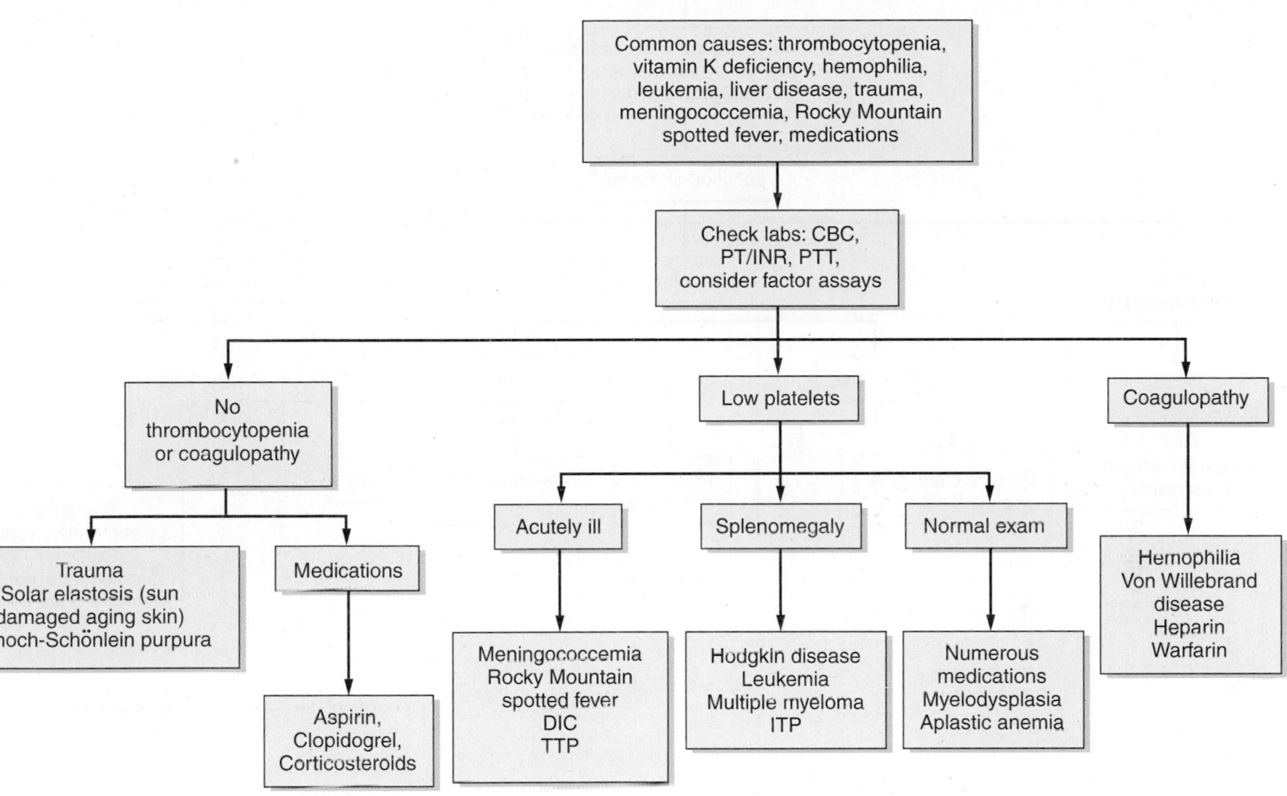

Robert A. Baldor, MD and Alan M. Ehrlich, MD

Arch Dermatol. 2010;146(1):94–5.

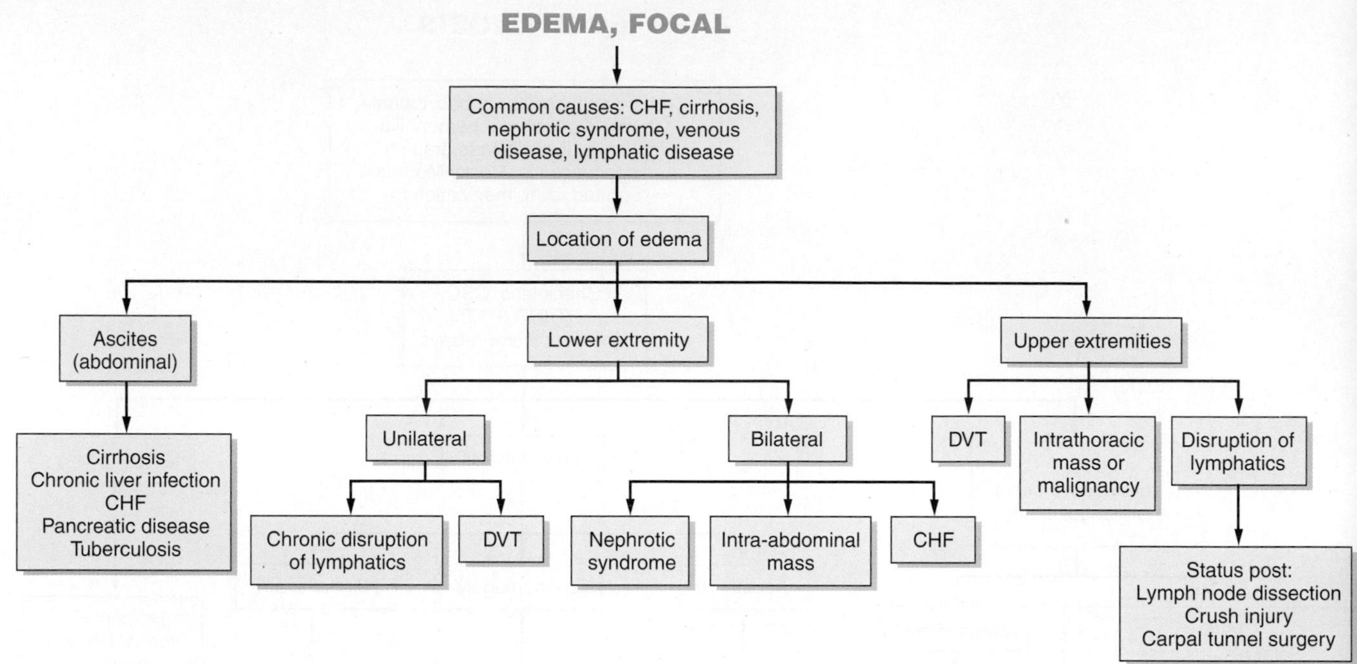

Robert A. Baldor, MD and Alan M. Ehrlich, MD

Am J Med. 2002;113(7):580–6.

ENURESIS

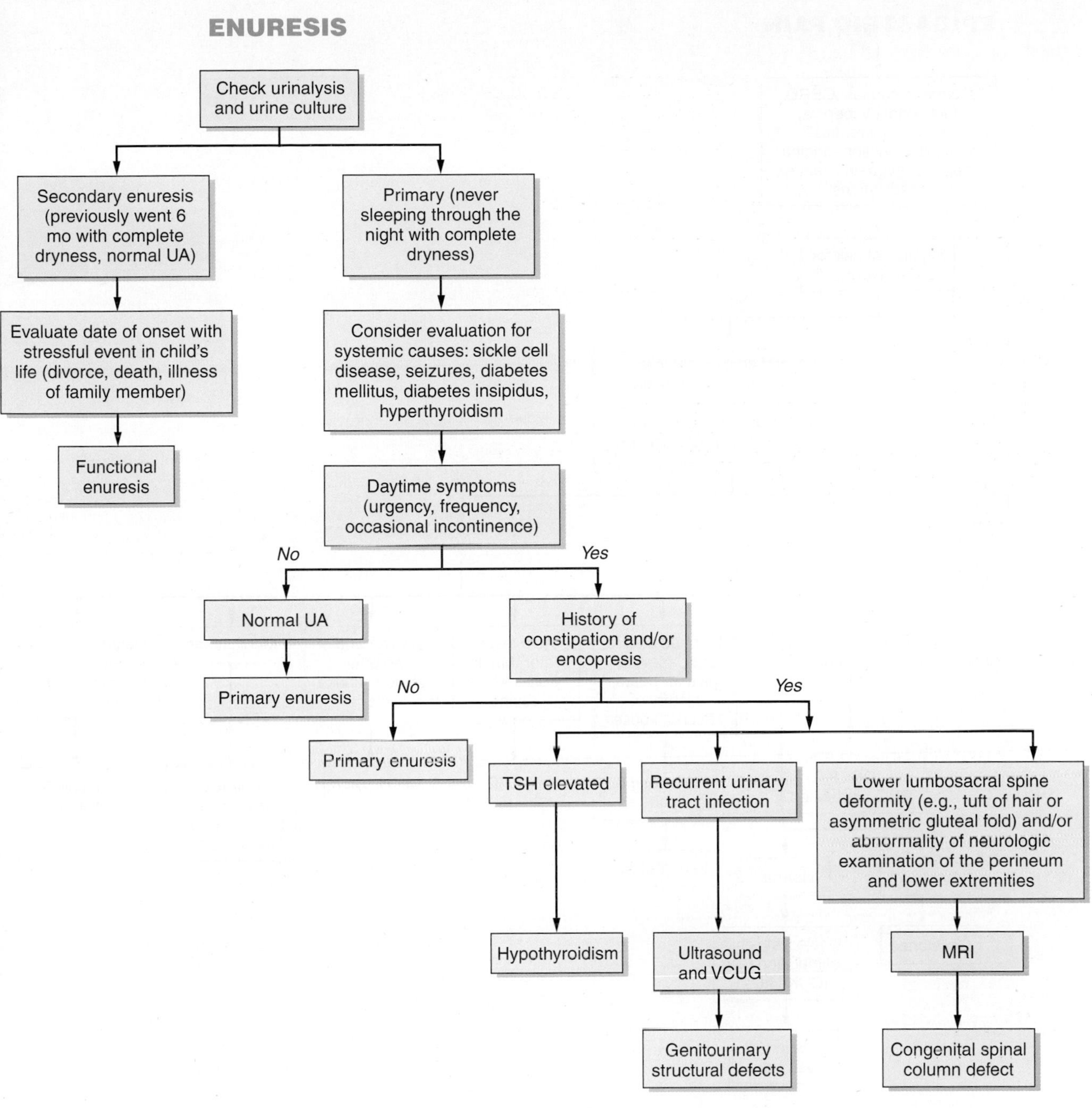

Robert A. Baldor, MD and Alan M. Ehrlich, MD

J Am Acad Child Adolesc Psychiatry. 2004;43(1).

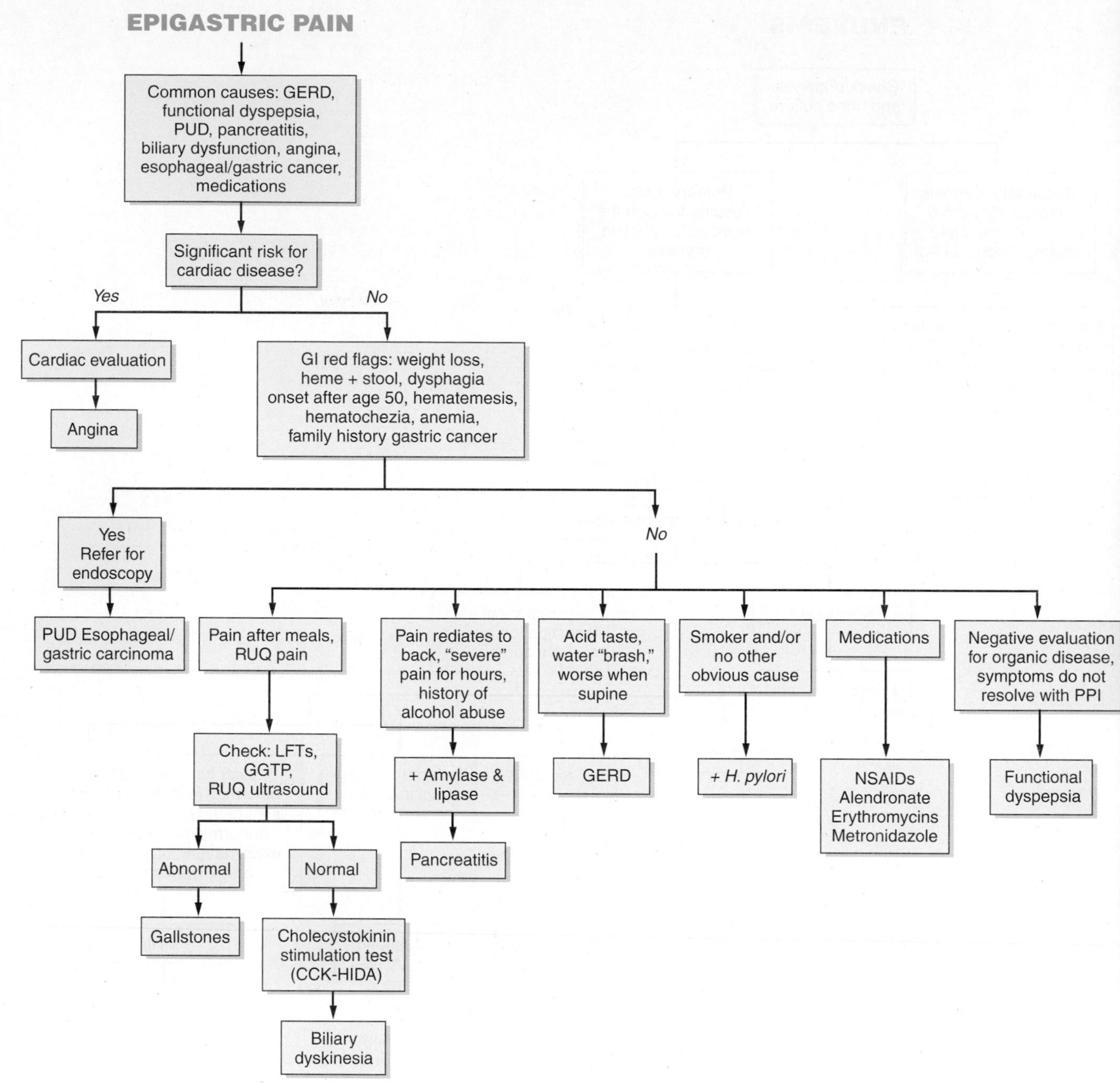

Robert A. Baldor, MD and Alan M. Ehrlich, MD

Curr Gastroenterol Rep. 2009;11(4):288–94.

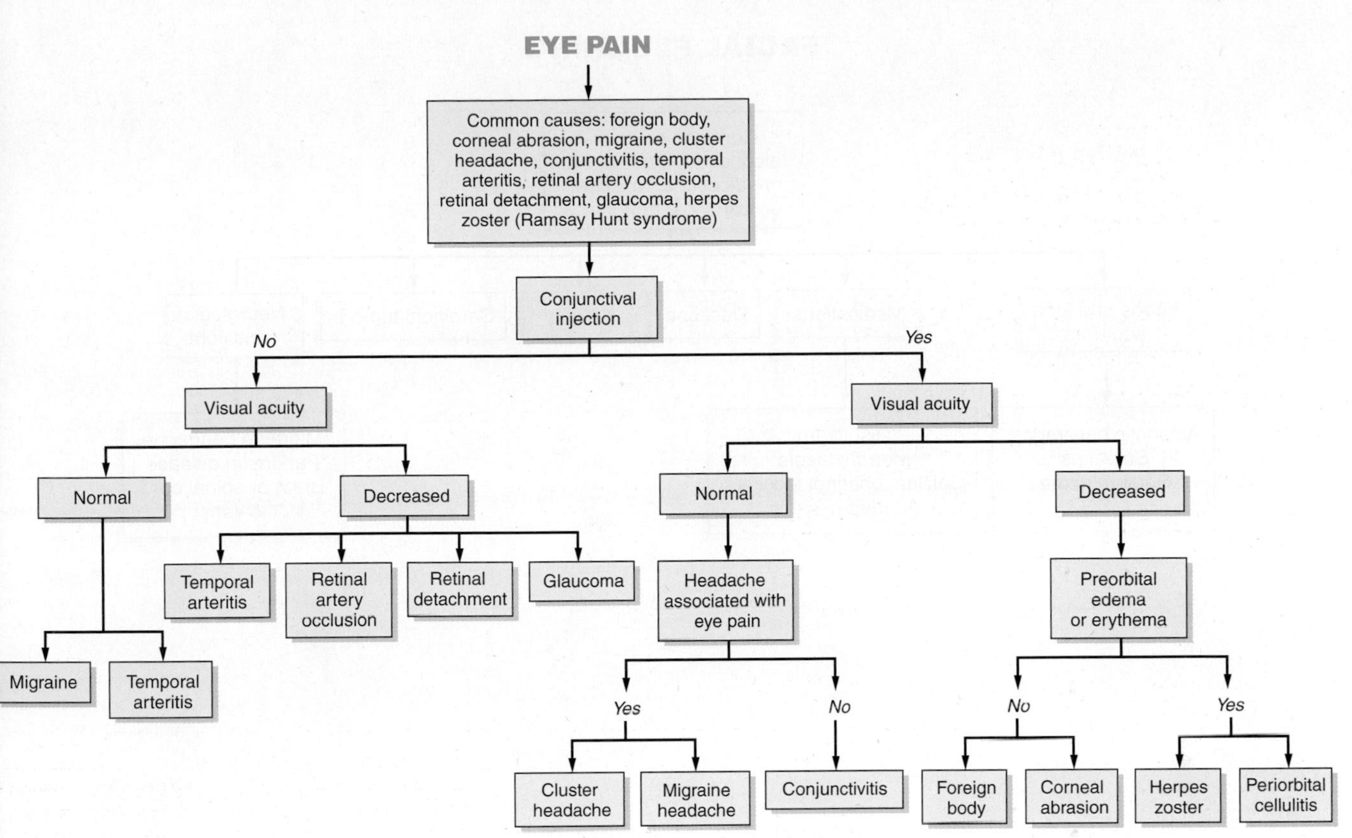

Robert A. Baldor, MD and Alan M. Ehrlich, MD

Curr Pain Headache Rep. 2008;12(4):296–304.

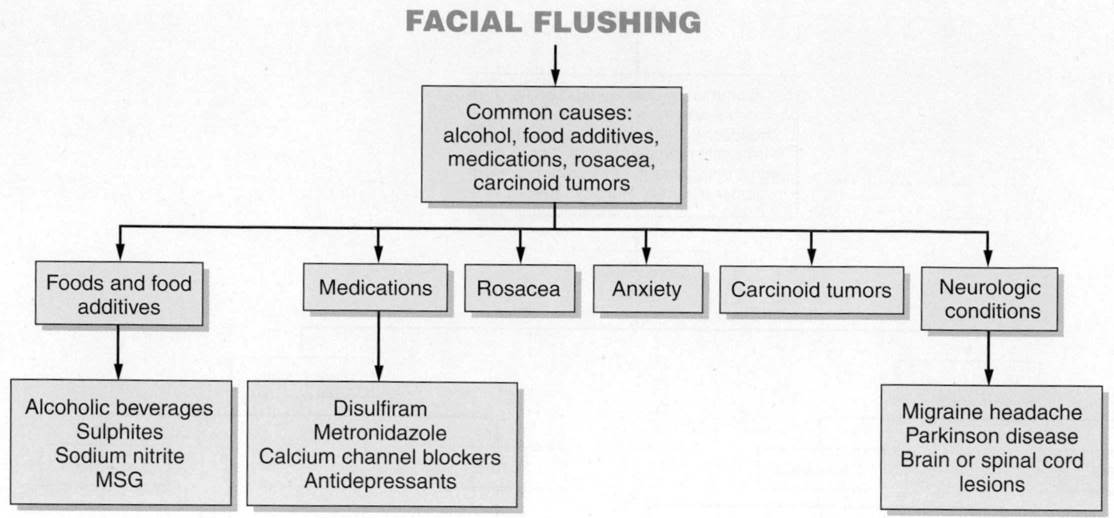

Robert A. Baldor, MD and Alan M. Ehrlich, MD

PLoS Med. 2009;6(3):e50.

FACIAL PARALYSIS

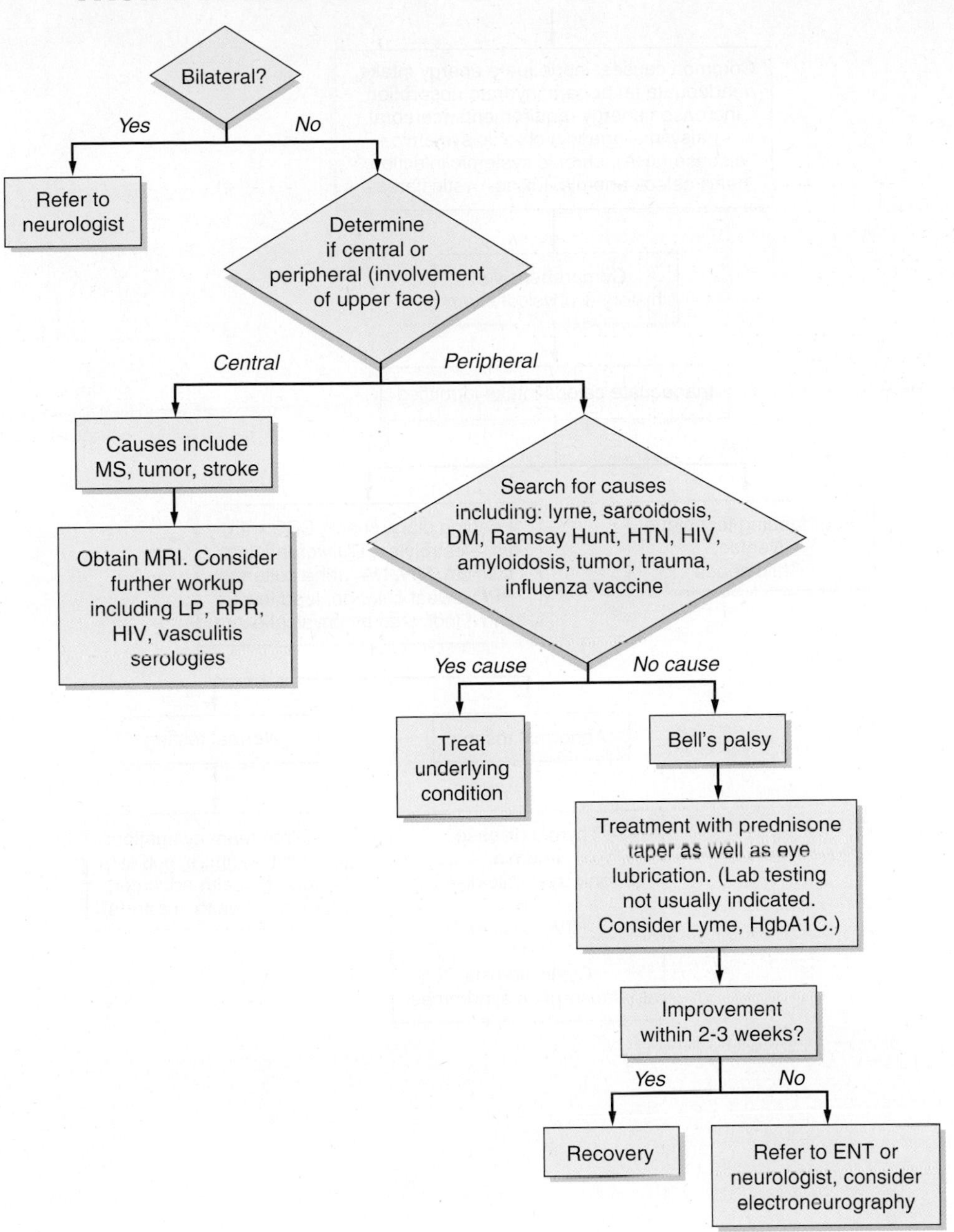

Laura Hagopian, MD and William A. Tosches, MD

Rev Med Intern. 2009;30(9):769–75.

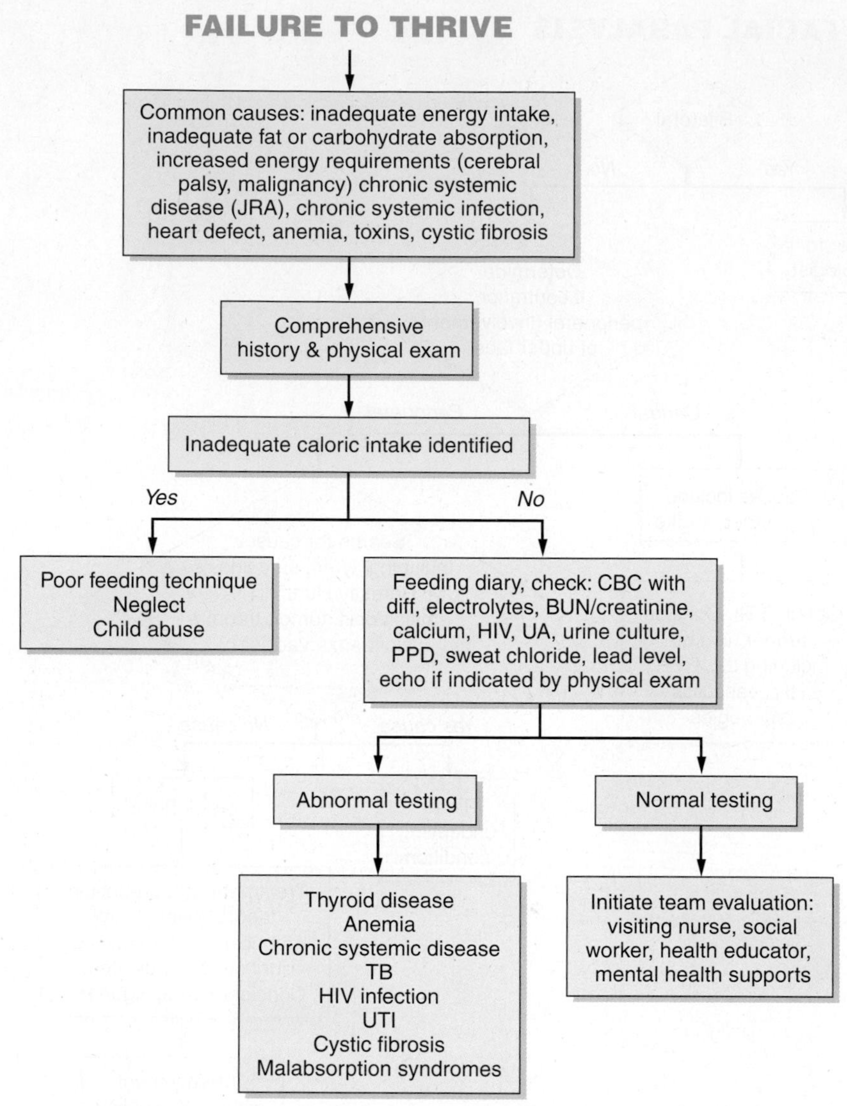
FAILURE TO THRIVE
Common causes: inadequate energy intake, inadequate fat or carbohydrate absorption, increased energy requirements (cerebral palsy, malignancy) chronic systemic disease (JRA), chronic systemic infection, heart defect, anemia, toxins, cystic fibrosis
Comprehensive history & physical exam
Inadequate caloric intake identified
Yes
No
Poor feeding technique
Neglect
Child abuse
Feeding diary, check: CBC with diff, electrolytes, BUN/creatinine, calcium, HIV, UA, urine culture, PPD, sweat chloride, lead level, echo if indicated by physical exam
Abnormal testing
Normal testing
Thyroid disease
Anemia
Chronic systemic disease
TB
HIV infection
UTI
Cystic fibrosis
Malabsorption syndromes
Initiate team evaluation: visiting nurse, social worker, health educator, mental health supports

Robert A. Baldor, MD and Alan M. Ehrlich, MD

Eur J Pediatr. 2009;168(7):839–45. Epub 2008 Oct 16.

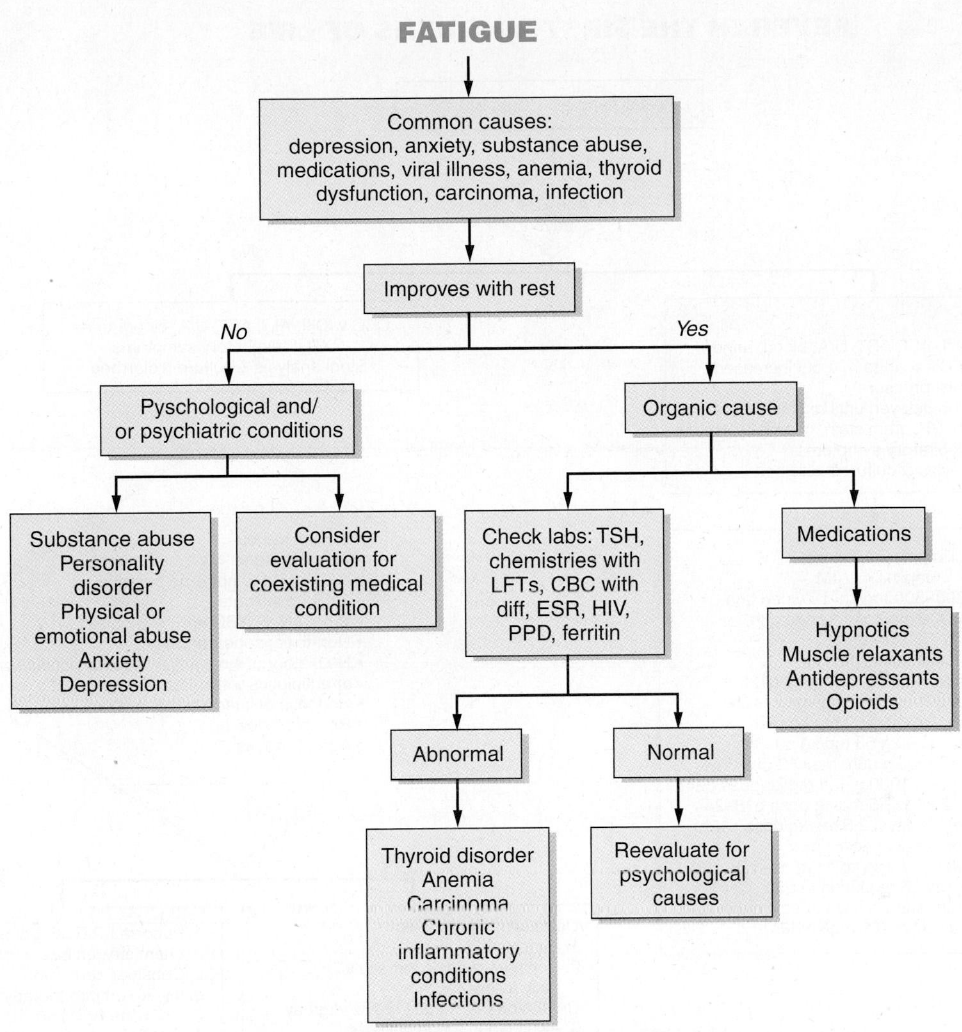

Robert A. Baldor, MD and Alan M. Ehrlich, MD

CMAJ. 2009;181(10):683–7. Epub 2009 Oct 26.

FEVER IN THE FIRST 3 MONTHS OF LIFE

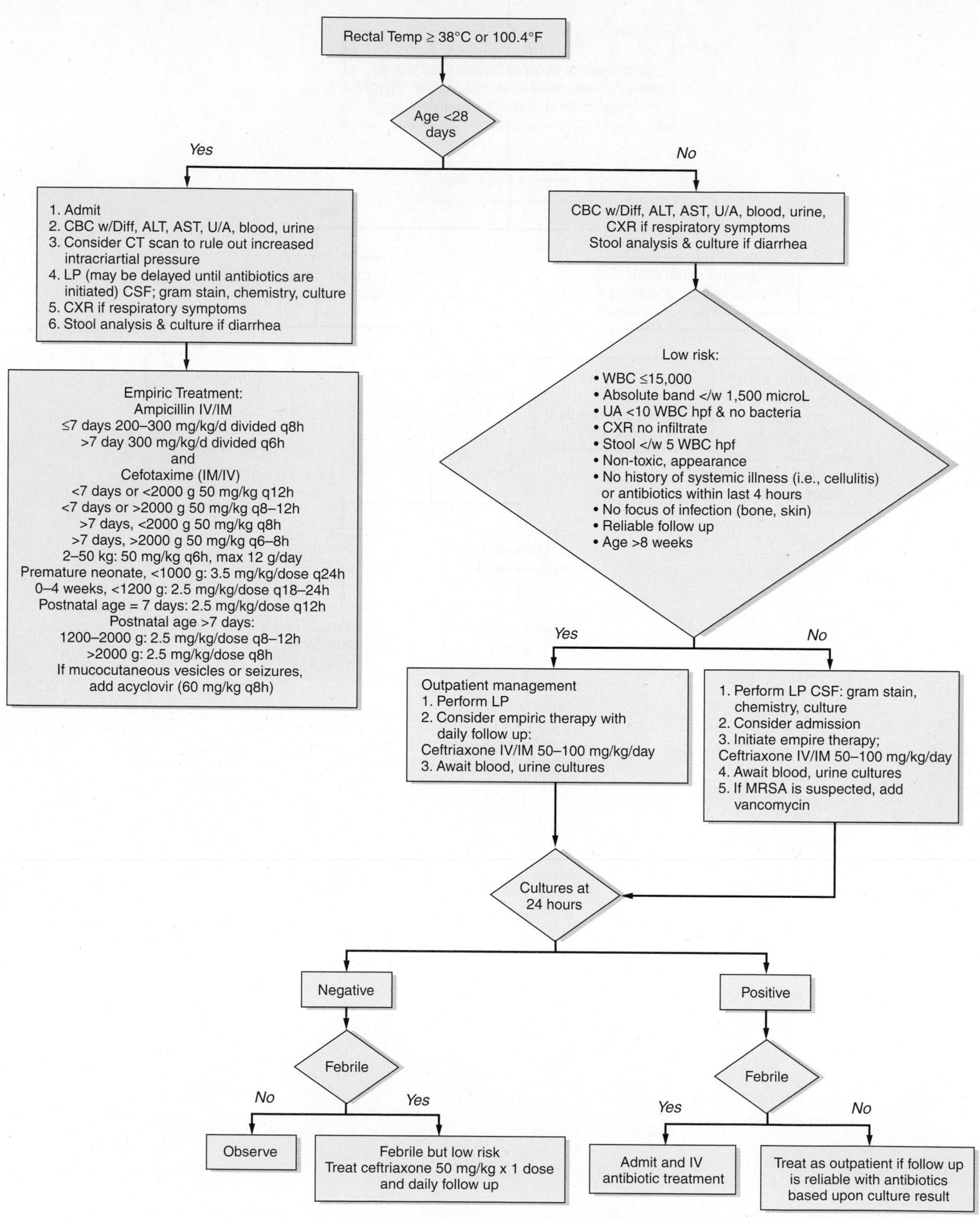
Rectal Temp ≥ 38°C or 100.4°F
Age <28 days
Yes
No
1. Admit
2. CBC w/Diff, ALT, AST, U/A, blood, urine
3. Consider CT scan to rule out increased intracriartial pressure
4. LP (may be delayed until antibiotics are initiated) CSF; gram stain, chemistry, culture
5. CXR if respiratory symptoms
6. Stool analysis & culture if diarrhea
Empiric Treatment:
Ampicillin IV/IM
≤7 days 200–300 mg/kg/d divided q8h
>7 day 300 mg/kg/d divided q6h
and
Cefotaxime (IM/IV)
<7 days or <2000 g 50 mg/kg q12h
<7 days or >2000 g 50 mg/kg q8–12h
>7 days, <2000 g 50 mg/kg q8h
>7 days, >2000 g 50 mg/kg q6–8h
2–50 kg: 50 mg/kg q6h, max 12 g/day
Premature neonate, <1000 g: 3.5 mg/kg/dose q24h
0–4 weeks, <1200 g: 2.5 mg/kg/dose q18–24h
Postnatal age = 7 days: 2.5 mg/kg/dose q12h
Postnatal age >7 days:
1200–2000 g: 2.5 mg/kg/dose q8–12h
>2000 g: 2.5 mg/kg/dose q8h
If mucocutaneous vesicles or seizures, add acyclovir (60 mg/kg q8h)
CBC w/Diff, ALT, AST, U/A, blood, urine, CXR if respiratory symptoms
Stool analysis & culture if diarrhea
Low risk:
• WBC ≤15,000
• Absolute band </w 1,500 microL
• UA <10 WBC hpf & no bacteria
• CXR no infiltrate
• Stool </w 5 WBC hpf
• Non-toxic, appearance
• No history of systemic illness (i.e., cellulitis) or antibiotics within last 4 hours
• No focus of infection (bone, skin)
• Reliable follow up
• Age >8 weeks
Yes
No
Outpatient management
1. Perform LP
2. Consider empiric therapy with daily follow up:
Ceftriaxone IV/IM 50–100 mg/kg/day
3. Await blood, urine cultures
1. Perform LP CSF: gram stain, chemistry, culture
2. Consider admission
3. Initiate empire therapy;
Ceftriaxone IV/IM 50–100 mg/kg/day
4. Await blood, urine cultures
5. If MRSA is suspected, add vancomycin
Cultures at 24 hours
Negative
Positive
Febrile
No
Yes
Observe
Febrile but low risk
Treat ceftriaxone 50 mg/kg x 1 dose and daily follow up
Febrile
Yes
No
Admit and IV antibiotic treatment
Treat as outpatient if follow up is reliable with antibiotics based upon culture result

Katharine Tumilty, MD, William J. Durbin, MD, and Mariann Manno, MD

Ann Emerg Med. 2003;42(4):530–45.

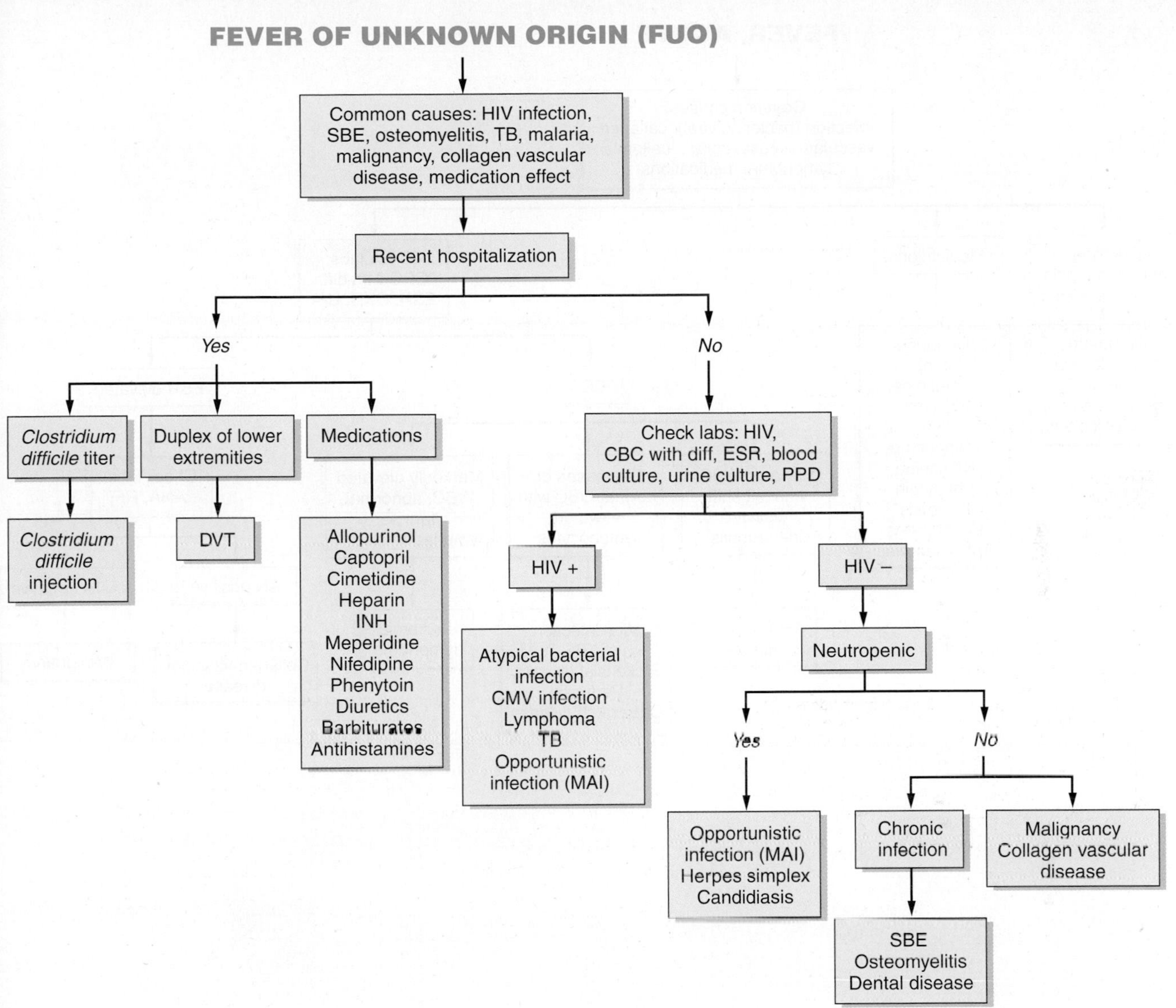
FEVER OF UNKNOWN ORIGIN (FUO)
Common causes: HIV infection, SBE, osteomyelitis, TB, malaria, malignancy, collagen vascular disease, medication effect
Recent hospitalization
Yes
No
Clostridium difficile titer
Duplex of lower extremities
Medications
Clostridium difficile injection
DVT
Allopurinol
Captopril
Cimetidine
Heparin
INH
Meperidine
Nifedipine
Phenytoin
Diuretics
Barbiturates
Antihistamines
Check labs: HIV, CBC with diff, ESR, blood culture, urine culture, PPD
HIV +
HIV –
Atypical bacterial infection
CMV infection
Lymphoma
TB
Opportunistic infection (MAI)
Neutropenic
Yes
No
Opportunistic infection (MAI)
Herpes simplex
Candidiasis
Chronic infection
Malignancy
Collagen vascular disease
SBE
Osteomyelitis
Dental disease

Robert A. Baldor, MD and Alan M. Ehrlich, MD

Pediatr Infect Dis J. 2009 Nov 25.

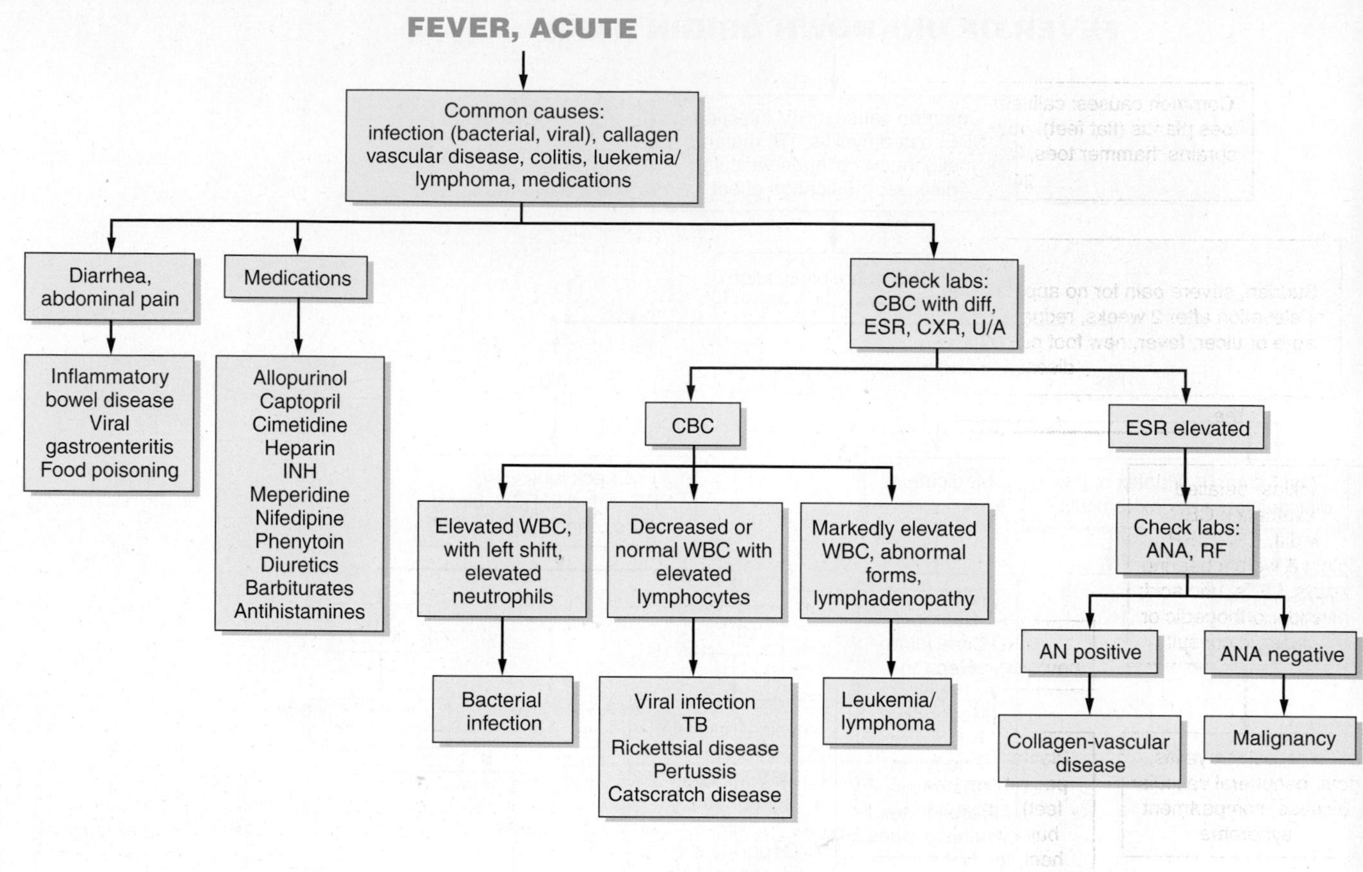
FEVER, ACUTE
Common causes: infection (bacterial, viral), callagen vascular disease, colitis, luekemia/ lymphoma, medications
Diarrhea, abdominal pain
Medications
Check labs: CBC with diff, ESR, CXR, U/A
Inflammatory bowel disease
Viral gastroenteritis
Food poisoning
Allopurinol
Captopril
Cimetidine
Heparin
INH
Meperidine
Nifedipine
Phenytoin
Diuretics
Barbiturates
Antihistamines
CBC
ESR elevated
Elevated WBC, with left shift, elevated neutrophils
Decreased or normal WBC with elevated lymphocytes
Markedly elevated WBC, abnormal forms, lymphadenopathy
Check labs: ANA, RF
Bacterial infection
Viral infection
TB
Rickettsial disease
Pertussis
Catscratch disease
Leukemia/ lymphoma
AN positive
ANA negative
Collagen-vascular disease
Malignancy

Robert A. Baldor, MD and Alan M. Ehrlich, MD

Crit Care Med. 2010;38(2):457–63.

FOOT PAIN

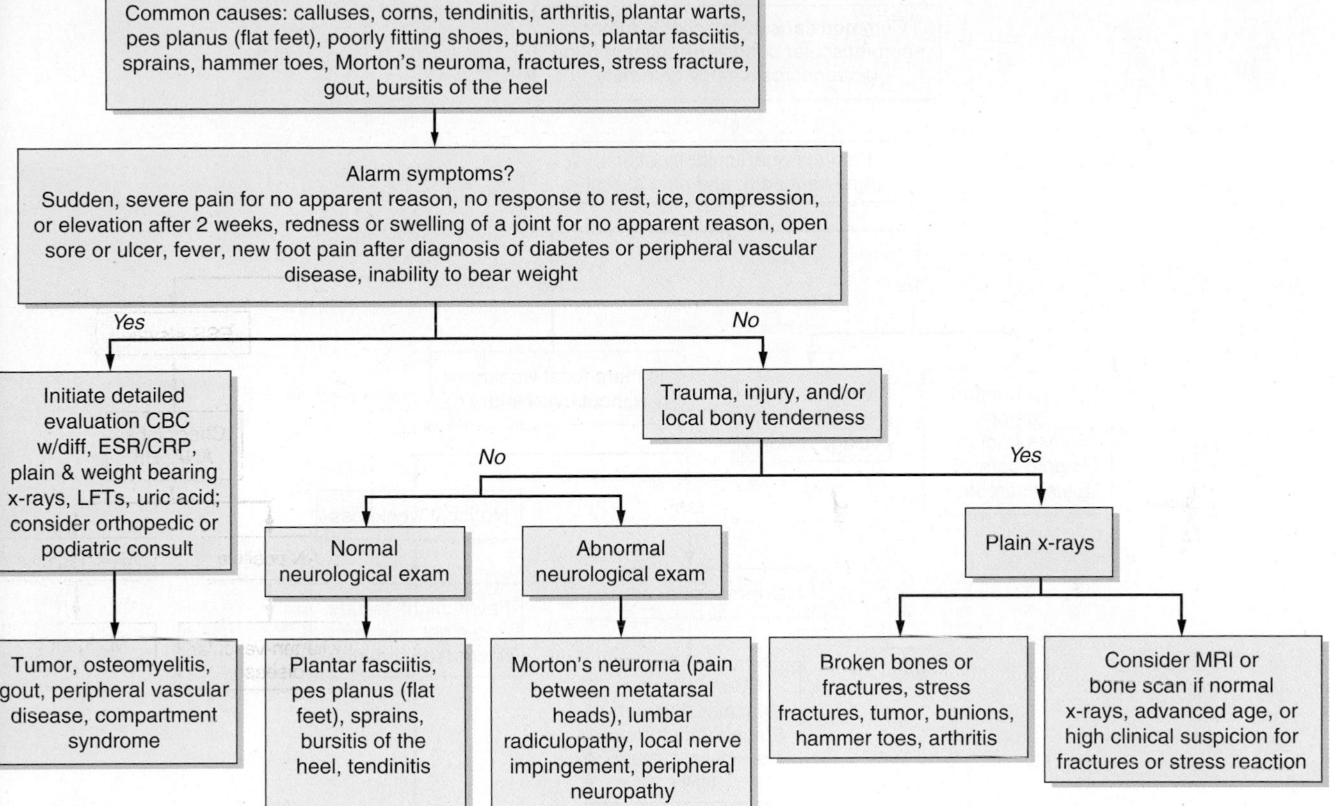

Common causes: calluses, corns, tendinitis, arthritis, plantar warts, pes planus (flat feet), poorly fitting shoes, bunions, plantar fasciitis, sprains, hammer toes, Morton's neuroma, fractures, stress fracture, gout, bursitis of the heel
Alarm symptoms?
Sudden, severe pain for no apparent reason, no response to rest, ice, compression, or elevation after 2 weeks, redness or swelling of a joint for no apparent reason, open sore or ulcer, fever, new foot pain after diagnosis of diabetes or peripheral vascular disease, inability to bear weight
Yes
No
Initiate detailed evaluation CBC w/diff, ESR/CRP, plain & weight bearing x-rays, LFTs, uric acid; consider orthopedic or podiatric consult
Trauma, injury, and/or local bony tenderness
No
Yes
Normal neurological exam
Abnormal neurological exam
Plain x-rays
Tumor, osteomyelitis, gout, peripheral vascular disease, compartment syndrome
Plantar fasciitis, pes planus (flat feet), sprains, bursitis of the heel, tendinitis
Morton's neuroma (pain between metatarsal heads), lumbar radiculopathy, local nerve impingement, peripheral neuropathy
Broken bones or fractures, stress fractures, tumor, bunions, hammer toes, arthritis
Consider MRI or bone scan if normal x-rays, advanced age, or high clinical suspicion for fractures or stress reaction

George Gunter A. Pujalte, MD

BMJ. 2003;326(7386):417.

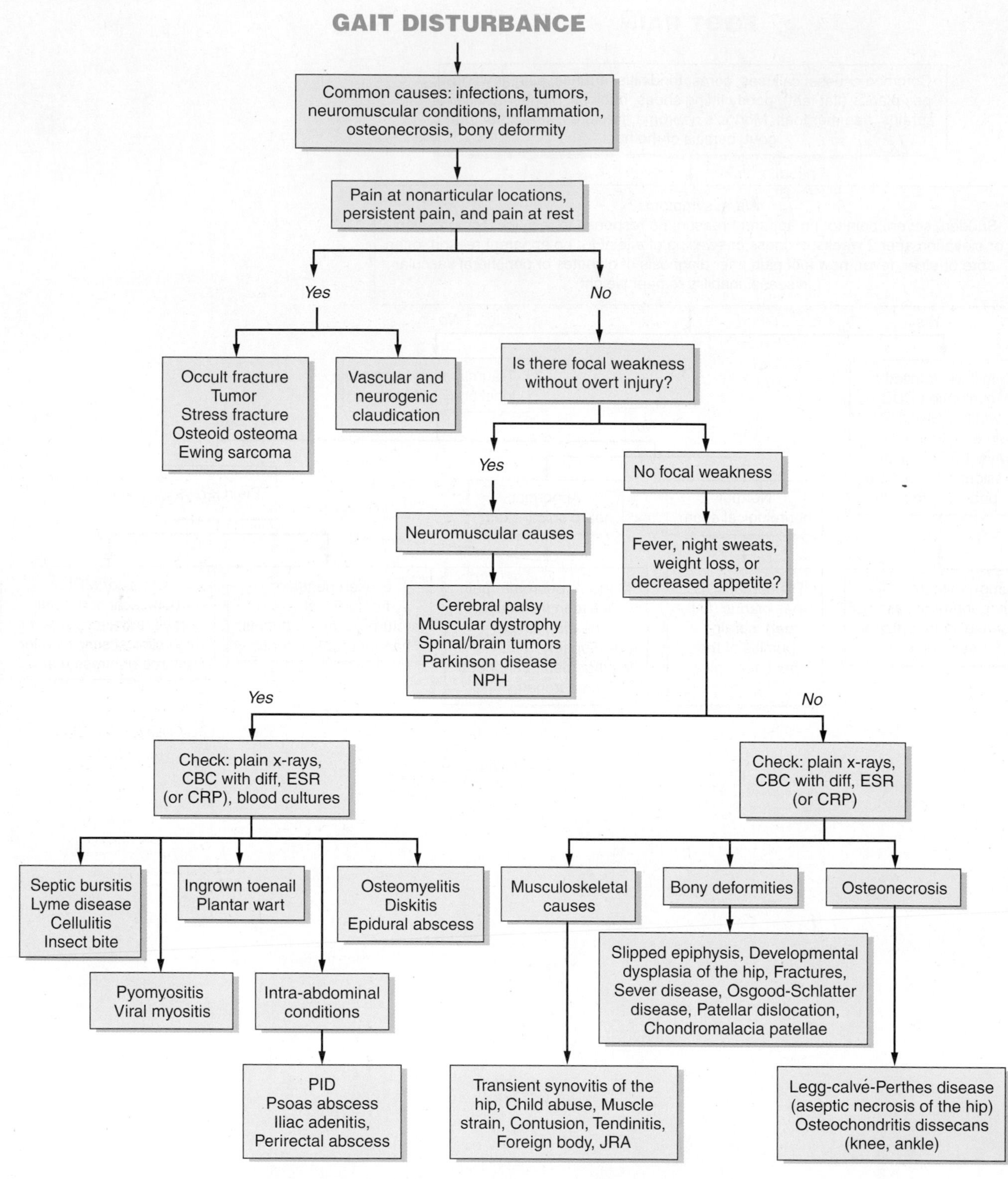

Robert A. Baldor, MD and Alan M. Ehrlich, MD

Stroke. 2009;40(12):3816–20.

GASTROESOPHAGEAL REFLUX DISEASE (GERD), TREATMENT

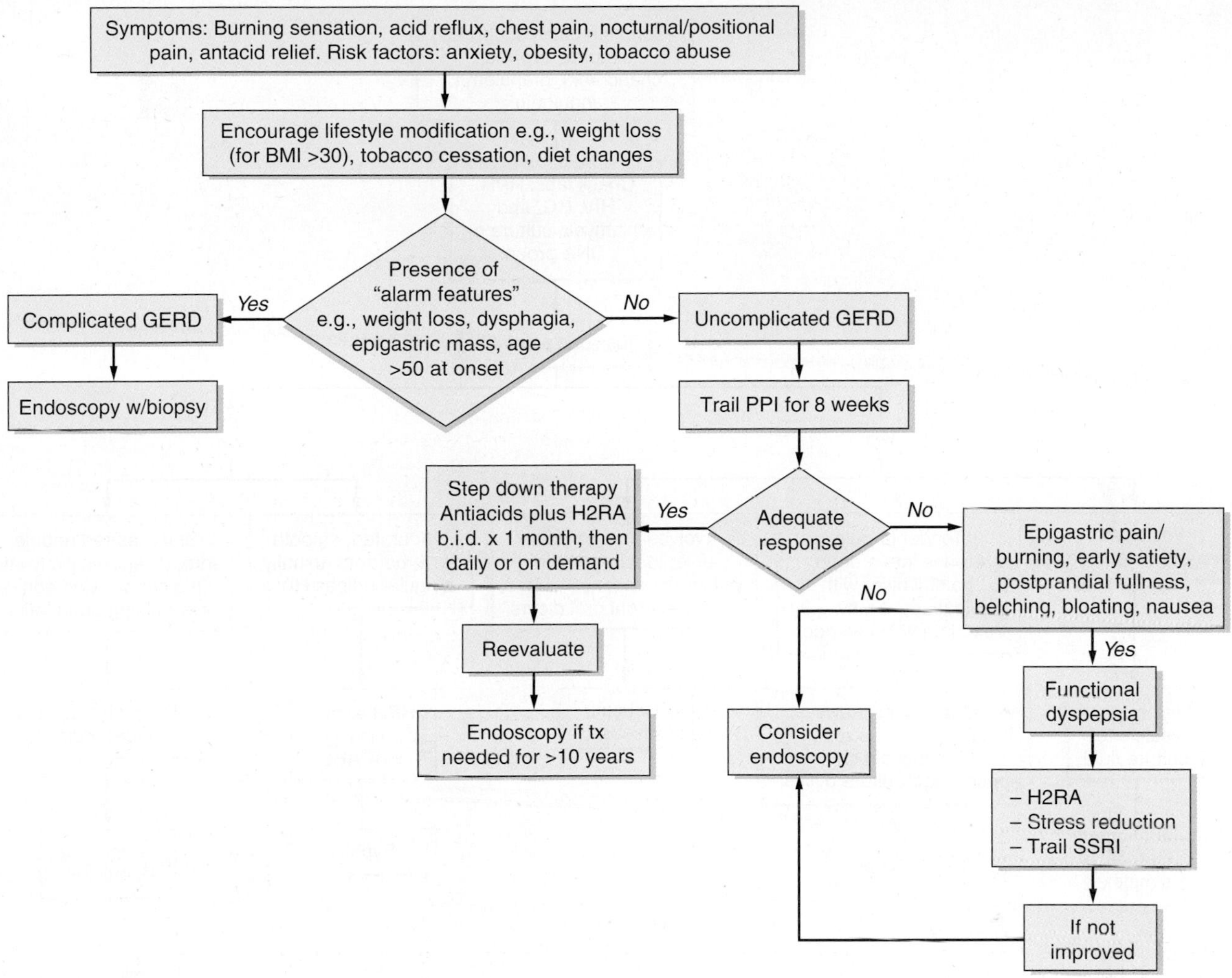

Richard E. Trowbridge, MD and Rebecca A. Frye, DO

Am J Med. 2010;123(7):583–92.

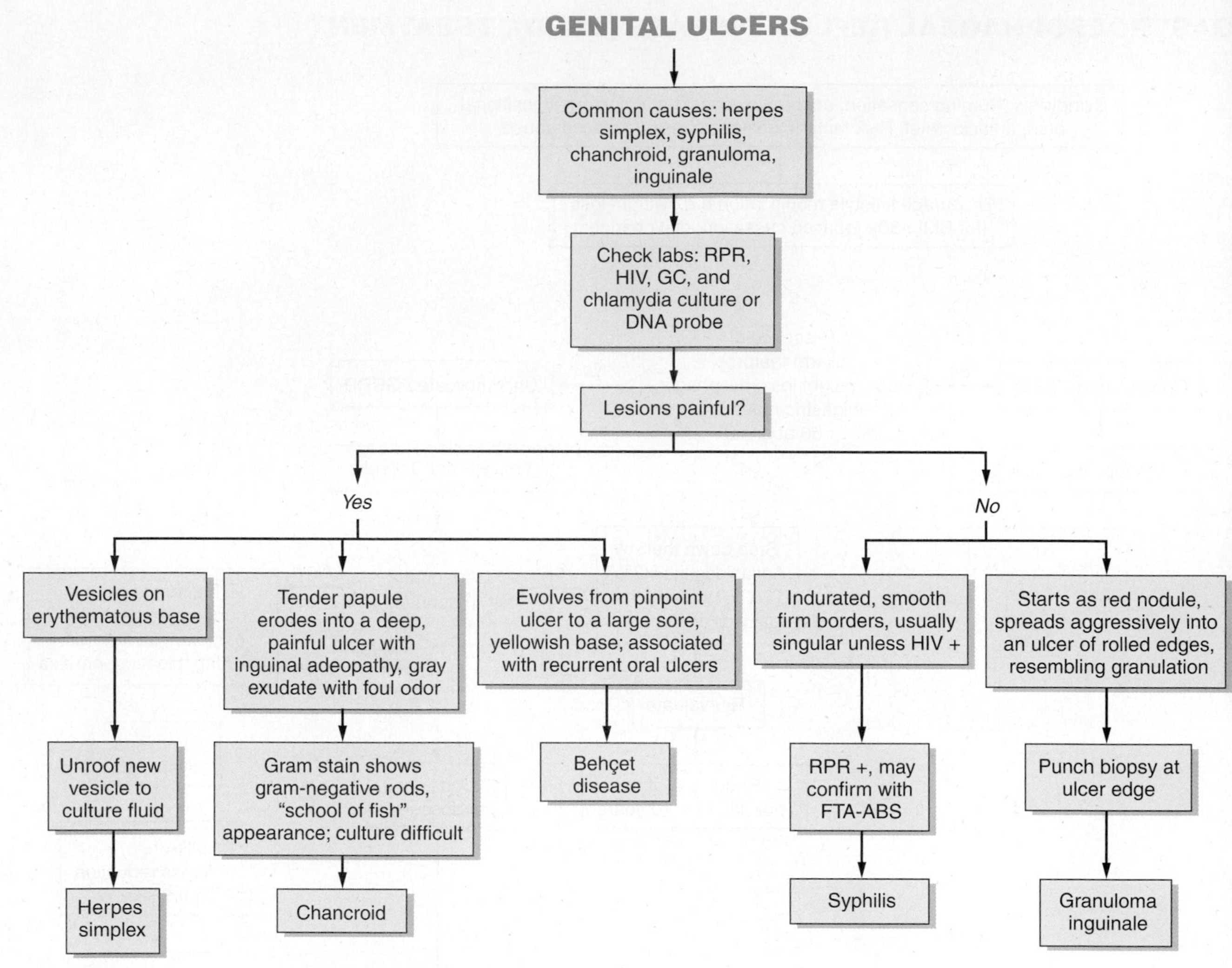
GENITAL ULCERS
Common causes: herpes simplex, syphilis, chancroid, granuloma, inguinale
Check labs: RPR, HIV, GC, and chlamydia culture or DNA probe
Lesions painful?
Yes
No
Vesicles on erythematous base
Tender papule erodes into a deep, painful ulcer with inguinal adeopathy, gray exudate with foul odor
Evolves from pinpoint ulcer to a large sore, yellowish base; associated with recurrent oral ulcers
Indurated, smooth firm borders, usually singular unless HIV +
Starts as red nodule, spreads aggressively into an ulcer of rolled edges, resembling granulation
Unroof new vesicle to culture fluid
Gram stain shows gram-negative rods, "school of fish" appearance; culture difficult
Behçet disease
RPR +, may confirm with FTA-ABS
Punch biopsy at ulcer edge
Herpes simplex
Chancroid
Syphilis
Granuloma inguinale

Robert A. Baldor, MD and Alan M. Ehrlich, MD

Sex Transm Dis. 2008;35(6):545–9.

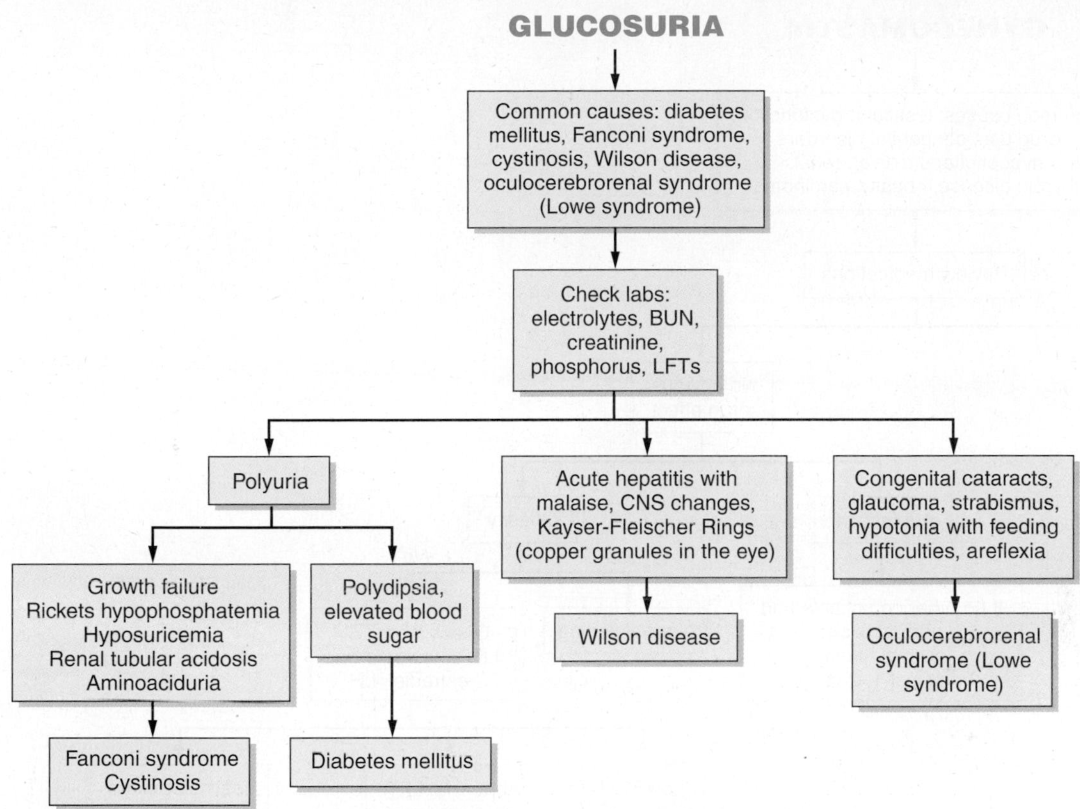

Robert A. Baldor, MD and Alan M. Ehrlich, MD

Scand J Clin Lab Invest. 2009;69(6):662–72.

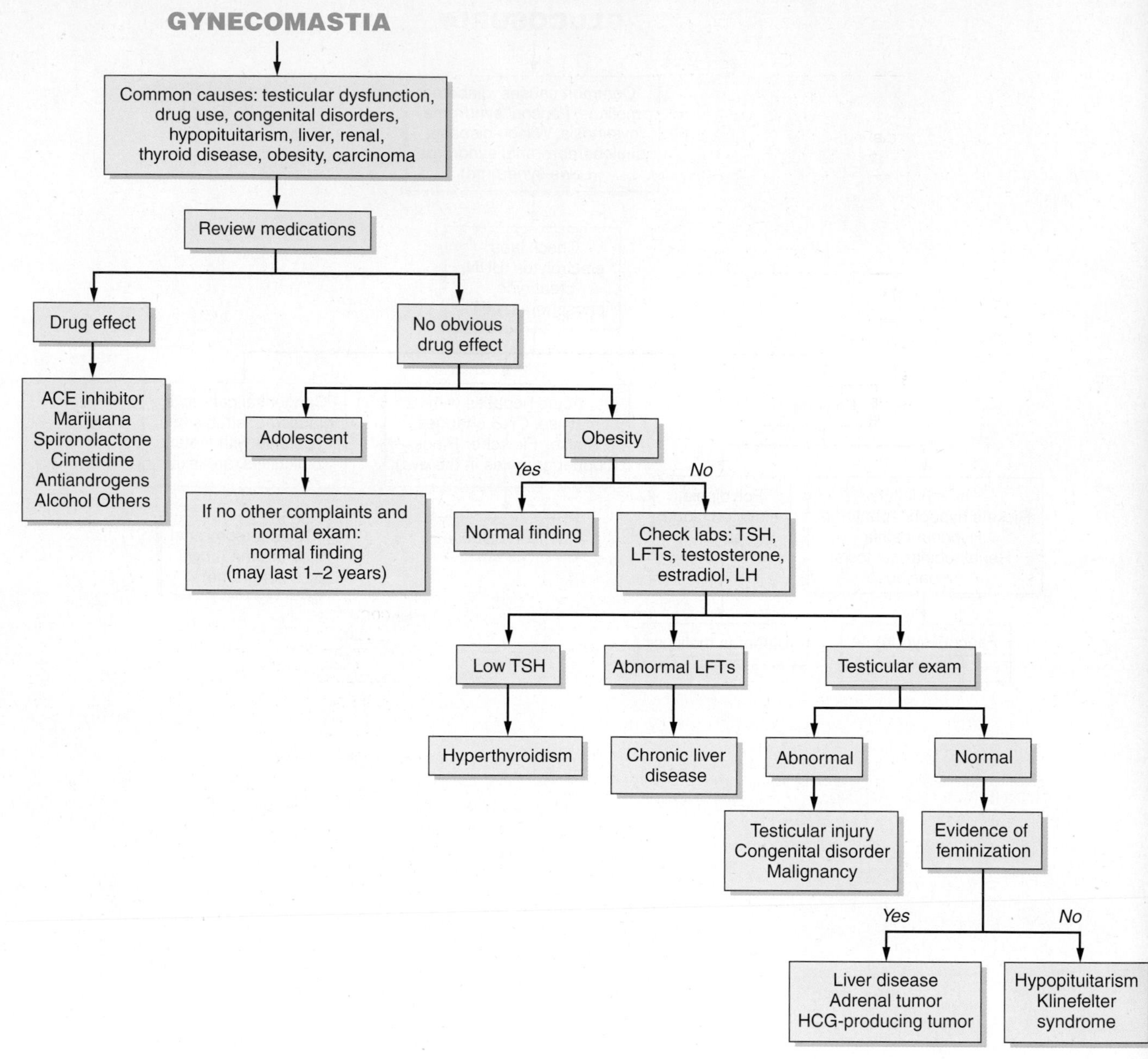

Robert A. Baldor, MD and Alan M. Ehrlich, MD

J Clin Endocrinol Metab. 2009;94(8):2975–8. Epub 2009 May 26.

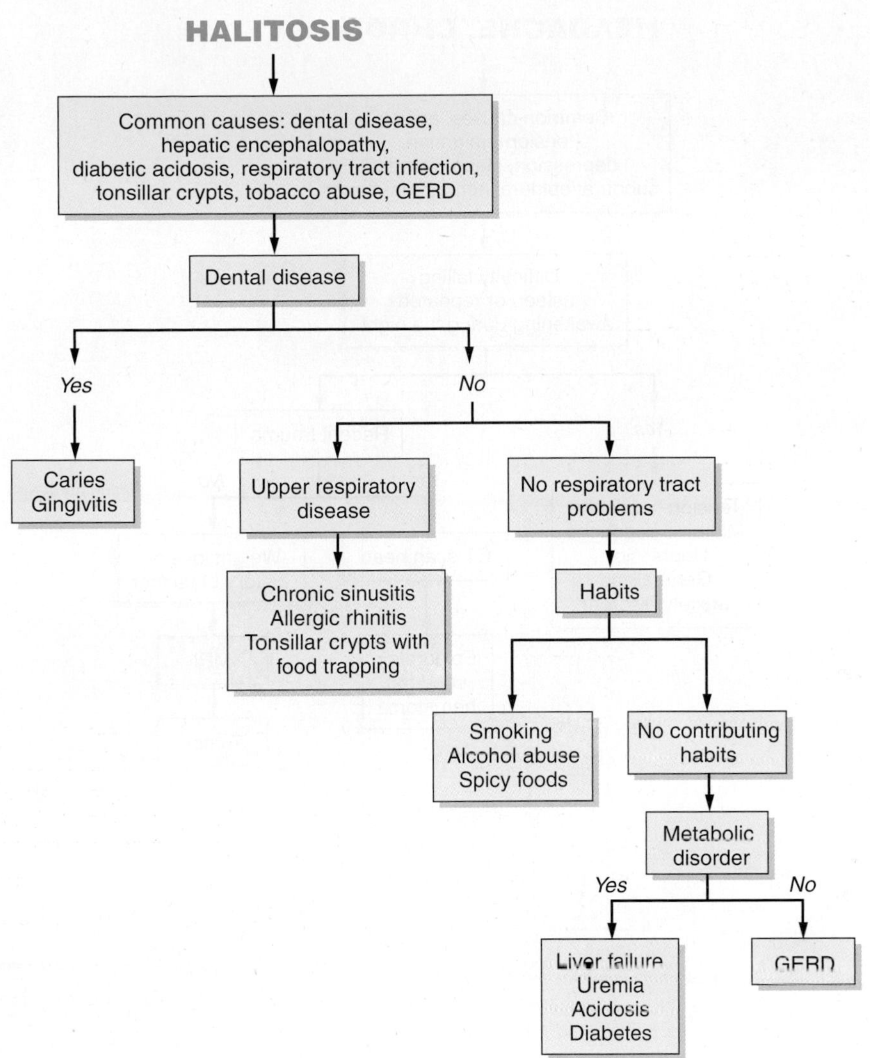

Robert A. Baldor, MD and Alan M. Ehrlich, MD

Oral Surg Oral Med Oral Pathol Oral Radiol Endod. 2008;106(3):384–8. Epub 2008 Jul 7.

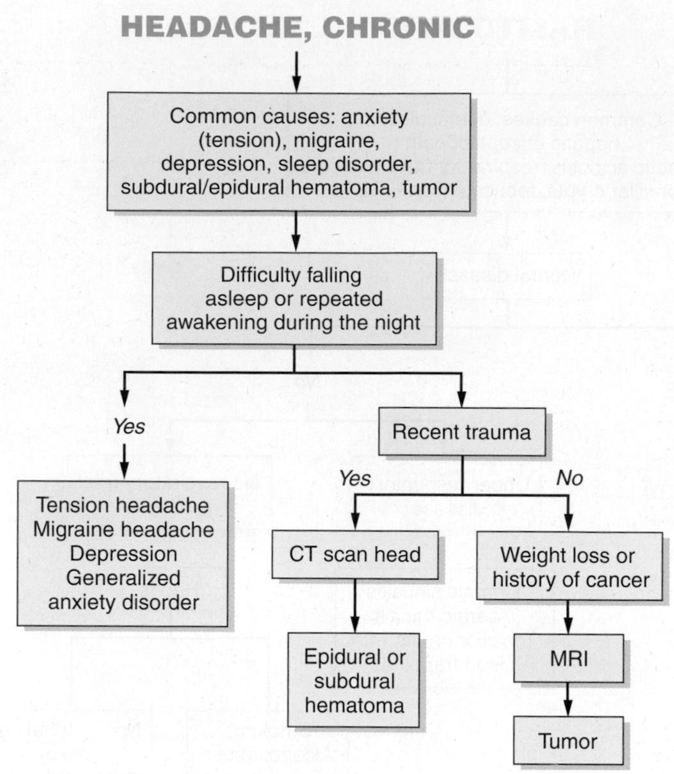

Robert A. Baldor, MD and Alan M. Ehrlich, MD

Acta Neurochir Suppl. 2010;107:65–9.

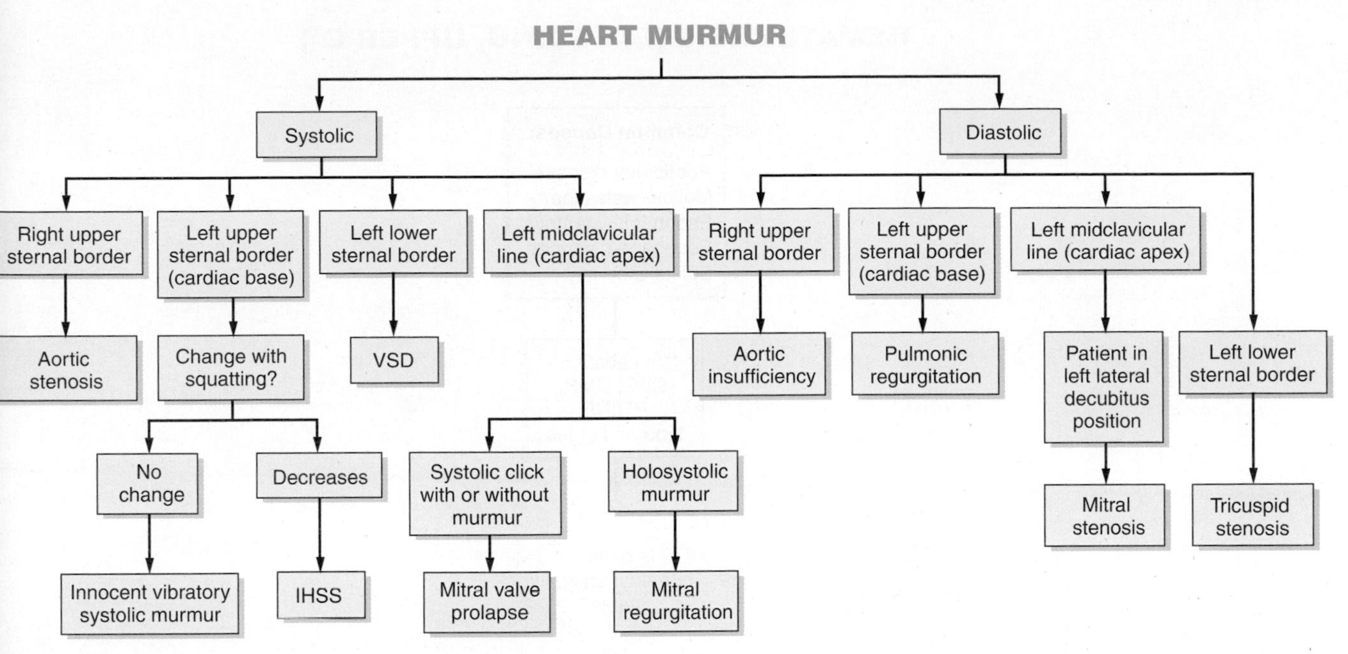

Robert A. Baldor, MD and Alan M. Ehrlich, MD

Pediatr Int. 2008;50(2):145–9.

HEMATEMESIS (BLEEDING, UPPER GI)

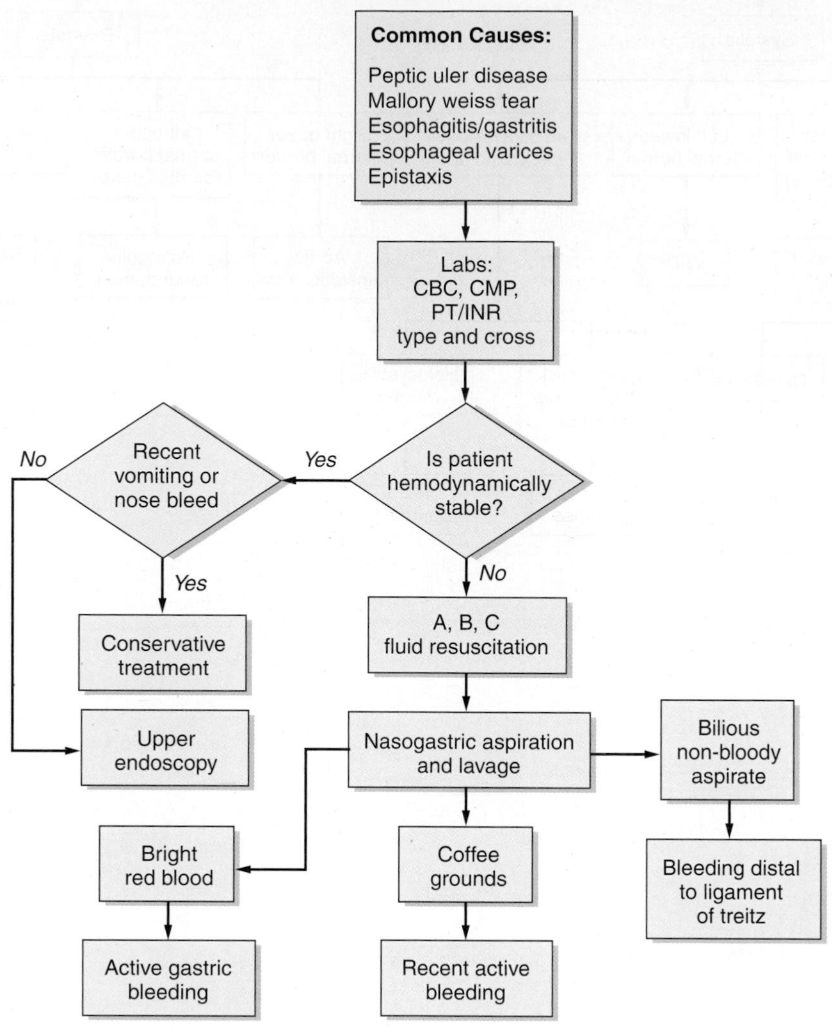

Sanjeev K. Sharma, MD and Kyle V. Contini, MD

Can J Gastroenterol. 2004;18(10):605–9.

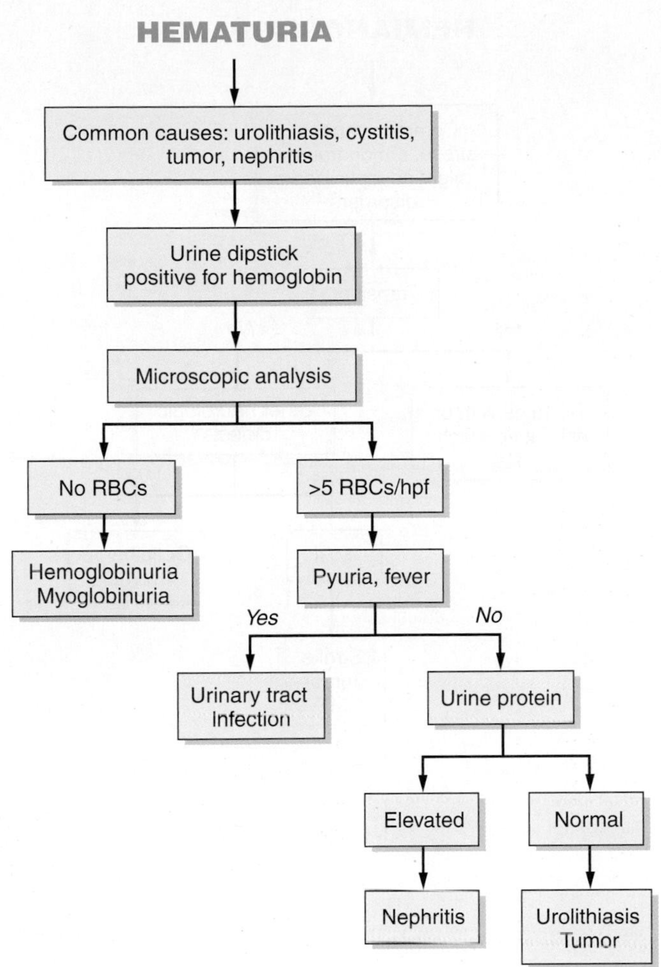

Robert A. Baldor, MD and Alan M. Ehrlich, MD

Med Clin North Am. 2004;88(2):329–43.

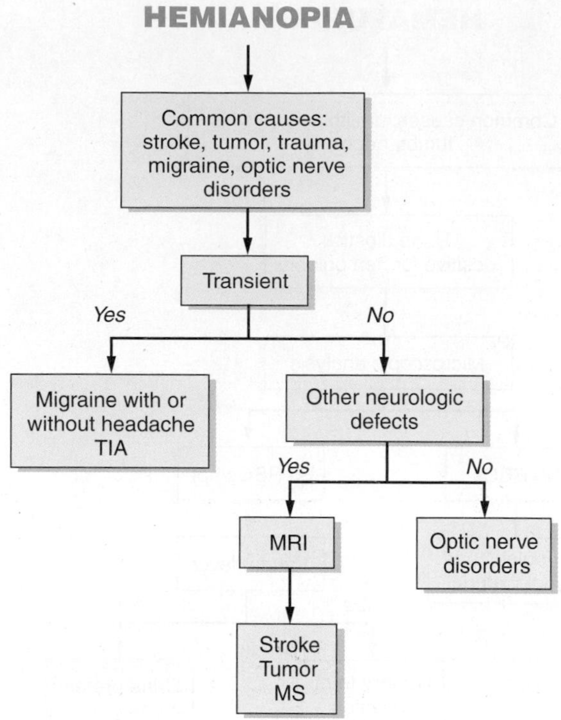

Robert A. Baldor, MD and Alan M. Ehrlich, MD

Stroke. 2010;41(2):e88–90.

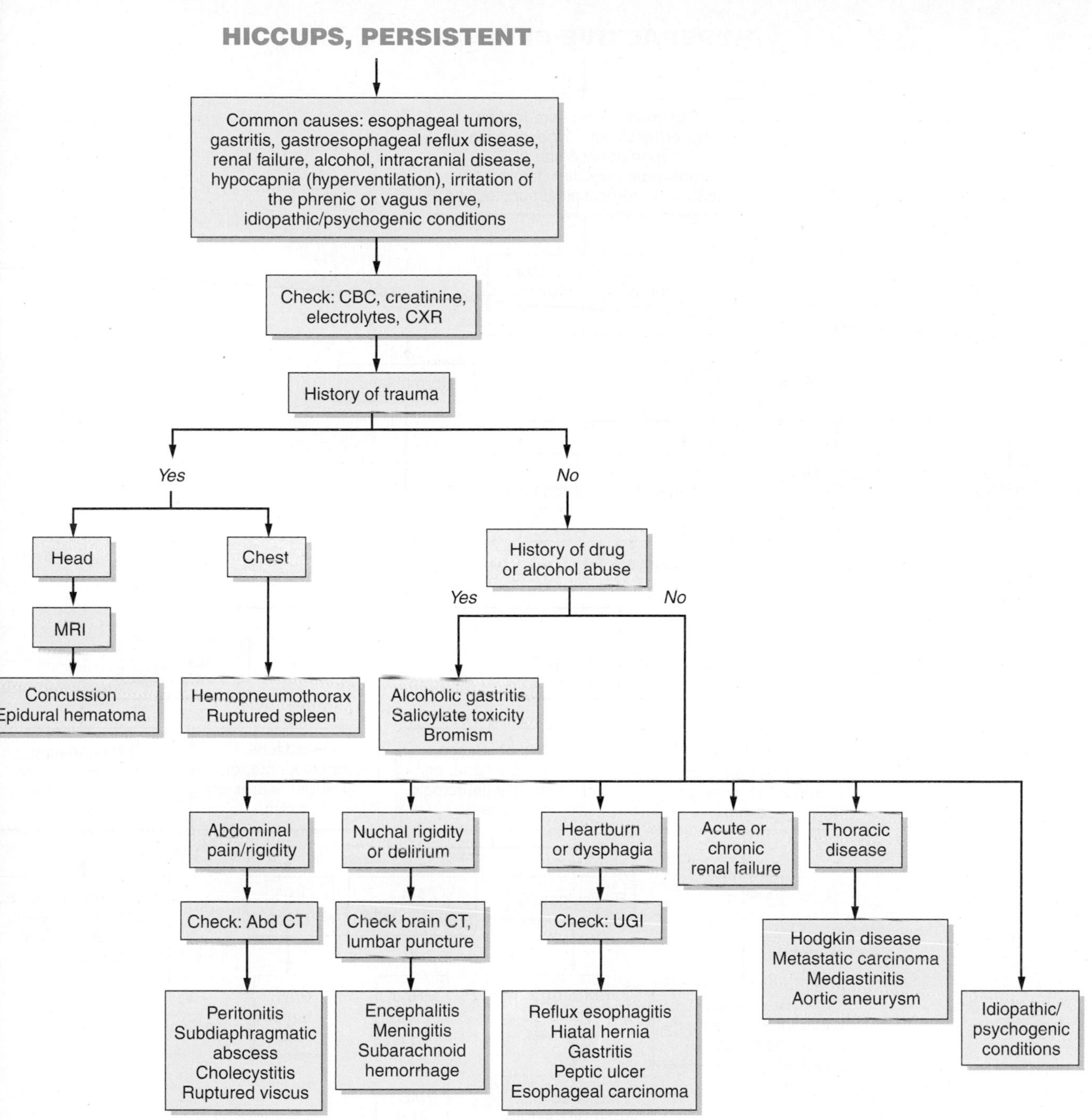

Robert A. Baldor, MD and Alan M. Ehrlich, MD

J Support Oncol. 2009;7(4):122–7, 130.

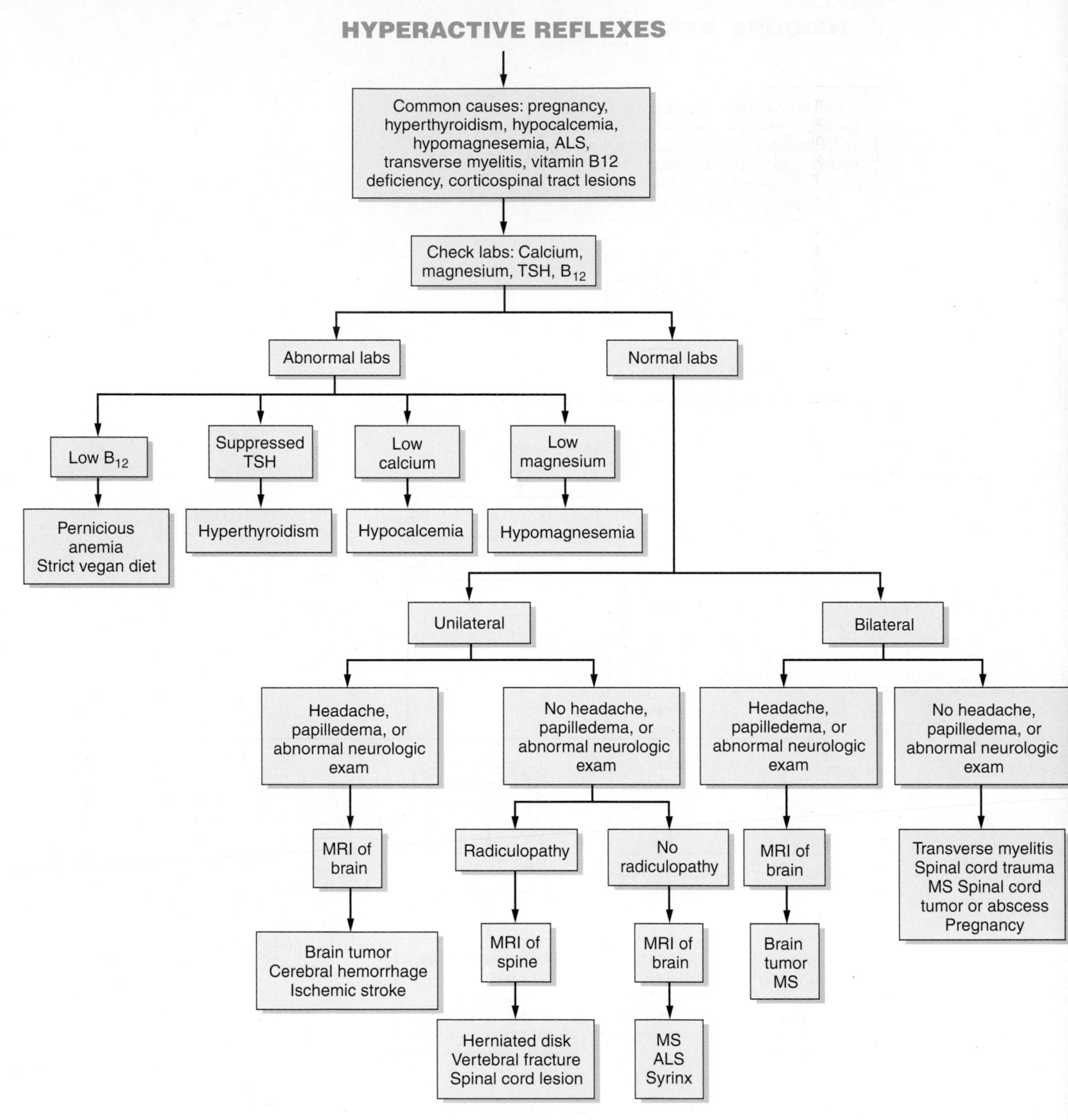
HYPERACTIVE REFLEXES
Common causes: pregnancy, hyperthyroidism, hypocalcemia, hypomagnesemia, ALS, transverse myelitis, vitamin B12 deficiency, corticospinal tract lesions
Check labs: Calcium, magnesium, TSH, B12
Abnormal labs
Normal labs
Low B12
Suppressed TSH
Low calcium
Low magnesium
Pernicious anemia
Strict vegan diet
Hyperthyroidism
Hypocalcemia
Hypomagnesemia
Unilateral
Bilateral
Headache, papilledema, or abnormal neurologic exam
No headache, papilledema, or abnormal neurologic exam
Headache, papilledema, or abnormal neurologic exam
No headache, papilledema, or abnormal neurologic exam
MRI of brain
Radiculopathy
No radiculopathy
MRI of brain
Transverse myelitis
Spinal cord trauma
MS Spinal cord tumor or abscess
Pregnancy
Brain tumor
Cerebral hemorrhage
Ischemic stroke
MRI of spine
MRI of brain
Brain tumor
MS
Herniated disk
Vertebral fracture
Spinal cord lesion
MS
ALS
Syrinx

Robert A. Baldor, MD and Alan M. Ehrlich, MD

Dev Med Child Neurol. 2009;51(2):128–35. Epub 2008 Oct 17.

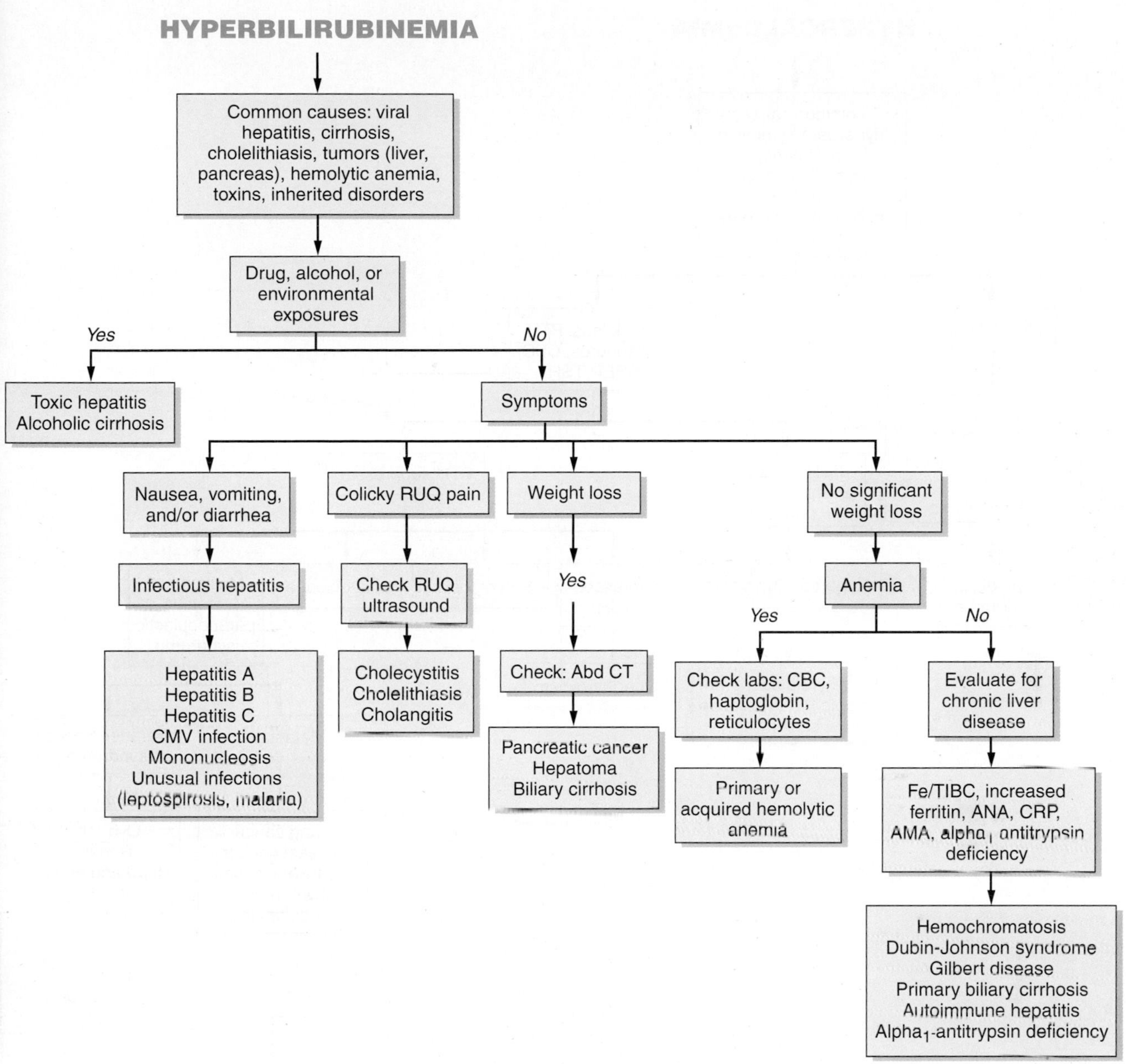

Robert A. Baldor, MD and Alan M. Ehrlich, MD

Am J Surg. 2009;198(2):193–8. Epub 2009 Mar 23.

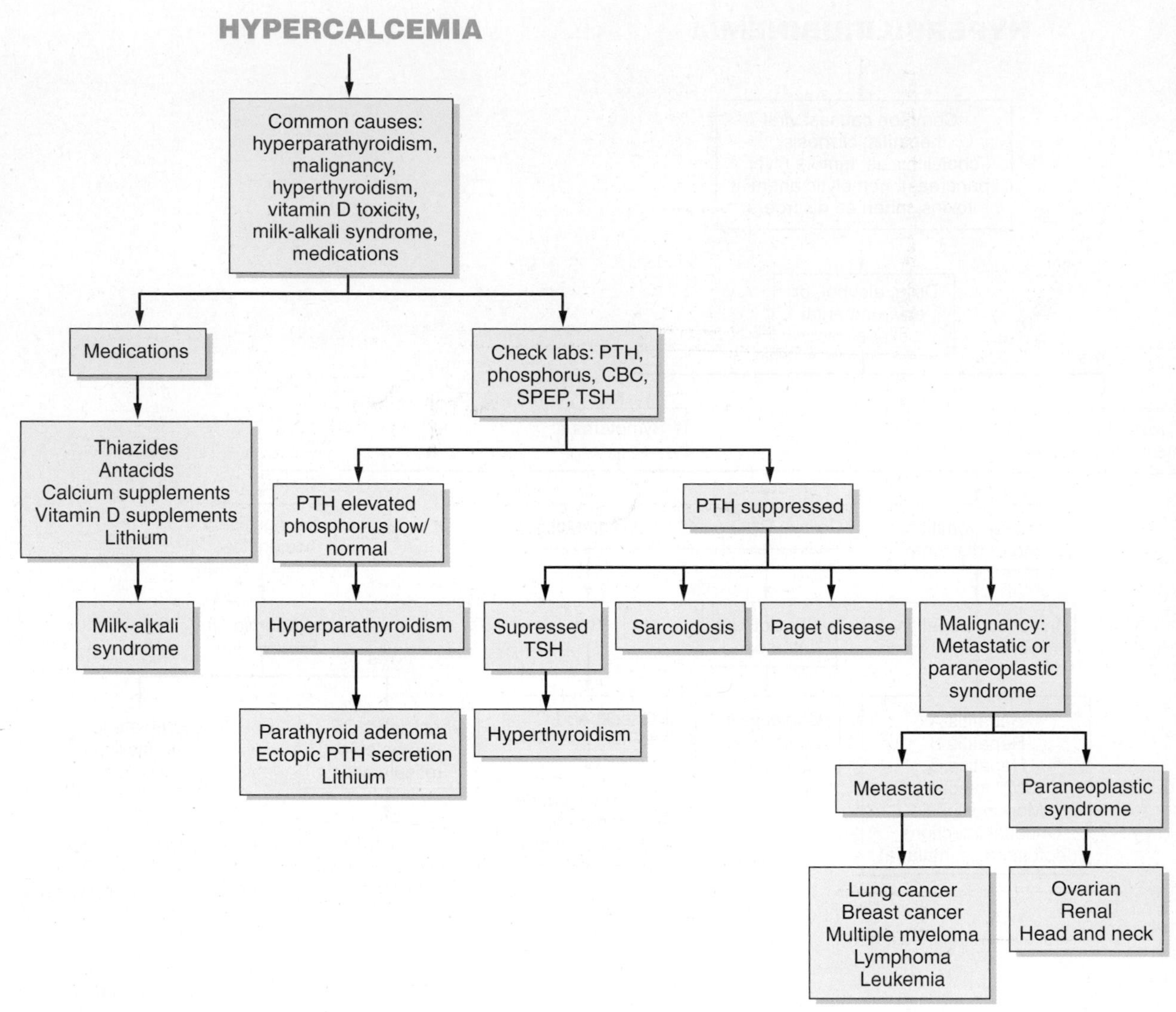

Robert A. Baldor, MD and Alan M. Ehrlich, MD

Iran J Kid. 2009;54(4):19–37.

HYPERCHOLESTEROLEMIA

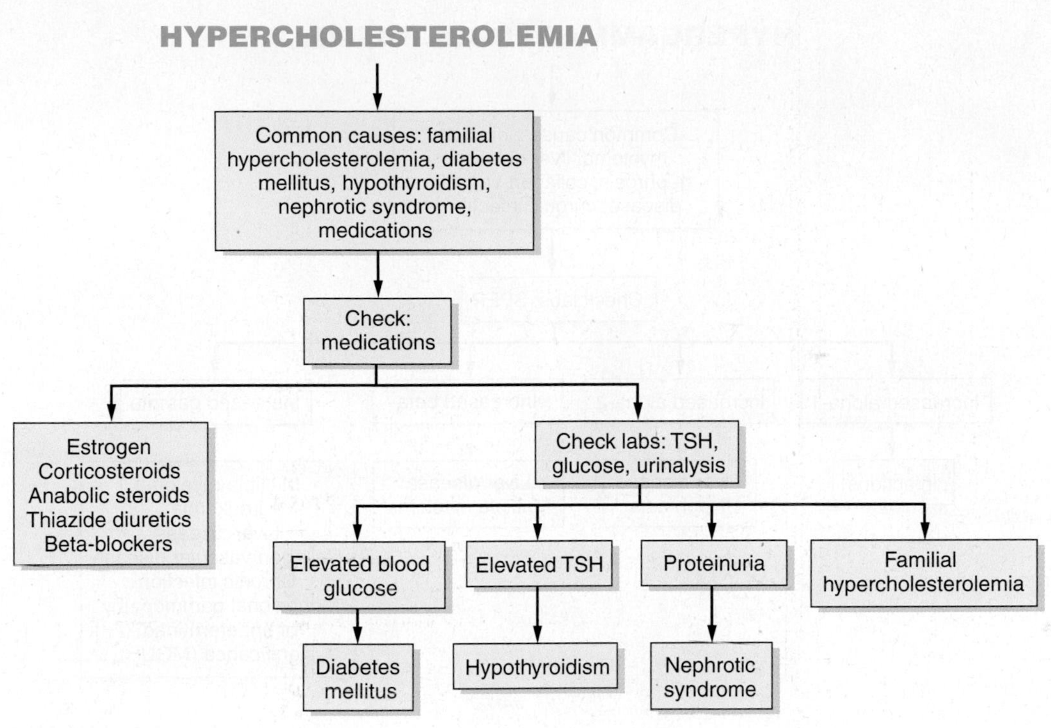

Robert A. Baldor, MD and Alan M. Ehrlich, MD

Curr Med Res Opin. 2009;25(2):431–47.

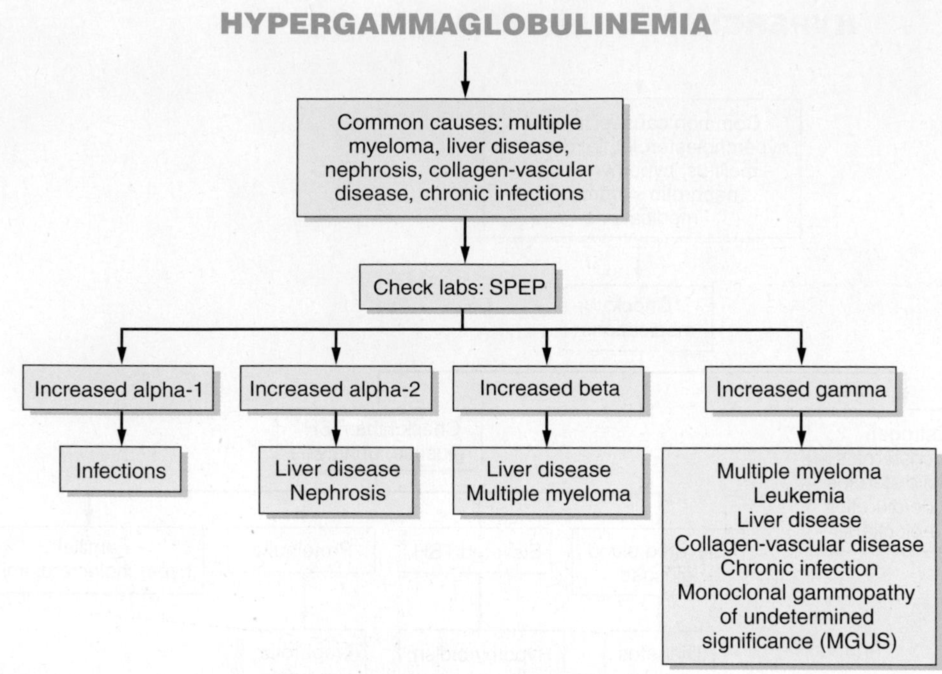

Robert A. Baldor, MD and Alan M. Ehrlich, MD

Medicine (Baltimore). 2009;88(5):284–93.

HYPERGLYCEMIA

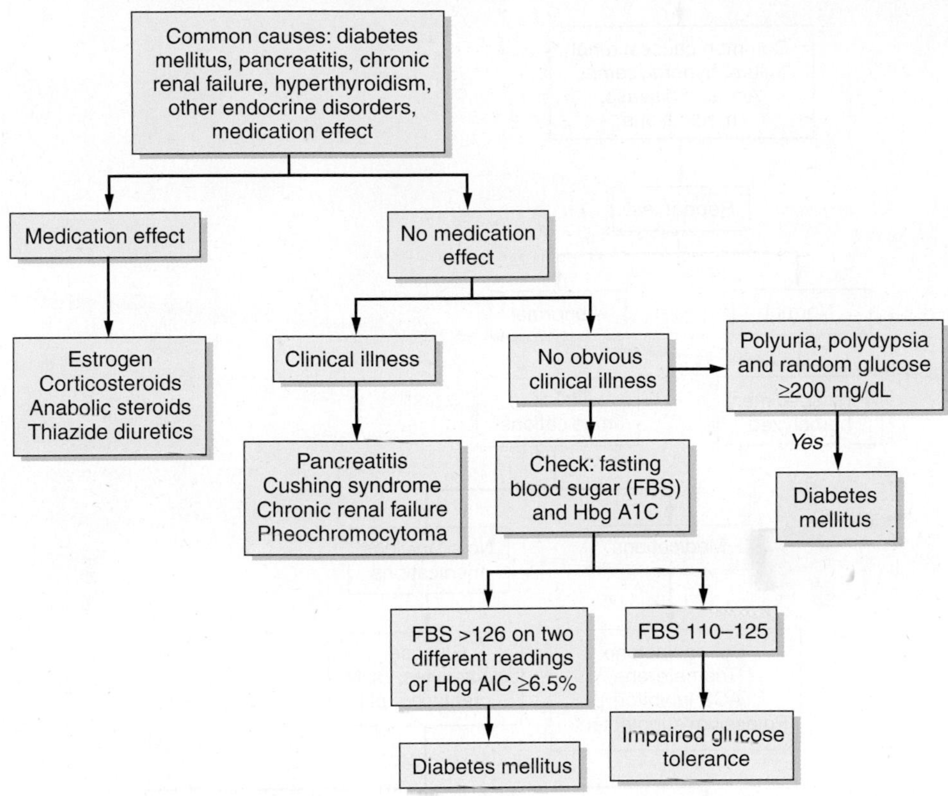

Robert A. Baldor, MD and Alan M. Ehrlich, MD

Crit Care Med. 2009;37(5):1769–76.

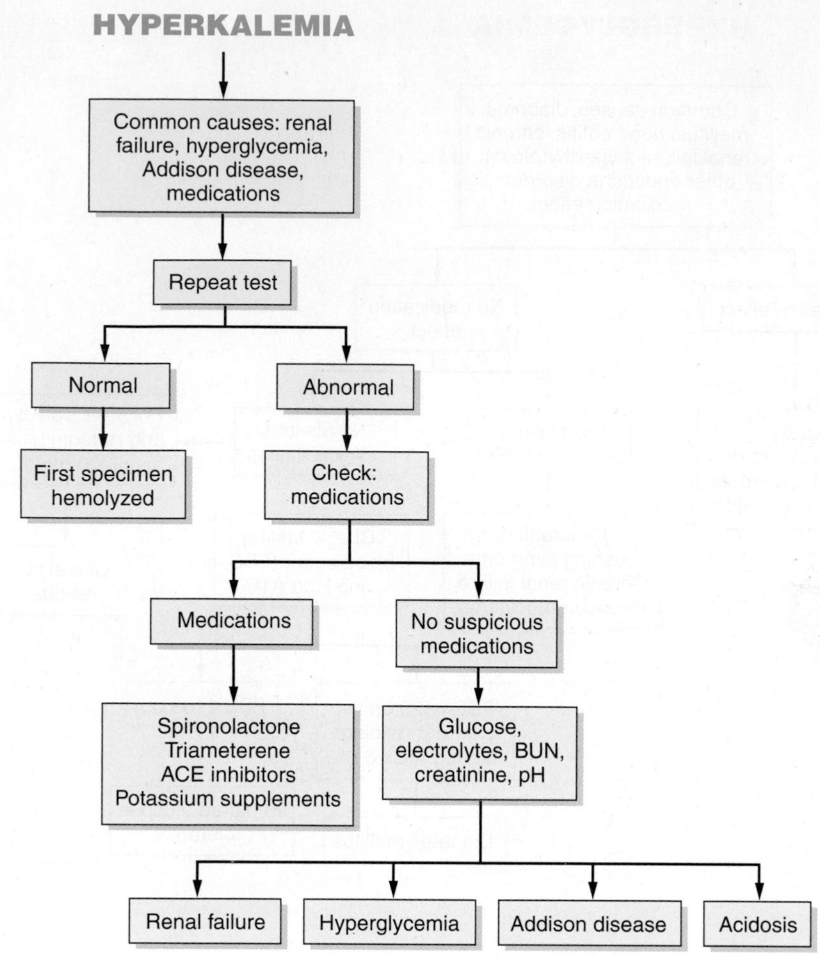

Robert A. Baldor, MD and Alan M. Ehrlich, MD

J Gen Intern Med. 2010.

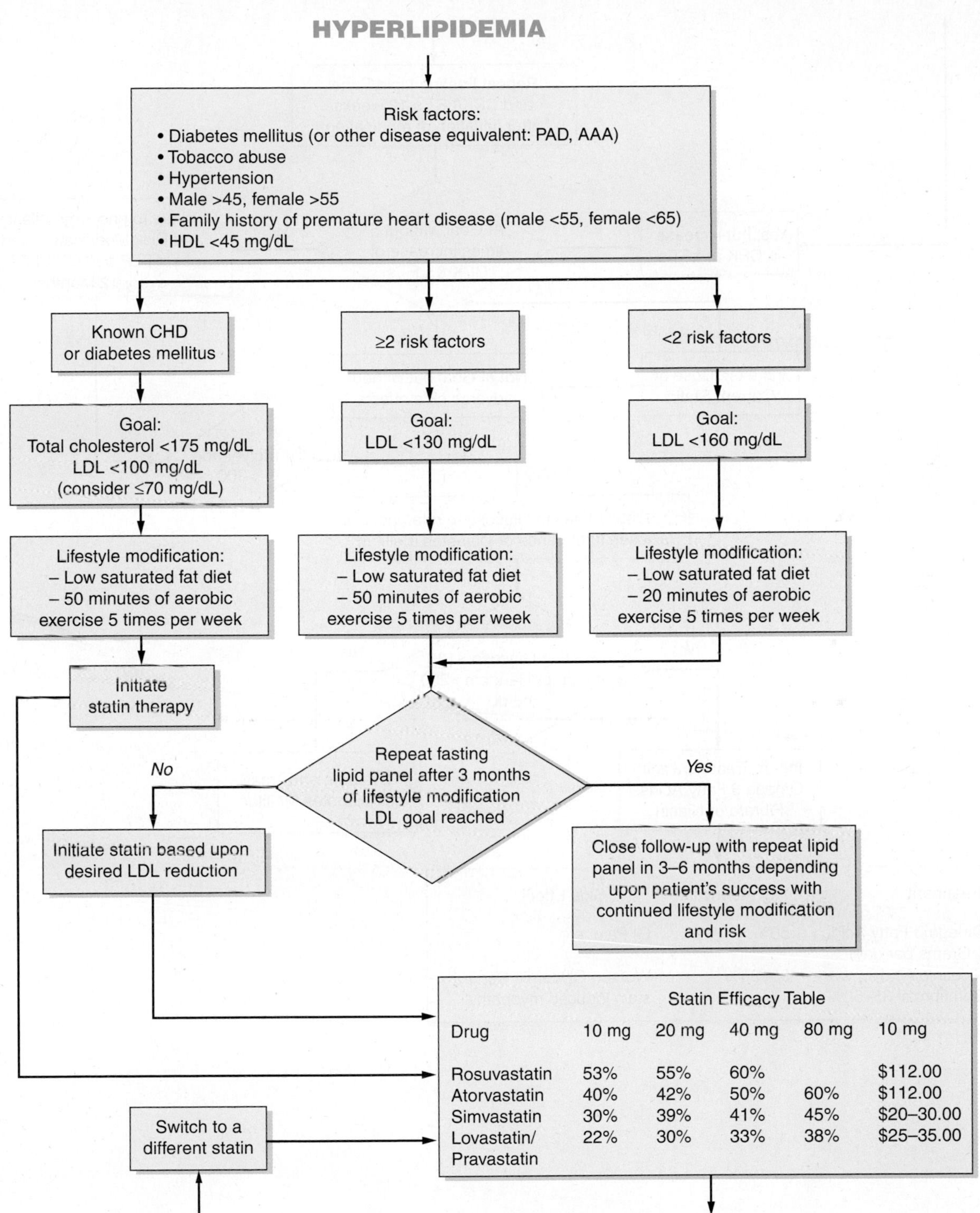
HYPERLIPIDEMIA
Risk factors:
• Diabetes mellitus (or other disease equivalent: PAD, AAA)
• Tobacco abuse
• Hypertension
• Male >45, female >55
• Family history of premature heart disease (male <55, female <65)
• HDL <45 mg/dL
Known CHD or diabetes mellitus
≥2 risk factors
<2 risk factors
Goal: Total cholesterol <175 mg/dL LDL <100 mg/dL (consider ≤70 mg/dL)
Goal: LDL <130 mg/dL
Goal: LDL <160 mg/dL
Lifestyle modification: – Low saturated fat diet – 50 minutes of aerobic exercise 5 times per week
Lifestyle modification: – Low saturated fat diet – 50 minutes of aerobic exercise 5 times per week
Lifestyle modification: – Low saturated fat diet – 20 minutes of aerobic exercise 5 times per week
Initiate statin therapy
Repeat fasting lipid panel after 3 months of lifestyle modification LDL goal reached
No
Yes
Initiate statin based upon desired LDL reduction
Close follow-up with repeat lipid panel in 3–6 months depending upon patient's success with continued lifestyle modification and risk
Switch to a different statin

Statin Efficacy Table

Drug	10 mg	20 mg	40 mg	80 mg	10 mg
Rosuvastatin	53%	55%	60%		$112.00
Atorvastatin	40%	42%	50%	60%	$112.00
Simvastatin	30%	39%	41%	45%	$20–30.00
Lovastatin/ Pravastatin	22%	30%	33%	38%	$25–35.00

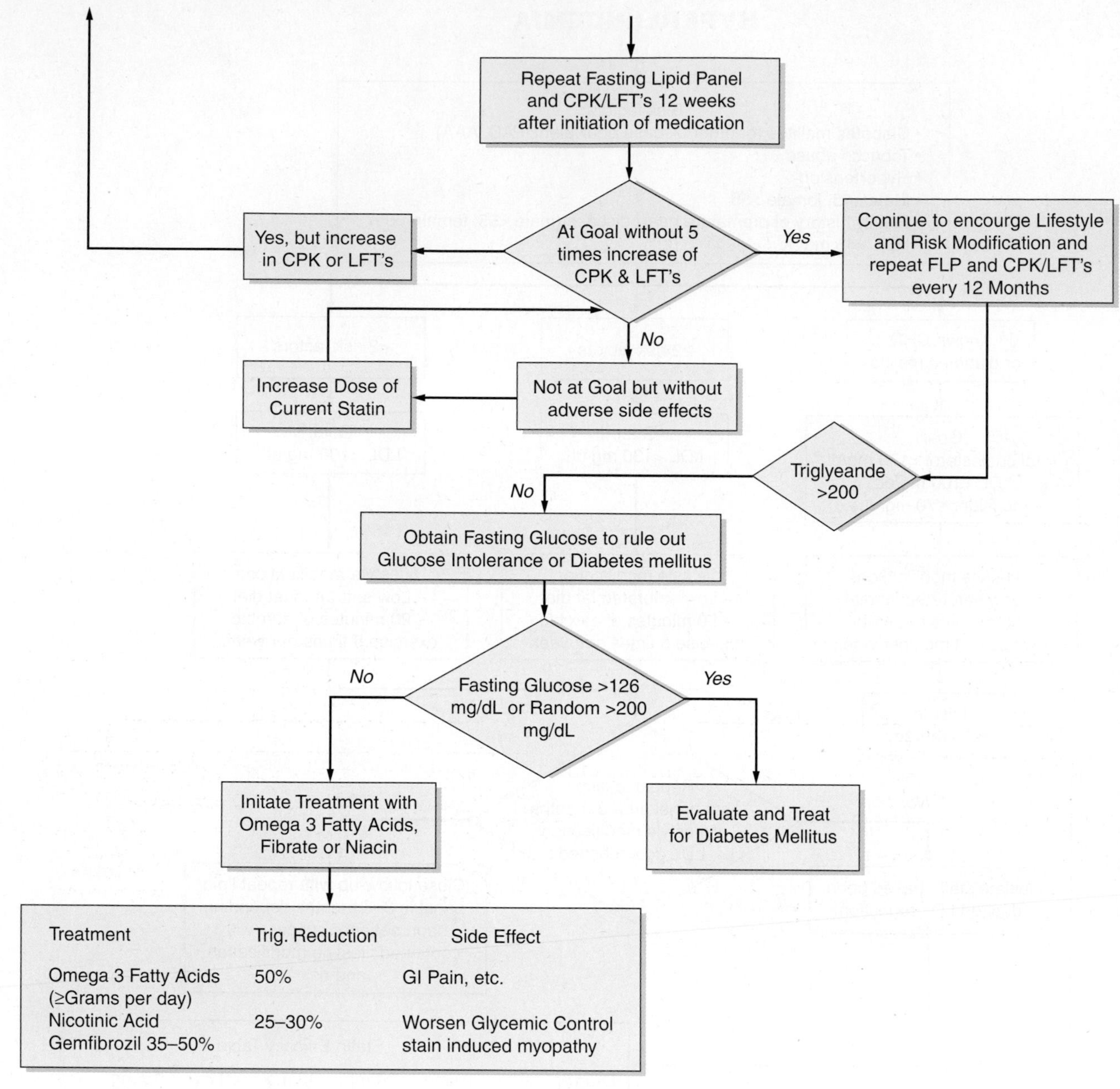

Rade N. Pejic, MD

Adv Ther. 2010;27(6):348–64.

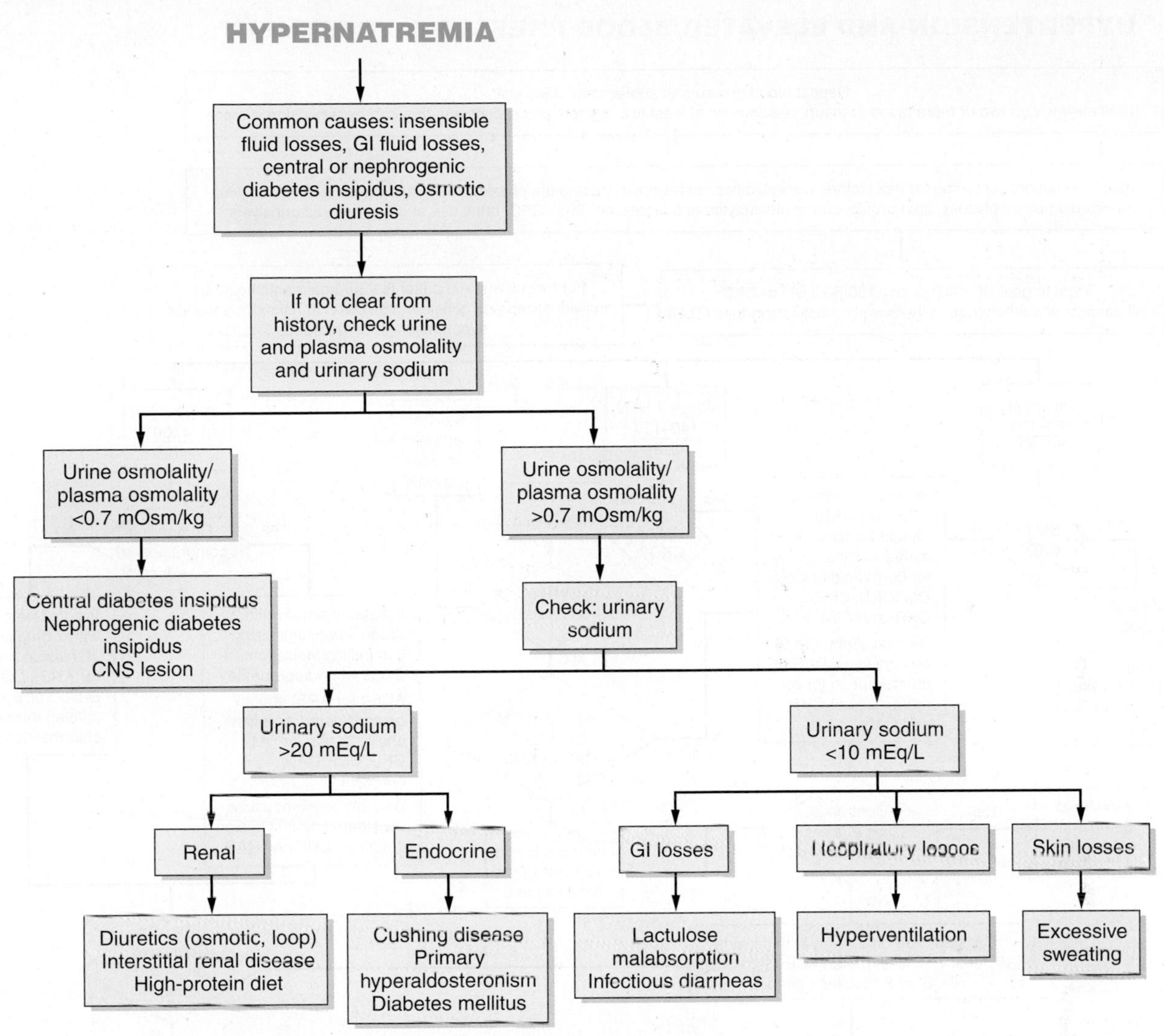
HYPERNATREMIA
Common causes: insensible fluid losses, GI fluid losses, central or nephrogenic diabetes insipidus, osmotic diuresis
If not clear from history, check urine and plasma osmolality and urinary sodium
Urine osmolality/ plasma osmolality <0.7 mOsm/kg
Central diabetes insipidus Nephrogenic diabetes insipidus CNS lesion
Urine osmolality/ plasma osmolality >0.7 mOsm/kg
Check: urinary sodium
Urinary sodium >20 mEq/L
Renal
Diuretics (osmotic, loop) Interstitial renal disease High-protein diet
Endocrine
Cushing disease Primary hyperaldosteronism Diabetes mellitus
Urinary sodium <10 mEq/L
GI losses
Lactulose malabsorption Infectious diarrheas
Respiratory losses
Hyperventilation
Skin losses
Excessive sweating

Robert A. Baldor, MD and Alan M. Ehrlich, MD

N Engl J Med. 2000;342(20):1493–9.

HYPERTENSION AND ELEVATED BLOOD PRESSURE, TREATMENT

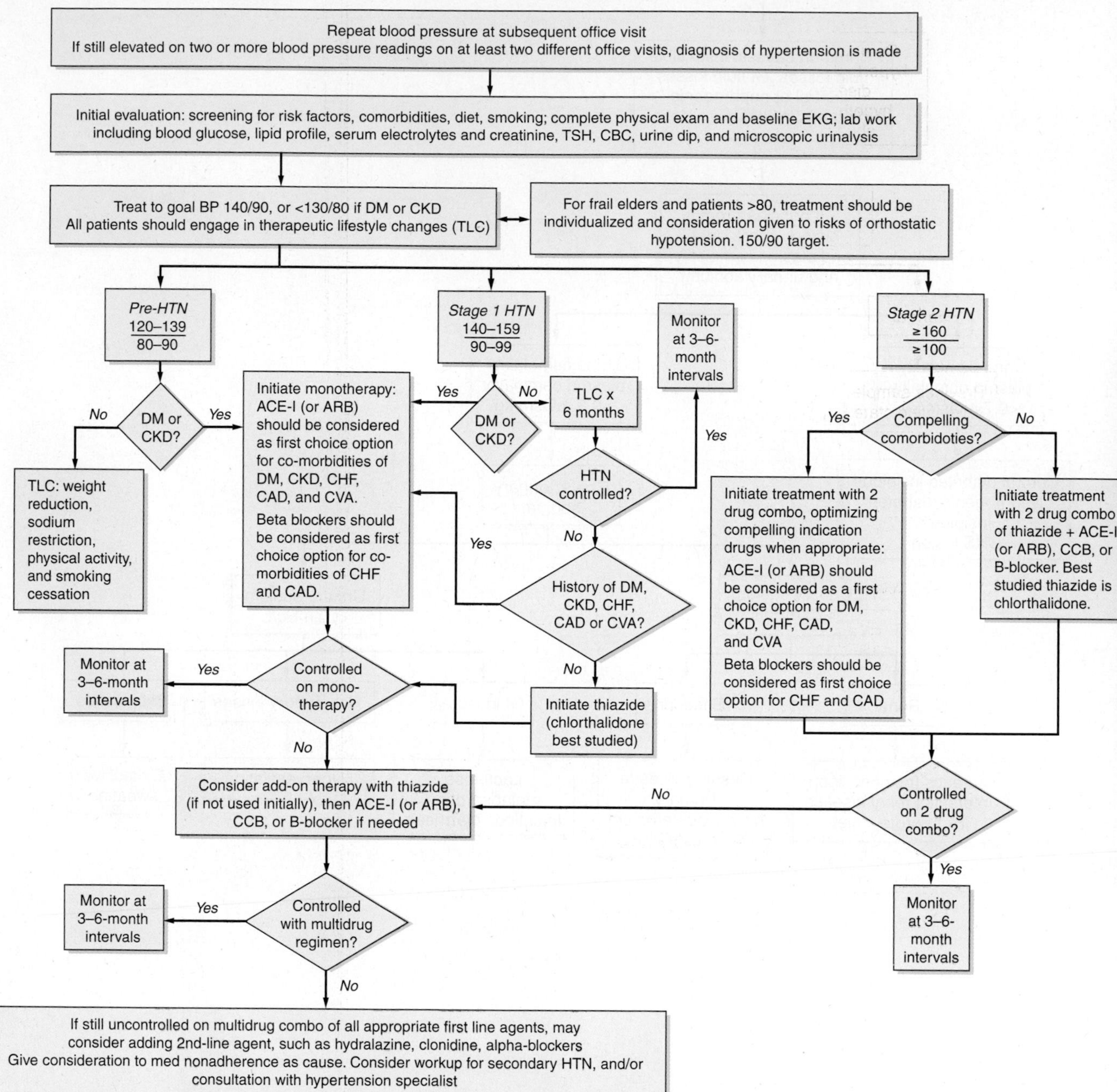
Repeat blood pressure at subsequent office visit
If still elevated on two or more blood pressure readings on at least two different office visits, diagnosis of hypertension is made
Initial evaluation: screening for risk factors, comorbidities, diet, smoking; complete physical exam and baseline EKG; lab work including blood glucose, lipid profile, serum electrolytes and creatinine, TSH, CBC, urine dip, and microscopic urinalysis
Treat to goal BP 140/90, or <130/80 if DM or CKD
All patients should engage in therapeutic lifestyle changes (TLC)
For frail elders and patients >80, treatment should be individualized and consideration given to risks of orthostatic hypotension. 150/90 target.
Pre-HTN
120–139
80–90
Stage 1 HTN
140–159
90–99
Stage 2 HTN
≥160
≥100
DM or CKD?
No
Yes
TLC: weight reduction, sodium restriction, physical activity, and smoking cessation
Initiate monotherapy: ACE-I (or ARB) should be considered as first choice option for co-morbidities of DM, CKD, CHF, CAD, and CVA.
Beta blockers should be considered as first choice option for co-morbidities of CHF and CAD.
Yes
No
DM or CKD?
TLC x 6 months
Monitor at 3–6-month intervals
Yes
HTN controlled?
No
Yes
History of DM, CKD, CHF, CAD or CVA?
No
Initiate thiazide (chlorthalidone best studied)
Monitor at 3–6-month intervals
Yes
Controlled on mono-therapy?
No
Yes
Compelling comorbidoties?
No
Initiate treatment with 2 drug combo, optimizing compelling indication drugs when appropriate: ACE-I (or ARB) should be considered as a first choice option for DM, CKD, CHF, CAD, and CVA
Beta blockers should be considered as first choice option for CHF and CAD
Initiate treatment with 2 drug combo of thiazide + ACE-I (or ARB), CCB, or B-blocker. Best studied thiazide is chlorthalidone.
Consider add-on therapy with thiazide (if not used initially), then ACE-I (or ARB), CCB, or B-blocker if needed
No
Controlled on 2 drug combo?
Yes
Monitor at 3–6-month intervals
Monitor at 3–6-month intervals
Yes
Controlled with multidrug regimen?
No
If still uncontrolled on multidrug combo of all appropriate first line agents, may consider adding 2nd-line agent, such as hydralazine, clonidine, alpha-blockers
Give consideration to med nonadherence as cause. Consider workup for secondary HTN, and/or consultation with hypertension specialist

B. Brent Simmons, MD

Hypertension. 2003;42:1206.

HYPERTRIGLYCERIDEMIA

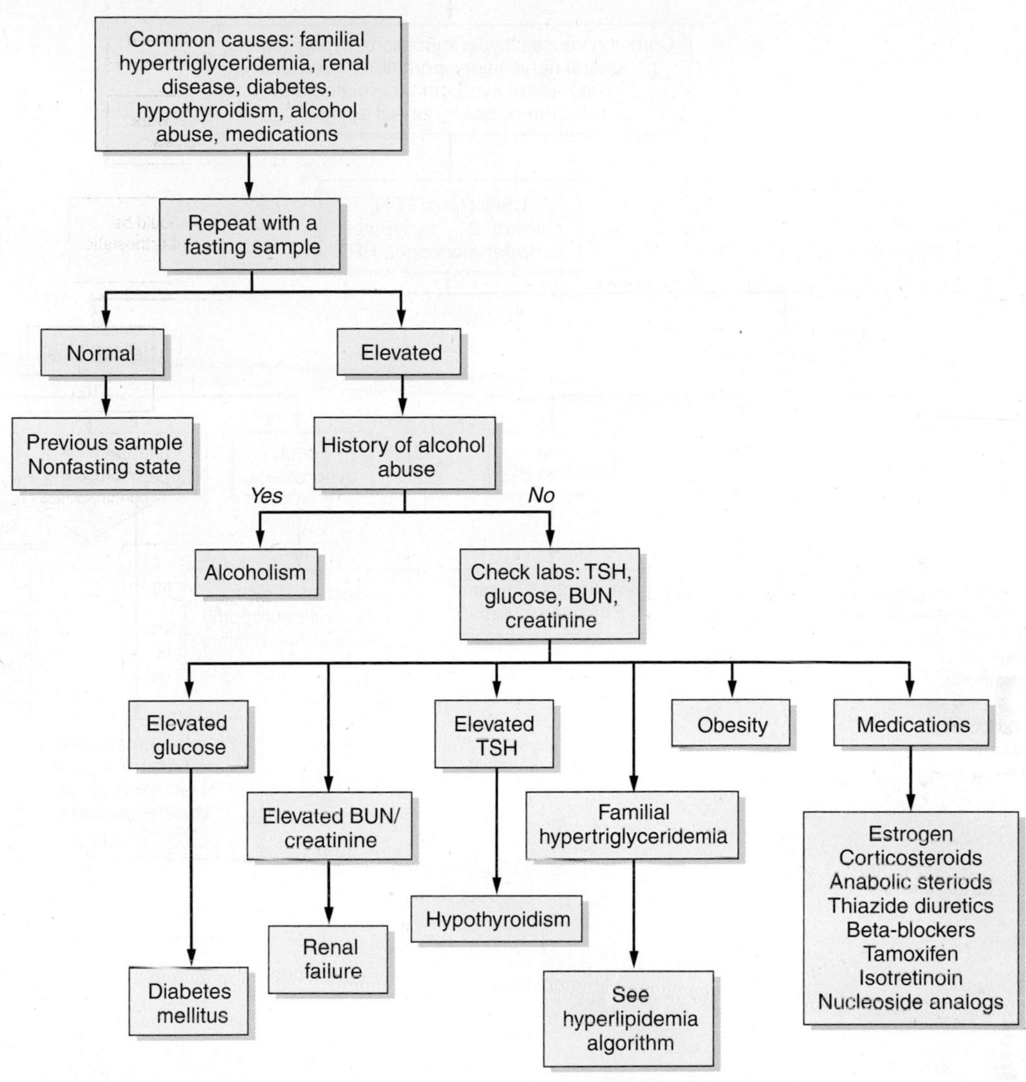

Robert A. Baldor, MD and Alan M. Ehrlich, MD

Am J Cardiol. 2001;87:1174.

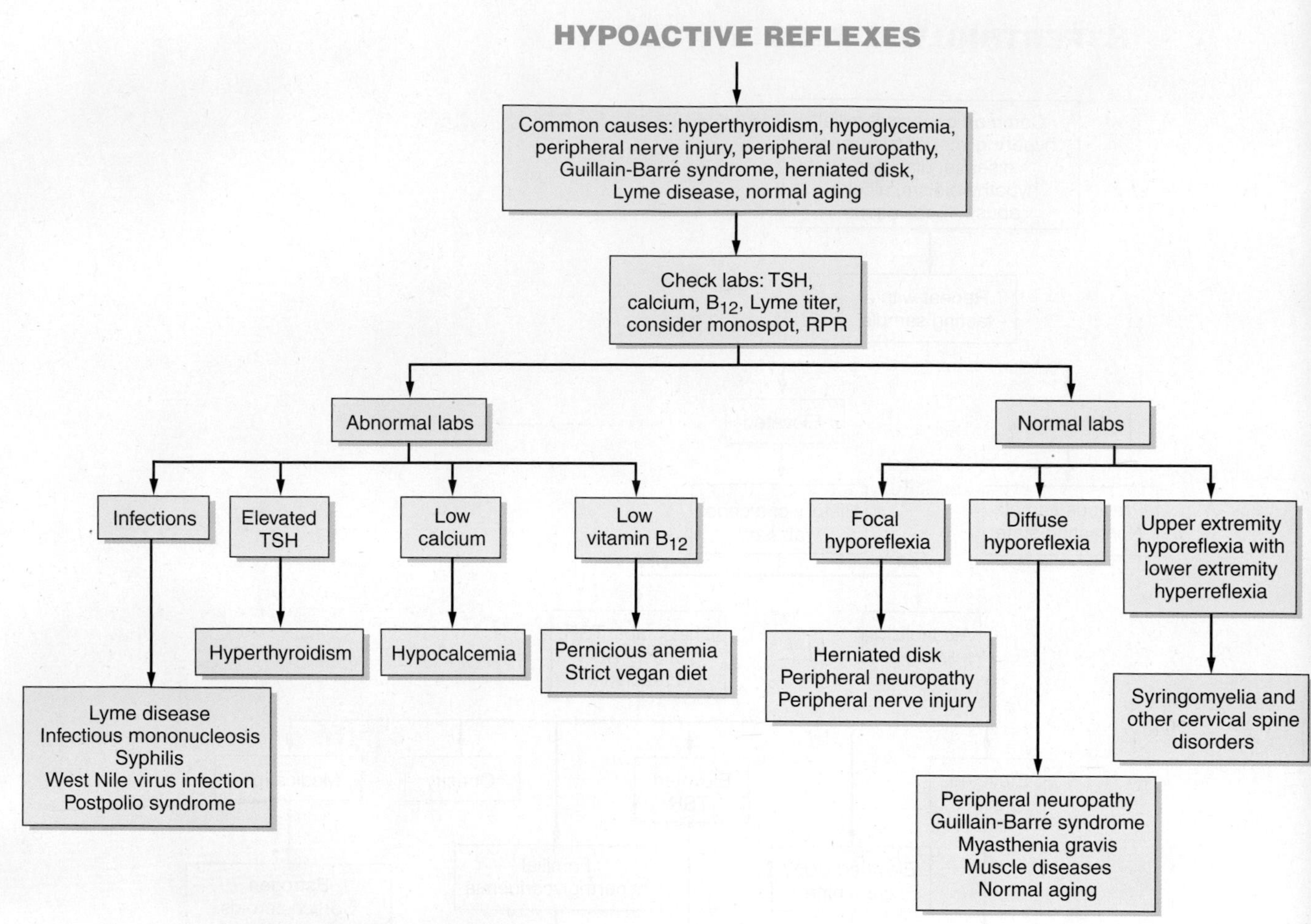

Robert A. Baldor, MD and Alan M. Ehrlich, MD

Med Clin North Am. 2009;93(2):317–42, vii–viii.

HYPOALBUMINEMIA

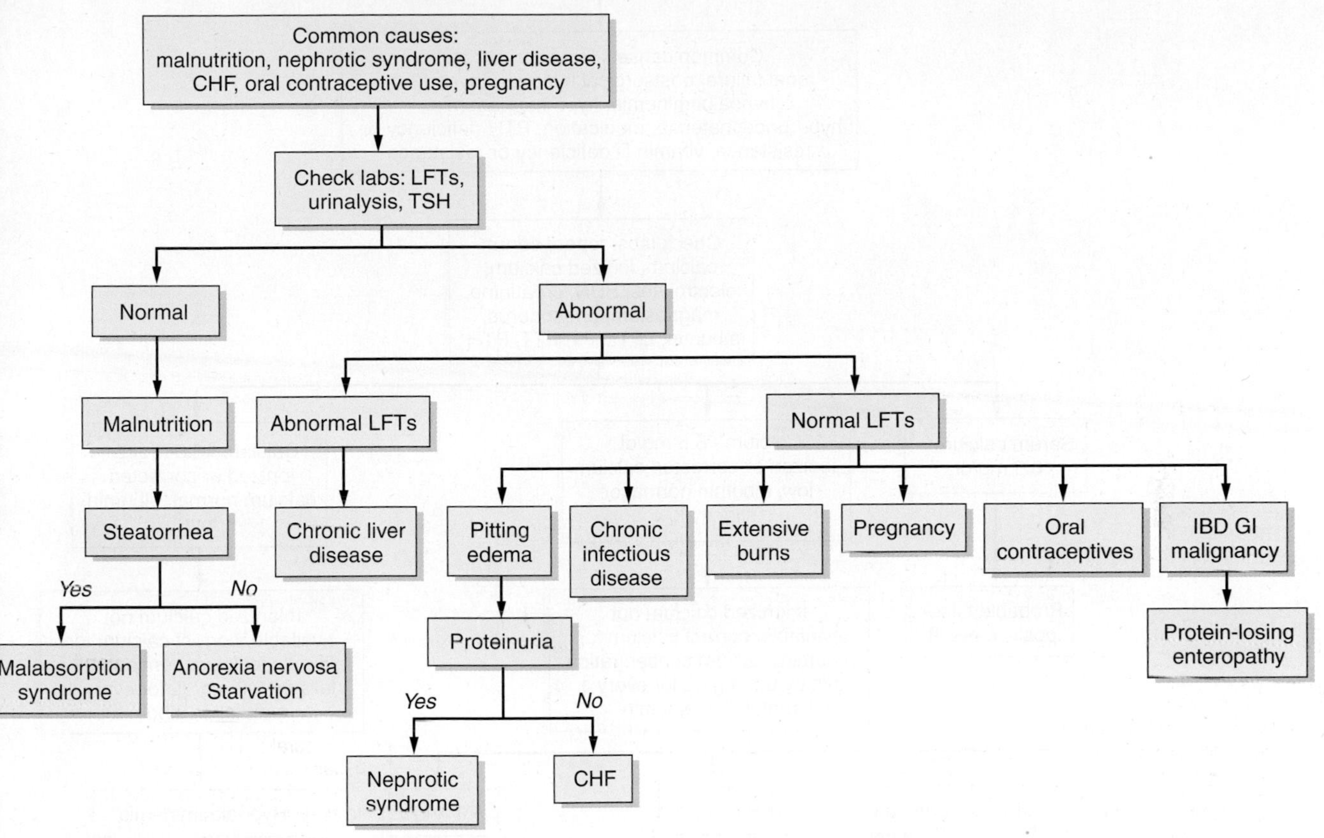

Robert A. Baldor, MD and Alan M. Ehrlich, MD

Am Fam Physician. 2009;80(10):1129–34.

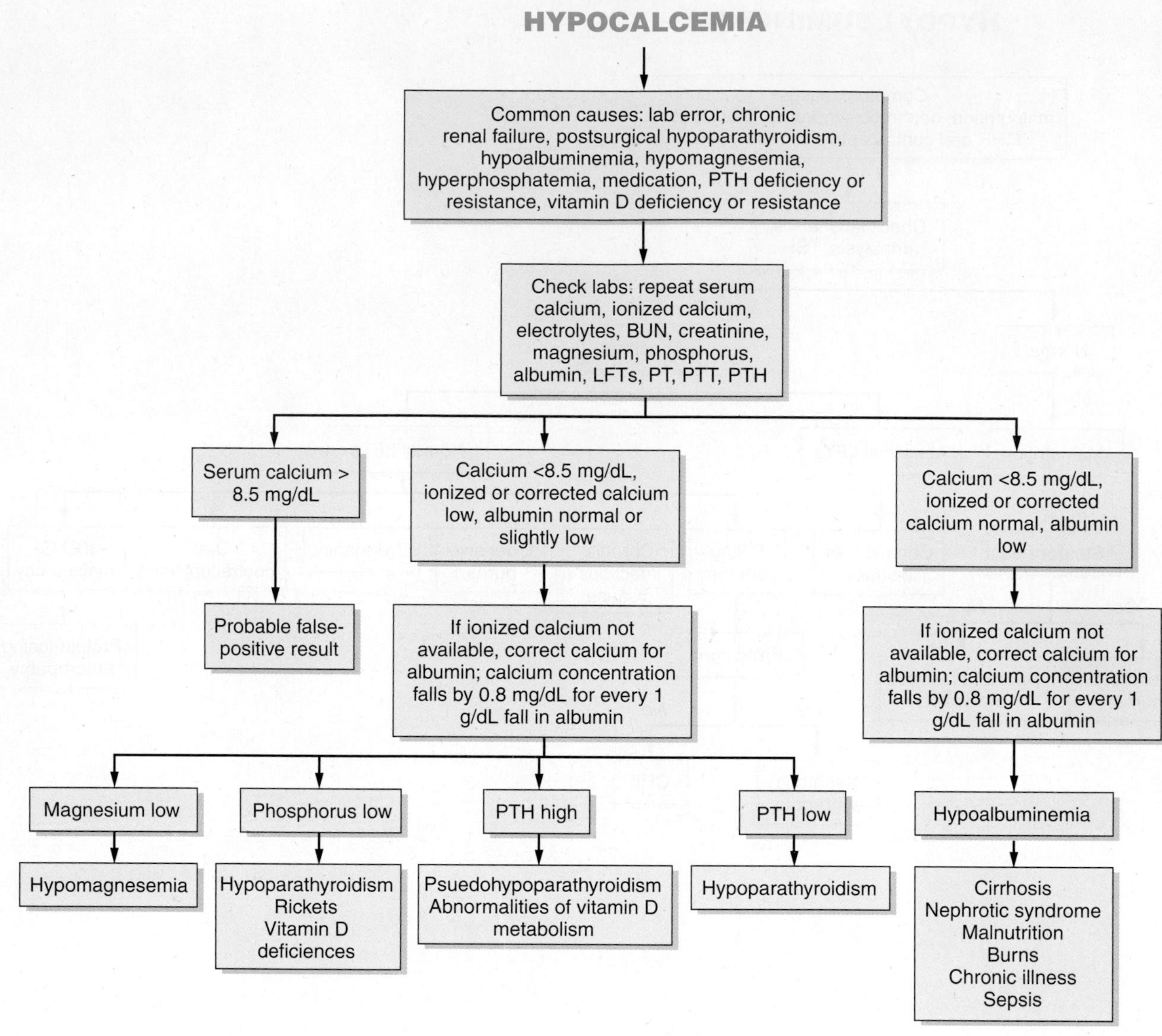

Robert A. Baldor, MD and Alan M. Ehrlich, MD

J Fam Pract. 2008;57(10):677–9.

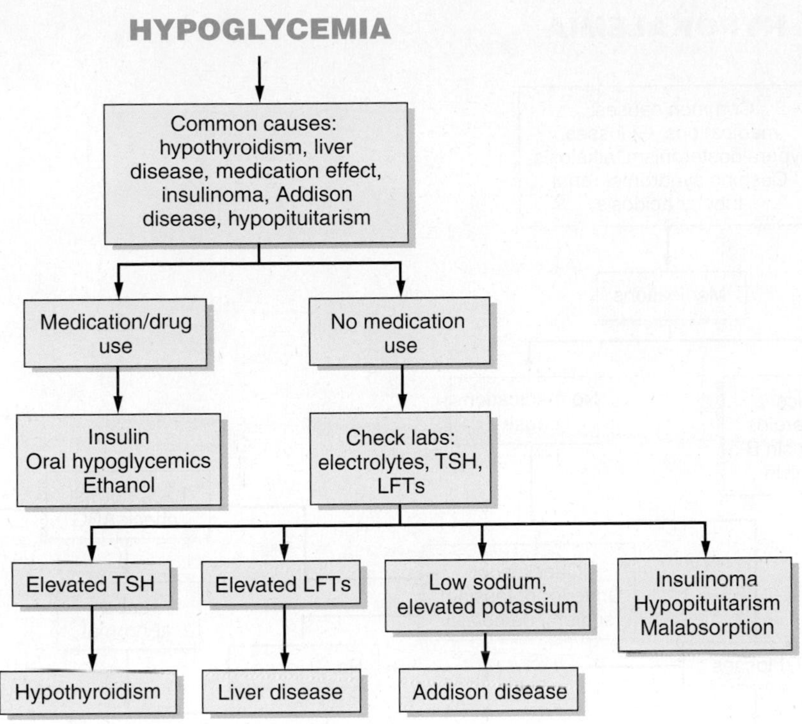

Robert A. Baldor, MD and Alan M. Ehrlich, MD

J Clin Endocrinol Metab. 2009;94(3):741–5. Epub 2008 Dec 16.

HYPOKALEMIA

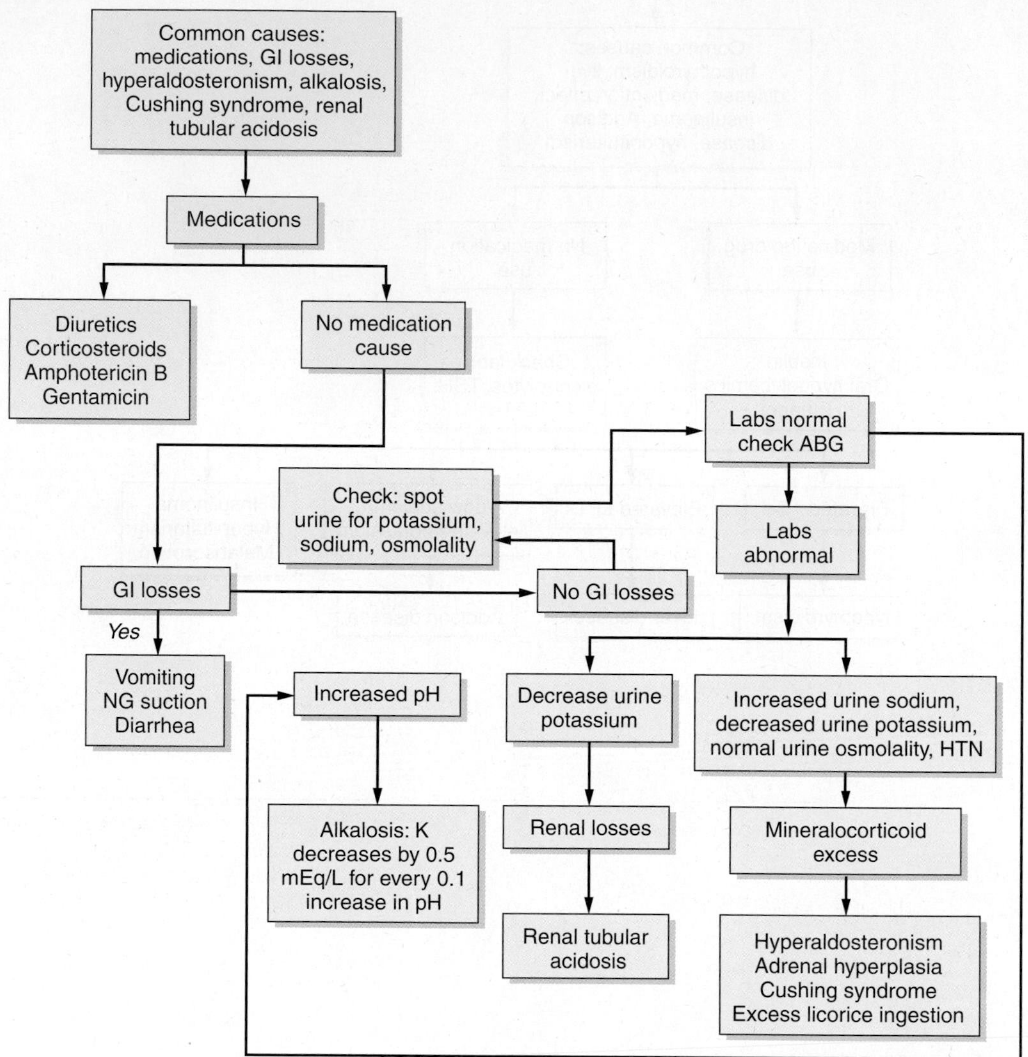

Robert A. Baldor, MD and Alan M. Ehrlich, MD

Ann Intern Med. 2009;150(9):619–25.

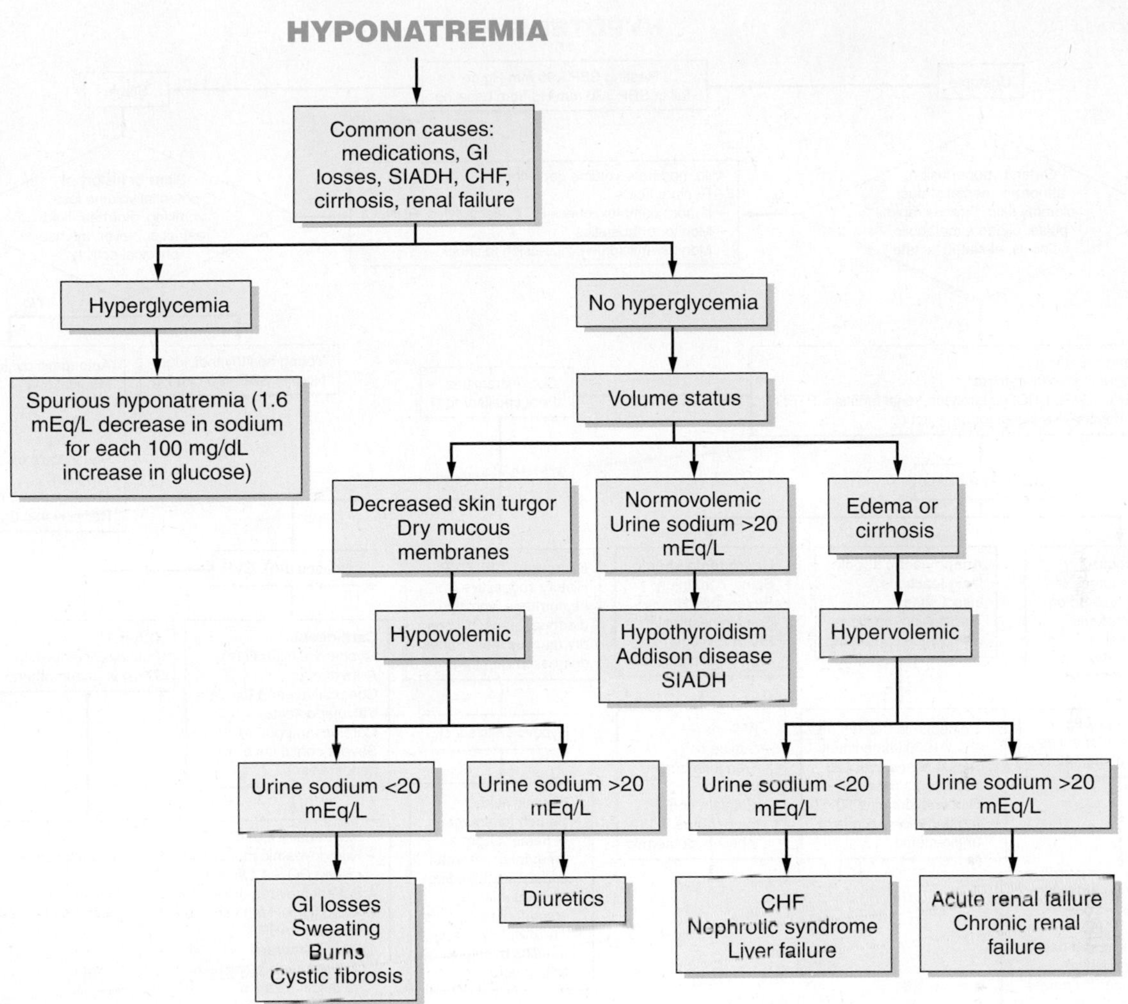
HYPONATREMIA
Common causes: medications, GI losses, SIADH, CHF, cirrhosis, renal failure
Hyperglycemia
No hyperglycemia
Spurious hyponatremia (1.6 mEq/L decrease in sodium for each 100 mg/dL increase in glucose)
Volume status
Decreased skin turgor Dry mucous membranes
Normovolemic Urine sodium >20 mEq/L
Edema or cirrhosis
Hypovolemic
Hypothyroidism Addison disease SIADH
Hypervolemic
Urine sodium <20 mEq/L
Urine sodium >20 mEq/L
Urine sodium <20 mEq/L
Urine sodium >20 mEq/L
GI losses Sweating Burns Cystic fibrosis
Diuretics
CHF Nephrotic syndrome Liver failure
Acute renal failure Chronic renal failure

Robert A. Baldor, MD and Alan M. Ehrlich, MD

Am J Med. 2007;120(8):653–8.

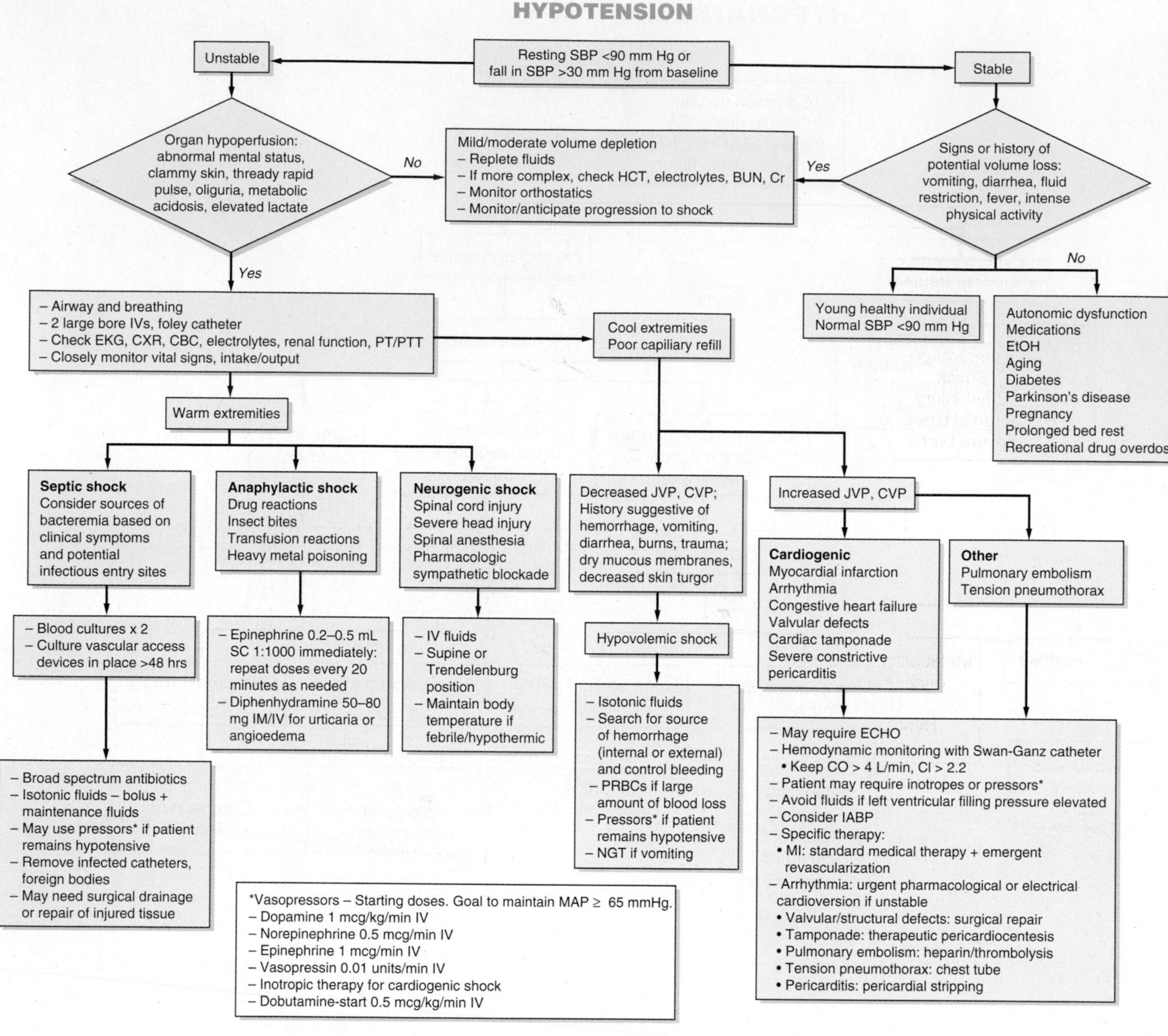

Martin A. Espinosa Ginic, MD and Bryan K. Moffett, MD

Arch Phys Med Rehabil. 2009;90(5):876–85.

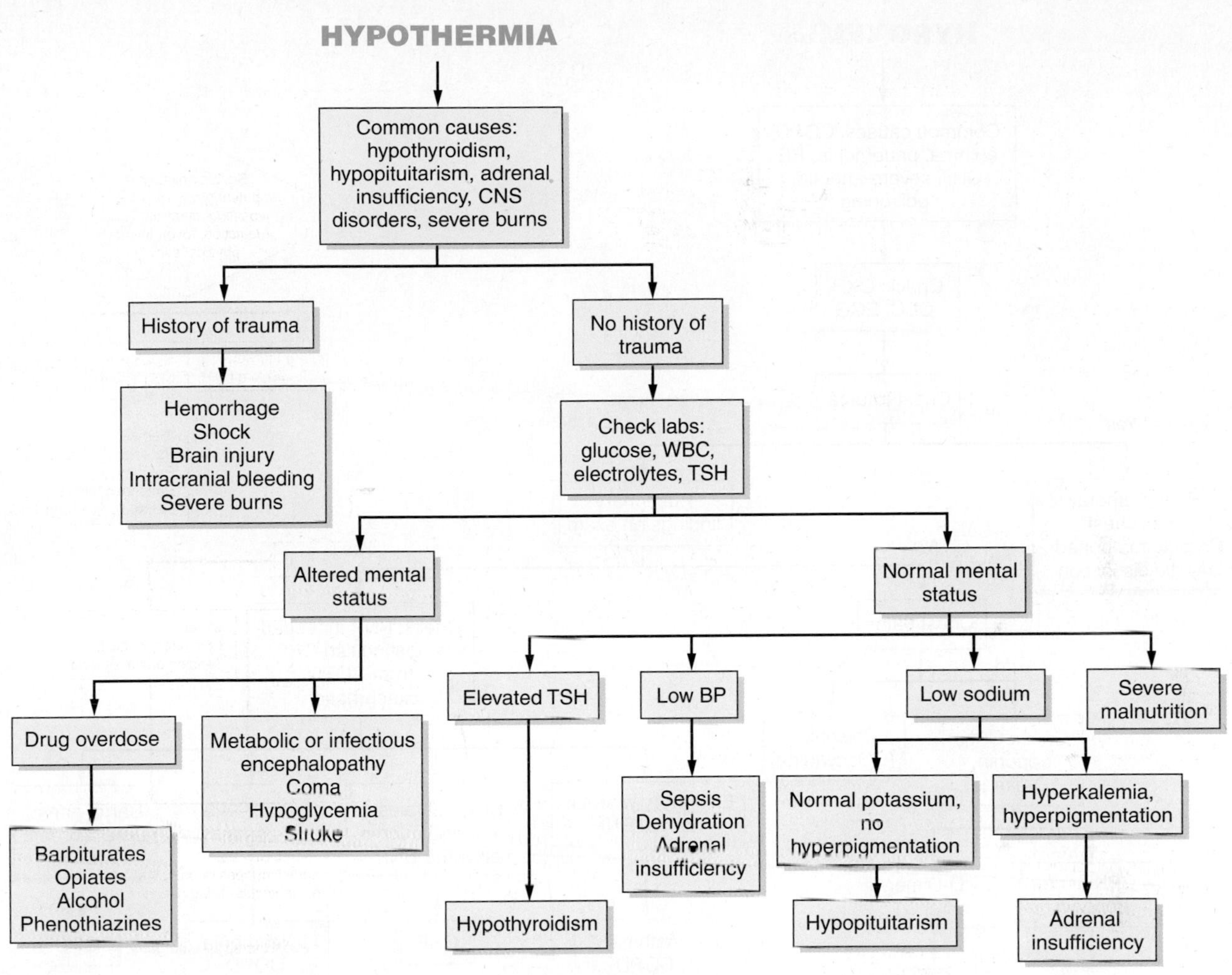

Robert A. Baldor, MD and Alan M. Ehrlich, MD

Am J Med. 2006;119(4):297–301.

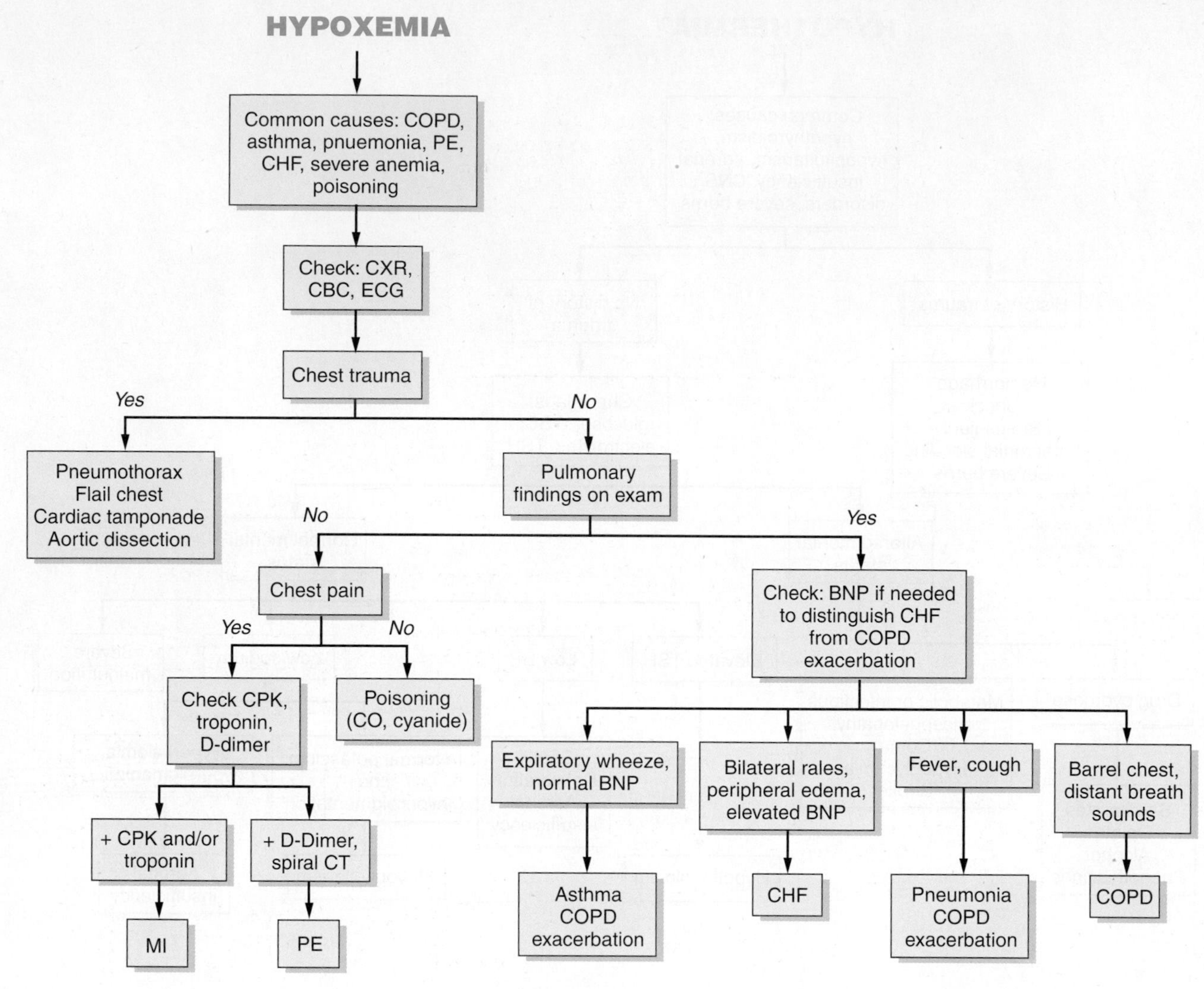

Robert A. Baldor, MD and Alan M. Ehrlich, MD

Lancet. 2009;374(9691):721–32.

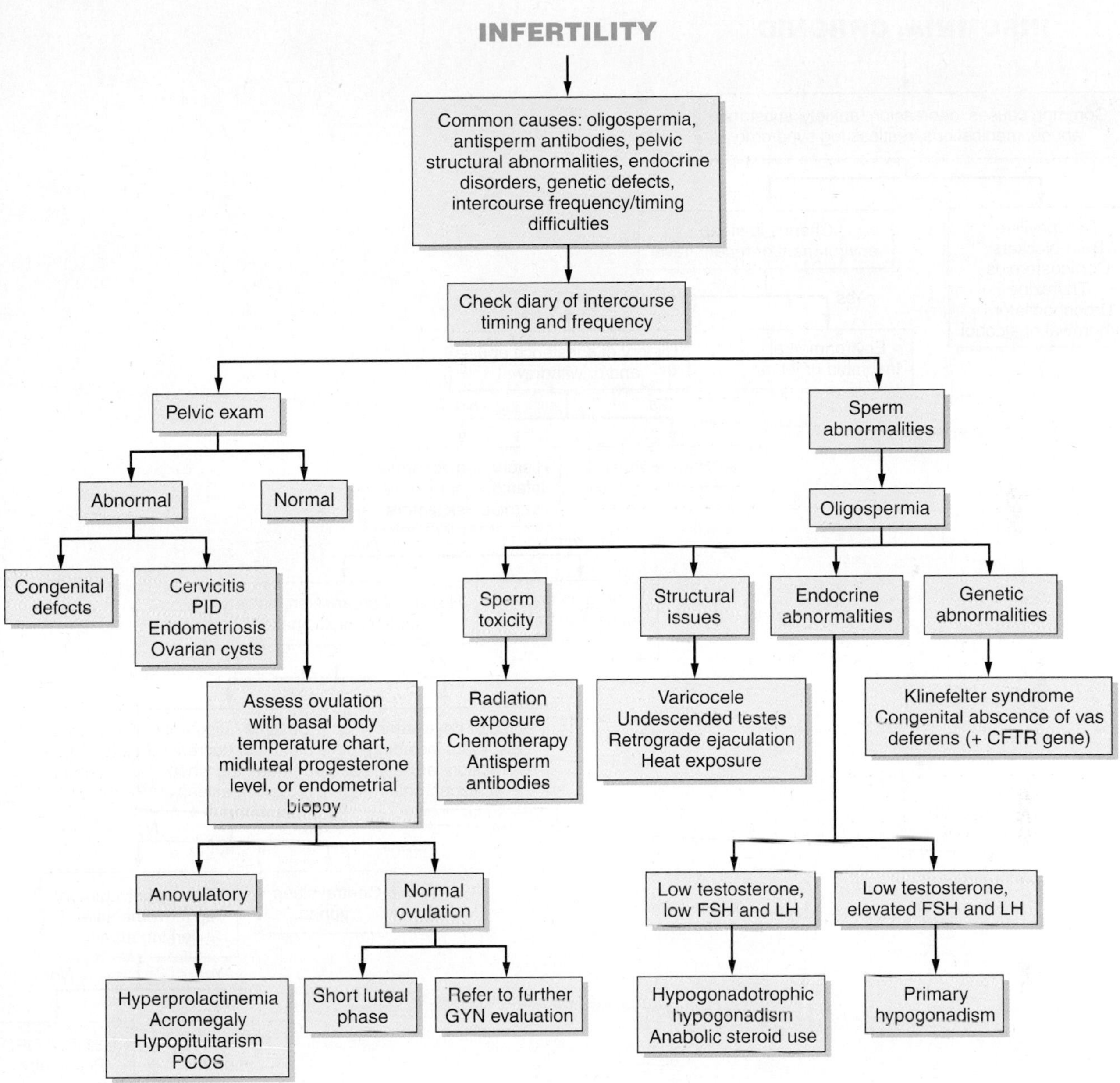
INFERTILITY
Common causes: oligospermia, antisperm antibodies, pelvic structural abnormalities, endocrine disorders, genetic defects, intercourse frequency/timing difficulties
Check diary of intercourse timing and frequency
Pelvic exam
Abnormal
Normal
Congenital defects
Cervicitis
PID
Endometriosis
Ovarian cysts
Assess ovulation with basal body temperature chart, midluteal progesterone level, or endometrial biopsy
Anovulatory
Normal ovulation
Hyperprolactinemia
Acromegaly
Hypopituitarism
PCOS
Short luteal phase
Refer to further GYN evaluation
Sperm abnormalities
Oligospermia
Sperm toxicity
Structural issues
Endocrine abnormalities
Genetic abnormalities
Radiation exposure
Chemotherapy
Antisperm antibodies
Varicocele
Undescended testes
Retrograde ejaculation
Heat exposure
Klinefelter syndrome
Congenital absence of vas deferens (+ CFTR gene)
Low testosterone, low FSH and LH
Low testosterone, elevated FSH and LH
Hypogonadotrophic hypogonadism
Anabolic steroid use
Primary hypogonadism

Robert A. Baldor, MD and Alan M. Ehrlich, MD

Med Clin North Am. 2008;92(5):1163–92, xi.

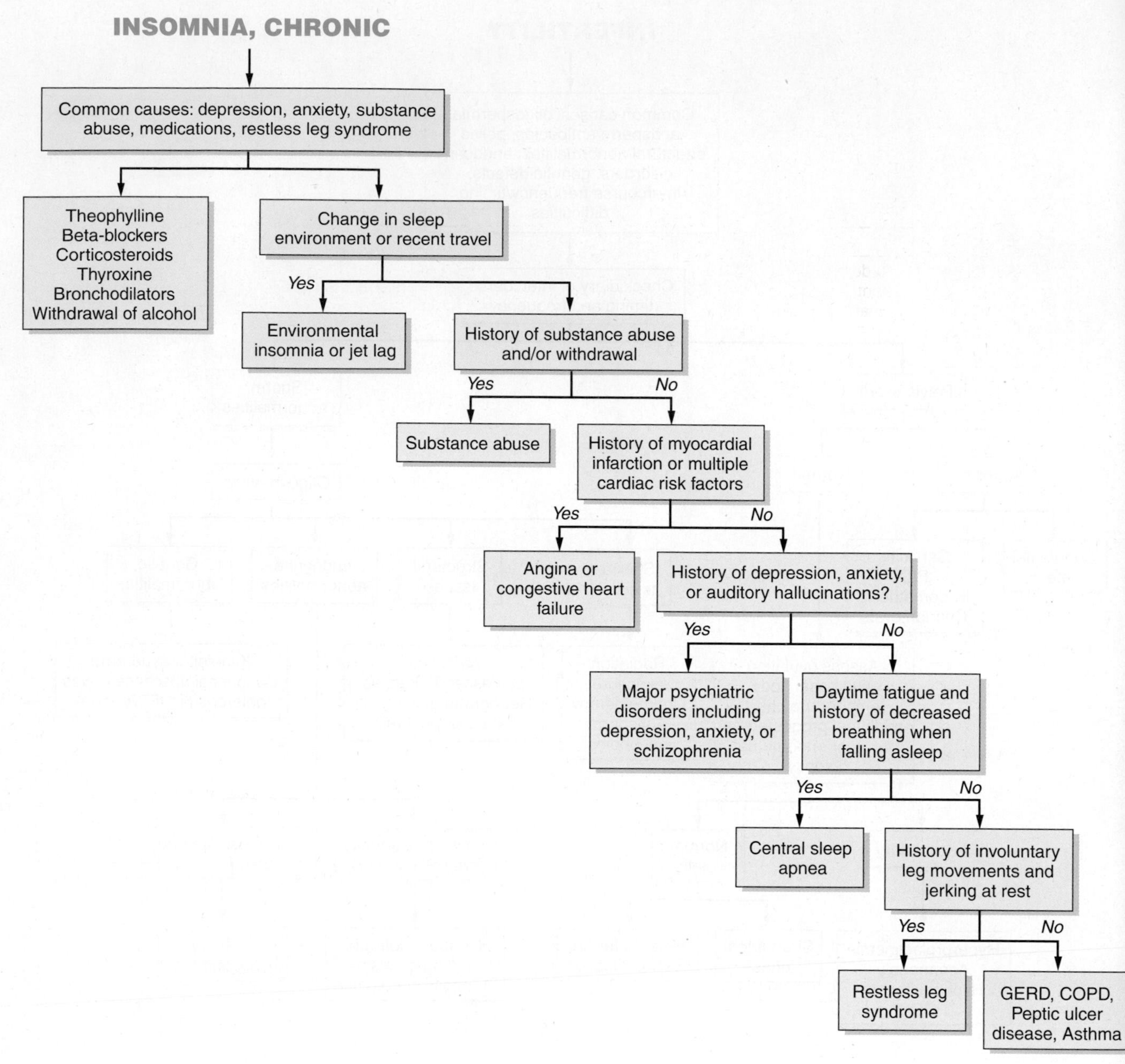

Robert A. Baldor, MD and Alan M. Ehrlich, MD

Am Fam Physician. 2007;76(4):517–26.

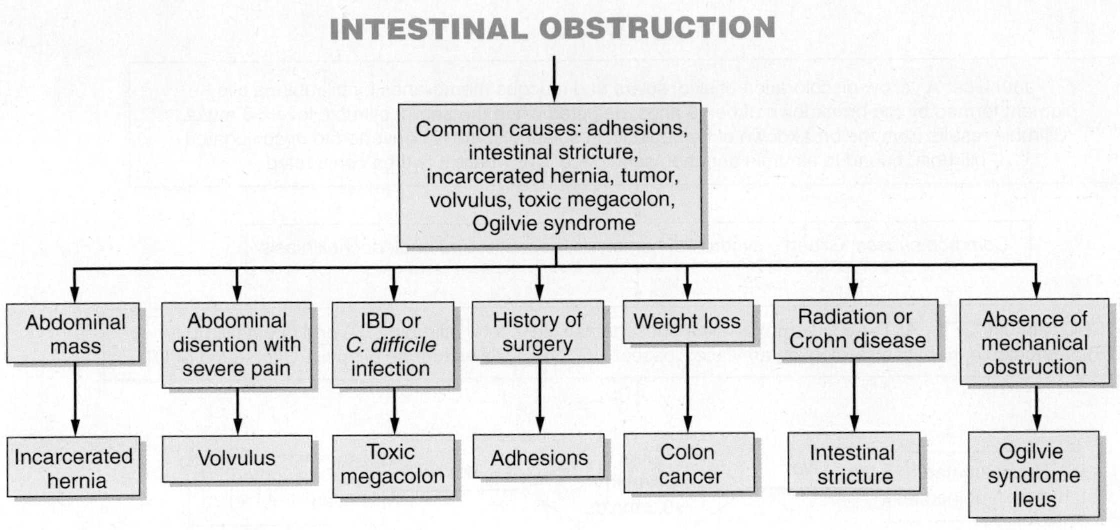

Robert A. Baldor, MD and Alan M. Ehrlich, MD

Med Clin North Am. 2008;92(3):575–97, viii.

JAUNDICE

Jaundice: A yellow discoloration of skin, sclera and mucous membranes by bilirubin, a bile pigment formed by the breakdown of heme rings; detected when the serum bilirubin level >3 mg/dL. Bilirubin results from the breakdown of hemoglobin in spleen. Heme is converted to unconjugated bilirubin, bound to albumin and then sent to the liver where it is then conjugated.

↓

Common causes: Gilbert's syndrome, hemolysis, hepatitis, and choledocholithiasis

↓

CBC with diff, LFTs: ALT, AST, serum alkaline phosphatase (AP), total bilirubin (TB) and direct bilirubin (DB), haptoglobin, hepatitis serologies, amylase, lipase, hCG, urinalysis with urine bilirubin. Ultrasound or CT

↓

Direct bilirubin >0.3 mg/dL
- *No* → Unconjugated hyperbilirubinemia
- *Yes* → Conjugated hyperbilirubinemia

Unconjugated hyperbilirubinemia → Elevated AP
- *Yes* → Intrahepatic
- *No* → Prehepatic

Conjugated hyperbilirubinemia → Obstruction on imaging
- *No* → Intrahepatic
- *Yes* → Extrahepatic

Prehepatic:

- **Hemolytic anemia**
- **Reabsorption of large hematoma**

Labs: Anemia, possible reticulocytosis, mild TB elevation (5 mg/dL), increased indirect bilirubin, normal DB levels and negative urine bilirubin. All other LTs are normal.

Intrahepatic:

Unconjugated hyperbilirubinemia

Enzyme defects:

- **Gilbert's syndrome:** Mild defect in UDP glucuronosyltransferase (UGT, responsible for conjugation of bilirubin)
- **Crigler-Najjar syndromes:** More severe defect in UGT, usually presents during infancy
- ***Conjugated hyperbilirubinemia***
- **Dublin-Johnson syndrome:** Defective secretion of conjugated bilirubin
- **Rotor's syndrome**

Both Conjugated & Unconjugated Hepatocellular injury:

- **Hepatitis:** Viral, alcohol, or autoimmune insult leading to inflammation which impedes or prevents transport/secretion of conjugated bilirubin
- **Medication/drug:** Acetaminophen
- **Cirrhosis**
- **Congestive heart failure:** Hypoxia/anoxia of hepatocytes leads to cellular injury.

- **Intrahepatic cholestasis:** (Elevated LTs, primarily AP. US shows normal sized bile duct(s).)

- **Medication/drug induced**
- **Total parenteral nutrition (TPN)**
- **Sepsis**
- **Sarcoidosis**
- **Pregnancy**

Extrahepatic:

Extrahepatic cholestasis (Labs: Elevated TB and DB, elevated AP and positive urine bilirubin. US shows dilated bile duct(s).

- Choledocholithiasis
- Chronic pancreatitis alcohol
- **Cholangitis:** Fever, pain and jaundice, altered mental status, sepsis
- **Biliary structure:** History of surgical/invasive procedure
- Primary biliary cirrhosis
- Primary sclerosing cholangitis
- **Biliary tract tumor/cholangiocarcinoma:** Hepatomegaly, weight loss, abdominal pain
- **Pancreatic tumor:** Painless jaundice, palpable gallbladder (rare)

Krunal Patel, MD and John K. Zawacki, MD

Am Fam Physician. 2004;60(2):200–305.

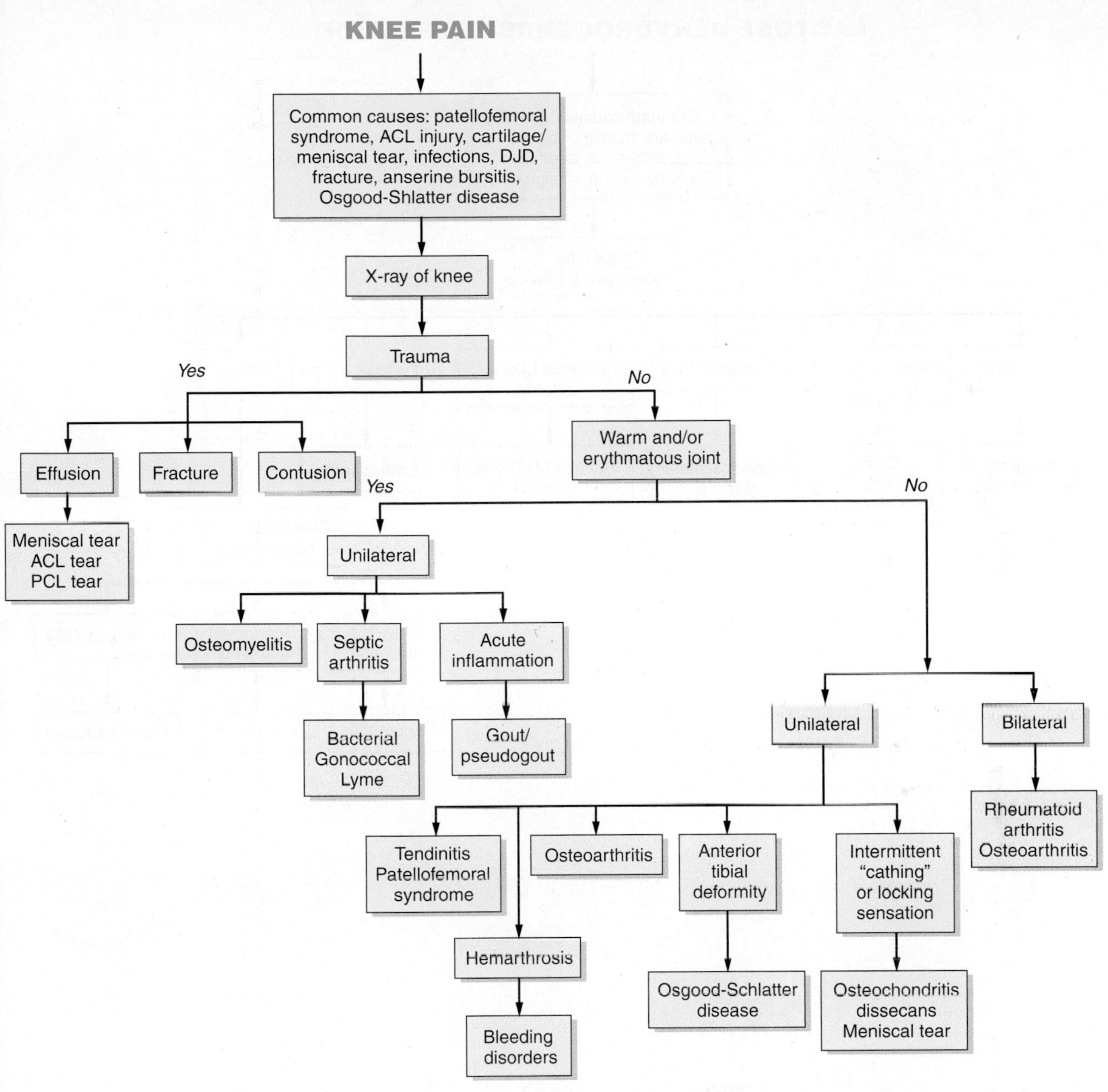
KNEE PAIN
Common causes: patellofemoral syndrome, ACL injury, cartilage/ meniscal tear, infections, DJD, fracture, anserine bursitis, Osgood-Shlatter disease
X-ray of knee
Trauma
Yes
No
Effusion
Fracture
Contusion
Meniscal tear ACL tear PCL tear
Warm and/or erythmatous joint
Yes
No
Unilateral
Osteomyelitis
Septic arthritis
Acute inflammation
Bacterial Gonococcal Lyme
Gout/ pseudogout
Unilateral
Bilateral
Rheumatoid arthritis Osteoarthritis
Tendinitis Patellofemoral syndrome
Osteoarthritis
Anterior tibial deformity
Intermittent "cathing" or locking sensation
Hemarthrosis
Osgood-Schlatter disease
Osteochondritis dissecans Meniscal tear
Bleeding disorders

Robert A. Baldor, MD and Alan M. Ehrlich, MD

J Fam Pract. 2008;57(2):116–8.

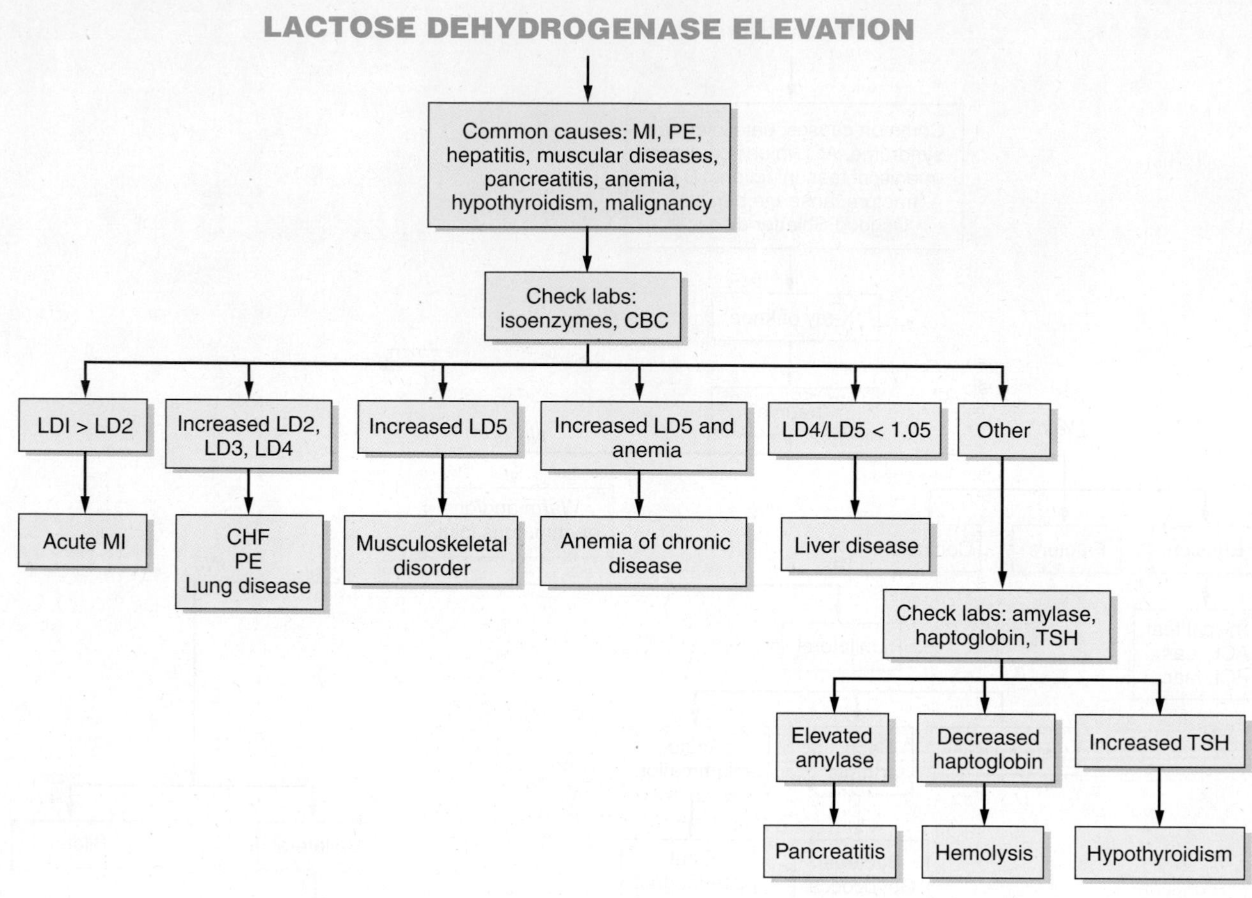

Robert A. Baldor, MD and Alan M. Ehrlich, MD

Ann Int Med. 1991;115(12):931–5.

LEG ULCER

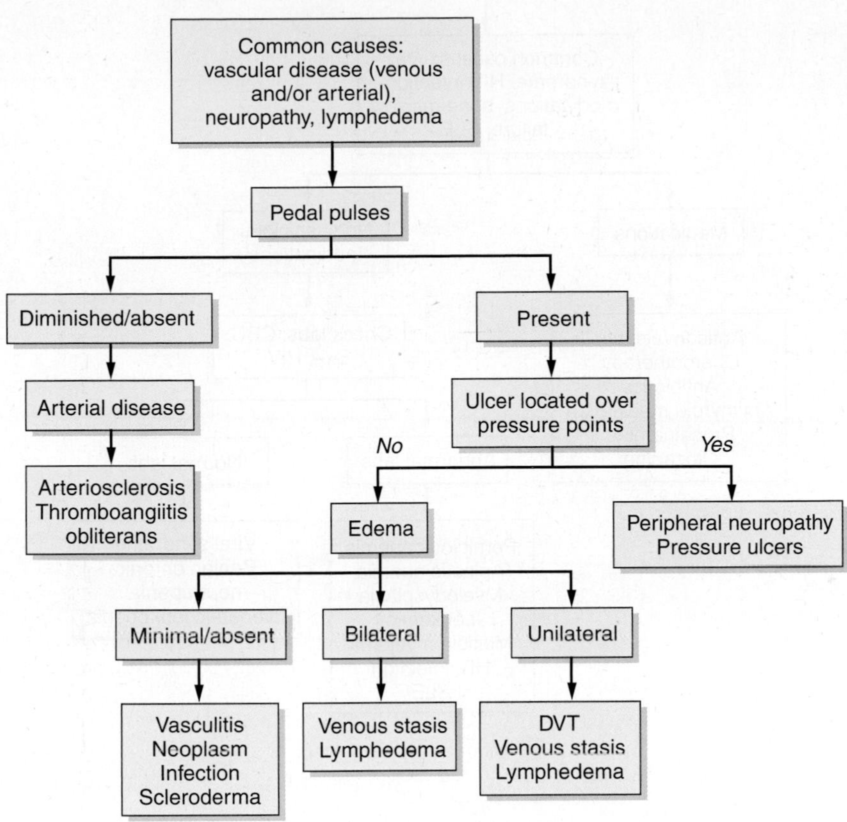

Robert A. Baldor, MD and Alan M. Ehrlich, MD

Surg Clin North Am. 2007;87(5):1149–77, x.

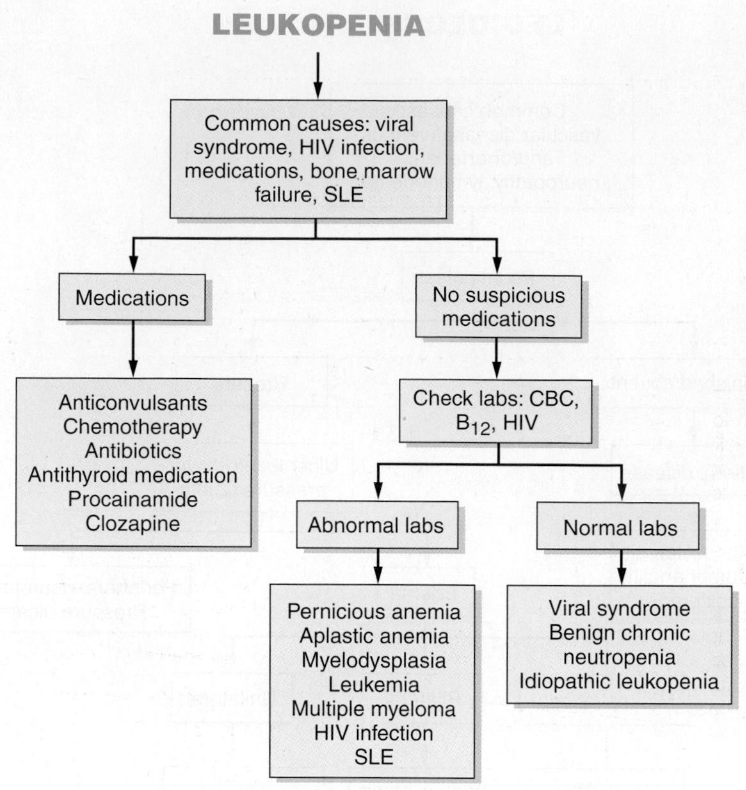

Robert A. Baldor, MD and Alan M. Ehrlich, MD

Mayo Clin Proc. 2005;80(7):923–36.

LOW BACK PAIN, ACUTE

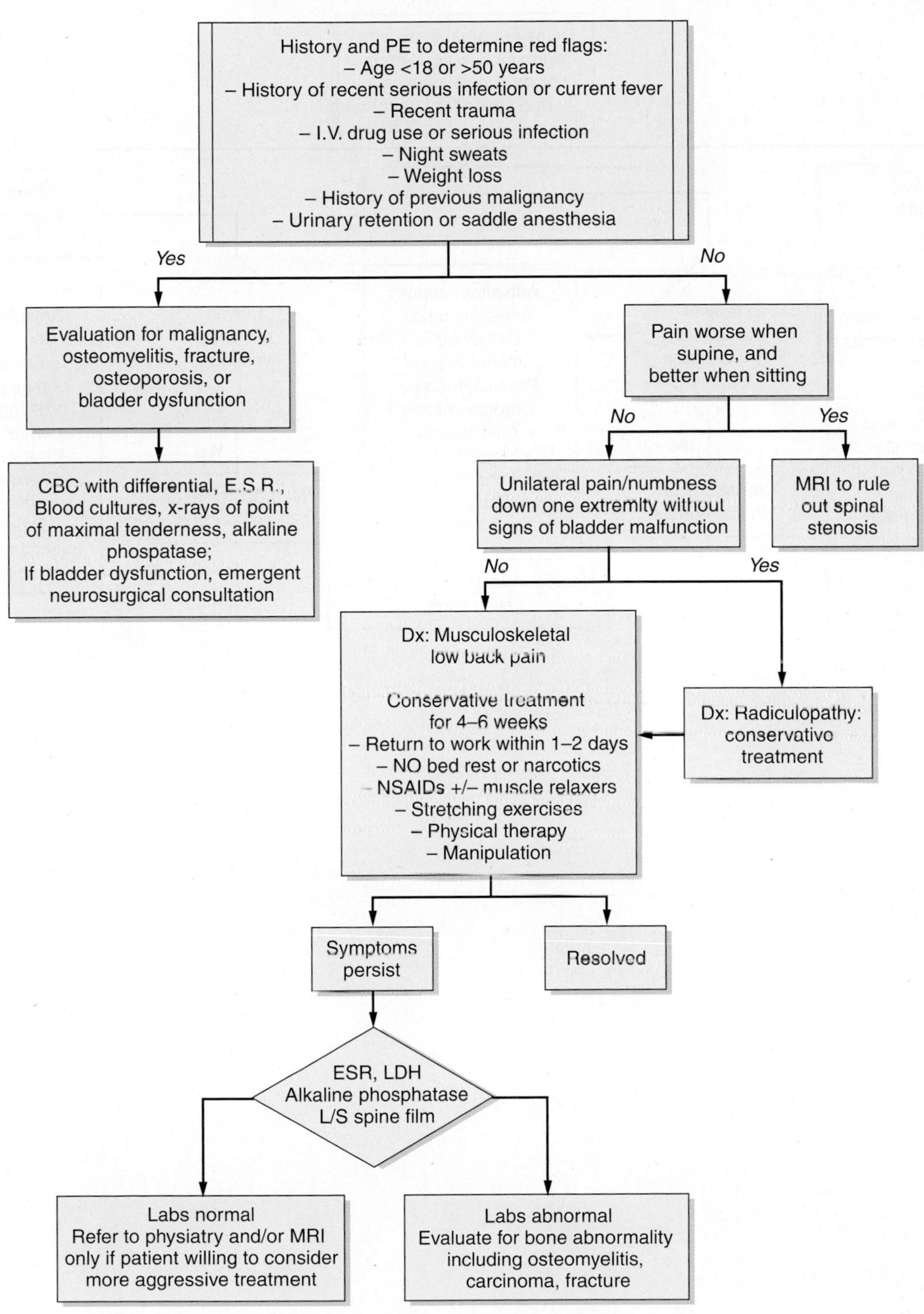

Patricia Bruno, MD

Med Clin North Am. 2009;93(2):477–501, x.

LOW BACK PAIN, CHRONIC

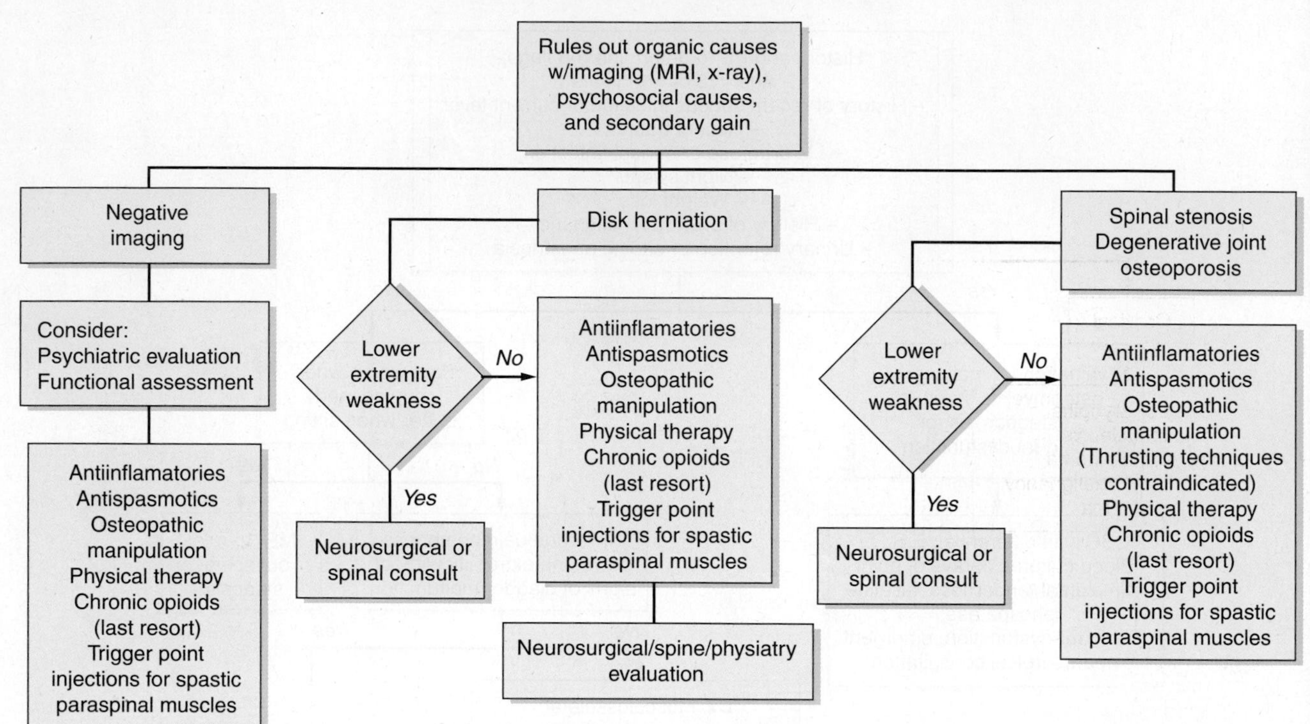

Patricia Bruno, MD

Spine. 2009;34(7):718–24.

LYMPHADENOPATHY

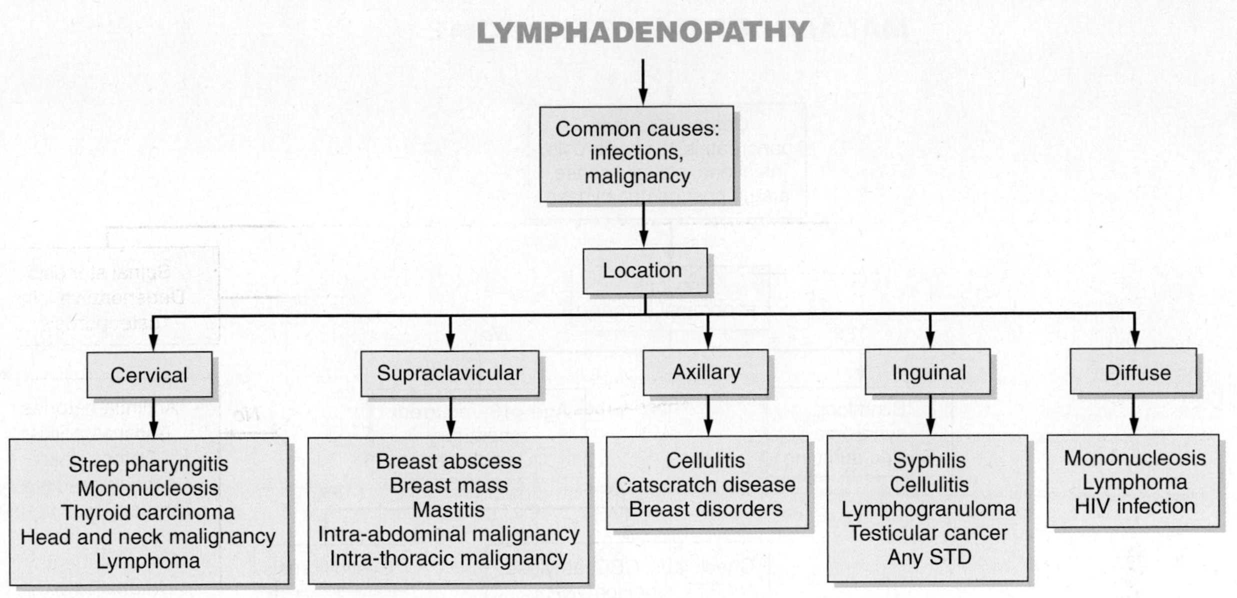

Robert A. Baldor, MD and Alan M. Ehrlich, MD

Radiol Clin North Am. 2008;46(2):175–98, vii.

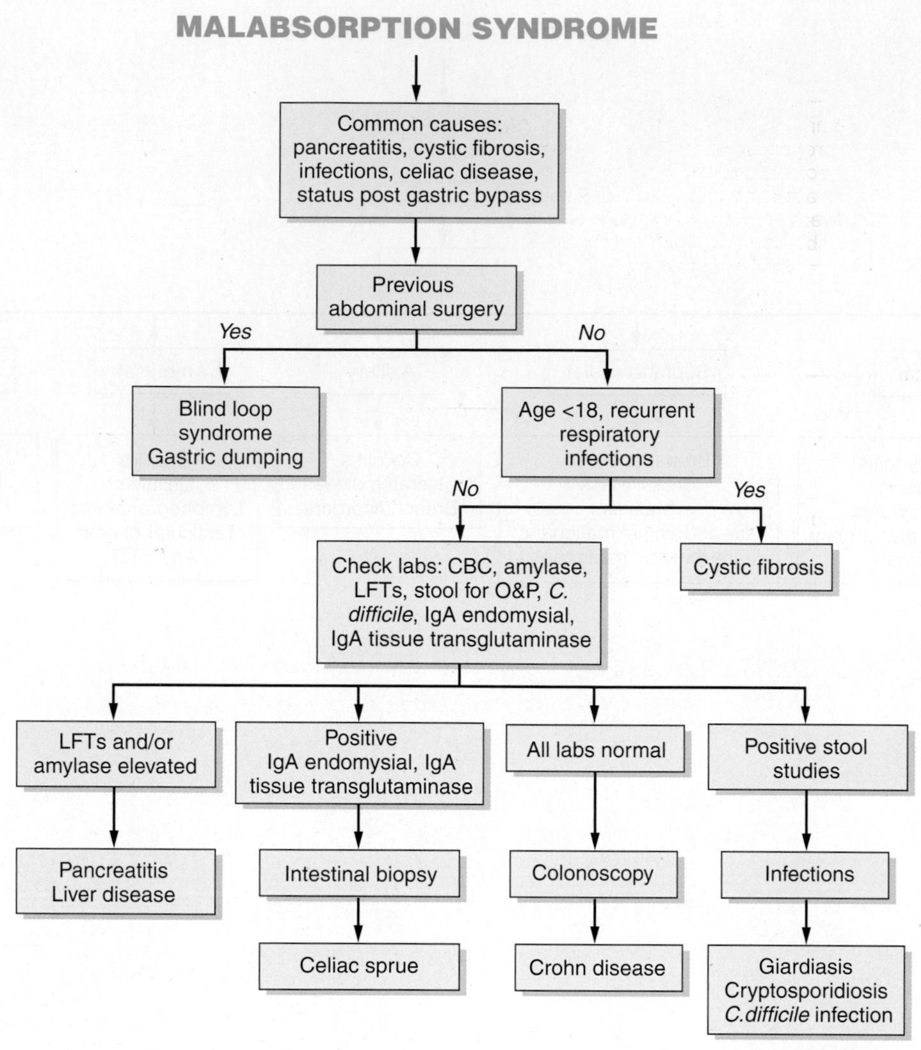

Robert A. Baldor, MD and Alan M. Ehrlich, MD

Pediatr Clin North Am. 2009;56(5):1105–21.

MENORRHAGIA (EXCESSIVE BLEEDING)

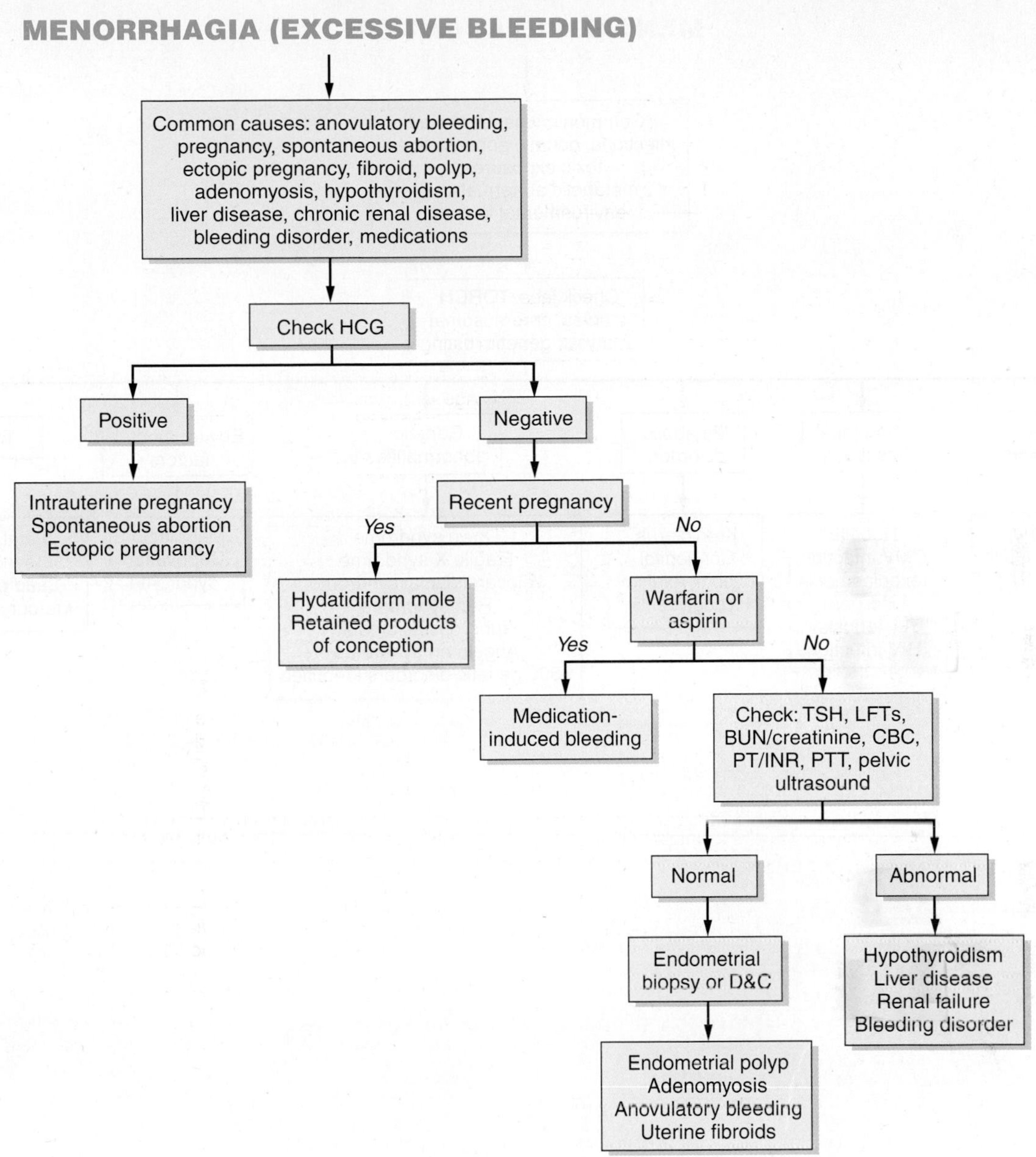

Robert A. Baldor, MD and Alan M. Ehrlich, MD

Am Fam Physician. 2004;69(8):1915–26.

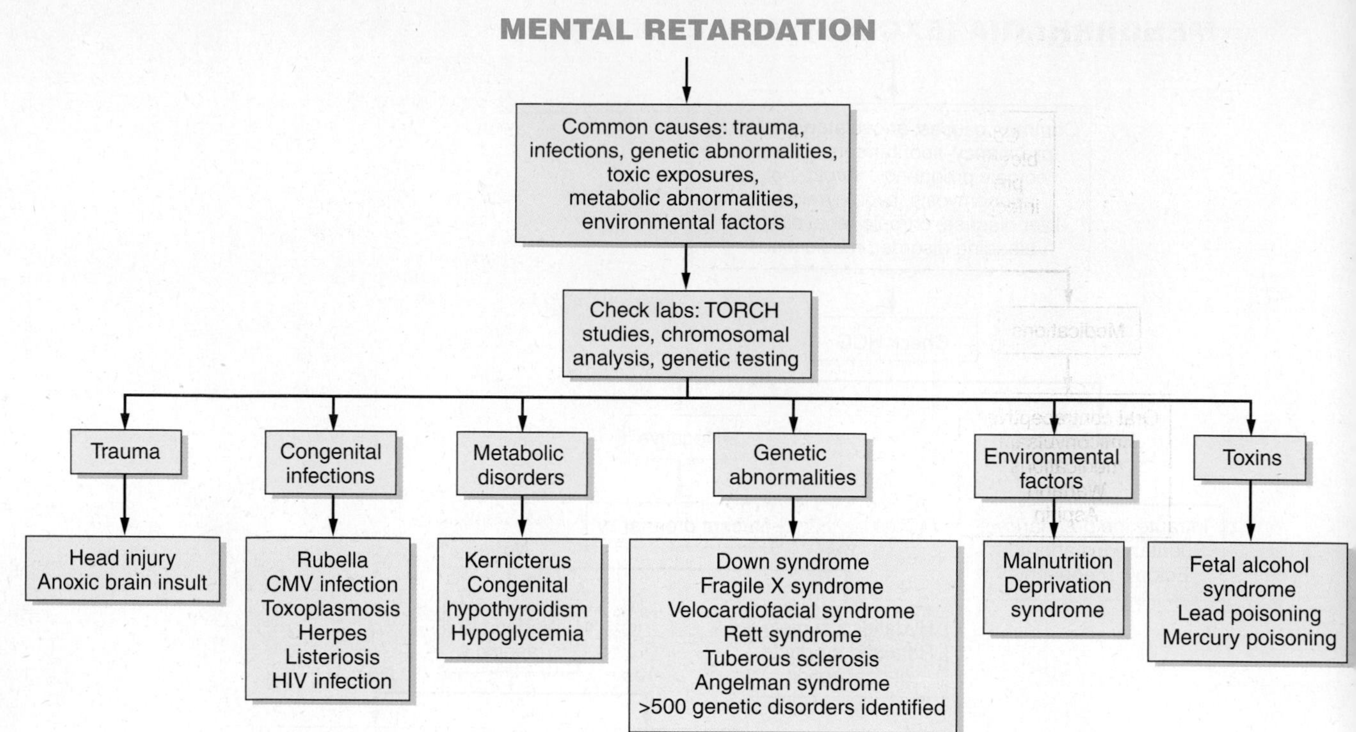
MENTAL RETARDATION
Common causes: trauma, infections, genetic abnormalities, toxic exposures, metabolic abnormalities, environmental factors
Check labs: TORCH studies, chromosomal analysis, genetic testing
Trauma
Head injury
Anoxic brain insult
Congenital infections
Rubella
CMV infection
Toxoplasmosis
Herpes
Listeriosis
HIV infection
Metabolic disorders
Kernicterus
Congenital hypothyroidism
Hypoglycemia
Genetic abnormalities
Down syndrome
Fragile X syndrome
Velocardiofacial syndrome
Rett syndrome
Tuberous sclerosis
Angelman syndrome
>500 genetic disorders identified
Environmental factors
Malnutrition
Deprivation syndrome
Toxins
Fetal alcohol syndrome
Lead poisoning
Mercury poisoning

Robert A. Baldor, MD and Alan M. Ehrlich, MD

Pediatr Clin North Am. 2008;55(5):1071–84, xi.

METORRHAGIA (INTERMENSTRUAL BLEEDING)

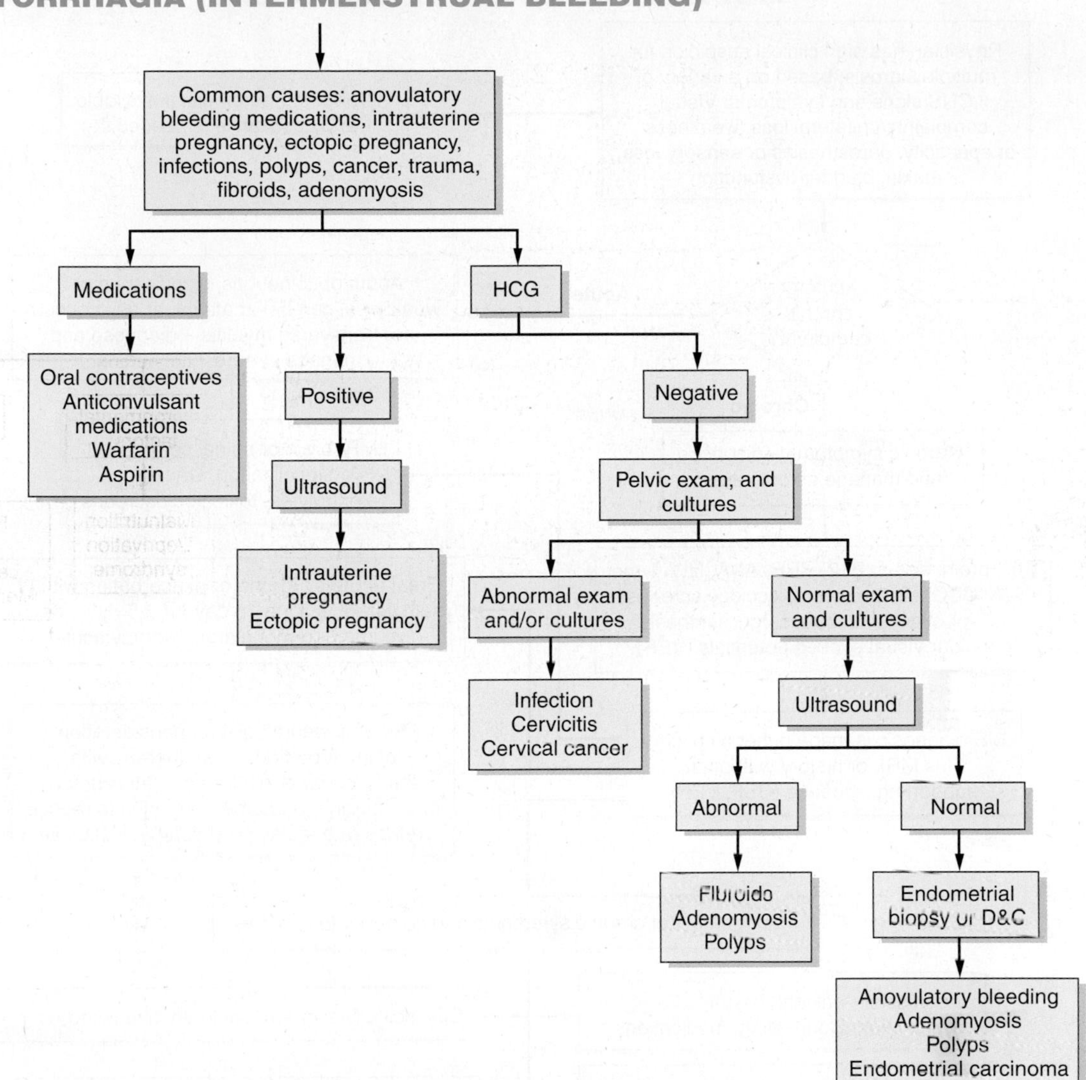

Robert A. Baldor, MD and Alan M. Ehrlich, MD

Am Fam Physician. 2004;69(8):1915–26.

MULTIPLE SCLEROSIS, TREATMENT

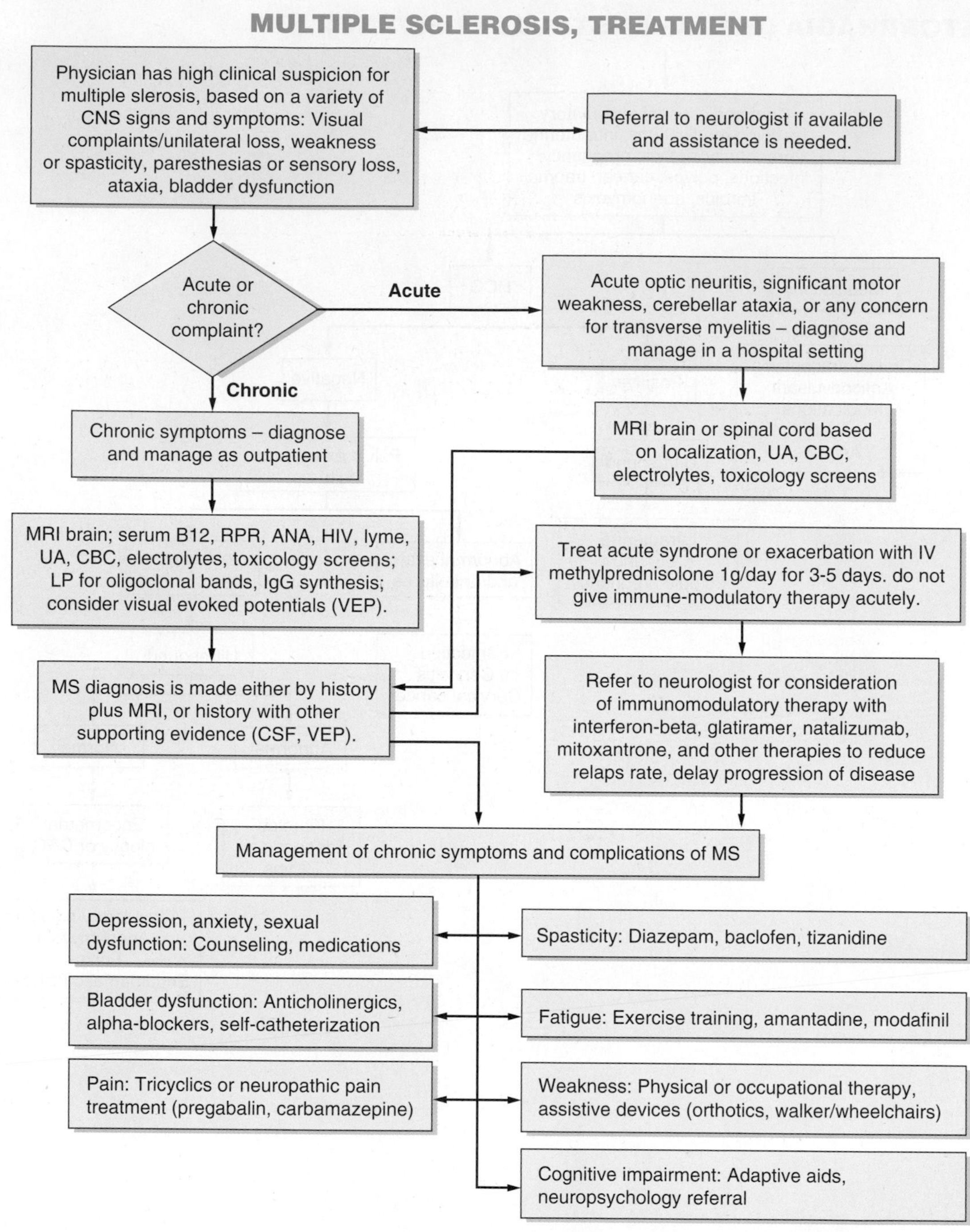
Physician has high clinical suspicion for multiple slerosis, based on a variety of CNS signs and symptoms: Visual complaints/unilateral loss, weakness or spasticity, paresthesias or sensory loss, ataxia, bladder dysfunction
Referral to neurologist if available and assistance is needed.
Acute or chronic complaint?
Acute
Acute optic neuritis, significant motor weakness, cerebellar ataxia, or any concern for transverse myelitis – diagnose and manage in a hospital setting
Chronic
Chronic symptoms – diagnose and manage as outpatient
MRI brain or spinal cord based on localization, UA, CBC, electrolytes, toxicology screens
MRI brain; serum B12, RPR, ANA, HIV, lyme, UA, CBC, electrolytes, toxicology screens; LP for oligoclonal bands, IgG synthesis; consider visual evoked potentials (VEP).
Treat acute syndrone or exacerbation with IV methylprednisolone 1g/day for 3-5 days. do not give immune-modulatory therapy acutely.
MS diagnosis is made either by history plus MRI, or history with other supporting evidence (CSF, VEP).
Refer to neurologist for consideration of immunomodulatory therapy with interferon-beta, glatiramer, natalizumab, mitoxantrone, and other therapies to reduce relaps rate, delay progression of disease
Management of chronic symptoms and complications of MS
Depression, anxiety, sexual dysfunction: Counseling, medications
Spasticity: Diazepam, baclofen, tizanidine
Bladder dysfunction: Anticholinergics, alpha-blockers, self-catheterization
Fatigue: Exercise training, amantadine, modafinil
Pain: Tricyclics or neuropathic pain treatment (pregabalin, carbamazepine)
Weakness: Physical or occupational therapy, assistive devices (orthotics, walker/wheelchairs)
Cognitive impairment: Adaptive aids, neuropsychology referral

Julie L. Roth, MD

Ann Neurol. 2005;58:840–6.

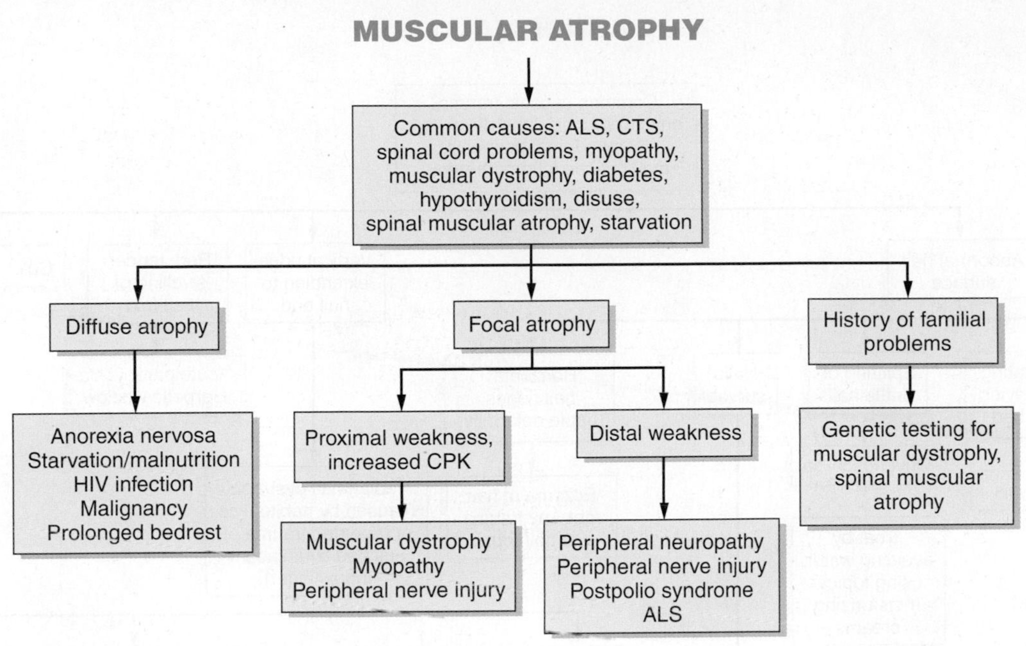

Robert A. Baldor, MD and Alan M. Ehrlich, MD

Lancet. 2007;369(9578):2031–41.

NAIL ABNORMALITIES

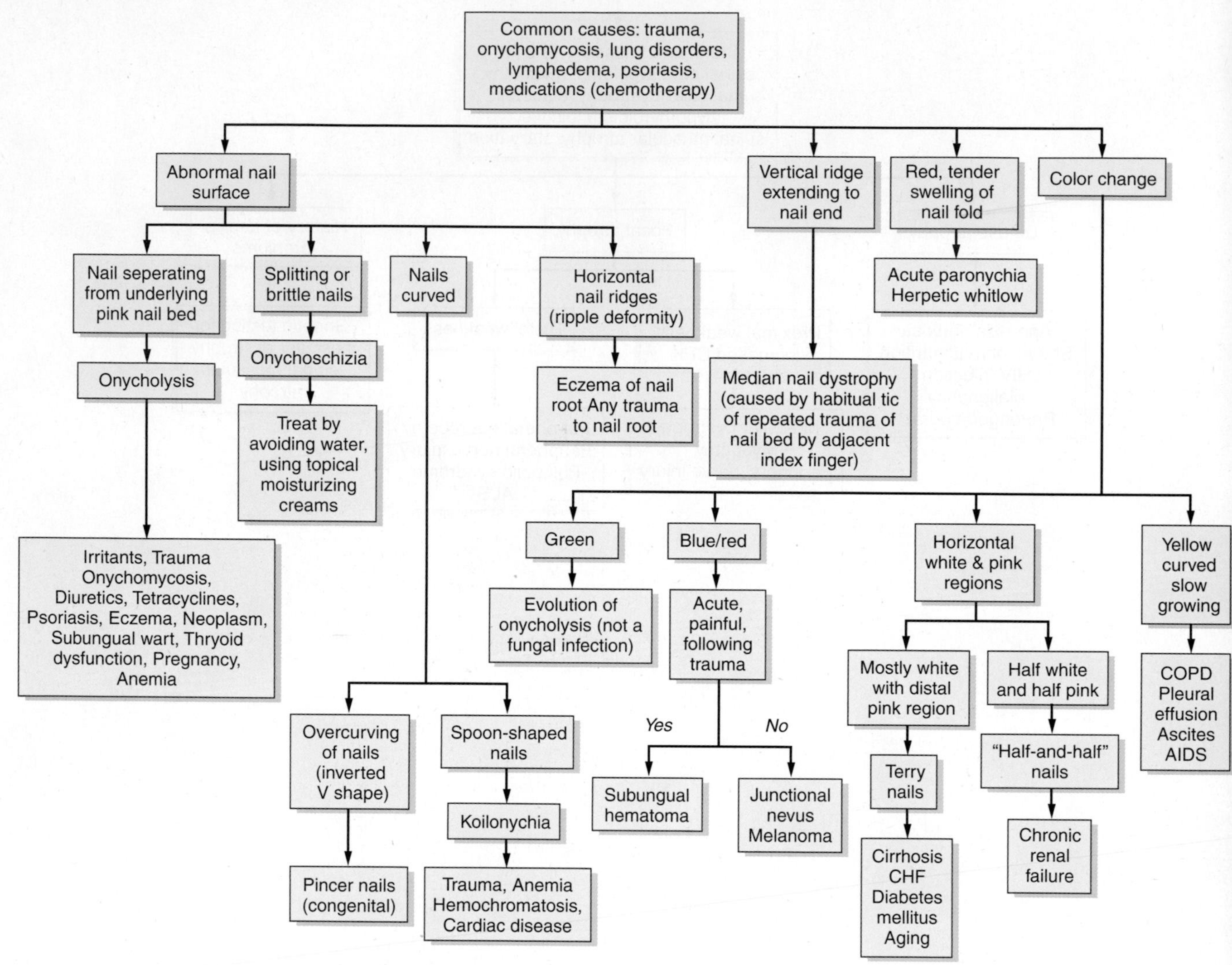

Robert A. Baldor, MD and Alan M. Ehrlich, MD

Am Fam Physician. 2004;69(6):1417–24.

NASAL DISCHARGE, CHRONIC

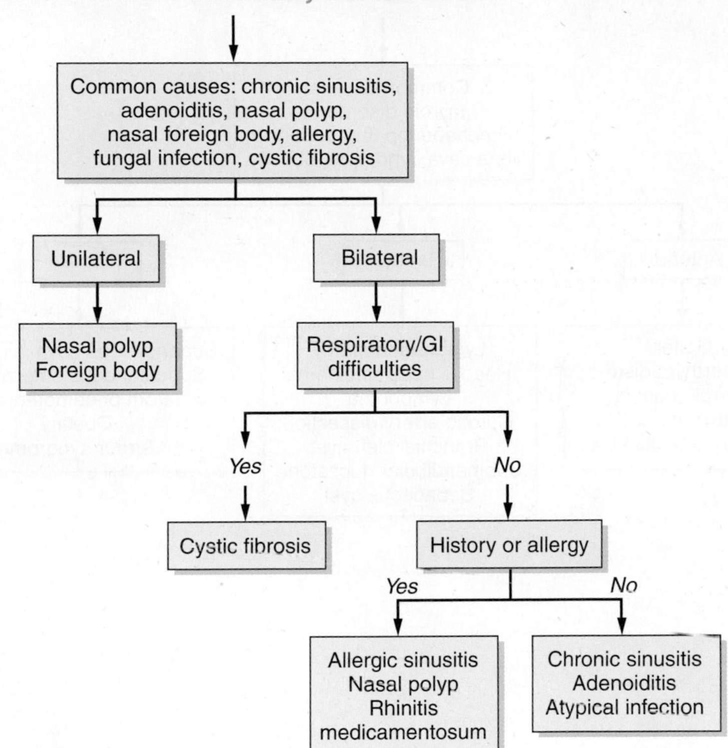

Robert A. Baldor, MD and Alan M. Ehrlich, MD

Postgrad Med. 2009;121(6):121–39.

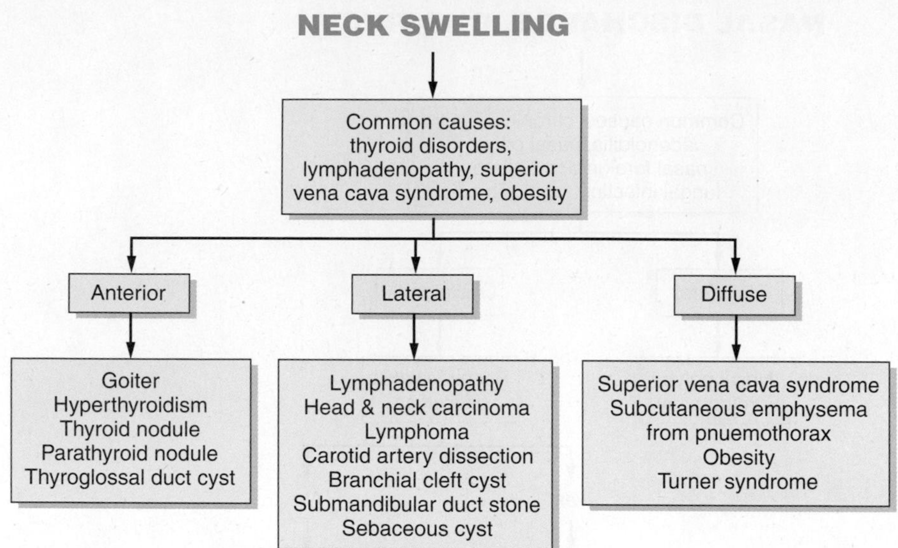

Robert A. Baldor, MD and Alan M. Ehrlich, MD

Am Fam Physician. 1995;51(8):1904–12.

NEPHROTIC SYNDROME

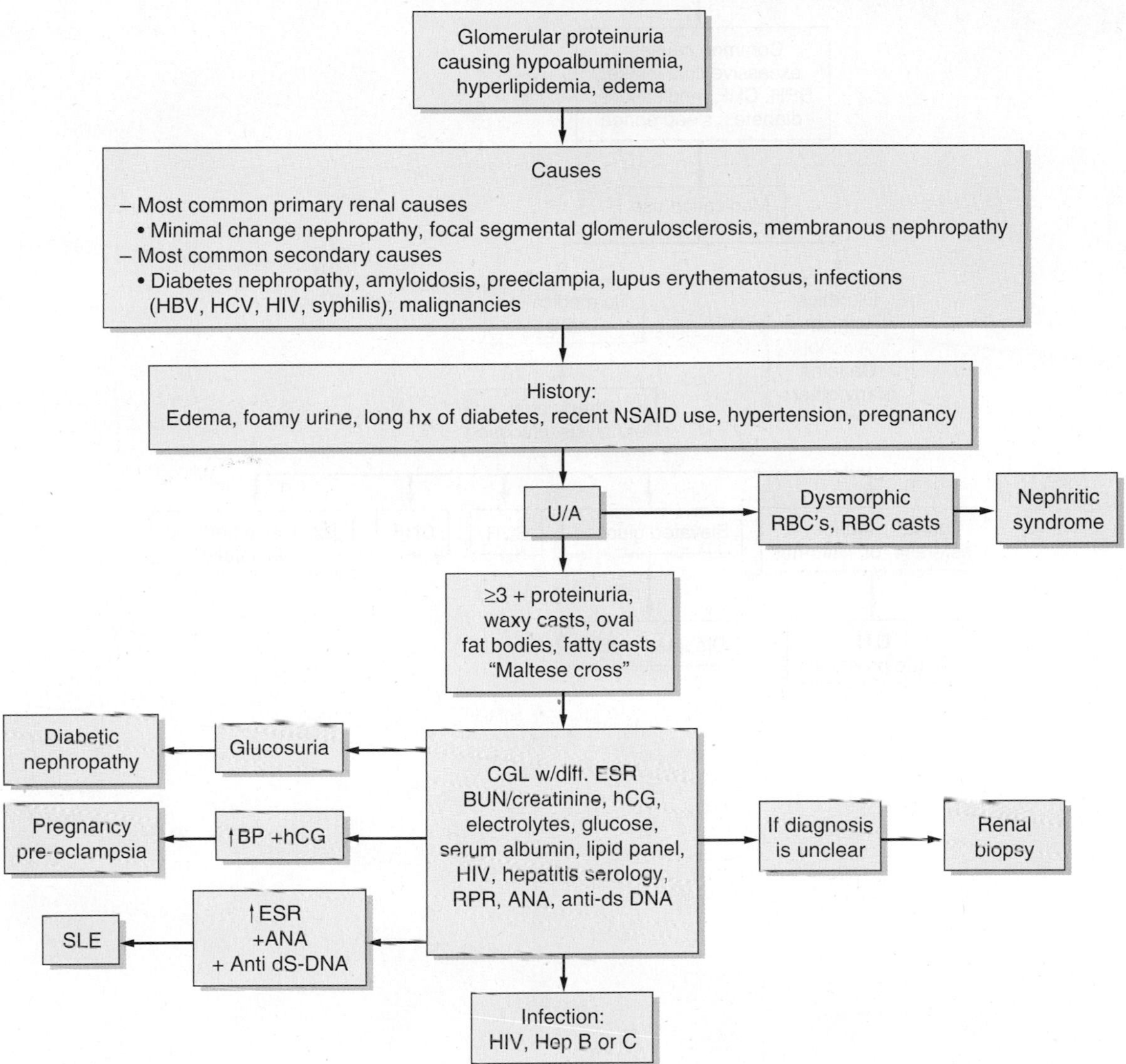

Jonathan Min, MD and Robert M. Black, MD

Cleve Clin J Med. 2006;73(2):161–7.

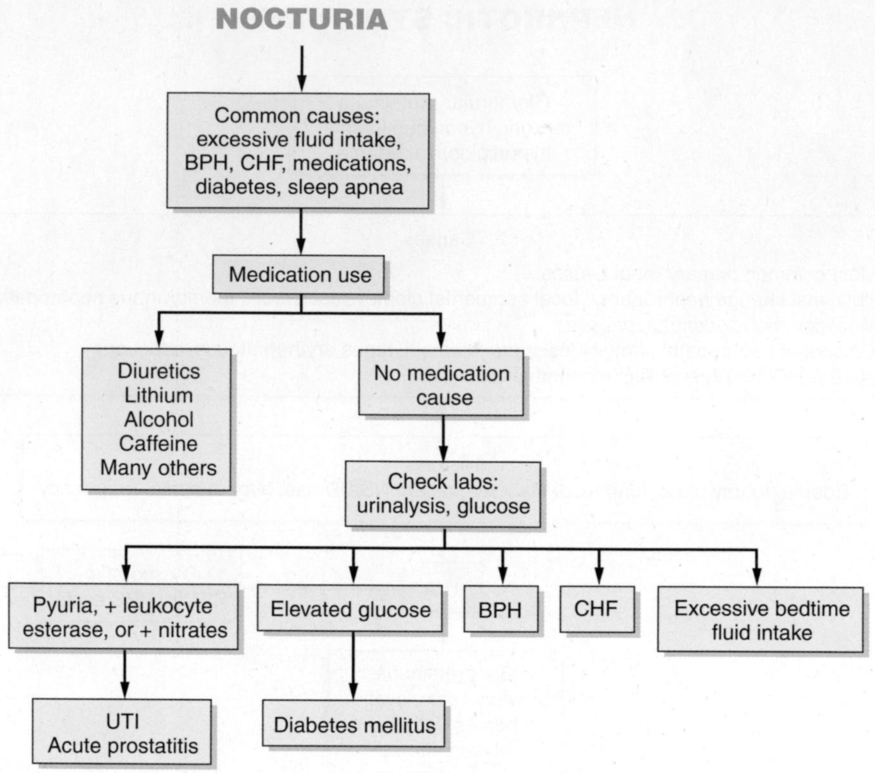

Robert A. Baldor, MD and Alan M. Ehrlich, MD

BMJ. 2004;328(7447):1063–6.

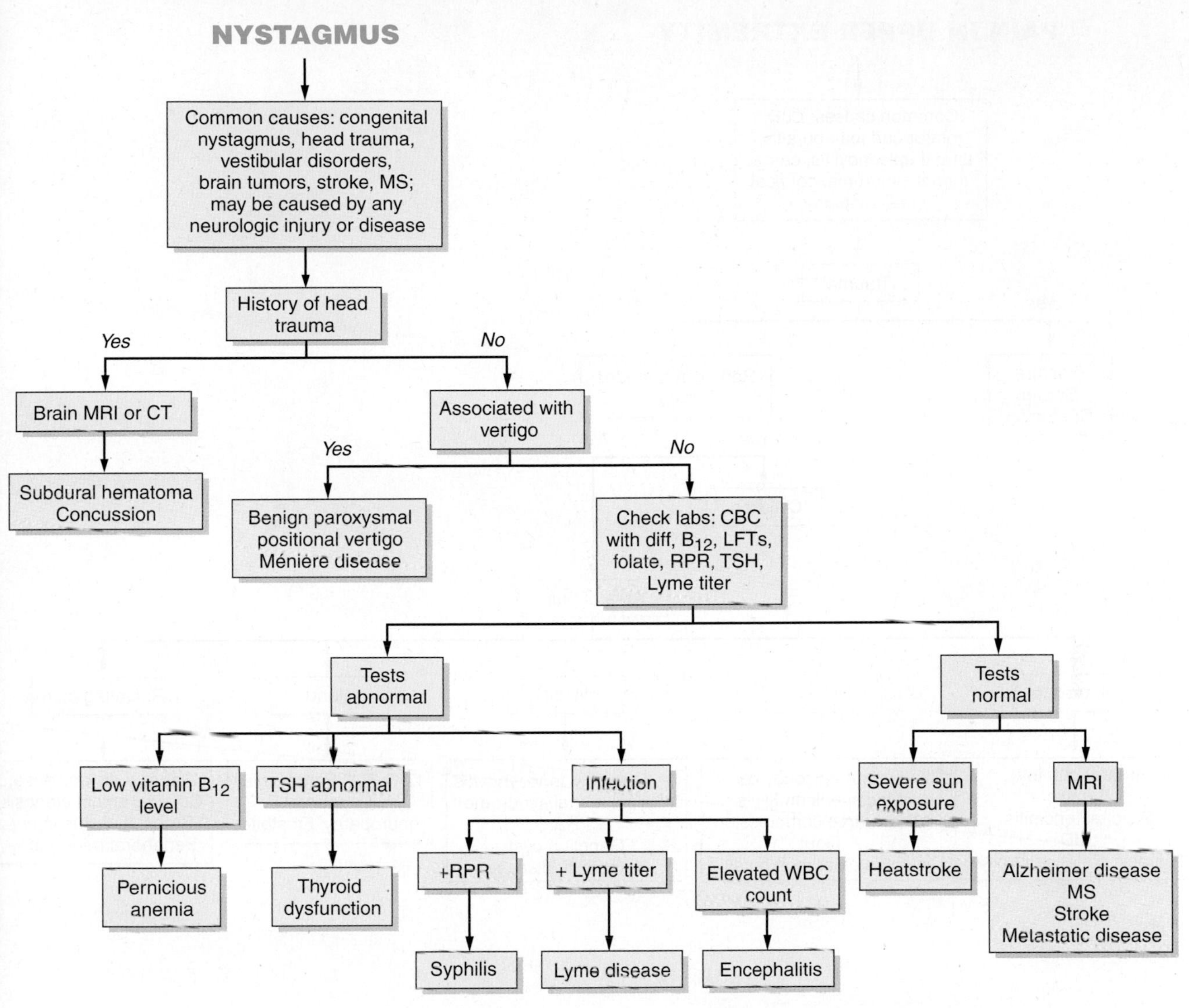

Robert A. Baldor, MD and Alan M. Ehrlich, MD

Med Clin North Am. 2009;93(2):263–71, vii.

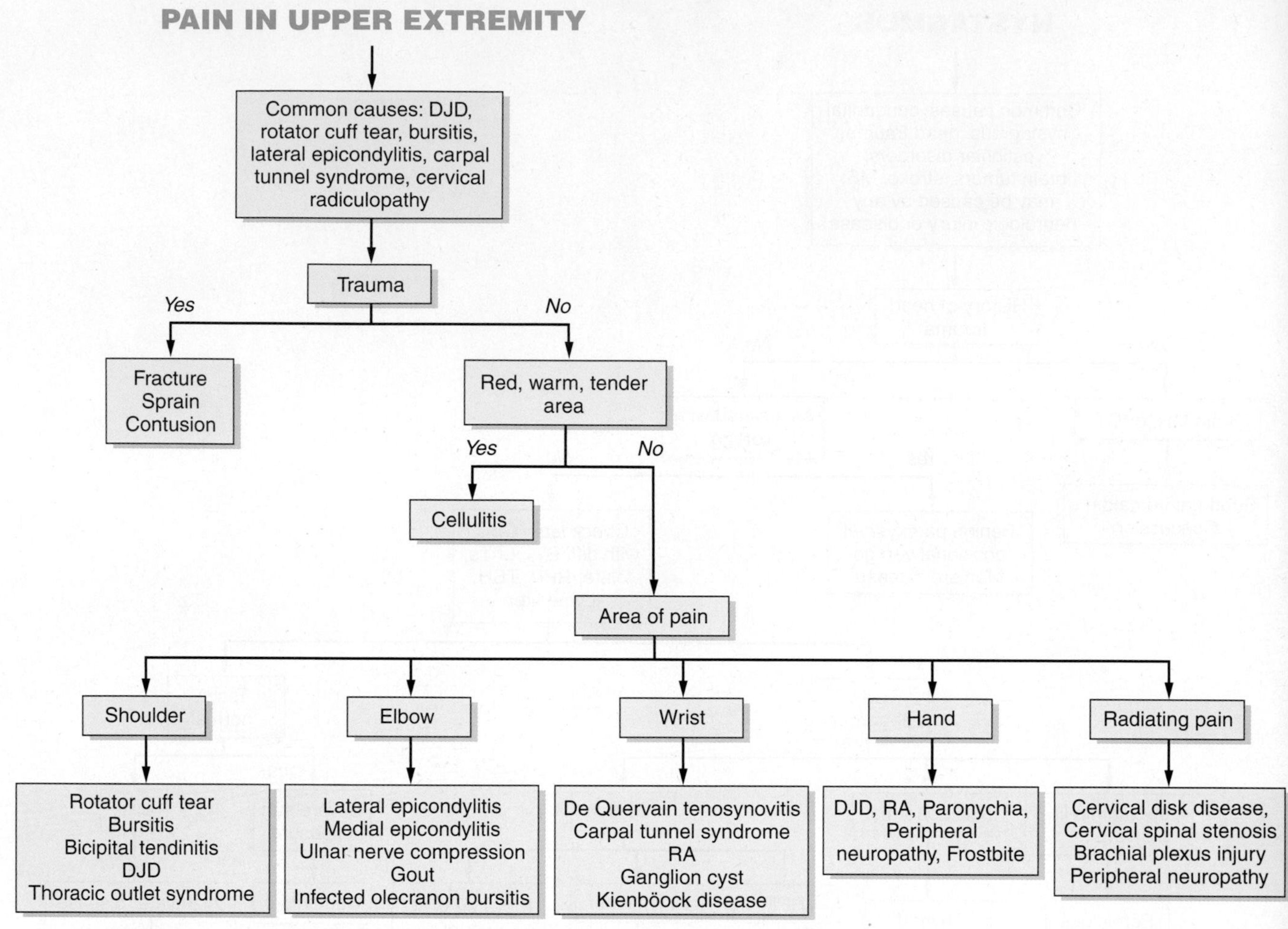
PAIN IN UPPER EXTREMITY
Common causes: DJD, rotator cuff tear, bursitis, lateral epicondylitis, carpal tunnel syndrome, cervical radiculopathy
Trauma
Yes
No
Fracture
Sprain
Contusion
Red, warm, tender area
Yes
No
Cellulitis
Area of pain
Shoulder
Elbow
Wrist
Hand
Radiating pain
Rotator cuff tear
Bursitis
Bicipital tendinitis
DJD
Thoracic outlet syndrome
Lateral epicondylitis
Medial epicondylitis
Ulnar nerve compression
Gout
Infected olecranon bursitis
De Quervain tenosynovitis
Carpal tunnel syndrome
RA
Ganglion cyst
Kienböock disease
DJD, RA, Paronychia, Peripheral neuropathy, Frostbite
Cervical disk disease,
Cervical spinal stenosis
Brachial plexus injury
Peripheral neuropathy

Robert A. Baldor, MD and Alan M. Ehrlich, MD

N Engl J Med. 2008;358(20):2138–47.

PALLOR, GENERALIZED

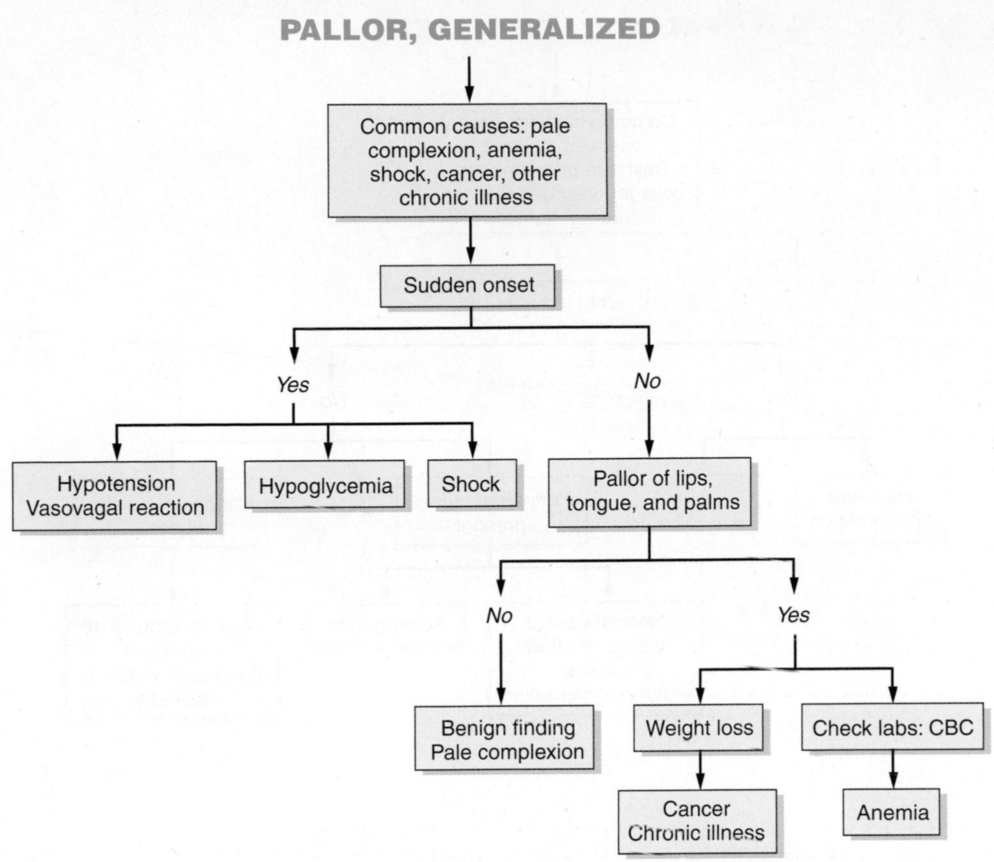

Robert A. Baldor, MD and Alan M. Ehrlich, MD

Am Fam Physician. 2007;75(5):671–8.

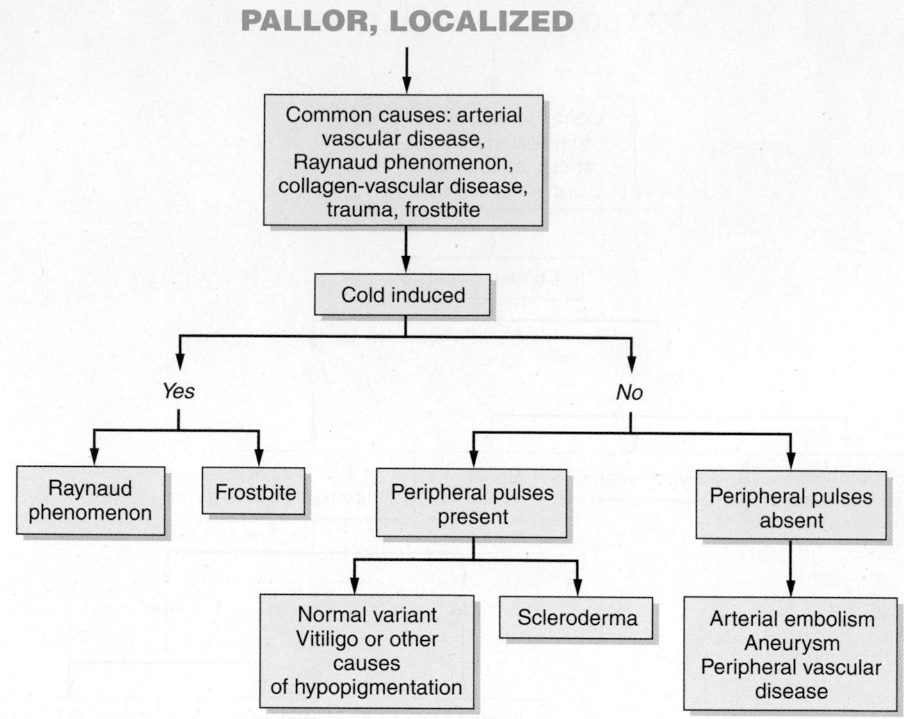

Robert A. Baldor, MD and Alan M. Ehrlich, MD

South Med J. 2009;102(11):1141–9.

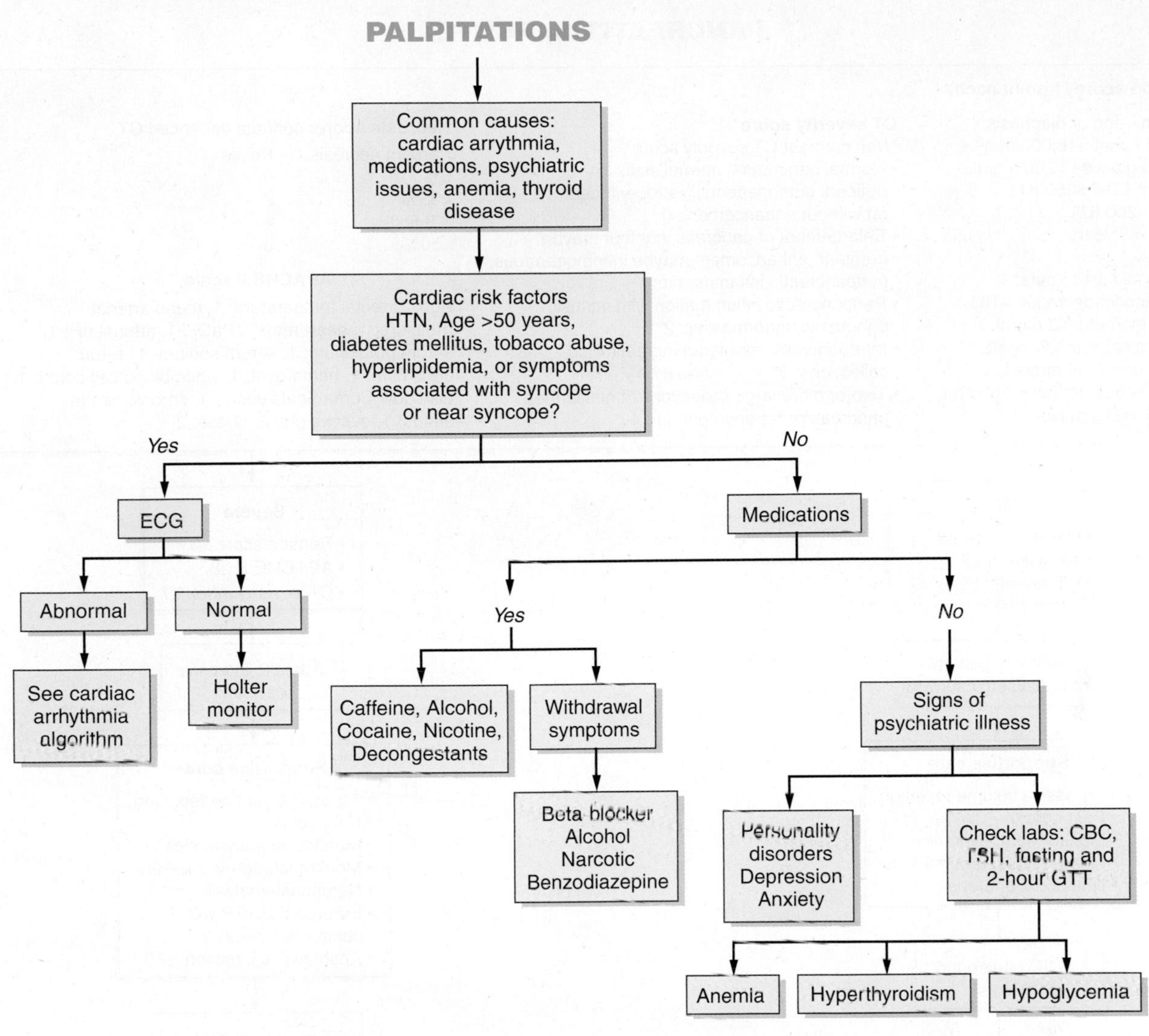

Robert A. Baldor, MD and Alan M. Ehrlich, MD

NEJM. 338(19):1369–73.

PANCREATITIS, ACUTE

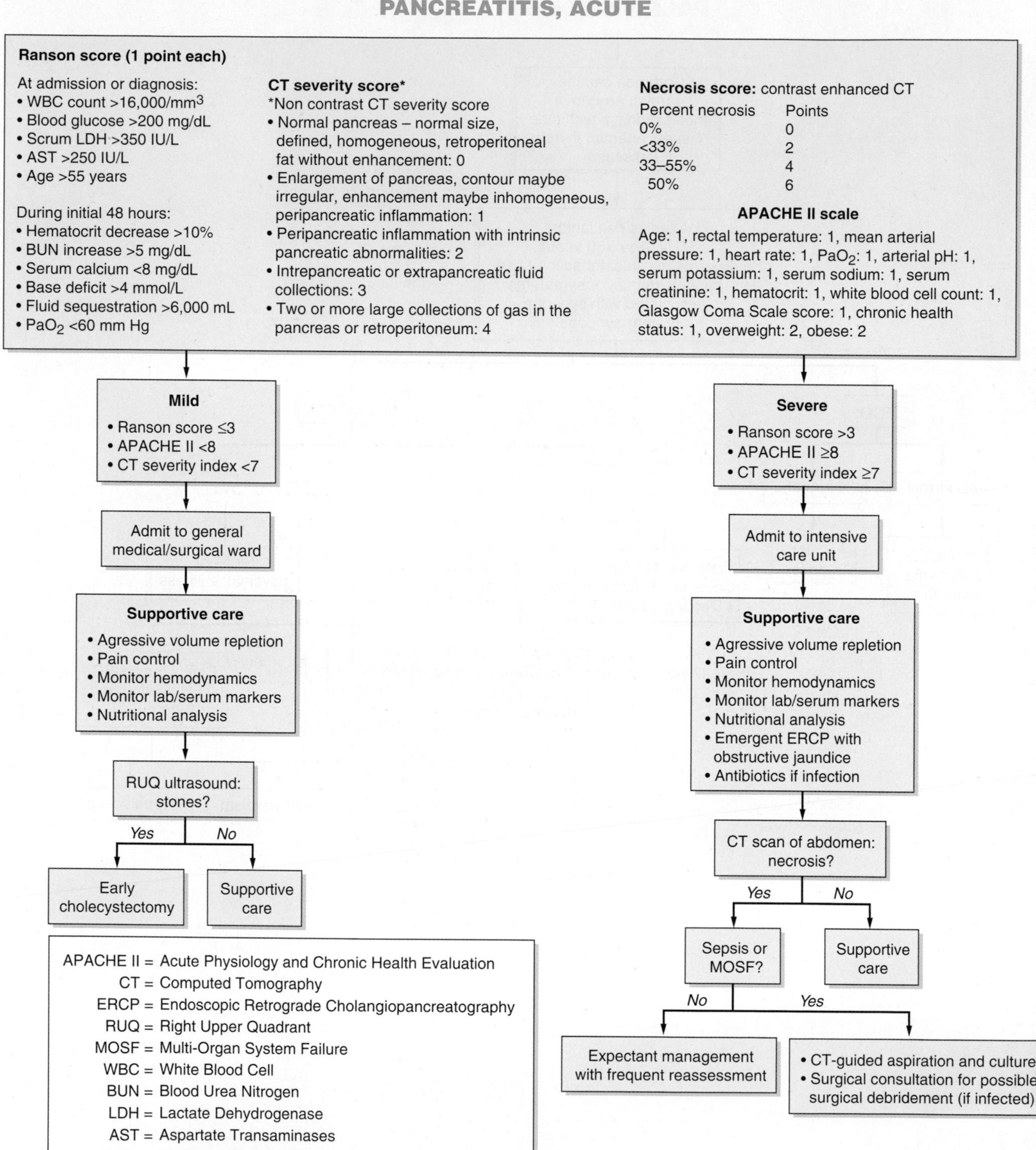
Ranson score (1 point each)
At admission or diagnosis:
• WBC count >16,000/mm3
• Blood glucose >200 mg/dL
• Scrum LDH >350 IU/L
• AST >250 IU/L
• Age >55 years
During initial 48 hours:
• Hematocrit decrease >10%
• BUN increase >5 mg/dL
• Serum calcium <8 mg/dL
• Base deficit >4 mmol/L
• Fluid sequestration >6,000 mL
• PaO2 <60 mm Hg
CT severity score*
*Non contrast CT severity score
• Normal pancreas – normal size, defined, homogeneous, retroperitoneal fat without enhancement: 0
• Enlargement of pancreas, contour maybe irregular, enhancement maybe inhomogeneous, peripancreatic inflammation: 1
• Peripancreatic inflammation with intrinsic pancreatic abnormalities: 2
• Intrepancreatic or extrapancreatic fluid collections: 3
• Two or more large collections of gas in the pancreas or retroperitoneum: 4
Necrosis score: contrast enhanced CT
Percent necrosis Points
0% 0
<33% 2
33–55% 4
50% 6
APACHE II scale
Age: 1, rectal temperature: 1, mean arterial pressure: 1, heart rate: 1, PaO2: 1, arterial pH: 1, serum potassium: 1, serum sodium: 1, serum creatinine: 1, hematocrit: 1, white blood cell count: 1, Glasgow Coma Scale score: 1, chronic health status: 1, overweight: 2, obese: 2
Mild
• Ranson score ≤3
• APACHE II <8
• CT severity index <7
Admit to general medical/surgical ward
Supportive care
• Agressive volume repletion
• Pain control
• Monitor hemodynamics
• Monitor lab/serum markers
• Nutritional analysis
RUQ ultrasound: stones?
Yes
No
Early cholecystectomy
Supportive care
Severe
• Ranson score >3
• APACHE II ≥8
• CT severity index ≥7
Admit to intensive care unit
Supportive care
• Agressive volume repletion
• Pain control
• Monitor hemodynamics
• Monitor lab/serum markers
• Nutritional analysis
• Emergent ERCP with obstructive jaundice
• Antibiotics if infection
CT scan of abdomen: necrosis?
Yes
No
Sepsis or MOSF?
Supportive care
No
Yes
Expectant management with frequent reassessment
• CT-guided aspiration and culture
• Surgical consultation for possible surgical debridement (if infected)
APACHE II = Acute Physiology and Chronic Health Evaluation
CT = Computed Tomography
ERCP = Endoscopic Retrograde Cholangiopancreatography
RUQ = Right Upper Quadrant
MOSF = Multi-Organ System Failure
WBC = White Blood Cell
BUN = Blood Urea Nitrogen
LDH = Lactate Dehydrogenase
AST = Aspartate Transaminases
PaO2 = Partial Arterial Oxygen Tension

Maurice F. Joyce, III, MD and Mitchell A. Cahan, MD

PAP (ABNORMAL), >21 YEARS OF AGE*

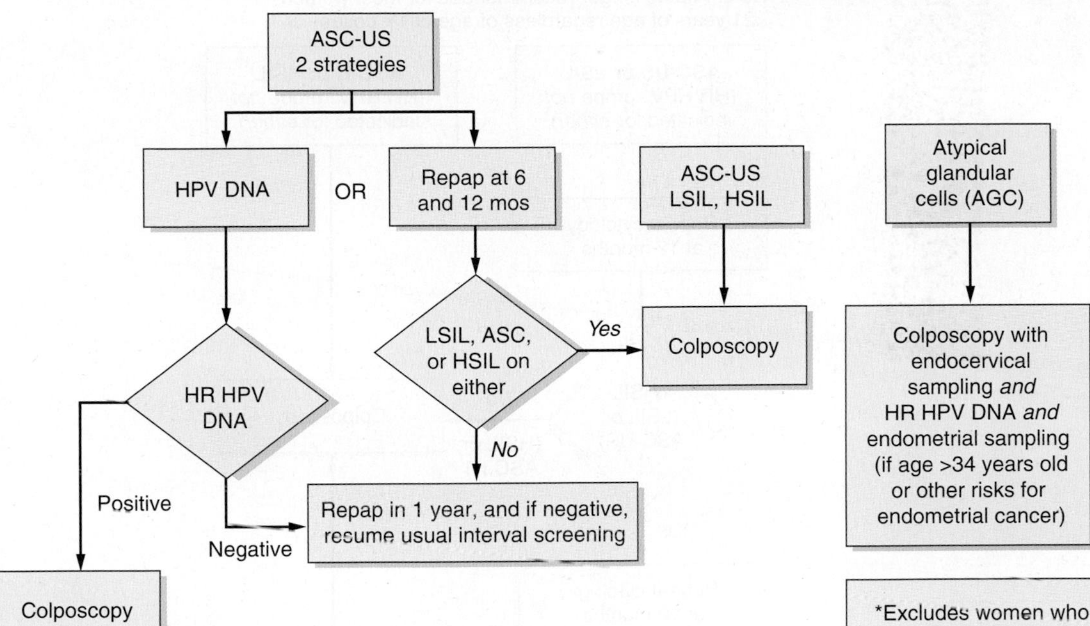

Pap smears: Recommended screening frequency [A]

Age	Recommended Frequency
<21	Screening not recommended
21–29	Every 2 years, either conventional or liquid-based
30–65	Every 3 years if either • Previous 3 paps (every 1–2 years) all normal *or* • Cytology negative and HR HPV DNA negative
>65	Discontinue screening if 3 previous paps normal and no abnormal results in past 10 years

Women of any age who had total hysterectomy for benign disease (and w/o history of high-grade CIN) do *not* require Pap smears

*Excludes women who are:
- HIV positive
- Immunosuppressed
- DES-exposed *in utero*
- Previously treated for CIN2,3 or cervical cancer

All above should have at least an *annual* screening

HR HPV DNA = probe for high-risk HPV strains

Jeremy Golding, MD

ACOG Practice Bulletin Number 109, December 2009.

PAP (ABNORMAL), ADOLESCENTS

Note: Pap no longer recommended for most women <21 years of age regardless of age of 1st coitus

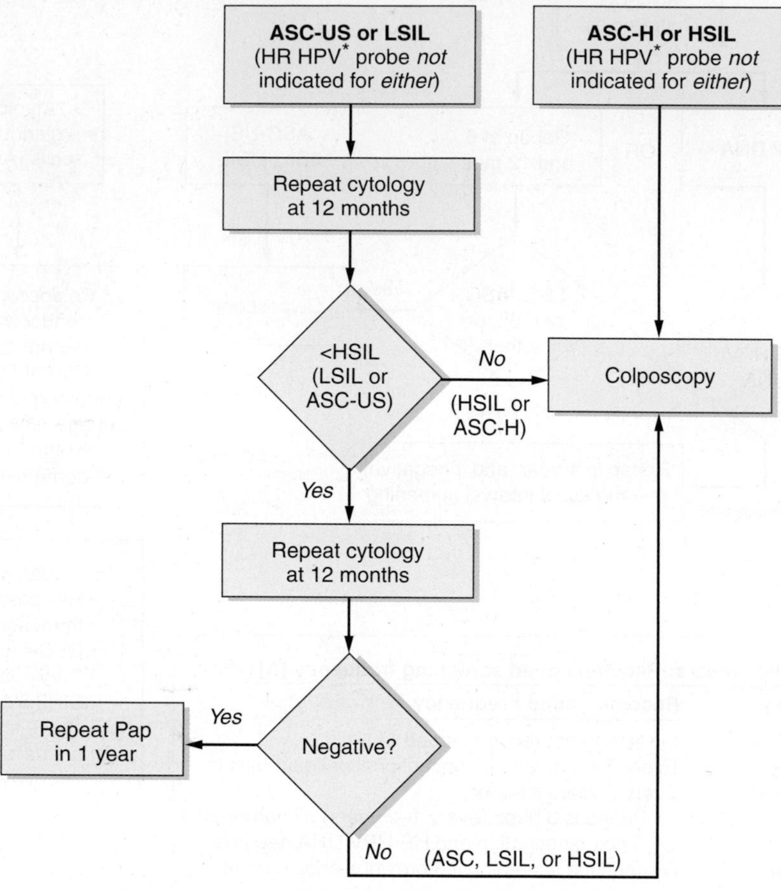

HR HPV DNA = probe for high-risk HPV strains

Jeremy Golding, MD

ACOG Practice Bulletin Number 109, December 2009.

PAP, USE OF HPV DNA TESTING IN WOMEN OVER 30*

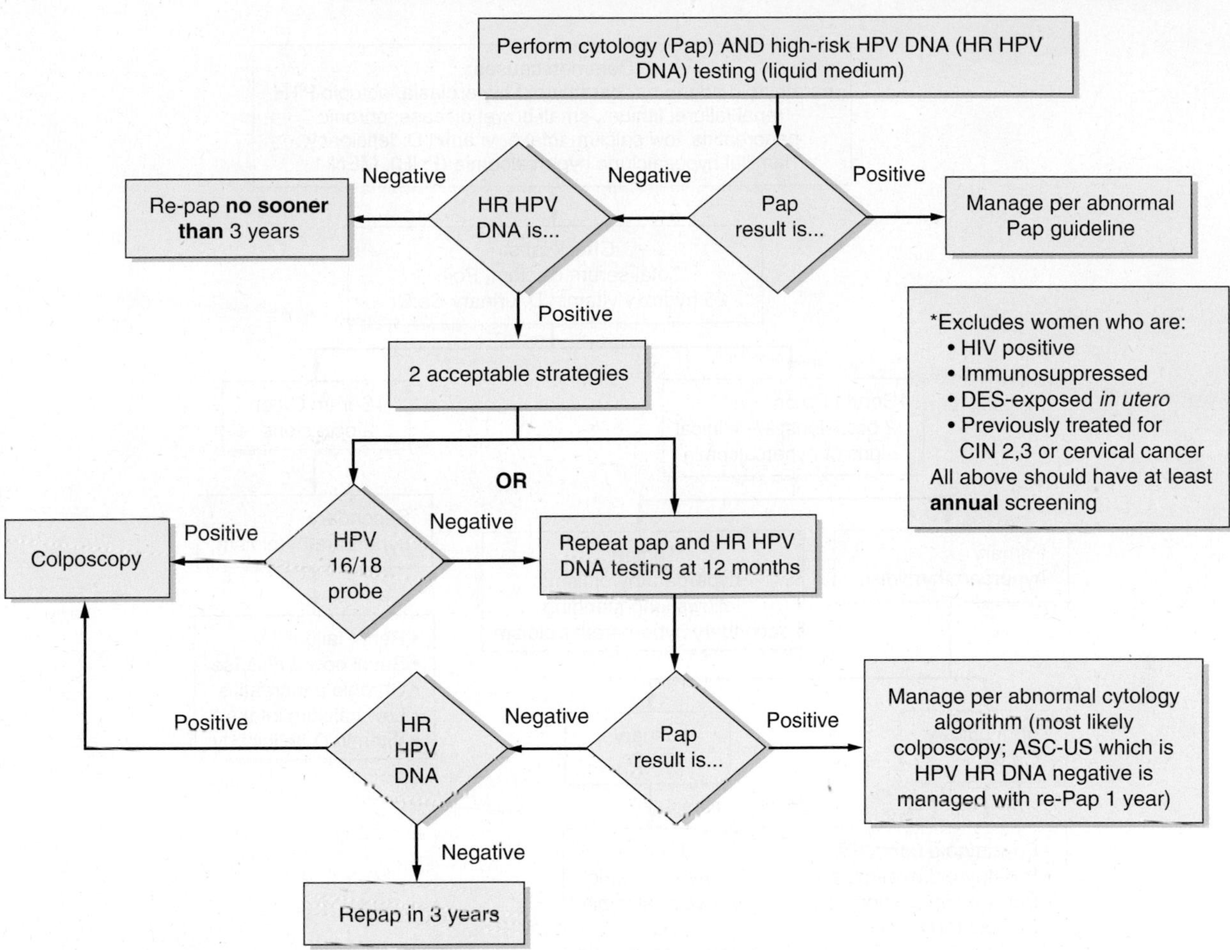

*Excludes women who are:
- HIV positive
- Immunosuppressed
- DES-exposed *in utero*
- Previously treated for CIN 2,3 or cervical cancer

All above should have at least **annual** screening

Jeremy Golding, MD

ACOG Practice Bulletin Number 109, December 2009.

PARATHYROID HORMONE, ELEVATED SERUM

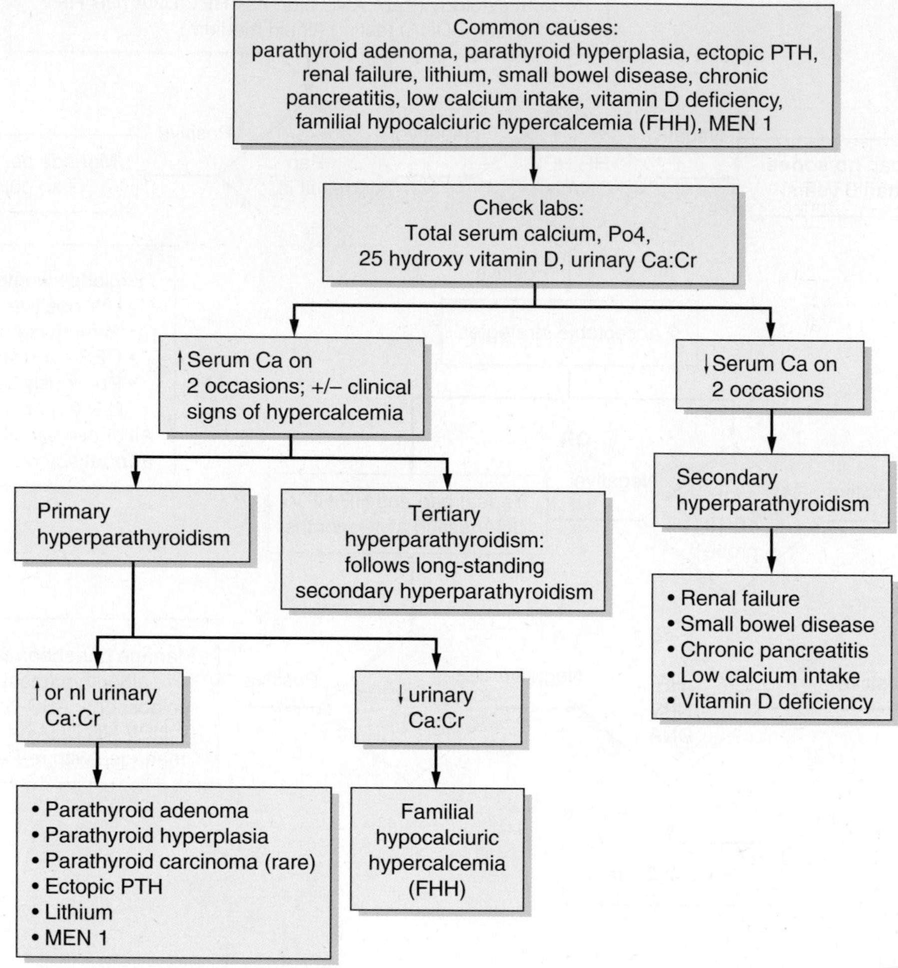

Andrew Gara, MD and Auguste Turnier, MD

JAMA. 2005;294(21):2700.

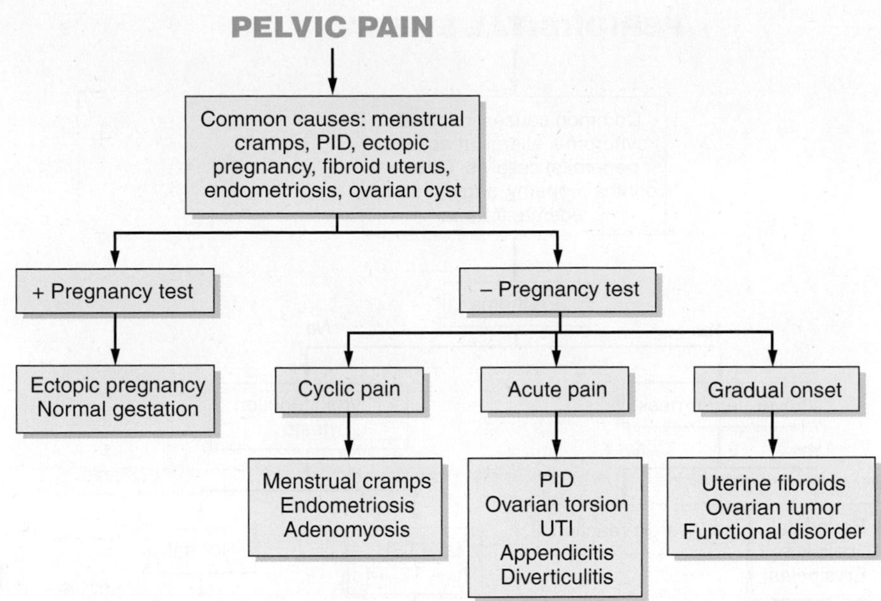

Robert A. Baldor, MD and Alan M. Ehrlich, MD

Am Fam Physician. 2008;77(11):1535–42.

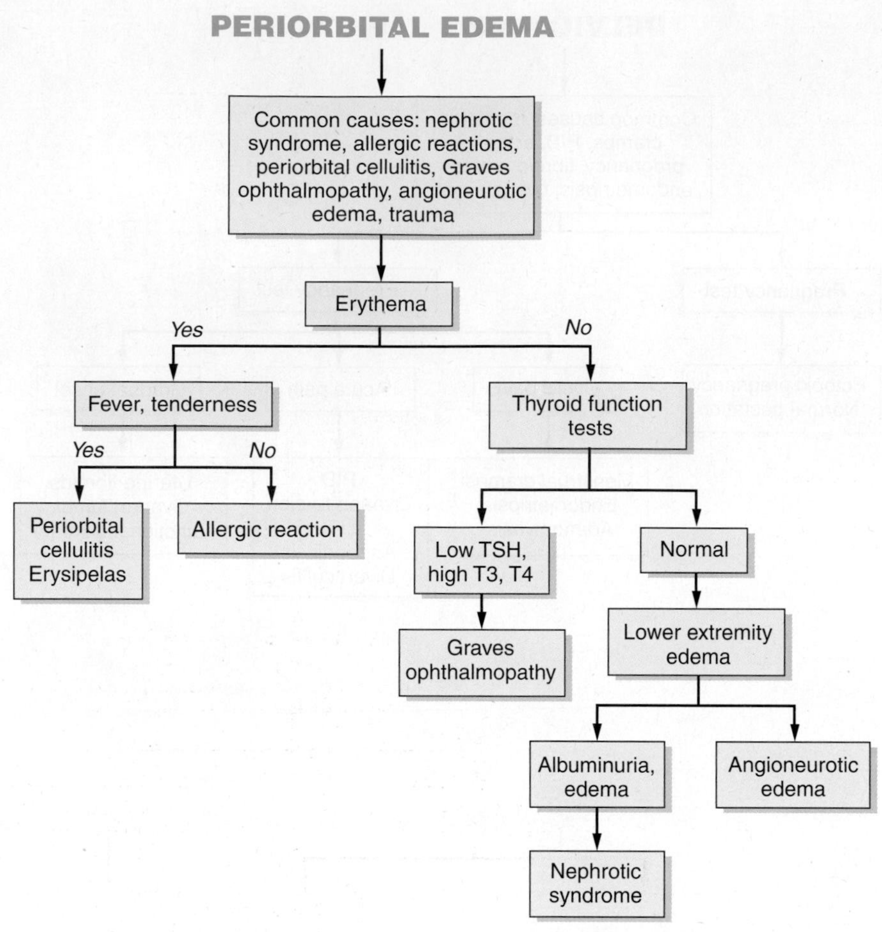

Robert A. Baldor, MD and Alan M. Ehrlich, MD

Infect Dis Clin North Am. 2007;21(2):393–408.

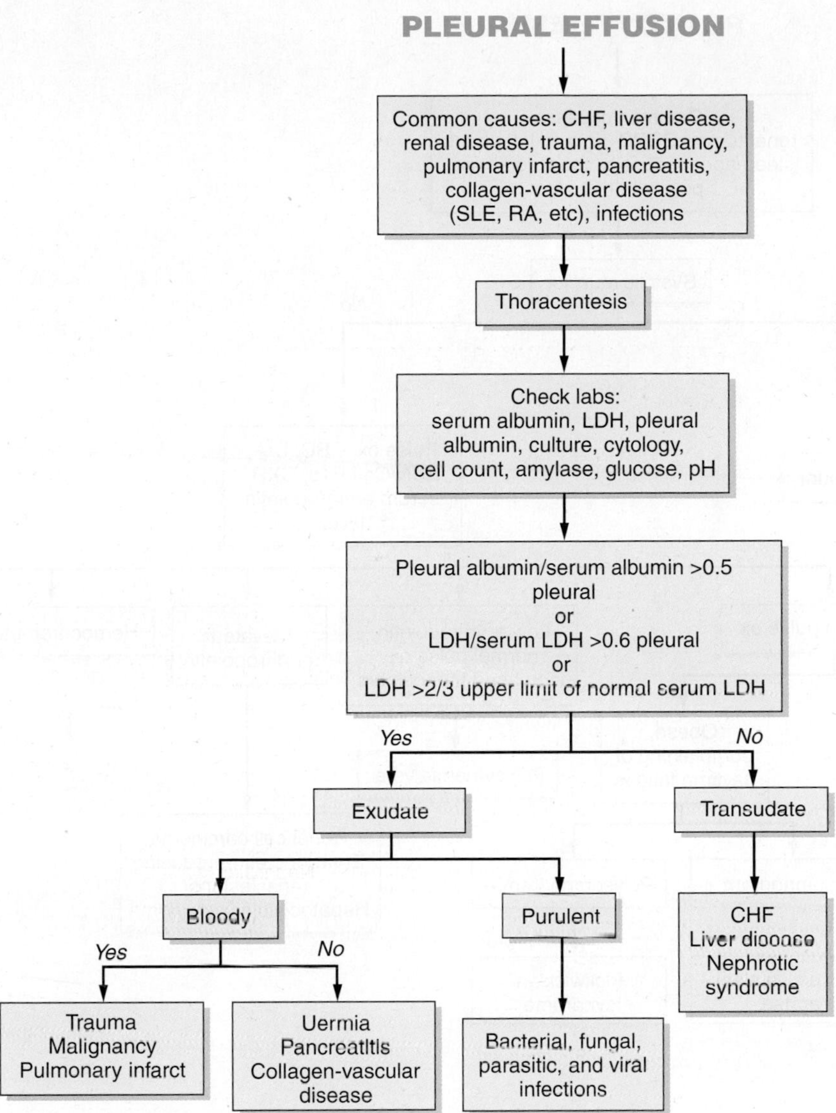

Robert A. Baldor, MD and Alan M. Ehrlich, MD

Am Fam Physician. 2006;73:1211–20.

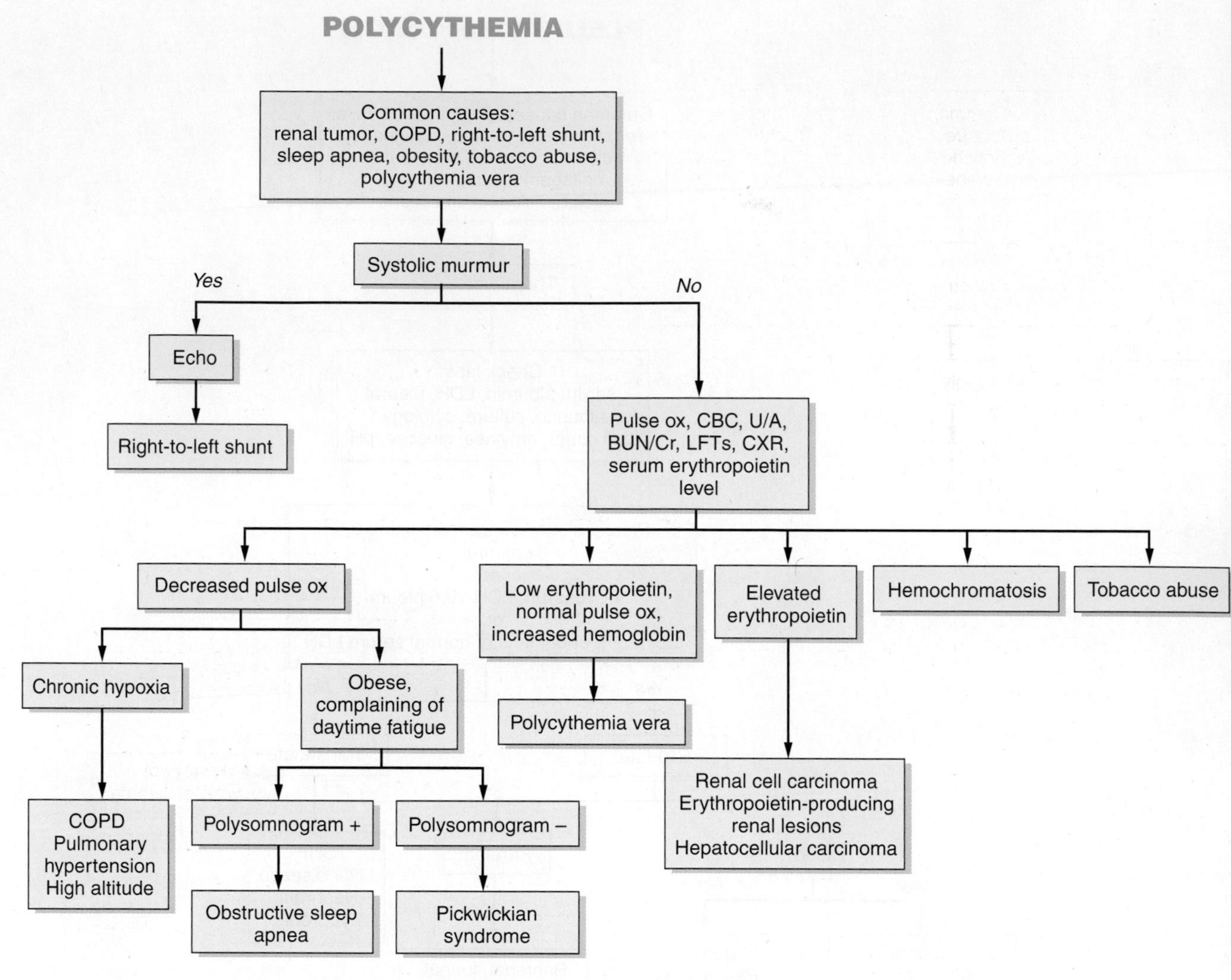
POLYCYTHEMIA
Common causes: renal tumor, COPD, right-to-left shunt, sleep apnea, obesity, tobacco abuse, polycythemia vera
Systolic murmur
Yes
No
Echo
Right-to-left shunt
Pulse ox, CBC, U/A, BUN/Cr, LFTs, CXR, serum erythropoietin level
Decreased pulse ox
Low erythropoietin, normal pulse ox, increased hemoglobin
Elevated erythropoietin
Hemochromatosis
Tobacco abuse
Chronic hypoxia
Obese, complaining of daytime fatigue
Polycythemia vera
Renal cell carcinoma
Erythropoietin-producing renal lesions
Hepatocellular carcinoma
COPD
Pulmonary hypertension
High altitude
Polysomnogram +
Polysomnogram –
Obstructive sleep apnea
Pickwickian syndrome

Robert A. Baldor, MD and Alan M. Ehrlich, MD

Mayo Clin Proc. 2005;80(7):923–36.

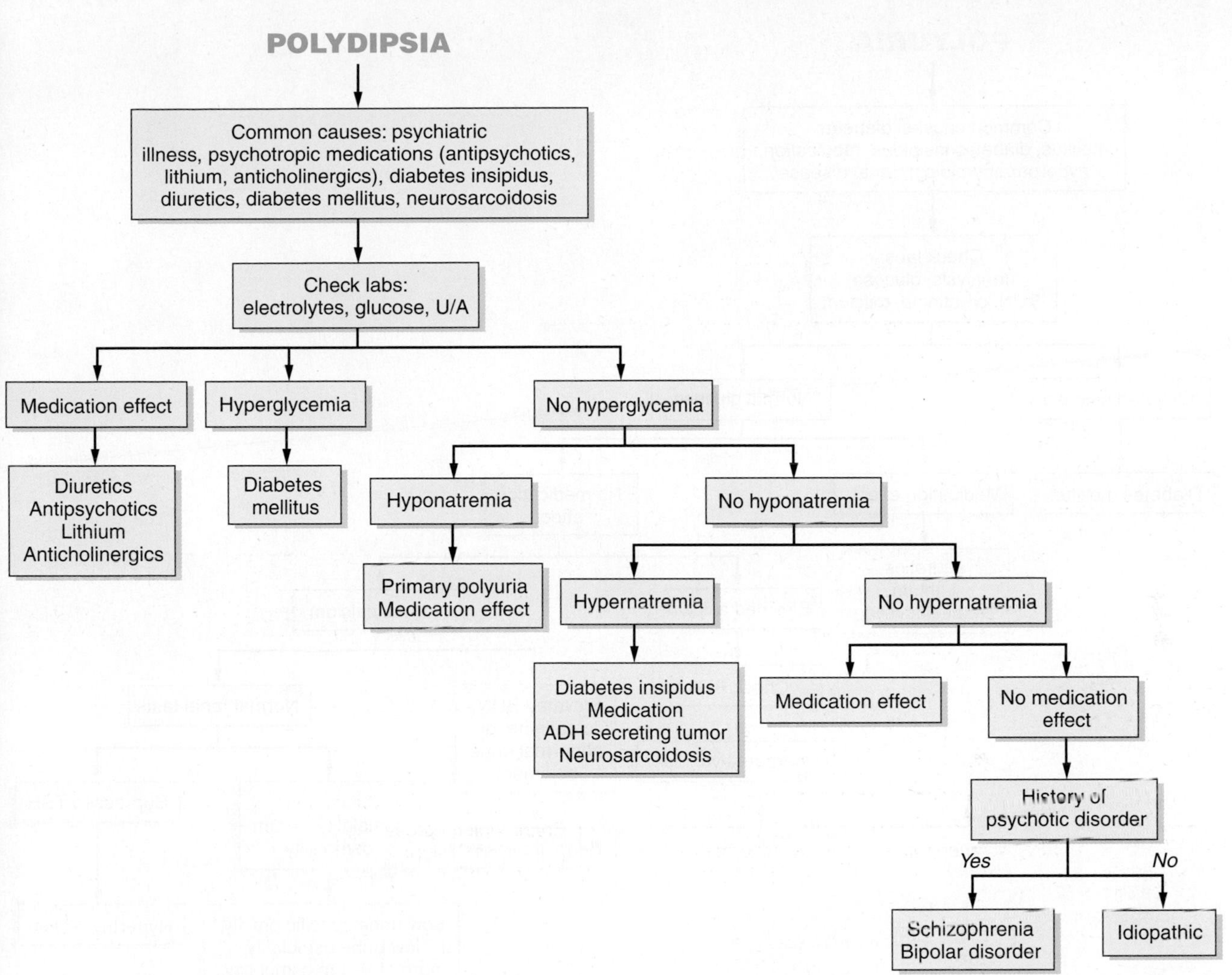

Robert A. Baldor, MD and Alan M. Ehrlich, MD

Nat Clin Proc Nephrol. 2007;3(7):374–82.

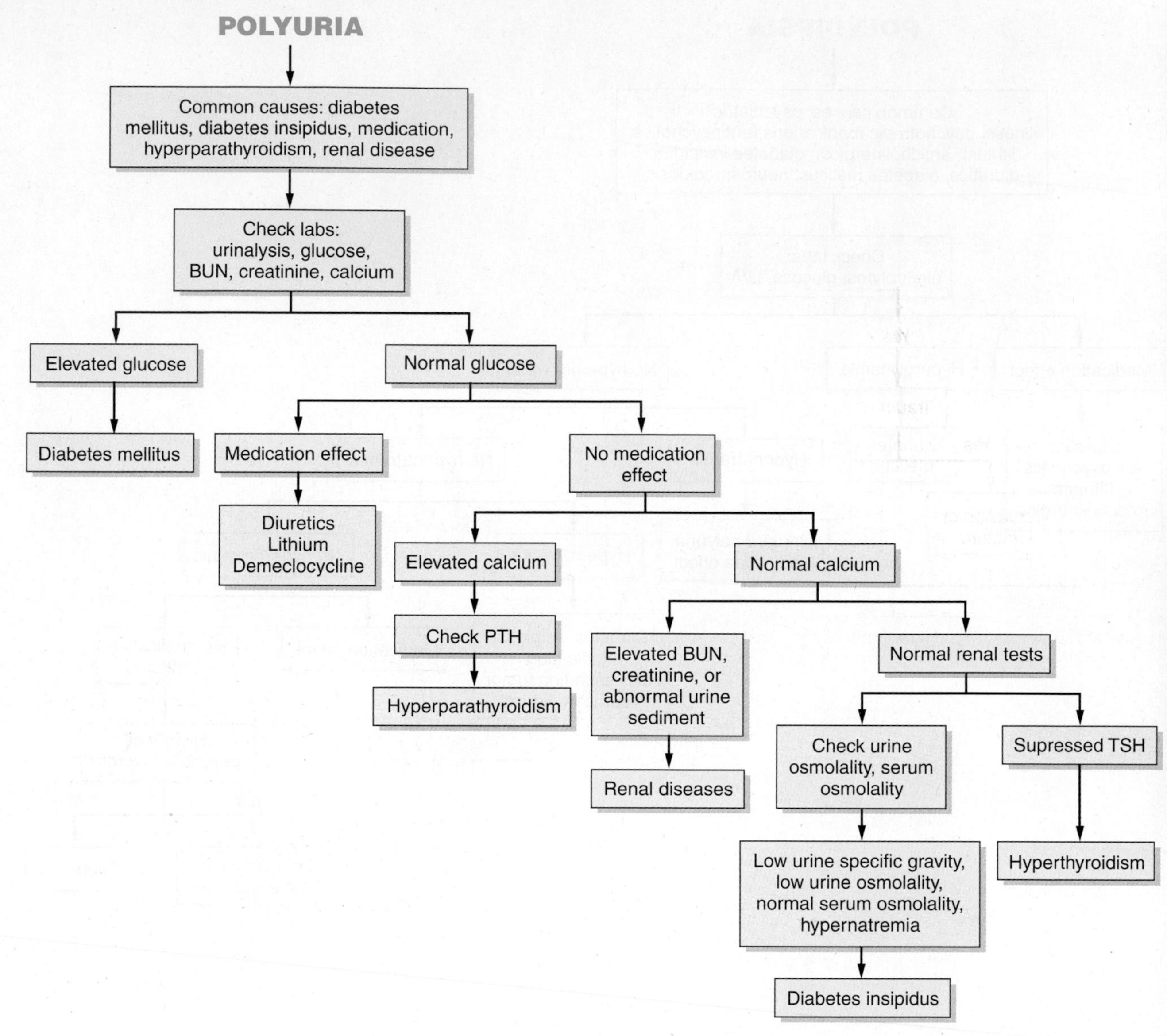
POLYURIA
Common causes: diabetes mellitus, diabetes insipidus, medication, hyperparathyroidism, renal disease
Check labs: urinalysis, glucose, BUN, creatinine, calcium
Elevated glucose
Diabetes mellitus
Normal glucose
Medication effect
Diuretics
Lithium
Demeclocycline
No medication effect
Elevated calcium
Check PTH
Hyperparathyroidism
Normal calcium
Elevated BUN, creatinine, or abnormal urine sediment
Renal diseases
Normal renal tests
Check urine osmolality, serum osmolality
Low urine specific gravity, low urine osmolality, normal serum osmolality, hypernatremia
Diabetes insipidus
Supressed TSH
Hyperthyroidism

Robert A. Baldor, MD and Alan M. Ehrlich, MD

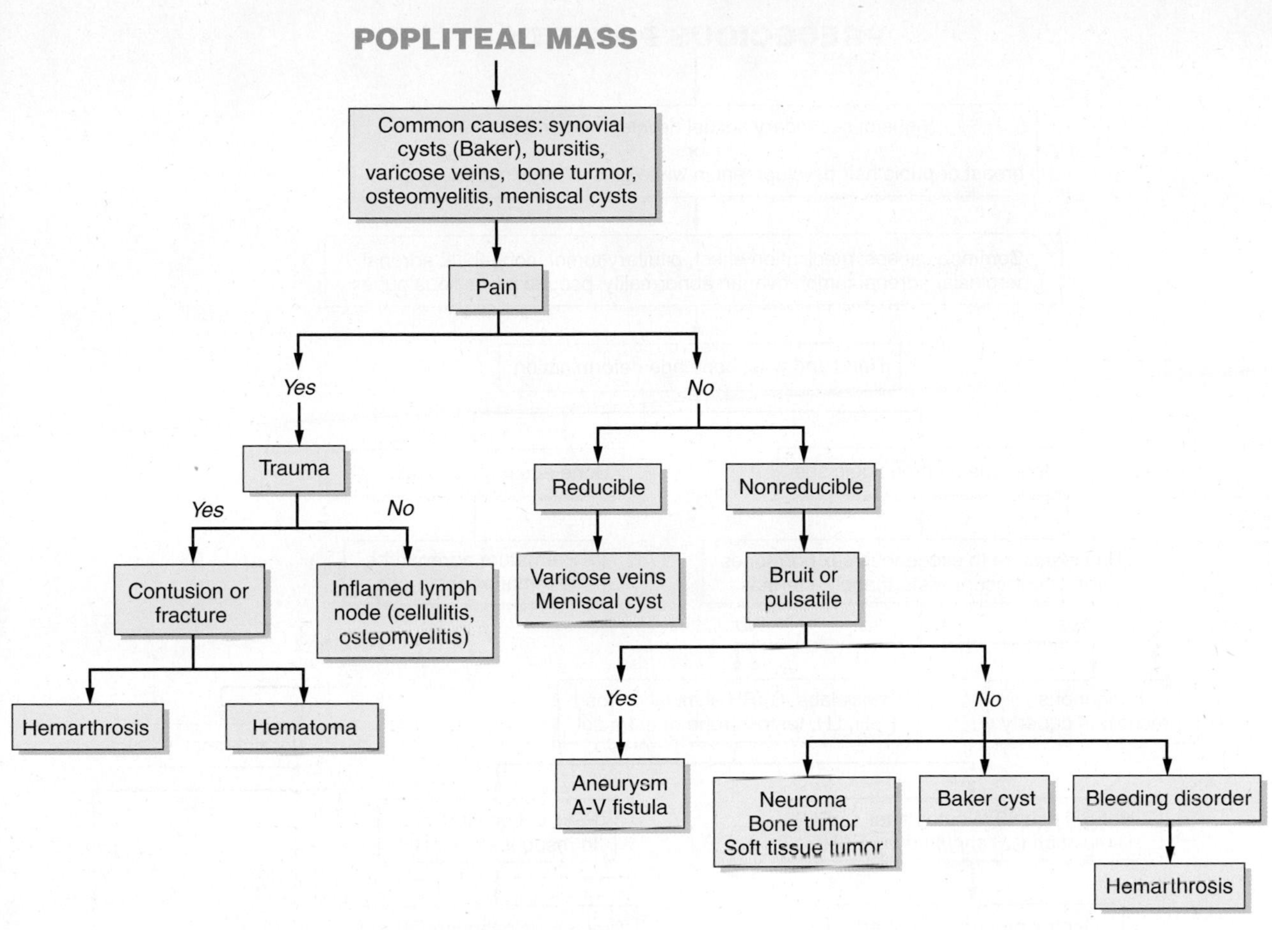

Robert A. Baldor, MD and Alan M. Ehrlich, MD

Am Fam Physician. 2003;68:917–22.

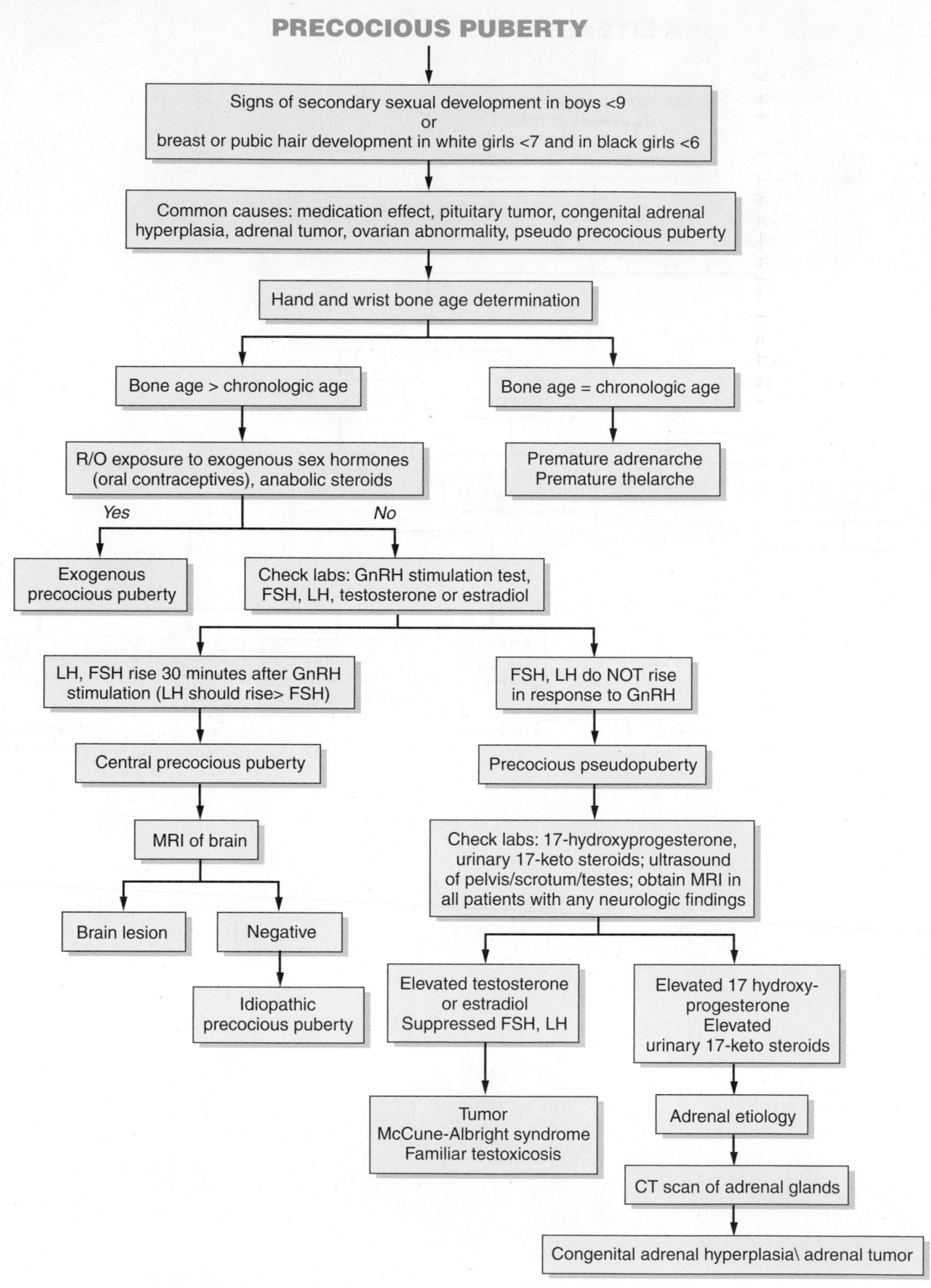
PRECOCIOUS PUBERTY
Signs of secondary sexual development in boys <9
or
breast or pubic hair development in white girls <7 and in black girls <6
Common causes: medication effect, pituitary tumor, congenital adrenal hyperplasia, adrenal tumor, ovarian abnormality, pseudo precocious puberty
Hand and wrist bone age determination
Bone age > chronologic age
Bone age = chronologic age
R/O exposure to exogenous sex hormones (oral contraceptives), anabolic steroids
Premature adrenarche
Premature thelarche
Yes
No
Exogenous precocious puberty
Check labs: GnRH stimulation test, FSH, LH, testosterone or estradiol
LH, FSH rise 30 minutes after GnRH stimulation (LH should rise> FSH)
FSH, LH do NOT rise in response to GnRH
Central precocious puberty
Precocious pseudopuberty
MRI of brain
Check labs: 17-hydroxyprogesterone, urinary 17-keto steroids; ultrasound of pelvis/scrotum/testes; obtain MRI in all patients with any neurologic findings
Brain lesion
Negative
Idiopathic precocious puberty
Elevated testosterone or estradiol Suppressed FSH, LH
Elevated 17 hydroxy-progesterone Elevated urinary 17-keto steroids
Tumor
McCune-Albright syndrome
Familiar testoxicosis
Adrenal etiology
CT scan of adrenal glands
Congenital adrenal hyperplasia\ adrenal tumor

Robert A. Baldor, MD and Alan M. Ehrlich, MD

Am Fam Physician. 2008;78(5):597–04.

PREOPERATIVE EVALUATION OF NONCARDIAC SURGICAL PATIENT

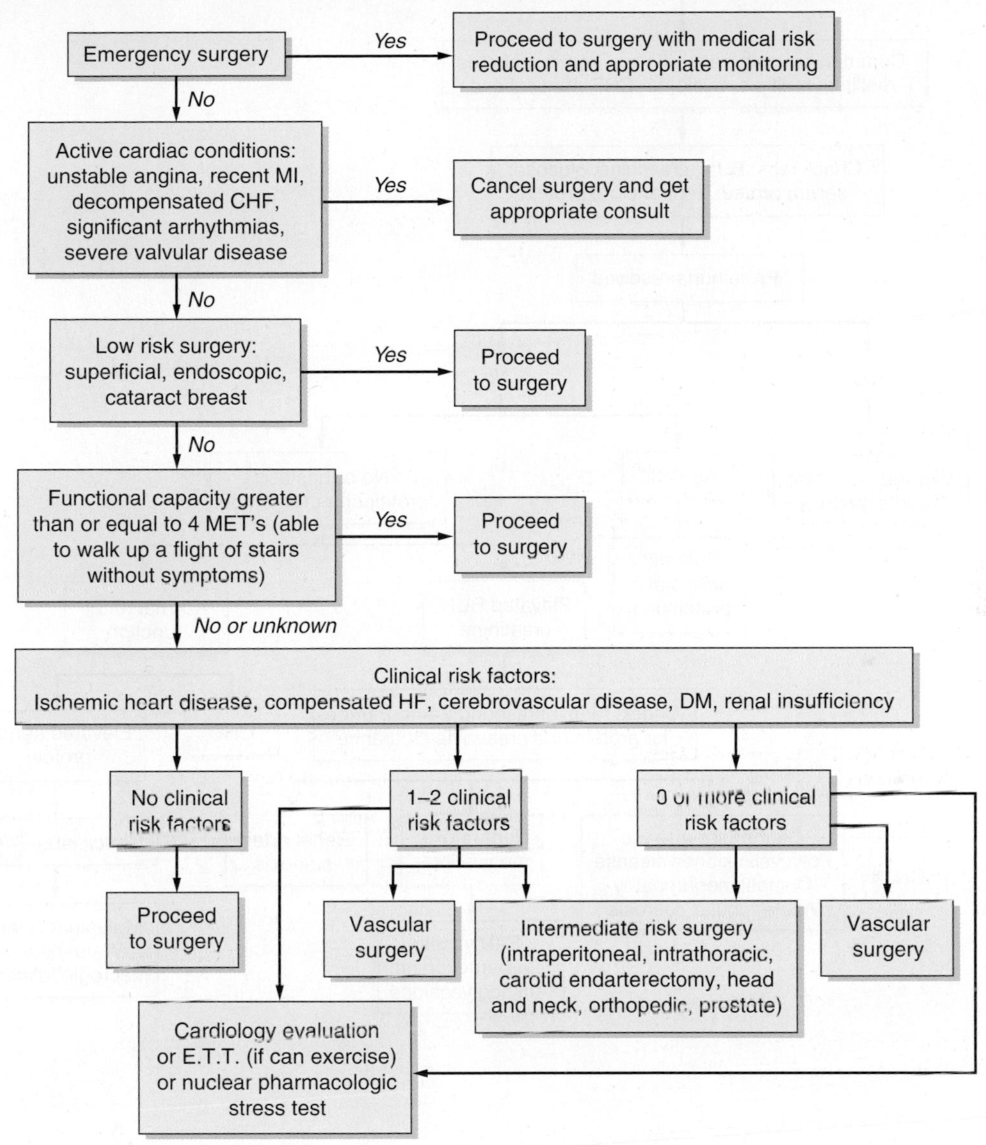

Drew Grimes, MD and Stacy Jones, MD

Circulation. 2007;116(17):e418–99.

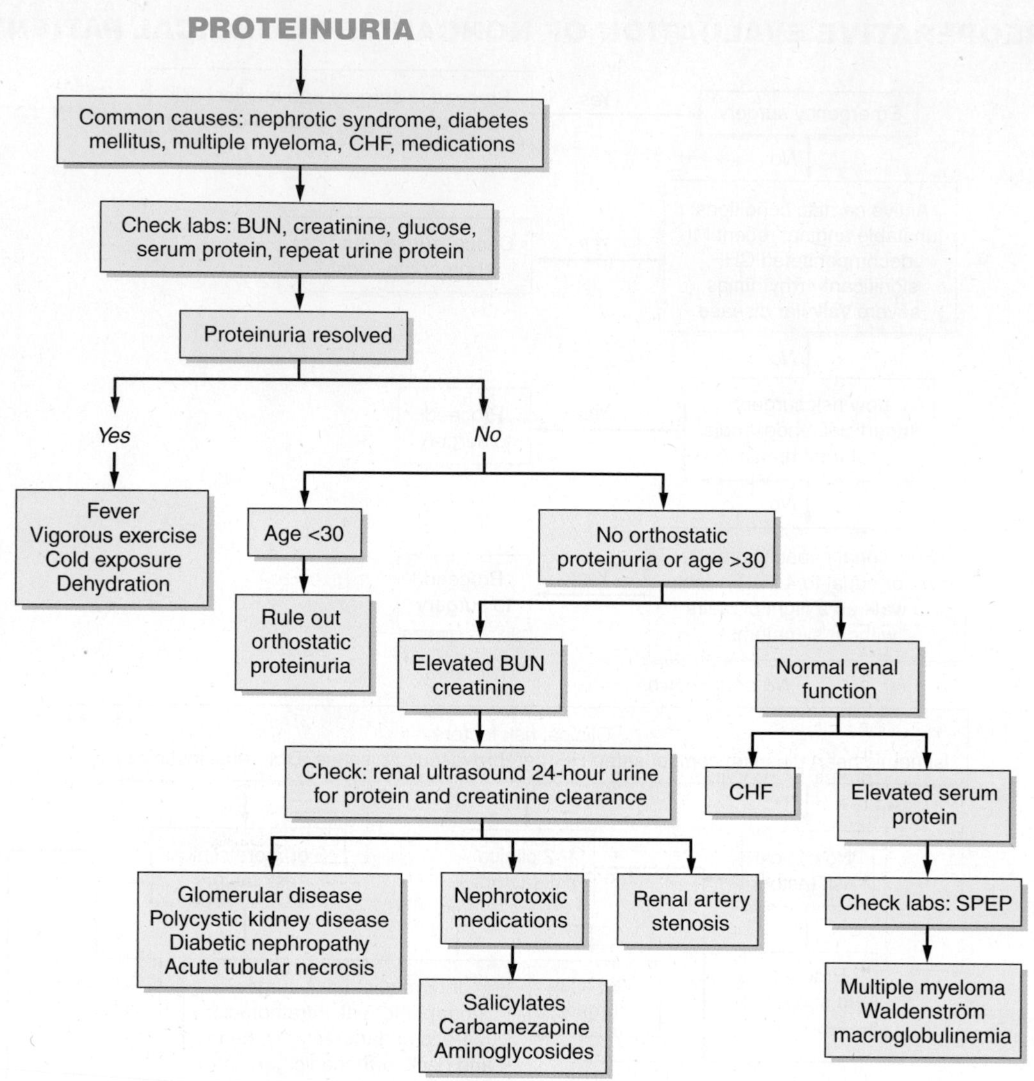
PROTEINURIA
Common causes: nephrotic syndrome, diabetes mellitus, multiple myeloma, CHF, medications
Check labs: BUN, creatinine, glucose, serum protein, repeat urine protein
Proteinuria resolved
Yes
No
Fever
Vigorous exercise
Cold exposure
Dehydration
Age <30
Rule out orthostatic proteinuria
No orthostatic proteinuria or age >30
Elevated BUN creatinine
Normal renal function
Check: renal ultrasound 24-hour urine for protein and creatinine clearance
CHF
Elevated serum protein
Glomerular disease
Polycystic kidney disease
Diabetic nephropathy
Acute tubular necrosis
Nephrotoxic medications
Renal artery stenosis
Check labs: SPEP
Salicylates
Carbamezapine
Aminoglycosides
Multiple myeloma
Waldenström macroglobulinemia

Robert A. Baldor, MD and Alan M. Ehrlich, MD

Am Fam Physician. 2000;62:1333–40.

PULMONARY EMBOLISM, DIAGNOSIS

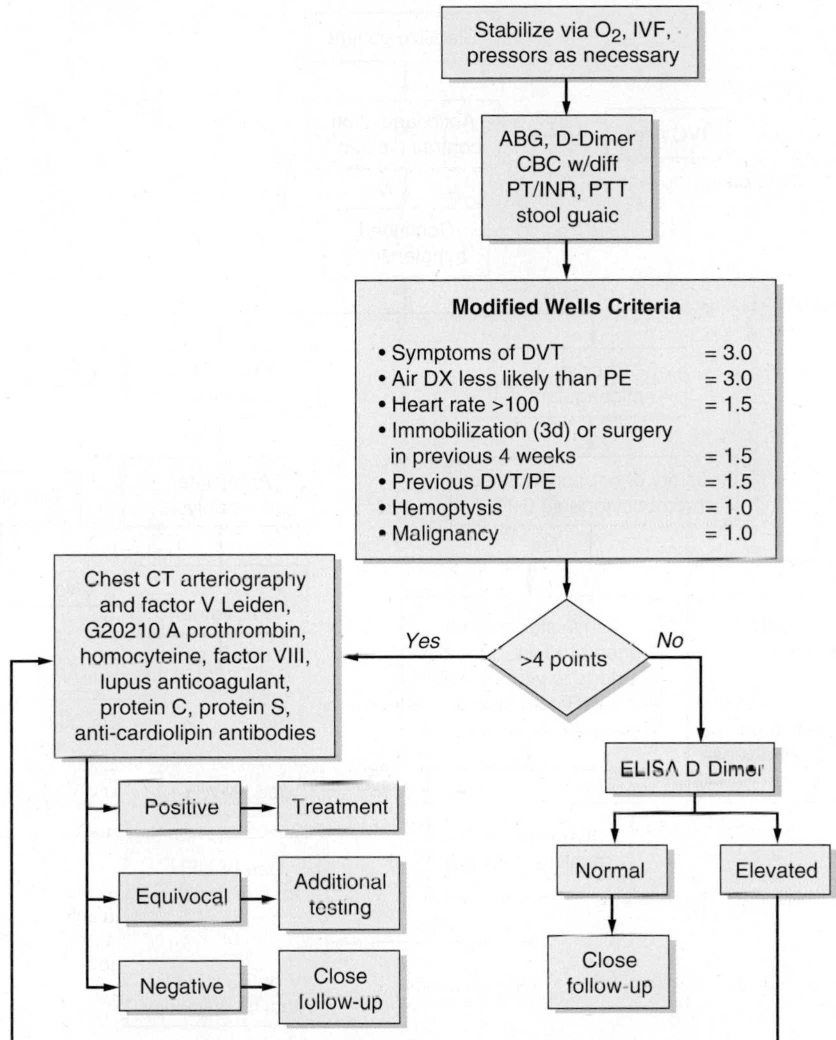

Parag Goyal, MD

Radiol Clin North Am. 2010;48(1):31–50.

PULMONARY EMBOLISM, TREATMENT

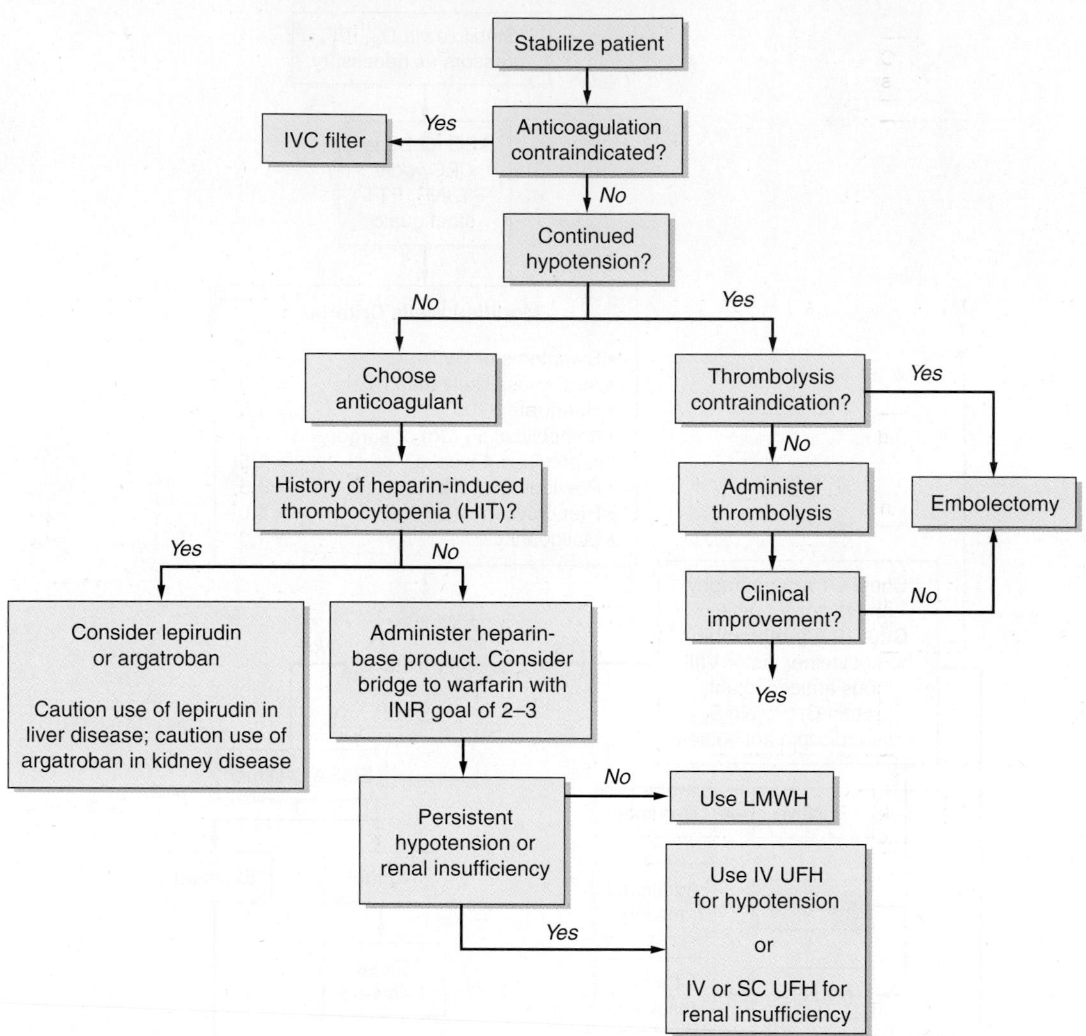

Parag Goyal, MD

NEJM. 2008;358(10):1037–52.

PUPIL ABNORMALITIES

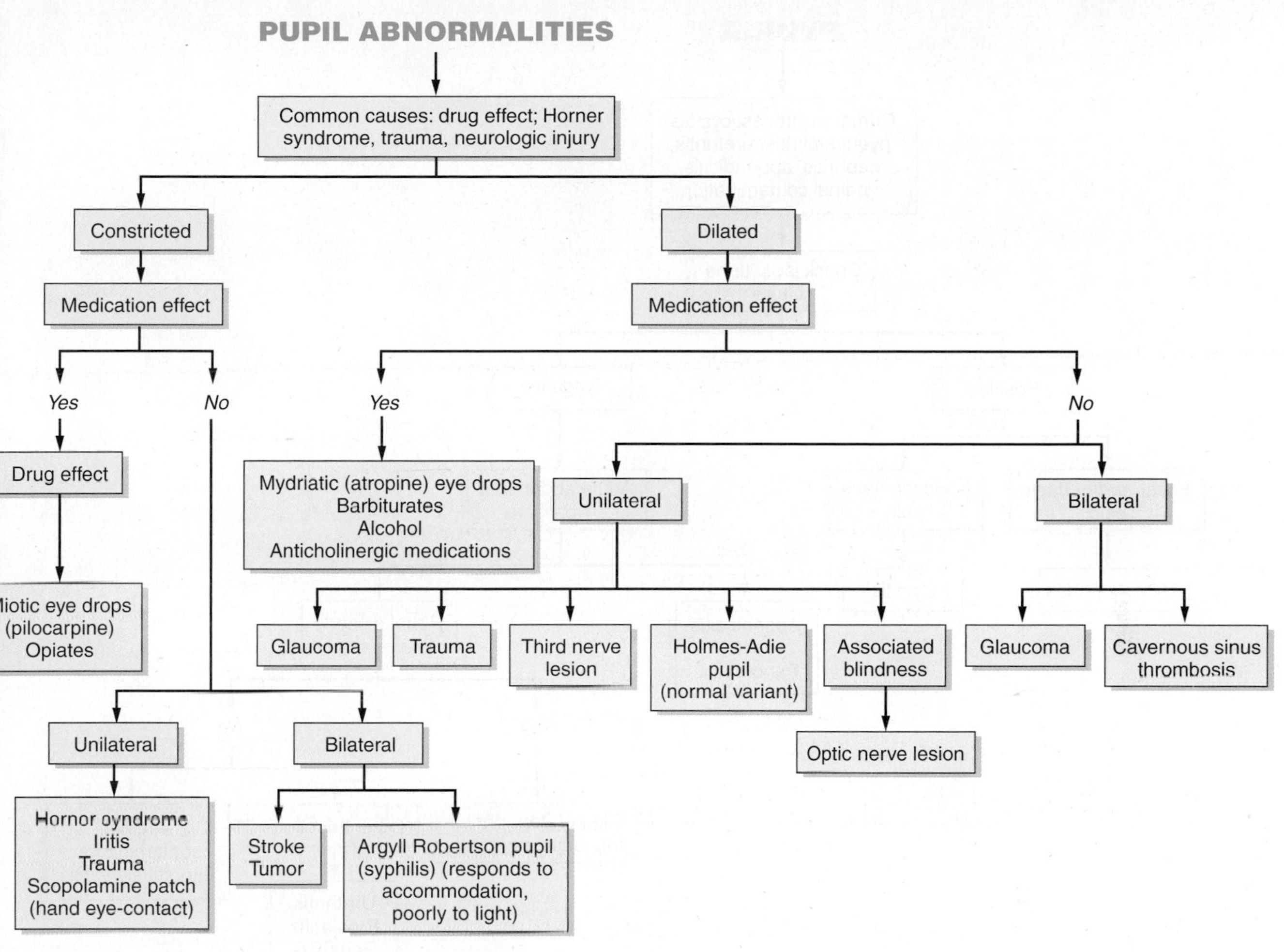

Robert A. Baldor, MD and Alan M. Ehrlich, MD

Vision Res. 2005;45(19):2549–63.

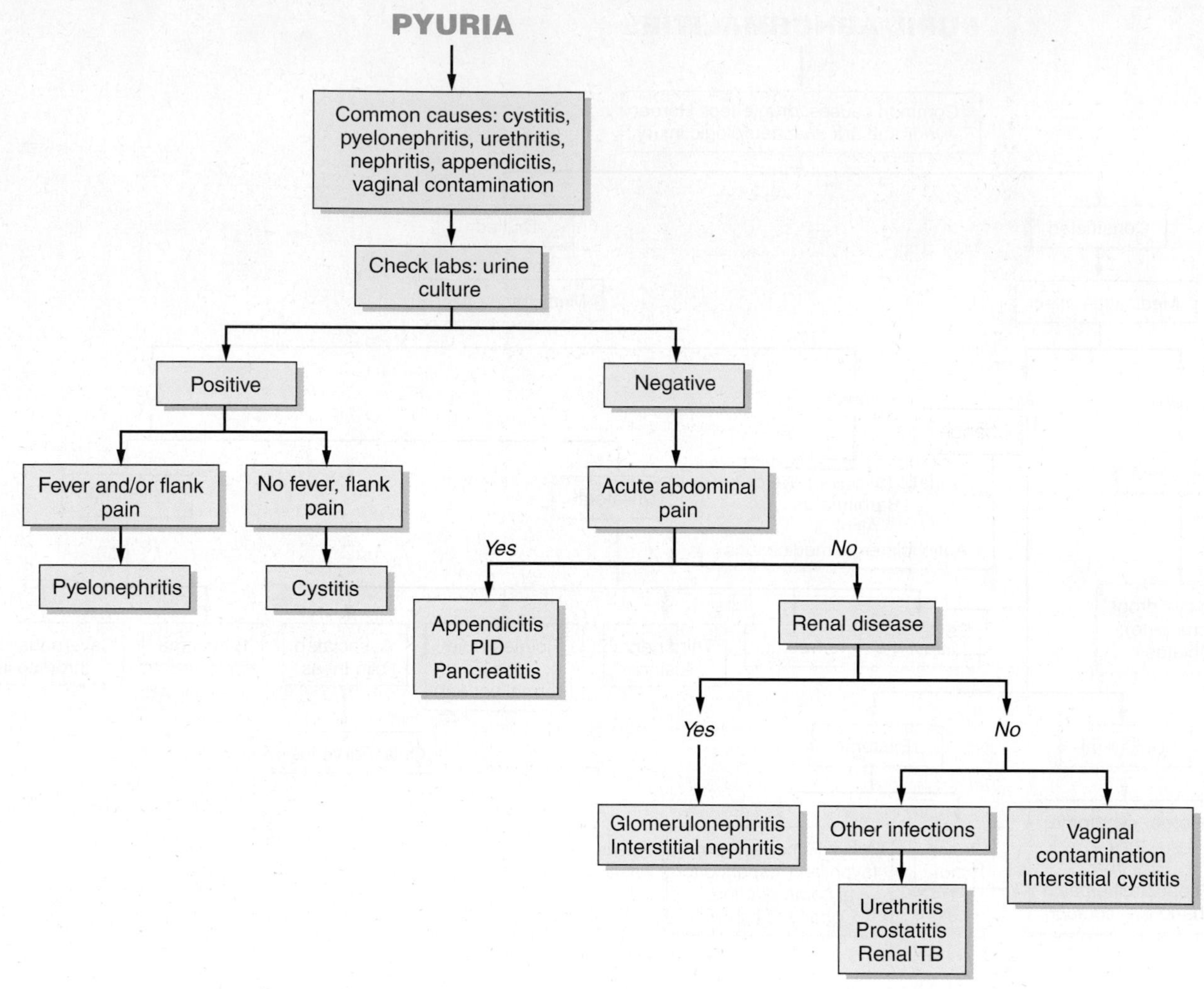

Robert A. Baldor, MD and Alan M. Ehrlich, MD

Am Fam Physician. 2005;71:1153–62.

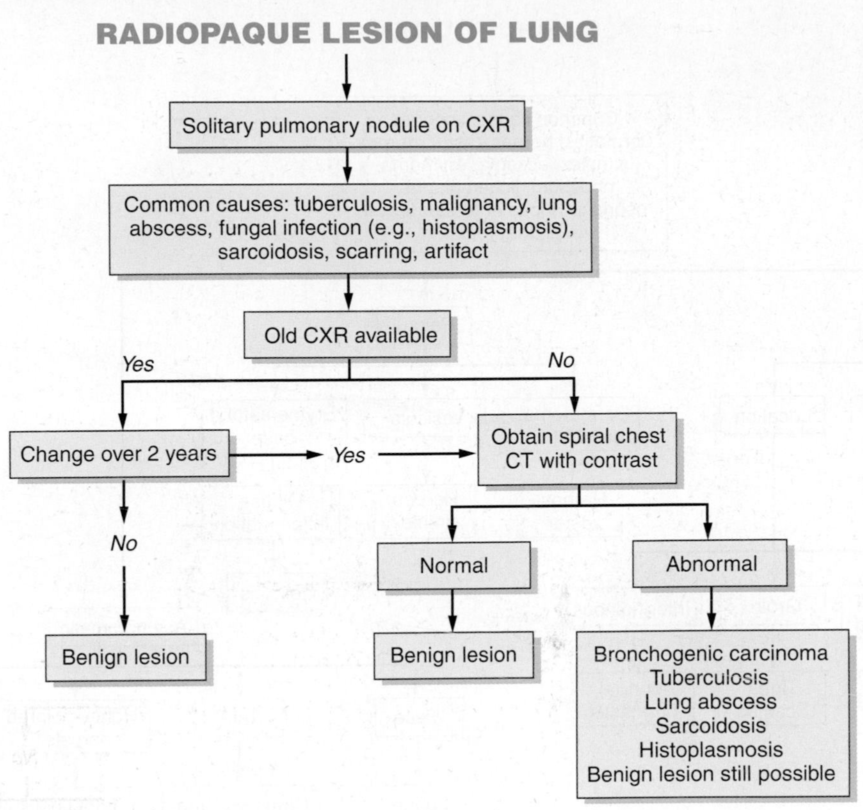

Robert A. Baldor, MD and Alan M. Ehrlich, MD

NEJM. 348(25):2535–42.

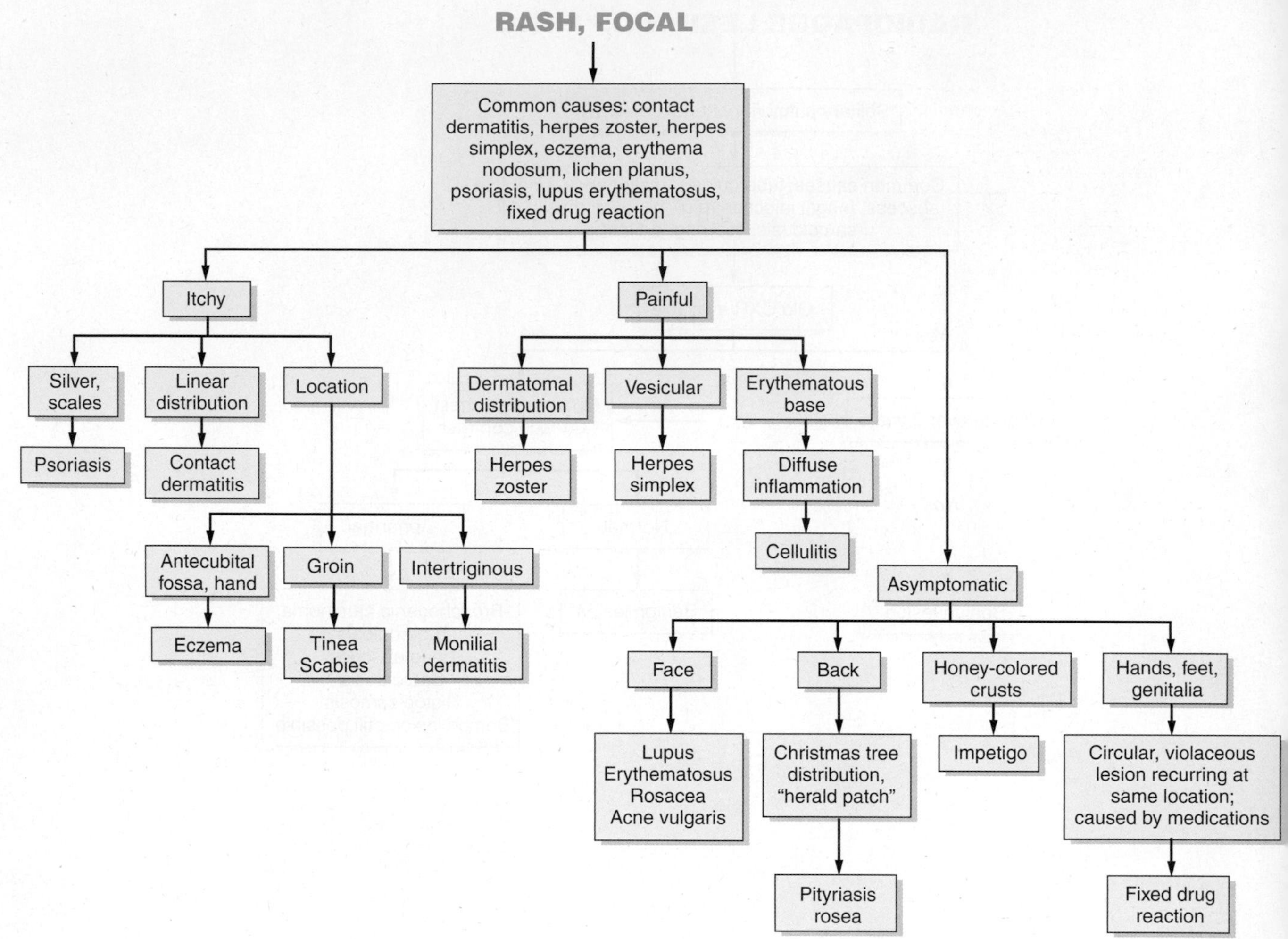
RASH, FOCAL
Common causes: contact dermatitis, herpes zoster, herpes simplex, eczema, erythema nodosum, lichen planus, psoriasis, lupus erythematosus, fixed drug reaction
Itchy
Painful
Silver, scales
Linear distribution
Location
Psoriasis
Contact dermatitis
Antecubital fossa, hand
Groin
Intertriginous
Eczema
Tinea Scabies
Monilial dermatitis
Dermatomal distribution
Vesicular
Erythematous base
Herpes zoster
Herpes simplex
Diffuse inflammation
Cellulitis
Asymptomatic
Face
Back
Honey-colored crusts
Hands, feet, genitalia
Lupus Erythematosus Rosacea Acne vulgaris
Christmas tree distribution, "herald patch"
Impetigo
Circular, violaceous lesion recurring at same location; caused by medications
Pityriasis rosea
Fixed drug reaction

Robert A. Baldor, MD and Alan M. Ehrlich, MD

Arch Dermatol. 2001;137(1):25–9.

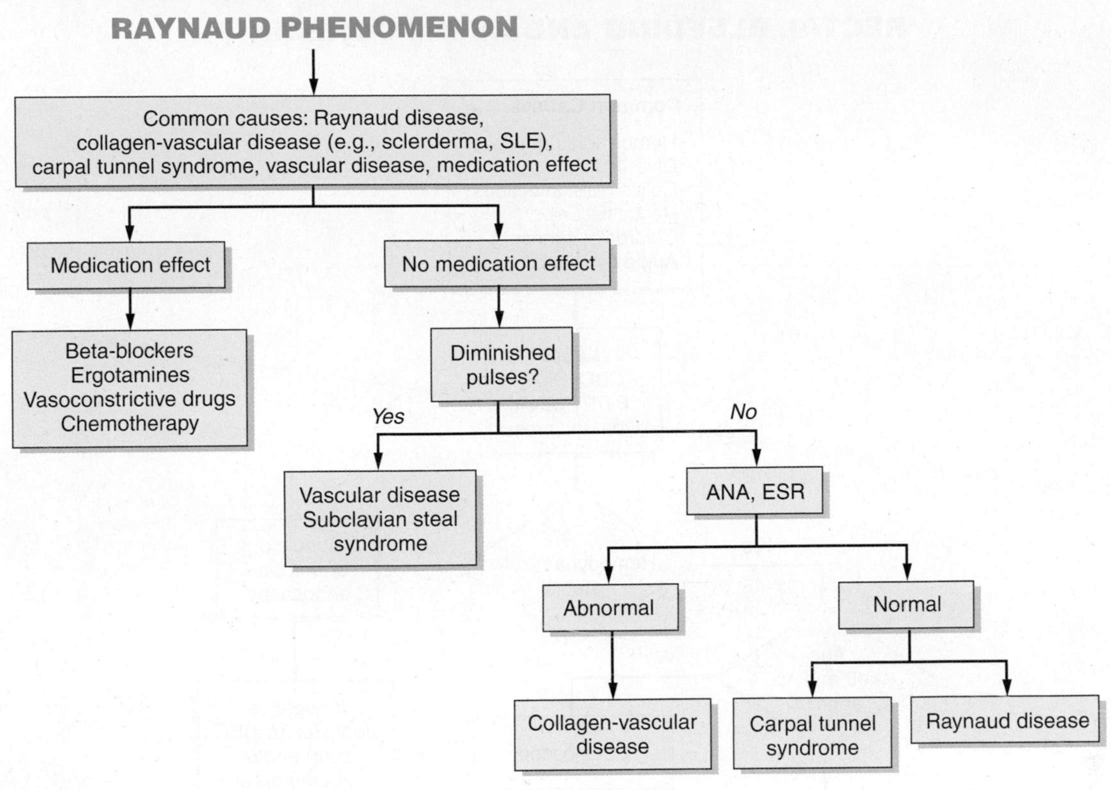

Robert A. Baldor, MD and Alan M. Ehrlich, MD

JFP. 2005 (54:6).

RECTAL BLEEDING AND HEMATOCHEZIA

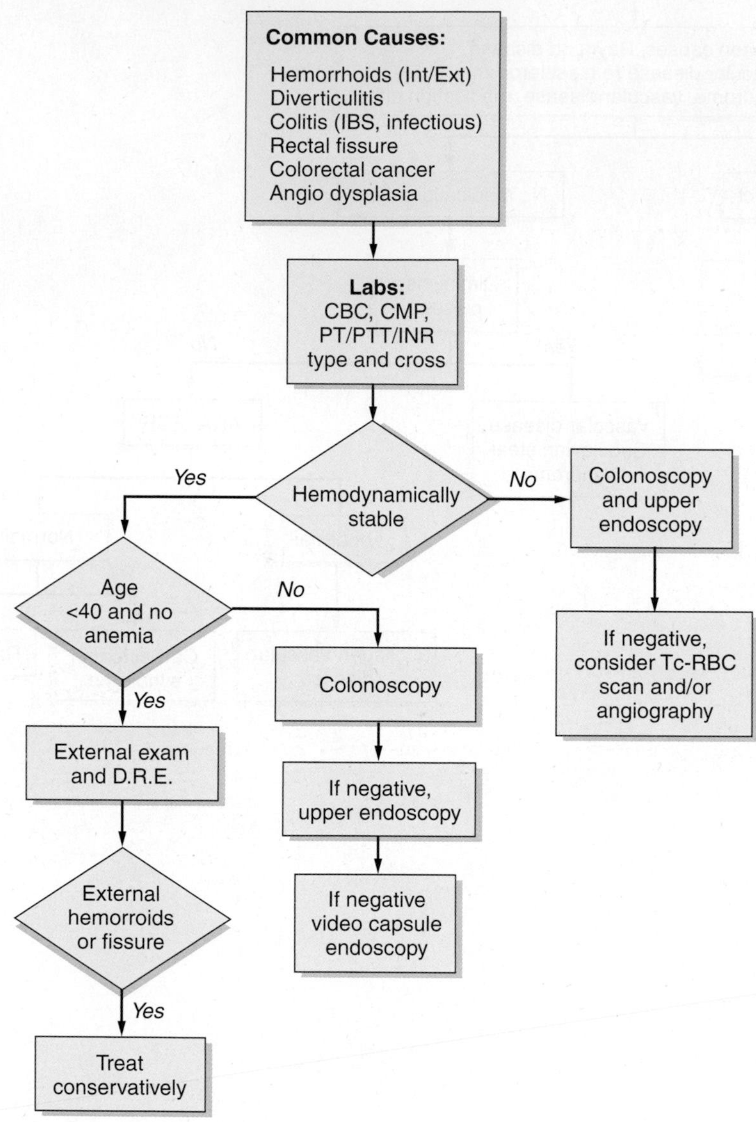

Mohammad Ansar Mughal, MD

Dis Colon Rectum. 2005;48(11):2010–24.

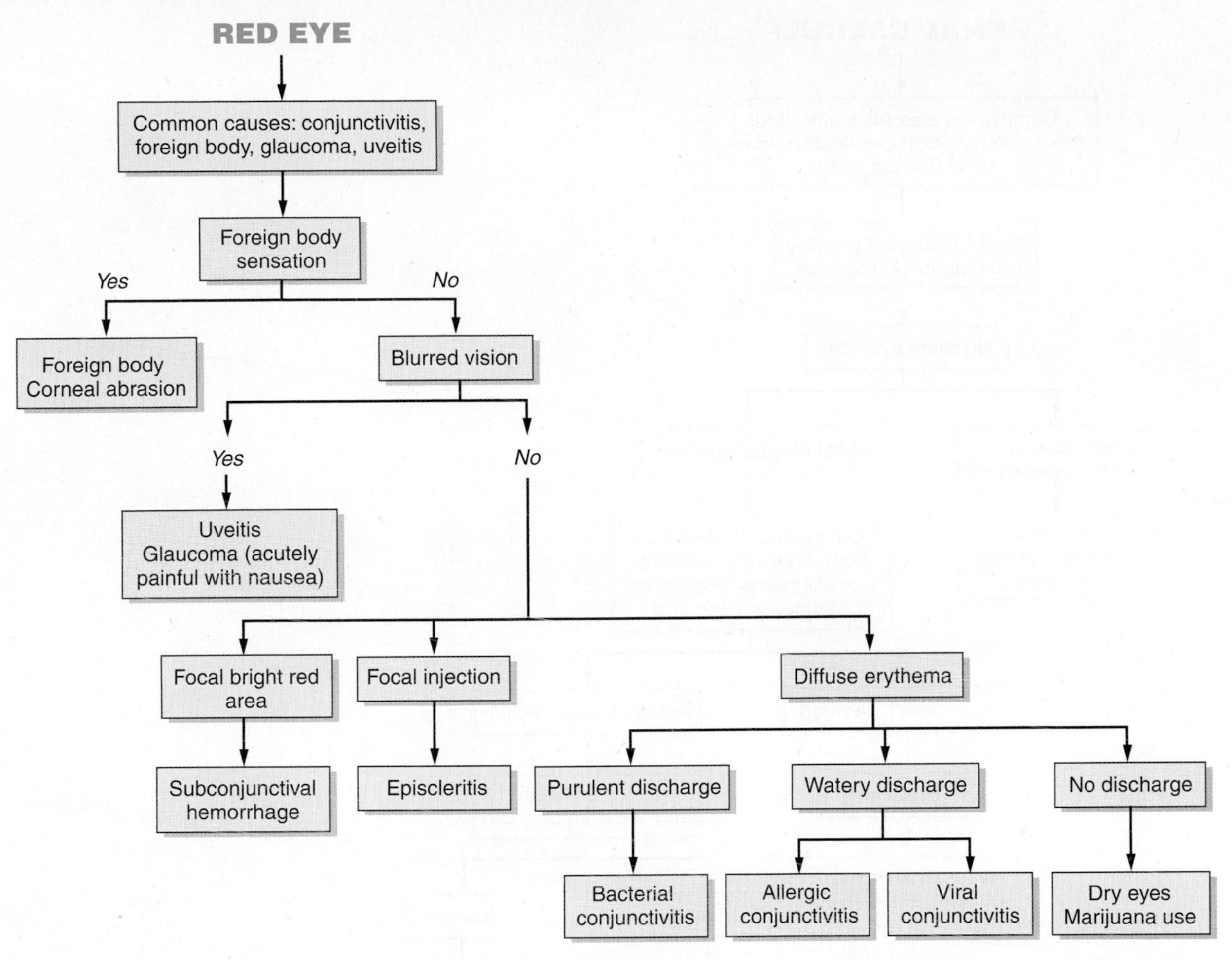

Robert A. Baldor, MD and Alan M. Ehrlich, MD

NEJM. 2000;343(5):345–51.

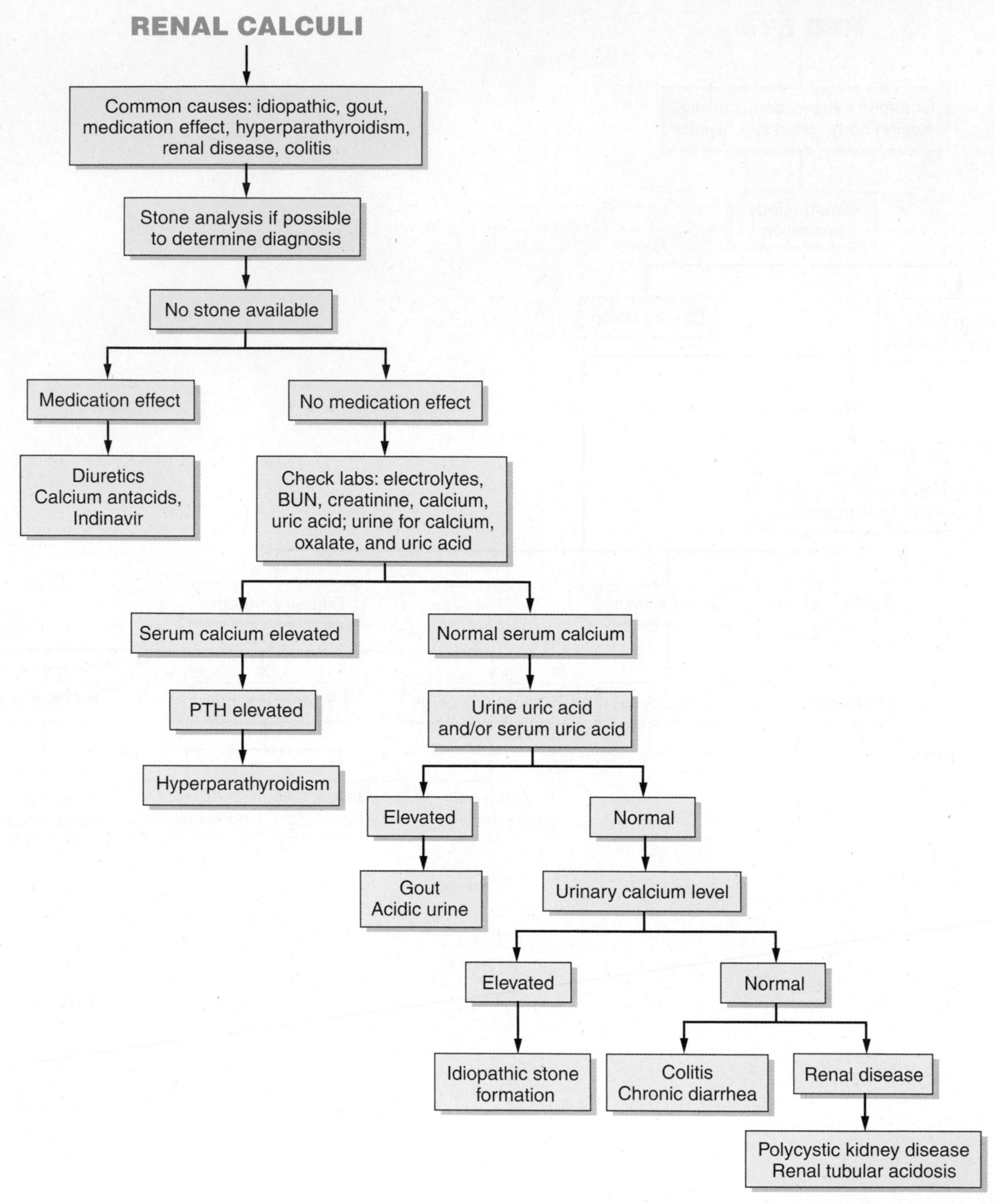
RENAL CALCULI
Common causes: idiopathic, gout, medication effect, hyperparathyroidism, renal disease, colitis
Stone analysis if possible to determine diagnosis
No stone available
Medication effect
No medication effect
Diuretics
Calcium antacids,
Indinavir
Check labs: electrolytes, BUN, creatinine, calcium, uric acid; urine for calcium, oxalate, and uric acid
Serum calcium elevated
Normal serum calcium
PTH elevated
Hyperparathyroidism
Urine uric acid and/or serum uric acid
Elevated
Normal
Gout
Acidic urine
Urinary calcium level
Elevated
Normal
Idiopathic stone formation
Colitis
Chronic diarrhea
Renal disease
Polycystic kidney disease
Renal tubular acidosis

Robert A. Baldor, MD and Alan M. Ehrlich, MD

Prim Care. 2008;35(2):369–91.

RENAL FAILURE, ACUTE

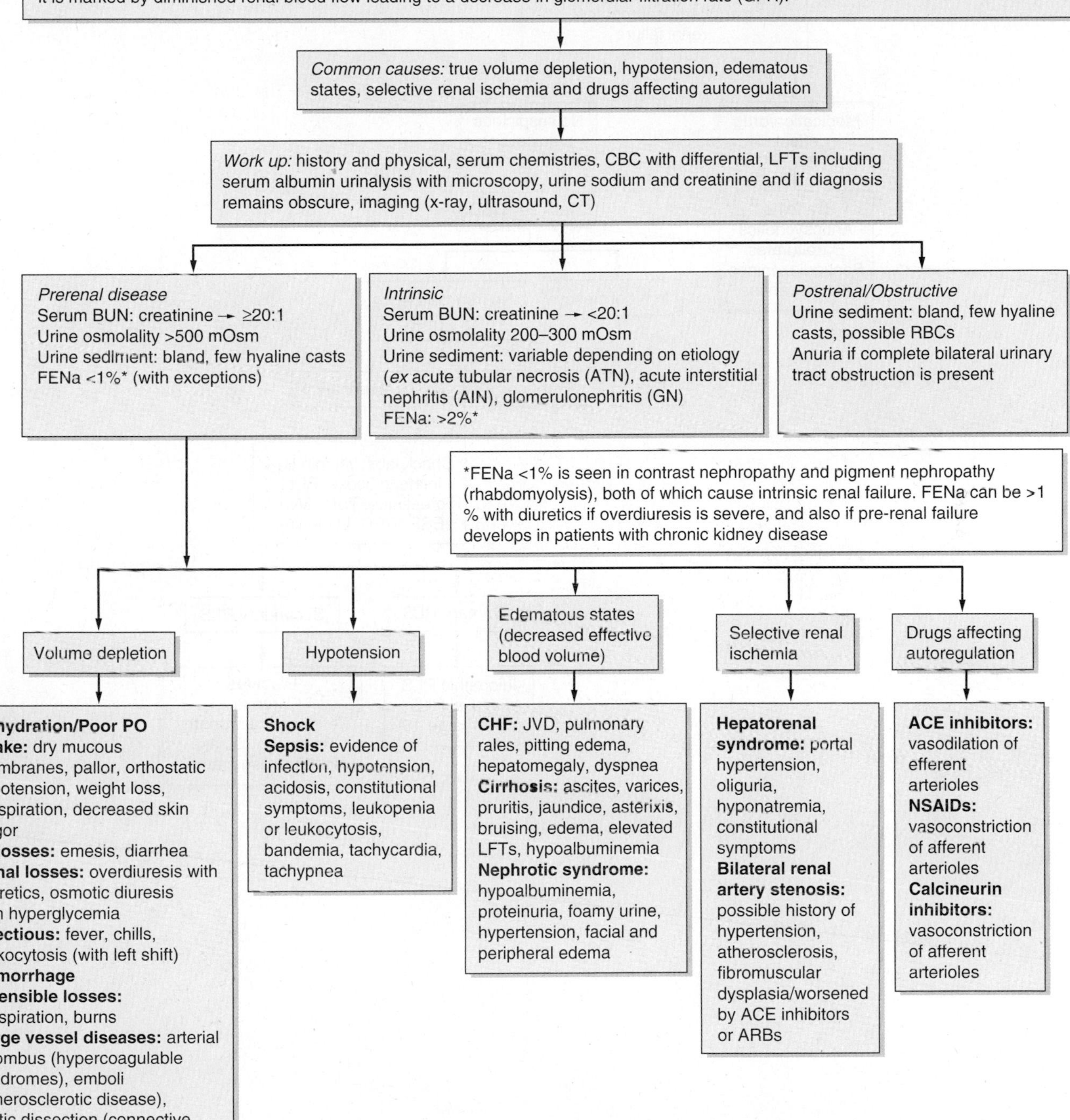

Acute kidney injury (AKI, previously called acute renal failure) is an acute loss of kidney function over days to weeks resulting in an inability to excrete nitrogenous wastes and creatinine. Patients are often asymptomatic, and are recognized by an increase in serum creatinine level (>0.5 mg/dL from baseline). Prerenal disease (PD) is one category of AKI where the injury occurs outside the nephron; it is marked by diminished renal blood flow leading to a decrease in glomerular filtration rate (GFR).
Common causes: true volume depletion, hypotension, edematous states, selective renal ischemia and drugs affecting autoregulation
Work up: history and physical, serum chemistries, CBC with differential, LFTs including serum albumin urinalysis with microscopy, urine sodium and creatinine and if diagnosis remains obscure, imaging (x-ray, ultrasound, CT)
Prerenal disease
Serum BUN: creatinine → ≥20:1
Urine osmolality >500 mOsm
Urine sediment: bland, few hyaline casts
FENa <1%* (with exceptions)
Intrinsic
Serum BUN: creatinine → <20:1
Urine osmolality 200–300 mOsm
Urine sediment: variable depending on etiology (*ex* acute tubular necrosis (ATN), acute interstitial nephritis (AIN), glomerulonephritis (GN)
FENa: >2%*
Postrenal/Obstructive
Urine sediment: bland, few hyaline casts, possible RBCs
Anuria if complete bilateral urinary tract obstruction is present
*FENa <1% is seen in contrast nephropathy and pigment nephropathy (rhabdomyolysis), both of which cause intrinsic renal failure. FENa can be >1 % with diuretics if overdiuresis is severe, and also if pre-renal failure develops in patients with chronic kidney disease
Volume depletion
Hypotension
Edematous states (decreased effective blood volume)
Selective renal ischemia
Drugs affecting autoregulation
Dehydration/Poor PO intake: dry mucous membranes, pallor, orthostatic hypotension, weight loss, perspiration, decreased skin turgor
GI losses: emesis, diarrhea
Renal losses: overdiuresis with Diuretics, osmotic diuresis with hyperglycemia
Infectious: fever, chills, leukocytosis (with left shift)
Hemorrhage
Insensible losses: perspiration, burns
Large vessel diseases: arterial thrombus (hypercoagulable syndromes), emboli (atherosclerotic disease), aortic dissection (connective tissue disease, trauma)
Shock
Sepsis: evidence of infection, hypotension, acidosis, constitutional symptoms, leukopenia or leukocytosis, bandemia, tachycardia, tachypnea
CHF: JVD, pulmonary rales, pitting edema, hepatomegaly, dyspnea
Cirrhosis: ascites, varices, pruritis, jaundice, asterixis, bruising, edema, elevated LFTs, hypoalbuminemia
Nephrotic syndrome: hypoalbuminemia, proteinuria, foamy urine, hypertension, facial and peripheral edema
Hepatorenal syndrome: portal hypertension, oliguria, hyponatremia, constitutional symptoms
Bilateral renal artery stenosis: possible history of hypertension, atherosclerosis, fibromuscular dysplasia/worsened by ACE inhibitors or ARBs
ACE inhibitors: vasodilation of efferent arterioles
NSAIDs: vasoconstriction of afferent arterioles
Calcineurin inhibitors: vasoconstriction of afferent arterioles

Krunal Patel, MD and Dagmar Klinger, MD

Am Fam Physician. 2005;72(9):1739–47.

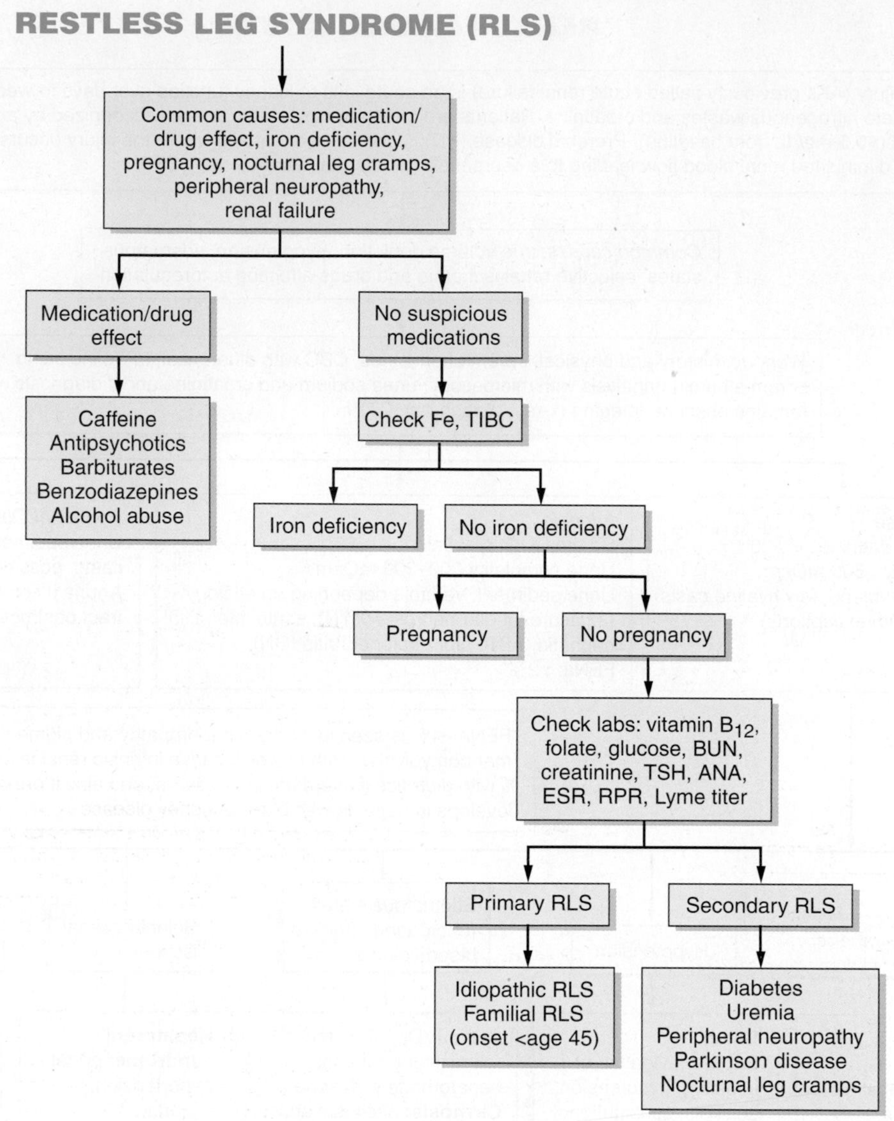

Robert A. Baldor, MD and Alan M. Ehrlich, MD

Am Fam Physician. 2000;62:108–14.

SEIZURE, NEW ONSET

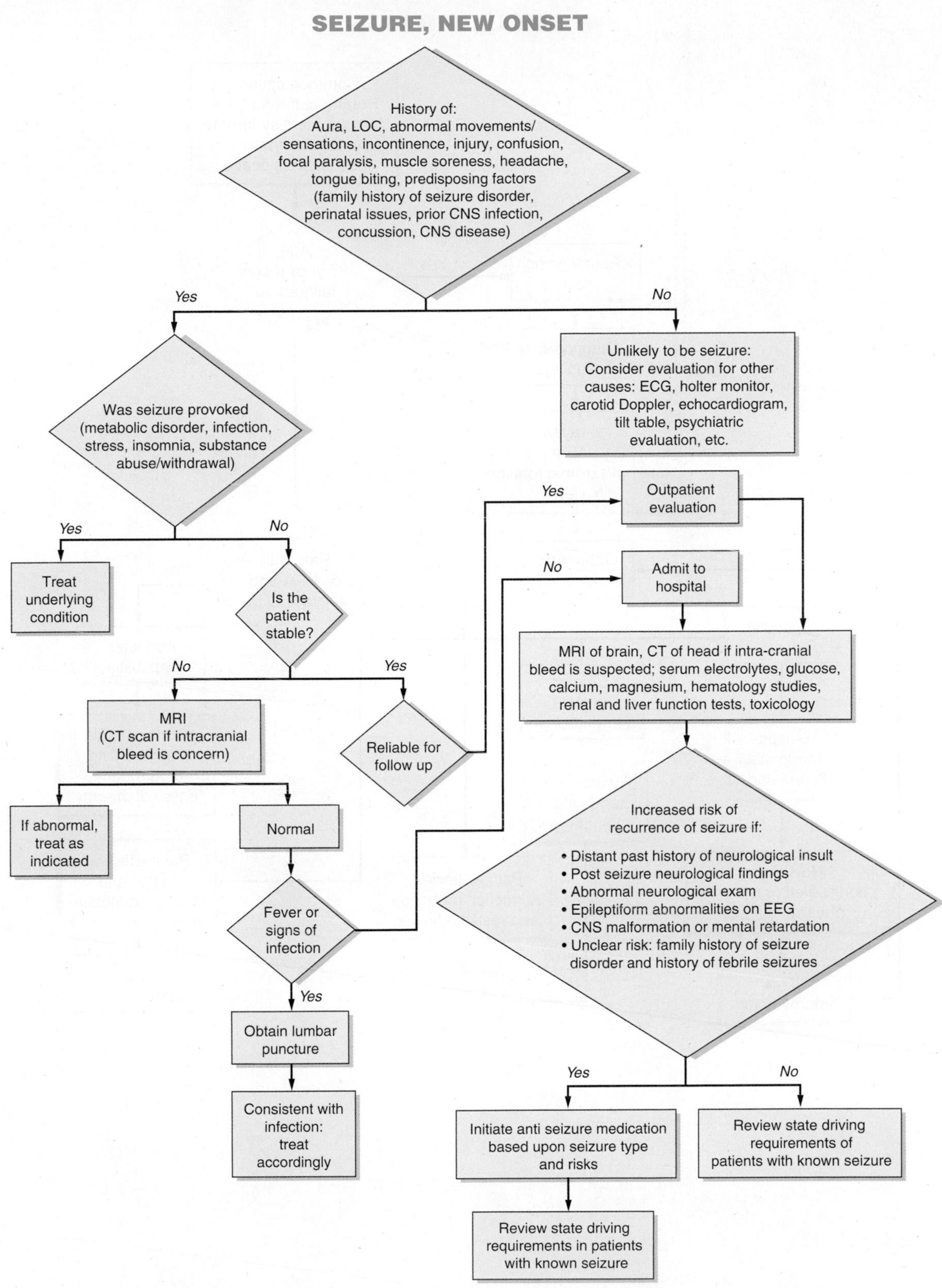

Neepa Patel, MD and Ioannis Karakis, MD

N Engl J Med. 2003;349:1257.

SHOULDER PAIN

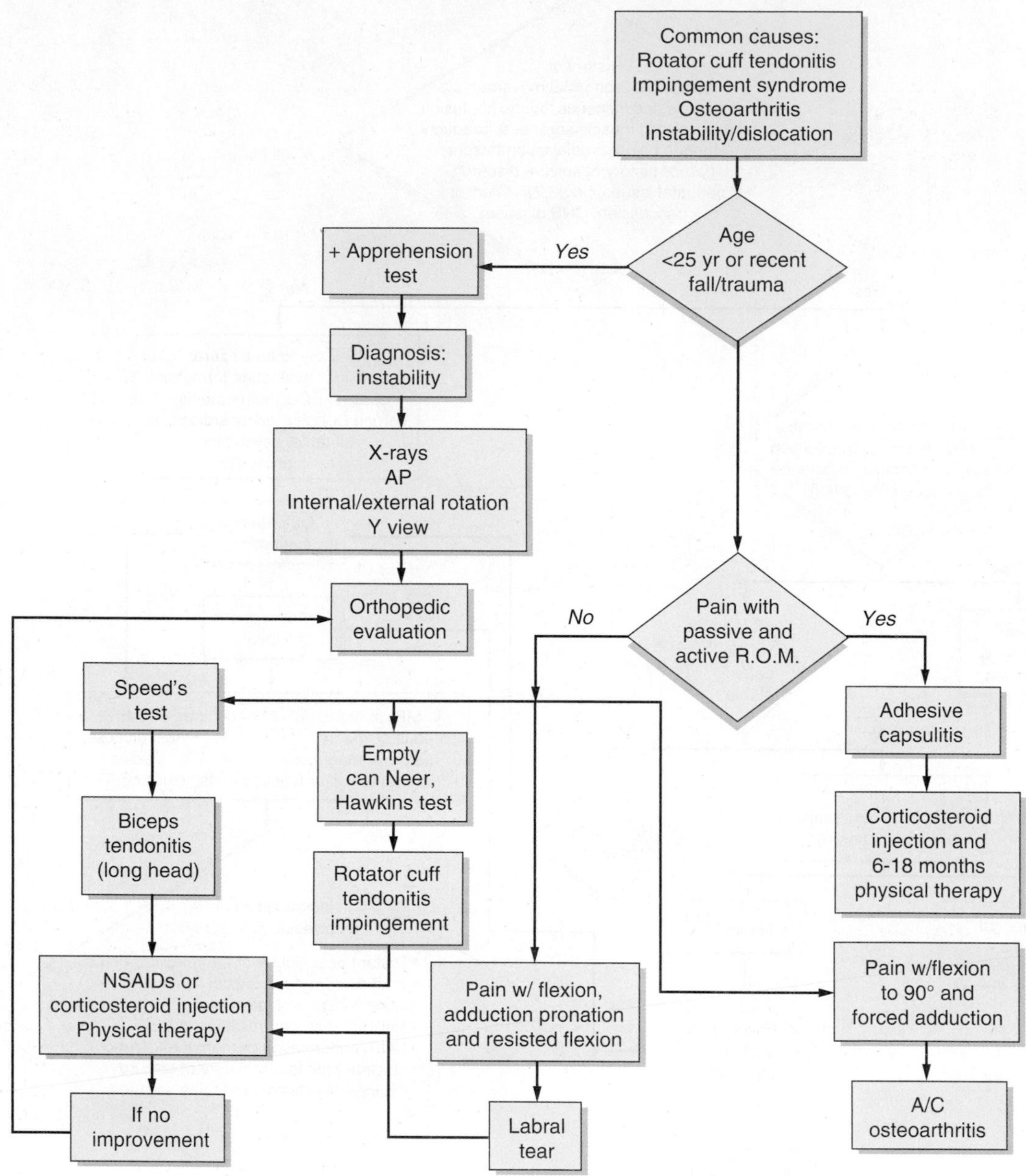

David W. Kruse, MD and Murat Mardirossian, MD

Am Fam Physician. 2000;61:3079–89.

SICKLE CELL ANEMIA, ACUTE COMPLICATIONS

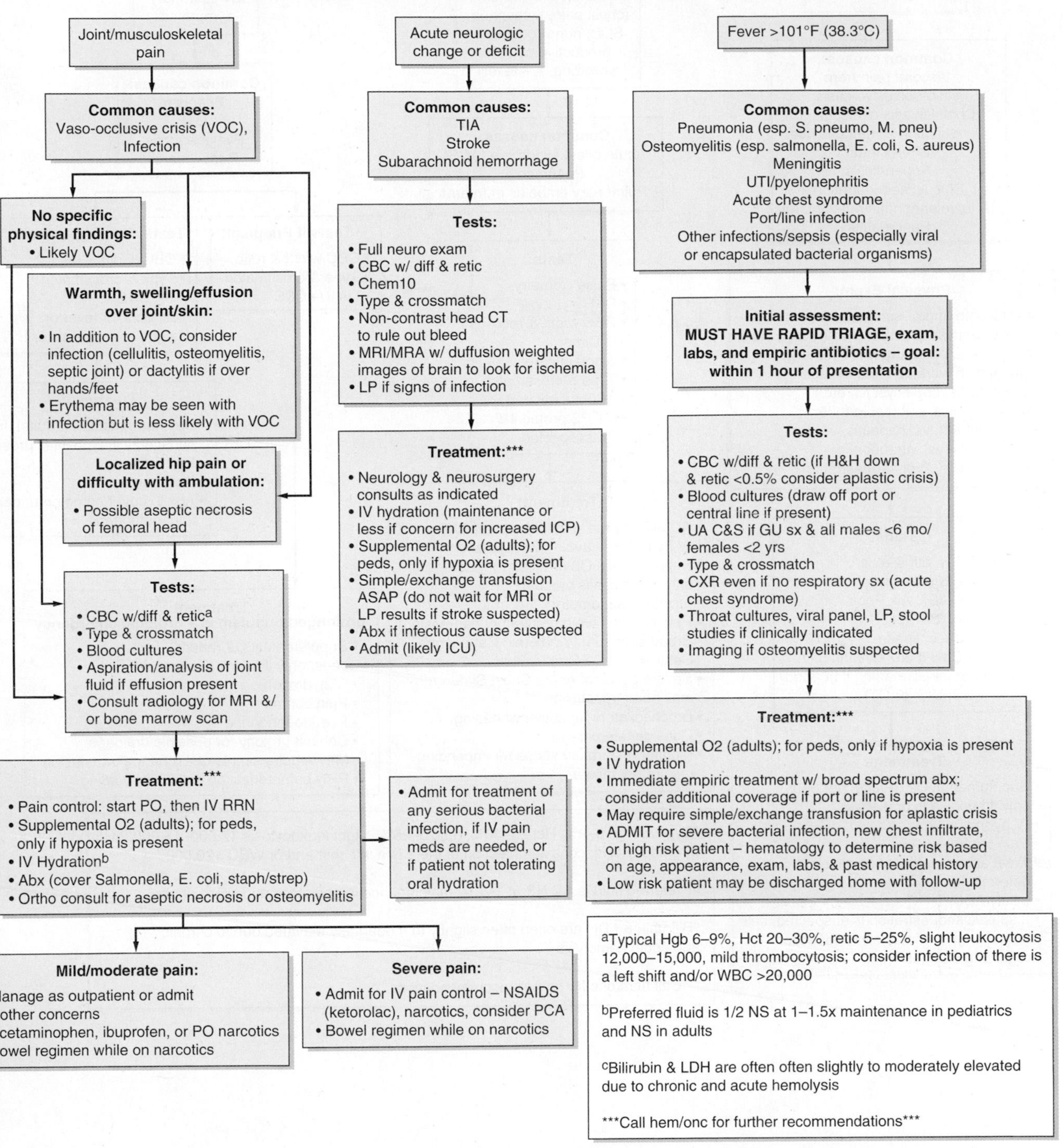
Joint/musculoskeletal pain
Common causes: Vaso-occlusive crisis (VOC), Infection
No specific physical findings: • Likely VOC
Warmth, swelling/effusion over joint/skin:
• In addition to VOC, consider infection (cellulitis, osteomyelitis, septic joint) or dactylitis if over hands/feet
• Erythema may be seen with infection but is less likely with VOC
Localized hip pain or difficulty with ambulation:
• Possible aseptic necrosis of femoral head
Tests:
• CBC w/diff & retic[a]
• Type & crossmatch
• Blood cultures
• Aspiration/analysis of joint fluid if effusion present
• Consult radiology for MRI &/ or bone marrow scan
Treatment:***
• Pain control: start PO, then IV RRN
• Supplemental O2 (adults); for peds, only if hypoxia is present
• IV Hydration[b]
• Abx (cover Salmonella, E. coli, staph/strep)
• Ortho consult for aseptic necrosis or osteomyelitis
• Admit for treatment of any serious bacterial infection, if IV pain meds are needed, or if patient not tolerating oral hydration
Mild/moderate pain:
• Manage as outpatient or admit if other concerns
• Acetaminophen, ibuprofen, or PO narcotics
• Bowel regimen while on narcotics
Severe pain:
• Admit for IV pain control – NSAIDS (ketorolac), narcotics, consider PCA
• Bowel regimen while on narcotics
Acute neurologic change or deficit
Common causes: TIA Stroke Subarachnoid hemorrhage
Tests:
• Full neuro exam
• CBC w/ diff & retic
• Chem10
• Type & crossmatch
• Non-contrast head CT to rule out bleed
• MRI/MRA w/ duffusion weighted images of brain to look for ischemia
• LP if signs of infection
Treatment:***
• Neurology & neurosurgery consults as indicated
• IV hydration (maintenance or less if concern for increased ICP)
• Supplemental O2 (adults); for peds, only if hypoxia is present
• Simple/exchange transfusion ASAP (do not wait for MRI or LP results if stroke suspected)
• Abx if infectious cause suspected
• Admit (likely ICU)
Fever >101°F (38.3°C)
Common causes:
Pneumonia (esp. S. pneumo, M. pneu)
Osteomyelitis (esp. salmonella, E. coli, S. aureus)
Meningitis
UTI/pyelonephritis
Acute chest syndrome
Port/line infection
Other infections/sepsis (especially viral or encapsulated bacterial organisms)
Initial assessment: MUST HAVE RAPID TRIAGE, exam, labs, and empiric antibiotics – goal: within 1 hour of presentation
Tests:
• CBC w/diff & retic (if H&H down & retic <0.5% consider aplastic crisis)
• Blood cultures (draw off port or central line if present)
• UA C&S if GU sx & all males <6 mo/ females <2 yrs
• Type & crossmatch
• CXR even if no respiratory sx (acute chest syndrome)
• Throat cultures, viral panel, LP, stool studies if clinically indicated
• Imaging if osteomyelitis suspected
Treatment:***
• Supplemental O2 (adults); for peds, only if hypoxia is present
• IV hydration
• Immediate empiric treatment w/ broad spectrum abx; consider additional coverage if port or line is present
• May require simple/exchange transfusion for aplastic crisis
• ADMIT for severe bacterial infection, new chest infiltrate, or high risk patient – hematology to determine risk based on age, appearance, exam, labs, & past medical history
• Low risk patient may be discharged home with follow-up

[a]Typical Hgb 6–9%, Hct 20–30%, retic 5–25%, slight leukocytosis 12,000–15,000, mild thrombocytosis; consider infection of there is a left shift and/or WBC >20,000

[b]Preferred fluid is 1/2 NS at 1–1.5x maintenance in pediatrics and NS in adults

[c]Bilirubin & LDH are often often slightly to moderately elevated due to chronic and acute hemolysis

Call hem/onc for further recommendations

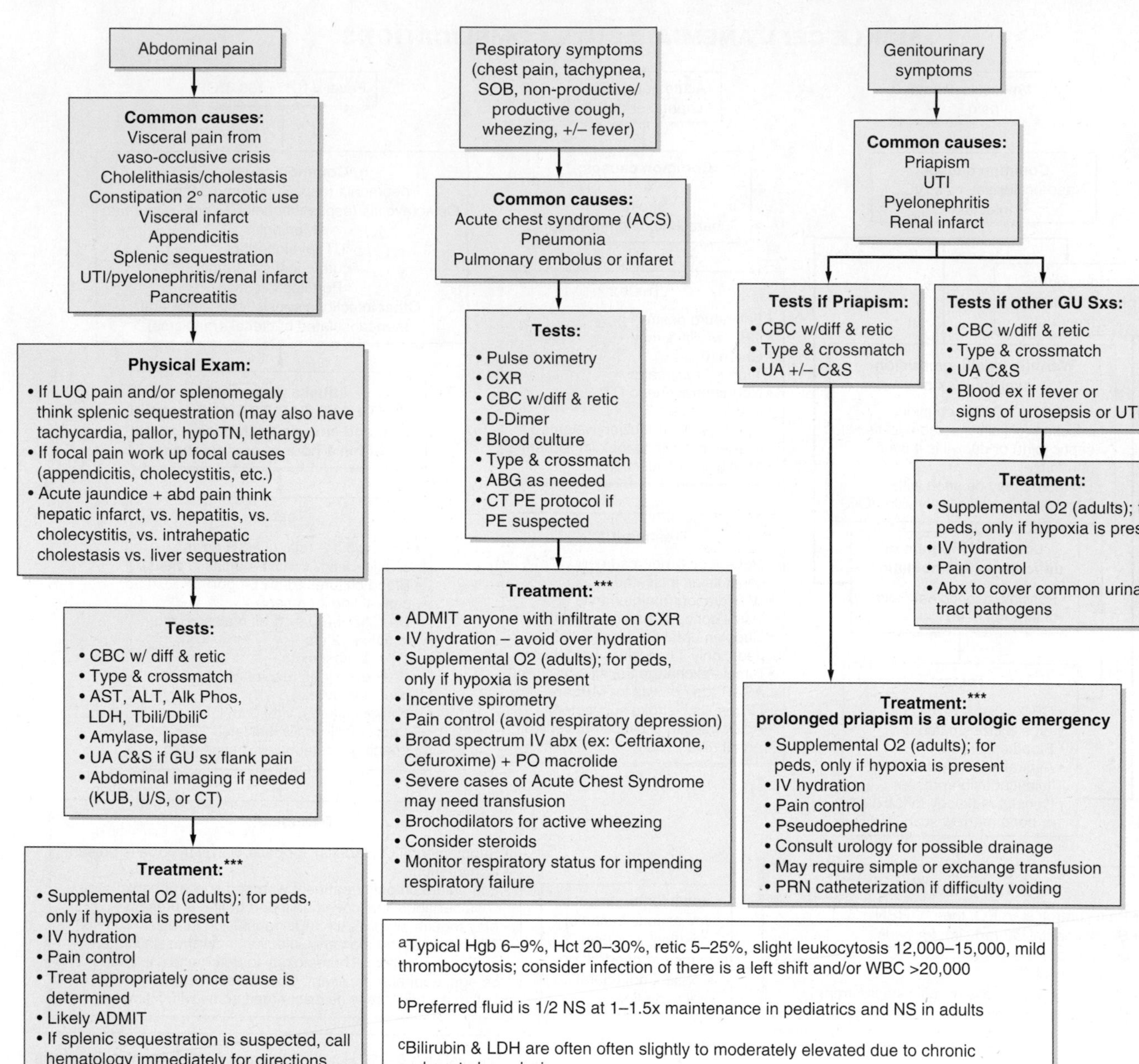
Abdominal pain
Common causes:
Visceral pain from vaso-occlusive crisis
Cholelithiasis/cholestasis
Constipation 2° narcotic use
Visceral infarct
Appendicitis
Splenic sequestration
UTI/pyelonephritis/renal infarct
Pancreatitis
Physical Exam:
• If LUQ pain and/or splenomegaly think splenic sequestration (may also have tachycardia, pallor, hypoTN, lethargy)
• If focal pain work up focal causes (appendicitis, cholecystitis, etc.)
• Acute jaundice + abd pain think hepatic infarct, vs. hepatitis, vs. cholecystitis, vs. intrahepatic cholestasis vs. liver sequestration
Tests:
• CBC w/ diff & retic
• Type & crossmatch
• AST, ALT, Alk Phos, LDH, Tbili/Dbili[c]
• Amylase, lipase
• UA C&S if GU sx flank pain
• Abdominal imaging if needed (KUB, U/S, or CT)
Treatment:***
• Supplemental O2 (adults); for peds, only if hypoxia is present
• IV hydration
• Pain control
• Treat appropriately once cause is determined
• Likely ADMIT
• If splenic sequestration is suspected, call hematology immediately for directions regarding transfusion
Respiratory symptoms (chest pain, tachypnea, SOB, non-productive/ productive cough, wheezing, +/– fever)
Common causes:
Acute chest syndrome (ACS)
Pneumonia
Pulmonary embolus or infaret
Tests:
• Pulse oximetry
• CXR
• CBC w/diff & retic
• D-Dimer
• Blood culture
• Type & crossmatch
• ABG as needed
• CT PE protocol if PE suspected
Treatment:***
• ADMIT anyone with infiltrate on CXR
• IV hydration – avoid over hydration
• Supplemental O2 (adults); for peds, only if hypoxia is present
• Incentive spirometry
• Pain control (avoid respiratory depression)
• Broad spectrum IV abx (ex: Ceftriaxone, Cefuroxime) + PO macrolide
• Severe cases of Acute Chest Syndrome may need transfusion
• Brochodilators for active wheezing
• Consider steroids
• Monitor respiratory status for impending respiratory failure
Genitourinary symptoms
Common causes:
Priapism
UTI
Pyelonephritis
Renal infarct
Tests if Priapism:
• CBC w/diff & retic
• Type & crossmatch
• UA +/– C&S
Tests if other GU Sxs:
• CBC w/diff & retic
• Type & crossmatch
• UA C&S
• Blood ex if fever or signs of urosepsis or UTI
Treatment:
• Supplemental O2 (adults); for peds, only if hypoxia is present
• IV hydration
• Pain control
• Abx to cover common urinary tract pathogens
Treatment:***
prolonged priapism is a urologic emergency
• Supplemental O2 (adults); for peds, only if hypoxia is present
• IV hydration
• Pain control
• Pseudoephedrine
• Consult urology for possible drainage
• May require simple or exchange transfusion
• PRN catheterization if difficulty voiding

[a]Typical Hgb 6–9%, Hct 20–30%, retic 5–25%, slight leukocytosis 12,000–15,000, mild thrombocytosis; consider infection of there is a left shift and/or WBC >20,000

[b]Preferred fluid is 1/2 NS at 1–1.5x maintenance in pediatrics and NS in adults

[c]Bilirubin & LDH are often often slightly to moderately elevated due to chronic and acute hemolysis

Call hem/onc for further recommendations

Stephanie Ruest, MD, Neil Grossman, MD and Doreen Brettler, MD

http://www.nepscc.org/index.html.

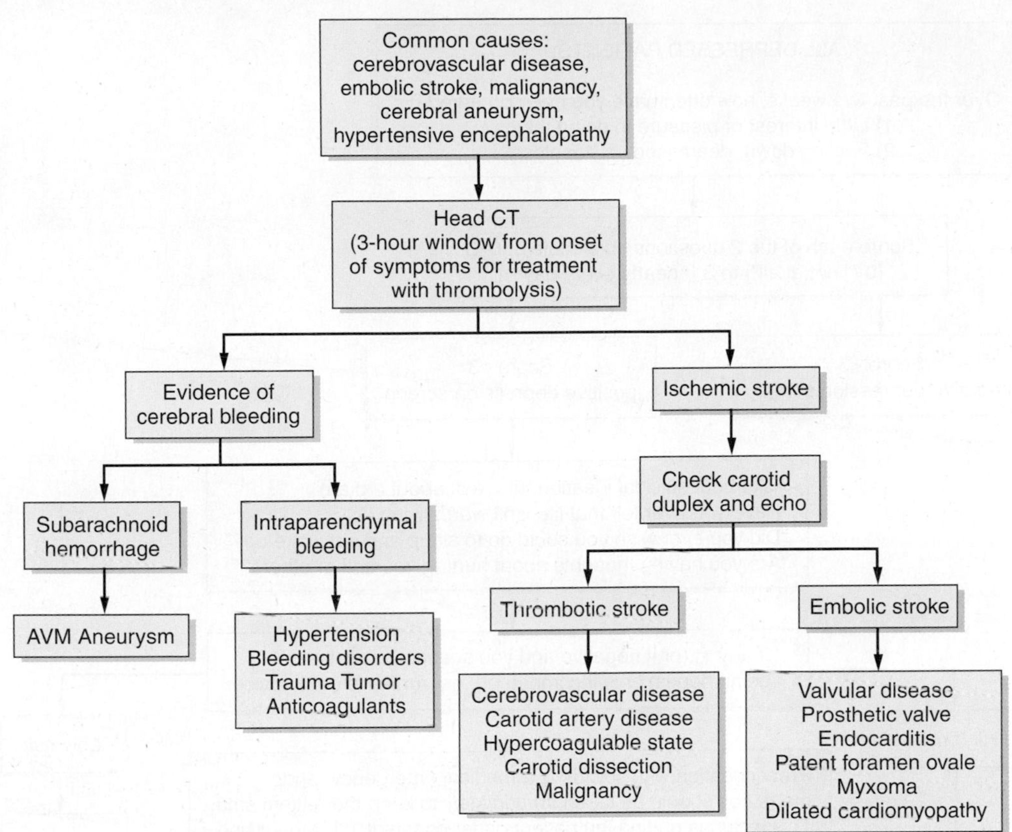

Robert A. Baldor, MD and Alan M. Ehrlich, MD

Stroke. 2007;38:1655–711.

SUICIDE, EVALUATING RISK FOR

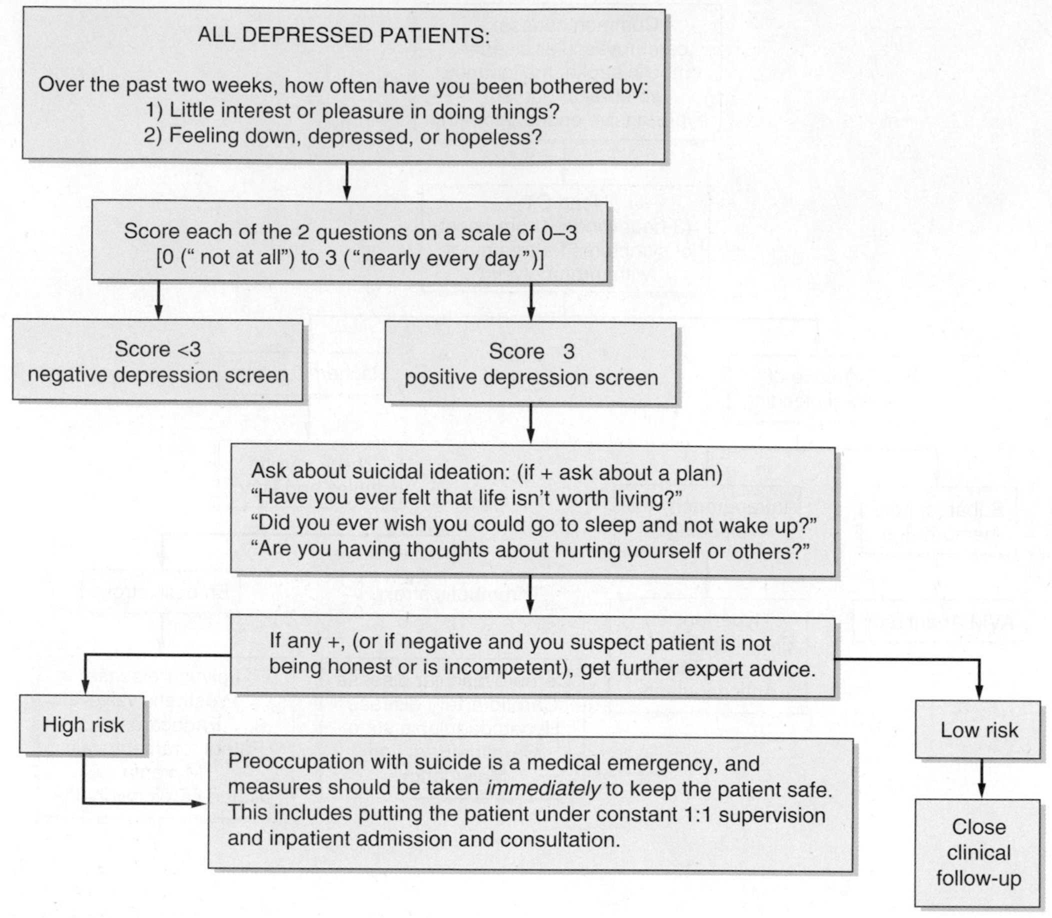

Irene C. Coletsos, MD and Harold J. Bursztajn, MD

Am J Psych. 2007;164:1035–43.

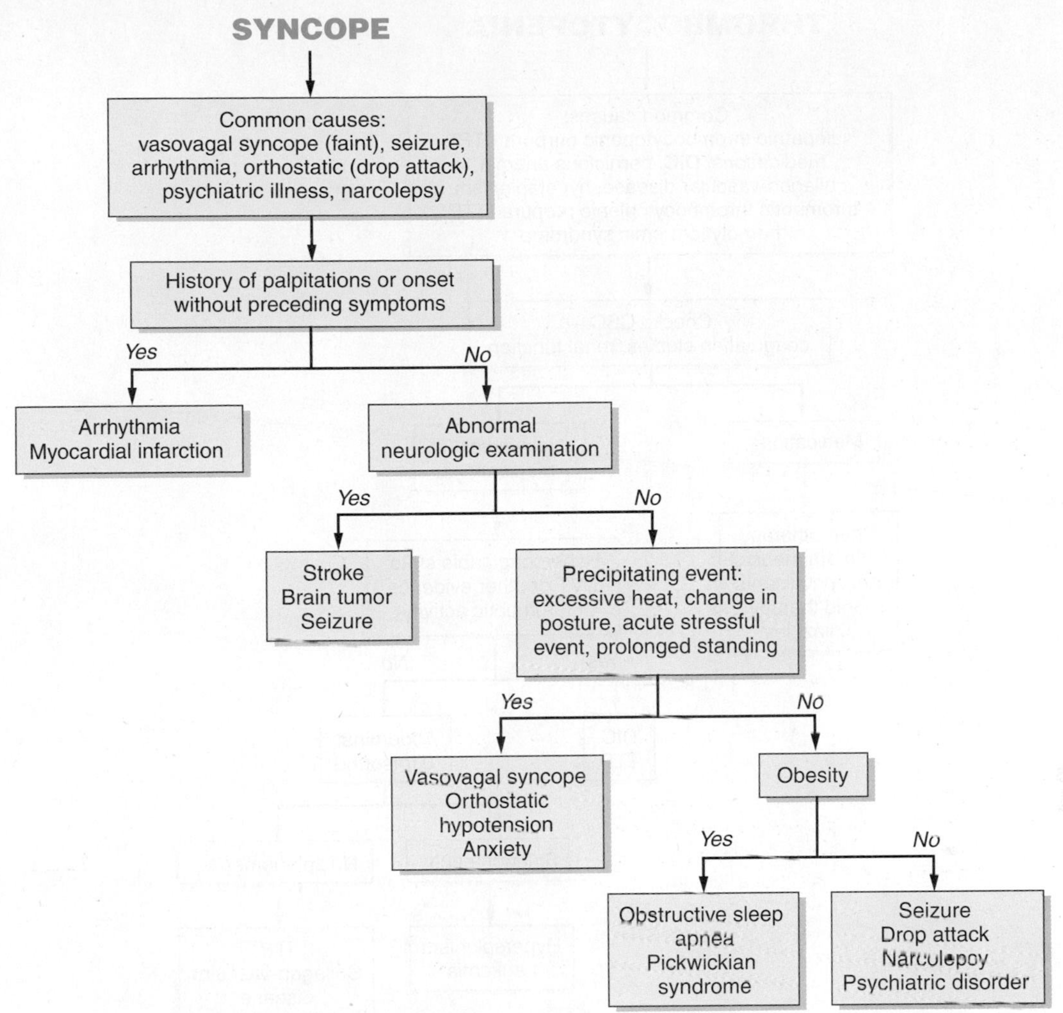

Robert A. Baldor, MD and Alan M. Ehrlich, MD

Med Clin North Am. 1995;79(5):1153–70.

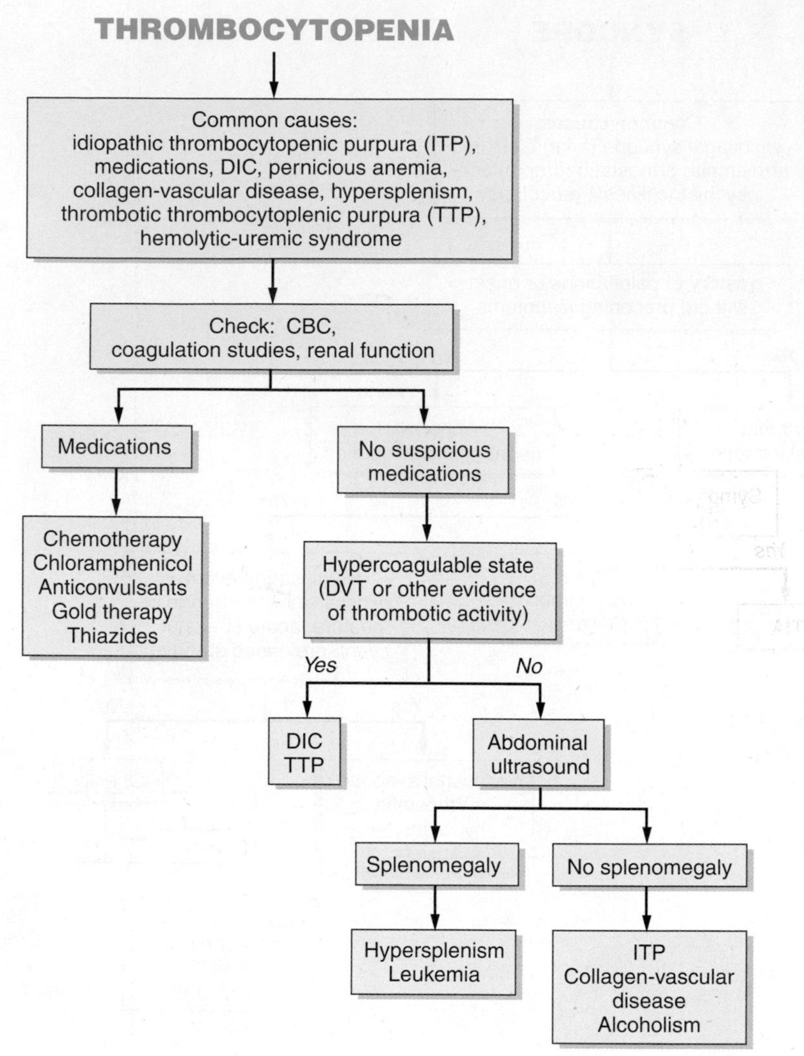
THROMBOCYTOPENIA
Common causes:
idiopathic thrombocytopenic purpura (ITP),
medications, DIC, pernicious anemia,
collagen-vascular disease, hypersplenism,
thrombotic thrombocytoplenic purpura (TTP),
hemolytic-uremic syndrome
Check: CBC,
coagulation studies, renal function
Medications
No suspicious
medications
Chemotherapy
Chloramphenicol
Anticonvulsants
Gold therapy
Thiazides
Hypercoagulable state
(DVT or other evidence
of thrombotic activity)
Yes
No
DIC
TTP
Abdominal
ultrasound
Splenomegaly
No splenomegaly
Hypersplenism
Leukemia
ITP
Collagen-vascular
disease
Alcoholism

Robert A. Baldor, MD and Alan M. Ehrlich, MD

Blood. 2005;106(7):2244–51.

TRANSIENT ISCHEMIC ATTACK AND TRANSIENT NEUROLOGIC DEFICIT

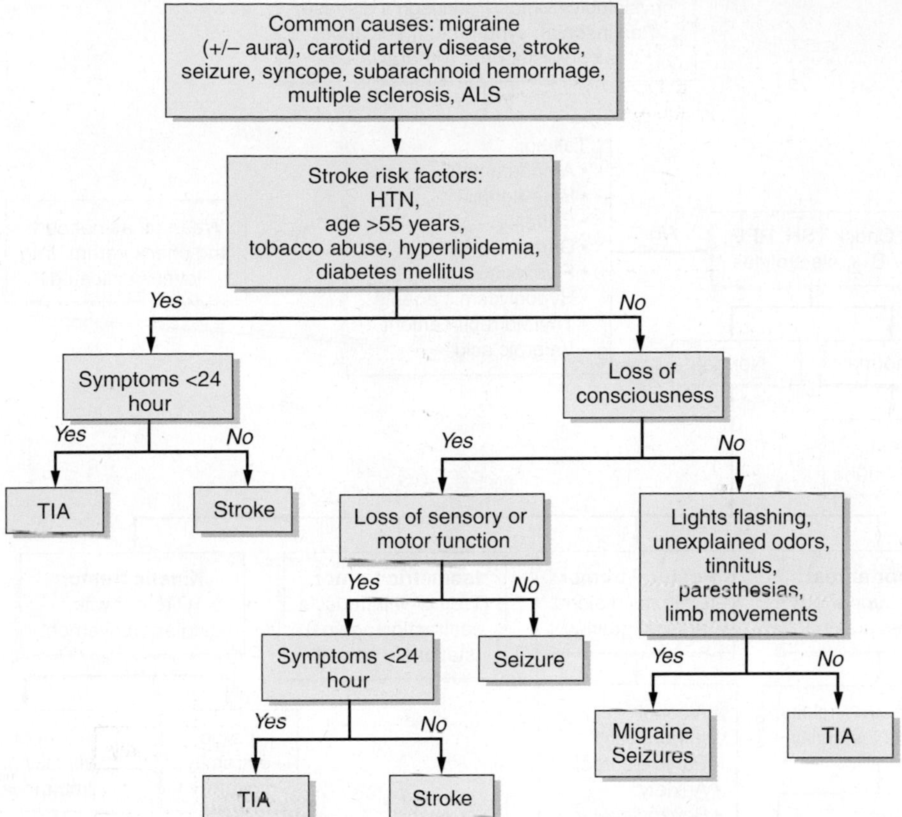

Robert A. Baldor, MD and Alan M. Ehrlich, MD

Am Fam Physician. 2004;69:1665–74, 1679–81.

TREMOR

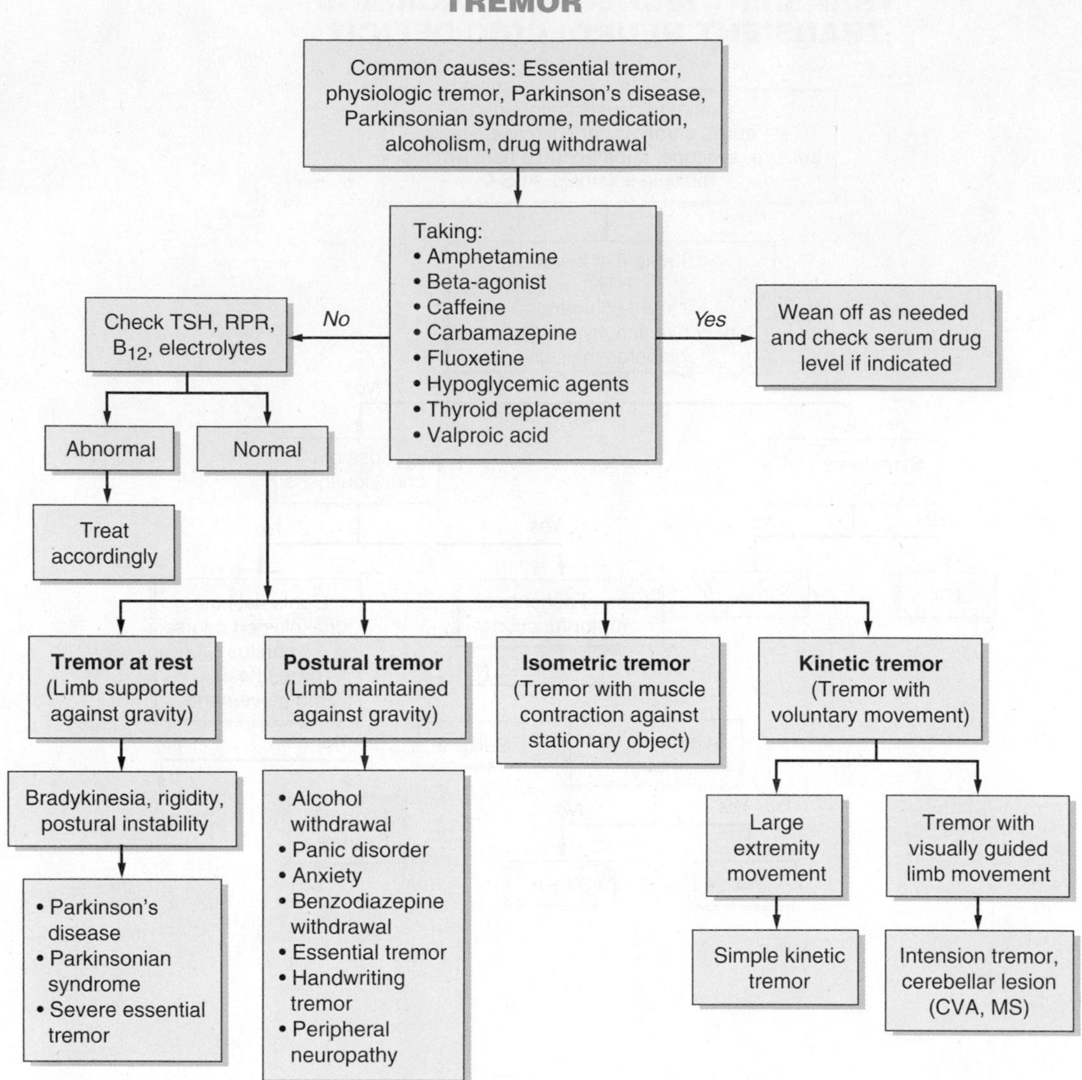
Common causes: Essential tremor, physiologic tremor, Parkinson's disease, Parkinsonian syndrome, medication, alcoholism, drug withdrawal
Taking:
• Amphetamine
• Beta-agonist
• Caffeine
• Carbamazepine
• Fluoxetine
• Hypoglycemic agents
• Thyroid replacement
• Valproic acid
No
Check TSH, RPR, B12, electrolytes
Yes
Wean off as needed and check serum drug level if indicated
Abnormal
Normal
Treat accordingly
Tremor at rest (Limb supported against gravity)
Postural tremor (Limb maintained against gravity)
Isometric tremor (Tremor with muscle contraction against stationary object)
Kinetic tremor (Tremor with voluntary movement)
Bradykinesia, rigidity, postural instability
• Parkinson's disease
• Parkinsonian syndrome
• Severe essential tremor
• Alcohol withdrawal
• Panic disorder
• Anxiety
• Benzodiazepine withdrawal
• Essential tremor
• Handwriting tremor
• Peripheral neuropathy
Large extremity movement
Tremor with visually guided limb movement
Simple kinetic tremor
Intension tremor, cerebellar lesion (CVA, MS)

Andrew J. Westwood, MD

Am Fam Physician. 2003;68(8):1545–52.

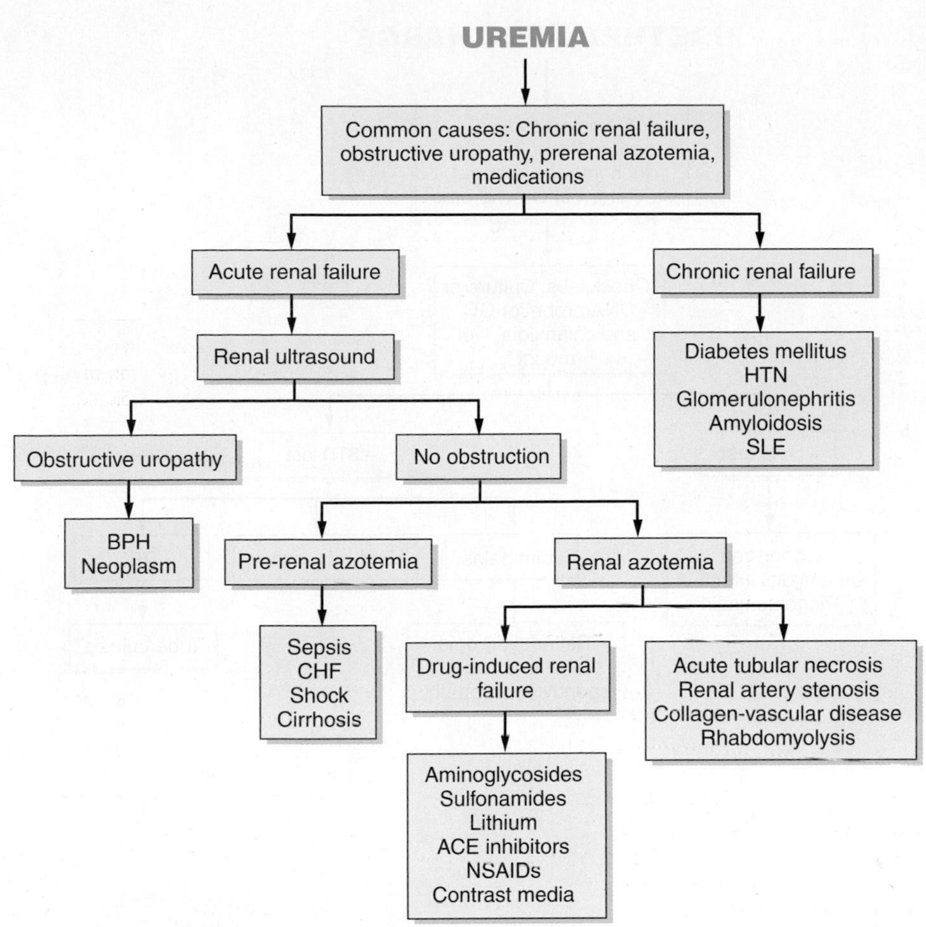

Robert A. Baldor, MD and Alan M. Ehrlich, MD

Diagnosis and management of adults with chronic kidney disease. Michigan Quality Improvement Consortium - Professional Association. 2006 Nov (revised 2008 Nov). 1 page. NGC:007054.

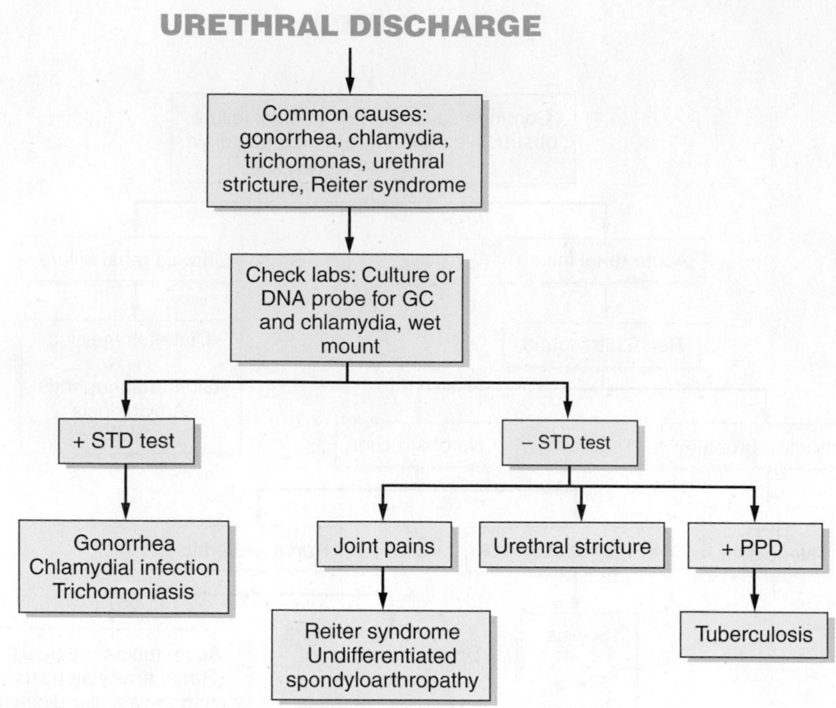

Robert A. Baldor, MD and Alan M. Ehrlich, MD

Sex Transm Infect. 1998;74(Suppl 1):S29–33.

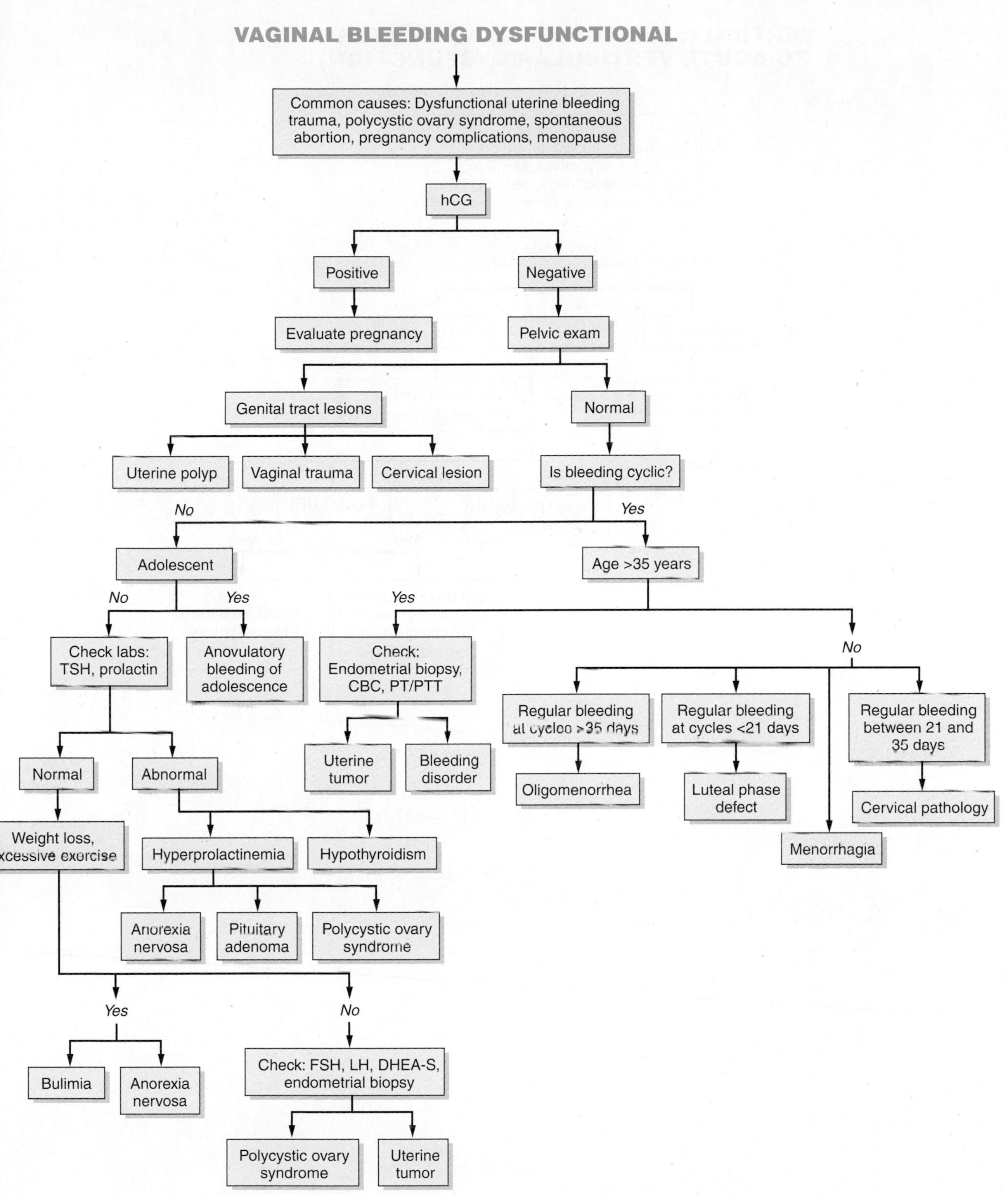

Robert A. Baldor, MD and Alan M. Ehrlich, MD

Am Fam Physician. 2004;69:1915–26;1931–3.

VERTIGO (SYMPTOM OF MOVEMENT DUE TO ACUTE VESTIBULAR DYSFUNCTION)

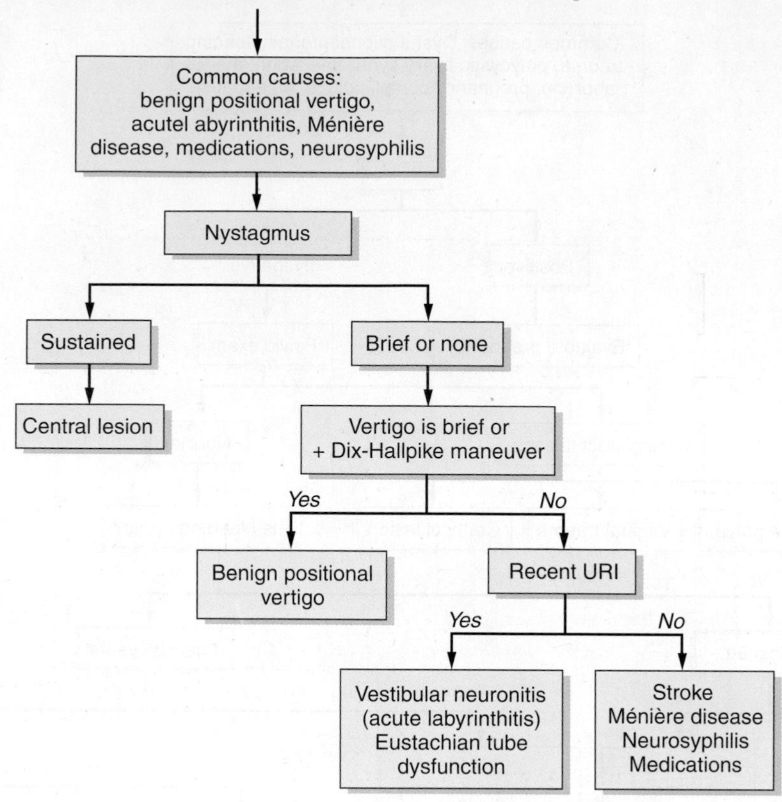

Robert A. Baldor, MD and Alan M. Ehrlich, MD

Am Fam Physician. 2006;73:244–51, 255.

WEIGHT LOSS

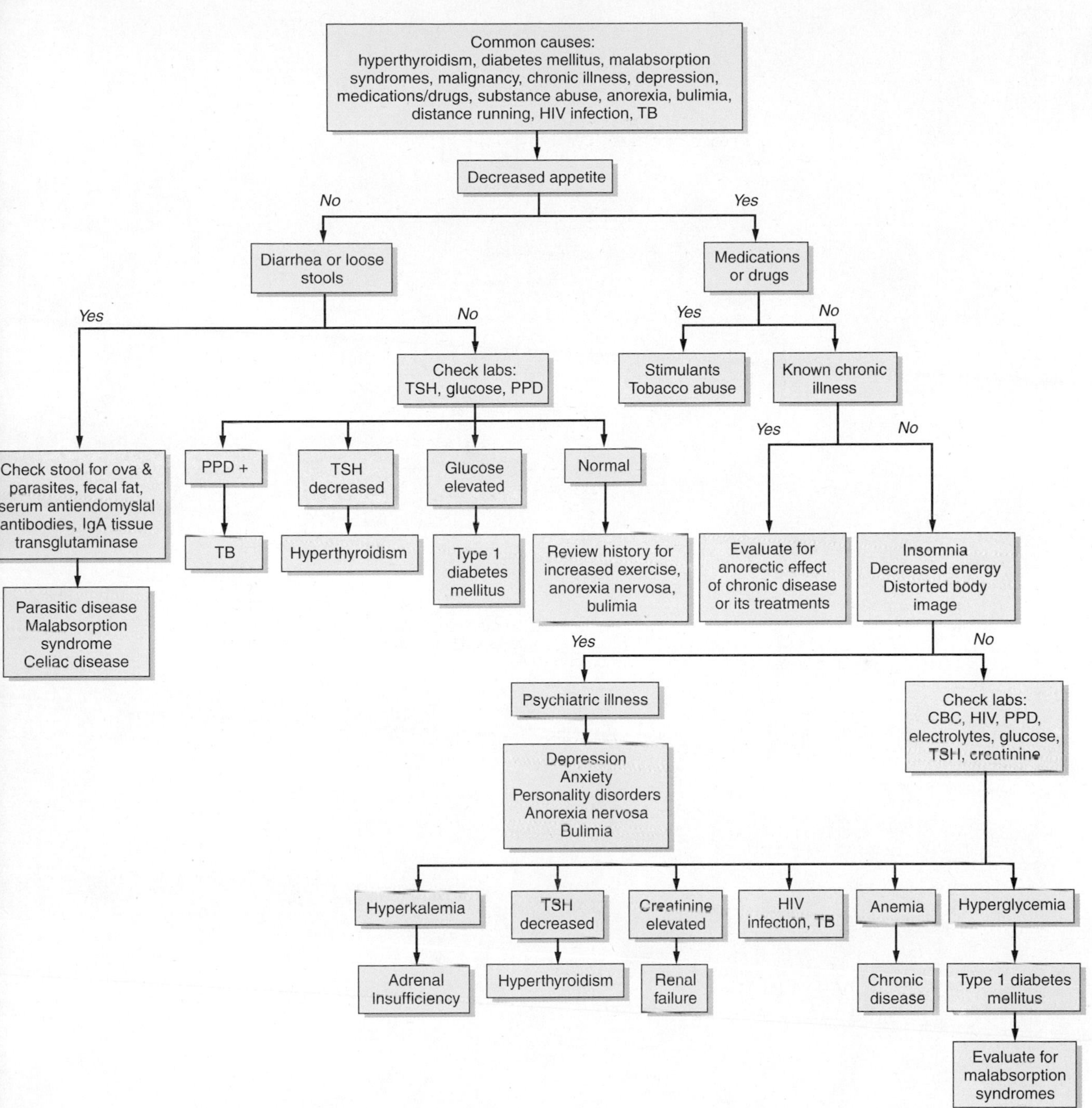

Robert A. Baldor, MD and Alan M. Ehrlich, MD

Am Fam Physician. 2002;65:640–51.

The 5-Minute Clinical Consult 2012

20TH EDITION

ABNORMAL PAP AND CERVICAL DYSPLASIA

Jeremy Golding, MD
Patricia Seymour, MD

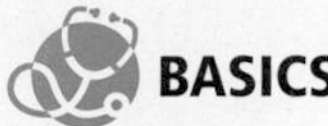

BASICS

DESCRIPTION

Cervical dysplasia: Precancerous epithelial changes in the transformation zone of the uterine cervix almost always associated with human papillomavirus (HPV) infections:

- Mild dysplasia (cervical intraepithelial neoplasia [CIN] I): Cellular changes are limited to the lower 1/3 of the squamous epithelium.
- Moderate dysplasia (CIN II): Cellular changes are limited to the lower 2/3 of the squamous epithelium.
- Severe dysplasia (CIN III or carcinoma in situ): Cellular changes involve the full thickness of the squamous epithelium.
- Pap smear:
  - Screening test for cervical cellular pathology. In many laboratories, automated cervical screening complements the Pap smear or supersedes it.
  - Abnormal cervical smear results can range from benign cellular changes to suggestion of invasive cancer.
- System(s) affected: Reproductive

ALERT

Cervical cancer arises from HPV, which is a sexually acquired disease. Good evidence that screening for cervical cancer with Pap smears reduces incidence of and mortality from cervical cancer (1)[A].

Geriatric Considerations

Natural progression of cervical dysplasia involves acquisition of HPV at or after first coitus with a small percentage of lesions progressing. See guidelines below.

Pregnancy Considerations

- Squamous intraepithelial lesions can progress during pregnancy, but often regress postpartum.
- Colposcopy only to rule out invasive cancer in high-risk women (2)

EPIDEMIOLOGY

- Predominant age: Can occur at any age
- Incidence of CIN III peaks between ages 25 and 29; invasive disease peaks 15 years later.

Incidence

- Low-grade squamous intraepithelial lesion ranges from 2–3% of all Pap smears.
- High-grade squamous intraepithelial lesion and invasive cancer present on 1% of Pap smears.
- Other reactive, reparative, and ASC-US (atypical squamous cells of undetermined significance) results are difficult to assess because of the lack of reporting mechanisms.

Prevalence

26.8% of women are HPV-positive.

RISK FACTORS

- Cigarette smoking
- Possible deficiency of antioxidants
- Early age at first coitus
- Multiple sexual partners
- Some correlation to low socioeconomic level
- Intercourse with a high-risk male partner
- HPV infection
- Immunosuppression

GENERAL PREVENTION

- HPV immunization of girls and women prior to first intercourse (e.g., Gardasil) 3 doses (0, 2, 6 months) (3)[C] reduces dysplasia due to covered and related HPV strains; long-term effect on cancer as yet uncertain. Role of immunization of boys and men not yet established.
- Delay first intercourse beyond early adolescence
- Monogamous relationship for both partners
- Smoking cessation
- Adequate antioxidant-rich food intake has been associated with decreased risk
- Obtain routine Pap smears (see guidelines below)
- Use barrier methods of birth control if in nonmonogamous relationship (likely decreases but does not eliminate HPV transmission)
- Screening guidelines:
  - Screening indicated for woman beginning at age 21
  - Frequency of screening recommendations vary:
    - United States Preventive Services Task Force: Every 3 years
    - American Cancer Society/American Congress of Obstetricians and Gynecologists: Every 2 years until age 30 then every 3 years if normal
    - May be beneficial to do combined cellular screening (Pap) and high-risk HPV test in women >age 30. If normal cytology and high-risk HPV negative, screening should be repeated in no less than 3 years. If cytology is normal but HPV is positive, repeat BOTH cytology and HPV in 1 year, and if HPV remains positive (or if abnormal cytology), proceed to colposcopy (2,4).
- Screen until age 65–70. May discontinue if 3 or more consecutive, satisfactory normal or negative smears, no abnormal smears in past 10 years, or until total hysterectomy for benign conditions (1,5)

PATHOPHYSIOLOGY

- HPV DNA is found in virtually all cervical carcinomas and precursor lesions worldwide.
- HPV viral types 16, 18, 31, 35, 45, 51, 52, 56, and 58 are common high-risk or oncogenic virus types for cervical cancer.
- HPV viral types 6, 11, 42, 43, and 44 are considered common low-risk types, and may cause genital warts.

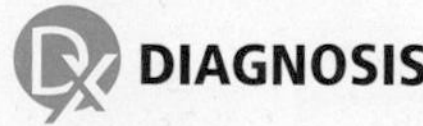

DIAGNOSIS

Frequently no symptoms

HISTORY

- Occasionally vaginal discharge related to sexually transmitted disease
- Rarely vaginal bleeding

PHYSICAL EXAM

Pelvic exam occasionally reveals external HPV lesion

DIAGNOSTIC TESTS & INTERPRETATIO

- ThinPrep is a fluid-based collection and thin-layer preparation for cervical cancer screening.
- Sensitivity of a single Pap smear for HSIL ~70%; specificity of ~90%

Lab

- Bethesda system for reporting Pap/cervical smear results (*cytologic grading*) (6)
- Specimen adequacy
- Presence of endocervical cells:
  - Negative for intraepithelial lesion or malignancy
  - Epithelial cell abnormalities:
    - ASC: Atypical squamous cells
    - ASC-US: ASC of undetermined significance
    - ASC-H: Atypical cells cannot exclude high-gra squamous intraepithelial lesion (SIL)
    - LSIL: Low-grade SIL (combines mild dysplasia (CIN I) with HPV)
    - HSIL: High-grade SIL (combines CIN II and III)
    - Squamous cell carcinoma
    - Glandular cells
    - AGC: Atypical glandular cells
    - AGCs of undetermined significance
    - Atypical glandular cells, favor neoplasia
    - Endocervical adenocarcinoma in situ
    - Adenocarcinoma

Diagnostic Procedures/Surgery

- Colposcopy with or without biopsy recommended for the following (2) (and see algorithms):
  - Initial Pap smear with LSIL (exception for adolescent, although screening of adolescents n longer recommended), HSIL; ASCUS that is + fo high-risk HPV types on (reflex) HPV hybrid captu 2 test.
  - ASC-US present on 2 Pap smears 6 months apar if HPV testing not available
  - ASC-H needs colposcopic evaluation.
  - Any abnormal or suspicious lesion of the cervix c vagina that is visualized by the eye
  - Atypical glandular cells (mandate colposcopy an uterine sampling)
- HPV viral typing:
  - Hybrid capture 2 test has 2 viral type probes: a low-risk probe and a high-risk probe.
  - High-risk (HR) probe can be used to identify patients with ASC-US who need colposcopy follow-up.

- HPV typing may be used in combination with Pap smear for women ≥30.
  - Low-risk women with negative cytology and who are negative for high-risk HPV may be followed every 3 years.
  - Women with negative cytology but positive (HR) probe may be approached with 1 of 2 strategies (optimal strategy uncertain): Repeat Pap and HPV in 1 year. If either Pap abnormal or HPV HR positive, then colposcopy. Order an HPV 16/18-specific probe on cytology fluid. If either probe for 16 or 18 is positive, evidence suggests the risk of a high-grade lesion is still similar to the risk for ASCUS/HPV+, and colposcopy is recommended. If HPV 16 and 18 are negative with a negative Pap and a high-risk HPV screen positive, the risk of a high-grade lesion is about 15-fold less, and repeat Pap plus HPV screen in 1 year is recommended. At 1 year, if either the Pap or the HPV test is NOT negative, then colposcopy is recommended.
- Little utility for low-risk viral type screening
- oop electrosurgical excision procedure (LEEP):
- "See and treat" for HSIL in nonadolescent age groups acceptable, but not for adolescents (as they should no longer be screened).
- :one biopsy
- :ervicography: Photographic evaluation of cervix

thological Findings

- typical squamous or columnar cells
- :oarse nuclear material
- ncreased nuclear diameter
- :oilocytosis (HPV hallmark)

FFERENTIAL DIAGNOSIS

- cute or chronic cervicitis
- :ervical squamous intraepithelial neoplasia
- :ervical glandular neoplasia
- nvasive cervical malignancy
- Jterine malignancy (rare)

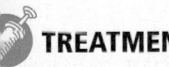

TREATMENT

dence-based management algorithms guide Pap ear and post-colposcopic diagnostics and rapeutics (2,4).

EDICATION

- nfective/reactive Pap smear:
  - Metronidazole 250 mg t.i.d. p.o. for 7 days
- :ondyloma acuminatum:
  - Cryotherapy
  - Podophyllin topically q1–2wk
  - Trichloroacetic acid, applied topically by a physician and covered for 5–6 days

DDITIONAL TREATMENT

eneral Measures

-)ffice evaluation and observation
- romote smoking cessation.
- romote protected intercourse.

JRGERY/OTHER PROCEDURES

- SILs and HSILs and carcinoma in situ can be treated vith outpatient surgery:
  - Cryotherapy, laser ablation, LEEP/large loop excision of transition zone, or cold-knife conization all effective, but requiring different training and with different side effects for patient
- f cervical malignancy, see Cervical Malignancy.

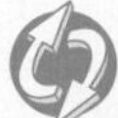

ONGOING CARE

FOLLOW-UP RECOMMENDATIONS

- LSIL/CIN1: Observation with Pap smear repeated every 6 months or high-risk HPV testing every year is appropriate for young women with LSIL, especially with confirmed CIN I.
- HPV-related CIN I typically resolves within 2–3 years.
- LSIL persisting beyond 2–3 years in a young woman is indication for colposcopy

DIET

Promote increased intake of antioxidant-rich foods.

PATIENT EDUCATION

- Promote HPV immunization.
- Promote smoking cessation.
- Promote protected intercourse.
- Promote regular Pap smears according to recognized guidelines.
- Reschedule follow-up consultation for any abnormality.

PROGNOSIS

- Generally excellent
- <50% of persistent infective, reactive, reparative, or ASC-US Pap/cervical smears will have more advanced lesions.
- Only a small percentage of LSILs will progress to more advanced lesion (80% or more of adolescent and young adult CIN I resolves in 2–3 years).
- Lesions discovered early are amenable to treatment, with excellent results and few recurrences.

COMPLICATIONS

- Minor abnormalities on Pap/cervical smears can mask more advanced lesions.
- HSIL does progress to invasive cancer. Best estimate of risk of CIN III progression to invasive cervical cancer is >50% (7).
- Aggressive cervical surgery may be associated with cervical stenosis, cervical incompetence, and scarring affecting cervical dilatation in labor.

REFERENCES

1. Guide to Clinical Preventive Services: Report of the US Preventive Services Task Force 2003. Accessed 4/22/2009 at www.ahrq.gov/clinic/3rduspstf/cervcan/cervcanrr.htm
2. Wright TC Jr, et al. 2006 Consensus Guidelines for the management of women with abnormal cervical cancer screening tests. *AJOG* 2007;346–56. Accessed 4/22/2009 at http://www.asccp.org/consensus.shtml.
3. Markowitz LE, Dunne EF, Saraiya M et al. Quadrivalent Human Papillomavirus Vaccine: Recommendations of the Advisory Committee on Immunization Practices (ACIP). *MMWR Recomm Rep*. 2007;56:1–24.
4. ICSI. Management of abnormal pap smear 2008. Accessed 4/22/2009 at http://guidelines.gov/summary/summary.aspx?doc_id=13311&nbr=006755&string=ICSI+AND+abnormal+AND+pap
5. Saslow D, Runowicz CD, Solomon D et al. American Cancer Society guideline for the early detection of cervical neoplasia and cancer. *CA Cancer J Clin*. 2002;52:342–62.
6. Solomon D, Davey D, Kurman R et al. The 2001 Bethesda System: terminology for reporting results of cervical cytology. *JAMA*. 2002;287:2114–9.
7. McCredie MR, Sharples KJ, Paul C et al. Natural history of cervical neoplasia and risk of invasive cancer in women with cervical intraepithelial neoplasia 3: a retrospective cohort study. *The Lancet Oncology* 2008;5(9):425–434.

ADDITIONAL READING

Dunne EF, Unger ER, Sternberg M et al. Prevalence of HPV infection among females in the United States. *JAMA*. 2007;297:813–9.

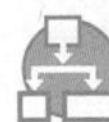

See Also (Topic, Algorithm, Electronic Media Element)

Cervical Malignancy; Condyloma Acuminata; Failure to Thrive; Trichomoniasis; Vulvovaginitis, Prepubescent
Algorithm: Abnormal Pap Smear in Adolescents, Pap smear in Women age 20–30, Pap Smear in Women >30 years of age

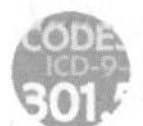

CODES

ICD9

- 622.10 Dysplasia of cervix, unspecified
- 622.11 Mild dysplasia of cervix
- 622.12 Moderate dysplasia of cervix

CLINICAL PEARLS

- A connection exists between HPV infection and abnormal Pap smears. HPV was defined as a "carcinogen" by World Health Organization in 1996. HPV is present in virtually all cervical cancers (99.7%).
- No evidence suggests that offering HPV immunization increases the likelihood of early sexual intercourse and acquisition of sexually transmitted infections.
- Preliminary data suggest that vaccine is much less effective for prevention of cervical dysplasia if offered after women are infected with HPV, and no effect on regression of existing CIN has been seen thus far in trials. Vaccine should therefore be offered prior to onset of any sexual activity (even nonintercourse activity) for maximum effectiveness.

ABORTION, SPONTANEOUS (MISCARRIAGE)

Elizabeth W. Patton, MD
Patricia K. Aronson, MD

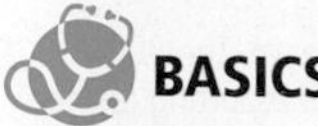

BASICS

DESCRIPTION

- Separation of products of conception from the uterus prior to the potential for fetal survival outside the uterus
- Spontaneous abortion (SAb):
  - Expulsion or extraction from the uterus of an embryo or fetus weighing ≤500 g
- Threatened abortion:
  - Vaginal bleeding early in pregnancy without dilatation of the cervix, rupture of the membranes, or expulsion of products of conception
- Inevitable abortion:
  - Cervical dilatation, rupture of membranes, or expulsion of products in the presence of vaginal bleeding
- Complete abortion:
  - Entire contents of uterus expelled; common before 12 weeks' gestation
- Incomplete abortion:
  - Abortion with retained products of conception, generally placental tissue; more common after 12 weeks' gestation
- Missed abortion:
  - In utero death of embryo/fetus prior to 20 weeks' gestation; products of conception retained
- Induced abortion:
  - Evacuation of uterine contents or products of conception medically or surgically
- Septic abortion:
  - Common complication of illegally performed induced abortions; a spontaneous or therapeutic abortion complicated by pelvic infection
- Habitual spontaneous abortion:
  - 2 or more consecutive pregnancy losses at <15 weeks' gestation
- Synonym(s): Miscarriage; Habitual abortion; Recurrent abortion; Involuntary pregnancy loss

EPIDEMIOLOGY

Predominant age: Increases with advancing age, especially >35 years; at age 40, the loss rate is twice that of age 20

Prevalence

- ~8–20% of all clinically recognized pregnancies end in spontaneous abortion, 80% of these in the first 12 weeks.
- When both clinical and biochemical (B-HCG detected) pregnancies are considered, up to 50% of pregnancies end in spontaneous abortion.

RISK FACTORS

Most cases of spontaneous abortion occur in patients without identifiable risk factors; however, risk factors listed in order of importance include:

- Chromosomal abnormalities
- Advancing maternal age
- Uterine abnormalities
- Maternal chronic disease (diabetes mellitus, polycystic ovarian syndrome, systemic lupus erythematosus, hypertension, antiphospholipid antibodies, thyroid disease, renal disease)
- Other possible contributing factors include smoking, alcohol, infection, and luteal phase defect, although conclusive data are currently lacking.

Genetics

~50–65% of 1st-trimester spontaneous abortions have significant chromosomal anomalies, with 1/2 of these being autosomal trisomies and the remainder being triploidy, tetraploidy, or 45X monosomies.

GENERAL PREVENTION

- Progestogens: Currently, there is no evidence that routine use of oral or IM progestogens prevents miscarriage in early to mid-pregnancy. However, there is some evidence that women with a history of recurrent miscarriage may benefit from this type of treatment (1)[A].
- Immunotherapy: No current evidence to support use of immunotherapy in patients with a history of recurrent miscarriage (2)[A]

ETIOLOGY

- Chromosomal anomalies
- Congenital anomalies
- Trauma
- Maternal factors: Uterine abnormalities, infection (toxoplasma, other viruses, rubella, cytomegalovirus, herpesvirus), maternal endocrine disorders, hypercoagulable state

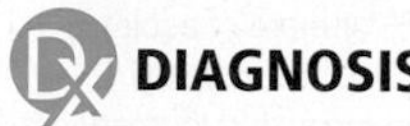

DIAGNOSIS

HISTORY

- Consider any reproductive-age woman with vaginal bleeding to be pregnant until proven otherwise.
- Vaginal bleeding:
  - Characteristics (amount, color, consistency, associated symptoms), onset (abrupt or gradual), duration, intensity/quantity, and exacerbating/precipitating factors
- Abdominal pain/uterine cramping
- Rupture of membranes
- Passage of products of conception
- Prenatal course: Toxic or infectious exposures, family or personal history of genetic abnormalities, past history of ectopic pregnancy or spontaneous abortion, endocrine disease, autoimmune disorder, bleeding/clotting disorder

PHYSICAL EXAM

- Any pregnant woman with vaginal bleeding needs immediate evaluation.
- Estimate hemodynamic stability:
  - Obtain orthostatic vital signs.
- Abdominal exam for tenderness (SAb), guarding, rebound, bowel sounds (peritoneal signs more likely seen with ectopic pregnancy)
- Pelvic exam for cervical dilation, blood, products of conception, uterine size/tenderness

DIAGNOSTIC TESTS & INTERPRETATION

Lab

Initial lab tests

- Urine human chorionic gonadotropin (HCG)
- Complete blood count
- Rh type
- Cultures: Gonorrhea/chlamydia
- Serial serum HCG measurements can assess viability of the pregnancy. Serum HCG should rise at least 67% every 48 hours in early pregnancy.

Pregnancy Considerations

HCG levels are particularly useful in cases where a intrauterine pregnancy (IUP) has not been documented by ultrasound.

Follow-Up & Special Considerations

- In the case of vaginal bleeding with no documen IUP, follow serum HCG levels weekly to zero to ensure complete expulsion of all products of conception.
- If levels plateau, suspect ectopic pregnancy or retained products of conception.

Imaging

Initial approach

- Ultrasound (US) exam to evaluate fetal viability a to rule out ectopic pregnancy:
  - HCG >2,000 U/L necessary to detect IUP via transvaginal US (TVUS), >6,500 U/L for abdominal ultrasound
- TVUS criteria for nonviable intrauterine gestation include 5-mm fetal pole without cardiac activity c 16-mm gestational sac without a fetal pole.

Follow-Up & Special Considerations

- If initial HCG level does not permit documentatio of IUP by TVUS, follow serum HCG in 48 hrs to ensure appropriate rise.
- Follow HGC and repeat US once HCG at a level commensurate with visualization on US (see abo
- Provide patient with ectopic precautions in interi

Diagnostic Procedures/Surgery

- Fetal heart tones can be auscultated with Dopple starting between 10–12 weeks' gestation from la menstrual period for a viable pregnancy.
- 90–96% of pregnancies with fetal cardiac activit and vaginal bleeding at 7–11 weeks' gestation result in continued pregnancy.

Pathological Findings

Products of conception, placental villi

DIFFERENTIAL DIAGNOSIS

- Ectopic pregnancy: Potentially life-threatening; m be ruled out with US in any woman of childbearir age with abdominal pain and vaginal bleeding
- Cervical polyps, neoplasias, and/or inflammatory conditions can cause vaginal bleeding.
- Hydatidiform mole pregnancy
- HCG-secreting ovarian tumor
- Physiologic bleeding in normal pregnancy (implantation bleeding)

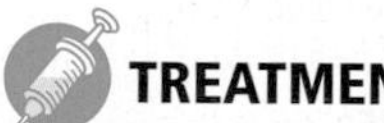

TREATMENT

MEDICATION

- Long-term conception rate and pregnancy outcon are similar for women who undergo medical or surgical evacuation.
- Postinfection rates lower with medical vs surgical management

st Line

isoprostol: Most common agent for inducing ıssage of tissue in missed or incomplete ɔortion:

Not approved by Food and Drug Administration for treatment of early pregnancy failure

Efficacy: Complete expulsion of products of conception in 71% by day 3, 84% by day 8

Efficacy depends on route of administration, gestational age of pregnancy, and dose

Recommended dose 800 μg vaginally (3)[A]; alternate regimens exist including World Health Organization regimen of 800 μg vaginally or 600 μg sublingually q.3 hours for up to 3 doses; multidose regimens and oral dosing may result in increased side effects

ommon adverse effects include abdominal ain/cramping, nausea, and diarrhea. Pain increases higher doses, but manageable with analgesia. No crease in nausea/diarrhea with higher dose.

ecommended for stable patients who decline ırgery but do not want to wait for spontaneous ıssage of products of conception

cond Line

negative patients should be given Rh immune ɔulin following spontaneous abortion (4)[C].

DITIONAL TREATMENT

neral Measures

lore any 1st-trimester vaginal bleeding.

ues for Referral

ents should be monitored for up to 1 year for the elopment of psychosomatic symptoms such as ression and anxiety (5)[A].

MPLEMENTARY AND ALTERNATIVE DICINE

min supplementation does not appear to prevent carriage (6)[A].

RGERY/OTHER PROCEDURES

terine aspiration (dilation and curettage or via ıcuum aspiration) is the conventional treatment.

dications: Septic abortion, heavy bleeding, potension, patient choice

isks: Anesthesia, uterine perforation, intrauterine dhesions, cervical trauma, infection that may lead infertility or increased risk of ectopic pregnancy

ırgical intervention leads to fewer days of vaginal eeding, with a lower risk of incomplete abortion nd heavy bleeding. It does carry a higher risk of fection (7)[A].

acuum aspiration may be less painful than latation and curettage (D & C), and does not quire general anesthesia (8)[B].

ata from induced abortions suggests that ntibiotic prophylaxis with doxycycline 100 mg i.d. substantially reduces postprocedure infection sk; however, data for incomplete abortions eated surgically is inconclusive (9)[A].

ɔr patients who desire contraception after ɔmpletion of a spontaneous abortion, immediate sertion of an intrauterine device is acceptable nd safe (10)[A].

PATIENT CONSIDERATIONS

tial Stabilization

atient with orthostatic vital signs, initiate ıscitation with IV fluids and/or blood products if ded

IV Fluids

Hemodynamically unstable patients may require IV fluids and/or blood products to maintain blood pressure.

ONGOING CARE

FOLLOW-UP RECOMMENDATIONS

All patients should be seen in 2–6 weeks to monitor for resolution of bleeding, reestablishment of menses, review of contraception plan, and psychosomatic symptoms.

Patient Monitoring

- Identification of products of conception within material expelled from the uterus or D & C specimen (important to distinguish villi and sac from decidua)
- If abortion is complete, observe the patient for further bleeding.
- Pelvic rest until 2 weeks after evacuation
- If spontaneous abortion occurs in setting of previously documented IUP and abortion is completed with resumption of normal menses, it is not necessary to check or follow serum HCG to 0.

DIET

n.p.o. if patient to undergo dilation and curettage

PATIENT EDUCATION

Patient pamphlet (no. AP090) available from the American College of Obstetricians and Gynecologists 409 12th St., SW, Washington, DC 20090-6290; (800) 762-2264 or online at http://www.acog.org

PROGNOSIS

- If bleeding ceases, prognosis is excellent.
- Habitual abortion:
  - Prognosis depends on etiology.
  - Prognosis is still excellent, with up to 70% rate of success with subsequent pregnancy.

COMPLICATIONS

- Potential complications of D & C include uterine perforation, bleeding, adhesions, cervical trauma, infection that may lead to infertility, or increased risk of ectopic pregnancy.
- Retained products of conception
- Psychological morbidity, including depression, anxiety, feelings of guilt

REFERENCES

1. Haas DM, Ramsey PS. Progestogen for preventing miscarriage. *Cochrane Database Syst Rev*. 2008; CD003511.
2. Porter TF, LaCoursiere Y, Scott JR. Immunotherapy for recurrent miscarriage. *Cochrane Database Syst Rev*. 2006;CD000112.
3. Neilson JP, Hickey M, Vazquez J. Medical treatment for early fetal death (less than 24 weeks). *Cochrane Database Syst Rev*. 2006;3: CD002253.
4. Prevention of Rho(D) alloimmunization. American College of Obstetricians and Gynecologists Practice Bulletin No 4. American College of Obstetricians and Gynecologists, Washington, DC: 1999.
5. Lok IH, Neugebauer R. Psychological morbidity following miscarriage. *Best Pract Res Clin Obstet Gynaecol*. 2007;21:229–47.
6. Rumbold A, Middleton P, Crowther CA. Vitamin supplementation for preventing miscarriage. *Cochrane Database Syst Rev*. 2005;CD004073.
7. Nanda K, Peloggia A, Grimes D et al. Expectant care versus surgical treatment for miscarriage. *Cochrane Database Syst Rev*. 2006;CD003518.
8. Forna F, et al. Surgical procedures to evacuate incomplete miscarriage. *Cochrane Database Sys Rev*. 2001;1:CD001993.
9. May W, Gülmezoglu AM, Ba-Thike K et al. Antibiotics for incomplete abortion. *Cochrane Database Syst Rev*. 2007;CD001779.
10. Grimes DA, Lopez LM, Schulz KF, Van Vliet HA, Stanwood NL et al. Immediate post-partum insertion of intrauterine devices. *Cochrane Database Syst Rev*. 2010;5:CD003036.

ADDITIONAL READING

- Harwood B, et al. Quality of life and acceptability of medical vs. surgical management of early pregnancy. *Br J Obstet and Gynaec*. 2008;115(4):501–8.
- Tam WH, Tsui MH, Lok IH et al. Long-term reproductive outcome subsequent to medical versus surgical treatment for miscarriage. *Hum Reprod*. 2005;20:3355–9.
- Zhang J, Gilles JM, Barnhart K, Creinin MD, Westhoff C, Frederick MM, National Institute of Child Health Human Development (NICHD) Management of Early Pregnancy Failure Trial et al. A comparison of medical management with misoprostol and surgical management for early pregnancy failure. *N Engl J Med*. 2005;353:761–9.

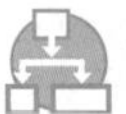

See Also (Topic, Algorithm, Electronic Media Element)

Ectopic Pregnancy

Algorithm: Abortion, Recurrent

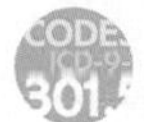

CODES

ICD9

- 632 Missed abortion
- 634.90 Spontaneous abortion, unspecified, without mention of complication
- 640.03 Threatened abortion, antepartum

CLINICAL PEARLS

- Any reproductive-age woman or pregnant woman with abdominal pain and vaginal bleeding must be evaluated. Ectopic pregnancy must be ruled out, and hemodynamic stability should be ensured.
- Patient preference should determine whether management is medical, expectant, or surgical, as all options have similar long-term outcomes.
- Assessment of psychological symptoms after spontaneous abortion should be an integral part of follow-up visits, with counseling, medication, and referral as appropriate.
- Patients and their partners should be reassured that there are no known interventions to prevent spontaneous abortion, and should be provided with appropriate medical explanations to reduce anxiety and guilt.

ABRUPTIO PLACENTAE

Mark J. Manning, DO, Med
Amy Ellingson-Itzin, MD

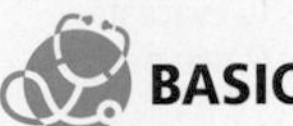

BASICS

DESCRIPTION

- Premature separation of an otherwise normally implanted placenta
- Grades:
  - Grade 1: Minimal or no bleeding; detected as retroplacental clot after delivery of viable fetus. Mild uterine irritability (40% of cases).
  - Grade 2: Viable fetus with bleeding and tender, irritable uterus. Mild-to-moderate bleeding; fibrinogen level decreased (45% of cases).
  - Grade 3: Type A with dead fetus and no coagulopathy; type B with dead fetus and coagulopathy (Types A and B = 15% of all cases)

EPIDEMIOLOGY

Incidence

- 0.5–1.2% of all deliveries:
  - Placental abruption is the most common cause of serious vaginal bleeding in late pregnancy (1).
- 15% if 1 prior abruption
- 25% if 2 or more prior abruptions
- 80% of cases occur prior to onset of delivery.
- Peaks at 24–26 weeks, then decreases with increasing gestation
- Rising in the US from 0.8% 1979–1981 to 1.2% 1999–2001

RISK FACTORS

- Prior abruption: Increases 15–20-fold (2)
- Increasing maternal age and parity
- Advanced maternal age
- Maternal smoking: dose–response relationship (2)
- Cocaine use and abuse
- Factor V Leiden and other thrombophilic disorders
- Hypertensive disorders
- Uterine anomalies
- Multiple-gestation pregnancies (3)[B]
- 1st- or 2nd-trimester bleeding
- Preeclampsia: Mild and severe
- Increased risk if hypertension and parity >3
- Preterm rupture of membranes (4)[B]
- Hydramnios
- Severe small-for-gestational-age birth
- Blunt trauma/motor vehicle accident

Genetics

- Genetic predisposition may be the cause of abruption in women with no other inciting factor discovered.
- Placental growth is primarily under control of paternally inherited fetal genes.

GENERAL PREVENTION

Eliminate risk factors when possible: Quit smoking and cocaine use, control hypertension, use seat belts, etc.

PATHOPHYSIOLOGY

Exact cause is unknown: Appears to be the final common clinical event secondary to a variety of causes

ETIOLOGY

- Acute:
  - Trauma of variable amounts, especially blunt abdominal trauma in which external signs of trauma may be incongruent with fetal injury
  - Sudden decompression of overdistended uterus, as in hydramnios or twin gestation
  - Vasospasm secondary to cocaine use
- Chronic (majority of cases):
  - Hypertensive disorders and growth restriction associated with chronic process
  - Early bleeding in pregnancy releases thrombin, which is a potent uterotonic agent

COMMONLY ASSOCIATED CONDITIONS

- Preeclampsia and other forms of hypertension in pregnancy
- Uteroplacental insufficiency
- Postpartum hemorrhage
- Disseminated intravascular coagulation (DIC)
- Rupture of membranes

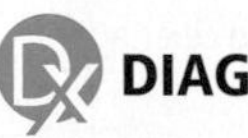

DIAGNOSIS

HISTORY

- Classic triad of vaginal bleeding, abdominal pain, and contractions
- Abruption in prior pregnancy
- Early trimester bleeding
- Recent trauma
- Cocaine or tobacco use
- Back pain
- Frequent or tetanic contractions
- May present in active labor

PHYSICAL EXAM

- Vital signs: Tachycardia, hypotension:
  - Because blood volumes increase in pregnancy, volume lost may exceed 30% before signs of shock or hypovolemia occur.
- Uterine tenderness, hypertonia, or high-frequency contractions
- Vaginal bleeding (not always present):
  - Clinical signs of shock may occur with little vaginal bleeding.
- Fetal distress or demise
- Idiopathic preterm labor with or without fetal distress

DIAGNOSTIC TESTS & INTERPRETATION

Lab

Initial lab tests

- Blood type, Rh, cross-match for possible transfusion:
  - RHoD immune globulin administered <12 weeks prior may affect antibody test.
- Complete blood count with platelet count
- Prothrombin time (PT)/partial thromboplastin time (PTT)
- Kleihauer-Betke test checks for evidence of fetal blood in maternal circulation; >30 mL fetal blood indicative of large fetal blood loss:
  - 300 μg dose of RhoGAM will cover up to 30 mL whole fetal blood in maternal circulation
- Bedside clot test: Red-top tube of maternal bloo with poor or nonclotting blood after 7–10 minut indicates coagulopathy.

Follow-Up & Special Considerations

- DIC can result from a large abruption. Best to stabilize patient without waiting for DIC labs. Thi typically a clinical diagnosis.
- Can send PT/PTT, fibrinogen levels at clinician discretion when stable or following resolution of DIC:
  - Fibrinogen levels climb to 350–550 mg/dL in 3 trimester and must fall to 100–150 mg/dL bef PTT will rise.
  - Fibrin split or degradation products are elevat pregnancy and are not specific in assessing DI

Imaging

Initial approach

- Placental abruption is a clinical diagnosis.
- Ultrasound can help to make the diagnosis, but low sensitivity and is only helpful in cases of a la abruption.

Follow-Up & Special Considerations

Ultrasound: Appearance depends on size and locat of the bleed:

- With acute bleed, nothing may be seen.
- Will fail to detect at least 50% of abruptions
- Retroplacental clot is diagnostic of abruption (2):
  - If incidental abruption is found in a patient at term, delivery is reasonable.
  - A preterm patient with an incidental abruption may be managed conservatively if stable.

Diagnostic Procedures/Surgery

- Tocometer often shows elevated baseline pressu and frequent low-amplitude contractions.
- External fetal monitoring may show recurrent lat decelerations, variable decelerations, sinusoidal f heart tracing, bradycardia, or decreased variability—all indicative of fetal stress.

Pathological Findings

- Placental examination after delivery may show a retroplacental clot, pathologic signs of early separation/inflammation
- Normocytic normochromic anemia with acute bleeding
- Elevated PT/PTT, fibrinogen levels <100–150 mg (1.0–1.5 g/L), platelets 20,000–50,000/μL if DI active
- Positive Kleihauer-Betke reaction if fetal–materna transfusion has occurred
- Positive antibody if RhoD isosensitization has occurred

DIFFERENTIAL DIAGNOSIS

- Placenta previa or vasa previa (1)
- Uterine rupture
- Bloody show associated with labor
- Cervical and vaginal infections (e.g., chlamydia o gonorrhea with bloody, friable cervix)
- Other painful abdominal conditions (e.g., appendicitis, pyelonephritis)
- Fibroid degeneration
- Ovarian pathology: Torsed ovary, ruptured cyst

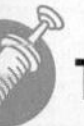

TREATMENT

EDICATION

'st Line

- ocolytics are generally contraindicated in presence f abruption:
  - Tocolytics, such as nifedipine or terbutaline, may be used in mild noncompromising preterm abruption (specific cases only, such as for fetal lung maturity)
- hoD immune globulin for RhoD-negative mother if ndelivered or indicated after delivery if leihauer-Betke is positive
- luid resuscitation as required for signs of shock

cond Line

- ransfuse packed red blood cells (PRBC) or other actors to stabilize patient as needed.
- teroids for fetal lung maturation, if fetus is viable

DDITIONAL TREATMENT

ues for Referral

- preterm and hemodynamically stable, refer to ertiary care center.
- lert anesthesia if delivery via cesarean section is kely.

RGERY/OTHER PROCEDURES

- lay need cesarean delivery after maternal tabilization if fetus is viable, remote from delivery, nd nonreassuring fetal heart tracing is present.
- ostpartum hemorrhage/DIC may be treated nedically or with uterine packing, embolization, or ysterectomy.

-PATIENT CONSIDERATIONS

tial Stabilization

- listory and physical exam with medical history, llergies, prior ultrasounds (present gestation), and me of last meal
- lanagement depends on presentation, gestational ge, and degree of maternal and fetal ompromise:
  - In general, severe abruption is best managed by delivery of fetus.
  - Grade 1: Usual labor protocol
  - Grade 2: Rapid delivery, most often by cesarean delivery (if mother stable)
  - Grade 3: Vaginal delivery preferable if mother stable

n trauma (2)[B], monitor in the inpatient setting for t least 4 hours for evidence of fetal insult, bruption, fetal–maternal transfusion. If ontractions or preterm labor occur, patient should e monitored for at least 24 hours. Risk factors for ontractions with trauma include:
- Gestational age >35 weeks
- Assaults and pedestrian/vehicular collisions, even without direct abdominal trauma
- Ejections from vehicle or lack of restraints

- arly aggressive restoration of maternal physiology o protect fetus and maternal organs from ypoperfusion/DIC
- tabilize vitals
- edrest with external fetal and labor monitoring, if etus is viable
- arge-bore, 16- to 18-gauge IV crystalloid infusion o maintain volume
- Transfusions of whole blood and PRBCs as necessary
- Fresh frozen plasma and platelet transfusions for coagulopathy, with cryoprecipitate and fibrinogen given if indicated
- Follow hemoglobin/hematocrit and coagulation status.
- Consider internal monitoring of fetus if patient is in active labor.
- Role of amniotomy to prevent amniotic fluid embolism is debatable, but may speed delivery
- Positioning on left side may enhance venous return and cardiac output
- Oxygen as needed

Admission Criteria

Patients with suspected placental abruption should be admitted for workup until deemed clinically stable and ready for discharge/outpatient follow-up or delivered for medical indication.

IV Fluids

Saline or Ringer's lactate to restore maternal vascular volume

Nursing

- Bed rest until status defined
- Frequent vital sign monitoring
- Record fluid ins and outs

Discharge Criteria

- 2nd trimester suspected abruption may be managed on outpatient basis if hemodynamically stable
- Viable patients may be discharged if maternal/fetal status is stable.

ONGOING CARE

FOLLOW-UP RECOMMENDATIONS

- Monthly growth ultrasonograms for those patients where conservative management is possible.
- Serial ultrasounds may also be used to follow regression or progression of abruption (2).

Patient Monitoring

Severe cases or unstable patients may require critical care unit admission.

DIET

n.p.o. until status is defined and possibility of immediate cesarean delivery ruled out

PATIENT EDUCATION

- Call physician or proceed to hospital whenever patient experiences vaginal bleeding or if severe uterine or back pain or decreased fetal movement occurs.
- Wear seat belts while in automobile.
- Discontinue use of cocaine, tobacco
- Visit Mayo Health: http://mayohealth.org

PROGNOSIS

- 0.5–1% fetal mortality and 30–50% perinatal mortality:
  - 1/2 of perinatal deaths due to preterm delivery
- With trauma and abruption, 1% maternal and 30–70% fetal mortality

COMPLICATIONS

- Maternal complications include anemia, stroke, myocardial infarction, DIC, and Sheehan's syndrome, and may include maternal death with severe hemorrhage.
- Surgical interventions and transfusion carry their own morbidity/mortality.
- Amniotic fluid embolism is rare, but may present with severe respiratory distress.

REFERENCES

1. Sakornbut E, Leeman L, Fontaine P. Late pregnancy bleeding. *Am Fam Physician*. 2007;75:1199–206.
2. Ananth CV, Getahun D, Peltier MR et al. Placental abruption in term and preterm gestations: evidence for heterogeneity in clinical pathways. *Obstet Gynecol*. 2006;107:785–92.
3. Salihu HM, Bekan B, Aliyu MH et al. Perinatal mortality associated with abruptio placenta in singletons and multiples. *Am J Obstet Gynecol*. 2005;193:198–203.
4. Ananth CV, Oyelese Y, Srinivas N et al. Preterm premature rupture of membranes, intrauterine infection, and oligohydramnios: risk factors for placental abruption. *Obstet Gynecol*. 2004;104:71–7.

ADDITIONAL READING

- *Creasy & Resnik's Maternal-Fetal Medicine, Principles and Practice*, 6th ed. Saunders Elsevier. 2009:731–737.
- Getahun D, et al. Acute and chronic respiratory diseases in pregnancy: Associations with placenta abruption. *Am J Obst Gynecol* 2006;195(4):1180–4.
- Oyelese Y, et al. Placental abruption. *Obst Gynecol* 2006;108:1005–16.
- Pressman EV. Imaging of the Placenta. *Ultrsound Clinics*. Volume 3, Issue 1. January 2008.
- Yang Q, Wen SW, Oppenheimer L et al. Association of caesarean delivery for first birth with placenta praevia and placental abruption in second pregnancy. *BJOG*. 2007;114:609–13.

CODES

ICD9

641.23 Premature separation of placenta, antepartum

CLINICAL PEARLS

- Placental abruption is the most common cause of serious vaginal bleeding in late pregnancy.
- Abruption is a clinical diagnosis. The classic triad is vaginal bleeding, abdominal pain, and contractions. Ultrasound can help to make the diagnosis, but has low sensitivity and is only helpful in cases of a large abruption.
- Because blood volumes increase in pregnancy, volume lost may exceed 30% before signs of shock or hypovolemia occur.
- Individualize management on a case-by-case basis, depending upon maternal and fetal considerations.

ACETAMINOPHEN POISONING

Lars C. Larsen, MD

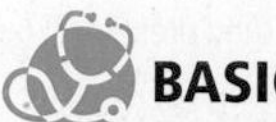

BASICS

DESCRIPTION

- A disorder characterized by hepatic necrosis following large ingestions of acetaminophen. Symptoms may vary from initial nausea, vomiting, diaphoresis, and malaise to jaundice, confusion, somnolence, coma, and death. The clinical hallmark is the onset of symptoms within 24 hours of ingestion of acetaminophen-only or combination products.
- Acetaminophen poisoning is most often encountered following large single ingestions of acetaminophen-containing medications. Usual toxic doses are above 10 g in adults and 150 mg/kg in children. However, poisoning also occurs after acute and chronic ingestions of lesser amounts in susceptible individuals, including those who regularly abuse alcohol, are chronically malnourished, or take medications that affect hepatic metabolism of acetaminophen.
- Therapeutic adult doses are 0.5–1 g q4–6h, up to a maximum of 4 g/d. Therapeutic pediatric doses are 10–20 mg/kg q4–6h.
- System(s) affected: Gastrointestinal; Cardiovascular; Renal/Urologic:
  – Multisystem organ failure can occur.
- Synonym(s): Paracetamol poisoning

Geriatric Considerations

Hepatic damage may be increased if taking hepatotoxic medications chronically.

Pediatric Considerations

Hepatic damage at toxic acetaminophen levels is decreased in children <6 years.

Pregnancy Considerations

- Increased incidence of spontaneous abortion, especially with overdose at early gestational age
- Incidence of spontaneous abortion or fetal death appears to be increased when *N*-acetylcysteine (NAC) treatment is delayed.
- The optimal route for administration of NAC in pregnant patients remains debatable, although IV NAC may offer greater bioavailability.

EPIDEMIOLOGY

- Predominant age: Children and adults
- Predominant sex: No reported association

Incidence

- More than 50,000 calls placed to poison control centers in 2007 related to possible acetaminophen overdoses.
- 74 deaths in 2006, none in children <6 years of age

Prevalence

Approximately 29% of single exposures are in children <6 years.

RISK FACTORS

- Age >6 years
- Concurrent poisoning with other substances
- Psychiatric illness
- Previous toxic ingestions or suicide attempts
- Regular ingestion of large amounts of alcohol

GENERAL PREVENTION

Parent/caregiver education essential:

- Education during well-child exams regarding poisoning prevention
- Emergency telephone numbers

ETIOLOGY

- Accidental or intentional ingestion of acetaminophen or combination medications containing acetaminophen
- Approximately 96% of ingested acetaminophen is metabolized in the liver with only 2% to 4% excreted unchanged in the urine. When taken in therapeutic doses, 90–95% of hepatic metabolism occurs via glucuronidation and sulfation and results in the formation of benign metabolites. 5–10% of hepatic metabolism is by oxidation through the cytochrome P_{450} enzyme system (CYP 3A4 and CYP 2E1) and results in the formation of the toxic metabolite *N*-acetyl-*p*-benzoquinoneimne (NAPQI). NAPQI is rapidly conjugated with glutathione to form a nontoxic metabolite. The metabolites are excreted in the urine along with the small amount of unchanged drug. Hepatocellular damage typically occurs when toxic doses of acetaminophen result in saturation of the glucuronidation and sulfation pathways with subsequent production of excessive amounts of NAPQI. Available glutathione stores become depleted, NAPQI accumulates, and hepatocellular damage occurs.

DIAGNOSIS

- Signs and symptoms develop over the 1st 24 hours following large ingestions, and may last as long as 8 days.
- May develop gradually following long-term ingestion of near maximal-therapeutic amounts of acetaminophen. Such patients may present in stages 1–3, without a history of ingestion of the usual toxic doses.
- Severe symptoms indicate large ingestions or coingestants:
  – Stage 1: 1st 24 hours after time of ingestion:
    ○ Nausea
    ○ Vomiting
    ○ Diaphoresis
  – Stage 2: 24–48 hours:
    ○ Right upper quadrant pain
    ○ Typically less nausea, vomiting, diaphoresis, and malaise than in stage 1
  – Stage 3: 72–96 hours:
    ○ Nausea, vomiting, malaise reappear
    ○ Severe poisonings may result in jaundice, confusion, somnolence, and coma.
  – Stage 4: 7–8 days:
    ○ Resolution of clinical signs in survivors
- Fulminant hepatic failure occurs in <1% of adults and is very rare in children <6 years of age.
- Patients with an unexplained rise in liver function tests (LFTs) with negative acetaminophen levels may be overdose patients presenting in stage 3.

HISTORY

Ingestion or suspected ingestion of acetaminophen-containing product

DIAGNOSTIC TESTS & INTERPRETATIO

Lab

- Plasma acetaminophen levels should be drawn o all patients 4 hours or more after ingestion (level prior to 4 hours not helpful).
- At least 1 additional acetaminophen level drawn 4–6 hours after the 1st level is recommended if t ingested acetaminophen is an extended-release product (e.g., Tylenol Extended Relief) or is not known to be an immediate-release product.
- If the 2nd level is higher than the 1st level or is cl to the "possible risk" level on the Rumack-Matth nomogram, it may be prudent to obtain additiona acetaminophen levels every 2 hours until the leve stabilize or decline.
- If coingestants include drugs that slow gastrointestinal (GI) motility, an acetaminophen level drawn 4–6 hours after the 2nd level may detect a late increase in serum acetaminophen concentration.
- Screens for suspected coingestants (aspirin, iron, and others) may be positive (especially when suic attempt is a possibility).
- With toxic ingestions, aspartate transaminase (AS serum glutamic-oxaloacetic transaminase), alanin transaminase (ALT; serum glutamic-pyruvic transaminase), and bilirubin levels begin to rise ir stage 2 and peak in stage 3. In severe poisonings the PT/INR will parallel these changes and should monitored.
- AST levels >1,000 IU/L are consistent with the diagnosis, and levels of 20,000 IU/L are not uncommon.
- Laboratory abnormalities usually resolve by stage
- Renal function abnormalities are common in patients with hepatotoxicity.
- Evidence of damage to the pancreas and heart m present following severe poisonings.
- Drugs that may alter lab results: None with clinica significant cross-reactivity with plasma acetaminophen assay
- Disorders that may alter lab results: Diseases or tc substances that damage the liver, particularly alcohol.

Initial lab tests

- Acetaminophen serum concentration: 4 hours aft ingestion and again per comments above (see General)
- AST, ALT (rise in first 72 hours, then slowly declin prothrombin time (PT)/international normalized ration (INR), bilirubin, LDH
- Electrolytes, glucose, blood urea nitrogen (BUN), creatinine
- Pregnancy screen in females (urine or serum)
- Urinalysis
- Consider arterial blood gas if pH disturbance suspected on clinical or lab grounds.

Follow-Up & Special Considerations

- Repeat 4 hours after ingestion and possibly every 2 hours thereafter if long-acting product is ingest or acetaminophen ingested with other agents tha slow GI passage.
- Arterial blood gas after hydration if pH is acidotic

Imaging

No specific imaging required

thological Findings

ntrilobular hepatic necrosis

FFERENTIAL DIAGNOSIS

- Consider presence of coingestants, especially alcohol and aspirin.
- Other ingested toxins that produce severe acute hepatic injury, including the mushroom *Amanita phalloides* and products containing yellow phosphorus or carbon tetrachloride

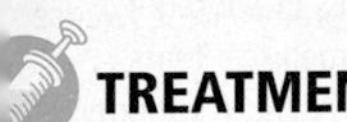

TREATMENT

- Contact a regional poison control center for management recommendations. In the US, a local poison control center can be reached by calling 800) 222-1222.
- NAC should be given when plasma acetaminophen concentrations measured 4 hours or more after ingestion are in the "possible risk" or higher levels on the Rumack-Matthew nomogram. This corresponds to acetaminophen levels >150 μg/mL 993 μmol/L), >75 μg/mL (497 μmol/L), and >37 μg/mL (244 μmol/L) at 4, 8, and 12 hours after ingestion, respectively. See http://www.ars-nformatica.ca/toxicity_nomogram.php?calc=acetamin or http://www.merck.com/mmpe/sec21/ch326/ch326c.html
- NAC should be started within 8 hours of ingestion for best chance of hepatic protection. Patients presenting near 8 hours should empirically receive NAC while waiting for labs.
- All patients with acetaminophen liver injury (even after 8 hours) should receive NAC.
- NAC therapy may be effective up to 36 hours or more after ingestion.
- Single dose activated charcoal can be used (especially in cases of coingestants) (1,2)[C],(3)[A] but not within 1 hour of administration of the antidote NAC. Never delay NAC for activated charcoal.
- NAC should be initiated within 8 hours of ingestion whenever possible.
- Ipecac and gastric lavage are no longer recommended for routine use at home or in health care facilities (4)[C].

EDICATION

rst Line

- Acetylcysteine (NAC, Mucomyst) should be initiated within 8 hours of ingestion whenever possible; single dose activated charcoal may be given 1 hour after oral NAC. NEVER delay oral NAC for activated charcoal.
- Acetylcysteine may be given p.o. or IV, depending on situation and availability: IV is often preferred, particularly if activated charcoal is given:
  - Currently, IV is the recommended form of administration:
    - Oral loading dose of 140 mg/kg, followed by 70 mg/kg q4h for 17 additional doses. IV loading dose of Acetadote 150 mg/kg over 15 to 60 minutes followed by an infusion of 50 mg/kg over 4 hours (12.5 mg/kg/hour); this is followed by an infusion of 100 mg/kg over the next 16 hours (6.25 mg/kg/hour).
- Contraindications: Medication allergies
- Precautions:
  - Oral NAC may cause significant nausea and vomiting due to its sulfur content; consider IV administration or by nasogastric tube.
  - Nausea can be treated with metoclopramide (Reglan), 0.5–1 mg/kg IV, or ondansetron (Zofran), 0.15 mg/kg IV (for age >4 years, usually 4 mg/dose).
  - IV NAC (Acetadote) may cause anaphylactoid reactions, including rash, bronchospasm, pruritus, angioedema, tachycardia, or hypotension (higher rates seen in asthmatics and those with atopic history) (5,6)[C].
- Reactions usually occur with loading dose. Slow or temporarily stop the infusion; may concurrently treat with antihistamines.
- Significant possible interactions: Activated charcoal given within 1 hour of oral NAC may adsorb the NAC, limiting its effectiveness.
- Activated charcoal: 1 g/kg p.o. for initial dose; preferably not within 1 hour of NAC administration. Additional concurrent use during NAC therapy is controversial.

Second Line

Oral racemethionine (methionine)

ADDITIONAL TREATMENT

Issues for Referral

- Psychiatric and psychological evaluation in emergency room and close follow-up for all after intentional ingestions
- Consider child abuse reporting if neglect led to overdose.

IN-PATIENT CONSIDERATIONS

Initial Stabilization

Aggressive age- and weight-appropriate IV hydration

Admission Criteria

- Toxic and intentional ingestions
- Any reported ingestion with increased LFTs, acidosis on arterial blood gas (ABG), elevated creatinine, etc.

ONGOING CARE

FOLLOW-UP RECOMMENDATIONS

- All patients should be evaluated at a health care facility.
- Patients with evidence of organ failure, increased LFTs, or coagulopathy should be evaluated for transfer to a site capable of liver transplant.
- Outpatient for nontoxic accidental ingestions
- Activity may be restricted if significant hepatic damage.

Patient Monitoring

Inquire as to possible ingestion by others (i.e., suicide pacts).

DIET

No special diet, except with severe hepatic damage

PATIENT EDUCATION

- Patients should be counseled to avoid Tylenol if already using combination product containing acetaminophen.
- Education of parents/caregivers during well-child visits
- Anticipatory guidance for caregivers, family, and cohabitants of potentially suicidal patients
- Patient brochure (item no. 1515), *Child safety: keeping your home safe for your baby*. American Academy of Family Physicians: www.familydoctor.org or http://familydoctor.org/online/famdocen/home/healthy/safety/kids-family/027.html
- Education of patients taking long-term acetaminophen therapy

PROGNOSIS

- Complete recovery with early therapy
- <1% of adult patients develop hepatic failure. King criteria (pH <7.3, PT >100 s [INR >65], creatinine >3.4 mg/dL [>300 μmol/L]) are associated with a poor prognosis and possible need for liver transplant (7)[C].
- Hepatic failure is very rare in children <6 years of age.

COMPLICATIONS

Rare following recovery from acute poisoning

REFERENCES

1. Gaudreault P. Activated charcoal revisited. *Clin Ped Emerg Med*. 2005;6:76–80.
2. Heard K. Gastrointestinal decontamination. *Med Clin North Am*. 2005;89:1067–78.
3. Brok J, Buckley N, Glud C. Interventions for paracetamol (acetaminophen) overdoses. *The Cochrane Database of Systematic Reviews* 2006 volume 1.
4. American Academy of Pediatrics Committee on Injury, Violence, and Poison Prevention. Poison treatment in the home. American Academy of Pediatrics Committee on Injury, Violence, and Poison Prevention. *Pediatrics*. 2003;112:1182–5.
5. Acetylcysteine (Acetadote) for acetaminophen overdosage. *Med Lett*. 2005;47:70–1.
6. Culley CM, Krenzelok EP. A clinical and pharmacoeconomic justification for intravenous acetylcysteine: a US perspective. *Toxicol Rev*. 2005;24:131–43.
7. O'Grady JG, Alexander GJ, Hayllar KM et al. Early indicators of prognosis in fulminant hepatic failure. *Gastroenterology*. 1989;97:439–45.

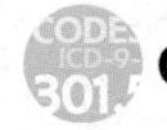

CODES

ICD9

965.4 Poisoning by aromatic analgesics, not elsewhere classified

CLINICAL PEARLS

- Contact a regional poison control center for management recommendations. In the US, a local poison control center can be reached by calling (800) 222-1222.
- NAC should be given when plasma acetaminophen concentrations measured 4 hours or more after ingestion are in the "possible risk" or higher levels on the Rumack-Matthew nomogram. This corresponds to acetaminophen levels >150 μg/mL (993 μmol/L), >75 μg/mL (497 μmol/L), and >40 μg/mL (265 μmol/L) at 4, 8, and 12 hours after ingestion, respectively.
- NAC should be started within 8 hours of ingestion for best chance of hepatic protection. Patients presenting near 8 hours should empirically receive NAC while waiting for labs.
- All patients with acetaminophen liver injury (even after 8 hours) should receive NAC.

ACL INJURY

J. Herbert Stevenson, MD

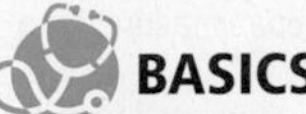

BASICS

DESCRIPTION

- The anterior cruciate ligament (ACL) is one of the major stabilizers of the knee. It prevents excessive anterior translation and internal rotation of the tibia on the femur. During dynamic movement, the ACL and PCL work together to stabilize the knee.
- ACL injuries are common and can occur through noncontact or contact mechanisms. >70% of ACL injuries are caused by noncontact forces (1,2).
- Partial tears of the ACL can occur, but complete tears are far more common.
- Female athletes are at 2–5 times higher risk of ACL tear, particularly in soccer, basketball, and skiing (2).
- ACL injury is associated with early onset of knee osteoarthritis, regardless of surgical or nonsurgical treatment (3,4)[B].

EPIDEMIOLOGY

Incidence

- 250,000 ACL injuries annually in the US (1)
- Female athletes incidence 2- to 5-fold > male athletes (2)
- Greater incidence of noncontact ACL injuries in sports requiring cutting, pivoting, and rapid deceleration, such as basketball and soccer.

Prevalence

- Young athletes aged 15–25 years sustain >50% of all ACL injuries (5).
- >2/3 of patients with complete ACL tear have associated menisci and/or articular cartilage injury (1).

Geriatric Considerations

Management is based on anticipated activity level, associated injuries, coexisting medical conditions, and acute versus long-standing ACL deficiency.

Pediatric Considerations

- Must be concerned about physeal injuries in the skeletally immature
- The incidence of ACL tears in patients with open physes has increased in recent years.
- ACL injury rates increase for both boys and girls beginning at age 11 years.

RISK FACTORS

- No single risk factor correlates directly with higher ACL injury rates in female athletes. Likely multifactorial etiology:
  - Sex hormones:
    - Increased rate may be due to monthly hormonal fluctuations.
    - No conclusive evidence linking a menstrual cycle phase
  - Anatomical gender differences:
    - Increased Q angle, increased genu valgum, narrower femoral notch size, smaller ACL
    - Neuromuscular imbalances (increased quadriceps activation, decreased hamstring activity during landings)
  - Movement patterns (sudden deceleration, change of direction cutting movements, landing from a jump in hyperextension)

Genetics

Familial tendency has been identified.

GENERAL PREVENTION

- Neuromuscular training with proprioceptive, plyometric, and strength exercises may reduce ACL injuries in female athletes (1,2,6)[B].
- No evidence that prophylactic knee bracing prevents ACL injuries (5)[C]
- Educate the patient about possible risk factors for ACL injury and provide instruction on neuromuscular training exercises.

ETIOLOGY

- Noncontact mechanisms (torsional or hyperextension forces)
- Direct trauma (player, object on playing field)

COMMONLY ASSOCIATED CONDITIONS

- Meniscal tear
- Collateral ligament tear
- PCL tear
- Tibia or femur fractures
- Osteochondral injury
- Loose bodies
- Early-onset degenerative joint disease

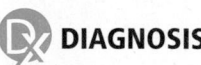

DIAGNOSIS

HISTORY

May recall mechanism:

- Noncontact:
  - Sudden deceleration
  - Cutting, sudden change in direction
  - Landing from a jump in extension
  - Combination of mechanisms
- Contact with player, object
- May recall sudden pop or snap
- Sudden pain and giving way
- Marked effusion/hemarthrosis within 4–12 hours

PHYSICAL EXAM

- Pain
- Effusion
- Decreased range of motion (ROM)
- Joint instability
- Giving way
- Difficulty bearing weight
- Inspect for malalignment (fracture, dislocation)
- Palpate for effusion
- Evaluate extensor mechanism integrity
- Evaluate ROM:
  - Deficits may be secondary to pain, effusion, mechanical blocks (meniscal tear, loose body, torn ACL stump).

DIAGNOSTIC TESTS & INTERPRETATION

- Lachman test: Most sensitive and highly specific diagnostic test for ACL injury, especially in acute setting (7)[A]:
  - Knee placed in 20–30° flexion. Tibia is pulled forward while femur is stabilized with opposite hand. Increased anterior translation compared with uninjured knee indicates injury. Lack of a solid endpoint indicates rupture.
- Pivot shift test: Lower sensitivity, but more specific for ACL tear than Lachman test (7)[B]:
  - Knee placed in extension. Knee is flexed while applying a valgus and internal rotation stress. A positive test is subluxation at 20–40° of flexion
- Anterior drawer test:
  - Low sensitivity for ACL integrity, especially in acute setting (7)[A]
- Posterior drawer test assesses PCL integrity.
- McMurray test assesses for meniscal tears.
- Valgus/varus stress test for MCL/LCL integrity

Imaging

- Radiographs to rule out associated bony injury
- AP, lateral, and tunnel views:
  - Segond fracture: Avulsion fracture of the lateral capsular margin of the tibia
  - Tibial eminence avulsion fracture
  - Fracture of proximal tibia or distal femur
  - Osteochondral injuries
- MRI is the gold standard for imaging ligamentous and intra-articular structures; MRI will reveal associated bone bruises.

Diagnostic Procedures/Surgery

Surgical management should be considered in the active population, young or old.

DIFFERENTIAL DIAGNOSIS

- Fracture
- Meniscal injury
- Patellar dislocation/subluxation
- Tendon disruption
- PCL injury
- Collateral ligament injury

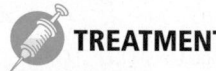

TREATMENT

MEDICATION

First Line

- NSAIDs:
  - Acute ligament sprains (8)[C]:
    - Ibuprofen: 200–800 mg t.i.d.
    - Naproxen: 375–500 mg b.i.d.
    - Indomethacin: 25–50 mg t.i.d.
- Acetaminophen
- Narcotics for severe pain (e.g., acetaminophen-hydrocodone)
- Contraindications/Precautions/Interactions: Refer to the manufacturer's profile of each drug.

ADDITIONAL TREATMENT

General Measures

- Acute injury: PRICEMM therapy: Protection, Relative rest, Ice, Compression, Elevation, Medications, Modalities
- Crutches may be indicated until patient is able to ambulate without pain.
- Knee immobilizer or brace may be used initially for comfort.
- Aspiration of large effusion may be indicated to alleviate pain and increase ROM.

ues for Referral

rgical management should be considered in the tive population.

dditional Therapies

Physical therapy is recommended if an athlete chooses nonsurgical or surgical treatment.
Nonsurgical PT is focused on restoring ROM, strength, and proprioception.
Preoperative phase:
- Increase ROM, minimize inflammation.

Early postoperative phase: Weeks 2–4:
- ROM full extension is the most important goal. Rehabilitation begins immediately.
- Progress to full weight bearing.

Intermediate postoperative phase: Weeks 4–12:
- ROM: Full flexion, hyperextension
- Quadriceps and hamstring strengthening proprioceptive training, normalize gait

Late postop phase: 2–3 months postop:
- Straight-line running
- Increased speed, duration over 6–8 weeks
- Progress to cutting and sport-specific drills.
- Strength and proprioceptive training

URGERY/OTHER PROCEDURES

Surgical versus conservative management depends on patient's activity level, age, associated injuries, and presence of OA.

Insufficient evidence for ACL reconstructive surgery versus conservative management in the skeletally immature patient (9)[A]

Insufficient evidence from randomized trials comparing surgical versus nonoperative management of ACL injuries in adults based on studies in the 1980s (10)[A]

Reconstruction techniques:
- Bone-patella tendon-bone autograft
- Hamstring autograft
- Allograft tendon

No consistent significant differences in outcome between patellar tendon and hamstring tendon autografts (11)[A]

Concomitant meniscal tears are repaired at the time of ACL reconstruction.

N-PATIENT CONSIDERATIONS

itial Stabilization

utpatient

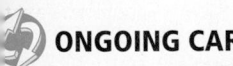

ONGOING CARE

OLLOW-UP RECOMMENDATIONS

ROM exercises to regain full flexion and extension
Advance activity as tolerated

atient Monitoring

ssess functional status, rehabilitative exercise ompliance, and pain control at follow-up visit.

PROGNOSIS

- Athletes typically are out of competitive play for 6–9 months after injury to undergo ACL reconstructive surgery and rehabilitation.
- High prevalence of OA, even in those with early ACL reconstruction (3,4)[B].
- Delay of surgical reconstruction of torn ACL raises risk of secondary meniscal injury.

COMPLICATIONS

- Instability
- Secondary meniscal and articular cartilage injury
- Early-onset degenerative arthritis
- Surgical risks:
  - Infection, PE, subsequent ACL graft rupture, laxity due to failure of graft remodeling

REFERENCES

1. Silvers HJ, Mandelbaum BR. Prevention of anterior cruciate ligament injury in the female athlete. *Br J Sports Med.* 2007;41 Suppl 1:i52–9.
2. Renstrom P et al. Non-contact ACL injuries in female athletes: an International Olympic Committee current concepts statement. *Br J Sports Med.* 2008;42:394–412.
3. Fithian DC, Paxton EW, Stone ML et al. Prospective trial of a treatment algorithm for the management of the anterior cruciate ligament-injured knee. *Am J Sports Med.* 2005;33:335–46.
4. Lohmander LS et al. Long term consequences of anterior cruciate ligament and meniscus injuries. *Am J Sports Med.* 2007;35:1756–69.
5. Griffin LY, Albohm MJ, Arendt EA et al. Understanding and preventing noncontact anterior cruciate ligament injuries: a review of the Hunt Valley II meeting, January 2005. *Am J Sports Med.* 2006;34:1512–32.
6. Hewett TE, Ford KR, Myer GD. Anterior cruciate ligament injuries in female athletes: Part 2, a meta-analysis of neuromuscular interventions aimed at injury prevention. *Am J Sports Med.* 2006;34:490–8.
7. Jackson JL, O'Malley PG, Kroenke K. Evaluation of acute knee pain in primary care. *Ann Intern Med.* 2003;129:575–88.
8. Mehallo CJ, Drezner JA, Bytomski JR. Practical management: Nonsteroidal anti-inflammatory drug use in athletic injuries. *Clin J Sports Med.* 2006;16:170–4.
9. Mohtadi N, Grant J. Managing anterior cruciate ligament deficiency in the skeletally immature individual: A systematic review of the literature. *Clin J Sports Med.* 2006;16:457–64.
10. Linko E, Harilainen A, Malmivaara A, Seitsalo S. Surgical versus conservative interventions for anterior cruciate ligament rupture in adults. *The Cochrane Database of Systematic Reviews* 2005 Issue 4.
11. Spindler KP, Kuhn JE, Freedman KB et al. Anterior cruciate ligament reconstruction autograft choice: bone-tendon-bone versus hamstring: does it really matter? A systematic review. *Am J Sports Med.* 2004;32:1986–95.

ADDITIONAL READING

Cascio BM, Culp L, Cosgarea AJ. Return to play after anterior cruciate ligament reconstruction. *Clin Sports Med.* 2004;23:395–408, ix.

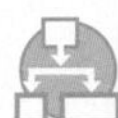

See Also (Topic, Algorithm, Electronic Media Element)

Algorithm: Knee pain

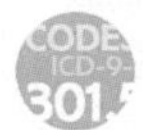

CODES

ICD9

844.2 Sprain of cruciate ligament of knee

CLINICAL PEARLS

- Lachman test: Most sensitive and highly specific diagnostic test for ACL injury, especially in acute setting (7)[A]
- Pivot shift test: Less sensitive but more specific for ACL tear than the Lachman test (7)[B]
- Anterior drawer test: Low sensitivity for ACL integrity, especially in acute setting (7)[A]
- 2/3 of complete ACL tears have associated meniscal or articular injuries.

ACNE ROSACEA

Adarsh K. Gupta, DO, MS

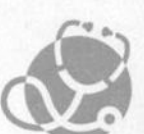

BASICS

DESCRIPTION

- Rosacea is a chronic condition characterized by recurrent episodes of facial flushing, erythema (due to dilatation of small blood vessels in the face), papules, pustules, and telangiectasia (due to increased reactivity of capillaries) in a symmetrical, facial distribution. Sometimes associated with ocular symptoms (ocular rosacea).
- System(s) affected: Skin/Exocrine
- Synonym(s): Rosacea

Geriatric Considerations

- Uncommon >60 years of age
- Effects of aging might increase the side effects associated with oral isotretinoin (at present, data is insufficient due to lack of clinical studies in elderly patients aged 65 and above).

EPIDEMIOLOGY

Prevalence

- Predominant age: 30–50 years
- Predominant sex: Female > Male. However, male will often progress to later stages.

RISK FACTORS

- Exposure to cold, heat, hot drinks
- Environmental trigger factors: Sun, wind, cold

Genetics

People of Northern European and Celtic background commonly afflicted

GENERAL PREVENTION

No preventive measures known

ETIOLOGY

- No proven cause
- Possibilities include:
  - Thyroid and gonadal disturbance
  - Alcohol, coffee, tea, spiced food overindulgence (unproven)
  - Demodex follicular parasite (suspected)
  - Exposure to cold, heat, hot drinks
  - Emotional stress
  - Dysfunction of the gastrointestinal tract

COMMONLY ASSOCIATED CONDITIONS

- Seborrheic dermatitis of scalp and eyelids
- Keratitis with photophobia, lacrimation, visual disturbance
- Corneal lesions
- Blepharitis
- Uveitis

DIAGNOSIS

HISTORY

- Usually have a history of episodic flushing with increases in skin temperature in response to heat stimulus in mouth (hot liquids), spicy foods, alcohol, sun (solar elastosis). Acne may have preceded the onset of rosacea by years; nevertheless, rosacea usually arises de novo without any preceding history of acne or seborrhea.
- Excessive facial warmth and redness is the predominant presenting complaint. Itching is generally absent.

PHYSICAL EXAM

- Rosacea has typical stages of evolution:
  - The rosacea diathesis: Episodic erythema, "flushing and blushing"
  - Stage I: Persistent erythema with telangiectases
  - Stage II: Persistent erythema, telangiectases, papules, tiny pustules
  - Stage III: Persistent deep erythema, dense telangiectases, papules, pustules, nodules; rarely persistent "solid" edema of the central part of the face (phymatous)
- Facial erythema, particularly on cheeks, nose, and chin. At times, entire face may be involved.
- Inflammatory papules are prominent, and there may be pustules and telangiectasia.
- Comedones are absent (unlike acne).
- Women usually have lesions on the chin and cheeks, whereas nose is commonly involved in men.
- Ocular findings (mild dryness and irritation with blepharitis, conjunctival injection, burning, stinging, tearing, eyelid inflammation, swelling, and redness) are present in 50% of patients.

DIAGNOSTIC TESTS & INTERPRETATION

Diagnosis is based on physical exam findings.

Pathological Findings

- Inflammation around hypertrophied sebaceous glands, producing papules, pustules, and cysts
- Absence of comedones and blocked ducts
- Vascular dilation and dermal lymphocytic infiltrate

DIFFERENTIAL DIAGNOSIS

- Drug eruptions (iodides and bromides)
- Granulomas of the skin
- Cutaneous lupus erythematosus
- Carcinoid syndrome
- Deep fungal infection
- Acne vulgaris
- Seborrheic dermatitis
- Steroid rosacea (abuse)
- Systemic lupus erythematosus

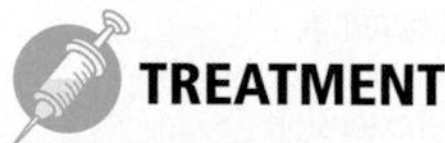

TREATMENT

MEDICATION

First Line

- Azelaic acid (Finacea) with oral doxycycline is very effective as initial therapy and then Azelaic acid topical alone is effective for maintenance (3,4)[A].

Precautions: Tetracycline may cause photosensitivity, sunscreen is recommended.
Significant possible interactions:

- Tetracycline: Avoid concurrent administration with antacids, dairy products, or iron.
- Broad-spectrum antibiotics: May reduce the effectiveness of oral contraceptives; barrier method is recommended.

Pediatric Considerations

- Tetracycline: Not for use in children <8 years

Pregnancy Considerations

Tetracycline: Not for use during pregnancy

- Isotretinoin: Teratogenic; not for use during pregnancy or in women of reproductive age who are not using reliable contraception

econd Line
- Topical erythromycin
- Topical clindamycin lotion preferred
- Possible utility of calcineurin inhibitors (tacrolimus 0.1%; pimecrolimus 0.1%)
- Permethrin 5% cream (5)[A] similar efficacy compared to metronidazole
- Topical steroids should not be used, as they may aggravate rosacea.
- For severe cases, isotretinoin p.o. for 4 months

ODITIONAL TREATMENT

eneral Measures
- Use of mild, nondrying soap is recommended; local skin irritants should be avoided.
- Reassurance that rosacea is completely unrelated to poor hygiene
- Treat psychological stress if present
- Avoid oil-based cosmetics:
  - Others are acceptable and may help women tolerate the symptoms.
- Electrodesiccation or chemical sclerosis of permanently dilated blood vessels
- Possible evolving laser therapy
- Support physical fitness

URGERY/OTHER PROCEDURES

ser treatment is an option for progressive angiectasias or rhinophyma.

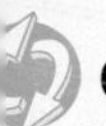

ONGOING CARE

OLLOW-UP RECOMMENDATIONS

utpatient treatment

atient Monitoring
- Occasional and as needed
- Close follow-up for women using isotretinoin

DIET

Avoid alcohol, excessive sun exposure, and hot drinks of any type.

PROGNOSIS
- Slowly progressive
- Subsides spontaneously (sometimes)

COMPLICATIONS
- Rhinophyma (dilated follicles and thickened bulbous skin on nose), especially in men
- Conjunctivitis
- Blepharitis
- Keratitis
- Visual deterioration

REFERENCES

1. Zuuren EJ, et al. Interventions for rosacea (Cochrane review). In: *The Cochrane Library* 2007 Issue 1. Chichester, UK: John Wiley and Sons, Ltd.
2. Del Rosso JQ, Webster GF, Jackson M et al. Two randomized phase III clinical trials evaluating anti-inflammatory dose doxycycline (40-mg doxycycline, USP capsules) administered once daily for treatment of rosacea. *J Am Acad Dermatol*. 2007;56:791–802.
3. Thiboutot DM, Fleischer AB, Del Rosso JQ, Rich P et al. A multicenter study of topical azelaic acid 15% gel in combination with oral doxycycline as initial therapy and azelaic acid 15% gel as maintenance monotherapy. *J Drugs Dermatol*. 2009;8:639–48.
4. Liu RH, Smith MK, Basta SA et al. Azelaic acid in the treatment of papulopustular rosacea: a systematic review of randomized controlled trials. *Arch Dermatol*. 2006;142:1047–52.
5. Koçak M, Ya?li S, Vahapo?lu G et al. Permethrin 5% cream versus metronidazole 0.75% gel for the treatment of papulopustular rosacea. A randomized double-blind placebo-controlled study. *Dermatology*. 2002;205:265–70.

ADDITIONAL READING

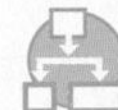

See Also (Topic, Algorithm, Electronic Media Element)

Acne Vulgaris; Blepharitis; Dermatitis, Seborrheic; Lupus Erythematosus, Discoid; Uveitis
Algorithm: Acne

CODES

ICD9

695.3 Rosacea

CLINICAL PEARLS

- Rosacea usually arises de novo without any preceding history of acne or seborrhea.
- Rosacea may cause chronic eye symptoms, including blepharitis.
- Avoid alcohol, sun exposure, and hot drinks.
- Medication treatment resembles that of acne vulgaris with oral and topical antibiotics.

ACNE VULGARIS

Gary I. Levine, MD

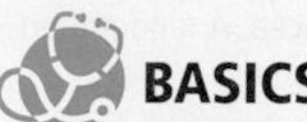

BASICS

DESCRIPTION

- Acne vulgaris is a disorder of the pilosebaceous units. It is a chronic inflammatory dermatosis notable for open/closed comedones and inflammatory lesions, including papules, pustules, or nodules.
- System(s) affected: Skin/Exocrine

Geriatric Considerations

Favre-Racouchot syndrome:

- Comedones on face and head due to sun exposure

Pregnancy Considerations

- May result in a flare or remission of acne
- Erythromycin can be used in pregnancy; use topical agents when possible.
- Isotretinoin is a teratogenic; Class X
- Avoid topical tretinoin, although no good evidence exists that its use is teratogenic.
- Contraindicated: Isotretinoin, tazarotene, tetracycline, doxycycline, minocycline

Pediatric Considerations

- Neonatal acne
- Infantile acne: Increased risk for severe teenage acne vulgaris
- Rare in ages 1–7 years:
  - Check for hyperandrogenemia of adrenal or ovarian origin.
  - Do not use tetracyclines <8 years of age

EPIDEMIOLOGY

- Predominant age: Early to late puberty, may persist into 4th decade
- Predominant sex:
  - Male > Female (adolescence)
  - Female > Male (adult)

Prevalence

- 17–50 million cases in the US
- Nearly 80–95% of adolescents affected. A smaller percentage will seek medical advice.
- 8% of adults aged 25–34 years, 3% of those aged 35–44 years

RISK FACTORS

- Increased endogenous androgenic effect
- Oily cosmetics: Cleansing creams, moisturizers, and oil-based foundations; pomade
- Rubbing or occluding skin surface (e.g., sports equipment such as helmets and shoulder pads), telephone, or hands against the skin
- Polyvinyl chloride, chlorinated hydrocarbons, cutting oil, tars
- Numerous drugs including androgenic steroids (e.g., steroid abuse, some birth control pills)
- Endocrine disorders: Polycystic ovarian syndrome, Cushing syndrome, congenital adrenal hyperplasia, androgen-secreting tumors, acromegaly
- Stress

Genetics

- Familial association in 50%
- If a family history exists, the acne may be more severe and occur earlier.

PATHOPHYSIOLOGY

- Immune changes and inflammatory responses may predate hyperkeratinization
- Androgens (testosterone and dehydroepiandrosterone [DHEA]) stimulate sebum production and proliferation of keratinocytes in hair follicles.
- Keratin plug obstructs follicle os, causing sebum accumulation and follicular distention.
- *Propionibacterium acnes*, an anaerobe, colonizes and proliferates in the plugged follicle.
- *P. acnes* promotes chemotactic factors and proinflammatory mediators, causing inflammation of follicle and dermis.

COMMONLY ASSOCIATED CONDITIONS

- Acne fulminans
- Pyoderma faciale
- Acne conglobata
- Hidradenitis suppurativa
- Pomade acne
- SAPHO syndrome: Synovitis, acne, pustulosis, hyperostosis, osteitis
- PAPA syndrome: Pyogenic sterile arthritis, pyoderma gangrenosum, cystic acne
- Behçet syndrome
- Apert syndrome
- Dark-skinned patients: 50% keloidal scarring and 50% acne hyperpigmented macules

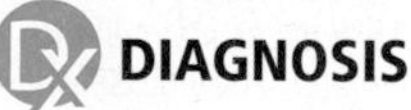

DIAGNOSIS

HISTORY

Ask duration, medications, cleansing products, stress, smoking, exposures, family history. Factors influencing symptomatology:

- Males later onset, greater severity
- Females may worsen prior to menses

PHYSICAL EXAM

- Closed comedones (whiteheads)
- Open comedones (blackheads)
- Nodules or papules
- Pustules ("cysts")
- Scars: Ice pick, rolling, boxcar, atrophic macules, hypertrophic, depressed, sinus tracts
- Grading system (American Academy of Dermatology, 1990):
  - *Mild:* Few papules/pustules; no nodules
  - *Moderate:* Some papules/pustules; few nodules
  - *Severe:* Numerous papules/pustules; many nodules
  - *Very severe:* Acne conglobata, acne fulminans, acne inversa
- Most common areas affected are: Face, chest, back, and upper arms (areas of greatest concentration of sebaceous glands)

DIAGNOSTIC TESTS & INTERPRETATION

Lab

Labs only indicated if there are additional signs of androgen excess; if so: Free testosterone, dehydroepiandrosterone sulfate (DHEA-S), luteinizing hormone, and follicle-stimulating hormone (1)[A]

DIFFERENTIAL DIAGNOSIS

- Folliculitis: Gram negative and gram positive
- Acne (rosacea, cosmetica, steroid-induced)
- Perioral dermatitis
- Chloracne
- Pseudofolliculitis barbae
- Drug eruption
- Verruca vulgaris and plana
- Keratosis pilaris
- Molluscum contagiosum
- Facial angiofibromas
- Sarcoidosis

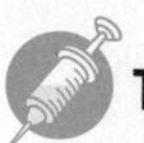

TREATMENT

- Topical retinoid plus a topical antimicrobial agent 1st-line treatment
- Topical retinoid plus antibiotic (topical or p.o.) is better than either alone (2,3)[A]
- Topical retinoids 1st-line agents for maintenance. Avoid antibiotics for maintenance.
- Comedonal acne (grade 1): Keratinolytic agent (2,3)[A]
- Mild inflammatory acne (grade 2): Benzoyl peroxide +/− topical antibiotic. Keratinolytic if needed (3,4)[A].
- Moderate inflammatory acne (grade 3): Add systemic antibiotic to grade 2 regimen.
- Severe inflammatory acne (grade 4): As in grade 3, or isotretinoin (2,3)[A]
- Recommended vehicle type:
  - Cream: Dry or sensitive skin
  - Gel or solution: Oily skin, humid weather
  - Lotion: Hair-bearing areas
- Mild soap daily to control oiliness; avoid abrasives
- Avoid drying agents with keratinolytic agents.
- Use of a gentle cleanser and noncomedogenic moisturizer helps decrease irritation from keratinolytic agents.
- Oil-free, noncomedogenic sunscreens
- Stress management if acne flares with stress

MEDICATION

Keratinolytic agents (side effects include dryness, erythema, scaling, and photosensitivity; start with lower strength; increase as tolerated) (1,2)[A]:

- Tretinoin (Retin-A, Retin A micro, Avita): Apply at bedtime; wash skin and let skin dry 30 minutes before topical application:
  - Retin-A Micro and Avita are less irritating, less phototoxicity
  - May cause an initial flare of lesions. May be eased by 14-day course of oral antibiotics.
- Adapalene (Differin): 0.1%, Apply topically at night:
  - Effective; less irritation than tretinoin or tazarotene (2,4)[A]
  - May be combined with benzoyl peroxide
- Tazarotene (Tazorac): Apply at bedtime:
  - Most effective and most irritating
  - Teratogenic
- Azelaic acid (Azelex, Finevin): 20% topically, b.i.d.:
  - Keratinolytic, antibacterial, anti-inflammatory
  - Reduces postinflammatory hyperpigmentation in dark-skinned individuals
  - Side effects: Erythema, dryness, scaling, hypopigmentation
  - Less effective in clinical use than in studies
- Salicylic acid: Less effective than tretinoin
- Alpha-hydroxy acids: Available over-the-counter

Topical antibiotics and anti-inflammatories (2)[A]:
- Topical benzoyl peroxide:
  - Bactericidal through direct toxic effect
  - No *P. acnes* resistance noted
  - 2.5% as effective as stronger preparations
  - When used with tretinoin, apply benzoyl peroxide in morning and tretinoin at night
  - Side effects: Irritation; may bleach clothes

Topical antibiotics (1,2)[A]:
- Erythromycin 2%
- Clindamycin 1%
- Metronidazole gel or cream: Apply once daily.
- Azelaic acid (Azelex, Finevin): 20% cream: Enhanced effect and decreased risk of resistance when used with zinc and benzoyl peroxide
- Benzoyl peroxide-erythromycin (Benzamycin): Especially effective with azelaic acid
- Benzoyl peroxide-clindamycin (BenzaClin, DUAC, Clindoxyl): Effective combined (4)[A]
- Sodium sulfacetamide (Sulfacet-R, Novacet, Klaron): Useful in acne with seborrheic dermatitis or rosacea

Oral antibiotics (1,2)[A]:
- Tetracycline: 500–2,000 mg/d b.i.d.–q.i.d.; high dose initially, taper in 6 months, as tolerated. Side effects: Photosensitivity, esophagitis:
  - Avoid use with antacids, iron
- Minocycline 50–200 mg/d, q.i.d.–b.i.d. Side effects: Photosensitivity, urticaria, gray-blue skin, vertigo, autoimmune hepatitis, pseudotumor cerebri, lupuslike syndrome. May be more effective than tetracycline (1)[A].
- Doxycycline 50–200 mg/d, given b.i.d.–q.i.d.; side effects include photosensitivity
- Erythromycin: 500–1,000 mg/d; given b.i.d.–q.i.d.; decreasing effectiveness as a result of increasing *P. acnes* resistance
- Trimethoprim-sulfamethoxazole (Bactrim DS, Septra DS); 1 daily or b.i.d.

Oral retinoids:
- Isotretinoin (Accutane) (1,2)[A]: 0.5–2.0 mg/kg/d b.i.d.; 60–90% cure rate; usually given for 12–20 weeks; maximum cumulative dose = 120–150 mg/kg; 20% of patients relapse and require retreatment:
  - Side effects: Numerous (see package insert). Highly teratogenic.
  - Avoid tetracyclines or vitamin A preparations during isotretinoin therapy.
  - Monitor for pregnancy, complete blood count, lipids, and liver function tests at baseline and every month.
  - Should be registered member of manufacturer's iPLEDGE program

Pregnancy Considerations

Isotretinoin is a teratogenic; Class X

Medications for women only:
- Oral contraceptives (1,2)[A]:
  - Norgestimate/ethinyl estradiol (Orth Tricyclen), norethindrone acetate/ethinyl estradiol (Estrostep), drospirenone/ethinyl estradiol (Yaz, Yasmin) are approved by Food and Drug Administration.
  - Levonorgestrel/ethinyl estradiol (Alesse) is also effective.
- Spironolactone (Aldactone); 25–200 mg/d; antiandrogen; reduces sebum production
- Flutamide (Eulexin) 250–500 mg/d; potentially hepatotoxic

ADDITIONAL TREATMENT

Acne hyperpigmented macules:
- Topical hydroquinones (1.5–10%)
- Azelaic acid (20%) topically
- Topical retinoids as above
- Corticosteroids: Low dose, suppresses adrenal androgens (1)[B]
- Dapsone 5% gel (Aczone): Topical, anti-inflammatory use in patients >12 years

Issues for Referral

Consider referral/consultation to dermatologist:
- Refractory lesions despite appropriate therapy
- Consideration of isotretinoin therapy
- Management of acne scars

Additional Therapies

- Light-based treatments
  - UVA/UVB, blue light, blue/red light, pulse dye laser, KTP laser, infrared laser
  - Photodynamic therapy for 30–60 minutes with 5-aminolevulinic acid × 3 sessions is effective for inflammatory lesions:
    - Greatest utility when used as adjunct to medications or in patient who can't tolerate medications
  - More data needed to define role of light-based therapies in treating acne

COMPLEMENTARY AND ALTERNATIVE MEDICINE

- Zinc gluconate 30 mg/d may reduce inflammatory lesions (2)[B]:
  - Topical zinc is ineffective.
- Topical tree oil is effective, but has slow onset (1)[B].

SURGERY/OTHER PROCEDURES

- Comedo extraction after incising the layer of epithelium over comedo (1)[C]
- Incision and drainage for abscesses
- Inject large cystic lesions with 0.05–0.3 mL triamcinolone (Kenalog 2–5 mg/mL); use 30-g needle to inject and slightly distend cyst (1)[C].
- Acne scar treatment: Retinoids, steroid injections, cryosurgery, electrodessication, microdermabrasion, dermabrasion, chemical peels, laser resurfacing, grafting, subcutaneous incision, punch excision, punch elevation, subcision, tissue augmentation injections

ONGOING CARE

FOLLOW-UP RECOMMENDATIONS

Use oral or topical antibiotics for 3 months; stop if inflammatory lesions resolve. Can switch abruptly from oral to topical without taper. Do not use topical and oral together.

Patient Monitoring

- Pretreatment and monthly lipids, liver function tests, and pregnancy tests when on isotretinoin
- Consider antibiotic resistance (60% overall) or gram-negative folliculitis if treatment fails.

DIET

Special diets do not diminish acne (1)[B].

PATIENT EDUCATION

- There may be a worsening of acne during 1st 2 weeks of treatment.
- Treatment takes a minimum of 4 weeks to show results.
- Topical agents can cause redness and drying of the skin.
- Picking at or popping lesions may increase inflammation and scarring.

PROGNOSIS

Gradual improvement over time (usually within 8–12 weeks after beginning therapy)

COMPLICATIONS

- Acne conglobata: Severe confluent inflammatory acne with systemic symptoms
- Facial and psychological scarring
- Gram-negative folliculitis: Superinfection due to long-term oral antibiotic use; treatment with ampicillin, trimethoprim-sulfa, or isotretinoin

REFERENCES

1. Strauss JS, Krowchuk DP, Leyden JJ et al. Guidelines of care for acne vulgaris management. *J Am Acad Dermatol*. 2007;56:651–63.
2. Feldman S, Careccia RE, Barham KL et al. Diagnosis and treatment of acne. *Am Fam Physician*. 2004;69:2123–30.
3. Webster G. Mechanism-based treatment of acne vulgaris: The value of combination therapy. *J Drugs and Dermatol*. 2005;4(3):281–8.
4. Haider A, Shaw JC. Treatment of acne vulgaris. *JAMA*. 2004;292:726–35.

ADDITIONAL READING

- Heymann WR. Oral contraceptives for the treatment of acne vulgaris. *J Am Acad Dermatol*. 2007;56:1056–7.
- Thiboutot D, et al. New insights into the management of acne: An update from the Global Alliance to Improve Outcomes in Acne Group. *Journal of the American Academy of Dermatology*. 2009;60(5 suppl1).

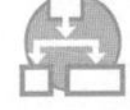

See Also (Topic, Algorithm, Electronic Media Element)

Acne Rosacea
Algorithm: Acne

CODES

ICD9

706.1 Other acne

CLINICAL PEARLS

- Expect worsening for the 1st 2 weeks. Full results take 8–12 weeks.
- Decrease topical frequency from b.i.d. to every day or every day to every other day for irritation; may also use a moisturizing soap and a moisturizer before treatment application.
- Acne resolves with age for most individuals, although 8% of 30-year-olds and 3% of 40-year-olds may have persistent lesions.
- Acne often appears more significant to adolescent than to doctor; may be "entry ticket" for other advice.

ACOUSTIC NEUROMA

Sam Seung Yeol Kim, MBBS, Mmed
Phillip Chang, MBBS

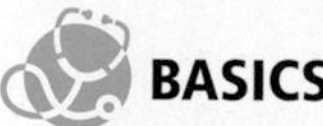

BASICS

DESCRIPTION
- Slow-growing benign tumor, most often arising from the vestibular division of 8th cranial nerve
- Originates from Schwann cells of the nerve sheath ("schwannoma")
- Usually arises in the internal auditory canal near the cerebellopontine angle
- Often has extracanalicular portion into the cerebellopontine angle, but may also stay purely intracanalicular
- Most are unilateral; bilateral only seen in neurofibromatosis type II

EPIDEMIOLOGY
- 6–10% of all intracranial tumors
- 80–90% of cerebellopontine angle tumors
- 95% of cases are unilateral.
- Present most commonly in the 5th–6th decade
- Female predominance
- Bilateral acoustic neuroma occurring in neurofibromatosis II present before age 30

Incidence
- 1/100,000 per year
- Asymptomatic lesions may be more common.

Prevalence
3,000 diagnosed annually in the US

RISK FACTORS
- Pregnancy and epilepsy may increase risk (1).
- Smoking may decrease the risk (1).

Genetics
- Unknown for unilateral acoustic neuroma (AN)
- Neurofibromatosis type II: Bilateral ANs:
  - Autosomal dominant
  - Gene located on chromosome 22q1

PATHOPHYSIOLOGY
- Exerts pressure on the surrounding structures
- Compression of acoustic and facial nerve when located within internal acoustic canal
- Compression of brainstem, 4th ventricle, and trigeminal nerve when tumor at the cerebellar pontine angle

ETIOLOGY
Unknown

COMMONLY ASSOCIATED CONDITIONS
- Neurofibromatosis type II
- Pregnancy may accelerate the growth of the tumor.

DIAGNOSIS

HISTORY
- Common:
  - Sensorineural hearing loss (unilateral), often progressive
  - Loss of speech discrimination
  - Tinnitus
  - Balance problems are common, but vertigo is less common.
- Less common:
  - Weakness/loss of facial muscle functions
  - Headache with hydrocephalus and increased intracranial pressure
  - Trigeminal nerve involvement when tumor is large and compressing on cranial nerve (CN) V
  - Ataxia due to cerebellar or brainstem compression from very large tumor

PHYSICAL EXAM
- Examination with otoscope to exclude other causes of hearing loss (e.g., middle ear effusion, infection, wax, cholesteatoma, or tympanic membrane rupture)
- Detailed neurologic exam concentrating on the cranial nerves
- Weber and Rinne tests to confirm sensorineural hearing loss
- Evaluation of the contralateral ear in patients <30 years; suspect neurofibromatosis type II

DIAGNOSTIC TESTS & INTERPRETATION

Lab
Initial lab tests
- Pure-tone and speech audiometry (asymmetrical, high-frequency sensorineural hearing loss)
- Speech discrimination
- Stacked auditory brainstem response (ABR): 95% sensitivity and 88% specificity (2). Can detect tumors <1 cm.
- Standard ABR: Can only detect tumors >1 cm

Imaging
Initial approach
- Magnetic resonance imaging (MRI) with gadolinium (gold standard):
  - 100% specificity
  - Detects tumors starting at 2 mm
  - Tumor has marked enhancement with gadolinium
- Noncontrast T2-weighted fast spin-echo MRI:
  - 98% specificity
  - Cheaper than MRI with gadolinium
- Computed tomography (CT):
  - Detect tumors as small as 1 cm
  - Up to 37% false-negatives
  - Provides good information of surrounding bony structures of the tumor

Pathological Findings
- Well-demarcated and encapsulated mass attached to neural structures without direct invasion
- Can be dense or cystic
- Microscopic: Densely packed spindle cells (Schwann cells) mixed in with myxoid and collagenous matrix:
  - Zones of alternatively dense and sparse areas of Antoni A and B

DIFFERENTIAL DIAGNOSIS
- Cerebellopontine lesions:
  - Meningioma
  - Glioma
  - Facial nerve schwannoma
  - Epidermoid
  - Hemangioma
  - Arachnoid cyst
- Sensorineural hearing loss:
  - Ménière disease
  - Ototoxicity
  - Presbycusis
  - Cerebellar pathology

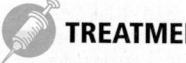

TREATMENT

MEDICATION
Chemotherapy has not yet been explored sufficiently

ADDITIONAL TREATMENT

General Measures
- Conservative management is suitable for elderly patients with contraindications to surgery and radiotherapy.
- Up to 57% of acoustic neuromas may show zero growth or shrinkage (3)[B].
- Up to 70% of extracanalicular tumors may never have growth rate exceeding 2 mm per year (4)[B].
- Growth rate of enlarging acoustic neuromas decreases over time:
  - From 4.9 mm/yr in the 1st year of detected growth to 0.75 mm in 4th year.
- Up to 20% of patients may eventually fail conservative management and require intervention
- More likely to preserve hearing than radiotherapy or surgery (5)[C]
- 69% of patients with 100% speech discrimination at diagnosis have maintained good hearing even after 10 years of observation (6)[B]

Issues for Referral
- Yearly MRI follow-up for slow-growing tumors
- If an asymptomatic tumor becomes symptomatic, this is often indication for intervention.

dditional Therapies

ereotactic radiosurgery:

Gamma knife single-dose stereotactic radiosurgery:
- Performed on an outpatient basis
- Alternative for those with smaller tumor (<3 cm) or contraindications to microsurgery
- No discernible significant difference between growth patterns of untreated tumors and those treated radiosurgically (7)[A]
- Lower-dose radiation has lower complication rates, but evidence is insufficient on whether as effective as high-dose radiation in tumor control (8)[A]
- Higher-dose radiation significantly influences hearing preservation rates (9)[C]
- Complications include trigeminal and/or facial nerve neuropathy from radiation damage.

Fractionated stereotactic radiosurgery:
- Conformal radiation delivers a higher dose of radiation within the tumor and less damage to surrounding healthy tissue.
- Requires multiple treatments and the total dose of radiation is higher compared to the single-dose radiation
- Suitable for all sizes of tumor

URGERY/OTHER PROCEDURES

Recommended definitive treatment (10)[A]
Lowest rate of recurrence, with up to 97.5% complete tumor removal (10)[A]

Intraoperative facial nerve monitoring is generally used.

3 standard approaches, all using operating microscopes:
- Retromastoid/retrosigmoid: For any size, especially tumor located mostly outside the internal auditory canal and adjacent to the brainstem. May require retraction of cerebellum.
- Middle cranial fossa: For small tumors with aim of preserving hearing. Involves retraction of temporal lobe and has higher risk of facial nerve injury.
- Translabyrinthine: For larger tumors. Hearing not preserved. Completely exposes the distal internal auditory canal and has more favorable facial nerve results.

Endoscopic approach used in some centers

Surgical complications:
- Hearing loss
- Cerebrospinal fluid leakage
- Facial nerve injury
- Headache
- Meningitis

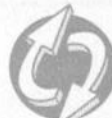

ONGOING CARE

FOLLOW-UP RECOMMENDATIONS

MRI and audiometric follow-up for those treated by radiotherapy and conservative management

COMPLICATIONS

Due to pressure effect of a large tumor:
- Cranial nerve compression
- Hydrocephalus
- Brainstem compression
- Cerebellar tonsil herniation

REFERENCES

1. Schoemaker MJ, Swerdlow AJ, Auvinen A et al. Medical history, cigarette smoking and risk of acoustic neuroma: an international case-control study. *Int J Cancer*. 2007;120:103–10.
2. Don M, Kwong B, Tanaka C et al. The stacked ABR: a sensitive and specific screening tool for detecting small acoustic tumors. *Audiol Neurootol*. 2005;10:274–90.
3. Smouha EE, Yoo M, Mohr K et al. Conservative management of acoustic neuroma: a meta-analysis and proposed treatment algorithm. *Laryngoscope*. 2005;115:450–4.
4. Stangerup SE, Caye-Thomasen P, Tos M et al. The natural history of vestibular schwannoma. *Otol Neurotol*. 2006;27:547–52.
5. Lin VY, Stewart C, Grebenyuk J et al. Unilateral acoustic neuromas: long-term hearing results in patients managed with fractionated stereotactic radiotherapy, hearing preservation surgery, and expectantly. *Laryngoscope*. 2005;115:292–6.
6. Stangerup SE, Thomsen J, Tos M, Cayé-Thomasen P et al. Long-term hearing preservation in vestibular schwannoma. *Otol. Neurotol*. 2010;31: 271–5.
7. Battaglia A, Mastrodimos B, Cueva R. Comparison of growth patterns of acoustic neuromas with and without radiosurgery. *Otol Neurotol*. 2006;27:705–12.
8. Weil RS, et al. Optimal dose of stereotactic radiosurgery for acoustic neuromas: A systematic review. *Brit J Neurosurg* 2006:195–202.
9. Combs SE, Welzel T, Schulz-Ertner D, Huber PE, Debus J et al. Differences in clinical results after LINAC-based single-dose radiosurgery versus fractionated stereotactic radiotherapy for patients with vestibular schwannomas. *Int. J. Radiat. Oncol. Biol. Phys*. 2010;76:193–200.
10. Kaylie DM, Horgan MJ, Delashaw JB et al. A meta-analysis comparing outcomes of microsurgery and gamma knife radiosurgery. *Laryngoscope*. 2000;110:1850–6.

CODES

ICD9

- 225.1 Benign neoplasm of cranial nerves
- 237.70 Neurofibromatosis, unspecified
- 237.71 Neurofibromatosis, type 1, von recklinghausen's disease

CLINICAL PEARLS

A bone-anchored hearing aid can restore hearing for those patients with sensorineural hearing loss that may be present before or after the surgery.

ADOPTION, INTERNATIONAL

Maya Leventer-Roberts, MD, MPH

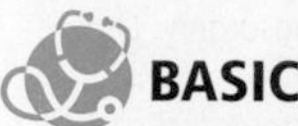

BASICS

DESCRIPTION

Adoption of children from foreign countries into the US has tripled in the past 15 years, and the demographics of those children and their homelands have also shifted significantly during that time. The diverse birth countries, disease exposures, and unknown health histories of these children make them a population that requires special attention (1).

EPIDEMIOLOGY

Incidence

- More than 20,000 international adoptions by US families every year
- >90% are from Asia, Central and South America, and Eastern Europe, with growing numbers from Africa and the Middle East

RISK FACTORS

- Unknown birth history, past medical history, and vaccination status
- Possible exposure to toxins and/or inadequate nutrition in utero
- Exposures to infectious diseases not commonly seen in the US
- Previous living conditions:
  - Overcrowding
  - Institutionalization (orphanages)
  - Environmental toxins
- History of neglect, deprivation, or abuse

GENERAL PREVENTION

- Required to be examined by a US State Department physician in their native country before immigration to the US (2)
- Should be examined by US physician within 3 weeks of arrival
- A follow-up visit 4–6 weeks after their post-adoption appointment is recommended.
- All internationally adopted children should be routinely screened for hearing, vision, growth, and developmental delays.

COMMONLY ASSOCIATED CONDITIONS

- Infectious diseases, including (2,3):
  - Hepatitis B
  - Intestinal parasites
  - Tuberculosis
  - Syphilis
- Emotional or behavioral problems
- Developmental delay
- Fetal alcohol syndrome
- Feeding difficulties
- Anemia
- Congenital conditions, including:
  - Cleft lip/palate
  - Orthopedic deformities
- Prematurity or low birth weight
- Malnutrition, rickets
- Inadequate immunizations
- Lead poisoning
- Sensorineural and conductive hearing loss
- Strabismus, blindness

DIAGNOSIS

HISTORY

- Immunization records and titers (most helpful when dates of administration are included) (4)
- Birth/prenatal history
- Known family history of birth parents
- Prenatal and perinatal disease or toxin exposures
- Documented history of emotional or nutritional deprivation, or physical or sexual abuse
- Duration of time, if any, spent in orphanage. (Studies have suggested every 3–5 months spent in orphanage is associated with 1 month delay in developmental milestones, although quality of care can vary widely.)
- Growth charts when available: Failure to gain weight appropriately (or weight loss) is earliest sign of malnutrition, followed by slowed linear growth, and finally lagging head circumference (brain growth).
- Development, behavior, attachment, parent stress, and parent-child interactions should also be routinely monitored.

PHYSICAL EXAM

- Age-appropriate complete physical exam, particular attention to growth, evaluation for microcephaly (red flag for fetal alcohol syndrome, genetic disorders, or perinatal brain injury), vision, and hearing
- Evaluate for signs of dental decay and refer for prompt treatment
- Developmental assessment, especially for those with unknown date of birth
- Skin exam for signs of scabies, pediculosis, and tinea

DIAGNOSTIC TESTS & INTERPRETATION

- Developmental screening: Denver II Test (±) PEDS parent questionnaire or other validated developmental screening tools at each visit to screen for potential developmental delay and to assess improvement, decline, and need for additional services
- Age-appropriate hearing screening
- Age-appropriate vision screening

Lab

Initial lab tests

- Obtain (5):
  - Hepatitis B (HBsAg, HBsAb, anti-HBc)
  - Hepatitis C
  - HIV
  - Rapid plasma reagin (RPR)
  - Tuberculin skin test
  - 3 stool specimens for ova and parasites, and single specimen for *Giardia lamblia* and *Cryptosporidium parvum* antigens
  - Complete blood count (CBC)
  - Lead
  - Thyroid-stimulating hormone (TSH)
  - Ca^{++}, PO_4, alkaline phosphate, and 25 vitamin D level (if signs of rickets)
  - Urinalysis
- >6 months old: Measure titers for antibodies to diphtheria and tetanus toxoids and poliovirus (regardless of immunization documentation).
- >12 months old: Measure titers for antibodies to diphtheria, tetanus toxoids, poliovirus, measles, mumps, rubella, and varicella (regardless of immunization documentation).

Follow-Up & Special Considerations

Follow-up testing (5):

- Hep B: Repeat at 6 months.
- Hep C: Required in children from China, Russia, Eastern Europe, and Southeast Asia (decision to te children from other countries depends on history and prevalence of infection)
- HIV: Transplacentally acquired maternal antibody may be present in uninfected infants up to 18 months, so will need to retest those with an initial positive result.
- Tuberculosis (TB): Positive test should NOT be attributed to BCG vaccine, and must be investigat further. Give preventive therapy if known exposure Consider repeat testing at 6 months because poor nutrition may result in false-negative (anergic) skir test.
- Gastrointestinal tract signs or symptoms occurring years after immigration: Test for intestinal parasite
- If anemia is detected with a normal lead level, ma consider G6PD deficiency in appropriate countries origin (Africa, Asia, Mediterranean, Middle Easterr and can test with rapid fluorescent spot test.
- Developmental screening: Repeat at each visit and follow progress. 50–90% of all internationally adopted children are delayed upon adoption; however, most of them have normal cognition at long-term follow-up.
- Social history screening: Behavioral concerns may first present during adolescence, even for children were adopted in infancy. (6)

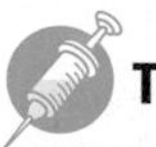

TREATMENT

MEDICATION

- Immunizations per Centers for Disease Control and Prevention schedule with catch-up as needed: http://www.cdc.gov/vaccines/recs/schedules/
- It is recommended that if the child does not have records, or has records that do not comply with the US or World Health Organization guidelines, then h or she should be treated as unimmunized and started on an appropriate catch-up immunization schedule.

ADDITIONAL TREATMENT

General Measures

- Regular diet for children who arrive malnourished should result in rapid weight gain to appropriate weight for height (or length).
- Monitor linear growth; American growth chart might not be applicable to all children.
- If developmental delay is diagnosed, consider early services (such as early intervention) or referral to developmental specialist, depending on the nature and severity of the delay.
- Recommend local support groups for parents.
- Attention to parental interactions: Post-adoption depression may occur.

Issues for Referral

- Many internationally adopted children show sensory-seeking behaviors early on that are sometimes thought to be related to the sensory-depriving orphanage experience of their past. These behaviors typically improve or abate without treatment, but may benefit from work with occupational therapy if the behaviors are significan Out of context, they may appear quite similar to autistic-like features on exam (hand-flapping, rocking, etc.), but as long as the child is otherwise developing normally (socially, emotionally), should not raise significant levels of concern (2).

If a child continues to have disruptive behaviors, or would rather self-soothe than seek nurturing human interaction, he or she warrants a complete and thorough developmental evaluation with a specialist (developmental/behavioral pediatrician or pediatric psychiatrist).

Persistent behavioral issues in the parent-child interactions should also be evaluated by a pediatric psychologist or psychiatrist.

Concerns about vision should be referred to pediatric ophthalmology for more extensive vision workup.

Concerns about hearing should be referred to audiology and/or ENT for more extensive workup for conductive vs sensorineural hearing loss.

Recommend pediatric dental evaluation by 12 months, sooner if signs of dental pathology.

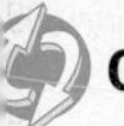

ONGOING CARE

OLLOW-UP RECOMMENDATIONS

atient Monitoring

- Regular well child visits, particularly within first months of entry into the US
- Close monitoring of developmental milestones, behavior, and individual attachment

IET

- Regular diet
- Weight catch-up will occur with a normal diet, barring other medical conditions, and eating habits should normalize using parenting methods discussed below.

ATIENT EDUCATION

- Eating: The recommended approach is to allow access to as much healthy food as the child wants, as often as he or she wants it, so that the child can learn the important self-regulatory behaviors of eating that may not have been learned in an institution (hunger, satiety) and can build trust with the parent(s) who feed him or her.
- Toileting: While some children may simply not be trained yet, others may have accidents in their new home because of regression. Time and positive reinforcement, avoiding punishment, will resolve this issue as the child becomes comfortable with his or her new surroundings.
- Sleeping: Children must learn to trust their new home and parents, and thus this is not a time for aggressive sleep rules (i.e., ferberization). Parents should be present, physically and emotionally, just enough to let the child know he or she is safe, establish a bedtime ritual upon arrival, and then should gently reinforce this ritual.
- Language: As the child experiences a myriad of changes, it may be helpful for the adoptive family to have learned some key phrases in the child's native language for the first few weeks post-adoption. Depending on the child's age and language proficiency, an interpreter may also be useful in the home and at medical appointments until English becomes more comfortably understood and familiar (2).
- Adopted children may experience grieving of lost family, relationships, and culture, which is normal and expected behavior.
- At 3–4 years old, adopted children will begin to recognize physical differences between themselves and adoptive family if they are of differing racial origin.
- Children and families should be encouraged to learn about the heritage and culture of the birth countries or ethnic groups.
- Relationships with others of the same racial or ethnic group may be very helpful to the adopted child.

PROGNOSIS

Long-term issues include (7,8):

- Children who experienced early neglect, deprivation, or loss prior to adoption are more likely to have developmental delay or behavioral or attachment problems.
- These issues decrease with time the child has spent within the adoptive family, although those with significant histories of deprivation are at risk for difficulties that may persist for life.
- Although most adopted children are healthy, as a group they have been found to have higher rates of moderate to severe physical and mental health problems, hearing and visual impairment, learning disability, developmental delay, or special health care needs when compared with biologic children of the same parents.
- Developmental delay, in particular, is reportedly found to be 2–3 times more likely in an internationally adopted child than in his or her nonadopted peers. However, recent studies show marked catch-up development reported after living in adoptive homes, with many children achieving normal-range development later in life (depending on length of time spent in an institution prior to adoption).
- Fortunately, international adoption pairs some of the most vulnerable, potentially high-risk children with the lowest-risk parents (usually financially stable, well-educated, with relatively extremely low divorce rates).
- Most families have found the process of international adoption deeply rewarding, while acknowledging the potential challenges.

REFERENCES

1. Dawood F, Serwint JR. International adoption. *Pediatr Rev*. 2008;29:292–4.
2. Schulte EE, Springer SH. Health care in the first year after international adoption. *Pediatr Clin North Am*. 2005;52:1331–49, vii.
3. Johnson DE. Long-term medical issues in international adoptees. *Pediatr Ann*. 2000;29: 234–41.
4. American Academy of Pediatrics Committee on Early Childhood, Adoption & Dependent Care: Initial medical evaluation of an adopted child. *Pediatrics*. 1991;88:642–4.
5. American Academy of Pediatrics. Medical evaluation of internationally adopted children for infectious diseases. In: Pickering LK ed. *Red Book: 2006 Report of the Committee on Infectious Diseases* – 27th Ed.
6. Hawk B, McCall RB et al. CBCL behavior problems of post-institutionalized international adoptees. *Clin Child Fam Psychol Rev*. 2010;13:199-211
7. Van Ijzendoorn MH, Bakermans-Kranenburg MJ, Juffer F. Plasticity of Growth in Height, Weight, and Head Circumference: Meta-analytic Evidence of Massive Catch-up After International Adoption. *J Dev Behav Pediatr*. 2007;28:334–43.
8. Weitzman C, Albers L. Long-term developmental, behavioral, and attachment outcomes after international adoption. *Pediatr Clin North Am*. 2005;52:1395–419, viii.

ADDITIONAL READING

- Borchers D, American Academy of Pediatrics Committee on Early Childhood, Adoption, and Dependent Care. Families and adoption: the pediatrician's role in supporting communication. *Pediatrics*. 2003;112:1437–41.
- http://www.travel.state.gov/pdf/Prospective_Adoptive_Parents_Guide.pdf.

CODES

ICD9

V70.3 Other general medical examination for administrative purposes

CLINICAL PEARLS

- Initial labs:
  - Hepatitis B (HBsAg, HBsAb, anti-HBc), hepatitis C IgG, HIV, RPR, CBC, TSH, lead, Ca, PO4, 25 OH vitamin D
  - Tuberculin skin test
  - 3 stool specimens for ova and parasites, and single specimen for *Giardia lamblia* and *Cryptosporidium parvum* antigens
  - Urinalysis
- >6 months old: Measure antibodies to diphtheria and tetanus toxoids and poliovirus (regardless of immunization documentation).
- >12 months old: Measure antibodies to diphtheria, tetanus toxoids, poliovirus, measles, mumps, rubella, and varicella (regardless of immunization documentation).
- Many internationally adopted children show sensory-seeking behaviors early on that are sometimes thought to be related to the sensory-depriving orphanage experience of their past. These behaviors typically improve or abate without treatment, but may benefit from work with occupational therapy if the behaviors are significant. Out of context, they may appear quite similar to autistic-like features on exam (hand-flapping, rocking, etc.), but as long as the child is otherwise developing normally (socially, emotionally), they should not raise significant levels of concern.

ALCOHOL ABUSE AND DEPENDENCE

Gennine M. Zinner, RNCS, ANP

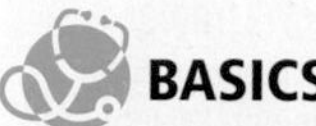

BASICS

DESCRIPTION
- Any pattern of alcohol use causing significant physical, mental, or social dysfunction; key features are tolerance, withdrawal, and persistent use despite problems
- Alcohol abuse: Maladaptive pattern of alcohol use manifested by 1 (or more) of:
  - Failure to fulfill obligations at work, school, or home
  - Recurrent use in hazardous situations
  - Recurrent alcohol-related legal problems
  - Continued use despite related social or interpersonal problems
- Alcohol dependence: Maladaptive pattern of use manifested by 3 (or more) of the following:
  - Tolerance
  - Withdrawal
  - Using more than intended
  - Persistent desire or attempts to cut down/stop
  - Significant amount of time obtaining, using, or recovering from alcohol
  - Social, occupational, or recreational activities sacrificed for alcohol use
  - Continued use despite physical or psychological problems
- National Institute on Alcohol Abuse and Alcoholism criteria for "at-risk" drinking: Men >14 drinks a week or >4 per occasion. Women: >7 drinks a week or >3 per occasion.
- System(s) affected: Nervous; Gastrointestinal
- Synonym(s): Alcoholism; Alcohol abuse; Alcohol dependence

Geriatric Considerations
- Common and underdiagnosed in elderly; less likely to report problem. May exacerbate normal age-related cognitive deficits and disabilities.
- Multiple drug interactions
- Signs and symptoms may be different or attributed to chronic medical problem or dementia.
- Assessment tools may be inappropriate.

Pediatric Considerations
- Children of alcoholics at high risk
- In 2004, 28% of persons 12–20 years reported use in past month, 1 in 5 binge drink; binge drinkers are 7 times more likely to report illicit drug use.
- Negative effect on maturation and development
- Early drinkers are 4 times more likely to develop a problem than those who begin >21.
- Depression, suicidal or disorderly behavior; family disruption; violence or destruction of property; poor school or work performance; sexual promiscuity; social immaturity; lack of interests; isolation; moodiness

Pregnancy Considerations
- Alcohol is teratogenic, especially during the 1st trimester; women should abstain during conception and throughout pregnancy.
- 10–50% of children born to women who are heavy drinkers will have fetal alcohol syndrome.
- Women experience harmful effects at lower levels and are less likely to report problems.

EPIDEMIOLOGY
- Predominant age: 18–25, but all ages affected
- Predominant sex: Male > Female (3:1)

Prevalence
- Lifetime prevalence: 13.6%
- 20% in primary care setting
- 48.2% of 21-year-olds in the US reported binge drinking in 2004.

RISK FACTORS
- Family history
- Depression (40% with comorbid alcohol abuse)
- Anxiety
- Other substance abuse
- Tobacco
- Male gender
- Low socioeconomic status
- Unemployment
- Peer/social approval
- Family dysfunction or childhood trauma
- Posttraumatic stress disorder
- Antisocial personality disorder
- Bipolar disorder
- Eating disorders
- Criminal involvement

Genetics
50–60% of risk is genetic.

GENERAL PREVENTION
Counsel with family history and risk factors

PATHOPHYSIOLOGY
Alcohol is a central nervous system depressant, facilitating γ-aminobutyric acid (GABA) inhibition and blocking N-methyl-d-aspartate receptors.

ETIOLOGY
Multifactorial: Genetic, environment, psychosocial

COMMONLY ASSOCIATED CONDITIONS
- Cardiomyopathy
- Atrial fibrillation
- Hypertension
- Peptic ulcer disease/gastritis
- Cirrhosis
- Fatty liver
- Cholelithiasis
- Hepatitis
- Diabetes mellitus
- Pancreatitis
- Malnutrition
- Upper gastrointestinal (GI) malignancies
- Peripheral neuropathy
- Seizures
- Abuse
- Violence
- Trauma (falls, motor vehicle accidents [MVAs])
- Severe psychiatric disorders (depression, bipolar, schizophrenia): >50% of patients with these disorders have a comorbid substance abuse problem.

DIAGNOSIS

HISTORY
- Behavioral issues:
  - Anxiety, depression, insomnia
  - Psychological and social dysfunction, marital problems
  - Social isolation/withdrawal
  - Domestic violence
  - Alcohol-related legal problems
  - Repeated attempts to stop/reduce
  - Loss of interest in nondrinking activities
  - Employment problems (tardiness, absenteeism, decreased productivity, interpersonal problems, frequent job loss)
  - Blackouts
  - Complaints about alcohol-related behavior
  - Frequent trauma, MVAs, emergency department visits
- Physical symptoms:
  - Anorexia
  - Nausea, vomiting
  - Abdominal pain
  - Palpitations
  - Headache
  - Impotence
  - Menstrual irregularities
  - Infertility

PHYSICAL EXAM
- Physical exam may be completely normal
- General: Fever, agitation, diaphoresis
- Head/eyes/ears/nose/throat: Plethoric face, rhinophyma, poor oral hygiene, oropharyngeal malignancies
- Cardiovascular: Hypertension, dilated cardiomyopathy, tachycardia
- Respiratory: Aspiration pneumonia
- GI: Stigmata of chronic liver disease, peptic ulcer disease, pancreatitis, esophageal malignancies, esophageal varices
- Genitourinary: Testicular atrophy
- Musculoskeletal: Poorly healed fractures, myopathy, osteopenia, bone marrow suppression
- Neurologic: Tremors, cognitive deficits (e.g., memor[y] impairment), peripheral neuropathy, Wernicke-Korsakoff syndrome
- Endocrine/metabolic: Hyperlipidemias, cushingoid appearance, gynecomastia
- Dermatologic: Burns (e.g., cigarettes), bruises, poor hygiene, palmar erythema, spider telangiectasias, caput medusa, jaundice

DIAGNOSTIC TESTS & INTERPRETATION
- CAGE Questionnaire: (Cut down, Annoyed, Guilty, and Eye opener): More than 2 "yes" answers is 74–89% sensitive, 79–95% specific for alcohol use disorder; less sensitive for white women, college students, elderly. Not an appropriate tool for less severe forms of alcohol abuse (1)[A].
- Alcohol Use Disorders Identification Test: 10 items, if >4: 70–92% sensitive (2)[A]
- Single Question for Screening: "How many times in the last year have you had X or more drinks in one day" (X = 5 for men, 4 for women); sensitive screen for unhealthy alcohol use; 81.8% sensitive, 79% specific for alcohol use disorders (3)

ab

- Blood alcohol concentration:
  - >100 mg/dL in outpatient setting
  - >150 mg/dL without obvious signs of intoxication
  - >300 mg/dL at any time
- Serum levels increased in chronic abuse:
  - AST/ALT ratio >2.0
  - γ-Glutamyl transferase (GGT)
  - Carbohydrate-deficient transferrin
  - Elevated mean corpuscular volume
  - Prothrombin time
  - Uric acid
  - Triglycerides
  - Cholesterol (total)
- Often decreased:
  - Calcium, magnesium, potassium, phosphorus
  - Blood urea nitrogen
  - Hemoglobin, hematocrit
  - Platelet count
  - Serum protein, albumin
  - Thiamine, folate

naging

- Radiograph: Multiple old rib fractures
- Computed tomography scan, magnetic resonance imaging of brain: Cortical atrophy, lesions in thalamic nucleus and basal forebrain
- Abdominal ultrasound: Ascites, periportal fibrosis, fatty infiltration, inflammation

athological Findings

- Liver: Inflammation or fatty infiltration (alcoholic hepatitis), periportal fibrosis (alcoholic cirrhosis occurs in only 10–20% of alcoholics)
- Gastric mucosa: Inflammation, ulceration
- Pancreas: Inflammation, liquefaction necrosis
- Heart: Dilated cardiomyopathy
- Immune system: Decreased granulocytes
- Endocrine organs: Elevated cortisol levels, testicular atrophy, decreased female hormones
- Brain: Cortical atrophy, enlarged ventricles

IFFERENTIAL DIAGNOSIS

- Other substance use disorders
- Depression
- Dementia
- Cerebellar ataxia
- Cerebrovascular accident (CVA)
- Benign essential tremor
- Seizure disorder
- Hypoglycemia
- Diabetic ketoacidosis
- Viral hepatitis

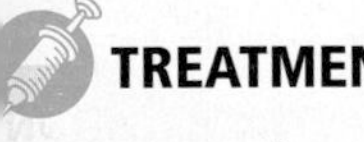

TREATMENT

or management of acute withdrawal, please see lcohol Withdrawal.

IEDICATION

irst Line

- Adjuncts to withdrawal regimens:
  - Naltrexone 50–100 mg/d p.o. or 380 mg IM once every 4 weeks: Opiate antagonist reduces craving and likelihood of relapse (IM route may enhance compliance and thus efficacy) (4,5)[A]
  - Acamprosate (Campral) 666 mg p.o. t.i.d. beginning after completion of withdrawal; reduces relapse risk (4)[A]
  - Topiramate (Topamax) 25–300 mg/d p.o. or divided b.i.d.; enhances abstinence (4)[B]
- Supplements to all:
  - Thiamine 100 mg/d (1st dose IV prior to glucose to avoid Wernicke encephalopathy)
  - Folic acid 1 mg/d
  - Multivitamin daily
- Contraindications:
  - Naltrexone: Pregnancy, acute hepatitis, hepatic failure
  - Monitor liver function tests.
- Precautions: Organic pain, organic brain syndromes
- Significant possible interactions: Alcohol, sedatives, hypnotics, naltrexone, and narcotics

ALERT
Treat acute symptoms if in alcohol withdrawal.

Second Line

- Disulfiram 250–500 mg/d p.o.: Unproven efficacy; may provide psychologic deterrent
- Selective serotonin reuptake inhibitors may be beneficial if comorbid depression exists.

ADDITIONAL TREATMENT

General Measures

- Brief interventions by primary care clinicians are effective for problem drinking (6)[A].
- Involve family, if feasible.
- Treat comorbid problems (sleep, anxiety, etc.); use caution if prescribing medications with cross-tolerance to alcohol (benzodiazepine).
- Group programs and/or 12-step programs may have benefit in helping patients accept treatment.

Issues for Referral

Addiction specialist, 12-step or long-term program, psychiatrist

IN-PATIENT CONSIDERATIONS

Assess medical and psychiatric condition.

Initial Stabilization

- Correct electrolyte imbalances, acidosis, hypovolemia (treat if in alcohol withdrawal)
- Thiamine 100 mg IM, followed by orally 100 mg, and folic acid 1 mg/day
- Benzodiazepines used to lower risk of alcohol withdrawal, seizures

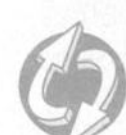

ONGOING CARE

FOLLOW-UP RECOMMENDATIONS

Patient Monitoring

- Outpatient detoxification: Daily visits
- Early outpatient rehabilitation: Weekly visits
- Detoxification alone is not sufficient.

PATIENT EDUCATION

- American Council on Alcoholism: (800) 527-5344 or http://www.aca-usa.org (treatment facility locator, educational information)
- National Clearinghouse for Alcohol and Drug Information: (800) 729-6686 or http://www.health.org
- Center for Substance Abuse Treatment: (800) 662-HELP or http://www.csat.samhsa.gov
- Alcoholics Anonymous: http://www.aa.org
- Rational Recovery: http://www.rational.org
- Secular Organizations for Sobriety: www.cfiwest.org/sos/index.htm
- http://www.alcoholanswers.org/list: An evidence-based Web site for those seeking credible information on alcohol dependence and online support forums.

PROGNOSIS

- Chronic relapsing disease; mortality rate > twice general population, death 10–15 years earlier
- Abstinence benefits survival, mental health, family, employment
- 12-step programs, cognitive behavior, and motivational therapies are effective during 1st year following treatment (2)[B].

COMPLICATIONS

- Cirrhosis (women sooner than men)
- GI malignancies
- Neuropathy
- Dementia
- Wernicke-Korsakoff syndrome
- CVA
- Ketoacidosis
- Infection
- Adult respiratory distress syndrome
- Depression
- Suicide
- Trauma

REFERENCES

1. Dhalla S, Kopec JA. The CAGE questionnaire for alcohol misuse: a review of reliability and validity studies. *Clin Invest Med*. 2007;30:33–41.
2. Enoch MA, et al. Problem drinking and alcoholism: Diagnosis and treatment. *Am Fam Phys* 2002;65: 441–8.
3. Smith PC, Schmidt SM, Allensworth-Davies D et al. Primary Care Validation of a Single Question Alcohol Screening Test. *J Gen Intern Med*. 2009;
4. Williams SH. Medications for treating alcohol dependence. *Am Fam Phys*. 2005;72(pt 9): 1775–80.
5. Pettinati HM, Gastfriend DR, Dong Q et al. Effect of Extended Release Naltrexone (XR-NTX) on Quality of Life in Alcohol-Dependent Patients. *Alcohol Clin Exp Res*. 2008.
6. Asplund CA, Aaronson JW, Aaronson HE. 3 regimens for alcohol withdrawal and detoxification. *J Fam Pract*. 2004;53:545–54.

ADDITIONAL READING

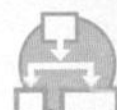

See Also (Topic, Algorithm, Electronic Media Element)

Substance Use Disorders; Alcohol Withdrawal

CODES

ICD9

- 303.90 Other and unspecified alcohol dependence, unspecified drinking behavior
- 305.00 Nondependent alcohol abuse, unspecified drinking behavior

CLINICAL PEARLS

Clinicians should avoid assumptions and adopt an "addiction-oriented" practice style, asking a few basic questions regarding substance use of all patients.

ALCOHOL WITHDRAWAL

Ryan Dono, MD
Erik J. Garcia, MD

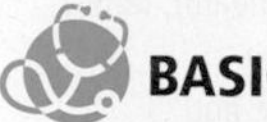

BASICS

DESCRIPTION

Alcohol withdrawal syndrome (AWS) is a spectrum of symptoms that results from abrupt cessation of alcohol in a dependent patient. Symptoms can begin within 5 hours of last drink and persist for 5–10 days, ranging in severity.

EPIDEMIOLOGY

Each year, 8.2 million Americans meet diagnostic criteria for alcohol dependence. It is more prevalent among men, whites, Native Americans, younger and unmarried adults, and those with lower socioeconomic status. Only 24.1% of those with alcohol dependence are ever treated.

RISK FACTORS

- Older age
- High tolerance, prolonged use, high quantities
- Previous alcohol withdrawal episodes, detoxifications, alcohol withdrawal seizures, and delirium tremens
- Symptoms of withdrawal in the presence of high blood alcohol level
- Serious medical problems
- Concomitant benzodiazepine dependence

Geriatric Considerations

- Geriatric populations dependent on alcohol are more susceptible to symptoms of alcohol withdrawal and often have chronic comorbid conditions placing them at higher risk of complications from withdrawal.

Pregnancy Considerations

- Hospitalization or inpatient detoxification is usually required for medical treatment and monitoring of acute alcohol withdrawal.

Genetics

There is some evidence for a genetic basis of alcohol dependence.

GENERAL PREVENTION

- The US Preventative Services Task Force recommends routine screening for alcohol misuse for all adults (1)[B].
- Screening for alcohol abuse during the office visit and appropriate follow-up with the CAGE or similar questionnaire:
  - Feeling the need to **C**ut down
  - **A**nnoyed by criticism about alcohol use
  - **G**uilt about drinking/behaviors while intoxicated
  - "**E**ye opener" to quell withdrawal symptoms
  - Useful to detect problematic alcohol use, positive screen is $\geq$2 "yes" responses
- 10-question AUDIT screening test is also useful to identify problem drinking.

PATHOPHYSIOLOGY

- Consumption of alcohol potentiates the effect of the inhibitory neurotransmitter GABA. With chronic alcohol ingestion, this repeated stimulation down-regulates the inhibitory effects of GABA.
- Concurrently, alcohol ingestion inhibits the stimulatory effect of glutamate on the central nervous system with chronic alcohol use up-regulating excitatory NMDA glutamate receptors.
- When alcohol is abruptly stopped, the combined effect of a down-regulated inhibitory neurotransmitter system (GABA-modulated) and up-regulated excitatory neurotransmitter system (glutamate-modulated)—no longer suppressed by alcohol—results in brain hyperexcitability; clinically seen as AWS.

COMMONLY ASSOCIATED CONDITIONS

- General: Poor nutrition, hyponatremia, hypomagnesemia, hypokalemia, low thiamine, dehydration
- Gastrointestinal: Hepatitis, cirrhosis, varices, GI bleed
- Heme: Splenomegaly, thrombocytopenia, macrocytic anemia
- Cardiovascular: Cardiomyopathy, hypertension, atrial fibrillation, other arrhythmias
- CNS: Trauma, seizure disorder, generalized atrophy, Wernicke-Korsakoff syndrome
- PNS: Neuropathy, myopathy
- Psychiatric: Depression, posttraumatic stress disorder, bipolar disease, polysubstance abuse

DIAGNOSIS

- The *Diagnostic and Statistical Manual (4th ed. - TR)* can be used to assess symptoms of AWS. AWS may be diagnosed when $\geq$2 of the following symptoms present within a few hours to several days after the cessation or reduction of heavy and prolonged alcohol ingestion:
  - Autonomic hyperactivity (sweating, tachycardia)
  - Increased hand tremor
  - Insomnia
  - Psychomotor agitation
  - Anxiety
  - Nausea
  - Vomiting
  - Grand mal seizures
  - Transient (visual, auditory, or tactile) hallucinations or illusions
  - These should cause clinically significant distress or impair functioning and not be secondary to an underlying medical condition or mental disorder.
  - There are 3 stages to AWS.
- Stage 1 (Minor withdrawal; onset 5–8 hours after cessation):
  - Mild anxiety, restlessness, and agitation
  - Mild nausea/GI upset and decreased appetite
  - Sleep disturbance
  - Sweating
  - Mild tremulousness
  - Fluctuating tachycardia and hypertension
- Stage 2 (Major withdrawal; onset 24–72 hours after cessation):
  - Marked restlessness and agitation
  - Moderate tremulousness with constant eye movements
  - Diaphoresis
  - Nausea, vomiting, diarrhea, anorexia
  - Marked tachycardia and hypertension
  - Alcoholic hallucinosis (auditory, tactile, or visual); may have mild confusion but can be reoriented
- Stage 3 (Delirium tremens; onset 72–96 hours after cessation):
  - Fever
  - Severe hypertension, tachycardia
  - Delirium
  - Drenching sweats
  - Marked tremors
- Alcohol withdrawal– associated seizures are often brief, generalized tonic-clonic seizures and can occ 6–48 hours after last drink.

HISTORY

Essential historical information should be:

- Duration and quantity of alcohol intake
- Time since last drink
- Previous episodes/symptoms of alcohol withdrawa
- Prior detox admissions
- Concurrent substance use
- Pre-existing medical and psychiatric conditions
- Prior seizure activity
- Social history: Living situation, social support, stressors, triggers, etc.

PHYSICAL EXAM

Should include assessment of conditions likely to complicate or that are exacerbated by AWS:

- Cardiovascular: Arrhythmias, congestive heart failure, coronary artery disease
- Gastrointestinal: GI bleed, liver disease, pancreatiti
- Neuro: Oculomotor dysfunction, gait ataxia, neuropathy
- Psych: Orientation, memory
- General: Hand tremor, infections

DIAGNOSTIC TESTS & INTERPRETATION

Lab

Initial lab tests

- Blood alcohol level
- Urine drug screen
- Complete blood count (CBC)
- Electrolytes
- Blood glucose
- Magnesium
- Liver function tests
- Renal function tests

Imaging

Initial approach

Low threshold for CNS imaging in any patient with acute mental status changes, given high incidence of traumatic brain injury.

DIFFERENTIAL DIAGNOSIS

- Cocaine, amphetamine intoxication
- Neuroleptic malignant syndrome
- Anticholinergic drug toxicity
- Liver failure
- CNS infection or hemorrhage
- Opioid withdrawal
- Mania, psychosis
- Thyroid crisis (2)[C]

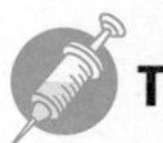

TREATMENT

- The goal of treatment is to reduce the likelihood of adverse clinically significant events (i.e., seizures, DTs, cardiovascular events). This is done mainly wit benzodiazepines that reduce withdrawal intensity and raise the seizure threshold.
  - Medical and psychiatric causes, along with withdrawal from other psychotropic substances, must be excluded first.
  - The patient should be provided a quiet, protective environment.

- The Clinical Institute Withdrawal Assessment for Alcohol Scale, Revised (CIWA-Ar) is useful for determining medication dosing and frequency of evaluation for AWS. The CIWA-Ar scale numerically rates the severity of 10 symptoms on a scale from 1–7, 1 being without the symptom and 7 the max score.

The 10 symptoms in the CIWA-Ar scale are:
- Nausea and vomiting
- Tremor
- Paroxysmal sweats
- Anxiety
- Agitation
- Tactile disturbances
- Auditory disturbances
- Visual disturbances
- Headache or fullness in head
- Orientation and clouding of sensorium

Frequent reevaluation with CIWA-Ar is crucial.

EDICATION

rst Line

Benzodiazepine (BZD) monotherapy remains the treatment of choice, and has been found to be effective against placebo (3)[A]:
- Long-acting BZDs (e.g., diazepam, chlordiazepoxide) are more effective at preventing seizures and delirium.
- Short-acting BZDs (e.g., lorazepam, oxazepam) preferable when severe hepatic insufficiency may impair metabolism; also preferable in elderly to limit oversedation (4)[A]

BZD amounts will vary from patient to patient. Medication can be given in symptom-triggered or fixed-schedule regimens. Symptom-triggered regimens have been found to require less BZD amounts and reduce hospitalization times, but require persistent observation (4)[A].

Example symptom-triggered regimen: Start with chlordiazepoxide 50–100 mg IV, repeat CIWA-Ar every hour and if score is ≥8, give additional dose of chlordiazepoxide 50 mg IV. Continue to reevaluate with CIWA-Ar hourly until adequate sedation achieved (score <8). May substitute chlordiazepoxide with respective doses of diazepam, lorazepam, or oxazepam (4)[C].

econd Line

β-blockers (e.g., atenolol) and $\alpha 2$ agonists (e.g., clonidine) help to control hypertension and tachycardia, and can be used in conjunction with BZDs (2)[C]. These should not be used as a monotherapy, due to their inability to prevent DTs and seizures.

Antiepileptic agents such as carbamazepine (Tegretol) have not shown clear benefit over BZDs (5)[B].

Thiamine 100 mg/d for at least 3 days:
- Note that IV glucose administered before treatment with thiamine may precipitate Wernicke's encephalopathy.

If patient exhibits significant agitation and alcoholic hallucinosis, an antipsychotic (haloperidol) can be used, but this requires close observation, as it lowers the seizure threshold (2)[C].

DDITIONAL TREATMENT

dditional Therapies

eripheral neuropathy and cerebellar dysfunction merit ıysical therapy evaluation.

IN-PATIENT CONSIDERATIONS

- Individuals in stages 1 and 2 of alcohol withdrawal can be treated safely in the outpatient setting unless medical comorbidities require inpatient observation. However, a reliable and supportive social environment should be in place with frequent, consistent follow-up.
- Individuals in or approaching stage 3 should always be treated as inpatients.

Admission Criteria

- CIWA score >15, or severe withdrawal
- Concurrent acute or chronic illness requiring inpatient treatment and monitoring
- Poor ability to follow up or no reliable social support
- Pregnancy
- Seizure disorder or history of severe alcohol-related seizures
- Suicide risk
- Concurrent benzodiazepine dependence
- High risk for severe withdrawal or delirium tremens
- >40 years old
- Prolonged heavy drinking >8 years
- Consumes >1 pint of alcohol or 12 beers per day
- Random blood alcohol level >200 mg/dL
- Elevated MCV, blood urea nitrogen
- Cirrhosis, liver failure

IV Fluids

IV hydration is required in withdrawal due to losses from autonomic hyperactivity.

Discharge Criteria

CIWA scores of <10 on 3 consecutive determinations

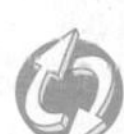

ONGOING CARE

FOLLOW-UP RECOMMENDATIONS

Arrangements for aftercare include discharge to a treatment facility (i.e., sober house or residential program), outpatient substance abuse counseling, peer support groups (Alcoholics Anonymous), the use of adjuvant treatment such as acamprosate (Campral), naltrexone (ReVia, Depade, Vivitrol), or topiramate (Topamax).

Patient Monitoring

Frequent patient follow-up is recommended to monitor for relapse.

PATIENT EDUCATION

- Alcoholics Anonymous at www.aa.org
- SMART Recovery (Self-Management and Recovery Training) at www.smartrecovery.org (not spiritually based)
- National Institute on Alcohol Abuse and Alcoholism at www.niaaa.nih.gov
- FamilyDoctor.Org: Alcoholism (Spanish resources available)

PROGNOSIS

Current mortality from severe withdrawal (delirium tremens) is 1–5%.

COMPLICATIONS

Complications may occur more frequently in individuals who have prior episodes of withdrawal or concomitant illnesses.

REFERENCES

1. Rockville MD. Screening and Behavioral Counseling Interventions in Primary Care to Reduce Alcohol Misuse, Topic Page USPSTF April 2004.
2. Bayard M, et al. Alcohol withdrawal syndrome. *Am Fam Phys*. 2004;69:1443.
3. Ntais C, Pakos E, Kyzas P, Ioannidis JP et al. Benzodiazepines for alcohol withdrawal. *Cochrane Database Syst Rev*. 2005;CD005063.
4. Mayo-Smith MF. Pharmacological Management of Alcohol Withdrawal: A Meta-Analysis and Evidence-Based Practice Guideline. *JAMA* 1997;278:144–151.
5. Polycarpou A, Papanikolaou P, Ioannidis JP et al. Anticonvulsants for alcohol withdrawal. *Cochrane Database Syst Rev*. 2005;CD005064.

ADDITIONAL READING

- Blondell RD. Ambulatory detoxification of patients with alcohol dependence. *Am Fam Phys*. 2005;71: 495–502, 509–10.
- Daeppen JB, Gache P, Landry U et al. Symptom-triggered vs fixed-schedule doses of benzodiazepine for alcohol withdrawal: a randomized treatment trial. *Arch Intern Med*. 2002;162:1117–21.
- Kosten TR, O'Connor PG. Management of drug and alcohol withdrawal. *N Engl J Med*. 2003;348: 1786–95.
- Lohr RH. Treatment of alcohol withdrawal in hospitalized patients. *Mayo Clin Proc*. 1995;70: 777–82.
- Mayo-Smith MF, Beecher LH, Fischer TL et al. Management of alcohol withdrawal delirium. An evidence-based practice guideline. *Arch Intern Med*. 2004;164:1405–12.
- Reoux JP, Miller K. Routine hospital alcohol detoxification practice compared to symptom triggered management with an Objective Withdrawal Scale (CIWA-Ar). *Am J Addict*. 2000;9:135–44.

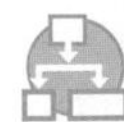

See Also (Topic, Algorithm, Electronic Media Element)

Substance Use Disorders

CODES

ICD9

- 291.0 Alcohol withdrawal delirium
- 291.81 Alcohol withdrawal
- 303.90 Other and unspecified alcohol dependence, unspecified drinking behavior

CLINICAL PEARLS

- Kindling phenomenon: Postulated that long-term exposure to alcohol affects neurons resulting in increased alcohol craving and progressively worse withdrawal episodes
- The CIWA-Ar is a useful tool for managing symptoms and treatment of alcohol withdrawal.
- Be sure to administer thiamine before patient receives glucose, so as not to precipitate Wernicke's encephalopathy.
- Frequent outpatient follow-up is recommended to monitor for relapse.

ALDOSTERONISM, PRIMARY

Amara Lai, MD

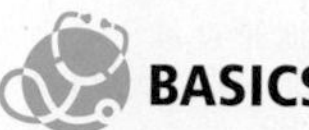

BASICS

DESCRIPTION

- Aldosterone secretion independent of the renin-angiotensin system, usually caused by:
  - a unilateral aldosterone-producing adenoma, treated with unilateral adrenalectomy, *or*
  - bilateral adrenal hyperplasia, treated with aldosterone antagonists
- Clinically manifested by hypertension, hypokalemia, normal or mildly elevated sodium, and metabolic alkalosis
- Systems affected: Endocrine/Metabolic
- Synonyms: Conn syndrome, hyperaldosteronism, aldosteronoma

Pregnancy Considerations

Can be associated with toxemia during pregnancy or persistent HTN following delivery. Treat HTN with agents safe during pregnancy; avoid spironolactone and ACE inhibitors.

EPIDEMIOLOGY

Prevalence

- Uncommon in the general population
- Approximately 5–10% of hypertensive patients
- 11.3% prevalence reported in a study of patients with resistant hypertension (1)
  - Resistant hypertension was defined as blood pressure >140/90 mm Hg despite 3 antihypertensive agents, including a diuretic.
- 14% prevalence reported in a study of patients with both type 2 diabetes and resistant hypertension (2)
  - Resistant hypertension was defined as blood pressure >140/90 mm Hg despite ≥3 antihypertensive agents.

RISK FACTORS

Genetics

Familial hyperaldosteronism is categorized as either glucocorticoid-remediable (autosomal dominant) or type II, and it is a rare finding.

PATHOPHYSIOLOGY

- Aldosterone secretion independent of renin-angiotensin stimulation
- Negative feedback loop suppresses renin.
- Increased aldosterone results in retention of sodium and excretion of potassium and hydrogen ions in the distal renal tubules.

ETIOLOGY

- Aldosterone-producing adenoma, APA (85% unilateral, <5% bilateral)
- Idiopathic bilateral adrenal hyperplasia (10–40%)
- Less common causes include unilateral hyperplasia, aldosterone-producing adrenocortical carcinoma, aldosterone-producing ovarian tumor, or familial hyperaldosteronism including glucocorticoid-remediable hyperaldosteronism.

COMMONLY ASSOCIATED CONDITIONS

Hypertension, especially treatment-resistant or severe

DIAGNOSIS

HISTORY

- Usually asymptomatic
- Can be associated with headaches, muscle weakness, fatigue, cramping, polyuria (hypokalemic nephropathy), nocturia, polydipsia, paresthesias, or tetany

PHYSICAL EXAM

- Hypertension
- Edema (uncommon)
- Fundoscopy: Benign or grade 1–2 hypertensive retinopathy
- Forceful and sustained apical impulse consistent with left ventricular hypertrophy, or cardiac arrhythmias (complications of primary aldosteronism)

DIAGNOSTIC TESTS & INTERPRETATION

Lab

- Patients should be screened for primary aldosteronism with laboratory testing if they are at higher risk (3)[C].
- Higher risk is variably defined as:
  - Hypertension (BP >140/90) resistant to treatment with 3 antihypertensive agents
  - Hypertension with hypokalemia
  - Hypertension in the presence of an adrenal incidentaloma
  - Hypertension that meets Joint National Commission criteria as stage 2 (BP >160/100)

Initial lab tests

- Serum aldosterone and plasma renin activity to determine the aldosterone-renin ratio (ARR) is recommended (3)[C], but no consensus cutoff value has been established at the time of this writing.
  - ARR values are affected by posture, time of day, and acute salt loading.
  - In one study, morning values obtained after 30 minutes in the seated position, in the absence of salt loading, suggest a cutoff value of 23.6 (using conventional units of ng/dL and ng/ml°h), which conveys a sensitivity of 96.8 [95% CI 83.2–99.5], specificity of 94.1 [95% CI 71.2–99.0], and positive LR of 16.45) (4)[B].
  - It is suggested that the most sensitive testing is performed in the morning, after 2 hours of upright posture, and being seated for 5–15 minutes, on patients with unrestricted dietary salt intake before testing, and the most commonly used cutoff with this method is 30 (using conventional units of ng/dL and ng/ml°h) (3)[C].
- Basic metabolic panel to determine serum sodium, potassium, chloride, and bicarbonate levels
  - Sodium may be high-normal or elevated.
  - Hypokalemia, although "classic," may be present in a minority of patients.
    - Reported as low as 9–37% (5)
  - Chloride-resistant metabolic alkalosis
- Urine analysis may reveal dilute urine.
- Urine potassium may demonstrate inappropriate kaliuresis, usually >30 mmol/L.

ALERT

Lab results may be altered by malignant HTN or certain drugs, such as diuretics, ACE inhibitors, and aldosterone antagonists.

Follow-Up & Special Considerations

- Patients with a positive ARR screen should underg confirmatory testing with one of the following (3)[C]:
  - Oral sodium loading test
    - Sodium intake of >200 mmol per day (~6 g p day) for 3 days
    - 24-hour urine aldosterone is measured from th morning of day 3 to the morning of day 4
    - Elevated urinary aldosterone (>12 mcg per 24 hours) make primary aldosteronism highly likely
    - Notes and precautions: Patients should receive adequate slow-release KCl supplementation to maintain plasma potassium in the normal rang This test should not be performed in patients with severe uncontrolled HTN, renal insufficiency, cardiac insufficiency, cardiac arrhythmia, or severe hypokalemia. There are currently two methods available for measuring the urinary aldosterone, with the HPLC-tandem mass spectrometry preferred over the RIA.
  - Saline infusion test
  - Fludrocortisone suppression test
  - Captopril challenge test
- Confirmed cases should then undergo CT scan and adrenal vein sampling (AVS) for subtype classification (3)[C].

Imaging

Initial approach

Adrenal CT with fine cuts for subtype testing and to exclude large masses that may represent adrenocortical carcinoma (3)[C]

Diagnostic Procedures/Surgery

Adrenal vein sampling should be performed to lateralize an aldosteronoma (6)[A],(7)[B].

- Post-ACTH stimulation values are the most accurate measurement for AVS lateralization (7)[B].

Pathological Findings

- Aldosteronoma usually solitary, benign
- Bilateral adrenal (zona glomerulosa) hyperplasia
- Aldosterone-producing adrenocortical carcinoma, rare

DIFFERENTIAL DIAGNOSIS

- Diuretic use
- Renovascular HTN
- Malignant HTN
- Pheochromocytoma
- Dexamethasone-suppressible hyperaldosteronism
- Congenital adrenal hyperplasia
- High-dose glucocorticoid therapy
- Exogenous mineralocorticoid
- Bartter syndrome
- Licorice (glycyrrhizinic acid) ingestion
- Edema secondary to other conditions (CHF, nephrotic syndrome, liver failure)

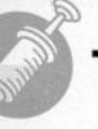

TREATMENT

Treat hypertension and electrolyte abnormalities, particularly hypokalemia, if present.
Unilateral laparoscopic adrenalectomy is the definitive treatment for patients with documented unilateral APA or hyperplasia.
Medical management with aldosterone antagonists is the treatment of choice for bilateral hyperplasia.

IEDICATION

irst Line

dosterone antagonist: spironolactone (Aldactone), eplerenone (Inspra) as an alternative

econd Line

Other potassium-sparing diuretics: amiloride (Midamor) or triamterene (Dyrenium)
Antihypertensive agents: Calcium channel antagonist, ACE inhibitor, angiotensin-II receptor antagonist, beta-blocker, or low-dose thiazide diuretic
Contraindications: Potassium-sparing agent and ACE inhibitors in renal failure, hyperkalemia, and pregnancy
Precautions: Monitor serum potassium closely after any adjustment in potassium replacement or potassium-sparing agent
Significant possible interactions: Lithium with diuretics, NSAIDs with diuretics, and ACE inhibitors with diuretics

DDITIONAL TREATMENT

sues for Referral

Endocrinology for confirmatory testing of an ARR suggestive of primary aldosteronism
Interventional radiology to perform AVS
General surgery to perform unilateral laparoscopic adrenalectomy in patients with confirmed unilateral APA or hyperplasia

URGERY/OTHER PROCEDURES

ne treatment of choice for patients with unilateral PA or hyperplasia is laparoscopic adrenalectomy.

N-PATIENT CONSIDERATIONS

nitial Stabilization

ontrol of any HTN

dmission Criteria

Hypertensive urgency/emergency
Refractory HTN
Severe hypokalemia
Cardiovascular events

V Fluids

s needed

Nursing

areful monitoring of BP

Discharge Criteria

Vhen hemodynamically stable

ONGOING CARE

FOLLOW-UP RECOMMENDATIONS

Follow BP and potassium

Patient Monitoring

- BP checks
- Serum potassium check
- 24-hour urine aldosterone following surgery

DIET

Low-sodium, high-potassium

PATIENT EDUCATION

- HTN teaching
- Medication management

PROGNOSIS

- Hypertension and hypokalemia can usually be controlled by doses of 25 to 100 mg spironolactone every 8 hours.
  - Chronic therapy in men may be limited by side effects of gynecomastia, decreased libido, and impotence.
- Surgical adrenalectomy resulted in hypertension cure or improvement in 77% of patients with unilateral adenoma (8).
- There is no further increased risk of complications of primary aldosteronism (see below) after treatment with either surgery or medical management (9,10).

COMPLICATIONS

- Increased GFR and albuminuria in untreated primary aldosteronism compared with essential hypertension (9)
- Increased prevalence of cardiovascular events in untreated primary aldosteronism compared with essential hypertension (35% vs 11%, OR 4.61) (10)[B]
- Left ventricular hypertrophy
- Cardiac arrhythmias if hypokalemia is severe

REFERENCES

1. Douma S, et al. Prevalence of primary hyperaldosteronism in resistent hypertension: a retrospective observational study. *Lancet*. 2008; 371:1921–1926.
2. Umpierrez GE, et al. Primary aldosteronism in diabetic subjects with resistant hypertension. *Diabetes Care*. 2007;30(7):1699.
3. Funder JW, et al. Case Detection, Diagnosis, and Treatment of Patients with Primary Aldosteronism: An Endocrine Society Clinical Practice Guideline. *J Clin Endocrinol Metab*. 2008;93(9):3266–3281.
4. Sau-Cheung Tiu et al. The Use of Aldosterone-Renin Ratio as a Diagnostic Test for Primary Hyperaldosteronism and Its Test Characteristics under Different Conditions of Blood Sampling. *J Clin Endorinol Metab*. 2005; 90(1):72–78.
5. Mulatero P, et al. Increased diagnosis of primary aldosteronism, including surgically correctable forms, in centers from 5 continents. *J Clin Endocrinol Metab*. 2004;89:045.
6. Kempers et al. Systematic Review: Diagnostic Procedures to Differentiate Unilateral from Bilateral Adrenal Abnormality in Primary Aldosteronism. *Ann Intern Med*. 2009;151(5): 329–337.
7. Mathur A, et al. Consequences of Adrenal Venous Sampling in Primary Hyperaldosteronism and Predictors of Unilateral Adrenal Disease. *Journal of the American College of Surgeons*. 2010.
8. Letavernier E, et al. Blood Pressure Outcome of Adrenalectomy in Patients with Primary Hyperaldosteronism with or without Unilateral Adenoma. *J Hypertens*. 2009;27(3):656–657.
9. Sechi LA, et al. Long-term renal outcomes in patients with primary aldosteronism. *JAMA*. 2006;295(22):2638–2645.
10. Catena C, et al. Cardiovascular outcomes in patients with primary aldosteronism after treatment. *Arch Intern Med*. 2008;168(1):80–85.

ADDITIONAL READING

Mansmann G, Lau J, Balk E et al. The clinically inapparent adrenal mass: update in diagnosis and management. *Endocr Rev*. 2004;25:309–40.

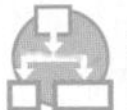

See Also (Topic, Algorithm, Electronic Media Element)

Algorithm: Aldosteronism

CODES

ICD9

255.10 Hyperaldosteronism, unspecified

CLINICAL PEARLS

- Patients with drug-resistant HTN, HTN plus hypokalemia, HTN plus adrenal incidentaloma, or stage 2 HTN are at increased risk for primary aldosteronism.
- Patients at increased risk should have testing with serum aldosterone and plasma renin activity, and the ARR should be calculated.
- Suggestive ARR values (in general, at least 20–30 in conventional units) should be referred for confirmatory testing.
- Confirmed primary aldosteronism warrants an adrenal CT and AVS for lateralization.
- Unilateral adrenalectomy is the treatment of choice for unilateral APA or hyperplasia; spironolactone for the treatment of bilateral hyperplasia.

ALOPECIA

Ann M. Rodden, DO, MS

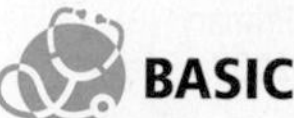

BASICS

DESCRIPTION

- Alopecia: Absence of hair from any areas where it normally exists:
  - Anagen hairs: Growing hairs
  - Telogen hairs: Dead, "resting" hairs
- Androgenic alopecia (male- or female-pattern hair loss): Hair loss along with miniaturization of hair follicles:
  - In men: Frontal recession, then vertex affected; over time, only has lateral and occipital hair
  - In women: Thinning across the crown, with frontal hair initially in place but later may be lost
- Alopecia areata: Patchy, nonscarring hair loss:
  - Alopecia totalis: Hair loss of the entire scalp
  - Alopecia universalis: Loss of all body hair
- Telogen effluvium: Diffuse hair loss that (usually) results in temporarily decreased hair density but not complete baldness:
  - Abnormal hair cycling leads to excessive loss of hairs in telogen phase.
  - Usually occurs 3 months after the trigger occurs
- Anagen effluvium: Diffuse shedding of hairs, including growing hairs, that may progress to complete baldness:
  - Growth arrest of hair in anagen phase and sheds
  - Begins days to weeks after inciting incident
- Cicatricial alopecia (scarring alopecia): Slick, smooth scalp without any evidence of follicular openings for hair
- Traction alopecia: Patchy, initially nonscarring hair loss usually due to physical stressors on hair:
  - Trichotillomania: Hair loss due to the person pulling hair out
- Tinea capitis: Patches of hair broken off close to the scalp, with or without associated inflammation, caused by fungal infection

Pediatric Considerations

Tinea capitis is more common among children.

Pregnancy Considerations

Telogen gravidarum: Hair loss 2 to 4 months after childbirth

EPIDEMIOLOGY

- Age:
  - Androgenic alopecia: May begin after puberty and increases in prevalence over time
- Predominant sex: Male > Female

Incidence

Alopecia areata: 0.1–0.2% incidence in all races

Prevalence

- Androgenic alopecia:
  - Men: 15% of adolescent males:
    - 50% of white men over 50 years old
  - Women: 6% under age of 50:
    - 38% of postmenopausal women
- Alopecia areata:
  - 1.7% of US population

RISK FACTORS

- Physiologic or psychologic stress
- Pregnancy
- Poor nutrition
- Use of certain medications/chemotherapy
- Tight living quarters
- Sharing hair products/supplies

Genetics

- Family history of early hair loss
- Polygenic inheritance of androgenic alopecia

GENERAL PREVENTION

- For traction alopecia: Minimize braids, coloring, bleaching, waving of hair, or hair styles that pull hair.
- For tinea capitis: Avoid sharing hats, combs, hairbrushes, hair ornaments, and pillows.

PATHOPHYSIOLOGY

- All hair follicles pass through stages of anagen and telogen.
- When many are in the telogen phase at one time, the hair loss becomes noticeable.
- Activity of hair follicles may diminish due to trauma, medications, or disease.

ETIOLOGY

- Androgenic alopecia:
  - Genetically predisposed
  - Polycystic ovarian syndrome
  - Adrenal hyperplasia
  - Pituitary hyperplasia
  - Drugs (testosterone, progesterone, danazol, adrenocorticosteroids, anabolic steroids)
- Alopecia areata (autoimmune process):
  - Autoimmune thyroiditis
- Telogen effluvium:
  - In most cases, no specific etiology is found.
  - Postpartum
  - Adding or changing medications (oral contraceptives, anticoagulants, anticonvulsants, selective serotonin reuptake inhibitors, retinoids, β-blockers, angiotensin-converting enzyme inhibitors, colchicine, cholesterol-lowering medications, cimetidine, levodopa, bromocriptine, chemotherapeutic agents, interferon, others)
  - Stress: Physical (fever, trauma, surgery) or psychologic
  - Chronic illness (systemic lupus erythematosus [SLE], syphilis, systemic amyloidosis, hepatic failure, chronic renal failure, inflammatory bowel disease, dermatomyositis, human immunodeficiency virus, lymphoproliferative disorders)
  - Hormonal (hypo/hyperthyroid, pituitary dysfunction)
  - Malnutrition (iron deficiency, zinc deficiency, caloric restriction/eating disorder)
  - Malabsorption (celiac disease, pancreatic disease)
  - Inflammatory skin disorders (psoriasis, seborrheic dermatitis, allergic contact dermatitis)
- Anagen effluvium:
  - Chemotherapy is most common trigger
  - Radiation to the area
  - Drugs (chemotherapeutic agents, allopurinol, colchicine)
  - Poisoning (mercury, thallium, bismuth, arsenic, gold, boric acid)
  - Severe protein malnutrition
- Cicatricial alopecia:
  - Physical agents/trauma (burns, freezing, radiation)
  - Congenital (aplasia cutis congenital, Conradi-Hunermann chondropysplasia punctata)
  - Lymphocytic (central centrifugal cicatricial alopecia, cutaneous discoid lupus erythematous, lichen planopilaris)
  - Neutrophilic (folliculitis decalvans, dissecting folliculitis)
  - Acne keloidosis
  - Infection (zoster, kerion, folliculitis)
  - Metastatic or primary neoplasm
- Traction alopecia:
  - Trichotillomania (direct self-pulling of the hair, obsessive-compulsive behavior)
  - Tight rollers or braids
- Tinea capitis (*Microsporum, Trichophyton*)

COMMONLY ASSOCIATED CONDITIONS

Alopecia areata:

- Down syndrome
- Autoimmune thyroiditis
- Vitiligo
- Diabetes

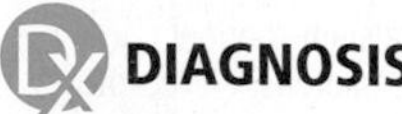

DIAGNOSIS

HISTORY

- Duration of hair loss
- Episodic or continuous
- Pattern of hair loss
- Medications
- Chronic disease, recent illness, surgeries, pregnancy
- Changes in health/medication in past 2–3 months
- Psychological stress
- Dietary history and weight changes
- Menstrual history
- Family history of hair loss or autoimmune disorders
- Radiation or exposure to heavy metals
- Pruritus (in tinea capitis)

PHYSICAL EXAM

- Pattern of hair loss:
  - Is hair loss generalized or local?
  - If local, is it symmetrical at the vertex and/or the hairline at the forehead?
- Scalp scaling, inflammation (in tinea capitis)
- Changes in the hair:
  - Hair-pull test: Pinch 25–50 hairs between thumb and forefinger, and exert slow, gentle traction while sliding fingers up:
    - Normal: 1–2 dislodge
    - Abnormal: ≥6 hairs dislodged (in effluvium, alopecia areata)
  - Broken hairs (tinea capitis, traction alopecia)
  - Broken-off hair at the borders of the patch that are easily removable (in alopecia areata)
  - Hair loss in circular pattern (in alopecia areata, tinea capitis)
- Clinical signs of thyroid disease, lupus, or other diseases
- Clinical signs of virilization: Acne, hirsutism, acanthosis nigrans, truncal obesity (in androgenic alopecia)

DIAGNOSTIC TESTS & INTERPRETATION

Lab

- Thyroid-stimulating hormone and free thyroxine (fT_4) (hypo- or hyperthyroidism)
- Complete blood count (anemia)
- Comprehensive metabolic panel (liver and renal disease)
- Free testosterone and dehydroepiandrosterone sulfate (hyperandrogenism)
- Serum ferritin and total iron-binding capacity (iron deficiency)

Serum zinc (deficiency)
Rapid plasma reagin test (syphilis)
Prolactin (pituitary hyperplasia)
ANA (SLE)

iagnostic Procedures/Surgery

Light hair-pull test:
- Pull on 25–50 hairs and ≥6 hairs dislodge is consistent with shedding (effluvium, alopecia areata)

Direct microscopic exam of the hair shaft:
- Anagen hairs: Elongated and possibly pigmented bulb with gelatinous root sheath
- Exclamation point hairs: At periphery of lesion and has club-shaped root with thinner proximal shaft that distally becomes normal in size (alopecia areata)

Daily hair counts: Collect hair in dated envelopes:
- More than 100 hairs per day is consistent with effluvium

Ultraviolet light fluorescence and potassium hydroxide prep (to rule out tinea capitis)

athological Findings

alp biopsy with routine microscopy will aid in the agnosis.

IFFERENTIAL DIAGNOSIS

earch for type of alopecia and then for reversible uses.

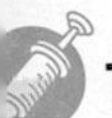

TREATMENT

IEDICATION

Androgenic alopecia:
- Minoxidil (Rogaine) 2% topical solution (1 mL b.i.d.) for women, 5% topical solution (1 ml b.i.d.) or foam (daily) for men (1)[A]
- Finasteride (Propecia), 1 mg/day p.o. for men (1)[A]
- Spironolactone (Aldactone) 100–200 mg/day in women who are hyperandrogenic (off-label) (1)[C]:
  - Diuretic with antiandrogen action
- Oral contraception pills with low levels of androgenic affect in women (Yasmin, Ortho-TriCyclen, Ortho-Cyclen, Ortho-Evra, Mircette) (off-label) (2)[C]
- Ketoconazole 2% shampoo with minoxidil 2% (1)[C]

Alopecia areata:
- Intralesional steroids: triamcinolone 2.5–10 mg/mL (3,4)[C]
  - First line in adults if <50% scalp involved
  - Repeat every 4–6 weeks
  - 0.5-inch, 30-gauge needle and inject 0.1 mL at each point at 1-cm intervals
  - If no improvement in 6 months, stop treatment
- If >50% scalp involved, refer to dermatologist (3)
- Topical midpotent corticosteroids for children (3)[C]
- Systemic glucocorticoids: May induce regrowth, but alopecia recurs after cessation of medication and risks may outweigh benefits for long-term use (3,4)[C]

Telogen effluvium: Remove offending medication (5)[C].

Tinea capitis: See appropriate section on tinea.

Side effects/precautions:
- Topical minoxidil:
  - Irritant dermatitis or contact allergic dermatitis
  - Hypertrichosis
  - Exacerbation of angina (rare)
- Intralesional steroids:
  - Local burning/stinging/pruritis/skin atrophy
- Spironolactone:
  - Menstrual cycle abnormalities
  - Postural hypotension
  - Electrolyte imbalance (hyperkalemia)
- Finasteride:
  - Caution in known liver disease
  - Sexual side effects
  - Monitor prostate-specific antigen (PSA): Will decrease PSA level by 50%

Pregnancy Considerations

Finasteride not indicated for use in women; pregnancy Category X. Women should not handle crushed or broken pills during childbearing years.

ADDITIONAL TREATMENT

General Measures

- Trial off medication that may have triggered the hair loss may resolve issue. If unsure it was the medication, may repeat trial with medication to determine if hair loss occurs again (if patient is willing).
- Traction alopecia:
  - Only with discontinuation of the hair pulling will the disorder resolve.
  - Psychologic or psychiatric intervention may be necessary.
  - Successful therapeutic approaches have included medications, behavior modification, and hypnosis.

COMPLEMENTARY AND ALTERNATIVE MEDICINE

Androgenic alopecia:
- Low-energy laser light: HairMax LaserComb (1)[C]: Safe alternative, but lacking research

SURGERY/OTHER PROCEDURES

- Hair transplantation
- Wigs/hairpieces
- Androgenic alopecia:
  - Surgical (hair transplantation, scalp reduction, transposition flap, and soft tissue expansion)
  - Medical tattooing of eyebrows
- Cicatricial alopecia:
  - The only effective treatment is surgical (graft transplantation, flap transplantation, or excision of the scarred area).

ONGOING CARE

DIET

If nutritional deficit noted, supplementation may be necessary.

PATIENT EDUCATION

National Alopecia Areata Foundation: www.naaf.org

PROGNOSIS

- Androgenic alopecia:
  - Prognosis depends on treatment
- Alopecia areata:
  - Usually regrows within 1 year even without treatment
  - Recurrence common
  - 10% have severe, chronic form
- Telogen effluvium:
  - Maximum shedding 3 months after the inciting event (medication, stress, nutritional deficiency) and recovery following correction of the cause
  - Usually subsides in 3–6 months
  - Rarely permanent baldness
  - Chronic effluvium uncommon
- Anagen effluvium:
  - Shedding begins days to a few weeks after the inciting event, with recovery following correction of the cause.
  - Rarely permanent baldness
- Cicatricial alopecia:
  - Hair follicles permanently damaged
- Traction alopecia:
  - Depends on behavior modification
- Tinea capitis:
  - Usually complete recovery

REFERENCES

1. Rogers NE, Avram MR. Medical treatments for male and female pattern hair loss. *J Am Acad Dermatol*. 2008;59:547–66; quiz 567–8.
2. Goh C, Zippin JH et al. Androgenetic alopecia: diagnosis and treatment with a focus on recent genetic implications. *J Drugs Dermatol*. 2009;8: 185–92.
3. Alkhalifah A, Alsantali A, Wang E, McElwee KJ, Shapiro J et al. Alopecia areata update: part II. Treatment. *J Am Acad Dermatol*. 2010;62:-
4. Mounsey AL, Reed SW et al. Diagnosing and treating hair loss. *Am Fam Physician*. 2009;80: 356–62.
5. Harrison S, Bergfeld W. Diffuse hair loss: its triggers and management. *Cleve Clin J Med*. 2009;76: 361–7.

ADDITIONAL READING

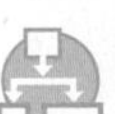

See Also (Topic, Algorithm, Electronic Media Element)

Tinea (Capitis, Corporis, Cruris); Syphilis; Systemic Lupus Erythematosus; Polycystic Ovarian Syndrome; Lichen Planus; Hyperthyroidism
Algorithm: Alopecia

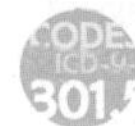

CODES

ICD9

- 704.00 Alopecia, unspecified
- 704.01 Alopecia areata
- 704.02 Telogen effluvium

CLINICAL PEARLS

- History and physical examination findings will usually determine type of alopecia.
- Treatment of underlying medical condition or removal of triggering medication in many types of alopecia will reinstate hair growth without the need of further interventions.
- Educating the patient about the nature of the condition and expectations is key to patient care.

ALTITUDE ILLNESS

Robert J. Hyde, MD

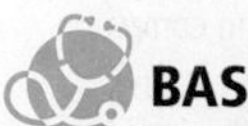

BASICS

DESCRIPTION

Altitude illness is a spectrum of medical problems ranging from mild discomfort to fatal illness that may occur on ascent to higher altitude [elevations >1,500 m (4,921 feet)]. It is divided into 3 categories: High, 1,500–3,500 m; very high, 3,500–5,500 m; and extreme, 5,500–8,850 m (1). It can affect anyone, including the most experienced and fit individual. For most, it is an unpleasant but self-limiting syndrome that will not require physician intervention.

- Acute mountain sickness (AMS): Symptoms associated with a physiologic response to a hypobaric, hypoxic environment. Onset occurs within 24 hours of arrival at altitude, often within 1–4 hours. Neurologic symptoms are predominant and range from mild-to-moderate headache and malaise to severe impairment.
- High-altitude pulmonary edema (HAPE): Noncardiogenic pulmonary edema. Onset 1–4 days at altitude. Rare <8,000 feet (2,438 m).
- High-altitude cerebral edema (HACE): A potentially fatal neurologic syndrome; considered the end stage of AMS. Onset within 3–5 days at elevation as low as 9,022 feet (2,750 m), but may be more abrupt at higher altitudes. Death results from brain herniation.
- System(s) affected: Nervous/Pulmonary
- Synonym(s): Mountain sickness

Geriatric Considerations

- Risk does not increase with age.
- Age alone should not preclude travel to high altitude; allow extra time to acclimate.
- Preexisting medical problems made worse are referred to as altitude-exacerbated conditions.

Pediatric Considerations

- Altitude illness seems to have the same incidence in children as in adults, but diagnosis may be delayed in younger children.
- Any child who experiences behavioral symptoms after recent ascent should be presumed to be suffering from altitude illness.

Pregnancy Considerations

- The risk during pregnancy is unknown.
- No evidence that exposure to high altitude (1,500–3,500 m) poses a risk to a pregnancy
- It may be prudent to advise a low-altitude dwelling for any pregnant woman experiencing complications.

EPIDEMIOLOGY

Most epidemiologic studies are limited to relatively homogenous populations of men.

Incidence

- AMS: 10–90% globally
- HAPE/HACE: 0.01–1% of sojourner ascents at typical mountain resorts, although incidence increases with rapid and higher ascents (2).

RISK FACTORS

- Rapid rate of ascent
- Maximum altitude attained
- Increased duration at high altitude
- Failure to acclimatize at lower altitude
- Higher altitude during sleep cycle
- Prior history of altitude illness
- Cardiac congenital abnormalities

GENERAL PREVENTION

- General guidelines:
  - Preacclimatization affords some protection against altitude illness.
  - Staged or graded ascent (rest every 600–1,200 m) and a slow ascent rate (maximum 600 m/d) should allow adequate time for acclimatization.
  - Sleeping elevation: "Climb high and sleep low" is a prudent practice for anyone going above 3,500 m.
  - Avoid heavy exertion for the 1st 1–3 days.
  - Avoid respiratory depressants such as alcohol and soporifics.
  - Preascent physical conditioning is not preventive.
- Drug prophylaxis:
  - Acetazolamide and dexamethasone (see below)
  - For HAPE only:
    - Consider nifedipine and beta agonists (see Treatment section).

PATHOPHYSIOLOGY

- Not completely understood
- Hypobaric hypoxia and hypoxemia are the pathophysiologic precursors to altitude illness.
- Symptoms of AMS may be the result of cerebral swelling, either through vasodilatation induced by hypoxia or through cerebral edema.
- Other mechanisms include impaired cerebral autoregulation, release of vasogenic mediators, and alteration of the blood–brain barrier.
- HAPE is a noncardiogenic pulmonary edema characterized by exaggerated pulmonary hypertension leading to vascular leakage through overperfusion, stress failure, or both.

ETIOLOGY

Individuals with a prior episode of HAPE have an increased risk of recurrence (3).

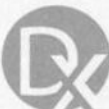

DIAGNOSIS

HISTORY

- AMS, mild-to-moderate symptoms:
  - Headache, plus at least 1 of the following:
    - Anorexia
    - Nausea or vomiting
    - Dizziness or lightheadedness
    - Insomnia
- AMS, severe symptoms:
  - Increased headache
  - Irritability
  - Marked fatigue
  - Dyspnea with exertion
  - Nausea and vomiting
  - HAPE (Lake Louise diagnostic criteria):
    - At least 2 of the following symptoms: Dyspnea at rest, cough, weakness, decreased exercise performance, chest tightness, congestion
    - AND at least 2 of the following signs: Crackles or wheezing in at least 1 lung field, central cyanosis, tachycardia, tachypnea. (Note: Fatigue may be pulmonary edema.)
  - HACE symptoms: Mental status changes (irrational behavior, lethargy, obtundation, coma)

PHYSICAL EXAM

- HAPE:
  - Lung crackles or wheezing
  - Central cyanosis
  - Tachycardia
  - Tachypnea
- HACE:
  - Abnormal mental status exam (behavioral change, lethargy, obtundation, coma)
  - Truncal ataxia
  - Papilledema, retinal hemorrhage, cranial nerve palsies
  - Focal neurologic deficits (rare)

DIAGNOSTIC TESTS & INTERPRETATION

Electrocardiogram may show sinus tachycardia or right-sided heart strain.

Lab

- AMS: Laboratory studies are nonspecific and rarely required for diagnosis.
- HAPE: Severe hypoxemia demonstrated with oximetry or blood gas analysis.

Imaging

No radiographic feature is specific to HAPE.

DIFFERENTIAL DIAGNOSIS

Onset of symptoms >3 days at a given altitude, the absence of headache, or the lack of rapid response to oxygen or descent suggest other diagnoses.

AMS/HACE:
- Subarachnoid hemorrhage, central nervous system (CNS) mass, cerebrovascular accident
- Migraine headache
- Dehydration
- Ingestion of toxins, drugs, or alcohol
- Carbon monoxide exposure
- CNS infection
- Acute psychosis

HAPE:
- Pneumonia
- Cardiogenic pulmonary edema
- Spontaneous pneumothorax
- Pulmonary embolism
- Asthma
- Bronchitis
- Myocardial infarction
- Hyperventilation syndrome

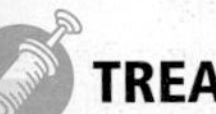

TREATMENT

MEDICATION

First Line

Oxygen: 2–15 L/min to maintain SaO_2 >90% until symptoms improve

Acetazolamide: (If patient has a history of problems at altitude and/or plans to ascend >500 m/d). Dosage is usually 125–500 mg p.o. b.i.d. starting 2 days before ascent and continued for 3 days at maximum altitude. Patients with a drug allergy to sulfonamides should avoid acetazolamide.
- Prevention of AMS: 125–500 mg p.o. b.i.d. starting 1 day before ascent and continued for 2 days at maximum altitude
- Treatment of AMS: 125–500 mg p.o. b.i.d. until symptoms resolve

Dexamethasone: May significantly reduce the incidence and severity of AMS. Dosage is 2–4 mg p.o. q6h, begun the day of ascent, continued for 3 days at the higher altitude, and then tapered over 5 days. Adverse side effects are rare:
- Prevention of AMS: 2 mg p.o. q6h or 4 mg p.o. q12h, starting 1 day before ascent and discontinued cautiously after 2 days at maximum altitude
- Treatment of AMS: 4 mg p.o./IV/IM q6h
- Treatment of HACE: 8 mg p.o./IV/IM initially, then 4 mg q6h

Nifedipine (reduces pulmonary arterial pressure):
- Prevention of HAPE: 20–30 mg extended-release p.o. b.i.d. starting 1 day prior to ascent and continued for 2 days at maximum altitude
- Treatment of HAPE: 10 mg, then 20–30 mg extended-release p.o. b.i.d.

Salmeterol:
- Prevention and possible treatment of HAPE: 125 μg inhaled b.i.d. starting 1 day before ascent and continued for 2 days at maximum altitude

Nonsteroidal anti-inflammatory drugs:
- Prevention and treatment of headache
- Aspirin 325 mg p.o. q4h for total 3 doses
- Ibuprofen 400–600 mg p.o.
- Prevention of AMS: Dose unknown. Begin 1–5 days before ascent.

- Antiemetics:
  - Prochlorperazine 10 mg p.o./IM q6–8h
  - Promethazine 25–50 mg p.o./IM/p.r. q6h

Second Line

Furosemide: Consider for treatment of AMS or HACE, 20–80 mg p.o./IV q12h for a total of 2 doses. Currently out of favor; not recommended for prophylaxis; not established for use in HAPE.

ADDITIONAL TREATMENT

General Measures

- Therapy must be tailored to fit disease severity.
- Early recognition is critical.
- Stop ascent, acclimatize at the same altitude, and/or descend if symptoms do not improve over 24 hours. Definitive treatment is to descend to a lower altitude. Dramatic improvement accompanies even modest reductions in altitude.
- Oxygen helps relieve symptoms. Give continuously by cannula or mask initially, and then titrate to SaO_2 >90%.
- AMS:
  - Acetazolamide is effective in reducing mild-to-moderate symptoms of AMS, but the optimum dosage is unknown. Consider 125–500 mg p.o. b.i.d. until symptoms resolve.
  - Dexamethasone may also be effective in treating moderate AMS. Consider 4 mg p.o./IM/IV q6h
  - Analgesics and antiemetics as needed for symptomatic relief
- HAPE:
  - Oxygen therapy
  - Minimize exertion and keep patient warm.
  - Immediate descent or evacuation to a lower altitude
  - Portable hyperbaric therapy (2–15 psi), such as the Gamow bag or Chamberlite, is an effective and practical alternative when descent is not possible.
  - Consider nifedipine 10 mg p.o., then 20–30 mg extended-release p.o. b.i.d.
- HACE:
  - Immediate descent
  - Supplemental oxygen (highest flow available; maintain SaO_2 >90%)
  - Dexamethasone 8 mg IV/IM/p.o. initially, then 4 mg q6h
  - Hyperbaric therapy if unable to descend

IN-PATIENT CONSIDERATIONS

Initial Stabilization

Outpatient treatment for mild cases

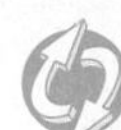

ONGOING CARE

FOLLOW-UP RECOMMENDATIONS

Patient Monitoring

- For mild cases, no follow-up is needed.
- For more severe cases, follow until symptoms subside.

PATIENT EDUCATION

Patients should be counseled about the risks of high-altitude travel and how to recognize high-altitude illnesses.

PROGNOSIS

Most cases of mild-to-moderate AMS are self-limiting and do not require physician intervention. Patients may resume ascent once symptoms subside. HAPE and HACE respond well to descent, evacuation, and/or pharmacologic treatment if identified early.

COMPLICATIONS

Patient may experience high-altitude retinal hemorrhage, which can cause visual changes, but is usually asymptomatic.

REFERENCES

1. Gallagher SA, Hackett PH. High-altitude illness. *Emerg Med Clin North Am*. 2004;22:329–55, viii.
2. Maloney JP, Broeckel U. Epidemiology, risk factors, and genetics of high-altitude-related pulmonary disease. *Clin Chest Med*. 2005;26:395–404, v
3. Basnyat B, Murdoch DR. High-altitude illness. *Lancet*. 2003;361:1967–74.

ADDITIONAL READING

- Barry PW, Pollard AJ. Altitude illness. *BMJ*. 2003;326:915–9.
- Dumont L, Mardirosoff C, Tramèr MR. Efficacy and harm of pharmacological prevention of acute mountain sickness: quantitative systematic review. *BMJ*. 2000;321:267–72.
- Hackett PH, Roach RC. High-altitude illness. *N Engl J Med*. 2001;345:107–14.
- Luks AM, Swenson ER. Medication and dosage considerations in the prophylaxis and treatment of high-altitude illness. *Chest*. 2008;133:744–55.
- Rodway GW, Hoffman LA, Sanders MH. High-altitude-related disorders–Part I: Pathophysiology, differential diagnosis, and treatment. *Heart Lung*. 2003;32:353–9.
- Rodway GW, et al. High altitude -related disorders: Part II. Prevention, special populations and chronic medical conditions. *Heart Lung*. 2003;33(1):3–12.

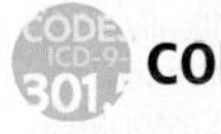

CODES

ICD9

993.2 Other and unspecified effects of high altitude

CLINICAL PEARLS

- Slow ascent and timely descent are important tenets in the prevention and treatment of high-altitude illnesses, respectively.
- High-flow oxygen, followed by oxygen titrated to maintain SaO_2 >90%, is the first-line treatment for all patients with more than mild illness.

ALVEOLAR PULMONARY PROTEINOSIS

Caitlin M. Connolly, MD
Jerry Balikian, MD

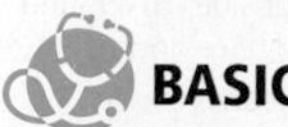

BASICS

DESCRIPTION

- Pulmonary alveolar proteinosis (PAP) is a rare disease characterized by accumulation of lipoproteinaceous (surfactantlike) material in the alveolar spaces, leading to impaired gas exchange. There are 3 recognized categories of PAP (1).
- Congenital PAP (2% of cases):
  - Congenital PAP results from several rare gene mutations (2).
- Secondary PAP (<10% cases):
  - Secondary PAP is associated with environmental exposures, immunodeficiency disorders, and hematologic disorders and malignancies (1).
- Primary or idiopathic PAP (90% of cases):
  - Primary PAP, which is discussed here, has recently been found to be associated with antigranulocyte-macrophage colony-stimulating-factor (GM-CSF) autoantibodies (2).
- Whole lung lavage, the standard treatment for PAP, has improved prognosis (94% 5-year survival) (3).
- Systems affected: Pulmonary

EPIDEMIOLOGY

- Seen worldwide with median age of onset at 39 years old (4)
- 2-3:1 Male:Female incidence; however, may be confounded by greater male smoking, a known association (3)

Incidence

Estimated 0.36 per million annually (5)

Prevalence

Estimated 3.7 per million (5)

RISK FACTORS

- Association between tobacco smoke exposure and primary PAP (3)
- Exposure to environmental dusts, specifically silica, aluminum, cement, titanium dioxide, nitrogen dioxide, and insulation fibers, has been associated with secondary PAP (2).

Genetics

- No genetic predilection in primary or secondary PAP.
- Congenital PAP mostly transmitted in autosomal recessive pattern (1)

Pediatric Considerations

- Congenital PAP leads to neonatal respiratory distress syndrome not responsive to surfactant or corticosteroids. Caused by mutation in surfactant protein B or C genes, or GM-CSF receptor beta or alpha chain abnormalities (2). Lung transplant is primary therapy, but prognosis is poor (1)[C].

GENERAL PREVENTION

No specific measure for prevention; avoid tobacco smoke exposure

PATHOPHYSIOLOGY

Primary PAP has recently been found to be associated with neutralizing anti-GM-CSF autoantibodies causing impaired functioning of alveolar macrophages, resulting in disruption in surfactant homeostasis (6). Surfactant accumulates in alveoli due to reduced clearance.

ETIOLOGY

Primary PAP: Autoimmune

COMMONLY ASSOCIATED CONDITIONS

No conditions commonly associated with primary PAP

DIAGNOSIS

HISTORY

- Diagnosis often delayed due to nonspecific presentation
- Occupational and exposure history to exclude secondary PAP
- Symptoms:
  - Progressive dyspnea with insidious onset (most common presentation)
  - Nonproductive cough (75%):
    - Less common
  - Fatigue
  - Weight loss
  - Low-grade fever (prominent fever should prompt search for complicating infection); hemoptysis or chest pain (<20%)

PHYSICAL EXAM

Often unremarkable:

- Fine crackles (50%)
- Clubbing or cyanosis (<20%)

DIAGNOSTIC TESTS & INTERPRETATION

Lab

Initial lab tests

- Complete blood count, liver and renal function tests to exclude systemic disorders
- Nonspecific:
  - Mild-moderate elevation in serum lactate dehydrogenase (LDH) (82%)
  - Serum levels of carcinoembryonic antigen, cytokeratin 19, and mucin KL-2 can be elevated.
  - Serum levels of surfactant protein-A, -B, and -D can be elevated.
  - Assay for anti-GM-CSF antibodies available at some centers (not commercially available) (2)

Follow-Up & Special Considerations

Serial serum LDH level can correlate with disease activity.

Imaging

Initial approach

- Chest x-ray: Bilateral, symmetric, central lung opacities (often appears worse than clinical symptoms)
- Chest computed tomography (CT): "Crazy-paving patchy ground-glass opacities with network of thickened reticular lines in a geographic pattern (7) is characteristic of PAP but not specific.

Follow-Up & Special Considerations

Posttheraputic brachioalveolar lavage (see Treatmen CT shows ground-glass opacities resolve, but thickened septal lines can persist (7).

Diagnostic Procedures/Surgery

Pulmonary function tests:

- Severe reduction of carbon monoxide diffusing capacity
- Restrictive ventilatory defect
- Arterial blood gas: Hypoxemia
- Bronchoalveolar lavage: Milky fluid with large, foamy alveolar macrophages and large, acellular eosinophilic bodies that stain with periodic acid-Schiff

Pathological Findings

Open-lung biopsy is gold standard for diagnosis, but not always required. Can have false negative due to mosaic pattern leading to sampling error (6)[C]:

- Normal alveolar architecture. Alveoli filled with granular, eosinophilic material that stains with periodic acid-Schiff (6)[C].

DIFFERENTIAL DIAGNOSIS

Primary PAP is diagnosis of exclusion; must exclude causes of secondary PAP:

- Differential for material in alveolar space includes pneumonia, cardiogenic pulmonary edema, acute respiratory distress syndrome, sarcoidosis, alveolar hemorrhage, hypersensitivity pneumonitis, bronchiolitis obliterans organizing pneumonia, bronchoalveolar carcinoma

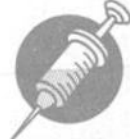

TREATMENT

MEDICATION

No specific medication

First Line

- Whole lung lavage is the standard treatment for symptomatic PAP; however, there are no randomized controlled trials on any treatment for PAP yet available (2)[C]:
  - Whole lung lavage is performed under general anesthesia with a dual-lumen endotracheal tube while ventilating the other lung.
  - Large volumes of saline are flushed until returnin fluid becomes clear.

– About 70% of patients with PAP become symptomatic enough to require whole lung lavage within 5 years of diagnosis.
– Most patients experience a return to normal exercise capacity after lavage; however, a subset of patients do not respond for unknown reason.
– Median duration of freedom from symptoms is 15 months, with many patients requiring repeat lavage (2)[C].

Patients with secondary PAP should have underlying disorder treated, or should avoid exposure to inciting environmental agent. Whole lung lavage can also be used for symptomatic secondary PAP (4)[C].

DDITIONAL TREATMENT

'eneral Measures

ıpportive measures such as supplemental oxygen, onchodilators, antibiotics for infection, smoking ıssation, and treatment of concurrent diseases that ıpair respiratory function can improve dyspnea mporarily. Respiratory support should be given when ɔpropriate:

Steroids should be avoided when possible due to interference with surfactant maturation and secretion (1)[C].

Pulmonary rehabilitation may be helpful (1)[C].

ssues for Referral

'atients with symptomatic PAP should be referred to ɛnters performing whole lung lavage, with ıesthesiologists skilled in management of ɔuble-lumen catheters (4)[C].

ıdditional Therapies

linical trials examining the usefulness of GM-CSF ıerapy in treating primary PAP are currently ongoing. ıitial trials appear to show that high doses of kogenous GM-CSF can overcome anti-GM-CSF eutralizing antibodies. Trials are studying dosage ɔutes of subcutaneous injection for a systemic ɔproach vs nebulized treatment for a localized ɔproach. These trials are still in the initial stages, and 'hole lung lavage remains standard therapy (8)[C]:

There is no role for GM-CSF therapy in secondary or congenital PAP, as they are not related to anti-GM-CSF antibodies.

URGERY/OTHER PROCEDURES

.ung transplantation has been used in congenital PAP ınd for PAP that is not responsive to whole lung ıvage (1)[C].

ONGOING CARE

FOLLOW-UP RECOMMENDATIONS

Patient Monitoring

Respiratory infections are a common complication of PAP, especially with atypical organisms such as *Norcardia*. Any sign of infection should lead to thorough search for organism, including bronchial washings and/or bronchoalveolar lavage (1).

PATIENT EDUCATION

The American Lung Association at http://www.lungusa.org/

PROGNOSIS

Prognosis for those who do not undergo whole lung lavage is 85% 5-year survival compared to 94% 5-year survival for those who do undergo therapeutic lavage (4). PAP can result in death from respiratory distress (80%) or infection (20%) (1):

- Congenital PAP has an especially poor prognosis.

COMPLICATIONS

Complications from PAP include respiratory failure and increased susceptibility to infection, especially *Norcardia* species:

- Whole lung lavage complications: Hypoxemia, pneumonia, sepsis, adult respiratory distress syndrome, pneumothorax (1)

REFERENCES

1. Ioachimescu OC, Kavuru MS et al. Pulmonary alveolar proteinosis. *Chron Respir Dis*. 2006;3: 149–59.
2. Huizar I, Kavuru MS et al. Alveolar proteinosis syndrome: pathogenesis, diagnosis, and management. *Curr Opin Pulm Med*. 2009;15: 491–8.
3. Presneill JJ, Nakata K, Inoue Y, Seymour JF et al. Pulmonary alveolar proteinosis. *Clin. Chest Med* 2004;25:593–613, viii.
4. Juvet SC, Hwang D, Waddell TK, Downey GP et al. Rare lung disease II: pulmonary alveolar proteinosis. *Can Respir J*. 2008;15:203–10.
5. Seymour JF, Presneill JJ et al. Pulmonary alveolar proteinosis: progress in the first 44 years. *Am J Respir Crit Care Med*. 2002;166:215–35.
6. Trapnell BC, Whitsett JA, Nakata K et al. Pulmonary alveolar proteinosis. *N Engl J Med*. 2003;349: 2527–39.
7. Frazier AA, Franks TJ, Cooke EO, Mohammed TL, Pugatch RD, Galvin JR et al. From the archives of the AFIP: pulmonary alveolar proteinosis. *Radiographics*. 2008;28:883–99; quiz 915.
8. Greenhill SR, Kotton DN et al. Pulmonary alveolar proteinosis: a bench-to-bedside story of granulocyte-macrophage colony-stimulating factor dysfunction. *Chest*. 2009;136:571–7.

ADDITIONAL READING

- Chung MJ, Lee KS, Franquet T, et al. Metabolic lung disease: imaging and histopathologic findings. *Eur J Radiol*. 2005;54:233–45.
- Wang BM, Stern EJ, Schmidt RA, Pierson DJ, et al. Diagnosing pulmonary alveolar proteinosis. A review and an update. *Chest*. 1997;111:460–6.

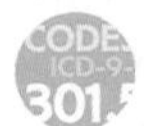

CODES

ICD9

516.0 Pulmonary alveolar proteinosis

CLINICAL PEARLS

- Pulmonary alveolar proteinosis is a rare disease characterized by accumulation of surfactantlike material in the alveolar spaces leading to impaired gas exchange.
- Nonspecific respiratory symptoms and physical exam findings often delay diagnosis.
- Chest CT finding of "crazy paving" is characteristic, but not specific.
- Whole lung lavage is standard therapy for symptomatic patients. 5 year survival is 94% with treatment.

ALZHEIMER DISEASE

Jill A. Grimes, MD
Linda H. Hatch, MD

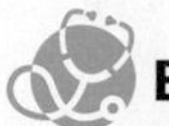

BASICS

DESCRIPTION
- Most common cause of dementia in the elderly
- Degenerative neurologic disease with progressive cognitive and behavioral impairment
- Usual course: Progressive and chronic
- System(s) affected: Nervous
- Synonym(s): Presenile dementia; senile dementia of the Alzheimer type

Geriatric Considerations
Asymptomatic screening is not recommended.

EPIDEMIOLOGY
- Predominant age: >60 years
- Predominant sex: Female > Male (slightly)

Incidence
40% of those >85 years of age are affected, which is 1,100/100,000 population.

Prevalence
5.3 million in US

RISK FACTORS
- Aging
- Low education level
- Down syndrome
- Positive family history
- Inheritance of the E4 allele of apolipoprotein E gene on chromosome 19 (E4 is much less of a risk factor for African Americans and Hispanics)
- Cardiovascular and carotid artery disease
- Smoking (2- to 4-fold increase) (1)

Genetics
Positive family history in 50% of the cases, but 90% of Alzheimer disease (AD) cases are sporadic.

GENERAL PREVENTION
- Studies show that nonsteroidal anti-inflammatory drugs (NSAIDs), estrogen, and vitamin E do NOT delay AD (2)[A].
- Hormone-replacement therapy (HRT) is not recommended (3)[A].
- Intellectual challenge (puzzles) and regular physical exercise may offer preventive benefit.
- Control vascular risks factors (e.g., hypertension). Statins and lowering cholesterol may retard pathogenesis of AD (4)[A].
- Ginkgo biloba may be beneficial in treatment for cognition, but not activities of daily living (5).
- Participation in physical activities and omega-3 fatty acids may help to prevent or delay cognitive decline (6).
- Ultrasound may help to identify asymptomatic patients at increased risk with chronic brain hypoperfusion secondary to cardiovascular or carotid artery pathology (7).

ETIOLOGY
- Unknown, but toxic β-amyloid deposits in neuritic plaques and arterial walls appear critical to pathogenesis.
- β-Amyloid precursor gene localized to chromosome 21

COMMONLY ASSOCIATED CONDITIONS
- Down syndrome
- Depression

DIAGNOSIS

HISTORY
- Include family members in interview (for accuracy and for behavioral assessment)
- Progressive and disruptive memory loss
- Depression, anhedonia, or apathy
- Intellectual decline; difficulty with calculations; multiple missed appointments
- Loss of interest, social withdrawal
- Date or time confusion
- Occupational dysfunction or personality change
- Restlessness and sleep disturbances

PHYSICAL EXAM
- Neurologic exam to rule out other causes
- Folstein Mini Mental Status Exam (MMSE): Copyrighted, but available (http://www.aafp.org/afp/20010215/703.html)
- No focal neurologic signs
- Short-term memory loss
- Acalculia (e.g., cannot balance checkbook)
- Agnosia: Inability to recognize objects
- Apraxia: Inability to carry out movements
- Confabulation
- Delusions
- Impaired abstraction
- Decreased attention to hygiene
- Visuospatial distortion
- Late signs: Psychotic features; mutism

DIAGNOSTIC TESTS & INTERPRETATION
Neuropsychologic testing (if clinical picture is confusing or to help determine level of independence for skills such as balancing checkbooks, driving, or managing medicines)

Lab
To help rule out other causes of dementia

Initial lab tests
- Complete blood count, erythrocyte sedimentation rate
- Chemistry panel
- Thyroid-stimulating hormone
- Folate and B_{12} levels
- VDRL or RPR
- HIV antibody (selected cases)

Follow-Up & Special Considerations

For genetic testing for E4 allele of apolipoprotein, discuss with genetic counselor (2)[A].

Imaging
Initial approach
- Controversy exists; consider MRI or CT scan if:
  - cognitive decline is recent; history of stroke; or focal neurologic signs
- Evidence is not sufficient to include resting electroencephalogram in routine clinical practice (8).

Follow-Up & Special Considerations
- CT scan/MRI: Moderate cortical atrophy, ventricular enlargement
- MRI: Hippocampal volumetry; positron-emission tomography (PET) and single-photon-emission computed tomography not indicated
- Medicare pays for PET to distinguish AD from frontotemporal dementia.

Pathological Findings
- Gross: Diffuse cerebral atrophy in hippocampus, amygdala, and some subcortical nuclei
- Micro:
  - Neuritic senile plaques
  - Neurofibrillary tangles
  - Pyramidal cell loss
  - Decreased cholinergic innervation (other neurotransmitters variably decreased)
  - Degeneration of locus ceruleus and basal forebrain nuclei of Meynert; amyloid angiopathy

DIFFERENTIAL DIAGNOSIS
- Vascular dementia, multi-infarct dementia
- Lewy body disease
- Dementia associated with Parkinson disease
- Normal-pressure hydrocephalus
- Creutzfeldt-Jakob disease
- End-stage multiple sclerosis
- Brain tumor: Primary or metastatic
- Subdural hematoma
- Progressive multifocal leukoencephalopathy
- Metabolic dementia (hypothyroidism)
- Drug reactions, alcoholism, other addictions
- Dementia pugilistica
- Depression
- Toxicity from liver and kidney failure
- Vitamin and other nutritional deficiencies
- Vasculitis
- Neurosyphilis

TREATMENT

MEDICATION
Memory enhancement and slowing progression of disease:

- Cholinesterase inhibitors (9)[A] (Equally effective; all have largely GI side effects):
  - Best in mild to moderate disease (Folstein MMSE scores 10–24); drugs *may* be effective in Lewy body dementia.
  - Donepezil (Aricept): Start at 5 mg p.o. daily; may increase to 10 mg daily after 1 month
    - Comes in tablets or orally disintegrating tabs
    - Generic available
    - Caution with digoxin or beta-blockers (can cause 3* heart block)
    - Aricept 23 mg tablet approved in 2010
  - Rivastigmine (Exelon): Start tabs at 1.5 mg p.o. b.i.d., increase by 1.5 mg b.i.d. every 2 weeks; maintenance 6-12 mg total daily
    - Capsule, solution, or patch (patch greatly reduces side effects)
    - Indicated for both AD and Parkinson dementia
  - Galantamine (Razadyne): Start 4 mg b.i.d. for 4 weeks, then increase by 4 mg b.i.d. every month with goal 16–24 mg daily dose
    - Tablets, solution, and extended release capsule (ER has daily dosing)
- NMDA receptor antagonists (for moderate to sever AD; MMSE 5–14)
  - Monotherapy or in combination with acetylcholinesterase inhibitors
  - Memantine (Namenda): Start at 5 mg daily, with starter pack titrating to target dose of 10 mg b.i. after 4 weeks
  - Often improves behavioral issues

rst Line

- Behavioral techniques and environmental modification help more than medications for wandering, restlessness, uncooperativeness, hoarding, and irritability.
- For depression (occurs in 1/3 of patients), use selective serotonin reuptake inhibitors (SSRIs).
- Insomnia:
  - Trazodone 25–100 mg at bedtime, zolpidem (Ambien) 5 mg at bedtime, zaleplon (Sonata) 5–10 mg at bedtime, ramelteon (Rozerem) 8 mg at bedtime
  - Avoid diphenhydramine in elderly males, which can cause urinary retention.
- Moderate anxiety/restlessness: Consider low-dose, short-acting benzodiazepines, buspirone, or SSRIs, but efficacy unproven.
- Severe aggressive agitation (especially if psychotic features present):
  - Memantine (Namenda) (9)[A]: 1st of new class of NMDA receptor antagonists; can be used as monotherapy or in combination with acetylcholinesterase inhibitors to enhance or preserve memory; shows efficacy in severe disease (Folstein MMSE score 5–14). Start at 5 mg daily, titrating to target dose of 10 mg b.i.d. after 4 weeks. Often improves behavioral issues.
  - Risperidone (Risperdal) 0.25–1.0 mg b.i.d., olanzapine 2.5 mg/d b.i.d.; other newer atypical antipsychotic agents may be preferred owing to fewer side effects (10)[A], but all are likely to increase mortality. Minimize use.
  - Carbamazepine (Tegretol) 100 mg b.i.d.–t.i.d., propranolol (Inderal) 10–40 mg b.i.d.–t.i.d., trazodone 200 mg daily, and valproic acid 250–1,500 mg daily
- Contraindications:
  - Avoid anticholinergic drugs, such as tricyclic antidepressants and antihistamines.
  - Ginkgo biloba: Avoid anticoagulants and aspirin.
- Precautions:
  - Benzodiazepines may produce paradoxical excitation or daytime drowsiness.
  - Triazolam (Halcion) can produce confusion, memory loss, and psychotic behavior.
  - Atypical antipsychotic agents are associated with hyperglycemia, ketoacidosis, increased stroke risk, and increased mortality in elders and dementia patients.
  - Cholinesterase inhibitors provide only modest benefit for 1–2 years, after which decline continues at somewhat lesser rate than placebo. Number needed to treat (NNT) = 7. No deterioration over 6–12 months is evidence of efficacy (9)[A].
- Significant possible interactions:
  - Antipsychotics: Lithium may induce extrapyramidal symptoms, disorientation.
  - Benzodiazepines may increase serum phenytoin concentration; cimetidine may increase benzodiazepine concentration.
  - Donepezil (Aricept): Use with caution with anticholinergic medication or in patients with sick sinus syndrome or a history of peptic ulcers.
  - Paroxetine causes increased donepezil levels.

econd Line

onflicting efficacy for selegiline 5 mg b.i.d., vitamin E 000 mg b.i.d., or NSAIDs in slowing the progression the disease (2)[A].

ADDITIONAL TREATMENT

General Measures

- Outpatient, day care, assisted living, skilled nursing facility
- Optimize treatment of associated comorbidities.
- Analyze environment for safety and security and avoid sudden changes in environment.
- Assess needs of spouse/caregiver.
- Advance directives planning

Issues for Referral

- Assess DRIVING SAFETY (vision, spatial relations, hearing, judgement)
  - http://www.nhtsa.gov/people/injury/olddrive/Driving%20Safely%20Aging%20Web/
- Visiting nurse or social worker
- Physical, occupational, or speech therapist
- Lawyer (living will, power of attorney)
- Support groups for patient and family

Additional Therapies

- Exercise to reduce restlessness
- Continued cognitive challenge

COMPLEMENTARY AND ALTERNATIVE MEDICINE

- Ginkgo biloba extracts (120 mg a day) show conflicting efficacy in treatment of AD but may be beneficial (5).
- Coenzyme Q_{10}, huperzine not effective
- Occupational therapy, music therapy (10)[B], aroma therapy (10)[B], pet therapy (10)[B]

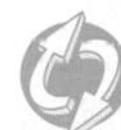

ONGOING CARE

FOLLOW-UP RECOMMENDATIONS

Patient Monitoring

- Schedule regular follow-up (every 3 months) to assess medical complications, provide support for family, and assess need for placement.
- Serial mental status testing is potentially helpful, but bedside tests (Folstein MMSE) offer wide variability and lack of sensitivity.

PATIENT EDUCATION

- Printed patient and family information: Alzheimer Association, 919 N. Michigan Ave., Suite 1000, Chicago, IL; (800) 272-3900; http://www.alz.org/
- Explain progressive nature of the disease and start advance directives planning as early as possible.
- Prenatal testing is available for the *PSEN1* mutation (which causes 30–70% of early-onset familial AD).

PROGNOSIS

Poor: Average survival from diagnosis is 4–6 years (diagnosis is often delayed).

COMPLICATIONS

- Behavioral: Hostility, agitation, wandering, uncooperative
- Metabolic: Infection, dehydration, drug toxicity, malnutrition
- Falls
- "Sundowning" (increase full-spectrum lights in evenings/winter)
- Depression (1/3 of patients)
- Suicide: Especially in early stages

REFERENCES

1. Cataldo JK, Prochaska JJ, Glantz SA, et al. Cigarette smoking is a risk factor for Alzheimer's Disease: an analysis controlling for tobacco industry affiliation. *J Alzheimers Dis*. 2010;19:465–480.
2. Patterson C, Feightner JW, Garcia A et al. Diagnosis and treatment of dementia: 1. Risk assessment and primary prevention of Alzheimer disease. *CMAJ*. 2008;178:548–56.
3. Hogervorst E, et al. Hormone replacement therapy for cognitive function in postmenopausal women. *Cochrane Database Syst Rev*. 2006;4:CD003799.
4. Scott, H Denman. Laake, Knut. Statins for the prevention of Alzheimer's disease and dementia. [Systematic Review] Cochrane Dementia and Cognitive Improvement Group. *Cochrane Database of Systematic Reviews*. 1, 2009.
5. Weinmann S, Roll S, Schwarzbach C, et al. Effects of Ginkgo biloba in dementia: systematic review and meta-analysis. *BMC Geriatr*. 2010;10:14.
6. Daviglus ML, Bell CC, Berrittini W, et al. NIH State-of-the-Science Conference: Preventing Alzheimer's Disease and Cognitive Decline. 2010.
7. de la Torre JC. Vascular risk factor detection and control may prevent Alzheimer's disease. *Ageing Res Rev*. 2010;10.
8. Jelic V, Kowalski J, et al. Evidence-based evaluation of diagnostic accuracy of resting EEG in dementia and mild cognitive impairment. *Clin EEG Neurosci*. 2009;40:129–42.
9. Raina P, Santaguida P, Ismaila A et al. Effectiveness of cholinesterase inhibitors and memantine for treating dementia: evidence review for a clinical practice guideline. *Ann Intern Med*. 2008;148:379–97.
10. Sink KM, Holden KF, Yaffe K. Pharmacological treatment of neuropsychiatric symptoms of dementia: a review of the evidence. *JAMA*. 2005;293:596–608.

See Also (Topic, Algorithm, Electronic Media Element)

Substance Use Disorders; Hypothyroidism, Adult; Depression

CODES

ICD9

- 290.0 Senile dementia, uncomplicated
- 290.10 Presenile dementia, uncomplicated
- 331.0 Alzheimer's disease

CLINICAL PEARLS

- Daily intellectual stimulation, such as puzzles, and moderate physical exercise may help prevent AD.
- Imaging studies have low yield in patients with a history typical of AD.
- Encourage families to join a chapter of the Alzheimer Association and to pursue advanced directive planning early in the course of the disease.
- Atypical antipsychotic medications increase mortality.

AMBLYOPIA

Robert M. Kershner, MD, MS

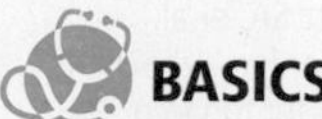

BASICS

DESCRIPTION

A reduction in visual acuity resulting from abnormal visual development in the absence of a structural or pathologic abnormality of the eye, which cannot be corrected by eyeglasses or contact lenses. The lesion is typically unilateral, although it may be bilateral:

- System(s) affected: Nervous
- Synonym(s): Lazy eye

Pediatric Considerations

More commonly seen in the pediatric age group early in life. The mean age at presentation is 3–6 years old.

EPIDEMIOLOGY

- Predominant age: The onset may be present from birth or in early childhood. The condition may go undiagnosed and be detected at any age.
- Predominant gender: Male = Female

Prevalence

~2–2.5% in the general population

RISK FACTORS

Preexisting refractive error, such as myopia, hyperopia, or astigmatism. More common with occlusion of the visual pathway. Conditions that cause anisometropia (refractive difference between the eyes) or obstruction to clear vision, i.e., cataract, corneal abnormalities, can lead to permanent amblyopia.

Genetics

Increased incidence in children with 1 parent with a history of amblyopia

PATHOPHYSIOLOGY

- Strabismic amblyopia is a loss of visual acuity in an individual with misalignment of the visual axis in 1 eye, due to suppression of the images from an eye that turns out or in.
- Anisometropic amblyopia is present when 1 eye has a significantly different refractive error from the fellow eye, leading to visual blurring and suppression of the image from that eye.
- Refractive amblyopia is due to uncorrected high refractive error, resulting in visual blurring in either or both eyes.
- Deprivation amblyopia (amblyopia ex anopsia) is due to relatively complete visual deprivation in 1 eye, which may be caused by a congenital abnormality such as a corneal scar or cataract.
- Deficiency amblyopia is also known as nutritional optic neuropathy or tobacco–alcohol amblyopia. Deficiencies of vitamin B_1 or B_{12} or riboflavin may be responsible.
- Amblyopia can only occur early in life. When the brain detects unequal images, for any reason, it is forced to ignore one. The ability of a brain to suppress the unwanted image can only occur when the development of neuroadaptive responses is in a critical "plastic" period, usually the first several years of life. If amblyopia has not developed after that period has passed, the individual will be unable to "suppress" the unwanted image and diplopia or double vision will result.

ETIOLOGY

Strabismus causes disparate retinal images whereby one eye sees the object of regard in the fovea and the other in a different part of the retina. Inability to fuse the 2 images results in the brain ignoring the less preferred image (this does not necessarily need to be the less clear image). Refractive errors such as anisometropia (a difference in refractive error between the 2 eyes) can cause the 2 retinal images to be of unequal clarity. An obstruction to the visual axis, such as cataracts, also causes unequal clarity of the retinal image. The result of one eye seeing better than the other is the interruption of development of fine visual perception, which can contribute to the development of amblyopia. Individuals with amblyopia do not have normal degrees of stereo vision and often complain of not appreciating 3D images.

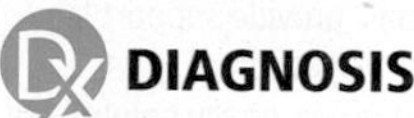

DIAGNOSIS

HISTORY

- Squinting one eye in bright light is the most common symptom, hence the alternative term for strabismus, "squint."
- Rubbing the eyes
- Sitting close to television or computer screen
- Problems in sports
- Preference for front-row seating
- Covering or closing an eye
- Eye turns in or out, wandering eye
- Poor vision in one eye without apparent explanation or a diagnosable organic cause
- Poor vision that does not correct with glasses

PHYSICAL EXAM

- Ophthalmologic exam to screen for unequal refractive error, outward or inward turning of the e (strabismic amblyopia), obstruction to the visual pathway. Vision testing of the eye under monocul conditions can reveal dissimilarities.
- All children should have complete visual exams pr to starting school, with each eye tested individual Children from families with a known history of amblyopia or strabismus should have dilated exam performed by an ophthalmologist.
- The corneal light reflex test (shining a light into th child's eyes and noting the location of the light in relation to the pupil) may be used to assess ocular alignment in young children. An abnormal test should prompt referral to an ophthalmologist.
- When a dilated examination is not possible, evaluation of the "red reflex" such as that seen wi flash photography may indicate an obstruction of vision that would warrant prompt evaluation by ar ophthalmologist.
- Any of the above conditions indicate prompt evaluation and referral. In a young child the earlie the diagnosis, the better the therapeutic outcome. Children with cataract may require cataract surger and unequal refractive errors need to be promptly treated with glasses or contact lenses to improve sight before amblyopia sets in.

DIFFERENTIAL DIAGNOSIS

The diagnosis of amblyopia can be confused with an organic lesion causing decreased visual acuity, and this must always be excluded before the diagnosis o amblyopia is considered. Intraocular tumors, glaucoma, and congenital abnormalities can result ir and be mistaken for amblyopia.

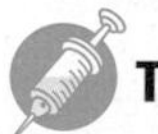

TREATMENT

ADDITIONAL TREATMENT

General Measures

- Correction of the underlying disorder should be instituted promptly as the condition may become irreversible if the child is more than 4–6 years of ag
- Patching of the stronger eye to encourage visual development of the amblyopic eye is warranted. There may be resistance of the child to the wearinc of a patch, which may lessen benefit. Various patching regimens have been studied (from 2–23 hours of patching per day for 4–6 months, and alternate patching). Close follow-up is necessary. Should the "good" eye be patched excessively, the risk of development of amblyopia i that eye increases.
- An alternative therapy to patching is pharmacologi blurring, usually achieved with atropine eye drops. Similar efficacy is achieved compared to patching, with improved compliance. The risk associated wit systemic effects from the antimuscarinic effects of the drug cannot be ignored (1)[A].

- :orrective lenses should be prescribed for refractive rrors.
- :orrection of anatomic obstructions, including ataracts or ptosis, may improve vision and minimize ecurrence.
- ›mblyopia never corrects itself spontaneously and vill always require treatment. Children do not utgrow amblyopia.
-)eficiency amblyopia: Balanced diet, vitamins, and voidance of alcohol and tobacco

:ues for Referral

struction of vision in the infant or toddler is a :ential medical emergency. Failure to refer can result rreversible loss of vision in an otherwise healthy :.

)MPLEMENTARY AND ALTERNATIVE EDICINE

ne. There are no effective homeopathic remedies amblyopia. Vision training can be an effective unct only if the underlying organic causes are dressed and patching therapy instituted.

JRGERY/OTHER PROCEDURES

·gical correction of an abnormal eye position, or ·aocular obstruction may be required.

ONGOING CARE

)LLOW-UP RECOMMENDATIONS

children diagnosed with amblyopia need to be owed for years to prevent recurrence.

tient Monitoring

ce the diagnosis of amblyopia is made, the patient ist be seen frequently until complete resolution of problem occurs.

TIENT EDUCATION

vise all parents to have children's eyes examined or to starting school.

PROGNOSIS

- A treatable condition in most cases if the diagnosis is made early:
  - Patching therapy, pharmacologic blurring, eyeglasses, and surgical correction of abnormal eye positions can result in near-normal vision when instituted early.
  - Visual development occurs during the first several years of life, and amblyopia therapy can be effective until 12 years of age.
- The risk of recurrence is 24% after 1 year; reinstitution of treatment is warranted.

COMPLICATIONS

Failure to institute early therapy may result in permanent unilateral visual loss. Unilateral amblyopia causes an increased risk of severe visual impairment due to loss of vision in the nonamblyopic eye. Psychosocial complications include difficulty in schooling, work, or physical activity, and an increased risk of depression and anxiety.

REFERENCES

1. Kushner BJ. Atropine vs patching for treatment of amblyopia in children. *JAMA*. 2002;287(16): 2145–6.
2. Levi DM, Li RW. Perceptual Learning as a potential treatment for amblyopia: a mini-review. *Vision Res*. 2009.

ADDITIONAL READING

- Li T, Shotton K et al. Conventional occlusion versus pharmacologic penalization for amblyopia. *Cochrane Database Syst Rev*. 2009;CD006460.
- Schmucker C, Grosselfinger R, Riemsma R et al. Diagnostic accuracy of vision screening tests for the detection of amblyopia and its risk factors: a systematic review. *Graefes Arch Clin Exp Ophthalmol*. 2009.
- Schmucker C, Kleijnen J, Grosselfinger R, Riemsma R, Antes G, Lange S, Lagrèze W et al. Effectiveness of early in comparison to late(r) treatment in children with amblyopia or its risk factors: a systematic review. *Ophthalmic Epidemiol*. 2010;17:7–17.
- Teed RG, Bui CM, Morrison DG, Estes RL, Donahue SP et al. Amblyopia therapy in children identified by photoscreening. *Ophthalmology*. 2010;117: 159–62.

See Also (Topic, Algorithm, Electronic Media Element)

Refractive Errors; Strabismus

CODES

ICD9

- 368.00 Amblyopia, unspecified
- 368.01 Strabismic amblyopia
- 368.02 Deprivation amblyopia

CLINICAL PEARLS

- Amblyopia typically presents between the ages of 3 and 6 years, but it needs to be diagnosed earlier if treatment is to be effective. It is never too early to refer if an inequality in visual appearance of the eyes or function is suspected.
- Due to increased incidence in families where there is a history of amblyopia, all related children should be screened by an ophthalmologist.
- Perceptual learning appears to be beneficial in older youth and adults diagnosed late with amblyopia (2)[A].

AMEBIASIS

Najmul H. Siddiqui, MBBS, MD
Naureen B. Rafiq, MBBS, MD

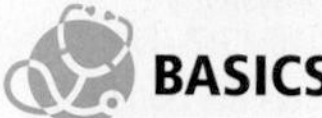

BASICS

DESCRIPTION

- Amebiasis is caused by *Entamoeba histolytica*, an intestinal protozoan found worldwide.
- Most common in developing countries, immigrants from or travelers to endemic regions, those who perform anal sex, and immunocompromised individuals.
- Most infected patients are asymptomatic or have minimal gastrointestinal symptoms (about 90%).
  - Severe infection (i.e., amebic colitis), can occur in very young patients, pregnant women, patients on steroid therapy, and malnourished individuals (1,2).
- Infection is spread by the feco-oral route and caused by the ingestion of *E. histolytica* cysts (infective form) in contaminated food (garden vegetables), fecally contaminated soil, or water. It is then followed by excystation in the terminal ileum or colon to form highly motile trophozoites (invasive form). The trophozoites then encyst and are excreted in the feces or invade the intestinal mucosal barrier and spread hematogenously via the portal circulation to the liver or other distant organs. The excreted cysts reach the environment to complete the cycle.
- Amebiasis is primarily an infection of the colon but extraintestinal (liver, kidney, bladder, skin, lung, brain, male or female genitalia) disease can occur. Amebic liver abscess is the most common complication of invasive amebiasis. It can develop during the acute attack or 1–3 months later.
- May play a substantial role in the clinical initiation and relapses of inflammatory bowel disease (3).
- The genus *Entamoeba* contains many species, including *E. histolytica, E. dispar, E. moshkovskii, E. polecki, E. coli* and *E. hartmanni*. Only *E. histolytica* has been clearly associated with disease; the others are considered nonpathogenic (4).
- System(s) affected: GI; Nervous; Renal/Urologic; Reproductive; Skin/Exocrine
- Synonym(s): Amebic colitis; Amebic dysentery

Geriatric Considerations

More severe in elderly

Pediatric Considerations

More severe in neonates

Pregnancy Considerations

More severe in pregnancy

EPIDEMIOLOGY

- Infection can affect patients of all ages.
- Amebic colitis affects both sexes equally (1).
- Amebic liver abscess incidence greater in men than women for unknown reasons.

Pediatric Considerations

Very young children seem to be predisposed to fulminant colitis.

Prevalence

- The overall prevalence of amebiasis in the United States is approximately 4% and approximately 10% of the world's population.
- Entamoeba infection is as high as 50% in areas of Central and South America, Africa, and Asia.

RISK FACTORS

- Low socioeconomic status
- Institutional living
- Male homosexuality
- Immunocompromised
- Invasive disease is more common in certain geographic locations, including some parts of Mexico, South Africa, and India.

GENERAL PREVENTION

- Eradication of fecal contamination of food and water through improved sanitation, hygiene, and water treatment.
- Individuals traveling to endemic areas should be advised on proper food and water handling. Water should be boiled for more than 1 minute and uncooked vegetables washed with a detergent soap or soaked in acetic acid or vinegar for 10–15 minutes before consumption.
- Avoiding sexual practices that involve fecal–oral contact with potential contamination of infective cysts
- Treatment of patients and close contacts, since reinfection is common
- Amebiasis does not confer lifelong immunity and thus individuals with previous infection are as susceptible to reinfection as other members of the population (2).

PATHOPHYSIOLOGY

- Invasion to the colonic mucosa is mediated by a galactose/N-acetylgalactosamine (GAL/GalNAc)-specific lectin, able to activate lytic and apoptotic pathways, and direct inhibition of the complement system by the trophozoite.
- Extraintestinal disease can result from hepatobiliary and/or hematogenous spread.

ETIOLOGY

Infection results from ingestion of *E. histolytica* cysts in contaminated food, water, or by direct fecal–oral transmission.

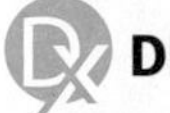

DIAGNOSIS

HISTORY

- Noninvasive infection (symptoms are often nonspecific):
  - Asymptomatic
  - Mild diarrhea
  - Abdominal discomfort
- Invasive infection (amebic colitis):
  - Gradual onset of bloody diarrhea
  - Abdominal pain
  - Fever (10–30%)
  - Weight loss and anorexia
  - Fulminant colitis with severe bloody diarrhea, worsening abdominal pain with peritonitis and fever. Risk factors include malnutrition, pregnancy, steroid use, and very young age.
- Extraintestinal infection:
  - Amebic liver abscess:
    - Fever (up to 90%), right upper quadrant (RUC pain <10 days duration
    - Subacute presentation is associated with mild fever, weight loss, and anorexia
    - Cough can occur. Jaundice not common.
    - Up to 70% can present without colitis.
    - Symptoms may start years after exposure.
  - Pleuropulmonary amebiasis: Pleuritic chest pain cough, and respiratory distress after rupture of amebic liver abscess through the diaphragm
  - Cerebral amebiasis: Headache, nausea, vomitin and rapid mental status change with rapid progression

PHYSICAL EXAM

- Amebic colitis:
  - Diffuse abdominal tenderness (12–85%)
  - Fever (10–30%)
  - Weight loss (40%)
  - Heme-positive stools (70–100%)
- Amebic liver abscess:
  - Fever (85–90%)
  - RUQ tenderness (85–90%)
  - Hepatomegaly (30–50%)
  - Weight loss (30–50%)

DIAGNOSTIC TESTS & INTERPRETATIO

Lab

Initial lab tests

- Microscopic stool examination for trophozoites fro a single sample is only 33–50% sensitive. Serial stool sampling $\times$ 3 in no more than 10 days increa detection to 85–95% but with poor specificity as cannot differentiate *E. histolytica* from nonpathogenic *E. dispar* and *E. moshkovskii* (1).
- ELISA to detect *E. histolytic*-specific antigens, with an overall sensitivity of 71–100% and specificity c 93–100%. Antigen testing from serum and liver aspirate in amebic liver abscess yields a sensitivity 96% and 100%, respectively.
- Serology assays are available for diagnosis measuring the presence of serum antilectin antibodies (IgG), with a sensitivity of 97.9% and specificity of 94.8% in *E. histolytica* infection with amebic liver abscess.
- Polymerase chain reaction (PCR) techniques are more sensitive for detection of *E. histolytica* in fec or liver aspirate samples, but are not routinely available in clinical laboratories.
- In bladder infections: Amoebae and/or cysts in urir
- Liver enzymes, alkaline phosphatase (80%), and erythrocyte sedimentation rate may be elevated, a anemia and leucocytosis without eosinophilia (80 may be present in amebic liver abscess.

Follow-Up & Special Considerations

Follow-up stool examination after completion of therapy to ensure intestinal eradication.

Imaging

Initial approach

Ultrasonography and computed tomography (CT) scanning are sensitive but nonspecific for amebic live abscess. Usually solitary lesions in the right hepatic lobe (70–80%).

agnostic Procedures/Surgery

Jltrasound or CT-guided needle aspiration for uspected amebic abscess with studies of aspirate

Colonoscopy with biopsy can be performed in highly uspicious cases with negative stool and antigen esting. It is contraindicated in fulminant colitis due o increased perforation risk.

thological Findings

Colon biopsy:
- Amebic invasion through the mucosa and into submucosa is the hallmark of amebic colitis, which gives the classical flask-shaped ulcers.
- Periodic acid–Schiff-stained trophozoites in magenta color
- Neutrophils at the periphery

Liver biopsy:
- Necrosis surrounded by a rim of trophozoites

Liver aspirate:
- Red-brown material (anchovy paste)

IFFERENTIAL DIAGNOSIS

Other infectious causes of colitis:
- Shigellosis
- Campylobacter infection
- Pseudomembranous colitis
- Occasionally salmonellosis or *Yersinia* infection
- Viral hepatitis

Noninfectious causes of colitis:
- Ulcerative colitis
- Crohn colitis
- Ischemic colitis in elderly
- Hepatocellular adenoma

Hepatic amebiasis must be distinguished from pyogenic liver abscess or superinfection of amebic abscess.

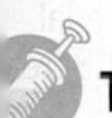

TREATMENT

Mostly treated as an outpatient but fulminant colitis with hypovolemia and complicated liver abscess require inpatient management.

Asymptomatic *E. histolytica* infection should be treated with luminal agent (iodoquinol, paromomycin) alone to eradicate infection as invasive infection may develop and also continuous shedding of cyst transmits infection through feco-oral route.

E. dispar and *E. moshkovskii* infections do not require treatment as they are nonpathogenic strains (2,4).

IEDICATION

irst Line

Noninvasive infection: Treat with luminal agents only.
- Paromomycin: Adult: 500 mg PO t.i.d. for 10 days; Pediatric: Administer as in adults

Invasive infection: Treat with nitroimidazole (metronidazole/tinidazole) followed by luminal agent.
- Metronidazole: Adult: 500–750 mg t.i.d PO for 10 days, Pediatric: 35–50 mg/kg PO divided tid for 10 days. It is then followed by a 20-day course of diiodohydroxyquin to eliminate intestinal carriage.
- Tinidazole: 2 g/d for 3 days with food for intestinal infection and 2 g/d for 3–5 days for liver abscess; better tolerated than metronidazole (5)[A]

- Contraindications:
  - Known allergy to given medication
  - Diiodohydroxyquin should be used with caution in patients with thyroid disease. It is contraindicated in renal and hepatic patients and may cause optic nerve and peripheral neuropathy.
- Precautions:
  - None of the agents has been proven safe during pregnancy, but pregnant women with invasive disease should still be treated.
- Significant possible interactions:
  - Metronidazole and tinidazole: Disulfiram reaction with concomitant use of ethanol.

Pregnancy Considerations

- Most agents are avoided in pregnancy (especially 1st trimester) because of concerns of teratogenicity, but invasive disease must still be treated.
  - Paromomycin is sometimes recommended for noninvasive disease because it is not absorbed.
- Infectious disease consultation should be obtained.

Second Line

- Luminal agent for noninvasive infection:
  - Diloxanide: Adult: 500 mg PO tid for 10 days; Pediatric: <2 years not recommended; >2 years 20 mg/kg PO divided tid for 10 days
  - Diiodohydroxyquin (also called iodoquinol): Adult: 650 mg tid PO for 20 days (if available); Pediatric: 10–13 mg/kg PO tid for 20 days
- Invasive infection:
  - Dehydroemetine (as effective as metronidazole, but cardiotoxic): 1–1.5 mg/kg/d IM for 5 days
  - Chloroquine (less effective): 600 mg base/day PO for 2 days, then 200 mg/day PO for 2–3 weeks (pediatric dose: 10 mg/kg/day up to maximum of 300 mg/d)
  - Treatment for invasive infection should be followed by a luminal agent.

ADDITIONAL TREATMENT

General Measures

- Fluids and nutrition
- Electrolyte management

SURGERY/OTHER PROCEDURES

- Surgery may be necessary in severe amebic colitis, peritonitis, and perforated viscus.
- Surgical drainage of uncomplicated amebic liver abscess should be avoided.

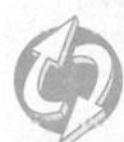

ONGOING CARE

FOLLOW-UP RECOMMENDATIONS

Patient Monitoring

- Patient signs and symptoms should be monitored.
- Stool studies should be repeated after the completion of therapy to ensure eradication since no regimen is completely effective.

DIET

As tolerated

PATIENT EDUCATION

Maintain good hygiene and avoid situations of re-exposure.

PROGNOSIS

- Untreated invasive amebiasis is frequently fatal.
- With treatment, improvement usually occurs within a few days.
- Some patients with amebic colitis have irritable bowel symptoms for weeks after successful treatment.
- Relapses possible

COMPLICATIONS

- Amebic colitis:
  - Fulminant or necrotizing colitis
  - Toxic megacolon
  - Ameboma
  - Rectovaginal fistula
- Amebic liver abscess:
  - Rupture to intraperitoneal, intrathoracic, or intrapericardial spaces with secondary bacterial infection
  - Direct extension to pleura or pericardium
  - Hematogenous dissemination and formation of brain abscess

REFERENCES

1. Fotedar R, Stark D, Beebe N et al. Laboratory diagnostic techniques for entamoeba species. *Clin Microbiol Rev*. 2007;20:511–32.
2. Stanley SL. Amoebiasis. *Lancet*. 2003;361: 1025–34.
3. Yamamoto-Furusho JK, Torijano-Carrera E et al. Intestinal protozoa infections among patients with ulcerative colitis: prevalence and impact on clinical disease course. *Digestion*. 2010;82:18–23.
4. Haque R, Huston CD, Hughes M et al. Amebiasis. *N Engl J Med*. 2003;348:1565–73.
5. Gonzales ML, Dans LF, Martinez EG. Antiamoebic drugs for treating amoebic colitis. *Cochrane Database Syst Rev*. 2009:CD006085.

ADDITIONAL READING

- Haque R, Kabir M, Noor Z, Rahman SM, Mondal D, Alam F, Rahman I, Al Mahmood A, Ahmed N, Petri WA et al. Diagnosis of amebic liver abscess and amebic colitis by detection of Entamoeba histolytica DNA in blood, urine, and saliva by a real-time PCR assay. *J Clin Microbiol*. 2010;48:2798–801.
- Stark D, van Hal S, Marriott D, Ellis J, Harkness J et al. Irritable bowel syndrome: a review on the role of intestinal protozoa and the importance of their detection and diagnosis. *Int J Parasitol*. 2007;37: 11–20.

See Also (Topic, Algorithm, Electronic Media Element)

Diarrhea, Acute; Diarrhea, Chronic

CODES

ICD9
- 006.0 Acute amebic dysentery without mention of abscess
- 006.3 Amebic liver abscess
- 006.4 Amebic lung abscess

CLINICAL PEARLS

- Most infected patients are asymptomatic or have minimal diarrheal symptoms.
- Untreated invasive disease is frequently fatal and treated cases may get relapses.
- Irritable bowel symptoms may persist for weeks despite successful treatment of infection.
- Nonpathogenic strains of Entamoeba species do not require treatment.

AMENORRHEA

Heidi L. Gaddey, MD

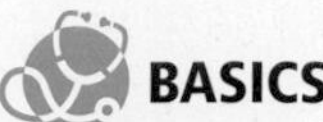

BASICS

DESCRIPTION
- Primary amenorrhea:
  - No menses by age 13–14 with absence of secondary sexual characteristics or
  - No menses by age 15–16 with normal secondary characteristics
- Secondary amenorrhea: Absence of menses for 3 months in a woman with previously normal menstruation or 6 months in a woman with a history of irregular cycles
- System(s) affected: Endocrine/metabolic; Reproductive

Pregnancy Considerations
Pregnancy is by far the most common cause of secondary amenorrhea.

EPIDEMIOLOGY
Prevalence
- Primary amenorrhea: <1% of female population
- Secondary amenorrhea: 3–5% of female population
- No evidence for race and ethnicity affecting prevalence
- Secondary amenorrhea more common than primary

RISK FACTORS
- Obesity
- Overtraining
- Eating disorders
- Malnutrition
- Anovulatory disorders
- Psychosocial crisis

Genetics
No known genetic pattern

GENERAL PREVENTION
Maintenance of proper body mass index (BMI) and healthy lifestyle with respect to food and exercise

PATHOPHYSIOLOGY
- Pathophysiology varies, depending on etiology.
- Primary amenorrhea should be evaluated in context of presence or absence of secondary sexual characteristics.
- Can result from dysfunction in hypothalamic–pituitary–gonadal axis, anatomic abnormalities, or other endocrine gland disorder

ETIOLOGY
- Primary amenorrhea:
  - Hypothalamic-pituitary abnormalities:
    - Constitutional delay of puberty
    - Isolated GnRH deficiency
    - Eating disorder
    - Stress/exercise
    - Central lesions (tumors, hypophysitis, granulomas)
    - Hyperprolactinemia
  - Gonadal abnormalities:
    - Chromosomal abnormalities (androgen insensitivity syndrome)
    - Euchromosomal gonadal agenesis or dysgenesis (Turner syndrome, Swyer syndrome, and pure gonadal dysgenesis)
    - Ovarian resistance syndrome
    - Abnormal gonadotropin function
    - Autoimmune gonadal failure
    - Idiopathic gonadal failure
  - Anatomic abnormalities:
    - Imperforate hymen
    - Transverse vaginal septum
    - Congenital absence of the cervix
    - Müllerian agenesis
- Secondary amenorrhea:
  - Pregnancy
  - Thyroid disease
  - Hyperprolactinemia (altered metabolism, ectopic production, breastfeeding/stimulation, hypothyroidism, medications, empty sella syndrome, pituitary adenoma)
  - After pregnancy, thyroid disease, and hyperprolactinemia are ruled out, other causes classified as:
    - Normogonadotropic amenorrhea: Hyperandrogenic anovulation (acromegaly, androgen secreting tumors, Cushing's disease, exogenous androgens, nonclassical congenital adrenal hyperplasia, PCOS); outflow tract obstruction (Asherman's syndrome, cervical stenosis, fibroids or polyps)
    - Hypergonadotropic hypogonadism. Postmenopausal ovarian failure; premature ovarian failure (autoimmune, chemotherapy, galactosemia, genetic, 17-hydroxylase deficiency, idiopathic, mumps oophoritis, pelvic radiation)
    - Hypogonadotropic hypogonadism (eating disorders, CNS tumors, chronic illness, cranial radiation, excessive weight loss/exercise/malnutrition, hypothalamic or pituitary destruction, Sheehan's syndrome)

COMMONLY ASSOCIATED CONDITIONS
- Premature ovarian failure may be associated with autoimmune abnormalities (autoimmune thyroiditis, type 1 diabetes).
- Polycystic ovarian syndrome associated with insulin-resistance and obesity

DIAGNOSIS

HISTORY
- Careful review of systems, including recent weight changes, symptoms of early pregnancy or menopause, virilizing changes, cyclic pelvic pain, galactorrhea, headaches, vision changes, fatigue, palpitations
- Growth and pubertal development history, including age of breast development, pubertal growth spurt, and adrenarche
- History of chronic illness, trauma, surgery, medications, prior chemotherapy or radiation
- Psychiatric history
- Social history, including diet and exercise history, drug abuse, and sexual history

PHYSICAL EXAM
- General appearance
- Vital signs, including height and weight, BMI: Hypotension, bradycardia, hypothermia (anorexia nervosa)
- HEENT exam: Evidence of dental erosions, trauma to palate (bulimia), visual field defect, fundoscopic changes, cranial nerve findings (prolactinoma), webbed neck (Turner syndrome), thyromegaly
- Skin exam: Evidence of androgen excess (acne, hirsutism), acanthosis nigricans (PCOS)
- Breast: State of development, evidence of galactorrhea (prolactinoma)
- Pelvic exam: Presence or absence of pubic hair (if sparse: Androgen insensitivity or deficiency); clitoromegaly (androgen excess); distention or bulging of external vagina (imperforate hymen); thin, pale vaginal mucosa without rugae (estroge deficiency and ovarian failure); presence of cervic mucus (evidence for estrogen production); blind vaginal pouch (müllerian agenesis, androgen insensitivity syndrome); ovarian enlargement (tumors, PCOS, autoimmune oophoritis)

DIAGNOSTIC TESTS & INTERPRETATIO
Lab
Initial lab tests
- Primary amenorrhea:
  - Serum prolactin (PRL) and thyroid stimulating hormone (TSH)
  - If no secondary sexual characteristics, measure serum follicle stimulating hormone (FSH) and luteinizing hormone (LH):
    - FSH/LH <5 IU per L suggests primary hypothalamic or pituitary etiology
    - FSH >20 and LH >40 IU per L suggests gonadal failure and karyotype analysis should be performed
  - If secondary sexual characteristics present, evaluate for anatomic abnormalities. If uterus absent or abnormal, perform karyotype analysis
- Secondary amenorrhea:
  - Exclude pregnancy with HCG
  - Serum TSH: Elevated in hypothyroidism, decreas in hyperthyroidism
  - Serum chemistry, complete blood count (CBC), urinalysis to rule out underlying disease
  - Serum prolactin (PRL):
    - >100 ng per mL suggests empty sella syndror or pituitary adenoma. Perform MRI for evaluation.
    - < 100 ng per mL, evaluate for other etiologie of which medications are most common
- If PRL and TSH are normal, perform progestin challenge (see Treatment):
  - If withdrawal bleed: Normogonadotropic amenorrhea related to hyperandrogenic chronic anovulation most commonly PCOS
  - If no withdrawal bleed: Follow up with estradiol priming (see Diagnostic Procedures/Other and Treatment) and repeat progestin challenge:
    - If no bleed: Consider outflow tract obstructior
    - If bleed occurs: Check FSH/LH: Elevated in hypergonadotropic hypogonadism, decreased pituitary tumors or hypogonadotropic hypogonadism
- If virilizing signs and significant acne present, measure free testosterone, DHEA-S, and 17-OH progesterone levels.

Follow-Up & Special Considerations
- Women <30 with ovarian failure (see below) shou have karyotype analysis and be investigated for premutations of FMR1 gene (fragile X syndrome) and for adrenal antibodies.
- If absence of uterus or foreshortened vagina, karyotype analysis should also be performed.

Imaging
- Imaging is not generally indicated as a 1st-line approach for amenorrhea.
- Ultrasound may show ovarian cysts (PCOS), presence or absence of uterus, and endometrial thickness.
- Magnetic resonance imaging (MRI) of the pelvis can clarify any uterine or vaginal anomalies suggested by ultrasound, or if pediatric patient is unable to tolerate transvaginal ultrasound probe.
- MRI of the sella turcica if prolactinoma suspected (elevated serum prolactin >100), and consider with functional hypothalamic amenorrhea (other adenomas)

Follow-Up & Special Considerations
- Laparoscopy: Diagnosis of the streak ovaries of Turner syndrome or PCOS (not often done)
- Hysterosalpingogram: To rule out Asherman syndrome and other etiologies of outflow obstruction

Diagnostic Procedures/Surgery
- Suspect constitutional delay: Obtain bone age.
- Hypothalamic amenorrhea from functional suppression: Consider dual-energy x-ray absorptiometry (DEXA) scan to assess for bone loss.

DIFFERENTIAL DIAGNOSIS
Includes all causes listed in Etiology

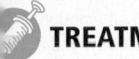

TREATMENT

MEDICATION
- Progesterone challenge and replacement: Medroxyprogesterone (Provera) 10 mg/d for 10 days will result in withdrawal bleed if hypothalamic–pituitary–gonadal axis intact
- Estrogen replacement: Cycling with a combination oral contraceptive (containing 35 or 50 mcg of estrogen) or conjugated estrogen (Premarin) 0.625 mg for 25 days with progesterone added as above for the last 10 days will result in a withdrawal bleed if the uterus and lower genital tract are normal.
- Use of hormonal therapies will not correct underlying problem. Other drugs might be required to treat specific conditions (e.g., bromocriptine for hyperprolactinemia).
- Use of hormonal replacement therapy is NOT recommended for long-term management of amenorrhea in older women (1)[A]:
  - It may be safe for symptom management in young women (1)[C].
  - Give to maintain secondary sex characteristics, prevent osteoporosis in adolescents and young women
- Combination estrogen/progesterone contraceptives (oral contraceptive pills [OCPs], patch, ring) replace estrogen and prevent pregnancy:
  - They also have a positive effect on bone mineral density in oligo-/amenorrheic women (2)[B].
  - Can decrease hirsutism in PCOS
- Calcium supplementation 1,500 mg/d if cause is hypoestrogenism
- Because PCOS is related to insulin resistance, metformin (Glucophage) has been used (often starting at 500 mg b.i.d.) in an effort to correct metabolic abnormalities, improve ovulation (3)[A], and restore normal menstrual patterns (3)[B].
- Contraindications to estrogen administration:
  - Pregnancy, thromboembolic disease, previous myocardial infarct or cerebrovascular accident, estrogen-dependent malignancy, severe hepatic impairment or disease
- Precautions:
  - Patients who are amenorrheic and wish to become pregnant should not be given hormone replacement therapy, but should receive treatment for infertility based on the specific cause.

ADDITIONAL TREATMENT

General Measures
- Definitive treatment depends on determining the cause of the amenorrhea.
- May not be necessary to treat all cases, especially if just temporary amenorrhea

Issues for Referral
Many causes of amenorrhea require referral to specialists in ob/gyn, endocrine, surgery, and/or psychiatry.

SURGERY/OTHER PROCEDURES
- Hymenectomy, done as a day surgery, required for those whose primary amenorrhea is due to imperforate hymen
- Lysis of adhesions in Asherman syndrome has been shown to be effective in restoring menstrual regularity and fertility.
- In patients with karyotype XY, gonads must be removed due to increased risk of gonadal tumors.
- Patients with müllerian agenesis and other congenital anatomical abnormalities of the vagina can undergo surgery to create a functioning vagina.

ONGOING CARE

FOLLOW-UP RECOMMENDATIONS
If overtraining is suspected, activity level should be reduced by 25–50%.

Patient Monitoring
- Depends on the cause and treatment chosen
- If hormonal replacement is used, discontinuation after 6 months is advised to assess spontaneous resumption of menses.

DIET
- Correct overweight or underweight by dietary management and behavior modification.
- If PCOS is the etiology, weight loss diet will help restore ovulation.

PATIENT EDUCATION
- Patient education consists of fully informing the patient of your findings, including the presence or absence of pregnancy, and of the underlying cause.
- Specific educational resources can be utilized as necessary (e.g., prenatal classes and menopause support groups).
- Specific information should be given about the expected duration of amenorrhea (temporary or permanent), effect on fertility, and the long-term sequelae of untreated amenorrhea (e.g., osteoporosis, vaginal dryness).
- Appropriate contraceptive advice should be given, as fertility returns before menses.
- Additional support may be needed if the amenorrhea is associated with a reduction in, or loss of, fertility.
- Society for Menstrual Cycle Research, 10559 N. 104th Place, Scottsdale, AZ 85258, (602) 451-9731.

PROGNOSIS
- Reflects the underlying cause
- In secondary amenorrhea from functional suppression of hypothalamic–pituitary–ovarian axis (stress, disordered eating, exercise), 1 study demonstrated 83% reversal rate in presence of obvious contributing factor

COMPLICATIONS
- Estrogen-deficiency symptoms (e.g., hot flashes, vaginal dryness)
- Osteoporosis in prolonged hypoestrogenic amenorrhea
- Increased risk of endometrial cancer in patients whose amenorrhea is secondary to anovulation with estrogen excess (obesity, PCOS)

REFERENCES

1. Farquhar CM, Marjoribanks J, Lethaby A et al. Long term hormone therapy for perimenopausal and postmenopausal women. *Cochrane Database Syst Rev*. 2005:CD004143.
2. Liu SL, Lebrun CM. Effect of oral contraceptives and hormone replacement therapy on bone mineral density in premenopausal and perimenopausal women: a systematic review. *Br J Sports Med*. 2006;40:11–24.
3. Andy C, Flake D, French L. Clinical inquiries. Do insulin-sensitizing drugs increase ovulation rates for women with PCOS? *J Fam Pract*. 2005;54:156, 159–60.

See Also (Topic, Algorithm, Electronic Media Element)
Diabetes Mellitus, Type 1; Diabetes Mellitus, Type 2; Hyperthyroidism; Hypothyroidism, Adult; Osteoporosis
Algorithms: Amenorrhea, Primary; Amenorrhea, Secondary; Delayed Puberty

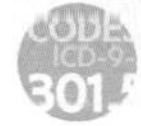

CODES

ICD9
626.0 Absence of menstruation

CLINICAL PEARLS

- There are both physiological and pathological causes of amenorrhea.
- Pregnancy is the most common cause of secondary amenorrhea.
- Among certain women with amenorrhea, a progestin challenge is a useful diagnostic tool.
- Use of hormonal replacement therapy is NOT recommended for long-term management of amenorrhea in older women.

AMNESTIC DISORDER

Jessica Lenore Wilson, MD
Noah S. Walman, MD

BASICS

- Memory is an arbitrary term that encompasses:
  - Knowledge of facts (*semantic* memory)
  - Knowledge of previous self-experiences (*episodic* memory)
  - Exercise of a learned skill (*procedural* memory)
  - Temporary knowledge for immediate use (*working* memory)
- Coded for by various regions of the brain, with significant involvement of the:
  - Medial temporal lobe, including:
    - Amygdaloid nucleus
    - Hippocampus
    - Parahippocampal region
  - Thalamus, especially the dorsomedial nuclei
  - Hypothalamus
  - Basal forebrain
- Amnestic disorder is a blanket statement to describe a deficit in any of these various memory types.

DESCRIPTION

- A single disease process can manifest with abnormalities in more than one memory system.
- For example, Alzheimer disease sufferers have a notable deficit in semantic memory, but can also have working memory deficits.
- Amnestic disorder, amnestic syndrome, or simply amnesia comes from the Greek for forgetfulness.
- Indicates a loss of, or gap in, one's memory, usually due to brain injury, shock, fatigue, repression, or illness
- Can be categorized based on amnesia for:
  - Events prior to the causative event, as in *retrograde*
  - Events after the causative event, as in *anterograde*
  - Information related to all senses and past experiences, as in *global* amnesia
- Unless otherwise stated, this topic will deal in particular with transient global amnesia (TGA).

EPIDEMIOLOGY

- Incidence and prevalence of amnesia is in direct proportion to the epidemiology of the primary cause.
- In transient global amnesia, incidence is greater among individuals over the age of 50.

Incidence

- In 1 study (1) in Rochester, Minnesota, TGA was found to be 5.2 cases per 100,000.
- The study further estimated 23.5 cases per 100,000 per year among 50+-year-olds.
- TGA recurrence rate is low, 4–5% in this study.

RISK FACTORS

- Evidence for and against established risk factors (1)
- Not a symptom of arteriosclerosis
- No higher risk of heart or cerebrovascular disease

Genetics

Recent evidence supports the possibility of a genetic predisposition (2).

PATHOPHYSIOLOGY

- Transient global amnesia is well studied, but not fully understood.
- Thought to have various mechanisms
- Findings from positron emission tomography, diffusion-weighted imaging magnetic resonance imaging (MRI), single photon emission computed tomography, and MR spectroscopy have demonstrated involvement of known memory-related structures in patients with TGA.
- Some theorize spreading depression of cortical electrical activity; that is, a wave of cellular depolarization and subsequent cellular edema.
- Others suggest that TGA is the result of:
  - Migraines
  - Venous congestion of the brain
  - Jugular valvular insufficiency

ETIOLOGY

- In general, metabolic or structural changes that cause an imbalance in the memory-related regions of the brain can cause an amnestic disorder
- Common causes include:
  - Thiamine deficiency
  - Hypothalamic tumors
  - Vertebrobasilar ischemia
- Less common are:
  - Neurodegenerative dementias such as Alzheimer disease
  - Bilateral damage to the medial temporal lobes
  - Head trauma
  - Chronic alcoholism
  - Nutritional disorders
  - In the case of dissociative amnesia, extreme psychological trauma causes the deficit.
- Transient global amnesia has been associated wit
  - Physical exertion
  - Emotional stress
  - Pain
  - Exposure to cold water
  - Sex
  - Valsalva maneuver

COMMONLY ASSOCIATED CONDITION

- Some relationship has been found between migraines and transient global amnesia.
- TGA patients were found to have a higher frequer of psychiatric disease relative to transient ischemi attack controls in 1 study.

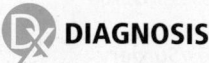

DIAGNOSIS

HISTORY

- In TGA, patients have confusion and global amnesia, usually for 6–12 hours.
- Retrograde, and to a lesser extent anterograde, memory deficits
- Complete resolution
- Social history and family history are important.
- TGA in women is associated with an emotional precipitating event, a history of anxiety, and a pathological personality.
- TGA in men occurs more after a physical precipitating event.
- There is a history of headaches among younger patients.
- No association with vascular risk factors

PHYSICAL EXAM

- If there are no focal abnormalities on exam, then transient global ischemia can be diagnosed.
- Loss of memory for recent events
- Difficulty with retaining new information
- If neurological exam demonstrates more than memory dysfunction, other differential diagnoses should be further explored.

AGNOSTIC TESTS & INTERPRETATION
GA is largely a clinical diagnosis.
hysical exam largely unremarkable

b
ial lab tests
omplete blood count with differential
asic metabolic profile
rothrombin time/partial thromboplastin time to ule out hypercoagulable state

aging
ial approach
I and/or computed tomography to rule out stroke

agnostic Procedures/Surgery
lectroencephalogram if seizure is suspected
lectrocardiogram if cardiac etiology is suspected

FFERENTIAL DIAGNOSIS
asilar artery thrombosis
ardioembolic stroke
omplex partial seizures
pilepsy of frontal or temporal lobe
acunar syndromes
ligraine variants
osterior cerebral artery stroke
yncope

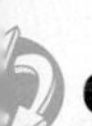

TREATMENT
upportive care for TGA
eassurance that recurrence of TGA is low (3)
there is an underlying disease process present .e., Alzheimer disease, herpes encephalitis), it hould be treated.

ONGOING CARE
edule at least 1 follow-up visit to a neurologist in a ient diagnosed with transient global amnesia.

ET
restrictions on diet

PROGNOSIS
TGA is a benign condition, with low risk of recurrence (3).

REFERENCES

1. Miller JW, Petersen RC, Metter EJ et al. Transient global amnesia: clinical characteristics and prognosis. *Neurology*. 1987;37:733–7.
2. Segers-van Rijn J, de Brujin SF et al. Transient global amnesia: a genetic disorder? *Eur. Neurol.* 2010;63:186-7
3. Hinge HH, Jensen TS, Kjaer M et al. The prognosis of transient global amnesia. Results of a multicenter study. *Arch Neurol*. 1986;43:673–6.

ADDITIONAL READING

- Agosti C et al. Recurrency in transient global amnesia: a retrospective study. *Eur J Neurol*. 2006;13(9):986–9.
- Budson A et al. Memory Dysfunction. *N Engl J Med*. 2005;352:7.
- Greer DM, Schaefer PW, Schwamm LH. Unilateral temporal lobe stroke causing ischemic transient global amnesia: role for diffusion-weighted imaging in the initial evaluation. *J Neuroimaging*. 2001;11: 317–9.
- Jenkins KG, Kapur N, Kopelman MD. Retrograde amnesia and malingering. *Curr Opin Neurol*. 2009.
- Piñol-Ripoll G, de la Puerta González-Miró I, Martínez L et al. [A study of the risk factors in transient global amnesia and its differentiation from a transient ischemic attack.] *Rev Neurol*. 2005;41: 513–6.
- Quinette P, Guillery-Girard B, Dayan J et al. What does transient global amnesia really mean? Review of the literature and thorough study of 142 cases. *Brain*. 2006.
- Sellal F. Transient amnesia in the elderly. *Psychol Neuropsychiatr Vieil*. 2006;4(1):31–8.
- Shekhar R. Transient global amnesia—a review. *Int J Clin Pract*. 2008.
- Zorzon M et al. Transient global amnesia and transient ischemic attack. Natural history, vascular risk factors, and associated conditions. *Stroke*. 1995;26(9):1536–42.

See Also (Topic, Algorithm, Electronic Media Element)
Algorithm: Amnesia

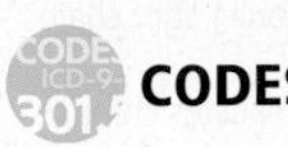

CODES

ICD9
- 291.1 Alcohol-induced persisting amnestic disorder
- 292.83 Drug-induced persisting amnestic disorder
- 294.8 Other persistent mental disorders due to conditions classified elsewhere

CLINICAL PEARLS
- Any patient with possible TGA should be ruled out for stroke, especially if stroke risk factors are present.
- In a patient diagnosed with TGA, reassurance and a follow-up appointment with a neurologist are appropriate management.
- Other than memory problems, the neurological exam of a TGA patient is most often normal.

AMYLOIDOSIS

Tara J. Rizvi, MD

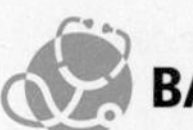

BASICS

DESCRIPTION
- A group of diseases characterized by extracellular deposition of insoluble protein fibrils in organs and tissues
- Classification is based on the nature of precursor plasma proteins that form fibril deposits (1):
  - Primary (AL): Plasma cell dyscrasia; deposition of protein derived from immunoglobulin light chain fragments
  - Secondary or reactive (AA): Complicates chronic infections or inflammatory diseases; deposition of serum amyloid A(SAA) protein
  - Heritable or familial (AF): Many different types of variant plasma proteins form amyloid deposits beginning in midlife; most common form is caused by mutations of transthyretin (ATTR)
  - Dialysis-related: Deposition of fibrils derived from β_2-microglobulin; predilection for osteoarticular structures
  - Senile systemic amyloidosis: Deposition of otherwise normal (wild-type) transthyretin in myocardium and other sites seen in elderly
  - Organ-specific amyloidosis: Deposition isolated to 1 organ, resulting in specific syndromes; most common is Alzheimer disease caused by cerebral amyloid plaques:
    - Localized amyloidosis: Results from local amyloid deposits in tracheobronchial tree, urinary tract, or skin, which are also derived from monoclonal light chains, but not due to underlying systemic plasma cell disorder

EPIDEMIOLOGY
Incidence
- AL: 1,275–3,200 new cases annually in US (2):
  - Easily missed, so incidence may be higher
- AA: Rare; occurs in <5% of patients with chronic inflammatory diseases, most commonly with rheumatoid arthritis (RA)

Prevalence
- AF: Rare, <1 per 100,000 population
- AL: Most common type in North America, 4.5 per 100,000 population (2)
  - Predominant age: 60–70
  - Predominant sex: Male > Female (2:1)
- AA is more prevalent in:
  - Japan, Finland, developing countries due to less adequate treatment of inflammatory and infectious diseases
  - Turkey, Middle East in association with familial Mediterranean fever (FMF)

RISK FACTORS
Depends on type of systemic amyloidosis:
- Age (senile systemic/Alzheimer)
- Heredity (AF/AA)
- Underlying plasma cell dyscrasia (AL)
- Untreated chronic inflammatory diseases (AA)
- Untreated chronic infections (AA)
- Long-term hemodialysis

Genetics
- Only familial amyloidosis can be inherited; usually autosomal-dominant inheritance.
- Three types of genetic abnormalities have been identified in amyloidogenic proteins: Polymorphisms, variant molecules, and genetically determined post-translational modifications.

GENERAL PREVENTION
Early detection and treatment of underlying disorders, such as plasma cell dyscrasias, chronic inflammatory conditions, chronic infections

PATHOPHYSIOLOGY
- Fibrillogenesis results from disorder of protein folding; cofactors may significantly modulate this.
- Soluble precursor proteins undergo transformation to a β-pleated fibrillar configuration.
- Amyloid fibrils thus formed are insoluble polymers composed of LMW subunits of a variety of proteins, many of which circulate as plasma constituents:
  - In AL, monoclonal Ig light chain deposits are predominantly composed of λ chains.
  - In AA, IL-1, IL-6, and TNF associated with chronic inflammation induce serum amyloid A protein (SAA), an acute-phase reactant.
- Fibril deposition in extracellular matrix results in damage to the structure and function of the tissues involved.

ETIOLOGY
Cause of amyloid production and its deposition in tissues is unknown.

COMMONLY ASSOCIATED CONDITIONS
- Primary amyloidosis (AL):
  - Multiple myeloma
  - Non-Hodgkin lymphoma
  - Rarely Waldenström macroglobulinemia
- Secondary amyloidosis (AA) (1):
  - Chronic inflammatory arthritides:
    - Most commonly seen in adult and juvenile RA
    - Spondyloarthropathies: Ankylosing spondylitis, psoriatic arthritis
    - Rarely in SLE, Sjögren, and vasculitides
  - Periodic fever syndromes:
    - FMF
    - TRAPS syndrome
    - Muckle–Wells syndrome
  - Chronic infections:
    - Bronchiectasis, tuberculosis, osteomyelitis
    - Pressure sores, UTIs, other infections seen in complications of paraplegia
  - Crohn disease
  - Due to IVDA
  - Neoplasms, particularly renal cell CA
  - Castleman disease

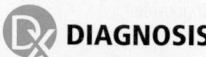

DIAGNOSIS

HISTORY
- Careful family history to assess for familial amyloidosis: ATTR can present as syndromes of:
  - Familial amyloidotic polyneuropathy
  - Familial amyloidotic cardiomyopathy
- Suspect secondary AA amyloidosis with a history long-standing inflammatory disease, uncontrolled for >5 years
- Symptoms are determined by the organ or system involved, and can often be obscured by the underlying disease:
  - Renal and cardiac involvement are most commo
  - Primary (AL) can affect all organs except CNS.
  - Heritable (ATTR) can present similar to AL, but with more peripheral and autonomic neuropath symptoms and less renal involvement.
  - Secondary AA: Mostly kidney, liver involved
- Symptom manifestations are nonspecific:
  - Initial: Fatigue, malaise, weight loss
  - Other: Nephrotic syndrome, CHF, dyspnea, abdominal pain, diarrhea, early satiety (due to autonomic neuropathy), malabsorption, carpal tunnel syndrome, arthralgias, arthritis, myalgias, symptoms due to hypothyroidism

PHYSICAL EXAM
- Renal involvement is most common and can prese as asymptomatic proteinuria or nephrotic syndrom particularly in AL-type amyloidosis. Microscopic hematuria is more prominent in AA type.
- Cardiac involvement is common and may present restrictive cardiomyopathy resulting in diastolic dysfunction, conduction abnormalities.
- Autonomic neuropathy: Postural hypotension
- Peripheral neuropathy: Carpal tunnel syndrome
- Hepatic amyloid deposition can lead to hepatomegaly but rarely jaundice
- GI amyloid may cause esophageal motility abnormalities, gastric atony, small and large intestinal motility abnormalities, malabsorption, bleeding, or pseudo-obstruction
- Thyromegaly due to infiltration of thyroid
- Amyloid arthropathy may mimic RA: Symmetrical polyarthritis, periarticular soft tissue swelling.
- Due to infiltration of soft tissue by amyloid:
  - Macroglossia: Pathognomonic for primary AL; occurs in 20%; and is characterized by a large, s tongue, frequently rimmed by teeth indentation
  - Shoulder pad sign
  - Nail dystrophy, alopecia
  - Hoarse, weak voice (vocal cord infiltration)
- Vascular infiltration can lead to raccoon eyes or spontaneous purpura with minimal trauma such a sneezing.
- Rarely, bleeding diathesis may occur with factor X deficiency.

AGNOSTIC TESTS & INTERPRETATION
b
tial lab tests
- BC, electrolytes, creatinine, calcium, U/A, TSH
- ssess for proteinuria, Bence-Jones proteins, renal nsufficiency, anemia, hypothyroidism

low-Up & Special Considerations
- rimary AL: Serum and urine protein electrophoresis with immunofixation for monoclonal protein spike
- econdary AA: Tests to assess underlying nflammatory disease:
  - ESR, CRP, RF, anti-CCP, ANA
  - Gene testing for FMF, TRAPS
- amilial (ATTR): Abnormal transthyretin protein may e isolated

aging
tial approach
- chocardiogram: Thickening of interventricular eptum and ventricular walls, restrictive pattern
- onsider renal U/S, bone scan as appropriate

low-Up & Special Considerations
- diolabeled serum amyloid P component (SAP) ntigraphy: Quantitatively monitors accumulation of yloid deposits. This is available only at specialized ters in Europe.

agnostic Procedures/Surgery
- onfirmation of diagnosis requires presence of myloid deposits on biopsy.
- ess invasive and 1st-line: Abdominal fat pad spirate, rectal, bone marrow, or skin biopsy
- f negative, biopsy of affected organs have higher ensitivity: Kidney, liver, sural nerve.

thological Findings
- ight microscopy: Demonstration of amyloid deposits as amorphous, nodular hyaline material
- ibrils bind to Congo red, leading to apple green birefringence under polarized light, and thioflavin T, producing intense yellow-green fluorescence.
- Electron microscopy: Fibrils are rigid, linear, nonbranching; measure 7.5–10 nm in width (3)[B].
- Bone marrow biopsy in AL may show clonal excess of plasma cells (λ or κ).

IFFERENTIAL DIAGNOSIS
- Distinguish different forms of amyloidosis from each other after biopsy by immunofluorescence, or immunohistochemical staining for SAA protein, TTR, κ/λ light chains.
- Particularly distinguish AL from genetic, senile, and localized amyloidosis, since management and prognosis vary considerably.

TREATMENT

IEDICATION
rst Line
- Primary AL (4,5)[A]:
  - High-dose melphalan followed by hemopoietic cell transplant (HCT): Improves quality of life and even results in remission in some cases
  - Melphalan and high-dose dexamethasone for patients who cannot tolerate HCT
  - Precautions with melphalan: Bone marrow suppression, cytopenias, infections
- Secondary AA:
  - Control of underlying inflammatory disease: Consider anticytokine therapy for autoimmune diseases (6)[A]
  - Colchicine for familial Mediterranean fever (3)[A]

Second Line
Primary AL (5)[B]:
- Lenalidomide with dexamethasone (7)[B]:
  - Precautions: Neutropenia, thrombocytopenia, rash, fatigue
- Bortezomib with dexamethasone

ADDITIONAL TREATMENT
General Measures
- Secondary AA: Treat underlying cause
- Familial (ATTR): Liver transplant
- Hemodialysis-related amyloidosis: Change to peritoneal dialysis

Issues for Referral
- Refer to specialized amyloidosis centers if diagnosis is unclear and/or for treatment failures.
- Consider referral to rheumatology, hematology, cardiology, and other specialties based on underlying disease association.

Additional Therapies
Investigational:
- Eprodisate for secondary AA (8)[B]:
  - Interferes with AA amyloid protein interaction with glycosaminoglycans, disrupting fibril formation
  - Shown to decrease the rate of deterioration in renal function (5)[A]
- Diflunisal for familial amyloidosis (5)[C]

SURGERY/OTHER PROCEDURES
For localized amyloidosis of lip, skin, nasopharynx, or urinary tract, removal or excision at site of occurrence may be sufficient.

IN-PATIENT CONSIDERATIONS
Admission Criteria
- Acute nephrotic syndrome/renal failure
- Cardiomyopathy/acute CHF
- Hepatic failure, pseudo-obstruction

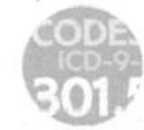

ONGOING CARE

FOLLOW-UP RECOMMENDATIONS
Patient Monitoring
- Routine monitoring of renal function
- Monitor adverse effects of medications.
- AA: Maintenance of low serum amyloid A protein levels correlates to better outcome (1)[B].
- AL: Prognostic indicators to follow are: NT-pro-BNP, cardiac troponin T and I, serum-free light chains.

DIET
- Low-protein, low-salt diet for patients with renal disease
- Low-salt, cardiac diet for CHF patients

PATIENT EDUCATION
- The Amyloidosis Support Network: http://www.amyloidosis.org
- Amyloid Research Group of Indiana University: http://www.iupui.edu/~amyloid/

PROGNOSIS
- In general, older patients do less well.
- Primary AL: Median survival is 1–2 years after diagnosis (2):
  - Cardiac involvement: 6 months
  - Renal involvement: 21 months
- Secondary AA: Based on underlying disease:
  - Mean survival = 133 months (1)
- ATTR: 5–15 years, based on precursor protein
- Senile (cardiac) amyloidosis: Survival is better than AL amyloid.

REFERENCES

1. Lachmann HJ, Goodman HJ, Gilbertson JA et al. Natural history and outcome in systemic AA amyloidosis. *N Engl J Med*. 2007;356:2361–71.
2. Falk RH, Comenzo RL, Skinner M. The systemic amyloidoses. *N Engl J Med*. 1997;337:898–909.
3. Rajkumar SV, Gertz MA. Advances in the treatment of amyloidosis. *N Engl J Med*. 2007;356:2413–5.
4. Jaccard A, Moreau P, Leblond V et al. High-dose melphalan versus melphalan plus dexamethasone for AL amyloidosis. *N Engl J Med*. 2007;357:1083–93.
5. Dember LM. Modern Treatment of Amyloidosis: Unresolved Questions. *J Am Soc Nephrol*. 2008.
6. Keersmaekers T, Claes K, Kuypers DR et al. Long-term efficacy of infliximab treatment for AA-amyloidosis secondary to chronic inflammatory arthritis. *Ann Rheum Dis*. 2009;68:759–61.
7. Sanchorawala V, Wright DG, Rosenzweig M et al. Lenalidomide and dexamethasone in the treatment of AL amyloidosis: results of a phase II trial. *Blood*. 2006.
8. Dember LM, Hawkins PN, Hazenberg BP et al. Eprodisate for the treatment of renal disease in AA amyloidosis. *N Engl J Med*. 2007;356:2349–60.

See Also (Topic, Algorithm, Electronic Media Element)
Multiple Myeloma

CODES

ICD9
277.30 Amyloidosis, unspecified

CLINICAL PEARLS
- Consider amyloidosis in patients with multiple myeloma, RA, JRA, familial Mediterranean fever, and other long-standing chronic inflammatory conditions.
- Biopsy for definitive diagnosis: Congo red stain demonstrates apple green birefringence under polarized light.
- Differentiate specific type based on immunohistochemical staining.
- Remember that treatment varies vastly depending on type of amyloidosis.

AMYOTROPHIC LATERAL SCLEROSIS

Mhd Basheer Rahmoun, MD
Dalia Sbat, PharmD

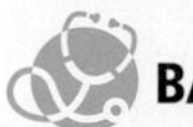

BASICS

Amyotrophic Lateral Sclerosis (ALS) is a degenerative disease that affects the upper and lower motor neurons (UMN and LMN).

DESCRIPTION

- Sporadic ALS is the most common form of the disease. It includes a number of overlapping syndromes, such as pseudobulbar palsy, progressive bulbar palsy, progressive muscular atrophy, and primary lateral sclerosis.
- Familial ALS is an autosomal-dominant or -recessive disease, which is clinically similar to sporadic ALS but probably represents a distinct entity pathologically and biochemically.
- Guam ALS and Parkinson-dementia complex is an ALS-like syndrome often, but not always, associated with Parkinson syndrome and dementia, which is prevalent among the Chamorro Indians of Guam and rare in the US.
- System(s) affected: Nervous
- Synonym(s): Motor neuron disease, MND, Lou Gehrig's disease, ALS

Pediatric Considerations

- Infantile and juvenile spinal muscular atrophies are conditions distinct from ALS, both clinically and pathologically.
- Symptoms of ALS may inappropriately be attributed to age.

Pregnancy Considerations

- Uncommon among affected individuals
- Pregnancy would be unwise in any individual suffering from a disease with poor prognosis.
- If pregnancy did occur, the only foreseeable difficulties would be related to weakness.

EPIDEMIOLOGY

Incidence

In Europe and North America, between 1.47 and 2.7 per 100,000/year

Prevalence

- Estimated prevalence rates range between 2.7 and 7.4 per 100,000.
- Predominant age: Uncommon before age 40
- Predominant sex: Male > Female in sporadic ALS:
  – After 65: Male = Female

RISK FACTORS

- Family history
- Age >40
- Smoking (in women) (1)[A]

Genetics

- Familial ALS (10% of cases) can be autosomal-dominant or -recessive; X-linked cases have been reported.
- Gene locus has been localized to the long arm of chromosome 21 and encodes the superoxide dismutase (SOD1) enzyme in 20% of familial ALS cases
- Mutation in the gene encoding fused in sarcoma (FUS) was identified in familial ALS type 6 (2).
- Mutations in the angiogenin gene (ANG) have been recently discovered to be associated with sporadic ALS (3,4).
- Mutations in TARDP region encoding TAR DNA-binding protein TDP-43 have also been identified in familial and sporadic ALS (5).

GENERAL PREVENTION

Genetic counselling is advised if there is a family history of ALS.

PATHOPHYSIOLOGY

Degeneration of the upper and lower motor neurons with their respective axons and with gliosis replacing lost neurons

ETIOLOGY

- Sporadic: Cause is unknown, but elevated levels of glutamate have been found in serum and cerebrospinal fluid (CSF).
- Familial ALS: A genetically transmitted degenerative disease
- Guam ALS and Parkinson-dementia complex: Possible relationship to ingestion of the cycad nut or to some other environmental toxin

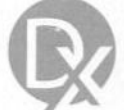

DIAGNOSIS

Diagnosis can be established according to Revised El Escorial World Federation of Neurology criteria

- The presence of:
  – Evidence of LMN degeneration by clinical, electrophysiological, or neuropathologic examination
  – Evidence of UMN degeneration by clinical examination
  – Progressive spread of symptoms or signs within a region or to other regions, as determined by history or examination
- The absence of:
  – Electrophysiological and pathological evidence of other disease processes that might explain the signs of LMN and/or UMN degeneration
  – Neuroimaging evidence of other disease processes that might explain the observed clinical and electrophysiological signs

HISTORY

ALS is suggested when symptoms are consistent with UMN and LMN dysfunction that worsen over time. Symptoms include:

- Loss of muscle strength and coordination
- Difficulty opening and closing the jaw, drooling
- Voice change, hoarseness
- Muscle cramps, difficulty breathing, difficulty swallowing, paralysis

PHYSICAL EXAM

Variable combinations of:

- Unexplained weight loss
- Limb weakness with variable symmetry and distribution
- Gait disorder (steppage-waddling)
- Slurring of speech
- Inability to control affect (inappropriate laughing, crying, yawning)
- Focal atrophy of muscle groups (initially in a myotomal distribution)
- Fasciculations (other than calves)
- Hyper-reflexia (including jaw jerk—Hoffman's sign)
- Babinski sign, present in 50% of patients
- Spasticity
- Sialorrhea
- Spares cognitive, oculomotor, sensory, and autonomic functions

DIAGNOSTIC TESTS & INTERPRETATIO

Lab

No simple reliable laboratory test is available that confirms the diagnosis.

Initial lab tests

- Elevated levels of glutamate in CSF and serum
- Anti-monosialoganglioside autoantibodies in low titer commonly found (of unclear significance)
- Possibly reduced levels of nerve growth factor

Imaging

Initial approach

MRI: To exclude other possible diagnoses in the evaluation of suspected ALS:

- MRI is usually normal in ALS, although increased signal in the corticospinal tracts on T2-weighted a FLAIR images and hypointensity of the motor cort on T2-weighted images has been reported (6).

Diagnostic Procedures/Surgery

- Electromyography: Denervation potentials (fibrillations-positive sharp waves) and often doublets are associated with prominent fasciculations, which suggest anterior horn cell dysfunction. Voluntary motor unit potentials have increased amplitude, long duration, and/or polyphasic pattern. The recruitment pattern is reduced for the force generated, and individual motor units have a high rate of discharge (7).
- Nerve conduction studies: Sensory and motor NCS are most often normal in ALS, although compounc motor action potential (CMAP) amplitudes may be reduced in severely atrophic and denervated muscl (7).
- Motor unit number estimation is a nerve conduction–based method that assesses the number of viable motor axons innervating small hand or foot muscles. In ALS, it drops prior to the onset of clinical weakness (8).
- Muscle biopsy: Not a routine part of the diagnostic evaluation of ALS, but may be performed if myopathy is suspected on clinical, electrodiagnosti or serologic grounds:
  – Muscle biopsy will show groups of shrunken angulated muscle fibers (grouped atrophy) amid other groups of fibers with a uniform fiber type (fiber type grouping).

Pathological Findings

- Loss of Betz cells in the motor cortex
- Atrophic or absent anterior horn cells of spinal cor
- Atrophic or absent neurons within the motor nucle of the medulla and pons
- Degeneration of the lateral columns of the spinal cord
- Atrophy of the ventral roots
- Grouped atrophy of muscle (motor units)

DIFFERENTIAL DIAGNOSIS

- Multifocal motor neuropathy
- Cervical radiculomyelopathy
- Cervical spondylosis
- Lead intoxication
- Spinal muscular atrophy (adult form)
- Primary lateral sclerosis
- Familial spastic paraparesis

- ·enign fasciculations
- yme disease
- ·pinal multiple sclerosis
- ropical spastic paraparesis
- Ayasthenia gravis

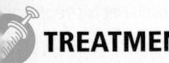

TREATMENT

EDICATION

ɪzole 50 mg PO b.i.d.: The only FDA-approved drug ALS. It produces a slight prolongation in life ɔectancy by decreasing the release of glutamate 10), and it slows the disease progression.

LERT

luzole withhold should be considered for patients ɘveloping fatigue.

DDITIONAL TREATMENT

ɘse drugs may be used to relieve severe spasticity:

- Baclofen 5 mg PO t.i.d. initially, followed by gradual increase of 5 mg per day every 4–7 days; not to exceed 80 mg per day divided q.i.d.
- Tizanidine 4–8 mg PO every 8 hours p.r.n.; not to exceed 36 mg per day

eneral Measures

- Outpatient may ultimately need nursing home placement or hospice.
- Supportive care is necessary for complicating emergencies (aspiration, respiratory failure). Use of a respirator is a major ethical dilemma.
- Consideration should be given to those with selective respiratory dysfunction.
- Discussion of advance directives, focusing on patient's specific values about which interventions to be used, is critical to meeting the patient's needs.
- Prosthetic devices

sues for Referral

- Multidisciplinary clinic referral to optimize health care delivery, prolong survival, and enhance quality of life
- Early exam by a neurologist can confirm diagnosis of ALS.
- Tracheostomy or G-tube placement may be performed by surgeon or gastroenterologist.
- Pulmonologist and respiratory therapist for ventilator assistance and management of intercurrent infections and tracheostomy

OMPLEMENTARY AND ALTERNATIVE EDICINE

- Research offering therapy with stem cells is evolving, providing a new approach in cellular replacement and support for patients (11,12)[A].
- Therapeutic trials of the efficacy of antioxidants (vitamin E and vitamin C and β-carotene), nerve growth factor, gabapentin, Myotrophin, and thyrotropin-releasing hormone, and creatine have been undertaken. Reports are not encouraging (13)[A].

URGERY/OTHER PROCEDURES

- Treatment for refractory sialorrhea
  - Botulinum toxin B
  - Low-dose radiation therapy to the salivary glands
- Percutaneous endoscopic gastrostomy (PEG) tube should be considered with early signs of malnutrition to stabilize weight and prolong survival.
- Noninvasive ventilation (NIV) can lengthen survival and improve quality of life.
- Elective tracheostomy should be considered in patients with early signs of respiratory difficulty.

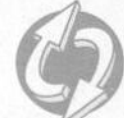

ONGOING CARE

FOLLOW-UP RECOMMENDATIONS

Patients should be involved in regular exercise and a physical therapy program.

Patient Monitoring

- Initially every 3 months; frequency to be increased as needed for symptomatic therapy
- Patients with a presumed diagnosis of ALS should have neuroimaging and electrodiagnostic studies.

DIET

- Evaluate swallowing to quantify any dysphagia.
- Modify the patient's diet to prevent aspiration.
- Consider a gastrostomy tube when patient cannot swallow fluids or soft foods (14).

PATIENT EDUCATION

Printed material for patients (and reference lists for physicians) available from:

- The Muscular Dystrophy Association: (520) 529-2000; (800) 572-1717; http://www.mdausa.org
- The ALS Association: (800) 782-4747; http://www.alsa.org
- Families of Spinal Muscular Atrophy: http://www.fsma.org

PROGNOSIS

- ALS usually results in death within 5 years.
- Patients who predominantly manifest progressive muscular atrophy have a better prognosis.
- There have been reports of spontaneous arrest of the disease.

COMPLICATIONS

- Aspiration pneumonia
- Pulmonary embolism
- Nutritional deficiency
- Complications from wheelchair-bound or bedridden states, including decubitus ulcers and skin infections

REFERENCES

1. Alonso A, Logroscino G, Hernán MA et al. Smoking and the risk of amyotrophic lateral sclerosis: a systematic review and meta-analysis. *Journal of Neurology, Neurosurgery, and Psychiatry*. 2010;
2. Vance C, Rogelj B, Hortobágyi T et al. Mutations in FUS, an RNA processing protein, cause familial amyotrophic lateral sclerosis type 6. *Science*. 2009;323:1208–11.
3. Conforti FL et al. A novel Angiogenin gene mutation in a sporadic patient with amyotrophic lateral sclerosis from southern Italy. *Neuromuscul Disord*. 2008;18:68.
4. Paubel A, Violette J, Amy M et al. Mutations of the ANG gene in French patients with sporadic amyotrophic lateral sclerosis. *Arch Neurol*. 2008; 65:1333–6.
5. Sreedharan J, Blair IP, Tripathi VB et al. TDP-43 mutations in familial and sporadic amyotrophic lateral sclerosis. *Science*. 2008;319:1668–72.
6. Oba H, Araki T, Ohtomo K et al. Amyotrophic lateral sclerosis: T2 shortening in motor cortex at MR imaging. *Radiology*. 1993;189:843–6.
7. Daube JR. Electrodiagnostic studies in amyotrophic lateral sclerosis and other motor neuron disorders. *Muscle Nerve*. 2000;23: 1488–502.
8. Olney RK, et al. Motor unit number estimation (MUNE): How may it contribute to the diagnosis of ALS? *Neurol Neurosurg Psychiatry*. 2000; 1(Suppl 2):S41–4.
9. Bensimon G, Lacomblez L, Meininger V. A controlled trial of riluzole in amyotrophic lateral sclerosis. ALS/Riluzole Study Group. *N Engl J Med*. 1994;330:585–91.
10. Riluzole for amyotrophic lateral sclerosis. *Med Lett*. 1995;37:113.
11. Lunn JS, Hefferan MP, Marsala M et al. Stem cells: comprehensive treatments for amyotrophic lateral sclerosis in conjunction with growth factor delivery. *Growth Factors*. 2009;1.
12. Kim SU, de Vellis J. Stem cell-based cell therapy in neurological diseases: A review. *J Neurosci Res*. 2009.
13. Pastula DM, Moore DH, Bedlack RS et al. Creatine for amyotrophic lateral sclerosis/motor neuron disease. *Cochrane Database Syst Rev*. 2010;6: CD005225.
14. Andersen PM, Borasio GD, Dengler R et al. Good practice in the management of amyotrophic lateral sclerosis: clinical guidelines. An evidence-based review with good practice points. EALSC Working Group. *Amyotroph Lateral Scler*. 2007; 8:195–213.

ADDITIONAL READING

- Miller RG, Jackson CE, Kasarskis EJ, et al. Practice parameter update: The care of the patient with amyotrophic lateral sclerosis: drug, nutritional, and respiratory therapies (an evidence-based review): report of the Quality Standards Subcommittee of the American Academy of Neurology *Neurology*. 2009;73(15):1218–26.
- Practice parameter update: The care of the patient with amyotrophic lateral sclerosis: multidisciplinary care, symptom management, and cognitive/ behavioral impairment (an evidence-based review): report of the Quality Standards Subcommittee of the American Academy of Neurology. *Neurology*. 2009;73(15):1227–33.

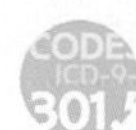

CODES

ICD9

335.20 Amyotrophic lateral sclerosis

CLINICAL PEARLS

- ALS is an upper and lower motor neuron disease.
- Diagnosis is made by history, physical exam, EMG, and NCS.
- Riluzole is the only available treatment that might increase survival.

ANAEROBIC AND NECROTIZING INFECTIONS

Ruben Peralta, MD
Packrisamy Kannan, MD

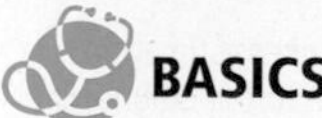

BASICS

DESCRIPTION

- Necrotizing infections of the skin and fascia are called necrotizing cellulitis and necrotizing fasciitis (NF), respectively.
- Necrotizing fasciitis is a rapidly spreading and potentially fatal soft tissue infection located in the fascia, with secondary necrosis of the subcutaneous tissue. Organisms spread from the subcutaneous tissue along the deep fascial planes, presumably facilitated by bacterial enzymes and toxins.
- Type I necrotizing fasciitis is a mixed infection caused by the synergistic effect of both aerobic and anaerobic bacteria; type II necrotizing fasciitis is a monomicrobial infection caused by group A β-hemolytic streptococci (*Streptococcus pyogenes*).
- Gas gangrene is a subset of necrotizing infection usually caused by the *Clostridium* sp. with gas formation within the tissue (type III), and type IV is commonly due to fungal infections.
- Necrotizing skin and soft tissue infections are associated with extensive tissue destruction, systemic toxicity, and loss of limb, and are potentially fatal.
- Synonym(s): Fournier gangrene; Cullen ulcer; Meleney ulcer; Flesh-eating infections

EPIDEMIOLOGY

- Predominant age: Any age
- Predominant sex: Male = Female

Incidence

Incidence of necrotizing fasciitis: 500–1,500 cases annually in the US (1)[B]

RISK FACTORS

Can occur in young, previously healthy persons without predisposing or precipitating risk factors. However, some cases are associated with the following:

- Predisposing risk factors:
  - Advanced age
  - Obesity
  - Malnutrition
  - Diabetes mellitus
  - Immune suppression (e.g., HIV, malignancies, alcoholism, steroid exposure)
  - Peripheral vascular disease
  - Inadequate tissue perfusion
- Precipitating risk factors:
  - Intravenous drug abuse
  - Trauma
  - Burns
  - Skin ulceration
  - Herpes zoster
- Prior surgical procedures
- Risk factors with patient undergoing surgical procedures includes:
  - Prior operations
  - Duration of operation
  - Hypoalbuminemia
  - History of chronic obstructive pulmonary disease

GENERAL PREVENTION

- Avoid tight orthopedic casts.
- Routine surgical principles for surgical procedures and skin closure (2)

ETIOLOGY

Most commonly due to polymicrobial infection, including both aerobic and anaerobic bacteria. Bacteria extend from subcutaneous tissue and proliferate along fascial planes. Bacterial toxins and surface proteins facilitate this process and can cause systemic toxicity with serious consequences (such as septic shock).

DIAGNOSIS

HISTORY

- Symptoms of malaise, anorexia, and fever progress rapidly over hours; rare cases with slower evolution over days.
- Some cases arise from previous trauma or infection (surgical wound from open or laparoscopic procedure, ulcers, burns, IV drug injection site, abscess).
- In >20%, a precipitant is never identified.
- Given the significant risk of delayed diagnosis, keep high index of suspicion if suggestive history but no clear risk factors (1)[B].

PHYSICAL EXAM

- The diagnosis of necrotizing fasciitis is made clinically. A high index of suspicion is necessary to make the diagnosis (1)[B].
- Not uncommonly, patients report pain out of proportion to physical exam.
- Fever, often low-grade early in the disease
- Tachycardia
- Hypotension
- Diaphoresis
- Foul odor
- Rapidly spreading skin lesions
- Skin changes, including localized erythema or discoloration, bullae, vesicles, ulceration, necrosis, edema
- Crepitus
- Bacterial toxins may trigger an inflammatory response leading to multiorgan failure or sepsis; in some advanced cases, this may be the presenting concern and necrotizing infection may not be immediately apparent.

DIAGNOSTIC TESTS & INTERPRETATION

Lab

- Hyponatremia, leukocytosis, anemia, hypocalcemia, acidosis, prolonged prothrombin time, elevated creatine kinase and serum glucose level
- Elevated liver function tests may result from release of bacterial toxins.
- Renal dysfunction may occur secondary to hypotension and myoglobinuria.
- Cultures and sensitivities are not diagnostic, but may be used to narrow initial broad-spectrum antibiotic treatment.
- Commonly associated pathogens:
  - Gram-positive anaerobes:
    - Cocci: Group A streptococci, *Peptostreptococcus* (anaerobic *Streptococcus*), or *Staphylococcus aureus*
    - Bacilli: *Clostridium perfringens* and other clostridia
  - Gram-negative aerobes: Bacilli: *Escherichia coli*, *Klebsiella pneumoniae, Enterobacter, Proteus*
- Gram-negative anaerobes: Bacilli: *Bacteroides fragilis* (usually with other gram-negative bacilli)
- Recently reported in salt water contaminated with *Vibrio* species (3)
- In the Far East, the Laboratory Risk Indicator for Necrotizing Fasciitis scoring system has been useful and incorporated in the clinical practice of some centers (4).

ALERT

Antibiotics given before cultures are performed may alter lab results.

Imaging

- Plain radiographs may show subcutaneous air (a rare finding that is specific but not sensitive).
- Computed tomography may reveal soft tissue swelling and presence of gas in tissues.

Pathological Findings

- Only frozen-section biopsy of the fascia is diagnostic. However, treatment should not be delayed while awaiting biopsy.
- Soft tissue necrosis, with polymorphonuclear cells and vascular thrombosis

DIFFERENTIAL DIAGNOSIS

Other soft tissue infection, including abscess and postsurgical wound infection

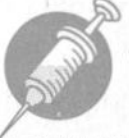

TREATMENT

MEDICATION

- Precautions: Without surgical debridement, antibiotics will not be effective (see General Measures).
- Important: Do not delay antibiotic treatment, even if smear, cultures, and tests are negative.
- Start with a broad-spectrum antibiotic regimen, then tailor antibiotics to organisms identified by blood and wound cultures and organism sensitivities (5)[B].
- Initial broad-spectrum coverage should include penicillin to cover *Streptococcus* and clindamycin, which works synergistically with penicillin when large bacterial load is present and also binds group A streptococci toxin.
- Aminoglycosides will cover enteric gram-negative organisms.
- Metronidazole is an alternative to clindamycin for treatment of anaerobic organisms.
- Retrospective studies suggest there may be a survival benefit with the use of IV immunoglobulin (IVIG) therapy. IVIG works by binding toxins and superantigens, which suppresses proinflammatory mediators (6)[B].

nlike *C. perfringens* and group A β-hemolytic treptococci, the *Aeromonas* sp. are uniformly esistant to penicillin-G, but are reported to be ighly sensitive to 3rd-generation cephalosporins.

DDITIONAL TREATMENT

eneral Measures

- rompt and wide surgical debridement is the ornerstone of treatment.
- nfectious disease consultation, if available
- yperbaric oxygen (HBO) is used as an adjunct to ntimicrobial agents and aggressive surgical ebridement. No survival benefit has been found.
- he results of studies on the use of HBO therapy in JF are inconsistent (7).
- o not delay surgical intervention for HBO.
- V fluids with electrolyte repletion, if indicated
- rophylaxis for tetanus

IRGERY/OTHER PROCEDURES

- Necrotizing soft tissue infections are a surgical mergency. Patients should be taken to the operating room as soon as the diagnosis is made or when there is high clinical suspicion.
- All necrotic tissue should be resected. Dissection hould be carried out along all involved fascial lanes. Adequate debridement should take priority over preservation of tissue.
- Limb amputation may be necessary because of extensive fascial and subcutaneous soft tissue necrosis and overwhelming systemic toxicity.
- Adequate surgical treatment can rarely be accomplished with a single operation. Repeated daily debridement may be necessary. Debridement should continue until all necrotic tissue is removed 8)[C].
- Negative-pressure suction dressing (i.e., vacuum assisted closure dressing) may be utilized to improve wound care and assist with postoperative fluid management.
- Reconstruction can be undertaken once systemic sepsis has been controlled and all nonviable tissue has been removed.

-PATIENT CONSIDERATIONS

ursing

- Following surgical debridement, patients often require intensive care unit (ICU) level of care.
- Close contacts of patients and health care workers do not require chemoprophylaxis with antibiotics 9)[B].

ONGOING CARE

DLLOW-UP RECOMMENDATIONS

atient Monitoring

- May require ICU-level critical care
- Diligence required to recognize spreading gangrene that would require repeated debridement
- As clinically indicated; may include following cultures, electrolytes, drug levels

IET

pends on clinical scenario; ranges from n.p.o. to et as tolerated

PROGNOSIS

- Mortality for necrotizing fasciitis ranges from 16–45%, and 1 publication has shown a decreased trend from nearly 28% in 1994 to 14% in 2002 (10).
- Increased mortality associated with age >60 years, male, IV drug abuse, malnutrition, significant medical comorbidities (e.g., cardiac or pulmonary disease), carcinoma, presence of bacteremia. Recent study suggests that Fournier's gangrene in females has an increased risk for mortality due in part to more aggressive inflammatory manifestations in the retroperitoneum and abdominal cavity (11).
- Independent predictors of mortality include:
  - Admission white blood cell count >30,000
  - Creatinine level >2 mg/dL within 48 hours of admission
  - Presence of clostridial infection
  - Presence of heart disease
- Independent predictors of limb loss include:
  - Shock (systolic pressure <90 mm) on admission
  - Clostridial infection
  - Presence of heart disease

COMPLICATIONS

- Tissue and functional losses
- Amputation
- Septic shock
- Death
- Physiologic derangement, as estimated by the Acute Physiology and Chronic Health Evaluation II score, is predictive of death (12)[B].

REFERENCES

1. Anaya DA, Dellinger EP. Necrotizing soft-tissue infection: diagnosis and management. *Clin Infect Dis*. 2007;44:705–10.
2. Kirby JP, Mazuski JE. Prevention of surgical site infection. *Surg Clin North Am*. 2009;89:365–89.
3. Tsai YH, Huang TJ, Hsu RW et al. Necrotizing soft-tissue infections and primary sepsis caused by Vibrio vulnificus and Vibrio cholerae non-O1. *J Trauma*. 2009;66:899–905.
4. Su YC, Chen HW, Hong YC, Chen CT, Hsiao CT, Chen IC et al. Laboratory risk indicator for necrotizing fasciitis score and the outcomes. *ANZ J Surg*. 2008;78:968-72
5. Dellinger RP, Carlet JM, Masur H et al. Surviving Sepsis Campaign guidelines for management of severe sepsis and septic shock. *Crit Care Med*. 2004;32:858–73.
6. Norrby-Telund A, et al. Group A streptococcal toxic syndrome and necrotizing fasciitis. *Curr Treat Opt Infect Dis*. 2003;5:419–29.
7. Jallali N, Withey S, Butler PE. Hyperbaric oxygen as adjuvant therapy in the management of necrotizing fasciitis. *Am J Surg*. 2005;189:462–6.
8. Marshall JC, Maier RV, Jimenez M et al. Source control in the management of severe sepsis and septic shock: an evidence-based review. *Crit Care Med*. 2004;32:S513–26.
9. Smith A. Invasive group A streptococcal disease: Should close contacts routinely receive antibiotic prophylaxis? *Lancet Inf Dis*. 2005;5:494–500.
10. Anaya DA, McMahon K, Nathens AB et al. Predictors of mortality and limb loss in necrotizing soft tissue infections. *Arch Surg*. 2005;140: 151–7; discussion 158.
11. Czymek R, Frank P, Limmer S, Schmidt A, Jungbluth T, Roblick U, Bürk C, Bruch HP, Kujath P et al. Fournier's gangrene: is the female gender a risk factor? *Langenbecks Arch Surg*. 2010;395: 173–80.
12. Gunter OL, Guillamondegui OD, May AK et al. Outcome of necrotizing skin and soft tissue infections. *Surg Infect (Larchmt)*. 2008;9:443–50.
13. Malangoni MA. Timing is everything. *Ann Surg*. 2009;250:17–8.
14. Steinberg JP, Braun BI, Hellinger WC et al. Timing of antimicrobial prophylaxis and the risk of surgical site infections: results from the Trial to Reduce Antimicrobial Prophylaxis Errors. *Ann Surg*. 2009;250:10–6.

ADDITIONAL READING

- de Lissovoy G, Fraeman K, Hutchins V et al. Surgical site infection: incidence and impact on hospital utilization and treatment costs. *Am J Infect Control*. 2009;37:387–97.
- Morgan MS et al. Diagnosis and management of necrotising fasciitis: a multiparametric approach. *The Journal of hospital infection*. 2010.

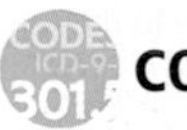

CODES

ICD9

- 041.84 Other specified bacterial infections in conditions classified elsewhere and of unspecified site, other anaerobes
- 728.86 Necrotizing fasciitis
- 785.4 Gangrene

CLINICAL PEARLS

- A necrotizing infection is a potentially life-threatening condition consisting of a soft tissue infection with rapidly progressive, widespread fascial necrosis.
- The symptom most commonly associated with necrotizing soft tissue infection is pain out of proportion to the physical exam.
- Necrotizing fasciitis may be an infection of 1 species of bacteria or may be polymicrobial.
- Prompt diagnosis and treatment are essential (13).
- Surgical debridement and antibiotic therapy are the primary treatment options.
- Be aware of antibiotic-resistant organisms (13,14).

ANAL FISSURE

Michael Rousse, MD, MPH

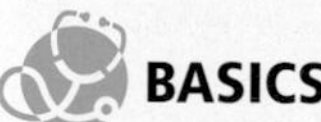

BASICS

DESCRIPTION

Anal fissure is a benign anorectal disease characterized by a knifelike tearing sensation on defecation. An anal fissure is a tear in the lining of the anal canal distal to the dentate line, most commonly in the posterior midline.

EPIDEMIOLOGY

Very common anorectal condition often confused with hemorrhoids

Incidence

Exact incidence is unknown. Patients often treat with home remedies and do not seek medical care.

ALERT

- Common in infants 6–24 months; not common in children; suspect abuse or trauma. Elderly are spared owing to lower resting pressure in the anal canal.
- Predominant sex: Male = Female, but women are more likely to get anterior midline tears (25% vs 8%).

Prevalence

- 80% of infants, usually self-limited
- 20% of adults, the majority of whom do not seek medical advice, have symptoms referable to the anorectum.

RISK FACTORS

Constipation, passage of hard or large-caliber stool, high resting tone of internal anal sphincter (prolonged sitting), trauma (anal sex), inflammatory bowel disease (Crohn's disease), syphilis, tuberculosis

Genetics

None known

GENERAL PREVENTION

Avoid constipation and prolonged sitting on toilet.

PATHOPHYSIOLOGY

High resting pressure within the anal canal can lead to ischemia of the anodermal tissues resulting in splitting of the tissues with passage of stool. Exposed internal sphincter muscle spasms causing the knifelike pain.

ETIOLOGY

Splitting of susceptible anodermal tissue

COMMONLY ASSOCIATED CONDITIONS

Constipation, Crohn's disease, tuberculosis, leukemia, and HIV

DIAGNOSIS

HISTORY

Severe rectal pain, often with and following defecation, but can be continuous; some will see bright red blood on the stool or when wiping. Occasionally, itch or perianal irritation is the presenting sign.

PHYSICAL EXAM

Gentle spreading of the buttocks will reveal a tear in the anodermal tissue, typically posterior midline, occasionally anterior midline, rarely eccentric to midline. Minimal swelling or bleeding. Hypertrophic papillae (*sentinel tag*) is seen in chronic fissure.

DIAGNOSTIC TESTS & INTERPRETATION

Diagnostic Procedures/Surgery

- Avoid anoscopy or endoscopy initially unless necessary for other diagnoses.
- Some patients may require exam under anesthesia to diagnose properly.

DIFFERENTIAL DIAGNOSIS

- Thrombosed external hemorrhoid: Swollen, painf[ul] mass; no fissure
- Perirectal abscess: Sinus tract with purulent drainage rather than a fissure
- Pruritus ani: Shallow excoriations rather than a fissure

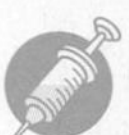

TREATMENT

The goal of treatment is to avoid repeated tearing o[f] the anal mucosa with resultant spasm of the intern[al] anal sphincter.

MEDICATION

First Line

- Stool softeners (docusate)
- Fiber supplements (psyllium)
- Topical analgesics (2% lidocaine gel)
- Warm sitz baths

Second Line

- Topical nitroglycerin ointment 2% diluted to 0.2% applied q.i.d., marginally but significantly better than placebo in healing (48.6% vs 37%), late recurrence was common (50%) (1)[A]; effect is to reduce resting anal pressure through the release [of] nitric oxide (2)[B]
- Calcium channel blockers (e.g., nifedipine, diltiazem), oral or topical; no better than nitrates but with fewer side effects (1)[A]; effect is to rela[x] the internal sphincter muscle, thereby reducing th[e] resting anal pressure (3)[B]
- Botulinum toxin 4 mL injected into the internal sphincter muscle; no better than topical nitrates but with fewer side effects (1)[A]; effect is to inhibit the release of acetylcholine from nerve endings to inhibit muscle spasm (3)[B]

DDITIONAL TREATMENT

eneral Measures

ash area with warm water; high-fiber diet; avoid nstipation

sues for Referral

- ate recurrence is common (50%).
- Medical therapy usually is tried for 90–120 days before referral (4)[B].

JRGERY/OTHER PROCEDURES

- Reserved for failure of medical therapy; involves division of the internal sphincter muscle
- Lateral internal sphincterectomy appears to be the surgical procedure of choice (5)[B].
- Risk for fecal incontinence: 45% short term, 6–8% long term (3)[C]
- Anal stretching/dilation: Unlikely to benefit (2)[C]

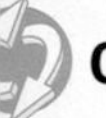

ONGOING CARE

IET

gh fiber

ATIENT EDUCATION

oid prolonged sitting during bowel movements; ink plenty of fluids; avoid constipation

PROGNOSIS

Medical therapy is less likely to be successful for chronic anal fissures; 40% failure rate (6)[A],(7)[B].

COMPLICATIONS

Fecal incontinence and incontinence to flatus; primarily associated with surgery (8)[B]

REFERENCES

1. Nelson RL. Non surgical therapy for anal fissure. *Cochrane Database of Systematic Reviews* 2006, Issue 4. Art. No.: CD003431. DOI:10.1002/14651858.CD003431.pub2.
2. Madoff RD, Fleshman JW. AGA Technical Review on the Diagnosis and Care of Patients with Anal Fissure. *Gastroenterology* 2003;124:235–245.
3. Breen E, Bleday R. *Anal Fissures*, Up To Date 18.1, updated Jan 29, 2010.
4. Essani R, Sarkisyan G, Beart RW, Ault G, Vukasin P, Kaiser AM et al. Cost-saving effect of treatment algorithm for chronic anal fissure: a prospective analysis. *J Gastrointest Surg*. 2005;9:-
5. Mousavi SR, Sharifi M, Mehdikhah Z et al. A comparison between the results of fissurectomy and lateral internal sphincterotomy in the surgical management of chronic anal fissure. *J Gastrointest Surg*. 2009;13:1279–82.
6. Shao WJ, Li GC, Zhang ZK et al. Systematic review and meta-analysis of randomized controlled trials comparing botulinum toxin injection with lateral internal sphincterotomy for chronic anal fissure. *Int J Colorectal Dis*. 2009;24:995–1000.
7. Mente BB, Irkörücü O, Akin M, Leventolu S, Tatliciolu E et al. Comparison of botulinum toxin injection and lateral internal sphincterotomy for the treatment of chronic anal fissure. *Dis Colon Rectum*. 2003;46:232–7.
8. Sileri P, Stolfi VM, Franceschilli L, Grande M, Di Giorgio A, D'Ugo S, Attina' G, D'Eletto M, Gaspari AL et al. Conservative and surgical treatment of chronic anal fissure: prospective longer term results. *J Gastrointest Surg*. 2010;14:773–80.

CODES

ICD9

565.0 Anal fissure

CLINICAL PEARLS

- Best chance to prevent recurrence is to avoid prolonged sitting on toilet and avoid constipation.
- No medical therapy approaches the cure rate of surgery.

ANAPHYLAXIS

Bobby X. Peters, MD

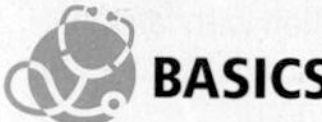

BASICS

DESCRIPTION

- An IgE-mediated, acute systemic reaction following antigen exposure in a sensitized person
- A non–IgE-mediated idiopathic anaphylactoid reaction also may occur. Anaphylactoid reactions are clinically indistinguishable from anaphylaxis and are treated in the same manner.
- System(s) affected: Cardiovascular; Endocrine/Metabolic; Gastrointestinal; Hematologic/Lymphatic/Immunologic; Pulmonary; and Skin/Exocrine
- Synonym(s): Anaphylactoid reactions

EPIDEMIOLOGY

- Predominant age: All ages
- Predominant sex: Male = Female

Incidence

- Up to 40,000 cases of idiopathic anaphylaxis with no identifiable cause occur each year.
- Drug-induced anaphylaxis occurs in 1/2,700 hospitalized patients.
- Anaphylaxis deaths: 0.3–0.7/100,000 per year
- Food allergic reactions constitute 1/3 to 1/2 of all anaphylactic reactions worldwide.
- Anaphylaxis may occur secondary to allergy skin testing.
- Asthmatics are more prone to anaphylaxis than nonasthmatics. Female asthmatics are at greater risk of anaphylaxis than their male counterparts.

RISK FACTORS

- Previous anaphylaxis
- History of atopy or asthma

Genetics

Genetic predisposition for sensitization to antigens

GENERAL PREVENTION

- Avoid inducing drugs and foods.
- Carry a prefilled epinephrine syringe. Keep a syringe at home, work/school, and in vehicle, although syringe should be protected from temperature extremes.
- Avoid areas where insect exposure is likely. Avoid wearing insect attractants (e.g., perfumes, colored clothing); avoid bare feet outdoors.
- Carry or wear a medical alert ID about the anaphylaxis-causing substance or event.
- When radiologic contrast is unavoidable, use of low osmolar contrast agents (e.g., iothalamate) reduces the risk of contrast reactions to 3.1%:
  - Only 0.22% were considered severe.
  - Stop beta blockers before administering contrast materials.
  - Pretreat with diphenhydramine (50 mg IV) and a steroid (e.g., methylprednisolone 60 mg IV q6h) until procedure. Start methylprednisolone the day before the procedure is scheduled.
  - Those with frequent (>6 per year) episodes of idiopathic anaphylaxis should be treated prophylactically with prednisone (40–60 mg/d in a single morning dose), hydroxyzine (25 mg tid), and albuterol (2 mg PO tid). The prednisone should be rapidly tapered to an every-other-day regimen.

ALERT

- Have a latex-free kit (gloves, etc.) available for the treatment of latex-allergic patients. Some latex-allergic patients will react to tropical fruits, such as kiwi, bananas, avocados, and chestnuts.
- Avoid beta-blockers.

ETIOLOGY

- IgE-mediated mast cell degranulation
- Complement activation (C3a, C4a, C5a) by antigen–antibody complexes that contain complement-fixing antibodies
- Other non–IgE-dependent anaphylaxis-like syndromes may be caused by modulators of arachidonic acid metabolism, sulfiting agents, exercise-induced anaphylaxis, and idiopathic recurrent anaphylaxis.
- Some important causes of anaphylaxis are:
  - Antimicrobials (e.g., penicillin)
  - Blood products (especially in IgA deficiency)
  - Iodinated contrast media
  - Ethylene oxide gas (dialysis tubing, other sterilized products)
  - Exercise
  - Foods (commonly, peanuts, nuts, fish, crustaceans, mollusks, cow's milk, eggs, and soy)
  - Immunotherapy
  - Insect stings (e.g., honeybees, wasps, kissing bugs, and deer flies)
  - Latex rubber (gloves, catheters)
  - Macromolecules (e.g., chymopapain, insulin, dextran, glucocorticoid, and protamine)
  - Vaccines

COMMONLY ASSOCIATED CONDITIONS

- Asthma
- Atopy

DIAGNOSIS

HISTORY

Rapid progression within minutes to hours of the signs and symptoms of anaphylaxis, with or without an obvious trigger, including but not limited to: Cutaneous symptoms (90% of cases), respiratory symptoms (70%), gastrointestinal symptoms (40%), and cardiovascular symptoms (35%)

PHYSICAL EXAM

- Pruritus, flushing, urticaria, angioedema
- Dyspnea, cough, rhonchi
- Rhinorrhea, bronchorrhea, wheezing, stridor
- Difficulty swallowing
- Nausea, vomiting, diarrhea, cramps, bloating
- Tachycardia, hypotension, shock, syncope
- Malaise, shivering
- Mydriasis

DIAGNOSTIC TESTS & INTERPRETATION

Lab

- Hypoxemia, hypercarbia, acidosis
- Acidosis may cause apparent hyperkalemia by moving potassium extracellularly
- Elevated serum tryptase, a mast cell enzyme for allergic and anaphylactic reactions (1)[B]
- Drugs that may alter lab results: Epinephrine and albuterol may cause apparent hypokalemia by shifting K+ intracellularly.

DIFFERENTIAL DIAGNOSIS

- Anaphylactoid reactions:
  - May occur after the 1st contact with substance such as polymyxin, pentamidine, radiographic contrast media, and aspirin
- Carcinoid syndrome
- Globus hystericus:
  - May mimic pharyngeal edema
- Hereditary angioedema:
  - C1q esterase deficiency with painless, pruritus-free angioedema without urticaria, flushing, or wheezing
- Pheochromocytoma:
  - Paradoxically, because of beta-2 stimulation, some patients have hypotensive attacks accompanied by tachycardia.
  - Urticaria, angioedema, and wheezing are absent
- Pseudoanaphylactic reaction:
  - After injection of procaine penicillin
    - Is a drug effect of procaine and not a penicillin allergy
- Scombroid poisoning:
  - From ingestion of dark meat fish (e.g., tuna, mackerel, and mahi-mahi)
  - Histamine-like mediator: Symptoms include flushing, sweating, nausea, vomiting, diarrhea, headache, palpitations, dizziness, rash, swelling of face and tongue, respiratory distress, and vasodilatory shock.
- Serum sickness:
  - Occurs several days after exposure
- Systemic mastocytosis:
  - Benign or malignant overgrowth of mast cells
  - Urticaria pigmentosa seen in the benign form and the presence of reddish-brown macular–papular cutaneous lesions, which urticate after trauma (Darier sign)
- Vasovagal reactions:
  - Bradycardia and hypotension without tachycardia, flushing, urticaria, angioedema, pruritus, and wheezing
- Pulmonary embolism, foreign body aspiration, and arrhythmia

TREATMENT

EDICATION

rst Line

:pinephrine:
- Less severe reaction: 0.3–0.5 mg (0.01 mg/kg in children) = (0.3–0.5 mL of a 1:1,000 solution, 0.01 mL/kg in children), SQ q20–30min as needed, up to 3 doses
- Life-threatening reactions: 0.5 mg (5 mL of a 1:10,000 solution) (for children: 0.05–0.1 mL/kg per dose) given intravenously, slowly: q5–10min as needed. If IV access is not possible, endotracheal or intraosseous may be effective.

)iphenhydramine: (SOR Grade A) an H_1 blocker: 25–50 mg intravenously (IM or PO:) q6h for 72 hours (children 1.25 mg/kg to 25 mg)

Cimetidine: an H_2 blocker: 300 mg IV over 3–5 minutes (children 5–10 mg/kg per dose) and then 400 mg PO bid is helpful and may be more effective than diphenhydramine.

Corticosteroids: No immediate effect and unclear if they prevent recurrence:
- Hydrocortisone sodium succinate: 250–500 mg IV q4–6h (4–8 mg/kg for children)
- Prednisone: 1 mg/kg in children, up to 60 mg
- Methylprednisolone: 60–125 mg IV in adults (1–2 mg/kg in children)

Bronchodilator, if persistent bronchospasm:
- Inhaled beta-2 agonists. Continuous nebulized albuterol of 10 mg/hour or 2.5 mg q15–20min is safe, effective, and preferable to aminophylline as a first line.

Laryngeal edema:
- Epinephrine: 5 mL 1:1,000 by nebulizer is more effective than racemic epinephrine and is usually available.

Persistent hypotension:
- Dopamine: 200 mg in 500 mL of dextrose in water given by infusion pump; titrate to BP (3–20 mcg/kg/min)
- Glucagon: May be beneficial for resistant hypotension caused by concurrent beta blockade therapy; 50 mcg/kg IV bolus over 1 min, or alternatively, give as continuous infusion at 5–15 mcg/min

Normal saline or Ringer's lactate: As necessary to maintain tissue perfusion

Oral antihistamines and steroids for 72 hours

eriatric Considerations

oinephrine may induce myocardial ischemia in those ith cardiac disease, but is the drug of choice. Be alert r anticholinergic and CNS side effects after giving phenhydramine or cimetidine.

ediatric Considerations

oinephrine could reduce the placental blood flow, but ay save the life of the mother and fetus. It also creases risk of congenital malformation.

econd Line

Several reports of tranexamic acid: 1,000 mg IV or sigma-aminocaproic acid for refractory anaphylaxis These drugs are not standard care; use only in patients who do not respond to other therapy.

Aminophylline: 5–6 mg/kg IV in 100 cc D_5W over 20 min, then maintenance at 1 mg/kg/h drip

- Anti-IgE monoclonal antibody may have a role in long-term management of food-induced anaphylaxis.
- Venom immunotherapy has been effective in the prevention of sting anaphylaxis, but with a high side-effect risk (2)[A].

ADDITIONAL TREATMENT

General Measures

- Treatment depends on severity
- Maintain a patent airway:
  - Endotracheal intubation and assisted ventilation may be necessary.
  - Possibly tracheostomy or needle cricothyrotomy in children <12 years
- Oxygen
- IV fluids (normal saline/lactated Ringer's)

Issues for Referral

- Allergist referral if anaphylaxis cause unclear
- Patients with anaphylaxis from insect stings benefit from desensitization immunotherapy.

IN-PATIENT CONSIDERATIONS

Admission Criteria

Moderate–severe anaphylaxis, admit for observation.

Discharge Criteria

Outpatient: Patients with cutaneous angioedema, urticaria, and minimal bronchospasm may be released when symptoms and signs have cleared.

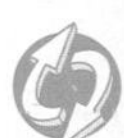

ONGOING CARE

FOLLOW-UP RECOMMENDATIONS

Bedrest until anaphylaxis clears and patient is hemodynamically stable

DIET

NPO until acute symptoms are controlled

PATIENT EDUCATION

- Asthma and Allergy Foundation of America, 1717 Massachusetts Avenue, Suite 305, Washington, DC 20036; (800)-7-ASTHMA or American Allergy Association, P.O. Box 7273, Menlo Park, CA 94026, (415) 322-1663
- Medic-Alert–type tags (Medic-Alert Foundation, Turlock, CA 95381-1009)
- Avoid beta-blockers, if possible.
- Instruct patient in the use of the bee sting kit.

PROGNOSIS

- Good prognosis if treated immediately; worse outcome with a delay of >30 minutes in administration of epinephrine.
- Of those with idiopathic anaphylaxis, 60% are free of anaphylactic episodes at 2.5 years; most others are steroid-free.

COMPLICATIONS

- Hypoxemia
- Cardiac arrest
- Death

REFERENCES

1. Brown SG, Blackman KE, Heddle RJ. Can serum mast cell tryptase help diagnose anaphylaxis? *EMA*. 2004;2:120–4.
2. Brown SG, Wiese MD, Blackman KE, Heddle RJ. Ant venom immunotherapy: A double-blind, placebo-controlled, crossover trial. *Lancet*. 2003;(361)9362:1001–6.

ADDITIONAL READING

- Arias K, Waserman S, Jordana M. Management of food-induced anaphylaxis: unsolved challenges. *Curr Clin Pharmacol* 2009;4(2):113–25.
- González-Pérez A, Aponte Z, Vidaurre CF, Rodríguez LA et al. Anaphylaxis epidemiology in patients with and without asthma: A United Kingdom database review. *The Journal of allergy and clinical immunology*. 2010;
- Pitsios C, Dimitriou A, Stefanaki EC, Kontou-Fili K et al. Anaphylaxis during skin testing with food allergens in children. *Eur J Pediatr*. 2010;169: 613–5.
- Sheikh A, Shehata YA, Brown SGA, Simons FER. Adrenaline (epinephrine) for the treatment of anaphylaxis with and without shock. *Cochrane Database of Systematic Reviews* 2008, Issue 4. Art. No.: CD006312. DOI:10.1002/14651858. CD006312.pub2.
- Sheikh A, ten Broek VM, Brown SGA, Simons FER. H1-antihistamines for the treatment of anaphylaxis with and without shock. *Cochrane Database of Systematic Reviews* 2007, Issue 1. Art. No.: CD006160. DOI:10.1002/14651858. CD006160.pub2.
- Tanus T, Mines D, Atkins PC et al. Serum tryptase in idiopathic anaphylaxis: a case report and review of the literature. *Ann Emerg Med*. 1994;24:104–7.
- Wittbrodt ET, Spinler A. Prevention of anaphylactoid reactions in high-risk patients receiving radiographic contrast media. *Ann Pharmacother*. 1994;28: 236–41.

See Also (Topic, Algorithm, Electronic Media Element)

Food Allergy; Insect Bites; Stings

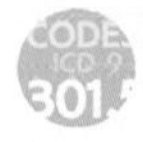

CODES

ICD9

- 989.5 Toxic effect of venom
- 995.0 Other anaphylactic shock, not elsewhere classified
- 995.60 Anaphylactic shock due to unspecified food

CLINICAL PEARLS

- Allergy to one species of legume (e.g., peanuts) or one type of seafood (e.g., shrimp) doesn't mean allergy to all products in that category. Skin testing is prudent.
- MMR vaccine can be safely administered to those with a history of egg allergy; most egg allergies are related to the albumin.
- Penicillin-allergic patients can generally tolerate 2nd- and 3rd-generation cephalosporins as well as monobactams (e.g., aztreonam). Generally, they will be allergic to carbapenems (e.g., imipenem) and 1st-generation cephalosporins.
- IgA-deficient patients should have washed red blood cells for transfusion.
- Those allergic to seafood are not allergic to iodine-based radiocontrast. Shellfish allergy is protein related.

ANEMIA, APLASTIC

Kerri Keslow, MD
Daniel T. Lee, MD

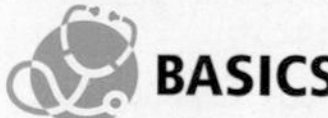

BASICS

DESCRIPTION

- Aplastic anemia is defined as pancytopenia in the setting of a hypocellular bone marrow without the presence of infiltrates or fibrosis. There are two forms: Acquired (much more common) and congenital.
- Acquired aplastic anemia has an insidious onset and is caused by an exogenous insult triggering an autoimmune reaction. This form is usually responsive to immunosuppressive agents.
- The congenital forms are rare and occur mostly in childhood. The exception is an atypical presentation of Fanconi syndrome later in adult life, into the 30s for males and up to age 48 years in females.
- The identification of specific mutations in genes of the telomere complex in patients with acquired aplastic anemia has blurred the distinction between the congenital and acquired forms.
- System(s) affected: Heme/Lymphatic/Immunologic
- Synonym(s): Hypoplastic anemia; panmyelophthisis; refractory anemia; aleukia hemorrhagica; toxic paralytic anemia

ALERT

- Early intervention for aplastic anemia greatly improves the chances of treatment success.
- Hematopoietic growth factors should not be used without close supervision in newly diagnosed patients.

Geriatric Considerations

The elderly are often exposed to large numbers of drugs and, therefore, may be more susceptible to acquired aplastic anemia.

Pediatric Considerations

- Congenital forms of aplastic anemia require different treatment regimens than the acquired forms.
- Acquired aplastic anemia is seen in children exposed to ionizing radiation or treated with cytotoxic chemotherapeutic agents.

Pregnancy Considerations

- Pregnancy appears to be a real but rare cause of aplastic anemia. Symptoms may resolve after delivery and have been shown to disappear with pregnancy termination.
- Complications in pregnant patients appear to be more likely with low platelet counts and paroxysmal nocturnal hemoglobinuria-associated aplastic anemia.

EPIDEMIOLOGY

- Predominant age: Biphasic 15–25 (more common) and over 60
- Predominant sex: Male = Female

Incidence

- 2–3 new cases per million per year in Europe and North America
- The incidence is 3-fold higher in Thailand and China, when compared to the Western world.

RISK FACTORS

- Treatment with high-dose radiation or chemotherapy
- Exposure to toxic chemicals
- Use of certain medications
- Certain blood diseases, autoimmune disorders, and serious infections
- Tumors of thymus (red cell aplasia)
- Pregnancy, rarely

Genetics

- Telomerase mutations have been found in a small number of patients with acquired and congenital forms. These mutations render carriers more susceptible to environmental insults.
- Mutations in genes called TERC and TERT were found in pedigrees of adults with acquired aplastic anemia who lacked the physical abnormalities or a family history typical of inherited forms of bone marrow failure. These genes encode for the RNA component of telomerase.
- HLA-DR2 is twice as frequent as in the normal population.

GENERAL PREVENTION

- Avoid possible toxic industrial agents.
- Use safety measures when working with radiation.

PATHOPHYSIOLOGY

- The immune hypothesis describes immune suppression through the activation of T cells with associated cytokine production leading to the destruction or injury of the hematopoietic stem cells. This leads to a hypocellular bone marrow in the absence of marrow fibrosis.
- The activation of T cells likely occurs because of both genetic and environmental factors. Exposure to specific environmental precipitants, diverse host genetic risk factors, and individual differences in the characteristics of the immune response likely account for variations in its clinical manifestations and patterns of responsiveness to treatment.
- Telomerase deficiency leads to short telomeres and a quantitative reduction in marrow progenitors and likely a qualitative deficiency in the repair capacity of hematopoietic tissue.
- Reduction of natural killer T cells in the bone marrow

ETIOLOGY

- Idiopathic (~70% of the cases)
- Drugs: Phenylbutazone, chloramphenicol, sulfonamides, gold, cytotoxic drugs, antiepileptics (felbamate, carbamazepine, valproic acid, phenytoin)
- Viral: HIV, Epstein-Barr virus (EBV), nontypeable postinfectious hepatitis (not A, B, or C), parvovirus B19 (mostly in the immunocompromised), atypical mycobacterium
- Toxic exposure (benzene, pesticides, arsenic)
- Radiation exposure
- Immune disorders (systemic lupus erythematosus, eosinophilic fascitis, graft-vs-host disease)
- Pregnancy (rare)
- Congenital (Fanconi anemia, dyskeratosis congenita, Shwachman-Diamond syndrome, amegakaryocytic thrombocytopenia)

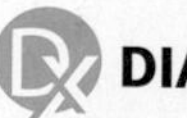

DIAGNOSIS

HISTORY

- Detailed solvent and radiation history, as well as family, environmental, travel, and infectious disea[se] history
- Patients are often asymptomatic but may complai[n] of frequent infections, fatigue, or bleeding.

PHYSICAL EXAM

- Mucosal hemorrhage, petechiae
- Pallor
- Fever
- Hemorrhage, menorrhagia, occult stool blood, melena, epistaxis
- Dyspnea
- Palpitations
- Progressive weakness
- Retinal flame hemorrhages
- Systolic ejection murmur
- Weight loss
- Signs of congenital aplastic anemia:
  - Short stature
  - Microcephaly
  - Nail dystrophy
  - Abnormal thumbs
  - Oral leukoplakia
  - Hyperpigmentation (café au lait spots) or hypopigmentation

DIAGNOSTIC TESTS & INTERPRETATION

Screening tests to exclude other etiologies:

- Complete blood count (CBC) and reticulocyte cour[nt]
- Blood smear exam
- Cytogenetic studies of peripheral lymphocytes if <35 to exclude Fanconi anemia
- Liver function test
- Viral serology: Hepatitis A, B, C; EBV; cytomegalovirus (CMV); HIV
- Vitamin B_{12} and folate levels
- Autoantibody screening ANA and anti-DNA
- Flow cytometry or Ham test for paroxysmal nocturnal hemoglobinuria
- Fetal hemoglobin in children
- Red cell adenosine deaminase (pure red cell aplasi[a])
- Cytogenetic analysis of bone marrow

Lab

- CBC: Pancytopenia, anemia (usually normocytic), leucopenia, neutropenia, thrombocytopenia
- Decreased absolute number of reticulocytes
- Increased serum iron secondary to transfusion
- Normal total iron binding capacity (TIBC)
- High mean corpuscular volume (MCV) >104
- CD 34+ cells decreased in blood and marrow
- Urinalysis: Hematuria
- Abnormal liver function tests (hepatitis)
- Increased fetal hemoglobin (Fanconi)
- Increased chromosomal breaks under specialized conditions (Fanconi)
- Molecular determination of abnormal gene (Fancon[i])

aging
:omputed tomography (CT) of thymus region if
hymoma-associated red blood cell (RBC) aplasia
uspected
ladiographs of radius and thumbs (congenital
nemia)
lenal ultrasound (to rule out congenital anemia or
nalignant hematologic disorder)
:hest x-ray to exclude infections such as
nycobacterial

agnostic Procedures/Surgery
ne marrow aspiration

thological Findings
Normochromic RBC
Bone marrow:
- Decreased cellularity (<10%): No fibrosis, no malignant cells seen
- Decreased megakaryocytes
- Decreased myelocytes
- Decreased erythroid precursors
- Prominent fat spaces and marrow stroma

FFERENTIAL DIAGNOSIS
:ludes other causes of bone marrow failure and
ncytopenia:
Marrow replacement:
- Acute lymphoblastic leukemia
- Lymphoma
- Hairy cell leukemia (increased reticulin and infiltration of hairy cells)
- Large granular lymphocyte leukemia
- Fibrosis

Megaloblastic hematopoiesis:
- Folate deficiency
- Vitamin B_{12} deficiency

Paroxysmal nocturnal hemoglobinuria, hemolytic anemia (dark urine), pancytopenia venous thrombosis (classically hepatic veins)
Systemic lupus erythematosus
Prolonged starvation or anorexia nervosa (bone marrow is gelatinous with loss of fat cells and increased ground substance)
Transient erythroblastopenia of childhood
Overwhelming infection:
- HIV with myelodysplasia
- Viral hemophagocytic syndrome

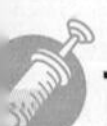

TREATMENT

rly treatment increases the chance of success. Two ajor treatment pathways: Immunosuppressive erapy and hematopoietic stem cell transplantation. eatment decisions are based on the age of the tient, the severity of the disease, and the availability an HLA-matched sibling donor for transplantation.

IEDICATION
nmunosuppressive therapy:
1st-line treatment is a combination of antithymocyte globulin (ATG) plus cyclosporine. ATG lyses lymphocytes, and cyclosporin blocks T cell function.
Antithymocyte globulin (ATG):
- A horse serum containing polyclonal antibodies against human T cells
- Treatment for patients >40 and patients without a compatible donor. Consider in patients 30–40.
- May be used as a single agent, but is more common in combination with cyclosporine

- Cyclosporine following initial ATG therapy for minimum of 6 months:
  - Monitor through blood levels. Normal values for assays vary.
- Granulocyte colony-stimulating factor (G-CSF):
  - Used in conjunction with ATG and cyclosporine
  - Shows faster neutrophil recovery, but survival is not improved
  - Treatment is costly and is disputed in two randomized trials.
- Note: Relapses may occur after the initial response to the immunosuppressive therapy if cyclosporine is discontinued too early.

ADDITIONAL TREATMENT

General Measures
- Supportive measures: RBC and platelet transfusions. Use only CMV-negative blood initially if patient is candidate for hematopoietic stem cell transplantation.
- Antibiotics, antifungals, antivirals when appropriate
- Oxygen therapy for severe anemia
- Good oral hygiene
- Control menorrhagia with norethisterone.
- Avoid causative agents/isolation if necessary.
- Human leukocyte antigen (HLA) testing on all patients and their immediate families
- Transfusion support (judiciously prescribed RBCs for severe anemia, consider leukocyte-depleted units; platelets for severe thrombocytopenia; white blood cells [WBCs]):
  - Transfuse when platelet count is $<10 \times 10^9$ or if $<20 \times 10^9$ with fever
- Immunosuppressive therapy (antithymocyte globulin [ATG] and cyclosporine) if no suitable donor

SURGERY/OTHER PROCEDURES
- Hematopoietic stem cell transplantation for patients with severe aplastic anemia and an HLA-identical donor, <30 years old. Consider in patients 30–40 in good general medical condition.
- Patients >45 have higher rates of graft-vs-host disease and graft rejection compared with children.
- Unrelated donor transplants, if other therapy fails and/or <16 without HLA-matched sibling
- Thymectomy for thymoma

IN-PATIENT CONSIDERATIONS

Initial Stabilization
Referral to an institution that has experience in treating these patients is recommended.

Nursing
If neutropenic, use antiseptic mouthwash such as chlorhexidine and give food low in bacterial content.

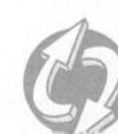

ONGOING CARE

FOLLOW-UP RECOMMENDATIONS
Activity: Isolation procedures if neutropenic

Patient Monitoring
Close monitoring for all treatments is recommended. Drugs and other forms of treatment have numerous and severe side effects.

DIET
If neutropenic, give food low in bacterial content.

PATIENT EDUCATION
Printed patient information available from Aplastic Anemia & MDS International Foundation, Inc., 800-747-2828. Web: www.aamds.org/aplastic

PROGNOSIS
- Hematopoietic stem cell transplantation with HLA-matched sibling:
  - Age <16, 91%
  - Age >16, 70–80%
- Immunosuppressive therapy using ATG and cyclosporine: Overall survival of 75%; 90% among responders at 5 years.

COMPLICATIONS
- Infection (fungal, sepsis)
- Graft-vs-host disease in bone marrow transplant recipients (acute 18%; chronic 26%)
- Side effects of immunosuppressant medications
- Hemorrhage
- Transfusion hemosiderosis
- Transfusion hepatitis
- Heart failure
- Development of secondary cancer: Leukemia or myelodysplasia (15–19% risk at 6–10 years)
- Refractory pancytopenia

ADDITIONAL READING

- Bacigalupo A, Passweg J. Diagnosis and Treatment of Acquired Aplastic Anemia. *Hematol Oncol Clin N Am*. 2009;23:159–70.
- Guinan EC. Acquired Aplastic Anemia in Childhood. *Hematol Oncol Clin N Am*. 2009;23:171–91.
- Rosenfeld S, Follman D, Nunez O, et al. Antithymocyte Globulin and Cyclosporine for Severe Aplastic Anemia: Association Between Hematologic Response and Long-term Outcome. *JAMA*. 2003; 289(9):1130–35.
- Scheinberg P, Wu CO, Nunez O, Young NS. Long-Term Outcome of Pediatric Patients with Severe Aplastic Anemia Treated with Antithymocyte Globulin and Cyclosporine. *J Pediatr*. 2008;153: 814–19.
- Young NS. Pathophysiologic Mechanisms in Acquired Aplastic Anemia. *Hematology*. 2006(1): 72–7.

See Also (Topic, Algorithm, Electronic Media Element)
Leukemia, Hairy Cell; Myelodysplastic Syndromes (MDS); Systemic Lupus Erythematosus
Algorithm: Anemia

CODES

ICD9
- 284.01 Constitutional red blood cell aplasia
- 284.89 Other specified aplastic anemias
- 284.9 Aplastic anemia, unspecified

CLINICAL PEARLS

- Acquired aplastic anemia has an insidious onset and is caused by an exogenous insult triggering an autoimmune reaction. This form is usually responsive to immunosuppressive agents.
- Immunosuppressive therapy using ATG and cyclosporine: Overall survival of 75%; 90% among responders at 5 years.

ANEMIA, AUTOIMMUNE HEMOLYTIC

Nathan T. Connell, MD

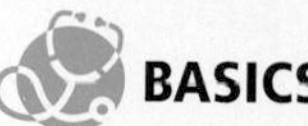

BASICS

DESCRIPTION

- Acquired anemia induced by antibodies binding to red blood cell (RBC) membrane antigens
- Three main types defined by maximal binding temperature of the autoantibodies:
  - Warm-reacting [37°C (98.6°F)] IgG antibody
  - Cold-reacting [0–4°C (32–39.2°F)] IgM antibody
  - Mixed type: Both warm-reacting IgG and cold-reacting C3 antibodies
- Drug-induced: Mostly warm-reacting IgG antibodies
- System(s) affected: Hematopoietic/Lymphatic/Immunologic

EPIDEMIOLOGY

Incidence

- Predominant age: <50 years
- Predominant sex: Female > Male
- Estimated incidence is 1/80,000 population per year (1).

RISK FACTORS

- Malignancy
- Autoimmune disorders
- Infection
- Medications
- Prior blood transfusion
- Prior hematopoietic cell transplant

Genetics

No known genetic predisposition

PATHOPHYSIOLOGY

- Warm autoimmune hemolytic anemia (AIHA): IgG attaches to erythrocytes, which are then ingested by macrophages of the spleen.
- Cold AIHA:
  - IgM binds erythrocyte surface temporarily, which then activates complement, causing deposition of C3 on cell surface. Erythrocytes then are ingested by macrophages of the liver.
  - Rarely, complete complement cascade is activated, with membrane attack complex insertion causing intravascular hemolysis.
- Mixed-antibody AIHA: Both warm IgG and cold C3 involved
- Drug-induced:
  - Hapten-induced: Drug attaches to erythrocyte membrane, inducing IgG production.
  - Immune complex: Drug–IgM immune complex binds erythrocyte membrane, activating complement.
  - Autoantibody: Drug induces production of anti-RBC IgG.

ETIOLOGY

- Warm antibody (48–70% cases):
  - Primary cause: Idiopathic
  - Secondary causes:
    - Lymphoproliferative disorders (chronic lymphocytic leukemia, Hodgkin disease, non-Hodgkin lymphoma)
    - Autoimmune disorders
    - Viral infection (especially in children)
- Cold antibody:
  - Cold agglutinin syndrome (CAS) (16–32%):
    - Acute: Infection (mycoplasma, mononucleosis, viral)
    - Chronic: Lymphoproliferative disorders (lymphoma) (2)
  - Paroxysmal cold hemoglobinuria: Infection
- Mixed type:
  - Idiopathic
  - Secondary to lymphoproliferative or autoimmune disorders
- Drug-induced:
  - Penicillin: Hapten-induced
  - Quinine: Immune complex
  - α-Methyldopa: Autoantibody-induced

COMMONLY ASSOCIATED CONDITIONS

- Evans syndrome (AIHA and idiopathic thrombocytopenic purpura)
- Systemic lupus erythematosus
- Chronic lymphocytic leukemia (CLL): AIHA is the most common autoimmune condition associated with CLL and occurs in 5–37% of patients with CLL (2,3).
- Diffuse lymphomas

DIAGNOSIS

HISTORY

- Weakness/fatigue
- Exertional dyspnea
- Dizziness
- Palpitations
- Malaise
- Association with cold (CAS)

PHYSICAL EXAM

- Pallor
- Jaundice
- Splenomegaly
- Hepatomegaly
- Tachycardia
- Flow murmur
- Blue-gray discoloration of acral surfaces (CAS)

DIAGNOSTIC TESTS & INTERPRETATION

Lab

Initial lab tests

- Direct Coombs [direct antiglobulin test (DAT)]: Positive test indicates presence of antibodies or complement on RBC surface.
- Complete blood count:
  - Anemia (normocytic, normochromic); may be sudden and life-threatening
  - Mild to moderate increase in mean corpuscular volume depending on level of reticulocytosis
  - Increased mean cell hemoglobin concentration
  - Spherocytosis
  - Poikilocytosis
  - Anisocytosis
  - Rouleaux
  - Reticulocytosis
  - Nucleated RBCs
  - Large polychromatophilic reticulocytes
- Hyperbilirubinemia (unconjugated)
- Decreased haptoglobin
- Elevated lactate dehydrogenase
- Hemoglobinemia
- Serology:
  - IgG antibody (warm, mixed, drug-induced, paroxysmal hemoglobinuria)
  - IgM antibody (cold)
- Urinalysis: Hemoglobinuria, hemosiderinuria

Pathological Findings

- Peripheral blood smear: Spherocytes, schistocytes
- Bone marrow biopsy: Bone marrow hyperplasia, increased marrow hemosiderin

DIFFERENTIAL DIAGNOSIS

- Other hemolytic anemias
- Evans syndrome
- Microangiopathic hemolytic disorders
- Aplastic anemia
- Megaloblastic anemia

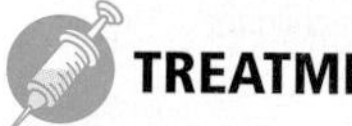

TREATMENT

MEDICATION

First Line

- Warm antibody:
  - Glucocorticoids: Prednisone 1 mg/kg/d PO in divided doses:
    - 70–80% patients improve within 3 weeks.
    - Taper gradually to 20 mg/d over 2 weeks.
    - May require maintenance dose of 10 mg every other day (4,5)
  - Precautions: Significant side effects with long-term use
- Cold antibody:
  - Malignancy-induced: Chemotherapy
  - Rituximab for cold AIHA owing to chronic lymphoproliferative disorders (3,4,5)[C]
- Mixed antibody: Prednisone as in warm AIHA

Second Line

- Warm antibody:
  - Immunosuppressive drugs: Recommended for patients who fail splenectomy, relapse after splenectomy, cannot tolerate corticosteroids, and nonsurgical candidates:
    - Cyclophosphamide 50 mg/kg/d × 4 days, followed by GCSF for those with refractory anemia (6)[C]
    - Precautions: Monitor for marrow suppression.
    - Azathioprine (Imuran) 1–2 mg/kg/d within 2 weeks of starting steroids if not responding (7)[C]
    - Cyclosporine 5–10 mg/kg/d in 2 divided doses
    - Rituximab (anti-CD20 monoclonal antibody) 375 mg/m^2 once weekly × 2–4 weeks for children and refractory cases (8)
    - Mycophenolate mofetil 500–1,000 mg/d in 2 divided doses; increase to 1–2 g daily (6)[C].
  - Other medical therapies for refractory cases:
    - Danazol 600–800 mg/d PO
    - Intravenous immunoglobulin (IVIG) (4)[C]
- Mixed antibody: Immunosuppressives if refractory to steroids and splenectomy

ADDITIONAL TREATMENT

General Measures

- Warm antibody:
  - Folic acid supplementation
  - Mild and moderate: See "Medication."
  - Severe:
    - Plasmapheresis as a temporizing measure for refractory or life-threatening anemia (4)[C]
    - Packed RBC transfusion for life-threatening anemia; difficult to cross-match; need special blood bank techniques; in emergency, use most compatible cross-match (6)[C].
- Cold antibody:
  - Cold agglutinin syndrome:
    - Avoid cold; maintain high temperatures indoors; wear additional clothing outdoors
    - Folic acid supplementation
    - Plasmapheresis as a temporizing measure for refractory or life-threatening anemia (9)[C]
    - Packed RBC transfusion for life-threatening anemia (6)[C]
- Paroxysmal cold hemoglobinuria: Supportive care
- Mixed: Steroids, splenectomy, and immunosuppressives as in warm AIHA
- Drug-induced:
  - Stop the offending drug.
  - Plasmapheresis/exchange transfusion for severe life-threatening cases

Issues for Referral

It is recommended that treatment be in consultation with an experienced hematologist.

SURGERY/OTHER PROCEDURES

- Warm antibody: Splenectomy is the preferred 2nd-line treatment for warm AIHA for those who have failed steroids.
  - 50% initial response rate
  - Patients may require low-dose maintenance prednisone <15 mg daily.
  - After splenectomy: Vaccinate against encapsulated organisms such as *Pneumonococcus* and *Meningococcus* (6)[A]. Patients who have had splenectomy are at increased risk for overwhelming postsplenectomy infection and should receive empirical antibiotics if they develop fever.
- Cold antibody: Surgery not recommended (3,9)
- Mixed antibody: Splenectomy

IN-PATIENT CONSIDERATIONS

Initial Stabilization

If patients start to develop symptoms related to the anemia (i.e., tachycardia, hypotension, chest pain, dyspnea), transfusion may be required.

Admission Criteria

Patients requiring plasmapheresis should be monitored in an ICU setting.

IV Fluids

Use only warmed IV fluids and blood products for cold AIHA in order to prevent further exacerbation of the condition.

ONGOING CARE

FOLLOW-UP RECOMMENDATIONS

Patient Monitoring

- Monitor carefully if a transfusion is essential.
- Use only warm IV fluids and blood products for cold AIHA.
- Avoid hypothermic surgical procedures for cold AIHA.
- Patients are at increased risk for venous thromboembolism, especially those with systemic lupus erythematosus. Consider prophylactic anticoagulation for patients at highest risk (i.e., those with other risk factors for venous thromboembolism, including immobilization, surgery, or concomitant malignancy) (10).

DIET

No special diet

PROGNOSIS

- Good with appropriate treatment
- Determined by course of the primary disease if secondary to an underlying disorder

COMPLICATIONS

- Shock (severe anemia)
- Venous thromboembolism
- Thrombocytopenic purpura (Evans syndrome)
- Lymphoproliferative disorders in warm AIHA
- Postsplenectomy sepsis syndrome

REFERENCES

1. Garratty G et al. Drug-induced immune hemolytic anemia. *Hematology Am Soc Hematol Educ Program*. 2009;73–9.
2. Zent CS, Ding W, Reinalda MS, Schwager SM, Hoyer JD, Bowen DA, Jelinek DF, Tschumper RC, Call TG, Shanafelt TD, Kay NE, Slager SL et al. Autoimmune cytopenia in chronic lymphocytic leukemia/small lymphocytic lymphoma: changes in clinical presentation and prognosis. *Leuk. Lymphoma*. 2009;50:1261–8.
3. Petz LD. Cold antibody autoimmune hemolytic anemias. *Blood Rev*. 2008;22:1–15.
4. Gehrs BC, Friedberg RC. Autoimmune hemolytic anemia. *Amer J Hematol*. 2002;69:258–71.
5. Dearden C et al. Disease-specific complications of chronic lymphocytic leukemia. *Hematology Am Soc Hematol Educ Program*. 2008;450–6.
6. King KE, Ness PM. Treatment of autoimmune hemolytic anemia. *Sem in Hematology*. 2005; 42:131–6.
7. Pruss A, Salama A, Ahrens N et al. Immune hemolysis-serological and clinical aspects. *Clin Exp Med*. 2003;3:55–64.
8. Bussone G, Ribeiro E, Dechartres A, Viallard JF, Bonnotte B, Fain O, Godeau B, Michel M et al. Efficacy and safety of rituximab in adults' warm antibody autoimmune haemolytic anemia: retrospective analysis of 27 cases. *Am J Hematol*. 2009;84:153–7.
9. Gertz MA et al. Management of cold haemolytic syndrome. *Br J Haematol*. 2007;138:422–9
10. Hoffman PC et al. Immune hemolytic anemia–selected topics. *Hematology Am Soc Hematol Educ Program*. 2006;13–8.

See Also (Topic, Algorithm, Electronic Media Element)

Lymphoma, Non-Hodgkin's; Leukemia; Systemic Lupus Erythematosus (SLE)
Algorithm: Anemia

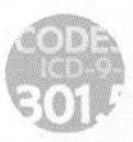

CODES

ICD9

283.0 Autoimmune hemolytic anemias

CLINICAL PEARLS

- Initial workup of suspected hemolytic anemia includes complete blood count, DAT, fractionated bilirubin, haptoglobin, lactate dehydrogenase, and urinalysis.
- It is important to distinguish between cold and warm antibody autoimmune hemolytic anemia because treatments are different.
- Have a low threshold to hospitalize patients or step up level of care to an ICU if indicated.
- Consultation with an experienced hematologist is recommended, especially for severe cases.

ANEMIA, CHRONIC DISEASE

Cheryl L. Gilmartin, PharmD
Claudia M. Lora, MD

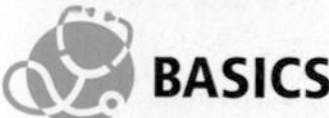

BASICS

DESCRIPTION

Anemia of chronic disease (ACD) is a normocytic, normochromic, hypoproliferative anemia associated with infectious, neoplastic, and inflammatory processes. The chronic immune activation accompanying these processes results in the production of inflammatory cytokines, which in turn create an anemic state by interfering with iron homeostasis and impairing erythropoiesis. ACD is the 2nd most common type of anemia and is the most common anemia found in hospitalized patients (1).

EPIDEMIOLOGY

Incidence

Incidence of anemia in cancer: 53.7% (2)

Prevalence

The estimated reports of ACD prevalence for individual conditions varies widely in the literature.

PATHOPHYSIOLOGY

Inflammatory cytokines (e.g., TNF-α, IFN-γ, IL-6) released by cells of the immune system in the setting of malignant, autoimmune, or infectious disease are the major mediators of anemia in ACD. They exert their effects in 3 main ways:

- Disrupted iron homeostasis:
  - Chronic inflammation, infection, malignancy → ↑ IFN-γ, LPS, TNF-α → ↑ iron uptake by and ↓ iron release from reticuloendothelial system (RES) cells → ↓ iron availability for heme biosynthesis and RBC production in the bone marrow
  - Chronic inflammation, infection, malignancy → ↑ IL-6, LPS → ↑ hepatocyte production of hepcidin, a major negative iron regulator → ↓ iron absorption in duodenum and ↓ iron release from RES cells → ↓ iron availability for RBC production
- Impaired erythropoiesis:
  - ↑ IFN-γ, TNF-α, IL-1 → down-regulation of erythropoietin (EPO) receptors on erythroid precursors, cytokine-induced apoptosis of erythroid precursors, ↓ hematopoietic growth factors in the marrow → impaired function, proliferation, and differentiation of erythroid cells → ↓ RBC production
  - ↑ IFN-γ, TNF-α, IL-1 → ↓ synthesis and diminished effect of EPO → ↓ RBC production
- RBC destruction:
  - ↑ TNF-α, IL-1 → ↑ phagocytosis of RBCs by RES cells → ↓ RBC half-life
  - ↑ IFN-γ, TNF-α, IL-1 → ↑ free radical formation → ↑ RBC destruction

ETIOLOGY

Inflammatory cytokines (e.g., TNF-α, IFN-γ, IL-6) released by cells of the immune system in the setting of infectious, inflammatory, or neoplastic diseases cause anemia by interfering with iron metabolism and RBC production.

COMMONLY ASSOCIATED CONDITIONS

- Autoimmune disease:
  - Rheumatoid arthritis
  - Systemic lupus erythematosus
  - Inflammatory bowel disease
  - Sarcoidosis
  - Vasculitis
- Infectious disease:
  - HIV and other viral infections
  - Chronic or subacute bacterial, fungal, parasitic infection
- Neoplastic disease:
  - Both solid and hematologic tumors
  - Chronic kidney disease
  - Chronic rejection post solid-organ transplantation

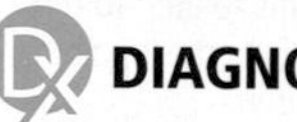

DIAGNOSIS

HISTORY

History or symptoms of an acute or chronic inflammatory, infectious, or neoplastic process and no clinical evidence for occult bleeding

PHYSICAL EXAM

Findings related to the underlying disease

DIAGNOSTIC TESTS & INTERPRETATION

Lab

Initial lab tests

- Hemoglobin: Mild (Hgb <10–12 g/dL) or moderate (Hgb 8–10 g/dL) or severe (Hgb <8 g/dL) anemia
- Reticulocyte production index: Inappropriately low or normal, <2%
- Absolute reticulocyte count: Low, <25,000/μL
- MCV: Normal, 80–100 fL (in the absence of coexistent additional cause of anemia)
- Peripheral smear: No evidence of other hematologic disorders
- Serum iron: Low (M: <65 μg/dL, F: <50 μg/dL)
- Transferrin or TIBC: Low
- Ferritin: Normal (M: 215–365 mg/dL, F: 250–380 mg/dL) or high in the absence of coexisting iron deficiency
- Soluble transferrin receptor: Normal
- Ratio of soluble transferrin receptor: Log ferritin <1
- Elevated levels ESR, CRP, fibrinogen, cytokines
- Rule out other causes of anemia with appropriate tests if doubt as to diagnosis. Additional tests might include TSH, Hgb electrophoresis, B_{12} and folate levels, direct and indirect Coombs tests, bone marrow aspiration.

DIFFERENTIAL DIAGNOSIS

- Iron deficiency anemia
- Thalassemia
- Myelodysplastic syndromes
- Hyperthyroidism or hypothyroidism
- Hypopituitarism
- Hyperparathyroidism

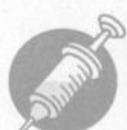

TREATMENT

- Treat the underlying disease. (1).
- The erythropoietic stimulating agents (ESA), recombinant erythropoietin (rEPO), and darbepoet (DARB) decrease the need for transfusions, increas hemoglobin levels in chronic kidney failure, and may improve quality of life in patients with CKD. According to the Food and Drug Administration, therapy should be initiated when hemoglobin leve (Hgb) are <10 g/dL and TSAT >20% (3). The National Kidney Foundation Kidney Disease Outcomes Quality Initiatives (KDOQI) recommend individual evaluation of the benefit of ESA utilization and maintaining the Hgb between 11–1 g/dL patients TSAT >20% and ferritin >100 ng/m in nondialysis CKD patients and >200 ng/mL in dialysis-treated CKD patients (4)[A].
- rEPO also increases Hgb levels in patients with ACD from HIV and chronic renal failure (5)[A].
- DARB has a simpler dosing schedule than rEPO (6
- Iron therapy given prior to or concurrently with ES improves response to ESA. IV iron is recommende for dialysis-treated CKD patients. Iron indices shou be evaluated prior to and during ESA use (4).
- Target Hgb levels in patients treated with ESA should not exceed 12 g/dL because of the increase risk of thromboembolic events at higher levels.
- Treatment with ESA should be reserved for symptomatic chemotherapy-induced anemia (CIA) in cancer treatment without curative intent. Treatment should be discontinued when chemotherapy is complete or if a rise in Hgb is not achieved within 8–9 weeks (7)[A].
- ESA therapy in patients with cancer has been associated with increased risk of venous thromboembolism and mortality (8).
- Iron studies and therapy for iron-deficient asymptomatic CIA cancer treatment without curative intent are recommended for absolute iron deficiency (7).

MEDICATION

- Epoetin α:
  - CKD start at 50–100 U/kg IV or SC 3 times a wee (TIW). ESA dosage should be adjusted according to the patient's Hgb level and response (4,9,10).
  - Cancer patients on chemotherapy start at 150 U/kg SC TIW or 40,000 U SC weekly; if no rise in Hgb >1 g/dL in 4 weeks, may increase to 300 U/kg TIW or 60,000 U SC weekly, respectively (7 Decrease dose by 25–50% if a rise in Hgb >1 g/dL in 2 weeks.

Darbepoetin α:
- CKD start at 0.45 μg/kg IV or SC weekly; alternative for CKD not on dialysis 0.75 μg/kg SC every 2 weeks. Dose adjustments are made similar to epoetin α (3,4).
- Cancer patients on chemotherapy start with 2.25 μg/kg weekly or 500 μg/kg every 3 weeks SC. If HgB rise $\leq$1 g/dL in 4 weeks, increase to 4.5 μg/kg SC weekly (7). Decrease dose by 25–50% if a rise in Hgb >1 g/dL in 2 weeks.

ALERT

With EPO/DARB use:
- CKD: Increased risk for death and serious cardiovascular events when dosed to Hgb $\geq$13 g/dL
- Cancer-related anemia and CIA with curative intent: ESA are not indicated. ESA therapy is only indicated in CIA without curative intent. Dose adjustments should be made to maintain the lowest Hgb to avoid transfusion.
- The FDA has included ESA therapy in CIA without curative intent in the Risk Evaluation and Mitigation Strategy (REMS) to assess the risk vs benefit for ESA use in this indication. To utilize ESA therapy physicians need to enroll in the **A**ssisting **P**roviders and cancer **P**atients with **R**isk **I**nformation for the safe use of **ES**As (APPRISE). Enrollment in the ESA Oncology APPRISE Program may be found at www.esa-apprise.com or by calling 1-866-284-8089.

ADDITIONAL TREATMENT

General Measures
- Most patients with ACD have a mild, asymptomatic anemia. However, if anemia becomes severe (Hgb <8 g/dL) and patients symptomatic, transfusion with PRBCs may become necessary, especially with a concurrent bleeding complication.
- Long-term transfusion therapy is not recommended in ACD patients with chronic kidney disease (1).

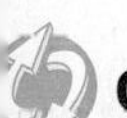

ONGOING CARE

FOLLOW-UP RECOMMENDATIONS

To minimize the risks of thromboembolic events, the lowest dose needed to avoid RBC transfusion should be utilized (3,7,9,10).

Patient Monitoring

Hgb or hematocrit levels should be followed, especially during therapy with ESA, when they should be checked biweekly until a stable dose, then monthly.

PROGNOSIS

Although ACD is chronic, it is usually not progressive.

COMPLICATIONS
- Anemia is associated with a worse prognosis in cardiovascular, chronic renal, and neoplastic disease (1).
- Treating anemia in these conditions improves quality of life (1) but may not improve length of life (and may shorten in some circumstances).

REFERENCES

1. Weiss G. Anemia of chronic disease. *N Engl J Med*. 2005;52:1011–23.
2. Ludwig H, Van Belle S, Barrett-Lee P et al. The European Cancer Anaemia Survey (ECAS): a large, multinational, prospective survey defining the prevalence, incidence, and treatment of anaemia in cancer patients. *Eur J Cancer*. 2004;40: 2293–306.
3. Product Information: ARANESP(R) injection, darbepoetin alfa injection. Amgen, Inc, Thousand Oaks, CA, 2007.
4. KDOQI, National Kidney Foundation. KDOQI Clinical Practice Guidelines and Clinical Practice Recommendations for Anemia in Chronic Kidney Disease. *Am J Kidney Dis*. 2006;47:S11–145.
5. Volberding P. Consensus statement: anemia in HIV infection–current trends, treatment options, and practice strategies. Anemia in HIV Working Group. *Clin Ther*. 2000;22:1004–1020; discussion 1003.
6. Vanrenterghem Y, Bárány P, Mann JF et al. Randomized trial of darbepoetin alfa for treatment of renal anemia at a reduced dose frequency compared with rHuEPO in dialysis patients. *Kidney Int*. 2002;62:2167–75.
7. National Comprehensive Cancer Network (NCCN.org). Jenkintown: NCCN Clinical Practice Guidelines in Oncology. Cancer- and Chemotherapy-Induced Anemia. V.2.2010. Accessed May 12, 2010 Fort Washington, PA: National Comprehensive Cancer Network; 2010, at http://www.nccn.org/professionals/physician_gls/PDF/anemia.pdf.
8. Bennett CL, Silver SM, Djulbegovic B et al. Venous thromboembolism and mortality associated with recombinant erythropoietin and darbepoetin administration for the treatment of cancer-associated anemia. *JAMA*. 2008;299:914–24.
9. Product Information: PROCRIT(R) injection, epoetin alfa injection. Ortho Biotech Products, LP, Raritan, NJ, 2005.
10. Product Information: EPOGEN(R) injection, epoetin alfa injection. Amgen, Inc, Thousand Oaks, CA, 2007.

ADDITIONAL READING

Nissenson AR, Swan SK, Lindberg JS et al. Randomized, controlled trial of darbepoetin alfa for the treatment of anemia in hemodialysis patients. *Am J Kidney Dis*. 2002;40:110–8.

See Also (Topic, Algorithm, Electronic Media Element)

Algorithm: Anemia

CODES

ICD9
- 285.21 Anemia in chronic kidney disease
- 285.22 Anemia in neoplastic disease
- 285.29 Anemia of other chronic disease

CLINICAL PEARLS
- ACD and iron-deficiency anemia (IDA) may coexist. The following parameters can generally distinguish them:
  - ACD-normocytic, ↓ or normal transferrin, ↑ or normal ferritin, normal soluble transferrin receptor levels (sTfR), ratio sTfR:log ferritin <1.
  - IDA-microcytic, ↑ transferrin, ↓ ferritin, ↑ sTfR levels, ratio sTfR:log ferritin >2.
- Anemia in ACD is usually symptomatic, although anemia is often mild or moderate. Patients with ACD always have an underlying disease, such as RA or chronic renal failure. These diseases will usually limit the patient's mobility, exercise capacity, or energy level, and typical symptoms of anemia (e.g., exertional dyspnea, fatigue, weakness) are attributed to the underlying disease.
- Iron sequestration and anemia may be an adaptive response when inflammation, infection, or neoplasia are present. When iron is hoarded in RES cells in ACD, rapidly proliferating micro-organisms or tumor cells do not have access to it, thereby limiting their growth. These rapidly proliferating cells also have increased oxygen demand, which is more difficult to meet in an anemic state.

ANEMIA, IRON DEFICIENCY

Pablo I. Hernandez Itriago, MD
Matthew A. Silva, PharmD, RPh, BCPS

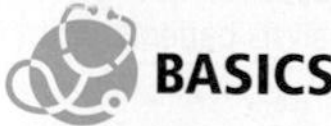

BASICS

DESCRIPTION

- A deficiency in red blood cells, hemoglobin, or blood volume due to decreased iron stores
- Onset may be acute with rapid blood loss or chronic with poor diet or slow blood loss.
- System(s) affected: Hemic/Lymphatic/Immunologic
- Synonym(s): Anemia of chronic blood loss; Hypochromic; Microcytic anemia; Chlorosis

Geriatric Considerations

60% of anemias in people >65 years

Pediatric Considerations

Frequent problem in infants whose major source of nutrition is unfortified cow's milk and/or juices

Pregnancy Considerations

Common during pregnancy unless iron supplements are included in the diet

EPIDEMIOLOGY

- Iron deficiency anemia (IDA) is the most common cause of anemia in the US.
- Predominant age: All ages, but especially toddlers and menstruating women
- Predominant sex: Female > Male
- More likely in the poor and in underimmunized children

Incidence

- Adults: Men 2%, women 15–20% annually
- Infants and toddlers: 3–5% annually
- Pregnant patients: 20%

Prevalence

- Infants and children <12: 4–7% (1)
- Males: 2–5% (1)
- Females: 9–16% (18–50% in menstruant blood donors) (1,2)

RISK FACTORS

- Female
- Frequent blood donor
- Pregnancy

GENERAL PREVENTION

- Screen asymptomatic pregnant women (3)[B].
- Supplementation in asymptomatic children 6–12 months if at increased risk for IDA (3)[B]

PATHOPHYSIOLOGY

Depletion of iron stores leads to decrease in reticulocyte count and decrease in production of hemoglobin.

ETIOLOGY

- Blood loss (e.g., menses, gastrointestinal [GI] bleeding, trauma)
- Poor iron intake
- Poor iron absorption (e.g., atrophic gastritis, postgastrectomy, celiac disease)
- Increased demand for iron (e.g., infancy, adolescence, and pregnancy)

COMMONLY ASSOCIATED CONDITIONS

- Hookworm infestation
- Pregnancy
- Gastric or colon carcinoma
- Hypermetrorrhagia

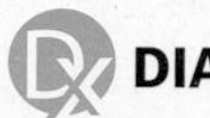

DIAGNOSIS

HISTORY

- Asymptomatic in most cases
- Weakness/fatigue
- Exertional dyspnea
- Palpitations
- Malaise
- Dizziness
- Headaches, inability to concentrate, irritability, listlessness
- Pica

PHYSICAL EXAM

- Pallor
- Cheilosis
- Tachycardia
- Tachypnea
- Koilonychia (spoon-shaped, brittle nails)

DIAGNOSTIC TESTS & INTERPRETATION

Lab

Initial lab tests

- Hemoglobin: <13 g in men and <12 g in women (4). Patients with higher premorbid hemoglobin (such as patients with chronic hypoxemia, smokers, living in high altitude) may be anemic at higher hemoglobin levels.
- Mean corpuscular volume (MCV): <80 fL
- Ferritin: <45 ng per mL. It is the best noninvasive test in adults, but may miss some deficient patients (e.g., cirrhosis), because ferritin is an acute-phase reactant.
- Transferrin saturation: <9 percent
- Total iron-binding capacity (TIBS): Increased
- Complete blood count (CBC) with differential, peripheral smear, reticulocyte count, and index. A peripheral smear usually shows hypochromia and microcytosis, but may be normal, and reticulocyte production index is low.
- Fe/total iron binding capacity (transferrin ratio) is usually not recommended, because it is less sensitive and less specific than ferritin.
- Stainable iron in bone marrow aspiration is the gold standard.
- Consider testing for G6PD deficiency: Assay at least 6 weeks after last drop in hemoglobin.
- Rule out thalassemia:
  - Review prior CBCs for persisting mild anemia and marked micro-ovalocytosis, elevated hemoglobin A2 or hemoglobin F, family history, and especially high or high normal red blood cell (RBC) count
  - A low RBC count in chronic bleeding helps to distinguish it from thalassemia trait where the count is high or high-normal
  - Microcytosis with ovalocytosis and anemia unresponsive to iron suggests the thalassemia trait.
- MCV may be normal in mild anemia or hidden by the population of larger cells (e.g., reticulocytes or macrocytes). Red cell distribution width (RDW) will be increased if a mixed population of cells is prese[nt] (e.g., mixed iron deficiency anemia and B12 deficiency)
- An empiric trial of iron at 3 mg/kg/d may be the be[st] way to diagnose decreased iron stores in infants an[d] children; reticulocytes become elevated in 7–10 days or hemoglobin increases >1.0 g/dL weekly, indicating Fe deficiency.
- Drugs that may alter lab results: Iron supplements o[r] multivitamin–mineral preparations that contain iro[n]
- Disorders that may alter lab results:
  - Elevated ferritin: Acute or chronic liver disease, Hodgkin disease, acute leukemia, solid tumors, fever, acute inflammation, renal dialysis
  - Elevated hemoglobin: Smoking, chronic hypoxemia, long-term residency at high altitude
  - Stool guaiac (2)[C]; if high index of suspicion of G[I] bleed, GI endoscopy. Under appropriate circumstances, stool for ova and parasites.
  - Rule out poor reutilization: Trial of iron, bone marrow aspiration, and iron stain
  - Rule out colorectal cancer and gastric carcinoma, especially in the elderly.

Diagnostic Procedures/Surgery

GI endoscopy to discover occult bleeding sites

Pathological Findings

- Absent marrow iron stores
- Marrow: Hyperplastic, micronormoblastic

DIFFERENTIAL DIAGNOSIS

- Gastritis
- Peptic ulcer disease
- GI bleeding
- Gastrointestinal carcinomas
- Defective iron utilization (e.g., thalassemia trait, sideroblastosis, G6PD deficiency)
- Defective iron reutilization (e.g., infection, inflammation, cancer, other chronic diseases)
- Hypoproliferation (e.g., decreased erythropoietin from hypothyroidism, renal failure)

TREATMENT

MEDICATION

- Ferrous sulfate 325 mg t.i.d. on an empty stomach [1] hour before meals provides 180 mg of elemental iron per day:
  - Reduce dose as needed for GI symptoms, which affect 15% of patients on standard iron therapy, or the dose can be taken with meals, which may reduce the delivery of iron by 50%. Constipation will occur in approximately 1 in 4 patients using various iron formulations (5).
  - Drugs that increase gastric pH (e.g., proton pump inhibitors [PPIs], H_2 antagonists) also reduce iron absorption (6).
  - Individuals with moderate anemia (Hg = 10 g/dL) need only a total of 1,500–2,000 mg of elementa[l] iron replacement; reducing the iron per dose as much as necessary to abate adverse effects will make parenteral iron therapy unnecessary in almost all cases.

– Special oral iron formulations and compounds are expensive and reduce symptoms only to the degree that they reduce the delivery of iron.

Liquid iron preparations are useful for children, with a recommended dose of 3 mg/kg/d; can also be used in adults when tablets are not absorbed or low tolerance requires a dose reduction.

Foods and beverages containing ascorbic acid (vitamin C) enhance iron absorption when taken simultaneously with the iron.

Continued bleeding and untreated hypothyroidism are causes for "failure to respond" to iron.

Consider parenteral iron for patients with an Hgb <6 g/dL, malabsorption, if higher oral doses and use of vitamin C fail:

– Anaphylaxis to parenteral iron therapy has occurred; ferric gluconate or iron sucrose may be safer alternatives to iron dextran (7,8)[B]

– Iron sucrose 200 mg IV × 5 doses over 2 weeks, or 500 mg IV q2 weeks × 2 doses (less experience with this regimen). Total dose is 1000 mg, then re-evaluate. 1 ml = 20 mg elemental iron. 100 mg IV × 10 weekly doses in hemodialysis-dependent patients.

Contraindications:
– Antacids concomitantly
– Dairy products concomitantly
– Tetracycline concomitantly

Significant possible interactions:
– Allopurinol
– Antacids
– Penicillamine
– Quinolones
– Tetracyclines
– Vitamin E

Precautions:
– Iron preparations may cause black bowel movements and constipation.
– Iron overdose is highly toxic; patients should be instructed to keep tablets and liquids out of the reach of small children.

ADDITIONAL TREATMENT

General Measures

Search for the cause and correct it.

Occult GI malignancy should be suspected in all older individuals with iron deficiency.

Avoid transfusions except in rare cases.

Issues for Referral

- Pregnant women with an Hgb <9 g/dL or failure to respond to a 4–6-week trial or oral iron therapy
- Nonpregnant women or other patients with an Hgb <6 g/dL

IN-PATIENT CONSIDERATIONS

Initial Stabilization

Outpatient

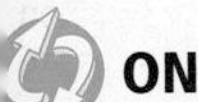

ONGOING CARE

FOLLOW-UP RECOMMENDATIONS

Patient Monitoring

- Regularly after Hgb returns to normal (in order to detect recurrences)
- Hgb increases 1 g/dL every 2–3 weeks.
- Iron stores may take up to 4 weeks to correct after Hgb returns to normal.

DIET

- Do not consume milk, other dairy products, antacids, quinolones, or tetracycline within 2 hours of iron supplement ingestion.
- Limit tea, coffee, and caffeinated beverages.
- Limit milk to 16 ounces per day (adults).
- Emphasize protein and iron-containing foods (meat, beans, and leafy green vegetables).
- Taking iron with orange juice or ascorbic acid increases absorption but decreases GI tolerability.
- Increase fluid and dietary fiber to decrease likelihood of constipation during iron replacement therapy.

PATIENT EDUCATION

National Heart, Lung & Blood Institute, Communications & Public Information Branch, National Institutes of Health, Building 31, Room 41-21, 9000 Rockville Pike, Bethesda, MD 20892; (301) 251-1222.

PROGNOSIS

- Can be resolved with iron therapy if the underlying cause can be discovered and appropriately treated
- Treat subclinical hypothyroidism and iron deficiency anemia together when these conditions co-exist. Failure to treat hypothyroidism results in poor response to iron therapy (9)[B].

COMPLICATIONS

- Neglecting to identify hidden bleeding points, particularly a bleeding malignancy
- Maternal iron deficiency negatively affects mother–child interactions. Iron supplementation protects against these negative effects (10).

REFERENCES

1. Iron Deficiency—United States, 1999–2000. *MMWR Morb Mortal Wkly Rep*. 2002;51:897–9.
2. Dubois RW, Goodnough LT, Ershler WB et al. Identification, diagnosis, and management of anemia in adult ambulatory patients treated by primary care physicians: evidence-based and consensus recommendations. *Curr Med Res Opin*. 2006;22:385–95.
3. U.S. Preventative Services Task Force (USPSTF). Screening for iron deficiency anemia—including iron supplementation for children and pregnant women. Rockville (MD): Agency for Healthcare Research and Quality (AHRQ); 2006. 12p.
4. Worldwide prevalence of anaemia 1993–2005: WHO global database on anaemia/Edited by Bruno de Benoist, Erin McLean, Ines Egli and Mary Cogswell.
5. Melamed N, Ben-Haroush A, Kaplan B et al. Iron supplementation in pregnancy–does the preparation matter? *Arch Gynecol Obstet*. 2007; 276:601–4.
6. Killip S, Bennett JM, Chambers MD. Iron deficiency anemia. *Am Fam Physician*. 2007;75:671–8.
7. Chertow GM, Mason PD, Vaage-Nilsen O et al. On the relative safety of parenteral iron formulations. *Nephrol Dial Transplant*. 2004;19:1571–5.
8. Chertow GM, Mason PD, Vaage-Nilsen O et al. Update on adverse drug events associated with parenteral iron. *Nephrol Dial Transplant*. 2006; 21:378–82.
9. Cinemre H, Bilir C, Gokosmanoglu F, Bahcebasi T et al. Hematologic effects of levothyroxine in iron-deficient subclinical hypothyroid patients: a randomized, double-blind, controlled study. *J. Clin. Endocrinol. Metab*. 2009;94:151–6
10. Murray-Kolb LE, Beard JL. Iron deficiency and child and maternal health. *Am J Clin Nutr*. 2009.

ADDITIONAL READING

- Andrews NC. Disorders of iron metabolism. *N Engl J Med*. 1999;341:1986–95.
- Auerbach M, Ballard H, Glaspy J. Clinical update: intravenous iron for anaemia. *Lancet*. 2007;369: 1502–4.
- Baker WF. Iron deficiency anemia in pregnancy, obstetrics and gynecology. *Hematol Oncol Clin North Am*. 2000;64(4):231–6.
- Iron Deficiency – United States, 1999–2000. *MMWR Morb Mortal Wkly Rep*. 2002;51(40): 897–9.
- Provan D, Weatherall D. Red cells II: acquired anaemias and polycythaemia. *Lancet*. 2000;355: 1260–8.
- Recommendations to prevent and control iron deficiency in the United States. *MMWR Morb Mortal Wkly Rep*. 1998;47(RR-3):1–36.
- Steensma DP, Tefferi A. Anemia in the elderly: How should we define it, when does it matter, and what can be done? [Review]. *Mayo Clinic Proc*. 2007; 82(8):958–66.
- Tefferi A, Hanson CA, Inwards DJ. How to interpret and pursue an abnormal complete blood cell count in adults. *Mayo Clin Proc*. 2005;80:923–36.

See Also (Topic, Algorithm, Electronic Media Element)

Algorithm: Anemia

CODES

ICD9

280.9 Iron deficiency anemia, unspecified

CLINICAL PEARLS

- Iron deficiency anemia is the most common type of anemia in the US.
- Blood loss and reduced iron stores due to malabsorption or poor utilization are major factors for iron deficiency anemia.
- Premenopausal women and children are at the greatest risk for iron deficiency anemia.
- Oral iron supplementation is the standard treatment option for patients with IDA.

ANEMIA, SICKLE CELL

Diane M. Haleem, PhD, RN
William V. Walsh, MD

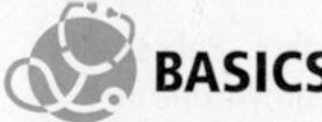

BASICS

DESCRIPTION

- Chronic hemoglobinopathy marked by moderately severe chronic hemolytic anemia, periodic acute episodes of painful "crises," and increased susceptibility to intercurrent infections. Hereditary, generally manifesting in 1st year of life.
- Sickle cells are abnormally shaped, fragile red blood cells. Increased red cell destruction causes an inability to maintain adequate hemoglobin levels and results in fatigue.
- The heterozygous condition (Hb A/S), sickle cell trait, is usually asymptomatic without anemia.
- System(s) affected: Hematologic; Lymphatic/Immunologic; Musculoskeletal
- Synonym(s): Sickle cell disease; Hb S disease

Pediatric Considerations

- Sequestration crises and hand–foot syndrome seen typically in infants/young children
- Adolescence/young adulthood:
  - Frequency of complications and organ/tissue damage increases with age (except for strokes, which occur mostly in childhood).
  - Psychological complications: Body image and sexual identity problems; interrupted schooling, career; restriction of activities; stigma of disease; low self-esteem
- Consider periodic transcranial Doppler ultrasound in all children ages 2–16.

Pregnancy Considerations

- Usually complicated and hazardous, especially 3rd trimester and delivery:
  - Fetal survival is >90% if the fetus reaches the 3rd trimester.
- Increased risk of pain rises, toxemia, infection, pulmonary infarction, phlebitis
- Fetal mortality 35–40%
- Partial exchange transfusion in 3rd trimester may reduce maternal morbidity and fetal mortality, but this is controversial.
- Chronic transfusions have been effective in diminishing pain episodes in pregnant women.

EPIDEMIOLOGY

Prevalence

- Almost 90,000 Americans have sickle cell disease and >2 million carry the trait. ~1/500 African Americans and 1/1,000 Hispanics have homozygous sickle cell anemia. Each year in the United States, about 1 in 400 African American infants are born with sickle cell disease.
- 10% of African Americans have sickle trait.
- To a lesser extent, people from the Middle East, Mediterranean area, and aboriginal tribes in India may be affected.

RISK FACTORS

- For vaso-occlusive crisis ("painful crisis"): Pain results from tissue ischemia and necrosis: Hypoxia, dehydration, fever, infection, acidosis, cold, anesthesia, strenuous physical exercise, smoking
- For aplastic crisis (suppression of RBC production): Severe infections, human parvovirus B19 infection, folic acid deficiency
- Hyperhemolytic crisis (accelerated hemolysis) (existence is controversial): Acute bacterial infections, exposure to oxidant drugs

Genetics

Autosomal recessive, mostly in African Americans. Homozygous presence of a variant hemoglobin, Hb S, or sickle hemoglobin (genotype SS). Heterozygous condition Hb AS.

GENERAL PREVENTION

- General: Genetic counseling
- Prevention of crises:
  - Avoid hypoxia, dehydration, cold, infection, fever, acidosis, and anesthesia.
  - Guidelines for prompt management of fever, infections, pain, and specific complications should be reviewed at each visit.
  - Stress importance of keeping well hydrated.
  - Avoid alcohol and smoking.
  - Avoid high-altitude areas. Traveling to a high-altitude area may trigger a crisis because of lower partial pressure of oxygen.
- Teach early recognition of possible complications, especially priapism.
- Stress importance of minimizing trauma; care using aseptic technique is imperative.

PATHOPHYSIOLOGY

Sickle cells express very late antigen (VLA)-4 on the surface. VLA-4 interacts with the endothelial cell adhesive molecule, vascular cell adhesive molecule (VCAM)-1. VCAM-1 is upregulated by hypoxia and inhibited by nitric oxide. Hypoxia also decreases nitric oxide production, thereby adding to the adhesion of sickle cells to the vascular endothelium. Nitric oxide is a vasodilator (1).

ETIOLOGY

- At molecular level: Substitution of valine for glutamic acid in the 6th amino acid position of the hemoglobin β-chain. As a result of the mutation, red blood cells (RBCs) change from biconcave to sickle shape when deoxygenated.
- At cellular level: Sickle RBCs are inflexible, which causes increased blood viscosity, stasis, mechanical obstruction of small arterioles and capillaries, and ischemia. Sickle RBCs are fragile, leading to hemolysis.
- At clinical level: Chronic anemia; crises:
  - Vaso-occlusive crisis ("painful crisis"): Pain results from tissue ischemia and necrosis. Progressive organ failure and tissue damage from repeated vaso-occlusive episodes.
  - Hand–foot syndrome: When vessel occlusion and ischemia affects small blood vessels in hands or feet, pain and swelling can result.
  - Aplastic crisis: Suppression of RBC production by severe infection or by parvoviral (and other viral) suppression of RBC production
  - Hyperhemolytic crisis: Accelerated hemolysis; increased RBC fragility/shortened lifespan
  - Sequestration crisis: Splenic sequestration of blood (only in infants/young children—occasionally seen in adults with sickle variants) causing acute anemia and acute splenic enlargement
- Susceptibility to infection: Impaired/absent splenic function; defect in the alternate pathway of complement activation

COMMONLY ASSOCIATED CONDITIONS

The psychosocial effects can result in low self-esteem, depression, and dependency.

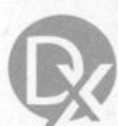

DIAGNOSIS

A chronic hemolytic anemia. Increased infection risk, (ex: pneumococcal sepsis and *Salmonella* osteomyelitis), with functional asplenia by ~5–6 year of age, and delayed physical/sexual maturation. Diagnosis now often made by newborn screening programs.

HISTORY

- >6 months of age, earliest symptoms are irritability and painful swelling of the hands and feet (hand–foot syndrome).
- Often asymptomatic in early months of life due to presence of fetal hemoglobin.
- Painful crises in bones, joints, abdomen, back, and viscera (account for 90% of all hospital admissions)
- Acute chest syndrome: Tachycardia, fever, bilateral infiltrates caused by decrease in hemoglobin and pulmonary infarction

PHYSICAL EXAM

- Fever, pale skin and nail beds, mild jaundice
- Acute chest syndrome: Tachycardia, fever, bilateral infiltrates caused by decrease in hemoglobin and pulmonary infarction

DIAGNOSTIC TESTS & INTERPRETATION

Lab

- Hb electrophoresis (diagnostic test of choice). Sickle cell anemia (FS pattern):
  - 80–100% Hb S, variable amounts of Hb F and no Hb A
  - Sickle cell trait (FS pattern): 20–40% Hb S, 60–80% Hb A1, minimal Hb F
- Screening tests: Sickledex test
- Hemoglobin ~8 g/dL (1.24 mmol/L); RBC indices usually normal, but mean corpuscular volume (MCV) <75/m^3 (<75 fL), reticulocytosis of 10–20%
- Leukocytosis; bands in absence of infection, and thrombocytosis
- Peripheral smear: Sickled RBCs, nucleated RBCs, Howell-Jolly bodies
- Serum bilirubin mildly elevated (2–4 mg/dL [34–68/mmol/L]); fecal/urinary urobilinogen high
- Erythrocyte sedimentation rate (ESR) low
- Serum lactate dehydrogenase (LDH) elevated, haptoglobin absent or very low

Imaging

Need for imaging depends upon clinical circumstances:

- Bone scan to rule out osteomyelitis
- Computed tomography (CT)/magnetic resonance imaging (MRI) to rule out cerebrovascular accident (CVA)
- Chest x-ray (CXR): May show enlarged heart; diffuse alveolar infiltrates in acute chest syndrome
- Transcranial Doppler: Start at age 2; repeat yearly (2,3)[B]. Transcranial Doppler ultrasound identifies children age 2-16 at higher risk of stroke. Those at increased risk may be treated with regular red blood cell transfusion to reduce risk of stroke.
- Electrocardiogram (ECG) to detect pulmonary hypertension (3)[C]

Pathological Findings

In moderate-to-severe cases, hyposplenism due to autosplenectomy is common.

Hypoxia/infarction in multiple organs

DIFFERENTIAL DIAGNOSIS

Anemia: Other hemoglobinopathies

Painful crises: Other causes of acute pain in bones, joints, and abdomen

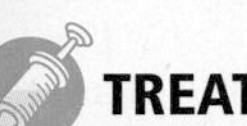

TREATMENT

MEDICATION

First Line

Supplemental oxygen

Painful crises (mild, outpatient):

- Non-narcotic analgesics (ibuprofen, tramadol) (2,3)[C]

Painful crises (severe, hospitalized) (2,3)[B]:

- Parenteral narcotics (e.g., morphine on fixed schedule); patient-controlled analgesia (PCA) pump may be useful.

Prevention of painful crisis:

- Hydroxyurea in adult patients with ≥3 crises/year. Start with 15 mg/kg/d single daily dose; titrate upward every 12 weeks if blood counts satisfactory:
  - Increase in 5 mg/kg increments to maximum of 35 mg/kg/d. Reduces crisis and chest syndrome 50%; long-term safety unknown.
  - Contraindicated in pregnancy (4)[A]
- Inhaled nitric oxide, arginine butyrate (may enhance availability of nitric oxide), and combination of erythropoietin with hydroxyurea (4)[B]

For infections prior to culture results (3), prescribe an antibiotic(s) that covers *S. pneumoniae*, *H. influenzae*, *Mycoplasma pneumoniae*, and *Chlamydia pneumoniae*—for example, ceftriaxone and azithromycin. If osteomyelitis, cover for *Staphylococcus aureus* and *Salmonella*—for example, ciprofloxacin. If the patient has an apparent pneumonia not promptly responding to antibiotics, consider diagnosis of acute chest syndrome and consider simple transfusions or exchange transfusion.

Prophylactic penicillin is indicated in all infants and children starting at 2 months (2,4)[A]: 2–6 months of age: 62.5 mg b.i.d. 6 months–3 years: 125 mg b.i.d. 3–5 years: 250 mg b.i.d. If no pneumococcal infections and no splenectomy, stop at 6 years; if high risk remains, continue until puberty. Alternative penicillin, benzathine IM 300,000 U/mo, ages 4 months–3 years, then 600,000 U/mo for 3–5 years. Rising pneumococcal resistance to penicillin may change future recommendations.

Precautions: Avoid high-dose estrogen oral contraceptives; consider Depo-Provera.

Second Line

Other nonsteroidal anti-inflammatory drugs (NSAIDs)

Folic acid supplements (2,3)[C]: 0–6 months: 0.1 mg/d; 6–12 months: 0.25 mg/d; 1–2 years: 0.5 mg/d; >2 years of age 1 mg/d

ADDITIONAL TREATMENT

Blood transfusions carry risk of iron overload, resulting in damage to heart, liver, and other organs. Consider chelation with Deferasirox, an oral agent, if transfusion therapy is necessary. This medication can be used in people older than 2.

- Transfusion needed with aplastic crises, severe complications (i.e., CVA), prophylactically before surgery, and as part of treatment for acute chest syndrome. However, there is a dearth of randomized trials in this area.

General Measures

- Infections/fever: Treat with antibiotics.
- Minimize factors that enhance sickling.
- Painful crises: Hydration, analgesics; oxygen regardless of whether the patient is hypoxic
- Transfusion needed with aplastic crises, severe complications (i.e., CVA), before surgery, and as treatment for acute chest syndrome
- Retinal evaluation starting at school age to detect proliferative sickle retinopathy
- Occupational therapy, cognitive and behavioral therapies, support groups
- Special immunizations (2,3)[B]:
  - Influenza vaccine yearly starting at age 2
  - Heptavalent conjugated pneumococcal vaccine at 2, 4, 6 months; booster at 15 months, 2 years, 5 years
  - 23-valent pneumococcal vaccine at 2 years; booster at age 5; always separate this by 8 weeks from heptavalent vaccine
- Meningococcal vaccine > 2 years of age

Additional Therapies

Physical therapy to include heat, massage, and exercise

COMPLEMENTARY AND ALTERNATIVE MEDICINE

Nicosan: This is an herbal treatment in early trials in the US. Nicosan has been used to prevent sickle crises in Nigeria.

SURGERY/OTHER PROCEDURES

Gene therapy experimental. Approaches under consideration: Replacement with a normal gene and attempts to inactivate Hgb S while reactivating Hgb F (fetal hemoglobin)

IN-PATIENT CONSIDERATIONS

Admission Criteria

Severe pain, suspected infection or sepsis

IV Fluids

The preferred maintenance IV fluid is 1/2 NS, as NS may theoretically increase the risk of sickling.

Nursing

- Psychosocial support
- Education about disease

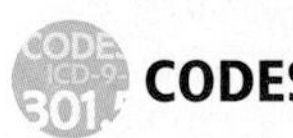

ONGOING CARE

FOLLOW-UP RECOMMENDATIONS

Bed rest with crises

Patient Monitoring

- Treat infections early. Parents and patients should be instructed that a temperature of ≥101°F (38.3°C) requires immediate medical attention.
- For patients who receive chronic transfusions, monitor for hepatitis and hemosiderosis.
- Begin periodic eye evaluations at age 5 to detect proliferative sickle retinopathy (2,3)[C].

DIET

Folic acid supplementation, avoid alcohol (leads to dehydration), maintain hydration

PATIENT EDUCATION

Sicklecellkids.org—Education Web site for children with sickle cell anemia: http://www.sicklecelldisease.org

American Sickle Cell Anemia Association: http://www.ascaa.org

PROGNOSIS

- In 2nd decade of life, fewer crises, but complications are more frequent. Median age of death is 42 for men and 48 for women. Common causes are infections, thrombosis, pulmonary emboli, pulmonary hypertension, and renal failure.
- Children become anemic in infancy and begin to have sickle cell crises at 1–2 years of age; some children die in their 1st year.

COMPLICATIONS

- Alloimmunization, bone infarct, aseptic necrosis of femoral head
- Cerebrovascular accidents (peak age 6–7), decreased intelligence, even without stroke
- Cholelithiasis/abnormal liver function
- Chronic leg ulcers, poor wound healing
- Impotence, priapism, hematuria/hyposthenuria, renal concentrating and acidifying defects
- Retinopathy, splenic infarction (by 10 years of age)
- Acute chest syndrome (infection/infarction) leading to chronic pulmonary disease
- Infections (pneumonia, osteomyelitis, meningitis, pyelonephritis); sepsis (leading cause of morbidity and mortality)
- Hemosiderosis (secondary to multiple transfusions). Substance abuse related to chronic pain.

REFERENCES

1. Marti-Carvajal AJ, Conterno LO, Kinght-Madden JM. Antibiotics for treating acute chest syndrome in people with sickle cell disease. *Cochrane Database of Systematic Reviews* 2007, Issue 2.
2. Section on Hematology/Oncology Committee on Genetics, American Academy of Pediatrics. Health supervision for children with sickle cell disease. *Pediatrics*. 2002;109:526–35.
3. National Institutes of Health. *The management of sickle cell disease*, 4th ed. 2002. NH Publ No. 02-2117.
4. Bonds DR. Three decades of innovation in the management of sickle cell disease: the road to understanding the sickle cell disease clinical phenotype. *Blood Rev*. 2005;19:99–110.

See Also (Topic, Algorithm, Electronic Media Element)

Algorithm: Anemia

CODES

ICD9

- 282.60 Sickle cell disease, unspecified
- 282.61 Hb SS disease without crisis
- 282.62 Hb SS disease with crisis

ANEMIA, SIDEROBLASTIC

Ekaterina Brodski-Quigley, MD

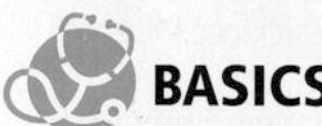

BASICS

DESCRIPTION

A subgroup of myelodysplastic syndromes, characterized by the presence of ringed sideroblasts in the bone marrow and impaired erythropoiesis. Peripheral blood smear may show micro-, macro-, or normocytic red blood cells (RBCs). Severity and course may range from severely progressive to indolent asymptomatic anemia; may be congenital or acquired (acquired is most prevalent in older males).

EPIDEMIOLOGY

- As a group, sideroblastic anemias (SAs) are uncommon, and specific incidence/prevalence is ill defined.
- Acquired forms are more common than hereditary forms (1) and usually occur in older adults; present in 25–30% of alcoholics with anemia, most commonly with folate and B_6 deficiency.
- Several hundred X-linked cases described
- Hereditary forms vary in severity, usually manifesting in childhood.

RISK FACTORS

- Male gender (X-linked SA)
- Family history of hereditary SA
- Chronic alcohol abuse
- Gastric bypass surgery (1 case report) (2)
- Family history of mitochondrial disorders (3,4)

Genetics

- Congenital form, usually X-linked:
  - Defect in aminolevulinic acid synthase (ALAS-2 mutation), the 1st and rate-limiting enzyme in heme biosynthesis
  - With congenital ataxia: hABC7 gene mutations (mitochondrial transport protein)
- Rarely autosomal-dominant or -recessive; gene(s) unknown
- Mitochondrial cytopathy:
  - Heterogeneous, involve deletions in mtDNA (4)
  - Unpredictable maternal inheritance
- See Etiology

GENERAL PREVENTION

Pyridoxine prophylaxis with INH therapy or as maintenance in congenital forms

PATHOPHYSIOLOGY

- Impaired heme biosynthesis within mitochondria
- Ineffective erythropoiesis despite abundance of iron in the body
- Increased gastrointestinal (GI) absorption of iron (Fe overload)
- Enhanced apoptosis in bone marrow
- Possibly, reactive oxygen species play a role.

ETIOLOGY

- Drugs and toxins:
  - Ethanol (related to associated folate and B_6 deficiency)
  - INH
  - Pyrazinamide
  - Chloramphenicol
  - Cycloserine
  - Azathioprine
  - D-penicillamine
  - Zinc toxicity (Cu deficiency)
- Nutritional deficiencies:
  - Pyridoxine deficiency
  - Copper deficiency:
    - Postgastrectomy
    - Prolonged parenteral nutrition
    - Prolonged zinc supplementation
- Hypothermia
- Acquired idiopathic sideroblastic anemia (AISA):
  - Pure sideroblastic anemia (PSA):
    - Only the erythroid line affected
  - Refractory anemia with ringed sideroblasts (RARS):
    - Myelodysplasia, other cell lines also affected
  - Associated with hematologic malignancies, myeloproliferative disorders
- Other:
  - X-linked
  - Autosomal dominant, recessive, maternal inheritance
  - Mitochondrial cytopathy:
    - Wolfram syndrome
    - Pearson syndrome
    - Kearns-Sayre syndrome (3)
- Disproportionately male, sporadic, mild to severe; kindreds too small to analyze inheritance

COMMONLY ASSOCIATED CONDITIONS

- Alcoholism
- According to mutation, e.g., severe congenital ataxia (hABC7 mutation), pancreatic dysfunction (Pearson syndrome)
- Iron overload or secondary hemochromatosis from transfused blood products
- Rarely, coexisting iron deficiency masks SA.
- Transformation into leukemia rare, 1–2%

DIAGNOSIS

- Often an incidental finding
- Moderate to severe anemia:
  - Fatigue
  - Dizziness or dyspnea
  - Diminished exercise tolerance
  - More symptomatic in older patients with comorbid conditions
- Specific to cause:
  - Pyridoxine deficiency (peripheral neuropathy, dermatitis)
  - Alcoholism
- Manifestations of iron overload

HISTORY

- Toxin, alcohol, or drug exposures
- Family history of anemia or myopathy, especially in men

PHYSICAL EXAM

- No pathognomonic physical findings
- Pallor
- Mild to moderate hepatosplenomegaly at diagnosis in 1/3–1/2 of patients with AISA

DIAGNOSTIC TESTS & INTERPRETATION

Lab

- Complete blood count (CBC):
  - Low mean corpuscular hemoglobin (MCH) and low mean corpuscular hemoglobin concentration (MCHC)
  - Low, normal or high MCV
  - Red cell distribution width (RDW) and hemoglobin (Hgb) highly variable
  - Siderocytes in peripheral smear (occasional)
  - White blood cell (WBC) normal; may be reduced hypersplenism, myelodysplasia
  - Platelets normal; may be reduced if hypersplenism, myelodysplasia
  - Low reticulocyte count
- Iron studies:
  - Ferritin increased
  - Transferrin saturation increased
  - Serum transferrin decreased
  - Reticuloendothelial iron increased
  - Total iron binding capacity (TIBC) normal
- Erythrogram of peripheral blood is predictive of bone marrow changes.
- Serum copper, ceruloplasmin, serum zinc if suspected as cause
- Liver enzyme derangements possible, depending on cause (EtOH, cirrhosis, Fe overload)
- Folate and B_{12} levels if EtOH-related malnutrition suspected

- Molecular studies identify specific mutations causing hereditary SA syndromes.
- Myelodysplasia: Morphologic and cytogenetic evaluation required for prognosis

iagnostic Procedures/Surgery

- Bone marrow biopsy confirms diagnosis.
- Liver biopsy is best; test to assess degree of iron overload.
- See Pathological Findings

athological Findings

- Bone marrow exam is the key diagnostic modality (1)[C]:
  - Normoblastic erythroid hyperplasia
  - Perls Prussian blue iron stain: Ringed sideroblasts, >10% of erythroblasts with increased number of abnormally large granules ringing the nucleus
  - Electron microscopy: Iron-overloaded mitochondria within erythroblasts
  - Iron-laden macrophages
- Liver biopsy:
  - Iron deposition as in hereditary hemochromatosis
- Micronodular cirrhosis by 3rd, 4th decade

IFFERENTIAL DIAGNOSIS

- Thalassemias
- Iron deficiency anemia
- Folate or B_{12} deficiency
- Anemia of chronic disease
- Myelodysplastic syndromes
- Lead toxicity with anemia
- Marrow dysplasia secondary to viral or drug toxicity (should be transient)

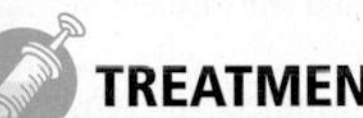

TREATMENT

IEDICATION

rst Line

- Trial of pyridoxine is indicated because it has few drawbacks and is very beneficial in responsive cases (1)[B]:
  - Pyridoxine 50–100 mg p.o. daily
  - Maintenance: Minimum dose to maintain acceptable Hgb
  - Supplement folate to compensate for increased erythropoiesis if effective.
  - Response likely if SA caused by alcohol abuse, pyridoxine antagonists, or some forms of hereditary X-linked SA
- Chelation therapy for iron overload (1)[B]
- Deferoxamine 40 mg/kg daily in continuous 12–24-hour daily infusions:
  - Limit ascorbate intake to 200 mg daily.
  - Auditory/visual toxicity very rare
- Deferasirox is an oral once-daily iron chelator:
  - No long-term safety data
  - Main complications skin rash, GI upset
- Goal is to maintain serum ferritin <500 μg/L

Second Line

- Myelodysplasia: PSA and RARS
- Treatment considerations as above, although no expected response to pyridoxine
- Some respond to combination of erythropoietin (EPO) and granulocyte colony-stimulating factor (G-CSF) (1)[C].
- Chemotherapeutic agents may have a role.

ADDITIONAL TREATMENT

General Measures

- Treatment is largely supportive:
  - Pyridoxine supplementation improves symptoms in responsive cases (1)[B].
  - Eliminate toxins and causative drugs.
  - Periodic transfusion: Maintain acceptable Hgb to alleviate symptoms and allow normal growth and development (children) (1)[B].
  - Prevent end-organ damage from severe iron overload (1)[B]:
    - Phlebotomy preferred modality if anemia is mild or moderate
- Iron chelation in patients with more severe anemia or requiring more transfusions

Issues for Referral

- Hematology consultation is helpful for diagnosis and management, particularly if no reversible cause is identified.
- Genetic counseling is important for patients with heritable cause of SA.

Additional Therapies

Allogeneic stem cell transplantation has been successful in a few cases in younger patients with myelodysplastic syndromes.

SURGERY/OTHER PROCEDURES

Splenectomy is contraindicated due to frequent postoperative thromboembolic complications.

IN-PATIENT CONSIDERATIONS

Admission Criteria

Generally managed in outpatient settings except for treatment of complications such as congestive heart failure (CHF), dysrhythmias

IV Fluids

RBC transfusion when necessary

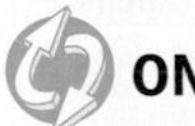

ONGOING CARE

FOLLOW-UP RECOMMENDATIONS

Patient Monitoring

- Yearly ferritin and transferrin saturation to monitor for Fe overload
- Follow response to treatment: Reticulocytosis within 2 weeks, improved Hgb within 1–2 months of response to pyridoxine, and correction of nutritional deficiency or withdrawal of reversible cause

DIET

Address relevant nutritional deficiencies. Address alcohol intake.

PROGNOSIS

- 2 methods of classification of myelodysplastic syndromes: French-American-British (FAB) and World Health Organization (WHO) (5)
- 75% of X-linked SA with ALAS-2 mutations are pyridoxine-responsive.
- Prognosis is better if iron overload is prevented.
- Acquired idiopathic SA:
  - RARS: Median survival 3–6 years, <10% progression to leukemia
  - When only the erythroid line is affected (PSA), course as in age-matched controls, transformation to leukemia not observed
- If SA follows treatment for malignancy, leukemic transformation is common.

COMPLICATIONS

- Iron overload causing organ damage:
  - Cardiac arrhythmia or CHF
  - Hepatic dysfunction
- Transfusion complications

REFERENCES

1. Alcindor T, Bridges KR. Sideroblastic anaemias. *Br J Haematol*. 2002;116:733–43.
2. Almhanna K, Khan P, Schaldenbrand M et al. Sideroblastic anemia after bariatric surgery. *Am J Hematol*. 2006;81:155–6.
3. Casas K, et al. Mitochondrial myopathy and sideroblastic anemia. *Am J Med Genetics*. 2004; 125A:201–4.
4. Matthes T, et al. Different pathophysiological mechanisms of intramitochondrial iron accumulation in acquired and congenital sideroblastic anemia caused by mitochondrial DNA deletion. *Eur J Haematol*. 2006;77:169–174
5. Müller-Berndorff H, Haas PS, Kunzmann R et al. Comparison of five prognostic scoring systems, the French-American-British (FAB) and World Health Organization (WHO) classifications in patients with myelodysplastic syndromes: Results of a single center analysis. *Ann Hematol*. 2006;85:502–13.

ADDITIONAL READING

Rovó A, Stüssi G, Meyer-Monard S et al. Sideroblastic changes of the bone marrow can be predicted by the erythrogram of peripheral blood. *Int J Lab Hematol*. 2009.

See Also (Topic, Algorithm, Electronic Media Element)

Algorithms: Anemia, Sideroblastic; Anemia

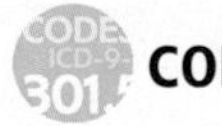

CODES

ICD9

285.0 Sideroblastic anemia

ANEURYSM OF THE ABDOMINAL AORTA

James J. Sullivan, Jr., MD, USN
Michael Gray, MD

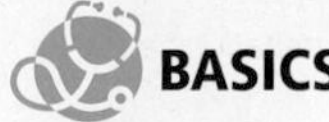

BASICS

DESCRIPTION

- An infrarenal aorta 3 cm in diameter or larger is considered aneurysmal.
- Types:
  - Fusiform aneurysm: Involves the whole circumference or wall of the artery
  - Saccular aneurysm: Does not involve the full circumference, often appears as an asymmetrical bleb or blister on the side of the aorta. Clinical presentation relates to aneurysm location, size, type, and comorbid factors affecting the patient. The majority are asymptomatic. May present with rupture, embolism, or thrombosis. Treatment and indications for surgical repair dictated by risk of rupture, risk of surgical repair, and estimated patient life expectancy.
- System(s) affected: Cardiovascular; Neurologic; Heme/Lymphatic/Immunologic
- Synonym(s): Aortic aneurysms; AAA

Geriatric Considerations

Incidence of AAA, risk of rupture, and operative morbidity and mortality all rise with age.

Pediatric Considerations

AAA in children is rare and may be associated with umbilical artery catheters, connective tissue diseases, arteritides, or congenital abnormalities.

EPIDEMIOLOGY

- Frequency increases >50 years of age
- Predominant sex: Male > Female (5:1)

Incidence

- >15,000 deaths per year in US
- 10th leading cause of death in men 65–75

Prevalence

- Depends on risk factors associated with AAA
- Prevalence of AAAs 2.9–4.9 cm in diameter ranges from 1.3% for men aged 45–54 to up to 12.5% for men aged 75–84 years of age. Data for women are 0% and 5.2%, respectively (1); however, when detected, women presented at an older age and were more likely to present with a ruptured AAA. Female sex is an independent risk factor for death from AAA .

RISK FACTORS

Older age, male, white, family history, smoking, hypertension (HTN), hyperlipidemia, peripheral vascular disease, peripheral aneurysms, chronic obstructive peripheral disease (COPD)

Genetics

- Familial aggregations exist: Aneurysms may develop at an earlier age.
- The frequency of AAA in 1st-degree relatives is 15–19% compared with 1–3% in unrelated patients.
- Marfan syndrome
- Ehlers-Danlos syndrome
- Polycystic kidney disease
- Tuberous sclerosis

GENERAL PREVENTION

- Address cardiovascular disease risk factors.
- Follow screening guidelines.

PATHOPHYSIOLOGY

- Vascular inflammatory degenerative disease with major role of matrix metalloproteinases and inflammatory markers that result in aortic medial degeneration (1)
- Gradual and/or sporadic expansion of aneurysm and accumulation of mural thrombus
- Aneurysms tend to expand over time. (Laplace law: T (wall tension) = pressure × radius. Wall tension directly related to blood pressure and the radius of the artery.) When wall tension exceeds wall tensile strength, rupture occurs.
- Average small AAA (<5.5 cm) grows at a rate of 2.6–3.2 mm/year. Larger aneurysms grew at a faster rate, as did increased tobacco use, but otherwise no identifiable risk factors to assess which small AAAs will advance to require further intervention (2).

ETIOLOGY

- Degenerative: Atherosclerotic (80%)
- Rare causes: Inflammatory diseases; trauma; connective tissue disorders; infection (Brucella, Salmonella, staph, tuberculosis)

COMMONLY ASSOCIATED CONDITIONS

- HTN, myocardial infarction (MI), heart failure, carotid artery, and/or lower extremity peripheral arterial disease
- Screening for thoracic aneurysm should also be considered.

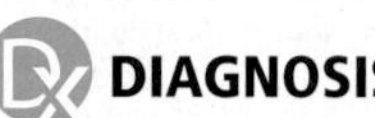

DIAGNOSIS

Screening: Recommended 1-time ultrasound for AAA in men 65–75 years of age who have ever smoked. Men >60 years old who are siblings or offspring of patients with AAA should undergo physical exam and ultrasound screening (1)[B]. US Preventative Services Task Force has recommended against routine screening for women (3):

- Most often asymptomatic: Discovered during exams for other complaints
- Symptomatic: Embolization, thrombosis, vague abdominal or back pain, syncope, lower extremity paralysis
- Rupture

ALERT

- The triad of shock, pulsatile mass, and abdominal pain always suggests rupture of AAA:
  - Shock may be absent if rupture is contained.
  - Palpable pulsatile mass may be absent in up to 50% of the patients with rupture.
  - Pain may radiate to the back, groin, flank, buttocks, or legs.
- Unusual presentations:
  - Primary aortoenteric fistula: Erosion/rupture of AAA into duodenum
  - Aortocaval fistula: Erosion/rupture of AAA into vena cava or left renal vein: 3–6%
  - Inflammatory aneurysm: Encasement by thick inflammatory rind; can cause chronic abdominal pain, weight loss, and elevated erythrocyte sedimentation rate. Surrounding viscera densely adherent.

HISTORY

Abdominal or back pain; AAA risk factors

PHYSICAL EXAM

- Pulsatile supraumbilical mass
- Vague abdominal tenderness: May radiate to the back or flank
- Encroachment by aneurysm:
  - Vertebral body erosion; gastric outlet obstructior ureteral obstruction
  - Lower extremity ischemia secondary to embolization of mural thrombus
- Rupture leads to tachycardia, hypotension, evidenc of shock and anemia, and possible flank contusion (Grey-Turner sign).
- Scrotal sign of Bryant: Painless scrotal ecchymosis rare manifestation of ruptured AAA.

DIAGNOSTIC TESTS & INTERPRETATION

Lab

Initial lab tests

If rupturing AAA being considered: Complete blood chemistry, chemistries, coags, type and cross, electrocardiogram

Follow-Up & Special Considerations

Evaluation for coronary artery disease is appropriate prior to elective AAA repair (i.e., cardiac clearance).

Imaging

Initial approach

- Ultrasonography: Simplest and least expensive diagnostic procedure
- Multiple studies have demonstrated high sensitivity (94–100%) and specificity (98–100%) of ultrasonographic diagnosis of AAA by emergency physicians.
- Although effective in detecting AAA, it is a poor te to show leakage or rupture if bleeding is into the retroperitoneal space.
- Screening: Ultrasound screening for detection of AAA in male patients, ages 65–75, who have ever smoked and men >60 who are siblings or offsprin of patients with AAA
- Surveillance of known asymptomatic aneurysm:
  - <3 cm: No further testing
  - 3–4 cm: Screen annually
  - 4–4.5 cm: Screen every 6 months
  - >4.5 cm: Refer to vascular specialist
- Computed tomography (CT) scans are the preferred pre-op study (caution w/IV contrast in renal failure)
- Magnetic resonance imaging/magnetic resonance angiography can also visualize AAA, but is often nc plausible in emergent situations.
- Aortography: Does not define outer dimensions of aneurysm
- Abdominal x-rays can be diagnostic if calcifications exist; not a diagnostic tool of choice
- Indications for vascular imaging:
  - Associated renovascular hypertension
  - Symptoms of visceral angina
  - Significant iliofemoral occlusive disease
  - Peripheral aneurysms
- Horseshoe or pelvic kidney

Diagnostic Procedures/Surgery

ALERT

Use clinical judgment: Patients with known AAA having abdominal or back pain symptoms may be rupturing despite a negative CT scan.

DIFFERENTIAL DIAGNOSIS

- Other abdominal masses
- Other causes of abdominal or back pain (e.g., peptic ulcer disease, renal colic, diverticulitis, appendicitis, incarcerated hernia, gastrointestinal hemorrhage, arthritis, metastatic disease)

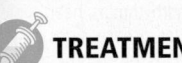

TREATMENT

- Emergent treatment in unstable or symptomatic patients is immediate vascular surgery consultation, adequate IV access and resuscitation, type and cross for multiple units, and rapid bedside ultrasound.
- Less acute treatment of AAA and prevention of rupture is elective repair and risk factor modification.

MEDICATION

- Beta-blockers may be initiated to reduce the rate of aneurysm expansion (1)[B].
- Beta-blockers should be used perioperatively in absence of contraindications (1)[A].
- Early studies suggest that statins may be beneficial both perioperatively and to inhibit further expansion.
- Doxycycline, and aspirin may also inhibit expansion, but further studies are needed. Early animal studies indicate a possible role for ACE-I/ARBs, mast cell stabilizers, prostaglandin inhibitors, and novel gene therapy, but no human studies yet (1,2).

ADDITIONAL TREATMENT

General Measures

- Treat atherosclerotic risk factors
- Medical optimization of cardiac, renal, and pulmonary conditions; smoking cessation

SURGERY/OTHER PROCEDURES

Current recommendations (4)[C]:

- Elective:
  - 5.5-cm diameter is the threshold for repair in "average" patient.
  - Younger, low-risk patients with long life expectancy may prefer early repair.
  - Women or AAA with high risk of rupture: Consider elective repair at 4.5–5 cm
  - Consider delayed repair in high-risk patients.
- High risk of rupture:
  - Expansion >0.6 cm/yr
  - Smoking/COPD severe/steroids
  - Family history multiple relatives
  - Hypertension poorly controlled
  - Shape nonfusiform
- High-risk patients for elective repair:
  - Risk factors for open repair include age >70 years, COPD, CRI, suprarenal clamp site with 1-year mortality if 0 risk factors present of 1.2% and 67% for all 4 risk factors present.
  - Other risk factors include inactive/poor stamina, congestive heart failure, significant coronary artery disease, liver disease, and family history of AAA.
- Emergent/symptomatic repair:
  - Traditionally has been open repair; however, candidates with appropriate anatomy can have endovascular repair, with an estimated mortality of 32% for endovascular vs 44% open.
- Open repair vs endovascular repair (EVAR):
  - Open repair indicated in patients who are good or average surgical candidates (1)[B].
  - EVAR for patients at high risk of complication based on cardiopulmonary or other comorbid illness: Periodic long-term surveillance indicated to monitor for endoleak, status of aneurysmal sac, and need for further intervention (1)[B]

IN-PATIENT CONSIDERATIONS

Risk of abdominal compartment syndrome after repair 4–12%; usually associated with large fluid resuscitation

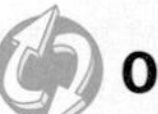

ONGOING CARE

FOLLOW-UP RECOMMENDATIONS

See surveillance recommendations

Patient Monitoring

Blood pressure and fasting lipid values: Control as would for atherosclerotic disease (1)[C]

DIET

Low-fat, low-salt, and low-caffeine diet

PATIENT EDUCATION

Smoking cessation (1)[B], aerobic exercise

PROGNOSIS

- Annual risk of rupture (5):
  - <4 cm diameter: ~0%
  - 4–4.9 cm: ~1%
  - 5–5.9 cm: ~11%
  - 6–6.9 cm: ~26%
  - >7 cm: ~32%
- Patients with AAAs measuring 5.5 cm or larger should undergo repair (1)[B], as should all patients with symptomatic AAA (1)[C].
- Only ~18% of patients with ruptured AAA survive.
- Although there is a 5:1 ratio of AAA between males and females, women have a higher mortality and morbidity associated with AAA, regardless of open or endovascular repair (6).

COMPLICATIONS

- Nonoperative:
  - Rupture, dissection, thromboembolization
- Elective operative (conventional):
  - Death 2–8%
  - All cardiac 10–12% (MI 2–8%)
- Pulmonary 5–10%; renal 5–7%; wound infection >5%; colon ischemia 1%; spinal cord ischemia <1%

REFERENCES

1. Hirsch AT, et al. ACC/AHA 2005 Practice Guidelines for Management of Patients With Peripheral Arterial Disease: A Collaborative Report. *Circulation*. 2006;113:e563–e601.
2. Baxter BT, et al. Medical management of small abdominal aortic aneurysms. *Circulation*. 2008;117(14):1883–9.
3. U.S. Preventive Services Task Force. Screening for Abdominal Aortic Aneurysm. *Ann Intern Med*. 2005;142:198–202.
4. Brewster DC, Cronenwett JL, Hallett JW et al. Guidelines for the treatment of abdominal aortic aneurysms. Report of a subcommittee of the Joint Council of the American Association for Vascular Surgery and Society for Vascular Surgery. *J Vasc Surg*. 2003;37:1106–17.
5. Lederle FA, Johnson GR, Wilson SE et al. Rupture rate of large abdominal aortic aneurysms in patients refusing or unfit for elective repair. *JAMA*. 2002;287:2968–72.
6. Abedi NN, Davenport DL, Xenos E et al. Gender and 30-day outcome in patients undergoing endovascular aneurysm repair (EVAR): An analysis using the ACS NSQIP dataset. *J Vasc Surg*. 2009.

ADDITIONAL READING

- Fleming C, Whitlock EP, Beil TL et al. Screening for abdominal aortic aneurysm: a best-evidence systematic review for the U.S. Preventive Services Task Force. *Ann Intern Med*. 2005;142:203–11.
- Hamerlynck JV, Legemate DA, Hooft L et al. [From the Cochrane Library: ultrasonographic screening for abdominal aortic aneurysm in men aged 65 years and older: low risk of fatal aneurysm rupture] *Ned Tijdschr Geneeskd*. 2008;152:747–9.

See Also (Topic, Algorithm, Electronic Media Element)

Aortic Dissection; Thoracic Aneurysms; Ehlers-Danlos; Giant Cell Arteritis; Marfan Syndrome; Polyarteritis Nodosa; Turner Syndrome

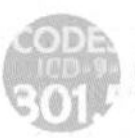

CODES

ICD9

- 441.3 Abdominal aneurysm, ruptured
- 441.4 Abdominal aneurysm without mention of rupture

CLINICAL PEARLS

- Major risk factors: Smoking, HTN, hyperlipidemia, family history, male gender, age
- Triad of hypotension/shock, pulsatile abdominal mass, and abdominal/back pain always suggests rupture, which requires emergent evaluation for surgery.
- 5.5 cm is the threshold diameter for elective surgical treatment (with some exceptions).
- Ultrasound is the procedure of choice for screening and initial diagnosis.

ANGINA PECTORIS, STABLE

Balakumar Pandian, MD

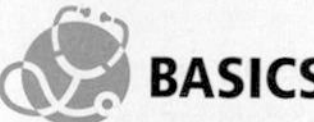

BASICS

DESCRIPTION

- Predictable and reproducible chest discomfort that occurs in a consistent pattern at a certain level of exertion or emotional stress and is relieved with rest or sublingual nitroglycerin
- Definitions:
  - Typical angina: A sense of choking or of pressure or heaviness deep to the precordium, frequently radiating to the jaw, arms, or epigastrium; usually brought on by exertion or anxiety and relieved by rest. Discomfort may be described with a clenched fist over the sternum (Levine sign).
  - Anginal equivalent: Occasionally, patients with angina will present without chest discomfort, but with nonspecific symptoms such as dyspnea, fatigue, belching, nausea, lightheadedness, indigestion
- Unstable angina: Anginal symptoms that are new or are changed in character to become more frequent, more severe, or both. Considered an acute coronary syndrome in the same continuum as non-ST segment elevation myocardial infarction (NSTEMI).
- System(s) affected: Cardiovascular

Geriatric Considerations

Elderly patients may present with atypical anginal symptoms. Maintain a high degree of suspicion during evaluation. They may also be very sensitive to the side effects of medications.

Pregnancy Considerations

Other diagnoses should be excluded and the patient managed closely by an obstetrician or family physician and cardiologist; the metabolic demands of pregnancy can exacerbate symptoms and directly interfere with treatment.

EPIDEMIOLOGY

- Predominant age: Most common in middle age and older men, postmenopausal women
- Predominant sex: Male > Female

Incidence

~500,000 new cases of stable angina occur yearly in the United States.

Prevalence

More than 10 million people in the United States suffer from angina.

RISK FACTORS

Risk factors for coronary artery disease include:

- Family history of premature CAD in 1st-degree relatives (in male relatives <55 yrs old or female relatives <65 yrs old)
- Obesity
- Hypercholesterolemia
- Elevated blood pressure
- Cigarette smoking
- Diabetes mellitus
- Male gender
- Advanced age

GENERAL PREVENTION

- Stop smoking.
- Low-fat/low-cholesterol diet
- Regular aerobic exercise program
- Weight loss (goal BMI <25)
- Blood pressure control (goal BP <140/90)
- Antilipidemics if indicated by current ATP guidelines or a risk-based approach
- Optimize glycemic control in those with diabetes mellitus.

PATHOPHYSIOLOGY

- Anginal symptoms occur during times of myocardial ischemia caused by a mismatch between coronary artery perfusion and myocardial oxygen demand. Sensory nerves from the heart travel up the sympathetic chain and enter the spinal cord at levels C7-T4, causing diffuse referred pain/discomfort in the associated dermatomes.
- Atherosclerotic narrowing of the coronary arteries (stenosis of >70%) is the most common pathology. Angina may occur in those with significant aortic valve disease or hypertrophic cardiomyopathy, even with normal coronary arteries.

ETIOLOGY

- Atherosclerosis of the coronary arteries (most common)
- Aortic stenosis
- Hypertrophic cardiomyopathy
- Aortic insufficiency
- Primary pulmonary HTN

COMMONLY ASSOCIATED CONDITIONS

- Hypercholesterolemia
- Peripheral vascular disease
- Hypertension
- Overweight
- Diabetes mellitus

DIAGNOSIS

- Predictable and reproducible anginal symptoms lasting 3–15 minutes brought on by exertion, emotional stress, meals, cold air, or smoking; symptoms relieved by rest or nitrates
- Careful history is important in eliciting symptoms of angina as listed above.
- Dyspnea on exertion may present as the only symptom.
- Atypical symptoms more likely in women, elderly, and diabetic patients.
- Canadian Cardiovascular Society grading of chronic stable angina severity:
  - Class 1: Ordinary physical activity does not cause angina; angina with strenuous or rapid or prolonged exertion
  - Class 2: Slight limitation of ordinary activity (walking rapidly or >2 blocks, climbing >1 flight of stairs, emotional stress)
  - Class 3: Marked limitation of ordinary physical activity.
  - Class 4: Inability to carry on any physical activity without discomfort. Angina may occur at rest.

HISTORY

- Quality of any previous anginal episodes and patte[rn] over time
- Underlying history of heart disease or valvular disease
- Family history of myocardial infarction, CAD, sudde[n] death

PHYSICAL EXAM

- Measure vital signs such as blood pressure, heart rate, respiratory rate, and oxygen saturation.
- Cardiac exam may reveal dysrhythmias, heart murmurs indicative of valvular disease, signs of ventricular hypertrophy, gallops, or signs of congestive heart failure.
- Vascular exam may show signs of peripheral vascular disease (diminished pulses, bruits, abdominal aneurysm)
- Pulmonary exam may reveal signs of obstructive or restrictive diseases, pulmonary edema
- May see signs of dyslipidemia (xanthomas, xanthelesma)
- Normal physical exam should not exclude cardiac causes of anginal symptoms.

DIAGNOSTIC TESTS & INTERPRETATION

- ECG:
  - May show evidence of prior myocardial infarctio[n]. However, ECG is frequently unremarkable when asymptomatic. May show signs of myocardial ischemia during symptomatic episodes.
  - Bundle branch block, Wolff Parkinson White syndrome, or intraventricular conduction delay may make stress ECG interpretation unreliable.
- Stress testing (exercise testing preferable):
  - Exercise testing for those who can physically exercise (≥5 METS):
    - Standard exercise ECG for those with normal baseline ECG
    - Exercise stress testing with echocardiography o[r] perfusion imaging for those with abnormal baseline ECG or in premenopausal women
  - In patients who cannot tolerate exercise, pharmacologic stress testing with adenosine, regadenoson, or dipyridamole. Dobutamine preferred if asthma or heart block (2° or 3°).
- Coronary angiography is the gold standard for confirmation and delineation of coronary disease and direction of interventional therapy or surgery.

Lab

- Total cholesterol and low-density lipoprotein (LDL) may be elevated and high-density lipoprotein (HDL) cholesterol may be reduced.
- CRP: Most useful for those individuals at intermediate risk of developing coronary artery disease (10–20% over 10 years by Framingham risk criteria) in whom an elevated CRP may suggest an increased likelihood of benefit from statin therapy)

Initial lab tests

Hematocrit, fasting lipid profile, fasting blood sugar, basic metabolic panel

Imaging

- Consider echocardiogram if valvular disease or hypertrophic cardiomyopathy is suspected.
- Stress imaging with echocardiogram or perfusion imaging (see section on stress testing)
- Consider chest radiography if signs of pulmonary disease

IFFERENTIAL DIAGNOSIS
Pulmonary disease
Deconditioning

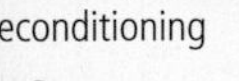

TREATMENT

IEDICATION
ʼrst Line
Anti-ischemic (anti-anginal) medications:
- Beta blockers decrease heart rate, blood pressure, and myocardial contractility:
  - Atenolol (25–100 mg/d), metoprolol (25–100 mg b.i.d.)
  - Adjust doses according to clinical response. Aim to maintain resting heart rate of 50–60 beats per minute.
  - Side effects may include fatigue, exercise intolerance, erectile dysfunction, bradycardia, or heart block.
  - Contraindications include decompensated CHF, severe bradycardia, advanced AV block, or severe lung disease.
- Nitrates dilate systemic veins and arteries (including coronary vessels) and cause decreased afterload and increased myocardial flow:
  - Sublingual nitroglycerin 0.4 mg SL. For acute anginal episodes. Repeat 2–3 times over a 10–15 minute period; if no relief, immediate medical attention must be sought.
  - Long–acting nitrates: Should be used with a drug–free interval of 8–12 hours to prevent tolerance. Side effects such as headaches and hypotension tend to clear with continued usage.
  - Concurrent use of phosphodiesterase inhibitors for erectile dysfunction (e.g. sildenafil, vardenafil, tadalafil) may cause life-threatening hypotension and are contraindicated.
- Calcium channel blockers (CCB) cause arterial vasodilation, decrease myocardial oxygen demand, and improve coronary blood flow. Only long-acting CCBs should be used:
  - Dihydropyridine CCBs such as nifedipine (30–90 mg/d), amlodipine (5–10 mg/d), or felodipine (2.5–10 mg/d) cause more vasodilation. Nondihydropyridine CCBs such as diltiazem (120–480 mg/d) or verapamil (120–480 mg/d). Amlodipine preferred in patients with low ejection fraction.
  - Side effects include constipation and peripheral edema. The nondihydropyridine CCBs may also cause bradycardia, heart block, and precipitate heart failure in those with severe systolic dysfunction.
- Ranolazine (500–1000 mg b.i.d.) likely works by improving left ventricular function, although the exact mechanisms are unclear:
  - Use as adjunctive therapy in those who are still symptomatic on optimal doses of β-blockers, nitrates, or amlodipine
  - Side effects may include nausea, constipation, dizziness, and headache.
  - Contraindications include combination with nondihydropyridine calcium channel blockers, prolonged QT, and medications that inhibit cytochrome P-450 system.

- Vasculoprotective therapies:
  - Antiplatelet therapy is indicated in all patients:
    - Aspirin (81–325 mg/d) is preferred
    - Clopidogrel (75 mg/d) may be used in patients with contraindications to aspirin.
    - Combination of aspirin and clopidogrel is indicated for those with stent placement to reduce rate of stent thrombosis (1 month for bare metal stents and ≥12 months for drug eluting stents)
  - Statins (e.g., simvastatin, atorvastatin, pravastatin, lovastatin) for hypercholesterolemia:
    - Most beneficial as secondary prevention in those with CAD. Decrease incidence of symptomatic CAD and reduce both myocardial infarction and death from MI.
    - LDL target <100 mg/dL for established CAD. Consider target <70 in high-risk patients.
    - Current ATP guidelines support using lipid-lowering drugs for those with suspected or documented CAD.
    - Side effects may include elevated transaminases, myalgias. May rarely cause myositis or rhabdomyolysis. Monitor labs with any changes in medication doses.
  - ACE inhibitors have been shown to reduce both cardiovascular death and MI. Indicated in patients with CAD or other vascular disease (1)[B], particularly in those with diabetes or left ventricular (LV) systolic dysfunction (1)[A]:
    - Angiotensin receptor blockers may be used in patients intolerant of ACE inhibitors.

ADDITIONAL TREATMENT
General Measures
Lifestyle modifications are very important:
- Blood pressure control
- Smoking cessation
- Minimize emotional stress
- Weight reduction in obese patients (2)[C]
- Daily physical activity (30–60 minutes) (3)[C]
- Annual influenza vaccination (3)[C]

COMPLEMENTARY AND ALTERNATIVE MEDICINE
Relaxation/stress reduction therapy may help reduce anginal episodes.

SURGERY/OTHER PROCEDURES
- Revascularization therapies: Consider if optimal medication management is inadequate in controlling symptoms:
  - Percutaneous coronary intervention (PCI):
    - Balloon angioplasty
    - Stent placement (with drug eluting or bare metal stent)
  - Coronary artery bypass grafting (CABG)
- For refractory angina (4):
  - Spinal cord stimulation
  - Enhanced external counterpulsation
  - Myocardial laser revascularization therapy

IN-PATIENT CONSIDERATIONS
Admission Criteria
Inpatient evaluation is warranted in any patient with new changes in their angina symptoms.

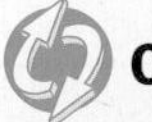

ONGOING CARE

FOLLOW-UP RECOMMENDATIONS
Lifestyle modifications should be stressed at every visit.

Patient Monitoring
Changes in severity or frequency of anginal symptoms need further evaluation.

DIET
Low-fat, low-cholesterol, low-salt diet

PROGNOSIS
Variable; depends on severity of symptoms, the extent of CAD, and LV function

COMPLICATIONS
- Unstable angina or myocardial infarction
- Arrhythmia
- Cardiac arrest
- Congestive heart failure (CHF)

REFERENCES

1. Yusuf S, Sleight P, Pogue J, Bosch J, Davies R, Dagenais G et al. Effects of an angiotensin-converting-enzyme inhibitor, ramipril, on cardiovascular events in high-risk patients. The Heart Outcomes Prevention Evaluation Study Investigators. *N Engl J Med*. 2000;342:145–53.
2. Gibbons RJ, et al. Committee on the Management of patients with chronic stable angina. ACC/AHA 2002 guideline update for the management of patients with chronic stable angina—summary article: a report of the American College of Cardiology/American Heart Association Task Force on Practice Guidelines. *Circulation*. 2003;107: 149–58.
3. Fraker TD, Fihn SD writing on behalf of the 2002 Chronic Stable Angina Writing Committee. 2007 Chronic Angina Focused Update of the ACC/AHA 2002 Guidelines for the Management of Patients with Chronic Stable Angina. *Circulation*. 2007; 116:2762–2772.
4. Khan SN, Dutka DP. A systematic approach to refractory angina. *Current Opinion in Supportive and Palliative Care*. 2008;2:247–251.

See Also (Topic, Algorithm, Electronic Media Element)
Algorithms: Chest Pain; Chest Pain/Acute Coronary Syndrome

CODES

ICD9
413.9 Other and unspecified angina pectoris

CLINICAL PEARLS
- Careful history taking is important in diagnosis, especially in the elderly.
- Maximize antianginal therapy by combining β blockers, CCB, and nitrates in those still symptomatic with monotherapy.
- Exercise testing may be useful diagnostically and to assess effectiveness of antianginal therapy.

ANGIOEDEMA

Michelle T. Martin, PharmD
Jamie Berkes, MD

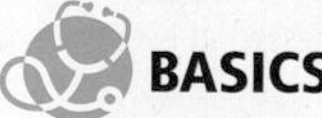

BASICS

DESCRIPTION
- Angioedema (AE) is an acute, localized swelling of skin, mucosa, and submucosa caused by extravasation of fluid into the affected tissues.
- Often resolves in hours to days but can be life-threatening if the upper airway is involved
- Usually involves the face, tongue, larynx, GI tract, and extremities
- Causes:
  - Idiopathic
  - Medications such as angiotensin-converting enzyme (ACE) inhibitors
  - Allergens such as foods, latex, or venom
  - Physical elements such as vibration or cold
- Hereditary AE (HAE) and acquired AE (AAE) are diseases of the complement cascade that result in recurrent episodes of AE of the skin, upper airway, and GI tract.
- System(s) affected: Skin/Exocrine
- Synonym(s): Angioneurotic edema; Quincke edema

EPIDEMIOLOGY
- Predominant age:
  - Allergen, medication, or other triggers can affect all ages.
  - HAE: Infancy to 2nd decade of life
  - AAE: Typically patients in 4th decade of life
- Predominant gender: Male = Female (except type III HAE affects more women than men)

Incidence
25% of ACE inhibitor–induced AE cases will occur within the 1st month of taking the medication; however, they are not limited to this period.

Prevalence
- AE occurs in about 15% of the population over a lifetime.
- AE: 0.1–2.2% of patients receiving ACE inhibitors: African Americans have a 4–5 times greater risk of ACE inhibitor–induced AE than Caucasians.
- HAE: 1:10,000–50,000 population in US

RISK FACTORS
- Consuming medications and foods that can cause allergic reactions
- Preexisting diagnosis of HAE or AAE

Genetics
- HAE types I and II are autosomal dominant, whereas type III is dominant X-linked.
- HAE occurs in 25% of patients as a result of spontaneous genetic mutations.

GENERAL PREVENTION
- Avoid known triggers.
- Avoid ACE inhibitors in patients with a history of AE.
- Do not use ACE inhibitors in patients with C1 esterase inhibitor (C1 INH) deficiency.

PATHOPHYSIOLOGY
- Type 1 hypersensitivity reaction
- Increase in vascular permeability secondary to IgE-mediated mast cell–stimulated histamine release or from activation of the complement system and an elevation in bradykinin (HAE)
- Attacks of HAE are triggered by prolonged mechanical pressure, cold, heat, trauma, emotional stress, menses, illness, and inflammation.
  - Type I HAE is the most common form, caused by decreased production of C1 esterase inhibitor (C1 INH), and has autosomal-dominant inheritance.
  - Type II HAE has functionally impaired C1 INH and autosomal-dominant inheritance.
  - Type III HAE involves an X-linked factor XII gene mutation (often estrogen-dependent, associated with estrogen administration).
- AAE is a rare condition.
  - Type I is associated with lymphoproliferative diseases or paraneoplastic diseases.
  - Type II is due to autoimmune disorders (anti-C1 INH antibody).
  - Affected patients have circulating antibodies directed either against specific immunoglobulins expressed on B cells (type I) or against C1 INH (type II).

ETIOLOGY
- Idiopathic
- Medication-induced:
  - ACE inhibitors cause 10–25% of AE cases, mostly occurring within the first 3–4 weeks of use of the medication. However, onset may be delayed years.
  - Angiotensin-receptor blockers (ARBs) also can cause AE, but more rarely than ACE inhibitors.
- Allergic triggers:
  - Food allergens such as shellfish, nuts, eggs, milk, wheat, soy
  - Medications such as aspirin, nonsteroidal anti-inflammatory drugs (NSAIDs), antibiotics, narcotics, and oral contraceptives
- Physically induced: Cold, heat, pressure, vibration, trauma, emotional stress, ultraviolet light
- Hereditary or acquired C1 INH deficiency
- Thyroid autoimmune disease–associated AE

COMMONLY ASSOCIATED CONDITIONS
- Quincke disease (AE of the uvula)
- Urticaria

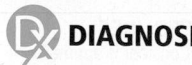

DIAGNOSIS

HISTORY
- Identify potential triggers, including medication history, recent exposure to allergens, physical elements, or trauma (1)[C].
- In comparison with urticaria, AE typically is nonpruritic, but it can cause a burning sensation.
- Obtain family medical history.

PHYSICAL EXAM
- Acute onset of asymmetric localized swelling, usually of the face (eyelids, lips, ears, nose) and less often of the extremities or genitalia
- GI tract involvement may manifest as intermittent unexplained abdominal pain.

ALERT
10–35% of patients present with severe respiratory compromise requiring endotracheal intubation.

DIAGNOSTIC TESTS & INTERPRETATIO
Lab
Initial lab tests
- If AE with urticaria and/or anaphylaxis, check for allergen-specific IgE to verify suspected trigger. Serum tryptase is elevated during acute AE (1)[C].
- Without a clear etiology and recurrence in AE and urticaria, check complete blood count (CBC) and erythrocyte sedimentation rate (ESR).
  - Macrocytosis implies a pernicious anemia.
  - Eosinophilia may imply atopy or, rarely, a parasit infection.
  - Elevated ESR may imply systemic disorders (1)[C
- In recurrent AE without a clear etiology and witho urticaria, consider ordering serum C4 level determination.
  - Low serum C4 is a sensitive but nonspecific screening test for hereditary and acquired C1 IN deficiency.
  - If C4 is normal, determine C1 INH level and function, and recheck C4 during an acute attack
  - If C4 level and C1 INH level and function are stil normal, consider other causes (i.e., medications HAE type III) for AE (2)[C].
  - If C4 level, C1 INH level, and C1 INH function ar low, this indicates HAE type I.
  - HAE type II is characterized by low C4 and low C INH function, but C1 INH level can be normal or elevated (2)[C].
  - C1q is decreased in AAE but normal in all types HAE (2)[C].

Follow-Up & Special Considerations
If C4 and C1q are low (as in AAE), neoplastic and autoimmune workup is warranted. CBC, a peripheral smear, protein electrophoresis, immunophenotyping lymphocytes, and imaging studies are often undertaken to rule out hematologic malignancies or cancer (2)[C].

Imaging
Initial approach
- Abdominal radiographs and CT scan can demonstrate GI angioedema or ileus.
- C1 INH deficiency may occur in association with internal malignancy, so angioedema rarely can be paraneoplastic disease. Imaging (CT scan, radiography, etc) then would be done as part of a neoplastic workup for patients with AAE.

Diagnostic Procedures/Surgery
Skin biopsy (may be nonspecific)

Pathological Findings
- Edema of deep dermis and subcutaneous tissue
- Variable perivascular and interstitial infiltrate

DIFFERENTIAL DIAGNOSIS
- Urticaria (with AE in 40–50% of patients)
- Allergic contact dermatitis
- Connective-tissue disease: Lupus, dermatomyositis
- Anaphylaxis
- Cellulitis, erysipelas
- Lymphedema
- Diffuse subcutaneous infiltrative process

TREATMENT

EDICATION

rst Line

- Acute allergic AE (with airway compromise):
  - Epinephrine 1:1,000, 0.3 mL IV or SC (1)[C]
  - Glucocorticoids (hydrocortisone 200 mg IV or Solu-Medrol 40 mg IV) (1)[C]
  - Diphenhydramine 50 mg IV
  - If medication-induced, stop the causative agent.
- Idiopathic recurrent AE:
  - 1st-generation antihistamines for acute AE (cause drowsiness)
  - Older children and adults: Hydroxyzine (Vistaril 5 mg/5 mL, 25-mg tablets) 10–25 mg t.i.d., or diphenhydramine (Benadryl) 25–50 mg q6h (3)[C]
  - Children <6 years of age: Diphenhydramine 12.5 mg (elixir) q6–8h (5 mg/kg/d) (3)[C]
  - 2nd-generation H_1 blockers: Fexofenadine (Allegra) 180 mg/d b.i.d., loratadine (Claritin) 10 mg/d, cetirizine (Zyrtec) 10 mg/d, desloratadine (Clarinex) 5 mg/d (3)[C]; use with caution in pregnancy and in the elderly.
- HAE chronic prophylaxis:
  - A nanofiltered plasma-derived C1 INH concentrate (Cinryze) is dosed at 1,000 units/10 mL IV at a rate of 1 mL/min (for 10 min) q3–7d (4)[B].
  - Attenuated androgens increase hepatic production of C1 INH: Danazol 50–200 mg/d or stanozolol 2–4 mg/d; danazol maximum dose 600 mg/d; use lowest effective dose. Side effects include headache, weight gain, liver dysfunction, hirsutism, and menstrual disturbances. Monitor CBC, liver function tests (LFTs), fasting lipid profile (FLP), and urinalysis every 6 months. Danazol is not to be used in children, during first 2 trimesters of pregnancy, during lactation, and in patients with prostate cancer (2)[C].
- HAE short-term prophylaxis:
  - Minor procedures (dental work): If C1 INH is available, no prophylaxis; otherwise: danazol 10 mg/kg/d (maximum 600 mg/d) or tranexamic acid [not approved by the Food and Drug Administration (FDA) in US] 75 mg/kg/d divided b.i.d. or t.i.d. × 4–5 days prior to and 2–4 days after event (2)[C]
  - Major procedures (including intubation): C1 INH 1 h prior with an additional dose on hand during procedure or 1–4 units fresh-frozen plasma (FFP) 1 day prior (for an adult)
- Acute HAE treatment:
  - C1 INH concentrate IV, dosed at 1,000 units if <50 kg; 1,500 units if 50–100 kg; 2,000 units if >100 kg (2)[C]; a pasteurized human plasma-derived C1 INH concentrate (Berinert P), dosed at 20 units/kg (available in 500 units/10 mL, to be infused at a maximum rate of 4 mL/min IV. Worsening of HAE pain was reported as the most severe adverse event (4,5)[B].
  - Kalbitor (Ecallantide), a kallikrein inhibitor, is dosed in patients ≥16 years old at 30 mg SC with 3 separate 10 mg/mL injections in the abdomen, thigh, or upper arm, and a 2nd 30-mg dose may be repeated within 24 h if needed. Injection-site rotation is not necessary but must be 2 in away from site of the attack. Anaphylaxis is a potential adverse event (4)[B].
  - Antihistamines and glucocorticoids typically do not benefit HAE patients.
- New therapies are in phase 3 clinical trials for HAE treatment:
  - A bradykinin receptor-2 antagonist (icatibant), dosed SC, was not approved by the FDA for use in the US in April 2008 and is currently undergoing further clinical trials. It was approved in the European Union under the trade name Firazyr (4)[C].
  - Other C1 INH replacement therapies, including a recombinant C1 INH isolated from the milk of transgenic rabbits (Rhucin), dosed IV (6)[C]
  - Cinryze is awaiting FDA approval for use during acute attacks (4)[C].
- Acute AAE treatment:
  - C1 INH concentrate and FFP
  - Treatment of underlying lymphoproliferative disease is often curative in AAE type I.
  - Immunosuppressive therapy to suppress antibody production
  - Clinical trials underway with recombinant human C1 INH (Rhucin) (4)[C]

Second Line

- HAE chronic prophylaxis: If patient cannot tolerate attenuated androgens, antifibrinolytic agents (plasmin inhibitors), such as tranexamic acid (not FDA approved in US) and ϵ-aminocaproic acid could be used. They are less effective than attenuated androgens and have many side effects. On rare occasions, they have been linked to (but not proven to cause) thrombophlebitis, embolism, or myositis (6).
- Acute HAE: FFP if C1 INH concentrate is not available, but it can potentially worsen attack (6).
- Idiopathic AE: Doxepin (Sinequan) may be effective for AE (10–25 mg at bedtime).
- H2RA: Ranitidine (Zantac) 150 mg/d b.i.d.

ADDITIONAL TREATMENT

General Measures

Intubation if airway is threatened

SURGERY/OTHER PROCEDURES

Tracheostomy if progressive laryngeal edema prevents endotracheal intubation

IN-PATIENT CONSIDERATIONS

Initial Stabilization

Ensure patent airway. If anaphylaxis, epinephrine (1:1,000) SC 0.3–0.5 mg q10–15min

IV Fluids

Given if needed to stabilize patient

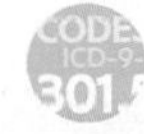

ONGOING CARE

FOLLOW-UP RECOMMENDATIONS

Patient Monitoring

- Diagnostic workup if symptoms are severe, persistent, or recurrent
- Protect airway if mouth, tongue, or throat is involved.

DIET

Avoid known dietary allergens.

PATIENT EDUCATION

Educate on avoidance of triggers (i.e., food, medication, other physical stimuli), types of treatment, when to seek emergency care, and wearing Medic Alert bracelet.

PROGNOSIS

- AE symptoms often resolve in hours to 2–3 days. If airway is compromised, AE can be life-threatening.
- Patients with HAE have an average of 20 attacks/year; each may last 3–5 days. Prophylaxis can decrease the frequency of events and number of missed days of school or work.

COMPLICATIONS

Anaphylaxis

REFERENCES

1. Temiño VM, Peebles RS. The spectrum and treatment of angioedema. *Am J Med*. 2008;121: 282–6.
2. Bowen T, Cicardi M, Farkas H et al. Canadian 2003 International Consensus Algorithm For the Diagnosis, Therapy, and Management of Hereditary Angioedema. *J Allergy Clin Immunol*. 2004; 114:629–37.
3. Frigas E, Park M. Idiopathic recurrent angioedema. *Immunol Allergy Clin North Am*. 2006;26:739–51.
4. Levy JH, Freiberger DJ, Roback J et al. Hereditary angioedema: current and emerging treatment options. *Anesth Analg*. 2010;110:1271–80.
5. Craig TJ, Levy RJ, Wasserman RL, Bewtra AK, Hurewitz D, Obtuowicz K, Reshef A, Ritchie B, Moldovan D, Shirov T, Grivcheva-Panovska V, Kiessling PC, Keinecke HO, Bernstein JA et al. Efficacy of human C1 esterase inhibitor concentrate compared with placebo in acute hereditary angioedema attacks. *J Allergy Clin Immunol*. 2009;124:801–8.
6. Craig T, Riedl M, Dykewicz MS, Gower RG, Baker J, Edelman FJ, Hurewitz D, Jacobs J, Kalfus I et al. When is prophylaxis for hereditary angioedema necessary? *Ann Allergy Asthma Immunol*. 2009;102:366–72.

See Also (Topic, Algorithm, Electronic Media Element)

Urticaria; Anaphylaxis

CODES

ICD9

995.1 Angioneurotic edema, not elsewhere classified

CLINICAL PEARLS

- Trigger identification and avoidance are key in the prevention of AE.
- New AE treatments are in development.
- Patients with a history of allergies and angioedema should be prescribed an epinephrine autoinjector.

ANKLE FRACTURES

Francesca L. Beaudoin, MS, MD
Kimberly Pringle, MD

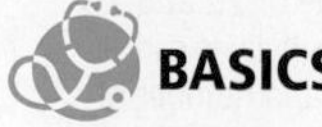

BASICS

- Bones: Tibia, fibula, talus
  - Mortise: Tibial plafond (horizontal surface of the tibia), medial malleolus, and lateral malleolus.
- Ligaments:
  - Syndesmotic ligaments: tibia-fibular ligaments
  - Lateral collateral ligaments: Posterior tibiofibular, calcaneofibular, lateral talocalcaneal, anterior talofibular
  - Medial collateral ligaments; "Deltoid ligament": Posterior tibiotalar, tibiocalcaneal, anterior tibiotalar, tibionavicular

DESCRIPTION

- Fractures involving the distal fibula (lateral malleolus) and/or distal tibia (medial malleolus and plafond)
- Two common classification systems useful for describing fractures, but neither address ankle stability or reliably describe prognosis (1)[B].
- Danis-Weber system (level of fibular fracture):
  - Type A: Below the level of syndesmosis (of tibiofibular joint); usually stable
  - Type B: At syndesmosis; usually stable
  - Type C: Above syndesmosis; usually unstable
    - Maisonneuve fracture: Proximal fracture of fibula from external rotation; partial or complete disruption of syndesmosis
- Lauge Hansen (theorized the type of fracture based on foot position and applied force):
  - Pronation-abduction rotation: Injury to medial malleolus or deltoid, injury to syndesmotic ligaments, fracture of the fibula
  - Pronation-external rotation: Transverse fracture of medial malleolus or deltoid ligament, rupture of anterior tibiofibular ligament, oblique/spiral fracture of fibula, tibiofibular ligament rupture
  - Supination-adduction: Transverse avulsion fracture of fibula below the level of the joint
    - Associated with osteochondral fractures of talus
  - Supination-external rotation: Oblique fracture at the level of the syndesmosis
- The most basic nomenclature refers to the number of fractures: Unimalleolar, bimalleolar, trimalleolar
- Pilon fracture: Fracture of the talar dome and the tibial plafond; usually axial loading mechanism; unstable

Pediatric Considerations

- Different injury pattern in children
- Injuries more likely to affect the growth plate
- Salter-Harris classification of fractures

EPIDEMIOLOGY

- Predominant ages: Even age distribution
- Predominant sex:
  - Age <50: Male > Female
  - Age >50: Female > Male
- Unimalleolar (fibular fractures) = 60–70%; bimalleolar = 15–20%; trimalleolar = 7–12%

Incidence

- 1–2 cases per 1,000 people per year
- Highest incidence in elderly women (2)[B]

RISK FACTORS

- Increased body mass index
- History of smoking or osteoporosis

GENERAL PREVENTION

- Proper shoe wear (i.e., flat, supportive shoes)
- Avoid, or use caution for, activities on uneven or slick surfaces.
- Avoid physical activity when fatigued.

PATHOPHYSIOLOGY

- The location and pattern of injury depend on foot position and the direction of force applied.
- Most commonly the foot is plantar flexed and inverted, and the force is external rotation.
- Axial loading can cause a tibial plafond or pilon fracture, an intra-articular fracture of the distal tibia where it articulates with the talus.

ETIOLOGY

- Fall or twisting injury to the ankle
- Alcohol involved in 1/3 injuries
- Slippery surfaces involved in 1/3 cases

COMMONLY ASSOCIATED CONDITIONS

- Ligamentous injury (sprains)
- Syndesmosis injury
- Ankle or subtalar dislocation
- Fractures of metatarsals, talus, or calcaneus
- Osteochondral fractures
- Posterior ankle impingement (Os trigonum)
- Peroneal tendon dislocation
- Compartment syndrome (rare)
- Neurovascular injury (rare)
- Other axial loading or shearing injuries:
  - Vertebral compression fractures
  - Contralateral pelvic fractures

DIAGNOSIS

HISTORY

- Location of pain
- Timing/Mechanism of injury
- Weight-bearing status at scene of injury
- Past history of ankle injuries or surgery
- Comorbidities (diabetes, coagulopathy)

Geriatric Considerations

- Assess for safety and fall risk
- More likely to require higher level of care

PHYSICAL EXAM

- Pain, swelling, and ecchymosis
- Inability to bear weight
- Possible deformity
- Find point of maximal tenderness
- Skin integrity: tenting, lacerations, or blistering
- Neurovascular status: Motor/Sensory exam of Foot/Ankle; Check dorsalis pedis and posterior tibial pulses
- Capillary refill
- Evaluate for compartment syndrome:
  - Swelling and pain with passive extension
- Palpate ankle, foot, leg, and knee
- Examine for other associated injuries (i.e., Pilon fractures: vertebral injuries, contralateral tibial plateau)

DIAGNOSTIC TESTS & INTERPRETATION

Imaging

- Plain radiographs are the standard
- Ottawa Ankle Rules (OAR) has a sensitivity 96.4–99.6% in adults (3)[B]:
  - X-rays indicated when malleolar pain AND:
    - Bone tenderness at the posterior edge or tip of the medial malleolus, or
    - Bone tenderness at the posterior edge or tip of the lateral malleolus, or
    - Inability to bear weight both immediately and in the emergency department, or
    - Pain at navicular or along 5th metatarsal
  - If OAR criteria not met but symptoms persist beyond 48–72 hours, obtain films
  - OAR performs well in children (missing ~1% of fractures) (3), but some experts have proposed alternate rules.
  - OAR are not valid in intoxicated patients, patients with multiple injuries, or sensory deficits (diabetics with neuropathy).
- Three standard views:
  - AP
  - Lateral: Instability depicted by talar dome and distal tibia incongruity
  - Mortise (15–25° internal rotation view): Look for parallel lines between joint spaces, and space between the medial malleolus and talus should not exceed 4 mm.
- CT useful for pilon fractures or fractures with intra-articular involvement; can find subtle injuries (i.e., stress fracture)
  - Newer 3-D reconstruction technology shows relationships between ligaments and bones.
- MRI sometimes used to explore Salter-Harris fractures or ligamentous injuries.

Diagnostic Procedures/Surgery

- Arthroscopy is an option in cases of persistent pain or suspicion of any cartilaginous lesions.
- Surgery is definitive in cases of instability (see Treatment).

DIFFERENTIAL DIAGNOSIS

- Stress fracture
- Ankle sprain
- Osteochondral fracture
- Talus fracture
- 5th metatarsal fracture
- Calcaneus fracture

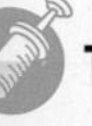

TREATMENT

edication, joint support, consultation, surgical repair, ysical therapy

EDICATION

general, ankle fractures are painful, particularly in e 1st 5–7 days following an injury. As the swelling creases, so does the pain.

rst Line

- Acetaminophen 1,000 mg QID
- NSAIDs
- Opioid analgesics

econd Line

onopioid analgesics (i.e., tramadol)

DDITIONAL TREATMENT

eneral Measures

- Assess the extent of all injuries
- Immobilization:
  - If there is a suspected open fracture, remove any debris from the wound, place a moist (Betadine) dressing over the wound
  - Noncircular cast; Short leg posterior splint stirrup
  - Jones compression bandage
  - Crutches
  - For suspected open fractures tetanus booster, broad-spectrum cephalosporin and aminoglycoside Penicillin G for farm injuries at risk for *Clostridium perfringens*
  - Do not reduce the fracture or dislocation unless neurovascular compromise is apparent.
- Ice and elevate the extremity.

sues for Referral

- Send to Emergency Department for surgical evaluation:
  - Neurovascular compromise
  - Tenting of skin/open fracture
  - Displaced fracture of malleoli
  - Intra-articular fracture
  - Bi- or trimalleolar
  - Pilon fracture
  - Unstable fracture
  - Signs of compartment syndrome
  - Instability
  - Pediatric Salter types III, IV, V
  - Maisonneuve fracture
- All other fractures orthopaedic follow-up within 1 week and be non-weight bearing EXCEPT:
  - Isolated avulsion fractures of the tip of the lateral malleolus may be weight bearing as tolerated.
  - Pediatric Salter I, II of the distal fibula

URGERY/OTHER PROCEDURES

- Surgical options:
  - Open reduction internal fixation
  - External fixation for comminuted distal tibia fractures
- Timing of surgery:
  - Within 6–8 hours for emergent cases (i.e., open fractures)
  - After swelling decreased in all other cases (preferably not >1 week)
- Length of recovery:
  - In general, 6–8 weeks for healing
  - 6–8 weeks in a cast or splint (longer if fracture involves both medial and lateral malleoli)
  - 2–4 months for syndesmotic injury
  - Orthopedist may allow range of motion after 4 weeks and place in removable cast boot (fracture pattern and surgeon dependent)
- Circular cast or protective boot
  - Isolated nondisplaced medial malleolar: non-weight bearing 3 weeks + 6–8 weeks in a cast
  - Posterior malleolar with no instability: 6-week cast
  - Bimalleolar: Surgery vs. cast; orthopedic follow-up

IN-PATIENT CONSIDERATIONS

Admission Criteria

Admit to the hospital if:

- Patient will require emergency surgery (e.g., open fracture, neurovascular injury, compartment syndrome)
- Cannot maintain non-weight bearing status and requires physical therapy consultation
- Concern of mechanism of injury (i.e., syncope, MI, head injury)

Nursing

- Apply ice
- Instruct patient to keep leg elevated.

Discharge Criteria

When patient has completed the following:

- Able to ambulate with walker/crutches
- Medical workup (if needed) is completed
- Appropriate orthopedic follow-up is arranged
- Elderly patients may require a short stay in a rehabilitation facility.

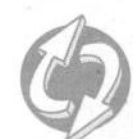

ONGOING CARE

FOLLOW-UP RECOMMENDATIONS

If the fracture does not require emergent orthopedic consultation, most ankle fractures require an orthopedic consultation within 1 week and close follow-up.

Patient Monitoring

- Orthopedic follow-up:
  - Serial x-rays should be performed weekly for 4 weeks if there is any question about stability.
  - Otherwise, x-rays should be performed at 2 weeks, 4 weeks, and 8 weeks or until the fracture is healed .
- Physical therapy: once begins healing
  - Encourage toe and knee motion as soon as possible.
  - Start ankle ROM.
  - Physical therapy for strength and proprioception critical for full recovery.

DIET

NPO if surgery is being considered

PATIENT EDUCATION

- It may take the bone 6–12 weeks to heal.
- Ice and elevate the affected leg for 2–3 weeks following the injury to decrease swelling.
- Prevent splint/cast from getting wet.
- Use crutches/cane as instructed.
- Call physician if:
  - Swelling increases
  - Toes become numb or painful
  - Burning pain under the cast
  - Pain increases and is not helped by elevation and pain medication

PROGNOSIS

- Good results can be achieved in many ankle fractures without surgery, provided the ankle mortise is maintained (4)[B].
- Long term, 30% of patients may develop ankle arthritis; timing is unpredictable.
- Effusion or pain can persist for up to 1 year.

COMPLICATIONS

Nonoperative and operative:

- Displacement of the fracture
- Malunion or nonunion
- Skin breakdown or necrosis (early)
- DVT (rarely pulmonary embolism)
- Complex regional pain syndrome
- Infection (osteomyelitis)
- Loss of fixation (post-op)
- Osteoarthritis (late)

REFERENCES

1. Michelson JD, et al. Clinical Utility of a Stability-Based Ankle Fracture Classification System. *J Orthop Trauma* 2007;21:301–307.
2. Court-Brown CM, McBirnie J, Wilson G. Adult ankle fractures–an increasing problem? *Acta Orthop Scand*. 1998;69:43–7.
3. Bachmann LM, Kolb E, Koller MT, Steurer J, ter Riet G, et al. Accuracy of Ottawa ankle rules to exclude fractures of the ankle and mid-foot: systematic review. *BMJ*. 2003;326:417.
4. Michelson JD. Ankle fractures resulting from rotational injuries. *J Am Acad Orthop Surg*. 2003;11:403–12.

ADDITIONAL READING

- Bucholz RW, Heckman JD, eds. *Rockwood and Green's Fractures in Adults* 5th ed. Philadelphia: Lippincott Williams & Wilkins Publishers; 2001.
- Stielll G, Greenberg GH, McKnight RD, et al. Decision rules for the use of radiography in acute ankle injuries: Refinement and prospective validation. *JAMA*. 1993;269:1127–32.

CODES

ICD9

- 824.0 Fracture of medial malleolus, closed
- 824.8 Unspecified fracture of ankle, closed
- 824.9 Unspecified fracture of ankle, open

CLINICAL PEARLS

- OAR have a near 100% sensitivity in adults for identifying ankle fractures.
- Ankle fractures mandating immediate surgical consultation include: Signs of compartment syndrome, neurovascular compromise, or skin compromise (open or tenting).

ANKYLOSING SPONDYLITIS

Sangeetha Balasubramanian, MD
Nancy Y. Liu, MD

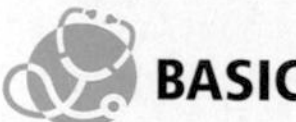

BASICS

DESCRIPTION

- Ankylosing spondylitis (AS) is a chronic inflammatory seronegative arthritis affecting mainly the axial skeleton and sacroiliac (SI) joints, but hips and shoulders may also be involved.
- System(s) affected: Musculoskeletal; Eyes; Cardiac; Neurological; Pulmonary
- Synonym: Marie-Strümpell disease

EPIDEMIOLOGY

- Predominant age: Onset usually in early 20s, rarely occurs after age 40
- Predominant sex: Male > Female (2–3:1)

Incidence

Age- and gender-adjusted rate of 6.3–7.3 per 100,000 person-years

Prevalence

0.1–1% in US

RISK FACTORS

- HLA-B27 (but only 1–8% of HLA-B27–positive adults have AS)
- Positive family history: A HLA-B27–positive child of a parent with AS has 10–30% risk of developing the disease.

Genetics

90–95% of Caucasian patients with AS are HLA-B27–positive.

PATHOPHYSIOLOGY

Inflammation at the insertion of tendons (enthesitis), ligaments and fasciae to bone, causing inflammation, erosion, and new bone formation

ETIOLOGY

Interaction between genetic factors and unknown trigger(s)

COMMONLY ASSOCIATED CONDITIONS

- Uveitis/iritis (up to 40%)
- Aortitis
- Cardiac conduction defects
- Spondylitis and sacroiliitis also seen in psoriatic arthritis, reactive arthritis, and arthropathy associated with inflammatory bowel disease

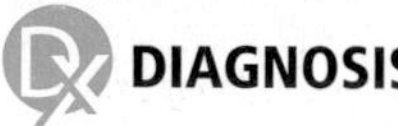

DIAGNOSIS

HISTORY

- Insidious onset of back pain
- Duration >3 months
- Morning stiffness in spine lasting more than 1 hour
- Frequent awakenings at night secondary to back pain
- Increased pain and stiffness with rest and improvement with activity
- Alternating buttock pain common symptom
- Constitutional symptoms (fatigue, weight loss, low-grade fever)

PHYSICAL EXAM

- Sacroiliac joint tenderness, loss of lumbar lordosis, and cervical spine rotation
- Diminished range of motion in the lumbar spine in all 3 planes of motion
- Modified Wright-Schober test for lumbar spine flexion is abnormal or <5 cm:
  - Mark the patient's back over the L5 spinous process (or at dimples of Venus) and measure 10 cm above and 5 cm below this point. Have the patient bend forward. The normal exam is at least 5 cm of expansion between these two marks.
- Thoracocervical kyphosis (rarely occurs before 10 years of symptoms)
- Chest pain with inspiration due to enthesitis at costochondral junction and chest wall expansion
- Measurement of respiratory excursion of chest wall:
  - Normal is >5 cm of maximal respiratory excursion of chest wall measured at 4th intercostal space
  - <2.5 cm is virtually diagnostic of ankylosing spondylitis.
- Aortic regurgitation murmur (1%)
- Acute anterior uveitis (usually unilateral on initial presentation but can recur on contralateral side)
- Achilles tendonitis
- Plantar fasciitis
- Peripheral oligoarthritis rare; seen mostly with psoriatic arthropathy, reactive arthritis, and arthropathy associated with inflammatory bowel disease
- Cauda equina syndrome is rare but well recognized late in the disease.

DIAGNOSTIC TESTS & INTERPRETATION

Lab

- Since up to 10% of Caucasian population and 4% of African American population is HLA-B27–positive, gene testing is not recommended as part of initial evaluation.
- Erythrocyte sedimentation rate (ESR) and c-reactive protein (CRP) may be mildly elevated or normal; if high, correlate poorly with disease activity and prognosis
- Absent rheumatoid factor
- Mild normochromic anemia (15%)
- Synovial fluid: mild leukocytosis

Imaging

- SI joints: Preferred position for imaging the SI joints with plain films is oblique projection:
  - X-ray changes may not be apparent for up to 10 years after disease onset. Magnetic resonance imaging (MRI) is more sensitive in documenting changes; increased signal from the bone and bone marrow suggesting osteitis and edema.
  - Sequential plain radiographic changes with time: Widening, erosions, sclerosis on both sides of joint not extending >1 cm from articular surface and finally ankylosis of sacroiliac joint
- Spine:
  - Early plain radiograph changes include "shiny corners" due to osteitis and sclerosis at site of annulus fibrosus attachments to the corners of vertebral bodies and "squaring" due to erosion and remodelling of vertebral body; contrast enhanced MRI imaging is more sensitive in revealing these early changes
  - Late changes include ossification of annulus fibrosis resulting in bony bridging between vertebral bodies (syndesmophytes) to give the classic "bamboo spine" appearance; ankylosis o apophyseal joints, ossification of spinal ligament and/or spondylodiscitis also occurs
- Peripheral joints:
  - Rare; asymmetric involvement of joints of lower extremities
  - Pericapsular ossification, sclerosis, loss of joint space, and erosions may occur.

Diagnostic Procedures/Surgery

- Electrocardiogram: Conduction defects
- Dual energy x-ray absorptiometry scan may reveal osteopenia/osteoporosis.

Pathological Findings

- Erosive changes coupled with new bone formation at the attachment of the tendons and ligaments to the bone, resulting in ossification of periarticular soft tissues
- Synovial hypertrophy and pannus formation, mononuclear cell infiltrate into subsynovium and subchondral bone marrow inflammation in the SI joint with erosions is followed by granulation tissue formation, and finally, obliteration of joint space by fusion of joint and sclerosis of para-articular bone

DIFFERENTIAL DIAGNOSIS

- Osteoarthritis of the axial spine
- Diffuse idiopathic skeletal hypertrophy (DISH)
- Psoriatic arthritis
- Reactive arthritis
- Spondylitis associated with inflammatory bowel disease
- Osteitis condensans illi: Benign sclerotic changes in the iliac portion of the SI joint found in women after pregnancies
- Infectious arthritis or discitis, especially unilateral sacroiliitis: Tuberculosis, brucellosis, bacterial (in IV drug users)

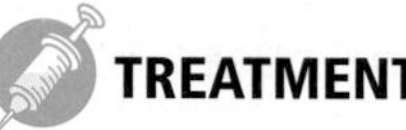

TREATMENT

Aggressive physical therapy, with referral to a physical therapist for daily home exercises, as well as group programs, is the most important nonpharmacological management.

MEDICATION

First Line

- Anti-inflammatory drugs:
  - Nonsteroidal anti-inflammatory drugs (NSAIDs) provide rapid and dramatic symptomatic relief, which can be virtually diagnostic of AS. NSAIDs chosen empirically but most importantly, in high doses
  - Injection of intra-articular corticosteroids into SI joints and esthesias can provide relief, but systemic corticosteroids are usually ineffective.

'recautions:
- All patients on long-term NSAIDs should have their hepatic and renal function monitored.
- NSAIDs may aggravate peptic ulcer disease or cause gastritis; such patients and all patients >60 years of age should receive prophylactic proton pump inhibitors (PPIs) or misoprostol while on NSAIDs.
- NSAIDs should be used with caution in patients with a bleeding diathesis or patients requiring anticoagulants
- Please refer to complete package insert with each drug for complete information on the individual drug.

econd Line

Disease-modifying agents:
- Used in those patients who have persistently high disease activity, fail, or become intolerant of NSAIDs
- Biologic disease-modifying agents: Anti-TNF-α-blocking agents that are approved by FDA for AS include: Etanercept (recombinant TNF receptor fusion protein) (1)[A], infliximab (chimeric monoclonal IgG1 antibody to TNF-α) (2)[A], adalimumab (fully humanized IgG1 monoclonal antibody to TNF-α) (3), and golimumab (human IgG1 kappa monoclonal antibody to TNF-α) (4).
- Pamidronate may also help function and decrease disease activity.
- Nonbiologic disease-modifying antirheumatic drugs such as methotrexate and sulfasalazine are ineffective for axial disease; sulfasalazine may be effective for peripheral arthritis.

Precautions:
- Anti-TNFs increase the risk for all infections.
- It is imperative to screen for latent tuberculosis before initiation of treatment.
- Screening for hepatitis B is also required.
- Monitoring for reactivation of tuberculosis in all patients and invasive fungal infections like histoplasmosis, especially with travel to or residence in endemic areas
- Please refer to complete package insert with each drug for complete information on individual drugs.

DDITIONAL TREATMENT

eneral Measures

Posture training and range-of-motion exercises for spine are essential.
Firm bed, sleep in supine position without a pillow
Breathing exercises 2–3 times a day
Smoking cessation

ssues for Referral

onfirmation of diagnosis before initiating any type of econd-line therapy

dditional Therapies

lay need treatment with antiresorptive medications if steopenia or osteoporosis is present

URGERY/OTHER PROCEDURES

Crucial to evaluate for c-spine ankylosis/instability before intubation
Total hip replacement should be considered to restore mobility and to control pain.
Vertebral osteotomy can improve posture for those patients with severe cervical or thoracolumbar flexion

ONGOING CARE

FOLLOW-UP RECOMMENDATIONS

- Maintaining physical activity and posture is critical in preventing disability.
- Swimming, tai chi, walking, and maintenance of active lifestyle are recommended.
- Avoid trauma/contact sports.
- Appropriate work ergonomics

Patient Monitoring

- Visits every 6–12 months to monitor posture and range of motion
- Counsel about risk of spinal fracture.

PATIENT EDUCATION

- Arthritis Foundation: http://www.arthritis.org
- Spondylitis Association of America: http://www.spondylitis.org

PROGNOSIS

- Extent and rapidity of progression of ankylosis are highly variable.
- Progressive limitation of spinal mobility necessitates lifestyle modification.

COMPLICATIONS

- Spine:
  - Spinal fusion causing kyphosis
  - Cervical spine fracture carries high mortality rate but fracture can occur at any level of ankylosed spine
  - C1–C2 subluxation
  - Cauda equina syndrome (rare)
- Pulmonary:
  - Restrictive lung disease
  - Upper lobe fibrosis (rare)
- Cardiac:
  - Conduction defects at atrioventricular (AV) node
  - Aortic insufficiency
  - Aortitis
  - Pericarditis extremely rare
- Uveitis and cataracts
- Renal:
  - IgA nephropathy
  - Amyloidosis (<1%)
- GI: Microscopic, subclinical ileal, and colonic mucosal ulcerations in up to 50% of patients, mostly asymptomatic

REFERENCES

1. Davis JC, van der Heijde DM, Braun J et al. Sustained durability and tolerability of etanercept in ankylosing spondylitis for 96 weeks. *Ann Rheum Dis*. 2005;64:1557–62.
2. Baraliakos X, Listing J, Brandt J et al. Radiographic progression in patients with ankylosing spondylitis after 4 yrs of treatment with the anti-TNF-alpha antibody infliximab. *Rheumatology (Oxford)*. 2007; 46:1450–3.
3. Haibel H, Rudwaleit M, Brandt HC et al. Adalimumab reduces spinal symptoms in active ankylosing spondylitis: clinical and magnetic resonance imaging results of a fifty-two-week open-label trial. *Arthritis Rheum*. 2006;54:678–81.
4. Inman RD, Davis JC, Heijde DV et al. Efficacy and safety of golimumab in patients with ankylosing spondylitis: Results of a randomized, double-blind, placebo-controlled, phase III trial. *Arthritis Rheum*. 2008;58:3402–12.
5. Sieper J, Rudwaleit M. Early referral recommendations for ankylosing spondylitis (including pre-radiographic and radiographic forms) in primary care. *Ann Rheum Dis*. 2005;64:659–63.

ADDITIONAL READING

- van der Heijde D, Maksymowych WP et al. Spondyloarthritis: state of the art and future perspectives. *Ann Rheum Dis*. 2010;69:949–54.
- Zochling J, van der Heijde D, Burgos-Vargas R, Collantes E, Davis JC, Dijkmans B, Dougados M, Géher P, Inman RD, Khan MA, Kvien TK, Leirisalo-Repo M, Olivieri I, Pavelka K, Sieper J, Stucki G, Sturrock RD, van der Linden S, Wendling D, Böhm H, van Royen BJ, Braun J, 'Assessment in AS' international working group, European League Against Rheumatism et al. ASAS/EULAR recommendations for the management of ankylosing spondylitis. *Ann Rheum Dis*. 2006;65:442–52.

See Also (Topic, Algorithm, Electronic Media Element)

Arthritis, Psoriatic; Arthritis, Rheumatoid; Crohn Disease; Reiter Syndrome; Ulcerative Colitis

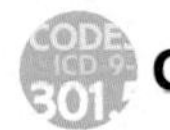

CODES

ICD9

720.0 Ankylosing spondylitis

CLINICAL PEARLS

- HLA-B27 antigen exists in 8–10% of Caucasians and 4% of African Americans in the general US population.
- Diagnosis is based on history of inflammatory back pain and morning stiffness for more than an hour, alternating buttock pain, and evidence of limitation of chest wall expansion and spinal movements in all planes; evidence of sacroiliitis and response to NSAIDs (5).
- HLA-B27 testing is an expensive and unnecessary test when clinical diagnosis is clear, but may help support the diagnosis when clinical features are less definitive.
- Plain radiography may fail to reveal changes of sacroiliitis or axial changes for up to 10 years.
- MRI is sensitive for detecting early changes of sacroiliitis or enthesitis in the axial spine.
- Physical therapy to maintain posture and mobility remains the most important nonpharmacological intervention.
- NSAIDs and TNF-α blockers are the mainstay of treatment and improve symptoms and function, but unfortunately, there is no current evidence that the latter treatment prevents bony ankylosis.

ANORECTAL ABSCESS

Timothy L. Black, MD

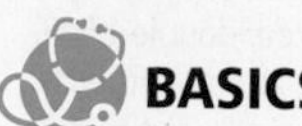

BASICS

DESCRIPTION

- Localized induration and fluctuance due to inflammation of the soft tissue near the rectum or anus
- 80% are perianal; the remainder are intrasphincteric or supralevator.
- System(s) affected: Gastrointestinal; Skin/Exocrine

Geriatric Considerations

A high pelvirectal abscess may cause minimal symptoms, such as lower abdominal pain and fever.

Pediatric Considerations

Common in 1st year of life

EPIDEMIOLOGY

- Predominant age: All ages (most common in infants) (1)[C]
- Predominant sex: Male > Female (4:1)

Incidence

Common

RISK FACTORS

- Inciting trauma:
  - Injections for internal hemorrhoids
  - Enema tip abrasions
  - Puncture wounds from eggshells or fish bones
  - Foreign objects
  - Prolapsed hemorrhoid
- Inflammatory bowel disease
- Chronic granulomatous disease (especially Crohn disease)
- Immunodeficiency disorders
- Hematologic malignancies (5–8% of these patients will have abscess at some time)
- Diabetes
- Chronic medical immunosuppression

GENERAL PREVENTION

- Avoid constipation.
- Avoid rectal thermometers, enemas, or suppositories whenever possible in immunocompromised patients.

ETIOLOGY

- Bacterial invasion of the anal glands found in the intersphincteric space, which may begin with an abrasion or tear in lining of anal canal, rectum, or perianal skin
- Organisms (usually mixed):
  - *Escherichia coli*
  - *Proteus vulgaris*
  - *Streptococci*
  - *Staphylococci* (especially methicillin-resistant variety)
  - *Bacteroides*
  - *Pseudomonas aeruginosa*

COMMONLY ASSOCIATED CONDITIONS

- Crohn disease
- Other inflammatory disease (e.g., appendicitis, salpingitis, diverticulitis)
- Possible perianal hidradenitis suppurativa or HIV infection in patients with recurring perianal or ischiorectal abscesses
- Anal fistula should be considered in patients with recurrent perianal abscesses in same location

DIAGNOSIS

HISTORY

- Pain on defecation
- Pain with sitting
- Spontaneous foul-smelling drainage

PHYSICAL EXAM

- Perirectal swelling for superficial abscesses
- Perirectal redness
- Perirectal tenderness
- Perirectal throbbing pain
- Fever and other toxic symptoms with deep abscesses
- If abscess is not accompanied by external swelling, digital rectal exam will reveal a swollen tender mass.
- Digital rectal examination is mandatory.

DIAGNOSTIC TESTS & INTERPRETATION

Lab

Complete blood count: Leukocytosis

Follow-Up & Special Considerations

Culture and sensitivity testing of purulent fluid may be important in guiding antibiotic treatment (especially in high or extensive abscess).

Imaging

- Barium enema (rarely needed)
- Computed tomography scan of pelvis and perine[um] indicated if horseshoe or ischiorectal abscess suspected (2)[C]

Diagnostic Procedures/Surgery

Only indicated if diagnosis in doubt:

- Sigmoidoscopy: Rule out unusual causes
- Proctoscopy: Redness, induration of anus; tender mass

Pathological Findings

- Inflammation of anal mucosa
- Pus
- Inflammatory tissue
- Possible fistula tract

DIFFERENTIAL DIAGNOSIS

- Carcinoma
- Retrorectal tumors
- Crohn disease
- Primary lesions of syphilis
- Tuberculous ulceration
- Thrombosed hemorrhoid

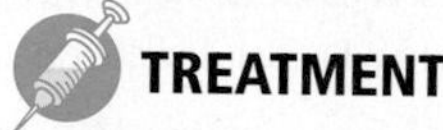

TREATMENT

MEDICATION

- Antibiotics (gram-negative and anaerobic coverag[e] based on culture results)
- Stool-softening laxatives

ADDITIONAL TREATMENT

General Measures

- Outpatient surgery with oral antibiotics (although some cases antibiotics may not be necessary) (3)[
- Inpatient surgery with IV antibiotics for supralevat[or] abscess or toxicity (2)[C]

SURGERY/OTHER PROCEDURES

- Perianal abscess:
  - Incise and drain abscess (3)[B].
  - Local anesthetic frequently appropriate with sm[all] abscesses
  - Pack wound with iodoform gauze (24–48 hours

schiorectal abscess:
- Incise and drain abscess (3)[B].
- General anesthetic usually required
- Pack wound with iodoform gauze or similar packing (removed gradually over several days).
- Fistulectomy may be done at the same time in selected cases.

upralevator abscess:
- Incise and drain abscess into lower rectum or anal canal (2)[C].
- General anesthesia required

reatment of anorectal fistula at time of abscess drainage may be performed (4)[C],(5):
- Recurrent abscess risk lower when fistula treated at same procedure
- Incontinence risk higher when fistula treated as delayed procedure
- Recommended in cases of subcutaneous, intersphincteric, or low trans-sphincteric fistula

After surgery:
- Sitz baths every 2–4 hours
- Heating pad, heat lamp, or warm compress as needed for pain
- Encourage moving legs as soon as possible
- Prevent constipation.

-PATIENT CONSIDERATIONS

dmission Criteria

- Fever
- Systemic toxicity
- Most supralevator abscesses

ONGOING CARE

OLLOW-UP RECOMMENDATIONS

esume work and normal activity as soon as possible

atient Monitoring

outine postoperative care with attention to wound ealing, which should progress from the inside out

IET

crease fiber and fluid intake.

PATIENT EDUCATION

- Provide sitz bath instructions.
- Provide diet instructions.
- Provide dressing change instructions.
- Stress length of time to heal.
- Stress physical cleanliness.
- Watch for possible development of fistula-in-ano.
- Stress stool regularity; avoid constipation.

PROGNOSIS

- Slow healing depending on extent of disease and concurrent illnesses; complete healing by 6 months if no complications
- Healing in infants may be complete in 1–3 weeks.
- Drainage alone results in cure rate of 50% or more.

COMPLICATIONS

- Possible anorectal fistula (in 25% of patients) (1,2)[C]
- Possible rectovaginal fistula
- Fecal incontinence due to rupture through sphincter muscle
- Recurrence of abscess if underlying cause not corrected
- Necrotizing infection with rapid progression, sepsis, and death (2)[C]

REFERENCES

1. Ziegler M, Azizkhan R, Weber T, et al., eds. *Operative Pediatric Surgery*. New York: McGraw-Hill, 2003.
2. Townsend C, Beauchamp RD, Evers BM, et al., eds. *Sabiston Textbook of Surgery*, 17 ed. Philadelphia: Elsevier Saunders, 2006.
3. Whiteford MH, Kilkenny J, Hyman N et al. Practice parameters for the treatment of perianal abscess and fistula-in-ano (revised). *Dis Colon Rectum*. 2005;48:1337–42.
4. Oliver I et al. Randomized clinical trial comparing simple drainage of anorectal abscess with and without fistula track treatment. *Int J Colorectal Dis*. 2003;18:107–10.
5. Malik AI, Nelson RL, Tou S. Incision and drainage of perianal abscess with or without treatment of anal fistula (Protocol). *Cochrane Database of Systematic Reviews*. 2007, Issue 4. Art. No.: CD006827. DOI: 10.1002/14651858.CD006827.

ADDITIONAL READING

Schubert MC, Sridhar S, Schade RR, Wexner SD et al. What every gastroenterologist needs to know about common anorectal disorders. *World J Gastroenterol*. 2009;15:3201–9.

See Also (Topic, Algorithm, Electronic Media Element)

Anorectal Fistula

CODES

ICD9

566 Abscess of anal and rectal regions

CLINICAL PEARLS

- Anorectal abscess should be treated as soon as possible after diagnosis.
- Any patient who has systemic signs of infection requires hospital admission for treatment. Most infants and children do not require admission.
- Incision and drainage with packing is the treatment of choice for perianal abscesses, and may be done under local anesthesia. Ischiorectal and supralevator abscesses usually require drainage under general anesthesia.

ANORECTAL FISTULA

Timothy L. Black, MD

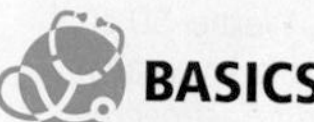

BASICS

DESCRIPTION

Inflammatory tract with 1 opening in the anal canal and another in perianal skin. Fistulas occur spontaneously or secondary to perirectal abscess. Most fistulas originate in the anal crypts at the anorectal junction:

- Goodsall rule:
  - If external opening is anterior to an imaginary line drawn horizontally through anal canal, fistula usually runs directly into anal canal. Positive predictive value is ~70%.
  - If external opening is posterior to line, fistula usually curves to posterior midline of anal canal. PPV is ~40%.
  - In children, tract is usually straight.
- Classification (1)[C]:
  - Intersphincteric: Fistula is confined to the intersphincteric plane (most common).
  - Trans-sphincteric: Fistula connects intersphincteric plane with ischiorectal fossa by perforating the external sphincter.
  - Suprasphincteric: Fistula connects intersphincteric plane with ischiorectal fossa but loops over external sphincter.
  - Extrasphincteric: Fistula connects rectum to perineal skin but passes external to sphincter.
- System(s) affected: Gastrointestinal; Skin/Exocrine
- Synonym(s): Fistula-in-ano; Anal fistula

Geriatric Considerations

Constipation is a common complication.

Pediatric Considerations

- Most common in infants
- More frequent in males

EPIDEMIOLOGY

- Predominant age: All ages
- Predominant sex: Male > Female

Incidence

Common

RISK FACTORS

- Injection of internal hemorrhoids, puncture wound from eggshells or fish bones, foreign objects, enema tip injuries
- Ruptured anal hematoma
- Prolapsed internal hemorrhoid
- Acute appendicitis, salpingitis, diverticulitis
- Inflammatory bowel disease (chronic ulcerative colitis, Crohn disease)
- Previous perirectal abscess
- Radiation treatment to perineum/pelvis
- Trauma, either internal or external
- Carcinoma

GENERAL PREVENTION

Prevention or prompt treatment of anorectal abscess

ETIOLOGY

- Erosion of anal canal
- Extension from infection from a tear in lining of anal canal
- Infecting organism is commonly *E. coli* (other enteric pathogens may also contribute to infection)

COMMONLY ASSOCIATED CONDITIONS

- Possibly associated with penetrating injury, intestinal tuberculosis, ulcerative colitis
- Hidradenitis suppurativa
- Crohn disease

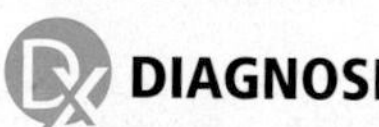

DIAGNOSIS

HISTORY

- History of perianal drainage
- History of perianal pain
- History of perianal abscesses in 26–37% (may be higher in recurrent abscesses) (2)[A]

PHYSICAL EXAM

- Constant or intermittent drainage or discharge (drainage may be purulent, bloody, or fecal)
- Firm, tender perianal mass
- External anal sphincter pain during and after defecation
- Spasm of external anal sphincter during and after defecation
- Anal bleeding
- Discoloration of skin surrounding fistula
- Fistulous opening frequently granulose or scarred
- Possible fever (uncommon)
- Perineal or perianal draining orifice
- Recurrent perianal abscesses in identical location
- Small palpable lesion sometimes identified on rectal exam at level of anal crypts

DIAGNOSTIC TESTS & INTERPRETATION

Lab

- Complete blood count (usually not indicated)
- Serologic testing using perinuclear antineutrophil cytoplasmic antibody and antisaccharomyces cerevisiae antibody if inflammatory bowel disease (i.e., Crohn disease) suspected
- Consider rapid plasma reagin for recurrent fistulas sexually active patients to rule out syphilis

Imaging

- Lower gastrointestinal series if inflammatory bowel disease suspected
- Pelvic magnetic resonance imaging or endorectal ultrasound may be useful in complex or recurrent fistulas.

Diagnostic Procedures/Surgery

- Proctoscopy or sigmoidoscopy
- Colonoscopy and esophagogastroduodenoscopy if Crohn disease suspected
- Probe inserted into tract to determine its course (be careful not to create an artificial opening); best done at time of surgery
- Injection of dilute methylene blue into abscess cavity at time of surgery may be helpful in demonstrating fistula (1)[C]

Pathological Findings

- Fistulous tract may be simple or multiple
- Fistulous tract has primary opening in anal crypt; secondary opening in anal skin, para-anal skin, perineal skin, or in rectal mucous membrane
- Anal sinus: Opens in anal crypt
- Termination of sinus is blind and located in para-anal or pararectal tissue.

DIFFERENTIAL DIAGNOSIS

- Pilonidal sinus
- Perianal abscess
- Urethroperineal fistulas
- Ischiorectal abscess
- Submucous or high muscular abscess
- Pelvirectal abscess (rare)
- Rule out: Crohn disease, carcinoma, retrorectal tumors

TREATMENT

EDICATION

Broad-spectrum antibiotic if active infection:
- Cephalexin (Keflex)
- Cefadroxil (Duricef)
- Ampicillin-sulbactam (Unasyn)
- Amoxicillin-clavulanate (Augmentin)
- Cefoxitin or piperacillin/tazobactam (Zosyn) for IV use

Stool-softening laxative

ODITIONAL TREATMENT

eneral Measures

Appropriate health care: Outpatient surgery

Sitz baths 3–4 times per day until definitive surgery

JRGERY/OTHER PROCEDURES

Fistulotomy:
- Surgical incision of entire length of fistula (unroofing) (3)[A]
- Mucosal tract should be cauterized or curetted.
- Consider fistulotomy at time of initial abscess drainage if fistula tract can be identified.
- Sphincterotomy

Fistulectomy:
- Complete excision of tract (rarely indicated because of extensive tissue loss)
- Sphincterotomy

Consider Seton stitch placement (especially for suprasphincteric or trans-sphincteric fistulas) (3)[A].

Endorectal advancement flap closure for complex fistulas (3)[A]

General anesthesia or regional anesthesia usually required (usually done as outpatient procedure in children)

Consider use of fibrin glue in selected cases of anal fistulas (3)[A],(4)[C].

Fistulas in Crohn disease (3)[A],(5)[B]:
- Asymptomatic fistulas may not need treatment.
- Simple fistulas treated with unroofing
- Complex fistulas treated with advancement flap or long term Setons
- Fibrin glue may be of benefit in patients with complex fistulae or Crohn disease (2)[A].
- May require a diverting stoma
- Occasional patients may require proctectomy.
- Aggressive treatment of Crohn disease

Postoperative: Sitz baths several times per day

Avoid constipation.

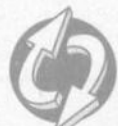

ONGOING CARE

FOLLOW-UP RECOMMENDATIONS

Resume work and normal activity as soon as possible.

Patient Monitoring

Frequent follow-up examinations following surgery to ensure complete healing and assess continence

DIET

Clear liquid diet until gastrointestinal function returns

PROGNOSIS

- Surgical results usually excellent
- Postoperative healing:
  - 4–5 weeks for perianal fistulas
  - 12–16 weeks for deeper fistulas
  - Less than 1/3 of patients with Crohn disease who have active proctitis demonstrate significant healing following surgical intervention (5)[B].
- Postoperative healing may occur within 2–3 weeks in children.
- Recurrence rates 2–9% in simple fistulas (3)[A]
- Healing may be significantly delayed in patients with Crohn disease.

COMPLICATIONS

- Constipation (urge to defecate may be suppressed due to pain)
- Rectovaginal fistula
- Partial incontinence of fecal material if sphincter is divided
- Delayed wound healing
- Low-grade carcinoma may develop in long-standing fistulas.
- Recurrent anorectal fistula if fistula is incompletely opened or excised
- Chronic intermittent infections
- Sepsis (rarely)

REFERENCES

1. Townsend C, Beauchamp RD, Evers BM, et al., eds. *Sabiston Textbook of Surgery*, 17th ed. Philadelphia: Elsevier Saunders; 2006.
2. Malik AI, Nelson RL et al. Surgical management of anal fistulae: a systematic review. *Colorectal Dis.* 2008;10:420–30.
3. Whiteford MH, Kilkenny J, Hyman N et al. Practice parameters for the treatment of perianal abscess and fistula-in-ano (revised). *Dis Colon Rectum.* 2005;48:1337–42.
4. Hammond TM, Grahn MF, Lunniss PJ. Fibrin glue in the management of anal fistulae. *Colorectal Dis.* 2004;6:308–19.
5. Lewis RT, Maron DJ et al. Anorectal Crohn's disease. *Surg Clin North Am.* 2010;90:83–97, Table of Contents

See Also (Topic, Algorithm, Electronic Media Element)

Anorectal Abscess; Crohn Disease

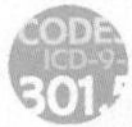

CODES

ICD9

565.1 Anal fistula

CLINICAL PEARLS

- Suspect anorectal fistula when patient complains of constant or intermittent perianal drainage or discharge (drainage may be purulent, bloody, or fecal).
- Surgery is the definitive treatment and usually produces excellent results.
- Antibiotics should be reserved for acute infection.

ANOREXIA NERVOSA

Pamela M. Williams, MD, Lt Col, USAF, MC
Jeffrey L. Goodie, PhD

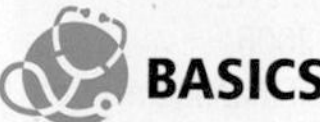

BASICS

DESCRIPTION
- Refusal to maintain normal body weight, with associated fear of weight gain, body-image disturbance, and amenorrhea
- Restricting and binge eating/purging subtypes
- System(s) affected: Cardiovascular; Endocrine; Metabolic; GI; Nervous; Reproductive

EPIDEMIOLOGY
- Predominant age: 13–20 years
- Predominant sex: Female > Male (20:1)
- Global distribution

Incidence
8–19 women, 2 men per 100,000 population per year

Prevalence
- 0.9% in women
- 0.3% in men (higher in gay and bisexual men)

RISK FACTORS
- Female gender
- Body dissatisfaction
- Perfectionism, obsessionality, rigidity
- Negative self-evaluation
- Academic and other achievement pressure
- Severe life stressors
- Participation in sports or artistic activities that emphasize leanness or involve subjective scoring: Ballet, running, wrestling, figure skating, gymnastics, cheerleading, weight lifting
- Type I diabetes mellitus
- Family history of substance abuse, affective disorders, or eating disorder

Genetics
- Underlying genetic vulnerability likely but not well understood
- 1st-degree female relative with eating disorder increases risk 6- to 10-fold.

GENERAL PREVENTION
Prevention programs can reduce risk factors and future onset of eating disorders (1)[C].
- Target adolescents and young women 15 years of age or older.
- Encourage realistic and healthy weight-management strategies and attitudes.
- Decrease body dissatisfaction.
- Promote self-esteem.
- Reduce focus on thin as ideal.
- Moderate overly high self-expectations.
- Decrease anxiety/depressive symptoms.
- Improve stress management.

PATHOPHYSIOLOGY
- Complex relationship between biologic, psychological, and social factors that results in an unrealistic perception of fatness
- Subsequent malnutrition leads to disorder of multiple organs.

ETIOLOGY
- Serotonin neuronal systems are implicated.
- Multifactorial with psychological, biologic, genetic, environmental, and social factors

COMMONLY ASSOCIATED CONDITIONS
- Mood disorder
- Social phobia, obsessive-compulsive disorder
- Substance abuse disorder
- High rates of cluster C personality disorders

DIAGNOSIS

- (DSM-IV-TR) criteria:
  - Refusal to maintain body weight at or above a minimally normal weight for age and height
  - Intense fear of gaining weight even though underweight
  - A disturbance in the way body weight/shape is experienced; undue influence of body on self-evaluation or denial of seriousness of low body weight
  - Specific types:
    - Restricting type: Not engaged in binge eating or purging behaviors
    - Binge eating/purging type: Regularly engages in binge eating or purging behaviors (see bulimia information related to these behaviors)
- Psychological self-report screening tools:
  - Eating Attitudes Test (EAT)
  - Eating Disorder Inventory (EDI)
  - Eating Disorder Screen for Primary Care (ESP)
  - SCOFF (sick, control, one, fat, food) questionnaire

HISTORY
- Patient unlikely to self-identify problem; corroborate with family or friends.
- Ascertain fear of weight gain and/or distorted body image.
- Onset may be insidious or stress-related.
- Report feeling fat even when emaciated
- Preoccupation with body size, weight control
- Elaborate food preparation and eating rituals
- Extensive exercise
- Amenorrhea (primary or secondary)
- Weakness, fatigue, cognitive impairment
- Cold intolerance
- Constipation, bloating, early satiety
- Growth arrest, delayed puberty
- Decreased bone density, fractures

PHYSICAL EXAM
- Often normal
- Vital signs: Hypothermia, bradycardia, orthostatic hypotension, body weight <85% of expected
- Cardiac: Dysrhythmias, midsystolic click of mitral valve prolapse
- Skin/extremities: Dry skin; lanugo hair on extremities, face, and trunk; hair loss; edema
- Neurologic and abdominal exams: To rule out other causes of weight loss and vomiting

DIAGNOSTIC TESTS & INTERPRETATION

Lab
- No specific test for anorexia nervosa (AN)
- Most findings are related directly to starvation and/or dehydration.
- All findings may be within normal limits.

Initial lab tests
- Low serum leuteinizing hormone, follicle-stimulat hormone; low serum testosterone in males
- Thyroid function tests: Low thyroid-stimulating hormone with normal T_3/T_4
- Liver function tests: Abnormal liver enzymes
- Chem 7: Altered blood urea nitrogen, creatinine clearance; electrolyte disturbances
- Hypoglycemia, hypercholesterolemia, hypercortisolemia, hypophosphatemia
- Low sedimentation rate
- Complete blood count: Anemia, leukopenia, thrombocytopenia
- 12-lead electrocardiogram to assess for prolongec QT interval

Imaging
Dual-energy x-ray absorptiometry (DEXA) of bone or if underweight for >6 months to assess for diminish bone density

Pathological Findings
- Osteoporosis/osteopenia, pathologic fractures
- Sick euthyroid syndrome
- Cardiac impairment

DIFFERENTIAL DIAGNOSIS
- Hyperthyroidism, adrenal insufficiency
- Inflammatory bowel disease, malabsorption
- Immunodeficiency, chronic infections
- Diabetes
- CNS lesion
- Bulimia; body dysmorphic disorder
- Depressive disorders with loss of appetite
- Anxiety disorder, food phobia
- Conversion disorder, schizophrenic disorder

ALERT
AN may exist concurrently with chronic medical disorders such as diabetes and cystic fibrosis.

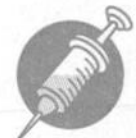

TREATMENT

- Most patients should be treated as outpatients using an interdisciplinary team (2,3)[C].
- Behavioral therapies (e.g., cognitive-behavioral, interpersonal, or family therapy) should be offered (2,4,5,6)[C].
- Pharmacotherapy should not be used as the sole treatment modality (2,3,7)[C].

MEDICATION

First Line
- No medications are available that effectively treat patients with AN, but pharmacotherapy may be used as an adjuvant to cognitive-behavioral therapies (2,3,6,7)[C].
- Selective serotonin reuptake inhibitors (SSRIs) may
  - Help to prevent relapse after weight gain
  - Treat comorbid depression or obsessive-compulsive disorder (2,3,6,7)[C].
- Studies using atypical antipsychotics are underway.
- Attend to black-box warnings concerning antidepressants, and conduct appropriate informed consent if prescribed.

cond Line

1anagement of osteopenia:
- Primary treatment is weight gain (3)[C].
- Elemental calcium 1,200–1,500 mg/d plus MVI containing 800 IU of vitamin D (3)[C]
- No indication for bisphosphonates in AN (3)[C]
- Weak evidence for use of hormone-replacement therapy (3)[C]

syllium (Metamucil) preparations (1 T) to prevent onstipation

DDITIONAL TREATMENT

eneral Measures

- nitial treatment goal geared to weight restoration; nost managed as outpatients
-)utpatient treatment:
  - Interdisciplinary team (primary care physician, mental health provider, nutritionist) (2,3)[C]
  - Average weekly weight gain goal: 0.5–1.0 kg (2,3)[C], with stepwise increase in calories
  - Cognitive-behavioral therapy, interpersonal psychotherapy, family-based therapy (2,4,5,6)[C]
  - Focus on health, not weight gain alone.
  - Build trust, treatment alliance.
  - Involve patient in establishing diet and exercise goals.
  - Challenge fear of uncontrolled weight gain; help the patient to recognize feelings that lead to disordered eating.
  - In chronic cases, goal may be to achieve a safe weight rather than a healthy weight.
- npatient treatment:
  - If possible, admit to specialized eating disorders unit (3)[C].
  - Assess risk for refeeding syndrome (weight loss >10% in 2–3 months; current weight <70% ideal body weight).
  - Monitor vital signs, electrolytes, cardiac function, edema, weight gain.
  - Initial bed rest with supervised meals may be necessary.
  - Stepwise increase in activity
  - Tube feeding or total parental nutrition is used only as a last resort.
  - Supportive symptomatic care as needed

sues for Referral

tients with AN require an interdisciplinary team rimary care physician, mental health provider, trilionist).

I-PATIENT CONSIDERATIONS

dmission Criteria

- Suggested physiologic values: Heart rate <40 beats/min, blood pressure <90/60 mm Hg, symptomatic hypoglycemia, potassium <3 mmol/L, temperature <97.0°F (36.1°C), dehydration, other cardiovascular abnormalities, weight <75% of expected, rapid weight loss, lack of improvement while in outpatient therapy
- Suggested psychological indications: Poor motivation/insight, lack of cooperation with outpatient treatment, inability to eat, need for nasogastric feeding, suicidal intent or plan, severe coexisting psychiatric disease, problematic family environment

Pediatric Considerations

- Children often present with nausea, abdominal pain, fullness, and inability to swallow.
- Additional indications for hospitalization: Heart rate <50 beats/min, orthostatic blood pressure, hypokalemia or hypophosphatemia, rapid weight loss even if weight not <75% below normal

Geriatric Considerations

Late-onset AN (>50 years of age) may be long-term disease or triggered by death of loved one, marital discord, or divorce.

Discharge Criteria

Lower relapse rate when discharged at expected healthy weight

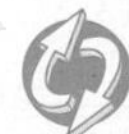

ONGOING CARE

FOLLOW-UP RECOMMENDATIONS

- Close follow-up until patient demonstrates forward progress in care plan
- Focus on enjoyable activities rather than goal-oriented ones.
- Emphasize importance of moderate activity for health, not thinness.

Patient Monitoring

- Level of exercise activity
- Weigh weekly until stable, then monthly.
- Depression, self-esteem, suicidal ideation

DIET

- Importance of adherence to prescribed diet
- Goal is stabilization at a healthy weight on a balanced diet with normal eating pattern.
- Diminished ruminations about calories, weight; increased enjoyment

PATIENT EDUCATION

- Provide patients and families with information on the diagnosis and its natural history, health risks, and treatment strategies.
- The National Alliance on Mental Illness has information at www.nami.org/helpline/anorexia.htm
- Also: familydoctor.org

PROGNOSIS

- Prognosis: ~50% recover; 30% improve; 20% are chronically ill.
- Mortality: 5%

COMPLICATIONS

- Refeeding syndrome
- Cardiac arrhythmia, cardiac arrest
- Cardiomyopathy, congestive heart failure
- Delayed gastric emptying, necrotizing colitis
- Seizures, Wernicke encephalopathy, peripheral neuropathy, cognitive deficits
- Osteopenia, osteoporosis

Pregnancy Considerations

- Fertility may be affected.
- Behaviors may persist, decrease, or recur in pregnancy and postpartum interval.
- Increased risk for preterm labor, operative delivery, and infants with low birth weight, smaller head circumference, and/or microcephaly; anemia; genitourinary infections; and labor induction; should be managed as high risk

REFERENCES

1. Stice E, Shaw H, Marti CN. A meta-analytic review of eating disorder prevention programs: encouraging findings. *Annu Rev Clin Psychol*. 2007;3:207–31.
2. NICE. Eating disorders—core interventions in the treatment and management of anorexia nervosa, bulimia nervosa and related eating disorders. NICE Clinical Guideline no 9. London: NICE, 2004 (accessed May 8, 2010).
3. American Psychiatric Association. Practice Guideline for the Treatment of Patients with Eating Disorders. 3rd ed. 2006 (accessed May 8, 2010).
4. Hay P, Bacaltchuk J, Claudino A, Ben-Tovim D, et al. Individual psychotherapy in the outpatient treatment of adults with anorexia. *Cochrane Database Syst Rev*. 2003 Issue 4:CD003909.
5. Fisher CA, Hetrick SE, Rushford N et al. Family therapy for anorexia nervosa. *Cochrane Database Syst Rev*. 2010;4:CD004780.
6. Bulik CM, Berkman ND, Brownley KA, Sedway JA, Lohr KN et al. Anorexia nervosa treatment: a systematic review of randomized controlled trials. *Int J Eat Disord*. 2007;40:310–20.
7. Claudino A, Hay P, Lima M, et al. Antidepressants for anorexia nervosa. *Cochrane Database Syst Rev*. 2006 Issue 1:CD04365.

ADDITIONAL READING

American Psychiatric Association. *Diagnostic and Statistical Manual of Mental Disorders DSM-IV-TR*, 4/e. American Psychiatric Publishing, Inc, 2000.

See Also (Topic, Algorithm, Electronic Media Element)

Amenorrhea; Osteoporosis; Bulimia Nervosa
Algorithm: Weight Loss

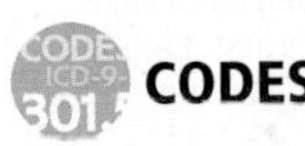

CODES

ICD9

307.1 Anorexia nervosa

CLINICAL PEARLS

- Particularly among young women with a risk factor, asking, "Are you satisfied with your eating patterns?" and/or "Do you worry that you have lost control over how you eat?" may help to screen those with an eating problem.
- In AN, there is a sustained and determined pursuit of weight loss resulting in a body weight <85% of expected.
- To care for a patient with AN, an interdisciplinary team that includes a medical provider, a dietician, and a behavioral health professional is the most accepted approach.

ANTHRAX

Gregory D. Gutke, MD, MPH
Richard J. Thomas, MD, MPH

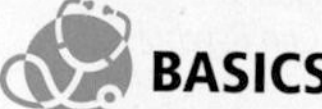

BASICS

DESCRIPTION

- Anthrax is a highly infectious disease of animals, especially ruminants (hooved animals such as cows, goats, and sheep) that is caused by the bacteria *Bacillus anthracis*. Cutaneous (95% of US cases), inhalational, and GI forms can be transmitted to humans by contact with the animals or their products (typically hair or hides).
- Synonym(s) for cutaneous anthrax: Charbon; Malignant pustule; Siberian ulcer; Malignant edema; Splenic fever; Milzbrand
- Synonym(s) for inhalational anthrax: Ragpicker disease; Woolsorter disease

EPIDEMIOLOGY

- Total of 235 anthrax cases (224 cutaneous and 11 inhalational) occurred in the US between 1955 and 1994, resulting in 20 fatalities.
- Cutaneous: 95% of cases in the US; cases of cutaneous anthrax without occupational risk should raise concern for bioterrorism.
  - ~5–20% of untreated cases result in death; case fatality rate is <1% with antibiotic therapy.
- GI: Very rare in the US (no documented case in the 20th century).
- Inhalational anthrax is very rare in US; must be considered a bioterrorist event in US until proven otherwise (the last US occupational case occurred in 1976):
  - Death results in 99% of untreated cases and in 45–80% of patients with severe symptoms who are treated in a state-of-the-art facility.
- Anthrax is most common in agricultural regions, where it occurs in animals. These regions include the Middle East, Asia, Southern and Eastern Europe, Africa, South and Central America, and the Caribbean.

RISK FACTORS

- Contact with infected animals or their products
- Bioterrorist event

GENERAL PREVENTION

- Anthrax vaccine protects against all forms of anthrax and is as safe as other vaccines, according to the FDA, CDC, and the National Academy of Sciences.
- A 2009 review by the Cochrane Infectious Disease Group concluded that the anthrax vaccine is effective in reducing the risk of contracting anthrax and has a low rate of adverse effects (1)[A]
- Anthrax vaccine should be effective against all known strains of *B. anthracis* as well as against any strains that might be bioengineered by terrorists or others.
- Vaccine schedule and route changed in late 2008: Route is now intramuscular (previously subcutaneous) and schedule is decreased from 6 doses down to 5 doses (0 and 4 weeks, and 6, 12, and 18 months) plus annual boosters. Intramuscular versus subcutaneous injection greatly reduces the incidence of injection-site adverse events (2):
  - Anthrax vaccine adsorbed (trade name BioThrax) is FDA approved for ages 18 through 65 and is pregnancy category D.
  - If you get behind schedule, do not start the series over; begin where you left off (delays do not reduce the resulting protection).
  - Individuals are not considered protected until they have completed the full vaccination series.
  - The most common (>10%) local (injection-site) adverse reactions observed in clinical studies were tenderness, pain, erythema, and arm motion limitation. The most common (>5%) systemic adverse reactions were muscle aches, fatigue and headache.
  - The Advisory Committee on Immunization Practices recommends vaccination for the following groups:
    - Persons who work directly with the organism in the laboratory
    - Persons who work with imported animal hides or furs in areas where standards are insufficient to prevent exposure to anthrax spores
    - Persons who handle potentially infected animal products in high-incidence areas
    - Military personnel deployed to areas with high risk for exposure to organisms (when used as a biologic warfare weapon)
    - Pregnant women should be vaccinated for anthrax only if absolutely necessary.
- Patients with a likely inhalational exposure history but no symptoms are candidates for postexposure prophylaxis with either ciprofloxacin 500 mg PO b.i.d. or doxycycline 100 mg PO b.i.d. for 60 days. Levofloxacin is also FDA approved for patients age 18 or older. CDC guidelines state patients should also receive 3 doses of Anthrax vaccine (0, 2 weeks, 4 weeks), but since BioThrax is not licensed for post-exposure prophylaxis or for a 3-dose series this would need to be conducted under an Investigational New Drug application. Prophylactic medications are not indicated for prevention of cutaneous anthrax.

PATHOPHYSIOLOGY

- *B. anthracis* is a spore-forming, gram-positive bacterium found in the soil worldwide. The word *anthracis* is derived from a Greek word meaning "coal," which is used to describe the cutaneous form of the disease that leads to a characteristic black lesion.
- *B. anthracis* has 3 known virulence factors: An antiphagocytic capsule and 2 protein toxins (known as edema factor and lethal factor):
  - The capsule provides resistance to phagocytosis.
  - Lethal factor and edema factor are named for the effects they induce when injected into experimental animals.
  - A protein called *protective antigen* binds to the host cell's surface; when cleaved by a protease on the cell surface it creates a site to which the lethal factor and edema factor can bind; protective antigen is required for the action of the 2 protein toxins.
- *B. anthracis* spores introduced into the host are ingested at the exposed site by macrophages and then germinate into vegetative forms that produce the virulence factors.

ETIOLOGY

- Cutaneous: Occurs when *B. anthracis* enters the sk through a cut or abrasion during the handling of animal products (such as meat, wool, or hides infected with *B. anthracis*)
- GI: Ingestion of bacillus-contaminated meat
- Inhalational: Inhalation of aerosolized *B. anthracis* spores

DIAGNOSIS

- Cutaneous: Incubation period is usually immediate up to 1 day. Begins as a pruritic spot, followed by red-brown papule that enlarges with peripheral erythema, vesiculation, and induration, followed b black eschar formation within 7–10 days of the initial lesion:
  - The papule, blister, and eschar are painless, and cutaneous symptoms may be accompanied by fever, malaise, and headache.
  - A black eschar with massive edema is nearly pathognomonic for cutaneous anthrax.
- GI: Incubation period is usually 1–7 days. Presents as 1 of 2 distinct syndromes—oropharyngeal and abdominal:
  - Oropharyngeal syndrome presentation can incluc fever, edema, ulcer, severe sore throat, and lymphadenopathy, resulting in marked unilateral or bilateral neck swelling.
  - Abdominal syndrome may present with fever, malaise, hematemesis, anorexia, severe abdominal pain, and hematochezia or melena. 2–4 days after onset of symptoms, pain begins tc subside and ascites develops, with shock and death within just a few days.
- Inhalational: Incubation period is usually less than one week, but may be up to 60 days. Biphasic presentation, with initial phase featuring nonspecifi influenzalike symptoms such as low-grade fever, chills, headache, nonproductive cough, diaphoresis, malaise, chest discomfort, nausea, vomiting, diarrhea, and abdominal pain:
  - This initial phase is followed by a 2nd fulminant phase that begins 1–5 days after onset of the initial phase symptoms. Signs and symptoms of the fulminant phase include abrupt onset of high fever, severe dyspnea, hypoxia, hypotension, and death within 24–36 hours.

HISTORY

- Cutaneous: Crucial clinical clues are rapid evolution of symptoms, lack of pain, occasional massive edema, and the near pathognomonic black eschar. Incubation period is usually immediate but may last up to 1 day.
- GI: Incubation period usually 1–7 days; 2–4 days after onset of symptoms, ascites develop as abdominal pain decreases. Shock and death occur within 2–5 days after onset of symptoms.

nhalational: Incubation period is usually <1 week out may be as long as 2 months. 2nd portion of the biphasic presentation begins 1–5 days after onset of initial symptoms. There may be a 1- to 3-day period of improvement after the 1st phase and before the 2nd phase begins. Shock and death occur within 24–36 hours after onset of the 2nd phase.

HYSICAL EXAM

Cutaneous: Red-brown papule, vesicles, or black eschar

GI: Acute abdomen with rebound tenderness may occur. Ascites present later in course.

Inhalational: Rhonchi may be present.

IAGNOSTIC TESTS & INTERPRETATION

ab

ram stain and culture. Obtain specimens for culture efore initiating antimicrobial therapy. *B anthracis* is asily isolated from blood cultures in <24 hours. A esumptive diagnosis can be made if gram-positive ds are present that are nonmotile, nonhemolytic, d encapsulated (usually seen with India ink). If tibiotics have been given for >24 hours, perform munohistochemical staining and/or PCR.

naging

Inhalational: Widened mediastinum on chest X-ray may be present; pleural effusions frequently present; infiltrates are rare.

GI: Mesenteric adenopathy on computed tomography scan is likely.

IFFERENTIAL DIAGNOSIS

Skin cellulitis
Brown recluse spider bite
Cat-scratch disease
Rat bite fever
Rickettsial spotted fever
Carbuncle
Cowpox
Bullous erysipelas
Tularemia vasculitides
Ecthyma gangrenosum
Orf (a transmissible viral disease of goats and sheep)

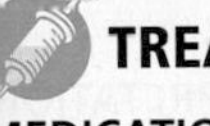

TREATMENT

MEDICATION

irst Line

Cutaneous: Ciprofloxacin 500 mg PO b.i.d. or doxycycline 100 mg PO b.i.d. for 7–10 days for localized or uncomplicated cases of naturally acquired cutaneous anthrax. Treat for 7–10 days with IV instead for severe cases of naturally acquired cutaneous anthrax with signs of systemic involvement, extensive edema, or lesions of the head and neck.

- If cutaneous case is localized or uncomplicated but is bioterrorism-related, the patient must be treated for 60 days with PO ciprofloxacin or doxycycline since they are at risk for inhalational anthrax.
- Patients with bioterrorism-related cutaneous anthrax who show signs of systemic involvement, massive edema, or lesions on the head or neck should be treated per inhalational anthrax recommendation (below) (3,4)[C].

- Inhalational and GI: Intravenous ciprofloxacin 400 mg q12h (1st line) or doxycycline 100 mg q12h (2nd line) and 1 or 2 additional antimicrobials such as rifampin, vancomycin, penicillin, ampicillin, chloramphenicol, imipenem, clindamycin, and clarithromycin
  - May switch to PO when clinically appropriate.
  - Must complete 60-day course (combined PO and IV) (3)[C].
  - Early and aggressive pleural fluid drainage is recommended for all inhalational anthrax patients (4)[C].

Second Line

Patients being treated for anthrax may also benefit from vaccination as part of their regimen (5)[C].

ADDITIONAL TREATMENT

General Measures

- Inhalational and GI anthrax are not known to spread from person to person, so communicability concerns are not an issue during management of the patient.
- Although cutaneous anthrax is also considered noncontagious, avoidance of contact with the wound or wound drainage seems prudent.

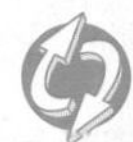

ONGOING CARE

FOLLOW-UP RECOMMENDATIONS

Patient Monitoring

Must monitor patient for 60 days to ensure completion of the treatment course

PROGNOSIS

- Cutaneous: Death in 5–20% of untreated cases, but the case fatality rate is <1% with antibiotic therapy
- GI: Mortality rates as high as 50% reported
- Inhalational: Death in 45–80% of patients with severe symptoms who are treated in a state-of-the-art facility; case fatality rate approaches 99% in untreated cases.

REFERENCES

1. Donegan S, Bellamy R, Gamble CL. Vaccines for preventing anthrax. *Cochrane Database of Systematic Reviews* 2009, Issue 2. Art. No.: CD006403. DOI:10.1002/14651858.CD006403.pub2.
2. Marano N, Plikaytis BD, Martin SW et al. Effects of a reduced dose schedule and intramuscular administration of anthrax vaccine adsorbed on immunogenicity and safety at 7 months: a randomized trial. *JAMA*. 2008;300:1532–43.
3. Centers for Disease Control and Prevention. Update: Investigation of bioterrorism-related anthrax and interim guidelines for exposure management and antimicrobial therapy, October 2001. *MMWR Morb Mortal Wkly Rep*. 2001;50: 909–19.
4. Stern EJ, Uhde KB, Shadomy SV et al. Conference report on public health and clinical guidelines for anthrax. *Emerg Infect Dis*. 2008;14.
5. Centers for Disease Control and Prevention. Use of anthrax vaccine in the US, ACIP Recommendations. *MMWR Recommendations & Reports*. 2000; 49(RR-15):1–20.

ADDITIONAL READING

- Centers for Disease Control and Prevention, Emergency Preparedness and Response. http://www.bt.cdc.gov/agent/anthrax/
- Durning SJ, Roy MJ. Anthrax. In: Roy MJ, ed. *Physician's guide to terrorist attack*. Totowa, NJ: Humana, 2003.
- Schwartz MN. Recognition and management of anthrax—an update. *N Engl J Med*. 2001;345:1621–1626.
- The anthrax vaccine immunization program. http://www.anthrax.mil

CODES

ICD9

- 022.0 Cutaneous anthrax
- 022.1 Pulmonary anthrax
- 022.2 Gastrointestinal anthrax

CLINICAL PEARLS

- Anthrax vaccine (only recommended for high-risk groups) protects against all forms of anthrax and is as safe as other vaccines, according to the FDA, CDC, and the National Academy of Sciences.
- Inhalational anthrax is very rare in US; must be considered a bioterrorist event until proven otherwise (last U.S. occupational case occurred in 1976).
  - Death results in 99% of untreated cases and in 45–80% of patients with severe symptoms who are treated in a state-of-the-art facility.
- Widened mediastinum on chest X-ray may be present; pleural effusions frequently present; infiltrates are rare.

ANTIPHOSPHOLIPID ANTIBODY SYNDROME

Shefali B. Khandwala, DO
Desiree Lie, MD

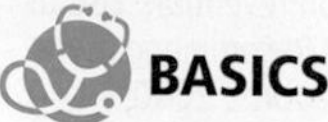

BASICS

DESCRIPTION

Antiphospholipid antibody syndrome (APS) is an autoimmune thrombotic syndrome characterized by the presence of antiphospholipid antibodies (APAs) in association with either recurrent venous or arterial thromboembolic events or repeated fetal loss. The antiphospholipid antibodies are directed against phospholipid-binding plasma proteins and cause an increased risk of clot formation.

- Types:
  - Primary (50%): Occurs in patients without clinical evidence of another autoimmune disease
  - Secondary: Occurs in association with another disease, most commonly systemic lupus erythematosus (SLE)
  - Catastrophic APS (<1%):
    - Differs from primary and secondary types in the caliber of vessels affected. Venous or arterial thrombosis of large vessels is less common, and patients present with acute thrombotic microangiopathy, the kidneys being the most commonly affected organ.
    - DIC, which does not occur in primary or secondary forms, is seen in up to 25% of patients with the catastrophic type
    - Has a high mortality, approaching 50% even with treatment
- Synonym(s): Hughes syndrome

Geriatric Considerations

Atherosclerosis and cancer are more frequent causes of thrombosis than is APS.

Pregnancy Considerations

- Increased frequency of recurrent fetal loss
- Increased risk of premature delivery due to pregnancy-related hypertension and uteroplacental insufficiency

EPIDEMIOLOGY

- No specific age or race predilection
- Equal frequency occurs among males and females for both primary and secondary forms in young pre-pubertal patients
- Female predilection for both primary and secondary forms because of the inclusion of pregnancy-related events in the classification criteria and because of the female predominance in autoimmune diseases such as SLE, respectively.

Incidence

- 15% of women with recurrent pregnancy loss have APS
- 5–21% of all patients with DVT have APS

Prevalence

APAs are present in 1–15% of the general population and in up to 70% of those with SLE. Of those with SLE who have APAs, 50–70% may develop this syndrome.

RISK FACTORS

The following may increase the likelihood of thrombosis in patients with APAs:

- Smoking
- Oral contraceptive use
- Surgery
- Immobilization
- Pregnancy

Genetics

Increased risk in relatives of individuals with APS, however, no specific genetic patterns isolated

GENERAL PREVENTION

- Modification of secondary risk factors for atherosclerosis includes control of HTN, diabetes, hyperlipidemia, and smoking cessation
- Avoidance of oral contraceptives in patients with known APA

PATHOPHYSIOLOGY

APAs may promote thrombosis in any organ by the following hypotheses:

- Increased platelet adhesion and aggregation due to interactions of the antibodies with platelet membrane phospholipids
- Oxidant-mediated injury of vascular endothelium
- Interference with the phospholipid-binding proteins involved in the regulation of coagulation

ETIOLOGY

- Mechanism by which APAs become generated is speculative, but may occur as a result of autoimmunity, as a response to inner membrane antigens exposed on apoptotic cells, or from cross-reactivity to exogenous antigens from infectious organisms
- The presence of APAs alone may not generate thrombosis, but the occurrence of a "second hit" via environmental factors or comorbidities may be required for activation

COMMONLY ASSOCIATED CONDITIONS

- SLE (most common rheumatic disease associated with APAs)
- Thrombotic thrombocytopenic purpura (TTP)
- Hemolytic-uremic syndrome (HUS)
- Malignant hypertension
- Acute renal failure
- Nephrotic syndrome
- HELLP syndrome (hemolysis, elevated liver enzymes, and low platelet count in association with pregnancy)
- DVT/pulmonary embolus (PE)
- Valvular disease
- Sneddon syndrome (APS variant syndrome in which livedo reticularis is associated with HTN and stroke)
- Malignant neoplasms
- Multiple bacterial, viral, and parasitic infections may result in transient increases in APAs
- Certain medications may be associated with APA production, including phenothiazines, hydralazine, procainamide, and phenytoin, but usually do not result in thrombotic events

DIAGNOSIS

- Sapporo criteria, revised 2006 (1):
- The presence of at least 1 of the following clinical criteria:
  - Vascular thrombosis:
    - ≥1 clinical episodes of arterial, venous, or small vessel thrombosis, occurring within any tissue or organ, confirmed by imaging studies, Doppler studies, or histopathology
  - Complications of pregnancy:
    - ≥1 unexplained deaths of morphologically normal fetuses at or after the 10th week of gestation OR
    - ≥1 premature births of morphologically norm neonates at or before the 34th week of pregnancy due to severe preeclampsia, eclampsia, or placental insufficiency OR
    - ≥3 unexplained consecutive spontaneous abortions before the 10th week of pregnancy unexplained by maternal or paternal chromosomal abnormalities or maternal anatomic or hormonal causes
- AND the presence of at least 1 of the following laboratory criteria on ≥2 occasions at least 12 weeks apart:
  - Lupus anticoagulant antibodies detected in the blood
  - Anticardiolipin IgG or IgM antibodies present a moderate or high levels in the blood via a standardized ELISA
  - Anti-B_2 glycoprotein-I IgG or IgM antibodies in blood at a titer >99th percentile via a standardized ELISA
  - Valid lab findings should occur no more than 5 years prior to clinical manifestations

HISTORY

- Personal history of thrombosis (DVT, PE, stroke)
- Obstetric history (especially pregnancy losses)
- Bleeding (from thrombocytopenia)
- Family history of rheumatologic illness
- Vaso-occlusive events can occur in any organ system, so perform thorough review of systems

PHYSICAL EXAM

- DVT of the legs (most common manifestation of APS)
- Skin exam may include findings of livedo reticulari (lacy, erythematous rash in net-like pattern, typica on wrists and knees), purpuric lesions, or ulceratio
- Insufficiency murmur of aortic or mitral valve
- Diverse neurologic symptoms: paresthesias, weakness, tremors, cognitive deficits, stroke/TIA

DIAGNOSTIC TESTS & INTERPRETATION

- May result in false-positive VDRL/RPR
- The risk of thrombosis may increase with the level APA detected and the number of APA types preser in one individual
- The clinical significance of other autoantibodies, including those directed against prothrombin, annexin V, phosphatidylserine, and phosphatidylinositol, remains unclear

Lab

"Lupus anticoagulant" (LA) is a misnomer since it results in an increased risk of thrombus, not an anticoagulant effect. The antibodies cause an increas in the aPTT in vitro, although they are associated wit hypercoagulable state in vivo.

Initial lab tests

- Clotting test for lupus anticoagulant
- ELISA test for anticardiolipin antibodies
- ELISA test for anti-β_2 glycoprotein-I antibodies
- CBC to determine if thrombocytopenia (platelet count usually 50,000–140,000/μL) or hemolytic anemia are present

Follow-Up & Special Considerations

LAs cannot be detected in patients treated with unfractionated heparin, but may be detected in

nxiety often comorbidly exists with attention eficit–hyperreactivity disorder (ADHD).

egnancy Considerations

uspirone: Category B: Secreted in breast milk; adequate studies to assess risk

enzodiazepines: Category D: May cause lethargy nd weight loss in nursing infants; avoid reast-feeding if the mother is taking chronically or high doses.

SRIs: If possible, taper and discontinue. After 0 weeks' gestation, there is increased risk of ulmonary hypertension; mild transient neonatal yndrome of CNS; and motor, respiratory, and GI igns.

- Paroxetine: Category D, conflicting evidence regarding the risk of congenital cardiac defects and other congenital anomalies
- Other SSRIs are category C.

ydroxyzine: Category C: Case reports of neonatal withdrawal exist.

LERT

ecautions:

Benzodiazepines: Advanced age (>65 years), hepatic insufficiency, respiratory disease/sleep apnea, renal insufficiency, suicidal tendency, contraindicated with narrow-angle glaucoma, precaution with open-angle glaucoma; sudden discontinuation increases the risk of seizures, especially with alprazolam. Long-term use has small potential for tolerance and dependence; use with caution in patients with history of substance abuse.

Buspirone: Hepatic and/or renal dysfunction; monoamine oxidase inhibitor (MAOI) treatment

TCAs: Advanced age, glaucoma, benign prostate hypertrophy, hyperthyroidism, cardiovascular disease, liver disease, urinary retention, MAOI treatment

DDITIONAL TREATMENT

dditional Therapies

ychological:

Cognitive-behavioral therapy (CBT): Has shown comparable benefit to medical management; also may improve comorbid conditions such as depression

Mindfulness-based cognitive therapy and stress-reduction studies have been limited. 2010 meta-analysis showed promise in reducing acute symptoms of anxiety in individuals diagnosed with anxiety disorders and in other populations with high anxiety (i.e., the chronically ill) (4).

Relaxation training: Historically, treatment of choice for GAD but limited evidence for objective benefit

Psychodynamic psychotherapy: Treatment is focused on patient discovering and verbalizing unconscious content of the psyche.

eneral Measures

All patients with GAD are at increased risk for suicidal ideation and attempts; risk increases with comorbid conditions.

Identify and treat coexisting substance abuse and other psychiatric conditions.

sues for Referral

oncomitant depression with GAD should prompt a sychiatric evaluation in light of increased suicide sk.

COMPLEMENTARY AND ALTERNATIVE MEDICINE

- Yoga and meditation may be helpful; additional studies are needed, but few adverse effects are known.
- Kava: Evidence for benefit over placebo in mild to moderate anxiety, but significant concern exists regarding potential for hepatotoxicity.
  - May consider for short-term use (up to 24 weeks) (5,6)
  - Studied doses 70–240 mg/d; up to 330 mg/d appears to be safe (7).
  - Must avoid concomitant use of alcohol or other medications metabolized via the liver (CYP 450 inhibitor)
  - Other adverse effects include dermatopathy (usually reversible), ataxia, hearing loss, and loss of appetite; dermatopathy is seen in doses much higher than recommended here.
- St. John's wort: Case reports of benefit in adults, but little evidence for use with anxiety in randomized, controlled trials
  - Drug interactions: CYP 450 3A4, 1A2, or 2E1 inducer; may activate P-glycoprotein
  - In combination with SSRI or buspirone, may lead to serotonin syndrome; otherwise, benign side-effect profile (rare photosensitivity or triggering of mania)
- Passionflower, valerian: Little evidence to support use; benign side-effect profile
- Inositol: Evidence for efficacy in panic disorder and obsessive-compulsive disorder; not studied in GAD

ONGOING CARE

FOLLOW-UP RECOMMENDATIONS

Patient Monitoring

- Continue to monitor for development of comorbid conditions.
- Monitor mental status on benzodiazepines, and avoid drug dependence.
- Monitor blood pressure, heart rate, and anticholinergic side effects of TCAs.
- Monitor all patients for suicidal ideation, but especially those on SSRIs, SNRIs, and imipramine.

DIET

- Limit caffeine intake.
- Avoid alcohol (drug interactions, high rate of abuse, potential for increased anxiety).

PATIENT EDUCATION

- Regular exercise may be beneficial for both anxiety and comorbid conditions.
- Continue with meditation, CBT, and other therapies that provide relief.
- Additional patient information is available at:
  - www.familydoctor.org
  - The National Institute of Mental Health (NIMH) Web site: www.nimh.nih.gov/health/publications/index.shtml

PROGNOSIS

- GAD is a chronic disease, with many patients experiencing continued symptoms or relapse.
- Successful treatment is possible but must be carried out over the long term.
- Relapse is more likely with the discontinuation of medications, particularly in the first year of treatment and during periods of increased stress.

REFERENCES

1. American Psychiatric Association. *Diagnostic and Statistical Manual of Mental Disorders*, 4e. Washington, DC: American Psychiatric Association, 2000:429–84.
2. Kavan MG, Elsasser GN, Barone EJ. Generalized Anxiety Disorder: Practical Assessment and Management. *Am Fam Physician*. 2009;79:785–91.
3. Davidson JR. First-line pharmacotherapy approaches for generalized anxiety disorder. *J Clin Psychiatry*. 2009;70(Suppl 2):25–31.
4. Hofmann SG, Sawyer AT, Witt AA, Oh D et al. The effect of mindfulness-based therapy on anxiety and depression: A meta-analytic review. *J Consult Clin Psychol*. 2010;78:169–83.
5. Saeed SA, Bloch RM, Antonacci DJ. Herbal and dietary supplements for treatment of anxiety disorders. *Am Fam Physician*. 2007;76:549–56.
6. Pittler MH, Ernst E. Kava extract for treating anxiety. *Cochrane Database Syst Rev*. 2003:CD003383.
7. Ernst E. The risk-benefit profile of commonly used herbal therapies: Ginkgo, St. John's Wort, Ginseng, Echinacea, Saw Palmetto, and Kava. *Ann Intern Med*. 2002;136:42–53.

ADDITIONAL READING

- Gorman JM. Treating generalized anxiety disorder. *J Clin Psychiatry*. 2003;64(Suppl 2):24–9.
- Shearer SL. Recent Advances in the Understanding and Treatment of Anxiety Disorders. *Prim Care*. 2007;34:475–504.
- Ströhle A. Physical activity, exercise, depression and anxiety disorders. *J Neural Transm*. 2008.
- Weisberg RB. Overview of generalized anxiety disorder: epidemiology, presentation, and course. *J Clin Psychiatry*. 2009;70(Suppl 2):4–9.

See Also (Topic, Algorithm, Electronic Media Element)

Algorithms: Depression, Adult; Anxiety

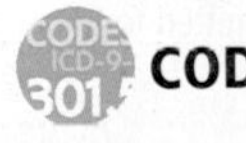

CODES

ICD9

- 300.00 Anxiety state, unspecified
- 300.02 Generalized anxiety disorder
- 300.09 Other anxiety states

CLINICAL PEARLS

- GAD is a chronic disease with a relapsing and remitting course for many patients; long-term treatment is required.
- Psychiatric comorbidities, especially depression, are extremely common with GAD.
- Patients are at increased risk for suicidality and should be screened accordingly.
- Antidepressants are the treatment of choice, although they require up to 4 weeks for full effect.
- Benzodiazepines may be used to relieve anxiety initially; they should be tapered and then withdrawn to avoid dependence and tolerance.
- CBT is comparable with medical management; mindfulness meditation and other techniques have shown initial promise.

AORTIC DISSECTION

Mia D. Sorcinelli, MD

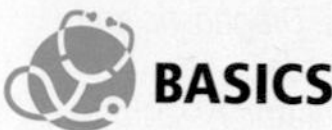

BASICS

DESCRIPTION

Intimal tear in the aorta resulting in hematoma formation. Accumulating blood in false lumen of arterial wall leads to propagation of dissection (1):

- Stanford classification (most widely used):
  - Type A: Involves ascending aorta and aortic arch regardless of site of intimal tear
  - Type B: Involves descending aorta
- DeBakey classification (based on origin site):
  - Type 1: Originates in ascending aorta, propagates at least as far as aortic arch
  - Type 2: Involves only ascending aorta
  - Type 3: Originates in descending aorta, may propagate proximately or distally
- Svensson:
  - Class 1: Classic dissection with true and false lumen
  - Class 2: Intramural hematoma or hemorrhage
  - Class 3: Subtle dissection without hematoma
  - Class 4: Atherosclerotic plaque rupture and ulceration
  - Class 5: Iatrogenic
- Synonym: Dissecting aneurysm

EPIDEMIOLOGY

- Predominant age varies with cause
- Type A dissection average age 60
- Type B dissection patients generally older
- Patients with Marfan syndrome have mean age 36
- Approximately 2/3 of patients are male
- Studies indicate peak time of day between 8 and 9 AM
- Some studies also report slightly higher incidence in winter months

Incidence

About 3 cases per 100,000 people per year

Prevalence

United States:

- Diagnosed in 1 in 10,000 patients admitted to hospital
- Found in 1:350 patients at autopsy
- Numbers may be slightly higher due to unexplained deaths at home or in hospital without autopsy

RISK FACTORS

- Most common associated factors:
  - Hypertension (about 70% of patients)
  - Old age
  - Atherosclerosis
  - Previous cardiovascular surgery, particularly repair of aneurysm or dissection
- Collagen abnormalities:
  - Marfan syndrome
  - Ehlers-Danlos syndrome
- Recreational drug use:
  - Smoking
  - Cocaine
- Inflammatory vasculitis:
  - Takayasu arteritis
  - Giant cell arteritis
- Chest trauma
- Turner syndrome
- Bicuspid aortic valve
- Uncommonly seen in infants following infection
- Also seen in infants during balloon dilation of aortic coarctation
- Reports of dissection in patients with untreated coarctation of the aorta

Genetics

Up to 20% of patients with thoracic aneurysm or dissection were found to have first-degree relatives with aneurysm or dissection. Studies have found the TGFBR1 and TGFBR2 genes are related to aneurysm and dissection in isolated cases and in patients with Marfan's syndrome. Other research has found ACTA2 gene mutations to be involved in isolated and familial dissections and aneurysms.

GENERAL PREVENTION

- Rigorous medical management of precipitating risk factors such as hypertension
- Surveillance of aortic root and replacement when appropriate in patients with collagen disorders (e.g., Marfan, Ehlers-Danlos)

PATHOPHYSIOLOGY

In most cases, dissection develops in the absence of aneurysm, but the false lumen that can be created during dissection can later expand to form an aneurysm. In patients with inherited connective tissue disease, abnormal and/or deficient proteins lead to weakening of vessel walls. Bicuspid aortic valves may also lead to an acquired dysfunction of vascular walls and smooth muscle cells. Histological investigation of postmortem and biopsy specimens reveal cystic medial necrosis, especially in those patients with known preexisting aneurysm

ETIOLOGY

Although the exact sequence of events is controversial, aortic dissection is likely the result of multiple pathological processes. Stress on the aortic wall from hypertension, intimal damage with subsequent tear, rupture or ulceration of atherosclerotic plaques, and involvement of vasa vasorum and intramural hematoma may be contributory.

COMMONLY ASSOCIATED CONDITIONS

See Risk Factors

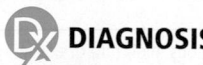

DIAGNOSIS

HISTORY

- High level of clinical suspicion is key to correct and prompt diagnosis
- Typical patient is a hypertensive man aged 60–80
- Positive family history raises index of suspicion
- Subjective complaints (2):
  - 85% of patients report abrupt onset of pain
  - Pain was more often described as sharp, less often as tearing or ripping
  - 90% of patients stated that the pain was "severe" or "worst ever"
  - Patients with type A dissections more often report chest pain
  - Patients with type B dissections more often report back and abdominal pain
  - Symptoms overlap between type A and type B dissections

PHYSICAL EXAM

- Hypotension and shock are more common with type A dissection.
- Hypertension is more common with type B dissection.
- Syncope or cerebrovascular accident symptoms
- Any pulse deficit
- Auscultation of aortic regurgitation
- Signs of congestive heart failure
- Limb ischemia
- Acute myocardial infarction/angina
- Spinal cord syndromes/deficits (3)
- Features of tamponade

DIAGNOSTIC TESTS & INTERPRETATION

- Important to use easily available testing to assist in prompt diagnosis
- Blood testing, EKG, chest x-ray, CT scans, and echocardiograms can all assist in diagnosis.
- A normal EKG and chest x-ray cannot be used to rule out the diagnosis if clinical suspicion is high.
- EKG may show (2):
  - Normal findings in up to 1/3 of patients
  - Nonspecific ST-T changes (about 40%)
  - Left ventricular hypertrophy (about 25%)
  - Ischemic changes (about 15%)
  - Acute MI (about 3%)
  - Old MI with Q waves (about 7%)

Lab

Possible novel markers for aortic dissection include a combination of D-dimer, elastin fragments, and smooth-muscle myosin heavy-chain protein. Presently none of these tests are used routinely as diagnostic tools, and several authors debate the use of D-dimer alone, with research being inconclusive as to its sensitivity and specificity.

Imaging

- Chest X-ray may show:
  - Normal findings in about 15% of patients
  - Widening of the mediastinum (about 60%)
  - Abnormal aortic outline (about 50%)
  - Abnormal cardiac silhouette (about 25%)
  - Calcified or displaced aorta (about 15%)
  - Pleural effusion (about 19%)
- Studies suggest that CT scan with IV contrast, transesophageal echocardiography, and MRI imaging all provide around 95% sensitivity and specificity for diagnosis:
  - MRI may be better for patients where clinical suspicion and pretest probability for aortic dissection are already high.
  - CT scan may be better to rule out dissection in those patients where clinical suspicion and pretest probability are both low.
  - Transesophageal echocardiography can be done at the bedside of an unstable patient in 15–20 minutes, and can offer additional information about heart function (4).
  - In reality, the ready availability and speed with which CT scans can be performed in many hospitals may outweigh the above considerations.
- Both MRI and CT scans can be used by clinicians to assess the extent, size, and location of the dissection, as well as involvement of the branches off the aorta, although some sources suggest MRI as the preferred modality for precise anatomic definition.

iagnostic Procedures/Surgery

ɔntrast angiography can be used specifically as a agnostic tool, especially when visceral perfusion efects are suspected. Angiography may also be used entry point into endovascular treatment of ssection.

athological Findings

~60% of intimal tears occur in the proximal ascending aorta. Remainder are between origin of left subclavian artery and ligamentum arteriosum, descending aorta (20%), aortic arch (10%), and abdominal aorta.
Although medial necrosis is found in aging aortas, it is more extensive in patients who develop aortic dissection.
Cystic medial necrosis is seen in patients with defects in elastin and connective tissue organization (e.g., Marfan, Ehlers-Danlos).
Death usually is due to rupture and tamponade.

IFFERENTIAL DIAGNOSIS

lyocardial infarction, pericarditis, pericardial mponade not from aortic dissection, angina or therosclerotic embolism, pulmonary embolism, neumonia, pleurisy, acute pancreatitis or olecystitis, penetrating duodenal ulcer, Mallory-Veiss tear or esophageal rupture, mediastinal athology, musculoskeletal pain

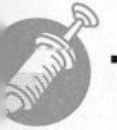

TREATMENT

ue to the acute nature of aortic dissection, there are o randomized controlled trials related to treatment nd management.

MEDICATION

ɔr uncomplicated dissection of descending aorta Stanford B), medical therapy is indicated.

irst Line

he cornerstone of medical management is blood ressure control using beta blockers, including ropranolol, metoprolol, labetalol, and esmolol

econd Line

For patients with severe asthma, calcium-channel blockers may be used
If hypertension is refractory to initial therapies, nitroprusside can be considered, but the patient should be evaluated for possible surgical intervention at that time

ADDITIONAL TREATMENT

General Measures

Patients should be monitored in intensive care units
Arterial BP monitoring is preferred, particularly in less stable patients
Pain control should involve the use of morphine
If surgical repair of aneurysm is indicated, do not delay repair to evaluate for CAD and valvular dysfunction
Prompt correction of hypotension, along with identification of the cause, are essential
Hemodynamically unstable patients will likely require intubation and mechanical ventilation

SURGERY/OTHER PROCEDURES

Stanford A type dissection:
- Surgery is the treatment of choice for dissections of the ascending aorta (80% treated surgically) to prevent aortic rupture and cardiac tamponade, while relieving any aortic regurgitation that may be present (2).
- Patients who are inappropriate surgical candidates (comorbid medical conditions, patient choice, very advanced age) have an in-hospital mortality of 50% after 30 days.
- Surgical correction aims to resect ascending aorta and arch, and replace them with a graft.
- Other procedures, including repair/replacement of aortic valves and coronary arteries, may be indicated depending on the extent of the dissection.
- Many different surgical options exist and depend on the extent of dissection.

- Stanford B type dissection:
  - Surgical resection of aorta for type B generally associated with worse outcomes than medical management.
  - Surgical indications for Stanford B include (2):
    - Continued aortic expansion
    - Impending aortic rupture
    - Occlusion of major aortic branch to renal, mesenteric, or iliac arteries
    - Persistent and recurrent chest pain
    - Periaortic or mediastinal hematoma
- Poor prognostic factors for surgical success:
  - Age >70 years
  - Abrupt-onset chest pain
  - Hypotension, shock, or tamponade at presentation
  - Renal failure
  - Pulse deficit
  - Abnormal ECG, ST segment elevation
  - History of aortic valve replacement
  - Renal and/or visceral ischemia
- Stenting of complicated type B dissections seems to be a reasonable and safe alternative to surgical management, although further follow-up is needed

IN-PATIENT CONSIDERATIONS

Initial Stabilization

- Admit to ICU
- Intubate hemodynamically unstable patients
- Control BP:
  - Systolic 100–120 mm Hg
  - IV beta blocker to achieve HR 60
  - Determine etiology of hypotension:
    - Blood loss
    - Tamponade
    - Heart failure
- Pain control

Admission Criteria

Low threshold for admission in presence of thoracic or abdominal pain, radiographic corroboration, or pulse deficit.

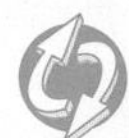

ONGOING CARE

FOLLOW-UP RECOMMENDATIONS

Patient Monitoring

- Maintain systolic BP at 120 mm Hg (16 kPa) or below, as tolerated
- Routine chest films and/or chest CT may be helpful for patient treated medically long term.
- During follow-up, pay careful attention to signs and symptoms of aortic insufficiency, chest or back pain, and development of saccular aneurysms as displayed on chest films.

DIET

NPO until surgical evaluation is complete and patient classified as medical therapy only.

PATIENT EDUCATION

Depending on etiology, emphasis must be placed on risk factors and prevention of recurrence:
- Smoking cessation
- Blood pressure control with beta blockers
- Diabetic control

PROGNOSIS

- Hospital survival estimate, treated medically and surgically: 70% (2)
- Data for Type A dissections treated surgically show a 90% survival rate at 3 years (5).
- Survival at 10 years similar for medically and surgically treated patients.
- Redissection risk:
  - 5 years: 13%
  - 10 years: 23%

COMPLICATIONS

Redissection, localized saccular aneurysm, cardiac tamponade, aortic valvular insufficiency, progressive aortic enlargement. Stent placement risks include paraplegia, stroke, embolization, side-branch occlusion, infection

REFERENCES

1. Golledge J, Eagle KA. Acute aortic dissection. *Lancet*. 2008;372:55 66.
2. Hagan PG, Nienaber CA, Isselbacher EM et al. The International Registry of Acute Aortic Dissection (IRAD): new insights into an old disease. *JAMA*. 2000;283:897–903.
3. Gaul C, Dietrich W, Friedrich I et al. Neurological symptoms in type A aortic dissections. *Stroke*. 2007;38:292–7.
4. Nair HC et al. Transesophageal echocardiography evaluation of thoracic aorta. *Ann Card Anaesth*. 2010;13:106.
5. Tsai TT, Evangelista A, Nienaber CA, Trimarchi S, Sechtem U, Fattori R, Myrmel T, Pape L, Cooper JV, Smith DE, Fang J, Isselbacher E, Eagle KA, International Registry of Acute Aortic Dissection (IRAD) et al. Long term survival in patients presenting with type A acute aortic dissection: insights from the International Registry of Acute Aortic Dissection (IRAD). *Circulation*. 2006;114: I350–6.

See Also (Topic, Algorithm, Electronic Media Element)

Hypertension; Ehlers-Danlos Syndrome; Marfan Syndrome

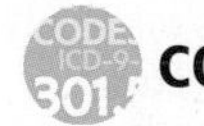

CODES

ICD9

- 441.00 Dissection of aorta, unspecified site
- 441.01 Dissection of aorta, thoracic

CLINICAL PEARLS

- 90% of patients with aortic dissection report acute pain, more often sharp than tearing, and located in the chest, abdomen, or back
- Maintain a high level of suspicion and act quickly if the diagnosis of aortic dissection is suspected.
- Survival at 10 years similar for medically and surgically treated patients.

AORTIC VALVULAR STENOSIS

Ajar Kochar, MD
Dawn Abbott, MD

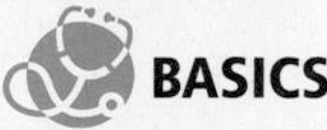

BASICS

DESCRIPTION

Aortic stenosis (AS) is a narrowing of the aortic valve area that causes an obstruction to left ventricular outflow. The disease has a long asymptomatic latency period, but development of severe obstruction or onset of symptoms such as syncope and angina as associated with a high mortality rate if surgical intervention is not accomplished promptly.

EPIDEMIOLOGY

- Most common valvular disease in developed countries
- >50% of patients with isolated aortic stenosis also have a congenitally malformed valve (1).
- Predominant age:
  - <30 years: Congenital
  - 30–70 years: Congenital or rheumatic fever
  - >70 years: Degenerative calcification of aortic valve

Prevalence

- 1.3% at 65–74 years old, 2.4% at 75–84 years old, 4% at >84 years old (1)
- Bicuspid aortic valve: 1–2% of population (1)

RISK FACTORS

- Congenital (1):
  - Bicuspid valve
    - Most commonly in men
    - AS occurs at younger age
    - Associated with coarctation of aorta
  - Unicommissural valve
- Acquired (1):
  - Rheumatic fever
  - Degenerative (CAD-related RF): Hypercholesterolemia [elevated LDL, lipoprotein (a)], smoking, male gender, age, hypertension, diabetes mellitus

PATHOPHYSIOLOGY

- Progressive stiffening of aortic valve results in LV outflow obstruction
- Obstruction causes increased afterload and decreased forward flow.
- Increased afterload is compensated for by development of concentric left ventricular hypertrophy (LVH).
- LVH preserves ejection fraction but adversely affects heart functioning:
  - LVH impairs coronary blood flow reserve by compression of coronary arteries and reduced capillary ingrowth into hypertrophied muscle.
  - LVH results in diastolic dysfunction by reducing ventricular compliance.
- Diastolic dysfunction mandates stronger left atrial (LA) contraction to augment pre-load and maintain stroke volume. Loss of LA contraction by atrial fibrillation (AFib) can induce acute deterioration.
- Angina: Myocardial demand is elevated due to increased left ventricular pressure. Myocardial supply is compromised due to LVH.
- Syncope (exertional): Ventricular contraction cannot augment cardiac output enough to match increase demands of exercise due to the fixed obstruction to LV outflow.
- Heart Failure: Eventually LVH cannot compensate for increasing afterload resulting in high LV Pressure and Volume which is accompanied with a rise in LA and Pulmonary pressures

ETIOLOGY

- Calcific aortic stenosis (2): Initiating insult is mechanical stress to valve leaflets:
  - Note bicuspid valves are at higher risk for shear stress
  - Early lesions: Subendothelial accumulation of oxidized LDL and macrophages and T-lymphocytes (inflammatory response)
  - Disease progression: Fibroblasts undergo transformation into osteoblasts. Protein production of osteopontin, osteocalcitonin, and BMP-2, which modulate calcification of leaflets
- Congenital: Unicuspid valve. Tricuspid valve with fusion of commissures, hypoplastic annulus
- Rheumatic Fever: Fusion of commissures and scarring

COMMONLY ASSOCIATED CONDITIONS

- Coronary artery disease (50% of patients)
- Hypertension (40% of patients) Results in "double-loaded" left ventricle (dual source of obstruction from AS and hypertension)
- Aortic regurgitation (common in calcified bicuspid valves and rheumatic disease)
- Mitral valve disease: 95% of patients with AS from rheumatic fever also have mitral valve disease.
- LV dysfunction and CHF
- Atrial fibrillation associated with CHF
- Acquired von Willebrand disease: Impaired platelet function and decreased vWF results in bleeding (ecchymosis and epistaxis) in 20% of AS patients. Severity of coagulopathy is directly related to severity of AS.
- Rarely: Calcific embolization to systemic organs

DIAGNOSIS

HISTORY

- Primary symptoms: Angina, syncope, and heart failure (3). Angina is most frequent symptom. Syncope is often exertional. Heart failure symptoms include: Fatigue, exertional dyspnea, orthopnea, paroxysmal nocturnal dyspnea, shortness of breath
- Palpitations
- Neurologic events (transient ischemic attack or cerebrovascular accident) owing to embolization
- Geriatric patients may have subtle symptoms such as fatigue and exertional dyspnea
- Note: Symptoms do not always correlate with valve area (severity of AS) but most commonly occur when AV area is <1.0 cm^2

PHYSICAL EXAM

- Auscultation (3):
  - Harsh, systolic crescendo-decrescendo murmur (grade 4/6):
    - Best heard at 2nd right sternal border
    - Radiates into carotid arteries
    - Peak of murmur correlates with severity of stenosis: Earlier peaking murmur suggests less severe narrowing
  - High-pitched diastolic blow, suggests associated aortic regurgitation
  - Paradoxically split S2 or absent A2
  - Note: Normally split S2 reliably excludes severe AS
  - S4
- Other associated signs: (3) Thrill (denotes more severe narrowing); Parvus et Tardus: Carotid upstrokes decreased in volume, delayed in rate. LV heave

DIAGNOSTIC TESTS & INTERPRETATION

Lab

BNP may be elevated (no cutoffs exist) (1). Values altered by obesity, pulmonary hypertension, renal disease

Imaging

Initial approach

- Chest x-ray (CXR) (1)
  - May be normal in compensated, isolated valvular aortic stenosis.
  - Boot-shaped heart reflective of concentric hypertrophy
  - Post-stenotic dilatation of ascending aorta
  - Calcification of aortic valve (seen on lateral PA CXR)
- Electrocardiogram (ECG):
  - Often normal ECG (ECG is non-diagnostic)
  - LV hypertrophy
  - Left atrial enlargement
  - Nonspecific ST and T-wave abnormalities
- Echo Indications:
  - Initial workup:
    - Doppler echocardiogram is mainstay of diagnosis
    - Severity of AS
    - Assess left ventricular wall thickness, size, function.
  - In known AS and changing signs/symptoms
  - In known AS and pregnancy due to hemodynamic changes of pregnancy
- Echo findings:
  - Aortic valve morphology, thickening, calcifications
  - Decreased aortic valve excursion
  - Aortic valve area
  - LV hypertrophy
  - LV ejection fraction
  - Chamber dimensions will often be normal.
  - Wall-motion abnormalities suggesting coronary artery disease (CAD)
  - Evaluate for concomitant mitral valve disease.
- Doppler echo adds information on:
  - Transvalvular gradient
  - Valve area
  - Diastolic function
  - Associated aortic regurgitation
- Aortic stenosis severity based on echo values (assumes normal cardiac output):
  - Normal: Area: 3–4 cm Gradient: 0 mm Hg Jet Vel. <2.5 m/s
  - Mild: Area: 1.5–2 cm Gradient: <25 mm Hg Jet Vel. 2.5–2.9 m/s
  - Mod: Area: 1–1.5 cm Gradient: 25–40 mm Hg Jet Vel. 3–4 m/s
  - Severe: Area: <1 cm Gradient: >40 mm Hg Jet Vel. >4 m/s

Patients with severe AS and low cardiac output may have a relatively low transvalvular pressure gradient (i.e., mean gradient less than 30 mm Hg)

Diagnostic Procedures/Surgery

Exercise stress testing:
- Asymptomatic patients (4)[B]: Helpful to uncover subtle symptoms or changes, abnormal blood pressure (increase less than 20 mm Hg), and EKG changes (ST depressions). 1/3 of patients develop symptoms with exercise testing – STOP testing at this point.
- Symptomatic patients (4)[B]: DO NOT perform exercise stress testing as may induce hypotension or ventricular tachycardia
- CHF patients (4)[B]: Dobutamine stress echocardiography is reasonable to evaluate patients with low-flow/low-gradient AS and LV dysfunction.

Cardiac catheterization: Perform Prior to AVR in patients with suspected CAD (4)[B]. Determines need for Coronary Artery Bypass Graft (CABG). If unambiguous diagnosis of AS, only perform coronary angiography.

Perform as diagnostic adjunct:
- Catheterization is gold standard for diagnosis
- Use if noninvasive testing is inconclusive.
- Use if discrepancy in severity of symptoms and findings on echo
- Perform complete right and left heart catheterization.
- Measure: Transvalvular flow, transvalvular pressure gradient, and effective valve area
- Hemodynamic measurements with infusion of dobutamine can be useful for evaluation of patients with low-flow/low-gradient AS and LV dysfunction

Pathological Findings

Aortic valve: nodular calcification on valve cusps (initially at bases), cusp rigidity, cusp thickening, and fibrosis

LV hypertrophy

Myocardial interstitial fibrosis

50% incidence of concomitant CAD

DIFFERENTIAL DIAGNOSIS

Mitral regurgitation: Either primary or secondary to underlying coronary artery disease or dilated cardiomyopathy. Usually an apical, high-frequency, pansystolic murmur, often radiating to axilla.

Hypertrophic obstructive cardiomyopathy: Also systolic crescendo-decrescendo murmur, but best heard at left sternal border and may radiate into axilla. Murmur intensity increases by changing from squatting to standing and/or by Valsalva maneuver.

Discrete fixed subaortic stenosis 50–65% have associated cardiac deformity (PDA, VSD, coarctation of aorta)

Aortic supravalvular stenosis Williams syndrome, homozygous familial hypercholesterolemia

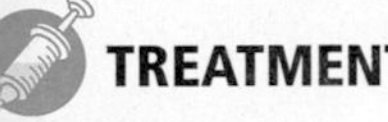

TREATMENT

MEDICATION

NO medical therapy for severe or symptomatic aortic stenosis

Prevention: Currently no recommended medical therapy. Statins may have a role if initiated during mild disease. Antibiotic prophylaxis against recurrent rheumatic fever is indicated for patients with rheumatic AS (Penicillin G 1,200,000 U IM every 4 weeks, duration varies with age and history of carditis). Antibiotic prophylaxis is no longer indicated for prevention of infective endocarditis (4).
- Complications: Decompensated heart failure responds rapidly to IV nitroprusside (dose titrated to MAP of 60–70); can be used as bridge therapy until surgery.
- Co-morbidities: Hypertension: ACE inhibitors, start with low dose and increase cautiously. Be cautious of vasodilators which may cause hypotension

ADDITIONAL TREATMENT

Percutaneous balloon aortic valvotomy or valvuloplasty (BAV)
- Percutaneous prosthetic valve implantation is under development and improves outcomes in patients that are not candidates for surgery. Poor surgical candidates: Advanced age, left ventricular dysfunction, numerous comorbidities
- In young adults and others without significantly calcified aortic valves and no AR, BAV is indicated in the following patients:
  - Symptoms of angina, syncope, dyspnea on exertion, and peak-to-peak gradients at catheterization greater than 50 mm Hg.
  - Asymptomatic adolescents or young adults who demonstrate ST or T-wave abnormalities in the left precordial leads on ECG at rest or with exercise and a peak-to-peak catheter gradient greater than 60 mm Hg (4)[C].
  - Asymptomatic adolescent or young adult with AS and a peak-to-peak gradient on catheterization greater than 50 mm Hg when the patient is interested in playing competitive sports or becoming pregnant (4)[C].
- In older adults with rheumatic or degenerative AS, BAV may be considered as a bridge to surgery in hemodynamically unstable adults with AS, adults at high risk for AVR, or when AVR cannot be performed secondary to significant comorbidities (4)[C].

SURGERY/OTHER PROCEDURES

Indications for aortic valve replacement (AVR):
- Symptomatic and severe AS (4)[B] should be performed rapidly due to high risk of sudden cardiac death
- Asymptomatic, severe AS and
  - Requires aortic root surgery or other valvular surgery (4)[C]
  - Requires coronary artery bypass grafting (CABG) (4)[C]
  - Ejection fraction (EF) (<50%) (4)[C]
  - Positive exercise stress testing findings (4)[C]
  - Risk of rapid progression (moderate-severe calcification, age, CAD) (4)[C]
- Asymptomatic, extremely severe AS (4)[C]: Aortic valve area <0.6 cm, gradient >60 mm Hg, or jet velocity >5 m/s
- Moderate stenosis and undergoing CABG or valvular surgery (4)[B]
- Mild AS and CABG and high risk of rapid progression (4)[C]. Note if AV Area >1.5 cm and gradient <15 mm Hg no benefit from AVR

ONGOING CARE

FOLLOW-UP RECOMMENDATIONS

- Advise patient to immediately report symptoms referable to AS.
- Asymptomatic patients: Yearly history and physical (4)[C]
- Serial echo: Recommendation (4)[B]: Yearly for severe AS, every 1–2 years for moderate AS, every 3–5 years for mild AS

PATIENT EDUCATION

Physical activity limitations:
- Asymptomatic mild AS: No restrictions, competitive sports are okay
- Asymptomatic moderate-to-severe AS: Avoid competitive sports that have high muscle demand. Milder exercise can be done safely. Consider exercise stress test prior to starting exercise program.

PROGNOSIS

- 25% mortality/year in symptomatic patients who do not undergo valve replacement; Average survival is 2–3 years without AVR surgery
- Median survival in symptomatic AS (3): Heart failure: 2 years syncope: 3 years angina: 5 years
- After aortic valve replacement, a patient's lifespan returns to near that of an unselected population
- Peri-surgical mortality AVR surgery has 4% mortality; AVR + CABG has 6.8% mortality
- Adverse postoperative prognostic factors: Age, HF NYHA III/IV, cerebrovascular disease, renal dysfunction, CAD

REFERENCES

1. Carabello BA, Paulus WJ et al. Aortic stenosis. *Lancet*. 2009;373:956–66
2. Otto CM et al. Calcific aortic stenosis–time to look more closely at the valve. *N Engl J Med*. 2008;359:1395–8.
3. Grimard BH, Larson JM et al. Aortic stenosis: diagnosis and treatment. *Am Fam Physician*. 2008;78:717–24.
4. Bonow RO, et al. ACC/AHA 2006 guidelines for the management of patients with valvular heart disease: a report of the American College of Cardiology/American Heart Association Task Force on Practice Guidelines *Circulation*. 2006;114:e84–231.

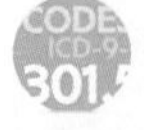

CODES

ICD9

- 395.0 Rheumatic aortic stenosis
- 424.1 Aortic valve disorders
- 746.3 Congenital stenosis of aortic valve

CLINICAL PEARLS

- Aortic stenosis is diagnosed on physical exam by a systolic crescendo-decrescendo murmur, and delayed and diminished pulses.
- Symptomatic AS most commonly presents as angina, syncope, and heart failure.
- Symptomatic AS has a very poor prognosis unless treated with surgical intervention.

APPENDICITIS, ACUTE

Francesca L. Beaudoin, MS, MD
Erik E. Wang, MD

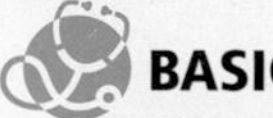

BASICS

DESCRIPTION

- Acute inflammation of the vermiform appendix, first described by Reginald Fitz in 1886
- Arising from the base of the cecum in right lower quadrant (RLQ); can be localized anterior, posterior, medial, lateral to the cecum, as well as in the pelvis
- Vascular supply by appendicular artery, a branch of the ileocolic artery
- Most common cause of the acute surgical abdomen

EPIDEMIOLOGY

- Predominant age: 10–30 years:
  - Rare in infancy
- Predominant sex: Slight male predominance:
  - Ages 10–30: Male > Female (3:2)
  - Age >30: Male = Female

Incidence

- 1 case per 1,000 people per year
- Lifetime incidence 1 in every 15 persons (7%)

Pregnancy Considerations

- Most common extrauterine surgical emergency
- 1 in 2,000 pregnancies

RISK FACTORS

- Adolescent males
- Familial tendency
- Intra-abdominal tumors

Genetics

1st-degree relative with history of appendicitis increases risk, although no direct genetic link has been found

PATHOPHYSIOLOGY

The initial event inciting appendicitis is thought to be obstruction of the appendiceal lumen. This leads to distention, ischemia, and bacterial overgrowth. Without intervention, most cases of appendicitis will lead to perforation and subsequently abscess formation or generalized peritonitis.

ETIOLOGY

Causes of obstruction:

- Fecaliths (most common)
- Lymphoid tissue hyperplasia (in children)
- Inspissated barium
- Vegetable, fruit seeds
- Other foreign bodies
- Intestinal worms (ascarids)
- Strictures, fibrosis
- Neoplasms

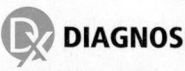

DIAGNOSIS

Diagnosis of acute appendicitis relies on the clinical integration of history, physical exam, and often laboratories and imaging. Scoring systems, including the Alvarado Score and the Pediatric Appendicitis Score, have been developed to help predict the likelihood of acute appendicitis, although diagnosis is still considered a clinical decision.

HISTORY

- The classic history is vague periumbilical pain, followed by anorexia/nausea/vomiting. Over the next 4–48 hours, pain then migrates to the right lower quadrant.
- Only 50% of patients present with this classic history.
- Pain before vomiting (~100% sensitive)
- Abdominal pain (~100%)
- Anorexia (~100%)
- Nausea (90%)
- Vomiting (75%)
- Pain migration (50%)
- Obstipation
- Atypical symptoms and pain with retrocecal and pelvic appendix

PHYSICAL EXAM

- Fever; temp >100.4°F (can be absent)
- Tachycardia
- RLQ tenderness
- Maximal tenderness at McBurney's point
- Voluntary and involuntary guarding
- Cutaneous hyperesthesia at T10–12
- Rovsing sign: RLQ pain with palpation of left lower quadrant
- Psoas sign: Pain with right thigh extension (retrocecal appendix)
- Obturator sign: Pain with internal rotation of flexed right thigh (pelvic appendix)
- Local and suprapubic pain on rectal exam (pelvic appendix)
- Pelvic and rectal exams necessary to explore other pathology (pelvic inflammatory disease, prostatitis, etc.)
- Serial exams can be useful in indeterminate cases.

Pediatric Considerations

- Decreased diagnostic accuracy
- Higher fever, more vomiting

Pregnancy Considerations

- Difficult diagnosis
- Appendix displaced by gravid uterus

Geriatric Considerations

Decreased diagnostic accuracy, atypical presentations

DIAGNOSTIC TESTS & INTERPRETATION

Lab

- Leukocytosis: white blood cells (WBC) >10,000/mm^3 (70%)
- Polymorphonuclear predominance or "left shift" (>90%)
- hCG (if negative, rules out ectopic pregnancy)
- Urinalysis:
  - Elevated specific gravity
  - Hematuria, pyuria (~30%)
- C-reactive protein:
  - Nonspecific inflammatory marker
  - When paired with an elevated WBC can increase the likelihood of appendicitis
- Drugs that may alter lab results:
  - Antibiotics
  - Steroids

Imaging

- Used in cases of suspected appendicitis when the diagnosis is not clear
- Helpful to detect complications (abscess)
- Computed tomography (CT) scan: Sensitivity ~91–98%; specificity 95–99%; imaging modality of choice.
- CT scan with IV contrast alone provides equivalent information to CT scan with rectal or oral contrast (1)[A].
- Ultrasound: Viable alternative in pregnant patients, children, and in women with suspected gynecologic pathology (2)[B]. Sensitivity ~86%; specificity ~81%. An initial ultrasound and, if negative, a CT scan has been shown to be an effective workup strategy for all patients (3)[B].
- Plain films: Little utility, nonspecific findings, may visualize fecalith
- Magnetic resonance imaging: May be helpful in pregnant patients
- Radioisotope-labeled WBC scans: May be used in patients with indeterminate CT scans and suspected appendicitis as an alternative to observation or surgery

Diagnostic Procedures/Surgery

Diagnostic laparoscopy useful in equivocal cases, especially in fertile women (1)[A]

Pathological Findings

- Acute appendiceal inflammation
- Local vascular congestion
- Obstruction
- Gangrene
- Perforation with abscess (15–30%)
- Fecalith

DIFFERENTIAL DIAGNOSIS

- Gastrointestinal:
  - Gastroenteritis
  - Inflammatory bowel disease
  - Diverticulitis
  - Ileitis
  - Cholecystitis
  - Pancreatitis
  - Intussusception
  - Volvulus
- Gynecologic:
  - Pelvic inflammatory disease
  - Ectopic pregnancy
  - Ovarian cyst, ovarian torsion
  - Endometriosis
  - Ruptured graafian follicle
- Urologic:
  - Testicular torsion, epididymitis
  - Kidney stones
  - Prostatitis, cystitis, pyelonephritis
- Systemic:
  - Diabetic ketoacidosis
  - Henoch Schönlein purpura
  - Sickle cell crisis
  - Porphyria

Other:
- Acute mesenteric lymphadenitis
- No organic pathologic condition
- Hernias
- Psoas abscess
- Rectus sheath hematoma
- Epiploic appendagitis
- Pneumonia (basilar)

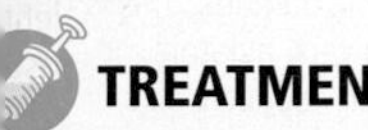

TREATMENT

EDICATION

rst Line

Uncomplicated acute appendicitis: Perioperative dose of broad-spectrum antibiotic (4)[A]:
- Cefoxitin (Mefoxin); cefotetan (Cefotan)

Gangrenous or perforating appendicitis:
- Broadened antibiotic coverage for aerobic and anaerobic enteric pathogens
- Fluoroquinolone and metronidazole typical
- Adjust dosage and choice of antibiotic based on intraoperative cultures.
- Continue antibiotics for 7 days postoperatively or until patient becomes afebrile with normal white blood cell count.

econd Line

Ampicillin-sulbactam (Unasyn)
Ticarcillin-clavulanate (Timentin)
Piperacillin-tazobactam (Zosyn)

DDITIONAL TREATMENT

eneral Measures

rgery (appendectomy) is still the standard of care. owever, nonoperative management with antibiotics s been studied as an alternative. Some literature ggests that antibiotic therapy alone may be initially successful as appendectomy, but this approach rries recurrent appendicitis rates of 14–20% in the st year (5). The possibility of recurrence or ogression to perforation must be weighed against e potential complications of surgery.

sues for Referral

cases of appendicitis require emergent surgical nsultation.

JRGERY/OTHER PROCEDURES

Inpatient surgery is appropriate measure
Patients presenting within 72 hours of onset:
- Immediate appendectomy; laparoscopic favored unless perforation (6)[A]
- Drainage of abscess, if present

Patients who present late (>4–5 days after symptom onset) may be treated initially with antibiotics, bowel rest, and drainage of any abscess. Later (4–10 weeks) appendectomy can then be performed in this subgroup only.

I-PATIENT CONSIDERATIONS

dmission Criteria

patients with appendicitis should be admitted.

Fluids

Fluid resuscitation with NS or LR
Correct fluid and electrolyte deficits

ursing

eoperative preparation

ischarge Criteria

lerating p.o.; return of bowel function; afebrile; rmal WBC

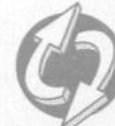

ONGOING CARE

FOLLOW-UP RECOMMENDATIONS

- Return to work is usually possible 1–2 weeks following most uncomplicated appendicitis.
- Restrict activity for 4–6 weeks after surgery: No heavy lifting (>10 lbs) or strenuous physical activity.

Patient Monitoring

Routine visits at 2 and 6 weeks after surgery

DIET

n.p.o. before surgery

PATIENT EDUCATION

Contact physician for postoperative development of:
- Anorexia
- Nausea
- Vomiting
- Abdominal pain
- Fever
- Chills

PROGNOSIS

- Generally uncomplicated course in young adults with unruptured appendicitis
- Factors increasing morbidity and mortality:
  - Extremes of age
  - Appendiceal rupture
- Morbidity rates:
  - Nonperforated appendicitis: 3%
  - Perforated appendicitis: 47%
- Mortality rates:
  - Unruptured appendicitis: 0.1%
  - Ruptured appendicitis: 3%
  - Patients >60 years of age: 50% of deaths from appendicitis
  - Older patients with ruptured appendix: 15%

Pediatric Considerations

- Rupture earlier
- Rupture rate: 15–50%

Pregnancy Considerations

Fetal mortality rate: 2–8.5%

Geriatric Considerations

Rupture rate: 67–90%

COMPLICATIONS

- Wound infection
- Intra-abdominal abscess; lower rate with antibiotic prophylaxis (1)[A]
- Intestinal fistulas
- Intestinal obstruction
- Incisional hernia
- Liver abscess (rare)
- Paralytic ileus
- Pyelophlebitis

REFERENCES

1. Mun S, Ernst RD, Chen K et al. Rapid CT diagnosis of acute appendicitis with IV contrast material. *Emerg Radiol*. 2006;12:99–102.
2. Old JL, Dusing RW, Yap W et al. Imaging for suspected appendicitis. *Am Fam Physician*. 2005;71:71–8.
3. Poortman P, Oostvogel HJ, Bosma E, Lohle PN, Cuesta MA, de Lange-de Klerk ES, Hamming JF et al. Improving diagnosis of acute appendicitis: results of a diagnostic pathway with standard use of ultrasonography followed by selective use of CT. *J Am Coll Surg*. 2009;208:434–41.
4. Andersen BR, Kallehaue FL, Andersen HK. Antibiotics versus placebo for prevention of postoperative infection after appendectomy. *Cochrane Database Syst Rev*. 2006;(1).
5. Hansson J, Körner U, Khorram-Manesh A et al. Randomized clinical trial of antibiotic therapy versus appendectomy as primary treatment of acute appendicitis in unselected patients. *Br J Surg*. 2009;96:473–81.
6. Sauerland S, Lefering R, Neugebauer EAM. Laparoscopic versus open surgery for suspected appendicitis. *Cochrane Database Syst Rev*. 2006;(1).

ADDITIONAL READING

- Anderson SW, Soto JA, Lucey BC, Ozonoff A, Jordan JD, Ratevosian J, Ulrich AS, Rathlev NK, Mitchell PM, Rebholz C, Feldman JA, Rhea JT et al. Abdominal 64-MDCT for suspected appendicitis: the use of oral and IV contrast material versus IV contrast material only. *AJR Am J Roentgenol*. 2009;193:1282–8.
- Hlibczuk V, Dattaro JA, Jin Z, Falzon L, Brown MD et al. Diagnostic accuracy of noncontrast computed tomography for appendicitis in adults: a systematic review. *Ann Emerg Med*. 2010;55:51–59.e1.
- Gaitini D, Beck-Razi N, Mor-Yosef D, Fischer D, Ben Itzhak O, Krausz MM, Engel A et al. Diagnosing acute appendicitis in adults: accuracy of color Doppler sonography and MDCT compared with surgery and clinical follow-up. *AJR Am J Roentgenol*. 2008;190:1300–6.

See Also (Topic, Algorithm, Electronic Media Element)

Algorithm: Abdominal Rigidity

CODES

ICD9

- 540.0 Acute appendicitis with generalized peritonitis
- 540.9 Acute appendicitis without mention of peritonitis
- 541 Appendicitis, unqualified

CLINICAL PEARLS

- Classic history of anorexia with periumbilical pain localizing to RLQ is the cornerstone of diagnosis for acute appendicitis.
- Diagnosis is much more challenging in children, pregnant patients, and the elderly due to varying symptoms and signs.
- CT of abdomen and pelvis is the diagnostic test of choice, although ultrasound in experienced hands has good sensitivity and avoids radiation exposure.
- Acute appendicitis is the most common surgical emergency during pregnancy.

ARTERIAL GAS EMBOLISM

Naida Cole, MD
Neha Raukar, MD

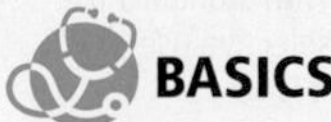

BASICS

DESCRIPTION

- Arterial gas embolism (AGE) is an uncommon, potentially fatal event caused by the entry of gas either directly into the arteries of the systemic circulation or indirectly into the pulmonary veins.
- Emboli can travel to any artery but the most serious consequences occur when they affect the cerebral or coronary circulation, as a result of the inherent vulnerability of the brain and heart to hypoxia.

EPIDEMIOLOGY

- Predominant age: Young adult
- Predominant sex: Male > Female

Incidence

Among divers, the incidence of AGE is <0.1%, but it is the cause of 18% of diving fatalities (based on Divers Alert Network America Report) (1).

RISK FACTORS

- Scuba diving is the most common cause of AGE. Arterial gas embolism is the most serious and rapidly fatal of all scuba diving injuries and is second only to drowning as the leading cause of death associated with sport diving. Two mechanisms may lead to arterial gas embolism:
  - Rapid ascent may lead to decompression sickness (the evolution of bubbles in blood or tissues from dissolved inert gas).
  - Breath holding during ascent may lead to pulmonary barotrauma and subsequent arterial gas emboli.
- Any right-to-left cardiac shunt is a risk factor for paradoxical embolism. These shunts include a patent foramen ovale, pulmonary arteriovenous malformation, or a septal defect. Divers with a patent foramen ovale have a greater than 4-fold increase in decompression illness events and sustain twice as many ischemic brain lesions than in divers without this condition.
- Diagnostic or therapeutic medical procedures can also introduce air directly into the arterial system. AGE most commonly occurs during radiologic procedures, cardiac bypass or coronary artery bypass graft surgery, and neurosurgical procedures.

GENERAL PREVENTION

- Scuba diving:
  - Adhere strictly to diver safety protocols.
  - Do not dive when dehydrated, after recent alcohol use, or with a dive injury or medical condition until evaluated and approved by a physician knowledgeable in diving medicine.
  - Avoid fatigue and hypothermia when diving and avoid rapid ascent with breath-holding.
  - Do not fly or travel to altitudes >700 feet within 24 hours of the last dive.
- Medical:
  - Minimize airway pressures in mechanically ventilated patients to prevent pulmonary barotrauma.
  - Avoid hypovolemia and low blood pressures in high-risk procedures.
  - Occlude the hub of the central venous catheter and ask patient to Valsalva/breath-hold during insertion and removal of a central venous catheter.
  - When flushing any arterial line, take extreme care to avoid air entering the fluid used to flush the line.
  - Place patient in Trendelenburg position when performing any procedure entering a large vein, in case of right to left shunt.

PATHOPHYSIOLOGY

- Two conditions must be present for AGE to occur:
  - Direct communication between arterial circulation and a source of gas
  - Pressure gradient favoring entry of gas into the arterial vessel (normally, arterial pressures exceed atmospheric pressure)
- Scuba diving:
  - AGE in divers occurs due to pulmonary barotrauma. Air in the lungs expands upon rapid ascent as predicted by Boyle's Law. This leads to overdistention and alveolar rupture. If the vascular parenchyma is also damaged, air can enter the arterial system and travel systemically.
- Medical:
  - AGE in the medical setting occurs when arterial blood is exposed to a pressure gradient that favors the flow of air from the atmosphere to the vasculature. This can be a result of pulmonary barotrauma (ventilator associated) or through direct introduction (surgery or central line placement).
  - AGE may also be the result of a paradoxical embolism.
- Emboli travel to all organs and if not absorbed, will eventually occlude end-arteries. Ischemic damage is most severe in brain and coronary arteries. Two separate mechanisms of damage exist (2):
  - Decreased perfusion leads to hypoxia and cell death (if bubble is large and cannot be quickly absorbed)
  - Local inflammatory response to the bubble leads to cytotoxic edema
    - Cerebral arterial gas embolism: Air bubbles occlude vasculature → unequal distribution of blood in brain → hyperemia and ischemia with focal deficits and increased ICP. In addition, bubbles irritate vascular wall → breakdown of blood-brain barrier → edema, increased ICP

ETIOLOGY

- Decompression illness
  - Pulmonary barotrauma: Pulmonary overpressurization causes alveolar rupture, which allows for gas to enter the pulmonary veins and then travel to the systemic circulation.
  - Rapid changes in pressure will cause the nitrogen in the bloodstream to come out of solution and create bubbles in the vascular system. These bubbles then travel systemically until they are lodged and cause ischemic damage. This is due to rapid ascent as seen in divers, aviators, or astronauts participating in "space walks."
- Ventilator-associated barotrauma
- Paradoxical embolism
- Diagnostic or therapeutic procedures, most commonly:
  - Cardiac surgery with extracorporeal bypass
  - Craniotomy with the patient in a seated position
  - Cesarean section

COMMONLY ASSOCIATED CONDITIONS

- Pulmonary barotrauma causing arterial gas embolism can lead to:
  - Pneumomediastinum
  - Subcutaneous emphysema
  - Pneumopericardium
  - Pneumothorax
  - Pneumoperitoneum
- Coronary arterial gas embolism leads to:
  - Temporary ischemia of myocardium
  - Labile blood pressure
  - Arrhythmias
  - Cardiac failure and/or arrest
- Cerebral arterial gas embolism leads to:
  - Focal or diffuse neurologic signs
  - Altered mental status, coma

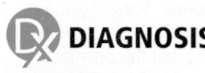

DIAGNOSIS

HISTORY

Rapid onset (usually within minutes) of new neurologic, cardiac, renal, or mucocutaneous symptoms after completion of a scuba dive or during or after a surgical procedure.

- Nonspecific symptoms
  - Nausea
  - Pain (e.g., joint pain "the bends")
  - Malaise
- Neurologic symptoms
  - Headache
  - Dizziness
  - Paresthesias
  - Weakness
  - Tinnitus
  - Visual disturbances, e.g., hemianopsia
- Cardiac symptoms
  - Chest pain
  - Palpitations

PHYSICAL EXAM

- Cerebral arterial gas embolism signs and symptoms
  - Altered mental status
  - Aphasia
  - Minor motor weakness
  - Paralysis
  - Seizures
  - Asymmetric pupils
  - Focal sensory deficits
  - Air in retinal vessels on ophthalmoscopic exam

Coronary arterial gas embolism signs and symptoms
– Arrhythmias
– Arrest

Renal arterial gas embolism signs and symptoms
– Hematuria
– Proteinuria
– Elevated blood urea nitrogen (BUN)/creatinine
– Elevated serum creatinine

Mucocutaneous signs and symptoms
– Cutis marmorata (cyanotic marbling of the skin)
– Focal area of pallor in the tongue

DIAGNOSTIC TESTS & INTERPRETATION

Lab

No tests are diagnostic for arterial gas embolism. Clinical evaluation is preferred.

Initial lab tests

Urinalysis and basic metabolic profile (to check for renal involvement)

Hb/Hct (to check for hemoconcentration; poor specificity)

Troponin (for myocardial ischemia)

Imaging

CXR (to rule out pneumothorax)

ECG (for signs of myocardial infarct)

CT scan: Changes are often very subtle, air may be visible (poor sensitivity)

MRI: Sometimes can show increased volume of water in injured tissue (poor sensitivity)

TTE or TEE: May show evidence of intracardiac shunt, or visible air embolism

DIFFERENTIAL DIAGNOSIS

Decompression sickness

Cerebral infarct

Intracerebral bleed

Coronary artery spasm

Myocardial infarction due to acute coronary syndrome

DVT/Pulmonary embolism

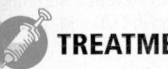

TREATMENT

Immediate measures:
– Lifesaving treatment and stabilization must take precedence: CPR, if required; clear the airway and prevent aspiration; intubate if somnolent or comatose.
– Ventilate with highest possible concentration of oxygen.
– Transfer to a hyperbaric oxygen chamber for recompression immediately.

When air transport is required, helicopter transport should be at an altitude <1,000 feet, and fixed-wing transfer should be limited to an aircraft that can maintain cabin pressure at 1 atm.

MEDICATION

Medication is used as an adjunct to 1st-line treatment; hyperbaric oxygen therapy (HBOT).

First Line

No medication is considered 1st-line treatment for arterial gas embolism.

Second Line

Aspirin

Adjunctive therapy with glucocorticoids, lidocaine, heparin, barbiturates or indomethacin: Efficacy unclear

ADDITIONAL TREATMENT

General Measures

- Place the patient supine. Placing the patient in the Trendelenburg position to capture the gas at the apex of the heart is considered controversial as this maneuver also increases intracranial pressure.
- Maintain hydration with IV fluids.
- Hyperbaric 100% oxygen recompression (3):
  – HBOT is treatment of choice for arterial gas embolism regardless of the cause; transport patient immediately to a hyperbaric chamber. There is no evidence that therapy >6 hours after insult has a negative impact on outcome.
  – Optimal strategy has yet to be determined; however, the most common regimen consists of 2.8 atm (284kPa) maximum pressure, with 100% oxygen for 4 hours 45 minutes.
  – Proposed mechanism of HBOT:
    ○ HBOT decreases bubble size (↑ambient pressure, so ↓volume and ↑surface area:volume ratio, therefore producing faster diffusion of nitrogen from the bubble).
    ○ Systemic hyperoxia creates a diffusion gradient favoring oxygen diffusion into bubble, and nitrogen out of bubble.
    ○ HBOT may prevent cerebral edema by causing vasoconstriction with ↓neutrophil influx and ↓vascular permeability, thereby supporting the blood-brain barrier.
  – For assistance and advice on locating the nearest treatment chamber in your area, call Divers Alert Network (DAN) at any hour (919) 684-9111. Worldwide contact information available at http://www.diversalertnetwork.org.

IN-PATIENT CONSIDERATIONS

IV Fluids

Goal: to achieve normovolemia. Colloids preferred in order to dilute any hemoconcentration.

ONGOING CARE

FOLLOW-UP RECOMMENDATIONS

None until after treatment

Patient Monitoring

Complete neurologic assessment at 1, 3, 6, and 12 months

DIET

Nothing to be consumed until after treatment

PATIENT EDUCATION

- Divers Alert Network: http://www.diversalertnetwork.org
- Medical emergencies: call Divers Alert Network/Duke University Medical Center hotline 24 hours a day, 7 days a week at +1-919-684-9111 or +1-919-684-4DAN (-4326) for collect calls.

PROGNOSIS

Complete recovery occurs in 91% of patients with decompression illness undergoing HBOT; residual deficits despite repeated HBOT occur in 67% (according to study of US military in Okinawa).

COMPLICATIONS

- Long-term serious neurologic impairments
- Death

REFERENCES

1. Vann RD, Denoble PJ, Dovenbarger JA. *2005 Report on Decompression Illness, Diving Fatalities and Project Dive Explorations*. 2003 Data Durham: Diving Alert Network. 2005:1–142.
2. van Hulst RA, Klein J, Lachmann B et al. Gas embolism: pathophysiology and treatment. *Clin Physiol Funct Imaging*. 2003;23:237–46.
3. Bennett MH, Lehm JP, Mitchell SJ, Wasiak J et al. Recompression and adjunctive therapy for decompression illness: a systematic review of randomized controlled trials. *Anesth Analg*. 2010;111:757–62.

ADDITIONAL READING

- Blanc P, Boussuges A, Henriette K, Sainty JM, Deleflie M et al. Iatrogenic cerebral air embolism: importance of an early hyperbaric oxygenation. *Intensive Care Med*. 2002;28:559–63.
- Muth CM, Shank ES et al. Gas embolism. *N Engl J Med*. 2000;342:476–82.
- Neuman TS et al. Arterial gas embolism and decompression sickness. *News Physiol Sci*. 2002;17:77–81.

See Also (Topic, Algorithm, Electronic Media Element)

Air Embolism

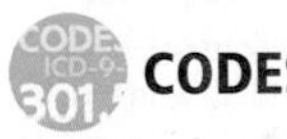

CODES

ICD9

958.0 Air embolism as an early complication of trauma

CLINICAL PEARLS

ALERT

- Any diver who has new symptom(s) or sign(s) after recently completing a self-contained underwater breathing apparatus (SCUBA) dive of any type, to any depth, for any period of time, should be considered for a dive-related injury.
- AGE should be considered in any patient undergoing central venous cannulation or invasive surgery, especially neurosurgical or radiological procedures, who suffer acute symptoms.
- Anesthesia and/or analgesics alter the symptomatology and may complicate evaluation of the patient's clinical status. Delayed recovery from general anesthesia may be a clue to cerebral arterial embolism.

ARTERIOSCLEROTIC HEART DISEASE

Felix B. Chang, MD
Jeremy Golding, MD

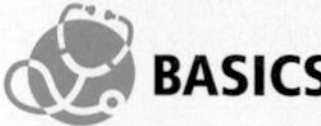

BASICS

The term *coronary artery disease* (CAD) is generally used to refer to a pathologic process affecting the coronary arteries (usually atherosclerosis).

DESCRIPTION

Arterio (athero) sclerosis progressively blocks coronary arteries and their branches.

EPIDEMIOLOGY

- Leading cause of death in the US and Europe
- Predominant sex: Male > Female
- Predominant age for peak clinical manifestations:
  - Men: 50–60 years
  - Women: 60–70 years
- In postmenopausal women, the risk for incident coronary disease is tripled compared with premenopausal women.
- Mortality from coronary heart disease (CHD) has fallen over the past four decades

Incidence

- Framingham data suggest that the age-adjusted annual incidence for men aged 35–64 is 12 per 1,000 per year, and for women, 5 per 1,000 per year. For men >65, the incidence is 27 per 1,000 per year, and for women, 16 per 1,000 per year.
- For persons aged 40 years, the lifetime risk of developing CHD is 49% in men and 32% in women. For those reaching age 70 years, the lifetime risk is 35% in men and 24% in women.

Prevalence

The 2010 Heart Disease and Stroke Statistics update of the American Heart Association reported that 17.6 million persons in the US have CHD, including 8.5 million with myocardial infarction (MI) and 10.2 million with angina pectoris.

RISK FACTORS

- Primary risk factors:
  - Diabetes mellitus
  - Male age >45; female >55
  - Family history of premature CHD (1st-degree relative: Male <55 years; female <65 years)
  - Blood pressure >140/90
  - Active cigarette abuse
  - High-density lipoprotein (HDL) cholesterol <40 mg/dL (HDL >60 mg/dL is a protective factor)
  - Elevated low-density lipoprotein (LDL) cholesterol
  - ESRD
- Secondary risk factors:
  - Obesity
  - Mild renal insufficiency
  - Estrogen deficiency
  - Inflammation
  - Depression and stress

Genetics

Family history is an independent risk factor.

GENERAL PREVENTION

- Lifestyle changes are indicated when lifestyle-related factors (obesity, physical inactivity, increased triglycerides, decreased HDL, or metabolic syndrome are present), regardless of LDL.
- HDL has antiatherogenic properties.

ETIOLOGY

- Atherosclerosis, inflammation, including autoimmunity
- Embolism compromising coronary arteries
- Subintimal atheromas in large and medium vessels

COMMONLY ASSOCIATED CONDITIONS

Cerebrovascular disease (ischemic stroke); peripheral arterial disease (claudication); aortic atherosclerosis (abdominal aortic aneurysm); metabolic syndrome

DIAGNOSIS

- Clinical manifestations:
  - Substernal chest pain, diaphoresis, palpitations
  - Exertional dyspnea
  - Orthopnea
  - Paroxysmal nocturnal dyspnea
  - Cardiac arrhythmias
  - Cardiomegaly
  - Pedal edema/fluid overload

Advanced obstructive CHD can exist with minimal or no symptoms, and can progress rapidly.

PHYSICAL EXAM

Focus on stigmata of vascular disease and manifestations of heart failure.

DIAGNOSTIC TESTS & INTERPRETATION

- ECG: Variable; may be normal or may see ST-segment elevation/depression and/or T-wave inversion, or Q waves from old infarction. 10–20% of acute MI have initially normal ECG.
- Exercise ECG testing is the most commonly used noninvasive test because it is simple and inexpensive, but sensitivity no better than 60–70%. Specificity is much higher.
- Stress testing (exercise, pharmacologic), with or without radionuclide or ECG imaging
- Echocardiography using either exercise or pharmacologic (dobutamine or dipyridamole) stress.
- Radionuclide myocardial perfusion imaging using either exercise or pharmacologic stress improves sensitivity somewhat (70–80%).
- Positron emission tomography
- Coronary artery calcium as measured by electron beam and multidetector row computed tomography and histologic, ultrasonographic, and angiographic measures of coronary disease.
- Cardiac computed tomography angiography is an emerging technique for examining coronary anatomy noninvasively.

Lab

- Fasting lipid profile.
- hs-CRP may be useful as an independent marker of prognosis in patients with stable CHD or in ACS.

Follow-Up & Special Considerations

- Specific changes in diet may reduce serum CRP.
- Hormone replacement therapy raises serum CRP in postmenopausal women.

Imaging

- Angiography: Narrowed coronary arteries
- Echocardiography: Possible wall-motion abnormalities

Pathological Findings

- Focal thickening of the intima with an increase in smooth muscle cells and extracellular matrix
- Accumulation of intracellular lipid deposits or extracellular lipids or both, which produce the fatty streak
- Development of fibrous plaques
- Advanced lesions become revascularized from both the luminal and medial aspects.

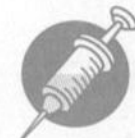

TREATMENT

The use of aspirin for primary prevention is controversial because of the difficulty determining benefits and risk for a given individual. Benefits in terms of reduction in risk of stroke and MI must be balanced against risk of hemorrhage:

- AHA: For men with >10%, 10-year risk of symptomatic CHD (Framingham risk score) (AHA) (1), consider 75–160 mg aspirin per day. A risk calculator is available online at http://hp2010.nhlbihin.net/atpiii/calculator.asp
- Low-risk diabetics (those aged <50 years with 1 c fewer additional risk factors) may not benefit from aspirin (AHA/ADA) for primary prevention.
- For high-risk women, aspirin (75–160 mg/dl) should be used unless contraindicated (AHA) (2)[A If intolerant of aspirin, clopidogrel should be substituted (2)[B].
- Women aged ≥65 years: Consider aspirin therapy (81 mg daily or 100 mg every other day) if blood pressure is controlled and benefit for ischemic stroke and MI prevention likely to outweigh risk of gastrointestinal bleeding and hemorrhagic stroke (2)[B]. Stroke risk calculator available at http://www.westernstroke.org/personalstrokerisk1.xls
- Consider in most diabetics aged >50 years with or more additional risk factors (cigarette smoking, hypertension, obesity, albuminuria, hyperlipidemia, or family history of CHD) (3)[C]. Recent trials failed to show a significant reduction in CVD end points (4).
- The 2009 USPTF statement on the use of aspirin fc the prevention of cardiovascular disease:
  - In women aged 55–79 years, when the potentia benefit of a reduction in ischemic stroke outweighs the risk of an increase in gastrointestinal hemorrhage (5).
  - In men aged 45–79, when the potential benefit a reduction in the rate of MI outweighs the risk c an increase in gastrointestinal hemorrhage (6). This occurs with 10-year MI risk of 10–20% in patients with average risk of GI bleeding.
- Aspirin is recommended for secondary prevention of CVD after acute MI and unstable angina, occlusive stroke, transient ischemic attack, stable angina, and coronary artery bypass surgery to reduce risk of MI, stroke and vascular death (7)[A].
- In secondary prevention, the absolute benefit is larg compared to the absolute risk of major bleeding.
- Statins:
- Primary prevention: Benefit depends more on overa risk than cholesterol levels
- Statins may reduce incidence of cardiovascular death, myocardial infarction and stroke in patients without cardiovascular disease, but number neede to treat is high and use is increasingly controversia especially since it is not clear that statins decrease overall death in primary prevention (8)[B].

WHO Cooperative Trial (clofibrate), Lipid Research Clinics Coronary Primary Prevention Trial (cholestyramine), and the Helsinki Heart Study (gemfibrozil) did not demonstrate a reduction in coronary mortality.
The ASCOT-LLA trial (atorvastatin) did not show statistically significant reductions in cardiovascular mortality.
condary Prevention:
Statins reduce mortality and myocardial infarction in adults with coronary heart disease (7) (SOR)[A].
Lipid-lowering therapy (primarily with statins) is recommended for most patients with diabetes (SOR) (3)[A].

EDICATION

rst Line

For established CAD: Aspirin/ASA: 75–160 mg/day; clopidogrel 75 mg PO daily, if ASA is contraindicated.
Angiotensin-converting enzyme (ACE) inhibitors in all with increased risk factors, diabetes mellitus (DM), or known CAD
Beta blockers for post-MI patients
Cholesterol-lowering agents:
- Data for mortality reduction best for HMG-CoA reductase inhibitor statins. Atorvastatin (10–80 mg PO once daily), initial dose 10–20 mg/d; fluvastatin (20–80 mg/d), initial dose 20–40 mg/dL; lovastatin (10–80 mg/d), initial dose 10–20 mg/dL; pravastatin (maintenance 10–80 mg/d), initial dose 40 mg/dL; simvastatin (20–40 mg once daily), maintenance 5–80 mg/dL; rosuvastatin (5–40 mg once daily), initial dose 10–20 mg/dL
- Statins also have anti-inflammatory and immunomodulatory effects, and effects on vascular tone and thrombogenicity.
  Average reduction % in LDL is dose-dependent: Atorvastatin 35–60%, fluvastatin 22–35%, lovastatin 21–42%; pravastatin 22–37%, rosuvastatin 45–63%, simvastatin 26–47%.

Fish oil and other γ-3 acid ethyl esters: 3 standard fish oil capsules daily supply approximately 1 g of EPA + DHA.
To increase HDL cholesterol (no proven benefit):
- Niacin: 2–6 g/d in divided doses
- Gemfibrozil: 600 mg 2 b.i.d.
- Fenofibrate: 67–200 mg/d
- Probucol: 500 mg 2 b.i.d.
- Colesevelam: 3.75–4.375 g/d

Average reduction % in triglyceride from baseline:
- Bile acid sequestrant: Cholestyramine 11–28%; colesevelam (no effect); colestipol 12–15%
- Fibric acid: Fenofibrate 28.9%; gemfibrozil 31%; niacin E 16–31%, niacin IR 18%
- Statin: Baseline TG levels >250 mg/dl 35–45%; baseline TG levels <250 mg/dl> <25%

Average increase % in HDL from baseline:
- Bile-acid sequestrant: Cholestyramine 4–8%; coleselevam 3–8%; colestipol, no effect
- Ezetimibe 3.5%
- Fibric acid: fenofibrate 1%; gemfibrozil: 6%
- Niacin ER 20–40%; Niacin IR 17%
- Statins: 5–10%

econd Line

ntiplatelet activity: Ticlopidine, dipyridamole, opidogrel

ADDITIONAL TREATMENT

General Measures

- Known CHD or CHD-risk equivalent (10-year risk >20%) has a LDL-C goal <100 mg/dL
- Prevention of further disease progression:
  - Smoking cessation, treatment of hypercholesterolemia (diet, drugs); increase HDL (diet, exercise); control of BP (<140/90; if DM or renal disease, <130/80); diabetes mellitus, exercise 30–40 minutes 5 times/week, moderate alcohol consumption, stress reduction, treatment of depression, diet changes, weight loss (body mass index <25).

ONGOING CARE

FOLLOW-UP RECOMMENDATIONS

For patients with type 2 diabetes taking statins, routine monitoring of liver function test or muscle enzymes is not recommended.

Patient Monitoring

- Monitor lipid panel.
- Preventive programs (weight loss, smoking cessation, diabetes nutritional education)

DIET

- Low fat: 20–30 g/d, and eliminate or reduce trans fats
- Weight loss diet if obesity a problem
- Increase soluble fiber and plant stanols.
- Reduce consumption of red meat; increase fish, olive oil, and nuts.
- Individuals who consume a healthy diet have significantly lower risks of CVD, including both CHD and stroke:
  - High intake of fruits and vegetables
  - High fiber intake, including cereals
  - Low glycemic index and low glycemic load
  - Monounsaturated fats rather than trans fatty acids or saturated fats
  - Limited intake of red or processed meats
  - Omega-3 fatty acids (from fish, fish oil supplements, or plant sources)

PATIENT EDUCATION

American Heart Association, 7320 Greenville Avenue, Dallas, TX 75231, (214) 373-6300.

PROGNOSIS

- In population studies, for every 10% reduction in serum cholesterol, CHD was reduced by 15%; and total mortality risk, by 11%
- The incidence of a MI is increased 6-fold in women and 3-fold in men who smoke at least 20 cigarettes per day.
- Current smoking was associated with a 50% increase in the progression of atherosclerosis versus nonsmokers.

COMPLICATIONS

- MI
- Ventricular fibrillation
- CHF
- Angina pectoris
- Sudden cardiac death

REFERENCES

1. AHA Guidelines for Primary Prevention of Cardiovascular Disease and Stroke: 2002 Update: Consensus Panel Guide to Comprenhensive Risk Reduction for Adult Patients Without Coronary of Other Atherosclerotic Vascular Diseases. American Heart Association Science Advisory and Coordinated Committee. *Circulation*. 2002;106(3):388–91.
2. Evidence-based guidelines for cardiovascular disease prevention in women: 2007 update. *Circulation*. 2007;115(11):1481–501.
3. Standards of Medical Care in diabetes. *Diabetes Care*. 2010;33(Suppl 1):S11–S61.
4. Belch J, MaqcCuish A, et al. The prevention of progression of arterial disease and diabetes (POPADAD) trial: factorial randomized placebo controlled trial of aspirin and antioxidants in patients with diabetes and asymptomatic peripheral arterial disease. *BMJ*. 2008;337:1840.
5. Aspirin for the prevention of cardiovascular disease: U.S. Preventive Services Tasks Force recommendation statement. *Ann Intern Med*. 2009;150(6):396–404.
6. Wolff T, Miller T, Ko S. Aspirin for the primary prevention of cardiovascular events: an update of the evidence for the U.S. Preventive Services Task Force. *Ann Intern Med*. 2009;150(6):405–10.
7. Becker RC, Meade T, et al. The primary and secondary prevention of coronary artery disease: American College of Chest Physicians Evidence-Based Clinical Practice Guidelines (8th Edition). *Chest*. 2008;133:776S.
8. Primary prevention of cardiovascular mortality and events with statin treatments: a network meta-analysis involving more than 65,000 patients. *J Am Coll Cardiol*. 2008;52(22):1469–81.

ADDITIONAL READING

- Aspirin for the prevention of cardiovascular disease. U.S. Preventive Services Task Force recommendation statement. *Ann Intern Med*. 2009;150(6):396–404.
- Framingham risk estimates: http://www.nhlbi.nih.gov/guidelines/cholesterol/index.htm

See Also (Topic, Algorithm, Electronic Media Element)

Angina; Atherosclerosis; Myocardial Infarction, ST-Segment Elevation (STEMI)
Algorithm: Chest_Pain/Acute Coronary Syndrome

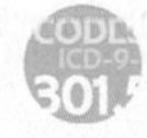

CODES

ICD9

414.00 Coronary atherosclerosis of unspecified type of vessel, native or graft

CLINICAL PEARLS

- Net benefit of aspirin increases with increasing cardiovascular risk.
- Insufficient evidence to recommend for or against aspirin for low-risk patients.
- Aspirin significantly reduced the relative risk of subsequent vascular events (nonfatal MI, nonfatal stroke, and vascular death) by approximately 22%.
- The CHD death rate increases at higher plasma concentrations of total and LDL-cholesterol, and statins for patients with known CAD reduce morbidity and mortality.

ARTERITIS, TEMPORAL

Jo Ellen Feugate, MD, PhD
Eric P. Gall, MD

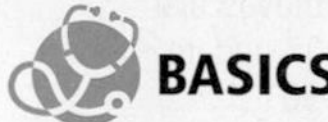

BASICS

DESCRIPTION

Also known as giant cell arteritis. A large vessel vasculitis affecting the elderly. Primarily involves the cranial branches of the carotid arteries and can cause visual loss.

EPIDEMIOLOGY

- Disease of the elderly, almost never seen in persons <50 years. Incidence increases with age
- Female > Male (2:1)

Incidence

More common in Northern Europe, esp. Scandinavia (20 per 100,000 per year) vs Southern Europe (10 per 100,000 per year). In the US, incidence in a largely white Minnesota cohort was 19 per 100,000 per year. It is likely less for the US as a whole. Temporal arteritis is very rare in populations of non-European ancestry.

RISK FACTORS

- Increasing age
- Polymyalgia rheumatica
- Atherosclerosis and smoking in women but not men

Genetics

- Some family clusters have been documented.
- HLA-DR4 and HLA-DRB1 are associated with temporal arteritis.

ETIOLOGY

Unclear, involves cell-mediated immune response and Il-6 production

COMMONLY ASSOCIATED CONDITIONS

Polymyalgia rheumatica

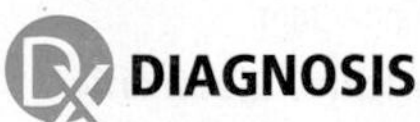

DIAGNOSIS

HISTORY

Usually gradual in onset but may be abrupt

- New or changed headache (usually unilateral temporal but may be generalized)
- Scalp and facial tenderness
- Jaw and tongue claudication with chewing (most specific symptom for temporal arteritis)
- Visual changes
  - Amaurosis fugax
  - Diplopia
  - Scotoma
  - Blindness
- Nonproductive cough
- Arm claudication
- Constitutional symptoms
  - Fever
  - Weight loss
  - Fatigue
  - Polymyalgia rheumatica (stiffness and aching in shoulder and hip girdles). Present in 50%.

PHYSICAL EXAM

- Prominent, tender, or pulseless temporal artery
- Scalp tenderness
- Cranial nerve palsies
- Visual field defect
- Abnormal retinal exam (cotton wool spots, pale edematous retina)
- Proximal muscle tenderness but no weakness

DIAGNOSTIC TESTS & INTERPRETATION

Lab

- ESR/CRP; usually very elevated (ESR >50). <10% have a normal ESR. If both ESR and CRP are normal, consider alternative diagnoses.
- Normocytic, normochromic anemia; usually mild
- Elevated acute phase reactants (platelets, LFTs, albumin)

Imaging

- Ultrasonography of the temporal artery can be up to 88% sensitive and 97% specific for diagnosing temporal arteritis but is quite operator dependent. It does not replace biopsy for definitive diagnosis. (1)
- MRI/MRA in patients with arm claudication or other evidence of aortic branch involvement. It also should be considered, esp. in patients with an aortic insufficiency murmur, to evaluate for presence of aortic aneurysm.

Diagnostic Procedures/Surgery

Temporal artery biopsy: The gold standard for the diagnosis of temporal arteritis

- Treatment prior to biopsy is unlikely to affect the biopsy results, but biopsy should be done within 2 weeks of commencing treatment.
- A segment >2 cm long is needed as there are often skip lesions.
- Serial sections should be done.
- Routine biopsy of both temporal arteries is not necessary; however, if the first biopsy is negative and clinical suspicion remains high, a contralateral biopsy could be considered.

Pathological Findings

Inflammatory infiltrate (either mononuclear cells or granulomas with giant multinucleated cells) seen in the intima and media of large vessels with resultant disruption of the internal elastic lamina. Lesions may be isolated (e.g., skip lesions).

DIFFERENTIAL DIAGNOSIS

- CNS vasculitis
- Embolic disease
- Temporomandibular joint syndrome
- Space-occupying lesion or other cause for new headache in the elderly
- Retinal disease
- CVA

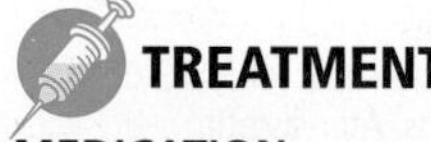

TREATMENT

MEDICATION

First Line

Prednisone:

- Due to the risk of irreversible vision loss, treatment with high-dose steroids should be starte on strong clinical suspicion of temporal arteritis, prior to the temporal biopsy being done. The initial dose of prednisone is 60 mg/day [B]. Steroids should not be in the form of alternate day therapy, as this is more likely to lead to a relapse of vasculitis.
- Pulsed dose intravenous methylprednisolone (1 g/day for 3 days) may be of benefit to patients who present with recent onset of visual symptoms (2)[C]. This is followed by prednisone 60 mg/day as above.
- At 6–8 weeks, prednisone can be tapered by 5 mg every 2 weeks to a dose of 25 mg/day. Then the taper is slowed to 2.5 mg every 2 weeks to a dose 10 mg/day. After that, the prednisone is very gradually weaned by 1 mg every 3–6 months. Dose reduction should be considered only in the absence of clinical symptoms, signs and laboratory abnormalities suggestive of active disease. Many patients may require a slower taper.
- Consider low-dose aspirin for all patients with giant cell arteritis (3)[C]
- Patients on corticosteroids should be on bone protection therapy unless they have contraindications

econd Line

- ethotrexate (10–15 mg/week) has a modest effect temporal arteritis and could be considered in tients who have not responded to glucocorticoids who have significant side effects from steroids [B].

ONGOING CARE

OLLOW-UP RECOMMENDATIONS

- Follow up in clinic at least monthly initially. When stable and steroids are being tapered, every 3 months.
- Disease relapse should be suspected in patients with new headaches, visual changes, fever, myalgias. A rise in ESR/CRP is usually seen with relapse. An increase in steroids by 10 mg/day is usually significant to control a relapse.

atient Monitoring

- Check ESR/CRP with each visit to monitor disease activity.
- Consider yearly CXR (to evaluate for aortic aneurysm) and biannual DEXA scans.

IET

- lcium and vitamin D supplementation

ATIENT EDUCATION

- Consequences of discontinuing steroids abruptly (adrenal suppression, disease relapse)
- Risks of long-term steroid use
- Importance of reporting new headaches and vision changes to provider immediately

ROGNOSIS

- Prior vision loss is unlikely to be recovered, but treatment resolves the other symptoms and prevents future vision loss and stroke.
- Average disease duration 3–4 years but may be up to 10 years.

OMPLICATIONS

- Sequelae of long-term steroid use (osteoporosis, diabetes, thinned skin, weight gain)
- Blindness
- Stroke
- Aortic aneurysm/dissection

REFERENCES

1. Karassa FB, Matsagas MI, Schmidt WA, Ioannidis JP et al. Meta-analysis: test performance of ultrasonography for giant-cell arteritis. *Ann Intern Med*. 2005;142:359–69.
2. Hayreh SS, Zimmerman B, Kardon RH et al. Visual improvement with corticosteroid therapy in giant cell arteritis. Report of a large study and review of literature. *Acta Ophthalmol Scand*. 2002;80:355–67.
3. Lee MS, Smith SD, Galor A et al. Antiplatelet and anticoagulant therapy in patients with giant cell arteritis. *Arthritis Rheum*. 2006;54:3306–9.
4. Mahr AD, Jover JA, Spiera RF, Hernández-García C, Fernández-Gutiérrez B, Lavalley MP, Merkel PA et al. Adjunctive methotrexate for treatment of giant cell arteritis: an individual patient data meta-analysis. *Arthritis Rheum*. 2007;56:2789–97.

ADDITIONAL READING

- Hunder GG, Bloch DA, Michel BA et al. The American College of Rheumatology 1990 criteria for the classification of giant cell arteritis. *Arthritis Rheum*. 1990;33:1122–8.
- Mukhtyar C, Guillevin L, Cid MC, Dasgupta B, de Groot K, Gross W, Hauser T, Hellmich B, Jayne D, Kallenberg CG, Merkel PA, Raspe H, Salvarani C, Scott DG, Stegeman C, Watts R, Westman K, Witter J, Yazici H, Luqmani R, European Vasculitis Study Group et al. EULAR recommendations for the management of large vessel vasculitis. *Ann Rheum Dis*. 2009;68:318–23.

See Also (Topic, Algorithm, Electronic Media Element)

Depression; Fibromyalgia; Headache, Cluster; Headache, Tension; Polymyalgia Rheumatica; Polymyositis/Dermatomyositis

CODES

ICD9

446.5 Giant cell arteritis

CLINICAL PEARLS

- Due to the risk of irreversible vision loss, treatment with high-dose steroids (prednisone 60 mg/day) should be started immediately in patients suspected of temporal artery.
- Temporal artery biopsy is the gold standard for diagnosis. Temporal artery biopsy is not likely to be affected by a few weeks of treatment.
- Treatment consists of a very slow steroid taper. Bone protection therapy and low dose aspirin should be considered.

ARTHRITIS, INFECTIOUS, BACTERIAL

Christopher J. Scola, MD
Raul Davaro, MD

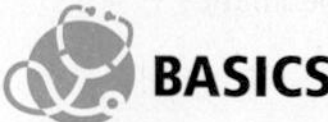

BASICS

DESCRIPTION

- Invasion of joints by pyogenic microorganisms. One of the curable causes of arthritis. May be part of systemic infection/disease.
- System(s) affected: Musculoskeletal
- Synonym(s): Suppurative arthritis; Septic arthritis; Pyarthrosis; Pyogenic arthritis; Bacterial arthritis

EPIDEMIOLOGY

- Predominant age:
  - Neisserial: Especially 15–40 years of age; can occur at any age
  - Nonneisserial (approximate):
    - Years <2: 60% *Staphylococcus*, 20% *Streptococcus*, 10% gram-negative rods, <5% miscellaneous
    - Years 2–14: 60% *Staphylococcus*, 30% *Streptococcus*, 5% *Haemophilus*, 5% other gram-negative rods, 5% miscellaneous
    - Adult: 60% *Staphylococcus*, 25% *Streptococcus*, <1% *Haemophilus*, and 15% other gram-negative rods
- Predominant gender:
  - Neisserial: Female > Male (4:1)
  - Nonneisserial: Male > Female (2:1)

Prevalence

- Neisserial:
  - Responsible for 50% of infectious arthritis
  - 0.6% of women with gonorrhea
  - 0.1% of men with gonorrhea
  - Arthritis occurs in 7% of individuals with *Neisseria meningitidis*
- Nonneisserial: Half as frequent as neisserial

RISK FACTORS

- Sexual exposure: Neisserial
- Inflammatory arthritis, e.g., rheumatoid arthritis
- Concurrent extra-articular infection
- Prior arthritis in affected joint
- Trauma
- Joint puncture or surgery
- Prosthetic joint (1)[A]
- Prior corticosteroid or immunosuppressive therapy
- Serious chronic systemic illness (e.g., diabetes, liver disease, malignancy, immunodeficiency)
- Defective phagocytic mechanisms (e.g., chronic granulomatous disease)
- Injection drug use
- Sickle cell anemia
- Complement deficiency
- Systemic infection; infection elsewhere
- Immunodeficiency; immunosuppression
- Dental procedures; poor dental/gingival hygiene
- Advanced age >80 years

GENERAL PREVENTION

- Prompt treatment of skin and soft tissue infections
- Condoms and limiting number of sexual partners for sexually transmitted disease protection

ETIOLOGY

- Hematogenous invasion (80–90%)
- Contiguous spread (10–15%)
- Direct penetration of microorganisms secondary to trauma or joint infection (5%)

COMMONLY ASSOCIATED CONDITIONS

- Serious chronic illness (e.g., rheumatoid arthritis, diabetes, liver disease, malignancy, primary immunodeficiency, complement deficiencies)
- Immunosuppressive therapy (disease-modifying antirheumatic drugs [DMARDs] agents, glucocorticoids, chemotherapy)
- Systemic infection associated with bacteremia, especially endocarditis

DIAGNOSIS

HISTORY

- Nongonococcal:
  - Predominantly monoarticular (90%)
- Fever: In 90% during course of infection
- Malaise
- Back pain: Subacute bacterial endocarditis
- Neisserial:
  - Bacteremic phase: Migratory polyarthritis, tenosynovitis, high fever, chills, pustules
  - Localized phase: Usually monoarticular with low-grade fever

PHYSICAL EXAM

- Limited or loss of joint use/motion
- Joint effusion, tenderness
- Joint warmth and redness: Present intenosynovitis; pustular skin lesions common for neisserial infection
- Hip and shoulder involvement may reveal severe pain on range of motion with less obvious joint swelling on exam.

DIAGNOSTIC TESTS & INTERPRETATION

Lab

Initial lab tests

- Synovial fluid (2)[A]:
  - Arthrocentesis prior to starting antibiotics increases diagnostic yield
  - Synovial fluid is usually cloudy with >50,000 white blood cells (WBC)/HPF.
    - Caveat: To be valid, cell count must be performed within 1 hour of obtaining specimen.
    - WBC count alone is not sufficient to rule in or rule out septic arthritis (3)[A]
  - Polymorphonuclear leukocytes usually predominate in synovial fluid, >90%.
  - Crystals (e.g., urate or calcium pyrophosphate) do not exclude infectious arthritis.
  - Joint fluid: For Gram stain (positive in 50%); culture (positive in 50–70%); usually negative in neisserial
- Cervical culture or urethral culture highest diagnostic yield for disseminated gonococcal infection in young adults

Pediatric Considerations

- There is no single lab test that can distinguish septic arthritis from transient synovitis (4)[A].
- The combination of fever, non-weight bearing, C-reactive protein >20 or erythrocyte sedimentation rate >40, and a white cell count >12 is suspicious of septic arthritis (4)[B].

Follow-Up & Special Considerations

- Bedside culture is recommended to enhance isolation of fastidious organisms.
- All cultures should be maintained and observed fo 3 days to 2 weeks (2,5)[A].
- Neisserial infection generally requires use of speci media (e.g., chocolate or Thayer Martin).
- Drugs that may alter lab results: Antibiotics

Imaging

Initial approach

- X-ray (5)[A]:
  - Soft tissue swelling
  - Juxta-articular osteoporosis
  - Radiolucent area (gas) in a joint space from gas-forming organisms (Caveat: May be normal as a "vacuum phenomenon")
  - Effacement of obturator fat pad (with hip involvement)
  - X-ray changes usually a late phenomenon
  - Rarefaction of subchondral bone may occur
  - Joint-space loss (secondary to cartilage destruction) may occur in 4–10 days.
  - Erosions
  - Joint destruction with ankylosis may occur.
- Other imaging techniques:
  - Technetium joint scans: Reveal distribution of inflammation; sensitive, not specific
  - Gallium WBC scan, indium scans: Reveal inflammation as well as infection
  - Computed tomography: To identify sequestratio
  - Magnetic resonance imaging: Effusion, perhaps early cartilage damage, osteomyelitis

Diagnostic Procedures/Surgery

Arthrocentesis with Gram stain and culture: Positive in 50–70% (6)[A]:

- Shoulder or hip joints may require image-guided aspiration.
- Must always be done when possibility of infectiou arthritis is considered
- Arthrocentesis should be performed prior to initiation of antibiotics whenever possible. Arthrocentesis approach must avoid contaminated tissue (e.g., overlying cellulitis) when possible.

Pathological Findings

Synovial biopsy will reveal polymorphonuclear leukocytes and possibly the causative organism, if synovial fluid and blood cultures are negative.

IFFERENTIAL DIAGNOSIS

Gout
Pseudogout (calcium pyrophosphate deposition disease)
Spondyloarthropathy (Reiter syndrome, psoriatic arthritis, ankylosing spondylitis, arthritis of inflammatory bowel disease)
Juvenile rheumatoid arthritis
Foreign-body synovitis
Rheumatoid arthritis
Rheumatic fever
Cellulitis
Palindromic rheumatism
Neuropathic arthropathy
Lyme arthritis
Granulomatous arthritis

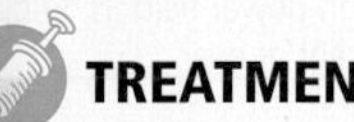

TREATMENT

EDICATION

rst Line

Neisserial (5)[A]:
- Ceftriaxone 1 g IM or IV every day for 14 days (and at least 7 days after symptoms resolve)
- Fluoroquinolone for 14 days; caveat resistance
- Concomitant treatment for *Chlamydia*

Nonneisserial (5)[A]:
- Gram-positive cocci in clusters: Empiric therapy: Vancomycin or linezolid IV. If methicillin-sensitive *Staphylococcus aureus* (MSSA), nafcillin or cefazolin IV
- Gram-positive cocci in chains: Ceftriaxone
- Gram-negative bacilli: Neonates: Cefotaxime, and gentamicin; ages 6 months to 4 years: 3rd-generation cephalosporin; adult: 3rd-generation cephalosporin plus gentamicin. No bacteria seen on smear: Vancomycin or linezolid plus 3rd-generation cephalosporin.

Precautions:
- Observe for allergic reactions

Significant possible interactions:
- Broad-spectrum antibiotics: May reduce effectiveness of oral contraceptives; barrier method recommended

econd Line

uoroquinolones (e.g., ciprofloxacin)

ODITIONAL TREATMENT

eneral Measures

Hospitalization for parenteral therapy
Outpatient treatment rarely possible for extremely compliant patient with known organism
Repeat (once) arthrocentesis if fluid reaccumulates. Next step is arthroscopic debridement and irrigation.
Avoid anti-inflammatory therapy to allow assessment of therapeutic response to antibiotic.

- If joint prosthesis is present in an infection, orthopedic surgery, to include possible removal of the prosthesis, must be considered.
- Continue treatment for 1–2 weeks after total resolution of all signs of inflammation, for a total of 4–6 weeks for most organisms, except Neisserial (2–3 weeks).
- Intra-articular antibiotics are not required.

Issues for Referral

Infectious disease and orthopedic consults strongly advised to supplement rheumatologist

SURGERY/OTHER PROCEDURES

- Arthroscopy indicated if fluid accumulated is loculated and/or not amenable to needle drainage
- Surgical drainage typically is required for shoulder or hip involvement.

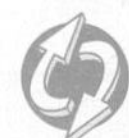

ONGOING CARE

FOLLOW-UP RECOMMENDATIONS

Patient Monitoring

- Repeat arthrocentesis (once) if fluid reaccumulates to verify sterilization of joint and reversion of inflammatory signs to normal.
- If no improvement within 24 hours, re-evaluate and consider arthroscopy.
- CBC, liver and kidney function, and urinalysis twice a week while on antibiotics (with creatinine when gentamicin used)
- Aminoglycoside levels
- Follow-up 1 week and 1 month after stopping antibiotics to detect any relapse.

PROGNOSIS

- Early treatment should allow cure.
- Delayed recognition/treatment complicated by morbidity and mortality

COMPLICATIONS

- Death (9–33% in elderly)
- Limited joint range of motion
- Secondary osteoarthritis
- Flail or fused or dislocated joint
- Septic necrosis
- Sinus formation
- Ankylosis
- Osteomyelitis
- Postinfectious synovitis
- Shortening of limb (in children)

REFERENCES

1. Zimmerli W, Trampuz A, Ochsner PE. Prosthetic-joint infections. *N Engl J Med*. 2004;351:1645–54.
2. Mathews CJ, Weston VC, Jones A, et al. Bacterial septic arthritis in adults. *Lancet*. 2010;375(9717): 846–55.
3. O'Malley A, Svinos H et al. Towards evidence based emergency medicine: Best BETs from the Manchester Royal Infirmary. BET 3: Is the white cell count of the joint aspirate sufficiently sensitive/ specific to rule in/out septic arthritis? *Emerg Med J*. 2009;26:435–7.
4. Taekema HC, Landham PR, Maconochie I et al. Towards evidence based medicine for paediatricians. Distinguishing between transient synovitis and septic arthritis in the limping child: how useful are clinical prediction tools? *Arch Dis Child*. 2009;94:167–8.
5. Margaretten ME, Kohlwes J, Moore D et al. Does this adult patient have septic arthritis? *JAMA*. 2007;297:1478–88.
6. Khachatourians AG, Patzakis MJ, Roidis N et al. Laboratory monitoring in pediatric acute osteomyelitis and septic arthritis. *Clin Orthop Relat Res*. 2003;186–94.

ADDITIONAL READING

- Mathews CJ, Coakley G. Septic arthritis: current diagnostic and therapeutic algorithm. *Curr Opin Rheumatol*. 2008;20:457–62.
- Ross JJ, Hu LT. Bacterial and Lyme arthritis. *Curr Infect Dis Rep* 2004;5:380–7.

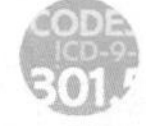

CODES

ICD9

- 040.89 Other specified bacterial diseases
- 711.40 Arthropathy, site unspecified, associated with other bacterial diseases

CLINICAL PEARLS

- Neisseria is the most common cause of septic arthritis in young adults.
- Acute onset of joint pain with redness and warmth is typical of nonneisserial infection.
- Crystalline process can mimic septic arthritis.
- Aspiration of joint prior to the initiation of antibiotics will optimize diagnostic yield.
- Synovial fluid appears inflammatory and is typically purulent.

ARTHRITIS, INFECTIOUS, GRANULOMATOUS

Christopher J. Scola, MD
Raul Davaro, MD

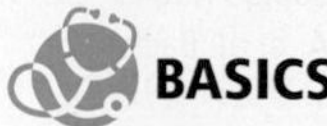

BASICS

DESCRIPTION
- Invasion of joints by microorganisms; may be part of systemic infection/disease
- One of the few curable causes of arthritis
- System(s) affected: Musculoskeletal
- Synonym(s): Fungal arthritis; Mycobacterial arthritis; Subacute bacterial arthritis

EPIDEMIOLOGY
- 1–3% of patients with tuberculosis (TB) infections
- 10–30% of extrapulmonary TB will present with musculoskeletal involvement
- Predominant age: Broad range
- Predominant gender:
  - Male > Female (*Brucella* and mycobacterial).
  - Female > Male (fungal).

Prevalence
1 in 3 million population

Pediatric Considerations
Infrequent in pediatric population

RISK FACTORS
- Acquired immune-deficiency disease (AIDS)
- Concurrent extraarticular infection
- Chronic inflammatory arthritis, such as rheumatoid arthritis (RA)
- Trauma, especially penetrating
- Prosthetic joint
- Prior antibiotic, corticosteroid, or immunosuppressive therapy
- Serious chronic systemic illness (e.g., diabetes mellitus, liver disease, malignancy, primary immunodeficiency)
- Defective phagocytic mechanisms (e.g., chronic granulomatous disease)
- Injection drug use
- Exposure (e.g., brucellosis, unpasteurized milk, farmers, butchers, veterinarians)
- Travel/habitat history
- Gardening (sporotrichosis)
- Aquatic exposure (e.g., fish hook puncture)

ETIOLOGY
- Hematogenous invasion is most common.
- Contiguous spread
- Direct penetration via trauma
- Fungal infections may disseminate from primary pulmonary involvement, particularly in immunocompromised hosts.

COMMONLY ASSOCIATED CONDITIONS
- Systemic infection
- Infection elsewhere
- Immunodeficiency/immunosuppression (e.g., from HIV/AIDS, lymphoma, transplantation, medications)

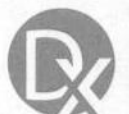

DIAGNOSIS

HISTORY
- Predominantly monarticular (90%)
- Fungal may present as a migratory polyarthritis, particularly with C. *immitis* and H. *capsulatum* owing to hypersensitivity reaction (1,2).
- Flare of arthritis in a single joint with preexisting joint disease
- Fever in 50% at some time during infection
- Fever of unknown origin (FUO) can be an early sign of brucellosis.
- Cutaneous lesions are seen with B. *dermatitidis* and S. *schenckii*.
- Back pain, especially in TB and brucellosis
- Sternal or rib involvement can occur with TB.
- Prosthetic joint infections owing to fungal infection can occur months to years after initial surgery (1).
- Prosthetic joint can present with subacute onset of pain and swelling.
- Fretfulness, in children

PHYSICAL EXAM
- Joint-line tenderness
- Joint effusion
- Synovial thickening (doughy consistency); may have only minimal tenderness
- Limited joint use/motion, especially in children
- Overlying warmth, redness; present in fewer than 50%
- Fungal joint infections can form draining sinus tracts.
- Spinal tenderness with TB (Pott disease) and with brucellosis
- Gibbous deformity with TB
- Tenosynovitis
- Dactylitis
- Erythema nodosum (*H. capsulatum* and TB) (2)
- Nodular skin lesions with mycobacterium and fungal
- Iritis (with mycobacterial arthritis)
- Brucellosis:
  - Hepatosplenomegaly
  - Lymphadenopathy

DIAGNOSTIC TESTS & INTERPRETATIO

Lab
Initial lab tests
- Arthrocentesis (3,4,5)[A]
- Bacterial: For Gram stain, silver, and acid-fast stai and culture, cell count and differential, glucose
- Mycobacterial: Acid-fast smear (positive in 20%), culture (positive in 80%); polymerase chain reacti (PCR)
- To be done in all patients when possibility of infectious arthritis is considered
- Synovial fluid usually cloudy with >20,000 white blood cell count (WBCs)/high-power field (HPF) bu may have fewer WBCs present or over 100,000/mm^3
- Synovial fluid analysis, including wet-mount prep, typically positive in *B. dermatidis* (1)
- Polymorphonuclear leukocytes usually predominat in synovial fluid, although granulomatous and vira arthritis may have a mononuclear cell predominanc
- Approach must avoid contaminated tissue during arthrocentesis (e.g., overlying cellulitis)
- Synovial membrane: Biopsy and culture
- Blood, urine, sputum cultures
- Fungal blood cultures or serologies (6)[C]
- All cultures should be held for 2 weeks; acid-fast cultures for 6 weeks.
- Drug susceptibility testing is recommended.
- The presence of crystals in the synovial fluid (e.g., urate or calcium pyrophosphate) does not exclude infectious arthritis.
- PCR for specific microorganisms
- Serum testing (i.e., cryptococcal antigen, *Brucella* antibody >1:160)
- PCR DNA analysis for TB
- Positive fungal tissue culture should not be disregarded as contaminated.

Imaging
Initial approach
- Radiographs (1,4,5,7)[A]
- X-ray changes usually a late phenomenon
- Soft tissue swelling
- Rarefaction of subchondral bone
- Joint-space loss
- Erosions
- Joint destruction with ankylosis
- Subchondral erosion with preservation of joint spa strongly suggests granulomatous infection.
- CT scan to identify sequestration
- MRI: T_2-weighted signals increase in affected soft tissue and bone (4,8)[A].

iagnostic Procedures/Surgery

novial biopsy or synovectomy is often needed to agnose specific pathogen.

athological Findings

novial biopsy may reveal granulomata and possibly e causative organism on microscopy or culture.

IFFERENTIAL DIAGNOSIS

Gout
Pseudogout (calcium pyrophosphate deposition disease)
Spondyloarthropathy (Reiter syndrome, psoriatic arthritis, ankylosing spondylitis, arthritis of inflammatory bowel disease)
Juvenile RA
Foreign-body synovitis (e.g., plant thorn synovitis)
RA
Pigmented villonodular synovitis (PVNS)
Palindromic rheumatism
Neuropathic arthropathy
Lyme arthritis
Sarcoidosis
Pyogenic arthritis

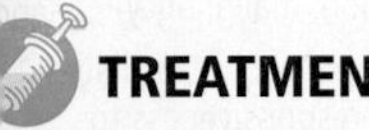

TREATMENT

IEDICATION

rst Line

Medications based on sensitivity of organisms

Mycobacterial infection (4,5,7,9)[A]:
- Use 4-drug combination initially: isoniazid, rifampin, pyrazinamide, and ethambutol.
- Continue therapy for 9–24 months.

Brucella: Tetracycline plus streptomycin (or gentamicin or trimethoprim-sulfamethoxazole or rifampin)

Fungal infection (5):
- Choice of medication depends on organism.
- Amphotericin B preparations
- Azoles

Contraindications: Tetracycline not for use in pregnancy or children <8 years

Precautions:
- Observe for allergic reactions/serum sickness.
- Tetracycline may cause photosensitivity; sunscreen is recommended.

Significant possible interactions:
- Tetracycline: Avoid concurrent administration with antacids, dairy products, or iron
- Azoles: Multiple drug interactions

econd Line

ıngal:

Azoles: Fluconazole, itraconazole

DDITIONAL TREATMENT

eneral Measures

Appropriate care:
- Fungal: Initial hospitalization for parenteral therapy
- Mycobacterial: Outpatient, once diagnosed
- *Brucella:* Outpatient, once diagnosed

- Repeat arthrocentesis if fluid reaccumulates.
- Infection associated with prosthetic joints may be difficult to eradicate without removal.
- For *Brucella* or fungal infections, continue treatment for 1–2 weeks after total resolution of all signs of inflammation and 6–8 weeks if joint was diseased previously (e.g., arthritis).
- Antimicrobic therapy requires a long program (i.e., in TB, fungal infection, brucellosis).
- Intraarticular antibiotics are not indicated.
- Infectious disease and rheumatology consultation helpful

SURGERY/OTHER PROCEDURES

- Arthrotomy is indicated only if fluid accumulated is loculated and/or not amenable to needle drainage.
- Prosthetic joints will require removal of hardware.
- Root joints, such as shoulder and hips, will require surgical intervention.

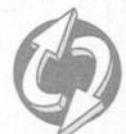

ONGOING CARE

FOLLOW-UP RECOMMENDATIONS

Patient Monitoring

- Verify sterilization of joint and reversion of inflammatory signs to normal.
- Treatment of mycobacterial arthritis requires monthly complete blood count, assessment of liver and kidney toxicity, and urinalysis.
- Essential to follow up frequently after stopping antibiotics to detect relapse.

PATIENT EDUCATION

Arthritis Foundation, 1314 Spring Street, NW Atlanta, GA 30309, (404) 872-7100.

PROGNOSIS

- Early initiation of treatment should allow cure.
- Delayed recognition/treatment is complicated by increased morbidity and mortality.

COMPLICATIONS

- Limited joint range of motion
- Flail or fused joint
- Carpal tunnel syndrome
- Septic necrosis
- Sinus formation
- Ankylosis
- Osteomyelitis
- Shortening of limb (in children)

REFERENCES

1. Kohli R, Hadley S. Fungal arthritis and osteomyelitis. *Infectious Dis Clin N Am.* 2005;19:831–51.
2. Kroot EJ, Hazes JM, Colin EM et al. Poncet's disease: reactive arthritis accompanying tuberculosis. Two case reports and a review of the literature. *Rheumatology (Oxford).* 2006.
3. Rothschild BM, Martin L. *Skeletal Impact of Disease Pathology.* Albuquerque, NM: New Mexico Museum of Natural History, 2006.
4. Fukushima M, Kakinuma K, Hayashi H et al. Detection and identification of Mycobacterium species isolates by DNA microarray. *J Clin Microbiol.* 2003;41:2605–15.
5. Hus C-Y, Shih TT-F. Tuberculous infection of the wrists: MRI features. *Am J Roentgenol.* 2004;183: 623–8.
6. Costa RO, de Mesquita KC, Damasco PS, Bernardes-Engemann AR, Dias CM, Silva IC, Lopes-Bezerra LM et al. Infectious arthritis as the single manifestation of sporotrichosis: serology from serum and synovial fluid samples as an aid to diagnosis. *Rev Iberoam Micol.* 2008;25:54–6.
7. Papagelopoulos PJ, Papadopoulos ECh, Mavrogenis AF et al. Tuberculous sacroiliitis. A case report and review of the literature. *Eur Spine J.* 2005;14: 683–8.
8. Leigh Moore S, Rafii M. Advanced imaging of tuberculosis arthritis. *Semin Musculoskelet Radiol.* 2003;7:143–53.
9. Yilmaz E, Parlak M, Akalin H et al. Brucellar spondylitis: review of 25 cases. *J Clin Rheumatol.* 2004;10:300–7.

ADDITIONAL READING

Sawlani V, Chandra T, Mishra RN et al. MRI features of tuberculosis of peripheral joints. *Clin Radiol.* 2003;58:755–62.

CODES

ICD9

- 711.00 Pyogenic arthritis, site unspecified
- 711.40 Arthropathy, site unspecified, associated with other bacterial diseases
- 711.50 Arthropathy, site unspecified, associated with other viral diseases

CLINICAL PEARLS

- Fungal infection of joint may present with synovial thickening and tenderness, but intense erythema and pain may not be present.
- Brucellosis can present initially as an FUO picture.
- TB can involve the spine, resulting in deformity.
- Synovial biopsy or synovectomy is often needed to diagnose specific pathogen.

ARTHRITIS, JUVENILE IDIOPATHIC

Caitlin Hurley, MD
Timothy Gibson, MD

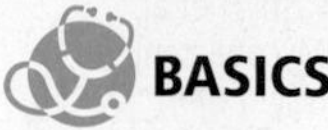

BASICS

DESCRIPTION

- Most common chronic rheumatic illness in children and a significant cause of short- and long-term disability
- General characteristics:
  - Age of onset <16 years
  - Signs of arthritis: Joint swelling, limitation of motion, pain, heat, or tenderness
  - >6 weeks of symptoms
- 7 subtypes exist, according to the International League of Associations for Rheumatology, determined by clinical characteristics seen in 1st 6 months of illness:
  - Systemic: Occurs in 10–20% of affected children; usually characterized by febrile onset and evanescent rash with multiple physical and laboratory abnormalities
  - Polyarticular RF (+): Occurs in 5–10% of affected children; multiple (≥5) joint involvement; large and small joints affected. RF positive 2x on tests at least 3 months apart
  - Polyarticular RhF (–) : Occurs in 30% of affected children; ≥5 joint involvement, large and small joints affected; RF negative
  - Oligoarticular: Occurs in 40–50% of affected children; involvement of ≤4 joints, usually larger joints, especially of lower extremities; risk for chronic uveitis in young girls and axial skeletal involvement in older boys
  - Psoriatic arthritis: Occurs in 2–15% of affected children. Arthritis with psoriasis or arthritis with at least 2 of following: dactylitis, nail pitting or onycholysis, psoriasis in 1st-degree relative.
  - Enthesitis arthritis: Occurs in 1–7% of affected children. Includes ankylosing spondylitis and inflammatory bowel disease–related arthritis. Peripheral and axial involvement.
  - Undifferentiated arthritis: Arthritis that does not fulfill above categories or fills 2 or more categories
- System(s) affected: Hematologic/Lymphatic/Immunologic; Musculoskeletal
- Synonym(s): Juvenile chronic arthritis; Juvenile arthritis; Juvenile rheumatoid arthritis (JRA); Still disease

EPIDEMIOLOGY

- Predominant age: 1–4 years and 9–14 years old
- Predominant sex:
  - Poly/oligoarticular: Female > Male
  - Systemic: Female = Male
  - Enthesitis: Male > Female

Incidence

1–22 per 100,000 children <16 years per year

Prevalence

8–150 per 100,000 children <16 years

Pediatric Considerations

Behavioral and compliance problems frequent in toddlers and teenagers

Pregnancy Considerations

Unpredictable effect on disease activity

RISK FACTORS

- Rheumatoid factor (RF) positivity increases risk for severe arthritis in polyarticular juvenile idiopathic arthritis (JIA).
- Antinuclear antibody (ANA) positivity increases risk for uveitis in oligo-JIA and poly-JIA.

Genetics

- Certain HLA class I and II alleles
- HLA-A2 in early-onset oligoarthritis in girls
- HLA-DRB1*11 confers increased risk of systemic and oligo-JIA.
- HLA-B27 risk of enthesitis-related arthritis
- HLA-DR4 associated with RF (+) polyarticular disease

GENERAL PREVENTION

No known preventive measures

ETIOLOGY

Multifactorial, including:

- Immunodysregulation
- Genetic predisposition
- Environmental triggers, possibly infectious:
  - Rubella or parvovirus B19 (1)
  - Heat shock proteins (1)
- Immunoglobulin or complement deficiency

COMMONLY ASSOCIATED CONDITIONS

- Other autoimmune disorders
- Chronic anterior uveitis (iridocyclitis)
- Nutritional impairment
- Growth disturbances (1)

DIAGNOSIS

Clinical diagnostic criteria: Age of onset <16 years and >6 weeks duration of objective arthritis in ≥1 joints, defined as swelling or limitation of motion of a joint accompanied by heat, pain, or tenderness

HISTORY

- Arthralgias, fever, fatigue, malaise, myalgias, weight loss, morning stiffness, rash, limp in patients with lower extremity involvement
- Arthritis for at least 6 weeks

PHYSICAL EXAM

- Arthritis: Swelling, effusion, limitation of motion, tenderness, pain on motion, warmth
- Rash, rheumatoid nodules, lymphadenopathy, hepato- or splenomegaly, enthesitis, dactylitis

DIAGNOSTIC TESTS & INTERPRETATION

Lab

Initial lab tests

- Complete blood count (CBC):
  - Leukocyte count normal or markedly elevated (systemic), lymphopenia
  - Reactive thrombocytosis
  - Anemia
- Joint-fluid aspiration and analysis helpful in excluding infection
- Inflammatory markers: Erythrocyte sedimentation rate and C-reactive protein may be elevated
- ANA positive (>1:80): 40% (polyarticular or oligoarticular): Increased risk of uveitis
- RF positive: 2–10% (usually polyarticular): Poor prognosis
- HLA-B27 positive: Enthesitis-related arthritis

Follow-Up & Special Considerations

- In polyarticular RF-positive variant, positivity shou be confirmed at least twice, 3 months apart (2).
- RF and ANA may be present in mixed connective tissue disease.

Imaging

Diagnostic radiography, magnetic resonance (MR) imaging, ultrasonography, and computed tomograp all play an important role in diagnosing or monitori juvenile idiopathic arthritis (JIA); no one modality ha evidence for superior diagnostic value (3)[A].

Initial approach

- Radiograph of affected joint(s)
- Early radiographic changes: Soft tissue swelling, periosteal reaction, juxta-articular demineralizatio
- Later changes include joint-space loss, articular surface erosions, subchondral cyst formation, sclerosis, joint fusion
- Electrocardiogram (pericarditis)
- Radionuclide scans (infection, malignancy)
- MRI can assess synovial hypertrophy, cartilage degeneration, and clinical responsiveness to treatment in peripheral joints in JIA (4)[B].

Follow-Up & Special Considerations

In interpreting results of dual energy x-ray photon absorptiometry scans, it is important to use pediatric not adult, controls as normative data.

Diagnostic Procedures/Surgery

- Synovial biopsy occasionally indicated
- Arthrocentesis

Pathological Findings

Synovium shows hyperplasia of synovial cells, hyperemia, and infiltration of small lymphocytes and mononuclear cells.

DIFFERENTIAL DIAGNOSIS

- Other rheumatic diseases:
  - Systemic lupus erythematosus, dermatomyositis, mixed connective tissue disease, sarcoidosis
- Musculoskeletal:
  - Legg-Calve-Perthes, toxic synovitis, growing pai
- Infectious:
  - Septic arthritis, osteomyelitis, Lyme disease
- Reactive arthritis:
  - Postinfectious, rheumatic fever, Reiter's syndrom
- Inflammatory bowel disease:
  - Crohn's disease and ulcerative colitis
- Hemoglobinopathies
- Malignancy:
  - Leukemia, bone tumors, neuroblastoma
- Vasculitis
- Kawasaki disease

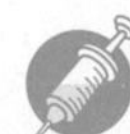

TREATMENT

MEDICATION

First Line

- Nonsteroidal anti-inflammatory drugs (NSAIDs) ar adequate in ~50% of patients, symptoms often improve within days, full efficacy 2–3 months
- Drugs for children include:
  - Ibuprofen (Motrin, Advil, Nuprin): 30–40 mg/kg divided q.i.d., max 800 mg t.i.d.
  - Naproxen (Naprosyn, Aleve): 10–20 mg/kg/d divided b.i.d., max dose of 500 mg b.i.d.

– Tolmetin sodium: 15–30 mg/kg/d; t.i.d. or q.i.d., max dose 600 mg t.i.d.
– Diclofenac 2–3 mg/kg, divided t.i.d., max of 50 mg t.i.d.
– Indomethacin 3 mg/kg/d, max of 200 mg/d

Contraindications to NSAIDs: Known allergies

Precautions: May worsen bleeding diatheses; use caution with all NSAIDs in renal insufficiency and hypovolemic states

Significant possible interactions: NSAIDs may lower serum levels of digitalis and anticonvulsants and blunt the effect of loop diuretics. NSAIDs may increase serum methotrexate levels.

Intra-articular long-acting corticosteroids especially for oligo-JIA. Immediately effective, local treatment. Improve synovitis, joint damage, contractures, and prevent leg length discrepancy (2)[B]:
– Triamcinolone hexacetonide

Glucocorticoids: Only in patients with extreme pain and functional limitation, while waiting for a 2nd-line agent to show some effect

Second Line

30–40% of patients will require addition of disease-modifying antirheumatic drugs (DMARDs), including methotrexate, sulfasalazine, leflunomide, and tumor necrosis factor antagonists (etanercept, infliximab, adalimumab). Newer biologic therapies including IL-1 and IL-6 receptor antagonists currently under investigation.

Methotrexate: Standard dose 8–12.5 mg/m^2/wk p.o. or SC. 10 mg/m^2/wk is most frequently used (2)[B]:
– Plateau of efficacy reached with 15 mg/m^2/wk; further increase in dosage is not associated with therapeutic benefit (5)

- Sulfasalazine: Oligoarticular and HLA B27 spondyloarthritis

Leflunomide: Not Food and Drug Administration approved for JIA

- Etanercept (Enbrel) 0.4 mg/kg, max of 25 mg, given SC twice weekly (2)[B]
- Infliximab 3–6 mg/kg q6–8 weeks
- Adalimumab 40 mg SC every 2 weeks (6)[B]
- Tocilizumab IL-6 antibody demonstrating efficacy in phase III open label trials, ongoing studies to evaluate efficacy and appropriate dosing regimen (2)
- Anakinra IL-1 receptor antibody under investigation with phase II and III clinical trials for systemic JIA (2)
- Alternative drugs:
  – Other NSAIDs and salicylates: Avoid salicylate therapy during serious viral illness, especially influenza or varicella, secondary to risk of Reye syndrome
- Analgesics for pain control, including narcotics

ADDITIONAL TREATMENT

General Measures

- Treatment goal: Control active disease and extra-articular manifestations to maintain musculoskeletal function as normal as possible.
- Outpatient care except for initial diagnostic workup of systemic JIA disease and complications for all subtypes
- All patients require regular (every 3–4 months for oligo-JIA and in ANA-positive patients) ophthalmic exams to uncover asymptomatic eye disease, at least for 1st 3 years.
- Moist heat, sleeping bag, or electric blanket to relieve morning stiffness
- Splints for contractures

Issues for Referral

- In general, a pediatric rheumatologist is best suited to manage juvenile idiopathic arthritis.
- Orthopedic surgeon: Need for surgery (joint replacement)
- Ophthalmologist: Uveitis
- Physical therapist for joint protection, to maintain range of motion, improve muscle strength, prevent deformities
- Occupational therapist to maintain and improve the normal life function
- Psychologists for coping

Additional Therapies

Physical therapy including daily home exercise program and orthotics for support

SURGERY/OTHER PROCEDURES

- Total hip and/or knee replacement may be needed for severe disease.
- Soft tissue release, if splinting, traction unsuccessful
- Limb length or angular deformity corrections
- Synovectomy is rarely performed.

IN-PATIENT CONSIDERATIONS

Admission Criteria

- Patient loses ambulatory ability
- Signs/symptoms of pericarditis
- Persistent fever

Discharge Criteria

Resolution of fever and swelling or serositis

ONGOING CARE

FOLLOW-UP RECOMMENDATIONS

Patient Monitoring

Determined by medication:

- NSAIDs: Periodic complete blood count (CBC), urinalysis, liver function tests (LFTs), renal function tests
- Aspirin and/or other salicylates: Transaminase and salicylate levels, weekly for 1st month, then every 3–4 months
- Methotrexate: Monthly LFTs, CBC, blood urea nitrogen, creatinine

DIET

Regular diet with special attention to adequate calcium, iron, protein, and caloric intake

PATIENT EDUCATION

- Ongoing education of patients and families with attention to:
  – Psychosocial needs
  – School issues, educational needs
  – Behavioral strategies for dealing with pain and noncompliance
  – Use of health care resources
- Printed and audiovisual information available from local arthritis foundation

PROGNOSIS

- 50–60% ultimately remit, but functional ability depends on adequacy of long-term therapy (disease control, maintaining muscle and joint function).
- Poorest prognosis in patients with RF + poly-JIA or patients with systemic JIA

COMPLICATIONS

- Blindness, band keratopathy, glaucoma
- Short stature
- Micrognathia if temporomandibular joint involvement
- Debilitating joint disease
- Disseminated intravascular coagulation; hemolytic anemia
- Patient on NSAIDs: Peptic ulcer, GI hemorrhage, central nervous system reactions, renal disease, leukopenia
- Patient on DMARD: Bone marrow suppression, hepatitis, renal disease, dermatitis, mouth ulcers, retinal toxicity (antimalarials, rare)
- Patients on tumor necrosis factor antagonists: Higher risk of infection
- Osteoporosis
- Macrophage activation syndrome:
  – Decreased blood cell precursors secondary to histiocyte degradation of marrow

REFERENCES

1. Weiss JE, Ilowite NT. Juvenile Idiopathic Arthritis. *Rheum Dis Clin N Am*. 2007;33:441–70.
2. Kahn P et al. Juvenile idiopathic arthritis–current and future therapies. *Bulletin of the NYU hospital for joint diseases*. 2009;67:291–302.
3. McKay GM, Cox LA, Long BW et al. Imaging juvenile idiopathic arthritis: assessing the modalities. *Radiol Technol*. 2010;81:318–27.
4. Miller E, Uleryk E, Doria AS. Evidence-based outcomes of studies addressing diagnostic accuracy of MRI of juvenile idiopathic arthritis. *AJR Am J Roentgenol*. 2009;192:1209–18.
5. Takken T, van der Net J, Helders P. Methotrexate for treating juvenile idiopathic arthritis. *The Cochrane Database of Systematic Reveiws*. 2009, Issue 1.
6. Lovell DJ, et al. Adalimumab with or without Methotrexate in Juvenile Rheumatoid Arthritis. *New Engl J Med*. 2008;359(8):810–20.

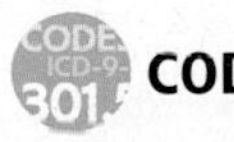

CODES

ICD9

- 714.30 Chronic or unspecified polyarticular juvenile rheumatoid arthritis
- 714.31 Acute polyarticular juvenile rheumatoid arthritis
- 714.32 Pauciarticular juvenile rheumatoid arthritis

CLINICAL PEARLS

- Consult pediatric rheumatologist
- High-titer RF correlates with severity
- ANA confers risk of uveitis
- No specific biomarker or test
- Diagnosis is one of exclusion

ARTHRITIS, OSTEO

Sergio A. Leon, MD
Jill A. Grimes, MD

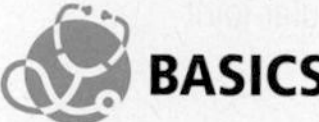

BASICS

DESCRIPTION

- Most common form of joint disease
- Involves progressive loss of articular cartilage and reactive changes at joint margins and in subchondral bone
- Primary:
  - Idiopathic: Divided into subsets depending on clinical features (i.e., localized, generalized, erosive)
- Secondary:
  - Posttraumatic
  - Childhood anatomic abnormalities (e.g., congenital hip dysplasia)
  - Inheritable metabolic disorders (e.g., Wilson disease, alkaptonuria, hemochromatosis)
  - Neuropathic arthropathy (Charcot joints)
  - Hemophilic arthropathy
  - Endocrinopathies: Acromegalic arthropathy, hyperparathyroidism, hypothyroidism
  - Paget disease
  - Noninfectious inflammatory arthritis (e.g., rheumatoid arthritis [RA], spondyloarthropathies)
  - Gout, calcium pyrophosphate deposition disease (pseudogout)
  - Septic or tuberculous arthritis
- System(s) affected: Musculoskeletal
- Synonym(s): Osteoarthrosis; Degenerative joint disease

EPIDEMIOLOGY

Predominant age:

- Symptomatic disease: >40 years old
- Leading cause of disability in those >65 years old
- Radiographic evidence (estimates): 33% to almost 90% in those >65 years old
- Predominant sex: Male = Female

Prevalence

- ~60 million patients
- Increases with age, almost universal >65 (by x-ray study but not clinically)

RISK FACTORS

- Increasing age: >50 years old
- Obesity (weight-bearing joints)
- Prolonged occupational or sports stress
- Injury to a joint from trauma, infection, or preexisting inflammatory arthritis
- Female gender (i.e., knee and hand osteoarthritis [OA])

Genetics

- OA has strong genetic factors, although they may be site- and gender-specific (i.e., hand OA in women).
- Up to 65% of OA may occur on a genetic basis.
- The genetic contribution may involve a combination of effects on structure (collagen), cartilage, or bone metabolism or inflammation.
- Failure of chondrocytes to maintain the balance between degradation and synthesis of extracellular matrix

ETIOLOGY

Biomechanical, biochemical, inflammatory, and immunologic factors all implicated in pathogenesis

DIAGNOSIS

HISTORY

- Slowly developing joint pain
- Pain that follows use of a joint
- Stiffness of <15 minutes duration (especially morning and after sitting)

PHYSICAL EXAM

- Joint bony enlargement (e.g., Heberden nodules of distal interphalangeal joints)
- Decreased range of motion with pain at the end of the range
- Tenderness usually absent; may occur along joint margin associated with synovitis
- Crepitation as late sign
- Weakness and wasting of the muscles acting on the joint
- Local pain and stiffness with OA of spine, with radicular pain (if compression of nerve roots present)

DIAGNOSTIC TESTS & INTERPRETATION

Lab

Initial lab tests

Usually not helpful in diagnosis (sedimentation rate not increased)

Follow-Up & Special Considerations

- May be useful in monitoring treatment with NSAIDs (renal insufficiency and GI bleeding)
- In secondary OA, underlying disorder may have abnormal lab results, e.g., hemochromatosis (abnormal iron studies).

Imaging

Initial approach

- X-ray films usually normal early
- Later often show:
  - Narrowed, asymmetric joint space
  - Osteophyte formation
  - Subchondral bony sclerosis
  - Cyst formation
- Erosions may occur on surface of distal and proximal interphalangeal joints when OA is associated with inflammation (erosive OA).

Diagnostic Procedures/Surgery

- Joint aspiration:
  - May be helpful in distinguishing from chronic inflammatory arthritis
  - OA: Cell count usually <500 cells/mm^3, predominantly mononuclear
  - Inflammatory: Cell count usually >2,000 cells/mm^3, predominantly neutrophils
- Calcium pyrophosphate dihydrate and/or apatite crystals may be seen in effusions.

Pathological Findings

- Characterized macroscopically by patchy cartilage damage and bony hypertrophy
- Histological phases:
  - Edema of the extracellular matrix and cartilage microcracks
  - Fissuring and pitting of the subchondral bone
  - Erosion and osteocartilaginous loose bodies
- Subchondral bone trabecular microfractures and sclerosis with osteophyte formation
- Degradation response produced by release of proteolytic enzymes, collagenolytic enzymes, prostaglandins, and immune responses

DIFFERENTIAL DIAGNOSIS

- Distinguish from other types of arthritis by:
  - Absence of systemic findings
  - Minimal articular inflammation
  - Distribution of involved joints (e.g., distal and proximal interphalangeal joints, not wrist and metacarpophalangeal joints)
- In spine, distinguish from osteoporosis, metastatic disease, multiple myeloma, or other bone diseases

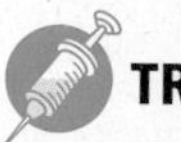

TREATMENT

MEDICATION

- Management of pain and inflammation:
  - Acetaminophen up to 1,000 mg q.i.d. Good evidence as most effective for pain relief in OA of knee or hip (1)[A].
  - A number of studies, mainly of knee osteoarthritis have shown short-term (<4 weeks) benefits from topical NSAID gels, creams, and ointments when compared to placebo. Topical NSAIDs should be core treatment for knee and hand OA.
  - If acetaminophen or topical NSAIDs are insufficient, then the addition or substitution by a oral NSAID/COX-2 inhibitor should be considered. They should be used at the lowest effective dose for the shortest possible period. Prolonged use is associated with renal insufficiency, hypertension (HTN), leg edema, and GI bleeding.
  - May use nonacetylated salicylates (e.g., salsalate choline-magnesium salicylate) or low-dose ibuprofen ≤1,600 mg/d.
  - Topical NSAIDs and capsaicin can be effective as adjunctives and alternatives to oral analgesic/ anti-inflammatory agents in knee OA (1)[A].
  - Other NSAIDs have similar efficacy.
- Contraindications:
  - All oral NSAIDs/COX-2 inhibitors have analgesic effects of a similar magnitude but vary in their potential GI and cardio-renal toxicity; therefore, the choice of agent and dose should take into account individual patient risk factors.
  - NSAIDs are contraindicated in patients with renal disease, CHF, HTN, active peptic ulcer disease, and previous hypersensitivity to an NSAID or aspirin (asthma, nasal polyps, hypotension, urticaria/ angioedema).
  - Combinations of NSAIDs are contraindicated due to risk of adverse reactions.
  - Avoid concomitant use of aspirin with NSAIDs.
  - In patients with increased cardiovascular risk, the combination of a nonselective NSAID, low-dose aspirin, and a proton-pump inhibitor (PPI) is preferred treatment.
  - Oral or parenteral corticosteroids are contraindicated.

recautions:
- If oral NSAID/COX-2 inhibitor is necessary for a patient aged >65 or a patient <65 with any increased GI risk factors, offer a PPI.
- Significant possible interactions:
  - NSAIDs reduce effectiveness of ACE inhibitors and diuretics.
  - Aspirin and NSAIDs (except COX-2 inhibitors) may increase effects of anticoagulants.
  - Increased hypoglycemic effects of oral hypoglycemics with aspirin
  - Salicylates reduce effectiveness of spironolactone (Aldactone) and uricosurics.
  - Corticosteroids and some antacids increase salicylate excretion, whereas ascorbic acid and ammonium chloride reduce salicylate excretion and may cause toxicity.

egnancy Considerations

ASA and NSAIDs: Some risk to fetus during 1st and 3rd trimesters of pregnancy
Compatible with breastfeeding

cond Line

A number of studies, mainly of knee OA, have shown short-term (<4 weeks) benefits from topical NSAID gels, creams, and ointments when compared to placebo. Topical NSAIDs should be a core treatment for knee and hand OA (2)[B].

Topical capsaicin should be considered as an adjunct therapy for knee and hand OA; may cause local burning.

Rubefacients are not recommended.

Opioid analgesics (e.g., codeine, oxycodone, propoxyphene): Evidence supporting their use in OA is extremely poor and should be restricted for treatment of acute episodes of pain.

Judiciously use intra-articular injections of corticosteroids for selected acute flare-ups of joints (no more than 3/year up to a maximum of 12 injections per joint). If used excessively, can accelerate joint deterioration.

Intra-articular viscosupplementation with hyaluronic acid preparations into a painful knee may provide relief of pain and improve function at earlier stages, though not statistically significant over injections with saline (placebo) (3)[B]. Definitive evidence is lacking in other joints. However, there are few randomized head-to-head comparisons of different products.

DDITIONAL TREATMENT

eneral Measures

Reassure patient of absence of generalized systemic disease, but recognize potential disability.

Weight reduction if obese and fitness program, including physical therapy (1)[A]

Walking aids instruction and proper footwear (1)[A]

Heat (e.g., local, tub baths) or cold applications

Physical therapy to maintain or regain joint motion and muscle strength. Quadriceps-strengthening exercises can relieve knee pain and disability.

Protect joints from overuse (e.g., cane, crutches, walker).

Assessment for bracing, joint supports, or insoles in those with biomechanical joint pain or instability

dditional Therapies

ddress psychosocial factors: Self-efficacy, coping kills, prevent, treat anxiety and depression, and nprove social support

COMPLEMENTARY AND ALTERNATIVE MEDICINE

- Nutritional supplements such as glucosamine and chondroitin sulfate may symptomatically benefit some patients and have low toxicity, but studies lack standardized case definition and outcome assessments. *If no response is apparent within 6 months, treatment should be discontinued.*
- A 2010 meta-analysis shows glucosamine, chondroitin, and their combination do not reduce joint pain or have an impact on narrowing of joint space compared with placebo (4)[A].
- TENS units and acupuncture may be beneficial (1)[A].

SURGERY/OTHER PROCEDURES

May be indicated in advanced disease (e.g., osteotomy, debridement, removal of loose bodies, joint replacement, fusion)

ONGOING CARE

FOLLOW-UP RECOMMENDATIONS

As active as tolerated

Patient Monitoring

- Follow range of motion and functional status at regular intervals.
- Watch for GI blood loss and follow cardiac, renal, and mental status in older patients on NSAIDs or aspirin.
- Periodic complete blood count, renal function tests, stool for occult blood

PATIENT EDUCATION

- American College of Rheumatology patient education overviews: http://www.rheumatology.org/public/factsheets/index.asp?aud=pat
- American Academy of Family Physicians Foundation: http://www.familydoctor.org.
- Arthritis Foundation: http://www.arthritis.org

PROGNOSIS

- Disease tends to be progressive
- Early in course, pain relieved by rest; later, pain may occur at rest and at night.
- Joint effusions may occur, especially in knees.
- Joint enlargement occurs later in course due to bony enlargement.
- Osteophyte (spur) formation, especially at joint margins, as disease progresses
- Advanced stage with full-thickness loss of cartilage down to bone

COMPLICATIONS

- One of the leading causes of pain and disability
- Decompensated CHF, GI bleeding, decreased renal function on NSAIDs or aspirin
- Hypoglycemic reactions (rare) in diabetic patients taking oral hypoglycemic agents:
  – Infection or accelerated cartilage loss with intra-articular corticosteroids

REFERENCES

1. Zhang W, Moskowitz RW, Nuki G, Abramson S, Altman RD, Arden N, Bierma-Zeinstra S, Brandt KD, Croft P, Doherty M, Dougados M, Hochberg M, Hunter DJ, Kwoh K, Lohmander LS, Tugwell P et al. OARSI recommendations for the management of hip and knee osteoarthritis, Part II: OARSI evidence-based, expert consensus guidelines. *Osteoarthr Cartil*. 2008;16:137–62.
2. Altman R, Barkin RL. Topical therapy for osteoarthritis: clinical and pharmacologic perspectives. *Postgrad Med*. 2009;121:139–47.
3. Kul-Panza E, Berker N et al. Is hyaluronate sodium effective in the management of knee osteoarthritis? A placebo-controlled double-blind study. *Minerva Med*. 2010;101:63–72
4. Wandel S, Jüni P, Tendal B, Nüesch E, Villiger PM, Welton NJ, Reichenbach S, Trelle S et al. Effects of glucosamine, chondroitin, or placebo in patients with osteoarthritis of hip or knee: network meta-analysis. *BMJ (Clinical research ed.)*. 2010;341:c4675.

ADDITIONAL READING

- Harvey WF, Hunter DJ et al. Pharmacologic intervention for osteoarthritis in older adults. *Clin Geriatr Med*. 2010;26:503–15.
- Hunter DJ, Lo GH. The management of osteoarthritis: an overview and call to appropriate conservative treatment. *Med Clin North Am*. 2009;93:127–43.
- Lane NE. Clinical practice. Osteoarthritis of the hip. *N Engl J Med*. 2007;357:1413–21.
- National Institute for Health and Clinical Excellence. *Osteoarthritis: national clinical guideline for care and management in adults*. London: NICE, 2008. http://www.nice.org.uk/CG059.
- Walsh NE, Hurley MV. Evidence based guidelines and current practice for physiotherapy management of knee osteoarthritis. *Musculoskeletal Care*. 2008.

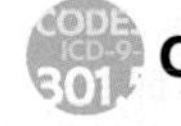

CODES

ICD9

- 715.10 Osteoarthrosis, localized, primary, involving unspecified site
- 715.20 Osteoarthrosis, localized, secondary, involving unspecified site
- 715.90 Osteoarthrosis, unspecified whether generalized or localized, involving unspecified site

CLINICAL PEARLS

- Morning stiffness lasts <15 minutes (vs an hour in rheumatoid arthritis)
- Distal predominance in hands
- Limit intra-articular steroid injections to 3 per year.

ARTHRITIS, PSORIATIC

Michael S. Krathen, MD
Amit Garg, MD

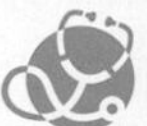

BASICS

Psoriatic arthritis (PsA) is a chronic destructive seronegative arthropathy seen most commonly in patients with long-standing psoriasis.

DESCRIPTION

- PsA is a seronegative spondyloarthropathy characterized by inflammatory arthritis and enthesitis.
- 5 patterns of arthritis in PsA include
  - Asymmetric oligoarthritis: Usually involves large joints
  - Distal interphalangeal (DIP) joint predominant: Often associated with nail psoriasis
  - Symmetric polyarthritis: May be indistinguishable from rheumatoid arthritis (RA)
  - Spondyloarthritis: Asymmetric and discontinuous, unlike ankylosing spondylitis (AS)
  - Arthritis mutilans: Destructive, resorptive arthritis; produces so-called opera-glass or telescoping digit
- Although psoriasis generally is present, it may be limited in extent.
  - Course of arthritis and extent of psoriasis do not appear to correlate.
  - Other extraarticular features, such as iritis, are less common.
  - Damaging joint disease may occur in 40–57%. Characteristic radiologic changes include joint erosions that begin marginally and move centrally ("pencil-in-cup deformity") and periostitis.
- Rheumatoid factor (RF) and cyclic citrullinated peptide (anti-CCP) antibody are usually negative. HLA-B27 may be positive.

EPIDEMIOLOGY

- Peak onset age: 35–40 years
- Predominant gender: Female = Male
- Polyarthritis is more common in women.
- Spondylitis in up to 25%, more common in males
- Psoriasis precedes arthritis in the majority by an average of 12 years. Arthritis may precede psoriasis in up to 15%, and this occurs more often in children. Arthritis and psoriasis also may present simultaneously.
- Psoriasis occurs in 2–3% of the US population; 6–42% of these individuals develop PsA (1).

Prevalence

Prevalence: 1–2/1,000 population (1)

RISK FACTORS

- Psoriasis
- Family history of PsA

Genetics

- 30–40% concordance in identical twins
- HLA-B27 in 15–50% with PsA (spondylitis pattern) vs 90% in AS
- Other HLA associations in psoriatic arthritis: HLA-B7, HLA-B38, HLA-B39, HLA-Cw6

GENERAL PREVENTION

There are no currently available prevention strategies. It is unknown if early systemic treatment of psoriasis prevents the onset of PsA.

PATHOPHYSIOLOGY

- CD4+/CD8+ T cells; tumor necrosis factor α (TNF-α); interleukins 1 (IL-1), 6, 8, and 10; and matrix metalloproteases present in synovial fluid (1)
- Osteoclast precursor cell upregulation

ETIOLOGY

Unknown. Probably multifactorial: Immunologic, genetic, environmental factors

COMMONLY ASSOCIATED CONDITIONS

Psoriasis

DIAGNOSIS

- Establishing a history of inflammatory arthritis, dactylitis, or enthesitis in a patient with existing psoriasis is usually adequate to establish the diagnosis. Nonetheless, differentiation from other inflammatory arthropathies such as RA can be difficult.
- The CASPAR criteria (2) comprise a validated instrument that may be used to screen patients for the presence of PsA. The sensitivity and specificity of the CASPAR criteria are 91.4% and 98.7%, respectively. To establish the presence of PsA, a patient must have inflammatory articular disease (joint, spine, or entheseal) with ≥3 points from the following five categories: (1) evidence of current psoriasis, a personal history of psoriasis, or family history of psoriasis (2 points), (2) typical psoriatic nail dystrophy, including onycholysis, pitting, and hyperkeratosis (1 point), (3) a negative rheumatoid factor, preferentially analyzed by enzyme-linked immunosorbent assay (1 point), (4) current dactylitis or a history of dactylitis (1 point), and (5) radiologic evidence of new bone formation (excluding osteophyte formation) on plain radiographs of the hand or foot (1 point).

HISTORY

- Long-standing (most often) psoriasis
- Morning stiffness of hands, feet, or low back for >45 minutes
- Discomfort or pain of involved joints
- Swelling or redness of peripheral joints
- Low back or buttock pain
- Ankle or heel pain
- Dactylitis, or uniform swelling of an entire digit

PHYSICAL EXAM

- Affected peripheral joints may have overlying erythema, warmth, and swelling.
  - Synovitis
  - Dactylitis
  - Swelling of tendons (e.g., Achilles tendon) and tenderness at insertion sites (e.g., calcaneus)
  - Limited range of motion of axial skeleton
  - Pain with stress on the sacroiliac joint
- Well-demarcated pink to red erythematous plaqu with a white silvery scale; common locations inc scalp, ears, trunk, buttocks, elbows and forearms knees and legs, and palms and soles.
- Nails may be dystrophic with pits, oil spots, crumbling, leukonychia, and red lunulae.

DIAGNOSTIC TESTS & INTERPRETATIO

History and physical examination may provide adequate data to establish the diagnosis of PsA. P radiographs may demonstrate characteristic change and aid in the diagnosis of PsA. Imaging allows assessment of current damage, disease progressior and response to therapy.

Lab

There is no specific blood test for PsA. Autoantiboc associated with RA or systemic lupus erythematosu for example, generally are not found.

Initial lab tests

- Serum RF is usually negative.
- Anti-CCP is usually negative.
- Antinuclear antibodies are usually negative.
- Acute-phase reactants (erythrocyte sedimentatior rate and C-reactive protein) may be elevated.
- HLA-B27 is noted in 50–70% with axial disease a <15% with peripheral disease.

Imaging

Juxtaarticular new bone formation (periostitis) and marginal joint erosions that may progress centrally form the "pencil-in-cup" erosions are the most characteristic plain radiographic features.

Initial approach

Baseline plain radiographs of affected joints

Follow-Up & Special Considerations

Follow-up radiographs; interval based on severity

Diagnostic Procedures/Surgery

Diagnosis is clinical.

Pathological Findings

Diagnosis is clinical, and biopsy of either skin or synovium is not usually required.

DIFFERENTIAL DIAGNOSIS

- Reactive arthritis
- Psoriasis and RA
- Psoriasis and osteoarthritis
- Psoriasis and polyarticular gout
- Psoriasis and AS

TREATMENT

ɜatment algorithms in PsA are based on severity of nt symptoms, extent of structural damage, and tent and severity of psoriasis (3)[A].

- is essential that the psychological burden of skin sease not be underestimated or discounted.
- onsteroidal anti-inflammatory drugs (NSAIDs) may considered for control of symptoms. Intraarticular ucocorticoid injections may be given judiciously to ntrol symptoms for persistent mono- or goarthritis.
- l patients with severe or moderate peripheral thritis should be started on disease-modifying tirheumatic drugs (DMARDs). DMARDs have the otential to reduce or prevent joint damage and eserve joint integrity and function.
- MARDs recommended as 1st-line therapy are lfasalazine, leflunomide, methotrexate, and closporine. No evidence supports the use of mbination DMARD therapy.
- tients who fail to respond to at least 1 standard MARD drug should be considered for anti-TNF-α erapy. Patients with poor prognosis could be nsidered for anti-TNF-α therapy even if they have ot failed a standard DMARD.

:DICATION

st Line

- IDs (4)[A]

cond Line

- ılfasalazine (4)[A]
- ethotrexate (4)[B]
- yclosporine (4)[B]
- zathioprine (4)[B]
- NF α inhibitors:
  - Adalimumab (4)[A]
  - Etanercept (4)[A]
  - Infliximab (4)[A]
- -12/23 inhibitor: Ustekinumab (5)[A]

LERT

ti TNF agents should not be used in the setting of tive infection, including patients with tuberculosis d hepatitis B infection, with concurrent live ccinations, with New York Heart Association YHA) class III–IV congestive heart failure, with alignancy, or with history of demyelinating sease.

egnancy Considerations

- void teratogenic medications (e.g., methotrexate, old, antimalarials, sulfasalazine, acitretin) during regnancy.
- dalimumab, etanercept, and infliximab are urrently listed as category B medications.

)DITIONAL TREATMENT

neral Measures

ysical therapy may be beneficial in all stages of ease.

ues for Referral

- heumatology
-)ermatology

SURGERY/OTHER PROCEDURES

Joint fusion or replacement for advanced destruction

ONGOING CARE

FOLLOW-UP RECOMMENDATIONS

Epidemiologic evidence suggests a relationship between psoriasis, the metabolic syndrome, myocardial infarction, and stroke. Periodic measurement of blood pressure, fasting lipids and glucose, cholesterol, and body mass index is recommended (6).

PATIENT EDUCATION

- Stress noncontagious nature of condition
- For a listing of sources for patient education materials favorably reviewed on this topic, physicians may contact:
  - American Academy of Family Physicians Foundation, P.O. Box 8418, Kansas City, MO 64114, (800) 274-2237, ext. 4400. Also see http://www.familydoctor.org.
  - National Psoriasis Foundation, 6600 SW 92nd Ave., Suite 300, Portland, OR 97223-7195. Also see http://www.psoriasis.org/about/psa.
  - Arthritis Foundation, 1314 Spring Street N.W., Atlanta, GA 30309, (404) 872-7100 or http://www.arthritis.org/conditions/diseasecenter/psoriatic_arthritis.asp.

PROGNOSIS

- Course: Insidious and chronic joint disease and recurring and remitting chronic skin disease
- More favorable than for RA (except for patients who develop arthritis mutilans)

COMPLICATIONS

- Chronicity
- Disability
- Psychosocial impact of psoriasis

REFERENCES

1. Gottlieb A, et al. Guidelines of care for management of psoriatic arthritis. *JAAD*. 2008;58:851–64.
2. Taylor W, Gladman D, Helliwell P, Marchesoni A, Mease P, Mielants H; CASPAR Study Group. Classification criteria for psoriatic arthritis: development of new criteria from a large international study. *Arthritis Rheum*. 2006;54(8):2665–73.
3. Menter A, et al. American Academy of Dermatology. Links Guidelines of care for the management of psoriasis and psoriatic arthritis. Section 3. Guidelines of care for the management and treatment of psoriasis with topical therapies. *J Am Acad Dermatol*. 2009;60(4):643–59.
4. Kavanaugh AF, Ritchlin CT, GRAPPA Treatment Guideline Committee. Systematic review of treatments for psoriatic arthritis: an evidence based approach and basis for treatment guidelines. *J Rheumatol*. 2006;33:1417–21.
5. Gottlieb A, Menter A, Mendelsohn A, Shen YK, Li S, Guzzo C, Fretzin S, Kunynetz R, Kavanaugh A et al. Ustekinumab, a human interleukin 12/23 monoclonal antibody, for psoriatic arthritis: randomised, double-blind, placebo-controlled, crossover trial. *Lancet*. 2009;373:633–40.
6. Gottlieb AB, Dann F et al. Comorbidities in patients with psoriasis. *Am J Med*. 2009;122:1150.e1–9.
7. Prey S, Paul C, Bronsard V, Puzenat E, Gourraud PA, Aractingi S, Aubin F, Bagot M, Cribier B, Joly P, Jullien D, Maitre ML, Richard-Lallemand MA, Ortonne JP et al. Assessment of risk of psoriatic arthritis in patients with plaque psoriasis: a systematic review of the literature. *J Eur Acad Dermatol Venereol*. 2010;24(Suppl 2):31–5.

ADDITIONAL READING

Ritchlin CT, Kavanaugh A, Gladman DD et al. Treatment recommendations for psoriatic arthritis. *Ann Rheum Dis*. 2008.

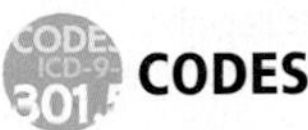

CODES

ICD9

696.0 Psoriatic arthropathy

CLINICAL PEARLS

- Severity of psoriasis may correlate with the likelihood of developing arthritis; however, severity of psoriasis does not correlate with severity of arthritis; 24% of psoriasis patients develop PsA (7)[A].
- Often overlooked locations of psoriasis include scalp, ears, umbilicus, and gluteal cleft.
- Other conditions may mimic or coexist with PsA: Osteoarthritis and polyarticular gout.
- The polyarticular pattern of PsA may mimic RA; however, the presence of enthesitis and recognition of psoriasis characterize PsA.
- Axial skeleton in PsA is asymmetric and discontinuous, in contrast to axial involvement in AS.

ARTHRITIS, RHEUMATOID (RA)

Sergio A. Leon, MD

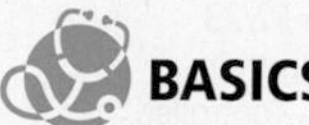

BASICS

DESCRIPTION

- RA is a chronic systemic inflammatory disease (typically joint-involving) of unknown cause.
- Articular inflammation may be remitting, but if continued, may result in joint damage and disability.
- Characteristic extra-articular manifestations include rheumatoid nodules, vasculitis, neuropathy, scleritis, pericarditis, and splenomegaly.
- System(s) affected: Musculoskeletal; Skin; Hematologic; Lymphatic; Immunologic; Muscular; Renal; Cardiovascular; Neurologic; Pulmonary

Geriatric Considerations

- Increased contribution/interaction of age-related comorbidities; pericarditis, septic arthritis, Sjögren syndrome are more common
- Less tolerance to drugs; increased incidence of hydroxychloroquine-associated maculopathy, D-penicillamine rash, and sulfasalazine-induced nausea/vomiting

Pregnancy Considerations

- Use effective contraception with disease-modifying antirheumatic drugs (DMARDs). Modify regimen with pregnancy or breast-feeding.
- Labor/delivery pose no serious problems, unless severe mechanical joint disease.
- >75% improve during pregnancy, but relapse in 6 months. 1st episodes may occur in pregnancy.

EPIDEMIOLOGY

Incidence

- Predominant age: 3rd–6th decades
- Predominant sex:
  - Female > Male (2–3:1; overall incidence and prevalence of articular manifestations)
  - Male > Female (systemic disease)

Prevalence

- US population: 0.5–1.5%
- Native Americans: >3.5–5.3%

RISK FACTORS

- HLA genes contribute to 30–50% genetic risk.
- Family history
- Native American ethnicity

Genetics

- 1st-degree relatives have 1.5-fold higher risk than the general population of developing RA.
- Twin studies show heritability of 60%.
- Seropositive RA aggregates in families.
- HLA-DR4+ person has increased relative risk of 4–5 x.

PATHOPHYSIOLOGY

Antibody-complement complex results in intra-articular inflammation

ETIOLOGY

- Genetic factors
- Host factors: Hormonal, immunologic, obesity
- Environmental: Socioeconomic, smoking

COMMONLY ASSOCIATED CONDITIONS

- Sjögren syndrome, Felty syndrome, Amyloidosis
- Increased incidence of infections, lymphomas, renal and cardiovascular disease

DIAGNOSIS

PHYSICAL EXAM

Evaluate specific joints and extra-articular involvement

DIAGNOSTIC TESTS & INTERPRETATION

Lab

Initial lab tests

- Hematocrit: Mild anemia (of chronic disease)
- ESR: Usually elevated
- C-reactive protein: Unspecific, direct measure of impact of IL-6 on liver cells
- Rheumatoid factor (RF): >1:80 in 70–80% of patients with RA (most commonly IgM Ab):
  - Poor screening tool
  - Disorders that may yield false-positive RF results: Sjögren syndrome, mixed cryoglobulinemia, parasitic infections (e.g., malaria), liver disease, endocarditis, acute viral infections.
- Anticyclic citrullinated peptide antibodies (Anti-CCP antibodies) are highly specific and present early. Linked to erosive RA.
- Antinuclear antibody: Present in 20–30%
- Electrolytes, creatinine, liver function, urinalysis to assess comorbid states

Follow-Up & Special Considerations

RF is not useful for monitoring course of illness

Imaging

Initial approach

- Radiographic abnormalities are very useful in the diagnosis and treatment.
- Periarticular osteopenia is the earliest change.
- More typical findings are juxta-articular bone erosions and symmetrical joint space narrowing.
- CT/MRI and ultrasound are useful in specific situations such as cervical-spine symptoms or detection of early joint erosions.
- Bone scan if suspected aseptic necrosis

Follow-Up & Special Considerations

Radiographs of the hands, wrists, and feet can be repeated to follow disease progression.

Diagnostic Procedures/Surgery

Synovial fluid:

- No pathognomonic findings
- Yellowish-white, turbid, poor viscosity
- WBC increased (3,500–50,000)
- Protein: ~4.2 g/dL (42 g/L)
- Serum-synovial glucose difference ≥30 mg/dL (≥1.67 mmol/L)

Pathological Findings

Synovial tissue is expanded by the recruitment and retention of inflammatory cells, with formation of villous projections and pannus that invades and destroys cartilage and bone.

DIFFERENTIAL DIAGNOSIS

- Other systemic connective tissue diseases: Sjögren syndrome, systemic lupus erythematosus, systemic sclerosis, adult Still disease, mixed
- Psoriatic arthritis
- Viral-induced arthritis: Parvovirus B19, hepatitis C (with cryoglobulinemia)
- Occult malignancy
- Vasculitis: Behçet syndrome
- Seronegative polyarthritis
- Erosive osteoarthritis
- Chronic infections: Lyme disease

TREATMENT

Goals: Controlling disease activity, relieving pain, maintaining or improving function, preventing or correcting impairments, and promoting self-management

MEDICATION

Disease-Modifying Anti-Rheumatic Drugs (DMARDs) are usually administered in combination following fo[r] general strategies: sequential monotherapy, step-up therapy, induction therapy or individualized targeted 'tight' control.

First Line

- Nonbiologic DMARDs:
  - Start DMARDs within 2 months of diagnosis if patient has ongoing active disease despite appropriate dose of aspirin or other NSAIDs.
  - Precautions: Offer proton pump inhibitors (PPIs) for chronic NSAID therapy; avoid NSAID combination.
  - Due to their greater convenience, lower toxicity profiles, and quicker onset of action, the initial therapy is a nonbiologic DMARD: Methotrexate, sulfasalazine, or leflunomide have shown evidence of comparable efficacy. Hydroxychloroquine is a less potent agent.
  - Combination DMARDs may be more effective tha[n] individual drugs.

– Bridging and/or low-dose corticosteroids, NSAIDs, and simple analgesics are often required to maximize symptoms management.
– Prednisone: 5–15 mg/d for severe disease or to minimize disease activity. Use only for short periods, or intermittently. Low-dose prednisolone is more effective than NSAIDs (1)[A].
– Methotrexate (MTX) (Rheumatrex): 7.5–25 mg per week PO. The DMARD with most predictable benefit. Many significant side effects, but the addition of folate reduces toxicity. 3–6-month trial. Monitor CBC, renal, and liver function every 8–12 weeks. Contraindicated in renal disease
– Sulfasalazine (SSZ): 500 mg/d, increase to 2 g/d over 1 month; max: 2–3 g/d; 6-month trial (2)[A]. Monitor CBC, liver enzymes every 8–12 weeks. Screen for G6PD deficiency.
– Leflunomide (Arava): Dose: 10–20 mg/d. Modifies T-cell function to decrease autoimmune activity, reduce structural damage. Response rate similar to SSZ and MTX. GI side effects and potentially teratogenic (3)[A]. Contraindicated in pregnancy.
– Antimalarials: Hydroxychloroquine (HCQ) (Plaquenil) 400 mg qhs for 2–3 months, then 200 mg at bedtime; 6-month trial usual (4)[A]. Usually to treat milder forms or in combination with other DMARDs. Yearly ophthalmologic exam. Adjust dose in renal insufficiency.

Biological DMARDs:
– Tumor necrosis factor (TNF) inhibitors: IV infliximab (Remicade), SC adalimumab (Humira), and SC etanercept (Enbrel). No evidence to suggest that one is superior to another. The combination with MTX appears to be the most effective regimen. Optimal dosage and duration of treatment unclear. Low toxicity. Costly. Check PPD prior to treatment and periodic CBC. Risk of lymphoma, CHF.
– Anakinra (Kineret), an IL-1 receptor antagonist. Injection site reaction, neutropenia, bacterial infections. Fewer clinical benefits than TNF inhibitors.
– Abatacept (Orencia) and rituximab (Rituxan) are approved for active moderate to severe RA with inadequate response to other DMARDs or failed anti-TNF agent.
– Two long-acting anti-TNF agents, Certolizumab pegol (Cimzia) and golimumab (Simponi), have been also approved in moderate-to-severe disease.

Other older nonbiologic DMARDs have been virtually abandoned in developed countries for the treatment of RA:
– Minocycline: In active mild/moderate disease.
– Auranofin (Ridaura): 6–10 mg/d PO. Slow onset of action. Poor GI tolerability.
– Injectable gold (Aurolate): Seldom used because of frequent toxicity
– D-Penicillamine: 250–1000 mg/d. Has dose-related side effects. Close monitoring.
– Protein A immunoadsorption (Prosorba): Removes antibodies. Costly.
– Cyclosporine: Inhibition of T-cell response. Incremental benefit combined with MTX.
– Azathioprine: Because of toxicity, reserved for persons not responsive to other DMARDs.

Second Line
- Intra-articular steroids: If disease is well controlled except for a single joint or two, after establishing that the joint is not infected
- Hyaluronate (Hyalgan): Hyaluronic acid substitute. For pain relief; exact role in RA unclear.

ADDITIONAL TREATMENT
Interdisciplinary care and management is necessary to minimize the consequences of loss of function, joint damage, maladaptive coping, and social isolation.

General Measures
- Complete remission of disease activity should be the ultimate goal
- Early, aggressive treatment is desirable to prevent structural damage and disability.
- Key elements include periodical evaluation of disease activity and extent of synovitis.
- Arthritis self-management education is a proven effective intervention in RA.

SURGERY/OTHER PROCEDURES
Surgical treatment, including synovectomy, tendon reconstruction, joint fusion, and joint replacement are powerful treatment modalities to prevent disability in advanced RA.

ONGOING CARE

The goals of comprehensive, interdisciplinary care are to stop the disease process, reduce pain, manage symptoms such as fatigue and stiffness, preserve joint integrity and function, and maintain social and occupational roles and quality of life.

FOLLOW-UP RECOMMENDATIONS
- Encourage full activity, but avoid heavy work or exercise during active phases.
- Emphasize exercise, mobility, and reduction of joint stress.
- Promote general health care and psychosocial functional status.

Patient Monitoring
- Address risk factors and evaluate for osteoporosis, a major comorbidity that can result from the disease itself or corticosteroids.
- Cardiovascular disease is the number one cause of death. Evaluate and manage CV risk factors, use low-dose aspirin as preventive.

DIET
No specific diet recommended

PATIENT EDUCATION
- American College of Rheumatology patient education overviews: www.rheumatology.org/public/factsheets/index.asp?aud=pat
- American Academy of Family Physicians Foundation: www.familydoctor.org.
- Arthritis Foundation: www.arthritis.org

PROGNOSIS
- Poor prognostic findings:
  – Persistent moderate-to-severe disease
  – Inheritance of shared epitope
  – Early or advanced age at disease onset
- 50% cannot function in primary job within 10 years of onset.

COMPLICATIONS
Extra-articular involvement: Pulmonary disease, vasculitis, pericarditis, nephropathy, nerve entrapment, muscle atrophy, eye disease, Felty syndrome, chronic anemia

REFERENCES

1. Gotzsche PC, Johansen HK. Short-term low-dose corticosteroids vs. placebo and NSAIDs in rheumatoid arthritis. *Cochrane Database Syst Rev.* 2006:1.
2. Suarez-Almazor ME, et al. Sulfasalazine for treating rheumatoid arthritis. *Cochrane Database Syst Rev.* 2006:1.
3. Osiri M, et al. Leflunomide for treating rheumatoid arthritis. *Cochrane Database Syst Rev.* 2006:1.
4. Suarez-Almazor ME, et al. Antimalarials for treating rheumatoid arthritis. *Cochrane Database Syst Rev.* 2006:1.

ADDITIONAL READING

- Aletaha D, Neogi T, Silman AJ et al. 2010 rheumatoid arthritis classification criteria: an American College of Rheumatology/European League Against Rheumatism collaborative initiative. *Ann Rheum Dis.* 2010;69:1580–8.
- Mertens M, Singh JA. Anakinra for Rheumatoid Arthritis: A Systematic Review. *J Rheumatol.* 2009.

CODES

ICD9
- 714.0 Rheumatoid arthritis
- 714.1 Felty's syndrome
- 714.2 Other rheumatoid arthritis with visceral or systemic involvement

CLINICAL PEARLS

- Females have more articular disease and males have more systemic presentations.
- Morning stiffness with symmetrical joint involvement of wrists, proximal interphalangeal and metacarpophalangeal joints.
- Start DMARDs early if patient still having symptoms despite adequate doses of NSAIDS or aspirin and use combination of DMARDs.

ASBESTOSIS

Ruben Peralta, MD

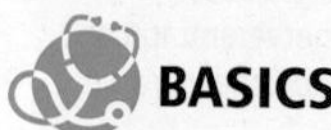

BASICS

DESCRIPTION

- Slowly progressive lung disease caused by inhalation of dust from fibrous silicate asbestos used in insulation, cement, and other building and construction materials
- Nodular interstitial fibrotic lung disease caused by cascade of inflammatory responses to inhaled asbestos fibers:
  - Pleural fibrosis, pleural plaques, and interstitial fibrosis develop.
  - Lung cancer risk is increased.
- Synonym(s): Asbestos pneumoconiosis

EPIDEMIOLOGY

- In the US, an estimated 1.3 million people who work in maintenance and construction are at risk for exposure (1).
- In a very large part of the world, data on mesothelioma are not available (2).
- Predominant age: Middle age (40–75 years)
- Predominant sex: Male > Female, owing to exposure pattern

RISK FACTORS

- Professional exposures most common in construction workers; those who mine, mill, or remove asbestos; ship builders; textile workers; railroad workers.
- Office workers, teachers, and students in buildings with asbestos in place have exposure significantly lower than those of construction workers.
- Dose-response phenomenon: Higher amounts of asbestos exposure are associated with higher risk of asbestosis (3,4,5).
- Cigarette smoking markedly increases risk of radiographic changes and eventual lung cancer risk:
  - Likely mechanism: Decreased clearance of asbestos fibers

Genetics

- Genetic polymorphisms have been implicated (6,7,8,9,10).
- Familial mesothelioma has been reported (11).

GENERAL PREVENTION

- In the US, asbestos is federally regulated by the Occupational Health and Safety Administration.
- Primary responsibility of employers is to provide safe work environment (3,12,13,14,15)
- Exposure control: Substitution of safer materials or adoption of control technologies
- During high-exposure periods, such as building repair, use fit-tested personal respirators for workers.
- To limit exposure to others in their household, those who work with asbestos should leave their clothing at work, if possible. Work clothes should be washed and stored separately from other clothing.

ETIOLOGY

- Asbestos fibers are inhaled. Macrophages engulf the fibers and release inflammatory mediators. Inflammatory mediators cause fibroblast proliferation, leading to fibrosis and remodeling of interstitial lung tissue, including intra-alveolar fibrosis and loss of alveolar capillary units (16).
- Disease continues to slowly progress over the course of years, even if exposure is not ongoing (14,17,18).
- Symptoms may be related to impaired gas exchange and/or a pattern of restrictive lung disease.

COMMONLY ASSOCIATED CONDITIONS

In addition to asbestosis, inhalation of asbestos is associated with several lung problems (11,18,19,20,21,22), including:

- Benign plaques
- Benign pleural effusions
- Lung cancer
- Malignant mesothelioma

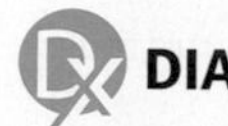

DIAGNOSIS

HISTORY

- Credible history of exposure (usually occupational) to asbestos fibers (3,4,5,17,23,24):
  - Ask about intensity and duration of exposure.
  - Aircraft or electrical maintenance
  - Shipyard workers
  - Those exposed to cement or building materials
  - Asbestos mining
  - People exposed to asbestos when it is disrupted during building maintenance
  - Family members of those who work with asbestos
- In addition to job type and activities and length of exposure, ask patients whether there was visible dust in air or on surfaces, visible dust in sputum, personal protective equipment used, and whether the workplace was cleaned during or after a shift (25).
- Common symptoms include:
  - Dyspnea upon exertion
  - Nonproductive cough (26,27,28)
- Delay from exposure to detection typically becomes clinically apparent 10–15 years after exposure.

PHYSICAL EXAM

- Insidious onset
- Progressive dyspnea is the most common symptom.
- Dry cough
- Progressive exercise intolerance
- Pleuritic chest pain
- Inspiratory crackles (may be best heard laterally)
- Wheeze with forced exhalation
- Digital clubbing and cyanosis in advanced disease
- Right-sided heart failure

DIAGNOSTIC TESTS & INTERPRETATION

Pulmonary function test:

- Not diagnostically specific
- Mainly restrictive pattern unless a smoker (29)
- Decreased total lung capacity and vital capacity
- Reduction in diffusing capacity to carbon monoxide (25)[B]
- Useful for following level of impairment

Lab

No pathognomonic lab findings

Imaging

- Chest x-ray (CXR) (sensitivity 90%, specificity 93%):
  - Most common findings are bilateral pleural thickening and circumscribed calcified pleural plaques
  - Pleural plaques usually posterior-lateral, may also involve diaphragm (30)
  - As disease progresses, small, irregular, linear opacities with a fine reticular pattern are seen
  - Less common: Rounded atelectasis (Blesovsky syndrome) when fibrosis of visceral pleura extends into parenchyma (31)
- Classification scheme available through International Labour Office (at http://www.ilo.org)
- High-resolution computed tomography (CT) may increase sensitivity to near 100%:
  - Improves detection of interstitial fibrosis
  - May show honeycombing in later stages of the disease
- Gallium scan with higher uptake even if the CXR and CT are normal

Pathological Findings

- Lung biopsy or bronchoalveolar lavage (BAL) can reveal asbestos fibers or asbestos bodies (25):
  - May help diagnostically in cases with history of minimal exposure or with atypical clinical or radiographic features
  - Transbronchial biopsy is less reliable than BAL or open-lung biopsy in establishing diagnosis.
- Pleural plaques are found in parietal pleura; made up of collagen bundles with rare inflammatory cells. Pleural thickening involves the visceral pleura (30).
- Asbestos bodies may be seen with iron staining in intra-alveolar macrophages.

DIFFERENTIAL DIAGNOSIS

Other pneumoconioses:

- Idiopathic pulmonary fibrosis
- Hypersensitivity pneumonitis
- Sarcoidosis
- Other pneumoconiosis, including mixed exposures

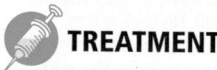

TREATMENT

MEDICATION

First Line

- No specific pharmacologic treatment
- Oxygen
- Bronchodilators for pulmonary toilet

Second Line

- Antibiotics for respiratory infections
- Diuretics if cor pulmonale develops

ADDITIONAL TREATMENT

General Measures

- As of now, there is no effective treatment to reverse the course of the disease.
- Clinical approach is directed at amelioration of symptoms, elimination of progression, and reduction of risk of associated disorders.
- Withdrawal from exposure (30)[B]:
  - Workers with no symptoms and only radiographic changes may make an informed choice to continue employment using maximum environmental and personal protection.
- Smoking cessation:
  - Cigarette smokers have more radiographic signs of disease and have a significantly increased risk for lung cancer.
- Pneumococcal and influenza vaccines (28)[B]
- Chest physiotherapy as needed
- Home oxygen as needed

Issues for Referral

All new cases must be reported to health authorities.

ONGOING CARE

•llow World Health Organization (WHO) commendations for regular health screening of :posed workers (32):

- CXR film at baseline
- For workers with <10 years since 1st exposure: CXR every 3–5 years
- >10 years: CXR every 1–2 years
- >20 years: CXR annually
- All workers: Annual respiratory symptom questionnaire, physical exam, and spirometry (alternatively can be done on CXR schedule)

OLLOW-UP RECOMMENDATIONS

atient Monitoring

- CXR
- Occasional pulmonary function tests
- Prompt treatment of infections

IET

igh-calorie, high-protein with advanced disease

ATIENT EDUCATION

- Smoking cessation counseling as needed
- In the US, asbestos has been federally regulated by the Occupational Health and Safety Administration since 1972: http://www.osha.gov.
- Printed patient information available from National Cancer Institute: http://www.cancer.gov/cancertopics/factsheet/Risk/asbestos
- Agency for Toxic Substances and Disease Registry: http://www.atsdr.cdc.gov

ROGNOSIS

- Severity depends on duration and intensity of exposure.
- Lung disease is irreversible.
- Increased risk for lung cancer (synergistic increase with cigarette smoking) and mesothelioma (25)[B]

COMPLICATIONS

- Mesothelioma:
  - Related to dose, time elapsed from exposure (usually 25–40 years after exposure)
  - Risk is higher with exposure to amphibole fibers rather than chrysotile fibers.
  - Pleural effusion in 80–95% (31)[B]
  - Insidious but progressive. Median survival for mesothelioma is 8–18 months (33)[B].
- Lung cancer risk is associated with asbestos exposure, whether asbestosis is present or not; synergistically increased risk in asbestos workers who smoke (13).
- Gastrointestinal cancer risk may also be increased with asbestos exposure.

REFERENCES

1. American Thoracic Society. Diagnosis and initial management of nonmalignant diseases related to asbestos. *Am J Respir Crit Care Med*. 2004;170: 691–715.
2. Bianchi C, Bianchi T. Malignant mesothelioma: global incidence and relationship with asbestos. *Ind Health*. 2007;45:379–87.
3. Lin RT, Takahashi K, Karjalainen A et al. Ecological association between asbestos-related diseases and historical asbestos consumption: an international analysis. *Lancet*. 2007;369:844–9.
4. Bhattacharya K, Dopp E, Kakkar P et al. Biomarkers in risk assessment of asbestos exposure. *Mutat Res*. 2005;579:6–21.
5. Chow S, Campbell C, Sandrini A et al. Exhaled breath condensate biomarkers in asbestos-related lung disorders. *Respir Med*. 2009.
6. Horská A, Kazimírová A, Barancoková M et al. Genetic predisposition and health effect of occupational exposure to asbestos. *Neuro Endocrinol Lett*. 2006;27(Suppl 2):100–3.
7. Franko A, Dolzan V, Arneri N et al. The Influence of Genetic Polymorphisms of GSTP1 on the Development of Asbestosis. *J Occup Environ Med*. 2008;50:7–12.
8. Helmig S, Belwe A, Schneider J. Association of Transforming Growth Factor beta1 Gene Polymorphisms and Asbestos-Induced Fibrosis and Tumors. *J Investig Med*. 2009.
9. Franko A, Dodic-Fikfak M, Arneri N et al. Manganese and extracellular superoxide dismutase polymorphisms and risk for asbestosis. *J Biomed Biotechnol*. 2009;2009:493083.
10. Neri M, Ugolini D, Dianzani I et al. Genetic susceptibility to malignant pleural mesothelioma and other asbestos-associated diseases. *Mutat Res*. 2008;659:126–36.
11. You B, Blandin S, Gérinière L et al. [Family mesotheliomas: genetic interaction with environmental carcinogenic exposure?] *Bull Cancer*. 2007;94:705–10.
12. Mueller TB. Tomorrow's causation standards for yesterday's wonder material: Reiter v. Acands, Inc. and Maryland's changing asbestos litigation. *J Contemp Health Law Policy*. 2009;25:437–61.
13. Dement J, Welch L, Haile E et al. Mortality among sheet metal workers participating in a medical screening program. *Am J Ind Med*. 2009.
14. Centers for Disease Control and Prevention (CDC). Asbestosis-related years of potential life lost before age 65 years—United States, 1968–2005. *MMWR Morb Mortal Wkly Rep*. 2008;57:1321–5.
15. Gehanno JF, Takahashi K, Darmoni S et al. Citation classics in occupational medicine journals. *Scand J Work Environ Health*. 2007;33:245–51.
16. Tercelj M, Salobir B, Simcic S et al. Chitotriosidase activity in sarcoidosis and some other pulmonary diseases. *Scand J Clin Lab Invest*. 2009;1–4.
17. Kurumatani N, Kumagai S. Mapping the risk of mesothelioma due to neighborhood asbestos exposure. *Am J Respir Crit Care Med*. 2008.
18. Mastrangelo G, Ballarin MN, Bellini E et al. Asbestos exposure and benign asbestos diseases in 772 formerly exposed workers: Dose-response relationships. *Am J Ind Med*. 2009.
19. Wagner GR. The fallout from asbestos. *Lancet*. 2007;369:973–4.
20. Wagner JC. The discovery of the association between blue asbestos and mesotheliomas and the aftermath. *Br J Ind Med*. 1991;48:399–403.
21. Wagner GR. Asbestosis and silicosis. *Lancet*. 1997;349:1311–5.
22. Toyokuni S. Mechanisms of asbestos-induced carcinogenesis. *Nagoya J Med Sci*. 2009;71:1–10.
23. Hansell A. Airborne environmental exposure to asbestos. *Am J Respir Crit Care Med*. 2008;178: 556–7.
24. Banks DE, Shi R, McLarty J et al. American College of Chest Physicians consensus statement on the respiratory health effects of asbestos. Results of a Delphi study. *Chest*. 2009;135:1619–27.
25. Costabel U, Uzaslan E, Guzman J. Bronchoalveolar lavage in drug-induced lung disease. *Clin Chest Med*. 2004;25:25–35.
26. Reid A, Berry G, de Klerk N et al. Age and sex differences in malignant mesothelioma after residential exposure to blue asbestos (crocidolite). *Chest*. 2007;131:376–82.
27. Wilson D, Takahashi K, Pan G et al. Respiratory symptoms among residents of a heavy-industry province in China: prevalence and risk factors. *Respir Med*. 2008.
28. O'Reilly KM, Mclaughlin AM, Beckett WS et al. Asbestos-related lung disease. *Am Fam Physician*. 2007;75:683–8.
29. Abejie BA, Wang X, Kales SN, Christiani DC et al. Patterns of pulmonary dysfunction in asbestos workers: a cross-sectional study. *J Occup Med Toxicol*. 2010;5:12.
30. Huggins JT, Sahn SA. Causes and management of pleural fibrosis. *Respirology*. 2004;9:441–7.
31. Cugell DW, Kamp DW. Asbestos and the pleura: a review. *Chest*. 2004;125:1103–17.
32. Welch LS, Haile E. Asbestos-related disease among sheet metal workers 1986–2004: Radiographic changes over time. *Am J Ind Med*. 2009.
33. Martino D, Pass HI. Integration of multimodality approaches in the management of malignant pleural mesothelioma. *Clin Lung Cancer*. 2004; 5:290–8.

ADDITIONAL READING

- Antonescu-Turcu AL, Schapira RM et al. Parenchymal and airway diseases caused by asbestos. *Curr Opin Pulm Med*. 2010;16:155–61
- Brody AR et al. Asbestos and lung disease. *Am J Respir Cell Mol Biol*. 2010;42:131–2.
- Kamp DW et al. Asbestos-induced lung diseases: an update. *Transl Res*. 2009;153:143–52.

CODES

ICD9

- 501 Asbestosis
- 515 Postinflammatory pulmonary fibrosis

CLINICAL PEARLS

- Associations between asbestos and all histologic subtypes of lung cancer have been observed.
- Higher amounts of asbestos exposure are associated with higher risk of asbestosis.
- Smoking cessation is particularly important because cigarette smokers have more radiographic signs of asbestosis and are at a synergistically increased risk for lung cancer.
- For those who work with asbestos, to limit exposure to others in their household, clothing should be left at work, if possible, or should be washed and stored separately from other clothing.

ASCITES

Anne M. Walsh, PA-C, MMSc
Auguste Turnier, MD

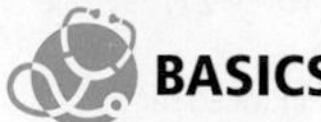

BASICS

DESCRIPTION

Pathologic accumulation of fluid in the abdominal cavity; may occur in any condition that causes generalized edema.

EPIDEMIOLOGY

- Children: Nephrotic syndrome and malignancy most common
- Adults: Cirrhosis, heart failure, nephrotic syndrome, peritonitis most common

RISK FACTORS

Those associated with possible causes

ETIOLOGY

- Peritoneal infection and inflammation:
  - Tuberculosis
  - Fungal disease
  - Bacterial infection (foreign body, fistula)
  - Perforated viscus
  - Granulomatous peritonitis (e.g., sarcoidosis)
  - Parasitic infection
- Metabolic diseases:
  - Cirrhosis
  - Prehepatic and posthepatic portal hypertension
  - Myxedema
  - Nephrogenous
  - Dialysis-related
  - Protein malnutrition (hypoalbuminemia <2 g/dL)
- Cardiac congestion:
  - CHF
  - Constrictive pericarditis
  - Tricuspid stenosis or insufficiency
- Trauma:
  - Pancreatic or biliary fistula
  - Lymphatic tear (chylous ascites)
  - Hemoperitoneum (trauma, ectopic pregnancy, tumor)
- Malignancy:
  - Peritoneal seeding: ovarian, colon, pancreas, others
  - Primary peritoneal carcinoma
  - Leukemia, lymphoma
- Mixed (more than one of the above causes, e.g., cirrhosis and cancer)
- Acute liver failure

DIAGNOSIS

HISTORY

- Abdominal pain
- Anorexia
- Nausea
- Early satiety
- Heartburn
- Flatulence
- Flank pain
- Weight gain
- Shortness of breath
- Dyspnea/orthopnea
- Edema

PHYSICAL EXAM

- Abdominal distention
- Bulging flanks
- Weight gain
- Abdominal fluid wave
- Shifting dullness or "puddle sign" (dullness over dependent abdomen)
- Penile/scrotal edema
- Umbilical/inguinal herniae
- Pleural effusion
- Pedal edema
- Rales
- Tachycardia
- Palmar erythema, spider angiomata in cirrhosis

DIAGNOSTIC TESTS & INTERPRETATION

Lab

Ascitic fluid should be sampled in all new-onset, new-to-treat, or hospitalized cases (1)[B].

- Obtain in all:
  - Total cell count
    - Polymorphonuclear leukocytes: $\geq$250 mm^3 suggests infection (even if culture is negative) requiring antibiotics
  - Albumin in both serum and ascites: Calculate serum-to-ascites albumin gradient (SAAG):
    - <1.1 g indicates exudate (i.e., inflammatory, biliary/pancreatic, carcinomatosis)
    - $\geq$1.1 g indicates transudate/portal hypertension
  - Protein: >2 g (some sources cite 2.5 g) indicates exudate
- Of use in specific circumstances:
  - Culture if infection suspected (fever, abdominal pain, hypotension, etc.)
  - Amylase, triglycerides, glucose
  - Lactate dehydrogenase
  - Acid-fast or fungal cultures/smears
  - Cytology only if exudate
- Blood tests:
  - BUN/creatinine
  - Electrolytes
- Urine tests:
  - Sodium levels in single sample:
    - <10 mEq/L (<10 mmol/L) diuretic response unlikely
    - >10–70 mEq/L (>10–70 mmol/L) diuretic response likely
    - >70 mEq/L (>70 mmol/L) diuretics unnecessary
- Other labs as indicated by underlying condition (liver enzymes, tumor markers, etc.)

Imaging

- Abdominal ultrasound highly sensitive
- CT scan to rule out intra-abdominal pathology
- MRI best for evaluation of liver disease and presence of hepatoma

Diagnostic Procedures/Surgery

- Diagnostic paracentesis
- Diagnostic laparoscopy

Pathological Findings

- Peritoneal biopsy may reveal tuberculosis or malignancy; of no value in other types of fluid
- Cytology may reveal malignant cells:
  - Typically adenocarcinoma (ovary, breast, GI tract)
  - Rarely primary peritoneal carcinoma

DIFFERENTIAL DIAGNOSIS

- Obesity
- Bowel obstruction
- Pregnancy in reproductive-age female
- If transudate, likely causes include:
  - Congestive heart failure
  - Constrictive pericarditis
  - Cirrhosis
  - Nephrotic syndrome
  - Protein malnutrition/hypoalbuminemia
- If exudate, likely causes include:
  - Neoplasm
  - Tuberculosis
  - Pancreatitis
  - Myxedema
  - Biliary pathology
  - Budd-Chiari syndrome

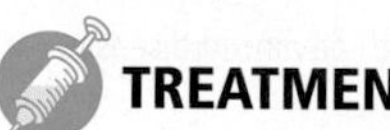

TREATMENT

Outpatient or inpatient, depending on physical condition

For all patients:

- Sodium restriction required (1)[A]:
  - 2 g/day until renal excretion improves, usually required 3–6 months
- Water restriction only necessary if serum sodium <120 mEq/L
- Persistent elevation of creatinine >2.5 mg/dL should lead to decreasing diuretic doses and therapeutic paracentesis
- Daily record of weight to monitor gains and losses

MEDICATION

ALERT

Carefully approach to diuresis as too aggressive treatment can induce hepatorenal syndrome. Monitor creatinine and electrolytes closely.

First Line

- Diuretics needed in nearly all patients:
  - Spironolactone 100–300 mg daily p.o. in single dose best for cirrhotic ascites; typical initial dose 100–200 mg given in AM
  - Furosemide 20–120 mg daily p.o. best for all other etiologies; typical initial dose is 40 mg given in AM
  - May use spironolactone and furosemide together
  - Dose should be sufficient to obtain net sodium loss in urine.
  - Discontinue NSAIDs except 81 mg dose of aspirin
  - Follow body weight daily. If there is a <2-pound loss in the next 4 days, increase either spironolactone by 100 mg or furosemide by 40 mg. If the 2-pound weight loss continues in the next 4 days, continue with the same dose. Emphasize sodium restriction.
  - Spot sodium in mEq/L × estimated urine output (1 L if no information) should equal estimated dietary sodium. Increase diuretics daily until this goal is attained. Measure serum electrolytes before each dose change.

Precautions:
– In hospital or in rapid diuresis, observe creatinine and electrolytes closely. NSAIDs may worsen or initiate oliguria or azotemia.
– Spironolactone or amiloride may increase potassium; monitoring necessary after 1st week of therapy and at least monthly thereafter.
– Observe patients closely for signs of volume depletion, encephalopathy, and renal insufficiency.
Significant possible interactions: Avoid concomitant potassium supplements if spironolactone used alone

econd Line

ternative diuretics unlikely to success if ›mbinations of spironolactone and furosemide fail or sult in increased BUN/creatinine:
Most commonly used in cases of GI intolerance or allergic reactions
Alternatives to spironolactone: Amiloride up to 10 mg/day; triamterene up to 200 mg/day in divided doses
Alternatives to furosemide: Torsemide up to 100 mg/day; ethacrynic acid 50 mg IV (may be effective when oral drugs cannot be used)

DDITIONAL TREATMENT

ieneral Measures

For ascites with edema:
– Salt restriction and diuretics usually effective
– Maximum weight loss of 5 lb/day
– Draw weekly serum electrolytes during rapid weight loss.

For ascites without edema:
– Dietary restrictions and diuretics as above
– Maximum weight loss of 2 lb/day

Refractory ascites:
– Confirm patient compliance with adequate sodium restriction (most common cause)

Diuretic-intractable ascites: worse despite max doses spironolactone (300 mg/day) and furosemide (160–200 mg/day) and sodium restriction OR progressive rise in creatinine to 2.0:
– Paracentesis 5–10 L per session:
  ○ Complications: Infection, hemodynamic collapse, renal failure
  ○ Replace albumin IV for all removals >5 L at rate of 8 g albumin for each liter removed
– Continue diuretics at 1/2 previous dose.

ssues for Referral

eferral for evaluation to liver transplant center in atients with cirrhosis and ascites may be appropriate. 2)[B]

COMPLEMENTARY AND ALTERNATIVE MEDICINE

aution patients to avoid herbs and other upplements unless approved by health care provider risk drug interactions, hepatotoxicity, coagulopathy).

SURGERY/OTHER PROCEDURES

Transjugular intrahepatic portosystemic shunt (TIPS) (2)[A]:
– TIPS is a transjugular conduit from the liver to the hepatic vein used for intractable ascites; placed by interventional radiologists under fluoroscopy.
  ○ At time of placement, measure portal pressure; should drop ≥20 mm Hg or to <12 mm Hg, and ascites should be readily controlled with diuretics. Conduct yearly ultrasonographic study to confirm functional shunt.
  ○ Dilation/replacement may be required after >2 years.
  ○ Encephalopathy is a known complication; however, no difference in mortality compared to paracentesis. (1)

- Surgical portacaval shunt: An 8–10 mm mesenteric caval shunt often is effective:
  – Significant operative mortality, morbidity, encephalopathy; most experts prefer TIPS, rarely used in the US due to its greater risks than TIPS (2)[C]
- When recurrent pleural effusion is present in patient with chronic ascites, fusing of pleural surfaces is sometimes used. Alternative is TIPS.
- Liver transplant referral should be considered in patients with decompensated liver disease, whether or not ascites is present/controlled.

ONGOING CARE

FOLLOW-UP RECOMMENDATIONS

Bed rest only if heart failure and/or prominent leg edema.

Patient Monitoring

- Daily body weight
- Closely follow creatinine and electrolytes when initiating diuresis and 1 week after change in dose/type of diuretic
- Mental status to assess for encephalopathy

DIET

Consultation with dietician helpful:
- Sodium restriction, 2 g/day, monitored
- Adequate nutrition
- Fluid restriction (1–1.5 L/day) only if dilutional hyponatremia (Na <120 mEq/L)
- Complete abstinence from alcohol if liver disease

PROGNOSIS

- Varies depending on underlying cause
- Rarely life-threatening in itself, but may be a sign of life-threatening disease (e.g., cancer, end stage liver disease):
  – Conservative therapy usually successful if cause is reversible or treatable (e.g., infection)

COMPLICATIONS

- Spontaneous bacterial peritonitis (SBP):
  – Ascitic fluid cell count ≥250, polymorphonuclear leukocytes, fever, clinical deterioration. Treat with 3rd-generation cephalosporin or comparable antibiotic; combined antibiotic treatment plus IV albumin results in improved survival in some patients (3)[B].
  – Lifetime antibiotic prophylaxis with norfloxacin or TMP/SMX is indicated in some patients who survive an episode of SBP (1)[A].
  – No antibiotic prophylaxis is necessary for patients with cirrhotic ascites and no GI bleeding as there is concern of developing resistant pathogens and transplant complication (1)[B]
  – GI bleeding and cirrhosis: IV ceftriaxone for 7 days to prevent bacterial infection (1)[A]
- Overly aggressive diuresis may lead to hypokalemia, worsening encephalopathy; intravascular volume depletion may lead to azotemia, renal failure, and death as a result of hepatorenal syndrome.
- Hepatorenal syndrome:
  – Acute renal failure secondary to decreased intravascular volume in ascites
  – May be induced by aggressive diuresis or paracentesis
  – Urine volume <500 mL/day, decreasing urine sodium, rising blood urea nitrogen, and creatinine >1.5 mg/dL:
    ○ Full discussion of hepatorenal syndrome, see Hepatorenal Syndrome
    ○ Stop all diuretics; IV fluid challenge of 1.5 L plasma expander after 1 day if no improvement.
    ○ Vasopressors (e.g., terlipressin IV every 4–6 hours) may resolve renal failure in 50% of patients (3)[B]
- Hydrothorax: Always on right side; cell and lab properties same as ascites. Treat ascites vigorously; if hydrothorax does not disappear, consider TIPS. Chest tube rarely helpful in acute setting.

REFERENCES

1. Runyon BA, Practice Guidelines Committee, American Association for the Study of Liver Diseases (AASLD). Management of adult patients with ascites due to cirrhosis. *Hepatology*. 2009;49:2087–2107.
2. Saab S, Nieto JM, Lewis SK, Runyon BA. TIPS versus paracentesis for cirrhotic patients with refractory ascites. *Cochrane Database of Systematic Reviews* 2006, Issue 4. Art. No.: CD004889. DOI: 10.1002/14651858.CD004889.pub2.
3. Talwalkar JA, Kamath PS. Influence of recent advances in medical management on clinical outcomes of cirrhosis. *Mayo Clin Proc*. 2005; 80:1501–8.

ADDITIONAL READING

Rössle M, Gerbes AL et al. TIPS for the treatment of refractory ascites, hepatorenal syndrome and hepatic hydrothorax: a critical update. *Gut*. 2010;59: 988–1000.

See Also (Topic, Algorithm, Electronic Media Element)

Cirrhosis of the Liver; Congestive Heart Failure; Nephrotic Syndrome; Hepatorenal Syndrome
Algorithm: Cirrhosis

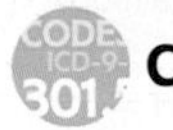

CODES

ICD9

- 789.51 Malignant ascites
- 789.59 Other ascites

CLINICAL PEARLS

- Diuretics are used for clinically significant ascites; spironolactone, alone or in combination with furosemide are highly effective treatments.
- Ultrasound is highly sensitive to detect ascites, but use CT to rule out intra-abdominal pathology and MRI if evaluating liver disease.
- Most common cause of "refractory ascites" is patient noncompliance with dietary sodium restriction.

ASTHMA

Fozia A. Ali, MD

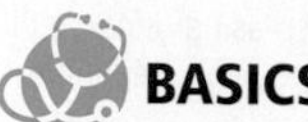

BASICS

DESCRIPTION

- Chronic, reversible inflammatory airway disease
- Four major classifications of asthma severity used primarily to initiate therapy (1,2):
  - Intermittent: Symptoms $\leq$2 days/week, night-time awakenings $\leq$2×/month, short-acting β-agonist use $\leq$2 days/week, no interference with normal activity, and normal FEV1 between exacerbations with FEV1 (predicted) >80% and FEV1/FVC >85%
  - Mild persistent: Symptoms >2 days/week but not daily, night-time awakenings 1–4×/month, short-acting β-agonist use >2 days/week but not daily, minor limitations in normal activity, and FEV1 (predicted) >80% and FEV1/FVC >80%
  - Moderate persistent: Daily symptoms, night-time awakenings 3–4×/month or $\geq$1×/week but not nightly, depending on age, daily use of short-acting β-agonist, some limitation in normal activity, and FEV1 (predicted) 60–80% and FEV1/FVC 75–80%
  - Severe persistent: Symptoms throughout the day, night-time awakenings >1×/week, short-acting β-agonist use several times a day, extremely limited normal activity, and FEV1 (predicted) <60% and FEV1/FVC <75%

EPIDEMIOLOGY

Prevalence

- One of the most common chronic diseases of childhood, affecting 6 million children
- In children, more common in boys than girls
- In adults, more common in women than men

Pregnancy Considerations

- In the US, 3.7–8.4% of pregnant women are affected. Maternal asthma complicates approximately 4–8% of all pregnancies.
- Prevalence of asthma in seniors (>age 65) is 5.3%

RISK FACTORS

- Host factors: Genetic predisposition, gender, race, body mass index
- Environmental exposures: Viral infections, airborne allergens, tobacco smoke, etc.
- Patients with food allergies and asthma are at increased risk for fatal anaphylaxis from those foods.

Genetics

- Inheritable component with complex genetics
- Active area of research: Treatments may be directed to specific genotypes.

GENERAL PREVENTION

- Eliminate or modify exposure to asthma triggers.
- Consider allergen immunotherapy when indicated.
- Treat comorbidities such as allergic rhinitis.
- Annual influenza vaccine (inactivated influenza vaccine) is recommended for all patients <6 months (3).
- Patients at risk for anaphylaxis should carry an EpiPen.

PATHOPHYSIOLOGY

- Inflammatory cell infiltration, sub-basement fibrosis, mucus hypersecretion, epithelial injury, smooth muscle hypertrophy, angiogenesis
- Remodeling of airways may occur (1).

ETIOLOGY

Host and environmental factors

COMMONLY ASSOCIATED CONDITIONS

- Atopy: Eczema, allergic conjunctivitis, allergic rhinitis
- Obesity (associated with higher asthma rates)
- Sinusitis
- Gastroesophageal reflux disease (GERD)
- Obstructive sleep apnea (OSA)
- Allergic bronchopulmonary aspergillosis (rare)
- Stress/depression

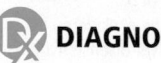

DIAGNOSIS

It is important to classify asthma severity.

HISTORY

Symptoms include:

- Cough (particularly if worse at night)
- Wheeze
- Chest tightness
- Difficulty breathing

PHYSICAL EXAM

- May be normal
- Focus on:
  - General appearance: Signs of respiratory distress such as use of accessory muscles
  - Upper respiratory tract: Rhinitis, nasal polyps, swollen nasal turbinates
  - Lower respiratory tract: Wheezing, prolonged expiratory phase
  - Skin: Eczema

DIAGNOSTIC TESTS & INTERPRETATION

Lab

Initial lab tests

- Spirometry: Does not rule out disease
- Peak expiratory flow rates are inappropriate for diagnosis.

Follow-Up & Special Considerations

- Bronchoprovocation (methacholine, histamine, cold air, or exercise) is only definitive diagnostic test.
- Asthma Action Plan: Patients monitor their own symptoms and/or peak flow measurements.

Imaging

Initial approach

Chest x-ray is used to exclude alternative diagnoses and to evaluate patients for complicating cardiopulmonary processes.

Diagnostic Procedures/Surgery

- Allergy skin testing may be considered to evaluate atopic triggers.
- Sweat testing if diagnosis of cystic fibrosis.
- Arterial blood gases is indicated for patients with respiratory distress and hypoxia.

Pathological Findings

Inflammatory cell infiltration, edema, goblet cell hyperplasia, smooth muscle hyperplasia, thickened basement membrane

DIFFERENTIAL DIAGNOSIS

- In children:
  - Upper airway diseases (allergic rhinitis or sinusitis)
  - Large airway obstruction (foreign-body aspiration, vocal cord dysfunction, vascular ring or laryngeal web, laryngotracheomalacia, lymph nodes or tumor)
  - Small airway obstruction (viral bronchiolitis, cystic fibrosis, bronchopulmonary dysplasia, heart disease)
  - Other causes (recurrent cough *not* due to asthma, aspiration/GERD)
- In adults:
  - Chronic obstructive pulmonary disease, congestive heart failure, pulmonary embolism, benign or malignant tumor, pulmonary infiltration with eosinophilia, drugs such as an angiotensin-converting enzyme inhibitor, vocal cord dysfunction

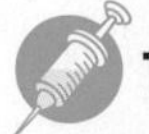

TREATMENT

MEDICATION

First Line

Short-acting β-agonist (SABA) for quick relief of acute symptoms and for prevention of exercise-induced bronchospasm

ALERT

- Delivery of SABA and other inhaled agents via "spacer" or holding chamber (AeroChamber, OptiChamber, others) provides increased efficacy with decreased side effects when compared to nebulized delivery. Reserve nebulized delivery of medication for those unable to use spacer (infants, those intubated, etc.).
- All short-acting agents are pregnancy Category C.
- Specific medicines include albuterol, levalbuterol (Xopenex), metaproterenol (Alupent) Pirbuterol (Maxair) (4)
- Anticholinergic agent:
  - Ipratropium bromide: Used in combination with SABA for added benefit in emergency situations
- Systemic corticosteroids can be used:
  - In moderate-to-severe asthma as adjunct
  - In patients with all but the mildest of acute asthma exacerbations (5)[A]
  - Steroids should be prescribed for up to 7 days in adults and for 3–5 days in children with no need for tapering.
  - Use corticosteroid doses of prednisolone 1–2 mg/kg/day or equivalent.

Second Line

For long-term control (4):

- Inhaled corticosteroids (ICS):
  - Preferred long-term controller therapy for children and adults with persistent asthma and persistent asthma during pregnancy

Pregnancy Considerations

- Most ICS agents are pregnancy Category C, except Budesonide which is category B.
- Long-acting β_2-agonists (LABA):
  - Should *not* be used as monotherapy
  - Salbutamol or formoterol
- Combination products, including a LABA and ICS, are available and offer additional control over ICS alone; preferred in moderate persistent asthma.
- Leukotriene receptor agonists: Alternative, not preferred for mild persistent asthma:
  - Montelukast or
  - Zafirlukast (patients $\geq$7 years)

- Lipoxygenase pathway inhibitor: Alternative not preferred for adjunctive treatment in adults
  – Zileuton (patients ≥12 years)
- Theophylline alternative not preferred as adjunctive therapy with inhaled corticosteroids
- Cromolyn sodium and nedocromil are alternatives, but not a preferred option
- Immunomodulators:
  – Omalizumab: Adjunctive not preferred therapy for patients ≥12 years with allergies and severe persistent asthma

ADDITIONAL TREATMENT

General Measures

- Identify triggers and control exposures.
- Identify patients at risk for reactions to aspirin and nonsteroidal anti-inflammatory drugs (NSAIDs), and avoid exposure.

Issues for Referral

Referral to an asthma specialist (either a pulmonologist or an allergist) should be considered:

- Diagnosis unclear
- Additional asthma education needed
- Comorbidities: Rhinitis, GERD, sinusitis, OSA
- Specialized testing (bronchoprovocation, skin testing, etc.)
- Specialized treatments (e.g., immunotherapy, anti-IgE therapy)
- Moderate-to-severe persistent asthma in adults
- Moderate-to-persistent asthma in children
- Not well controlled or very poorly controlled asthma: Multiple emergency room visits, for asthma

Additional Therapies

- Allergen immunotherapy
- Omalizumab (Xolair): Anti-IgE therapy

COMPLEMENTARY AND ALTERNATIVE MEDICINE

Patients should be cautioned regarding the potential for harmful ingredients and for interactions with recommended asthma medications.

IN-PATIENT CONSIDERATIONS

Initial Stabilization

- Supplemental oxygen to correct hypoxemia
- Repeated doses or continuous administration of SABA (1)[A]
- Ipratropium bromide may be used in the emergency room, but is not recommended for inpatient treatment (1)[B].
- Systemic corticosteroids for moderate or severe exacerbations or poor response to SABA (1)[A]
- Adjunctive therapy with $MgSO_4$ or Heliox may be considered in severe cases, but not routinely (1,6)[B].

Admission Criteria

No single measure is predictive:

- Dyspnea
- Hypoxia
- Poor or no response to SABA
- PEFR or FEV_1 <40%
- Decision for admission should be based on duration and severity of symptoms, severity of airflow obstruction, response to emergency department treatment, course and severity of prior exacerbations, access to medical care and medication, and adequacy of home condition. (1)

IV Fluids

- Avoid aggressive hydration in older children and adults.
- Monitor electrolytes.

Nursing

- Careful respiratory monitoring, including vital signs, pulse oximetry, response and duration of response to SABA, and, when possible, an objective measure of lung function such as PEF or FEV1
- Asthma education

Discharge Criteria

- Minimal or absent asthma symptoms
- Hypoxia has resolved
- FEV1 or PEF ≥70% predicted or personal best
- Bronchodilator response sustained ≥60 minutes

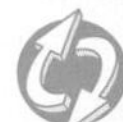

ONGOING CARE

FOLLOW-UP RECOMMENDATIONS

Smoking cessation counseling or elimination of secondhand smoke, if applicable

Patient Monitoring

- Quality-of-life measures: Impact on activities, sleep, emergency visits, hospitalizations, etc.
- Pharmacotherapy: Efficacy, compliance, side effects, technique
- Lung function: Peak flow is an inexpensive and easily available monitoring device once the diagnosis of asthma has been established.

DIET

Food allergies and sulfites (in food and wine) can precipitate symptoms for some patients. GERD precautions may be helpful with both symptomatic reflux and in those who are asymptomatic for reflux but with poorly controlled or nocturnal asthma.

PATIENT EDUCATION

- Patients' technique for using inhaled medications should be reviewed at every visit.
- American Academy of Allergy, Asthma & Immunology: 1-800-822-2762 or http://www.aaaai.org
- American Lung Association: http://www.lungusa.org
- Food Allergy & Anaphylaxis Network: http://www.foodallergy.org
- Asthma and Allergy Foundation of America: 1-800-727-8462 or http:www.aafa.org

PROGNOSIS

- Risk factors for persistent asthma (in children <3 years of age with ≥4 episodes of wheezing in preceding year): Either history of asthma in ≥1 parent or documented atopic dermatitis or aeroallergen sensitivity
- Alternatively, ≥2 of the following will also place these children at increased risk:
  – Food sensitivity
  – ≥4% peripheral eosinophilia
  – Wheezing episodes unrelated to upper respiratory tract infections
- Asthma worsens in 1/3 of women during pregnancy and improves in another 1/3.

COMPLICATIONS

- Atelectasis
- Pneumonia
- Air leak syndromes: Pneumomediastinum, pneumothorax
- Medication-specific side effects/adverse effects/interactions
- Respiratory failure
- Death: Approximately 50% of asthma deaths occur in the elderly (age >65 years), and mortality is increasing in that population (7).

REFERENCES

1. National Asthma Education and Prevention Program Expert Panel Report 3, Guidelines for the Diagnosis and Management of Asthma. No. 08-5846 Washington DC: NIH, Oct 2007.
2. Reddel HK, Taylor DR, Bateman ED et al. An official American Thoracic Society/European Respiratory Society statement: asthma control and exacerbations: standardizing endpoints for clinical asthma trials and clinical practice. *Am J Respir Crit Care Med*. 2009;180:59–99.
3. Centers for Disease Control and Prevention, Recommended adult immunization schedule – United States 2009 *MMWR*. 2008;57(53).
4. Fanta CH. Asthma. *N Engl J Med*. 2009;360: 1002–14.
5. Doherty S. Prescribe systemic corticosteroids in acute asthma. *BMJ*. 2009;338:b1234.
6. McGarvey JM, Pollack CV. Heliox in airway management. *Emerg Med Clin North Am*. 2008;26:905–20, viii.
7. Stupka E, deShazo R. Asthma in seniors: Part 1 evidence for underdiagnosis, undertreatment and increasing morbidity and mortality. *Am J Med*. 2009;122(1):6–11.

ADDITIONAL READING

- Busse, WW, NHLBI: NAEPP asthma & Pregnancy Working Group. NAEPP Expert Panel report: Managing asthma during pregnancy: Recommendations for pharmacologic treatment - 2004 update, *J Allergy Clin Immunol*. 2005;115:34–46.
- Dombrowski M, ACOG Practice Bulletin, Clinical Management Guidelines for Obstetrician-Gynecologists. *Asthma in Pregnancy*. 2008;111(2 Part 1): 457–64.
- Global Strategy for Asthma Management and prevention, 2006. At: http://www.ginasthma.org

See Also (Topic, Algorithm, Electronic Media Element)

http://www.ala.org

Algorithm: Asthma Exacerbation, Pediatric Acute

CODES

ICD9

- 493.00 Extrinsic asthma, unspecified
- 493.90 Asthma, unspecified
- 493.92 Asthma, unspecified, with (acute) exacerbation

CLINICAL PEARLS

- Asthma is a chronic, reversible inflammatory airway disease whose exacerbations are characterized by reversible bronchoconstriction, airway hyper-responsiveness, and airway edema.
- Short-acting β-agonist (SABA) is the most effective rescue therapy for acute asthma symptoms.
- Inhaled corticosteroids (ICS) are the preferred long-term control therapy for patients of all ages.
- Peak flow is an inexpensive and easily available monitoring device once the diagnosis of asthma has been established.

ATHEROSCLEROSIS

Manoj Singh, MD

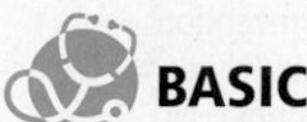

BASICS

DESCRIPTION
Atherosclerosis is the common form of arteriosclerosis in which deposits of yellowish plaques (atheromas) containing cholesterol, lipoid material, and lipophages are formed within the intima and inner media of large and medium-sized arteries.

Geriatric Considerations
- Atherosclerosis happens to all who live long enough.
- Effects and complications can be minimized and/or delayed by avoiding all risk factors possible.

Pediatric Considerations
Fatty streaks and deposits in the intima of the aortas of all children begin as early as 3 years of age.

EPIDEMIOLOGY
- Incidence/prevalence in the US:
  - Common, but declining steadily
  - The effects on the brain, heart, kidneys, extremities, and other vital organs form the leading cause of morbidity and mortality in the US and most Western countries.
  - Complications of atherosclerosis account for 1/2 of all deaths and 1/3 of the deaths in persons 35–65 years of age.
- Predominant age: 35 and older
- Predominant sex: Male > Female

RISK FACTORS
- Modifiable:
  - Hypertension
  - Tobacco smoking
  - Diabetes mellitus (risk factor for death or myocardial infarction [MI] considered equivalent to established coronary heart disease [CHD])
  - Obesity
  - Physical inactivity
  - Decreased high-density lipoprotein (HDL) cholesterol
  - Increased low-density lipoprotein (LDL) cholesterol
  - Comorbidities that may increase risk:
    - Hypothyroidism
    - Elevated homocysteine levels
    - High testosterone levels in women
    - Low testosterone levels in men
- Nonmodifiable:
  - Male gender
  - Increasing age
- Family history of *premature* atherosclerosis

Genetics
There is a probable genetic link; many risk factors for atherosclerosis (lipid metabolism, hypertension, and diabetes) are clearly inheritable. Inheritance is polygenic.

GENERAL PREVENTION
Treat or control modifiable risk factors.

ETIOLOGY
- Biochemical, physiologic, environmental factors that lead to inflammation, thickening, and occlusion of the lumen of arteries
- Aging (some degree of atherosclerosis is universal)
- 1 or more of the risk factors listed under Risk Factors

COMMONLY ASSOCIATED CONDITIONS
- Essential hypertension
- Coronary arteriosclerosis
- Heart failure (congestive heart failure [CHF])
- Cerebrovascular accident
- Atrial arrhythmias
- Ventricular arrhythmias
- Renal failure, chronic
- Aortic dissection
- Thrombosis and embolism, arterial
- Atherosclerotic occlusive disease

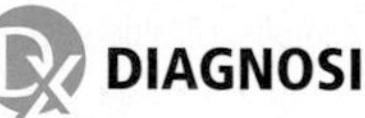

DIAGNOSIS

- Characteristically silent until atheromas produce:
  - Stenosis
  - Thrombosis
  - Aneurysm
  - Embolus
- For lists of possible symptoms, see the following topics:
  - Essential hypertension
  - Coronary arteriosclerosis
  - CHF
  - Cerebrovascular accident
  - Atrial arrhythmias
  - Renal failure, chronic
  - Dissecting aneurysm
  - Thrombosis and embolism, arterial

DIAGNOSTIC TESTS & INTERPRETATION

Lab
- Associated with elevated serum cholesterol
- Elevated LDL and low HDL
- Inflammation plays an as-yet incompletely defined role.

Imaging
Extensively calcified atherosclerotic plaques may be identified in major blood vessels on radiography.

Diagnostic Procedures/Surgery
- Arterial Doppler studies (carotid, renal)
- Angiography
- Ankle–brachial index

Pathological Findings
- Early changes (simple), potentially reversible:
  - Accumulation of lipid-laden cells in the intimal layer of the artery (usually monocytes/macrophages from circulating blood)
  - Lipid streaks in aorta and coronary arteries
- Late changes (complicated) usually reversible:
  - Atheromatous plaques with necrosis, fibrosis, calcification
  - Weakening of elastic lamellae
  - Neovascularization
  - Arterial obstruction
  - Thrombosis
- Oxidized low-density lipoprotein induces vascular smooth-muscle cell apoptosis and cell death.
- Alteration of endothelial function involving mostly nitrous oxide pathways promotes platelet adhesion and aggregation, local clotting, and vascular growth, and alters vascular tone.
- Decrease in elastin with aging along with collagen degeneration and increased intima-media thickness of arterial wall

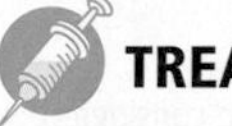

TREATMENT

MEDICATION

First Line
HMG-CoA reductase inhibitors (statins) have multiple effects in addition to lipid-lowering effects (they improve endothelial function, enhance the stability of atherosclerotic plaque, decrease oxidative stress and inflammation, and inhibit thrombogenic response). It is likely that these so-called pleiotropic effects of statins are clinically important, perhaps even more so than their absolute lipid-lowering effect.

Second Line
- Bile acid sequestrants
- Fibric acid derivatives
- Ezetimibe (lowers LDL effectively, but no outcomes data currently support use)
- Niacin

ADDITIONAL TREATMENT

General Measures
Treat hypertension, hypothyroidism (if present), and diabetes.

COMPLEMENTARY AND ALTERNATIVE MEDICINE
Good evidence exists showing the following do not lower atherosclerotic risk:
- Omega-3 fatty acids (1)
- Vitamin E (2)
- Lowering homocysteine levels (3)
- Chelation therapy (4)
- Anticoagulation (5)
- Garlic (6)
- No evidence that testosterone treatment is beneficial for aortic atherosclerosis (7)

URGERY/OTHER PROCEDURES

- Angioplasty (8)[A]
- Stent (9)[A]
- Carotid endarterectomy: For symptomatic patients, NNT 15 if severe (>70%) blockage, NNT 21 if blockage less severe (50–69%) (10)[A]
- Rotational atherectomy (in selected cases where angioplasty and stent may be ineffective) (11)[C]

N-PATIENT CONSIDERATIONS

nitial Stabilization

- Outpatient until complications occur
- Emphasis on prevention

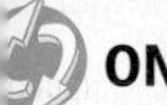

ONGOING CARE

OLLOW-UP RECOMMENDATIONS

ncourage physical fitness, as this may prevent rogression (12)[B].

DIET

merican Heart Association Dietary recommendations e controversial and have not been proven effective lowering atherosclerotic risk:

- Initial diet, step 1:
  - Total fat: <30% of total calories; saturated fat: <10%
  - Carbohydrates: 50–60% of total calories
  - Protein: 10–20% of total calories
  - Cholesterol: <300 mg/d
  - Total calories: Amount required to achieve and maintain desirable weight
  - Sodium: 1,650–2,400 mg
  - Alcohol: <30 g
- Initial diet, step 2:
  - Total fat: <30% of total calories; saturated fat: <7%
  - Carbohydrates: 50–60% of total calories
  - Protein: 10–20% of total calories
  - Cholesterol: <200 mg/d
  - Total calories: Amount required to achieve and maintain desirable weight
  - Sodium: 1,650–2,400 mg
  - Alcohol: <30 g
- A "Mediterranean" diet consisting of a low-salt, low red-meat diet with liberal amounts of fresh fruit and vegetables and whole grains, and regular consumption of fish, olive oil, and nuts is likely to be beneficial in preventing and treating atherosclerosis. Moderate consumption of red wine may also be of benefit.

PATIENT EDUCATION

- Crucial parts of preventing and treating atherosclerosis involve nutrition, fitness, and smoking cessation, and treating modifiable risk factors.
- Extensive educational materials are available from many agencies (e.g., American Heart Association, US Government Printing Office, National Cholesterol Education Program). Use these to help teach patients how to avoid or eliminate risk factors.

PROGNOSIS

Modifying risk factors has greatly decreased mortality rates in the last decade.

COMPLICATIONS

- Coronary artery disease
- Renal failure
- Cerebrovascular accidents
- Dissecting or ruptured aneurysms
- CHF
- Arterial thrombosis
- Gangrene
- Cardiac arrhythmias
- Sudden death

REFERENCES

1. Sommerfield T, Price J, Hiatt WR. Omega-3 fatty acids for intermittent claudication. *Cochrane Database of Systematic Reviews* 2007, Issue 4. Art. No.: CD003833. DOI:10.1002/14651858.CD003833.pub3.
2. Kleijnen J, Mackerras D. Vitamin E for intermittent claudication. *Cochrane Database of Systematic Reviews* 1998, Issue 1. Art. No.: CD000987. DOI:10.1002/14651858.CD000987.
3. Hansrani M, Stansby GP. Homocysteine lowering interventions for peripheral arterial disease and bypass grafts. *Cochrane Database of Systematic Reviews* 2002, Issue 3. Art. No.: CD003285. DOI:10.1002/14651858.CD003285.
4. Dans AL, Tan FN, Villarruz-Sulit EC. Chelation therapy for atherosclerotic cardiovascular disease. *Cochrane Database of Systematic Reviews* 2002, Issue 4. Art. No.: CD002785. DOI:10.1002/14651858.CD002785.
5. Cosmi B, Conti E, Coccheri S. Anticoagulants (heparin, low molecular weight heparin and oral anticoagulants) for intermittent claudication. *Cochrane Database of Systematic Reviews* 2001, Issue 2. Art. No.: CD001999. DOI:10.1002/14651858.CD001999.
6. Jepson RG, Kleijnen J, Leng GC. Garlic for peripheral arterial occlusive disease. *Cochrane Database of Systematic Reviews* 1997, Issue 2. Art. No.: CD000095. DOI:10.1002/14651858.CD000095.
7. Price J, Leng GC. Steroid sex hormones for lower limb atherosclerosis. *Cochrane Database of Systematic Reviews* 2001, Issue 3. Art. No.: CD000188. DOI:10.1002/14651858.CD000188.
8. Fowkes G, Gillespie IN. Angioplasty (versus non surgical management) for intermittent claudication. *Cochrane Database of Systematic Reviews* 1998, Issue 2. Art. No.: CD000017. DOI:10.1002/14651858.CD000017.
9. Bachoo P, Thorpe PA, Maxwell H, Welch K. Endovascular stents for intermittent claudication. *Cochrane Database of Systematic Reviews* 2010, Issue 1. Art. No.: CD003228. DOI:10.1002/14651858.CD003228.pub2.
10. Cina C, Clase C, Haynes RB. Carotid endarterectomy for symptomatic carotid stenosis. *Cochrane Database of Systematic Reviews* 1999, Issue 3. Art. No.: CD001081. DOI:10.1002/14651858.CD001081.
11. Villanueva E, Wasiak J, Petherick E. Percutaneous transluminal rotational atherectomy for coronary artery disease. *Cochrane Database of Systematic Reviews* 2003, Issue 4. Art. No.: CD003334. DOI:10.1002/14651858.CD003334.
12. Nordstrom CK, Dwyer KM, Merz CN et al. Leisure time physical activity and early atherosclerosis: the Los Angeles Atherosclerosis Study. *Am J Med*. 2003;115:19–25.

See Also (Topic, Algorithm, Electronic Media Element)

- Aortic Dissection; Arterial Embolus and Thrombosis; Atherosclerotic Occlusive Disease; Congestive Heart Failure; Hypertension, Essential; Renal Failure, Chronic; Stroke
- Algorithm: Chest Pain/Acute Coronary Syndrome

CODES

ICD9

440.9 Generalized and unspecified atherosclerosis

CLINICAL PEARLS

- Atherosclerosis is a generalized condition, affecting multiple organ systems.
- It is very likely that improvement in diet and exercise, control of hypertension, and elimination of risk factors like smoking can effectively stave off or at least delay the development of this condition.
- Statins control atherosclerosis via multiple mechanisms in addition to their lipid-lowering effects.

ATRIAL FIBRILLATION

Michael K. Chen, MD

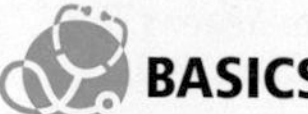

BASICS

This topic covers both atrial fibrillation (Afib) and atrial flutter (Aflut).

DESCRIPTION

- Afib: Continuous or paroxysmal arrhythmia characterized by chaotic atrial electrical activity and an irregularly irregular ventricular response
- In some patients, ventricular response is rapid (>110 bpm), because AV node is bombarded with nearly continuous atrial electrical impulses.
- Aflut: Continuous or paroxysmal arrhythmia with regular atrial electrical activity, typical atrial rate 250–350, manifested as sawtooth flutter waves on ECG. A 2:1 or 4:1 conduction through the AV node to the ventricle is common, so the ventricular response is frequently regular at a rate of 150 or 75 bpm.
- Clinical pattern:
  - Persistent: Sustained >7 days, usually requiring pharmacologic or DC cardioversion to restore sinus rhythm
  - Paroxysmal (PAF): Self-terminating episodes, usually <7 days
  - Permanent: Sinus rhythm cannot be restored; cardioversion has failed or has not been attempted.

EPIDEMIOLOGY

- Incidence/prevalence increases with age.
- Predominant gender: Male > Female

Incidence

- Afib: Age <40, <0.1%/year; >80, >1.5%/year, less for atrial flutter
- Lifetime risk: 25% for those ≥40 years

Prevalence

- Estimated 0.4–1% of general population <60
- ~2–5%, 7th decade; 5–10%, 8th decade

RISK FACTORS

In US, hypertension/coronary disease most common. See Etiology.

Genetics

Familial forms rare, but do exist. Multiple culprit genes have been identified.

GENERAL PREVENTION

Ethanol may trigger AF in some; so-called "holiday heart syndrome." Adequate HTN control may prevent development of AF due to hypertensive heart disease.

PATHOPHYSIOLOGY

- In patients with PAF and no/minimal structural heart disease, triggering premature atrial beats and/or bursts of tachycardia emanate from the pulmonary venous ostia or other sites.
- In patients with persistent/permanent AF and significant structural heart disease, multiple reentrant wavelets within atria may be the cause.

ETIOLOGY

- Cardiac: Hypertensive heart disease, valvular/rheumatic disease, CAD, acute MI, cardiomyopathy, CHF, pericarditis, infiltrative heart disease, sick sinus syndrome
- Pulmonary: Pulmonary embolism, COPD, pneumonia
- Ingestion: (e.g., ethanol in holiday heart), digoxin toxicity (AFlut)
- Endocrine: Hyperthyroidism
- Postoperative (e.g., cardiothoracic surgery)
- Idiopathic: Including lone AF (<60 without clinical or electrocardiogram [EKG] evidence of cardiopulmonary disease, including HTN)

COMMONLY ASSOCIATED CONDITIONS

- Sick sinus syndrome.
- Afib and Aflut are frequently associated with each other. Aflut tends to be a more unstable rhythm and tends to not last as long.

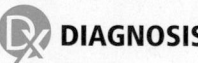

DIAGNOSIS

HISTORY

- Symptoms vary from none–mild (palpitations, lightheadedness, fatigue, poor exercise capacity) to severe (angina, dyspnea, syncope). Symptoms frequently more serious in patients with structural heart disease.
- In patients with Wolff-Parkinson-White syndrome and other types of bypass tracts, Afib may lead to an extremely rapid ventricular rate that may swiftly degenerate into ventricular fibrillation.

PHYSICAL EXAM

- Afib: Irregularly irregular pulse, frequently tachycardic
- Aflut: Regular pulse, frequently tachycardic

DIAGNOSTIC TESTS & INTERPRETATION

- Afib: EKG is diagnostic; low-amplitude fibrillatory waves without discrete P waves; irregularly irregular pattern of QRS complexes
- Aflut: Sawtooth P-waves are the classic sign. Narrow complex QRS. Frequent tachycardia.
- Holter monitor and event monitor helpful in diagnosing PAF and monitoring for recurrence.

Lab

Initial lab tests

TSH, CMP, cardiac enzymes, PT/INR (if anticoagulation is contemplated), consider digoxin level (if appropriate) and CBC

Follow-Up & Special Considerations

Occasional Holter monitoring and/or exercise stress testing to assess for adequacy of rate control

Imaging

- Chest x-ray (CXR) for cardiopulmonary disease
- EKG for structural heart disease, signs of ischemia, heart blocks, and other arrhythmias
- Spiral chest computed tomography (CT) (or other tests such as D-dimer, ventilation-perfusion scan, or pulmonary angiography) if pulmonary embolus possible etiology for new-onset disease
- Transesophageal echocardiogram to detect left atrial appendage thrombus if cardioversion planned

Diagnostic Procedures/Surgery

Electrophysiologic studies should be considered in patients with recurrent Aflut to map the source of the arrhythmia for possible ablation.

Pathological Findings

- Atrial dilatation and fibrosis
- Atrial injury (chronic or acute)
- Atrial thrombus, especially in atrial appendage
- Sclerosis/fibrosis of sinoatrial node
- Coronary artery disease, valvular/rheumatic disease, cardiomyopathy, pulmonary embolus
- Tachycardia-induced cardiomyopathy

DIFFERENTIAL DIAGNOSIS

- Multifocal atrial tachycardia
- Sinus tachycardia with frequent atrial premature beats
- Atrial flutter/atrial fibrillation

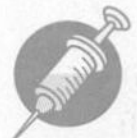

TREATMENT

MEDICATION

- Anticoagulation guidelines (same for Afib and Aflut):
  - Unless contraindicated, patients with AF with any high-risk factors for stroke (prior transient ischemic attack (TIA)/cerebrovascular accident (CVA)/thromboembolism, mitral stenosis, prosthetic valve) should receive warfarin to maintain INR of 2.0–3.0. Patients with mechanical valves should maintain INR >2.5.
  - CHADS2 score: Patients with ≥2 moderate risk factors (**C**HF, **H**TN, **A**ge >75 and/or **D**M), should receive warfarin (INR 2.0–3.0) unless contraindicated.
  - Patients with 1 moderate risk factor should be treated with warfarin (INR 2.0–3.0) or aspirin (81–325 mg/d). Discuss with patient risks and benefits.
  - Patients at low risk of thromboembolic complications or in whom warfarin is contraindicated should receive aspirin (81–325 mg/d) or clopidogrel.
  - Anticoagulation recommendations are independent of AF pattern (paroxysmal, persistent, permanent).
- So-called "rate control" and "rhythm control" strategies have approximately equivalent outcomes in terms of mortality. Rhythm control tends to have more adverse reactions.
- Control of ventricular rate:
  - Nondihydropyridine calcium channel blockers:
    - Diltiazem (Cardizem)
    - Class contraindications: Hypotension, documented sensitivity, 2nd- or 3rd-degree AV block, severe CHF, sick sinus syndrome
    - Precautions: Use caution with CHF, left ventricular (LV) dysfunction, liver or kidney disease. Adverse reactions: Hypotension, CHF, peripheral edema, AV block.
    - Interactions: May increase digoxin levels; with amiodarone or beta-blockers, may severely decrease cardiac output, trigger complete heart block
  - Beta-blockers:
    - Metoprolol (Lopressor)
    - Contraindications: Hypotension, documented sensitivity, 2nd- or 3rd-degree AV block, severe CHF, sick sinus syndrome
    - Precautions: Use caution with CHF, LV dysfunction, kidney disease, asthma
    - Interactions: Bradycardia with digoxin; with amiodarone or calcium channel blockers, may severely decrease cardiac output or trigger complete heart block
    - Adverse reactions: Hypotension, CHF, peripheral edema, AV block

- Digoxin (Lanoxin):
  - Indicated for CHF, hypotension
  - Contraindications: Documented sensitivity, sick sinus syndrome, hypertrophic cardiomyopathy
  - Precautions: Use caution with electrolyte abnormalities (especially hypokalemia, hypercalcemia), impaired renal function, thyroid disease, acute myocardial infarction (MI), AV block
  - Interactions: Unpredictable effects with many antiarrhythmics; additive bradycardia with calcium channel blockers, beta-blockers
  - Adverse reactions: AV block, bradycardia, mental disturbances, nausea
  - Rate control usually achieved in 4 hours (1).

Conversion to/maintenance of sinus rhythm:
- DC cardioversion
- Caution: Antiarrhythmic therapy for chemical cardioversion and maintenance of sinus rhythm following cardioversion may be proarrhythmic.
- Ibutilide, an IV type III agent, for chemical cardioversion of AF and flutter of short duration (<90 days)
- If duration of AF is >24–48 hours or unknown, treat with warfarin for ≥3 weeks before cardioversion. Or, once anticoagulation is established, perform transesophageal EKG. If no atrial thrombus, may cardiovert. Anticoagulation should be continued for ≥4 weeks following cardioversion.
- Long-term, perhaps indefinite, anticoagulation should be considered in patients with thromboembolic risk factors with chronic or recurrent AF.

Chronic oral antiarrhythmic therapy to suppress AF recurrences:
- Type IA (procainamide, disopyramide, quinidine): Generally not used
- Type IC (flecainide, propafenone) in patients with structurally normal hearts or mild hypertensive heart disease. Concomitant use of β-blocker recommended.
- Type III (sotalol, amiodarone, dofetilide)

Contraindications:
- Type IC drugs are contraindicated in patients with coronary artery disease, cardiomyopathy, and significant LVH.
- Type IA and III drugs should not be used in patients with torsade de pointes history or long QT. The risk of torsade de pointes increases with the extent of QT interval prolongation (the QTc), so these medications should be used with great caution, if at all, in patients on medications that prolong the QT.

Precautions: Avoid hypokalemia and hypomagnesemia.

With type IC drugs, stress testing to exclude exercise-induced arrhythmia or QRS widening

With amiodarone, careful surveillance for hepatic, thyroid, pulmonary, skin, ophthalmologic adverse effects

In many patients, adequate medical therapy of AF will cause bradycardia, necessitating a permanent pacemaker.

- According to a recent Cochrane Review, several class IA, IC, and III drugs are effective in maintaining sinus rhythm but increase adverse events, including pro-arrhythmia, and disopyramide and quinidine are associated with increased mortality. Any benefit on clinically relevant outcomes (embolisms, heart failure, mortality) remains to be established (1).

ADDITIONAL TREATMENT

Issues for Referral

AF refractory to medical therapy (unable to achieve adequate rate control or significant bradycardia) should be considered for more definitive therapy such as pacemaker +/−AV node ablation. Antiarrhythmic therapy should be prescribed by experienced practitioners.

SURGERY/OTHER PROCEDURES

- Current guidelines reserve catheter ablation in Afib to highly symptomatic patients who have failed at least 1 course of antiarrhythmic drug therapy [C]. It is the treatment of choice for patients who are in chronic Aflut, with a number needed to treat (NNT) of 2.2 to prevent rehospitalization, vs antiarrhythmics.
- Catheter ablation success rates vary with the type of Afb (paroxysmal > persistent > permanent) and the presence of structural heart disease, particularly left atrial enlargement. May require ≥2 ablation procedures to achieve clinical success.
- Cardiac surgery (e.g., the maze procedure or minimally invasive epicardial procedures) may be considered in severely symptomatic, medically refractory patients.
- Permanent dual-chamber pacing may reduce incidence of new-onset AF and reduce frequency of PAF episodes in patients with sick sinus syndrome.

IN-PATIENT CONSIDERATIONS

Initial Stabilization

Acute therapy for hemodynamically compromised patients:
- Heparin for anticoagulation (not generally necessary; may just initiate warfarin without "bridge" therapy)
- IV β- or calcium channel blocker for control of ventricular rate if blood pressure (BP) adequate
- Urgent cardioversion if hemodynamically unstable:
  - DC cardioversion is best treatment (2)[C].
  - Begin with dose of 50 J (with biphasic defibrillator) or 200 J (with monophasic defibrillator) and increase as needed (2)[C].
  - Atrial overdrive pacing also effective

Admission Criteria

- Inpatient if:
  - Significant symptoms
  - Extremely rapid ventricular rate
  - Initiating antiarrhythmic therapy
  - AF triggered by acute process (acute myocardial infarction, congestive heart failure [CHF], pulmonary embolus)
  - High risk for stroke (rheumatic heart disease, prior TIA/stroke)
- Outpatient management for low-risk patients with controlled ventricular rates

Discharge Criteria

Adequate rate or rhythm control without symptoms. Long-term plan for anticoagulation established.

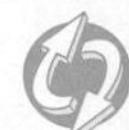

ONGOING CARE

There continues to be debate about whether rate or rhythm control is best for treating patients with chronic Afib/Aflut. Mortality is the same for both. Risk of stroke is higher for electrical cardioversion, but there are some measures of symptom control and quality of life that appear to be improved. Pharmacologic cardioversion is associated with more adverse events and hospitalization in elderly patients. Take into account the patient with their associated health conditions when deciding what path to take (3,4).

FOLLOW-UP RECOMMENDATIONS

Patient Monitoring

- Monitor warfarin levels.
- EKG to monitor QTc interval if on antiarrhythmic therapy

DIET

Avoid potential triggers: Ethanol, caffeine, nicotine

PROGNOSIS

Warfarin anticoagulation reduces annual embolic stroke rate from ~5% to 1–2%. Aspirin reduces risk to 3–4% annually. AF increases risk of morbidity and mortality, but prognosis is a function of underlying heart disease.

COMPLICATIONS

- Embolic stroke
- Peripheral arterial embolization
- Bleeding with anticoagulation
- Tachycardia-induced cardiomyopathy with prolonged periods of inadequate rate control

REFERENCES

1. Lafuente-Lafuente C, Mouly S, Longas-Tejero MA, Bergmann JF et al. Antiarrhythmics for maintaining sinus rhythm after cardioversion of atrial fibrillation. *Cochrane Database Syst Rev*. 2007;CD005049.
2. Fuster, Rydén LE, Cannom DS, et al. ACC/AHA/ESC 2006 guidelines for the management of patients with atrial fibrillation. *Circulation*. 2006;114: e257–354.
3. Mead GE, Elder AT, Flapan AD, Kelman A et al. Electrical cardioversion for atrial fibrillation and flutter. *Cochrane Database Syst Rev*. 2005; CD002903.
4. Cordina J, Mead G et al. Pharmacological cardioversion for atrial fibrillation and flutter. *Cochrane Database Syst Rev*. 2005;CD003713.

CODES

ICD9

- 427.31 Atrial fibrillation
- 427.32 Atrial flutter

CLINICAL PEARLS

- There continues to be debate about whether rate or rhythm control is best for treating patients with chronic Afib/Aflut. Mortality is the same for both. When in doubt and in absence of other contraindications, rate control appears to have the best outcome data.
- AF with rapid ventricular rates may be the initial presentation of tachy/brady syndrome with underlying sinus node dysfunction, particularly in the elderly. Exercise caution when initiating AV nodal-blocking agents in the elderly patient with rapid AF.

ATRIAL FLUTTER

Michael K. Chen, MD

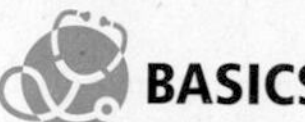

BASICS

DESCRIPTION

Atrial flutter (A. flutter) is a cardiac arrhythmia resulting in a (usually) narrow QRS rhythm, often tachycardia with an atrial rate of 250–350 beats per minute:

- "Saw-toothed" P-waves are classic.
- Ventricular rate is dependent upon AV node conduction (see Pathophysiology).
- System(s) affected: Cardiac

EPIDEMIOLOGY

Incidence

- Age: 5 per 100,000 person-years in people <50 years of age. 587 per 100,000 person-years in people >80 years of age.
- Sex: Male > Female (2.5:1)

RISK FACTORS

- Heart disease (e.g., left ventricular [LV] dysfunction), LV hypertrophy, hypertension [HTN], valvular heart disease (especially rheumatic), coronary artery disease, acute myocardial infarction [MI], atrial fibrillation [A. fib], pericarditis, history of congenital heart disease, recent cardiac surgery, atrial scarring
- Pulmonary disease (e.g., chronic obstructive pulmonary disease [COPD], pulmonary embolism, pneumonia)
- Hyperthyroidism
- Obesity

Genetics

Although several genes have been identified that may predispose to A. fib, there is no definite association of these genes with A. flutter.

GENERAL PREVENTION

Risk factor avoidance

PATHOPHYSIOLOGY

Most commonly caused by a rapid re-entrant circuit around the tricuspid valve (specifically, the cavotricuspid isthmus):

- AV node conduction is variable:
  - 2:1 most common (~150 bpm); 3:1, 4:1 possible, 1:1 more rare (>~200 bpm)
  - Variable conduction ratios can cause irregularly irregular pulse, mimicking A. fib.

ETIOLOGY

- Most cases associated with a predisposing factor (see Risk Factors)
- Lone A. flutter; no predisposing factor:
  - 1.7% of patients with A. flutter
- Digitalis toxicity; rare cause

COMMONLY ASSOCIATED CONDITIONS

- See Risk Factors.
- Atrial fibrillation patients frequently go in and out of atrial flutter.

DIAGNOSIS

HISTORY

- Common:
  - Palpitations, shortness of breath, fatigue, lightheadedness
- Less common:
  - Chest pain, near-syncope
  - Insidious onset with fatigue or worsening of a chronic cardiac/pulmonary disease
- Rare:
  - Syncope
  - Symptoms/signs of acute embolic stroke

PHYSICAL EXAM

- Common: Often normal exam
  - Tachycardia: May be regular or irregularly irregular
  - Mild dyspnea
  - Evidence of a predisposing factor
- Less common:
  - Moderate dyspnea
  - CHF: More common in elderly or with prior history
- Rarely, hemodynamic compromise occurs:
  - Hypotension
  - Severe dyspnea or respiratory failure
  - Hypoxia with cyanosis or pallor
  - Decreased level of consciousness

DIAGNOSTIC TESTS & INTERPRETATION

Lab

Initial lab tests

Complete blood count (CBC), BMP, cardiac enzymes, thyroid-stimulating hormone (TSH), digoxin level (as indicated), prothrombin time (PT)/international normalized ratio (INR) (if anticoagulated or anticoagulation being considered)

Imaging

Initial approach

- Chest x-ray to evaluate for acute cardiopulmonary disease
- Electrocardiogram (ECG) to evaluate for signs of ischemia, heart blocks, intervals, and for diagnosis of atrial flutter

Follow-Up & Special Considerations

- For new-onset atrial flutter, transthoracic echocardiogram is helpful in assessing atrial size, ejection fraction, valvular function, and evaluating right-sided pressures (acute pulmonary embolism).
- Transesophageal echocardiogram may be necessary if thrombus suspected before cardioversion.

Diagnostic Procedures/Surgery

When clinically indicated:

- Holter monitor: If symptoms are concerning but rhythm not present at time of evaluation
- Electrophysiologic studies should be considered in patients with recurrent A. flutter to map the source of the arrhythmia for possible ablation.

DIFFERENTIAL DIAGNOSIS

- Paroxysmal supraventricular tachycardia
- Sinus tachycardia
- Junctional tachycardia
- Multifocal atrial tachycardia (MAT)
- Wolff-Parkinson-White syndrome

TREATMENT

MEDICATION

First Line

- Rate-control agents useful in the initial management, but generally not efficacious in controlling chronic or recurrent arrhythmia (1)[C]
- Nondihydropyridine calcium channel blockers:
  - Diltiazem (Cardizem):
    - Initial dose: 0.25 mg/kg IV × 1, may give 0.35 mg/kg IV × 1 after 15 min if needed
    - Maintenance: 5–15 mg/h IV up to 24 hours
  - Verapamil (Isoptin, Calan, Verelan):
    - As efficacious as diltiazem; increased hypotension (1)
  - Class contraindications: Hypotension, documented sensitivity, 2nd- or 3rd-degree AV block, severe CHF, sick sinus syndrome
  - Precautions: Use caution with CHF, left ventricular (LV) dysfunction, liver or kidney disease
  - Interactions: May increase digoxin levels; with amiodarone or beta-blockers, may severely decrease cardiac output, trigger complete heart block
  - Adverse reactions: Hypotension, CHF, peripheral edema, AV block
- Beta-blockers:
  - Metoprolol (Lopressor):
    - Initial: 5 mg IV, repeat q5min; max, 15 mg
    - Maintenance: 5–15 mg IV q3–6h
  - Esmolol (Brevibloc):
    - Initial dose: 500 mcg/kg IV over 1 minute, repeat q4min to total of 3 doses if needed
    - Maintenance: 50 mcg/kg/min, increased by 50 mcg/kg/min q4min p.r.n.; max of 200 mcg/kg/min
    - Half-life ~8 min; good choice for patients at risk for complications
  - Contraindications: Hypotension, documented sensitivity, 2nd- or 3rd-degree AV block, severe CHF, sick sinus syndrome
  - Precautions: Use caution with CHF, LV dysfunction, kidney disease, or asthma.
  - Interactions: Bradycardia with digoxin; with amiodarone or calcium channel blockers may severely decrease cardiac output or trigger complete heart block
  - Adverse reactions: Hypotension, CHF, peripheral edema, AV block
- Digoxin (Lanoxin):
  - Indicated for CHF, hypotension
  - Initial dose: 0.75–1.25 mg p.o. or 0.5–1 mg IV divided 50% initially, then 25% × 2 q6–12h
  - Maintenance: 0.125–0.5 mg/d p.o. or 0.1–0.4 mg/d IV
  - Therapeutic level: 0.8–2 ng/mL
  - Contraindications: Documented sensitivity, sick sinus syndrome, hypertrophic cardiomyopathy
  - Precautions: Use caution with electrolyte abnormalities (especially hypokalemia, hypercalcemia), impaired renal function, thyroid disease, acute myocardial infarction (MI), and AV block.

– Interactions: Unpredictable effects with many antiarrhythmics; additive bradycardia with calcium channel blockers, beta-blockers
– Adverse reactions: AV block, bradycardia, mental disturbances, nausea
– Rate control usually achieved in 4 hours (1).

Second Line

Pharmacologic cardioversion is 2nd-line to electrical cardioversion in restoring sinus rhythm.

Pure class III antiarrhythmics:

– Ibutilide (Corvert) IV:
  ○ Initial dose: <60 kg, 0.01 mg/kg over 10 minutes; 60 kg, 1 mg over 10 minutes; may repeat in 10 minutes p.r.n.
– Dofetilide (Tikosyn) Oral:
  ○ Dosing: Dependent on QTc interval and creatinine clearance; see package insert
– Contraindications: Documented sensitivity, QTc >440 ms, use of a class I or III antiarrhythmic within 4 hours, structural heart disease, sinus node disease
– Precautions: Correct hypokalemia and hypomagnesium prior to use; use caution in AV block, CHF, QT prolongation, renal/hepatic disease, and elderly patients.
– Interactions: Many antiarrhythmics have unpredictable effects with digoxin; additive bradycardia with calcium channel blockers and beta-blockers.
– Adverse reactions: Polymorphic VT/torsades de pointes (1.5–3%), AV block, QT prolongation, CHF, renal failure, allergy, hypotension, HTN, headache (4%)
– Efficacy = 60–70% (1)

ADDITIONAL TREATMENT

General Measures

Identify and treat underlying causes first.

A. flutter often self-resolves within days:

– Watchful waiting may be appropriate in hemodynamically stable patients, particularly with a reversible predisposing cause and normal left atrial size.

Restoration of normal sinus rhythm is generally the goal of therapy (1)[C]:

– Self-limited A. flutter related to an underlying cause rarely requires chronic therapy (1)[C].
– >50% of patients with chronic or recurrent A. flutter experience recurrence within 1 year of successful cardioversion (2).

Issues for Referral

Cardiology referral recommended for refractory cases and for ablation.

Additional Therapies

- Anticoagulation for cardioversion: If >48 hrs duration, recommend warfarin anticoagulation (INR 2–3) 3 weeks before and 4 weeks after cardioversion (3)[B].
- If immediate cardioversion needed for hemodynamic instability in A. flutter >48 hrs or unknown, bridge with heparin (regular or LMWH) until warfarin therapeutic. Treat for 4 weeks. None needed for <48 hrs (3)[C].
- If TEE (–) for thrombus, no prior anticoagulation needed, but heparin bridge to 3–4 weeks of warfarin therapy (2)[B]. If (+) then treat as if >48 hrs. Longer post-cardioversion AC (3)[C].

SURGERY/OTHER PROCEDURES

Catheter ablation is the treatment of choice for patients with recurrent or chronic A. flutter (1)[A]. 80% remain in sinus rhythm at 21 months compared to 36% with antiarrhythmics (1). To prevent rehospitalization with ablation compared to antiarrhythmics, NNT is 2.2 (1). Catheter ablation results in improved symptoms and improved quality of life (1).

IN-PATIENT CONSIDERATIONS

Initial Stabilization

1st priority is to determine stability of patient:

- Hemodynamically stable:
  – Consider calcium channel blocker or beta-blocker for rate control (1)[C].
- Hemodynamically unstable (see Physical Exam: Hemodynamic compromise):
  – DC cardioversion is best treatment (1)[C].
  – Begin with dose of 50 J (with biphasic defibrillator) or 200 J (with monophasic defibrillator) and increase as needed (1)[C].
  – Atrial overdrive pacing also effective (1)[C]

Admission Criteria

- Most patients with 1st diagnosis of persistent A. flutter require admission for cardiac monitoring.
- All patients who cannot be rate-controlled in the outpatient setting should be admitted.
- Patients with hemodynamic compromise may require intensive care unit (ICU) admission.

IV Fluids

- If hemodynamic unstable, use fluid boluses to maintain blood pressure (BP).
- Caution in LV dysfunction: Avoid CHF.
- If n.p.o., use appropriate maintenance fluid.

Nursing

Strict I/O

Discharge Criteria

Patients can be discharged if rate-controlled, but typically they are when back in NSR.

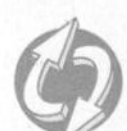

ONGOING CARE

FOLLOW-UP RECOMMENDATIONS

Patient Monitoring

Telemetry

DIET

n.p.o. until rate controlled

COMPLICATIONS

- Incidence of embolization with A. flutter is similar to that of A. fib: 1.7–7% (1).
- Hemodynamic instability, CHF

REFERENCES

1. Blomström-Lundqvist C, Scheinman MM, Aliot EM et al. ACC/AHA/ESC guidelines for the management of patients with supraventricular arrhythmias–executive summary. a report of the American college of cardiology/American heart association task force on practice guidelines and the European society of cardiology committee for practice guidelines (writing committee to develop guidelines for the management of patients with supraventricular arrhythmias) developed in collaboration with NASPE-Heart Rhythm Society. *J Am Coll Cardiol*. 2003;42:1493–531.
2. Crijns HJ, Van Gelder IC, Tieleman RG et al. Long-term outcome of electrical cardioversion in patients with chronic atrial flutter. *Heart*. 1997; 77:56–61.
3. Fuster V, Ryden L, et al. ACC/AHA/ESC Guidelines for the management of Patients with Atrial Fibrillation. *Circulation*. 2006;114:257–354.

ADDITIONAL READING

Scholten MF, Thornton AS, Mekel JM et al. Anticoagulation in atrial fibrillation and flutter. *Europace*. 2005;7:492–9.

See Also (Topic, Algorithm, Electronic Media Element)

Atrial Fibrillation

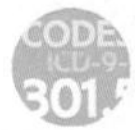

CODES

ICD9

427.32 Atrial flutter

CLINICAL PEARLS

- Atrial flutter is an unstable rhythm and will sometimes spontaneously resolve.
- Goals of care should be stabilization and rate control.
- Catheter ablation is the treatment of choice for recurrent or chronic atrial flutter.

ATRIAL SEPTAL DEFECT (ASD)

Jonathan Min, MD
Darshak Sanghavi, MD

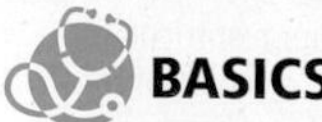

BASICS

DESCRIPTION

- Congenital defect or opening in the atrial septum allowing flow of blood between the 2 atria
- Shunting:
  - Typically left to right; occurs in late ventricular systole and early diastole
  - Degree depends on size of the defect and relative compliance (pressures) of the 2 ventricles
  - There can be minimal right-to-left shunting in early ventricular systole, especially during inspiration.
- Asymptomatic early in life. Exertional dyspnea or fatigue. Late cyanotic shunt.
- Types by location in the interatrial septum:
  - 75%: Ostium secundum defect occurs in the fossa ovalis region; most common and most amenable to percutaneous device closure
  - 10%: Sinus venosus defect occurs in the superior-posterior atrial septum near the orifice of the superior vena cava; usually associated with partial anomalous right upper pulmonary venous return
  - 15%: Ostium primum occurs in the inferior portion of the atrial septum, often associated with cleft mitral valve and failure of endocardial cushion development. Ostium primum also seen with incomplete persistent common atrioventricular canal.
- Definitive diagnosis is by transthoracic echocardiography:
  - Symptomatic patients or patients with a high degree of shunt flow should undergo closure to reduce subsequent morbidity (right ventricular dysfunction and failure, atrial tachyarrhythmias, or stroke) and mortality. The risk of arrhythmias may not be decreased unless the atrial septal defect (ASD) is detected and corrected during childhood.
  - Surgery is the only option for ostium primum and sinus venosus defects.
  - Percutaneous closure is an alternative to surgical repair for patients with secundum ASD.
- System(s) affected: Cardiovascular; Pulmonary

Pediatric Considerations

- Most cases of ASD are detected in the pediatric population and corrected at that time.
- Infants/children may just be small for their age, even in the absence of other symptoms.

EPIDEMIOLOGY

Incidence

- Predominant age: Newborn, but may be diagnosed at any age
- Predominant sex: Female > Male (2:1)
- No race predilection
- 4 per 10,000 births, or 1,574 cases per year, based on reporting on 11 US states 1999–2001 (1)

Prevalence

- Accounts for 10% of congenital heart defects, and accounts for 25–30% of congenital heart defects detected in adulthood
- Prevalence of asymptomatic patent foramen ovale in cohort of 2,291 adult patients undergoing cardiothoracic surgery—17.3% (2)[B]

RISK FACTORS

- Other congenital heart defects
- Family history
- Thalidomide, alcohol

Genetics

- 5% chromosomal abnormalities
- Ostium primum in Down syndrome

PATHOPHYSIOLOGY

- Flow across ASD based on relative compliance of left and right ventricles; therefore, usually left-to-right shunt because of higher left-sided pressures
- Symptoms typically occur due to right ventricular and pulmonary vascular volume overload, sometimes with resultant pulmonary hypertension.

COMMONLY ASSOCIATED CONDITIONS

- ASDs often may occur in the setting of other complex cardiac structural defects.
- Important to exclude anomalous pulmonary venous return
- Occasionally can indicate underlying genetic syndromes:
  - Holt-Oram syndrome: Secundum defect with bony abnormalities of forearms + hands
  - Ellis-von-Creveld syndrome: Chondroectodermal dysplasia + ASD
  - VACTERL:
    - V = vertebral abnormalities
    - A = anorectal malformation
    - C = congenital cardiac defects
    - T = tracheoesophageal fistula/esophageal atresia
    - R = renal–urinary defects
    - L = limb defects

DIAGNOSIS

HISTORY

- Easy fatigability, dyspnea on exertion, heart failure (late), palpitations, frequent respiratory tract infections
- Stroke due to paradoxical emboli
- Can be initially asymptomatic
- Symptoms can include (but not limited to) easy fatigability, dyspnea on exertion, right heart failure (later during course of disease), palpitations, and frequent respiratory tract infections.
- Other symptoms include stroke or unexplained end-organ infarcts due to paradoxical emboli.

PHYSICAL EXAM

Signs vary according to extent of shunting:

- Prominent precordial bulge
- Right ventricular lift
- Palpable pulmonary artery pulse
- Fixed, widely split S2
- Pulmonic flow murmur: Systolic ejection murmur
- Low-pitched diastolic murmur at left lower sternal border
- Cyanosis and clubbing (with severe pulmonary hypertension: Eisenmenger syndrome, jugular venous distention, edema)
- Key physical finding: *Fixed widely split S2*
- May have systolic ejection murmur (pulmonic flow murmur)
- Prominent precordial lift
- Low-pitched diastolic murmur at left lower sternal border

DIAGNOSTIC TESTS & INTERPRETATION

Lab

Oximetry: Cyanosis may suggest Eisenmenger syndrome (right-to-left shunting)

Initial lab tests

Electrocardiogram (ECG) findings:

- General findings for secundum ASDs:
  - Right axis deviation
  - Right atrial enlargement
  - Right ventricular conduction delay
  - Q wave in lead V1
  - Mild PR prolongation
- ECG findings for specific types of ASD:
  - Sinus venosus: Leftward axis, inverted P wave in lead III
  - Ostium primum: Leftward axis

Imaging

Initial approach

- Chest x-ray: Varying degrees of cardiac enlargement, increased pulmonary vascular workings, right ventricle and pulmonary artery enlargement
- Echocardiography: Type and size of ASD, pulmonary arterial and right ventricular dilatation and anterior systolic (paradoxical) septal motion

Follow-Up & Special Considerations

- Cardiac catheterization (indicated in select patients) demonstrates right ventricle enlargement and location of the shunt or if pulmonary hypertension suspected.
- Left ventricular angiography: Identifies prolapse of the mitral valve and allows assessment of the magnitude of the mitral regurgitation that might be present
- Transesophageal echocardiography might be required to define ASD morphology and to locate the pulmonary veins.

Follow-Up & Special Considerations

- Cardiac catheterization can be diagnostic (to assess anatomy, shunt fraction, and pulmonary vascular resistance) and therapeutic (for device closure).
- Transesophageal echocardiography might be required to define ASD morphology and to locate the pulmonary veins, often as adjunct to percutaneous closure.

Diagnostic Procedures/Surgery

- Echocardiography is the preferred noninvasive modality, unless patient body habitus prohibits adequate imaging.
  - A saline-contrast ("bubble") study is needed only for diagnosis of patent foramen ovale (PFO), rather than hemodynamically significant ASD
- Cardiac magnetic resonance allows excellent imaging and quantitation of shunt fraction.
- Ultrafast computed tomography scans can also define ASDs, but with significant radiation exposure

Pathological Findings

- Gross defect in atrial septum
- Dilated right atrium, right ventricle
- Enlarged pulmonary artery

IFFERENTIAL DIAGNOSIS

Other congenital heart disease
Right bundle branch block (for widely split S2)

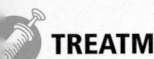

TREATMENT

EDICATION

rst Line

Consider catheter or surgical closure of the significant ASD if pulmonary hypertension is not present.
May require antiarrhythmic medications for atrial fibrillation or supraventricular tachycardia
Respiratory tract infections should be treated promptly.
Proper treatment of heart failure

econd Line

There are no data to support antibiotic prophylaxis against infective endocarditis; however, when a device or patch is placed, prophylaxis is recommended until complete neoendothelialization of the foreign material occurs (usually 6 months).
To prevent thrombus formation after device deployment, aspirin 325 mg daily for 6 months and clopidogrel 75 mg for a month

DDITIONAL TREATMENT

eneral Measures

5% of small ASDs (less than 8 mm) will close ontaneously by 18 months of age; however, close llow-up is warranted (3)[B]. Likelihood of ontaneous closure mainly dictated by diameter of efect: >10 mm at time of diagnosis—unlikely ontaneous closure (4)[B].

sues for Referral

ppropriate health care. Referral to a cardiologist for aluation

URGERY/OTHER PROCEDURES

Closure via percutaneous transcatheter device or surgery (particularly when the pulmonary systemic flow ratio is ≥1.5:1 or evidence of right heart enlargement)

Percutaneous transcatheter device closure of secundum atrial septal defects and patent foramen ovale is now considered a standard and low-risk procedure that has largely replaced the surgical approach (5)[A].

Secundum ASDs that are suitable for percutaneous closure should be 35 mm or less in stretched balloon diameter and should have a sufficient rim of surrounding atrial tissue.

In children, closure is usually delayed until preschool age (2–4 years), except for symptomatic defects (poor growth or exercise intolerance).

In general, PFOs are treated differently from ASDs with significant shunt burden, and the benefits of PFO closure are unclear. Consultation with a neurologist and cardiologist may be considered prior to device closure. Closure in adult patients with stroke reduces the risk of further neurologic events (6)[B]:
- PFO diagnosed intraoperatively not associated with any increase in risk of complications; closure at that time, however, increases risk of postoperative stroke vs unrepaired (7)[B].
- Some evidence suggests possible symptomatic migraine relief following patent foramen ovale closure (8)[B], although this remains controversial and unproven.

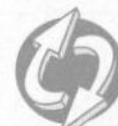

ONGOING CARE

FOLLOW-UP RECOMMENDATIONS

Echocardiography follow-up

Patient Monitoring

- In otherwise asymptomatic healthy children, follow until defect has closed or become negligible in size.
- Appropriate evaluation and management for atrial tachyarrhythmias in patients with long-term follow-up
- If ASD repaired as an adult, periodic long-term follow-up indicated
- ASDs repaired in childhood generally do not have late complications.
- Female patients with unrepaired ASD and Eisenmenger syndrome: Pregnancy not recommended due to increased risk of maternal and fetal mortality

DIET

Cardiac diet in patients with symptoms of cardiac failure, ascites, or edema

PATIENT EDUCATION

For patient education materials on this topic, contact American Heart Association, 7320 Greenville Avenue, Dallas, TX 75231, (214) 373-6300.

PROGNOSIS

- ASD closure in asymptomatic or minimally symptomatic adults reduces morbidity but not mortality (9)[A].
- ASD closure before age 25 in symptomatic adults improves morbidity and likely reduces mortality, and some benefits may occur even in older patients. However, if ASD repair is deferred until after adolescence, the long-term risk of future atrial arrhythmias may not be decreased.
- 50% mortality by age 50 in untreated symptomatic patients with large defects

COMPLICATIONS

- Congestive heart failure
- Late-onset arrhythmias 10–20 years after surgery (5%)
- Stroke
- Pulmonary hypertension
- Eisenmenger syndrome
- Infective endocarditis (ostium primum defects > ostium secundum defects)
- Perioperative atrial tachyarrhythmias occurred in 10–13% of patients.
- Device embolization (1%), cardiac perforation, thrombus formation, endocarditis, supraventricular arrhythmias postpercutaneous closure

REFERENCES

1. Improved National Prevalence for 18 Selected Major Birth Defects – United States, 1999–2001. *MMWR*. 2006;54(51–54):1301.
2. Hart SA, Krasuski RA et al. Incidence of asymptomatic patent foramen ovale according to age. *Ann Intern Med*. 2009;150:431–2.
3. McMahon CJ, Feltes TF, Fraley JK et al. Natural history of growth of secundum atrial septal defects and implications for transcatheter closure. *Heart*. 2002;87:256–9.
4. Hanslik A, Pospisil U, Salzer-Muhar U, Greber-Platzer S, Male C et al. Predictors of spontaneous closure of isolated secundum atrial septal defect in children: a longitudinal study. *Pediatrics*. 2006; 118:1560–5.
5. Holzer R, Hijazi ZM. Interventional approach to congenital heart disease. *Curr Opin Cardiol*. 2004;19:84–90.
6. Onorato E, Melzi G, Casilli F et al. Patent foramen ovale with paradoxical embolism: mid-term results of transcatheter closure in 256 patients. *J Interv Cardiol*. 2003;16:43–50.
7. Krasuski RA, Hart SA, Allen D, Qureshi A, Pettersson G, Houghtaling PL, Batizy LH, Blackstone E et al. Prevalence and repair of intraoperatively diagnosed patent foramen ovale and association with perioperative outcomes and long-term survival. *JAMA*. 2009;302:290–7.
8. Morandi E, Anzola GP, Angeli S et al. Transcatheter closure of patent foramen ovale: a new migraine treatment? *J Interv Cardiol*. 2003;16:39–42.
9. Attie F, Rosas M, Granados N et al. Surgical treatment for secundum atrial septal defects in patients >40 years old. A randomized clinical trial. *J Am Coll Cardiol*. 2001;38:2035–42.

ADDITIONAL READING

Lindsey J, Hillis L. Clinical update: atrial septal defect in adults. http://www.thelancet.com Vol 369 April 14, 2007.

See Also (Topic, Algorithm, Electronic Media Element)

Aortic Valvular Stenosis; Coarctation of the Aorta; Patent Ductus Arteriosus; Pulmonic Valvular Stenosis; Tetralogy of Fallot; Ventricular Septal Defect

CODES

ICD9

- 745.5 Ostium secundum, type atrial septal defect
- 745.60 Endocardial cushion defect, unspecified type
- 745.61 Ostium primum defect

CLINICAL PEARLS

- ASD is often missed due to subtle clinical presentation.
- Ideally, hemodynamically significant ASDs should be closed in early childhood, though some benefit from closure also is present in older patients.
- Many ASDs can be treated by catheter-directed percutaneous closure, rather than open-heart surgery.
- Routine endocarditis prophylaxis is not recommended for isolated ASDs.
- PFOs, unlike large ASDs, are very common and generally require no treatment in asymptomatic people.

ATTENTION DEFICIT/HYPERACTIVITY DISORDER

Laura L. Novak, MD

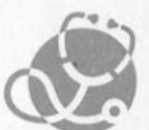

BASICS

DESCRIPTION

- Attention deficit hyperactivity disorder (ADHD) is a behavior problem characterized by a short attention span, distractibility, low frustration tolerance, impulsivity, and hyperactivity.
- ADHD is divided into 3 subsets: predominantly hyperactivity-impulsive, predominantly inattentive, or both.
- System affected: Nervous
- Synonym(s): Attention deficit disorder; Hyperactivity

EPIDEMIOLOGY

- Predominant age: Onset <7 years old; lasts into adolescence and adulthood; 50% meet diagnostic criteria by age 4 years.
- Predominant sex: Male > Female (5:1); predominantly inattentive type may be more common in girls.

Incidence

5% of school-aged children

RISK FACTORS

- Family history
- Comorbid conditions (associated with, but not caused by):
  - Learning disabilities
  - Mood disorders
  - Oppositional defiant disorder
  - Conduct disorder

Genetics

Familial pattern

GENERAL PREVENTION

- Children are at risk for abuse, depression, and social isolation.
- Parents need regular support and advice.
- Parents should establish contact with teacher each school year.

COMMONLY ASSOCIATED CONDITIONS

See Risk Factors

DIAGNOSIS

- American Academy of Pediatrics (AAP) guidelines recommend using the *DSM-IV* criteria to establish the diagnosis.
- Children undergoing extreme stress (divorce, illness, homelessness, abuse) may demonstrate ADHD behaviors secondary to stress. This can be assessed using the American Academy of Child and Adolescent Psychiatry (AACAP) screening tool, if needed.
- If diagnostic behaviors are noted in only one setting, explore the stressors in that setting.
- The diagnostic behaviors are more noticeable in tasks that require concentration or boredom tolerance than in free play or office situations.
- *DSM-IV* criteria: 6 or more inattention criteria and/or 6 or more hyperactivity/impulsivity criteria. Symptoms must begin by age 7 years, be present for >6 months, and be noticed in 2 settings (e.g., home and school). Teachers and caretakers should fill out assessments in addition to parents.
- Inattention:
  - Careless mistakes in tasks
  - Difficulty in sustaining attention
  - Does not seem to listen
  - Does not follow through or finish tasks
  - Difficulty in organizing tasks
  - Avoids tasks that require sustained mental effort
  - Loses things
  - Easily distracted
  - Forgetful
- Hyperactivity/impulsivity:
  - Fidgets
  - Difficulty in remaining seated
  - Runs or climbs excessively
  - Difficulty in playing quietly
  - Acts as if "driven by a motor"
  - Talks excessively
  - Blurts out answers before question is complete
  - Has difficulty in awaiting turn
  - Interrupts others

HISTORY

- Birth and development history
- Comprehensive psychosocial evaluation of home environment
- School performance history

DIAGNOSTIC TESTS & INTERPRETATION

Behavioral testing:

- Behavior rating scales (Connors, others) should be completed by parents and teachers. They are repeated after therapy is started to gauge differences (*DSM-IV* criteria can be used).
- An ADHD toolkit with forms is available from www.nichq.org/adhd.html
- Testing for learning disability (e.g., dyslexia) through the school

Lab

Rarely needed; check lead level if high risk

Diagnostic Procedures/Surgery

- Electroencephalogram not needed unless symptoms are highly suggestive of seizure disorder (e.g., absence seizures).
- Patients with a personal or family history of congenital heart disease or sudden death should be screened with an electrocardiogram (EKG) and possible cardiology consultation before beginning stimulant medication (1).

Pathological Findings

Motor tics can be present (e.g., cough, noises, twitching).

DIFFERENTIAL DIAGNOSIS

- Activity level appropriate for age
- Hearing or vision disorder
- Lead poisoning
- Medication reaction (decongestant, antihistamine, theophylline, phenobarbital)
- Dysfunctional family situation
- Learning disability (e.g., dyslexia)
- Pervasive developmental delay (autism)
- Asperger syndrome: High-functioning autism
- Oppositional/defiant disorder (see *DSM-IV*)
- Conduct disorder (see *DSM-IV*)
- Tourette syndrome: Motor and verbal tics
- Absence seizures (attention deficit only)

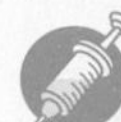

TREATMENT

MEDICATION

First Line

The 2001 AAP guideline recommends (1)[C] the use stimulant medications as 1st-line in treatment. A 2n type of stimulant should be tried if the 1st treatment fails.

ALERT

The Food and Drug Administration (FDA) has considered applying a "black box" warning to stimulants based on some reported cases of sudder death seen in patients using stimulant medications. It recommends that patients with a personal or family history of congenital heart disease or sudden death be screened with an EKG and possible cardiology consultation before beginning stimulant medication.

- Stimulant:
  - Methylphenidate (Ritalin, Concerta, Metadate C Ritalin LA, others):
    - Short-acting: Ritalin 5–20 mg in the morning, noon, and at 4 p.m.; maximum dose, 60 mg/d
    - Long-acting: Concerta 18, 36, 54 mg in the morning; Metadate CD 40 mg in the morning; Ritalin LA 20, 30, 40 mg in the morning
    - Methylphenidate patch (Daytrana): Apply to hi for up to 9 hours daily. Begin at 10 mg and titrate upward weekly as needed. Available as 10, 15, 20, and 30 mg.
  - Amphetamines:
    - Adderall: 2.5–20 mg q4–6h
    - Adderall XR: 5–30 mg every morning; ≥6 year
- Precautions:
  - If not responding, check compliance and conside another diagnosis (1)[C].
  - Some children experience withdrawal (tearfulnes agitation) after a missed dose or when medicatic wears off.
  - Stimulants are drugs of abuse and should be monitored carefully.
  - Drug holidays should be given only if family/peer relationships are not harmed.
- Significant possible interactions:
  - Stimulants may increase levels of anticonvulsants selective serotonin reuptake inhibitors (SSRIs), tricyclics, and warfarin.

Pregnancy Considerations

Medications used in ADHD are Category C: Caution i pregnancy.

Second Line

- Nonstimulant:
  - Atomoxetine carries a "black box" warning regarding potential exacerbation of suicidality (similar to selective serotonin reuptake inhibitors). Because of this, the manufacturer recommends weekly visits for 4 sessions, then every-other-wee visits for 4 sessions, then every-12-weeks visits. Atomoxetine has also been associated with hepatic injury in a small number of cases, and the manufacturer recommends checking liver enzyme if symptoms (jaundice, fatigue, malaise) develop.

- Atomoxetine (Strattera): Selective norepinephrine reuptake inhibitor; 0.5–2 mg/kg/d every morning (10 mg, 18 mg, 25 mg, 40 mg, 60 mg). Maximum dose, 1.4 mg/kg/d or 100 mg/d, whichever is less:
  - Slower onset of efficacy; gastrointestinal side effects and sedation. Not addictive.
- Atomoxetine interacts with paroxetine (Paxil), fluoxetine (Prozac), and quinidine.

Other nonstimulant drugs (e.g., clonidine, tricyclic antidepressants, SSRIs): Owing to the mixed efficacy and high side effects of these drugs, they are not recommended for use without a consultant.

DDITIONAL TREATMENT

Medication alone or combined with behavioral therapy produced better results than behavioral therapy alone.

Behavioral therapy may be useful in cases where parents object to medication (2).

eneral Measures

Parent/school/patient education (2)

Work closely with teacher.

Avoid unproven therapies.

OMPLEMENTARY AND ALTERNATIVE IEDICINE

Surveys have shown that parents of children with ADHD use herbals and complementary treatments frequently (20–60%) (3,4).

Many herbals have been assessed for efficacy, but studies are small and brief and, therefore, difficult to translate into clinical recommendations.

Dietary and nutritional supplements have also been assessed:
- Omega-3 fatty acids (found in fish oil and some supplements) showed improvement in rating scales in 2 double-blind, placebo-controlled studies of 116 and 130 patients

Rapid eye training and biofeedback have contradictory results and can be costly.

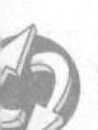

ONGOING CARE

ne "toolkit for physicians" may be useful: http://www.nichq.org/adhd.html

OLLOW-UP RECOMMENDATIONS

atient Monitoring

Parent/teacher rating scales initially, 2 weeks after an intervention such as starting medication, and regularly

Office visits to monitor side effects and efficacy: Endpoints are improved grades, improved rating scales, acceptable family interactions, and improved peer interactions.

Monitor growth (especially weight gain) and blood pressure.

IET

Insufficient evidence exists to suggest that dietary terventions improve the symptoms of ADHD in hildren" (5).

PATIENT EDUCATION

- Key points for parents:
  - 50% of children with ADHD have 1 parent with ADHD; modify education sessions with parents accordingly.
  - Behavioral interventions such as token systems may be helpful (1)[A].
  - Find things child is good at and emphasize these.
  - Reinforce good behavior (with rewards and attention).
  - Make eye contact with each request.
  - Give one task at a time.
  - Stop behavior before it escalates.
  - Some families benefit from "parent training" and family therapy.
  - Coordinate homework with teachers using daily assignment notebook.
  - Refer to advocacy and support groups.
- Schools are required by law to provide necessary testing and Individualized Educational Plans (IEPs) or 504 plans to accommodate the child's educational needs
- Support groups:
  - Children and Adults with Attention Deficit Disorder (CHADD): chadd.org; 800-233-4050
  - Attention Deficit Disorder Warehouse: addwarehouse.com; 800-233-9273
  - Learning Disabilities Association (LDA): LDAlearning.com
  - National Information Center for Children and Youth with Disabilities: www.nichcy.org

PROGNOSIS

- May last into adulthood
- The hyperactivity component may become easier to control with increasing age.
- Encourage career choices that allow autonomy and mobility.
- With treatment, there is no increased incidence of delinquency unless other comorbid features exist (e.g., conduct disorder).
- Encourage parents to subtract 2 years from their child's chronological age when allowing privileges (e.g., treat a 16-year-old like a 14-year-old, delay driving until age 18).

COMPLICATIONS

- Untreated ADHD can lead to failing school, parental abuse, social isolation, and poor self-esteem.
- Some children experience withdrawal (tearfulness, agitation) after a missed medication dose or when medication wears off.
- If appetite is poor as a side effect of stimulant medication, offer small frequent meals.

REFERENCES

1. American Academy of Pediatrics. Subcommittee on Attention-Deficit/Hyperactivity Disorder and Committee on Quality Improvement. Clinical practice guideline: treatment of the school-aged child with attention-deficit/hyperactivity disorder. *Pediatrics*. 2001;108:1033–44.
2. Laforett DR, Murray DW, Kollins SH. Psychosocial treatments for preschool-aged children with Attention-Deficit Hyperactivity Disorder. *Dev Disabil Res Rev*. 2008;14:300–10.
3. Sawni A. Attention-deficit/hyperactivity disorder and complementary/alternative medicine. *Adolesc Med State Art Rev*. 2008;19:313–26, xi.
4. Weber W, Newmark S. Complementary and alternative medical therapies for attention-deficit/hyperactivity disorder and autism. *Pediatr Clin North Am*. 2007;54:983–1006; xii.
5. Sinn N. Nutritional and dietary influences on attention deficit hyperactivity disorder. *Nutr Rev*. 2008;66:558–68.

ADDITIONAL READING

- *American Psychiatric Association. Diagnostic and Statistical Manual of Mental Disorders*. 4th ed. Revised. Washington, DC: American Psychiatric Association, 2000.
- Barkley RA. *ADHD: A Handbook for Diagnosis and Treatment*. 2nd ed. New York: Guilford Press, 1998.
- Brown RT, Amler RW, Freeman WS, et al. Treatment of attention deficit/hyperactivity disorder: Overview of the evidence. *Pediatrics*. 2005;115(6): e749–e757.
- Ghuman JK, Arnold LE, Anthony BJ. Psychopharmacological and other treatments in preschool children with attention-deficit/hyperactivity disorder: Current Evidence and Practice. *J Child Adolesc Psychopharmacol*. 2008.
- Pliszka S, AACAP Work Group on Quality Issues. Practice parameter for the assessment and treatment of children and adolescents with attention-deficit/hyperactivity disorder. *J Am Acad Child Adolesc Psychiatry*. 2007;46:894–921.
- Rader R, McCauley L, Callen EC. Current strategies in the diagnosis and treatment of childhood attention-deficit/hyperactivity disorder. *Am Fam Physician*. 2009;79:657–65.
- Rappley, MD. attention deficit-hyperactivity disorder. *N Engl J Med*. 2005;352(2):165–73.
- Rostain AL. Attention-deficit/hyperactivity disorder in adults: evidence-based recommendations for management. *Postgrad Med*. 2008;120:27–38.
- Soileau EJ. Medications for adolescents with attention-deficit/hyperactivity disorder. *Adolesc Med State Art Rev*. 2008;19:254–67, viii–ix.

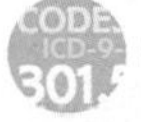

CODES

ICD9

- 314.00 Attention deficit disorder of childhood without mention of hyperactivity
- 314.01 Attention deficit disorder of childhood with hyperactivity

CLINICAL PEARLS

- Children undergoing extreme stress (divorce, illness, homelessness, abuse) may demonstrate ADHD behaviors secondary to stress.
- 50% of ADHD children have a parent with ADHD.
- AAP recommends the use of stimulant medications as the 1st-line treatment.

AUTISM SPECTRUM DISORDERS

Macario C. Corpuz, Jr., MD
Alphonsus K. Kung, MD

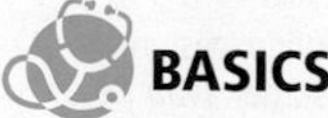

BASICS

DESCRIPTION
Group of neurodevelopmental disorders of early childhood
- Includes autistic disorder, Rett disorder, childhood disintegrative disorder, Asperger disorder, and pervasive developmental disorder not otherwise specified (PDD-NOS)
- Autistic disorder includes classic autism and childhood autism.
- Rett disorder involves mutations in the MECP2 gene. Mostly in females with initial normal development until approximately 18 months of age with microcephaly and dementia.
- Childhood disintegrative disorder: Regression after at least 2 years of normal development
- Asperger disorder: Better development with mechanics of verbal expression, higher levels of cognition and interest in social activity
- PDD-NOS: Meet some, but not all of DSM-IV-TR criteria for autistic disorder
- Characterized by:
  - Impairment of effective social skills
  - Absent or impaired communication skills
  - Repetitive and/or stereotyped behaviors and interests, especially in inanimate objects
  - System(s) affected: Nervous

EPIDEMIOLOGY
- Predominant age: Onset in early childhood
- Predominant sex: Male > Female (4:1) except for Rett disorder

Pediatric Considerations
Symptom onset seen in children <3 years (except for childhood disintegrative disorder)

Prevalence
Estimated 1/100 to 1/500 children

RISK FACTORS
Siblings with autism have shown to have a 5× greater risk of developing autism. Prevalence ranging from 2% to 8%.

Pregnancy Considerations
Siblings with autism have shown to have a 5× greater risk of developing autism. Prevalence ranging from 2% to 8%.

Genetics
- High concordance in monozygotic twins
- Increased recurrence risk (3–7%) in subsequent siblings

GENERAL PREVENTION
- Early screening for early treatment = better prognosis.
- Some ASDs such as Rett disorder are known to be caused by genetic mutations.

PATHOPHYSIOLOGY
Pathophysiology is incompletely understood.

ETIOLOGY
- No single cause has been identified.
- General consensus: A genetic abnormality leads to altered neurologic development.
- Research continues to investigate the links between heredity, genetics, and medical problems.
- No documented scientific evidence exists that proves vaccines or thimerosal cause ASDs.

COMMONLY ASSOCIATED CONDITIONS
- Mental retardation
- Attention deficit/hyperactivity disorder (ADHD)
- Phenylketonuria (PKU), tuberous sclerosis, fragile X syndrome, Angelman syndrome, and fetal alcohol syndrome (rare)
- Anxiety
- Depression
- Obsessive behavior
- Seizures (increased risk if severe mental retardation)

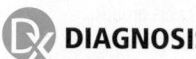

DIAGNOSIS

HISTORY
- Impairment in social interaction:
  - Impairment in nonverbal behaviors such as eye-to-eye gaze, facial expression
  - Unable to develop peer relationships
  - Does not smile nor share emotions
  - Loss of social or emotional reciprocity
- Communication impairment:
  - Delay or lack of development in language skills
  - Inability to initiate or sustain conversation
  - Stereotyped and repetitive use of language
  - Preoccupation with parts of toys or body parts
- Repetitive and stereotyped patterns of behavior:
  - Excessively lines up toys or other objects
  - Unusually attached to 1 particular toy or object
  - Repetitive odd movements (toe walking, hand flapping)
  - Adherence to specific routines or rituals
- Asperger disorder does not have clinically significant delays in cognitive development, language acquisitions, nor learning/adaptive skills.
- Rett disorder is predominantly in females without macrocephaly.
- Childhood disintegrative disorder with normal development until 2 years of age
- PDD-NOS does not meet DSM-IV-TR criteria for autism.
- Prenatal, neonatal, and developmental history
- Seizure disorder
- Family history of autism, genetic disorders, learning disabilities, psychiatric illness, neurological disorders, genetic disorders, or mental retardation

PHYSICAL EXAM
- Macrocephaly in 25% (except in Rett syndrome); head circumference growth peaks at age 6 months and begins to decline by 1 year.
- Dysmorphic features consistent with genetic disorder (fragile X syndrome)
- Hypotonia can occur in autism, but neurological deficit is a sign that imaging may be needed.
- Wood lamp skin exam to rule out tuberous sclerosis

DIAGNOSTIC TESTS & INTERPRETATION
- Checklist for Autism in Toddlers (CHAT) to screen for ASDs at 18 months of age. (To order: http:// www.nas.org.uk/nas/jsp/polopoly.jsp.)
- The Pervasive Developmental Disorders Screening Test-II (PDDST-II) to screen for ASDs beginning at 18 months
- Modified Checklist for Autism in Toddlers (M-CHAT) to screen for ASDs at 16–30 months
- Social Communication Questionnaire (SCQ) (formerly Autism Screening Questionnaire)—used with children age 4 years and older—the gold-standard diagnostic interview used in research studies

Lab
- Lead screening
- PKU screening
- Karyotype and DNA analysis (fragile X, PKU, tuberous sclerosis, and others)
- Metabolic testing if signs of:
  - Lethargy, limited endurance
  - Hypotonia
  - Recurrent vomiting and dehydration
  - Developmental regression
  - Unusual habits
  - Specific food intolerance

Follow-Up & Special Considerations
- Hearing tests: Audiometry and BAERS
- Comprehensive speech and language evaluation
- Evaluation by multidisciplinary team: Includes a psychiatrist, neurologist, psychologist, speech therapist, and other autism specialists
- Intellectual level needs to be established and monitored, as it is one of the best measures of prognosis.
- Test used to follow autism are:
  - Autism Behavior Checklist (ABC)
  - Gilliam Autism Rating Scale (GARS)
  - Childhood Autism Rating Scale (CARS)
  - Autism Diagnosis Interview-Revised (ADI-R)
  - Autism Diagnostic Observation Schedule-Generic (ADOS-G) Imaging

Imaging
Initial approach
Magnetic resonance imaging (MRI) useful only if focal neurologic symptoms

Diagnostic Procedures/Surgery
Electroencephalogram (EEG) only if history of seizure or spells

DIFFERENTIAL DIAGNOSIS
Other mental and central nervous system (CNS) disorders:
- Obsessive-compulsive disorder
- Elective mutism
- Language disorder/hearing impairment
- Intellectual disability/global developmental delay
- Stereotyped movement disorder
- Severe early deprivation/reactive attachment disorder
- Anxiety disorder
- Developmental language disorder

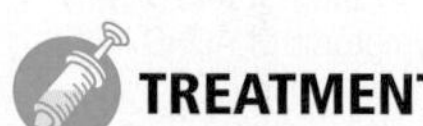

TREATMENT

MEDICATION
Medical causes of autistic-like behavior should be excluded with behavioral management maximized prior to considering medication with symptom-specific therapy, as pharmacological therapy data are scant.

First Line
- No true 1st-line medical therapy
- Stimulant medications (such as methylphenidate): Efficacious in treating concomitant symptoms of attention deficit disorder, such as impulsiveness,

yperactivity, and inattention; however, the agnitude of response is less than in typically eveloping children, and adverse effects are more equent.

elective serotonin reuptake inhibitors (SSRIs) have own some help in reducing ritualistic behavior nd improving mood and language skills. Initial oice for anxiety and depressive mood. Also dministered for dysregulated mood (1).

speridone (an atypical antipsychotic) has been own to be effective for short-term treatment of ntrums, aggression, and self-injurious behavior. nprovements in stereotyped behavior, hyperactivity, itability, repetitious behaviors, and social ithdrawal have also been noted (2)[A].

ecautions: Causes weight gain as an adverse fect. Associated with sedation, dry mouth, gitation enuresis, dyspepsia, diarrhea, onstipation, and tremor.

cond Line

min B6 and magnesium with inconclusive ence in improving speech and language (3,4)[C].

DITIONAL TREATMENT

neral Measures

omprehensive structured educational programming a sustained and intensive design, most commonly pplied behavioral analysis therapy

ore features of a successful education program:
- High staff–student ratio 1:2 or less
- Individualized programming
- Specialized teacher training with ongoing evaluation of teachers and programs
- 25 hours a week minimum of specialized services
- A structured routine environment that emphasizes attention, imitation, communication, socialization, and play interactions
- Functional analysis of behavioral problems
- Transition planning and involvement of the family

urrently no cure for ASDs. Early diagnosis and itiation of multidisciplinary intervention help nhance functioning in later life.

arly intervention for ages 3 and under

chool-based special education for older children

nd alternative methods of communication: Sign nguage; picture exchange communication system

ues for Referral

efer early to:
- Early learning for evaluation of behavior and language
- Genetic counseling
- Audiology

onsider referrals to psychiatry, ophthalmology, tolaryngology, neurology, and nutrition

efer family members to parent support groups and spite programs

MPLEMENTARY AND ALTERNATIVE DICINE

lusic therapy has been shown to improve ommunication skills in autistic patients with limited ata (5)[B].

uditory integration training is used for autistic ildren with sound sensitivity (6)[B].

steopathic manipulative therapy (OMT) has been own to improve sensory and motor performance ith neurological problems, including autism. eatment that starts before the age of 2 years owed the greatest effect (7)[C].

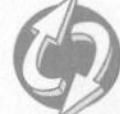

ONGOING CARE

FOLLOW-UP RECOMMENDATIONS

Patient Monitoring

- Constant by caregivers
- Reevaluation every 6–12 months by physician for seizures, sleep and nutritional problems, and prescribed medical management
- Intellectual and language testing every 2 years in childhood

DIET

Gluten- and casein-free diets show some reduction in autistic traits; however, large-scale, good-quality randomized controlled trials are needed (8).

PATIENT EDUCATION

- Autism Society of America: http://www.autismsociety.org.
- The Centers for Disease Control and Prevention, Autism Info. Center: http://www.cdc.gov/ncbddd/autism/index.htm
- The Centers for Disease Control and Prevention, "Learn the Signs. Act Early": http://www.cdc.gov/ncbddd/autism/actearly
- First Signs: http://www.firstsigns.org
- Autism Speaks: http://www.autismspeaks.org/index2.php
- Supplemental security income: http://www.socialsecurity.gov/ssi/index.htm
- Autism and vaccines: http://www.aap.org/immunization/families/faq/VaccineStudies.pdf

PROGNOSIS

- Those who begin treatment at a young age (2–4 years) have significantly better outcomes.
- Prognosis is closely related to initial intellectual abilities, with only 20% functioning above the mentally retarded level.
- Communicative language development before 5 years is also associated with a better outcome.
- The general expected course is for a lifelong need for supervised structured care.

COMPLICATIONS

- Increasing incidents of seizure disorders in up to 1 in 4 children.
- Increased risk for physical and sexual abuse
- If pica, increased risk of lead poisoning
- Limited variety of food consumed due to dietary obsessions
- Increased risk for gastrointestinal symptoms, including weight abnormalities and abnormal stool patterns

REFERENCES

1. Selective serotonin reuptake inhibitors (SSRIs) for autism spectrum disorders (ASD). Williams, Katrina. Wheeler, Danielle M. Silove, Natalie. Hazell, Philip. *Cochrane Developmental, Psychosocial and Learning Problems Group Cochrane Database of Systematic Reviews*. 8, 2010.
2. Risperdone for autistic spectrum disorder. Jesner, Ora S. Aref-Adib, Mehrnoosh. Coren, Esther. *Cochrane Developmental, Psychosocial and Learning Problems Group Cochrane Database of Systematic Reviews*. 1, 2009.
3. Vitamin B6 for cognition. Malouf, Reem. Grimley Evans, John. *Cochrane Dementia and Cognitive Improvement Group Cochrane Database of Systematic Reviews*. 1, 2009.
4. Combined vitamin B6-magnesium treatment in autism spectrum disorder. Nye, Chad. Brice, Alejandro. *Cochrane Developmental, Psychosocial and Learning Problems Group Cochrane Database of Systematic Reviews*. 1, 2009.
5. Music therapy for autistic spectrum disorder. Gold, Christian. Wigram, Tony. Elefant, Cochavit. *Cochrane Developmental, Psychosocial and Learning Problems Group Cochrane Database of Systematic. Reviews*. 1, 2009.
6. Auditory integration training and other sound therapies for autism spectrum disorders. Sinha, Yashwant. Silove, Natalie. Wheeler, Danielle M. Williams, Katrina J. *Cochrane Developmental, Psychosocial and Learning Problems Group Cochrane Database of Systematic Reviews*. 1, 2009.
7. Frymann VM, Carney RE, Springall P. Effect of osteopathic medical management on neurologic development in children. *J Am Osteopath Assoc*. 1992;92:729–44.
8. Gluten- and casein-free diets for autistic spectrum disorder. Millward, Claire. Ferriter, Michael. Calver, Sarah J. Connell-Jones, Graham G. *Cochrane Developmental, Psychosocial and Learning Problems Group Cochrane Database of Systematic Reviews*. 1, 2009.

See Also (Topic, Algorithm, Electronic Media Element)

Algorithm: Mental Retardation

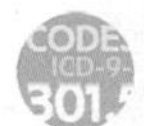

CODES

ICD9

- 299.00 Infantile autism, current or active state
- 299.10 Disintegrative psychosis, current or active state
- 299.80 Other specified early childhood psychoses, current or active state

CLINICAL PEARLS

ALARM mnemonic from the American Academy of Pediatrics (AAP):

- Autism spectrum disorder is prevalent (screen ALL children between 18–24 months).
- Listen to parents when they feel something is wrong.
- Act early: Screen all children who fall behind in language and social developmental milestones (use early learning to help with evaluation).
- Refer to multidisciplinary teams (speech and language evaluation, genetic screening, social support groups).
- Monitor support for patient and families.

AUTONOMIC DYSREFLEXIA

Shashidhara Nanjundaswamy, MD, MBBS, MRCP, DM
Madaiah Lokeshwari, MD

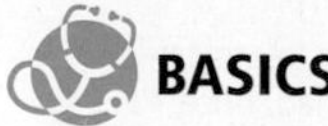

BASICS

DESCRIPTION

A medical emergency characterized by a sudden, dangerously elevated blood pressure (BP) due to a massive sympathetic/catecholamine surge in patients with spinal cord injury (SCI) above the level of T6 in response to a noxious stimulus below the level of injury.

EPIDEMIOLOGY

Incidence

- 16% of children and adolescents with SCI
- 50–90% of adults with SCI above level of T6; more common with complete SCI; rarely seen with lesions down to T10.
- Occurs 4 times more frequently in men:
  - Can occur as early as 2 months and as late as 12 years after the SCI
  - Occurs most often in the 1st year after SCI
  - Frequency varies from daily to once in a few years.

Pediatric Considerations

- Because of lower incidence of SCI in children, autonomic dysreflexia (AD) is often unrecognized or inappropriately treated.
- Recommendations include giving the nationally standardized guidelines to the child's primary care physician and school, along with the child's baseline BP and a description of AD (1)[A].

Pregnancy Considerations

- Occurs during labor in 2/3 of pregnancies in patients with SCI at or above T6 level.
- AD can occur in antepartum, intrapartum, and postpartum periods. AD should be recognized and treated early by all health care providers dealing with pregnant women to minimize the risk of intracranial bleeding and death.

RISK FACTORS

Spinal cord lesion at or above level T5–6, rarely as low as T10:

- Any unpleasant stimulus below the lesion can cause AD.
- Bladder distention (most common cause):
  - Urinary retention/blocked catheter
  - Detrusor sphincter dyssynergia
  - Urinary tract infection
  - Urinary calculi
  - Instrumentation
  - Cystoscopy
  - Urodynamics
  - Bladder irrigation
- Fecal impaction (2nd most common cause):
  - Bowel impaction
  - Anal fissure
  - Rectal digital disimpaction
  - Rectal exam
  - Enema administration
- Other:
  - Ingrown toe nails
  - Painful stimulus of any etiology
  - All causes of acute abdomen
  - Burns
  - Labor
  - Sexual intercourse
  - Pressure sore
  - Testicular torsion
  - Fracture dislocation
  - Heterotopic ossification
  - Pregnancy
  - Electroejaculation for sperm retrieval

GENERAL PREVENTION

- Good bladder and bowel care
- Use lubricant for catheter insertion or fecal digital disimpaction.
- Lubricants for instrumentation
- Use of local anesthetics for procedures below the level of SCI even if patient does not feel pain.

PATHOPHYSIOLOGY

- In AD, a disconnect occurs between the sympathetic and parasympathetic nervous systems.
- AD does not occur during the spinal shock phase. It occurs once the spinal shock phase is over and the spinal reflexes start returning. Any noxious stimulus below the level of SCI creates a volley of impulses that are transmitted via the intact peripheral nerves through the spinothalamic and posterior columns to the sympathetic neurons in the intermediolateral cell column of the thoracic spinal cord. Inhibitory responses from the cerebral vasomotor centers, although increased, are blocked by the SCI. The unopposed sympathetic outflow (as the parasympathetic outflow cannot reach below the level of SCI) causes massive release of neurotransmitters norepinephrine, dopamine-b-hydroxylase, dopamine, which result in piloerection, skin pallor, and severe vasoconstriction of the arterial vasculature, thus resulting in sudden elevation of BP and vasodilatation above the level of injury.
- Baroreceptors located in the cerebral vessels, carotid sinus, and aorta detect the rising BP and attempt to trigger visceral and peripheral vasodilatation, but the impulses cannot pass through the damaged spinal cord. The parasympathetic response is limited to vagal slowing of the heart rate and vasodilatation, flushing, nasal congestion, and diaphoresis above the level of spinal cord injury.
- SCI below the T6 level very rarely causes AD as the intact splanchnic innervation allows compensatory dilatation of the splanchnic vascular bed.

ETIOLOGY

SCI above the T5–6 level

DIAGNOSIS

AD is a clinical diagnosis and hence all personnel dealing with SCI patients should be aware of the clinical symptomatology/presentation.

HISTORY

- Pounding headache (due to elevated BP and vasodilatation of pain-sensitive intracranial vasculature)
- Piloerection (goose bumps above the level of lesio less often below the level
- Profuse sweating above the level of lesion could b the 1st sign.
- Flushing above the level of lesion
- Nasal congestion
- Chest pain
- Palpitations
- Dyspnea due to neurogenic pulmonary edema
- Nausea and malaise secondary to parasympathetic/vagal stimulation
- Blurred vision
- Mydriasis
- Rarely, absent symptoms
- Triad of bitemporal throbbing headache, head and neck sweating, and systolic hypertension.

PHYSICAL EXAM

- BP 20–40 mm Hg above range for the patient
- BP 15–20 mm Hg above baseline in adolescents
- BP 15 mm Hg above baseline in children
- Normal BP for a quadriplegic could be 90/60 mm Hg, hence even 120/80 mm Hg could indicate AD.
- Mild increase in BP initially and if untreated
- Further elevation to 200/100 or higher when it becomes a life-threatening medical emergency
- Systolic BP as high as 250–300 mm Hg and diasto pressure as high as 200–220 mm Hg have been reported.
- Reflex bradycardia secondary to vagal stimulation, usually a relative bradycardia with heart rate in the normal range
- Piloerection
- Tachycardia, rarely
- Profuse sweating above the level of the lesion
- Flushing, red skin above the level due to vasodilatation
- Nasal congestion
- Cold, pale skin due to vasoconstriction below the level of the injury
- Blotchy skin above the level of the lesion
- Blurred vision
- Retinal hemorrhages
- Minimal or no symptoms despite an elevated BP (silent AD)
- Rarely, seizures

DIAGNOSTIC TESTS & INTERPRETATION

No diagnostic lab test or imaging makes the diagnos of AD. Clinical suspicion and physical exam are paramount in making a diagnosis of this rare, potentially reversible life-threatening condition.

maging

ead CT scan if patient complains of worst headache his life or is in altered sensorium or has new focal urologic deficits, as abrupt increase in BP could use cerebral hemorrhage

IFFERENTIAL DIAGNOSIS

Spinal cord plaque above T6 in multiple sclerosis
Coexisting catecholamine-secreting tumor in SCI patients (symptoms similar to AD related to catecholamines released from the tumor)
Eclampsia

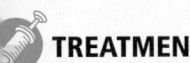

TREATMENT

onpharmacologic treatment must be tried mediately: Removing noxious stimuli, sitting patient), and loosening clothing.

IEDICATION

ntihypertensive agents with rapid onset and short uration of action, while sorting out the etiology or if e SBP is >150 mm Hg. BP should be lowered ithout causing hypotension, prior to checking for cal impaction or digital stimulation. BPs above 40 mm Hg in an adolescent, 130 mm Hg in children -12 years old, or 120 mm Hg in children <5 years d will necessitate initiation of medications (2,3)[A].

irst Line

Nifedipine immediate-release form, 10-mg cap initially; bite and swallow is the mainstay of therapy (3)[A].
- However, severe hypotension can be caused by the short-acting form of nifedipine.
- This hypotension can be avoided by using a pin or needle to puncture the nifedipine capsule and administering the liquid medication 1 drop at a time to titrate to effectiveness.
- The dose of nifedipine can be repeated in 15 minutes if needed. Care should be exercised to avoid hypotension, especially in older patients, and with coronary artery as well as cerebrovascular disease.

Nitrates: Sublingual 0.4-mg spray; second most commonly used drug in patients with SCI (2)[B]
2% nitroglycerine ointment, 0.5- to 1-inch strip to chest wall (above the level of the lesion) and titrate as needed; this is safer but slower.
Nitroglycerine: 0.15- to 0.6-mg tab SL
Nitrates are contraindicated if patient has taken any phosphodiesterase inhibitors such as sildenafil (Viagra), vardenafil (Levitra) within the past 24 hours or tadalafil (Cialis) within the previous 48 hours.

econd Line

Prazosin 0.5–1 mg PO q8h prn for prophylaxis of AD (3)[A]
Captopril 25 mg PO sublingually during AD (2)[B]
Terazosin (3)[A]
Clonidine: 0.1–0.3 mg PO q 8h to a maximum of 0.8 mg

DDITIONAL TREATMENT

ssues for Referral

regnant women with a SCI at T6 or above with atures of AD should be referred to an obstetrician if:
Life-threatening AD
1st episode of AD
AD in the 3rd trimester
- Vaginal bleeding or suspected labor
- Persistent symptoms despite treatment
- Choice of antihypertensive therapy

Additional Therapies

- Physical therapy
- Therapists should be aware of AD, its manifestations, and general measures of treatment.
- When AD suspected, patient should be supported to sit upright.
- If stretching exercise evoked the episode of AD, it should be stopped.

SURGERY/OTHER PROCEDURES

Transurethral sphincterotomy for chronic form of AD that is related to detrusor sphincter dyssynergia and overdistention of bladder

IN-PATIENT CONSIDERATIONS

Initial Stabilization

- Treatment should be initiated as quickly as possible.
- Most important step is removal of the causative noxious stimulus:
  - Patient should be helped to sit upright as venous pooling helps reduce the BP.
  - Loosen any constrictive clothing or devices.
  - Pressure relief should be tried.
  - Check the urinary catheter to make sure it is not kinked and is draining.
  - Irrigate a blocked catheter to reestablish drainage and irrigate bladder with 60 mL of 2% lidocaine. If unsuccessful, remove the catheter, insert 2% lidocaine jelly into the urethra; 30 minutes later insert a new catheter.
  - Do not allow bag to get full.
  - Gentle rectal exam using lidocaine jelly, as rectal exam of a spastic anal sphincter can aggravate AD.
  - Rectal disimpaction if constipated, using lidocaine jelly (unless procedure started AD)
  - If BP is significantly elevated, it may need to be lowered before checking for fecal impaction or digital stimulation.

Admission Criteria

- Poor response to treatment
- Undetermined precipitant of AD
- Obstetrical complications
- Transfer to ICU if antihypertensive measures fail, for IV hypotensive agents, including nitroprusside, 0.5 mcg/min IV (contraindicated with previous sildenafil use) and possibly spinal anesthesia.
- Epidural anesthesia in pregnant woman with AD during labor (4)

Nursing

Monitor BP frequently, every 5 minutes until normal, and then every 30 minutes for 4 hours, as BP tends to fluctuate during AD.

Discharge Criteria

- BP and pulse back to patient's norm
- Asymptomatic, no signs of cardiac failure or raised intracranial pressure
- Etiology of the AD is ascertained.

ONGOING CARE

FOLLOW-UP RECOMMENDATIONS

- Detailed medical evaluation if recurrent AD
- Patient and family education regarding early recognition of AD and its prevention
- For recurrent AD, consider the alpha blocker prazosin.

Patient Monitoring

Monitor symptoms and BP for at least 2 hours after resolution of AD because of risk of developing hypotension.

PATIENT EDUCATION

- Most important strategy is to prevent AD.
- All patients prone to develop AD should be counseled about the causes, manifestations, prevention, and treatment of AD.
- Optimal bladder and bowel care
- Patients should carry a Medic Alert bracelet informing of their risk of developing AD.
- Patients should carry AD emergency medical card summarizing the causes of AD and its treatment.
- Educate all health professionals who deal with SCI patients.

PROGNOSIS

Life-threatening if unrecognized and untreated due to massive elevation in BP

COMPLICATIONS

- Retinal, cerebral, and subarachnoid hemorrhage
- Myocardial infarction
- Seizures
- Cardiac arrest secondary to vagal overreactivity and death.

REFERENCES

1. McGinnis KB, Vogel LC, McDonald CM et al. Recognition and management of autonomic dysreflexia in pediatric spinal cord injury. *J Spinal Cord Med*. 2004;27(Suppl 1):S61–74.
2. Consortium for Spinal Cord Medicine. *Acute management of autonomic dysreflexia*, 2nd ed. Clinical Practice Guidelines, 2001.
3. Krassioukov A, Warburton DE, Teasell R, Eng JJ, Spinal Cord Injury Rehabilitation Evidence Research Team et al. A systematic review of the management of autonomic dysreflexia after spinal cord injury. *Arch Phys Med Rehabil*. 2009;90:682–95.
4. Pereira L. Obstetric management of the patient with spinal cord injury. *Obstet Gynecol Surv*. 2003;58:678–87.

ADDITIONAL READING

- Gall A, Turner-Stokes L, Guideline Development Group. Chronic spinal cord injury: management of patients in acute hospital settings. *Clin Med*. 2008;8:70–4.
- Weaver LC, Marsh DR, Gris D, Brown A, Dekaban GA et al. Autonomic dysreflexia after spinal cord injury: central mechanisms and strategies for prevention. *Prog Brain Res*. 2006;152:245–63.

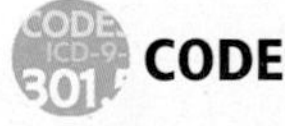

CODES

ICD9
337.3 Autonomic dysreflexia

CLINICAL PEARLS

- AD is a potentially life-threatening but reversible disorder, so early recognition and prevention is vital.
- Normal BP for a quadriplegic could be 90/60 mm Hg; hence even 120/80 mm Hg could indicate AD.

AVIAN FLU

Sheila M. Seed, PharmD, MPH
Walter K. Goljan, MD

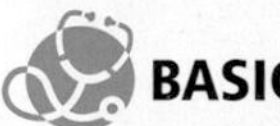

BASICS

DESCRIPTION

- Avian influenza A subtype H5N1 is a highly pathogenic and aggressive form of influenza.
- Presents with influenzalike symptoms, with lower respiratory tract symptoms (limited upper respiratory tract symptoms)
- High mortality rate in elderly and very young

EPIDEMIOLOGY

Incidence

- More than 490 confirmed human cases (60% fatality rate); primarily in Asia
- Predominate age: All age groups

Prevalence

Rare

RISK FACTORS

- Direct contact with H5N1 virus
- Contact with infected poultry
- Close contact with infected person
- Travel to affected country within 10 days of symptom onset

GENERAL PREVENTION

- Consider with any patient with influenzalike symptoms who has had close contact with H5N1 or ill poultry
- 2007: Food and Drug Administration approved a vaccine for adults 18–65. Currently only available from the government.
- Chemoprophylaxis with antivirals should be considered if H5N1 is circulating in the community.
- Ongoing environmental screening is more accessible now with availability of avian fecal testing (1)[B].

ETIOLOGY

- Infected poultry (domesticated ducks, turkeys, chickens)
- Low incidence of human-to-human transmission in household clusters and health care workers
- Incubation period: 7 days (range 2–3 days)

COMMONLY ASSOCIATED CONDITIONS

Severe respiratory distress (common in severe cases)

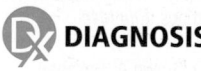

DIAGNOSIS

- Primary phase (2,3)[A]:
  - Influenzalike symptoms with lower respiratory tract symptoms
  - Temp >100.4°F (38°C)
  - Cough
  - Sore throat
  - Shortness of breath
  - Diarrhea (watery without blood)
  - Pleuritic pain
  - Bleeding of nose and gums
  - Conjunctivitis (rare)
- Secondary acute phase:
  - Severe respiratory distress
  - Pneumonia not responsive to antibiotics
  - Multiorgan dysfunction
- Respiratory (2,3)[A]:
  - Respiratory distress
  - Tachypnea
  - Inspiratory crackles

HISTORY

- Known close contact with suspected or confirmed case
- Close contact with infected poultry
- Travel within 10 days in high-risk area

DIAGNOSTIC TESTS & INTERPRETATION

Lab

Initial lab tests

- Complete blood count (CBC) with differential
- Liver profile
- Chemical profile
- Blood culture
- Lab abnormalities (2,4)[A]:
  - Leukopenia (mainly lymphopenia)
  - Thrombocytopenia (mild-to-moderate)
  - Elevated aminotransferases (slight-to-moderate)
  - Decreased leukocyte, platelet, and lymphocyte counts are associated with increased risk of death.

Imaging

Initial approach

Chest x-ray (CXR): Consolidation bilateral and multifocal (2,3)[A]:

- After 7 days: Patchy lobar and interstitial infiltrates
- Pleural effusions with cavitation (less common)

Follow-Up & Special Considerations

- Admit to negative-pressure room; if not available, cohort with other confirmed cases.
- Supplemental oxygen is essential to keep SaO_2 >90% (3)[A].

Diagnostic Procedures/Surgery

Lab confirmation of H5N1 virus is done case-by-case and requires 1 of the following (2,5)[A]:

- Positive influenza A/H5 (Asian lineage) virus real-time reverse transcription polymerase chain reaction (PCR) (Laboratory Response Network labs)
- Positive immunofluorescence test for antigen with use of monoclonal antibody against H5
- Positive isolation of H5N1 virus
- 4-fold rise in H5-specific antibody titer in paired serum samples

DIFFERENTIAL DIAGNOSIS

- Acute respiratory syndrome
- Influenza
- Pneumonia
- Severe acute respiratory syndrome

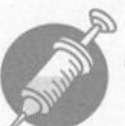

TREATMENT

All patients should receive neuraminidase inhibitors as soon as possible pending results of diagnostic lab tests (within 24–48 hours after exposure).

MEDICATION

ALERT

The use of amantadine (Symmetrel) and rimantadine (Flumadine) is not considered beneficial unless access to newer agents is unavailable. Vaccine is available only through US Strategic National Stockpile to be distributed by public health officials.

First Line

- Treatment of mild-to-moderate cases (2,3)[C]: Oseltamivir (Tamiflu) 75 mg p.o. b.i.d. for 5 days
- Treatment of severe cases (2,3)[C]: Oseltamivir (Tamiflu) 150 mg b.i.d. for 7–10 days
- Postexposure prophylaxis (2,3)[C]: Oseltamivir (Tamiflu) 75 mg p.o. once a day for 7–10 days
- Adverse effects: Neuropsychiatric events (hallucinations, delirium, and abnormal behavior) have been reported. Monitor for abnormal behavior. Nausea, vomiting, diarrhea, abdominal pain, insomnia, bronchitis, vertigo.
- Drug interactions: Not metabolized by CYP 450; drug interactions with drugs metabolized by this system are unlikely. Does not affect metabolism of acetaminophen.
- Higher doses may be considered case-by-case if present with pneumonic illness.
- Monitor for resistance; some H5N1 viruses isolated show resistance to oseltamivir.

Pediatric Considerations

- Pediatric treatment is weight-based. Safety and efficacy not established for children <1 year of age (2,3)[C]:
  - Oseltamivir 30 mg p.o. b.i.d. for 5 days ≤15 kg
  - Oseltamivir 45 mg p.o. b.i.d. for 5 days >15–23 kg
  - Oseltamivir 60 mg p.o. b.i.d. for 5 days >23–40 kg
  - Oseltamivir 75 mg p.o. b.i.d. for 5 days >40 kg
- Postexposure prophylaxis (2,3)[C]:
  - Dosing is weight-based as above but administered once daily for 7–10 days.

Geriatric Considerations

- Renal impairment (2,3)[C]:
  - Creatinine clearance 10–30 mL/min
    - Treatment: Oseltamivir 75 mg/d p.o.
    - Postexposure prophylaxis: Oseltamivir 75 mg p.o. every other day or 30 mg p.o. daily
- Hepatic impairment (2,4)[C]:
  - No dosage adjustment needed

Pregnancy Considerations

- Oseltamivir is Category C
- Use with caution only if potential benefits outweigh possible risk
- Unknown if distributed in breast milk

Second Line

- Zanamivir (Relenza) is considered 2nd-line agent. Not recommended for patients with underlying respiratory disease (asthma, chronic obstructive pulmonary disease) (3)[C].
- Treatment (ages 13 to ≥65 years):
  - Zanamivir 10 mg (2 inhalations) b.i.d. for 5 days
- Postexposure prophylaxis (ages 13 to ≥65):
  - Zanamivir 10 mg (2 inhalations) once daily for 7–10 days.
- Adverse effects:
  - Hypersensitivity reactions: Bronchospasms and allergiclike reactions have occurred.
  - Diarrhea, nausea, vomiting, headache, dizziness, sinusitis, cough, throat infections
  - Some adverse effects due to lactose in powder of inhaler
- Drug interactions: Not metabolized by CYP 450; drug interactions with drugs metabolized by this system are unlikely.

Pediatric Considerations

- Zanamivir is not licensed for use in children <7 years of age for treatment and <5 years for prophylaxis (3)[C]
- Treatment (7–13 years of age): Zanamivir 10 mg (2 inhalations) b.i.d. for 5 days
- Prophylaxis (5–13 years of age): Zanamivir 10 mg (2 inhalations) once daily 7–10 days

Geriatric Considerations

No dosage adjustment for renal or hepatic impairment (3)[C]

Pregnancy Considerations

- Zanamivir is Category C
- Use with caution only if potential benefits outweigh possible risk
- Unknown if distributed in breast milk
- Other medications (2,4)[C]:
  - Broad-spectrum antibiotics: Follow hospital protocols for community-acquired pneumonia.
- High-dose corticosteroids use associated with increased mortality.
- Immunomodulating drugs: No clear evidence of benefits, not recommended

ADDITIONAL TREATMENT

General Measures

Ventilatory support within 48 hours (2,6)[B]

IN-PATIENT CONSIDERATIONS

Initial Stabilization

- Broad-spectrum antibiotics, antiviral agents, with or without corticosteroids until lab confirmation of H5N1 virus (3)[A]
- Ventilatory support within 48 hours (2,6)[B]

Admission Criteria

If known H5N1 activity in the community, or if patient has traveled to country with H5N1 activity, admit if patient presents with:

- Severe acute respiratory illness
- Serious unexplained illness (encephalopathy or diarrhea)

Nursing

- Use standard and droplet precautions.
- N-95 masks

Discharge Criteria

- If discharged early, family requires education of proper hand hygiene and infection-control measures (surgical mask).
- Postexposure prophylaxis given to family members

ONGOING CARE

FOLLOW-UP RECOMMENDATIONS

Patient Monitoring

Clinical deterioration is rapid.

PATIENT EDUCATION

Hand hygiene, cough etiquette

PROGNOSIS

Mortality rate is high. Median time to death was 9 days (range 6–17 days) with or without treatment.

COMPLICATIONS

- Multiorgan failure, acute (2,4,5,6)[C]
- Renal dysfunction
- Cardiac compromise
- Cardiac dilatation, supraventricular
- Tachyarrhythmias
- Ventilator-associated pneumonia
- Pulmonary hemorrhage
- Pneumothorax
- Pancytopenia
- Reye syndrome
- Sepsis syndrome without documented bacteremia

REFERENCES

1. Pannwitz G, Wolf C, Harder T. Active surveillance for avian influenza virus infection in wild birds by analysis of avian fecal samples from the environment. *J Wildl Dis*. 2009;45:512–8.
2. Beigel JH, et al. Avian influenza A (H5N1) infections in humans. *N Engl J Med*. 2005;350:1374–1385.
3. World Health Organization. WHO Intermin Guidelines for Avian Influenza Case Management. 2007. Accessed 4/12/2010 at http://www.searo.who.int/LinkFiles/Publication_CD-167-Interim-guidelines-AI.pdf.
4. World Health Organization. Clinical management of human infection with avian influenza A (H5N1) virus. August 15, 2007. Accessed 4/11/2010 at http://who.int/csr/disease/avian_influenza/guidelines/Clinical Management07.pdf.
5. Tran TH, Nguyen TL, Nguyen TD et al. Avian influenza A (H5N1) in 10 patients in Vietnam. *N Engl J Med*. 2004;350:1179–88.
6. Chotpitayasunondh T, Ungchusak K, Hanshaoworakul W et al. Human disease from influenza A (H5N1), Thailand, 2004. *Emerg Infect Dis*. 2005;11:201–9.

ADDITIONAL READING

Centers for Disease Control and Prevention CDC: Key facts about Avian Influenza (Bird Flu) and Avian Influenza (H5N1) Virus. Accessed 4/11/2010 at http://www.cdc.gov/flu/avian/gen-info/facts.

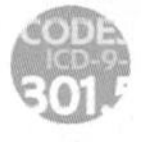

CODES

ICD9

- 488.01 Influenza due to identified avian influenza virus with pneumonia
- 488.02 Influenza due to identified avian influenza virus with other respiratory manifestations
- 488.09 Influenza due to identified avian influenza virus with other manifestations

CLINICAL PEARLS

- Consider avian influenza in the differential diagnosis for patients presenting with acute febrile respiratory illness and recent travel to high-risk areas (especially Asia) or who have spent time on poultry farms.
- Oseltamivir is considered 1st-line antiviral treatment: May need double usual dosage in patients with pneumonia.
- Perform: CBC, CXR, rapid tests for Ag detection, nasopharyngeal swabs for PCR, blood cultures, AST/ALT/CD4.

BABESIOSIS

Eleftherios Mylonakis, MD
Vassiliki P. Syriopoulou, MD

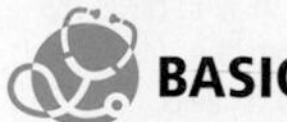

BASICS

DESCRIPTION

- Tickborne hemolytic disease that is caused by intraerythrocytic protozoan parasites of the genus *Babesia*
- Rarely reported outside the US:
  - Sporadic cases have been reported from a number of countries, including France, Italy, the former Yugoslavia, the United Kingdom, Ireland, the former Soviet Union, and Mexico.
  - In US, infections have been reported in many states, but most endemic areas are islands off the coast of Massachusetts (including Nantucket and Martha's Vineyard), New York (including Long Island, Shelter Island, and Fire Island), and in Connecticut. In these areas, asymptomatic human infection seems to be common.
- Incubation period of babesiosis varies from 5–33 days. Most patients do not recall recent tick exposure. After an infected blood transfusion, the incubation period can be up to 9 weeks.
- System(s) affected: Cardiovascular; Gastrointestinal; Hemic/Lymphatic/Immunologic; Musculoskeletal; Nervous; Pulmonary; Renal/Urologic

Geriatric Considerations

Morbidity and mortality are higher in patients >65.

EPIDEMIOLOGY

Predominant age: All ages; most patients present in their 40s or 50s.

Incidence

- Between 1968 and 1993, >450 *Babesia* infections were confirmed in US by blood smears or serologic testing. Prevalence is difficult to estimate because of lack of surveillance and because infections are often asymptomatic (1).
- In a recent 1-year seroconversion study of patients in New York State who were at high risk for tickborne diseases, antibodies to *B. microti* were seen in 7 of 671 participants (1%).

RISK FACTORS

- Exposure to endemic areas
- Transfusion-associated babesiosis and transplacental/perinatal transmission have been reported.
- High-level parasitemia is more common in asplenic patients. Such patients have been treated successfully with exchange transfusion in addition to drugs.

GENERAL PREVENTION

- Avoid endemic regions during the peak transmission months of May–September (especially relevant for asplenic or immunocompromised persons, in whom babesiosis can be a devastating illness).
- Using insect repellant is advised during outdoor activities, especially in wooded or grassy areas:
  - Products with 10–35% N-diethyl-meta-toluamide (DEET) will provide adequate protection under most conditions.
- Early removal of ticks is important; the tick must remain attached for at least 24 hours before the transmission of *B. microti* occurs. Daily self-examination is recommended for persons who engage in outdoor activities in endemic areas.
- Pets must be examined for ticks because they may carry ticks into the home.

ETIOLOGY

- *B. microti* (in US) and *B. divergens* and *B. bovis* (in Europe) cause most infections in humans. Recently, 1 case of *B. divergens* was reported in US.
- A previously unknown species of *Babesia* (WA-1) was isolated from an immunocompetent man in Washington State who had clinical babesiosis. Researchers also described another probable new *Babesia* species (MO1) associated with the 1st reported case of babesiosis acquired in Missouri. MO1 is probably distinct from *B. divergens*, but the two share morphologic, antigenic, and genetic characteristics.
- Ixodid (or hard-bodied) ticks, in particular, *Ixodes dammini (Ixodes scapularis)* and *I. ricinus*, are the vectors of the parasite.

COMMONLY ASSOCIATED CONDITIONS

- Coinfection with *Borrelia burgdorferi* and *B. microti* is relatively common in endemic areas.
- Coinfection with *Ehrlichia* sp. may also be seen. 3 species of *Ehrlichia* have been described that infect humans: *E. chaffeensis*, *E. phagocytophila*, and *E. ewingii*:
  - Typically, patients have a nonspecific febrile illness.
  - Rash is uncommon with human granulocytic ehrlichiosis, but common with human monocytic ehrlichiosis.
  - Laboratory findings often include leukopenia, thrombocytopenia, and increases in serum hepatic enzyme activities (2).

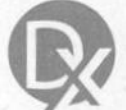

DIAGNOSIS

HISTORY

- High fever [up to 40°C (104°F)]
- Chills
- Diaphoresis
- Gastrointestinal (anorexia, nausea, abdominal pai vomiting, diarrhea)
- Generalized weakness
- Fatigue
- Myalgia
- Respiratory (cough, shortness of breath)
- Headache

PHYSICAL EXAM

- Hepatomegaly and splenomegaly or evidence of shock
- Rash (uncommon)
- Central nervous system involvement includes headache, photophobia, neck and back stiffness, altered sensorium, emotional lability
- Jaundice and dark urine may develop later in cours of illness.

DIAGNOSTIC TESTS & INTERPRETATION

Lab

Initial lab tests

- Mild-to-severe hemolytic anemia (common nonspecific finding)
- Normal-to-slightly depressed leukocyte count (common nonspecific finding)
- Typical morphologic picture on the blood smear
- A Wright- or Giemsa-stained peripheral blood sme is most commonly used to demonstrate the presen of intraerythrocytic parasites.
- Rarely, tetrads of merozoites are visible.
- Serologic evaluation with the indirect immunofluorescent antibody test with use of *B. microti* antigen is available in a few laboratories
  - The cut-off titer for determination of a positive result varies with the particular laboratory protoc used, but in most laboratories, titers of >1:64 ar considered consistent with *B. microti* infection.
  - 10–20-fold higher titers can be observed in the acute setting, with a gradual decline over weeks to months:
    - The correlation between the level of the titer and the severity of symptoms is poor.
- Detection of B. microti by PCR is more sensitive an equally specific for the diagnosis of acute cases, in comparison with direct smear examination and hamster inoculation. PCR-based methods may also be indicated for monitoring of the infection.

Follow-Up & Special Considerations

Monitoring the degree of intraerythrocytic parasitemi can help guide treatment.

B

agnostic Procedures/Surgery
sed on typical morphologic picture on the blood ear in conjunction with epidemiologic information

FFERENTIAL DIAGNOSIS
- Bacterial sepsis
- Hepatitis
- Lyme disease
- Ehrlichiosis
- Leishmaniasis
- Malaria

TREATMENT

EDICATION

rst Line

ovaquone (Mepron): Suspension 750 mg b.i.d. plus thromycin (Zithromax) 500–1,000 mg/d (3)[B]

cond Line

Combination of quinine sulfate (Quinamm): 650 mg orally t.i.d. and clindamycin (Cleocin) 600 mg orally t.i.d., or 1.2 g parenterally b.i.d. for 7–10 days is the most commonly used treatment. (Pediatric: Dosage s 20–40 mg/kg/d for quinine and 25 mg/kg/d for clindamycin.)

Several other drugs have been evaluated, including tetracycline, primaquine, sulfadiazine (Microsulfon), and pyrimethamine (Fansidar). Results have varied.

Pentamidine (Pentam) has proved to be moderately effective in diminishing symptoms and decreasing parasitemia.

Precautions: Clindamycin can lead to *Clostridium difficile*-associated diarrhea.

DDITIONAL TREATMENT

eneral Measures

n areas endemic for Lyme disease and ehrlichiosis, it may be advisable to add doxycycline (Vibramycin) 100 mg b.i.d. p.o. in the management of patients with babesiosis until serologic testing is completed. Note that some resistance is emerging to standard treatment in patients with severe immunocompromise (4).

sues for Referral

change transfusion, together with antibabesial emotherapy, may be necessary in critically ill tients. This treatment is usually reserved for patients 10 are extremely ill (blood parasitemia >10%, assive hemolysis, and asplenia).

ONGOING CARE

FOLLOW-UP RECOMMENDATIONS
- When left untreated, silent babesial infection may persist for months or even years.
- 139 hospitalized cases in New York State between 1982 and 1993:
  - 9 patients (6.5%) died.
  - 25% of the patients were admitted to the intensive care unit.
  - 25% of the patients required hospitalization for >14 days.
- Alkaline phosphatase levels >125 U/L, white blood cell counts $>5 \times 10^9$/L, history of cardiac abnormality, history of splenectomy, presence of heart murmur, and parasitemia values of 4% or higher were associated with disease severity.

Patient Monitoring

Monitor for complications (congestive heart failure [CHF], etc.) and follow parasitemia as needed.

COMPLICATIONS
- CHF
- Disseminated intravascular coagulation
- Acute respiratory distress syndrome (can occur even a few days after the onset of effective antimicrobial treatment)
- Renal failure and myocardial infarction also have been associated with severe babesiosis.

REFERENCES

1. Persing DH, Herwaldt BL, Glaser C, et al. Infection with a babesia-like organism in northern California. *N Engl J Med*. 1995;332:298–303.
2. Mylonakis E. When to suspect and how to monitor babesiosis. *Am Fam Physician*. 2001;63:1969–74.
3. Krause PJ, Lepore T, Sikand VK, et al. Atovaquone and azithromycin for the treatment of babesiosis. *N Engl J Med*. 2000;343:1454–8.
4. Wormser GP, Prasad A, Neuhaus E, Joshi S, Nowakowski J, Nelson J, Mittleman A, Aguero-Rosenfeld M, Topal J, Krause PJ et al. Emergence of resistance to azithromycin-atovaquone in immunocompromised patients with Babesia microti infection. *Clin Infect Dis*. 2010;50:381–6.

ADDITIONAL READING

- Beattie JF, Michelson ML, Holman PJ. Acute babesiosis caused by Babesia divergens in a resident of Kentucky. *N Engl J Med*. 2002;347:697–8.
- Berman KH, Blue DE, Smith DS, et al. Fatal case of babesiosis in postliver transplant patient. *Transplantation*. 2009;87:452–3.
- Gelfand JA. Babesia species. In: Mandell GL, et al., eds. *Mandell, Douglas, and Bennett's Principles and Practice of Infectious Diseases*, 6th ed. New York: Churchill Livingstone, 2005:3209–15.
- Gubernot DM, Lucey CT, Lee KC, et al. Babesia Infection through Blood Transfusions: Reports Received by the US Food and Drug Administration, 1997-2007. *Clin Infect Dis*. 2008.
- Gutman JD, Kotton CN, Kratz A. Case records of the Massachusetts General Hospital. Weekly clinicopathological exercises. Case 29-2003. A 60-year-old man with fever, rigors, and sweats. *N Engl J Med*. 2003;349:1168–75.
- Krause PJ, Gewurz BE, Hill D, et al. Persistent and relapsing babesiosis in immunocompromised patients. *Clin Infect Dis*. 2008;46:370–6.
- Wormser GP, Dattwyler RJ, Shapiro ED, et al. The clinical assessment, treatment, and prevention of lyme disease, human granulocytic anaplasmosis, and babesiosis: clinical practice guidelines by the Infectious Diseases Society of America. *Clin Infect Dis*. 2006;43:1089–134.

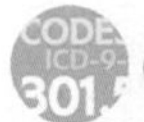

CODES

ICD9

088.82 Babesiosis

CLINICAL PEARLS

- High-level parasitemia is more common in asplenic patients.
- 1st-line treatment is atovaquone plus azithromycin.
- Coinfection with *B. burgdorferi* is relatively common in endemic areas. Coinfection with *Ehrlichia* species may also be seen. In areas endemic for Lyme disease and ehrlichiosis, it may be advisable to add doxycycline in the management of patients with babesiosis until serologic testing is completed.
- When left untreated, silent babesial infection may persist for months or even years.
- Tick must remain in place for 24 hours to transmit infection, so daily self-screening of skin is protective.

BACK PAIN, LOW

Christopher Garofalo, MD

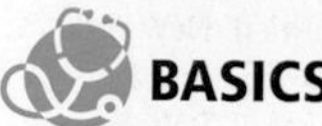

BASICS

DESCRIPTION

- Mechanical low back pain (LBP) is generally a benign and self-limiting condition responsive to conservative measures that include maintaining activity while using short-term pharmacologic therapy.
- Patients typically present with pain, muscle tension, or stiffness at the posterior belt line with occasional referred pain to the buttocks and/or posterior thighs; symptoms are often the result of the mechanical stresses and functional demands placed on the low back area by everyday activities.
- For most patients, pain is of short duration, and complete recovery is expected within 6 weeks.
- The primary goal is to rule out red-flag symptoms that may be indicative of possible underlying spinal pathology or nerve root problems; when such symptoms are absent, the patient is considered to have nonspecific LBP.
- System(s) affected: Musculoskeletal; Nervous
- Synonym(s): Low back syndrome; Lumbar strain/sprain; Lumbago

Geriatric Considerations

Tumors, degenerative conditions, fractures, and stenosis are common.

Pediatric Considerations

The presence of LBP is considered a red-flag symptom. A thorough workup is imperative.

Pregnancy Considerations

Pregnancy is commonly associated with LBP and/or sciatica; treatment is conservative.

EPIDEMIOLOGY

Incidence

- 90% of Americans experience mechanical LBP some time in their life.
- LBP is one of the most common primary-care complaints.
- Repetitive episodes are common.
- Predominant age: $\geq$25 years
- Predominant sex: Male = Female

RISK FACTORS

- Age
- Activity (e.g., heavy lifting, bending, twisting)
- Smoking
- Obesity
- Vibration (e.g., driving motor vehicles)
- Sedentary lifestyle
- Psychosocial factors such as increased stress, anxiety, or depressed mood

GENERAL PREVENTION

- Maintaining physical fitness
- Weight loss
- Smoking cessation
- Stress reduction
- Avoidance of aggravating tasks (e.g., heavy lifting, bending, twisting, sudden unexpected movements, or any combination of these tasks)

ETIOLOGY

- Normal aging process of musculoskeletal system aggravates an acute event.
- Degenerative joint disease of LS spine
- In primary-care setting, <15% of LBP patients have identifiable underlying disease.

COMMONLY ASSOCIATED CONDITIONS

- Deconditioning, obesity
- Psychosocial disease
- Compression fracture

DIAGNOSIS

HISTORY

- Onset of pain begins either suddenly after injury or gradually over the next 24 h.
- Occasional radiation of pain to buttocks and/or posterior thighs stopping at knees
- Pain pattern is referred rather than radicular.
- Back pain is worse than leg pain.
- Pain is aggravated by back motion, sitting, standing, lifting, bending, and twisting.
- Pain is relieved by rest.
- Bowel and bladder function are preserved.
- Psychosocial stressors at work and/or home may be present.
- Medical history and previous injuries should be noted.
- Red flags (possible etiology):
  - Age >50 years or <20 years (neoplastic)
  - History of cancer (carcinoma recurrence)
  - Night sweats or weight loss (neoplasm, rheumatologic)
  - Incontinence or saddle anesthesia (nerve compromise/cauda equina syndrome)
  - Recent bacterial infection (infectious)
  - Pain worse when supine (rheumatologic, nerve compromise)
  - History of trauma (fracture)

PHYSICAL EXAM

- Observation reveals preferred posture, facial expressions, and pain behaviors.
- Normal motor, sensory, and reflex examinations
- Decreased lumbar range of motion, paraspinous musculature tenderness, and spasm
- Nerve root stretch tests are often negative.
- Straight-leg raise (causing spinal motion) may increase LBP, but not leg pain.

DIAGNOSTIC TESTS & INTERPRETATION

Lab

Initial lab tests

- Not typically indicated on initial presentation (1)
- For those with red flags, pain that worsens, persists for >6 weeks, and/or is recalcitrant to conservative treatment measures, consider the following:
  - CBC with differential
  - Erythrocyte sedimentation rate (ESR)
  - Alkaline and acid phosphatase
  - Serum calcium
  - Serum protein electrophoresis
- Special tests: System-directed investigation

Imaging

Initial approach

- Plain radiographs:
  - Not recommended in the absence of red flags (2)[B]
  - Indicated for persistent symptoms (>6 weeks), age >50 years, systemic symptoms, presence c neurologic deficits or trauma, history of cancer, use of immunosuppressants, IV drug abuse, or abnormalities such as ankylosing spondylitis ar suspected
  - Anteroposterior, lateral, spot lateral of L5–S1, oblique films are included in routine lumbosac series.
- Bone scan (scintigraphy): Technetium-99m-labele phosphorus to rule out fractures, infections, or metastases

Diagnostic Procedures/Surgery

MRI and CT scan indicated only for persistent symptoms, neurologic deficits, and/or suspected infection or malignancy:

- MRI is useful for visualization of soft tissue.
- CT scan is useful for visualization of bony anaton

DIFFERENTIAL DIAGNOSIS

- Structural:
  - Lumbar strain/sprain
  - Herniated lumbar intervertebral disk
  - Degenerative disk disease
  - Degenerative segmental instability
  - Spinal stenosis
  - Spondylolisthesis
  - Congenital disease: Severe kyphosis, severe scoliosis
  - Fractures
- Inflammatory:
  - Ankylosing spondylitis and related inflammator spondylopathies
  - Infection: Vertebral osteomyelitis
  - Rheumatoid arthritis
- Neoplastic:
  - Primary tumors
  - Metastases
- Referred pain:
  - Orthopedic: Osteoarthritis of hip
  - Sacroiliac joint disease
  - GI: Duodenal ulcer, chronic pancreatitis, cholecystitis, irritable bowel syndrome, diverticulitis
  - Genitourinary: Pyelonephritis, nephrolithiasis, prostatism
  - Gynecologic: Pregnancy, endometriosis, ovarian cystic disease, pelvic inflammatory disease
  - Cardiovascular: Abdominal aortic aneurysm, vascular claudication

TREATMENT

IEDICATION

rst Line

Nonsteroidal anti-inflammatory drugs (NSAIDs):

- Agents are considered equally effective (3)[A]:
  - Ibuprofen: 800 mg PO q6h × 10 days, then as needed (maximum 3,200 mg/d)
  - Naproxen: 500 mg PO b.i.d. × 10 days, then as needed (maximum 1,500 mg/d)
- Adverse reactions: Fluid retention, rash, GI discomfort, dizziness, GI bleeding, acute renal failure
- Contraindications: Treatment of perioperative pain in the setting of coronary artery bypass grafting (CABG); aspirin allergy
- Precautions: High risk of cardiovascular event, high risk of GI bleeding, history of ulcer disease, elderly, renal disease
- Possible interactions: Antiplatelets, ACE inhibitors, lithium, low-molecular-weight heparin

COX-2 inhibitors are as effective as traditional NSAIDs and have fewer side effects (3)[A]. Precautions: Patients with cardiovascular concerns

Muscle relaxants:

- Use with caution (avoid alcohol, no driving or operating heavy machinery); comparative efficacy to NSAIDs is unknown (4)[A]:
  - Cyclobenzaprine (Flexeril): 10 mg PO at bedtime or q8h (maximum 60 mg/d)
  - Carisoprodol (Soma): 350 mg PO t.i.d. and at bedtime
  - Metaxalone (Skelaxin): 800 mg PO t.i.d.–q.i.d.
- Adverse reactions: Sedation, N/V, dizziness
- Contraindications:
  - Cyclobenzaprine: Arrhythmias, congestive heart failure, hyperthyroidism, concomitant monoamine oxidase inhibitors
  - Carisoprodol: Acute intermittent porphyria
  - Metaxalone: Anemia, renal or hepatic impairment
- Precautions: Concomitant use of CNS depressants; history of substance abuse
- Possible interactions: CNS depressants

econd Line

ıort-acting combination opioid analgesic products ıould be considered only for moderate–severe pain ɔt controlled with NSAIDs and/or muscle relaxants one (5)[B].

ALERT

Jse of narcotics in acute LBP may increase risk of ɔrogression to chronic LBP.

DDITIONAL TREATMENT

ieneral Measures

Outpatient management is appropriate.

Activity modification as appropriate

Short-term nonopioid analgesics at fixed time intervals: NSAIDs and/or muscle relaxants

Avoid short-acting combination opioid analgesic products (e.g., Vicodin); associated with inducing chronic LBP.

Use of opioid analgesics does not improve return-to-work status.

Issues for Referral

Refer patients with progressive motor and sensory symptoms and/or evidence of infection, tumor, or fracture to a neurosurgeon or ER for further evaluation.

Additional Therapies

There is strong evidence that an intensive individual education session is as effective as other interventions in short- and long-term return to work (6)[A].

COMPLEMENTARY AND ALTERNATIVE MEDICINE

- Chiropractic manipulation (5)[B]
- Devil's claw, white willow bark, and capsaicin have demonstrated efficacy versus placebo for acute episodes of chronic LBP (7)[B].

IN-PATIENT CONSIDERATIONS

Admission Criteria

Limit to patients who require surgical procedures for underlying causes.

ONGOING CARE

FOLLOW-UP RECOMMENDATIONS

- Bed rest is *not* recommended (5)[A].
- Restricted activities for 3–6 weeks.
- Back-specific exercises should be avoided.
- Activities of daily living should be resumed as soon as possible (5)[A].

Patient Monitoring

- Estimated duration of care is 1–6 weeks.
  - Schedule follow-up at 2–4 weeks.
  - Assess the following at each follow-up visit: Pain, functional status, and medication-related adverse effects.
- Reevaluate for possible underlying causes if relief does not occur.
- Patients should be encouraged to maintain normal levels of activity.
- Consider ongoing physical therapy.

DIET

Weight reduction, if appropriate

PATIENT EDUCATION

Advise the patient to stay active, use medication as prescribed, and discuss adverse drug effects.

PROGNOSIS

- Usually self-limiting; recovery is expected within 6 weeks in 90% of patients (4).
- Symptoms can recur in 50–80% of patients within the 1st year.
- Adverse psychosocial factors to resolving back pain:
  - Pending litigation or compensation
  - Prolonged use of habit-forming medications or alcohol
  - Poor coping strategies, depressed or hostile patient
  - Job dissatisfaction

COMPLICATIONS

- Chronic LBP
- Persistent psychosocial impairment

REFERENCES

1. Chou R, Qaseem A, Snow V, et al. Diagnosis and treatment of low back pain: a joint clinical practice guideline from the American College of Physicians and the American Pain Society. *Ann Intern Med*. 2007;147:478–91.
2. Jarvik JG, Deyo RA. Diagnostic evaluation of low back pain with emphasis on imaging. *Ann Intern Med*. 2002;137:586–97.
3. Roelofs PDDM, Deyo RA, Koes BW et al. Non-steroidal antiinflammatory drugs for low back pain. *Cochrane Database of Systematic Reviews*. 2008; 1:CD000396. DOI:10.1002/14651858.CD000396.pub3.
4. van Tulder MW, Touray T, Furlan AD et al. Muscle relaxants for non-specific low back pain. *Cochrane Database of Syst Rev*. 2006;(3).
5. Koes BW, van Tulder MW, Thomas S. Diagnosis and treatment of low back pain. *BMJ*. 2006;332:1430–4.
6. Engers AJ, Jellema P, Wensing M et al. Individual patient education for low back pain. *Cochrane Database of Systematic Reviews*. 2008(1): CD004057. DOI:10.1002/14651858.CD004057.pub3.
7. Gagnier JJ, van Tulder MW, Berman B, et al. Herbal medicine for low back pain. *Cochrane Database Syst Rev*. 2006;19(2).

See Also (Topic, Algorithm, Electronic Media Element)

Lumbar (intervertebral) disk disorders

Algorithm: Low Back Pain, Acute

CODES

ICD9

724.2 Lumbago

CLINICAL PEARLS

- Red flags include age <20 years or >55 years, nonmechanical pain, night sweats and/or weight loss, temperature >38°C, history of cancer, history of trauma, presence of neurologic deficits, and pain worse when supine.
- Bed rest is not recommended; patients are encouraged to maintain activity.
- NSAIDs are beneficial and should be considered as 1st-line therapy.

BAKER CYST

Chris Wheelock, MD

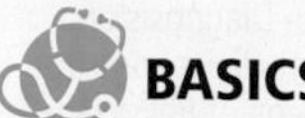

BASICS

DESCRIPTION

- A fluid-filled synovial sac arising in the popliteal fossa
- Distention of the gastrocnemial-semimembranous bursa
- Can be unilateral or bilateral
- Primary cysts are a distention of the bursa arising independently without an intra-articular disorder
- Secondary cysts occur if a communication exists between the bursa and knee joint, allowing articular fluid to fill the cyst. Pathologic joint processes can also be transmitted in this manner.
- Associated with synovial inflammation
- Synonym: Popliteal cyst

EPIDEMIOLOGY

Incidence

- Bimodal distribution: Children ages 4–7, and adults increasing with age
- Primary cysts usually seen in children under 15 years of age
- Secondary cysts seen in the adult population

Prevalence

- Varies by study
- Studies report a prevalence of 19–47% in symptomatic knees, 2–5% in asymptomatic knees
- In children, 6.3% in symptomatic knees, 2.4% in asymptomatic knees

RISK FACTORS

- Osteoarthritis of knee (most common) (1)[B]
- Rheumatoid arthritis
- Meniscal degeneration or tear
- Advancing age
- Ligamentous insufficiency

PATHOPHYSIOLOGY

- Extension or herniation of synovial membrane of the knee joint capsule or connection of normal bursa with the joint capsule
- May be the result of increased intra-articular pressure
- Commonly seen with knee effusions
- Direct trauma to the bursa likely the primary cause in children since there is no communication between the bursa and the joint in children
- A valve-like mechanism allowing one-way passage of fluid from the joint to the bursal connection has been described.

ETIOLOGY

Associated intra-articular pathological findings include:

- Meniscal tears, posterior horn
- ACL insufficiency
- Degenerative articular cartilage lesions
- Rheumatoid arthritis
- Osteoarthritis
- Osteochondritis
- Other potential factors: Infectious arthritis, polyarthritis, villonodular synovitis, and connective tissue diseases

COMMONLY ASSOCIATED CONDITIONS

Any condition causing knee joint effusion

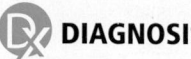

DIAGNOSIS

HISTORY

- Painless mass arising in the popliteal fossa
- Most cysts are asymptomatic
- Painful if cyst ruptures
- May report restricted range of motion or tightness with knee flexion
- Large cysts may cause entrapment neuropathy of the tibial nerve.
- Vascular compression, most commonly of the popliteal vein, may produce claudication or thrombophlebitis.
- Activity will alter the cyst size.

PHYSICAL EXAM

- Examine in full extension and 90° of flexion
- Foucher sign: Mass increases with extension and disappears with flexion.
- Most commonly found in medial aspect of popliteal fossa lateral to the head of the gastrocnemius and medial to the neurovascular bundle.
- Mass may be fluctuant or tender.
- Transillumination can distinguish cyst from solid mass.
- Ruptured cyst typically painful with associated swelling over calf and medial malleolus, pseudothrombophlebitis

DIAGNOSTIC TESTS & INTERPRETATION

Lab

Initial lab tests

- CBC, sedimentation rate if suspicious of septic arthritis
- Send aspirate for cell count to determine nature of effusion: Infectious, inflammatory, or mechanical.

Follow-Up & Special Considerations

In children, consider observation before invasive testing.

Imaging

Initial approach

- Ultrasound confirms presence and size; with Doppler can differentiate Baker cysts from popliteal vessel aneurysms or soft tissue tumors (2)[B].
- MRI is useful to assess for causal derangements of internal joint structures.
- Radiographs may show soft tissue density posteriorly.
- Arthrography may demonstrate communication with joint capsule, or rupture.
- CT–arthrography together is superior in visualizing cystic details and can help separate lipomas, aneurysms, and malignancies from cysts.

B

FFERENTIAL DIAGNOSIS
- nfection/abscess
- ipoma
- iposarcoma
- ibroma
- ibrosarcoma
- lematoma
- Deep venous thrombosis
- /ascular tumor
- opliteal vein varices
- Xanthoma
- Aneurysm (rare)
- Ganglion cyst
- Any condition causing synovitis
- Thrombophlebitis
- Muscular herniation (rare, related to trauma)

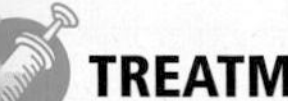

TREATMENT

EDICATION
- Once etiology is identified from cellular fluid examination, treat the underlying condition
- Analgesics, NSAIDS for symptomatic relief

ODDITIONAL TREATMENT
eneral Measures
- No treatment if cyst is asymptomatic
- Compressive wrap or sleeve may be used for comfort

dditional Therapies
- Physical therapy improves knee range of motion and strength, particularly with coexisting pathology
- Temporary relief with needle aspiration, recurrence common
- mprovement in joint range of motion, knee pain, swelling, accompanied reduction in bursa size has been shown after intra-articular or intracystic corticosteroid injection (2)[B]
- Sclerotherapy injections of ethanol or dextrose/sodium morrhuate shown to have good results in studies with small sample sizes (3)[B]

SURGERY/OTHER PROCEDURES
- Consider excision when symptoms persist despite treatment or no etiology is found.
- Recurrence after standard surgery is common and is highest when chondral lesions are present (4)[B].
- A modified surgical technique in children has been proven effective without recurrence (5)[B].
- Excision via arthroscopy or open procedure often requires concomitant treatment of underlying pathology (6)[B].

ONGOING CARE

PROGNOSIS
- Variable
- Many cysts remain asymptomatic.
- Some will regress or resolve with treatment of underlying etiology
- In children, most resolve without treatment.

COMPLICATIONS
- Compartment syndrome in ruptured cyst
- Thrombophlebitis from compression of the popliteal vein
- Infection of popliteal cyst
- Hemorrhage into cyst if on anticoagulants

REFERENCES

1. Chatzopoulos D, Moralidis E, Markou P, et al. Baker's cysts in knees with chronic osteoarthritic pain: a clinical, ultrasonographic, radiographic and scintigraphic evaluation. *Rheumatol Int*. 2008 Jun 27.
2. Acebes JC, Sanchez-Pernaute O, Diaz-Oca A, et al. Ultrasonographic Assessment of Baker's Cysts after Intra-articular Corticosteroid Injection in Knee Osteoarthritis. *J Clin Ultrasound*. 2006;34:113–7.
3. Centeno CJ, Schultz J, Freeman M, et al. Sclerotherapy of Baker's Cyst with Imaging Confirmation of Resolution. *Pain Physician*. 2008;11:257–61.
4. Rupp S, Seil R, et al. Popliteal cysts in adults: Prevalence, associated intraarticular lesions, and results after arthroscopic treatment. *Am Sport Med*. 2002;30(1):112–5.
5. Chen J-C, Cheng-Chang L, Lu Y-M, et al. A modified surgical method for treating Baker's cyst in children. *The Knee*. 2008;15:9–14.
6. Handy JR. Popliteal cysts in adults: A review. *Semin Arthritis Rheu*. 2001;31(2):108–18.

ADDITIONAL READING

- Fritschy D, Fasel J, Imbert J, et al. The popliteal cyst. *Knee Surg Sports Traumatol Arthosc*. 2006;14: 623–8.
- Marra MD, Crema MD, Chung M, et al. MRI features of cystic lesions around the knee. *The Knee*. 2008 Jun 16.
- Seil R, Rupp S, et al. Prevalence of popliteal cysts in children: A sonographic study and review of the literature. *Arch Ortho Traum Su*. 1999;119:73–5.
- Van Rhijn L, Jansen E, Pruijs H. Long term follow up of conservatively treated popliteal cysts in children. *Journal of Pediatric Orthopedics Part B*. 2000;9: 62–64.

See Also (Topic, Algorithm, Electronic Media Element)

Algorithm: Knee Pain

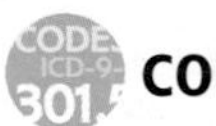

CODES

ICD9
727.51 Synovial cyst of popliteal space

CLINICAL PEARLS
- In children, it is acceptable to wait and observe.
- Treat underlying cause.
- Pain and swelling over the medial malleolus is classic for cyst rupture, also known as pseudothrombophlebitis.

BALANITIS

James P. Miller, MD
Timothy L. Black, MD

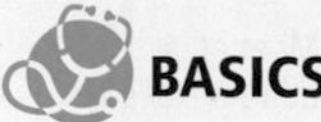

BASICS

DESCRIPTION

- Balanitis is an inflammation of the glans penis.
- Posthitis is an inflammation of the foreskin.
- Balanitis xerotica obliterans (BXO) is lichen sclerosis of the glans penis (uncommon).
- System(s) affected: Reproductive; Skin/Exocrine

Geriatric Considerations

Condom catheters can predispose to balanitis.

Pediatric Considerations

Oral antibiotics predispose male infants to *Candida balanitis.*

EPIDEMIOLOGY

- Predominant age: Adult
- Predominant gender: Male only

RISK FACTORS

- Presence of foreskin
- Morbid obesity
- Poor hygiene
- Diabetes
- Nursing home environment

GENERAL PREVENTION

- Proper hygiene and avoidance of allergens
- Circumcision

ETIOLOGY

- Allergic reaction (condom latex, contraceptive jelly)
- Infections (*C. albicans, Borrelia vincentii,* streptococci, *Trichomonas*)
- Fixed-drug eruption (sulfa, tetracycline)
- Plasma cell infiltration (Zoon balanitis)
- Autodigestion by activated pancreatic transplant exocrine enzymes

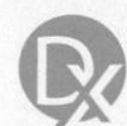

DIAGNOSIS

HISTORY

- Pain
- Drainage
- Dysuria

PHYSICAL EXAM

- Erythema
- Edema
- Discharge
- Ulceration
- Plaque

DIAGNOSTIC TESTS & INTERPRETATION

Lab

- Microbiology culture
- Wet mount
- Serology for syphilis
- Serum glucose

Initial lab tests

- Gram stain
- Wet prep

Diagnostic Procedures/Surgery

Biopsy, if persistent

Pathological Findings

Plasma cells infiltration with Zoon balanitis

DIFFERENTIAL DIAGNOSIS

- Leukoplakia
- Lichen planus
- Psoriasis
- Reiter syndrome
- Lichen sclerosus et atrophicus
- Erythroplasia of Queyrat
- Balanitis xerotica obliterans (BXO)

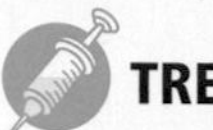

TREATMENT

MEDICATION

- Antifungal:
  - Clotrimazole (Lotrimin), 1% b.i.d.
  - Nystatin (Mycostatin), b.i.d.–q.i.d.
  - Fluconazole, 150-mg single dose (1)[B]
- Antibacterial:
  - Bacitracin, q.i.d.
  - Neomycin-polymyxin B-bacitracin (Neosporin), q.i.d.
  - If cellulitis, cephalosporin or sulfa drug PO or parenteral:
    - Dermatitis: Topical steroids q.i.d.
    - Zoon balanitis: Topical steroids q.i.d.
- BXO:
  - 0.05% betamethasone b.i.d. (2)[B]
  - 0.1% tacrolimus b.i.d. (3)[C]

DDITIONAL TREATMENT

eneral Measures

Appropriate health care: Outpatient
Warm compresses or sitz baths
Local hygiene

sues for Referral

current infections or development of meatal nosis

JRGERY/OTHER PROCEDURES

nsider circumcision as preventive measure.

I-PATIENT CONSIDERATIONS

dmission Criteria

Uncontrolled diabetes
Sepsis

ursing

propriate hygiene if condom catheters are used

ischarge Criteria

solution of problem

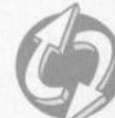

ONGOING CARE

FOLLOW-UP RECOMMENDATIONS

Patient Monitoring

- Every 1–2 weeks until etiology has been established
- Persistent balanitis may require biopsy to rule out malignancy or BXO.

DIET

Weight reduction, if obese

PATIENT EDUCATION

- Need for appropriate hygiene
- Avoidance of known allergens

PROGNOSIS

Should resolve with appropriate treatment

COMPLICATIONS

- Meatal stenosis
- Premalignant changes from chronic irritation
- Urinary tract infections

REFERENCES

1. Stary A, Soeltz-Szoets J, Ziegler C, et al. Comparison of the efficacy and safety of oral fluconazole and topical clotrimazole in patients with candida balanitis. *Genitourin Med*. 1996;72:98–102.
2. Kiss A, Csontai A, Pirót L, et al. The response of balanitis xerotica obliterans to local steroid application compared with placebo in children. *J Urol*. 2001;165:219–20.
3. Pandher BS, Rustin MH, Kaisary AV. Treatment of balanitis xerotica obliterans with topical tacrolimus. *J Urol*. 2003;170:923.

See Also (Topic, Algorithm, Electronic Media Element)

Reiter Syndrome

CODES

ICD9

- 112.2 Candidiasis of other urogenital sites
- 607.1 Balanoposthitis

CLINICAL PEARLS

- With recurrent infections and a plaque, a biopsy should be done to rule out BXO or malignancy.
- If there is a true phimosis that interferes with appropriate hygiene, treatment of the phimosis with steroids or circumcision should be performed to help with hygiene.

BAROTRAUMA OF THE MIDDLE EAR, SINUSES, AND LUNG

Michele Roberts, MD, PhD
Jeremy Golding, MD

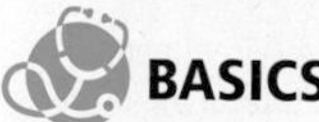

BASICS

DESCRIPTION

- Physical damage to tissue lining an enclosed body cavity resulting from an imbalance between ambient pressure and pressure within the cavity.
- Cavities at greatest risk for barotrauma include the middle ear (otic barotrauma), paranasal sinuses (sinus barotrauma), and lungs (pulmonary barotrauma).
- Otic and sinus barotrauma are associated with rapid or extreme changes in environmental pressure, as might result from air travel, mountain climbing, or scuba diving, especially in the presence of nasal congestion or eustachian tube dysfunction of any etiology:
  - Pressure changes with failure of eustachian tube to equilibrate pressure may distort the tympanic membrane (TM), causing discomfort and injury.
  - Rupture of round or oval membrane may cause inner ear barotrauma, vertigo, and sensorineural hearing loss.
- Pulmonary barotrauma:
  - An iatrogenic complication of mechanical ventilation
  - Also a complication of scuba diving
- Dental barotrauma is seen occasionally in scuba divers in whom small pockets of air trapped in dental work can cause rupture of teeth
- System(s) affected: Ear/Nose/Throat (ENT); Pulmonary
- Synonym(s): Dysbarism; aerotitis; otitic barotrauma; middle ear barotrauma

ALERT

- Dizziness and sensorineural hearing loss warrant immediate ENT referral for inner ear involvement.
- Valsalva maneuver can spread nasopharyngeal infection into the middle ear.
- Vertigo and hearing loss may cause disorientation.

EPIDEMIOLOGY

- Predominant age: All ages
- Predominant sex: Male = Female

Incidence

- Pulmonary barotrauma is the 2nd leading cause of death among divers.
- Otic barotrauma is common in air travel, especially among flight personnel.
- Pulmonary barotrauma is noted in 3% of mechanically ventilated patients.

Pediatric Considerations

- Children have difficulty opening the eustachian tube and have frequent upper respiratory infections. This combination results in higher risk for otic or sinus barotraumas at small pressure changes, as compared with adults.
- Mechanical ventilation of neonates is associated with barotrauma contributing to bronchopulmonary dysplasia.

Pregnancy Considerations

Increased nasal congestion in pregnancy increases risk of barotitis media.

RISK FACTORS

- Otic or sinus:
  - Participation in high-risk activities without adequate pressure equilibration:
    - Scuba diving, especially with rapid ascent or breath-holding
    - Airplane flight (especially high performance)
    - Sky diving
    - High-altitude travel or elevator rides
    - Underwater employment
    - High-impact sports: Boxing, soccer, water skiing
  - Upper respiratory infection: Sinusitis, rhinitis, tonsillitis, adenoiditis, otitis media
  - Nasal congestion or allergic rhinitis
  - Any cause of eustachian tube dysfunction
  - Exposure to blasting
  - Pregnancy (associated nasal congestion)
  - Anatomic obstruction in the nasopharynx:
    - Deviated nasal septum
    - Nasal polyps
    - Congenital anomalies, including cleft palate
  - Trauma to ear
- Pulmonary:
  - Iatrogenic:
    - Mechanical ventilation, especially in the presence of asthma, chronic interstitial lung disease, acute respiratory distress syndrome
    - Hyperbaric oxygen therapy
  - Scuba diving or other underwater activities
  - Air travel in people with preexisting pulmonary pathology

GENERAL PREVENTION

- Pulmonary barotrauma:
  - Judicious use of mechanical ventilation and hyperbaric oxygen therapy
  - In scuba diving, avoidance of breath-holding during ascent
- Otic barotrauma:
  - Avoidance of altitude changes or scuba diving when at risk for eustachian tube dysfunction
  - Treatment of upper respiratory congestion
- Equilibration of pressure by Valsalva, yawning, swallowing, drinking, chewing gum

ETIOLOGY

- For any gas at a constant temperature, the volum of the gas varies inversely with the pressure. Whe gas is trapped in a confined space such as the middle ear, paranasal sinus, or lungs, a sudden decrease in ambient pressure causes expansion o the gas within the cavity.
- Otalgia and hearing loss occur as a result of stretching and deformation of the TM.
- Sudden pressure differential between middle and inner ear may lead to rupture of round or oval window and consequent labyrinthine fistula and leakage of perilymph. Damage to inner ear may b permanent.
- When transalveolar pressure disrupts the structura integrity of the alveolus, the alveolar wall ruptures leading to interstitial emphysema, followed by pneumothorax, pneumomediastinum.

DIAGNOSIS

- Otic (middle ear) barotrauma:
  - Otalgia, sensation of fullness or pressure in ear
  - Conductive hearing loss
  - Vertigo secondary to cold water entering middle ear
  - Transient facial paralysis
  - With TM rupture, discharge of fluid from ear
  - Abnormality of TM
- All patients with middle ear barotrauma should be evaluated for inner ear barotrauma:
  - Sensorineural hearing loss
  - Tinnitus
  - Vertigo
  - Disorientation
- Sinus barotrauma: Facial pain, sensation of fullnes or pressure
- Pulmonary barotrauma:
  - Chest pain, dyspnea
  - Hypoxia, hypotension

HISTORY

- Otic barotrauma: History of high-risk activity
- Pulmonary barotrauma: Scuba diving, mechanical ventilation, air travel with preexisting lung disease

PHYSICAL EXAM

- Otic barotrauma:
  - Otoscopic exam
  - Assess patient's balance and hearing.
  - Palpate eustachian tube for tenderness.
- Pulmonary barotrauma:
  - Auscultation, percussion
- Assessment of respiratory distress

IAGNOSTIC TESTS & INTERPRETATION

ab

itial lab tests

ılmonary: Arterial blood gas

naging

itial approach

Otic or sinus: Imaging to rule out nasopharyngeal tumor or sinusitis, if indicated

Pulmonary:
- Chest radiograph
- Chest computed tomography (CT) if chest x-ray (CXR) not informative

Ultrasound

iagnostic Procedures/Surgery

Otic barotrauma:
- Tympanometry
- Audiometry: Conductive (middle ear) vs sensorineural (inner ear) hearing loss
- Surgical exploration to rule out inner ear involvement if suspected

Pulmonary barotrauma: Chest tube insertion if indicated for pneumothorax.

athological Findings

TM retraction or bulging:
- Teed 0: No visible damage
- Teed 1: Congestion around umbo (2 psi)
- Teed 2: Congestion of entire TM (2–3 psi)
- Teed 3: Hemorrhage into middle ear
- Teed 4: Extensive middle ear hemorrhage; TM may rupture
- Teed 5: Entire middle ear filled with deoxygenated blood

Inner ear involvement with rupture of the round or oval windows, perilymphatic fistula, and leakage of perilymph into the middle ear

Pulmonary barotrauma:
- Alveolar rupture may progress to interstitial emphysema, pneumoperitoneum, pneumothorax

IFFERENTIAL DIAGNOSIS

Acute and chronic otitis media

Otitis externa

Temporomandibular joint syndrome

Pulmonary: Other causes of decompensation on mechanical ventilation

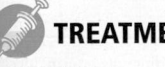

TREATMENT

MEDICATION

Treatment of predisposing conditions, upper respiratory congestion prior to air travel:
- Oral decongestants
- Nasal decongestants
- Antihistamines

Antibiotics are not indicated for middle ear effusion secondary to barotrauma.

Analgesics for pain control

Tinnitus can be treated with high-dose steroids if given within 3 weeks of onset (1)[C].

ADDITIONAL TREATMENT

General Measures

- Prevention/avoidance is best: Avoid flying or diving when risk factors are present.
- Autoinflate the eustachian tube during pressure changes:
  - Valsalva method (2)[B] during ascent and descent in air travel
  - Infants: Breast-feeding or sucking on pacifier or bottle
  - ≥4 years: Chewing gum
  - ≥8 years: Blowing up a balloon
  - Adults: Chewing gum, sucking hard candy, swallowing, or yawning
- Nasal balloon (2)[B]
- For inner ear barotrauma:
  - Bed rest with head elevated to avoid leakage of perilymph
  - Tympanotomy and repair of round or oval window may be necessary.
- Treatment of pneumothorax:
  - Removal of air from pleural space
- Adjustment of iatrogenic cause (adjustment of mechanical ventilation)

Issues for Referral

- Refer to otolaryngology if inner ear is exposed, perilymphatic fistula, or sensorineural hearing loss.
- Chest tube placement

SURGERY/OTHER PROCEDURES

- If necessary, myringotomy or tympanoplasty
- Tympanotomy and repair of round or oval window may be necessary in inner ear barotrauma.
- Tube thoracostomy for persistent pneumothorax

IN-PATIENT CONSIDERATIONS

Admission Criteria

- Patients with complicating emergencies (e.g., incapacitating pain requiring myringotomy, large tympanic perforation requiring tympanoplasty)
- Inner ear barotrauma with hearing loss
- Management of pneumothorax

ONGOING CARE

FOLLOW-UP RECOMMENDATIONS

- No flying or diving until complete resolution of all signs and symptoms, and Valsalva succeeds in equalizing pressure.
- Complete bed rest for inner ear barotrauma
- No high-risk activities or air travel until pneumothorax is completely resolved.

Patient Monitoring

- Otoscopic exams until symptoms clear
- In severe cases, audiograms

PATIENT EDUCATION

- Teach Valsalva maneuver.
- Educate on how to create allergy-free environment.
- American Academy of Pediatrics Travel Safety Tips: http://www.aap.org
- Divers Alert Network of Duke University Medical Center information line: (919) 684-2948

PROGNOSIS

- Mild barotitis media may resolve spontaneously.
- Tympanic rupture: Recovery within weeks–months
- Hearing loss may be permanent in barotitis externa.
- Prognosis of pulmonary barotrauma depends on underlying pathology.

COMPLICATIONS

- Permanent hearing loss
- Ruptured TM
- Chronic tinnitus, vertigo
- Fluid exudate in middle ear
- Perilymphatic fistula
- Sensorineural hearing loss

REFERENCES

1. Duplessis C, Hoffer M. Tinnitus in an active duty navy diver: a review of inner ear barotrauma, tinnitus, and its treatment. *Undersea Hyperbaric Med*. 2006;33(4):223–30.
2. Stangerup SE, et al. Point prevalence of barotitis and its prevention and treatment with nasal balloon inflation: a prospective, controlled study. *Otol Neurol*. 2004;25(2):89–94.

ADDITIONAL READING

- Mirza S, Richardson H. Otic barotrauma from air travel. *J Laryngol Otol*. 2005;119:366–70.
- Plötz FB, Slutsky AS, van Vught AJ, et al. Ventilator-induced lung injury and multiple system organ failure: a critical review of facts and hypotheses. *Intensive Care Med*. 2004;30:1865–72.

See Also (Topic, Algorithm, Electronic Media Element)

Algorithm: Ear Pain

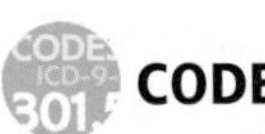

CODES

ICD9

- 993.0 Barotrauma, otitic
- 993.1 Barotrauma, sinus

CLINICAL PEARLS

- Small children can equalize eustachian tube pressure by sucking on bottles or pacifiers. Crying also serves as autoinflation.
- Pulmonary barotrauma is the 2nd leading cause of death among divers.
- Otic barotrauma is common in air travel, especially among flight personnel.
- Pulmonary barotrauma is noted in 3% of mechanically ventilated patients.

BARTONELLA INFECTIONS

Michael K. Chen, MD

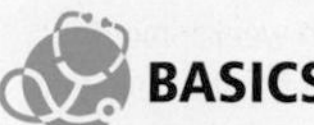

BASICS

DESCRIPTION

- Fastidious intracellular anaerobic gram-negative bacilli:
  - At least 20 distinct species, 8 known to cause disease in humans
  - *Bartonella henselae* and *B. quintana* ("trench fever") most common in North America
- Infections manifest in 2 broad categories:
  - Localized skin lesions and prominent regional lymphadenitis (cat scratch disease [CSD])
  - Bacteremia with localized vascular lesions in various organs and potential for persistent disseminated infection
- System(s) affected: Cardiovascular; Gastrointestinal; Heme/Lymphatic/Immunologic; Musculoskeletal; Nervous; Pulmonary; Skin/Exocrine; Ocular; Renal (rare)
- Synonym(s): Bartonellosis

EPIDEMIOLOGY

Incidence

- Carrion disease: 12.7/100 person-years in endemic areas
- CSD: Estimated 9.3/100,000 in US (~25,000 cases annually)
- Endocarditis: Estimated 3–4% of cases, up to 1/3 of "culture-negative" cases
- Others: Unknown

Prevalence

- Worldwide
- Seroprevalence studies of *B. henselae* suggest many childhood infections are asymptomatic.
- Seroprevalence studies of domestic cats show 25–51%.
- Studies of *B. quintana* in homeless populations suggest seroprevalence of 10%.

RISK FACTORS

- Vector exposure with cutaneous inoculation:
  - *B. henselae*: Domestic cat (especially scratch/bite from kitten), transmitted horizontally from cat fleas
  - *B. bacilliformis*: *Lutzomyia* sandflies, limited to Andean South America, cause of carrion disease
  - *B. quintana*: Human body louse, typically in alcoholic, homeless men
- Cell-mediated immune dysfunction (particularly in bacillary angiomatosis/bacillary peliosis):
  - HIV infection, especially with CD4+ lymphocyte count <100/mcL
  - Chronic steroid, immunosuppressant, or alcohol use

Genetics

No known genetic predisposition

GENERAL PREVENTION

Vector avoidance

PATHOPHYSIOLOGY

- Erythrocyte and endothelial cell invasion
- In immune-competent hosts, progresses to granulomatous and suppurative disease mainly in lymph nodes
- In immune-compromised hosts, leads to angiogenesis with mixed inflammatory cell infiltrate

DIAGNOSIS

HISTORY

- Carrion disease (aka bartonellosis); usually has 2 distinctive stages:
  - Oroya fever (acute bacteremia): In severe cases, abrupt onset 3 weeks after inoculation. Profound anemia, many complications, may be fatal.
  - Verruga peruana: Crops of nodular angiomatous skin lesions months after Oroya fever; mucosal and internal lesions also; involute in months to years
  - Asymptomatic persistent bacteremia: <15% of untreated Oroya fever survivors
- Typical cat scratch disease (up to 90% of cases):
  - Days after inoculation 2–3-mm nontender papules develop at the trauma site; progress to reddened then crusted vesicles
  - Tender regional adenopathy 1–8 weeks postinoculation; fever, malaise, headache
  - Usually involves nodes of upper extremities, neck, head, or groin; suppuration of nodes common, but only 10% require drainage
  - Resolution in 2–4 months for majority
- A typical cat scratch disease:
  - Parinaud oculoglandular syndrome: Unilateral granulomatous conjunctivitis and preauricular lymphadenitis
  - Neuroretinitis: Abrupt, painless unilateral vision loss; macular star exudate, papilledema; self-limited, full recovery
  - Encephalopathy: Rapid progression from headache to lethargy, coma, and seizure
  - Other manifestations self-limited, sequelae rare: Granulomatous hepatitis/splenitis, osteolysis, atypical pneumonitis, fever of unknown origin, mononucleosis-type syndrome, others
- Bacteremia (short-term mortality uncommon):
  - *B. quintana* (urban trench fever, Wolhynia fever, shinbone fever, quintan fever): Incubation days–weeks; sudden onset of fever, headache, leg pain; self-limited illness may be brief (4–5 days), prolonged (2–6 weeks), most commonly paroxysmal (3–5 episodes of 5 days duration). Insidious course in HIV.
  - *B. henselae*: If HIV-infected, insidious onset of fatigue, malaise, aches, weight loss, recurring fevers, headache; localizing findings uncommon. If HIV-uninfected, abrupt onset of fever (may persist or relapse), myalgias, arthralgias, headache; localizing findings unusual; may persist without symptoms.
- Endocarditis: Fever, dyspnea, murmur, embolic phenomena; aortic valve involvement most commc
- Bacillary angiomatosis: Mostly immunocompromise hosts (e.g., HIV-infected); involves skin (crops of subcutaneous or dermal nodules and/or skin-colore to purple papules; may ulcerate with serous or bloody drainage and crusting), regional lymph nodes, internal organs
- Bacillary peliosis: Involves liver and spleen in immunosuppressed persons; can involve lymph nodes; nonspecific clinical manifestations
- Neurologic syndromes in HIV: Cognitive dysfunctio behavioral disturbances; may be mistaken for dementia, psychiatric disease
- Pseudomalignancy: Increasing numbers of reports literature; sometimes confused with lymphoma, ca reports of breast nodules

PHYSICAL EXAM

See History.

DIAGNOSTIC TESTS & INTERPRETATION

Lab

- Nonspecific typical lab findings
- Skin testing reagents: Not recommended
- Giemsa-stained blood smear may show *B. bacilliformis* adherent to erythrocytes.
- Non-*bacilliformis* species:
  - Indirect fluorescent antibody (IFA) and enzyme immunoassay tests are available:
    - Interpretation complicated by variable correlation between titers and disease stage, lack of uniformity among serologic tests, and cross-reactivity among *Bartonella* species and other bacteria (1)[C]
    - In general, IFA IgG titers <1:64 suggest no current infection and >1:256 suggest active or recent infection. Immune-compromised patient may not develop adequate titers.

ALERT

- Advise lab if *Bartonella* infection is suspected so that blood, tissue, and cerebrospinal fluid cultures are prepared with appropriate media under optimal conditions; prolonged incubation required.
- Polymerase chain reaction (PCR) of valve tissue can aid diagnosis of endocarditis; otherwise, less helpful clinically.
- Antibiotics may result in false-negative culture.

Imaging

Initial approach

Ultrasound, computed tomography, transesophageal echocardiogram (as indicated)

Diagnostic Procedures/Surgery

Biopsy of lymph nodes for histology and culture. Consider biopsy of involved organs.

Pathological Findings

- Verruga peruana: Neovascular proliferation; bacteria uncommonly are identified.
- CSD: Granulomas, stellate necrosis, mixed inflammatory infiltrates; bacilli in tissue may be demonstrable by silver impregnation stains (e.g., Warthin-Starry).
- Endocarditis: Warthin-Starry-stained bacilli may be seen in vegetations.
- Bacillary angiomatosis:
  - Lobular proliferations of small blood vessels are seen, containing cuboidal endothelial cells interspersed with inflammatory cells, mostly neutrophils.
  - Warthin-Starry stain or electron microscopy may show clusters of bacilli.
- Bacillary peliosis: Blood-filled cystic structures. Warthin-Starry stain may show surrounding clumps of bacilli.

DIFFERENTIAL DIAGNOSIS

- Typical CSD: Sporotrichosis, histoplasmosis, plague, tularemia, brucellosis, mycobacteria, staphylococci, streptococci, other agents associated with injection drug use; lymphoma; metastatic malignancy
- Atypical CSD: Non-*bacilliformis* bacteremia syndromes:
  - Immunocompromised: *Cryptococcus neoformans*, *Histoplasma capsulatum*, *Coccidioides immitis*, *Mycobacterium avium*-complex
  - Arthropod exposure: Rickettsial infections, tularemia, plague, babesiosis, borreliosis
  - Cat/dog scratch/bite: Pasteurella
  - Influenza, infectious mononucleosis, hepatitis
- Endocarditis: Other slow-growing bacteria (*Haemophilus*, *Actinobacillus*, *Cardiobacterium*, *Eikenella*, *Kingella*, *Coxiella*)
- Bacillary angiomatosis/bacillary peliosis: Kaposi's sarcoma, pyogenic granuloma, hemangioma
- Neurologic syndrome in HIV: Tertiary syphilis, cryptococcal meningitis, toxoplasmosis, progressive multifocal leukoencephalopathy, alcohol or drug abuse

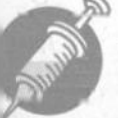

TREATMENT

MEDICATION

- Antibiotic choice depends on clinical situation; much data are secondary to case studies, as opposed to randomized controlled trial (RCT) data.
- Oroya fever: Chloramphenicol 500 mg (pediatric dose 50–75 mg/kg/d) p.o./IV q.i.d. + B-lactam (IV: PCN G 3 million U q4h (40K units/kg q4h for peds)/p.o.: PCN V recommended 500 mg q.i.d. or 20 mg/kg q.i.d. for peds) for 14 days (2)[B]
- Verruga peruana: Rifampin 10/mg/kg/d (not to exceed 600 mg/d in children) for 10–14 days (2)[B]
- Typical CSD: No clear benefit, although oral azithromycin may speed resolution of extensive lymphadenopathy: Adults and children >45.5 kg: 500 mg on day 1; 250 mg daily on days 2–5; children ≤4 5.5 kg: 10 mg/kg on day 1; 5 mg/kg daily on days 2–5 (2)[A]
- Retinitis: Doxycycline 100 mg p.o. b.i.d. (in peds <8 y/o, consider erythromycin 20 mg/kg/d to max daily dose of 2 g/d) + rifampin 300 mg p.o. b.i.d. for 4–6 weeks (2)[B]. Some data show that retinitis is self-limited, so some authors suggest no antibiotics are needed.
- Trench fever or chronic *B. quintana* bacteremia: Doxycycline 200 mg p.o. daily for 4 weeks + gentamicin 3 mg/kg IV daily for 2 weeks (2)[A]
- Bacillary angiomatosis/peliosis: Erythromycin 500 mg (pediatric dose 40 mg/kg/d to maximum daily dose of 2 g/d) p.o. q.i.d. or doxycycline 100 mg p.o. b.i.d. for 3 months (4 months for peliosis); consider longer course if immunocompromised (2)[B].
- Endocarditis (culture-positive): Gentamicin 1 mg/kg IV t.i.d. for 2 weeks + doxycycline 100 mg p.o. b.i.d. for 6 weeks (2)[B]. Add ceftriaxone 2 g IV/IM daily for 6 weeks for culture-negative.

ADDITIONAL TREATMENT

Issues for Referral

Cardiac surgery if endocarditis

SURGERY/OTHER PROCEDURES

Valve replacement if indicated in endocarditis

IN-PATIENT CONSIDERATIONS

Initial Stabilization

ABCs, high degree of clinical suspicion, and awareness of local infection risk. Blood transfusions if symptomatic severe anemia.

Admission Criteria

Consider admission for patients who are immune-compromised, hemodynamically unstable, or may not have access to appropriate antibiotics.

Discharge Criteria

Patients may be discharged when stable on p.o. antibiotics or receiving IV antibiotics through a peripherally inserted central catheter line.

ONGOING CARE

FOLLOW-UP RECOMMENDATIONS

Patient Monitoring

Immune-compromised patients at increased risk for relapse. Extended periods of antibiotics recommended

DIET

No diet modifications needed

PATIENT EDUCATION

Vector avoidance information

PROGNOSIS

- CSD: Spontaneous resolution usually in 2–4 months without specific therapy
- Other syndromes: With proper treatment, full resolution; if relapse, consider long-term suppressive antibiotics after retreatment
- Oroya fever: If untreated >40% mortality

COMPLICATIONS

Disseminated disease can present with specific organ-related findings such as focal seizures or renal microabscesses (3,4)[C]

REFERENCES

1. Vermeulen MJ, Verbakel H, Notermans DW et al. Evaluation of sensitivity, specificity and cross-reactivity in Bartonella henselae serology. *J Med Microbiol*. 2010;59:743–5.
2. Rolain JM, Brouqui P, Koehler JE et al. Recommendations for treatment of human infections caused by Bartonella species. *Antimicrob Agents Chemother*. 2004;48:1921–33.
3. Salehi N, Custodio H, Rathore MH et al. Renal microabscesses due to Bartonella infection. *Pediatr Infect Dis J*. 2010;29:472–3.
4. Farooque P, Khurana DS, Melvin JJ et al. Persistent focal seizures after cat scratch encephalopathy. *Pediatr. Neurol*. 2010;42:215–8.

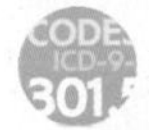

CODES

ICD9

- 041.84 Other specified bacterial infections in conditions classified elsewhere and of unspecified site, other anaerobes
- 078.3 Cat-scratch disease
- 083.1 Trench fever

CLINICAL PEARLS

- Bartonella infection and its various clinical manifestations can be difficult to identify, unless there is a high degree of clinical suspicion and awareness of local infection risks.
- CSD will resolve by itself in most immune-competent patients. Systemic lymphadenopathy will resolve faster with azithromycin.
- Immune-compromised patients are at increased risk for developing occult infections, but tend to have more dramatic response to antibiotics.

BARTTER'S SYNDROME

Maricarmen Malagon-Rogers, MD

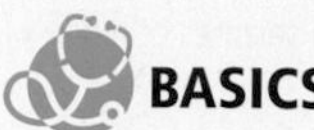

BASICS

- Bartter's syndrome and Bartter's-like syndrome are a group of rare autosomal, recessive, salt-wasting nephropathies characterized by polyuria, hypokalemia, metabolic alkalosis, and normotension with hyperreninemic-hyperaldosteronism (1).
- Traditionally they have been divided into two main disorders according to where the defect is located in the renal tubule, but since genetic classification has been available there are more subtypes (2).
- Bartter (Furosemide type) with 5 subtypes and Gitelman (Thiazide type) with 2 subtypes and combinations of the two.

DESCRIPTION

Bartter's disorders have diverse genetic origins, with a common pathological mechanism of a severe reduction in salt reabsorption by the thick ascending limb of Henle (TAL) and/or the distal convoluted tubule (DCT).

EPIDEMIOLOGY

Prevalence

Gitelman's prevalence is calculated at 1:40000. Heterozygote state in Caucasians: 1% (3)

RISK FACTORS

Consanguinity

Genetics

Autosomal recessive

PATHOPHYSIOLOGY

- Bartter type is caused by inactivating mutations in one of several genes encoding membrane proteins in charge of transporting Na, Cl, K, and sometimes Ca in the loop of Henle where 25% of the filtered solute load is reabsorbed. This causes large urinary losses of Na, Cl, K, Mg, and Ca. It resembles the effect of large doses of furosemide, which results in hypovolemia with activation of the renin aldosterone system without any hypertension. According to which transporter is compromised, the disease will be more or less severe and it will start sooner or later. When it starts in utero it causes polyhydramnios because of fetal polyuria. There is also secondary stimulation of prostaglandin E2 (PGE2) production with worsening of salt losses (2).
- In the Gitelman type the inactivating mutations are in the distal convoluted tube where 5% of the filtered Na is reabsorbed. It resembles the effect of thiazides and causes urinary losses of Na, Cl, K, and Mg, but not Ca. It is clinically less severe (2).

ETIOLOGY

- The inactivating mutations in Bartter syndrome are in type I. The Na^{+}-K-$2Cl^{-}$ cotransporter (*SLC12A1* encoding NKCC2), in type II the apical inward-rectifying potassium channel (*KCNJ1* encoding ROMK), in type III the basolateral chloride channel (*ClCNK* encoding ClC-Kb), and in type IV the *BSND*, a protein that acts as an essential activator β-subunit for ClC-Ka and ClC-Kb chloride channels. Type V is a gain-of-function mutations in the extracellular calcium ion-sensing receptor (CaSR) that cause a variant with hypocalcemia (12).
- In Gitelman the inactivating mutations are in the *SLC12A3* gene encoding the thiazide sensitive Na-Cl cotransporter, or NCCT (23).

COMMONLY ASSOCIATED CONDITIONS

- Polyhydramnios, prematurity
- Nephrocalcinosis, rickets, growth retardation
- Hyperprostaglandin levels
- Sensoneural deafness, mental retardation in type IV
- Cardiac problems (4)
- Gallstones (5)
- Constipation

DIAGNOSIS

HISTORY

- Polyuria and polydipsia are always present. History of episodes of dehydration.
- In types I, II, IV, and V the presentation is usually prenatal with polyhydramnios, prematurity, and postnatally there is failure to thrive, dehydration, muscle weakness, seizures, tetany, and paresthesia This type has been called Neonatal Bartter of In Bartter there is always hypercalciuria with normomagnesemia. Nephrocalcinosis is present in type I and II. Type II can show hyperkalemia at birth and less hypokalemia than the other subtypes.
- Type III is variable and can present later in early childhood with no nephrocalcinosis.
- Gitelman usually presents later with muscle weakness and hypokalemia, hypomagnesemia, and hypocalciuria.

PHYSICAL EXAM

- Premature AGE, normotension, and failure to thrive later on
- Dysmorphic features, including triangular facies, protruding ears, large eyes, and drooping mouth.
- Tetany, hypotonia.

DIAGNOSTIC TESTS & INTERPRETATION

Lab

- Hypokalemia of <2.5 mEq/L with metabolic alkalosis is almost universal. Only in type II hypokalemia may not be as severe and it may even have hyperkalemia in the newborn period.
- Prenatal testing of amniotic fluid may be diagnostic (6).

tial lab tests

Na, K, Cl, tCO2, Ca, and Mg in serum and in urine. There will be hypokalemia with elevated tCO2 and normomagnesemia with hyperkaluria, hyperchloruria, and hypercalciuria in Bartter, while in Gitelman there will be hypomagnesemia and decreased urinary calcium.

Renin and aldosterone will always be elevated and Prostaglandin E2 will be elevated in Bartter but not in Gitelman.

llow-Up & Special Considerations

Electrolytes need to be followed very frequently until they stabilize and then monthly. Urinary random Ca/Cr should be followed at least twice a year.

Creatinine and BUN should be followed because there can be renal failure mainly from nephrocalcinosis (7).

Cardiac studies are indicated (4).

naging

enal ultrasound is indicated always in Bartter ecause of the presence of nephrocalcinosis. It should done about every 2 years.

athological Findings

enal biopsy shows hyperplasia of the juxtaglomerular pparatus.

IFFERENTIAL DIAGNOSIS

Chronic diuretic abuse

Chronic vomiting

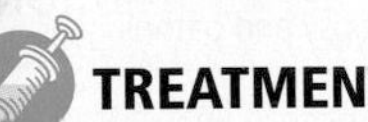

TREATMENT

The main goal in the neonatal period is to keep patients hydrated with correction of hypokalemia.

In Gitelman, correction of hypomagnesemia is also important.

EDICATION

on-steroidal antiinflammatory drugs (NSAIDs) should e used in Bartter's (8).

irst Line

Bartter: NSAIDs, potassium and sodium supplementation, spironolactone

Gitelman: Potassium and magnesium supplementation. NSAIDs are not useful.

econd Line

2 blockers or proton-pump inhibitors when using SAIDs

ONGOING CARE

DIET

High in salt, potassium, and water

PROGNOSIS

Good in general. With adequate management patients can grow normally (8).

COMPLICATIONS

Nephrocalcinosis, gastric ulcers, chronic kidney disease (1)

REFERENCES

1. Chadha V, Alon US et al. Hereditary renal tubular disorders. *Semin Nephrol*. 2009;29:399–411.
2. Seyberth HW et al. An improved terminology and classification of Bartter-like syndromes. *Nature clinical practice. Nephrology*. 2008;4:560–7.
3. Knoers NV, Levtchenko EN et al. Gitelman syndrome. *Orphanet J Rare Dis*. 2008;3:22.
4. Scognamiglio R, Calò LA, Negut C et al. Myocardial perfusion defects in Bartter and Gitelman syndromes. *Eur J Clin Invest*. 2008;38:888–95.
5. Shin JI, Lee JS et al. Comment on: Bartter syndrome and cholelithiasis in an infant: is this a mere coincidence? (*Eur J Pediatr* 2008;167(1):109–110). *Eur J Pediatr*. 2009;168.
6. Garnier A, Dreux S, Vargas-Poussou R et al. Bartter syndrome prenatal diagnosis based on amniotic fluid biochemical analysis. *Pediatr Res*. 2010;67:300–3.
7. Lin CM, Tsai JD, Lo YF et al. Chronic renal failure in a boy with classic Bartter's syndrome due to a novel mutation in CLCNKB coding for the chloride channel. *Eur J Pediatr*. 2009;168:1129–33.
8. Puricelli E, Bettinelli A, Borsa N et al. Long-term follow-up of patients with Bartter syndrome type I and II. *Nephrol Dial Transplant*. 2010;25:2976–81.

ADDITIONAL READING

- Brochard K, Boyer O, Blanchard A et al. Phenotype-genotype correlation in antenatal and neonatal variants of Bartter syndrome. *Nephrol Dial Transplant*. 2009;24:1455–64.
- Nozu K, Iijima K, Kanda K et al. The pharmacological characteristics of molecular-based inherited salt-losing tubulopathies. *J Clin Endocrinol Metabol*. 2010.

CODES

ICD9

255.13 Bartter's syndrome

CLINICAL PEARLS

Bartter's and Bartter's-like syndromes are autosomic recessive hypokalemic salt-losing nephropathies that mimic diuretic effects.

BASAL CELL CARCINOMA

Aleema Patel, MD
Leslie Robinson-Bostom, MD

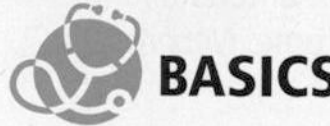

BASICS

Incidence in US: ~1,000,000 cases/year and is increasing about 10% each year

DESCRIPTION

Basal cell carcinoma (BCC) is the most common cancer, originating from the basal cell layer of the skin appendages:

- Rarely metastasizes, but capable of local tissue destruction

Geriatric Considerations

- Greater frequency in geriatric patients (ages 55–75 have 100 times incidence of age <20)
- The incidence is rapidly increasing in 20–40-year-olds.

Pediatric Considerations

Rare in children, but childhood sun exposure is important in adult disease.

EPIDEMIOLOGY

Worldwide, the most common form of cancer.

Incidence

- Incidence in US: 1,000,000 cases/year and is increasing about 10% each year
- Predominant age: Generally >40, but incidence is increasing in younger populations
- Predominant sex: Male > Female (although incidence is increasing in females)
- Lifetime risk of white North Americans: 30%

RISK FACTORS

- Chronic sun exposure (UV radiation)
- Most common in the following phenotypes:
  - Light complexion: Skin type I (burns but does not tan) and skin type II (usually burns, sometimes tans)
  - Red or blond hair
  - Blue or green eyes
- Tendency to sunburn
- Male sex, although increasing risk in women due to lifestyle changes such as tanning beds
- History of nonmelanoma skin cancer:
  - After initial diagnosis of skin cancer, 35% risk of new nonmelanoma skin cancer at 3 years and 50% at 5 years.
- Family history of skin cancer
- 3–4 decades after chronic arsenic exposure
- 2 decades after therapeutic radiation
- Chronic immunosuppression: Transplant recipients (10 times higher incidence), patients with HIV or lymphomas

Genetics

Several genetic conditions increase the risk of developing BCC:

- Albinism (recessive alleles)
- Xeroderma pigmentosum (autosomal recessive)
- Bazex syndrome (rare, x-linked dominant)
- Nevoid basal cell carcinoma syndrome/Gorlin syndrome (rare, autosomal dominant)
- Cytochrome P-450 CYP2D6 and glutathione S-transferase detoxifying enzyme gene mutations (especially in truncal basal cell carcinoma, marked by clusters of basal cell carcinomas and a younger age of onset)

GENERAL PREVENTION

- Use broad-spectrum sunscreens of at least SPF 30 daily and reapply after swimming or sweating.
- Avoid overexposure to the sun by seeking shade between 10 a.m. and 4 p.m. as well as wearing wide-brimmed hats and long-sleeved shirts.
- Avoid tanning and sunburns (including tanning salons).

PATHOPHYSIOLOGY

- UV-induced inflammation and cyclooxygenase activation in skin
- Mutation of PTCH1 (patched homolog 1), a tumor-suppressor gene that inhibits the hedgehog signaling pathway
- Mutation of the SMO (smoothened homolog) gene, which is also involved in the hedgehog signaling pathway
- UV-induced mutations of the TP53 (tumor protein 53), a tumor-suppressor gene
- Activation of BCL2, an antiapoptosis proto-oncogene

COMMONLY ASSOCIATED CONDITIONS

- Cosmetic disfigurement since head and neck most often affected
- Loss of vision with orbital involvement
- Loss of nerve function due to perineural spread or extensive and deep invasion
- Ulcerating neoplasms are prone to infections.

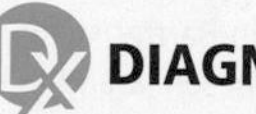

DIAGNOSIS

HISTORY

Exposure to risk factors, family history

PHYSICAL EXAM

- 80% on face and neck, 20% on trunk and lower limbs (mostly women) (1)[B]
- Nodular: Most common (60%); presents as pinkish pearly papule, plaque, or nodule often with telangiectatic vessels, ulceration, and a rolled periphery usually on face:
  - Pigmented: Presents as a translucent papule with "floating pigment"; more commonly seen in darker skin types
- Superficial: (30%); light red, scaly papule or plaque with atrophic center, ringed by translucent micropapules, usually on trunk or extremities; more common in men
- Morpheaform: (5–10%); firm, smooth, flesh-colored, scarlike papule or plaque with ill-defined borders

DIAGNOSTIC TESTS & INTERPRETATION

Diagnostic Procedures/Surgery

- Clinical diagnosis and histological subtype are confirmed through skin biopsy and pathological examination.
- Shave biopsy is typically sufficient; however, punch biopsy is more useful to assess depth of tumor and perineural invasion.
- If a genetic disorder is suspected, additional tests may be needed to confirm it.

Pathological Findings

- Nodular BCC:
  - Extending from the epidermis are nodular aggregates of basaloid cells.
  - Tumor cells are uniform; rarely have mitotic figures; and have large, oval, hyperchromatic nuclei with little cytoplasm, surrounded by a peripheral palisade.
  - Early lesions are usually connected to the epidermis, unlike late lesions.
  - Increased mucin in dermal stroma:
    - Cleft formation (retraction artifact) common between BCC "nests" and stroma due to mucin shrinkage during fixation and staining.
- Superficial BCC:
  - Appear as buds of basaloid cells attached to undersurface of epidermis
  - Peripheral palisading

Morpheoform BCC:
- Thin cords and strands of basaloid cells, embedded in dense, fibrous, "scarlike" stroma
- Less peripheral palisading and retraction, greater subclinical involvement

Infiltrating BCC:
- Like morpheoform BCC, but no "scarlike" stroma and thicker, more spiky, irregular strands
- Less peripheral palisading and retraction, greater subclinical involvement

Micronodular BCC:
- Small, nodular aggregates of tumor cells
- Less retraction artifact and higher subclinical involvement than nodular BCC

DIFFERENTIAL DIAGNOSIS

- Sebaceous hyperplasia
- Epidermal inclusion cyst
- Intradermal nevi (pigmented and nonpigmented)
- Molluscum contagiosum
- Squamous cell carcinoma
- Nummular dermatitis
- Psoriasis
- Melanoma (pigmented lesions)
- Atypical fibroxanthoma
- Rare adnexal neoplasms

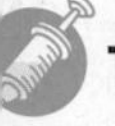

TREATMENT

MEDICATION

- May be especially useful in those who cannot tolerate surgical procedures and in those who refuse to have surgery
- 5-fluorouracil cream inhibits thymidylate synthetase, interrupting DNA synthesis for superficial lesions in low-risk areas; primary treatment only 5% applied b.i.d. for 3–10 weeks
- Imiquimod (Aldara) cream approved for treatment of low-risk superficial BCC; daily dosing for 6–12 weeks; 90% histologic cure

ADDITIONAL TREATMENT

- Radiation therapy:
  - Useful for patients who cannot or will not undergo surgery
  - Used following surgery, particularly if margins of tumor were not cleared
  - Cure rate is approximately 90%.
  - Tumors that recur in areas previously treated with radiation are harder to treat, and the area is more difficult to reconstruct.
- Photodynamic therapy (PDT) (2)[A]:
  - 5-aminolevulinic acid, a photosensitizer, is activated by specific wavelengths of light, creating singlet oxygen radicals that destroy local tissue (no damage to surrounding or deep tissues).
  - Useful in areas where tissue preservation is cosmetically or functionally important

SURGERY/OTHER PROCEDURES

- Generally 1st choice; specific treatment selection varies with extent and location of lesion as well as tumor border demarcation (3)[A]
- High-risk areas:
  - Inner canthus, nasolabial sulcus, philtrum, preauricular area, retroauricular sulcus, lip, temple
- Curettage and electrodesiccation:
  - If nodular lesion <1 cm, in low-risk area, not deeply invasive
- Excision:
  - Useful for lesions in high-risk areas
  - Not as dependent on lesion size
- Cryosurgery:
  - Reserved for small lesions in low-risk areas
  - May want pre- and post-treatment biopsies
- Mohs surgery:
  - Preferred microsurgically controlled surgical treatment for lesions in high-risk areas, recurrent lesions, and lesions exhibiting an aggressive growth pattern
  - Requires referral to appropriately trained dermatologic surgeon

IN-PATIENT CONSIDERATIONS

Outpatient unless extensive lesion

ONGOING CARE

FOLLOW-UP RECOMMENDATIONS

- Avoid sun exposure.
- Oral retinoids may prevent the development of new basal cell carcinomas in patients with Gorlin syndrome, renal transplant patients, and patients with severe actinic damage.

Patient Monitoring

- Every month for 3 months, then twice yearly for 5 years; yearly thereafter
- Increased risk of other skin cancers (4)[C]

PATIENT EDUCATION

- Teach patient appropriate sun-avoidance techniques, sunscreens, etc.
- Monthly self skin exam
- Educate patients concerning adequate calcium and vitamin D intake.

PROGNOSIS

- Proper treatment yields 90–95% cure.
- Most recurrences happen within 5 years.
- Development of new BCCs: Patients (36%) will develop a new lesion within 5 years.

COMPLICATIONS

- Local recurrence and spread
- Usually, recurrences will appear within 5 years.
- Metastasis: Rare (<0.1%), but metastatic disease usually fatal within 8 months

REFERENCES

1. Wong CS, Strange RC, Lear JT. Basal cell carcinoma. *BMJ*. 2003;327:794–8.
2. Soler AM, Angell-Petersen E, Warloe T, et al. Photodynamic therapy of superficial basal cell carcinoma with 5-aminolevulinic acid with dimethylsulfoxide and ethylendiaminetetraacetic acid: a comparison of two light sources. *Photochem Photobiol*. 2000;71:724–9.
3. Bath FJ, Bong J, Perkins W, et al. Interventions for basal cell carcinoma of the skin. *Cochrane Database Syst Rev*. 2003;CD003412.
4. Friedman GD, Tekawa IS. Association of basal cell skin cancers with other cancers (United States). *Cancer Causes Control*. 2000;11:891–7.

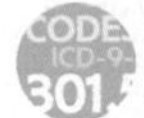

CODES

ICD9

- 173.0 Other malignant neoplasm of skin of lip
- 173.1 Other malignant neoplasm of skin of eyelid, including canthus
- 173.2 Other malignant neoplasm of skin of ear and external auditory canal

CLINICAL PEARLS

- Use diagnostic keys above to differentiate between BCC and cutaneous squamous cell carcinoma (SCC). SCC arises from actinic keratosis in 60% of cases and generally presents as an asymptomatic hyperkeratotic lesion. If unsure, biopsy or refer to a specialist.
- Some hyperpigmented BCCs may appear similar to melanoma. Remember the ABCDEs of melanoma recognition: *A*symmetry, *B*order irregularities, *C*olor variability, *D*iameter >6 mm, *E*nlargement. If unsure, refer to a specialist.
- The USPSTF concludes there is insufficient evidence to recommend for or against routine total body skin exams for melanoma, BCC, or SCC. Exams should be based on risk factors, including exposures and family and prior medical history. All patients may receive education about risks and self-exam.

BEHAVIORAL PROBLEMS, PEDIATRIC

Elizabeth Bade, MD

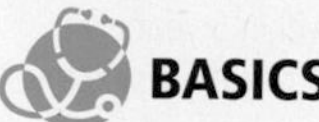

BASICS

DESCRIPTION

Behavior that disrupts ≥1 areas of psychosocial functioning but not seriously enough to receive an official DSM-IV diagnosis; most commonly reported behavioral problems are

- Noncompliance: Purposeful refusal (active/passive) to do what is requested by parent or other adult authority figure
- Temper tantrums: Loss of internal control believed to be provoked by overtiredness, physical discomfort, or fear that leads the child to exhibit behaviors such as crying, whining, breath holding, or in extreme cases, acts of aggression
- Sleep disorders: Sleep patterns that are distressing to parents, child, or physician; this can be further broken down into 2 categories based on polysomnograph:
  - Primary sleep disorders have abnormal polysomnograph. Examples include sleepwalking and night terrors.
  - Secondary sleep disorders have normal polysomnograph and are the most common sleep disorders. Examples include night awakenings and bedtime resistance.
- Nocturnal enuresis: Enuresis that occurs only at night in children >5 years of age with no medical problems
  - Primary: Nocturnal enuresis in a child who has never been dry at night
  - Secondary: Nocturnal enuresis in a child who has been dry at night for at least 6 months

EPIDEMIOLOGY

- Noncompliance: More common in children <1 year of age, especially as they develop autonomy; boys have a modestly greater likelihood of being noncompliant. Noncompliant behavior decreases with age.
- Temper tantrums: 70% of 18- to 24-month-old children; 75.3% of 3- to 5-year-old children; in children with severe tantrums, 52% have other non-tantrum-related behavioral/emotional problems (1).
- Sleep disorders (secondary): 25% of children between 1 and 5 years of age and 20–30% of infants, toddlers, and preschoolers
- Nocturnal enuresis:
  - At least 20% of children in the 1st grade wet the bed occasionally, and 4% wet 2 or more times per week; more common in boys than in girls (2):
    - Enuresis in boys aged 7 and 10 years is 9% and 7%, respectively.
    - Enuresis in girls aged 7 and 10 years is 6% and 3%, respectively.

RISK FACTORS

Genetics

- Genetic components contribute to the pathogenesis of primary nocturnal enuresis. One locus was assigned to chromosome 13q (3).
- Major genes are involved in a large proportion of enuresis families. Linkage results suggest that such a gene is located on chromosome 12q.
- Nocturnal enuresis is a genetic and heterogeneous disorder. The associations between genotype and phenotype are complex and are susceptible to environmental influences (4).

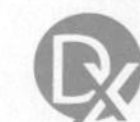

DIAGNOSIS

HISTORY

- Noncompliance: Complete history taken from parents and teachers; direct observation of child or child–parent interaction:
  - Criteria: Is problematic for at least some adults in child's life, leading to stressful/difficult interactions for minimum period of 6 months
  - Reduces child's ability to take part in structured activities
  - Creates stressful interactions and relationships with compliant children
  - Disrupts academic progress; places child at risk for physical injury
- Temper tantrums: History with focus on development, family depression, or violence:
  - Criteria: May consist of stiffening limbs and arching back, dropping to the floor, shouting, screaming, crying, pushing/pulling, stamping, hitting, kicking, throwing, or running away (1)
  - Screening for depression with the Preschool Feelings Checklist (5)
- Sleep disorders: Screening questions about sleep during well-child visit; complete history, including questions about snoring (6)
- Nocturnal enuresis: Complete history specifically asking about urine output/fluid intake/bowel movements; consider asking parent to keep a voiding diary.

PHYSICAL EXAM

- Nocturnal enuresis: Physical exam should focus on abdomen, spine, genitalia, and perineum, followed by a neurologic exam. Specifically, evaluate for
  - Abdomen: Enlarged bladder, kidneys, or fecal masses
  - Spine: Dimpling or tufts of hair on sacrum
  - Genital urinary exam:
    - Males: Meatal stenosis, hypospadias, epispadias, phimosis
    - Females: Vulvitis, vaginitis, labial adhesions, ureterocele at introitus; wide vaginal orifice with scar or healed laceration may be evidence of abuse.
- Rectal exam: Tone and constipation
- Neurologic exam: Focused on the lower extremities

DIAGNOSTIC TESTS & INTERPRETATION

Lab

Initial lab tests

For nocturnal enuresis: Urinalysis and urine culture

Follow-Up & Special Considerations

Sleep studies should be performed in children if there is a history of snoring and daytime attention-deficit hyperactivity disorder (ADHD)–type symptoms.

Diagnostic Procedures/Surgery

- General screening tools: Child Behavioral Checklist
- Pediatric Symptom Checklist (www. brightfutures.org/mentalhealth/pdf/professionals/ped_symptom_chklst.pdf)
- NICHQ Vanderbilt Assessment (ADHD screen; www.myadhd.com/vanderbiltparent6175.html

Pathological Findings

Certain tantrum behaviors are more likely to be indicative of a serious illness such as major depression or other DSM-IV diagnosable disorders such as ADHD, oppositional defiant disorder (ODD), etc. These behaviors include (5)

- Self-injurious behaviors
- Slow recovery time from tantrums
- More tantrums in the home than outside the home
- More aggressive behaviors toward others, including oral aggression

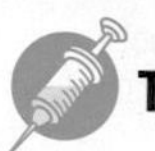

TREATMENT

- General: Educate parent about the specific behavioral problem (2).
- Noncompliance: In the case of extreme child disobedience, consider parent training programs. Child may need to be screened for ADHD, ODD, or conduct disorder (CD).
- Temper tantrums: Remind parent(s) that this is a normal aspect of childhood.
  - If tantrum is set off by external factors such as hunger or overtiredness, then correct.
  - Other methods for dealing with a tantrum include 1 of the following:
    - Ignoring the tantrum
    - Removing the child and placing him or her in time-out (1 minute for each year of age)
    - Holding child/restraining child until he or she calms down
    - Giving child clear, firm, and consistent instructions as well as enough time to obey
- Sleep disorders: Aside from parent education, other interventions include
  - Extinction: Child goes to bed at designated time, and cries/tantrums are ignored while monitoring child for safety.
  - Graduated extinction: Parent ignores cries/tantrums for specified period. Parent can check at a fixed time or check at increasing intervals.
  - Studies show that parent education and extinction are the most effective approaches (6).

- Nocturnal enuresis:
  - Bedwetting alarm: Continue for at least 2–3 months.
  - Little evidence from clinical trials, but good empirical evidence for behavioral training, including positive reinforcement (small reward for each dry night), or responsibility training (if old enough, child is responsible for changing or washing sheets), encouraging daily bowel movements, and frequent bladder emptying during the day (2).
  - If behavioral therapy fails: Desmopressin if child >6 years of age.
  - If behavioral and medical therapy fail, then refer to a specialist.

MEDICATION

Most pediatric behavioral issues respond well to nonpharmacologic therapy.

- Sleep disorders:
  - For certain delayed sleep onset disorders, after behavioral methods are exhausted, melatonin at low doses can be tried while behavior modification is continued (7). However, this is not approved by the Food and Drug Administration (FDA) for pediatric patients.
  - Melatonin has been used in pediatric patients in doses of 0.5–10 mg PO given at night.
- Nocturnal enuresis (also see topic Enuresis):
  - If behavioral therapy fails: Desmopressin is the only medicine approved as 1st-line therapy if child >6 years of age.
    - As of 2007, the FDA recommends against use of intranasal formulations in children owing to reports of severe hyponatremia resulting in seizures and death in children using intranasal formulations of desmopressin
    - Oral desmopressin (DDAVP): Dose-dependent; begin with 0.2-mg tablet taken at bedtime on empty stomach; may titrate to 0.6 mg
    - Maximally effective in 1 hour; cleared within 9 hours
    - Give nightly for 6 months; then stop for 2 weeks for test of dryness.
    - Suspend dose in children who experience acute condition affecting fluid/electrolyte balances (i.e., fever, vomiting, diarrhea, vigorous exercise).
    - Potential risks include water intoxication with hyponatremia.
    - 10–60% success; safe even when used for >12 months; high relapse rate after discontinuation without a structured withdrawal program

ADDITIONAL TREATMENT

Issues for Referral

A patient who exhibits self-injurious behaviors, slow recovery time from tantrums, more tantrums in the home than outside the home, or more aggressive behaviors toward others (including oral aggression) may require referral to a neurodevelopmental or psychiatric specialist.

COMPLEMENTARY AND ALTERNATIVE MEDICINE

- The EPA portion of omega-3 fatty acids has been shown to be useful in treating depression and mood disorders in the pediatric population (8). For patients >8 years of age, 1 g of fish oil is recommended daily, <8 years old, 700 mg/d is recommended.
- For irritability, there is some limited evidence for calcium at 400–800 mg/d and magnesium at 200–400 mg/d, B complex vitamins at 50 mg/d, vitamin C at 1,000 mg/d if younger than 8 years of age and 500 mg/d if over 8 years of age (8)[C].

ONGOING CARE

DIET

- Nutrition is very important in behavioral issues. Avoiding high-sugar foods and providing balanced, whole meals has been shown to decrease aggressive and noncompliant behaviors in children.
- Eliminate caffeine and increase protein.

PATIENT EDUCATION

- A few examples of parent training programs are
  - The Oregon Social Learning Center program: www.oslc.org
  - Forehand and McMahon program: Helping the Noncompliant Child (ages 3–8 years): www.strengtheningfamilies.org/html/programs_1999/02_HNCC.html
  - The BASIC program by Webster-Stratton: www.incredibleyears.com
- Also check local community organizations for parenting classes.

REFERENCES

1. Potegal M, Davidson RJ. Temper tantrums in young children: 1. Behavioral composition. *J Dev Behav Pediatr*. 2003;24:140–7.
2. Robson WL. Clinical practice. Evaluation and management of enuresis. *N Engl J Med*. 2009; 360:1429–36.
3. Arnell H, Hjälmås K, Jägervall M, et al. The genetics of primary nocturnal enuresis: inheritance and suggestion of a second major gene on chromosome 12q. *J Med Genet*. 1997;34:360–5.
4. von Gontard A, Schaumburg H, Hollmann E, et al. The genetics of enuresis: a review. *J Urol*. 2001;166:2438–43.
5. Belden AC, Thomson NR, Luby JL. Temper tantrums in healthy versus depressed and disruptive preschoolers: defining tantrum behaviors associated with clinical problems. *J Pediatr*. 2008;152:117–22.
6. Mindell JA, Kuhn B, Lewin DS, et al. Behavioral treatment of bedtime problems and night wakings in infants and young children. *Sleep*. 2006;29: 1263–76.
7. Gringras P. When to use drugs to help sleep. *Arch Dis Child*. 2008.
8. Shannon S et al. Integrative approaches to pediatric mood disorders. *Altern Ther Health Med*. 2009; 15(5):48–53.

ADDITIONAL READING

- Albrecht SJ, Dore DJ, Naugle AE. Common behavioral dilemmas of the school-aged child. *Pediatr Clin North Am*. 2003;50:841–57.
- Brown P, Schnall JG, Hallgren JD. When (and how) should you evaluate a child for obstructive sleep apnea? *J Fam Pract*. 2007;56:317–20.
- Caldwell PHY, et al. Bedwetting and toileting problems in children. *JAMA*. 2005;182:190–5.
- Kalb LM, Loeber R. Child disobedience and noncompliance: a review. *Pediatrics*. 2003;111: 641–52.
- Luby JL, Heffelfinger A, Koenig-McNaught AL, et al. The Preschool Feelings Checklist: a brief and sensitive screening measure for depression in young children. *J Am Acad Child Adolesc Psychiatry*. 2004;43:708–17.
- Miller JW. Screening children for developmental behavioral problems: principles for the practitioner. *Prim Care Clin Office Pract*. 2007;34:177–201.
- Thiedke CC. Sleep disorders and sleep problems in childhood. *Am Fam Physician*. 2001;63:277–84.

See Also (Topic, Algorithm, Electronic Media Element)

Enuresis

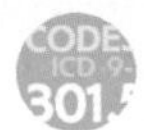

CODES

ICD9

- V40.3 Other behavioral problems
- 312.9 Unspecified disturbance of conduct

CLINICAL PEARLS

- Most commonly reported pediatric behavioral problems are noncompliance, temper tantrums, sleep disorders, and nocturnal enuresis.
- Well-child visits provide opportunities to systematically screen for these common conditions.
- Parental education is a key component of treatment.
- Nutrition is an important factor in behavior disorders and should be screened at the well-child visit.

BEHÇET SYNDROME

Prachaya Nitichaikulvatana, MD
Sangeetha Balasubramanian, MD

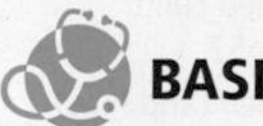

BASICS

DESCRIPTION

- Multisystem, chronic disease characterized by oral and genital mucocutaneous ulcerations, skin rashes, arthritis, thrombophlebitis, uveitis, colitis, and neurologic symptoms
- Rare in US and northern Europe, endemic in Japan, Middle East, and Mediterranean region (along "Silk Route")
- Rare in pediatric and geriatric populations
- Synonym(s): Mucocutaneous ocular syndrome; Franceschetti-Valero syndrome

Pregnancy Considerations

- Thalidomide for treatment contraindicated in pregnancy
- Possible increase in thrombosis and fetal demise

EPIDEMIOLOGY

- Predominant age: 3rd–4th decades
- Predominant gender: Male = Female, with males affected more severely and more in the Middle East

Prevalence

- 1/100,000 population in US
- In other countries, per 100,000:
  - Japan: 10
  - Iran: 16–100
  - Northern Europe: 0.3
  - Saudi Arabia: 20

RISK FACTORS

HLA-B51-positive

Genetics

One report in a mother and newborn

ETIOLOGY

Unknown: Classified as systemic vasculitis; associated with HLA-B51; possible immune response to ubiquitous heat-shock protein; possible infectious causes: herpes simplex virus (HSV), *Streptococcus*; report associated with HIV infection; possible environmental toxin: heavy metals, pesticides, possibly English walnuts or ginkgo nuts

COMMONLY ASSOCIATED CONDITIONS

- Amyloid
- Myelodysplastic syndrome and trisomy 8

DIAGNOSIS

HISTORY

- GI: Recurrent painful stomatitis or aphthous ulcers (nearly all cases); at least 3 crops in 12 months; spontaneous healing without scar, abdominal pain, melena
- Genital: Recurrent, painful ulcers with scarring
- Musculoskeletal: Myositis (rare), morning stiffness (1/3 of patients), arthralgias
- Ocular: Painful, red eyes
- Neurologic: Headache, weakness, numbness, cranial nerve palsy, seizures

PHYSICAL EXAM

- GI: Painful, shallow, or deep oral ulcers with central yellowish necrotic base and punched-out, clean margin; commonly on tongue, lips, buccal mucosa, and gingivae; ulceration in terminal ileum, cecum, ascending colon
- Genital: Painful, scarring ulcers
- Dermal: Papulopustular (acneiform) lesions, erythema nodosum, pyoderma
- Musculoskeletal: Self-limited, nonerosive arthritis mostly mono- or oligoarthritis predominantly affecting lower extremities, rarely polyarthritis
- Ocular: Anterior uveitis with hypopyon, iridocyclitis, chorioretinitis, retinal vasculitis, vitreous hemorrhage, papilledema, secondary glaucoma, optic atrophy
- Thrombophlebitis: Peripheral, pulmonary, cerebral, Budd-Chiari syndrome
- Neurologic: Parenchymal involvement, common in brain stem; cranial nerve palsy, hemiplegia, intracranial hypertension, meningoencephalitis and recurrent meningitis, confusional state (1)
- Pulmonary infiltrates, possibly related to thrombosis, noncavitating mass lesion
- Vascular: Peripheral gangrene, aneurysms
- Renal: Glomerulonephritis, epididymitis (rare)

DIAGNOSTIC TESTS & INTERPRETATION

- Pathergy phenomenon: Hallmark of this condition: Nonspecific cutaneous hypersensitivity reaction—formation of sterile pustules and/or papules along sites of puncture or needle track
- Normal to mildly elevated erythrocyte sedimentation (ESR) and C-reactive protein (CRP)
- Circulating immune complexes detected by Raji cell and C1q solid-phase assays and elevated interleukin 1 (IL-1), IL-8, and tumor necrosis factor α (TNF-α), but not clinically useful
- Hypergammaglobulinemia
- Depression of plasma antithrombin III levels with active disease
- Increased fibrinolytic activity during attacks; demyelinating antibodies in neurologic Behçet syndrome
- Anticardiolipin antibodies (rare), lupus anticoagulants
- Antiendothelial antibodies

Lab

Initial lab tests

- ESR and CRP
- If elevated or high clinical suspicion, order additional tests noted earlier.

Follow-Up & Special Considerations

- Periodic ophthalmologic examinations
- A careful history and examination, with attention to the vascular and neurologic systems

Diagnostic Procedures/Surgery

- Careful history and physical examination, with frequent reevaluations
- Synovial fluid: Inflammatory effusion
- Arteriography: For aneurysms or thrombosis

Pathological Findings

- May be no recognizable changes; neutrophilic perivascular infiltration ± fibrinoid necrosis
- Picture of leukocytoclastic vasculitis in older lesions
- Neutrophilic dermatitis (Sweet syndrome) (rarely)

DIFFERENTIAL DIAGNOSIS

- Reactive arthritis and other forms of seronegative spondyloarthropathy
- Inflammatory bowel disease (Crohn disease and ulcerative colitis)
- Syphilis and other venereal diseases
- Multiple sclerosis
- Aphthous stomatitis
- Herpes simplex
- Stevens-Johnson syndrome
- Other systemic vasculitides
- Relapsing polychondritis (MAGIC syndrome)
- Coxsackievirus and echovirus infection
- Mollaret meningitis
- Sarcoidosis

TREATMENT

EDICATION

rst Line

- Colchicine: 0.6 mg b.i.d. for mucocutaneous and oint symptoms
- Topical steroids for ocular and genital lesions
- Prednisone: 1 mg/kg for severe involvement, especially central nervous system
- Dapsone: 50–150 mg/d (2)[B]
- Azathioprine: 2–3 mg/kg/d PO
- Methotrexate: Use lowest possible dose; perhaps 7.5 mg per week. Monitor LFT.
- Cyclosporine: 1–4 mg/kg, but monitor liver function, creatinine, magnesium, and lipids every 2 weeks for 3 months, then every month
- Sulfasalazine 2–6 g/day for GI involvement
- Resistant cases may require:
  - Tacrolimus (FK 506) 0.09–0.15 mg/kg/d
  - Thalidomide 100 mg/d or 300 mg/d (3)[A]: Regulated prescription, teratogenic, refer to manufacturer's literature
  - Interferon alpha for severe ocular and mucocutaneous syndrome (4)[A] and GI manifestations
  - Anticoagulants for patients with anticardiolipin antibodies: Warfarin (Coumadin) to establish PT international normalized ratio 3.0 to 3.5
  - Precautions:
    - Absorption of drugs such as amitriptyline, diazepam, carbamazepine, phenytoin, and acetaminophen may be reduced in Behçet syndrome

econd Line

- Levamisole: 100–150 mg 2 days per week
- Chlorambucil: But concern with respect to toxicity, especially its malignant potential
- Cyclophosphamide: 2–2.5 mg/kg/day PO for severe cutaneous, arterial, pulmonary vasculitic or aneurysmal manifestations, risk of hemorrhagic cystitis with drug
- Tumor necrosis factor inhibitors: Infliximab (5)[A] etanercept (6)[A]
- Stem cell transplantation
- Anti-CD52 antibody
- Topical sucralfate suspension (7)[A]

ADDITIONAL TREATMENT

Issues for Referral

Ophthalmologic, neurological, gastrointestinal, vascular surgery referrals as appropriate

IN-PATIENT CONSIDERATIONS

Initial Stabilization

- Usually outpatient
- Inpatient usually required for neurologic complication or GI perforation

ONGOING CARE

FOLLOW-UP RECOMMENDATIONS

Patient Monitoring

Depends on severity of system involvement and medication monitoring

DIET

No special diet

PATIENT EDUCATION

American Behçet Association, 421 21st Avenue SW, Rochester, MN 55902; (507) 281-3059

PROGNOSIS

- Normal life expectancy, except with neurologic involvement, ruptured aneurysms, and catastrophic GI involvement
- Remissions and exacerbations of disease activity, with severity abating with time

COMPLICATIONS

- Death
- Blindness (most serious morbidity)
- Paralysis
- Embolism/thrombosis [pulmonary, vena cava, peripheral, intracardiac (rare)]
- Aneurysms
- Amyloidosis
- Thrombotic events, especially when anticardiolipin antibodies present
- Intestinal perforation

REFERENCES

1. Al-Araji A, Kidd DP et al. Neuro-Behçet's disease: epidemiology, clinical characteristics, and management. *Lancet Neurol*. 2009;8:192–204.
2. Lin P, Liang G et al. Behçet disease: recommendation for clinical management of mucocutaneous lesions. *J Clin Rheumatol*. 2006; 12:282–6.
3. Hamuryudan V, Mat C, Saip S, Ozyazgan Y, Siva A, Yurdakul S, Zwingenberger K, Yazici H et al. Thalidomide in the treatment of the mucocutaneous lesions of the Behçet syndrome. A randomized, double-blind, placebo-controlled trial. *Ann Intern Med*. 1998;128:443–50.
4. Alpsoy E, Durusoy C, Yilmaz E, Ozgurel Y, Ermis O, Yazar S, Basaran E et al. Interferon alfa-2a in the treatment of Behçet disease: a randomized placebo-controlled and double-blind study. *Arch Dermatol*. 2002;138:467–71.
5. Tugal-Tutkun I, Mudun A, Urgancioglu M, Kamali S, Kasapoglu E, Inanc M, Gül A et al. Efficacy of infliximab in the treatment of uveitis that is resistant to treatment with the combination of azathioprine, cyclosporine, and corticosteroids in Behçet's disease: an open-label trial. *Arthritis Rheum*. 2005;52:2478–84.
6. Melikoglu M, Fresko I, Mat C, Ozyazgan Y, Gogus F, Yurdakul S, Hamuryudan V, Yazici H et al. Short-term trial of etanercept in Behçet's disease: a double blind, placebo controlled study. *J Rheumatol*. 2005;32:98–105.
7. Alpsoy E, Er H, Durusoy C, Yilmaz E et al. The use of sucralfate suspension in the treatment of oral and genital ulceration of Behçet disease: a randomized, placebo-controlled, double-blind study. *Arch Dermatol*. 1999;135:529–32.

ADDITIONAL READING

Alpsoy E, Akman A et al. Behçet's disease: an algorithmic approach to its treatment. *Arch Dermatol Res*. 2009;301:693–702.

CLINICAL PEARLS

- Nonsuperficial oral or genital ulcers suggest Behçet syndrome rather than reactive arthritis (previously called *Reiter syndrome*). The combination of oral and genital ulcers is especially suggestive.
- The pathergy phenomenon (a cutaneous hypersensitivity reaction—formation of sterile pustules and/or papules along sites of puncture or needle track) is helpful if present but is insufficiently sensitive to rule out Behçet syndrome if absent.
- Colchicine is the 1st-line of therapy for Behçet syndrome.
- IgG, IgM, and IgA assays for anticardiolipin antibody tests are indicated for vascular complications in Behçet syndrome.

BELL PALSY

Dylan C. Kwait, MD

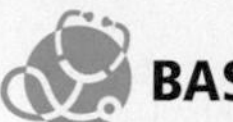

BASICS

DESCRIPTION

A peripheral lower motor neuron facial palsy, usually unilateral, which arises secondary to inflammation and subsequent swelling and compression of the 7th (facial) cranial nerve and the associated vasa nervorum.

EPIDEMIOLOGY

- Affects 0.02% of the population annually (1)[B]:
  - Most patients recover, but as many as 30% are left with facial disfigurement and pain (2)[B]
- Accounts for 60–75% of all cases of unilateral facial paralysis (3)[A]
- Predominant age:
  - Median age of onset is 40 years, but affects all ages (4)[A]
- Predominant sex: Male = Female (4)[A]

Incidence

- US: 20–30 cases per 100,000 people per year (4)[A]
- Lowest in children ≤10 years of age; highest in people ≥70 (4)[A]
- Higher among pregnant women (3)[A]
- Occurs with equal frequency on the left and right sides of the face (4)[A]

Prevalence

Affects 40,000 Americans every year (5)[A]

RISK FACTORS

- Pregnancy
- Diabetes mellitus
- Age >30
- Exposure to cold temperatures
- Upper respiratory infection (e.g., coryza, influenza)

Genetics

A genetic predisposition may be associated with Bell palsy, but it is unclear which factors are inherited.

ETIOLOGY

- Results from damage to the 7th (facial) cranial nerve
- Inflammation of the 7th nerve causes swelling and subsequent compression of both the nerve and the associated vasa nervorum
- May arise secondary to reactivation of latent herpes virus (HSV type 1 and herpes zoster virus) in cranial nerve ganglia (3)[A]
- May arise secondary to ischemia from arteriosclerosis associated with diabetes mellitus (4)[A]

COMMONLY ASSOCIATED CONDITIONS

- Herpes simplex virus
- Lyme disease
- Diabetes mellitus
- Hypertension
- Herpes zoster virus
- Ramsay-Hunt syndrome
- Sjögren syndrome
- Sarcoidosis
- Eclampsia
- Amyloidosis

DIAGNOSIS

HISTORY

- Time course of the illness (rapid onset)
- Any predisposing factors (e.g., recent viral infection, trauma, new medications, hypertension, diabetes mellitus)
- Presence of hyperacusis or history of recurrent Bell palsy (both associated with poor prognosis)
- Any associated rash (suggestive of herpes zoster, Lyme disease, or sarcoid)
- Weakness on affected side of face, often sudden in onset
- Pain in or behind the ear in 50% of cases (may precede the palsy in 25% of cases) (4)[A]
- Subjective numbness on the ipsilateral side of the face
- Alteration of taste on the ipsilateral anterior 2/3 of the tongue (chorda tympani branch of the facial nerve)
- Hyperacusis (nerve to the stapedius muscle)
- Decreased tear production

PHYSICAL EXAM

- Neurologic:
  - Determine if the weakness is due to a problem in either the central or peripheral nervous systems
  - Flaccid paralysis of muscles on the affected side, *including the forehead:*
    - Impaired ability to raise the ipsilateral eyebrow
    - Impaired closure of the ipsilateral eye
    - Bell phenomenon: Upward diversion of the eye with attempted closure of the lid
    - Impaired ability to smile, grin, or purse the lips
  - Patients may complain of numbness, but on sensory testing, no deficit is present
  - Examine for involvement of other cranial nerves
- HEENT:
  - Carefully examine head, neck, and oropharynx to exclude masses
  - Perform pneumatic otoscopic exam
- Skin:
  - Examine for erythema migrans (Lyme disease) and vesicular rash (herpes zoster virus)

DIAGNOSTIC TESTS & INTERPRETATION

Lab

Initial lab tests

- Lyme titer and IgM, IgG, and IgA for *B. burgdorferi*
- Salivary PCR for HSV1 or herpes zoster virus (these tests are largely reserved for research purposes) (3)[A]
- IgM, IgG, and IgA titers for varicella zoster virus, cytomegalovirus, rubella, hepatitis A, hepatitis B, and hepatitis C
- ESR
- Blood glucose level
- CBC
- RPR test
- HIV test

Follow-Up & Special Considerations

CSF analysis:

- Not routinely indicated
- CSF protein is elevated in 1/3 of cases
- CSF cells show mild elevation in 10% of cases with a mononuclear cell predominance.

Imaging

Initial approach

- Facial radiographs:
  - Rule out fractures.
- CT:
  - Rule out fractures.
  - Rule out stroke.
- Brain MRI:
  - Not routinely indicated
  - Rule out central pontine, temporal bone, and parotid neoplasms (4)[A].

Diagnostic Procedures/Surgery

- EMG:
  - Nerve conduction on affected and nonaffected sides can be compared to determine extent of nerve injury.
- Electroneurography:
  - Evoked potentials of affected and nonaffected sides can be compared.

Pathological Findings

Invasive diagnostic procedures are not indicated because biopsy could further damage the 7th cranial nerve.

DIFFERENTIAL DIAGNOSIS

- Infectious:
  - Lyme disease
  - Herpes zoster (Ramsay-Hunt syndrome)
  - Acute or chronic otitis media
  - Malignant otitis externa
  - Osteomyelitis of the skull base
  - Infectious mononucleosis
  - Leprosy
- Trauma:
  - Temporal bone fracture
  - Mandibular bone fracture
- Neoplastic (onset of palsy is usually slow and progressive, and accompanied by additional cranial nerve deficits and/or headache) (3)[A]:
  - Tumors of the parotid gland
  - Cholesteatoma
  - Skull-base tumor
  - Carcinomatous meningitis
  - Leukemic meningitis
- Cerebrovascular:
  - Brainstem stroke involving anteroinferior cerebellar artery
  - Aneurysm involving carotid, vertebral, or basilar arteries
- Other:
  - Multiple sclerosis
  - Myasthenia gravis (should be considered in cases of recurrent or bilateral facial palsy) (4)[A]
  - Guillain-Barré syndrome (may also present with bilateral facial palsy) (4)[A]
  - Sjögren syndrome
  - Sarcoidosis
  - Amyloidosis
  - Melkersson-Rosenthal syndrome
  - Polyneuritis

TREATMENT

IEDICATION

Debate had existed over whether pharmacologic intervention with anti-inflammatory and/or antiviral agents is any more beneficial than watchful waiting for the treatment and prevention of long-term effects.

Recent randomized control trials demonstrate definitively that corticosteroids decrease inflammation and limit nerve damage, thereby reducing the number of patients with residual facial weakness (6)[A].

Evidence now shows that antivirals targeting herpes simplex are no more effective than placebo at producing full recovery (7)[A].

- Antivirals are also less likely to produce full recovery than corticosteroids (1)[B].
- A combination of valacyclovir and steroids provides minimal added benefit over steroid use alone (1)[B].

Corticosteroids:

- Prednisone (8)[B]: Total from 410 mg over 10 days to 760 mg PO over 16 days, tapering dose (adults only)
  - Treatment should begin immediately after onset, and should not be instituted if symptoms have been present for >7 days.
  - May reduce edema around the 7th cranial nerve.
- Prednisolone (9)[B]: Total of 500 mg over 10 days, 25 mg PO b.i.d.:
  - Prednisolone alone may be an effective treatment.
  - Should be instituted within 72 hours of symptom onset

Antivirals in combination with corticosteroids:

- Valacyclovir (1)[B]: 1000 mg × 5 days plus prednisone 60 mg/day × 5 days then 30 mg/day × 3 days then 10 mg/day × 2 days

Contraindications:

- Documented hypersensitivity
- Preexisting infections, including TB and systemic mycosis

Precautions: Use with discretion in pregnancy, peptic ulcer disease, and diabetes

Significant possible interactions: Measles-mumps rubella, oral polio virus vaccine, and other live vaccines

Pregnancy Considerations

teroids should be used cautiously in pregnancy; onsult with an obstetrician.

ADDITIONAL TREATMENT

General Measures

Artificial tears should be used to lubricate the cornea.

The ipsilateral eye should be patched and taped shut at night to avoid drying and infection.

Issues for Referral

atients may need to be referred to an ENT specialist r a neurologist.

Additional Therapies

Physical therapy: No evidence of significant benefit or harm, but there is a possibility that facial exercises may reduce time to recover and/or sequelae (10)[A].

Electrostimulation has limited evidence of effect; more studies needed (11)[B].

SURGERY/OTHER PROCEDURES

- Surgical treatment of Bell palsy remains controversial and is reserved for intractable cases (3)[A].
- The 7th cranial nerve is surgically decompressed at the entrance to the meatal foramen where the labyrinthine segment and geniculate ganglion reside (4)[A].
- Decompression surgery should not be performed >14 days after the onset of paralysis because severe degeneration of the facial nerve is likely irreversible after 2–3 weeks (4)[A].

ONGOING CARE

FOLLOW-UP RECOMMENDATIONS

Patient Monitoring

- Patients should start treatment immediately and be followed for 12 months.
- Patients who do not recover complete facial nerve function should be referred to an ophthalmologist for tarsorrhaphy.

DIET

No restrictions

PROGNOSIS

- Most achieve complete spontaneous recovery within 2 weeks (5)[A]
- 85% of untreated patients will experience the 1st signs of recovery within 3 weeks of onset (8)[C].
- Over 80% recover within 3 months (5)[A].
- 16% are left with a partial palsy, motor synkinesis, and autonomic synkinesis (3)[A].
- 5% experience severe sequelae, and a small number of patients experience permanent facial weakness and dysfunction (3)[A].
- Poor prognostic factors include:
  - Age >60 years
  - Complete facial weakness
  - HTN
  - Ramsay-Hunt syndrome
- Absence of recovery at 3 weeks

COMPLICATIONS

- Corneal abrasion or ulceration
- Steroid-induced psychological disturbances; avascular necrosis of the hips, knees, and/or shoulders
- Steroid use can unmask subclinical infection (e.g., TB)

REFERENCES

1. Worster A, Keim SM, Sahsi R, Pancioli AM, Best Evidence in Emergency Medicine (BEEM) Group et al. Do either corticosteroids or antiviral agents reduce the risk of long-term facial paresis in patients with new-onset Bell's palsy? *J Emerg Med*. 2010;38:518–23.
2. De Diego-Sastre JI, Prim-Espada MP, Fernández García F. [The epidemiology of Bell's palsy] *Rev Neurol*. 2005;41:287–90.
3. Holland NJ, et al. Recent developments in Bell's palsy. *Br Med J*. 2004;329:553–7.
4. Gilden DH. Clinical practice. Bell's Palsy. *N Engl J Med*. 2004;351:1323–31.
5. Holten KB. How should we manage Bell's palsy? *J Fam Pract*. 2004;53:797–8.
6. Salinas RA, Alvarez G, Daly F, Ferreira J et al. Corticosteroids for Bell's palsy (idiopathic facial paralysis). *Cochrane Database Syst Rev*. 2010; 3:CD001942.
7. Lockhart P, Daly F, Pitkethly M, Comerford N, Sullivan F et al. Antiviral treatment for Bell's palsy (idiopathic facial paralysis). *Cochrane Database Syst Rev*. 2009;CD001869.
8. Peitersen E. The natural history of Bell's palsy. *Am J Otol*. 1982;4(2):107–11.
9. Madhok V, Falk G, Fahey T, et al. Prescribe prednisolone alone for Bell's palsy diagnosed within 72 hours of symptom onset. *BMJ*. 2009;338:b255.
10. Teixeira LJ, et al. Physical therapy for Bell's palsy (idiopathic facial paralysis). *Cochrane Database Syst Rev*. 2008;16(3):CD006283.
11. Alakram P, Puckree T et al. Effects of electrical stimulation on House-Brackmann scores in early Bell's palsy. *Physiother Theory Pract*. 2010; 26:160–6.

See Also (Topic, Algorithm, Electronic Media Element)

Amyloidosis; Herpes Simplex; Herpes Zoster; Sarcoidosis; Amyloidosis; Lyme Disease; Diabetes Mellitus Type 1; Diabetes Mellitus Type 2; Ramsay-Hunt Syndrome; Sjögren Syndrome; Melkersson-Rosenthal Syndrome

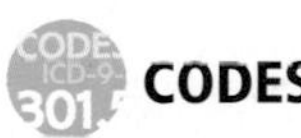

CODES

ICD9

351.0 Bell's palsy

CLINICAL PEARLS

- Steroids must be initiated immediately after onset of symptoms.
- Look closely at the voluntary movement on the upper part of the face on the affected side; in Bell palsy, all of the muscles are involved (weak or paralyzed), whereas in a stroke, the upper muscles are spared (due to bilateral innervation).
- Remember to protect the affected eye with lubrication and taping.
- In areas with endemic Lyme disease, Bell palsy should be considered to be Lyme disease until proven otherwise.

BIPOLAR I DISORDER

Laurie A. Carrier, MD

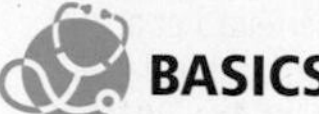

BASICS

DESCRIPTION

- Bipolar I (BP-I) is a mood disorder characterized by at least 1 manic or mixed episode, often alternating with episodes of major depression, that causes marked impairment and/or hospitalization.
- Symptoms are not caused by a substance (e.g., drug), a general medical condition, or a medication.

Geriatric Considerations

New onset in older patients (>50 years of age) requires a workup for organic or chemically induced pathology.

Pediatric Considerations

There is overlap with symptoms of attention-deficit hyperactivity disorder (ADHD) and oppositional defiant disorder (ODD). Children and adolescents experience more rapid cycling and mixed states. Depression often presents as irritable mood.

Pregnancy Considerations

- Potential teratogenic effects of commonly used medications (e.g., lithium, valproic acid)
- Symptoms may be exacerbated in the postpartum period.

EPIDEMIOLOGY

- Most common onset is between 15 and 30 years of age.
- More common in single and divorced persons
- Less common in college graduates
- Higher than average incidence in higher socioeconomic groups

Prevalence

- 1.0–1.6% lifetime prevalence
- Equal among men and women (manic episodes more common in men; depressive episodes more common in women)
- Women are more likely to be rapid cyclers (4 or more mood episodes per year)
- Equal among races; however, clinicians tend to misdiagnose schizophrenia in African-American patients with BP-I.

RISK FACTORS

Genetics, major life stressors (especially loss of parent or spouse), or substance abuse

Genetics

- Monozygotic twin concordance 40–70%
- Dizygotic twin concordance 5–25%
- 50% of patients have at least one parent with a mood disorder.
- 1st-degree relatives of people with BP-I are approximately 7× more likely to develop BP-I than the general population.

GENERAL PREVENTION

Treatment adherence and education can help to prevent relapses.

PATHOPHYSIOLOGY

Dysregulation of biogenic amines or neurotransmitters (particularly serotonin, norepinephrine, and dopamine). MRI findings suggest abnormalities in prefrontal cortical areas, striatum, and amygdala that predate illness onset (1).

ETIOLOGY

Genetic predisposition and major life stressors can trigger initial and subsequent episodes.

COMMONLY ASSOCIATED CONDITIONS

Substance abuse (60%), ADHD, anxiety disorders, and eating disorders

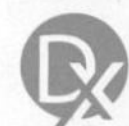

DIAGNOSIS

- The diagnosis of BP-I requires at least 1 manic or mixed episode (simultaneous mania and depression). Although a depressive episode is not necessary for the diagnosis, 80–90% of people with BP-I also experience depression.
- Manic episode, DSM-IV-TR criteria:
  - Distinct period of abnormally and persistently elevated, expansive, or irritable mood lasting at least 1 week (or any duration if hospitalization is necessary)
  - During the period of mood disturbance, 3 or more of the "DIG FAST" symptoms must persist (4 if the mood is only irritable) and must be present to a significant degree:
    - *D*istractibility (attention too easily drawn to unimportant or irrelevant external stimuli)
    - *I*nsomnia, decreased need for sleep (e.g., feels rested after only 3 hours of sleep)
    - *G*randiosity or inflated self-esteem
    - *F*light of ideas or subjective experience that thoughts are racing
    - *A*gitation or increase in goal-directed activity (socially, at work or school, or sexually)
    - *S*peech pressured/more talkative than usual
    - *T*aking risks: Excessive involvement in pleasurable activities that have a high potential for painful consequences (e.g., financial or sexual)
- Major depressive episode: See "Bipolar II Disorder" for DSM-IV-TR criteria (*Note:* A depressive episode is not necessary for the diagnosis of BP-I.)
- Mixed episode: Criteria are met for both a manic and major depressive episode nearly every day during at least a 1-week period, and the mood disturbance causes significant impairment in functioning.
- Signs and symptoms more likely in bipolar than in unipolar depression (2): Agitation/restlessness, suicidal ideation/planning, increased frequency of depressive episodes, melancholia, psychomotor retardation, younger age of onset, hyperphagia, hypersomnia, family history of bipolar disorder, subsyndromal hypomanic symptoms (particularly increased goal-directed activity)

HISTORY

- Collateral information makes diagnostics more complete and is often necessary for a clear history.
- History: Safety concerns (e.g., Suicide/homicide ideation? Safety plan? Psychosis present?); Physical well-being (e.g., Number of hours of sleep? Appetite? Substance abuse?); Personal history (e.g., Told life of the party? Talkative? Speeding? Spending sprees or donations? Credit-card or gambling debt? Promiscuous? Other risk-taking behavior? Legal trouble? Religious infatuation?)

PHYSICAL EXAM

- Mental status exam in acute mania:
  - General appearance: Bright clothing, excessive makeup, disorganized or discombobulated, psychomotor agitation
  - Speech: Pressured, difficult to interrupt
  - Mood/affect: Euphoria, irritability/expansive, labi
  - Thought process: Flight of ideas (streams of thought occur to patient at rapid rate), easily distracted
  - Thought content: Grandiosity, paranoia, hyperreligious
  - Perceptual abnormalities: 3/4 of manic patients experience delusions, grandiose or paranoid
  - Suicidal/homicidal ideation: Irritability or delusio may lead to aggression toward self or others; suicidal ideation is common with mixed episode.
  - Insight/judgment: Poor/impaired
- See "Bipolar II Disorder" for an example of a ment status exam in depression.
- With mixed episodes, patients may exhibit a combination of manic and depressive mental states

DIAGNOSTIC TESTS & INTERPRETATION

- BP-I is a clinical diagnosis.
- Mood Disorder Questionnaire is a self-assessment screen for bipolar disorders (sensitivity 73%, specificity 90%) (3).
- Patient Health Questionnaire-9 helps to determine the presence and severity of a depressive episode.

Lab

- Thyroid-stimulating hormone (TSH), complete blooc count (CBC), CMP, liver function tests (LFTs), antinuclear antibody, RPR, human immunodeficienc virus, erythrocyte sedimentation rate, UDS
- Drug/alcohol screen with each presentation
- Dementia workup if new onset in seniors (e.g., TSH RPR, vitamin B_{12}, brain imaging)

Imaging

Consider brain imaging (CT scan, MRI) with initial onset of mania to rule out organic cause (e.g., tumor, infection, or stroke), especially with onset in elderly and if psychosis is present.

Diagnostic Procedures/Surgery

Consider electroencephalogram if presentation suggests temporal lobe epilepsy (hyperreligiosity, hypergraphia).

DIFFERENTIAL DIAGNOSIS

- Other psychiatric considerations: Unipolar depression ± psychotic features, schizophrenia, schizoaffective disorder, personality disorders (particularly antisocial, borderline, histrionic, and narcissistic), attention-deficit disorder ± hyperactivity, substance-induced mood disorder
- Medical considerations: Epilepsy (e.g., temporal lobe), brain tumor, infection (e.g., AIDS, syphilis), stroke, endocrine (e.g., thyroid disease), multiple sclerosis
- In children, consider ADHD and ODD

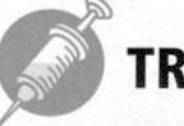

TREATMENT

- Ensure safety
- Medication management
- Psychotherapy (e.g., cognitive-behavioral therapy, social rhythm therapy)
- Stress reduction
- Patient and family education

IEDICATION

ʼrst Line

Treatment may consist of 1–4 of the following mood stabilizers or other psychotropic medications. When combining these agents, consider adding different classes (e.g., an atypical antipsychotic and/or an antiseizure medication and/or lithium).

Lithium (Lithobid, Eskalith, generic): *Dosing:* 600–1,200 mg/day divided bid–qid; start 600 mg PO tid in acute mania, and titrate based on blood levels. *Warning:* Use caution in kidney and heart disease; use can lead to diabetes insipidus, thyroid disease. Use caution in sodium-depleted patients (e.g., those using diuretics or ACE inhibitors); dehydration can lead to toxicity (seizures, encephalopathy, arrhythmias). Pregnancy category D (Ebstein anomaly). *Monitor:* Check electrocardiogram (ECG) >40 years, TSH, blood urea nitrogen, creatine, lytes at baseline and every 6 months; check level 5 days after initiation or dose change, then every 1–2 weeks ×3, then every 2–3 months (Goal: 0.8–1.2 mmol/L).

Antiseizure medications:

- Divalproex sodium, valproic acid (Depakote, Depakene, generic): *Dosing:* Start 250–500 mg bid–tid; maximum 60 mg/kg/day. *Black box warnings:* Hepatotoxicity, pancreatitis, thrombocytopenia, pregnancy category D (neural tube defects). *Monitor:* CBC, LFTs at baseline and every 6 months; check VPA level 5 days after initiation and dose changes (Goal: 50–125 μg/mL).
- Carbamazepine (Carbatrol, Equetro, Tegretol, generic): *Dosing:* 800–1,200 mg/day PO divided bid–qid; start 100–200 mg PO bid and titrate to lowest effective dose. *Warning:* Do not use with tricyclic acid or within 14 days of a monoamine oxidase inhibitor. Use caution with kidney/heart disease; risk of aplastic anemia/agranulocytosis, enzyme inducer; pregnancy category D. *Monitor:* CBC, LFTs at baseline and every 3–6 months; check level 4–5 days after initiation and dose changes (Goal: 4–12 μg/mL).
- Lamotrigine (Lamictal): *Dosing:* 200 mg/day; start 25 mg/day × 2 weeks, then 50 mg/day × 2 weeks, then 100 mg/day × 1 week (*Note:* Use different dosing if adjunct to valproate). *Warning:* Titrate slowly (risk of Stevens-Johnson syndrome); use caution with kidney/liver/heart disease; pregnancy category C.
- Oxcarbmazepine (Trileptal), gabapentin (Neurontin), and topiramate (Topamax) are also used in BP-I but are not approved by the Food and Drug Administration (FDA).

Atypical antipsychotics (AAs):

- Side effects of AAs: Orthostatic hypotension, metabolic side effects (glucose and lipid dysregulation, weight gain), tardive dyskinesia, NMS, prolactinemia (except Abilify), increased risk of death in elderly with dementia-related psychosis, pregnancy category C
- Monitor: LFTs, lipids, glucose at baseline, 3 months, and annually; check for EPS with AIMS and assess weight (with abdominal circumference) at baseline, at 4, 8, and 12 weeks, and then every 3–6 months; monitor for orthostatic hypotension 3–5 days after starting or changing dose.
- Aripiprazole (Abilify): *Dosing:* 15 mg/day, max. 30 mg/day; less likely to cause metabolic side effects
- Olanzapine (Zyprexa, Zydis): *Dosing:* 5–20 mg/day; most likely to cause metabolic side effects (weight gain, diabetes)
- Symbyax (olanzapine + fluoxetine): *Dosing:* 6/25 mg, FDA approved for BP depression
- Quetiapine (Seroquel): *Dosing:* In mania, 200–400 mg bid; in bipolar depression, 50–300 mg qhs. *Caution:* Cataracts
- Risperidone (Risperdal): *Dosing:* 1–6 mg/day divided qid–bid. Generic and every 2 weeks IM preparations available
- Ziprasidone (Geodon): *Dosing:* 40–80 mg bid; less likely to cause metabolic side effects. *Caution:* QTc prolongation (>500 ms) has been a/w use (0.06%). Consider ECG at baseline.

Second Line

- Antidepressants (in addition to mood stabilizers)
- Benzodiazepines (for acute agitation with mania, associated anxiety)
- Sleep medications

ADDITIONAL TREATMENT

General Measures

- Psychotherapy (e.g., cognitive-behavioral therapy, social rhythm therapy) in conjunction with medications is key (4).
- Regular exercise, a healthy diet, and sobriety have been shown to help prevent worsening of symptoms.

Issues for Referral

Comfort level of doctor, stability of patient, patients benefit from a multidisciplinary team, including a primary care physician and a psychiatrist.

Additional Therapies

- Electroconvulsive therapy can be helpful in acute mania and depression.
- Light therapy for seasonal component to depressive episodes (use with caution because it can precipitate manic episode)

COMPLEMENTARY AND ALTERNATIVE MEDICINE

Omega-3 fatty acids may help.

IN-PATIENT CONSIDERATIONS

Admit if acutely dangerous to self or others.

Admission Criteria

To admit a patient (>18 years of age) to a psychiatric unit involuntarily, the patient must have a psychiatric diagnosis (e.g., BP-I) or present a danger to him- or herself or others, or their mental disease must be inhibiting them from obtaining their basic needs (e.g., food, clothing, etc.).

Nursing

Alert staff to potentially dangerous or agitated patients. Acute suicidal threats need continuous observation.

Discharge Criteria

Determined by safety

ONGOING CARE

FOLLOW-UP RECOMMENDATIONS

- Regularly scheduled visits support adherence with treatment.
- Frequent communication among primary care doctor, psychiatrist, and therapist

Patient Monitoring

Mood charts are helpful to monitor symptoms.

PATIENT EDUCATION

National Alliance on Mental Illness (NAMI): http://www.nami.org/

PROGNOSIS

- Frequency and severity of episodes are related to medication adherence, consistency with therapy, amount of sleep, and support systems.
- 40–50% of patients experience another manic episode within 2 years of the 1st episode.
- 25–50% attempt suicide, and 15% die.
- Substance abuse, unemployment, psychosis, depression, and male sex are associated with a worse prognosis.

REFERENCES

1. Fornito A, Yücel M, Wood SJ, et al. Anterior cingulate cortex abnormalities associated with a first psychotic episode in bipolar disorder. *Br J Psychiatry.* 2009;194:426–33.
2. Perlis RH, Brown E, Baker RW, et al. Clinical features of bipolar depression versus major depressive disorder in large multicenter trials. *Am J Psychiatry.* 2006;163:225–31.
3. Hirschfeld RM, Holzer C, Calabrese JR, et al. Validity of the mood disorder questionnaire: a general population study. *Am J Psychiatry.* 2003;160:178–80.
4. Depp CA, Moore DJ, Patterson TL, et al. Psychosocial interventions and medication adherence in bipolar disorder. *Dialogues Clin Neurosci.* 2008;10:239–50.

ADDITIONAL READING

- American Psychiatric Association. Practice guideline for the treatment of patients with bipolar disorder (revision). *Am J Psychiatry.* 2002;159:1–50.
- McAllister-Williams RH. Relapse prevention in bipolar disorder: a critical review of current guidelines. *Psychopharmacol.* 2006;20(2 Suppl):12–6.

See Also (Topic, Algorithm, Electronic Media Element)

Algorithm: Depression, Adult

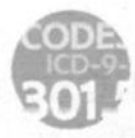

CODES

ICD9

- 296.40 Bipolar affective disorder, manic, unspecified degree
- 296.50 Bipolar affective disorder, depressed, unspecified degree
- 296.7 Bipolar I disorder, most recent episode (or current) unspecified

CLINICAL PEARLS

- Bipolar I is characterized by at least 1 manic or mixed episode, often alternating with episodes of major depression, that causes marked impairment.
- 25–50% of BP-I patients attempt suicide, and 15% die by suicide.
- There is no way to prevent the onset of BP-I, but treatment adherence and education can help to prevent further episodes.

BIPOLAR II DISORDER

Laurie A. Carrier, MD

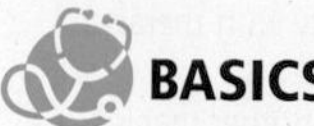

BASICS

DESCRIPTION

Bipolar II (BP-2) is a mood disorder characterized by at least 1 episode of major depression and at least 1 episode of hypomania, a milder form of mania.

Geriatric Considerations

New onset in older patients (>50) requires a workup for organic or chemically induced pathology.

Pediatric Considerations

- Large overlap with symptoms of attention deficit hyperactivity disorder (ADHD) and oppositional defiant disorder (ODD)
- Depression often presents as irritable mood.

Pregnancy Considerations

- Counsel women of childbearing age about potentially teratogenic effects of commonly used medications (e.g., lithium, valproic acid).
- Symptoms may be exacerbated in the postpartum period.

EPIDEMIOLOGY

More common in women

Prevalence

0.5–1.1% lifetime prevalence

RISK FACTORS

Genetics

Heritability estimate: >77%

GENERAL PREVENTION

There is no way to prevent the onset of BP-2, but treatment adherence and education can help to prevent further episodes.

PATHOPHYSIOLOGY

Dysregulation of biogenic amines or neurotransmitters (particularly serotonin, norepinephrine, and dopamine)

ETIOLOGY

- Genetics
- Major life stressors (especially loss of parent or spouse)

COMMONLY ASSOCIATED CONDITIONS

Substance abuse or dependence, ADHD, anxiety disorders, and eating disorders

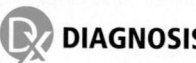

DIAGNOSIS

- DSM-IV-TR criteria: Patient must experience at least 1 hypomanic episode and at least 1 major depressive episode. The symptoms have caused *some* distress or impairment in social, occupational, or other areas of functioning. There can be no history of full manic or mixed episodes.
- Hypomania is a distinct period of persistently elevated, expansive, or irritable mood, different from usual nondepressed mood, lasting at least 4 days:
  - The episode must include at least 3 of the "DIG FAST" symptoms below (4 if the mood is only irritable):
    - **D**istractibility
    - **I**nsomnia, decreased need for sleep
    - **G**randiosity or inflated self-esteem
    - **F**light of ideas or subjective experience that thoughts are racing
    - **A**gitation or increase in goal-directed activity (socially, at work or school, or sexually)
    - **S**peech pressured/more talkative than usual
    - **T**aking risks: Excessive involvement in pleasurable activities that have high potential for painful consequences (e.g., sexual or financial)
  - The symptoms are not severe enough to cause *marked* impairment in functioning or hospitalization, and there is no associated psychosis as with BP-1.
- Major depression:
  - Depressed mood or diminished interest and 4 or more of the "SIG E CAPS" symptoms are present during the same 2-week period:
    - **S**leep disturbance (e.g., trouble falling asleep, early morning awakening)
    - **I**nterest: Loss or anhedonia
    - **G**uilt (or feelings of worthlessness)
    - **E**nergy, loss of
    - **C**oncentration, loss of
    - **A**ppetite changes, increase or decrease
    - **P**sychomotor changes (retardation or agitation)
    - **S**uicidal/homicidal thoughts
  - BP-2 with rapid cycling is diagnosed when a patient experiences at least 4 episodes of a mood disturbance in a 12-month period (either major depression or hypomania).
- Signs, symptoms, and history seen more often in BP-2 than in unipolar depression (1):
  - Agitation, hyperphagia, hypersomnia, melancholia, psychomotor retardation, suicidal ideation/planning, increased frequency of depressive episodes, younger age of onset, family history of bipolar disorder, subsyndromal hypomanic symptoms (especially overactivity) (2)
- Note: If symptoms have *ever* met criteria for a full manic episode or hospitalization was necessary secondary to manic/mixed symptoms or psychosis was present, then the diagnosis changes to bipolar I disorder (BP-1).

HISTORY

Collateral information makes diagnostics more complete and is often necessary for a clear history.

PHYSICAL EXAM

- Mental status exam in hypomania:
  - General appearance: Usually appropriately dressed, with psychomotor agitation
  - Speech: May be pressured, talkative, difficult to interrupt
  - Mood/affect: Euphoria, irritability/congruent or expansive
  - Thought process: May be easily distracted, difficulty concentrating on 1 task
  - Thought content: Usually positive with "big" plans
  - Perceptual abnormalities: None
  - Suicidal/homicidal ideation: Low incidence of homicidal or suicidal ideation
  - Insight/judgment: Usually stable/may be impaired by their distractibility
- Mental status exam in acute depression:
  - General appearance: Unkempt, psychomotor retardation, poor eye contact
  - Speech: Low, soft, monotone
  - Mood/affect: Sad, depressed/congruent, flat
  - Thought process: Ruminating thoughts, generalized slowing
  - Thought content: Preoccupied with negative or nihilistic ideas
  - Perceptual abnormalities: 15% of depressed patients experience hallucinations or delusions.
  - Suicidal/homicidal ideation: Suicidal ideation is very common.
  - Insight/judgment: Often impaired

DIAGNOSTIC TESTS & INTERPRETATION

- BP-2 is a clinical diagnosis.
- Mood disorder questionnaire, self-assessment screen for BP, sensitivity 73%, specificity 90% (3)
- Hypomania checklist-32 distinguishes between BP-2 and unipolar depression (sensitivity 80%, specificity 51%) (4)
- Patient health questionnaire-9 helps to determine the presence and severity of depression.

Lab

- Rule out organic causes of mood disorder during initial episode.
- Drug/alcohol screen is prudent with each presentation.
- Dementia workup if new onset in seniors (e.g., thyroid-stimulating hormone [TSH], rapid plasma reagin [RPR], B_{12}, brain imaging).

Initial lab tests

With initial presentation: Consider complete blood count (CBC), chem 7, TSH, liver function tests (LFTs), antinuclear antibody, RPR, HIV, erythrocyte sedimentation rate

Imaging

Consider brain imaging (computed tomography, magnetic resonance imaging) with initial onset of hypomania to rule out organic cause (e.g., tumor, infection, stroke), especially with onset in elderly.

DIFFERENTIAL DIAGNOSIS

- Other psychiatric considerations:
  - Bipolar 1 disorder, unipolar depression, personality disorders (particularly borderline, antisocial, and narcissistic), attention deficit disorder +/– hyperactivity, substance-induced mood disorder
- Medical considerations:
  - Epilepsy (e.g., temporal lobe), brain tumor, infection (e.g., AIDS, syphilis), stroke, endocrine (e.g., thyroid disease), multiple sclerosis
- In children, consider ADHD and ODD.

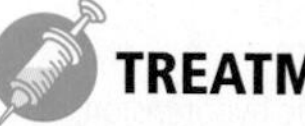

TREATMENT

- Ensure safety
- Medication management
- Psychotherapy (e.g., cognitive behavioral therapy [CBT], social rhythm therapy)
- Stress reduction
- Patient and family education

MEDICATION

- Less research has been conducted on the appropriate treatment of BP-2, but current consensus is to treat with the same medications as BP-1.
- Antidepressant medications must be used with caution during depressive episodes, as they may precipitate hypomanic episodes (less common than with BP-1).

ʳst Line

- ⁺merican Psychological Association guidelines state ˡthium or lamotrigine as first-line treatment for ›ipolar depression.
- ˈreatment may consist of 1–4. When combining ›nood stabilizers, consider adding different classes ›e.g., an atypical antipsychotic and/or an antiseizure ›nedication and/or lithium).
- .ithium (Lithobid, Eskalith, generic): Dosing ›00–1200 mg/day divided b.i.d.–q.i.d., titrate based ›n blood levels:
  - Selected warnings: Caution in kidney or heart disease; use can lead to diabetes insipidus, thyroid disease; caution sodium-depleted patients (diuretics, angiotensin-converting enzyme inhibitors); dehydration can lead to toxicity, which may cause seizures, encephalopathic syndrome, arrhythmias, pregnancy category D (Ebstein anomaly with 1st trimeter use)
  - Monitor: Check electrocardiogram (EKG) >40 y, TSH, blood urea nitrogen, creatinine, lytes at baseline and q6 months; check level 5 days after initiation or dose change, then q1–2 wk × 3, then q2–3 mo (goal: 0.8–1.2 mmol/L)
- Antiseizure medications:
  - Valproic acid, divalproex sodium (Depakene, Depakote, generic): Dosing: Start 250 500 mg b.i.d.–t.i.d., max 60 mg/kg/day. Selected warnings: Hepatotoxicity, pancreatitis, thrombocytopenia, pregnancy category D (neural tube defects). Monitor: CBC, LFTs at baseline and q6 mo; check valproic acid level 5 days after initiation and dose changes (goal: 50–125 mcg/mL).
  - Carbamazepine (Carbatrol, Equetro, Tegretol, generic): Dosing: 800–1200 mg/day p.o. div b.i.d.–q.i.d., start 100–200 mg p.o. b.i.d. and titrate to lowest effective dose. Selected warnings: Do not use with tricyclic antidepressants or within 14 d of monoamine oxidase inhibitor; caution with kidney or heart disease, may cause aplastic anemia/agranulocytosis, pregnancy category D. Monitor: CBC, LFTs at baseline and q3–6 mo; check level 4–5d after initiation and dose changes (goal: 4–12 mcg/mL).
  - Lamotrigine (Lamictal): Dosing: 200 mg a day, start 25 mg × 2 wk, then 50 mg × 2 wk, then 100 mg × 1 wk (Note: Different dosing if adjunct to valproate). Selected warnings: Titrate slowly (risk of Stevens-Johnson syndrome); caution with kidney, liver, or heart impairment; pregnancy category C. Monitor: Patient to monitor for rash.
  - Oxcarbmazepine (Trileptal), gabapentin (Neurontin), and topiramate (Topamax) are also used in BP but are not Food and Drug Administration (FDA)-approved.
- Atypical antipsychotics (AAs):
  - Side effects of AAs: Orthostatic hypotension, negative metabolic side effects (effect glucose and lipid regulation, weight gain), tardive dyskinesia, neuroleptic malignant syndrome, prolactinemia (except Abilify), increased risk of mortality in elderly with dementia-related psychosis, pregnancy category C
  - Monitor: LFTs, lipids, glucose at baseline, 3 months and annually; check for extrapyramidal symptoms with AIMS and assess weight (with abdominal circumference) at baseline, then 4, 8, and 12 weeks, then q3–6 m; monitor for orthostatic hypotension 3–5 days after starting or changing dose
  - Aripiprazole (Abilify) Dosing: 15 mg/day, max 30 mg/day, less likely to cause metabolic side effects
  - Olanzapine (Zyprexa, Zydis): Dosing: 5–20 mg/day, most likely AA to cause metabolic side effects (weight gain, diabetes mellitus)
  - Symbyax (olanzapine + fluoxetine): Dosing: 6/25 mg, FDA-approved for bipolar depression
  - Quetiapine (Seroquel): Dosing: Hypomania 200–400 mg b.i.d. Depression 50–300 mg q.h.s. Caution: Cataracts, sedation.
  - Risperidone (Risperdal): Dosing: 1–6 mg/day every day-b.i.d. Generic and q2 wk IM preparations available.
  - Ziprasidone (Geodon): Dosing: 40–80 mg b.i.d. Less likely to cause metabolic side effects, Warnings: QTc prolongation (>500 msec) has been associated with use (0.06%), consider EKG at baseline.

Second Line

- Antidepressants (in addition to mood stabilizers)
- Benzodiazepines (for acute agitation, anxiety)
- Sleep medications

ADDITIONAL TREATMENT

General Measures

- Psychotherapy (e.g., CBT, social rhythm therapy) in conjunction with medications is key.
- Regular exercise, a healthy diet, and sobriety have shown to help prevent worsening of symptoms.

Issues for Referral

- Experience and comfort level of physician
- Stability of patient
- Patients may benefit from care by a multidisciplinary team, including a primary care physician and a psychiatrist.

Additional Therapies

- Electroconvulsive therapy with severe depression (may precipitate hypomania)
- Light therapy if there is seasonal component to depressive episodes (may precipitate hypomania)

IN-PATIENT CONSIDERATIONS

If hypomanic symptoms are severe enough to necessitate hospitalization, the patient automatically meets criteria for mania and BP-1.

Initial Stabilization

- Medications for stabilization with acute depression
- Safety plan reviewed and safe environment assured

Admission Criteria

To admit a patient (>18) to a psychiatric unit involuntarily, they must have a psychiatric diagnosis (e.g., major depression) and present a danger to themselves or others, or their mental disease must be inhibiting them from providing their basic needs (e.g., food, clothing, and/or shelter).

Nursing

Acute suicidal threats need closer observation.

Discharge Criteria

Determined by safety

ONGOING CARE

FOLLOW-UP RECOMMENDATIONS

- Regularly scheduled visits support treatment adherence.
- Frequent communication between primary care doctor, psychiatrist, and therapist ensures comprehensive care.

Patient Monitoring

Mood charts are helpful adjuncts to care.

PATIENT EDUCATION

- Support groups for patients and families
- National Alliance on Mental Illness: http://www.nami.org/

PROGNOSIS

- Frequency and severity of problematic episodes are related to medication adherence, consistency with psychotherapy, sleep, support systems, regularity of daily activities, and social history.
- Substance abuse, unemployment, persistent depression, and male sex are associated with a worse prognosis.
- Although data are limited, evidence indicates that patients with BP-2 may be at greater risk of both attempting and completing suicide than with BP-1 and unipolar depression.

REFERENCES

1. Perlis RH, Brown E, Baker RW, et al. Clinical features of bipolar depression versus major depressive disorder in large multicenter trials. *Am J Psychiatry*. 2006;163:225–31.
2. Benazzi F. A prediction rule for diagnosing hypomania. *Prog Neuropsychopharmacol Biol Psychiatry*. 2009;33:317–22.
3. Hirshfeld RM. Validation of the Mood Disorder Questionnaire. *Bipolar Depression Bulletin*. 2004.
4. Angst J, Adolfsson R, Benazzi F, et al. The HCL-32: towards a self-assessment tool for hypomanic symptoms in outpatients. *J Affect Disord*. 2005; 88:217–33.

ADDITIONAL READING

- Benazzi F. Bipolar disorder–focus on bipolar II disorder and mixed depression. *Lancet*. 2007; 369:935–45.
- Benazzi F. Bipolar II disorder: epidemiology, diagnosis and management. *CNS Drugs*. 2007; 21:727–40.
- Edvardsen J, Torgersen S, Røysamb E, et al. Heritability of bipolar spectrum disorders. Unity or heterogeneity? *J Affect Disord*. 2007.

See Also (Topic, Algorithm, Electronic Media Element)

Algorithm: Depression, Adult

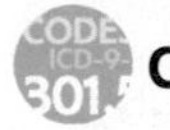

CODES

ICD9

296.89 Other manic-depressive psychosis

CLINICAL PEARLS

- BP-2 is characterized by at least 1 episode of major depression and 1 episode of hypomania.
- Patients are often resistant to treatment during a hypomanic episode, as they enjoy the elevated mood and productivity.
- Evidence indicates that patients with BP-2 may be at greater risk of both attempting and completing suicide than with BP-1 and unipolar depression.

BITES

Jennifer S. Daly, MD

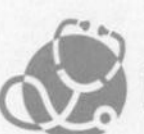

BASICS

DESCRIPTION

- Animal bites to humans from dogs (85–90%), cats (5–10%), rodents (2–3%), humans (2–3%), and other animals, including snakes
- System(s) affected: Potentially any

Geriatric Considerations

Increased risk of infection if patient is >50.

Pediatric Considerations

Young children are more likely to have severe bites.

EPIDEMIOLOGY

- Predominant age: All ages, but children > adults
- Predominant gender: Dog bites: Male > Female; cat bites: Female > Male

Incidence

- 4–5 million dog bites per year in US
- Account for 1% of all emergency room visits
- 20% of bites will require medical attention, 10,000 will require hospital admission, and an average of 19 victims will die from the bites annually (1).

Prevalence

50% of all Americans are bitten during their lifetime.

RISK FACTORS

- Male dogs are more likely to bite.
- Clenched-fist human bites are frequently associated with the use of alcohol.
- Patients presenting >8 hours following the bite are at greater risk of infection.

GENERAL PREVENTION

- Instruct children and adults about animal hazards and strongly enforce animal control laws.
- Educate dog owners.

PATHOPHYSIOLOGY

- Animal bites can cause tears, punctures, scratches, avulsions, or crush injuries.
- Contamination of wound with flora from the mouth of the biting animal or from the broken skin of the victim can lead to infection.

ETIOLOGY

- Most bite wounds are from a domestic pet known to the victim.
- 89% of cat bites are provoked.
- Pit bull terriers, German shepherds, Rottweilers, and mixed breeds are most commonly associated with bites.
- Human bites are often the result of 1 person striking another in the mouth with a clenched fist. They can also occur incidentally in the case of paronychia due to nail biting or thumb sucking or "love nips" to the face, breasts, or genital areas.

DIAGNOSIS

HISTORY

Obtain detailed history of the incident (provoked or unprovoked), the type of animal and vaccine status, the site of the bite, and the geographic setting.

PHYSICAL EXAM

- Dog bites (85–90% of bites):
  - Hands and face most common site of injury in adults and children, respectively
  - More likely to have associated crush injury
- Cat bites (5–10% of bites):
  - Predominantly involve the hands, followed by lower extremities, face, and trunk
  - Twice as likely to lead to infection as dog bites (due to puncture nature of wounds), with higher risk of osteomyelitis, tenosynovitis, and septic arthritis
- Human bites (2–3% of bites):
  - Intentional bite: Semicircular or oval area of erythema and bruising, with or without break in skin
  - Clenched-fist injury: Small wounds over the metacarpophalangeal joints from striking the fist against another's teeth
- Signs of wound infection include fever, erythema, swelling, tenderness, purulent drainage, lymphangitis

Pediatric Considerations

If human bite mark on child has intercanine distance >3 cm, bite probably came from an adult and should raise concerns about child abuse.

DIAGNOSTIC TESTS & INTERPRETATION

Lab

Initial lab tests

- Drainage from infected wounds should be Gram-stained and cultured:
  - If wound fails to heal, add cultures for atypical pathogens and ask lab to keep cultures for 7–10 days (some pathogens are slow-growing).
- 85% of bite wounds will yield a positive culture, with an average of 5 pathogens.
- Blood cultures should be obtained if bacteremia suspected (e.g., fever)

Follow-Up & Special Considerations

Previous antibiotic therapy may alter culture results.

Imaging

Initial approach

- If bite wound is near a bone or joint, a plain radiograph is needed to check for bone injury and to use for comparison later if osteomyelitis is subsequently suspected.
- Radiographs are needed to check for fractures in clenched-fist injuries.

Follow-Up & Special Considerations

Subsequent suspicion of osteomyelitis warrants comparison plain radiograph or magnetic resonance imaging (MRI).

Diagnostic Procedures/Surgery

Surgical exploration may be needed to ascertain extent of injuries, especially in serious hand wounds.

Pathological Findings

- Dog bites:
  - *Pasteurella* sp. is present in 50% of bites.
  - Also found: *Viridans streptococci, Staphylococcus aureus, Staphylococcus intermedius, Bacteroides, Capnocytophaga canimorsus, Fusobacterium*
- Cat bites:
  - *Pasteurella* sp. is present in 75% of bites.
  - Also found: *Streptococcus* spp. (including *Streptococcus pyogenes*), *Staphylococcus* spp. (including methicillin-resistant *Staphylococcus aureus* [MRSA]), *Fusobacterium* spp., *Bacteroides* spp., *Porphyromonas* spp., *Moraxella* spp.
- Human bites:
  - *Streptococcus* species, *S. aureus, Eikenella corrodens*, and various anaerobic bacteria (e.g., *Fusobacterium, Peptostreptococcus, Prevotella*, and *Porphyromonas* spp.)
  - Although rare, case reports have suggested transmission of viruses such as hepatitis, HIV, and herpes simplex (2)[C].
- Reptile bites:
  - In addition to snake venom tissue necrosis: *P. aeruginosa, Proteus* spp., *Salmonella, Bacteroides fragilis*, and *Clostridium* spp.
- Rodent bites:
  - *Streptobacillus moniliformis* or *Spirillum minor*, which cause rat-bite fever

ALERT

Asplenic patients and those with underlying hepatic disease are at risk of bacteremia and fatal sepsis after dog bites infected with *Capnocytophaga canimorsus* (gram-negative rod).

TREATMENT

MEDICATION

- Consider need for antirabies therapy: Rabies immune globulin and human diploid cell rabies vaccine for those bitten by wild animals (in US, primary vector is bat bite), rabid pets, or unvaccinated pets, or if animal cannot be quarantined for 10 days (3)[A].
- Tetanus toxoid for those previously immunized, but >5 years since their last dose and tetanus immune globulin and tetanus vaccination in patients without a full primary series of immunizations (4)[A]
- A patient negative for anti-HBs antibodies and bitten by an HBsAg-positive individual should receive both hepatitis B immune globulin (HBIG) and hepatitis B vaccine.
- HIV postexposure prophylaxis is generally not recommended for human bites, given the extremely low risk for transmission.
- Prophylactic antibiotics are only recommended for human bites and all penetrating animal bites to the hand (5,6)[A].
- For prophylaxis and for empiric treatment of established infection, amoxicillin-clavulanate is 1st line (3)[B]:
  - Adults: 500 mg p.o. t.i.d. or 875 mg p.o. b.i.d.
  - Children: <3 months: 30 mg/kg/d p.o. q12h; ≥3 months and <40 kg: 45 mg/kg/d q12h; >40 kg, use adult dosing

- Duration of therapy: Prophylaxis: 3–5 days; treatment: cellulitis/skin abscess: 5–10 days; bacteremia: 10–14 days. Antibiotic and duration of therapy should be adjusted based on culture results and clinical improvement:
  - Adults: Clindamycin (300 mg p.o. q.i.d.) plus either TMP-SMX (1 DS tablet p.o. b.i.d.–t.i.d.) or ciprofloxacin (500 mg p.o. b.i.d.) (3)[B]; moxifloxacin (Avelox) 400 mg q24h × 7–21 days
  - Children: Clindamycin (5–10 mg/kg IV [to a maximum of 600 mg] followed by 10–30 mg/kg/d in 3–4 divided doses to a maximum of 300 mg per dose) plus trimethoprim-sulfamethoxazole (8–10 mg/kg of trimethoprim) or cefoxitin IM/IV until culture results obtained

ʻregnancy Considerations
ʻenicillin-allergic pregnant women:
- Azithromycin 250–500 mg p.o. every day (3)[B]

Observe closely and note potential increased risk of failure.

ALERT
- 1st-generation cephalosporins (e.g., cephalexin), penicillinase-resistant penicillins (e.g., dicloxacillin), macrolides (e.g., erythromycin), and clindamycin (when not administered with another agent) lack activity against *P. multocida* (dog/cat bites) and *Eikenella corrodens* (human bites), and should be avoided (3)[B].
- Consider community-acquired MRSA as possible pathogen (from human skin or colonized pet). If high suspicion, doxycycline or trimethoprim-sulfamethoxazole provide good coverage (4)[A].
- Adverse reaction: Amoxicillin-clavulanate should be given with food to decrease gastrointestinal (GI) side effects.
- Precautions: Dose antibiotics by body weight and renal function.
- Significant possible interactions: Antibiotics may decrease efficacy of oral contraceptives.

ADDITIONAL TREATMENT
General Measures
- Elevation of the injured extremity to prevent swelling
- Contact the local health department regarding the prevalence of rabies in the species of animal involved (highest in bats).
- Snake bite: If venomous, patient needs rapid transport to facility capable of definitive evaluation. If envenomation has occurred, patient should receive antivenom. Be sure patient is stable for transport; consider measuring and/or treating coagulation and renal status along with any anaphylactic reactions before transport.

Issues for Referral
Deep wounds to the hand and face should be referred to a hand surgeon or plastic surgeon, respectively.

SURGERY/OTHER PROCEDURES
- Copious irrigation of the wound with normal saline via a catheter tip is needed to reduce risk of infection.
- Devitalized tissue needs debridement.
- Debridement of puncture wounds is not advised.
- Primary closure can be considered if the wound is clean after irrigation and bite is <12 hours old, and in bites to the face (cosmesis) (7)[B].
- Infected wounds and those at risk of infection (cat bites, human bites, bites to the hand, crush injuries, presentation >12 hours from injury) should be left open (8)[B].
- Delayed primary closure in 3–5 days is an option for infected wounds.
- Splint hand if it is injured.
- Large, gaping wounds should be reapproximated with widely spaced sutures or Steri-Strips.

IN-PATIENT CONSIDERATIONS
Initial Stabilization
ABCs for associated trauma or severe infection

Admission Criteria
- Patients with deep or severe wound infections, systemic infections requiring IV antibiotics, those requiring surgery, and the immunocompromised
- If hospitalized with established infection (animal or human bite):
  - Adults: Ampicillin/sulbactam 1.5–3 g IV q6h or piperacillin/tazobactam 3.375 g q6h or 4.5 g IV q8h or ticarcillin/clavulanate 3.1 g IV q4–6h (3)[B]
  - Children: Ampicillin/sulbactam 100–200 mg/kg/d IV given in 4 divided doses to maximum of 3 g per dose

Discharge Criteria
Pending clinical improvement

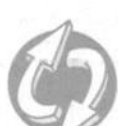

ONGOING CARE

FOLLOW-UP RECOMMENDATIONS
Patient Monitoring
- Patient should be rechecked in 24–48 hours if not infected at time of 1st encounter (9)[B].
- Daily follow-up is warranted for infections.
- Subsequent revisions of empiric antibiotic therapy should be based on the culture results and the clinical response.

PATIENT EDUCATION
- Educate parents at well-child checks about how to avoid animal bites.
- AAFP: http://familydoctor.org/online/famdocen/home/healthy/safety/kids family/668.html

PROGNOSIS
Wounds should steadily improve and close over by 7–10 days.

COMPLICATIONS
- Septic arthritis
- Osteomyelitis
- Extensive soft tissue injuries with scarring
- Hemorrhage
- Gas gangrene
- Sepsis
- Meningitis
- Endocarditis
- Post-traumatic stress disorder
- Death

REFERENCES

1. Langley RL. Human fatalities resulting from dog attacks in the United States, 1979–2005. *Wilderness Environ Med*. 2009 Spring;20(1):19–25.
2. Bartholomew CF, Jones AM. Human bites: a rare risk factor for HIV transmission. *AIDS*. 2006;20:631–2.
3. Stevens DL, Bisno AL, Chambers HF, et al. Practice guidelines for the diagnosis and management of skin and soft-tissue infections. *Clin Infect Dis*. 2005;41:1373–406.
4. Oehler RL, Velez AP, Mizrachi M, et al. Bite-related and septic syndromes caused by cats and dogs. *Lancet Infect Dis*. 2009;9:439–47.
5. Medeiros I, et al. Antibiotic prophylaxis for mammalian bites. *Cochrane Database Syst Rev*. 2008;2:CD001738.
6. Rittner AV, Fitzpatrick K, Corfield A. Best evidence topic report. Are antibiotics indicated following human bites? *Emerg Med J*. 2005;22:654.
7. Stefanopoulos PK, Tarantzopoulou AD. Facial bite wounds: management update. *Int J Oral Maxillofac Surg*. 2005;34:464–72.
8. Benson LS, Edwards SL, Schiff AP, et al. Dog and cat bites to the hand: treatment and cost assessment. *J Hand Surg [Am]*. 2006;31:468–73.
9. Okonkwo U, et al. Animal bites: Practical tips for effective management. *J Emerg Nursing*. 2008;34(3):225–6.

ADDITIONAL READING

Daly JS, et al. Bites and stings of terrestrial and aquatic life. In Fitzpatrick TB, Eisen AZ, Wolff K, et al. (eds). *Dermatology in General Medicine*, 6th ed. New York: McGraw Hill, 2008.

See Also (Topic, Algorithm, Electronic Media Element)
Cellulitis; Rabies; Snake Envenomations; Bartonella Infections

CODES

ICD9
- 879.8 Open wound(s) (multiple) of unspecified site(s), without mention of complication
- 879.9 Open wound(s) (multiple) of unspecified site(s), complicated

CLINICAL PEARLS
- Wound cleansing, debridement, and culture are essential. Most wounds should be left open.
- Prophylaxis is recommended for human bites and bites to the hand.
- Consider rabies and tetanus vaccination.
- Patients bitten by animals or humans require close follow-up to monitor for infection.

BLADDER CANCER

Margaret E. Thompson, MD

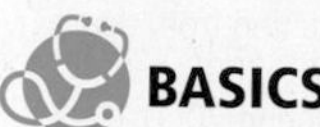

BASICS

DESCRIPTION

- Primary malignant neoplasms arising in the urinary bladder
- Most common type is transitional cell carcinoma (90%)
- Other types include adenocarcinoma, small cell carcinoma, squamous cell carcinoma
- Rhabdomyosarcoma of the bladder may occur in children.

EPIDEMIOLOGY

Incidence

- Increases with age (median age at diagnosis is 73 years)
- More common in Caucasians than in Asians or African Americans
- Male > Female (4:1)
- 37.2 per 100,000 men per year (1)
- 9.2 per 100,000 women per year (1)
- 21.1 per 100,000 men and women per year (1)

Prevalence

As of January 1, 2007, 535,236 cases in US (1)

RISK FACTORS

- Smoking is the single greatest risk factor (increases risk 4-fold) (2).
- Other risk factors:
  - Occupational carcinogens in dye, rubber, paint, plastics, metal, and automotive exhaust
  - Schistosomiasis in Mediterranean (squamous cell) cancer
  - History of pelvic irradiation
  - Chronic lower urinary tract infection (UTI)
  - Chronic indwelling urinary catheter
  - Cyclophosphamide exposure
  - High-fat diet
  - Chronic low fluid intake
  - Slight increase in risk with prostate cancer

ALERT

Any patient who smokes and presents with microscopic or gross hematuria, or irritative voiding symptoms such as urgency and frequency not clearly due to UTI, should be evaluated by cystoscopy for the presence of a bladder neoplasm.

Genetics

Hereditary transmission is unlikely, although transitional cell carcinoma pathophysiology is related to oncogenes.

GENERAL PREVENTION

Avoid smoking and other risk factors.

PATHOPHYSIOLOGY

- 70–80% is superficial (in lamina propria or mucosa):
  - Usually highly differentiated with long survival
  - Initial event seems to be activation of an oncogene on chromosome 9 in superficial cancers
- 20% of tumors are invasive (deeper than lamina propria) at presentation:
  - Tend to be high-grade with worse prognosis
  - Associated with other chromosome deletions

ETIOLOGY

Unknown, other than related to risk factors

DIAGNOSIS

HISTORY

- Hematuria
- Urinary symptoms (frequency, urgency)
- Abdominal or pelvic pain in advanced disease
- Exposures (see Risk Factors)

PHYSICAL EXAM

- Normal in early cases
- Pelvic or abdominal mass in advanced disease
- Wasting in systemic disease

DIAGNOSTIC TESTS & INTERPRETATION

Lab

Initial lab tests

- Urinalysis is the initial test in patients presenting with gross hematuria or urinary symptoms such as frequency, urgency, and dysuria.
- Macroscopic hematuria (55% sensitivity, positive predictive value [PPV] 0.22 for urologic cancer) (3)[C]

Follow-Up & Special Considerations

- Urine cytology 54% sensitivity overall (lower in less advanced tumors), 94% specific (4)[A]
- Other urine markers:
  - NMP22: 67% sensitive, 78% specific (4)[A]
  - Bladder tumor-associated antigen stat: 70% sensitive, 75% specific (4)[A]
  - Fluorescent in situ hybridization assay: 69% sensitive, 78% specific (PPV 27.1, negative predictive value 95.3) for all tumors, more sensitive and specific for higher grade (5)[B]
- Bottom line: None of the urine markers are sensitive enough to rule out bladder cancer on its own.
- Liver function tests, alkaline phosphatase if metastasis suspected

Imaging

Initial approach

- Done for staging and evaluating extent of disease but not for diagnosis itself:
  - Computed tomography (CT) urogram replacing to image upper tracts if there is suspicion of disease there
  - Diffusion-weighted magnetic resonance (MR) imaging and multidimensional CT scan are undergoing study for use in diagnosis and staging of bladder tumors.
  - For invasive disease, metastatic workup should include chest x-ray.
  - Bone scan should be performed if the patient has bone pain or if alkaline phosphatase is elevated (6)[B].
- Urologic CT scan (abdomen, pelvis, with and without contrast) or MRI 40–98% accurate, with MRI slightly more accurate (6)[B], is recommended if metastasis is suspected.

Diagnostic Procedures/Surgery

- Cystoscopy with biopsy is the gold standard for diagnosis, but 1 study showed that 33% of patients had residual tumor after transurethral resection of superficial tumor (TURBT) (6)[B].
- TURBT with bladder washings: Sensitivity of cytology on bladder washings for carcinoma in situ is nearly 100%.

Pathological Findings

- Characterized as superficial or invasive
- 70–80% present as superficial lesion
- Superficial lesions:
  - Carcinoma in situ: Flat lesion, high grade
  - Ta: Noninvasive papillary carcinoma
  - T1: Extends into submucosa, lamina propria
- Invasive cancer:
  - T2: Invasion into muscle:
    - pT2a: Invasion into superficial muscle
    - pT2b: Invasion into deep muscle
  - T3: Invasion into perivesical fat:
    - pT3a: Microscopic
    - pT3b: Macroscopic
  - T4: Invasion into adjacent organs:
    - aT4a: Invades prostate, uterus, or vagina
    - aT4b: Invades abdominal or pelvic wall
  - N1–N3: Invades lymph nodes
- M: Metastasis to bone or soft tissue

DIFFERENTIAL DIAGNOSIS

- Other urinary tract neoplasms
- UTI
- Prostatism
- Bladder instability
- Interstitial cystitis
- Urolithiasis
- Interstitial nephritis
- Papillary urothelial hyperplasia

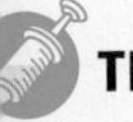

TREATMENT

r superficial bladder cancer, the treatment is ·nerally removal via cystoscopic surgery. For ıscle-invasive cancer, a radical cystectomy is ·eferred.

EDICATION

·rst Line

There is insufficient evidence to show that cisplatin-based neoadjuvant chemotherapy in patients with locally advanced bladder cancer improves survival (7)[A].

Intravesical bacillus Calmette-Guérin (BCG) after TURBT in high-grade lesions has been shown to decrease recurrence in Ta and T1 tumors (8)[A].

econd Line

ıemotherapy is the 1st-line treatment for metastatic adder cancer: Methotrexate-vinblastine-)xorubicin-cisplatin (MVAC) is the preferred regimen.

DDITIONAL TREATMENT

sues for Referral

ıtients with microscopic or gross hematuria not :herwise explained or resolving should be referred to urologist for cystoscopy.

dditional Therapies

adiotherapy:

In US, used for patients with muscle-invasive cancer who are not surgical candidates

Preoperative (radical cystectomy) radiotherapy also an option

Treatment of choice for muscle-invasive cancer in some European and Canadian centers:
- 65–70 Gy over 6–7 weeks is standard

URGERY/OTHER PROCEDURES

Surgery is definitive therapy for superficial and invasive cancer:
- Superficial cancer: TURBT sometimes followed by intravesical therapy

Invasive cancer:
- Radical cystectomy for invasive disease that is confined to the bladder is more effective than radical radiotherapy (9)[A]. Urine is diverted via an ileal loop with ostomy or neobladder constructed with intestine.

N-PATIENT CONSIDERATIONS

dmission Criteria

leed for surgery or intensive therapy

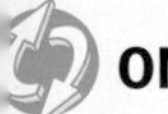

ONGOING CARE

OLLOW-UP RECOMMENDATIONS

Superficial cancers:
- Urine cytology alone has not been shown to be sufficient for follow-up.
- Cystoscopy every 3 months for 18–24 months, every 6 months for the next 2 years, then annually

Follow-up for invasive cancers depends on the approach to treatment.

Patients treated with BCG require lifelong follow-up.

)IET

:ontinue adequate fluid intake.

PATIENT EDUCATION

Smoking cessation

PROGNOSIS

- 5-year relative survival rates:
  - Localized: 93.7%
  - Regional metastasis: 46.0%
  - Distant metastasis: 6.2%
- Superficial bladder cancer:
  - BCG treatment prevents recurrence vs TURBT alone; difference 30%, NNT 3.3 (9)[A]
  - BCG prevents progression vs TURBT alone, difference 8%
- Invasive cancer:
  - T2 disease: Radical cystectomy results in 60–75% 5-year survival.
  - T3 or T4 disease: Radical cystectomy results in 20–40% 5-year survival.
  - Neoadjuvant chemotherapy with cystectomy has led to varying degrees of increased survival.
  - Radiation with chemotherapy has led to varying degrees of increased survival.
- Metastatic cancer:
  - MVAC resulted in mean survival of 12.5 months.

COMPLICATIONS

- Superficial bladder cancer:
  - Local symptoms:
    - Dysuria, frequency, nocturia, pain, passing debris in urine
    - Bacterial cystitis
    - Perforation
  - General symptoms:
    - Flulike symptoms
    - Systemic infection
- Invasive cancer:
  - Symptoms related to definitive treatment, including incontinence, bleeding
  - Patients with neobladder at risk for azotemia and metabolic acidosis

REFERENCES

1. Altekruse SF, Kosary CL, Krapcho M, et al. (eds). *SEER Cancer Statistics Review, 1975–2007*, National Cancer Institute. Bethesda, MD, http://seer.cancer.gov/csr/1975_2007/, based on November 2009 SEER data submission, posted to the SEER web site, 2010.
2. Kaplan M, Cologlu M. Bladder Tumors. In *Essential Evidence Plus*, John Wiley and Sons, Ltd, 2009, http://www.essentialevidenceplus.com/content/eee/480, accessed 4/26/10.
3. Buntinx F, Wauters H. The diagnostic value of macroscopic haematuria in diagnosing urological cancers: a meta-analysis. *Fam Pract*. 1997;14:63–8.
4. Glas AS, Roos D, Deutekom M, et al. Tumor markers in the diagnosis of primary bladder cancer. A systematic review. *J Urol*. 2003;169:1975–82.
5. Sarosdy MF, Kahn PR, Ziffer MD, et al. Use of a multitarget fluorescence in situ hybridization assay to diagnose bladder cancer in patients with hematuria. *J Urol*. 2006;176:44–7.
6. Kirkali Z, Chan T, Manoharan M, et al. Bladder cancer: epidemiology, staging and grading, and diagnosis. *Urology*. 2005;66:4–34.
7. Advanced Bladder Cancer Meta-analysis Collaboration. Neoadjuvant Cisplatin for advanced bladder cancer (Cochrane Review). In *the Cochrane Library Issue* 1, 2009. Chichester, UK: John Wiley and Sons, Ltd.
8. Shelley M, Court JB, Kynaston H, et al. Intravesical Bacillus Calmette-Guerin in Ta and T1 bladder cancer (Cochrane Review). In: *The Cochrane Library*, Issue 3, 2010. Chichester, UK: John Wiley and Sons, Ltd.
9. Shelley MD, et al. Surgery versus radiotherapy for muscle invasive bladder cancer (Cochrane Review). In: *The Cochrane Library*, Issue 4, 2005. Chichester, UK: John Wiley and Sons, Ltd.
10. U.S. Preventive Services Task Force. Screening for bladder cancer in adults: Recommendation statement. Rockville, MD: Agency for Healthcare Research and Quality; 2004.

ADDITIONAL READING

Vale C. Neoadjuvant chemotherapy for invasive bladder cancer (Cochrane Review). In: *The Cochrane Library* Issue 1, 2007. Chichester, UK: John Wiley and Sons, Ltd.

See Also (Topic, Algorithm, Electronic Media Element)

Hematuria
Algorithm: Hematuria

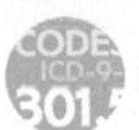

CODES

ICD9

188.9 Malignant neoplasm of bladder, part unspecified

CLINICAL PEARLS

- Gross hematuria in smokers should be evaluated with complete urologic workup.
- The United States Preventive Services Task Force recommends against routine screening for bladder cancer (10)[A].

BLADDER INJURY

Kyle D. Wood, MD
Ilya Gorbachinsky, MD

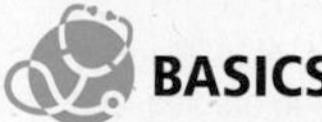

BASICS

DESCRIPTION

- Bladder injury can be the result of:
  - Blunt or penetrating trauma
  - Bladder rupture secondary to a full bladder or blunt injury
  - Surgical complication (iatrogenic injury)
- Classified as either intraperitoneal or extraperitoneal rupture
- Bladder contusion is injury to the mucosa or muscularis without full-thickness loss; without urine extravasation
- Often associated with ureter/urethral injury and/or other non-urological injuries

EPIDEMIOLOGY

Incidence

- ~0.5% of civilian trauma patients (1)
- 12% of civilian injuries in Iraq, mostly due to gunshot wounds (2)
- Blunt trauma with bladder injury is associated with other injuries 94% of the time (3); pelvic fracture being the most common followed by lower abdominal impact in the presence of a full bladder (4).
- During pelvic surgery, it is the most commonly damaged organ (5).

Pediatric Considerations

Children are more prone to rupture and are more likely to have intraperitoneal ruptures than adults (1).

RISK FACTORS

- High-energy mechanism (fall, motor vehicle accident [MVA])
- Pelvic fracture
- Penetrating wound
- Prior bladder/pelvic surgery
- Pelvic radiotherapy

GENERAL PREVENTION

Seat belts:

- Voiding prior to automobile travel

PATHOPHYSIOLOGY

- Bladder is often protected by its deep location in the bony pelvis.
- Contusion: Damage sustained to bladder mucosa and muscularis without loss of wall continuity (5)
- Intraperitoneal rupture: Increases in intravesical pressure can lead to rupture at the most weak and mobile portion, the bladder dome (6,7)
- Extraperitoneal rupture: Disruption of bony pelvis can tear bladder at fascial attachments while this or other bony protrusions can perforate the bladder (6).

Pediatric Considerations

Children <6 years old are more prone to bladder injury as the organ still lacks protection from the pubic symphysis (7).

ETIOLOGY

- The cause of injury is usually high-energy trauma (motor vehicle accidents, falls).
- Rupture due to increased pressure in nondistensible (full) bladder
- Laceration due to bone fragment or penetrating object (knife, bullet)
- Surgical complications: Gynecologic, general surgery, and urologic operations are the most common reported causes of iatrogenic bladder injury, in decreasing order of frequency (8).

ALERT

Rare instances of intravesical vascular graft erosion have recently been reported up to 8 years post-op (9).

COMMONLY ASSOCIATED CONDITIONS

- Pelvic fracture
- Urethral injury; almost exclusively males

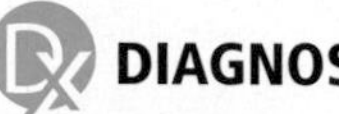

DIAGNOSIS

HISTORY

- Isolated bladder injury is rare. Typically, patient has other serious injuries.
- High mechanism deceleration injury (fall, MVA)
- Penetrating trauma
- Recent abdominal/pelvic surgery
- Urinary retention
- Preexisting bladder outlet obstruction
- Anatomical abnormalities
- Inability to void or oliguria
- Pain in the genital area or abdomen

PHYSICAL EXAM

- Abdominal exam: Suprapubic tenderness to palpation, guarding, distention, decreased bowel sounds, bruising
- Genitourinary exam: Blood at meatus, gross hematuria, clots in the urine, scrotal/urethral hematoma, free floating or high riding prostate, unstable pelvis

ALERT

Peritonitis is unusual in bladder injury.

DIAGNOSTIC TESTS & INTERPRETATION

Lab

Initial lab tests

- Immediate catheterization will likely demonstrate gross hematuria (3).
- Urinalysis will demonstrate blood.
- Basic metabolic panel: Serum blood urea nitrogen (BUN), creatinine, chloride, and potassium levels may be elevated and sodium and bicarbonate may be decreased in intraperitoneal ruptures secondary to peritoneal absorption. An increase in BUN/creatinine ratio may also be observed (5).
- Serum labs are unchanged in extraperitoneal ruptures (6).

Follow-Up & Special Considerations

If blood at the meatus or if the catheter does not pass easily, consider urethral injury and need for retrograde urethrography.

Imaging

Initial approach

- 2 types of imaging are acceptable:
  - Plain film cystography: Fill bladder until patient has sense of discomfort or fill with 350 mL. Use 3-film technique capturing before filling, when full, and after drainage.
    - Contusion: No extravasation but may see distortion of bladder outline with contrast.
    - Intraperitoneal: Contrast may be seen in cul-de-sac and paracolic gutters. Bowel loops may also be outlined.
    - Extraperitoneal: Flame-shaped perivesical stranding of contrast (5)
  - CT cystography: High-resolution computed tomography (CT) cystogram is also acceptable. C or radiology with only excreted contrast is not sensitive (6). Dilute contrast material.
- Absolute indication for immediate cystography: Gross hematuria with pelvic fracture as 29% of these patients will have a bladder injury (10).
- Relative indications: Gross hematuria without pelvi fracture, microhematuria with pelvic fracture, isolated microscopic hematuria (10)

ALERT

During plain film cystography, a post-void view is mandatory as contrast in the bladder may mask extravasation. This is not required with CT cystogram.

Follow-Up & Special Considerations

- Retrograde urethrography must be performed befo placing a Foley catheter when urethral injury is suspected.
- Other signs of bladder injury can include free intraperitoneal fluid on CT scan or ultrasound

Pathological Findings

- Perivesicular hematoma
- Perforation at dome of bladder (in trigone, near urachus)
- Jagged tear in bladder
- Intraoperative clues (11)
  - Appearance of Foley catheter/balloon or urine in the operative field
  - Presence of gas in catheter bag (during laparoscopy)

DIFFERENTIAL DIAGNOSIS

- Isolated urethral injury
- Isolated pelvic fracture
- Isolated ureteral injury
- Other visceral rupture

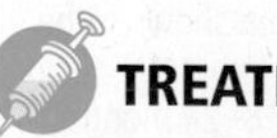

TREATMENT

- Contusion: Observation or 20–22 French Foley catheter for 10–14 days (6)[B]
- Intraperitoneal rupture: Immediate surgical repair (6)[C]
  - Often intraoperative damage falls under this heading and can also be treated immediately.
- Extraperitoneal rupture: 20–22 French Foley catheter for 10–14 days (6)

EDICATION

- Analgesics
- Antibiotics
- Antispasmodics

rst Line

- Narcotic pain control (i.e., morphine, hydromorphone); titrate to effect
- Broad-spectrum antibiotics like ciprofloxacin 500 mg b.i.d.
- Oxybutynin 5–10 mg t.i.d. for spasm

econd Line

- Broad-spectrum antibiotics
- Antispasmodics (i.e., flavoxate)

ALERT

here is concern about fluoroquinolones causing damage to cartilage in children.

DDITIONAL TREATMENT

- If uncomplicated extraperitoneal bladder rupture:
  - Can be treated with urethral catheter alone (use large bore catheter [22 French])
  - Exception: In pediatric patients, consider placing a suprapubic catheter as small catheters through urethra will clot and larger catheters through urethra risk future urethral stricture
  - Catheter should remain in place for 2 weeks. Cystography is necessary prior to removal of catheter.
  - Antibiotics should be given on day of injury and continued for 3 days after catheter removal.
- If a complicated extraperitoneal bladder rupture:
  - Needs to be treated with open repair
  - Complicated rupture is considered when there is coexisting bladder neck injury, vaginal injury, or rectal injury. Also if open pelvic fracture, or bone fragments are present.
  - Consider open repair if patient is scheduled for exploratory laparotomy or internal fixation of pelvic fracture (prevents urine leak on hardware).
- If an intraperitoneal bladder rupture or penetrating injury:
  - Urgent operative management is necessary.
  - Cystography should be repeated 7–10 days after surgery.
  - Antibiotics are needed for 3 days .
  - No need for suprapubic catheter as urethral catheter is sufficient, except in pediatric population (3)
- During pelvic surgery, iatrogenic full thickness defects are likely to be intraperitoneal, so can fix immediately with 2-layer (mucosa and muscularis) closure via absorbable suture
  - Prior to repair, be sure to confirm that ureters were not damaged concomitantly either with IV indigo carmine administration and visulation of blue dye expulsion from the ureteral orifices (UO) or by confirming easy placement of ureteral catheters through the UO (11).

General Measures

- Place Foley catheter
- Pain control
- Antibiotics
- Antispasmodics (Ditropan)
- Obtain imaging diagnosis

Issues for Referral

A urologist or trauma surgeon should be involved with all bladder injury management.

SURGERY/OTHER PROCEDURES

- Urgent surgery is indicated for intraperitoneal or bladder neck rupture
- Extraperitoneal rupture is usually manageable with 10–14 days of catheter drainage (20–22 French).

IN-PATIENT CONSIDERATIONS

Initial Stabilization

- Cervical spine precautions
- Stabilize hemodynamics
- Stabilize pelvis
- Follow advanced trauma life support protocols

Admission Criteria

All bladder injuries require admission for monitoring renal function and hemodynamic stability.

IV Fluids

Lactated Ringer's for initial resuscitation, unless contraindicated (i.e., concomitant head injury)

Nursing

- Foley to gravity
- Hourly urine output recorded

Discharge Criteria

- Stable for transfer to rehabilitation or home if can perform activities of daily living
- Extraperitoneal ruptures controlled with indwelling Foley catheter if rupture not healed
- Able to void if no catheter in place
- No evidence of infection
- Pain controlled

ONGOING CARE

FOLLOW-UP RECOMMENDATIONS

Patient Monitoring

- Hourly urine output
- Hemodynamic monitoring
- Progressive abdominal distention

DIET

No restrictions

PATIENT EDUCATION

- Regular lifestyle is expected
- Use of seat belts
- No special instructions needed

PROGNOSIS

Full return to normal function

COMPLICATIONS

- Infection
- Urine leak and/or urinoma
- Abscess formation
- Peritonitis or sepsis
- Bladder calculi
- Vesicocutaneous or other fistulas
- Stricture is a rare complication
- Death; usually from other injuries

REFERENCES

1. Inaba K, McKenney M, Munera F, et al. Cystogram follow-up in the management of traumatic bladder disruption. *J Trauma*. 2006;60:23–8.
2. Ramani AP, Ryndin I, Veetil RT, et al. Novel technique for removal of misdirected laparoscopic Weck clips. *Urology*. 2007;70:168–9.
3. Parry NG, Rozycki GS, Feliciano DV, Tremblay LN, Cava RA, Voeltz Z, Carney J et al. Traumatic rupture of the urinary bladder: is the suprapubic tube necessary? *J Trauma*. 2003;54:431–6.
4. Tezval H, Tezval M, von Klot C, Herrmann TR, Dresing K, Jonas U, Burchardt M et al. Urinary tract injuries in patients with multiple trauma. *World J Urol*. 2007;25:177–84.
5. Gomez RG, Ceballos L, Coburn M, Corriere JN, Dixon CM, Lobel B, McAninch J et al. Consensus statement on bladder injuries. *BJU Int*. 2004;94: 27–32.
6. Corriere JN, Sandler CM. Diagnosis and management of bladder injuries. *Urol Clin North Am*. 2006;33:67–71, vi.
7. Kessler DO, Francis DL, Esernio-Jenssen D et al. Bladder rupture after minor accidental trauma: case reports and a review of the literature. *Pediatr Emerg Care*. 2010;26:43–5.
8. Armenakas NA, Pareek G, Fracchia JA et al. Iatrogenic bladder perforations: longterm followup of 65 patients. *J Am Coll Surg*. 2004;198:78–82.
9. Nakamura LY, Ferrigni RG, Stone WM, Fowl RJ et al. Urinary bladder injuries during vascular surgery. *J Vasc Surg*. 2010;52:453–5.
10. Morey AF, Iverson AJ, Swan A, Harmon WJ, Spore SS, Bhayani S, Brandes SB et al. Bladder rupture after blunt trauma: guidelines for diagnostic imaging. *J Trauma*. 2001;51:683–6.
11. Sharp HT, Swenson C et al. Hollow viscus injury during surgery. *Obstet Gynecol Clin North Am*. 2010;37:461–7.

ADDITIONAL READING

- ATLS Protocol from the Committee on Trauma of the American College of Surgeons, http://www.facs.org/trauma/atls/.
- Eastern Association for the Surgery of Trauma, Management of Genitourinary Trauma, 2004, http://www.east.org/tpg/GUmgmt.pdf.

See Also (Topic, Algorithm, Electronic Media Element)

Algorithm: Hematuria

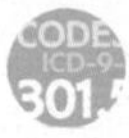

CODES

ICD9

- 596.6 Rupture of bladder, nontraumatic
- 596.9 Unspecified disorder of bladder
- 867.0 Injury to bladder and urethra without mention of open wound into cavity

CLINICAL PEARLS

- Foley should remain in place for 10–14 days. After this point, 85% of patients have healed all injuries.
- A cystogram must be performed before Foley removal to verify no extravasation of fluid. If extravasation continues, recheck every 3–5 days.
- An intraoperative consult to urology is indicated if an inadvertent bladder perforation occurs during another procedure. If urology is not available, the bladder must be examined intravesically, generally by increasing the size of the wound and searching for another occult injury. Do not delay repair.
- Repair bladder injuries in 2 layers with absorbable suture and place a Foley catheter.

BLEPHARITIS

Joshua J. Spooner, PharmD, MS
A. Raquel Mateo-Bibeau, MD

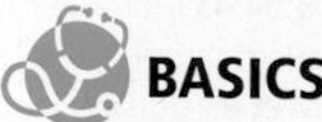

BASICS

DESCRIPTION

- An inflammatory reaction of the eyelid margin:
  - Usually occurs as seborrheic or staphylococcal blepharitis
  - Multiple types may coexist.
- System(s) affected: Skin/Exocrine
- Synonym(s): Granulated eyelids

EPIDEMIOLOGY

Incidence

- One of the most common ocular disorders
- Predominant age: Adult
- Predominant sex: Male = Female

RISK FACTORS

- Seborrheic dermatitis
- Contact dermatitis
- Herpes simplex dermatitis
- Varicella-zoster dermatitis
- Acne rosacea
- Diabetes mellitus
- Immunocompromised state (e.g., AIDS, chemotherapy)
- Isotretinoin use
- Dry eye syndromes

ETIOLOGY

- Seborrheic:
  - Accelerated shedding of skin cells with associated sebaceous gland dysfunction
  - *Malassezia furfur* (formerly *Pityrosporum ovale*) yeasts often colonize.
- Staphylococcal:
  - Superinfection of Zeis glands of lid margin and meibomian glands posterior to lashes with *Staphylococcus aureus*
  - Usually part of mixed blepharitis
- Meibomian gland dysfunction: Obstruction and inflammation of the meibomian glands; associated with acne rosacea, acne vulgaris, and oral retinoid therapy
- Other types of blepharitis:
  - Ulcerative blepharitis: More severe blepharitis with small marginal ulceration and destruction of the hair follicles
  - Contact dermatitis/blepharitis:
    - Develops from type IV hypersensitivity; common causes include ocular medications, topical anesthetics, antivirals, and cosmetics.
    - May occur with secondary *Staphylococcus* infection.
  - Eczematoid blepharitis:
    - Caused by hypersensitivity reaction to exotoxins and antigens from local flora
    - Strong association with eczema, asthma
    - Staphylococcal infection common
  - Angular blepharitis: Often caused by *Staphylococcus* or *Moraxella* infection.

COMMONLY ASSOCIATED CONDITIONS

See Risk Factors and Differential Diagnosis.

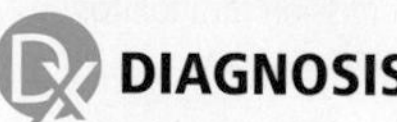

DIAGNOSIS

HISTORY

- Duration of symptoms
- Unilateral or bilateral presentation
- Note any exacerbating conditions (e.g., smoke, allergens, wind, contact lenses, etc.).
- Symptoms related to systemic diseases
- Current and recent medication use
- Recent exposure to infected individuals
- Frequently reported in all types of blepharitis:
  - Burning
  - Itching
  - Eyelid erythema
  - Conjunctival infection (red eyes)
  - Lacrimation, tearing
  - Tear deficiency
  - Foreign-body sensation
  - Photophobia (light sensitivity)
  - Impaired vision

PHYSICAL EXAM

- Test of visual acuity
- External exam (skin and eyelids):
  - Staphylococcal:
    - Recurrent stye (external or internal hordeolum)
    - Missing, broken, or misdirected eyelashes (trichiasis)
    - Eyelid deposits: Matted, hard scales; collarettes (ringlike formation around the lash shaft)
    - Ulcerations at base of eyelashes (rare)
    - Eyelid scarring may occur
  - Seborrheic blepharitis:
    - Eyelid deposits: Dry flakes, oily or greasy secretions on lid margins and/or lashes
    - Associated dandruff of scalp, eyebrows
  - Meibomian gland dysfunction:
    - Eyelash misdirection may occur with long-standing disease
    - Eyelid deposits: Fatty deposits; may be foamy
    - Eyelid margin thickening
    - Plugged meibomian gland orifices
    - Chalazion (sometimes multiple)
    - Eyelid scarring with long-term disease
  - Mixed blepharitis: Signs and symptoms of >1 type of blepharitis may be present.

DIAGNOSTIC TESTS & INTERPRETATION

Lab

Follow-Up & Special Considerations

- Cultures in atypical blepharitis
- Biopsy in atypical cases for carcinoma

Imaging

Initial approach

Slit-lamp biomicroscopy:

- Examine tear film, eyelid margins, eyelashes, tarsal and bulbar conjunctivae, and cornea.
- Reveals loss of lashes (madarosis), whitening of the lashes (poliosis), trichiasis, crusting, eyelid margin ulcers, and lid irregularities

DIFFERENTIAL DIAGNOSIS

Masquerade syndrome:

- Persistent inflammation and thickening of eyelid margin may indicate squamous cell, basal cell, or sebaceous cell carcinoma masquerading as blepharitis. These carcinomas also may mimic styes or chalazia.
- Sebaceous carcinoma of the eyelid has a 22% fatality rate. Up to 1/2 of these potentially fatal sebaceous cell carcinomas may resemble benign inflammatory diseases, particularly chalazia and chronic blepharoconjunctivitis.
- Consider this in all cases of recurrent, persistent, or atypical chalazion; chronic unilateral unresponsive blepharoconjunctivitis; diffuse or nodular tumors of the eyelid; orbital mass developing after removal of an eyelid or caruncular tumor; and any tumor developing in a person with a history of ocular radiotherapy (1)[C].

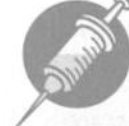

TREATMENT

MEDICATION

First Line

- Topical treatment to lid, if *Staphylococcus* likely: Bacitracin 500 μg/g or (2nd choice) erythromycin 0.5% ophthalmic ointment:
  - Apply with a cotton-tipped applicator.
  - The frequency and duration of treatment are guided by the severity (2)[C].
- Topical corticosteroids (short term) may be useful for eyelid or ocular surface inflammation. The minimum effective dose should be used; long-term use should be avoided if possible (2,3)[C].
- For patients with meibomian gland dysfunction inadequately controlled with eyelid hygiene, consider doxycycline 100 mg/d or tetracycline 1,000 mg/d in divided doses, tapered after clinical improvement (2–4 weeks) to doxycycline 50 mg/d or tetracycline 250–500 mg/d (2)[C].
- Since aqueous tear deficiency is common in blepharitis, use twice-daily artificial tears in addition to eyelid hygiene and medications.

:ontraindications: Allergy to medication; etracyclines are not for use in pregnancy, nursing vomen, or children <8 years of age.
'recautions: Tetracyclines may cause hotosensitivity; sunscreen is recommended.
:orticosteroids may increase intraocular pressure nd risk of cataract.

cond Line

'opical fluoroquinolones (e.g., gatifloxacin 0.3%, evofloxacin 0.5%, or moxifloxacin 0.5%) may be elpful for persistent or recurrent staphylococcal lepharitis or for those patients who prefer a olution.
eborrheic blepharitis may respond to antifungal gents such as a short course of itraconazole (4)[C].

DDITIONAL TREATMENT

eneral Measures

'romote proper eyelid hygiene (2)[C]:
- Apply warm compresses for several minutes once daily to soften adherent encrustations.
- The eyelid margins then are scrubbed gently with eyelid cleanser or diluted baby shampoo twice a day to remove adherent material and clean the meibomian gland orifices (5)[C].

3rief, gentle massage of the eyelids can help to express meibomian secretions in patients with neibomian gland dysfunction (2)[C].
)iscontinue soft contact lenses use during an acute case of blephartis.

sues for Referral

ronic recurrent blepharitis requires referral to an hthalmologist for evaluation as to whether patient ould continue soft lens use.

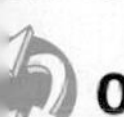

ONGOING CARE

)LLOW-UP RECOMMENDATIONS

tient Monitoring

Patients should schedule a return visit if their condition worsens despite treatment.
Return visit intervals for patients with severe disease vary.
If corticosteroid is prescribed, reevaluate within a few weeks to measure intraocular pressure and determine response to therapy.

PATIENT EDUCATION

- "Blepharitis Fact Sheet" from the American Academy of Ophthalmology
- Advise patient that blepharitis is a chronic condition, prone to recurrence if eyelid hygiene is not maintained after antibiotic treatment is discontinued.

PROGNOSIS

- Symptoms frequently can be improved but rarely are eliminated.
- Long-term eyelid hygiene is required for control.

COMPLICATIONS

- Stye and chalazion
- Scarring of eyelid margin
- Corneal infection

REFERENCES

1. Tsai T, O'Brien JM. Masquerade syndromes: malignancies mimicking inflammation in the eye. *Int Ophthalmol Clin*. 2002;41:115–31.
2. American Academy of Ophthalmology Cornea/External Disease Panel, Preferred Practice Patterns Committee. Preferred Practice Pattern: *Blepharitis*. San Francisco: AAO. 2003.
3. Abelson MB, et al. Blepharitis Hiding in plain sight. *Rev Ophthalmol*. May 15, 2004.
4. Ninomiya J, Nakabayashi A, Higuchi R, et al. A case of seborrheic blepharitis; treatment with itraconazole. *Nippon Ishinkin Gakkai Zasshi*. 2002;43:189–91.
5. McCulley JP, Shine WE. Changing concepts in the diagnosis and management of blepharitis. *Cornea*. 2000;19:650–8.

ADDITIONAL READING

- Lemp MA. Contact lenses and associated anterior segment disorders: dry eye, blepharitis, and allergy. *Ophthalmol Clin North Am*. 2003;16:463–9.
- McCulley JP, Shine WE. Eyelid disorders: the meibomian gland, blepharitis, and contact lenses. *Eye Contact Lens*. 2003;29:S93–5; discussion S115–8, S192–4.

See Also (Topic, Algorithm, Electronic Media Element)

Conjunctivitis, Acute; Dry Eye Syndrome (Keratoconjunctivitis Sicca)

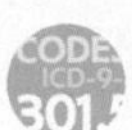

CODES

ICD9

373.00 Blepharitis, unspecified

CLINICAL PEARLS

- Blepharitis is often a chronic condition; symptoms frequently can be improved but rarely are eliminated.
- Promote proper eyelid hygiene.
- Bacitracin ophthalmic ointment is the 1st-line treatment if *Staphylococcus* is suspected.

BODY DYSMORPHIC DISORDER

Dawn S. Tasillo, MD

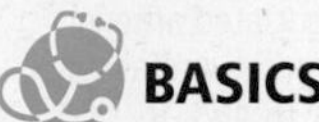

BASICS

DESCRIPTION

Body dysmorphic disorder (BDD) is a dysmorphic disorder in which patients have a pervasive subjective feeling of ugliness of some aspect of their appearance despite a normal or near-normal appearance:
- Diagnostic criteria according to the *DSM-IV*:
  - Preoccupation with an imagined defect in appearance. If there is a minor physical anomaly, the concern is excessive.
  - The preoccupation causes clinically significant distress or impairment in social, occupational, or other important areas of function.
  - The preoccupation is not accounted for by another mental disorder.

EPIDEMIOLOGY

- High comorbidity with depressive disorders
- Usually begins during adolescence, with a common average age of onset between 15 and 30 years
- Women are affected somewhat more often than men.
- Affected patients are likely to be unmarried.
- Different cultural beliefs may influence or amplify preoccupations:
  - Adolescents usually present similar to adults.
  - Can present in childhood, often with refusing to attend school or planning suicide
- Onset can be gradual or abrupt.
- Often a delay in diagnosis until 10–15 years after the onset

Prevalence

- <1% in general population
- More common in women than men
- 5–40% in individuals with anxiety or depressive disorders
- 6–15% in cosmetic surgery patients and in dermatologic clinics

RISK FACTORS

- Genetic predisposition
- Shyness, perfectionism, or anxious temperament
- Childhood adversity:
  - Teasing or bullying
  - Poor peer relationships
  - Social isolation
  - Lack of support of family
  - Sexual abuse
- History of dermatologic or other physical stigmata
- Being more aesthetically sensitive than average
- Low self-esteem

PATHOPHYSIOLOGY

- Not well understood
- A cognitive behavioral model has been described in which an external representation of the person's appearance (i.e., a photograph or mirror reflection) creates a distorted mental image. Through selective attention, awareness of the image and its specific features is increased. The affected individual becomes preoccupied by the distorted image; this is maintained by various safety and submissive behaviors meant to decrease scrutiny by others, but which may increase the individual's abnormal self-image and thus reinforces the behavior.
- Magnetic resonance imaging studies note left cerebral hemisphere hyperactivity, which may imply abnormal visual information processing, leading to selective recall of details and perception of distortions that do not exist (1).

ETIOLOGY

Not known, but likely multifactorial involving genetic, biological, and environmental factors

COMMONLY ASSOCIATED CONDITIONS

- Depression
- Social phobia
- Bipolar disorder
- Eating disorders
- Obsessive-compulsive disorder
- Suicide (up to 25%)
- Delusional disorder (27–39%)

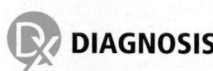

DIAGNOSIS

HISTORY

- Determine and validate the patient's concern.
- Determine the severity of the disorder.
- Quantify the amount of time spent worrying about the "distorted" appearance.
- Determine what is done to hide or eliminate the problem.
- Determine the degree to which the defect affects school, job, or social life.
- Rule out other psychiatric disorders.
- Signs and symptoms may include:
  - Preoccupation that $\geq$1 features are unattractive, ugly, or deformed
  - Can involve any part of the body, but usually involves the skin, hair, or facial features:
    - Women are more likely to be preoccupied with their weight, hips, legs, and breasts.
    - Men are more likely to be preoccupied with their height, body hair, body build, and genitals.
- Nature of the preoccupation can change with time
- Have little insight
- Tend to display delusions of reference
- Large amounts of time are consumed by behavior to examine the perceived defect repeatedly, disgu[ise] it, or improve it:
  - Mirror gazing
  - Excessive grooming
  - Camouflaging the "defect"
  - Skin picking
  - Reassurance seeking
  - Dieting
  - Pursuing dermatologic treatment or cosmetic surgery
- Tend to avoid social interactions
- Trouble staying in school, maintaining a job, or maintaining significant relationships:
  - Tend to be unhappy with results of dermatologi[c] and cosmetic procedures

PHYSICAL EXAM

- Important to do a mental status examination:
  - Look for:
    - Depression
    - Suicidal ideation
    - Anxiety
  - Rule out organic factors by reviewing:
    - Orientation
    - Memory
    - Ability to concentrate
- Rule out actual physical pathology.

DIAGNOSTIC TESTS & INTERPRETATION

- Several modules have been developed to assist wi[th] the diagnosis and severity rating of BDD (1).
- Administered by a trained clinician, these include:
  - The BDD Examination
  - Yale Brown Obsessive–Compulsive Scale modifi[ed] for BDD

DIFFERENTIAL DIAGNOSIS

- Normal concerns about appearance
- Eating disorders: BDD differs from an eating disorc[der] in that an eating disorder involves a preoccupation with overall body shape and weight, and with BDD the preoccupation is with only a specific body part
- Obsessive–compulsive disorder (OCD): While BDD may be a version of OCD, the diagnosis differs in that in OCD, the obsessions and compulsions are not just restricted to appearance, as they are in BD[D]
- Gender identity disorder
- Major depressive episode
- Narcissistic personality disorder
- Avoidant personality disorder
- Social phobia
- Schizophrenia
- Trichotillomania
- Hypochondriasis
- Delusional disorder, somatic type
- Koro: A culture-related syndrome seen in Southeas[t] Asia that involves a preoccupation that the genita[ls] (penis, labia, nipples, or breast) are shrinking and disappearing into the abdomen

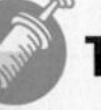

TREATMENT

n any patient with a coexisting mental disorder, such as a depressive or anxiety disorder, the coexisting disorder should be treated with the appropriate psychotherapy or pharmacotherapy.

Cognitive behavior therapy has been shown to be very effective (2,3)[A]:
- Behavioral experiments
- Graded exposure tasks
- Imagery rescripting
- Cognitive restructuring
- Reverse role-playing
- Relaxation

Support groups

Psychotherapy may be effective.

Therapy with and for family members, spouses, or significant others

EDICATION

Results from the small number of available randomized controlled trials suggest that selective serotonin reuptake inhibitors (SSRIs) may be useful in treating patients with BDD (2)[A].

SSRIs are currently considered the medication of choice for BDD (4).

rst Line

RI:

Not an approved use by the FDA

Patients with and without a delusional disorder did equally well with an SSRI.

Maximum tolerated dose should be taken for at least 12–16 weeks

Dosages may need to be higher than typically recommended for an eating disorder.

econd Line

dd a low-dose antipsychotic drug to an SSRI if there failure to respond to >2 SSRIs.

DDITIONAL TREATMENT

sues for Referral

Referral to a psychiatrist for diagnosis and therapy can be helpful and necessary for difficult cases.

Regular counseling

URGERY/OTHER PROCEDURES

Studies investigating the rate of BDD among persons who seek appearance-enhancing treatments suggest that approximately 5–15% of individuals who seek these treatments suffer from BDD (5).

Retrospective reports suggest that persons with BDD rarely experience improvement in their symptoms following these treatments, leading some to suggest that BDD is a contraindication to cosmetic surgery and other treatments.

ONGOING CARE

FOLLOW-UP RECOMMENDATIONS

Patient Monitoring

Many patients have substantial improvement in core BDD symptoms, psychosocial functioning, quality of life, suicidality, and other aspects of BDD when treated with appropriate pharmacotherapy that targets BDD symptoms (4).

PATIENT EDUCATION

- Phillips KA. *The Broken Mirror: Understanding and Treating Body Dysmorphic Disorder*. Revised and expanded. New York: Oxford University Press, 2005.
- Butler Hospital's Body Dysmorphic Disorder and Body Image Program at http://www.butler.org/body.cfm?id=123

PROGNOSIS

- Continuous course with periods of waxing and waning in the intensity of symptoms
- The longer the duration and the more severe the symptoms, the less the chance of partial or full remission.

COMPLICATIONS

- Repeated surgical or dermatologic procedures
- Inability or limited ability to function in society
- Comorbid conditions
- Poor social relations
- Poor self-esteem
- Suicide

REFERENCES

1. Feusner et al. Abnormalities of visual processing and frontostriatal systems in body dysmorphic disorder. *Arch Gen Psychiatry*. 2010;67(2):197–205.
2. Ipser JC, Sander C, Stein DJ. Pharmacotherapy and psychotherapy for body dysmorphic disorder. *Cochrane Database Syst Rev*. 2009;CD005332.
3. Buhlmann U, Reese HE, Renaud S, et al. Clinical considerations for the treatment of body dysmorphic disorder with cognitive-behavioral therapy. *Body Image*. 2008.
4. Phillips KA, Hollander E. Treating body dysmorphic disorder with medication: evidence, misconceptions, and a suggested approach. *Body Image*. 2008.
5. Sarwer DB, Crerand CE. Body dysmorphic disorder and appearance enhancing medical treatments. *Body Image*. 2008.
6. Albertini RS, Philips KA. Thirty-three cases of body dysmorphic disorder in children and adolescents. *J Am Acad Child Psy*. 1999;38:453–9.

ADDITIONAL READING

- *American Psychiatric Association: Diagnostic and Statistical Manual of Mental Disorders*, Fourth Edition, *Text Revision*. Washington, DC: American Psychiatric Association. 2000:507–10.
- Philips KA, et al. Predictors of remission from body dysmorphic disorder: a prospective study. *J Ner Ment Dis*. 2005;193:564–7.
- Phillips KA. *The Broken Mirror: Understanding and Treating Body Dysmorphic Disorder. Revised and expanded*. New York: Oxford University Press, 2005.
- Phillips KA. The presentation of body dysmorphic disorder in medical settings. *Prim Psychiatry*. 2006;13:51–9.
- Rief W, Buhlmann U, Wilhelm S, et al. The prevalence of body dysmorphic disorder: a population-based survey. *Psychol Med*. 2006;36:877–85.
- Sadock BJ, Sadock VA. *Kaplan & Sadock's Synopsis of Psychiatry*, 9th ed. Philadelphia: Lippincott Williams & Wilkins. 2003:653–5.
- Slaughter JR, Sun AM. In pursuit of perfection: a primary care physician's guide to body dysmorphic disorder. *Am Fam Physician*. 1999;60:1738–42.

CODES

ICD9

300.7 Hypochondriasis

CLINICAL PEARLS

- An eating disorder involves a preoccupation with overall body shape and weight, while in body dysmorphic disorder, the preoccupation is with only a specific body part (6).
- In obsessive-compulsive disorder, the obsessions and compulsions are not just restricted to appearance, as in body dysmorphic disorder.
- If the patient insists she has a physical defect and wants it surgically corrected but you don't appreciate a physical defect, after validating the patient's concerns, refer to a psychiatrist for further evaluation before performing the procedure. Most patients with body dysmorphic disorder are not content after the procedure, and their concerns persist.

BONE TUMOR, PRIMARY MALIGNANT

Nathan P. Falk, MD
Ashley Falk, MD

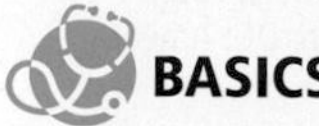

BASICS

DESCRIPTION
- Primary malignant bone tumors are rare.
- Osteogenic sarcomas arise from mesenchymal cells capable of differentiating into bone, cartilage, or fibrous tissue. Three histologic types:
  – Osteosarcoma: Characterized by the production of osteoid or immature bone by the malignant cells; has multiple subtypes
  – Chondrosarcoma: Cellular cartilaginous tumor with abundant binucleate cells, myxoid areas, pushing borders; lacks osteoid
  – Fibrosarcoma: Spindle cells and collagen; no osteoid
- Ewing sarcoma: Small, round blue-cell neoplasm
- Malignant fibrous histiocytoma (MFH): Pleomorphic sarcoma of storiform (starlike) pattern without differentiation; 10-year survival 20% for high grade, 90% for low grade
- Giant cell tumor of bone: Has both benign (90%) and malignant forms; often recurs
- Chordoma: Develops from remnants of primitive notochord at base of skull or sacrum; rare; slowly progressive; recurrent; cure possible

EPIDEMIOLOGY
Incidence
- Rare: 2,380 primary bone tumors diagnosed per year in US; 1,470 deaths (1)
- Osteosarcoma most common; chondrosarcoma, 2nd; Ewing sarcoma, 3rd
- Predominant age:
  – Bone tumors account for 6% of childhood malignancies.
  – Osteosarcoma: Bimodal: Ages 13–16 and >65 years
  – Chondrosarcoma: 3rd–7th decades
  – Fibrosarcoma: 2nd–6th decades
  – Ewing sarcoma: Children and teenagers usually 10–15 years old (70% of Ewing patients <20 years of age)
  – MFH: Adults and elderly
  – Chordoma: >30 years of age
- Predominant gender:
  – For most, Male = Female.
  – Osteosarcoma, Male > Female (1.5:1), and chondrosarcoma, Male > Female (2:1).
- Race:
  – Ewing sarcoma is significantly more common in Caucasian than in African-American children (2).
  – Osteosarcoma is slightly more common in African-American than in Caucasian children.

RISK FACTORS
- Previous irradiation is a risk factor for osteosarcoma and MFH.
- Rapid bone growth, teenage growth spurt
- Fibrous dysplasia

Genetics
- Genetic risk factors include
  – Bone dysplasias:
    ○ Paget disease risk factor for osteosarcoma
    ○ Multiple hereditary exostosis: Chondrosarcoma
    ○ Multiple enchondromatosis (Ollier disease): Chondrosarcoma
    ○ Enchondromatosis and hemangiomatosis (Maffucci syndrome)
  – Germ-line retinoblastoma, especially after radiation: Osteosarcoma
  – Li-Fraumeni syndrome (germ-line *p53* mutation)
  – Rothmund-Thomson syndrome (autosomal recessive association of congenital bone defects, hair and skin dysplasias, hypogonadism, and cataracts)
- Tumor genetics:
  – Ewing sarcoma has chromosomal translocation t(11;22)(q24;q12) in 90% of tumors and resulting EW5-FLI1 fusion protein.
  – Ewing sarcoma breakpoint region *EWSR1* gene encodes a putative ribonucleic acid (RNA)–binding protein.
  – Ewing sarcoma caveolin-1 overexpression is necessary for malignant tumor growth (3).
  – Osteosarcoma shows loss of retinoblastoma and *p53* suppressor genes and amplification of the genes *C-myc*, *mdm-2*, *SAS*, and *cyclin-dependent kinase*.

GENERAL PREVENTION
Irradiation is the only known environmental risk factor.

ETIOLOGY
- Generally unknown
- Malignant fibrous histiocytoma often follows irradiation or arises in old bone infarct.
- Osteosarcoma has association with loss of suppressor retinoblastoma and *p53* genes.
- Chondrosarcoma may arise in preexisting enchondroma or exostosis.

COMMONLY ASSOCIATED CONDITIONS
- Genetic conditions listed previously
- Patients with enchondromatosis more often die of gastrointestinal (GI) malignancies than of metastatic chondrosarcoma.

DIAGNOSIS

HISTORY
- Pain with weight bearing, at rest, and at night; often dull or aching
- Swelling
- Tenderness
- Fracture with minor trauma (pathologic fracture present in 10–15% of cases)
- Minor injury may bring attention to lesion.

PHYSICAL EXAM
- Bone tenderness
- Palpable bony or soft tissue mass
- Rectal exam, if risk for prostate cancer, should be done to exclude prostate nodules.

DIAGNOSTIC TESTS & INTERPRETATIO
Lab
Initial lab tests
- Calcium, phosphate, alkaline phosphatase, lactate dehydrogenase (LDH)
- 50% of osteosarcomas have an elevated alkaline phosphatase.
- Ewing sarcoma may be associated with an elevate erythrocyte sedimentation rate (ESR) and LDH.
- Prostate-specific antigen to exclude prostatic carcinoma
- Thyroid function tests to exclude thyroid carcinom
- Elevated ESR and white blood cells (WBCs) in osteomyelitis
- Serum protein electrophoresis and urine electrophoresis to exclude myeloma

Imaging
Initial approach
- Plain films provide important information regardin the nature of the lesion and guide further testing.
- Classic plain-film findings include "onion skin" for Ewing sarcoma and Codman triangle formation ar soft tissue "sunburst" for osteosarcoma.
- Bone scan is done prior to biopsy to look for other lesions.
- CT scan for cortical destruction and internal calcification or ossification
- MRI determines the extent of marrow involvement and associated soft tissue mass.
- Osteosarcoma: Location of lesion important: Surfa osteosarcomas often may be cured by surgery alor
- Chest radiograph and CT scan for metastatic disea
- Abdominal CT scan, MRI, or renal ultrasound
- Mammogram to exclude breast carcinoma

Diagnostic Procedures/Surgery
- Open biopsy or needle biopsy: Needle biopsies ma not provide enough tissue.
  – Frozen section problematic if calcified
  – Touch prep
  – Permanent section
  – Snap freezing
  – Electron microscopy
  – Cytogenetic and molecular studies
  – DNA indices
  – Immunoperoxidase staining
  – Immunophenotyping to rule out lymphoma
- Biopsy tract should be excised in continuity with th tumor at the time of resection (4).
- Biopsy of associated soft tissue mass may lessen th risk of pathologic fracture.

Pathological Findings
- Histology and special studies in combination with radiographic findings confirm the diagnosis.
- 90% of osteosarcomas are high-grade intramedullary tumors.
- Conventional osteosarcomas have histologic subtypes: Osteoblastic, chondroblastic, or fibroblastic depending on the predominant cellular component, but all are managed similarly.

- Osteosarcoma may express *Her-2/neu*, indicating, if present, a more aggressive tumor, but one that may respond more favorably to trastuzumab (Herceptin).
- Ewing sarcoma expresses MIC-2 protein (CD99).
- Electron microscopy: Glycogen granules in Ewing sarcoma

DIFFERENTIAL DIAGNOSIS

- Metastatic cancer: Breast, prostate, thyroid, lung, kidney
- Hematologic malignancy:
  – Myeloma, especially in patients >40 years of age
  – Lymphoma at any age
- Benign bone tumors: Endochondroma, osteochondroma, nonossifying fibroma, chondroblastoma, osteoid osteoma, osteoblastoma, periosteal chondroma, (benign) giant cell tumor, chondromyxoid fibroma
- Other space-occupying lesions: Aneurysmal bone cyst, unicameral bone cyst, fibrous dysplasia, eosinophilic granuloma
- Infection (osteomyelitis)
- Metabolic bone disease (osteopenia, Paget, hyperparathyroidism)
- Synovial diseases (pigmented villonodular synovitis, synovial chondromatosis, degenerative or inflammatory synovitis)
- Myositis ossificans and repair reaction to trauma
- Avascular necrosis

TREATMENT

MEDICATION

- Neoadjuvant chemotherapy treats micrometastatic disease, allows time for ordering replacement prosthesis and bone graft, and allows in vivo assessment of response to chemotherapy (5,6)[C].
- Osteosarcoma:
  – Standard agents: Doxorubicin, cisplatin, ifosfamide, and methotrexate (MTX)
  – Recurrent disease: High-dose (HD) MTX, doxorubicin, and cisplatin
- Chondrosarcoma is not likely to respond to chemotherapy.
- MFH: Less histologic response to chemotherapy than conventional osteosarcoma; survival similar
- Ewing sarcoma response to induction chemotherapy important prognostic factor:
  – A dramatic decrease in size of Ewing sarcoma usually occurs after initial chemotherapy.
  – Adjuvant chemotherapy improves cure rate dramatically; cure rate is 10–20% with surgery or radiation alone.
  – Standard agents: Vincristine, doxorubicin, and cyclophosphamide, alternating with ifosfamide, etoposide
- Precautions:
  – Left ventricular dysfunction with doxorubicin; cumulative dose >450 mg/m^2 increases risk.
  – With HD MTX, hydration, alkalinization of the urine, and close monitoring of plasma levels are needed.
- Significant adverse effects:
  – Myelosuppression
  – Renal tubular dysfunction with ifosfamide
  – Renal and hepatic dysfunction and GI mucositis with MTX
  – Nephrotoxicity and ototoxicity with cisplatin

SURGERY/OTHER PROCEDURES

- Complete surgical resection with adequate margins is crucial (7)[C].
- Chondrosarcoma in the extremities should be treated exclusively by surgery, unless it is of the mesenchymal or dedifferentiated high-grade variety.
- Ewing sarcoma is radiosensitive; however, surgery with limb salvage is increasingly accepted.
  – Surgery is preferred if lesion is resectable.
  – Despite irradiation, local recurrence is common in up to 25% with pelvic lesions.
  – After neoadjuvant chemotherapy, reassess resectability of lesion; either surgery or irradiation.
  – Nonresectable tumors may be irradiated.
  – Adjuvant radiotherapy is used for Ewing sarcoma only in some circumstances.
- Limb salvage is employed whenever a safe margin can be obtained.
  – Primary goal is eradication of disease.
  – Secondary goal is preservation of function.
- In selected patients, limb salvage does not increase risk of death.
- Limb-sparing surgery may require endoprosthesis or bone graft (allograft or homograft).
- Rotation-plasty is a procedure used when tumor dictates resection of the distal femur.
  – Lower leg is spared and rotated 180 degrees; tibia is fused to femur.
  – Reattached, reversed ankle serves as knee joint. Prosthesis is fitted to (reversed) foot.

ONGOING CARE

FOLLOW-UP RECOMMENDATIONS

Patient Monitoring

- Blood counts for myelosuppression
- Serial electrocardiograms (ECGs) when Adriamycin is being used; granulocyte colony-stimulating factor (G-CSF) is often used to minimize neutropenia.
- Chest radiographs should be obtained every 2 months for the 1st year, every 3 months for the 2nd year, and every 4 months for the 3rd year.
- CT scans of the lungs are repeated every 6 months during the 1st 2 years.
- Ewing sarcoma may recur >5 years after diagnosis.

PATIENT EDUCATION

Refer to local branch of American Cancer Society for information and support groups.

PROGNOSIS

- With amputation alone, 80% of patients with osteosarcoma had pulmonary metastatic disease by 2 years. With chemotherapy, the 5-year disease-free survival rate is 50–85% (8)[C].
- Favorable prognostic factors for MFH and osteosarcoma include responsiveness to chemotherapy, distal portions of the extremities, small size, and age >10 years.
- Most chondrosarcomas are of lower grade and have a low risk of metastatic spread and low incidence of local recurrence after adequate surgery.
- MFH, osteosarcoma, and Ewing sarcoma have an overall 50% survival with combined treatment modalities.

COMPLICATIONS

- For limb salvage with any primary malignant bone tumor, potential complications include leg-length discrepancy, infection, wound dehiscence, skin-coverage problems, and artery and nerve injury.
- Nonunion of bone grafts and mechanical loosening of prosthetic implants
- Local recurrence risk for osteosarcoma with limb salvage is <10%.
- Micrometastatic disease may have occurred by the time of presentation and can appear at any time during the course of treatment or follow-up.
- Thoracotomy and continued chemotherapy are often recommended for metastatic disease to the lung.
- Ewing sarcoma metastatic to the lung is often diffuse and not amenable to resection.

REFERENCES

1. Jemal A, Siegel R, Ward E, et al. Cancer statistics, 2008. *CA Cancer J Clin*. 2008;58:71–96.
2. Heare T, Hensley MA, Dell'Orfano S. Bone tumors: osteosaroma and Ewing's sarcoma. *Current Opinion in Pediatrics*. 2009;21:365–372.
3. Lewis VO. What's new in musculoskeletal oncology. *J Bone Joint Surg Am*. 2007;89:1399–407.
4. Schajowicz F, McGuire MH. Diagnostic difficulties in skeletal pathology. *Clin Orthop Rel Res*. 1991;240:281–310.
5. Longhi A, Pasini E, Bertoni F, et al. Twenty-year follow-up of osteosarcoma of the extremity treated with adjuvant chemotherapy. *J Chemother*. 2004;16:582–8.
6. Mendelsohn J. Jeremiah Metzger Lecture. Targeted cancer therapy. *Trans Amer Clin Climatol Assoc*. 2000;111:95–110.
7. Siegel HJ, Pressey JG. Current concepts on the surgical and medical management of osteosarcoma. *Expert Rev Anticancer Ther*. 2008;8:1257–69.
8. Bruland OS, Høifødt H, Saeter G, et al. Hematogenous micrometastases in osteosarcoma patients. *Clin Cancer Res*. 2005;11:4666–73.

CODES

ICD9

- 170.0 Malignant neoplasm of bones of skull and face, except mandible
- 170.1 Malignant neoplasm of mandible
- 170.9 Malignant neoplasm of bone and articular cartilage, site unspecified

CLINICAL PEARLS

- Osteosarcoma variants, such as parosteal, periosteal, and intraosseous osteosarcoma, are lower-grade lesions with a more favorable prognosis; they often do not require chemotherapy.
- Other variants and postirradiation and post-Paget osteosarcoma metastasize early.

BORDERLINE PERSONALITY DISORDER

Heath A. Grames, PhD
W. Jeff Hinton, PhD

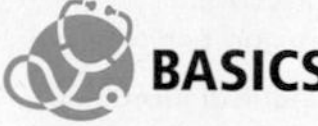

BASICS

DESCRIPTION

Beginning no later than adolescence or early adulthood, borderline personality disorder (BPD) is a consistent and pervasive pattern of an unstable affect and sense of self, impulsivity, and volatile interpersonal relationships (1):

- Common behaviors and variations:
  - Self-mutilation (pinching, scratching, cutting)
  - Suicide (ideation, history of attempts, plans)
  - Splitting (idealizing then devaluing people and relationships)
  - Presentation of helplessness or victimization
  - Emotional pain (may look for physical diagnoses)
  - May be high utilizer of medical services
  - High rate of associated mental disorders (see Associated Conditions)
- Patients with this disorder typically display little insight into their behavior.

Geriatric Considerations

Illness (both acute and chronic) may exacerbate BPD behaviors and may lead to intense feelings of fear and helplessness. Manifestations may decrease with age.

Pediatric Considerations

Diagnosis is rarely made in children. Must first rule out Axis I disorders and behavior related to a general medical condition or to the developmental cycle of the child.

Pregnancy Considerations

Physical and social changes may induce stress or increased fears, resulting in possible escalation of borderline behaviors.

EPIDEMIOLOGY

- Predominant age: Onset no later than adolescence or early adulthood (may go undiagnosed for years)
- Predominant sex: Female > Male

Prevalence

- General population: 2%
- Estimated lifetime prevalence: 10–13%
- 20–30% of patients in primary care outpatient settings have a personality disorder.
- 20% of patients in psychiatry inpatient settings have BPD.

RISK FACTORS

- Biological relatives with the disorder
- Childhood sexual and/or physical abuse and neglect
- Physical illness and external social factors may exacerbate borderline personality behaviors.

Genetics

1st-degree relatives are at greater risk for this disorder (undetermined whether due to genetic or psychosocial factors).

GENERAL PREVENTION

- Tends to be a multigenerational problem
- Children, caregivers, and significant others should have some time and activities away from the borderline individual, which may protect them.

ETIOLOGY

Undetermined, but generally accepted that PDs are due to a combination of the following:

- Hereditary temperamental traits
- Environment (i.e., history of childhood sexual and/or physical abuse, history of childhood neglect, ongoing conflict in home)
- Developmental traits

COMMONLY ASSOCIATED CONDITIONS

Other psychiatric disorders, including:

- Co-occurring PDs, frequent
- Mood disorders, common
- Anxiety disorders, common
- Substance-related disorders, common
- Eating disorders, common
- Post-traumatic stress disorder, common

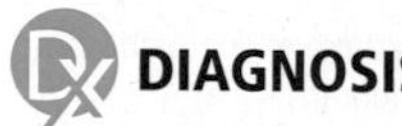

DIAGNOSIS

- The comprehensive evaluation should focus on (2):
  - Comorbid conditions
  - Functional impairments
  - Needs/goals
  - Adaptive/maladaptive coping styles
  - Psychosocial stressors
  - Patient strengths
- Initial assessment should focus on determining treatment setting (2):
  - Establish treatment agreement with patient and outline treatment goals.
  - Assess suicide ideation and self-harm behavior.
  - Assess for psychosis.
  - Hospitalization is necessary if patient presents a threat of harm to self or others.

HISTORY

- Clinic visits for problems that do not have biological findings
- Problems with medical staff members
- Idealizing or unexplained anger at physician
- History of unrealistic expectations of physician (e.g., "I know you can take care of me." "You're the best, unlike my last provider.")
- Obtain collateral information (i.e., from family, partner) about patient behaviors.

PHYSICAL EXAM

Possible scarring from self-mutilation (look on arms and legs where hidden by clothing, but can occur on other parts of the body)

DIAGNOSTIC TESTS & INTERPRETATION

- Consider age of onset. To meet criteria for BPD, borderline pattern will be present from adolescence or early adulthood.
- Formal psychological testing
- Rule out personality change due to a general medical condition (GMC) (1):
  - Traits may emerge due to the effect of a GMC on the central nervous system.
- Rule out symptoms related to chronic substance use.
- If symptoms begin later than early adulthood or are related to trauma (e.g., after a head injury), a GMC, or substance use, then consider other diagnoses.
- Increased diagnostic accuracy may be facilitated by utilizing the Structured Clinical Interview for DSM-IV Axis II disorders (SCID-II) (3).

Diagnostic Procedures/Surgery

Patient must meet at least 5 of the following criteria (1):

- Attempt to avoid abandonment
- Volatile interpersonal relationships
- Identity disturbance
- Impulsive behavior:
  - In ≥2 areas
  - Impulsive behavior is self-damaging.
- Suicidal or self-mutilating behavior
- Mood instability
- Feeling empty
- Is unable to control anger, or finds it difficult
- Paranoid or dissociative when under stress

DIFFERENTIAL DIAGNOSIS

- Mood disorders:
  - Look at baseline behaviors when considering BP vs mood disorder.
  - BPD symptoms increase the likelihood of misdiagnosing bipolar disorder (4).
- Psychotic disorder:
  - With BPD, only occurs under intense stress and i not characteristic of disorder
- Other PD:
  - Consider patient's thoughts, feelings, and behavior to differentiate borderline from other PDs.
  - High co-occurrence of borderline and other PDs
- General medical condition (GMC):
  - Traits may emerge due to the effect of a GMC or the central nervous system.
- Chronic substance abuse

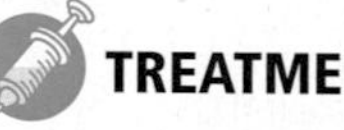

TREATMENT

- Patient may need to be placed on suicide watch.
- Inpatient hospitalization is ineffective in changing Axis II disorder behaviors.
- Inpatient hospital services for conditions related to Axis II disorder should be limited and of short duration to decrease dependence. Hospitalization should be considered for:
  - Adjusting medications
  - Implementing psychotherapy for crisis interventic
  - Stabilizing patient (psychosocial stressors)
- Extended inpatient hospitalization should be considered for the following reasons (2)[C]:
  - Persistent/severe suicidal ideation or risk to othe
  - Nonadherence to outpatient or partial hospitalization treatments
  - Comorbid Axis I disorders that may increase threa to life for the patient (i.e., eating disorders, mooc disorders)
  - Comorbid substance abuse or dependence that is unresponsive to outpatient or partial hospitalization treatments

MEDICATION

- While there are no specific medications approved by the U.S. Food and Drug Administration (FDA) to treat BPD, American Psychiatric Association (APA) guidelines recommend pharmacotherapy to manage symptoms (2)[B].
- Treat symptoms (5)[C].

- Treat Axis I disorders (2)[B].
- Consider high rate of self-harm and suicidal behavior in patients with BPD when prescribing (6)[C].
- Depression/anxiety (7)[A]:
  - SSRIs
- Impulsive, aggressive, or history of bipolar disorder (5)[C]:
  - Mood stabilizer
- Psychosis, paranoid or hostile behavior, debilitating anxiety (5)[C]:
  - Atypical antipsychotic
- APA guideline recommendations (2)[B]:
  - Affective dysregulation: SSRI and monoamine oxidase inhibitors (MAOIs)
  - Impulsive-behavioral control: SSRIs and mood stabilizers
  - Cognitive-perceptual symptoms: Antipsychotics

ADDITIONAL TREATMENT

General Measures

- Focus on patient management rather than on "fixing" behaviors.
- Schedule consistent appointment follow-ups to relieve patient anxiety.
- Meet with and rely on treatment team to avoid splitting of team by patient and to provide opportunity for team to discuss issues with patient.
- Psychotherapy (referral to mental health therapist) is considered treatment of choice (2,8,9)[A].

Issues for Referral

- If hospitalized, probably for suicide risk, mood or anxiety disorders, or substance-related disorders
- Urgency for scheduled follow up depends on community resources (i.e., Do outpatient day programs for suicidal patients exist? What substance abuse programs are available?):
  - With increased risk for self-harm or self-defeating behaviors and low community resources, the patient can/will use increased need for frequent visits.
- Treatment of Axis II disorder should include psychotherapy and/or psychiatry (2)[B].

Additional Therapies

Consider referring patient for specialty mental health behavioral services, including (2,10):

- Dialectic behavioral therapy (DBT)
- Psychoanalytic-oriented day hospital therapy
- Transference-focused psychotherapy

IN-PATIENT CONSIDERATIONS

Hospitalization is necessary if patient presents a threat of harm to self or others.

Initial Stabilization

- Assess suicidal ideation.
- Consider inpatient treatment if crisis intervention is warranted.
- If psychotic, consider antipsychotic medications (5).

Admission Criteria

Refer to inpatient or outpatient psychiatry services if harm to self or others is expressed:

- Call police or admit for inpatient services immediately if patient is psychotic and/or presents risk of harm to self or others.

Nursing

Nurses can be helpful in managing patient and calling the patient as needed (contact with the patient helps relieve patient stress).

Discharge Criteria

- Patient should not present risk of harm to self or others.
- Patient should have safety plan.
- Routine follow-up should be scheduled with psychiatrist, mental health therapist, or primary care provider.

ONGOING CARE

FOLLOW-UP RECOMMENDATIONS

- Schedule routine follow-up with patient (relieves patient anxiety about medical care relationship with physician).
- Focus primarily on medical conditions and comorbid Axis I disorders.
- Exercise to decrease stress
- Find time to relax: Remove self from daily problems (teaches self-management).

Patient Monitoring

Monitor for suicidal or other self-harm behaviors.

PATIENT EDUCATION

As appropriate, provide patient education about the disorder, treatment, and self-care (2).

PROGNOSIS

- Borderline behaviors may decrease with age (1) and over time (9).
- Treatment is complex and takes time.
- Medical focus is on patient management and caring for medical and Axis I disorders (11).

REFERENCES

1. American Psychiatric Association. *Diagnostic and Statistical Manual of Mental Disorders*. 4th ed. Washington, DC: American Psychiatric Association; 1994.
2. American Psychiatric Association: *Practice guideline for the treatment of patients with borderline personality disorder*. Arlington, VA: American Psychiatric Association, 2001.
3. First MB, Gibbon M, Spitzer RL, Williams JBW, Benjamin LS. *Structured Clinical Interview for DSM-IV Axis II Personality Disorders, (SCID-II)*. Washington, D.C.: American Psychiatric Press, Inc., 1997.
4. Ruggero CJ, Zimmerman M, Chelminski I, Young D. Borderline personality disorder and the misdiagnosis of bipolar disorder. *Journal of Psychiatric Research*. 2010;44:405–408.
5. Ward RK. Assessment and management of personality disorders. *Am Fam Phys*. 2004;70:1505–12.
6. Makela EH, Moeller KE, Fullen JE, et al. Medication utilization patterns and methods of suicidality in borderline personality disorder. *Ann Pharmacother*. 2006;40:49–52.
7. Binks CA, Fenton M, McCarthy L, et al. Pharmacological interventions for people with borderline personality disorder. *Cochrane Database Syst Rev*. 2006;1. Art. No.: CD005653. DOI:10.1002/14651858.CD005653.
8. Kraus G, Reynolds DJ. The "A-B-C's" of the cluster B's: identifying, understanding, and treating cluster B personality disorders. *Clin Psychol Rev*. 2001;21:345–73.
9. Oldham JA. *Guideline watch: practice guideline for the treatment of patients with borderline personality disorder*. Arlington, VA: American Psychiatric Association, 2005.
10. Binks CA, Fenton M, McCarthy L, et al. Psychological therapies for people with borderline personality disorder. *Cochrane Database Syst Rev*. 2006;1. Art. No.: CD005652. DOI:10.1002/14651858.CD005652.
11. Koenigsberg HW, Woo-Ming AM, Siever LJ. Pharmacological treatments of personality disorders. In: Nathan PE, Gorman JM, eds. *A Guide to Treatments that Work*. 2nd ed. New York: Oxford University Press, 2002:625–41.

ADDITIONAL READING

- Battle CL, Shea MT, Johnson DM, et al. Childhood maltreatment associated with adult personality disorders: findings from the Collaborative Longitudinal Personality Disorders Study. *J Personal Disord*. 2004;18:193–211.
- Bellino S, Paradiso E, Bogetto F. Efficacy and tolerability of pharmacotherapies for borderline personality disorder. *CNS Drugs*. 2008;22:671–92.

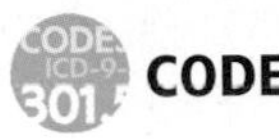

CODES

ICD9

301.83 Borderline personality disorder

CLINICAL PEARLS

- Borderline PD should be viewed as a chronic condition.
- Borderline PD patients are at increased risk for suicide attempts.
- If there are problems with the patient disrespecting the physician or support staff, clear guidelines should be established with the treatment team and then with the patient.
- If you are considering terminating your relationship with the patient, the patient may improve if he or she is warmly confronted about certain behaviors and is given clear guidelines on how to behave in the clinic. As it is the patient's job to follow the guidelines, it is you and your team's job to enforce the guidelines. Finally, designate a case management nurse or well-trained support staff person who can be the primary contact person for the patient.
- Have an agenda when you visit with PD patients. Be cordial—they deserve the same professionalism any patient gets. Help your patient understand that she can have 1 to 2 issues discussed per clinic visit. Frequently scheduled visits can help with this.
- Patients will benefit from regularly scheduled psychotherapy treatment in conjunction with or in addition to regularly scheduled office visits. Psychotherapy can help maximize physician performance by becoming the "home" for mental health treatment, leaving the physician to focus on the patient's immediate physical/medical issues.

BOTULISM

Payal S. Patel, DO

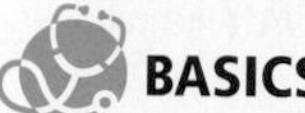

BASICS

DESCRIPTION

- Botulism is a muscle-paralyzing illness caused by a neurotoxin made by the bacterium *Clostridium botulinum*.
- Characterized by acute onset of bilateral cranial nerve involvement (diplopia, difficulty swallowing or speaking) associated with symmetric descending weakness, intact mental state, no fever, and no sensory dysfunction
- 7 types of *C. botulinum* (A–G) are distinguished by their antigenic characteristics. Types A, B, E, and, in rare cases, F, cause disease in humans.
- Forms include:
  - Foodborne: Caused by ingestion of preform toxin
  - Infant botulism: Caused by ingestion of *C. botulinum* that produce toxin in the gastrointestinal (GI) tract
  - Wound: Caused by wound infection with *C. botulinum* that secretes the toxin
  - Aerosolized/inhalational botulinum: Bioterrorism attack potential because of high toxicity; $<1\ \mu g$ is lethal human dose
  - Injection related: Rare
  - Adult colonization botulism: Rare
- System(s) affected: Neuromuscular; Respiratory; GI
- Diagnosis is made through history and clinical exam.
- Laboratory confirmation demonstrates presence of toxin in serum, stool, or wound; or culturing *C. botulinum* from stool, wound, or food
- Treatment should not wait for laboratory confirmation.
- Synonym(s): Sausage poisoning; Kerner disease
- A purified and diluted form of Type A neurotoxin is used to produce Botox injections.

EPIDEMIOLOGY

Incidence

- Average of 110 cases of botulism reported annually in US
- ~20% of cases are foodborne; 30–40% wound-related; 65% infant botulism
- Wound botulism incidence increasing due to IV heroin use and cocaine abuse
- Hidden or intestinal: More common in disorders of the GI tract, such as prior surgery, Crohn disease, or recent antibiotic use
- Inhalation: Only a single incident involving 3 laboratory workers has been described.

Prevalence

- Predominant age:
  - Foodborne: Mean age is 46 years; range of 3–78 years
  - Infantile: Mean age of onset 13 weeks, with range of 1–63 weeks
  - Wound: Median age is 41 years with a range of 23–58 years
- Predominant gender:
  - Foodborne and infantile: Male = Female
  - Wound: Female > Male

RISK FACTORS

- Foodborne: Ingestion of home-canned or prepared contaminated foods
- Infantile: From ingestion of honey or corn syrup; breastfeeding (controversial)
- Wound: IV drug use (black tar heroin; IM/SC) or "skin popping"

GENERAL PREVENTION

- Foodborne: Proper handling, processing, preparation (heating), and storage of food; avoid eating food from bulging cans and food that smells/looks spoiled.
- Infant: Avoid honey before 1 year of age.
- Wound: Proper wound care
- Health care providers: Standard precautions
- If meningitis is suspected in patients with flaccid paralysis, medical personnel should use droplet precautions.
- Heat potentially contaminated food or drink to an internal temperature of 85°C for at least 5 minutes.
- After exposure to *C. botulinum* toxin, clothing and skin should be cleaned with soap and water.
- Contaminated objects or surfaces should be cleaned with 0.1% bleach solution. All food suspected of contamination should be promptly removed from potential consumers.

PATHOPHYSIOLOGY

- Disease results from hematogenous spread of toxin from mucosal surface (stomach, small intestine) or from an infected wound.
- The toxin prevents acetylcholine release at presynaptic membranes, blocking neuromuscular transmission in cholinergic nerve fibers.

ETIOLOGY

- Toxin produced by *C. botulinum*, an encapsulated, anaerobe, gram-positive, spore-forming, rod-shaped bacillus
- Ingestion of *C. botulinum* neurotoxins (A, B, and E most common)
- Foodborne, usually from home-canned vegetables, prepared foods, or foods incubated in anaerobic conditions
- Infantile from ingestion of spores in environment or occasionally in honey
- Wound due to contamination with toxin-producing *C. botulinum*
- Inadvertent: IM injections of botulinum toxin

DIAGNOSIS

HISTORY

- Foodborne:
  - Incubation: Typically 12–36 hours after toxin ingestion. Rare case as late as 10 days after ingestion.
  - Wound and infant botulism: Incubation time cannot be ascertained.
  - Inhalational: Same as foodborne botulism
- Adults: Acute onset of symmetric neuropathies. Difficulty in swallowing or speaking, dry mouth. Diplopia, blurred vision, dilated or nonrelated ptosis (drooping eyelids).
- Symmetric descending, flaccid paralysis in oriented, afebrile patient
- Respiratory dysfunction
- Infant botulism: Disease presentation and severity variable:
  - Constipation, shortly followed by weakness, feeding difficulties, descending or global hypotonia, drooling, anorexia, irritability, and weak cry
- Ask about diet, travel, drug use, and other person with same symptoms.

PHYSICAL EXAM

- General appearance: Oriented, flaccid, may complain of malaise, dizziness, nausea, vomiting
- Vital signs, afebrile (fever may occur in wound botulism due to secondary infection), normal bloo pressure
- Head, eyes, ears, nose, throat: Dry mouth
- Chest/lungs: Respiratory muscle weakness, respiratory dysfunction, paralysis
- Heart: Normal or slow rate
- Abdomen: Distention, constipation (early sign in infant form); may be absent in wound form
- Genitourinary: Urinary retention
- Neurologic:
  - Symmetrical descending weakness beginning wi the cranial nerves
  - Ptosis; extraocular muscle paresis; fixed, dilated pupils; dysphagia
  - Infant botulism: Poor muscle tone (loss of head control and facial expression), poor feeding (loss of suck), drooling, feeding difficulties, weak cry
  - Diminished or absent deep tendon reflexes

DIAGNOSTIC TESTS & INTERPRETATION

Lab

Initial lab tests

- Laboratory confirmation is done by demonstrating the presence of toxin in serum or stool, or by culturing *C. botulinum* from stool, wounds, or food
- Mouse neutralization assay confirmation:
  - Standard method of diagnosis (1)[B]
  - Available from Centers for Disease Control and some state laboratories; takes ~4 days for result
- Routine tests (complete blood count, electrolytes, liver function tests, urinalysis) generally not helpful/show no characteristic abnormalities
- Cerebrospinal fluid testing: Normal helps differentiate from Guillain-Barré syndrome. Occasionally a borderline elevation in protein is seen
- Toxin detected in gastric contents, serum, stool, and suspected food and containers:
  - PCR tests are also available for rapid detection of clostridia in food samples (2)[B].
- A normal Tensilon test helps to differentiate botulism from myasthenia gravis; borderline can occur in botulism

Imaging

CT or MRI to rule out neurologic pathology

Diagnostic Procedures/Surgery

Electrophysiology testing:

- Presumptive evidence in patients with negative bioassay studies (3)[C]
- Brief, small-amplitude motor potential with incremental response on repetitive nerve stimulation

B

IFFERENTIAL DIAGNOSIS

Adult botulisms:
- Guillain-Barré syndrome
- Encephalitis, meningitis
- Tick paralysis
- Myasthenia gravis
- Eaton Lambert myasthenic syndrome
- Cerebrovascular accident: Basilar artery stroke
- Congenital neuropathy or myopathy
- Sepsis
- Hypokalemic periodic paralysis
- Poliomyelitis
- Other poisonings (organophosphate, shellfish, *Amanita* mushrooms, atropine, and aminoglycosides)
- Miller-Fisher variant of Guillain-Barré syndrome
- Diphtheritic neuropathy
- Carbon monoxide intoxication
- Hypermagnesemia

Infant botulism:
- Sepsis
- Meningitis
- Electrolyte–mineral imbalance
- Reye syndrome
- Congenital myopathy
- Leigh disease
- Werdnig-Hoffman disease

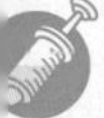

TREATMENT

IEDICATION

irst Line

Antitoxin therapy with trivalent A-B-E antitoxin:
- Call CDC Assistance (770) 488-7100
- Initiating botulinum antitoxin therapy is primarily based on symptoms and physical examination findings that are consistent with botulism (4)[B].
- Early administration is important (4)[B].
- Horse serum derived. Up to 20% reaction incidence. Consider skin testing or pretreatment with steroids or antihistamines.

Infantile:
- Treatment with human botulism immune globulin (BIG-IV or Baby BIG) for botulism types A and B (5)[B]
- Available only through the California State Health Department (510) 540-2646 or (510) 231-7600

Wound:
- Antitoxin therapy with trivalent A-B-E antitoxin, 1 vial IV and 1 vial IM, repeat in 2–4 hours if persistent symptoms
- Antibiotics unproven by clinical trial, but widely used and recommended:
  - Penicillin G (3 million units IV q4h in adults)
  - Metronidazole (500 mg IV q8h) for penicillin-allergic patients
- Vaccine: Pentavalent vaccine available:
  - Efficiency in terrorist attack is unknown
  - Newer vaccines being developed

Second Line

Supportive care, including mechanical ventilation (6)[C]

Pregnancy Considerations

Safety of botulism antitoxin during pregnancy and breastfeeding unknown or controversial (6)

ADDITIONAL TREATMENT

Issues for Referral

- Nutrition: For hyperalimentation and later, tube feeding
- Physical/occupational therapy: Including swallow evaluation

Additional Therapies

- Stress ulcer and deep vein thrombosis prophylaxis
- Pulmonary and physical rehabilitation

SURGERY/OTHER PROCEDURES

Wound excision/debridement

IN-PATIENT CONSIDERATIONS

Initial Stabilization

Hospital admission with meticulous airway management

Admission Criteria

All suspected cases must be admitted.

IV Fluids

Keep patient well hydrated.

Nursing

- Prevent decubitus ulcer, IV line infections, other nosocomial infections
- Before administration of antitoxin, skin testing should be performed for sensitivity.

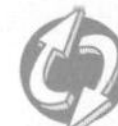

ONGOING CARE

FOLLOW-UP RECOMMENDATIONS

Outpatient follow-up with physical/occupational therapy, nutrition specialist, and psychiatry as needed

Patient Monitoring

- Pulmonary function testing
- Cardiorespiratory monitoring

DIET

Nasogastric feedings, if needed

PATIENT EDUCATION

- Spores destroyed by pressure cooking at 250°F (120°C) for 30 minutes
- Toxin destroyed by boiling for 10 minutes or cooking at 175°F (80°C) for 30 minutes
- Avoid honey in 1st year of life.
- Avoid IV drug use.
- Do not eat/sample foods that look and smell rotten or come from bulging cans.

PROGNOSIS

- Delay in administering antitoxin: Most important factor affecting clinical course and outcome (4)[B]
- Mortality: Overall 7–10%; <5% if infection is treated, but approaches 60% if untreated (6)
- Mortality for patients >60 years is twice that of younger patients
- Full recovery may take months.
- Significant health, functional, and social limitations several years after infection (7)[C]:
  - Recovery follows the regeneration of new neuromuscular connections.
  - 2–8 weeks of ventilator support may be required in more severe cases.
- Dyspnea with severe ptosis and pupil abnormality has been shown to correlate with severe illness and respiratory failure (8)[C].
- Increased incubation time has been shown to correlate with better outcomes (8)[C].

COMPLICATIONS

- Nosocomial infections, including aspiration pneumonia and ventilator-associated pneumonia
- Hypoxic tissue damage
- Death

REFERENCES

1. Lindström M, Korkeala H. Laboratory diagnostics of botulism. *Clin Microbiol Rev*. 2006;19:298–314.
2. Fach P, Micheau P, Mazuet C, et al. Development of real-time PCR tests for detecting botulinum neurotoxins A, B, E, F producing Clostridium botulinum, Clostridium baratii and Clostridium butyricum. *J Appl Microbiol*. 2009;107:465–73.
3. Bayrak A, et al. Electrophysiologic findings in a case of severe botulism. *J Neurol Sci*. 2006;23:49–53.
4. Dembek ZF, Smith LA, Rusnak JM. Botulism: cause, effects, diagnosis, clinical and laboratory identification, and treatment modalities. *Disaster Med Public Health Prep*. 2007;1:122–34.
5. Arnon SS, Schechter R, Maslanka SE, et al. Human botulism immune globulin for the treatment of infant botulism. *N Engl J Med*. 2006;354:462–71.
6. O'Brien KK, Higdon ML, Halverson JJ. Recognition and management of bioterrorism infections. *Am Fam Physician*. 2003;67:1927–34.
7. Gottlieb SL, Kretsinger K, Tarkhashvili N, et al. Long-term outcomes of 217 botulism cases in the Republic of Georgia. *Clin Infect Dis*. 2007;45: 174–80.
8. Witoonpanich R, Vichayanrat E, Tantisiriwit K, et al. Survival analysis for respiratory failure in patients with food-borne botulism. *Clin Toxicol (Phila)*. 2010;48:177–83.
9. Botulism Facts for Healthcare Providers. Accessed 5/30/2010 at http://emergency.cdc.gov/agent/botulism/hcpfacts.asp.

See Also (Topic, Algorithm, Electronic Media Element)

Food Poisoning, Bacterial

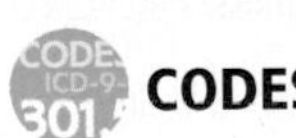

CODES

ICD9

- 005.1 Botulism food poisoning
- 040.42 Wound botulism

CLINICAL PEARLS

- Botulinum antitoxin should be administered as soon as possible; don't wait for lab results.
- Medical care providers who suspect botulism in a patient should immediately call their state health department's emergency 24-hour telephone number.
- A helpful mnemonic to recall progression of symptoms is the "dozen D's": Dry mouth, diplopia, dilated pupils, droopy eyes, droopy face, diminished gag reflex, dysphagia, dysarthria, dysphonia, difficulty lifting head, descending paralysis, and diaphragmatic paralysis (9)

BRAIN ABSCESS

Nathan Weldon, MD

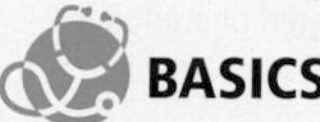

BASICS

DESCRIPTION
- Single or multiple abscesses within the brain, usually occurring secondary to a focus of infection outside the central nervous system
- May mimic brain tumor, but generally evolves more rapidly (over days to weeks)
- Starts as a cerebritis, becomes necrotic, and subsequently becomes encapsulated
- Synonym(s): Cerebral abscess

Geriatric Considerations
Age does not affect outcome as much as the abscess size and state of neurologic dysfunction at presentation.

Pediatric Considerations
- About 1/3 of the cases in pediatric age group
- Rarely found in infants <1 year of age
- Cyanotic congenital heart disease frequently associated

EPIDEMIOLOGY
- Predominant age: Median age 30–40 years, although brain abscess occurs at all ages
- Predominant sex: Male > Female (2:1)

Incidence
Infrequent, but increasing due to increase in immune-suppressed individuals, opportunistic pathogens, and resistance to antibiotics (1)

RISK FACTORS
- HIV/AIDS
- Immunocompromised state
- IV drug abuse

Genetics
No known genetic pattern

GENERAL PREVENTION
- Adequate treatment of otitis media, mastoiditis, sinusitis, dental abscess, other ear/nose/throat (ENT) infections
- Prophylactic antibiotics after compound skull fracture or penetrating head wound

ETIOLOGY
- Hematogenous source is most common overall for single or multiple cerebral abscesses.
- Direct extension from otitis, mastoiditis, sinusitis, or dental infection
- Cranial osteomyelitis
- Penetrating skull trauma
- Prior craniotomy
- Bacteremia from lung abscess, pneumonia
- Bacterial endocarditis
- Fungal infection of the nasopharynx
- *Toxoplasma gondii* (in AIDS patients)
- Cyanotic congenital heart disease
- IV drug use
- No source found in 20%.
- Most common infective organisms: Streptococci, staphylococci (especially after neurosurgery), enteric gram-negative bacilli and anaerobes (usually same as source of infection), *Nocardia*
- Brain abscess associated with HIV infection is assumed to be due to *T. gondii*.
- The frontal lobe of the brain is the most common site for an abscess.

COMMONLY ASSOCIATED CONDITIONS
- AIDS
- Congenital heart disease

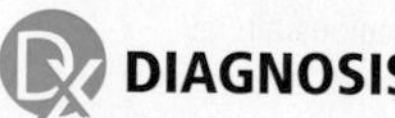

DIAGNOSIS

HISTORY
- Recent onset of headache becoming severe
- New focal neurological deficit
- Altered mental status progressing to stupor and coma
- Nausea and vomiting
- Seizures

PHYSICAL EXAM
- Afebrile or low-grade fever
- Papilledema
- Neck stiffness
- Focal neurologic signs depending on location

DIAGNOSTIC TESTS & INTERPRETATION
Abscess culture: Predominant organisms include *Toxoplasma* (AIDS), *Staphylococcus* (trauma), aerobic or anaerobic bacteria, fungi (rare).

ALERT
- Lumbar puncture often contraindicated
- Prior administration of antibiotics may alter lab results.

Lab
Initial lab tests
- White blood cell (WBC) count may be normal or mildly elevated.
- Blood studies: Mild PMN leukocytosis; elevated erythrocyte sedimentation rate (ESR)
- Culture and susceptibilities of the abscess material

Imaging
- Search for primary source of infection, depending on suspected source.
- Solitary intracerebral abscess suggests a direct contiguous source such as sinus or ear infection.
- Multiple cerebral abscesses suggest hematological spread.
- Head computed tomography (CT) and magnetic resonance imaging (MRI) are the diagnostic methods of choice. Specific findings are dependent on stages of the abscess (2)[B].
- CT provides sufficient diagnostic information in most cases (3)[B], including skull fracture, sinus infection, or otic source.
- Consider cardiac echo, chest x-ray, and chest CT if cardiac or pulmonary source suspected
- Radionuclide ^{117}In-labeled leukocytes may distinguish abscess from neoplasm.

Diagnostic Procedures/Surgery
- Lumbar puncture often contraindicated
- Surgical burr hole with aspiration to make a specif[ic] bacteriologic diagnosis

Pathological Findings
- Suppuration, liquefaction, or encapsulation, depending on stage of evolution
- Fibrosis

DIFFERENTIAL DIAGNOSIS
- Brain tumors
- Cysticercosis
- Stroke
- Resolving intracranial hemorrhage
- Subdural empyema
- Extradural abscess
- Encephalitis

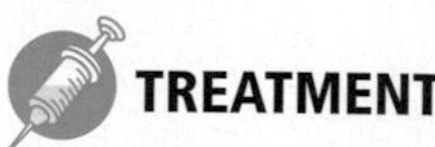

TREATMENT

Immediate neurosurgical consult is indicated for suspected CNS abscess.

MEDICATION
- Antibiotics according to organism and sensitivities, [if] known
- Initial empiric treatment according to suspected source
- Hematogenous sources should cover MRSA initially and should include vancomycin, and may be broadened to include metronidazole and a 3rd-generation cephalosporin.
- For dental source, penicillin G and metronidazole ar[e] reasonable initial choices.
- For otogenic or sinus source, coverage should include metronidazole and either ceftriaxone or cefotaxime.
- For gastrointestinal or genitourinary source, conside[r] a 3rd-generation cephalosporin such as cefotaxime to cover gram negatives.
- For traumatic source, consider vancomycin plus either ceftriaxone or cefotaxime.
- Hospital-acquired sources, including postsurgical abscess, consider vancomycin and cefepime or ceftazidime
- If MSSA is isolated, change vancomycin to oxacillin or nafcillin.
- Use vancomycin in penicillin-sensitive patients.
- Generally a 6–8-week course of parenteral antibiotics is required.
- If brain abscess associated with HIV/AIDS:
  - Daily doses of sulfadiazine and pyrimethamine
  - Lifelong therapy in AIDS patients
- Anticonvulsants:
  - Phenytoin until abscess resolves or perhaps longe[r]
  - Monitor anticonvulsant levels.
- Following a neurosurgical procedure, use corticosteroids such as dexamethasone to reduce edema. Taper rapidly. Use is usually limited to 1 week.
- Contraindications: Sensitivity or allergy to any prescribed medications

recautions:
- Sulfadiazine is poorly water-soluble. Patients must maintain adequate hydration or risk developing crystalluria.
- Decrease dosage of penicillin in patients with renal dysfunction.
- Monitor serum levels of anticonvulsants.
- A dose of pyrimethamine is required for the treatment of toxoplasmosis, which may approach toxic levels. The patient should be observed for folic acid deficiency and treated with folinic acid (leucovorin) 5–15 mg (p.o., IM, IV) if necessary.

ignificant possible interactions: Refer to the nanufacturer's literature.

DDITIONAL TREATMENT

eneral Measures

Palliative and supportive

Treatment of brain abscess requires a combination of antimicrobial agents, surgical intervention, and eradication of the primary foci of infection (4)[A].

nitial medical therapy includes broad-spectrum antibiotics pending determination of the causative organism.

Determination of point of entry and source of nfection is critical to effective treatment (5).

Medical therapy only may be indicated:
- For surgically inaccessible lesions or multiple abscesses
- For abscesses in early cerebritis stage
- For small (<2.5 cm) abscesses

Antibiotic therapy may be directed toward most ikely organism if no specific organism is identified.

Monitor clinical response to antibiotic therapy.

sues for Referral

eurosurgery for all patients. Consider infectious sease and neurology consultations if available.

JRGERY/OTHER PROCEDURES

Mandatory when neurologic deficits are severe or progressive

Often used when the abscess is in the posterior fossa or is the result of trauma

Type of surgical treatment used depends on the patient's clinical status, the neuroradiographic characteristics of the abscess, and the experience of the surgeon(s) carrying out the procedure (4).

Abscess drainage via a needle under stereotactic CT guidance through a burr hole under local anesthesia is the most rapid and effective surgical method of treatment and may be repeated if needed.

Craniotomy: If abscess is large or multilocular

In general, similar outcomes for stereotactic-guided drainage or craniotomy (6)

N-PATIENT CONSIDERATIONS

nitial Stabilization

patient care for close observation, diagnostic valuation, and specialty consultation (neurology, eurosurgery, or infectious disease)

dmission Criteria

pon diagnosis for close monitoring, IV antibiotics, nd possible surgery. A brain abscess often requires dmission to an intensive care unit (ICU), and may e the complication of ICU patients with neurologic jury, contributing significantly to morbidity and ortality (7)[B].

/ Fluids

/ fluids if nausea and vomiting present

Discharge Criteria

When patient is asymptomatic, afebrile, and responding to therapy as determined by serial imaging studies

ONGOING CARE

FOLLOW-UP RECOMMENDATIONS

- Bed rest until infection controlled and abscess evacuated or resolving, then as tolerated
- May need long-term rehabilitative care

Patient Monitoring

- Postsurgical monitoring as needed
- Serial CT or MRI for at least 3 months to evaluate the therapeutic response, confirm progressive resolution, detect new lesions, and manage complications.

DIET

IV fluids if significant nausea and vomiting

PATIENT EDUCATION

- Brain Research Foundation, 208 S. LaSalle Street, Suite 1426, Chicago, IL 60604; (312) 782-4311.
- Pri-Med Patient Education Center: Brain Abscess at http://www.patienteducationcenter.org/aspx/HealthELibrary/HealthETopic.aspx?cid=210320

PROGNOSIS

- The route of spread, the type and virulence of the organism, thickness of the capsule, location and number of abscesses in the brain, and immune status of the host are important determinants of outcome (1).
- Survival: >80% with early diagnosis and treatment
- In 1 retrospective analysis, 80% of patients recovered fully or had minimal incapacity and 10% died (3)[B].
- Patients with underlying cranial neoplasms or medical conditions have worse outcomes than those with a contiguous focus of infection or posttraumatic abscess (3)[B].

COMPLICATIONS

- Permanent neurologic deficits
- Surgical complications
- ICU-related complications
- Recurrent abscess
- Seizures
- Death

REFERENCES

1. Sundaram C, Lakshmi V. Pathogenesis and pathology of brain abscess. *Indian J Pathol Microbiol*. 2006;49:317–26.
2. Foerster BR, Thurnher MM, Malani PN, et al. Intracranial infections: clinical and imaging characteristics. *Acta Radiol*. 2007;48:875–93.
3. Carpenter J, Stapleton S, Holliman R. Retrospective analysis of 49 cases of brain abscess and review of the literature. *Eur J Clin Microbiol Infect Dis*. 2007;26:1–11.
4. Lu CH, et al. Strategies for the management of bacterial brain abscess. *J Clin Neurosci*. 2006;13(10):979–85. Epub 2006 Oct 23.
5. Bernardini GL. Diagnosis and management of brain abscess and subdural empyema. *Curr Neurol Neurosci Rep*. 2004;4:448–56.
6. Smith SJ, Ughratdar I, MacArthur DC et al. Never go to sleep on undrained pus: a retrospective review of surgery for intraparenchymal cerebral abscess. *Br J Neurosurg*. 2009;23:412–7.
7. Ziai WC, Lewin JJ. Update in the diagnosis and management of central nervous system infections. *Neurol Clin*. 2008;26:427–68, viii.

ADDITIONAL READING

- Alangaden G, Chandrasekar PH et al. Case 10-2010: a woman with weakness and a mass in the brain. *N Engl J Med*. 2010;363:395; author reply 395–6.
- Chang YT, Lu CH, Chuang MJ, Huang CR, Chuang YC, Tsai NW, Chen SF, Chang CC, Chang WN et al. Supratentorial deep-seated bacterial brain abscess in adults: clinical characteristics and therapeutic outcomes. *Acta Neurol Taiwan*. 2010;19:174–9.
- Mace SE et al. Central nervous system infections as a cause of an altered mental status? What is the pathogen growing in your central nervous system? *Emerg Med Clin North Am*. 2010;28:535–70.
- Patron V, Orsel S, Caire F, Aubry K, Jégoux F et al. Transethmoidal Drainage of Frontal Brain Abscesses. *Surgical innovation*. 2010;
- Shachor-Meyouhas Y, Bar-Joseph G, Guilburd JN, Lorber A, Hadash A, Kassis I et al. Brain abscess in children—epidemiology, predisposing factors and management in the modern medicine era. *Acta Paediatr*. 2010,99:1163–7.

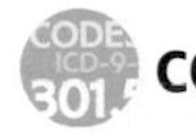

CODES

ICD9

324.0 Intracranial abscess

CLINICAL PEARLS

- Headache and altered mental status are common presenting symptoms of a brain abscess.
- Determination of point of entry and source of infection is essential for adequate treatment.
- Treatment of brain abscess may require a combination of antimicrobial agents for 6–8 weeks, surgical intervention, and eradication of the primary foci of infection.
- Serial head CTs for at least 3 months can help to evaluate a patient's response to therapies.

BRAIN INJURY, TRAUMATIC

Dana M. Collaguazo, MD

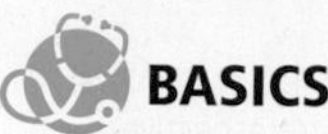

BASICS

DESCRIPTION
- A dynamic process with initial bleeding followed by secondary injury due to cerebral edema, continued bleeding
- Frequently related to rapid deceleration, as in motor vehicle or diving accidents, or blunt trauma
- System(s) affected: Cardiovascular; Endocrine/Metabolic; Nervous
- Synonym(s): Head injury

EPIDEMIOLOGY
Incidence
- 1.7 million per year
- 1,365,000 emergency department visits per year
- 275,000 hospitalizations per year
- 52,000 deaths per year

Prevalence
- Predominant age: 0–4, 15–19, and over 65 years
- Predominant gender: Male > Female

RISK FACTORS
Alcohol, prior head injury, contact sports; "heading" soccer balls may cause long-term cognitive loss.

Geriatric Considerations
Subdural hematomas are common after fall or blow; symptoms may be subtle.

GENERAL PREVENTION
- Safety education
- Seat belts, bicycle and motorcycle helmets
- Protective headgear for contact sports

PATHOPHYSIOLOGY
Initial intracranial bleeding followed by secondary injury due to cerebral edema, continued bleeding, etc.

ETIOLOGY
- Motor vehicle accident (17%)
- Falls (35%)
- Assault
- Child abuse:
  - Consider if dropped or fell <4 feet (e.g., off bed, couch) and significant injury present or any retinal hemorrhages

COMMONLY ASSOCIATED CONDITIONS
Alcohol and drug abuse

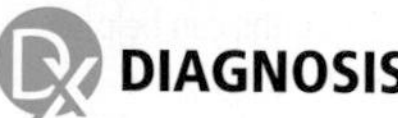

DIAGNOSIS

HISTORY
- Loss of consciousness (LOC)
- Headache
- Vomiting
- Amnesia
- Epidural hemorrhage from blunt trauma is generally acute, 30% with a "lucid interval" (initial LOC followed by recovery of consciousness, then LOC recurs and persists)
- Subdural hemorrhage usually has a slower onset and may present weeks after the initial injury, especially in the elderly.

PHYSICAL EXAM
- Focal neurologic signs and symptoms
- Evidence of increased intracranial pressure (ICP) (elevated BP, decreased pulse rate, or slow or irregular breathing [Cushing triad]—only 30% have all 3)
- Decorticate or decerebrate posturing (bad prognostic signs)
- Seizures
- Signs of basilar skull fracture: Raccoon eyes, battle sign, hemotympanum, CSF rhinorrhea or otorrhea (see Diagnostic Procedures)
- Unilateral dilated pupil in an alert patient is not consistent with impending herniation, as such patients are always unconscious.

DIAGNOSTIC TESTS & INTERPRETATION
Lab
Initial lab tests
- Evaluate for coagulopathy.
- Type and screen for possible surgical intervention.
- Perform drug and alcohol screening.

Imaging
Initial approach

CT, noncontrast, is study of choice to review bone windows, tissue windows, and subdural space:
- NEXUS II study (1)[B] demonstrated 8 clinical criteria that indicate a low likelihood of significant TBI when absent:
  - Evidence of significant skull fracture (depressed, basilar, or diastatic)
  - Altered level of alertness
  - Neurologic deficit
  - Persistent vomiting
  - Presence of scalp hematoma
  - Abnormal behavior
  - Coagulopathy
  - Age >65

Follow-Up & Special Considerations

Skull radiographs are not helpful in most cases, but can be done to document child abuse.

Diagnostic Procedures/Surgery
- CSF rhinorrhea:
  - Contains glucose; nasal mucus does not
  - Check for the double-halo sign: If nasal discharge contains CSF and blood, 2 rings appear when placed on filter paper—a central ring followed by a paler ring.
- Placement of ICP monitor when indicated
- Serial neurologic exams
- Neuropsychometric testing when able

Pathological Findings
- Epidural, subdural, or intraparenchymal hemorrhage
- Coup or contrecoup injury
- Evolving, diffuse axonal injury is a principal cause of neurologic sequelae with mild head trauma.

DIFFERENTIAL DIAGNOSIS
Other causes of altered mental status (e.g., toxicologic, infectious, metabolic, vascular causes)

TREATMENT

MEDICATION
First Line
- Pain: Morphine 1–2 mg IV p.r.n. with caution as c[an] depress mental status further and alter serial neurologic evaluations
- Increased ICP:
  - Mannitol: 0.25–2 g/kg (0.25–1 g/kg in children) given over 30–60 minutes in patients with adequate renal function; should not be used unless there is evidence of increased ICP; prophylactic use is associated with worse outcomes
  - Lasix: 20–40 mg IV to promote diuresis:
    - Neither furosemide nor mannitol should be given to a hypotensive patient.
  - Hypertonic saline: 2 mL/kg IV decreases ICP without adverse hemodynamic status and may have beneficial effects on immune system and excitatory neurotransmitters (2)[B].
- Sedation:
  - Propofol: Preferred due to short duration of action, which allows serial neurologic exams
- Seizures:
  - Phenytoin (Dilantin): 15 mg/kg IV (1 mg/kg/min not to exceed 50 mg/min). Stop infusion if QT interval increases by >50%.
  - Lorazepam (Ativan): 1–2 mg (0.1 mg/kg in children) IV
  - Phosphenytoin (Cerebyx): 15 mg/kg IV, not to exceed 150 mg/min. May give IM.
  - Levetiracetam (Keppra): May be desirable; lower complication rates, but prospective studies are needed. Use at neurosurgeon's instruction (3)[C].
- Contraindications: Allergy

Second Line
- Diuretics and IV β-blockers (e.g., esmolol or labetalol) can be used to maintain mean arterial pressure between 130 and 70 mm Hg.
- Nitrates may be helpful; however, may increase ICP.
- Antibiotics (e.g., cefazolin): Given if penetrating trauma is present; prophylactic antibiotics are not useful in basilar skull fractures.

ADDITIONAL TREATMENT
General Measures
- Acute management depends on severity of injury. Most patients need no interventions.
- Immediate goal: Determine who needs further therapy, imaging studies (CT), and hospitalization t[o] prevent further injury.
- For the severely injured patient:
  - Avoid hypotension or hypoxia. Head injury cause[s] increased ICP secondary to edema, and perfusion pressure must be maintained.
  - Hyperventilation is controversial. Prophylactic hyperventilation for those without signs or symptoms of increased ICP is contraindicated and may cause additional injury secondary to vasoconstriction (4)[B].

– Hypothermia: Although no difference is seen in mortality, may have marginal benefit, especially in patients with elevated ICP refractory to other methods (5)[B].
– Seizure prophylaxis does not change outcomes (such as death rates) but may prevent seizures. Consider phenytoin or levetiracetam for 1 week postinjury.

Manage breakthrough seizures with lorazepam.

Brain tissue oxygen probes can measure brain tissue hypoxia (<10 mm Hg is associated with worse outcomes) and may help define treatment parameters in acute traumatic brain injuries (6)[A].

ssues for Referral

:onsult neurosurgery for:

All penetrating head trauma
All abnormal head CTs

;URGERY/OTHER PROCEDURES

)epends on neurosurgical consult

N-PATIENT CONSIDERATIONS

nitial Stabilization

ABCs take priority over head injury.
C-spine immobilization should be considered in all head trauma.

Admission Criteria

- Abnormal CT
- Abnormal Glasgow coma scale
- Clinical evidence of basilar skull fracture
- Persistent neurologic deficits (e.g., confusion, somnolence)
- Patient with no competent adult at home for observation
- Possibly admit: LOC, amnesia, etc.

V Fluids

Jse normal saline for resuscitation fluid.

Discharge Criteria

Normal CT with return to normal mental status and responsible adult to observe patient at home (see Patient Monitoring)

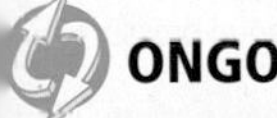

ONGOING CARE

FOLLOW-UP RECOMMENDATIONS

- Schedule regular follow-up within a week to determine return to activities.
- Rehabilitation indicated following a significant acute injury. Set realistic goals.

Patient Monitoring

Any patient discharged should have "head injury instructions" to watch for symptoms indicating need for further intervention (e.g., changing mental status, worsening headache, focal findings). Give to a competent adult who will observe the patient. A patient who deteriorates is not likely to remember or act on any instructions.

DIET

As tolerated

PATIENT EDUCATION

Proper counseling, symptomatic management, and gradual return to normal activities are essential to prevent a posttraumatic neurosis that can become refractory to treatment.

PROGNOSIS

- Gradual improvement for many
- 30–50% of severe head injuries may be fatal.
- Prolonged coma may be followed by satisfactory outcome.
- Predicting outcome is difficult, and patients may improve for years.

Geriatric Considerations

- Poorer prognosis with increasing age. Patients 75 and older have the highest rate of TBI hospitalizations and death.

Pediatric Considerations

- Outcome is more positive, except in severe TBI.

COMPLICATIONS

- Delayed hematomas
- Chronic subdural hematoma, which may follow even "mild" head injury, especially in the elderly. Often presents with headache and decreased mentation.
- Delayed hydrocephalus
- Emotional disturbances and psychiatric disorders resulting from head injury may be refractory to treatment.
- Seizure disorders: In 50% of penetrating head injuries, in 20% of severe closed head injuries, and in <5% of head injuries overall. Hematomas significantly increase risk of epilepsy.
- The postconcussion syndrome can follow mild head injury without LOC and includes headaches, dizziness, fatigue, and subtle cognitive or affective changes.
- 2nd-impact syndrome occurs when the CNS loses autoregulation. An individual with a minor head injury is returned to a contact sport and, following even minor trauma (e.g., whiplash), the patient will lose consciousness and herniate within 1–2 minutes, with a 50% mortality. A similar syndrome of "malignant edema" can occur in children with even a single injury.
- Increased risk for Alzheimer disease, Parkinson disease, and other brain disorders whose prevalence increases with age

REFERENCES

1. Mower WR, Hoffman JR, Herbert M, et al. Developing a decision instrument to guide computed tomographic imaging of blunt head injury patients. *J Trauma*. 2005;59:954–9.
2. Vincent JL, Berré J. Primer on medical management of severe brain injury. *Crit Care Med*. 2005;33:1392–9.
3. Szaflarski JP, Meckler JM, Szaflarski M, et al. Levetiracetam use in critically ill patients. *Neurocrit Care*. 2007;7:140–7.
4. Stocchetti N, Maas AI, Chieregato A, et al. Hyperventilation in head injury: a review. *Chest*. 2005;127:1812–27.
5. Henderson WR, Dhingra VK, Chittock DR, et al. Hypothermia in the management of traumatic brain injury. A systematic review and meta-analysis. *Intensive Care Med*. 2003;29:1637–44.
6. Maloney-Wilensky E, Gracias V, Itkin A, et al. Links brain tissue oxygen and outcome after severe traumatic brain injury: A systematic review. *Crit Care Med*. 2009 Apr 20. [Epub ahead of print].

ADDITIONAL READING

- Faul M, Xu L, Wald MM, Coronado VG. *Traumatic brain injury in the United States: emergency department visits, hospitalizations, and deaths.* Atlanta GA: Centers for Disease Control and Prevention, National Center for Injury Prevention and Control, 2010.
- Meloney-Wilensky E, Gracias V, Itkin A et al. Brain tissue oxygen and outcome after severe traumatic brain injury: a systematic review. *Crit Care Med.* 2009;37(6):2057–63.

See Also (Topic, Algorithm, Electronic Media Element)

Brain Injury–Post Acute Care Issues; Postconcussive Syndrome; Seizure Disorders

CODES

ICD9

- 852.00 Subarachnoid hemorrhage following injury, without mention of open intracranial wound, with state of consciousness unspecified
- 853.00 Other and unspecified intracranial hemorrhage following injury, without mention of open intracranial wound, with state of consciousness unspecified
- 854.00 Intracranial injury of other and unspecified nature, without mention of open intracranial wound, with state of consciousness unspecified

CLINICAL PEARLS

- Head injury is a dynamic process: Initial bleeding followed by secondary injury due to cerebral edema, continued bleeding, etc.
- Patients with history of head injury should have imaging if any of the following are present: Evidence of skull fracture, altered consciousness, neurologic deficit, persistent vomiting, scalp hematoma, abnormal behavior, coagulopathy, age >65
- Patient with normal head CT who has returned to normal mental status may be discharged to home with a competent adult observer for 24 hours.
- Strict criteria exist for patients to return to normal sport activity following head injury to avoid the 2nd-impact syndrome, which has 50% mortality.
- Predicting outcome is difficult, and patients may improve for years.

BRAIN INJURY–POST ACUTE CARE ISSUES

Maria I. Aguilar, MD

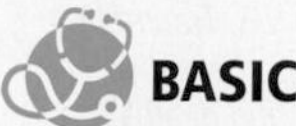

BASICS

DESCRIPTION

Traumatic brain injury (TBI) is a brain injury due to externally inflicted trauma; may result in significant impairment of an individual's physical, cognitive, and psychosocial functioning. TBI: leading mortality cause in North America for ages 1–45.

EPIDEMIOLOGY

- Predominant age: Highest incidence in the very young (ages 0–4), in persons 15–24 years of age and those >75 years old
- Predominant sex: Male > Female (2:1)

Incidence

- 1.2–1.7 million Americans sustain TBI per year.
- 50,000 deaths per year
- 80,000–90,000 sustain long-term disabilities

Prevalence

5.3 million Americans are living with TBI-related disabilities for which they require long-term assistance with activities of daily living.

RISK FACTORS

- High risk: Male, age 15–34
- Moderate risk <5 years and >60 years
- Lower socioeconomic status (head injury)

GENERAL PREVENTION

Improved safety standards and programs designed to minimize injury from vehicular-related events (motor vehicle, motorcycle, bicycle, pedestrian), falls, violence, sports, and recreation provide best prevention against TBI (1)[C].

PATHOPHYSIOLOGY

- Cortical contusions due to coup–contrecoup injuries. While axonal rupture from shear and tensile forces can occur at the time of severe head injury, milder degrees of axonal damage may play a role in mild TBI.
- Disruption of axonal neurofilament organization impairs axonal transport, leading to axonal swelling, Wallerian degeneration, and transection.
- Release of excitatory neurotransmitters acetylcholine, glutamate, and aspartate, and generation of free radicals may contribute to secondary injury.

ETIOLOGY

- Leading causes of TBI: falls and motor vehicle accidents (MVA). Violence-related TBI has increased during the past decade and accounts for about 10% of all cases. Sports and recreation injuries are also an important cause of TBI, especially in teenagers and young adults.
- As the conflict in the Middle East continues, the number of soldiers returning to the US with diagnosed and undiagnosed blast-related TBI will continue to increase.

COMMONLY ASSOCIATED CONDITIONS

- Psychosis
- Suicide attempts
- Substance abuse
- Attention deficit disorder

DIAGNOSIS

HISTORY

- Non-neurologic complications: Pulmonary, metabolic and endocrinologic, nutritional, GI, musculoskeletal, genitourinary, dermatologic, chronic pain
- Most neurologic complications are apparent within the 1st days following injury. Long-term sequelae include seizures, headache, hydrocephalus, visual defects, neuroendocrine abnormalities, and movement and sleep disorders.
- Cognitive consequences: Memory impairment, difficulties in attention and concentration, language deficits, visual perception problems, and poor problem-solving, reasoning, insight, judgment, and information processing
- Behavioral problems: Decreased ability to initiate responses, verbal and physical aggression, agitation, learning difficulties, shallow self-awareness, altered sexual functioning, impulsivity, social disinhibition
- Psychological consequences: Mood disorders, personality changes, altered emotional control, depression, anxiety
- Social consequences: Risk of suicide, divorce, unemployment, economic strain, alcohol/substance abuse.

Pediatric Considerations

Interactions of physical, cognitive, and behavioral sequelae interfere with new learning. Effects of early TBI may not become apparent until later in the child's development.

PHYSICAL EXAM

- TBI's severity is classified based on the Glasgow Coma Scale (GCS) as follows: Mild injury GCS 13–15; moderate injury GCS 9–12; severe injury GCS 8 or less.
- Glasgow Coma Scale (GCS). For all 3 categories, score best response:

Verbal response	Score
Oriented	5
Confused	4
Inappropriate words	3
Incomprehensible speech	2
No response	1
Eye opening	
Spontaneous	4
To speech	3
To pain	2
No response	1
Motor response	
Obeys commands	6
Localizes pain	5
Withdraws from pain	4
Abnormal flexion to pain	3
Abnormal extension to pain	2
No response	1

DIAGNOSTIC TESTS & INTERPRETATION

- Evoked potentials (auditory, visual, somatosensory)
- Behavioral assessment, neuropsychological testing, vocational assessment
- Cognitive test for orientation and arousal; use Western Neuro Sensory Stimulation Profile or Galveston Orientation Amnesia Test
- Electroencephalograph (EEG)

Lab

Initial lab tests

As needed for suspected metabolic complications

Imaging

Initial approach

- Bone scan: Heterotopic ossification
- CT: Hydrocephalus, atrophy, hematoma
- Video fluoroscopic swallowing study
- MRI to evaluate diffuse axonal injury
- EEG: To evaluate subclinical seizure activity. Limited predictive value in the setting of acute TBI.

Pathological Findings

- Evidence of microscopic axonal injury, axon retraction bulbs, and microglial clusters
- Hydrocephalus with periventricular edema
- Joint contractures result in collagen cross-linking: Decreased range of motion
- Heterotopic ossification: Disorganized osteoid calcification in soft tissue

DIFFERENTIAL DIAGNOSIS

- The diagnosis of pain following TBI can be difficult in light of limitations imposed by cognitive, language, and behavioral deficits.
  - Dysautonomia: Tachypnea, hypertension, painful posturing/contractions, diaphoresis
  - Neuropathic pain: Burning, shocklike, or pins and needles; allodynia/hyperpathia. 3 most common: Complex regional pain syndrome, central pain syndrome, and peripheral neuropathy.
  - Spasticity or spastic dystonia
  - Headache: Posttraumatic headache, hydrocephalus, increased intracranial pressure
  - Myofascial pain syndrome
  - Neurogenic heterotopic ossification: Bone formation in soft tissue
  - Deep vein thrombosis
  - Constipation and urinary retention
  - Trauma: Fractures, musculoskeletal injuries
  - Shoulder: Subluxation, acromioclavicular separation, rotator cuff tendonitis/tear
- Chronic infection, depression, hypothyroidism, hydrocephalus, intracerebral hemorrhage, seizures, fractures, tracheal stricture, pain, alcohol, drugs, polypharmacy, and/or central nervous system depressant

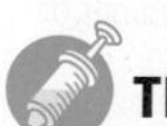

TREATMENT

MEDICATION

- Psychostimulants may affect speed of cognitive processing, mood, and behavior:
  - Methylphenidate 20–40 mg/d in 2 divided doses; dextroamphetamine [B]
  - Also likely to improve memory, attention, concentration, and mental processing in children/adults (2)[A]

- Agitation:
  - Treat epilepsy or depression 1st.
  - Minimize the use of antipsychotics and benzodiazepines, as they worsen cognition.
  - β-Blockers have best evidence for efficacy in agitation/aggression (3)[A].
  - Antidepressants (SSRIs) and AEDs in the context of an affective disorder or epilepsy, respectively, may help agitation/aggression (4)[B].
  - If necessary, use antipsychotics of the atypical class (clozapine, olanzapine, quetiapine, risperidone, and ziprasidone) (5)[B].
- Abulia (lack of initiative): Amantadine (Symmetrel), bromocriptine, methylphenidate, levodopa (5)[C]
- Epilepsy: American Academy of Physical Medicine and Rehabilitation does not recommend AEDs for preventing late (>7 days post TBI) posttraumatic seizures (6)[B]. If epilepsy occurs, avoid phenobarbital; too sedating (6).
- Spasticity caution: Be aware of potential negative consequences of all agents:
  - Use dantrolene sodium 25–200 mg/d divided t.i.d.; baclofen; intrathecal baclofen; diazepam, clonidine, tizanidine, and gabapentin; botulinum toxin injections for focal spasticity (7)[B].
- Neurogenic bladder: Oxybutynin 2.5 mg t.i.d.–10 mg q.i.d. if bladder pressures low and/or postvoid residuals low (1)[B]
- Bowel routine: Stool softener such as docusate sodium (daily) combined with laxative (night before suppository), high-fiber diet, and suppository (every other day) (1)[C]
- Heterotopic ossification: Indomethacin 25–50 mg t.i.d. If severe, progressive, or history of GI ulceration, then etidronate (Didronel) 20 mg/kg for 6 months or alendronate 20 mg/d (1)[C].
- Neurobehavioral problems: Weak evidence supports psychostimulants as effective in treatment of inattention, apathy, and slowness; high-dose β-blockers in treatment of agitation and aggression; and anticonvulsants and antidepressants in treatment of agitation and aggression with an affective disorder (4)[B].
- Precautions: Medications may have significant adverse effects in persons with TBI and can impede rehabilitation progress.

ADDITIONAL TREATMENT

General Measures

- Diminished level of arousal: Identify best modality for communication, assess functional skills (proper seating, hand function) with behaviorist/neuropsychologist.
- Social work (family education and long-term planning) and nursing
- Reduce sedatives
- Neurogenic bladder—treat urinary tract infection:
  - If postvoid residual <50 mL, then try regular voiding routine q2h
  - If still incontinent, add oxybutynin
  - If still incontinent, try condom catheter during the day; incontinence pads at night.
  - If high postvoid residuals or high pressure bladder or dyssynergic bladder on urodynamics: Intermittent catheter q4–6h
- Neurogenic bowel: Regular bowel routine
- Contractures and spasticity; stretching:
  - If no progress after 4 weeks, consider serial casting or custom-made orthotic
  - Contractures >45°: Consider tendon release.
- Heterotopic ossification: Stretch soft tissue to decrease maturation of osteoid, consider orthotics/splinting, bone scan at baseline
- Skin: Turn patient q2h; avoid sitting such as in bed at 45°, observe for erythema around tube sites, and rule out latex allergy.
- Respiratory: Night humidification for tracheotomy
- Endocrine: Monitor fluid balance
- Dental: Assessment and radiographs
- Rehabilitative practices: Rehabilitative programs should be interdisciplinary, comprehensive, and include cognitive and behavioral assessment and intervention (1)[C]

Issues for Referral

- Refer to multidisciplinary rehabilitation programs.
- Suicide attempts and ideation (SI) are more prevalent in people with TBI, even after controlling for psychiatric disorders (8)[C]. Assess hopelessness and SI proactively.

COMPLEMENTARY AND ALTERNATIVE MEDICINE

- Cognitive exercises (including computer-assisted strategies), compensatory devices (memory books, paging systems), psychotherapy, behavior modification, vocational rehabilitation, school rehabilitation, nutritional support, music and art therapy, therapeutic recreation
- Hyperbaric oxygen therapy (HBOT) cannot be routinely recommended for patients with TBI because of few trials, methodologic shortcomings, and poor reporting (9)[A].

ONGOING CARE

FOLLOW-UP RECOMMENDATIONS

Patient Monitoring

Patients make slow, steady gains; review medical status monthly.

DIET

- Ensure adequate hydration; 2–2.5 L of water/d.
- Bolus feeds preferred if fed by gastrostomy.
- Upright and quiet for 1/2 hour following feeds, as aspiration can occur even with a g-tube
- Early feeding is associated with trend toward better survival and disability outcomes (10)[A].

PATIENT EDUCATION

- For information and family support groups:
  - Brain Injury Information Network www.tbinet.org/
  - Brain Injury Association of America www.biausa.org/
- Families need support, advocacy, education, information (verbally and written), opportunity to have input regarding priorities and treatment plans, and to discuss limits of treatment for patient (advance directive).

PROGNOSIS

- Most rapid return of function is during 1st 2 years, but some improve slowly for 5–10 years
- Highly variable (80% of individuals with severe injuries become independent in dressing and self-care at 1 year)
- Negative prognostic factors:
  - Age >40 years old
  - Abnormal pupillary responses or extraocular eye movements
  - Prolonged coma
- Abnormal evoked potentials
- Accurate prediction of return to work is not feasible, with rates in the 12–70% range.

COMPLICATIONS

Major affective disorder (depression, psychosis) in up to 50% of patients, family and caregiver burnout, substance abuse, social isolation, dental caries, osteoporosis, aspiration pneumonia, pressure ulcers, dysphagia, esophagitis, bladder incontinence, contractures/spasticity

REFERENCES

1. Consensus conference. Rehabilitation of persons with traumatic brain injury. NIH Consensus Development Panel on Rehabilitation of Persons With Traumatic Brain Injury. *JAMA*. 1999;282: 974–83.
2. Siddall OM. Use of methylphenidate in traumatic brain injury. *Ann Pharmacother*. 2005;39: 1309–13.
3. Fleminger S, et al. Pharmacological management for agitation and aggression in people with acquired brain injury. *Cochrane Database Syst Rev*. 2003/2006;(1):CD003299.
4. Deb S, Crownshaw T. The role of pharmacotherapy in the management of behaviour disorders in traumatic brain injury patients. *Brain Inj*. 2004;18:1–31.
5. Elovic EP, et al. The use of atypical antipsychotics in traumatic brain injury. *J Head Trauma Rehab*. 2003;18(2):177–95.
6. Bushnik T, et al. Medical and social issues related to posttraumatic seizures in persons with traumatic brain injury. *J Head Trauma Rehab*. 2004;19(4):296–304.
7. Zafonte R, et al. Acute care management of post-TBI spasticity. *J Head Trauma Rehab*. 2004;19(2):89–100.
8. Simpson G, Tate R, et al. Suicidality in people surviving a traumatic brain injury: prevalence, risk factors and implications for clinical management. *Brain Inj*. 2007;21:1335–51.
9. Bennett M, Heard R. Hyperbaric oxygen therapy for multiple sclerosis. *Cochrane Database Syst Rev*. 2004:CD003057.
10. Perel P, Yanagawa T, Bunn F, et al. Nutritional support for head-injured patients. *Cochrane Database Syst Rev*. 2006:CD001530.

CODES

ICD9

- 339.20 Post-traumatic headache, unspecified
- 854.00 Intracranial injury of other and unspecified nature, without mention of open intracranial wound, with state of consciousness unspecified
- 907.0 Late effect of intracranial injury without mention of skull fracture

CLINICAL PEARLS

- TBI can cause both neurologic and non-neurologic manifestations.
- Best approach to treatment includes multi- and interdisciplinary team member participation.
- TBI can lead to devastating sequelae; prevention is key.

BRANCHIAL CLEFT FISTULA

Timothy L. Black, MD

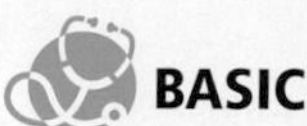

BASICS

DESCRIPTION

- A congenital, abnormal tract connecting the skin of the neck with an internal structure, resulting from failure of closure of 1 of the 4 branchial clefts
- May involve branchial clefts I–IV, which develop in the 4th gestational week
- System(s) affected: Skin/Exocrine

Pediatric Considerations

Almost all occur in the pediatric age group.

EPIDEMIOLOGY

- Predominant age: By definition, all are present at birth, although they may remain unnoticed for some time. (Branchial cleft cysts may not present until later childhood.) (1)[C]
- Predominant sex: Unknown

Incidence

Unknown

Prevalence

Unknown

RISK FACTORS

Positive family history

Genetics

10% have family history.

PATHOPHYSIOLOGY

- Both respiratory and squamous epithelium alone or in combination may line branchial anomalies (2)[C].
- Squamous epithelium is found more commonly in cysts.
- Ciliated, columnar epithelium is found more commonly in sinuses and fistulae.

ETIOLOGY

- The 1st branchial cleft contributes to the tympanic cavity and eustachian tube. Related fistulae are very rare and tend to be infra- or retroauricular. (Preauricular cysts and sinuses are not thought to be of branchial cleft origin.) The first branchial cleft anomalies enter the external auditory canal and/or the middle ear
- The 2nd branchial cleft forms the hyoid bone and tonsillar fossa. Related fistulae (most common variant) course between the internal and external carotid arteries. Internal opening usually at level of tonsillar fossa. External opening along anterior border of sternocleidomastoid muscle (1)[C]. 2nd branchial cleft lesions represent 90% or more of all branchial cleft lesions.
- 3rd and 4th branchial clefts form parathyroid glands, thymus, and portions of thyroid (parafollicular cells). Fistulae are rare; those from third cleft course posterior to carotid artery; both should have external ostia on lower anterior neck. Sinus tracts (also called pyriform sinuses) originate in the pyriform sinus and course adjacent to the thyroid cartilage (3)[C]. 3rd branchial cleft anomalies represent 2–8% of all branchial anomalies.

COMMONLY ASSOCIATED CONDITIONS

Microtia and aural atresia occur with failure of development of 1st branchial cleft.

DIAGNOSIS

HISTORY

- History of drainage from cervical area
- Neck abscess or suppurative thyroiditis

PHYSICAL EXAM

- Presence of tiny external opening usually on mid-to-lower neck along anterior border of sternocleidomastoid muscle
- Spontaneous mucoid drainage
- External openings may also be marked by a skin tag or cartilage.
- Infection may rarely be the presenting sign, with erythema, swelling, pain, or fever.
- 10% are bilateral.
- Small orifices located in the mid-neck, most commonly along the anterior border of the sternocleidomastoid muscle (less commonly in the lower neck or postauricular)
- Third branchial cleft anomalies are predominantly left-sided (89%) (4)[B].

DIAGNOSTIC TESTS & INTERPRETATION

Lab

Culture if signs of infection

Imaging

- Computed tomography (CT) of neck with IV contrast occasionally beneficial in 3rd and 4th branchial cleft fistulas/sinus (3)[C].
- CT may demonstrate fistula tract in up to 64% of cases (2)[C].
- Magnetic resonance imaging and ultrasound may occasionally be useful.
- Barium esophagogram may demonstrate the fistula (may have a sensitivity rate of 50–80% when used to evaluate 3rd and 4th branchial anomalies (2)[C].

agnostic Procedures/Surgery

- Sinogram or fistulogram may be done, but is of little value.
- Pharyngoscopy may occasionally be useful.

thological Findings

- Lined by stratified squamous epithelium; may contain hair follicles, sweat glands, sebaceous glands, or cartilage
- Some are lined by ciliated columnar epithelium.

FFERENTIAL DIAGNOSIS

- External sinuses
- Cystic hygroma
- Dermoid cysts
- Lymphadenopathy

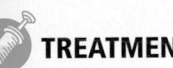

TREATMENT

- Surgical excision
- Outpatient status usually appropriate

JRGERY/OTHER PROCEDURES

- Small transverse incision at external ostium with careful dissection of fistula (1)[C]
- Stepladder incisions may be needed.
- End of fistula ligated flush with pharyngeal mucosa.
- 1st branchial cleft lesions may require larger incision (1)[C].
- Methylene blue injection into fistula may be useful.
- Drains are not used.
- Antibiotics only for infection
- Patients with abscess related to 3rd branchial cleft anomalies frequently require initial incision and drainage (4)[B]:
  - Incision and drainage failure rate of 94% at 1st attempt
  - Virtually all require resection.
  - Those with acute suppurative thyroiditis may require partial thyroidectomy with resection.
- Endoscopic cauterization of the internal orifice has been successfully used in some cases.

ONGOING CARE

FOLLOW-UP RECOMMENDATIONS

Patient Monitoring

- Follow at weekly intervals if infected until resolution, then excision
- Postoperative visit at 2 weeks

PROGNOSIS

Good

COMPLICATIONS

- Facial nerve injury
- Hypoglossal nerve injury
- Spinal accessory nerve injury
- Vagus nerve injury
- Infection
- Carotid artery injury
- Possible recurrence if any epithelium remains
- Neoplastic degeneration of branchial remnants (about 250 reported cases) if not resected

REFERENCES

1. Roback SA, Telander RL. Thyroglossal duct cysts and branchial cleft anomalies. *Sem Ped Surg.* 1994;3:142–46.
2. Waldhausen JH et al. Branchial cleft and arch anomalies in children. *Semin Pediatr Surg.* 2006;15:64–9.
3. Liberman M, Kay S, Emil S, et al. Ten years of experience with third and fourth branchial remnants. *J Ped Surg.* 2002;37:685–90.
4. Nicoucar K, Giger R, Jaecklin T, Pope HG, Dulguerov P et al. Management of congenital third branchial arch anomalies: a systematic review. *Otolaryngol Head Neck Surg.* 2010;142:21–28.e2.

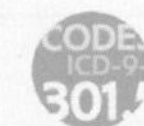

CODES

ICD9

744.41 Branchial cleft sinus or fistula

CLINICAL PEARLS

- Most common: 2nd branchial cleft; results in an opening in the mid-neck at the anterior border of the sternocleidomastoid muscle, together with a history of an occasional droplet of fluid, is diagnostic. Radiographic confirmation is not needed; surgical excision as an outpatient is both diagnostic and therapeutic.
- Branchial cleft remnants, sinuses, and cysts are the result of failure of branchial cleft to complete its normal development.

BREAST ABSCESS

Anya S. Koutras, MD

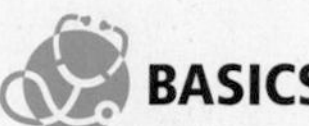

BASICS

DESCRIPTION
- Collection of pus, usually localized
- Can be associated with lactation or fistulous tracts secondary to squamous epithelial neoplasm or duct occlusion
- System(s) affected: Skin/Exocrine
- Synonym(s): Mammary abscess; peripheral breast abscess; subareolar abscess; puerperal abscess

Pregnancy Considerations
Most commonly associated with postpartum lactation

EPIDEMIOLOGY
Predominant age:
- Puerperal abscess: Premenopausal
- Subareolar abscess: Postmenopausal
- Predominant sex: Female

Incidence
- 0.1–0.5% of breast-feeding women
- Puerperal abscess rare after 1st 6 weeks of lactation

RISK FACTORS
- Puerperal mastitis: 5–11% go on to abscess (most often due to inadequate therapy). Risk factors for mastitis are those that result in milk stasis (infrequent feeds, missing feeds).
- Poor latch, damaged nipple, illness in mother or baby, rapid weaning, breast pressure, blocked nipple pore or duct, maternal stress or fatigue, maternal malnutrition
- General factors: Diabetes, rheumatoid arthritis
- Steroids, silicone/paraffin implants, lumpectomy with radiation, heavy cigarette smoking
- Nipple retraction

GENERAL PREVENTION
- Prevention of mastitis
- Early treatment of mastitis with milk expression and cold compresses
- Early treatment with antibiotics

ETIOLOGY
- Delayed treatment of mastitis
- Puerperal abscesses: Blocked lactiferous duct
- Subareolar abscess: Squamous epithelial neoplasm with keratin plugs or ductal extension with associated inflammation
- Peripheral abscess: Stasis of the duct

DIAGNOSIS

- Tender breast lump, fluctuant, usually unilateral
- Systemic malaise (though usually less malaise than with mastitis)
- Fever

HISTORY
Tender breast lump, usually unilateral

PHYSICAL EXAM
- Erythema
- Draining pus
- Local edema
- Nipple and skin retraction
- Proximal lymphadenopathy

DIAGNOSTIC TESTS & INTERPRETATION

Lab
- Leukocytosis
- Elevated sedimentation rate
- Culture and sensitivity of drainage to identify pathogen, usually *Staphylococci* or *Streptococci*. *E. coli* is 3rd most common. Nonlactational abscess associated with anaerobic bacteria.

Imaging
- Ultrasound
- Mammogram

Diagnostic Procedures/Surgery
- Aspiration for culture
- Fine-needle aspiration not accurate to exclude carcinoma

Pathological Findings
- Squamous metaplasia of the ducts
- Intraductal hyperplasia
- Epithelial overgrowth
- Fat necrosis
- Duct ectasia

DIFFERENTIAL DIAGNOSIS
- Carcinoma (inflammatory or primary squamous ce
- Tuberculosis (may be associated with HIV infectior
- Actinomycosis
- Typhoid
- Sarcoid
- Granulomatous disease
- Syphilis
- Foreign body reactions (e.g., to silicone and paraff
- Mammary duct ectasia
- Hydatid cyst
- Sebaceous cyst

TREATMENT

MEDICATION

- Combine antibiotics with drainage for cure
- Culture midstream sample of milk for mastitis, abscess fluid for breast abscess
- NSAIDs
- Dicloxacillin 500 mg q.i.d. for 10–14 days
- If no response in 24–48 hours, switch to cephalexin 500 mg q.i.d. for 10–14 days:
  - Or amoxicillin-clavulanate (Augmentin) 250 mg t.i.d.
- Clindamycin 300 mg t.i.d. if anaerobes suspected
- Contraindications: Allergy to the antibiotic
- Precautions: Refer to manufacturer's profile for each drug
- New techniques include percutaneous intracavitary urokinase irrigation for large abscesses in nonlactating women (1)[C]

ADDITIONAL TREATMENT

General Measures

- Cold compresses for pain control
- Important to continue to breast-feed or express milk

COMPLEMENTARY AND ALTERNATIVE MEDICINE

Lecithin supplementation

SURGERY/OTHER PROCEDURES

- Aspiration under ultrasound (1,2)[B],(3)[C]
- Needle aspiration alone (without antibiotics) may be effective for small breast abscesses (4)[A].
- If aspiration and antibiotics fail, incision and drainage with removal of loculations
- Biopsy of all nonpuerperal abscesses to rule out carcinoma
- Open all fistulous tracts, especially in nonlactating abscesses

IN-PATIENT CONSIDERATIONS

Initial Stabilization

Outpatient, unless systemically immunocompromised or septic

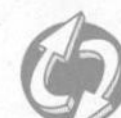

ONGOING CARE

FOLLOW-UP RECOMMENDATIONS

Patient Monitoring

Ensure resolution to exclude carcinoma.

PATIENT EDUCATION

- Care of wound
- Breast-feeding precautions

PROGNOSIS

- Complete healing expected in 8–10 days
- Subareolar abscesses frequently recur, even after I&D and antibiotics; may require surgical removal of ducts.

COMPLICATIONS

Fistula

REFERENCES

1. Schwarz RJ, Shrestha R. Needle aspiration of breast abscesses. *Am J Surgery*. 2001;182:117.
2. Dener C, Inan A. Breast abscesses in lactating women. *World J Surgery*. 2003;27:130.
3. Christensen AF, Al-Suliman N, Nielsen KR, et al. Ultrasound-guided drainage of breast abscesses: results in 151 patients. *Br J Radiol*. 2005;78:186–8.
4. Thirumalaikumar S, Kommu S et al. Best evidence topic reports. Aspiration of breast abscesses. *Emerg Med J*. 2004;21:333–4.

ADDITIONAL READING

- Berná-Serna JD, Berná-Mestre JD, Galindo PJ, et al. Use of urokinase in percutaneous drainage of large breast abscesses. *J Ultrasound Med*. 2009;28:449–54.
- Dabbas N, Chand M, Pallett A, Royle GT, Sainsbury R et al. Have the organisms that cause breast abscess changed with time?–implications for appropriate antibiotic usage in primary and secondary care. *Breast J*. 2010;16:412–5.
- Jahanfar S, Ng CJ, Teng CL et al. Antibiotics for mastitis in breastfeeding women. *Cochrane Database Syst Rev*. 2009;CD005458.

CODES

ICD9

- 611.0 Inflammatory disease of breast
- 675.14 Postpartum abscess of breast

CLINICAL PEARLS

- 5–11% of cases of puerperal mastitis go on to abscess (most often due to inadequate therapy for mastitis). Risk factors for mastitis are those that result in milk stasis (infrequent feeds, missing feeds).
- Abscess not associated with lactation should prompt coverage with antibiotics that cover anaerobic bacteria.
- Treatment is antibiotic and aspiration, with I&D, with breakup of loculations reserved for those failing more conservative management.

BREAST CANCER

Susan E. Donohue, MD
David S. Shepro, MD

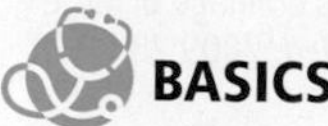

BASICS

DESCRIPTION

Common malignant tumor that originates from epithelial cells of breast tissue

EPIDEMIOLOGY

Incidence

- 123 cases per 100,000 women per year in 2006 (1)
- Invasive cancer new cases in 2009: Women: 194,280
- In situ cancer new cases in 2009: 62,280 (85% ductal carcinoma in situ)
- Breast cancer (BC) deaths: 40,480
- Lifetime risk BC: 1 in 8 (12%)
- Lifetime risk BC death: 1 in 35
- Most common malignancy in women in US, second only to lung cancer as cause of cancer death (2)

Prevalence

2.5 million women in the US

RISK FACTORS

- Female, family history, nulliparity and/or older age at first live birth, early menarche, delayed menopause, increasing patient age, personal history of BC
- Prior chest radiation (lymphoma), DES
- Prolonged hormone replacement therapy (HRT), high ethyl alcohol (ETOH) use, high body mass index (BMI), physical inactivity

Genetics

- BRCA1 and BRCA2
- Other genes: ATM, CHEK2, p53
- Cowden syndrome (PTEN): Hamartomas skin, mucosa, bones, central nervous system (CNS), thyroid (benign and malignant)
- Li-Fraumeni syndrome (TP53): Autosomal dominance, Ca in CNS, leukemia, sarcoma, adrenal cortex
- Criteria for additional risk evaluation/gene testing:
  - BC at age ≤50 years
  - 2 breast primaries of breast/ovary cancer in single patient or ≥2 breast primary cancers or breast + ovary cancer same side of family
  - Clustering of BC with thyroid Ca, sarcoma, adrenal cortex, endometrial, pancreas, CNS, leukemia/lymphoma same side of family
  - FH BC susceptibility gene
  - Ashkenazi Jewish with breast/ovary cancer at any age
  - Any male breast cancer
  - Ovarian cancer in family

GENERAL PREVENTION

- Avoid risk factors when possible.
- Selective estrogen receptor modulators
- For hereditary breast and/or ovarian cancer (3):
  - Begin at age 18–25: BSE (beginning at 18 years), clinical breast exam, yearly mammogram and breast magnetic resonance imaging (MRI) (at 25)
  - Discuss risk-reducing mastectomy. Counsel, suggest risk-reducing salpingo-oophorectomy ideally between 35 and 40 or after completion of child-bearing.

PATHOPHYSIOLOGY

- Estrogen/progesterone induce cyclin D1 and c-myc expression
- Bcl-2 commonly overexpressed
- Estrogen receptor (ER) not expressed in 1/3 BC:
  - Mutations of cell adhesion molecules
  - Epidermal growth factors (EGF, c-erb-B2 [HER2])
  - IGF family
  - TGF-β family
  - BRCA1 and BRCA2 may function in cell cycle progression and in DNA repair.

DIAGNOSIS

HISTORY

- Mass, pain, redness, nipple retraction, nipple discharge
- Symptoms of metastatic disease
- Family history

PHYSICAL EXAM

- Careful clinician breast exam:
  - Evidence suggests that clinical exam of breast produces a reduction in breast cancer mortality.
- Regional lymph node exam
- Evaluate possible metastatic disease.
- Psychosocial evaluation

DIAGNOSTIC TESTS & INTERPRETATION

Lab

Initial lab tests

New BC:

- Complete blood count, liver function tests/alkaline phosphatase
- Chest imaging
- Optional bone scan, computed tomography (CT) abdomen/pelvis
- Tumor markers usually not indicated for early BC

Imaging

Initial approach

- Screening for BC:
  - X-ray mammography decreases BC mortality
  - Digital mammography may benefit. Computer-aided detection (CAD) increases sensitivity and decreases specificity.
  - MRI: BRCA1 or 2, lifetime breast cancer risk of ≥20%, prior chest radiation, other factors increasing risk
  - Ultrasound: Limited data in women with dense breasts
- Diagnosis of BC:
  - X-ray, ultrasound-guided biopsy/aspirate
  - MRI commonly used to define disease in breast and presence of multifocal/multicentric ipsilateral disease

Follow-Up & Special Considerations

Staging of BC:

- CT, bone scan (back pain)
- MRI especially if CNS/spinal cord symptoms

Diagnostic Procedures/Surgery

- Primary tumor: Fine-needle aspiration, biopsy
- Genomic assay on formalin-fixed tissue for select ER-positive/node-negative (Oncotype DX)

Pathological Findings

- Histology:
  - Ductal/lobular/other
  - Benign/malignant
  - Tumor size
  - Inflammatory component
  - Invasive/noninvasive
  - Margins
  - Nodal involvement
  - Nodal micrometastases: Increased risk of disease recurrence
- Estrogen receptor
- Progesterone receptor
- HER-2 assay

DIFFERENTIAL DIAGNOSIS

- Benign breast disease
- Infection

B

TREATMENT

EDICATION

'revention:
- Risk assessment tool at http://www.cancer.gov/bcrisktool/
- Assertive screening/surveillance
- Risk-reducing mastectomy
- Risk-reducing bilateral salpingo-oophorectomy for breast and ovary cancer
- Surgery
- Chemoprevention/hormone therapy:
  - Risk reduction for ER-positive tumors
  - No demonstration of increased survival

Hormone therapy for ER-positive tumors:
- Tamoxifen
- Ovarian ablation
- Aromatase inhibitors

Adjuvant:
- Hormone therapy for ER-positive tumors:
  - Tamoxifen
  - Ovarian ablation with surgery or gonadotropin-releasing hormone agonists/antagonism
  - Aromatase inhibitors
- Cytotoxic therapy:
  - Anthracyclines, alkylating agents, taxanes, antimetabolites
  - Pre-op (neoadjuvant) vs post-op (adjuvant)
  - Combinations of above
  - Dose-dense versus non–dose-dense
- Anti-HER2/neu antibody in select HER2/neu-positive patients:
  - Monitor cardiac toxicity, especially with anthracycline.

Advanced disease:
- Hormone therapy
- Cytotoxic therapy
- Bisphosphonates to decrease skeletal complications
- Antivascular endothelial growth factor (VEGF) antibody
- Anti-HER2/neu antibody in select HER2/neu-positive patients

DDITIONAL TREATMENT

dditional Therapies

evention therapy discussed in Treatment section

OMPLEMENTARY AND ALTERNATIVE IEDICINE

esearch before prescribing

URGERY/OTHER PROCEDURES

Breast-conserving partial mastectomy/lumpectomy therapy if possible:
- Negative margins
- Tumor usually <5 cm
- No prior breast radiation

Mastectomy:
- Large tumors
- Young women with known BRCA
- Consider immediate or delayed reconstruction.

Radiation therapy should be initiated without delay:
- After breast-conserving therapy
- Postmastectomy in select high-risk patients
- Palliation of metastatic disease

ONGOING CARE

FOLLOW-UP RECOMMENDATIONS

- Interval history/physical every 4–6 months for 1st year and while receiving adjuvant therapy, then yearly (4):
  - Recognize increased risk of ovarian cancer
  - Rare: AML (therapy-induced), angiosarcoma (radiation), endometrial cancer (tamoxifen/postmenopause)
- Other signs/symptoms to monitor/manage related to chemo, hormone, radiation:
  - Hot flashes
  - Sexual dysfunction
  - Arthralgias (aromatase)
  - Cognitive dysfunction
  - Depression
  - Fatigue
  - BMI
  - Osteopenia or osteoporosis
  - Cardiovascular disease, congestive heart failure
  - Deep vein thrombosis
  - No evidence to support the use of "tumor markers" for BC/routine bone scan, CT scans, MRI, positron emission tomography (PET), ultrasound in the symptomatic patient
- Mammogram/imaging every 12 months (and 6–12 months postradiation therapy if breast conserved)
- Assess bone health.
- Gynecologic exam for women on tamoxifen every 12 months

Patient Monitoring

- Continue screening mammograms.
- Bone density
- Annual gynecologic exam if uterus present and on tamoxifen

DIET

- Evidence that certain lifestyle characteristics are risk factors for BC (obesity, increased alcohol consumption)
- No evidence that lifestyle modification changes BC risk

PROGNOSIS

- Influenced by age, menopausal status, stage of disease, ER and PR status, many other characteristics
- Risk of BC recurrences are maintained for life and are not limited by number of years postdiagnosis/therapy.
- Some patients with limited metastatic disease have a better prognosis.

COMPLICATIONS

- Spinal cord compression
- Hypercalcemia
- Visceral metastatic disease
- Emotional issues, especially depression and body-image alteration
- Postoperative lymphedema
- Therapy-induced toxicity

REFERENCES

1. National Cancer Institute, US National institutes of Health. 2009/2010 Update http://progressreport.cancer.gov/doc_detail.asp?pid=1&did=2009&chid=93&coid=920&mid=.
2. The NCCN Practice Guidelines in Oncology (Version 1. 2009) © 2009 Breast Cancer National Comprehensive Cancer Network, Inc. Accessed 6/14/2009 at http://www.nccn.org.
3. Robson M, Offit K. Clinical practice. Management of an inherited predisposition to breast cancer. *N Engl J Med*. 2007;357:154–62.
4. Hayes DF. Clinical practice. Follow-up of patients with early breast cancer. *N Engl J Med*. 2007;356: 2505–13.

ADDITIONAL READING

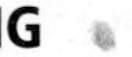

Pruthi S, Brandt KR, Degnim AC, et al. A multidisciplinary approach to the management of breast cancer, part 1: prevention and diagnosis. *Mayo Clin Proc*. 2007;82:999–1012.

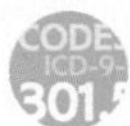

CODES

ICD9

- 174.0 Malignant neoplasm of nipple and areola of female breast
- 174.1 Malignant neoplasm of central portion of female breast
- 174.9 Malignant neoplasm of breast (female), unspecified site

CLINICAL PEARLS

- Pursue/refer all abnormal breast PE/imaging findings.
- Normal mammography does not exclude possibility of cancer with a palpable mass.

BREAST-FEEDING

Julie Scott Taylor, MD, MSc
Kathy Mariani, MD

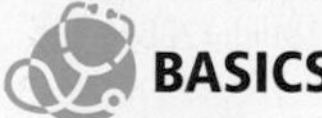

BASICS

- Breast-feeding is the natural process of feeding an infant human milk directly from the breast.
- Breast milk feeding is the process of feeding a child human milk that has been expressed either by hand or by pump.
- The American Academy of Pediatrics (AAP), the American Academy of Family Physicians, and other medical organizations recommend exclusive breast-feeding for approximately the 1st 6 months of life and support for breast-feeding for the 1st year and beyond as long as mutually desired by mother and child (1).

DESCRIPTION

- Maternal benefits (as compared to mothers who do not breast-feed) include: (2)
  - Decreased postpartum bleeding (due to oxytocin release)
  - Decreased risk of postpartum depression
  - Easier postpartum weight loss
  - Delayed postpartum fertility
  - Decreased risk of breast and ovarian cancer
  - Decreased risk of type 2 diabetes
  - Increased sense of well-being (endorphin response)
  - Increased bonding
  - Convenience
  - Cost
- Infant benefits (as compared with children who are formula-fed) include: (2)
  - Ideal food: Easily digestible, nutrients well absorbed, less constipation
  - Lower rates of virtually all infections via maternal antibody protection
    - Fewer respiratory and gastrointestinal infections
    - Decreased incidence of otitis media
    - Decreased severe lower respiratory infection
  - Decreased incidence of obesity
  - Decreased incidence of allergies and atopic dermatitis in childhood
  - Decreased incidence of type I and 2 diabetes
  - Decreased risk of childhood leukemia
  - Decreased risk of sudden infant death syndrome
  - Decreased mortality
  - Increased attachment between mother and baby

EPIDEMIOLOGY

Incidence

According to the most recent National Immunization Survey, for births in the US in 2007(3):

- Any breast-feeding: 75.0%
- Breastfeeding at 6 months: 43.0%
- Breastfeeding at 12 months: 22.4%
- Exclusive breast-feeding at 3 months: 33.0%
- Exclusive breast-feeding at 6 months: 13.3%

RISK FACTORS

Breast surgery, especially reduction surgery, prior to pregnancy may disrupt breast milk production in the future.

GENERAL PREVENTION

Maternal avoidance diets during lactation not recommended to prevent allergic disease (4)[B]

PATHOPHYSIOLOGY

The overarching mechanism of milk production is based on supply and demand.

- Stimulation of areola causes secretion of oxytocin.
- Oxytocin is responsible for let-down reflex when milk is ejected from cells into milk ducts.
- Sucking stimulates secretion of prolactin, which triggers milk production. Thus, milk is made in response to nursing and increases supply.
  - Endocrine/Metabolic: Thyroid dysfunction may cause delayed lactation or decreased milk production.

COMMONLY ASSOCIATED CONDITIONS

- Breast milk jaundice should be considered if jaundice persists for greater than 1 week in an otherwise healthy, well-hydrated newborn. It peaks at 10–14 days.
- Other causes, such as hypothyroidism and infection, should be considered.

DIAGNOSIS

PHYSICAL EXAM

- Examine breasts, ideally during pregnancy, looking for scars or inverted nipples.
- Breast cancer incidence low but possible in premenopausal women.
  - A breast lump should be followed to complete resolution or worked up if present and not just attributed to changes from lactation.

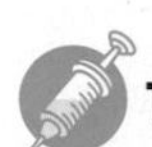

TREATMENT

ADDITIONAL TREATMENT

General Measures

- Flat or inverted nipples:
  - When stimulated, inverted nipples will retract inward, flat nipples remain flat; check for this on initial prenatal physical.
  - Nipple shells, a doughnut-shaped insert, can be worn inside the bra during the last month of pregnancy to gently force the nipple through the center opening of the shell.
  - Babies can nurse successfully even if the shell does not correct the problem before birth.
- Contraindications to breast-feeding are few:
  - Maternal HIV infection
  - Active tuberculosis
  - Substances of abuse and some medications that will pass into human milk (5)[B]
  - Infants with galactosemia should not be fed with breast milk.
  - Maternal hepatitis is not a contraindication to breast-feeding.

Issues for Referral

- Refer to trained physician, nurse, or lactation consultant for inpatient and/or outpatient teaching.
- Frequent follow-up if having problems with latching, sore nipples, or inadequate milk production.

COMPLEMENTARY AND ALTERNATIVE MEDICINE

Fenugreek may increase breast milk production. Suggested dose: 3 tablets t.i.d. Safety is not established.

IN-PATIENT CONSIDERATIONS

Initial Stabilization

- Initiate breast-feeding immediately after birth, ideally placing the infant at the mother's breast in the delivery room.
- Get mother in a comfortable position, usually sitti or reclining with the baby's head in crook of her arm.
  - Side-lying position often useful following cesarean-section delivery.
- Bring baby to mother to decrease stress on mothe back.
- Baby's belly and mother's belly should face each other or touch ("belly to belly"). Initiate the rootir reflex by tickling baby's lips with nipple or finger. baby's mouth opens wide, mother guides her nipp to back of her baby's mouth while pulling the bab closer. This will ensure that the baby's gums are sucking on the areola, not the nipple (6)[C].
- Feed every 2–4 hours, 20 minutes per side.
- Rooming-in to encourage on-demand feeding (6)
- Observation of a nursing session by an experience physician, nurse, or lactation consultant
- Avoid supplementation with formula or water.
- Review expectations, techniques, and feeding cue
- Be very encouraging.

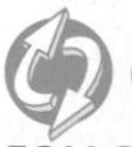

ONGOING CARE

FOLLOW-UP RECOMMENDATIONS

- See mother and baby within a few days of hospita discharge.
- Primary care-initiated interventions to promote breast-feeding have been shown to be successful with respect to child and maternal health outcome

Patient Monitoring

- Monitor infant's weight and output closely.
- Supplementation with infant formula recommende only if infant has lost 7% or more of birth weight, shows signs of dehydration such as decreased urir output, or has less than 3 small stools a day.
- Given that the mechanism of milk production is supply and demand, supplementation without persistent and regular breast stimulation with frequent feedings or breast pump use will decreas milk production and decrease breast-feeding success.

DIET

- For mothers:
  - Continue prenatal vitamins.
  - Drink plenty of fluids: 12.5 cups or 3.0 L of fluid per day.
  - Breast-feeding mothers require 1,800–2,300 calories per day; ~500 more than pre-pregnanc needs.
  - Gassy foods such as cabbage may cause baby to have colic.
  - American Academy of Pediatrics (AAP) suggests limiting maternal caffeine to 300 mg/day.
  - Alcohol should be avoided. 1–2 drinks/week of alcohol may be okay, but mothers should avoid nursing 2–3 hours after a drink. Only <2% of alcohol is passed to baby via breast milk.

For infants:
- In 2008, the AAP increased its recommended daily intake of vitamin D in infants to 400 IU. For exclusively breast-fed babies, this will require taking a vitamin supplement such as Poly-Vi-Sol or Vi-Daylin vitamin drops, 0.5 cc/day, beginning at 2 months of age.
- In 2010, the AAP recommended adding supplementation for breast-fed infants with oral iron 1 mg/kg per day beginning at age 4 months (7).
  - Preterm infants fed human milk should receive an iron supplement of 2 mg/kg per day by 1 month of age, and this should be continued until the infant is weaned to iron-fortified formula or begins eating complementary foods that supply the 2 mg/kg of iron.
- Fluoride supplement unnecessary until 6 months of age.

PATIENT EDUCATION

The US Preventive Services Task Force (USPSTF) recommends structured breast-feeding education and behavioral counseling programs to promote breast-feeding.

Regular promotion of advantages of breast-feeding (8)[C]

Emphasize importance of exclusive breast-feeding for 1st 4 weeks of life to allow adequate buildup of sufficient milk supply.

Discuss woman's postpartum plans (i.e., if going to work). Emphasize possibility of nursing part-time after returning to work or nursing until weaning the week before returning to work.

Immediate breast-feeding after the birth.

Milk will not come in before 3rd day postpartum.

Frequent nursing (8–12 feedings per 24 hours) will lead to milk coming in sooner and in greater quantities.

Baby should have 5–8 wet diapers per day and 2–5 bowel movements per day.

After day 4 of life, should gain 4–7 oz per week

See in office within a few days of discharge, especially if 1st time breastfeeding

Signs of adequate nursing:
- Breasts become hard before and soft after feeding.
- 6 or more wet diapers in 24 hours
- Baby satisfied; appropriate weight gain (average 1 oz/day in 1st few months)

Growth spurts: Anticipate these ~10 days, 6 weeks, 3 months, and 4–6 months. Baby will nurse more often at these times for several days. This will increase milk production to allow for further adequate growth.

The AAP recommends supplementation with vitamin D starting at age 2 months and iron starting at age 4 months (7,9).

Weaning:
- Exclusive breast milk is optimal food for 1st 6 months.
- Solid food may be introduced at 6 months.
- For mothers going to work, start switching the baby to breast milk feeding or formula feeding during the hours mother will be gone about a week ahead of time. Do this by dropping a feeding every few days and substituting pumped breast milk or formula, preferably given by another caregiver.

- Family planning:
  - Lactational amenorrhea method (LAM): Breast-feeding may be used as effective birth control option if (1) infant is less than 6 months old, (2) infant is exclusively breast-feeding, and (3) mother is amenorrheic (10).
  - Other options include barrier methods, implants, Depo-Provera, oral contraception, and intrauterine devices.
  - Most providers use progesterone-only birth control pills in the early postpartum period.
- The Academy of Breastfeeding Medicine (ABM), a worldwide organization of physicians dedicated to the promotion, protection and support of breastfeeding and human lactation. www.bfmed.org
- La Leche League at www.llli.org
- Protecting, Promoting and Supporting Breastfeeding: The Special Role of Maternity Services, a joint WHO/UNICEF statement published by the World Health Organization. http://www.unicef.org/newsline/tenstps.htm
- Thomas Hale's Medications and Mother's Milk: A Manual of Lactational Pharmacology.

COMPLICATIONS

- Plugged duct:
  - Mother is well except for sore lump in 1 or both breasts without fever
  - Use moist, hot packs on lump prior to and during nursing.
  - More frequent nursing on affected side; ensure good technique
- Mastitis (see topic Mastitis):
  - Sore lump in 1 or both breasts plus fever and/or redness on skin overlying lump
  - Use moist, hot packs on lump prior to and during nursing; more frequent nursing on affected side.
  - Antibiotics covering for *Staphylococcus aureus* (the most common organism) for at least 7 days (11)
  - Other possible sources of fever should be ruled out, endometritis, pyelonephritis in particular.
  - Mother should get increased rest; use acetaminophen (Tylenol) as necessary.
  - Fever should resolve within 48 hours or consider changing antibiotics. Lump should also resolve. If it continues, an abscess may be present, requiring surgical drainage.
- Milk supply inadequate:
  - Check infant weight gain.
  - Review signs of adequate supply; technique, frequency, and duration of nursing.
  - Check to see if mother has been supplementing, thereby decreasing her own milk production.
- Sore nipples:
  - Check technique.
  - Baby should be taken off the breast by breaking the suction with a finger in the mouth.
  - Air-dry nipples after each nursing and/or coat with expressed breast milk.
  - Do not wash nipples with soap and water.
  - Check for signs of thrush in baby and on mother's nipple. If affected, treat both.
- Engorgement:
  - Usually develops after milk 1st comes in (day 3 or 4)
  - Signs are warm, hard, sore breasts.
  - To resolve, offer baby more frequent nursing
    - May have to hand express a little milk to soften areola enough to let baby latch on.
    - Breast-feed long enough to empty breasts.
  - Generally resolves within a day or 2.

REFERENCES

1. http://www.aap.org/advocacy/releases/feb05breastfeeding.htm
2. *Breastfeeding and Maternal and Infant Health Outcomes in Developed Countries [Structured Abstract]*. Rockville, MD: Agency for Healthcare Research and Quality, 2007. Available at: http://www.ahrq.gov/clinic/tp/brfouttp.htm.
3. http://www.cdc.gov/breastfeeding/pdf/BreastfeedingReportCard2010.pdf
4. U.S. Department of Health and Human Services. *Healthy People 2010*, Conference ed. Vols I and II. Washington, DC: U.S. Department of Health and Human Services, Public Health Service, Office of the Assistant Secretary for Health, January 2000.
5. Berlin CM, Briggs GG. Drugs and chemicals in human milk. *Semin Fetal Neonatal Med*. 2005;10:149–59.
6. Sinusas K, Gagliardi A. Initial management of breast-feeding. *Am Fam Phys*. 2001;15;64:981–8.
7. http://www.aap.org/pressroom/Ironfinal.pdf
8. Chung M, Raman G, Trikalinos T, Lau J, Ip S et al. Interventions in primary care to promote breastfeeding: an evidence review for the U.S. Preventive Services Task Force. *Ann. Intern. Med.* 2008;149:565–82.
9. Casey CF, Slawson DC, Neal LR et al. Vitamin D supplementation in infants, children, and adolescents. *Am Fam Physician*. 2010;81:745–8.
10. http://www.llli.org/ba/Aug93.html
11. Jahanfar S, Ng CJ, Teng CL et al. Antibiotics for mastitis in breastfeeding women. *Cochrane Database Syst Rev*. 2009;CD005458.

ADDITIONAL READING

- Cramton R, Zain-Ul-Abideen M, Whalen B et al. Optimizing successful breastfeeding in the newborn. *Curr Opin Pediatr*. 2009;21:386–96.
- Grummer-Strawn LM, Shealy KR et al. Progress in protecting, promoting, and supporting breastfeeding: 1984–2009. *Breastfeeding medicine: the official journal of the Academy of Breastfeeding Medicine*. 2009;4 (Suppl 1):S31–9.

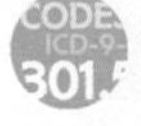

CODES

ICD9

V24.1 Postpartum care and examination of lactating mother

CLINICAL PEARLS

- Breast milk is the optimal food for infants with myriad health benefits for mothers and children.
- USPSTF recommends structured education to promote breast-feeding.
- Vitamin D and iron supplementation should begin at 2 and 4 months of age, respectively, for exclusively breast-fed infants.

BREECH BIRTH

Kimberle Vore, MD

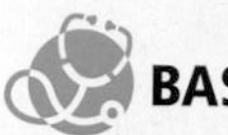

BASICS

DESCRIPTION

At the time of delivery, the fetal buttocks or lower limbs are the presenting part in the maternal pelvis:

- Frank breech: Fetal hips flexed and knees extended with feet near the shoulders (45–60% of breech presentations at term)
- Footling or incomplete breech: Foot or knee presenting (25–35% of breech presentations)
- Complete breech: Hips and knees flexed (as if squatting) (5–15% of breech presentations)

EPIDEMIOLOGY

Prevalence

- 3–4% of singleton term deliveries and up to 15–30% of low-birth-weight infants (<2,500 g)
- Breech presentation is common in early pregnancy. At 25–26 weeks, ~20–30% of singleton fetuses are in breech position, but this decreases near term.

RISK FACTORS

- Previous history of breech birth
- Fetal anomalies; see Genetics.
- Low-birth-weight or premature infant
- Oligohydramnios
- Uterine anomalies, including bicornate uterus
- Uterine relaxation associated with great parity
- Uterine overdistention as in polyhydramnios or multiple gestation
- Placenta previa
- Placental implantation in cornual-fundal region
- Pelvic contractures or irregularly shaped pelvis, such as android or platypelloid pelvis
- Pelvic tumors

Genetics

Fetal anomalies, including anencephaly, hydrocephalus, trisomy 21 and 18, Potter syndrome, and myotonic dystrophy, have higher incidences of breech birth.

GENERAL PREVENTION

- Antenatal folate therapy to decrease risk of neural tube defects
- Prevention of fetal anomalies by tight glucose control in diabetics

COMMONLY ASSOCIATED CONDITIONS

- See Risk Factors.
- Congenital hip dislocation has higher incidence in infants with breech presentation at term.

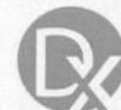

DIAGNOSIS

HISTORY

Mother reports kicking in lower abdomen

PHYSICAL EXAM

- Anus palpable on digital vaginal exam
- Leopold maneuver reveals ballottable head in fundal region.
- Presenting part not palpable in pelvis near term

DIAGNOSTIC TESTS & INTERPRETATION

Imaging

Initial approach

Ultrasound confirms presenting part

Diagnostic Procedures/Surgery

- Near-term women should be examined to determine presenting part.
- If breech is suspected, an ultrasound should be done to confirm presenting part.
- When breech presentation is confirmed, the options of external version or elective cesarean section should be discussed with the patient.

Pathological Findings

Congenital malformation among term breech infants: Overall incidence 6–9%

DIFFERENTIAL DIAGNOSIS

- Face vs. breech presentation on vaginal exam
- In breech presentation, greater trochanter and anus form a straight line. In face presentation, mouth and malar bones form a triangle.

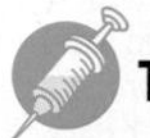

TREATMENT

ADDITIONAL TREATMENT

General Measures

- Continuous electronic fetal monitoring during labor
- Breech presentation may be converted to vertex by external version.
- American College of Obstetricians and Gynecologists (ACOG) recommends external version at term. Decision for mode of delivery should depend on the experience of the health provider, with planned cesarean delivery for persistent breech presentation likely to be preferred.
- In 2000, the Term Breech Trial showed decreased perinatal and neonatal morbidity and mortality in planned breech cesarean delivery (1) [NNT 30] vs. planned breech vaginal delivery. There was no difference in maternal morbidity or mortality (1)[B].
- In 2005, a large observational prospective study showed no difference in neonatal outcomes when vaginal breech candidates were carefully selected and followed strict protocols (2).

Additional Therapies

External cephalic version:

- Conversion of breech to vertex can be attempted after 36 weeks of gestation and, if successful, allows for vaginal vertex delivery. Success rates 48–78%, with reversion rates back to breech of 2% (3)[B].
- External cephalic version associated with risk (1–2%) of umbilical cord entanglement, abruptio placenta, preterm labor, premature rupture of membranes, fetal brachycardia, fetal–maternal hemorrhage, and severe maternal discomfort.
- Prior to procedure, tocolytics are usually administered and RhoGAM is given to Rh-negative mothers (3)[B].
- External cephalic version should be attempted only with continuous fetal heart monitoring in the delivery suite, where immediate cesarean delivery can be done (3)[C].
- Contraindications to external cephalic version include multiple pregnancy, nonreassuring fetal monitoring, placenta previa, premature rupture of membranes, placental abruption, uterine malformation, oligohydramnios, or major fetal anomalies.
- Predictors of successful external cephalic version include multiparity, relaxed abdominal wall, adequate amniotic fluid, nonfrank breech, floating presenting part, posterior placenta, and average maternal body weight.

SURGERY/OTHER PROCEDURES

- Breech delivery is accomplished either vaginally or by cesarean section (4).
- Most physicians and patients opt for elective cesarean delivery for breech presentation near term which is usually planned for the 39th week of pregnancy.
- When a patient presents in labor with the fetus in breech position, a decision about a trial of labor or immediate cesarean section must be made. Ideally this decision is made prior to onset of labor.
- Obtain ultrasound to document fetal presentation, check for fetal abnormalities, and estimate fetal weight in deciding candidacy for vaginal delivery.
- Vaginal breech delivery may be appropriate in the following situations:
  - Breech presentation in advanced labor
  - Delivery of a 2nd twin in nonvertex presentation
  - Fetus too immature to survive
  - Fetus with congenital defects incompatible with life
  - Multiparous mother, estimated fetal weight not greater than that of siblings delivered by uncomplicated SVD

Cesarean section procedure:
- Prepare for cesarean section by starting IV fluids and obtaining blood type and screen, in all patients, in case needed for emergency.
- A low transverse cesarean section may need to be extended vertically if there is difficulty with head entrapment (this extension produces a weak scar).
- General anesthesia with isoflurane can rapidly relax the uterus and allow delivery of an entrapped after-coming head.
- Delivery is usually accomplished with spinal anesthesia.
- Cord blood gases should be obtained following delivery.

Vaginal delivery procedures:
- The candidate for vaginal delivery needs to be attended by a birth attendant skilled in breech delivery, a scrubbed assistant, an anesthesiologist capable of rapid induction of general anesthesia, and an individual skilled in neonatal resuscitation.
- Epidural is preferred anesthesia.
- Leave membranes intact as long as possible to prevent possible cord prolapse.
- The patient should not push until fully dilated due to risk of partial delivery through a cervix that is not fully dilated, which can lead to head entrapment.
- Consider cutting a large episiotomy to allow sufficient room for delivery.
- Use abdominal guidance of fetal head to keep it flexed as it descends into the pelvis.
- The infant should not be touched before the umbilicus crosses the maternal perineum. Traction prior to this point constitutes a complete breech extraction and is associated with higher risk of perinatal morbidity and mortality.
- With the fetal back anterior, maintain downward traction while grasping the fetal hips until the scapula becomes visible.
- Check for nuchal arm.
- As 1 axilla becomes visible, rotate the infant until the shoulders are oriented anteriorly and posteriorly, allowing their delivery.
- The fetal head is delivered in a face-down position with either piper forceps or manual flexion of the head.
- Cord blood gases should be obtained following delivery.

N-PATIENT CONSIDERATIONS

Admission Criteria

- For planned C-section
- For labor and delivery

V Fluids

Maintain IV access and hydration status with lactated Ringer's or saline solution.

Discharge Criteria

- After delivery once stable
- 1–4 days after delivery depending on vaginal vs. breech delivery

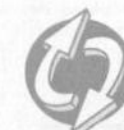

ONGOING CARE

FOLLOW-UP RECOMMENDATIONS

Routine postpartum care

Patient Monitoring

Continuous electronic fetal monitoring during labor

DIET

NPO

PATIENT EDUCATION

Educate patient about increased risk of fetal distress and fetal trauma in both cesarean and vaginal breech delivery compared to vaginal vertex delivery.

PROGNOSIS

- Perinatal morbidity and mortality are much higher in breech births. A large proportion of the deaths are related to congenital abnormalities.
- Successful external cephalic version at term significantly lowers cesarean rate (15)[A].
- For infants 750–1,500 g or <32 weeks gestational age, a much higher rate of cerebral hemorrhage and perinatal death is associated with vaginal compared to cesarean delivery.

COMPLICATIONS

- Trauma to the head, soft tissue, brachial plexus, and spinal cord; not always prevented by cesarean
- Entrapment of fetal head
- Asphyxia secondary to cord compression or prolapse
- Congenital hip dislocation

REFERENCES

1. Hannah ME, Hannah WJ, Hewson SA et al. Planned caesarean section versus planned vaginal birth for breech presentation at term: a randomised multicentre trial. Term Breech Trial Collaborative Group. *Lancet*. 2000;356:1375–83.
2. Goffinet F, Carayol M, Foidart J et al. Is planned vaginal delivery for breech presentation at term still an option? Results of an observational prospective survey in France and Belgium. *Am J Obstet Gynecol*. 2006;194:1002–11.
3. American College of Obstetricians and Gynecologists. External cephalic version. Practice Bulletin No. 13. February, 2000.
4. American College of Obstetricians and Gynecologists, Committee on Obstetric Practice. ACOG committee opinion. Mode of term singleton breech delivery. Practice Bulletin No. 340. July, 2006. American College of Obstetricians and Gynecologists.
5. Tan JM, Macario A, Carvalho B et al. Cost-effectiveness of external cephalic version for term breech presentation. *BMC Pregnancy Childbirth*. 2010;10:3.

ADDITIONAL READING

Kotaska A, Menticoglou S, Gagnon R et al. Vaginal delivery of breech presentation. *J Obstet Gynaecol Can*. 2009;31.

See Also (Topic, Algorithm, Electronic Media Element)

Placenta Previa; Preterm Labor

CODES

ICD9

- 652.10 Breech or other malpresentation successfully converted to cephalic presentation, unspecified as to episode of care
- 652.20 Breech presentation without mention of version, unspecified as to episode of care
- 652.80 Other specified malposition or malpresentation, unspecified as to episode of care

CLINICAL PEARLS

- Vaginal breech delivery is associated with increased risk of prolapsed cord and/or cord compression; fetal hypoxia; nuchal arm, with attendant risk of trauma, including humerus fracture, clavicle fracture, and nerve palsies; and entrapment of fetal head.
- External version after 36 weeks gestation may allow for vaginal vertex delivery with decreased risk of infant and maternal morbidity.
- If a patient goes into labor prior to a planned elective cesarean breech delivery, which is usually scheduled at 39–40 weeks gestation, she should go immediately to the hospital.
- Risks of cesarean delivery include infection, bleeding, and possible damage to maternal bladder or bowel; there is a slightly increased risk of maternal mortality compared with vaginal vertex delivery. Maternal recovery time is almost always longer with cesarean delivery.

BRONCHIECTASIS

Dylan C. Kwait, MD

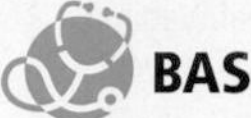

BASICS

DESCRIPTION

- Bronchiectasis is an irreversible dilation of 1 or more airways accompanied by recurrent transmural bronchial infection/inflammation and chronic mucopurulent sputum production.
- Generally classified into cystic fibrosis (CF) and noncystic fibrosis (non-CF) bronchiectasis.

EPIDEMIOLOGY

- Predominant age: Most commonly presents in 6th decade of life (1)
- Predominant sex: Female > Male (1)

Incidence

Incidence has decreased in the US for 2 reasons:

- Widespread childhood vaccination against pertussis (2)
- Effective treatment of childhood respiratory infections with antibiotics (1)

Prevalence

- Prevalence in adult US population estimated to be >110,000 affected individuals (1)
- Internationally, prevalence increases with age from 4.2 per 100,000 persons aged 18–34 years to 271.8 per 100,000 among those aged 75 years or older (3).

RISK FACTORS

- Nontuberculous mycobacterial infection is both a cause and a complication of non-CF bronchiectasis (4).
- Severe respiratory infection in childhood (measles, adenovirus, influenza, pertussis, or bronchiolitis)
- Systemic diseases (e.g., rheumatoid arthritis and connective tissue disorders)
- Chronic rhinosinusitis
- Recurrent pneumonia
- Aspirated foreign body
- Immunodeficiency

GENERAL PREVENTION

- Routine immunizations against pertussis, measles, Haemophilus influenza type B, influenza, and pneumococcal pneumonia
- Genetic counseling where congenital condition may increase likelihood of bronchiectasis
- Smoking cessation counseling

PATHOPHYSIOLOGY

Vicious circle hypothesis: Transmural infection, generally by bacterial organisms, causes inflammation and obstruction of airways. Damaged airways and dysfunctional cilia foster bacterial colonization, which leads to further inflammation and obstruction (2)[A].

ETIOLOGY

- CF bronchiectasis: Bronchiectasis due to cystic fibrosis
- Non-CF bronchiectasis:
  - Most cases are idiopathic.
  - Most commonly associated with non-CF bronchiectasis is childhood infection (2).

COMMONLY ASSOCIATED CONDITIONS

- Mucociliary clearance defects:
  - Primary ciliary dyskinesia
  - Young syndrome (secondary ciliary dyskinesia)
  - Kartagener syndrome
- Other congenital conditions:
  - α1-Antitrypsin deficiency
  - Marfan syndrome
  - Cartilage deficiency (Williams-Campbell syndrome)
- Chronic obstructive pulmonary disease
- Postinfectious conditions:
  - Bacteria (*H. influenzae* and *P. aeruginosa*)
  - Mycobacterial infections (TB and MAC)
  - Whooping cough
  - Aspergillus species
  - Viral (HIV, adenovirus, measles, influenza virus)
- Immunodeficient conditions:
  - Primary: Hypogammaglobulinemia
  - Secondary: Allergic bronchopulmonary aspergillosis, post-transplantation
- Sequelae of toxic inhalation or aspiration (e.g., chlorine, luminal foreign body)
- Rheumatic/chronic inflammatory conditions:
  - Rheumatoid arthritis
  - Sjögren syndrome
  - Systemic lupus erythematosus
  - Inflammatory bowel disease
- Miscellaneous:
  - Yellow nail syndrome

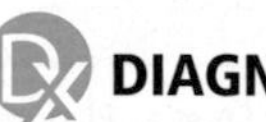

DIAGNOSIS

- Typical symptoms include chronic productive cough, wheezing, and dyspnea.
- Symptoms are often accompanied by repeated respiratory infections (5).
- Once diagnosed, investigation of possible causes and associated conditions is essential.

HISTORY

- Time course of illness
- Any predisposing factors (congenital, infectious, and/or exposure-related)
- Immunization history

PHYSICAL EXAM

Symptoms are commonly present for many years and include (1,2):

- Chronic cough (90%)
- Sputum may be copious and purulent (90%).
- Rhinosinusitis (60–70%)
- Fatigue may be a dominant symptom (70%).
- Dyspnea (75%)
- Chest pain may be pleuritic (20–30%).
- Hemoptysis (20–30%)
- Wheezing (20%)
- Bibasilar crackles (60%)
- Rhonchi (44%)
- Digital clubbing (3%)

DIAGNOSTIC TESTS & INTERPRETATION

- Spirometry:
  - Limited use in diagnosis
  - Characterized by moderate airflow obstruction and hyperresponsive airways (1)
  - FEV1 <80% predicted and FEV1/FVC <0.7 (6)
- Special tests:
  - Ciliary biopsy by electron microscopy

Lab

- Sputum culture (1):
  - *H. influenzae*, nontypeable form (42%)
  - *P. aeruginosa* (18%)
  - Cultures may also be positive for *S. pneumoniae*, *M. catarrhalis*, MAC, and *Aspergillus*.
  - 30–40% of all isolates will show no growth.
- Special tests:
  - Sweat test for CF
  - PPD test for TB
  - Skin test for *Aspergillus*
  - HIV
  - Serum immunoglobulins to test for humoral immunodeficiency

Imaging

- Chest radiograph:
  - Nonspecific findings; sensitivity and specificity are too low to confirm the diagnosis (6).
  - Increased lung markings (1)
  - May appear normal
- Chest CT:
  - Noncontrast high-resolution chest CT is most important diagnostic tool (2).
  - Bronchi are dilated and do not taper.
  - Varicose constrictions and balloon cysts may also be appreciated (2).

Diagnostic Procedures/Surgery

Interventional bronchoscopy may be used to obtain cultures and evacuate sputum.

Pathological Findings

Bronchoscopy findings include (2):

- Dilation of airways
- Thickened bronchial walls with necrosis of bronchial mucosa
- Peribronchial scarring

DIFFERENTIAL DIAGNOSIS

- CF
- Chronic obstructive pulmonary disease
- Asthma
- Chronic bronchitis
- Pulmonary TB
- Allergic bronchopulmonary aspergillosis

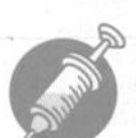

TREATMENT

- Non-CF bronchiectasis: Determining cause of exacerbations, promoting good bronchopulmonary hygiene via daily airway clearance, and surgical resection of damaged lung if necessary
- Medical management: Reduce morbidity by controlling symptoms and preventing disease progression.
- Patients with non-CF bronchiectasis may not respond to CF treatment regimens in the same way as patients with CF (4)[A].

MEDICATION

- Treat acute exacerbations with short courses of antibiotics.
- Frequent exacerbations may be treated with prolonged and aerosolized antibiotics (5)[A].
- The role of mucolytics, anti-inflammatory agents, and bronchodilators is still unclear (5)[A].

rst Line

Antibiotics:

- Useful in acute exacerbations
- Chronic therapy decreases sputum volume and purulence, but does not diminish the frequency of exacerbations (7)[A].
- Patients may require twice usual dose and longer treatment (7–14 days) (6)[B].
- Sputum culture and sensitivity should direct therapy; antibiotic selection complicated by wide range of pathogens and resistant organisms.
- Should be administered IV in cases of severe infection:
  - Augmentin (6)[B]: 500 mg p.o. every 8–12 hours for 7–10 days. Pediatric: Base dosing on amoxicillin content.
  - Trimethoprim/sulfamethoxazole (6)[B]: 160 mg TMP/800 mg SMX p.o. every 12 hours for 10–14 days. Pediatric: ≥2 months, 8 mg/kg TMP and 40 mg/kg SMX p.o. per 24 hours, administered in 2 divided doses every 12 hours for 10 days
  - Doxycycline and cefaclor given orally are also effective (6)[B].
  - Nebulized aminoglycosides (tobramycin): 300 mg by aerosol b.i.d. (8)[B]
  - Macrolides: Appear to have immunomodulatory benefits (1)[A]

Bronchodilators:

- Chronic use of β_2–agonists (e.g., albuterol) reverses airflow obstruction (1)[A].

Inhaled corticosteroids:

- There is insufficient evidence to recommend use of inhaled steroids in adults with stable-state bronchiectasis (9)[A].
- A therapeutic trial of inhaled steroids may be justified in adults with difficult-to-control symptoms and in certain subgroups (9)[A].
- Decrease sputum and tend to improve lung function (6)[B]:
  - Fluticasone: 110–220 μg inhaled b.i.d.

econd Line

ther broad-spectrum antimicrobials, including ntipseudomonals

DDITIONAL TREATMENT

eneral Measures

Dry powder mannitol improves tracheobronchial clearance (1)[A].

Maintain hydration (nebulized saline may be used) (2)[A].

Noninvasive positive-pressure ventilation (2)[A]

ssues for Referral

ay require pulmonologist for bronchoscopy and/or ng-term management

dditional Therapies

utum clearance techniques, including physiotherapy ercussion and postural drainage) and pulmonary habilitation (improves exercise tolerance) (1)[A]

URGERY/OTHER PROCEDURES

Surgery if area of bronchiectasis is localized and symptoms remain intolerable despite medical therapy or if disease is life-threatening (5)[A]

Surgery effectively improves symptoms in 80% of these cases (1)[A].

IN-PATIENT CONSIDERATIONS

For non-CF bronchiectasis, determine cause of exacerbations, promoting good bronchopulmonary hygiene via daily airway clearance, and surgical resection when necessary.

Initial Stabilization

Hemoptysis, although rare, may occur and can be life-threatening.

ONGOING CARE

Long-term outpatient treatment recommendations for bronchiectasis in children (10)[B]:

- Children with CF- and non–CF-related bronchiectasis should be treated by comprehensive interdisciplinary chronic disease management programs.
- Pathogen-directed aerosolized tobramycin treatment should be used long term on a regular basis to improve the course of CF-related bronchiectasis.
- Oral macrolide antibiotic use short term (up to 6 months) improves lung function among children with CF-related bronchiectasis.
- Long-term antibiotic use (oral or aerosolized) in children with non–CF-related bronchiectasis has not been studied enough to warrant routine use.
- Hypertonic saline administered by inhalation used long term (48 weeks) improves lung function and is safer when used with pretreatment bronchodilator therapy among children who have CF.
- Nebulized dornase improves multiple pulmonary outcomes of children who have CF and is indicated for long-term use.
- The risks for long-term oral corticosteroid use outweigh pulmonary benefits in the treatment of CF-related bronchiectasis.
- High-dose ibuprofen therapy reduces the rate of decline among children with mild CF-related bronchiectasis and is indicated for long-term use.
- Mucolytic agents, airway hydrating treatments, anti-inflammatory therapy, CPT, and bronchodilator therapy have not been studied sufficiently long term in children with non–CF-related bronchiectasis to merit their routine use.

FOLLOW-UP RECOMMENDATIONS

Regular exercise is recommended.

Patient Monitoring

- Serial spirometry, every 2–5 years, to monitor the course of the disease (1)[A]
- Routine microbiological sputum analysis (1)[A]

PATIENT EDUCATION

American Lung Association, 1740 Broadway, New York, NY 10019; (212) 315-8700, http://www.lungusa.org

PROGNOSIS

- Mortality rate (death due directly to bronchiectasis) is 13% (1).
- *Pseudomonas* infection is associated with poorer prognosis (1).

COMPLICATIONS

- Hemoptysis
- Recurrent pulmonary infections
- Pulmonary hypertension
- Cor pulmonale
- Lung abscess

REFERENCES

1. King P, Holdsworth S, Freezer N, et al. Bronchiectasis. *Intern Med J*. 2006;36:729–37.
2. Barker AF. Bronchiectasis. *N Engl J Med*. 2002;346:1383–93.
3. Pappalettera M, Aliberti S, Castellotti P, et al. Bronchiectasis: an update. *Clin Respir J*. 2009;3:126–34.
4. Bilton D. Update on non-cystic fibrosis bronchiectasis. *Curr Opin Pulm Med*. 2008;14:595–9.
5. ten Hacken NH, Wijkstra PJ, Kerstjens HA. Treatment of bronchiectasis in adults. *BMJ*. 2007;335:1089–93.
6. Bradley J, Lavery K, Rendall J, et al. Managing bronchiectasis. *Practitioner*. 2006;250:194, 197, 199–200 passim.
7. Evans DJ, Bara AI, Greenstone M. Prolonged antibiotics for purulent bronchiectasis. *Cochrane Database Syst Rev*. 2006;4:CD00284.
8. Lobue PA. Inhaled tobramycin: not just for cystic fibrosis anymore? *Chest*. 2005;127:1098–101.
9. Kapur N, Bell S, Kolbe J, et al. Inhaled steroids for bronchiectasis. *Cochrane Database Syst Rev*. 2009:CD000996.
10. Redding GJ. Bronchiectasis in children. *Pediatr Clin North Am*. 2009;56:157–71,xi.

ADDITIONAL READING

Pasteur MC, Bilton D, Hill AT, British Thoracic Society Bronchiectasis non-CF Guideline Group, et al. British Thoracic Society guideline for non-CF bronchiectasis. *Thorax*. 2010;65(Suppl 1):i1–58.

See Also (Topic, Algorithm, Electronic Media Element)

Cystic Fibrosis; Chronic Obstructive Pulmonary Disease; Asthma; Pulmonary Tuberculosis; Aspergillosis; Kartagener Syndrome

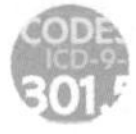

CODES

ICD9

- 494.0 Bronchiectasis without acute exacerbation
- 494.1 Bronchiectasis with acute exacerbation

CLINICAL PEARLS

- Symptoms of bronchiectasis include chronic productive cough, wheezing, and dyspnea, often accompanied by repeated respiratory infections.
- CXR has poor sensitivity and specificity for the diagnosis; noncontrast high-resolution chest CT is the most important diagnostic tool.
- Treat acute exacerbations with short courses of antibiotics; frequent exacerbations may be treated with prolonged and aerosolized antibiotics.

BRONCHIOLITIS

Dennis E. Hughes, DO

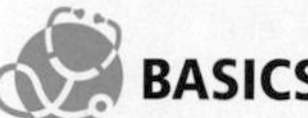

BASICS

DESCRIPTION

- Inflammation and obstruction of small airways and reactive airways generally affecting infants and young children
- May be seasonal (winter and spring) and often occurs in epidemics
- Usual course: Insidious, acute, progressive
- Leading cause of hospitalizations in infants and children
- Predominant age: Newborn–2 years (peak age <6 months). Neonates are not protected despite transfer of maternal antibody.
- Predominant sex: Male > Female

EPIDEMIOLOGY

Incidence

- 21% in North America
- 18.8% (90,000 annually) of all pediatric hospitalizations (excluding live births) in children <2 years of age
- Incidence increasing since 1980

RISK FACTORS

- Smoking exposure
- Low birth weight
- Immunodeficiency
- Formula feeding (not breastfed)
- Contact with infected person (primary mode of spread)
- Children in daycare environment
- Heart-lung transplantation patient
- Adults: Exposure to toxic fumes, connective tissue disease

GENERAL PREVENTION

- Handwashing
- Contact isolation of infected babies
- Persons with colds should keep contacts with infants to a minimum
- Palivizumab (Synagis), a monoclonal product, administered monthly, October–May, 15 mg/kg IM; used for respiratory syncytial virus prevention in high-risk patients (1):
  - 32–35-week gestation and <3 months old at the start of RSV season with at least 1 risk factor: Either attending daycare or with a sibling <5 years old at home
  - 28–32-week gestation and <6 months old
  - <28 weeks gestation and <12 months old
  - Moderately severe bronchopulmonary dysplasia and up to 2 years old
  - Hemodynamically significant congenital heart disease (until age 6 months)
  - Once begun, continue through end of season regardless of age attained
- Respiratory syncytial virus immune globulin, a human blood product, can also be used in at-risk patients. Monthly infusions of 750 mg/kg, October–May.

PATHOPHYSIOLOGY

- Infection results in necrosis and lysis of epithelial cells and subsequent release of inflammatory mediators.
- Edema and mucus secretion that, combined with accumulating necrotic debris and loss of cilia clearance, results in luminal obstruction.
- Ventilation-perfusion mismatching resulting in hypoxia
- Air trapping is due to dynamic airways narrowing during expiration, which increases work of breathing.

ETIOLOGY

Respiratory syncytial virus accounts for 70–85% of all cases, but parainfluenza virus, adenovirus, rhinovirus, influenza virus, *Mycoplasma pneumoniae*, and *Chlamydia pneumoniae* have all been implicated.

Pediatric Considerations

Prior infection does not seem to confer subsequent immunity.

COMMONLY ASSOCIATED CONDITIONS

- Upper respiratory congestion
- Conjunctivitis
- Pharyngitis
- Otitis media
- Diarrhea

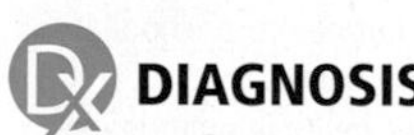

DIAGNOSIS

Consensus is that history and physical examination should be the basis for the diagnosis of bronchiolitis (2).

HISTORY

- Irritability
- Anorexia
- Fever
- Noisy breathing (due to rhinorrhea)
- Cough
- Grunting
- Cyanosis
- Apnea
- Vomiting

PHYSICAL EXAM

- Tachypnea
- Retractions
- Rhinorrhea
- Wheezing
- Upper respiratory findings: Pharyngitis, conjunctivitis, otitis

DIAGNOSTIC TESTS & INTERPRETATION

Routine laboratory and other ancillary testing not warranted

Lab

Initial lab tests

- Arterial oxygen saturation by pulse oximetry (<94 significant)
- Rapid respiratory viral antigen testing (not usually necessary during respiratory syncytial virus [RSV] season because the disease is managed symptomatically, but may be useful for epidemiologic, hospital cohorting purposes, or in the very young to reduce unnecessary other workup):
  - Sensitivity 87–91%; specificity 96–100% (2)

Imaging

Initial approach

Chest x-ray (CXR):

- Increased anteroposterior diameter
- Flattened diaphragm
- Air trapping
- Patchy infiltrates
- Focal atelectasis: Right upper lobe common
- Peribronchial cuffing

Pathological Findings

- Abundant mucous exudate
- Mucosal: Hyperemia, edema
- Submucosal lymphocytic infiltrate, monocytic infiltrate, plasmacytic infiltrate
- Small airway debris, fibrin, inflammatory exudate, fibrosis
- Peribronchiolar mononuclear infiltrate

DIFFERENTIAL DIAGNOSIS

- Other pulmonary infections such as pertussis, croup, or bacterial pneumonia
- Aspiration
- Vascular ring
- Foreign body
- Asthma
- Heart failure
- Gastroesophageal reflux
- Cystic fibrosis

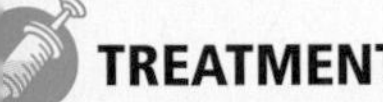

TREATMENT

ainstay of therapy is supportive to prevent hypoxia d dehydration.

IEDICATION

rst Line

- Oxygen
- Nebulized albuterol (0.15 mg/kg) is often tried for acute symptoms; a trial of therapy may be reasonable in the presence of a bronchospastic component, but no benefit noted in several high-quality studies (3)[B].
- Epinephrine aerosols (0.5 mL of 2.25% solution in 3 mL NS) also may be tried. Benefit remains unproved, but some studies support short-term improvement in outpatient settings (4,5)[B].
- Corticosteroids:
  – Oral dexamethasone (1 mg/kg loading dose, then 0.6 mg/kg b.i.d. for 5 days) reduced subsequent hospitalization. A recent multiple-center trial found no difference in admission rates or respiratory assessment scores in children treated with 1 mg/kg dexamethasone (6)[B].
  – Nebulized dexamethasone (2–4 mg in 3 mL NS) may have anecdotal benefit; studies show mixed results.

econd Line

- Antibiotics only if secondary bacterial infection present (rare) (7)[B]
- Heliox therapy (70% helium–30% oxygen) may be of benefit early in moderate-to-severe bronchiolitis to reduce amount of respiratory distress (8).
- Ribavirin (palivizumab):
  – Updated AAP guidelines for use (for prevention in high-risk children)
  – Inhaled antiviral agent active against RSV
  – Nebulize via small-particle aerosol generator.
  – Pregnant women should not be exposed.

DDITIONAL TREATMENT

- Nebulized hypertonic (3%) saline has recently been studied and may decease LOS in hospitalized patients (5).
- Positive pressure ventilation (PPV) in the form of CPAP can be used in cases of respiratory failure. There is limited clinical evidence other than observational studies (5).
- Leukotriene receptor antagonists currently show no sustained benefit (5).

N-PATIENT CONSIDERATIONS

ronchiolitis can be associated with apnea.

nitial Stabilization

upplemental oxygen for pulse oximetry <94% on oom air

Admission Criteria

- Respiratory rate >45/min with respiratory distress or apnea
- Hypoxia is common; evidence-based cutoff requiring admission is not available (only "D" level-expert opinion), so clinical criteria are more helpful.
- Ill or toxic appearance
- Underlying heart, respiratory condition, or immune suppression
- High risk for apnea (<30 days of age, preterm birth [<37 weeks]) (7)[B]
- Dehydrated or unable to feed
- Uncertain home care
- Use of Respiratory Distress Assessment Instrument can aid in determining admission vs discharge. Scoring based on quantification and quality of wheezes, retractions, and respiratory rate (6).

IV Fluids

Indicated only if tachypnea precludes oral feeding. Weight-based maintenance rate plus insensible losses

Discharge Criteria

Normal respiratory rate and no oxygen requirement (recent small studies suggest that after a period of observation, children can be safely discharged on home oxygen)

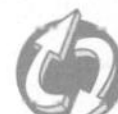

ONGOING CARE

FOLLOW-UP RECOMMENDATIONS

Patient Monitoring

- Hospitalization is usually only required if oxygen is a requirement or unable to feed/drink.
- For a hospitalized patient, monitor as needed depending on the severity of the infection.
- If the patient is receiving home care, follow daily by telephone for 2–4 days; the patient may need frequent office visits.

PATIENT EDUCATION

- American Academy of Pediatrics: http://www.aap.org
- American Academy of Family Physicians: http://www.familydoctor.org

PROGNOSIS

- In most cases, recovery is complete within 7–14 days.
- Mortality statistics differ, but probably <1%.
- High-risk infants (bronchopulmonary dysplasia, congenital heart disease) may have a prolonged course.

COMPLICATIONS

- Bacterial superinfection
- Bronchiolitis obliterans
- Apnea
- Respiratory failure
- Death
- Increased incidence of development of reactive airway disease (asthma)

REFERENCES

1. *REDBOOK: Report of the Committee on Infectious Disease*. American Academy of Pediatrics. 2009
2. Cincinnati Children's Hospital Medical Center. Evidence-based clinical practice guideline for medical management of bronchiolitis in children less than 1 year of age presenting with a first time episode. Cincinnati (OH): Cincinnati Children's Hospital Medical Center; 2006. May. 13p (85 references)
3. Patel H, et al. A randomized, controlled trial of the effectiveness of nebulized therapy with epinephrine compared with albuterol and saline in infants hospitalized for acute viral bronchiolitis. *J Ped*. 2002;141(6):818–24.
4. Mull CC, Scarfone RJ, Ferri LR, et al. A randomized trial of nebulized epinephrine vs albuterol in the emergency department treatment of bronchiolitis. *Arch Pediatr Adolesc Med*. 2004;158:113–8.
5. Petruzella FD, Gorelick MH et al. Current therapies in bronchiolitis. *Pediatr Emerg Care*. 2010;26: 302–7.
6. Corneli HM, Zorc JJ, Majahan P, et al. A multicenter, randomized, controlled trial of dexamethasone for bronchiolitis. *N Engl J Med*. 2007;357:331–9.
7. Spurling GKP, et al. Antibiotics for bronchiolitis in children. *Cochrane Database Syst Rev*. 2007;1: CD005189. DOI:10.1002/14651859, CD005189.pub2.
8. Liet JM, Ducruet T, Gupta V, Cambonie G et al. Heliox inhalation therapy for bronchiolitis in infants. *Cochrane Database Syst Rev*. 2010;4:CD006915.

ADDITIONAL READING

- Bush A, Thomson AH. Acute bronchiolitis. *BMJ*. 2007;335:1037–41
- Everard ML. Acute bronchiolitis and croup. *Pediatr Clin North Am*. 2009;56:119–33, x–xi.
- Worrall G. Bronchiolitis. *Can Fam Physician*. 2008;54:742–3.
- Yanney M, Vyas H. The treatment of bronchiolitis. *Arch Dis Child*. 2008;93:793–8.

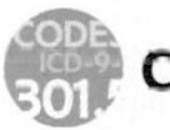

CODES

ICD9

466.19 Acute bronchiolitis due to other infectious organisms

CLINICAL PEARLS

- Bronchiolitis is the leading cause of hospitalizations in infants and children.
- Treatment is primarily supportive.
- Antibiotics not helpful in the majority of cases
- Parental education of expected course of illness important
- Be aware of new Synagis treatment guidelines for premature infants.

BRONCHITIS, ACUTE

Alan J. Cropp, MD

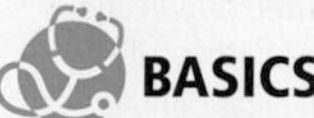

BASICS

DESCRIPTION

- Inflammation of trachea, bronchi, and bronchioles resulting from a respiratory tract infection or chemical irritant (1,2)
- Cough is the predominant symptom (3).
- Generally self-limited, with complete healing and full return of function
- Most infections are viral if no underlying cardiopulmonary disease is present.
- Synonym(s): Tracheobronchitis, chest cold

Geriatric Considerations

Can be serious, particularly if part of influenza, with underlying chronic obstructive pulmonary disease (COPD) or congestive heart failure (CHF) (3)

Pediatric Considerations

- Usually occurs in association with other conditions of upper and lower respiratory tract (trachea usually involved) (4)
- If repeated attacks occur, child should be evaluated for anomalies of the respiratory tract, including immune deficiencies or for chronic asthma.
- When acute bronchitis is caused by respiratory syncytial virus (RSV), it may be fatal.

EPIDEMIOLOGY

- Predominant age: All ages
- Predominant gender: Male = Female.

Incidence

- ~5% of adults per year (3)
- A common cause of infection in children (4)

Prevalence

Results in 10–12 million office visits per year (3)

RISK FACTORS

- Infants
- Elderly
- Air pollutants
- Smoking
- Secondhand smoke
- Environmental changes
- Chronic bronchopulmonary diseases
- Chronic sinusitis
- Tracheostomy
- Bronchopulmonary allergy
- Hypertrophied tonsils and adenoids in children
- Immunosuppression:
  - Immunoglobulin deficiency
  - HIV infection
  - Alcoholism
- Gastroesophageal reflux disease (GERD)

Genetics

No known genetic pattern

GENERAL PREVENTION

- Avoid smoking.
- Control underlying risk factors (i.e., asthma, sinusitis, and reflux).
- Avoid exposure, especially day care.
- Pneumovax, influenza immunization

PATHOPHYSIOLOGY

Acute bronchitis causes an injury to the epithelial surfaces, resulting in an increase in mucous production (2) and thickening of the bronchiole wall (1).

ETIOLOGY

- Viral infections, such as adenovirus, influenza A and B, parainfluenza virus, coxsackievirus, RSV, rhinovirus, coronavirus (types 1–3), herpes simplex virus
- Bacterial infections, such as *Chlamydia pneumoniae* [Taiwan acute respiratory (TWAR) agent], *Mycoplasma, Bordetella pertussis, Haemophilus influenzae, Streptococcus pneumoniae, Moraxella catarrhalis,* and *Mycobacterium tuberculosis*
- Secondary bacterial infection as part of an acute upper respiratory infection
- Possibly fungal infections
- Chemical irritants

COMMONLY ASSOCIATED CONDITIONS

- Allergic rhinitis
- Sinusitis
- Pharyngitis
- Epiglottitis (rare but can be rapidly fatal)
- Coryza
- Croup
- Influenza
- Pneumonia
- Asthma
- COPD/emphysema
- GERD

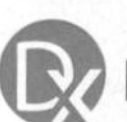

DIAGNOSIS

HISTORY

- Sudden onset of cough and no evidence of pneumonia, asthma, exacerbation of COPD, or the common cold (3)
- Cough is initially dry and unproductive, then productive; later, mucopurulent sputum, which may indicate secondary infection
- Dyspnea, wheeze, fever, and fatigue may occur.
- Possible contact with others who have respiratory infections (1)

PHYSICAL EXAM

- Fever
- Tachypnea
- Pharynx injected
- Rales, rhonchi, wheezing
- No evidence of pulmonary consolidation

DIAGNOSTIC TESTS & INTERPRETATION

Lab

Initial lab tests

- Sputum culture/sensitivity if purulent
- Influenza titers (if appropriate for time of year)
- White blood cell (WBC)

Follow-Up & Special Considerations

- Arterial blood gases: Hypoxemia (rarely)
- Pulmonary function tests (seldom needed during acute stages): Increased residual volume, decrease maximal expiratory rate (2)

Imaging

Initial approach

Chest radiograph:

- Lungs normal if uncomplicated
- Helps to rule out other diseases (pneumonia) or complications

DIFFERENTIAL DIAGNOSIS

- Common cold
- Acute sinusitis
- Bronchopneumonia
- Influenza
- Bacterial tracheitis
- Bronchiectasis
- Asthma
- Reactive airways dysfunction syndrome (RADS)
- Allergy
- Eosinophilic pneumonitis
- Aspiration
- Retained foreign body
- Inhalation injury
- Cystic fibrosis
- Bronchogenic carcinoma
- Heart failure
- GERD

TREATMENT

MEDICATION

ALERT

Antibiotics are usually not recommended (1,3,5)[A] unless a treatable pathogen has been identified or significant comorbidities are present.

First Line

- Amantadine or rimantadine therapy if influenza A is suspected; most effective if started within 24–48 h of development of symptoms [also consider oseltamivir (Tamiflu) or zanamivir (Relenza)]
- Decongestants if accompanied by sinus condition (
- Antipyretic analgesic, such as aspirin, acetaminophen, or ibuprofen
- Antibiotics if a treatable cause (i.e., pertussis) is identified (5)[A]:

– Amoxicillin 500 mg q8h or trimethoprim-sulfamethoxazole DS q12h for routine infection
  ○ Penicillins and trimethoprim-based regimens seem to be equivalent in terms of effectiveness and toxicity for acute bacterial exacerbations of chronic bronchitis (ABECB) (6)[B].
  ○ Clarithromycin (Biaxin) 500 mg q12h or azithromycin (Zithromax) Z-pack for penicillin allergy or *Mycoplasma* infection: In patients with acute bronchitis of a suspected bacterial cause, azithromycin tends to be more effective in terms of lower incidence of treatment failure and adverse events than amoxicillin or amoxycillin-clavulanicacid (7)[B].
– Doxycycline 100 mg/d × 10 days if *Moraxella, Chlamydia*, or *Mycoplasma* suspected
– Quinolone for more serious infections or other antibiotic failure or in elderly or patients with multiple comorbidities
– Macrolide for pertussis (1)[A]

Cough suppressant for troublesome cough (not with COPD); guaifenesin with codeine or dextromethorphan (3)[A]

Inhaled beta agonist (e.g., albuterol) or in combination with steroids for cough with bronchospasm (2,3)[B]

Consider steroids for bronchospasm

Contraindication(s): Doxycycline should not be used during pregnancy or in children.

Precautions:
– Watch for theophylline toxicity with macrolides and quinolones.
– Multiple antibiotics have the potential to interfere with the effectiveness of oral contraceptives.

econd Line

Other antibiotics if indicated by sputum culture (*Moraxella* needs a different set of antibiotics)

Antivirals

Other macrolides or quinolones based on pathogen and sensitivity

DDITIONAL TREATMENT

eneral Measures

Rest

Stop smoking/avoid smoke.

Steam inhalations

Vaporizers

Adequate hydration

Antitussives

Antibiotics are usually not recommended (1,3,5)[A].

Treat associated illnesses (e.g., GERD).

ssues for Referral

Complications, such as pneumonia or respiratory failure

Comorbidities, such as COPD

Cough lasting longer than 3 months

dditional Therapies

ntipyretic for fever (e.g., acetaminophen, aspirin, or uprofen)

COMPLEMENTARY AND ALTERNATIVE MEDICINE

Throat lozenges for pharyngitis

IN-PATIENT CONSIDERATIONS

Initial Stabilization

- Outpatient, unless elderly or complicated by severe underlying disease
- May require supplemental oxygen in selected patients
- Bronchodilators if patient is bronchospastic

Admission Criteria

- Hypoxia
- Severe bronchospasm
- Exacerbation of underlying disease

IV Fluids

May be helpful if patient is dehydrated

Nursing

- Ensure patient comfort and monitor for signs of deterioration, especially if underlying lung disease exists.
- May need to follow oxygen saturation in patients with underlying lung disease

Discharge Criteria

Improvement in symptoms and comorbidities

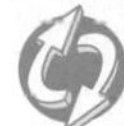

ONGOING CARE

FOLLOW-UP RECOMMENDATIONS

- Usually a self-limited disease not requiring follow-up
- Cough may linger for several weeks.
- In children, if recurrent, need to consider other diagnoses, such as asthma (4)

Patient Monitoring

- Oximetry until no longer hypoxemic
- Recheck for chronicity.

DIET

Increased fluids (3–4 L/d) while febrile

PATIENT EDUCATION

- For patient education materials favorably reviewed on this topic, contact the American Lung Association, 1740 Broadway, New York, NY 10019, (212) 315-8700; www.lungusa.org.
- American Academy of Family Physicians: www.familydoctor.org

PROGNOSIS

- Usual: Complete resolution
- Can be serious in the elderly or debilitated
- Cough may persist for several weeks after an initial improvement (1,2).
- Postbronchitic reactive airways disease (rare)
- Bronchiolitis obliterans and organizing pneumonia (rare)

COMPLICATIONS

- Superinfection such as bronchopneumonia
- Bronchiectasis
- Hemoptysis
- Acute respiratory failure
- Chronic cough

REFERENCES

1. Wenzel RP, Fowler AA. Clinical practice. Acute bronchitis. *N Engl J Med*. 2006;355:2125–30.
2. Knutson D, Braun C. Diagnosis and management of acute bronchitis. *Am Fam Physician*. 2002;65:2039–44.
3. Braman SS. Chronic cough due to acute bronchitis: ACCP evidence-based clinical practice guidelines. *Chest*. 2006;129:95S–103S.
4. Fleming DM, Elliot AJ. The management of acute bronchitis in children. *Expert Opin Pharmacother*. 2007;8:415–26.
5. Fahey T, et al. Antibiotics for acute bronchitis. *Cochrane Database Syst Rev*. 2004;4:CD000245. DOI:10.1002/14651858.CD000245.pub2.
6. Korbila IP, Manta KG, Siempos II, et al. Penicillins vs trimethoprim-based regimens for acute bacterial exacerbations of chronic bronchitis: Meta-analysis of randomized controlled trials. *Can Fam Physician*. 2009;55:60–7.
7. Panpanich R, Lerttrakarnnon P, Laopaiboon M. Azithromycin for acute lower respiratory tract infections. *Cochrane Database Syst Rev*. 2008; CD001954.

See Also (Topic, Algorithm, Electronic Media Element)

Asthma; Chronic Obstructive Pulmonary Disease and Emphysema

Algorithm: Cough

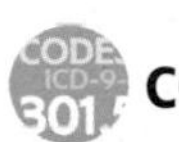

CODES

ICD9

466.0 Acute bronchitis

CLINICAL PEARLS

- Acute bronchitis is a common and generally self-limited disease.
- Usually does not require treatment with antibiotics
- Cough may linger for several weeks.
- Recurrent or seasonal episodes may suggest another disease process, such as asthma.

BRUCELLOSIS

Nancy J. Snapp, MD, MPH

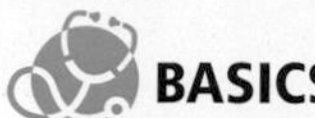

BASICS

DESCRIPTION

- Systemic bacterial infection caused by *Brucella sp.* in infected animal products or vaccine
- Incubation period usually 5–60 days, but highly variable and may be several months
- Characterized by intermittent or irregular fevers, with symptoms ranging from subclinical disease to infection of almost any organ system
- Bone and joint involvement common
- May be chronic or recurrent
- System(s) affected: Cardiovascular; Endocrine/Metabolic; GI; Musculoskeletal; Nervous; Pulmonary; Renal/Urologic; Skin/Exocrine
- Synonym(s): Undulant fever; Malta fever

Pediatric Considerations

May be mild, subclinical

Pregnancy Considerations

High rates of miscarriage or abortion (can occur in subclinical cases). Early antibiotic treatment is preventive.

EPIDEMIOLOGY

- Predominant age: All ages, but especially 20–60 years (occupational exposure), sometimes children (milk-related outbreaks)
- Predominant gender:
  - Male > Female (occupational exposure)
  - Female ≥ Male (milk exposure)

Incidence

~100 per year (0.34/100,000), but probably underreported (1,2)

Prevalence

- Common in developing countries; consider in immigrants
- Highest rates in Hispanic population along US–Mexico border
- Considered a potential biologic terror agent in aerosolized form
- Reportable in all states except Nevada

RISK FACTORS

- In US, from occupational exposure to infected animals (especially cattle, sheep): Veterinarians, meat processors, farm workers who may experience accidental exposure to vaccine
- Consumer exposure to unpasteurized milk products, cheese, especially Hispanics along US–Mexico border
- Exposure while traveling in countries where endemic (Mediterranean, Middle East, North and East Africa, central Asia, India, Mexico, Central and South America)
- Worse in chronically ill, immunosuppressed, and malnourished
- Iron deficiency increases susceptibility.

Genetics

- Some evidence for intrauterine transmission
- Some complications may have genetic predisposition (2).

GENERAL PREVENTION

- Avoid infected dairy products.
- For occupational exposure, use caution, animal vaccination, protective goggles, protective gloves. Possibility exists for future human vaccine.
- Postexposure prophylaxis same as treatment in large-scale exposure such as bioterrorism
- Susceptible to heat, disinfectant, but can survive in dust, soil, or water for weeks

ETIOLOGY

- *Brucella* ingestion from tissue or milk
- Worst disease: *B. melitensis, B. suis*; also *B. canis, B. abortus*; enters through mucous membrane or broken skin; occasionally inhaled
- Facultative intracellular parasite
- Person-to-person transmission rare; sexual, vertical, and possibly breast milk; case report of neonatal brucellosis from a blood transfusion
- Potential airborne biologic weapon

DIAGNOSIS

PHYSICAL EXAM

- Fever (may be undulant, increased in afternoon and evening, maximum 101–104°F daily), weakness, headache, sweating, chills, generalized aching, arthralgia (90%) (2)[A]
- Also common: Weight loss, depression, irritability, hepatosplenomegaly (20–30%)
- Hepatic dysfunction (abnormal liver function test): 30–60%
- GI symptoms (unusual)
- Lymphadenopathy, especially cervical, inguinal (12–21%)
- Orchitis, epididymitis (normal urinalysis) (2–40%)
- Nephritis, prostatitis (rare)
- Cystitis
- Pulmonary: Cough or other pulmonary symptoms; radiograph may be normal (15–25%)
- Cutaneous: Many transient, nonspecific rashes have been described; also, purpura from thrombopenia (5%)
- Visual disturbances, eye pain
- Chronic fatigue syndrome and various neuropsychiatric symptoms described. Relationship is unclear.
- Also localized suppurative infections (see Complications)
- Malodorous perspiration (2)
- Noncaseating granulomas (1); possibly some

DIAGNOSTIC TESTS & INTERPRETATION

Lab

Initial lab tests

- Isolation of organism from blood, discharge, bone, or other tissue: Bone marrow is gold standard (3)[A]:
  - Fastidious and slow growing
  - Watch for 3–4 weeks, with periodic subcultures
  - Automated systems shorten time, but not all recognize brucellosis.
  - Polymerase chain reaction (PCR) accurate, including nonblood samples, but not available in most clinical labs (3)[A]
  - Skin tests not standardized; not recommended for diagnosis
- Acute illness: Blood culture positive 70%, bone marrow 90%
- May have thrombocytopenia, disseminated intravascular coagulation, granulopenia, lymphopenia, lymphocytosis
- 30–60% with abnormal liver function test
- Up to 70% may have normal labs.
- Serology: Use at least 2 tests to confirm (4)[A]:
  - *Brucella* standard tube agglutination paired sera >1:160 or 4× rise (cheapest)
  - Easy, accurate, and rapid dipstick for IgM now exists for developing countries.
- More effective enzyme linked immunosorbent assa (ELISA), indirect fluorescent antibody test, Coombs tests, immunocapture-agglutination (*Brucella* apt). With ELISA, IgM, IgG, or IgA may be present at lo levels >1 year even if treated.
- IgM increases initially for several weeks, declines b 3 months
- IgG begins to rise in 2 weeks, may stay up (low levels) for >1 year if treated or not treated (although IgM increase may be lower or gone by 6 months if treated; can also persist >1 year at low levels). IgG titer rises again with reinfection or reactivation. IgG and IgA titer >1:160 at 1 year implies ongoing disease (4)[A].
- New research: Gene cloning and amplification for discriminatory markers detection and strain differences; PCR-ELISA
- Drugs that may alter lab results: None
- Disorders that may alter lab results:
  - Serologic cross-reaction with *F. tularensis, Yersin enterocolitica, V. cholerae*, or vaccinated patient
  - Has been misdiagnosed in culture as *Moraxella phenylpyruvica*

Imaging

- Bone scan, computed tomography, depending on location
- Chest x-ray: Pleural effusion, lung cavitation
- Joint radiographs frequently normal, requiring scan or magnetic resonance imaging

Diagnostic Procedures/Surgery

Bone marrow biopsy, biopsy of affected area

Pathological Findings

- Facultative intracellular gram-negative coccobacillus; can survive inside phagocytic cells, circulation lymph nodes, and into circulation
- Immune reaction in arthritis, including elevated C3, C4; antinuclear antibody, and rheumatoid factor
- Variable tissue reaction depending on site, organisms; causes local microabscesses

FFERENTIAL DIAGNOSIS

Many nonspecific systemic febrile illnesses; a great mimic
Tularemia
Psittacosis
Rickettsial disease
Tuberculosis
Visceral leishmaniasis
Other disease of infected organs
HIV infection

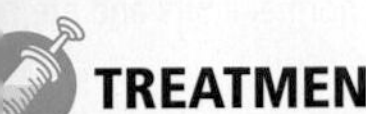

TREATMENT

EDICATION

rst Line

Optimal therapy includes 2 drugs, at least 1 with good intracellular penetration. In some cases, 3 drugs may give a better long-term cure.
Longer courses (months) may improve relapse rate in complicated disease.
Rifampin 600–1,200 mg and doxycycline 200 mg given together every day for at least 6 weeks (possibly for several months with severe complications):
- 5–10% relapse rate, not related to drug resistance; use same drugs for relapse
- Usual cause is localized sequestration of organisms or noncompliance with medication (5)[A]

Steroids in Herxheimer reaction, severe illness, and pancytopenia
Contraindications:
- Avoid doxycycline in children and pregnant women (affects bone).

Precautions:
- May get Herxheimer reaction when therapy initiated

Significant possible interactions:
- Rifampin is a potent inducer for the hepatic P450 enzyme system, and may increase metabolism of many drugs metabolized by the liver. Doxycycline: Antacids, anticoagulants, barbiturates, carbamazepine, hydantoins, cimetidine, digoxin, insulin, iron salts, lithium, methoxyflurane, oral contraceptives, penicillins, sodium bicarbonate

econd Line

Doxycycline orally b.i.d. and streptomycin by injection is very effective (streptomycin currently not available in the US except by special request from Centers for Disease Control); slightly more effective than doxycycline/rifampin, especially with spondylitis, but more toxic and less convenient (5).

In children and pregnant women, rifampin 15 mg/kg for 4–5 weeks plus cotrimoxazole for 6 weeks or gentamicin for 7 days or netilmicin 5–6 mg/kg IM. Significant cotrimoxazole resistance in some countries (1)[A].
Ofloxacin or ciprofloxacin plus rifampin effective in a recent study, but not as effective as 1st-line treatment (6)[A],(7)[B].
Sensitivities don't reflect in vivo action (2)[A].

ADDITIONAL TREATMENT

General Measures

- Supportive care
- In milk-related or occupational outbreak, look for other cases.
- Bed rest during febrile periods and restricted activity in acute cases

Issues for Referral

Need for procedures

SURGERY/OTHER PROCEDURES

Specific complications may require surgical drainage or valve replacement (endocarditis).

IN-PATIENT CONSIDERATIONS

Admission Criteria

- Outpatient in mild cases, hospitalization in severe illness
- Cardiac care unit for patients with complicating cardiac disease

ONGOING CARE

FOLLOW-UP RECOMMENDATIONS

Patient Monitoring

- Check serology at 6 months and 1 year for chronic disease (difficult to evaluate if continuing exposure).
- Investigate any suspicion of recurrence.
- PCR recently shown to be sensitive and specific for monitoring treatment relapse

DIET

- No special diet
- May need to provide supplemental foods, such as milkshakes, to counter weight loss

PATIENT EDUCATION

- Food Safety and Inspection Service, Office of Public Awareness, Department of Agriculture, Room 1165-S, Washington, DC 20205; (202)720-9904; http://www.fsis.usda.gov/
- Education about exposure

PROGNOSIS

- Untreated case fatality < 2%
- Most cases resolve with treatment in 2–3 weeks in acute uncomplicated cases, but at least 6 weeks treatment recommended

COMPLICATIONS

- Relapse rate overall: 5–10%
- Complications present: 10–15% (4)[A]
- Localized suppurative infections: Osteoarticular (20–85%). Includes arthritis (possibly also immune effect), bursitis, tenosynovitis, osteomyelitis, sacroiliitis, vertebral or paraspinous abscess
- Endocarditis: Rare, but main cause of death in brucellosis
- Thrombophlebitis
- Neurobrucellosis: Most are meningeal. Also peripheral neuritis (usually single; bilateral is possible), encephalitis, myelitis, radiculopathy. Possibly neuropsychiatric symptoms.
- Intrinsic ocular lesions: Uveitis, retinal thrombophlebitis, nummular keratitis
- Pneumonitis with pleural effusion
- Hepatitis
- Cholecystitis
- Chronic infection: Persistent (>1 year) signs of infection, elevated titers, occasional bacteria in blood or tissue. Chronic fatigue syndrome with everything negative is controversial.

REFERENCES

1. Sauret JM, Vilissova N. Human brucellosis. *J Am Board Fam Pract.* 2002;15:401–6.
2. Pappas G, et al. Brucellosis. *N Eng J Med.* 2005; 352(22):2325–36.
3. Al Dahouk S, Tomaso H, Nöckler K, et al. Laboratory-based diagnosis of brucellosis–a review of the literature. Part I: Techniques for direct detection and identification of Brucella spp. *Clin Lab.* 2003;49:487–505.
4. Al Dahouk S, Tomaso H, Nöckler K, et al. Laboratory-based diagnosis of brucellosis–a review of the literature. Part II: serological tests for brucellosis. *Clin Lab.* 2003;49:577–89.
5. Pappas G, et al. New approaches to the antibiotic treatment of brucellosis. *Intl J Antimicrob Ag.* 2005;26(2):101–5.
6. Skalsky K, Yahav D, Bishara J, et al. Treatment of human brucellosis: systematic review and meta-analysis of randomised controlled trials. *BMJ.* 2008;336:701–4.
7. Keramat F, Ranjbar M, Mamani M, Hashemi SH, Zeraati F, et al. A comparative trial of three therapeutic regimens: ciprofloxacin-rifampin, ciprofloxacin-doxycycline and doxycycline-rifampin in the treatment of brucellosis. *Trop Doct.* 2009;39:207–10.

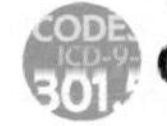

CODES

ICD9
023.9 Brucellosis, unspecified

CLINICAL PEARLS

- Infection is caused by infected animal products or animal vaccine. More common outside US. In US, most cases result from occupational exposure to infected animals (especially cattle, sheep): Veterinarians, meat processors, and farm workers who may experience accidental exposure to vaccine and ingestion of raw milk.
- Characterized by intermittent or irregular fevers, with symptoms ranging from subclinical disease to infection of almost any organ system
- Concern that this may become a weaponized bioterrorism agent

BULIMIA NERVOSA

Jeffrey L. Goodie, PhD
Pamela M. Williams, MD, Lt Col, USAF, MC

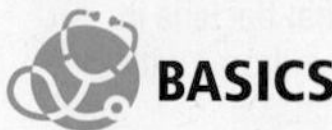

BASICS

DESCRIPTION
- A pattern of discrete periods of uncontrolled eating, followed by compensatory behaviors
- System(s) affected: Oropharyngeal; Endocrine/Metabolic; Gastrointestinal; Dermatologic; Cardiovascular; Nervous

EPIDEMIOLOGY
- Predominant age: Adolescents and young adults
- Mean age of onset: 18–21 years
- Predominant sex: Female > Male (10–20:1)

Incidence
28.8 women, 0.8 men per 100,000 per year

Prevalence
- 1–3% in women 16–35 years old
- 0.5% in young men (higher among gay and bisexual men)

RISK FACTORS
- Female gender
- History of obesity and dieting
- Body dissatisfaction
- Critical comments by family or others about weight, body shape, or eating
- Severe life stressor
- Low self-esteem
- Perceived pressure to be thin
- Perfectionist or obsessive thinking
- Poor impulse control, alcohol misuse
- History of anorexia nervosa (AN)
- Environment stressing high achievement, competition, thinness, or physical fitness (e.g., armed forces, ballet, cheerleaders, gymnastics, or models)
- Family history of substance abuse, affective disorders, eating disorder, or obesity
- Early feeding problems
- Low birth weight for gestational age
- Hyporeactivity at birth
- Type I diabetes
- Sexual abuse is not causally related to bulimia.

GENERAL PREVENTION
- Prevention programs can reduce risk factors and future onset of eating disorders (1)[C].
- Target adolescents and young women 15 years or older.
- Encourage realistic and healthy weight management strategies and attitudes.
- Decrease body dissatisfaction.
- Promote self-esteem.
- Reduce focus on thin as ideal.
- Moderate overly high self-expectations.
- Decrease anxiety/depressive symptoms.
- Improve stress management.

ETIOLOGY
Combination of biological, psychological, environmental, and social factors. Unique contribution of any specific factor remains unclear.

COMMONLY ASSOCIATED CONDITIONS
- Major depression and dysthymia
- Anxiety disorders
- Substance abuse/dependence
- Bipolar disorder
- Obsessive-compulsive disorder
- Borderline personality disorder
- Schizophrenic disorder

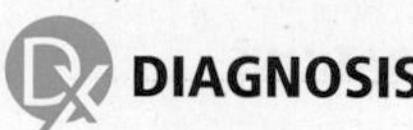

DIAGNOSIS

DSM-IV-TR criteria:
- Recurrent episodes of binge eating (2 times per week for 3 months):
  - Eating in a discrete period more than most people would eat during that time
  - Perceived lack of control during binges
- Recurrent inappropriate compensatory behavior (2 times per week for 3 months)
- Purging and nonpurging subtypes:
  - Purging: Often by self-induced vomiting, laxatives, diuretics
  - Nonpurging: Binges followed by sharply restricted diet and/or vigorous exercise
- Body shape and weight significantly affect self-evaluation.
- Does not occur during AN episodes
- Psychological self-report screening tests:
  - Eating Attitudes Test
  - Eating Disorder Inventory
  - Eating Disorder Screen for Primary Care
  - Bulimia Test (revised)
  - Bulimia Investigatory Test Edinburgh
  - SCOFF (sick, control, one, fat, food)

HISTORY
- Patients unlikely to self-identify binge eating or purging behaviors; corroborate with parent/relative
- Unhappiness and/or preoccupation with weight and diet attempts
- Pattern of restricting diet, binge eating, and purging behaviors:
  - Binge is context-specific; amount can vary
  - Vomiting (often with little effort)
  - Vigorous aerobic exercise
  - Distress/shame related to loss of control
- Depressed mood and self-depreciation following the binges
- Relief and increased ability to concentrate following the purges
- Other possible signs and symptoms:
  - Requesting weight loss help and mildly underweight to overweight
  - Diet pill, diuretic, laxative, ipecac, and thyroid medication use/abuse
  - Menstrual disturbance
  - Fatigue and lethargy
  - Abdominal pain, bloating, constipation, diarrhea, rectal prolapse
  - Sore throat
  - Frequent fluctuations in weight
  - Omission/underdosing insulin in diabetes patients

PHYSICAL EXAM
- Often normal
- Bradycardia
- Eroded tooth enamel
- Asymptomatic, noninflammatory parotid gland enlargement
- Epigastric tenderness to palpation
- Calluses, abrasions, bruising on hand, thumb
- Peripheral edema

DIAGNOSTIC TESTS & INTERPRETATION
All lab results may be within normal limits and are n[ot] necessary for diagnosis.

Lab
- Blood work:
  - Hypokalemia, hypochloremia
  - Hypomagnesemia, hyponatremia, hypocalcemia, hypophosphatasemia
  - Alkalosis
  - Elevated blood urea nitrogen
  - Hypoglycemia
- Urinalysis:
  - Increased urine-specific gravity

Diagnostic Procedures/Surgery
Electrocardiogram:
- Bradycardia or arrhythmias
- Conduction defects
- Depressed ST segment due to hypokalemia

Pathological Findings
- Esophagitis
- Acute pancreatitis
- Cardiomyopathy and muscle weakness due to ipecac abuse
- Delayed or arrested skeletal growth
- Stress fracture
- Irreversible dental erosions
- Osteopenia/osteoporosis

DIFFERENTIAL DIAGNOSIS
- Anorexia, binge eating/purging type
- Major depressive disorder
- Anxiety disorders
- Psychogenic vomiting
- Malabsorption
- Addison disease
- Celiac disease
- Diabetes mellitus
- Hyperthyroidism; hypothyroidism
- Hyperpituitarism
- Hypothalamic brain tumor
- Kleine-Levin syndrome
- Body dysmorphic disorder
- Borderline personality disorder

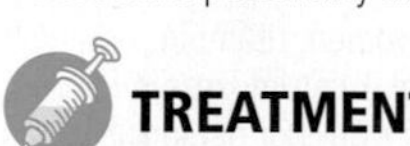

TREATMENT

- Cognitive behavioral therapy (CBT) should be considered as 1st-line treatment (2,3,4)[A].
- Guided self-help therapies may be effective (3,4)[B]

MEDICATION

First Line
- Selective serotonin reuptake inhibitors (SSRIs), particularly fluoxetine (Prozac) at 60 mg, are effective in reducing symptoms with relatively few side effects. Higher doses than standard doses for depression are often needed (3,5,6)[B]:

– Combination of medication and CBT has been shown to have added benefit over medication or therapy alone (6).

To prevent relapse, maintain antidepressant at full therapeutic dose for at least 1 year.
Bupropion not recommended due to its association with seizures in patients who purge.
Misrepresentation and nonadherence may be more likely in this population.
Precautions:
– Serious toxicity following overdose is common.
– Patients may vomit medications.

econd Line

Ondansetron (Zofran) 4–8 mg t.i.d. between meals can help prevent vomiting.
Psyllium (Metamucil) preparations, 1 tbs q.h.s. with glass of water, can prevent constipation during laxative withdrawal.

DDITIONAL TREATMENT

ost patients can be treated as outpatients.

ieneral Measures

Psychotherapies should be employed as 1st-line treatments.
Multidisciplinary team:
– Primary care physician, behavioral health provider, nutritionist
Build trust; increase motivation for change.
Assess psychological and nutritional status.
Consider evidence-based self-help program.

Cognitive behavioral therapy for bulimia nervosa (2,3,4,5)[A]:
– 16–20 50-minute appointments
– Involve patient in establishing goals.
Self monitoring of food intake, frequency of binges/purges, related antecedents, consequences, thoughts, and emotions
– Self-monitoring of weight once per week
– Educate about ineffectiveness of purging for weight control and adverse outcomes.
– Establish prescribed eating plan to develop regular eating habits; realistic weight goal.
– Gradually introduce feared foods into diet.
– Problem-solve how to cope with triggers.
– Decrease ruminations about calories, weight, and purging.
– Challenge fear of loss of control.
– Establish relapse prevention plan.
– Gradual laxative withdrawal
Interpersonal therapy (2,3)[B]:
– May act more slowly than CBT

Transdiagnostic cognitive-behavioral therapy
Dialectical behavior therapy
Family therapy for adolescents
Nutritional education, relaxation techniques
Educate patient to brush teeth and use baking soda to rinse mouth after vomiting.

ssues for Referral

'atients with bulimia require a multidisciplinary team, ıcluding a primary care physician, behavioral health provider, and a nutritionist.

COMPLEMENTARY AND ALTERNATIVE MEDICINE

Bright light therapy may help (3).

N-PATIENT CONSIDERATIONS

If possible, admit to a specialized eating disorders unit.
Supervised meals and bathroom privileges

- Monitor weight and physical activity.
- Monitor electrolytes.
- Gradually shift control to patients as they demonstrate responsibility.

Admission Criteria

Hospitalize if severe malnutrition, dehydration, electrolyte disturbances, cardiac dysrhythmia, uncontrolled binging and purging, psychiatric emergency, or if outpatient treatment failed

ONGOING CARE

FOLLOW-UP RECOMMENDATIONS

Patient Monitoring

- Binge-purge activity, including antecedents and consequences
- Level of exercise activity
- Self-esteem, comfort with body and self
- Ruminations and depressive symptoms
- Repeat any abnormal lab values weekly or monthly until stable.

DIET

- Balanced diet, normal eating pattern
- Reintroduce feared foods.

PATIENT EDUCATION

The following books may be useful for guided self-help treatment programs:

- Fairburn CG. *Overcoming Binge Eating*. New York, NY: Guilford Press; 1995.
- McCabe RE, McFarlane TL, Olmstead MP. *Overcoming Bulimia: Your Comprehensive, Step-by-Step Guide to Recovery*. Oakland, CA: New Harbinger; 2003.

PROGNOSIS

- After effective cognitive behavioral treatment:
  – In the short-term, 50% of treated individuals do not meet criteria for diagnosis.
  – In the long-term (2–10 years), 70% may be asymptomatic.
  Symptomatic individuals may demonstrate remissions, relapses, subclinical, or other eating-related behaviors.
- Untreated:
  – Likely to remain chronic/relapsing problem
- Greater weight fluctuations, other impulsive behaviors, and personality disorder diagnoses may predict poor prognosis.

COMPLICATIONS

- Drug and alcohol abuse
- Osteopenia/osteoporosis
- Stress fracture
- Gastric dilatation
- Mallory-Weiss tears
- Spontaneous pneumomediastinum
- Potassium depletion; cardiac arrhythmia; cardiac arrest
- Suicide

Pregnancy Considerations

Maternal and fetal problems if pregnant:

- Binging/purging behaviors may persist, increase, or decrease with pregnancy.
- Increased risk for preterm delivery, operative delivery, and infants with low birth weight, smaller head circumference, and/or microcephaly; should be managed as high risk

REFERENCES

1. Stice E, Shaw H, Marti CN. A meta-analytic review of eating disorder prevention programs: encouraging findings. *Annu Rev Clin Psychol*. 2007;3:207–31.
2. Hay PP, Bacaltchuk J, Stefano S, Kashyap P et al. Psychological treatments for bulimia nervosa and binging. *Cochrane Database Syst Rev*. 2009; CD000562.
3. Shapiro JR, Berkman ND, Brownley KA, et al. Bulimia nervosa treatment: a systematic review of randomized controlled trials. *Int J Eat Disord*. 2007;40:321–36.
4. NICE. *Eating disorders–core interventions in the treatment of anorexia nervosa, bulimia nervosa, and related eating disorders*. NICE Clinical Guideline no 9. London: NICE, 2004: Available at: http://www.nice.org.uk. Accessed July 17, 2008.
5. *Practice guideline for the treatment of patients with eating disorders*, 3rd edition. American Psychiatric Association. Available at http://www.psych.org. Accessed February 22, 2007.
6. Bacaltchuk J, Hay P, Trefiglio R. Antidepressants versus psychological treatments and their combination for bulimia nervosa. *Cochrane Database Sys Rev*. 2001(4):CD003385.

ADDITIONAL READING

- McElroy SL, Guerdjikova AI, Martens B, et al. Role of antiepileptic drugs in the management of eating disorders. *CNS Drugs*. 2009;23:139–56.
- Powers PS, Bruty H. Pharmacotherapy for eating disorders and obesity. *Child Adolesc Psychiatr Clin N Am*. 2009;18:175–87.

See Also (Topic, Algorithm, Electronic Media Element)

Anorexia Nervosa; Hyperkalemia; Laxative Abuse; Salivary Gland Tumors
Algorithm: Weight Loss

CODES

ICD9

307.51 Bulimia nervosa

CLINICAL PEARLS

- Particularly among young women with a risk factor, asking "Are you satisfied with your eating patterns?" and/or "Do you worry that you have lost control over how much you eat?" may help to screen for those with an eating problem. A brief, standardized screening measure (e.g., SCOFF, ESP, EAT) will help to identify those who may need a broader assessment.
- Binging and purging behaviors can be seen in anorexia nervosa as well.
- Consider using a stepped-care approach. Start with a guided self-help program using instructional aids, next begin cognitive behavioral therapy (e.g., 16–20 sessions over 4–5 months).
- SSRIs, particularly fluoxetine (60 mg daily), may be helpful as a 1st step or as an adjunctive treatment.

BUNION

Linda Sinclair, MD
Jason Kittler, MD, PhD, JD

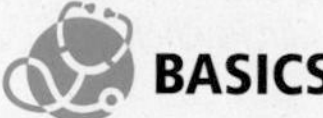

BASICS

DESCRIPTION

- Commonly known as a bunion, a hallux valgus deformity consists of a lateral deviation of the great toe (hallux) with medial deviation of the first metatarsal. There is often lateral rotation of the toe such that the nail faces medially (eversion) (1).
- Pressure at the head of the first metatarsal forces it to move medially. The hallux is forced laterally and a misalignment between the first metatarsal and the hallux develops. This results in a medial prominence of the first metatarsophalangeal (MTP) joint and a potentially painful and/or debilitating deformity.
- Strain on the medial collateral ligament along the MTP joint leads to loss of tensile strength, and eventually rupture, which decreases the medial stabilization of the joint (2).
- Changes in muscle positioning and tightening of the lateral collateral ligament can allow for the adductor hallucis muscle to pull unopposed, which can lead to hallux rotation (1).
- System(s) affected: Musculoskeletal/Skin

EPIDEMIOLOGY

- Predominant age: More common in adults
- Predominant sex: Female > Male
- Prevalence increases with age.

RISK FACTORS

- Familial predisposition
- Abnormal anatomy/mechanics
- Joint hypermobility or laxity
- Pronation of hindfoot
- Achilles tendon contracture
- Pes planus (fallen arches)
- Metatarsus primus varus
- Amputation of 2nd toe
- Inflammatory joint disease
- Neuromuscular disorders
- Exacerbated by improper footwear, especially tight-fitting or pointed shoes (3)

GENERAL PREVENTION

No known effective prevention exists, given that the etiology is poorly understood.

ETIOLOGY

The exact etiology of hallux valgus is unknown, but the disease is thought to be multifactorial. The risk factors listed above may all contribute to the development of the disease.

COMMONLY ASSOCIATED CONDITIONS

- Medial bursitis of the 1st MTP joint (most common)
- Hammertoe deformity of the second phalanx
- Plantar callus
- Central metatarsalgia
- Metatarsalgia of MTP joint
- Degeneration of 1st metatarsal head cartilage
- Pronated feet
- Ankle equinus
- Ingrown toenail
- Entrapment of the medial dorsal cutaneous nerve
- Synovitis of the MTP joint (1,3)

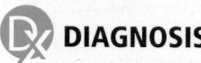

DIAGNOSIS

- Most often made on clinical exam
- Radiography for staging purposes

PHYSICAL EXAM

- Pain or deformity at the 1st digit (great toe)
- Increased valgus angle at the 1st MTP joint
- Medial eminence of 1st metatarsal
- Bursal inflammation/ulceration over medial surface
- Painful callus development on 2nd toe
- Displacement of the 1st digit above/below 2nd digit
- Lateral deviation of other digits
- Impaired gait
- To perform a complete exam, the physician should:
  - Observe the patient in sitting and standing positions, as weight bearing often accentuates the deformity.
  - Assess the magnitude of hallux valgus deformity, including any rotation of the 1st digit.
  - Measure the active/passive range of motion of the 1st MTP joint.
  - Assess the congruency of the 1st MTP joint by passive correction of the deformity.
  - Assess for pain and/or crepitus with movement of 1st MTP joint (may indicate degenerative osteoarthritis and change management).
  - Assess the neurovasculature of the foot.
  - Assess the gait of the patient (3)[C].

DIAGNOSTIC TESTS & INTERPRETATION

Imaging

Weight-bearing anteroposterior, lateral, and oblique radiographs may be obtained. The radiographs are used to make the following measurements:

- Hallux abductus (HA) angle: Created by the bisection of the longitudinal axis of the hallux and the longitudinal axis of the first metatarsal.
  - A normal angle is <20° (1).
  - Deformity is considered severe when HA angle is >40° (2).
- Intermetatarsal (IM) angle: Created by the bisectio of the longitudinal axes of the first and second metatarsals.
  - A normal angle is <9° (1).
  - Deformity is considered severe when IM angle is >16° (2).
- Medial prominence of the 1st metatarsal head: No erosions or squaring.
- MTP joint congruency: A congruent joint displays n lateral subluxation of the proximal phalanx on the metatarsal head.

DIFFERENTIAL DIAGNOSIS

- Trauma:
  - Turf toe
  - Sesamoiditis
  - Stress fracture
- Infection:
  - Osteomyelitis
  - Septic arthritis
- Joint disorder:
  - Osteoarthritis
  - Rheumatoid arthritis
  - Gout
- Tendon disorder:
  - Tendinosis
  - Tenosynovitis
  - Tendon rupture
- Other:
  - Bursitis
  - Ganglia
  - Foreign-body granuloma

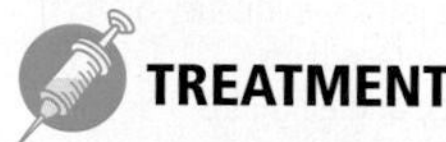

TREATMENT

Hallux valgus deformity will not resolve without treatment. Surgical treatment is more effective in improving patient outcomes than conservative therapy, although evidence is limited (4)[A].

MEDICATION

While no medication is available to treat the underlying cause of hallux valgus, nonsteroidal anti-inflammatory agents can be used for relief of pai and swelling (5)[C]. As with the use of any medicatior patients should be evaluated for contraindications an monitored for adverse reactions.

ᴐDITIONAL TREATMENT

nservative treatments (e.g., orthoses and night ints) did not appear to be any more beneficial in proving outcomes and preventing progression than treatment (4). Evidence suggests that custom-made hoses are a safe intervention that may slightly crease pain at 6 and 12 months (but no continued crease in pain after 12 months) compared to no atment; however, this improvement is less than that en with surgical interventions (see below) (6).

eneral Measures

spite the lack of strong evidence supporting the nical efficacy of conservative therapy, a number of noperative modalities have been recommended to tempt to alleviate symptoms and decrease the rates progression of hallux valgus deformity before rgical referral (5)[C]:

Shoe modification: Low-heeled, wide shoes to alleviate pressure on MTP joint
Orthoses: Shoe inserts may alter abnormal foot rotation
Night splinting: May help balance supporting ligaments
Stretching to improve intrinsic foot muscle strength
Bunion pads: To decrease friction on the MTP joint
Ice: To reduce inflammation

OMPLEMENTARY AND ALTERNATIVE IEDICINE

arigold ointment may reduce pain and soft tissue velling over an 8-week period (7)[C].

URGERY/OTHER PROCEDURES

urgery is indicated if patient has severe pain, ysfunction, or symptoms that do not improve with nservative therapy. Surgery is shown to be more eneficial than conservative therapy, and patient ould be referred to a podiatric foot and ankle urgeon (5)[A]. More than 150 different surgical chniques have been performed, but evidence is too nited to show which form of surgery is more fective (4)[A]. It is important that patients have alistic expectations about surgical outcomes. atients may not be able to fit into smaller shoes ter surgery, and the great toe may not appear raight. Choice of surgical technique will depend on everity of disease. Examples include:

Arthrodesis: Fusion of the 1st MTP joint
Arthroplasty: Removing the joint or replacing it with a prosthesis
Exostectomy/bunionectomy: Removing the medial bony prominence of the MTP joint
Lapidus procedure: Fusion at the 1st metatarsocuneiform joint
Soft-tissue procedure: To alter the function of surrounding ligaments and tendons
Osteotomy and realignment
Keller's arthroplasty: Removal of the medial eminence on the metatarsal head and removal of part of the proximal phalanx, leaving a flexible joint

ONGOING CARE

FOLLOW-UP RECOMMENDATIONS

Activity after surgery is indicated to decrease joint stiffness. Post-operative treatment may include physical therapy, physiotherapy, use of supportive shoe, continuous passive motion or manual manipulation. Although there is little evidence to support clinical efficacy, physical therapy and gait training after surgery may improve ability to weight bear and ambulate after surgery (8) and passive motion may improve time to recovery and range of motion of MTP (4). Early weight bearing has not been found to be detrimental to final outcome (4). Refer to specific recommendation made by patient's surgeon.

PROGNOSIS

Patient outcome varies depending on individual factors, severity, and treatment modality used. The radiological HA angle is a predictor of surgical correction; patients with a HA angle <37° have a higher chance of having the deformity corrected with surgery compared to patients with a HA angle >37° (9).

COMPLICATIONS

All surgery carries the risk of wound infection or poor wound healing. Additional complications may include:

- Early swelling
- Hallux varus
- Recurrence of bunion
- Decreased sensation over the 1st metatarsal or phalanx (5)

REFERENCES

1. Ferrari J, et al. Hallux valgus deformity (bunion). *Article from UpToDate*. Lasted updated 2/22/2010.
2. Glasoe WM, Nuckley DJ, Ludewig PM et al. Hallux valgus and the first metatarsal arch segment: a theoretical biomechanical perspective. *Phys Ther*. 2010;90:110–20.
3. Coughlin MJ. Hallux valgus. *J Bone Joint Surg Am*. 1996;78:932–66.
4. Ferrari J, et al. Interventions for treating hallux valgus (abductovalgus) and bunions. *Cochrane Database of Systematic Reviews*. 1, 2009.
5. Vanore JV, Christensen JC, Kravitz SR et al. Diagnosis and treatment of first metatarsophalangeal joint disorders. Section 1: Hallux valgus. *J Foot Ankle Surg*. 2003;42:112–23.
6. Hawke F, et al. Custom-made foot orthoses for the treatment of foot pain. *Cochrane Database of Systematic Reviews*. 1, 2009.
7. Khan MT. The podiatric treatment of hallux abducto valgus and its associated condition, bunion, with Tagetes patula. *J Pharm Pharmacol*. 1996;48:768–70.
8. Schuh R, Hofstaetter SG, Adams SB et al. Rehabilitation after hallux valgus surgery: importance of physical therapy to restore weight bearing of the first ray during the stance phase. *Phys Ther*. 2009;89:934–45.
9. Deenik AR, de Visser E, Louwerens JW et al. Hallux valgus angle as main predictor for correction of hallux valgus. *BMC Musculoskelet Disord*. 2008;9:70.

ADDITIONAL READING

- Ashman CJ, Klecker RJ, Yu JS. Forefoot pain involving the metatarsal region: differential diagnosis with MR imaging. *Radiographics*. 2001;21:1425–40.
- Klosok JK, Pring DJ, Jessop JH, et al. Chevron or Wilson metatarsal osteotomy for hallux valgus. A prospective randomised trial. *J Bone Joint Surg Br*. 1993;75:825–9.

CODES

ICD9

727.1 Bunion

CLINICAL PEARLS

- When bunions occur in children or adolescents, the condition may be termed juvenile or adolescent hallux valgus, respectively, and is thought to have an etiology different from that in the adult population.
- Also known as a bunionette, a tailor's bunion is a lateral prominence of the 5th metatarsal head.
- Patients should avoid any footwear with high heels, pointed toe boxes, or inadequate space for the toes to reduce the risk of bunions. Women's high-heeled shoes and cowboy boots often fall into this category.

BURNS

Timothy L. Black, MD
James P. Miller, MD

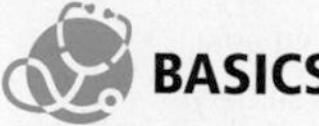

BASICS

DESCRIPTION

- Tissue injuries caused by application of heat, chemicals, electricity, or irradiation to the tissue
- Extent of injury (depth of burn) is result of intensity of heat (or other exposure) and duration of exposure.
  - 1st degree involves superficial layers of epidermis.
  - 2nd degree involves varying degrees of epidermis (with blister formation) and part of the dermis.
  - 3rd degree involves destruction of all skin elements (full thickness) with coagulation of subdermal plexus.
- System(s) affected: Endocrine/Metabolic; Skin/Exocrine

Geriatric Considerations

- Prognosis is poorer for severe burns.
- Patients >60 years of age account for 11% of burns.

Pediatric Considerations

Consider child abuse or neglect when dealing with hot-water burns in children.

EPIDEMIOLOGY

- Predominant age: 30 years; 13% infants; 11% >60 years of age
- Predominant gender: Males account for 70%

Incidence

Per year in US:

- 1.2–2 million burns, 700,000 emergency room visits, 45,000–50,000 hospitalizations, 3,900 deaths owing to burn-related complications
- In children: 250,000 burns, 15,000 hospitalizations, 1,100 deaths
- Estimated total cost of $2 billion annually for burn care
- 75% of deaths owing to house fires

RISK FACTORS

- Water heaters set too high
- Workplace exposure to chemicals, electricity, or irradiation
- Young children and older adults with thin skin are more susceptible to injury.
- Carelessness with burning cigarettes: Related to 18% of fatal fires in 2006
- Inadequate or faulty electrical wiring
- Lack of smoke detectors: Lacking or nonfunctioning smoke alarms are implicated in 63% of residential fires.
- Arson: Cause of 27% of fires that resulted in fatalities in 2006

GENERAL PREVENTION

- Home safety education should be a key mechanism for injury prevention.
  - Home education families were more likely to have safe hot-water temperatures.
  - Home education results in more families having functioning smoke alarms and increased use of fire guards.
  - There is no evidence that home education results in increasing the chance of possessing a fire extinguisher.
  - Home education did not improve the odds of keeping hot drinks or food out of reach of children and did not increase the safe storage of matches.
  - There is a lack of evidence that home safety education with or without the provision of safety equipment results in a reduction of thermal injuries.
- Skin grafts or newly epithelialized skin is highly sensitive to sun exposure and thermal extremes.

ETIOLOGY

- Open flame and hot liquid are most common (heat usually ≥45°C): Flame burns more common in adults; scald burns more common in children.
- Caustic chemicals or acids (may show little signs or symptoms for the 1st few days)
- Electricity (may have significant injury with very little damage to overlying skin)
- Excess sun exposure

COMMONLY ASSOCIATED CONDITIONS

Smoke inhalation syndrome:

- May involve thermal burn to respiratory mucosa (e.g., trachea, bronchi) as well as carbon monoxide inhalation
- Occurs within 72 h of burn
- Should be suspected in all burns occurring in an enclosed space

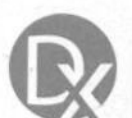

DIAGNOSIS

HISTORY

- History of source of burn
- In children, check for consistency between the history and the burn's physical characteristics.

PHYSICAL EXAM

- 1st degree:
  - Erythema of involved tissue
  - Skin blanches with pressure.
  - Skin may be tender.
- 2nd degree:
  - Skin is red and blistered.
  - Skin is very tender.
- 3rd degree:
  - Burned skin is tough and leathery.
  - Skin is not tender.
- Rule of nines (1)[C]:
  - Each upper extremity: Adult and child 9%
  - Each lower extremity: Adult 18%; child 14%
  - Anterior trunk: Adult and child 18%
  - Posterior trunk: Adult and child 18%
  - Head and neck: Adult 10%; child 18%
- Careful documentation of extent of burn and the estimated depth of burn
- Check for any signs suggestive of potential airway involvement: Singed nasal hair, facial burns, carbonaceous sputum, progressive hoarseness, or tachypnea.

DIAGNOSTIC TESTS & INTERPRETATION

- Children: Glucose (hypoglycemia may occur in children because of limited glycogen storage)
- Smoke inhalation: Arterial blood gas, carboxyhemoglobin
- Electrical burns: Electrocardiogram (ECG), urine myoglobin, creatine kinase isoenzymes

Lab

- Hematocrit
- Type and cross
- Electrolytes, including blood urea nitrogen (BUN) and creatinine
- Urinalysis

Imaging

- Chest radiograph
- Xenon scan useful in suspected smoke inhalation

Diagnostic Procedures/Surgery

Bronchoscopy may be necessary in smoke inhalation to evaluate lower respiratory tract.

TREATMENT

- Prehospital care (1)[C]:
  - Remove patient from source of burn.
  - Extinguish and remove all burning clothing.
  - Remove all rings, watches, and jewelry.
  - Room-temperature water may be poured onto burn, but only in the 1st 15 minutes following burn exposure.
  - Wrap patient to prevent hypothermia.
  - All patients to receive 100% O_2 via face mask
- Hospitalization for all serious burns:
  - 2nd-degree burns >10% of body surface area (BSA)
  - Any 3rd-degree burn
  - Burns of hands, feet, face, or perineum
  - Electrical/lightning burns
  - Inhalation injury
  - Chemical burns
  - Circumferential burn
- Transfer to burn center for (1)[C]
  - 2nd- and 3rd-degree burns >10% of BSA in patients <10 years and >50 years of age
  - 2nd-degree burns >20% of BSA and full-thickness burns >5% BSA in any age range
  - Burns of hands, feet, face, or perineum
  - Electrical or lightning burns
  - Inhalation injury
  - Chemical burns
  - Circumferential burn

MEDICATION

First Line

- Morphine: Small, frequent IV doses (0.1 mg/kg per dose in children; 2.5–20 mg q2–6h in adults)
- Silver sulfadiazine (Silvadene): Apply topically to burn site (can cause leukopenia).
- Neosporin or bacitracin ointment: Apply to facial burns.
- Mupirocen: Has potent inhibitory activity against methicillin-resistant *Staphylococcus aureus* (MRSA) (2)[B]
- Acticote A.B. (a dressing consisting of two sheets of high-density polyethylene mesh coated with nanocrystalline silver) has a more controlled, prolonged release of silver, allowing less frequent dressing changes (2)[B].

B

- Electrical burn with myoglobinuria will require alkalinization of urine and mannitol.
- No indication for prophylactic antibiotics.
- Consider H_2 blockers or proton-pump inhibitors (e.g., cimetidine, ranitidine, famotidine, lansoprazole, or nizatidine) for stress ulcer prophylaxis in severely burned patients.
- Tetanus toxoid/tetanus immunoglobulin
- There is no clear indication for prophylactic systemic antibiotics (2)[B].
- Use of VAC system may result in a low-protease environment with higher levels of angiogenic factor [vascular endothelial growth factor (VEGF)] during wound healing, leading to more chaotic, hyperkeratinized, thickened epidermis when compared with a standard hydrocolloid dressing (3)[C].

Second Line

- Mafenide (Sulfamylon) for full-thickness burn (*Caution:* Metabolic acidosis)
- Silver nitrate 0.5% (messy, leaches electrolytes from burn, causes water toxicity)
- Povidone–iodine (Betadine) may result in iodine absorption from burn and "tan eschar." Makes débridement more difficult.
- Travase (enzymatic débridement)

ADDITIONAL TREATMENT

General Measures

- Based on depth of burns and accurate estimate of total BSA involved (rule of nines)
- Quick estimate (for smaller burns): The surface area of the patient's hand is ~1% of the BSA.
- Tetanus prophylaxis (if not current)
- Remove all rings, watches, and other items from injured extremities to avoid tourniquet effect
- Remove clothing, and cover all burned areas with dry sheets.
- Flush area of chemical burn (for ~2 h).
- 100% oxygen administration for all major burns; consider early intubation.
- Do not apply ice to burn site.
- Nasogastric tube (high risk of paralytic ileus)
- Foley catheter
- Pain relief:
  - IV meperidine (Demerol), morphine, or methadone for severe pain
  - Oral analgesics, such as acetaminophen (Tylenol) with codeine, acetaminophen with oxycodone (Percocet), or acetaminophen with hydrocodone (Lortab) for moderate pain
- ECG monitoring in 1st 24 h following electrical burn
- Whirlpool hydrotherapy followed by silver sulfadiazine (Silvadene) occlusive dressings in severe burns
- Daily or b.i.d. cleansing with dressing changes
- Epilock or Elasto-Gel may be used as dressing in selected patients (especially useful for outpatient treatment of minor burns).

- Burn fluid resuscitation (1)[C]:
  - Calculate fluid resuscitation from time of burn, not from time treatment begins.
  - 2–4 mL Ringer's lactate × body weight (kg) × % BSA burn (1/2 given in 1st 8 hours, in 2nd 8 hours, and in 3rd 8 hours); in children, this is given in addition to maintenance fluids and is adjusted according to urine output and vital signs.
  - Colloid solutions are not recommended during the 1st 12–24 h of resuscitation (1)[C],(4)[A].
- Other: Use of biologic membranes or skin substitutes may be indicated for burn coverage.
- Inhalation injury:
  - Intubation, ventilation with positive end-expiratory pressure assistance
  - Hyperbaric oxygen treatment may be useful in patients with carbon monoxide levels >25%, patients with coma, focal neurologic deficit, ischemic ECG changes, and pregnant patients (1)[C].

SURGERY/OTHER PROCEDURES

- Escharotomy may be necessary in constricting circumferential burns of extremities or chest.
- Tangential excision with split-thickness skin grafts
- Early excision of burns results in a significant reduction in mortality (excluding patients with inhalational injury) and a significant decrease in hospital length of stay (5)[B].

ONGOING CARE

FOLLOW-UP RECOMMENDATIONS

Early mobilization is the goal.

DIET

- High-protein, high-calorie diet when bowel function resumes
- Nasogastric tube feedings may be required in early postburn period.
- Total parenteral nutrition if n.p.o. expected for >5 days

PATIENT EDUCATION

- Use of sunscreen
- Access to electrical cords/outlets
- Isolate household chemicals
- Use low-temperature setting for water heater (below 54°C)
- Household smoke detectors with special emphasis on maintenance
- Family/household evacuation plan
- Proper storage and use of flammable substances
- Burn management: www.aafp.org/afp/20001101/2029ph.html
- Burn prevention: www.aafp.org/afp/20001101/2032ph.html

PROGNOSIS

- 1st-degree burn: Complete resolution
- 2nd-degree burn: Epithelialization in 10–14 days (deep 2nd-degree burns probably will require skin graft)
- 3rd-degree burn: No potential for reepithelialization; skin graft required
- Length of hospital stay and need for ICU care depend on extent of burn, smoke inhalation, and age.
- A 50% survival rate can be expected with a 62% burn in patients aged 0–14 years, 63% burn in patients aged 15–40 years, 38% burn in patients aged 40–65 years, and 25% burn in patients >65 years of age (1)[C].
- 90% of survivors can be expected to return to an occupation as remunerative as their preburn employment.

COMPLICATIONS

- Gastroduodenal ulceration (curling ulcer)
- Marjolin ulcer: Squamous cell carcinoma developing in old burn site
- Burn wound sepsis: most commonly *S. aureus* (including MRSA), vancomycin-resistant enterococci, and gram-negative organisms (2)[B]
- Pneumonia
- Decreased mobility with possibility of future flexion contractures
- Hypertrophic scarring common with burns

REFERENCES

1. Teague H, Sweneki SA, Tang A. The burned patient: assessment, diagnosis, and management in the ED. *Trauma Reports*. 2005;6:1–12.
2. Church D, Elsayed S, Reid O, Winston B, Lindsay R, et al. Burn wound infections. *Clin Microbiol Rev*. 2006;19:403–34.
3. Caulfield RH, Tyler MP, Austyn JM, et al. The relationship between protease/anti-protease profile, angiogenesis and re-epithelialisation in acute burn wounds. *Burns*. 2008;34:474–86.
4. Roberts I, Alderson P, Bunn F, et al. Colloids versus crystalloids for fluid resuscitation in critically ill patients (Review). *Cochrane Database Sys Rev*. 2006; Vol 1.
5. Ong YS, Samuel M, Song C. Meta-analysis of early excision of burns. *Burns*. 2006;32:145–50.

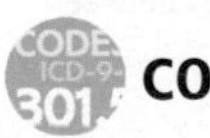

CODES

ICD9

949.0 Burn of unspecified site, unspecified degree

CLINICAL PEARLS

- 1st degree:
  - Erythema of involved tissue
  - Skin blanches with pressure.
  - Skin may be tender.
- 2nd degree:
  - Skin is red and blistered.
  - Skin is very tender.
- 3rd degree:
  - Burned skin is tough and leathery.
  - Skin is not tender.

BURSITIS

J. Herbert Stevenson, MD

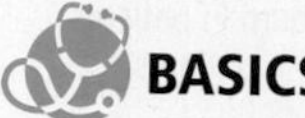

BASICS

DESCRIPTION

A *bursa* is a sac that is formed or found in areas subject to friction, such as locations where tendons pass over bony landmarks. Most common sites are subdeltoid, olecranon, prepatellar, trochanteric, and radiohumeral. Bursae essentially lubricate the region with synovial fluid:

- Large bursae usually communicate with joints and are responsible for retaining the synovial fluid in place.
- Bursae are fluid-filled sacs that serve as a cushion between tendons and bones.
- E.G. Bywaters, an English rheumatologist, found at least 78 bursae symmetrically placed on each side of the body.
- System(s) affected: Musculoskeletal

Pediatric Considerations

- Bursitis is less common in the pediatric population.

EPIDEMIOLOGY

Predominant age:

- 15–50 years (most common in skeletally mature)
- Traumatic bursitis more likely in patients < 35 years of age

Incidence

- Common
- Trochanteric pain: 1.8/1,000 per year (1)[B]

RISK FACTORS

Individuals who engage in repetitive and vigorous training or others who suddenly increase their level of activity (e.g., "weekend warriors")

GENERAL PREVENTION

- Appropriate warm-up and cool-down maneuvers, avoidance of overuse, or inadequate rest between workouts
- Range-of-motion exercises
- Maintain high level of fitness and general good health

ETIOLOGY

- Bursitis may be acute or chronic
- Many types of bursitis, including infectious, traumatic, inflammatory, and gouty
- Less often rheumatoid disease or tuberculosis as well as gout and pseudogout

COMMONLY ASSOCIATED CONDITIONS

- Tendinitis
- Sprains, strains
- Associated stress fractures

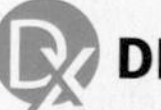

DIAGNOSIS

PHYSICAL EXAM

- Pain/tenderness
- Decreased range of motion of affected region (rare except at shoulder)
- Erythema if infection present
- Swelling
- Crepitus sometimes found

DIAGNOSTIC TESTS & INTERPRETATION

Consider ECG (if left shoulder pain mimics cardiac pain)

Lab

- The following may help in differentiating soft tissue disease from rheumatic and connective tissue disease:
  - CBC
  - ESR
  - Serum protein electrophoresis
  - Rheumatoid factor
  - Serum uric acid
  - Phosphorus
  - Alkaline phosphatase
  - Blood testing for syphilis
  - Joint fluid analysis and culture (when indicated)
- Drugs that may alter lab results:
  - ESR rate may be increased with coexistent use of methyldopa, methysergide, penicillamine, theophylline, vitamin A.
  - ESR may be decreased with coexistent use of quinine, salicylates, and drugs that cause a high glucose level.

Imaging

- MRI may prove beneficial if diagnosis is unclear.
- Calcific deposits may be seen on plain radiograph
- Ultrasound (2)[B]

Diagnostic Procedures/Surgery

- Aspiration of swollen bursa and evaluation of synovial fluid; the clinician must differentiate infected from inflammatory bursitis:
  - Fluid WBC 2–5,000/uL imply inflammatory, whereas >5,000 imply infectious cause.
  - Fluid analysis, Gram-stain, culture, and crystal analysis required to make the diagnosis.
- If the Gram-stain and culture yield an infective cause, treat with appropriate antibiotics. If the etiology is inflammatory, give local care.

Pathological Findings

- Acute with early inflammation: Bursa is distended with watery or mucoid fluid.
- Infection: Purulent fluid on aspiration
- Chronic:
  - Bursal wall is thickened, and inner surface is shaggy and trabeculated.
  - The space is filled with granular, brown, inspissated blood admixed with gritty, calcific precipitations.
  - Upper extremity tendinitis and bursitis are usuall the result of repetitive microtrauma, probably resulting in disruption of fibers, leading to pain, spasm, and disability.

DIFFERENTIAL DIAGNOSIS

- Septic arthritis
- Gout, pseudogout
- Rheumatic disorders
- Osteoarthritis
- Tendinitis, strains, and sprains
- Lyme arthritis

B

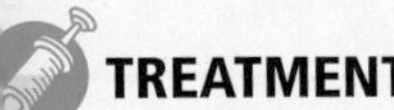

TREATMENT

utpatient; refer only difficult cases

MEDICATION

First Line

- NSAIDs or aspirin (3,4)[C]
- Antibiotic therapy if infection present; cover for staph and strep species (most common) (5)[B]
- Contraindications: Refer to manufacturer's profile of each drug.
- Precautions: Refer to manufacturer's profile of each drug.
- Significant possible interactions: Refer to manufacturer's profile of each drug.

Second Line

- Injectable corticosteroids once infectious etiology ruled out (3)[C],(4)[B],(6)[C],(7)[B]
- Systemic steroids provide limited short-term benefit (8)[B]

ADDITIONAL TREATMENT

General Measures

- Conservative therapy consists of rest, ice, and local care; elevation, gentle compression (often referred to as RICE therapy [rest-ice-compression-elevation])
- Compression with Ace wrap or neoprene sleeve
- Bursa aspiration
- Corticosteroid injection if infectious etiology ruled out
- Treatment of any underlying infection

SURGERY/OTHER PROCEDURES

Surgical excision in severe cases unresponsive to conservative treatments (5)[B]

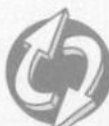

ONGOING CARE

FOLLOW-UP RECOMMENDATIONS

Rest and elevation of affected extremity

Patient Monitoring

- Discontinue NSAIDs as soon as possible to avoid side effects.
- Some patients may require repeated injections (usually no more than 3) of a corticosteroid and lidocaine (3,6)[C].

DIET

Consider changes if bursitis is directly related to obesity/crystalline deposition.

PROGNOSIS

- Most bouts of bursitis heal without sequelae.
- Repetitive acute bouts may lead to chronic bursitis, necessitating repeated joint/bursal aspirations or, eventually, surgical excision of involved bursa.

COMPLICATIONS

- Septic bursitis may extend to the nearby joint.
- Acute bursitis may progress to chronic.
- Severe long-range limitation of motion

REFERENCES

1. Lievense A, Bierma Zeinstra S, Schouten B, et al. Prognosis of trochanteric pain in primary care. *Br J Gen Pract*. 2005;55:199–204.
2. Finlay K, Friedman L. Ultrasonography of the lower extremity. *Orthop Clin North Am*. 2006;37: 245–75, v.
3. Talia AH, Cardone D. Diagnostic and therapeutic injection of the shoulder region. *Am Fam Phys*. 2003;67(6):1271–8.
4. McFarland EG, Gill HS, Laporte DM, et al. Miscellaneous conditions about the elbow in athletes. *Clin Sports Med*. 2004;23:743–63, xi–xii.
5. Small LN, Ross JJ. Suppurative tenosynovitis and septic bursitis. *Infect Dis Clin North Am*. 2005;19: 991–1005, xi.
6. Cardone D, Tallia AH. Diagnostic and therapeutic injection of the hip and knee. *Am Fam Phys*. 2003;67(10):2147–53.
7. Buchbinder R, et al. Corticosteroid injection for shoulder pain. *Cochrane Database Sys Rev*. 2003; Issue Jan. 1.
8. Buchbinder R, Hoving JL, Green S, et al. Short course prednisolone for adhesive capsulitis (frozen shoulder or stiff painful shoulder): a randomised, double blind, placebo controlled trial. *Ann Rheum Dis*. 2004;63:1460–9.

ADDITIONAL READING

Cardone D, Tallia AH. Diagnostic and therapeutic injection of the elbow. *Am Fam Phys*. 2002;66(11): 2097–3100.

See Also (Topic, Algorithm, Electronic Media Element)

Tendinitis
Video: Olecranon Bursitis Aspiration

CODES

ICD9

727.3 Other bursitis disorders

CLINICAL PEARLS

Remember RICE acronym for conservative therapy:

- Rest affected area
- Ice inflammed bursa
- Compression (with Ace wrap or neoprene sleeve)
- Elevate joint

CANDIDIASIS

Brock D. Lutz, MD
Ronald A. Greenfield, MD

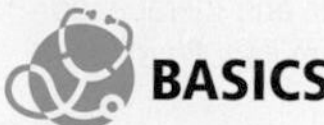

BASICS

DESCRIPTION

Candida albicans and related species cause a variety of infections:

- Cutaneous syndromes include erosio interdigitalis blastomycetica, folliculitis, balanitis, intertrigo, paronychia, onychomycosis, diaper rash, perianal candidiasis, and the syndromes of chronic mucocutaneous candidiasis.
- Mucous membrane infections include oral candidiasis (thrush), esophagitis, and vaginitis.
- The most serious manifestations of candidiasis are candidemia and hematogenously disseminated invasive candidiasis. This article discusses candidemia and hematogenously disseminated candidiasis.

EPIDEMIOLOGY

- Predominant age: All ages are susceptible to hematogenously disseminated candidiasis; premature neonates are at particularly high risk.
- Predominant sex: Male = Female (hematogenously disseminated candidiasis)

Incidence

≥20/100,000 persons per year

Prevalence

Data not available

RISK FACTORS

- Neutropenia
- Corticosteroid treatment
- HIV infection
- Diabetes mellitus
- Mucocutaneous colonization/infection
- Broad-spectrum antibacterial chemotherapy
- Recent chemotherapy or radiation
- Indwelling intravascular access devices
- Cardiothoracic or abdominal surgery
- Parenteral nutrition
- Prolonged hospital stay
- Intensive care unit (ICU) stay
- Burns
- End-stage renal disease
- Bone marrow or solid organ transplant recipient
- Cancer
- Premature birth

GENERAL PREVENTION

- Polyenes, azoles, and echinocandins reduce the incidence of candidiasis in patients undergoing induction therapy for acute leukemia or bone marrow or stem cell transplantation (1)[A].
- Fluconazole prophylaxis in high-risk ICU patients reduces the incidence of invasive candidiasis (2)[A]. See Medications.

PATHOPHYSIOLOGY

An acute suppurative infection in which polymorphonuclear host defense is the critical element

ETIOLOGY

- *Candida albicans* is the most frequent pathogen. Other important human pathogens include *C. tropicalis*, *C. krusei*, *C. stellatoidea*, *C. pseudotropicalis*, *C. guilliermondi*, *C. parapsilosis*, *C. lusitaniae*, *C. rugosa*, *C. lambica*, and *C. glabrata*.
- *Candida* species colonize human mucocutaneous surfaces; most infections are endogenously acquired from this reservoir.
- Human-to-human transmission of *Candida* occurs in some settings.

COMMONLY ASSOCIATED CONDITIONS

See Risk Factors.

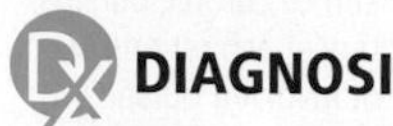

DIAGNOSIS

HISTORY

- Several days of fever that is unresponsive to broad-spectrum antibiotics
- Prolonged intravenous catheterization
- A history of several key risk factors
- Be alert to organ system dysfunction.

PHYSICAL EXAM

- Fever
- Malaise
- Tachycardia
- Hypotension
- Altered mental status
- Hepatosplenomegaly
- Maculopapular or nodular skin rash

Pediatric Considerations

- For an infant with thrush, be sure to also check for candidal diaper dermatitis. Also, there is often a concomitant infection.
- Fever
- Macronodular skin lesions (10%)
- Candidal endophthalmitis (10–28%)
- Generally patients are ill and may manifest septic shock.

DIAGNOSTIC TESTS & INTERPRETATION

- The diagnosis is established by isolating the causative organism from blood cultures or other normally sterile body sites or by demonstration of organisms in histopathologic specimens of normally sterile tissues.
- Isolation of *Candida* from multiple sites should raise the diagnostic suspicion of hematogenously disseminated invasive candidiasis.
- *Candida* species isolated from a normally sterile site should be identified to the species level (1)[A].
- Because fluconazole-resistant *C. albicans* and particularly nonalbicans species are reported with increasing frequency, fluconazole susceptibility testing should be performed before treatment with fluconazole (1)[B].

Imaging

- Generally not specifically useful in diagnosis of hematogenously invasive disseminated candidiasis. However, multisite metastasis of infection is common.
- In the syndrome of hepatosplenic candidiasis (chronic systemic candidiasis), imaging of the liver and spleen by liver scan, ultrasound, computed tomography (CT), or magnetic resonance imaging (MRI) may suggest this syndrome as the cause of persistent fever and liver dysfunction in patients who have recently recovered from neutropenia.

Diagnostic Procedures/Surgery

- If blood cultures remain consistently negative, aspiration or excisional biopsy of sites of focal infection may be useful in diagnosis.
- Aspiration and biopsy of skin lesions occasionally seen with hematogenously disseminated candidiasi are also useful.

Pathological Findings

Characteristic histopathology of lesions of *Candida* invasion of visceral organs is microabscess formation.

DIFFERENTIAL DIAGNOSIS

Includes a variety of cryptic bacterial infections and, in the neutropenic host, multiple opportunistic infections

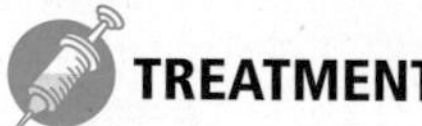

TREATMENT

Inpatient for hematogenously disseminated invasive candidiasis

MEDICATION

- Echinocandins (3)[A]:
  - An initial therapy of choice for any patient with candidemia (1)[A]
  - Patients with initial echinocandin therapy may have a survival advantage.
  - Caspofungin: Administer 70 mg IV dose on day 1 followed by 50 mg/d IV for 2 weeks after last positive sterile site culture if no evident metastatic infection.
  - Modify dose for severe hepatic insufficiency.
  - *C. parapsilosis* has reduced sensitivity to echinocandins.
  - The echinocandins anidulafungin and micafungin have similar efficacy.
- Fluconazole:
  - An initial therapy of choice for some patients (1)[A]
  - Because it is fungistatic rather than fungicidal, it should not be used for treatment of patients with severe neutropenia or severe immunosuppression.
  - It should only be used after confirmation of in vitro susceptibility in patients with azole therapy in prior 3 months.
  - Should be used empirically only in institutions with a very low prevalence of resistance
  - Useful for switch therapy after demonstration of in vitro susceptibility after initial therapy with an echinocandin or amphotericin

- For 1st week, administer 400–800 mg/d IV, followed by additional IV or oral therapy at the same dose for ≥2 weeks after the last positive blood culture or last evidence of infection. Higher doses of fluconazole may be required if non-*Albicans* species are known or suspected, because they carry a higher likelihood of drug resistance.
- *C. krusei* and many *C. glabrata* are resistant to fluconazole.

Liposomal amphotericin B:
- Can be used as an initial therapy for any patient with candidemia (1)[A]. Cautious use is indicated given relative risks of toxicity compared to alternative therapies.
- Usual dosage is 3 mg/kg/d IV.
- *C. lusitaniae* may be resistant.
- Consider higher doses for *C. krusei* or *C. glabrata* (5–10 mg/kg/d).

Other azole antifungals, depending on activity and safety (itraconazole and voriconazole)

Contraindications:
- The safety of amphotericin B therapy in pregnant patients has not been established.
- Echinocandins are pregnancy Category C.

Precautions:
- Liposomal amphotericin B:
  - The toxicity is less common than with conventional amphotericin B, but may still be formidable. Acute reactions (fever, rigors, and hypotension) may occur during the initiation of therapy. Ameliorate or eliminate by premedication with acetaminophen or ibuprofen. Use meperidine if needed to abort rigors.
  - Azotemia may occur. Maintenance of optimal fluid status and prevention of dehydration help minimize the risk of azotemia. "Sodium loading" with 1 L half-normal saline daily may decrease renal toxicity.
  - Significant hypokalemia and renal tubular acidosis may develop. Significant hypomagnesemia may worsen hypokalemia.
  - Anemia commonly develops in patients on protracted therapy, but is almost always reversible.
  - Headache and phlebitis are common. Use central venous access for administration.
  - Leukopenia, thrombocytopenia, and liver function abnormalities are rare.

- Itraconazole, voriconazole, caspofungin, anidulafungin, and micafungin do not enter the urinary stream in sufficient concentrations to treat urinary tract infections (UTIs).
- Significant possible drug-drug interactions:
  - Echinocandins:
    - Potentially important interactions with carbamazepine, phenytoin, cyclosporine, tacrolimus, sirolimus, non-nucleoside reverse transcriptase inhibitors, and rifampin.
  - Liposomal amphotericin B:
    - Concomitant therapy with cyclosporine or other nephrotoxic agents, such as aminoglycosides or vancomycin, may increase the risk of amphotericin-induced nephrotoxicity.
  - Fluconazole and other azoles:
    - Potentially important drug-drug interactions may occur in patients receiving oral hypoglycemics, coumarin-type anticoagulants, phenytoin, cyclosporine, rifampin, theophylline, or terfenadine or astemizole.
    - These drug-drug interactions are more likely with itraconazole and voriconazole than with fluconazole.

ADDITIONAL TREATMENT

General Measures
- Fluid and electrolyte therapy are often required.
- Hemodynamic and respiratory support may be required in seriously ill patients.
- The removal of potentially infected intravascular access devices is imperative.

Issues for Referral
Invasive *Candida* infections should be managed with the assistance of an infectious disease specialist.

SURGERY/OTHER PROCEDURES
Drainage of abscess (by any means clinically feasible) is necessary for resolution. Removal of any indwelling contaminated device or catheter is necessary.

IN-PATIENT CONSIDERATIONS

IV Fluids
Generally necessary in critically ill patients

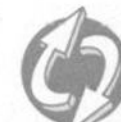

ONGOING CARE

FOLLOW-UP RECOMMENDATIONS
Patients should receive follow-up visit ~6 weeks after end of therapy and be screened for metastatic infection complications by history and physical exam.

Patient Monitoring
- Evaluate complete blood count (CBC), serum electrolytes, and serum creatinine at least twice weekly in patients on liposomal amphotericin B therapy.
- If blood cultures are positive, they should be repeated until negative. Therapy must be extended in this case.

DIET
Popular literature has reports of diet being linked to yeast overgrowth and subsequent chronic fatigue; randomized controlled trials suggest following a low-sugar, low-yeast diet has no benefit over general healthy eating for symptoms of fatigue (4)[B].

PATIENT EDUCATION
Advise patients of the nature of the infection and the toxicities associated with therapy.

PROGNOSIS
Overall mortality for patients with hematogenously disseminated candidiasis is 40–75%, with mortality attributable to candidemia being 15–37%.

COMPLICATIONS
- Systemic inflammatory response syndrome
- Pyelonephritis
- Endophthalmitis
- Endocarditis, myocarditis, pericarditis
- Arthritis, chondritis, osteomyelitis
- Pneumonitis
- Central nervous system infection

REFERENCES

1. Spellberg BJ, Filler SG, Edwards JE. Current treatment strategies for disseminated candidiasis. *Clin Infect Dis*. 2006;42:244–51.
2. Vardakas KZ, Samonis G, Michalopoulos A, et al. Antifungal prophylaxis with azoles in high-risk, surgical intensive care unit patients: a metaanalysis of randomized, placebo-controlled trials. *Crit Care Med*. 2006;34:1216–24.
3. Sucher AJ, Chahine EB, Balcer HE. Echinocandins: The Newest Class of Antifungals (October) (CE). *Ann Pharmacother*. 2009.
4. Hobday RA, Thomas S, O'Donovan A, et al. Dietary intervention in chronic fatigue syndrome. *J Hum Nutr Diet*. 2008;21:141–9.

ADDITIONAL READING

- Benjamin DK, Stoll BJ, Fanaroff AA, et al. Neonatal candidiasis among extremely low birth weight infants: risk factors, mortality rates, and neurodevelopmental outcomes at 18 to 22 months. *Pediatrics*. 2006;117:84–92.
- Golan Y, Wolf MP, Pauker SG, et al. Empirical anti-Candida therapy among selected patients in the intensive care unit: a cost-effectiveness analysis. *Ann Intern Med*. 2005;143:857–69.
- Ha JF, Italiano CM, Heath CH, et al. Candidemia and invasive candidiasis: a review of the literature for the burns surgeon. *Burns: Journal of the International Society for Burn Injuries*. 2010.
- Ostrosky-Zeichner L, Pappas PG. Invasive candidiasis in the intensive care unit. *Crit Care Med*. 2006;34:857–63.
- Worthington HV, Clarkson JE, Khalid T, et al. Interventions for treating oral candidiasis for patients with cancer receiving treatment. *Cochrane Database Syst Rev*. 2010;7:CD001972.

See Also (Topic, Algorithm, Electronic Media Element)
Vulvovaginitis, Candidal

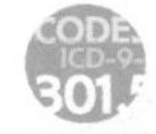

CODES

ICD9
- 112.0 Candidiasis of mouth
- 112.1 Candidiasis of vulva and vagina
- 112.2 Candidiasis of other urogenital sites

CLINICAL PEARLS
- Fluconazole prophylaxis in high-risk ICU patients reduces the incidence of invasive candidiasis.
- Caspofungin or another of the echinocandins is initial therapy of choice for any patient with candidemia (1)[A].

CANDIDIASIS, MUCOCUTANEOUS

Sheila O. Stille, DMD, MAGD
Hugh J. Silk, MD

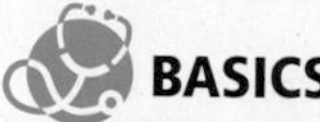

BASICS

DESCRIPTION

- A mucocutaneous disorder caused by infection with various *Candida* sp.
- Areas include:
  - GI
    - Oropharyngeal candidiasis: Mouth, pharynx
    - Angular cheilitis: Fissures at mouth corners
    - Candida esophagitis: Esophagus
    - GI candidiasis: Gastritis, +/− ulcers, associated with thrush; in tract or perianal
  - Non-Gastrointestinal
    - Candida vulvovaginitis: Vaginal mucosa and/or cutaneous aspects of the vulva
    - Candidal balanitis: Glans penis
    - Candidal paronychia: Nail bed of a digit
    - Folliculitis: Hair follicles
    - Interdigital candidiasis: Webs of the digits
- System(s) affected: Oropharynx; GI; Skin/Exocrine; Genitourinary
- Synonym(s): Monilia; thrush; yeast

ALERT
Vaginal antifungal creams and suppositories can weaken condoms and diaphragms.

Pregnancy Considerations

No known fetal complications of maternal *Candida*

EPIDEMIOLOGY

- Common in the US, very common with immunodeficiency and/or uncontrolled diabetes
- Predominant age: None:
  - Infants and seniors: Thrush and cutaneous infections (infant diaper rash)
  - Women of childbearing age: Vaginitis
  - Prepubertal or postmenopausal: Yeast vaginitis uncommon
  - Predominant sex: Female > Male (because of vaginitis)

Incidence

Not well studied, but some estimate 50/100,000

Prevalence

Candida colonization: >50% of US population

RISK FACTORS

- Immunosuppression
- Hormonal fluctuations in females
- Antibacterial therapy, especially broad-spectrum antibiotics
- Douches, chemical irritants, and other vaginitides can predispose to yeast vaginitis
- Dentures
- Birth control pills
- Hyperglycemia

Genetics

Chronic mucocutaneous candidiasis is a heterogeneous, genetic syndrome; usually presents in childhood, but mode of inheritance has not been clarified.

GENERAL PREVENTION

- Minimize antibiotic use
- Minimize inhaled and systemic steroid use; rinse mouth after inhaled steroid use
- Avoid douching, chemicals (i.e., spermicides)
- Treat other vaginitides
- Minimize moist environments (e.g., wear cotton underwear)
- Clean dentures appropriately; have new, well-fitting dentures fabricated
- Control diabetes (if present)

ETIOLOGY

C. albicans predominant (responsible for 80–92% vulvovaginal candidiasis and 70–80% oral isolates)

COMMONLY ASSOCIATED CONDITIONS

- HIV and other leukopenias
- Diabetes mellitus
- Cancer and other immunosuppressive disorders
- Disorders requiring corticosteroids (1) or other immunosuppressive chemotherapy

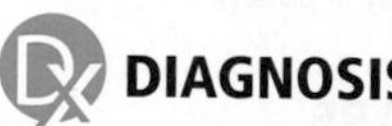

DIAGNOSIS

- NOTE: *Candida* is normal flora, in very small amounts, in oral cavity, GI tract, and female genital tract.
- In children:
  - Oral: White, raised, painless, distinct patches within the mouth; can be wiped off to reveal red base, sometimes with pinpoint bleeding
  - Perineal: Erythematous maculopapular rash with satellite pustules or papules
  - Angular cheilitis: Painful fissures in mouth corners, often cracked and bleeding
- In adults:
  - Vulvovaginal lesions; thin to thick whitish cottage cheese-like discharge; red patches in vagina or perineum; symptoms range from none to intense pruritus/burning
- In immunocompromised hosts:
  - Oral: White, raised, painless, distinct patches; red, slightly raised patches; thick, dark-brownish coating; deep fissures
  - Esophagitis: Dysphagia, odynophagia, retrosternal pain; usually with thrush
  - GI symptoms: Ulcerations, pain
  - Balanitis: Erythema, linear erosions, scaling; possible dysuria
  - Angular cheilitis (see In children)
  - Folliculitis: Follicular pustules
  - Interdigital: Redness, itchiness at base of fingers and/or toes susceptible to maceration

DIAGNOSTIC TESTS & INTERPRETATION

Imaging

Barium swallow: Esophageal candidiasis may reveal a cobblestone appearance, fistulas, or esophageal dilatation (from denervation)

Diagnostic Procedures/Surgery

- KOH prep: A sample of the discharge or coating of the infected area or ulcer is needed.
- Esophagitis may require biopsy.
- Oral hyperplastic candidiasis should be biopsied to rule out carcinoma.
- HIV seropositivity plus thrush with dysphagia relieved by antifungal treatment are acceptable criteria for diagnosis of *Candida* esophagitis.

Pathological Findings

- Slide preparation: Mycelia (hyphae) or pseudomycelia (pseudohyphae) yeast forms; *Candida* does not induce an increased PMN leukocyte response.
- Biopsy: Epithelial parakeratosis with PMNs in superficial layers; PAS staining reveals presence of candidal hyphae.

DIFFERENTIAL DIAGNOSIS

- For oral candidiasis:
  - Leukoplakia
  - Lichen planus
  - Geographic tongue
  - Herpes simplex
  - Erythema multiforme
  - Pemphigus
- Baby formula or breast milk can mimic thrush
- Hairy leukoplakia: Does not rub off to erythematou[s] base; usually on lateral tongue
- Angular cheilitis from vitamin B or iron deficiency, staph infection, or edentulous over closure
- *Bacterial vaginosis* and *Trichomonas vaginalis* tend to have more odor, itch, and have a different discharge, but symptoms that are similar to those c[of] *Candida vaginalis* include:
  - Marked vulvar irritation
  - Labial erythema
  - External dysuria
  - Vaginal tenderness

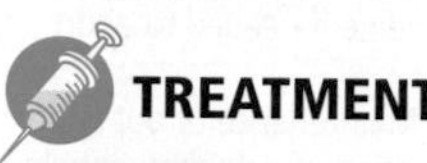

TREATMENT

MEDICATION

First Line

- Vaginal (choose 1):
  - Miconazole (Monistat) 2% cream: 1 applicator or 1 100–200-mg suppository, intravaginally q.h.s. for 7 days
  - Clotrimazole (Gyne-Lotrimin, Mycelex): Intravaginal tablets (100 mg q.h.s. for 6–7 days, 200 mg q.h.s. for 3 days; 500 mg daily for 1 day), or 1% cream (1 applicator q.h.s. for 6–7 days)
  - Fluconazole 150 mg PO in 1 dose.
  - Nystatin (Mycostatin, Nilstat): 100,000 U/g cream (1 applicator) or 100,000 U tablets (1 tablet) intravaginally 1 × day for 7–14 days
- Oropharyngeal:
  - Mild disease:
    - Clotrimazole (Mycelex): 10 mg troche, suck on over 20 minutes 5 times a day for 7–14 days, o[r]
    - Nystatin suspension: 100,000 U/ml given 4–6 times daily, or
    - Nystatin pastilles: 200,000 U each, administered 4 times daily for 7–14 days (2)[B]
    - Denture wearers:
      - Nystatin ointment: 100,000 U/g on fitting surfaces of denture and corners of mouth for 3 weeks
      - Remove dentures at night; clean twice weekly with diluted (1:20) bleach
  - Moderate to severe disease:
    - Fluconazole : 100–200 mg (3 mg/kg) daily for 7–14 days

C

Esophagitis:
- Fluconazole: 100 mg/d for 14–21 days, load with 200 mg
- Itraconazole (Sporanox):
  - Solution: 1–200 mg daily for 7–14 days
  - Capsules: 200 mg/d (take with food) for 2–3 weeks

GI: Therapy not well defined

Any site during pregnancy

Pregnancy Considerations

Miconazole is usually the drug of choice.

Second Line

Vaginal:
- Terconazole (Terazol): Recurrent cases: 0.4% cream (1 applicator q.h.s. for 10–14 days of induction therapy); 0.8% cream/80-mg suppositories (1 applicator or 1 suppository q.h.s. for 3 days)
- Prophylaxis: fluconazole, 150 mg once per week for 6 months to prevent recurrent infections

Oropharyngeal:
- Clotrimazole troches at a dosage of 10 mg 5 times daily
- Nystatin oral suspension (100,000 U/mL):
  - Children: 5–10 mL 4 times daily for 10 days directly to oral lesions
  - Infants: 0.5 mL in each cheek 4 times daily for 10 days
  - Adults: Swish for as long as reasonable and swallow 5–10 mL 4 times daily for 14 days; prophylaxis is achieved with above dosages 2–5 times a day.
- Fluconazole: 100 mg/d for 7–14 days (load immunocompromised patient with 200 mg)
- Itraconazole (Sporanox) suspension: 200 mg (20 mL) daily; swish and swallow for 7–14 days; capsules: 200 mg/d (take with food) for 2–4 weeks
- Miconazole oral gel (20 mg/mL): q.i.d., swish for as long as reasonable and swallow
- Amphotericin B (Fungizone) oral suspension (100 mg/mL): 1 mL 4 times daily, swish for as long as reasonable and swallow; use between meals
- Ketoconazole: 200–400 mg PO daily for 14–21 days

- Esophagitis:
  - Oral fluconazole at a dosage of 200–400 mg (3–6 mg/kg) daily for 14–21 days
  - Amphotericin B (variable dosing) i.v. dose of 0.3–0.7 mg/kg daily, or an echinocandin should be used for patients who cannot tolerate oral therapy
- Continue all treatments until 2 days after disappearance of infection:
  - Contraindications:
    - Ketoconazole, itraconazole, or nystatin (if swallowed): Severe hepatotoxicity
    - Amphotericin B: Renal failure
  - Precautions:
    - Miconazole: Can potentiate the effect of warfarin, but drug of choice in pregnancy
    - Fluconazole: Renal excretion; rare hepatotoxicity; resistance frequent
    - Itraconazole: Doubling the dosage results in ~3-fold increase in itraconazole plasma concentrations
- Possible interactions (rarely seen with creams, lotions, or suppositories):
  - Fluconazole:
    - Rifampin: Decreased fluconazole concentrations
    - Tolbutamide: Decreased tolbutamide concentrations
    - Warfarin, phenytoin, cyclosporine: Altered metabolism; check levels
  - Itraconazole: Potent CYP 3A4 inhibitor. Carefully assess all coadministered medications.

ADDITIONAL TREATMENT

General Measures

Screen severely immunodeficient patients at routine visits.

Issues for Referral

- Patients without obvious reasons for recurrent superficial candidal infections
- GI candidiasis

Additional Therapies

- For infants with thrush: Boil pacifiers and bottle nipples; assess mom's breasts/nipples for candida infections as well
- For denture-related candidiasis, disinfection of the denture, in addition to antifungal therapy

COMPLEMENTARY AND ALTERNATIVE MEDICINE

Probiotics: *Lactobacillus* and *Bifidobacterium* may inhibit *Candida sp* (3).

IN-PATIENT CONSIDERATIONS

Nursing

Staff for the elderly patients should be properly trained in oral hygiene. Protocols for brushing, proper denture care, and moistening the oral cavity can reduce candidal infections in the elderly.

ONGOING CARE

FOLLOW-UP RECOMMENDATIONS

Patient Monitoring

Immunocompromised persons may benefit from regular symptom evaluation plus routine KOH preps during vaginal and oral exams.

DIET

Active-culture yogurt or other live lactobacillus may decrease colonization; indeterminate evidence

PATIENT EDUCATION

- Advise patients at risk for recurrence about antibacterial therapy overgrowth (1)[B]
- "zole-type" medications are Category C

PROGNOSIS

- For immunocompetent individuals: Benign course, excellent prognosis
- For immunosuppressed persons: *Candida* may become an AIDS-defining illness, and chronicity may cause much morbidity

COMPLICATIONS

In immunosuppressed persons, complications depend on the severity of the immune status. In HIV infection, moderate immunosuppression (e.g., CD4 200–500 cells/mm^3) may be associated with chronic candidiasis. In severe immunosuppression (e.g., CD4 $<$100 cells/mm^3), thrush may lead to esophagitis, then a full-systemic infection involving every organ system, particularly renal.

REFERENCES

1. Kyrmizakis DE, Papadakis CE, Lohuis PJ, et al. Acute candidiasis of the oro- and hypopharynx as the result of topical intranasal steroids administration. *Rhinology*. 2000;38:87–9.
2. Pappas PG, Kauffman CA, Andes D, et al. Clinical practice guidelines for the management of candidiasis: 2009 update by the Infectious Diseases Society of America. *Clin Infect Dis*. 2009;48:503–35.
3. Strus M, Kucharska A, Kukla G, et al. The in vitro activity of vaginal Lactobacillus with probiotic properties against Candida. *Infect Dis Obstet Gynecol*. 2005;13:69–75.

ADDITIONAL READING

- Achkar JM, Fries BC, et al. Candida infections of the genitourinary tract. *Clin Microbiol Rev*. 2010;23:253–73.
- Pappas PG, Kauffman CA, Andes D, et al. Clinical practice guidelines for the management of candidiasis: 2009 update by the Infectious Diseases Society of America. *Clin Infect Dis* 2009;48(5):503–35. PubMed.
- Terai H, Shimahara M. Tongue pain: burning mouth syndrome vs Candida-associated lesion. *Oral Dis*. 2007;13:440–2.

See Also (Topic, Algorithm, Electronic Media Element)

Candidiasis; HIV Infection and AIDS

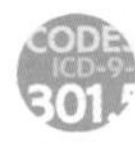

CODES

ICD9
- 112.0 Candidiasis of mouth
- 112.1 Candidiasis of vulva and vagina
- 112.2 Candidiasis of other urogenital sites

CLINICAL PEARLS

- The diagnosis of candidiasis is generally made clinically, but may include KOH. Rarely, a culture of skin scrapings or even a biopsy is needed for resistant strains or to explore the differential.
- Transmission from person to person is rare. Rarely, *Candida* vaginitis may be sexually transmitted.
- If tongue pain continues after treatment, consider burning mouth syndrome.
- Topical antifungals rarely cause problems, but oral medications may have hepatic side effects.
- Amphotericin B can cause nephrotoxicity.

CARBON MONOXIDE POISONING

Robert De Marco, MD

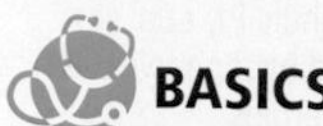

BASICS

DESCRIPTION

Carbon monoxide (CO) is the leading cause of poisoning death in the US. CO is an odorless, tasteless, colorless gas produced by combustion of carbon-containing compounds:

- CO inhalation leads to displacement of oxygen from binding sites on hemoglobin.
- Detrimental effects are related to tissue hypoxia from decreased oxygen content and a shift of the oxyhemoglobin dissociation curve to the left.
- CO binds to cytochrome oxidase, impairing mitochondrial function, and to cytochrome oxidase, affecting muscle function.
- CO binding to myoglobin affects muscle activity.
- System(s) affected: Cardiovascular; Musculoskeletal; Nervous

Pregnancy Considerations

Tissue hypoxia includes the fetus. CO poisoning may cause significant fetal abnormalities, depending on the developmental stage. Also, adult hemoglobin holds oxygen less tightly than does fetal hemoglobin. Therefore, a pregnant mother potentially may be unaffected while the fetus is affected.

EPIDEMIOLOGY

Incidence

- 40,000 emergency department visits annually
- 5,000–6,000 deaths annually in the US
- Inadvertent CO poisoning likely causes 500 deaths annually.
- Intentional CO poisoning is approximately 10 times higher.
- Unintended poisoning is most common during winter months in cold climates.
- 10,000 individuals miss 1 or more days of work due to CO poisoning.

RISK FACTORS

- Smoke inhalation
- Being in a closed space with a faulty furnace or stove or running engine
- Cigarette smoking
- Employment in a coal mine, as an auto mechanic, paint stripper, or in the solvent industry
- Improperly vented fuel-burning devices:
  - Kerosene heaters, charcoal grills, camping stoves, gasoline-powered generators, wood stoves
  - Open-air exposure to motorboat exhaust
- Underground utility electrical cable fires produce large amounts of CO, which can seep into adjacent buildings and homes.

GENERAL PREVENTION

- Appropriate ventilation, especially where there are fuel-burning devices
- Use of CO monitors
- Public education
- Determining the mechanism of exposure is critical in cases of accidental poisoning in order to limit future risk

PATHOPHYSIOLOGY

- CO is rapidly absorbed in lungs.
- CO has ~250 times the affinity for hemoglobin that oxygen has.
- CO binds to hemoglobin to form carboxyhemoglobin (COHb), resulting in impaired oxygen-carrying capacity, utilization, and delivery:
  - Leftward shift of the oxyhemoglobin dissociation curve occurs.
  - CO interferes with peripheral oxygen utilization by inactivating cytochrome oxidase.
- Delayed neurologic sequelae, probably due to lipid peroxidation by toxic oxygen species generated by xanthine oxidase.
- The half-life of CO while the patient is breathing room air is ~300 minutes, while breathing high-flow oxygen via a nonrebreathing face mask is ~90 minutes, and with 100% hyperbaric oxygen is ~30 minutes.

ETIOLOGY

- CO inhalation
- Inhaled or ingested methylene chloride (from paint remover [dichloromethane]) is metabolized to CO by the liver, causing CO toxicity in the absence of ambient CO.

COMMONLY ASSOCIATED CONDITIONS

CO and cyanide poisoning can occur simultaneously following smoke inhalation (synergistic effect).

DIAGNOSIS

- Acute CO poisoning is suggested by history, physical examination, and an elevated COHb.
- Chronic CO intoxication is difficult to diagnose.
- Pulse oximetry cannot screen for CO exposure because it does not differentiate carboxyhemoglobin from oxyhemoglobin.

HISTORY

- Tinnitus
- Headaches
- Dizziness, nausea, vomiting, or diarrhea
- Weakness or fatigue
- Flushing
- Syncope
- Angina

PHYSICAL EXAM

- "Cherry red" appearance of the lips and skin
- In absence of trauma or burns, look for altered mental status.
- Impaired judgment, respiratory depression, arrhythmias, hypotension
- Cyanosis or tachypnea
- A careful neurologic examination is crucial.
- Visual-field defects, blindness, papilledema, or nystagmus
- Central nervous system depression
- Ataxia
- Seizures
- Coma
- Angina
- Tachycardia or cardiac dysrhythmias
- Cardiopulmonary arrest

DIAGNOSTIC TESTS & INTERPRETATION

Lab

Initial lab tests

- Measurement of COHb
- Check CO level via co-oximetry of arterial or venous blood (some authors question their accuracy).
- Check acid-base status on blood gas.
- Electrocardiogram (EKG) in all patients
- Cardiac enzymes in:
  - ≥65 years
  - Patient with cardiac risk factors

Follow-Up & Special Considerations

Think of CO poisoning in younger patients with chest pain or symptoms suggestive of ischemia.

Imaging

Head computed tomography scan is helpful to rule out other causes of neurologic decompensation.

DIFFERENTIAL DIAGNOSIS

- Cyanide toxicity
- Acute viral syndrome
- Other causes of mental status changes: Metabolic, drugs, infectious, trauma

TREATMENT

MEDICATION

- Prompt removal from the source of CO
- Institution of 100% oxygen by high-flow mask or endotracheal tube
- 100% normobaric oxygen for all suspected victims of CO poisoning, regardless of pulse oximetry or arterial PO_2(1)[B]

ADDITIONAL TREATMENT

General Measures

- Removal from source
- Rapid reduction in tissue hypoxia with 100% oxygen to reduce the half-time of elimination of CO to 90 minutes
- Supportive care as necessary
- Intubation and mechanical ventilation may be necessary for severe intoxication. All patients who are comatose or have severely impaired mental status should be intubated and mechanically ventilated without delay (1)[B].
- Volume resuscitation

Additional Therapies

- 100% oxygen by tight-fitting nonrebreathing mask
- Hyperbaric oxygen for severe poisoning or in the following conditions (2)[B]:
  - CO level >20% in a pregnant patient
  - Loss of consciousness
  - Severe metabolic acidosis (pH <7.1)
  - Possible end-organ ischemia (EKG changes, chest pain, altered mental status)
- For mild poisoning (carboxyhemoglobin levels <30%); no signs or symptoms of cardiovascular or neurologic dysfunction:
  - Treatment: Admission if carboxyhemoglobin >25%
  - Symptomatic medication for headache
  - 100% oxygen by nonrebreathing mask until carboxyhemoglobin <5%
  - Patients with underlying heart disease should be admitted, regardless of level of carboxyhemoglobin
- For moderate poisoning (carboxyhemoglobin 30–40%); no signs or symptoms of cardiovascular or neurologic dysfunction:
  - Treatment: Admission
  - Cardiovascular status should be followed closely, even in the absence of clear cardiac effects
  - Determination of acid–base status: Corrected by oxygen
  - 100% oxygen by nonrebreathing mask until carboxyhemoglobin <5%
- For severe poisoning (carboxyhemoglobin >40%); cardiovascular or neurologic functional impairment at any carboxyhemoglobin level:
  - Treatment: Admission
  - Cardiovascular function monitoring
  - Acid–base status monitoring
  - 100% oxygen by nonrebreathing mask until carboxyhemoglobin <5%
  - Hyperbaric oxygen immediately if available; if unavailable, treat as in moderate poisoning
- If no improvement occurs in cardiovascular or neurologic function within 4 hours, transport the patient to the nearest facility with hyperbaric oxygen, regardless of distance.

IN-PATIENT CONSIDERATIONS

Patients often present in clusters, with similar symptoms and a common environment.

Initial Stabilization

- Emergency department (ED) for mild poisoning
- Inpatient treatment for moderate or severe poisoning

Admission Criteria

Patients whose symptoms do not resolve, who demonstrate EKG or laboratory evidence of severe poisoning, or who have other medical or social cause of concern should be hospitalized.

Discharge Criteria

Patients with mild symptoms from accidental poisoning can be managed in the ED and safely discharged.

ONGOING CARE

FOLLOW-UP RECOMMENDATIONS

Rest until carboxyhemoglobin reduced and symptoms abate

Patient Monitoring

- Measurement of carboxyhemoglobin levels
- Arterial blood gases
- Psychiatric evaluation and follow-up for intentional exposure

PATIENT EDUCATION

- Professional installation and maintenance of combustion devices: 1-800-638-2772; Consumer Products Safety Commission hotline
- CO detector installation in homes, especially near bedrooms and potential sources

PROGNOSIS

Most survivors recover completely, with only a minority developing chronic neuropsychiatric impairment.

COMPLICATIONS

- Myocardial infarction
- Pulmonary edema (congestive heart failure)
- Pneumonia (aspiration)
- Anoxic encephalopathy
- Long-term neuropsychiatric complications:
  - Intellectual deterioration
  - Memory impairment
- Dysrhythmia
- Shock
- Rhabdomyolysis, personality changes:
  - Irritability
  - Aggressiveness
  - Violence
- Moodiness

Geriatric Considerations

- Higher incidence of cardiovascular and neurologic disease, increasing complications
- Atherosclerosis with chronic exposure

REFERENCES

1. Hampson NB, Scott KL, Zmaeff JL. Carboxyhemoglobin measurement by hospitals: implications for the diagnosis of carbon monoxide poisoning. *J Emerg Med*. 2006;31:13–6.
2. Kao LW, Nañagas KA. Carbon monoxide poisoning. *Emerg Med Clin North Am*. 2004;22:985–1018.

ADDITIONAL READING

- Insufficient evidence to establish usefulness of hyperbaric oxygen for carbon monoxide poisoning. *Cochrane Library*. 2005;1:CD002041.
- Internet resources available at: http://www.cpsc.gov.
- Juurlink DN, Buckley NA, Stanbrook MB, et al. Hyperbaric oxygen for carbon monoxide poisoning. *Cochrane Database Syst Rev*. 2005:CD002041.
- Satran D, Henry CR, Adkinson C, et al. Cardiovascular manifestations of moderate to severe carbon monoxide poisoning. *J Am Coll Cardiol*. 2005;45:1513–6.
- World Health Organization's List of International Poison Control Centers www.who.int/ipcs/poisons/centre/directory/en.

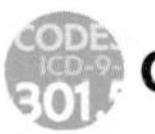

CODES

ICD9

986 Toxic effect of carbon monoxide

CLINICAL PEARLS

- The most appropriate intervention in the management of a CO-poisoned patient is a prompt removal from the source of CO and institution of 100% oxygen by high-flow face mask or endotracheal tube.
- Consider CO poisoning in younger patients with chest pain or ischemia.

CARDIAC ARREST

Aman D. Sabharwal, MD
Marc Grossman, MD

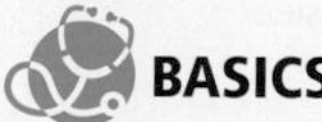

BASICS

DESCRIPTION

- The absence of effective mechanical cardiac activity
- This section is not a substitute for an AHA-approved Advanced Cardiac Life Support (ACLS) course and is intended only as a quick reference.
- Synonym(s): Code blue in many institutions

Geriatric Considerations

Low rate of survival and poor long-term outcome. Be aware of Do Not Resuscitate orders on patients at risk.

Pediatric Considerations

Bradycardia is linked to hypoxia. Bradycardia is the most common initial form of cardiac arrest and is often the response to hypoxia. Adequate oxygenation and ventilation are critical.

Pregnancy Considerations

- Displace the uterus to the left either manually or by placing a rolled towel under the right hip. If the patient cannot be resuscitated within 5–15 minutes, consider emergency C-section to relieve uterine obstruction and increase blood return to the heart. This may also be done to save the fetus if fetus has reached gestational age of viability.
- Consider amniotic fluid embolism or eclampsia-related seizures as precipitating factors.

EPIDEMIOLOGY

- Predominant age: Risk increases with age
- Predominant sex: Male > Female

Incidence

0.5–1.5/1,000 persons per year

RISK FACTORS

- Male gender
- Advanced age
- Hypercholesterolemia
- HTN
- Cigarette smoking
- Family history of atherosclerosis
- Diabetes
- Cardiomyopathy
- Prolonged QT

ETIOLOGY

- Asystole (confirm in 2 leads)
- Ventricular fibrillation (VF)
- Pulseless ventricular tachycardia (VT)
- Pulseless electrical activity (PEA, previously known as electrical mechanical dissociation [EMD])
- Consider possible reversible causes (5 Hs and 4 Ts):
  - Hypoxia, severe hypovolemia, hyper- and hypokalemia [H+] (acidosis), hypothermia
  - Cardiac tamponade, tension pneumothorax, thrombosis (pulmonary embolism, myocardial infarction), tablets (medications and overdoses)

COMMONLY ASSOCIATED CONDITIONS

- Coronary artery disease/ACS (cardiac arrest may be presenting symptom)
- Valvular heart disease
- HTN

DIAGNOSIS

- Loss of consciousness secondary to CNS hypoperfusion
- Absence of pulses in large arteries
- Apnea or agonal breathing
- Cyanosis or pallor

HISTORY

- Witnessed or unwitnessed
- Seizure activity
- History or risk factors
- Associated trauma

PHYSICAL EXAM

- Check pupils: May indicate drug overdose. Cannot interpret if patient has received atropine.
- Check pulse.
- Check lungs (i.e., did patient have respiratory decline prior to cardiac decline?).
- Check for dialysis shunt: Patients on dialysis are at increased risk for electrolyte imbalance causing arrest (especially hyperkalemia).

DIAGNOSTIC TESTS & INTERPRETATION

Lab

- Fingerstick glucose
- ABG
- Cardiac enzymes (troponin, CK, CK-MB); consider serial enzymes
- Chemistry and/or electrolyte panel
- CBC with platelets
- Drug levels (toxicology screen, acetaminophen/aspirin levels, history of specific medication (e.g., digoxin, antiepileptics)
- Blood type and cross, if indicated

Imaging

- CXR for endotracheal tube (ET) placement, pneumothorax; consider emergency echocardiogram for pericardial effusion and assessment of cardiac motion.
- Once stabilized, consider CT scan of brain.

Diagnostic Procedures/Surgery

- ECG
- 2-dimensional echocardiogram
- Airway management/intubation
- Peripheral IV access as close to central circulation as possible; intraosseous if no venous access. Avoid placement of central line during CPR. If must place during CPR, use femoral approach. Many medications may be administered by endotracheal tube if access otherwise unobtainable (double dose and flush with saline).
- Pericardiocentesis for cardiac tamponade
- Needle decompression/chest tube for pneumothorax

TREATMENT

- Prompt initiation of CPR, particularly chest compressions (push hard, push fast, and don't interrupt!), and immediate defibrillation (in witnessed VF and pulseless VT but not in PEA) are 1st priority (1)[A]:
  - In unwitnessed arrest, complete 1–2 minutes of CPR before attempting defibrillation (2)[A].
- Establishing IV access, intubation, and medications are 2nd priority.
- Continue CPR for 1–2 minutes following return of a potentially perfusing rhythm before stopping for pulse check, except for witnessed arrest with prompt return of rhythm following defibrillation.

MEDICATION

First Line

- Vascular access for medications: IV or intraosseous
- Consider medications after initiation of CPR and defibrillation attempt. Medications should be administered during CPR as soon as possible following a rhythm check.
- Epinephrine: 1 mg IV q3–5 min (1)[B] *OR* vasopressin 40 U IV single dose (1)[B] can be used once in lieu of the 1st or 2nd dose of epinephrine in VT or VF, but not in PEA:
  - Vasopressin is not recommended in children.
  - Pediatric dose of epinephrine: 0.01 mg/kg
- Atropine for asystole; consider in PEA with absolute bradycardia: 1 mg q3–5 min IV push to total dose of 3 mg (1)[C]:
  - Pediatric dose: 0.02 mg/kg
  - Minimum dose: 0.1 mg; maximum single dose is 0.5 mg in child, 1.0 mg in adolescent
- Magnesium sulfate: 1–2 g diluted in 10 mL D_5W IV push in suspected torsades de pointes (1)[B]:
  - Magnesium is relatively contraindicated in renal failure, but given the consequences of not correcting this rhythm, contraindication is only relative in this setting.
- Antiarrhythmics:
  - Consider if VT/VF unresponsive to 2–3 shocks and 1st dose of vasopressor
  - Amiodarone is drug preferred by AHA. Dosing: 300 mg IV push followed by 2nd dose of 150 mg IV (1)[B]
  - Amiodarone for perfusing tachyarrhythmias: Loading dose of 5 mg/kg IV or IO over 20–60 minutes, maximum dose 15 mg/kg/d
  - Lidocaine: Initial dose, 1–1.5 mg/kg IV; repeat loading dose of 1–1.5 mg/kg can be given at 5–10-minute intervals if VT/VF persist to maximum dose of 3 mg/kg (1)[C], then followed by drip if perfusing rhythm recovered

Endotracheal medications (NAVEL): Narcan, atropine, vasopressin (and Valium), epinephrine, or lidocaine. Each may be placed in 5–10 mL of normal saline or sterile water and given by ET followed by bagging. Dosage should be 2–2.5 times recommended IV dose. IV or IO is preferred.

econd Line

Procainamide: 30 mg/min IV in refractory VF/VT (maximum dose: 17 mg/kg) is permissible. However, because the time to a useful level by infusion is so long, it is unlikely to be of benefit in cardiac arrest, but may be useful in perfusing tachycardias (1)[C].

Calcium: May be useful in hyperkalemia, ionized hypokalemia secondary multiple transfusions, and Ca+ channel blocker toxicity; otherwise, no clear benefit is shown

High-dose epinephrine: No survival benefit is seen with high dose (0.1 mg/kg), but may be considered in exceptional situations, such as β-blocker or calcium channel blocker overdose.

Bicarbonate: 1 mEq/kg IV only in known preexisting bicarbonate-responsive acidosis, hyperkalemia, or to alkalinize the urine in known responsive overdoses (i.e., tricyclics, aspirin). Also may be considered in patients with prolonged or unknown down-time (1)[C].

ADDITIONAL TREATMENT

General Measures

Perform CPR: Fast (100/min) and hard, with minimal interruptions (1)[B]

80–100 bpm without interruption of CPR

Sequence should be:
- CPR
- Rhythm check
- Resume CPR
- Shock/meds (charge defibrillator and administer drugs during CPR)
- Continue CPR (after shocking) for 5 cycles before rechecking rhythm (repeat as needed) (1)[B]

In VF/pulseless VT, 1 shock should be delivered, and continue sequence above (1)[B]:
- Monophasic automatic external defibrillators (AEDs) initial and subsequent shocks at 360 J
- Biphasic AEDs:
  - 150–200 J for biphasic truncated exponential waveform
  - 120 J for rectilinear biphasic waveform
  - If not specified on the biphasic defibrillator, use default of 200 J
- Subsequent shocks should be same or higher energy
- Pediatric manual defibrillation energy should be 2 J/kg for 1st attempt and 4 J/kg for following attempts.

- Consider possible causes of VT/VF, including hypoxia, hyperkalemia, hypokalemia, preexisting acidosis, drug overdose, and hypothermia.
- Administer 100% oxygen by bag-valve-mask or ET.
- IV and IO are preferred methods of medication administration, followed by ET tube.
- Start IV lines as close to the heart as possible. Large-bore peripheral lines can deliver fluid more quickly than a triple-lumen catheter (avoid central line placement during CPR).
- Use an end-tidal CO_2 monitor to assess gas exchange, if available. Esophageal intubation will produce a very low end-tidal CO_2 and requires proper reintubation (1). Use of sodium bicarbonate will increase ET-CO_2 levels.
- Consider termination of efforts if no reversible underlying cause is found.

Issues for Referral

- Consider communication with medical examiner's office.
- Consider communication with organ/tissue bank.

Additional Therapies

Consider mild therapeutic hypothermia after resuscitation (to 32–34°C for 12–24 hours if initial rhythm was VF). Most benefit is seen in VF as initial rhythm and short down-time (less than 25 minutes) but may be considered with any patient with return of spontaneous circulation (ROSC) and coma state.

IN-PATIENT CONSIDERATIONS

Initial Stabilization

- Decreasing the EMS response interval increases survival (1)[A].
- Home use of automatic external defibrillators does not improve survival (3).

ONGOING CARE

FOLLOW-UP RECOMMENDATIONS

Patient Monitoring

Admit to ICU or CCU on continuous monitoring

PROGNOSIS

- Outcome is related to underlying disease, age, duration of arrest, and other factors.
- Outcome is poor if:
  - >4 minutes to CPR or >8 minutes to ACLS
  - Arrest occurs out of hospital
  - Resuscitation effort >30 minutes
- ~17% survive in-hospital arrest.
- ~1-10% survive to leave the hospital in out-of-hospital arrest, varying by geographic region.
- ~10-15% of those with VF survive.
- If arrest is out-of-hospital without return of vital signs from ALS prehospital care, patient is unlikely to respond to ED resuscitation efforts.
- If ROSC with coma, strongly consider induced hypothermia to improve neurologic outcome (number needed to treat in VF = 6).

COMPLICATIONS

- Significant neurologic, hepatic, renal, or cardiac ischemic injury
- Rib fractures, hemopneumothorax, abdominal organ injury from CPR

REFERENCES

1. Hypothermia after Cardiac Arrest Study Group. Mild therapeutic hypothermia to improve the neurologic outcome after cardiac arrest. *N Engl J Med*. 2002;346:549–56.
2. Wik L, Hansen TB, Fylling F, et al. Delaying defibrillation to give basic cardiopulmonary resuscitation to patients with out-of-hospital ventricular fibrillation: a randomized trial. *JAMA*. 2003;289:1389–95.
3. Bardy GH, Lee KL, Mark DB, et al. Home use of automated external defibrillators for sudden cardiac arrest. *N Engl J Med*. 2008;358:1793–804.

ADDITIONAL READING

2005 American Heart Association Guidelines for Cardiopulmonary Resuscitation and Emergency Cardiovascular Care. *Circulation*. 2005;112(Suppl I): IV-1–IV-203.

See Also (Topic, Algorithm, Electronic Media Element)

Algorithm: Coronary Syndrome, Acute

CODES

ICD9

427.5 Cardiac arrest

CLINICAL PEARLS

- Prompt initiation of CPR, particularly chest compressions (*push hard, push fast, and don't interrupt!*), and immediate defibrillation (in witnessed VF and pulseless VT but not in PEA) are 1st priority.
- In unwitnessed arrest, complete 1–2 minutes of CPR before attempting defibrillation.
- Get ECG following return of circulation to evaluate for acute coronary syndrome.
- Epinephrine is the first drug to give in any case requiring CPR:
  - Avoid use of central lines during CPR; intraosseous and endotracheal routes are preferred if peripheral access is not attainable.

CARDIAC TAMPONADE

Parag Goyal, MD
Rishi Vohora, DO

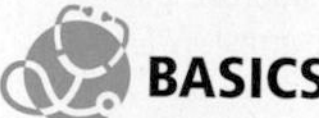

BASICS

DESCRIPTION

- A rapid or slow accumulation of fluid within the pericardium that causes compression of the chambers of the heart, impairing diastolic filling and ultimately leading to cardiovascular collapse.
- Tamponade can be acute or subacute, depending on the etiology:
  - Acute: Rapid accumulation (usually blood) within a stiff, noncompliant pericardium
  - Subacute: Gradual increase of a preexisting effusion, with limited accommodative pericardial stretch
- Variants include low-pressure and regional tamponade:
  - Low-pressure: Occurs when left- and right-sided pressures equalize at lower pressures; occurs when a decrease in intravascular volume makes an unchanged preexisting effusion hemodynamically significant (1)
  - Regional: Occurs when a loculation or hematoma limits diastolic filling

EPIDEMIOLOGY

Incidence

Difficult to assess due to absence of population-based studies

Prevalence

Difficult to assess due to absence of population-based studies

PATHOPHYSIOLOGY

- As a pericardial effusion accumulates, it overcomes the pericardium's intrinsic compliance yielding increased intrapericardial pressure. This pressure eventually exceeds intracardiac diastolic pressures, compresses the chambers of the heart, and limits diastolic filling with subsequent reduction of cardiac output.
- Diastolic filling is decreased first in the more compliant right-sided chambers (RA, then RV), followed by decrease of the left side. Tamponade is defined as the critical point at which diastolic equalization of the left and right ventricles occurs, total venous return drops, and cardiac output falls.
- The hemodynamic significance of the effusion depends on:
  - Rate of accumulation
  - Compliance of the pericardium to accommodate the enlarging effusion

ETIOLOGY

- Acute tamponade (most commonly from a rapidly accumulating hemopericardium, with sometimes as little as 50–100 mL of fluid):
  - Penetrating or blunt trauma
  - Iatrogenic instrumentation (cardiac surgery, central lines, pacer wire migration, peripherally inserted central catheter lines)
  - Aortic dissection
  - Rupture of cardiac free wall, ventricular aneurysm, or coronary artery. These most commonly occur during the postmyocardial infarction (MI) period.
- Subacute tamponade (any condition that causes a pericardial effusion) (2):
  - Idiopathic pericarditis (20%)
  - Iatrogenic effusions (16%) (see above)
  - Malignancy (13%): Breast, lung, lymphoma, leukemia, or radiation pericarditis
  - Idiopathic effusion (9%)
  - Acute MI (8%): Can complicate 15% of MIs and <1% of MIs treated with thrombolysis (2)
  - End-stage renal disease (ESRD) (6%): Usually blood urea nitrogen >60 mg/dL, but hemodialysis is an independent risk factor
  - Congestive heart failure (CHF) (5%): Effusions seen in 14% of CHF
  - Collagen vascular disease (5%): Systemic lupus erythematosus, rheumatoid arthritis (RA)
  - Infection (4%):
    - HIV
    - Bacterial infection: *Staphylococcus aureus*, *Mycobacterium tuberculosis*, *Streptococcus pneumoniae* (rare)
    - Fungal infection: *Histoplasmosis capsulatum*
    - Viral infection: Coxsackie group B, influenza, enteric cytopathogenic human orphan, herpes
  - Hypothyroidism with myxedema
  - Massive fluid resuscitation
  - Coagulopathies
- Low-pressure tamponade:
  - Patients with preexisting effusions who receive hemodialysis or diuretics thus reducing intravascular volume
- Regional tamponade:
  - Localized hematomas after cardiac surgery or post-MI

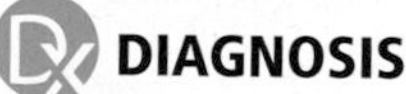

DIAGNOSIS

HISTORY

- Dyspnea: Most sensitive symptom (88%) (2)
- Vague chest pain or an overall subjective sense of discomfort
- Syncope or presyncopal symptoms
- Altered mentation from poor perfusion
- Nausea or abdominal pain from hepatic venous engorgement
- In acute presentations, look for history of recent trauma, surgery, vascular instrumentation
- In subacute presentations, patients may have histories of known preexisting effusions with new or worsening exertional dyspnea.

PHYSICAL EXAM

- Only sign may be pulseless electrical activity
- Beck triad: Distant heart sounds, hypotension, distended neck veins:
  - Pertains specifically to acute tamponade
  - Subacute tamponade: Beck triad is often absent, and blood pressure (BP) may be normal or elevated (2).
- Most sensitive physical findings on exam (2):
  - Pulsus paradoxus (82%).
  - Tachypnea (80%)
  - Tachycardia (77%)
  - Jugular venous distention (76%)
- Pulsus paradoxus: Defined as an exaggerated drop in systolic blood pressure (SBP) (usually >10 mm Hg) during inspiration:
  - This is due to the fact that the normal transmission of pressure from the intrapleural to intrapericardial cavity does not occur. Therefore, with inspiration, there is a relative decrease in th pressures across the pulmonary vascular bed wit a relatively fixed left atrial pressure. This leads to decreased pulmonary venous drainage into the left atrium and therefore a decrease in left-sided stroke volume with inspiration (3).
  - Likelihood ratio (LR) for >12 mm Hg: 5.9; likelihood ratio (LR) for >10 mm Hg: 3.3
  - Can be absent in the settings of hypovolemia, severe AI, severe LV dysfunction, ASD, or in patients with positive-pressure ventilation (4)
  - Can also be seen in the setting of acute pulmonary embolus, RV infarction, and COPD
  - Can be false positive in severe lung disease
  - Performed best via sphygmomanometer by the following steps:
    - Insufflate cuff >20 mm Hg beyond systolic pressure.
    - Slowly deflate cuff and record pressure at whic Korotkoff sounds are slightly audible at expiration only.
    - Further deflate cuff and record pressure at which Korotkoff sounds are equally audible at inspiration and expiration.
    - If these 2 pressures differ by >10 mm Hg, pulsus paradoxus is present.
- Respiratory distress, but with surprisingly little or nc pulmonary edema
- Jugular venous distention with a rapid systolic (X) descent and absent diastolic (Y) descent
- Narrow pulse pressure (due to limited stroke volum and increased peripheral vascular resistance)
- Signs of cardiogenic shock: Low BP with poor mentation and cool, poorly perfused extremities
- Kussmaul sign (elevation of jugular venous distention with inspiration caused by increased right-sided pressure)
- Increased peripheral (right-sided) edema due to impaired venous return
- Right upper quadrant tenderness due to hepatic engorgement
- Increased area of cardiac dullness outside the apical point of maximum impulse

DIAGNOSTIC TESTS & INTERPRETATION

Electrocardiogram (ECG):

- Sinus tachycardia
- Low-voltage QRS, defined as <5 mm in limb leads and <10 mm in precordial leads; sensitivity of 42%
- Signs of pericarditis (except in uremic pericarditis): Initially diffuse ST segment elevation and PR segment depression of pericarditis; later stages exhibit T-wave inversions that may be transient or permanent
- Electrical alternans (QRS and/or P-wave beat-to-beat variation in axis and/or amplitude) is only seen in 10–20% of cases of tamponade. However, it is the most specific ECG finding for tamponade (4).

Lab

Initial lab tests

- Acute tamponade (trauma and preoperative labs):
  - Complete blood count (CBC), serum chemistries, coagulation panel, ethanol, drugs of abuse, UA

Subacute tamponade (evaluate cause of the effusion):
– CBC, serum chemistries, erythrocyte sedimentation rate, cardiac enzymes, antinuclear antibodies, rheumatoid factor
– Fluid analysis of glucose, protein, cell count, lactate dehydrogenase, amylase, cholesterol, cytology, complement levels, Gram stain, and cultures (including bacterial, viral, acid-fast bacilli, and fungal cultures)

Imaging

Initial approach

- Chest radiograph:
  – May show enlargement of cardiac shadow (if >200 mL fluid present)
  – Cardiomegaly is 89% sensitive.
- Echocardiography (5):
  – Diastolic chamber collapse: RA collapse in late diastole (more sensitive 55–60%, less specific 50–68%) and RV collapse in early diastole (less sensitive 38–48%, more specific 84–100%) (3)
  – Doppler flow: An exaggerated increase through tricuspid valve (>40% variation) and exaggerated decrease (>25% variation) through mitral valve. High sensitivity (75%) and specificity (91%).
  – Inferior vena cava (IVC) distention with <50% collapse during inspiration (3)
  – Compression of pulmonary trunk
  – Paradoxical motion of interventricular septum
  – Swinging heart
- CT: Helpful in evaluating cause (i.e., aortic dissection) and characterizing the effusion (i.e., blood, pus, serous). A pericardial effusion with any of the following is suggestive of tamponade (3):
  – IVC diameter 2 × aorta
  – Reflux of contrast into IVC and/or azygous vein
  – Compression of coronary sinus
  – Flattening of anterior surface of heart and concave chamber deformity
  – Bowing of the IV septum into the LV
- MRI (3):
  – Can detect fluid collection as small as 30 mL
  – Highly effective in evaluating the composition of pericardial effusion
  – Use is limited due to emergent nature of tamponade.

Diagnostic Procedures/Surgery

Right heart catheterization:

- Diastolic pressures of RA and RV are increased and eventually equalize with the left-sided chambers and the intrapericardial pressure (usually at 15–20 mm Hg) (4).
- The dip and plateau pattern of constriction or restriction pericardial disease is absent.

DIFFERENTIAL DIAGNOSIS

- Any condition causing obstructive or cardiogenic shock, such as massive pulmonary embolism, tension pneumothorax, anterior wall MI, MI with valve rupture or dysfunction, or constrictive/restrictive pericarditis
- Of note, effusive-constrictive pericarditis can be especially difficult to distinguish from tamponade because it involves an effusion that is present with chamber collapse but is not the reason for the collapse. Differentiation can be made on echo by close examination of the diastolic filling patterns:
  – In tamponade, chamber filling is decreased but continuous throughout diastole.
  – In constrictive pericarditis, there is a surge of filling at the beginning of diastole, but is minimal during the rest of the diastolic cycle.

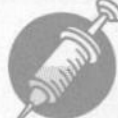

TREATMENT

MEDICATION

First Line

Fluid resuscitation:

- Fluid bolus is temporizing in acute setting.
- In subacute tamponade, most agree that while all patients do not universally benefit from fluid, those with hypotension do (6)[B].

Second Line

- Vasopressors if necessary: Dobutamine thought to maintain better cardiac output and delivery of oxygen than does norepinephrine.
- Benefit of inotropes is unclear.
- High-dose anti-inflammatory medications for pericarditis

ADDITIONAL TREATMENT

General Measures

- Maintain hemodynamic stability until definitive drainage.
- ICU monitoring
- Consider Swan-Ganz catheter if time allows.

Additional Therapies

- Hemodialysis for ESRD if patient is not in extremis (volume overload can be a cause for increasing pericardial effusions in ESRD)
- Minimize positive end expiratory pressure and pressure support if mechanically ventilated to preserve cardiac filling (4)[A].

SURGERY/OTHER PROCEDURES

Drainage is the definitive treatment (7)[A]. For acute traumatic tamponade: Prepare operating room for definitive cardiac repair via subxiphoid pericardotomy or full surgical thoracotomy. Pericardiocentesis is NOT the definitive treatment, as coagulated blood within the pericardium makes aspiration limited and hemorrhage from the cardiac injury usually refills the sac immediately. However, if there is hypotension despite fluid, a pericardiocentesis can be attempted in the emergency room (ER). For subacute tamponade: Pericardiocentesis may be guided by CT (98% success rate), fluoroscopy (93%), or ultrasound (93% for effusions >10 mm, only 58% in smaller effusions). Blind approach may be necessary in sudden cardiovascular collapse (73% success rate). An 18-G spinal needle is used, and, with the aid of a guide wire, a pigtail catheter can be introduced into the pericardium to prevent reaccumulation (7)[A]. The catheter can usually be pulled once it is draining <50 mL/d (4)[A]. If pericardiocentesis is unsuccessful in the setting of cardiovascular collapse, an immediate thoracotomy in ER is indicated (8)[B].

IN-PATIENT CONSIDERATIONS

Admission Criteria

Requires ICU-level monitoring

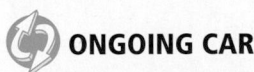

ONGOING CARE

FOLLOW-UP RECOMMENDATIONS

Follow-up echocardiogram may be used to evaluate for recurrence of effusions (7)[A].

PROGNOSIS

Acute traumatic tamponade: 70–80% survival rate quoted for level-1 trauma centers (8).

COMPLICATIONS

- Chamber lacerations
- Pneumothorax
- Ventricular tachycardia

REFERENCES

1. Sagristà-Sauleda J, Angel J, Sambola A, et al. Low-pressure cardiac tamponade: clinical and hemodynamic profile. *Circulation*. 2006;114: 945–52.
2. Roy CL, Minor MA, Brookhart MA, et al. Does this patient with a pericardial effusion have cardiac tamponade? *JAMA*. 2007;297:1810–8.
3. Restrepo CS, Lemos DF, Lemos JA, et al. Imaging findings in cardiac tamponade with emphasis on CT. *Radiographics*. 2007;27:1595–610.
4. Spodick DH. Acute cardiac tamponade. *N Engl J Med*. 2003;349:684–90.
5. Wann S, Passen E et al. Echocardiography in pericardial disease. *J Am Soc Echocardiogr*. 2008;21:7–13.
6. Sagristà-Sauleda J, Angel J, Sambola A, et al. Hemodynamic effects of volume expansion in patients with cardiac tamponade. *Circulation*. 2008;117:1545–9.
7. Cheitlin MD, Armstrong WF, Aurigemma GP, et al. ACC/AHA/ASE 2003 guideline update for the clinical application of echocardiography: summary article: a report of the American College of Cardiology/American Heart Association Task Force on Practice Guidelines (ACC/AHA/ASE Committee to Update the 1997 Guidelines for the Clinical Application of Echocardiography). *Circulation*. 2003;108:1146–62.
8. Fitzgerald M, et al. Definitive management of acute cardiac tamponade secondary to blunt trauma. *Emerg Med Australasia*. 2005;17:494–9.

ADDITIONAL READING

Hoit BD et al. Pericardial disease and pericardial tamponade. *Crit Care Med*. 2007;35:S355–64.

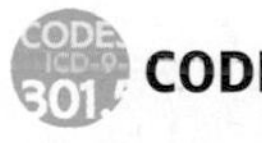

CODES

ICD9

423.3 Cardiac tamponade

CLINICAL PEARLS

- Pericardial tamponade is a potentially reversible cause of pulseless electrical activity: Perform emergent pericardiocentesis as diagnostic and therapeutic maneuver.
- Checking for pulsus parodoxicus may be a useful bedside maneuver with reasonable sensitivity in most cases, although nonspecific.
- Acute tamponade from trauma or intrapericardial rupture presents with much more rapid clinical deterioration than does subacute tamponade due to sudden rises in pericardial pressure and inability of the pericardium to stretch to accommodate the effusion.

CARDIOMYOPATHY, END STAGE

Timothy P. Fitzgibbons, MD

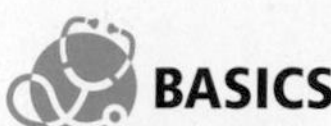

BASICS

DESCRIPTION

In 1995, the World Health Organization (WHO) defined cardiomyopathy as a "disease of the myocardium associated with cardiac dysfunction." The WHO proposed a classification system based on pathophysiology. Each class may be caused by many disorders, and some disorders may overlap classes:

- Classification of cardiomyopathy:
  - Dilated (systolic):
    - Characterized by dilation and reduced systolic function of 1 or both ventricles
  - Hypertrophic (diastolic):
    - Left and/or right ventricular hypertrophy with normal to reduced end diastolic volumes
    - May include asymmetric septal hypertrophy
    - Cause of sudden cardiac death in young athletes
  - Restrictive (diastolic):
    - Restrictive filling and reduced diastolic volume of either or both ventricles
    - Systolic function may be near normal.
    - Etiology: Idiopathic, amyloidosis, etc.
  - Arrhythmogenic right ventricular (RV) dysplasia:
    - Fibrofatty replacement of the RV
    - May present with arrhythmia or sudden cardiac death in the young
  - Unclassified:
    - Cases that do not fit easily into 1 group (i.e., noncompacted myocardium)
  - Specific: Includes patients with cardiomyopathy in association with a known systemic disorder:
    - Ischemic
    - Valvular
    - Hypertensive
    - Inflammatory
    - Metabolic
    - Peripartum
- End-stage cardiomyopathy patients have stage D heart failure or severe symptoms at rest refractory to standard medical therapy.
- System(s) affected: Cardiovascular; Renal

Pediatric Considerations

Etiology: Idiopathic, viral, congenital heart disease, and familial

Pregnancy Considerations

May occur in women postpartum

EPIDEMIOLOGY

Predominant age: Ischemic cardiomyopathy is the most common etiology; predominantly patients >50 years. Consider uncommon causes in young.

Incidence

- 60,000 patients <65 die each year from end-stage heart disease.
- 35,000–70,000 people might benefit from cardiac transplant or chronic support.

Prevalence

Most rapidly growing form of heart disease

RISK FACTORS

- Hypertension
- Hyperlipidemia
- Obesity
- Diabetes mellitus
- Smoking
- Physical inactivity
- Excessive alcohol intake
- Dietary sodium
- Obstructive sleep apnea
- Chemotherapy

Genetics

Hypertrophic, dilated cardiomyopathy, and arrhythmogenic RV dysplasia may present as familial syndromes with autosomal-dominant inheritance.

GENERAL PREVENTION

Reduce salt and water intake; home blood pressure (BP) and daily weight measurement

ETIOLOGY

The most frequent causes are in bold:

- **Ischemic heart disease: Most common etiology; up to 66% of patients**
- **Hypertension**
- **Familial cardiomyopathies**
- Congenital heart disease
- Peripartum/postpartum
- Toxic/metabolic causes:
  - **Alcoholism**
  - Radiation
  - Beriberi
  - Cobalt
  - Selenium deficiency
  - Thyrotoxicosis
- Infectious causes:
  - **Viral** (e.g., HIV, Coxsackie virus)
  - Diphtheria
  - Toxoplasmosis
  - Trichinosis
  - Trypanosomiasis
  - Acute rheumatic fever
- Inherited disorders of metabolism:
  - Glycogen storage disease
  - Pompe disease
  - Hurler syndrome
  - Hunter syndrome
  - Fabry disease
- Inherited neuromuscular disorders:
  - Duchenne muscular dystrophy
  - Friedreich ataxia
- Drugs:
  - Chemotherapy: Anthracyclines, cyclophosphamide, Herceptin
- Inflammatory/infiltrative causes:
  - Giant cell myocarditis
  - Loeffler eosinophilia
  - Sarcoidosis
  - Amyloidosis
  - Hemochromatosis
- Idiopathic
- Other causes:
  - **Tachycardia-mediated cardiomyopathy**
  - Valvular heart disease
  - Endomyocardial fibrosis

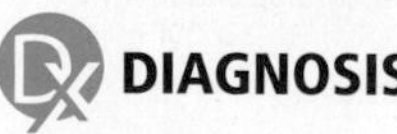

DIAGNOSIS

HISTORY

- Dyspnea at rest or with exertion
- Paroxysmal nocturnal dyspnea
- Orthopnea
- Postprandial dyspnea
- Right upper quadrant pain or bloating
- Fatigue
- Syncope
- Edema

PHYSICAL EXAM

- Tachypnea
- Low pulse pressure
- Cool extremities
- Jugular venous distention
- Bibasilar rales
- Tachycardia
- Displaced point of maximal impulse (PMI)
- S3 gallop
- Blowing systolic murmur
- Hepatosplenomegaly
- Ascites
- Edema

DIAGNOSTIC TESTS & INTERPRETATION

- Electrocardiogram: Left ventricular (LV) hypertrophy, interventricular conduction delay, atrial fibrillation, evidence of prior Q-wave infarction
- Cardiopulmonary exercise testing: Maximal oxygen consumption <10 mL/kg/mm correlates with 50% 1-year mortality, and >18 mL/kg/mm correlates with >90% 1-year survival. Used in stable outpatients to estimate prognosis and prior to cardiac transplant referral.

Lab

- Hyponatremia
- Prerenal azotemia
- Anemia
- Mild elevation in troponin
- Elevated B-type natriuretic peptide (BNP) or pro-BNP
- Mild hyperbilirubinemia
- Elevated liver function tests
- Elevated uric acid

naging

Chest radiograph:
- Cardiomegaly
- Increased vascular markings to the upper lobes
- Pleural effusions may or may not be present.

Echocardiography:
- In dilated cardiomyopathy, 4-chamber enlargement and global hypokinesis are present.
- In hypertrophic cardiomyopathy, severe left ventricular (LV) hypertrophy is present.
- Segmental contraction abnormalities of the LV are indicative of previous localized myocardial infarction.

Cardiac magnetic resonance imaging:
- May be useful to characterize certain nonischemic cardiomyopathies

iagnostic Procedures/Surgery

ardiac catheterization:
Helpful to rule out ischemic heart disease
Characterize hemodynamic severity
Pulmonary artery catheters may be reasonable in patients with refractory heart failure (HF) to help guide management (1)[C].

IFFERENTIAL DIAGNOSIS

Severe pulmonary disease
Primary pulmonary hypertension
Recurrent pulmonary embolism
Constrictive pericarditis
Hypothyroidism
Some advanced forms of malignancy
Anemia
Chronic illness

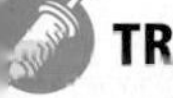

TREATMENT

ee "Congestive Heart Failure" for detailed treatment rotocols.

IEDICATION

irst Line

Systolic failure syndromes:
- Angiotensin-converting enzyme (ACE) inhibitors:
  - Lisinopril, 5–40 mg/d or captopril, 6.25–50 mg t.i.d. (1)[A]
- Loop diuretics:
  - May need to be given IV initially and then orally as patient stabilizes
  - Furosemide 40–120 mg/d or t.i.d. (1)[A]
- β-blockers:
  - Use with caution in acutely decompensated or low cardiac output states.
  - Metoprolol succinate, 12.5–200 mg/d; carvedilol, 3.125–25 mg b.i.d.; or bisoprolol, 1.25–10 mg/d (1)[A]
- Aldosterone antagonists:
  - Patients with New York Heart Association (NYHA) III-IV congestive heart failure (CHF), ejection fraction (EF) <35%, on standard therapy; spironolactone, 12.5–25 mg/d (2)[A]
- Digoxin, 0.125–0.250 mg/d for symptomatic patients on standard therapy (1)[A]

- Diastolic failure:
  - Few evidence-based therapies for diastolic heart failure. Empiric management goals include:
    - Management of hypertension
    - Reduction of congestive states (i.e., diuretics)
    - Prevention of progression of left ventricular hypertrophy (i.e., renin-angiotensin-aldosterone system blockade)
    - Maintenance of sinus rhythm
- Contraindications:
  - β-blockers: Low cardiac output, 1st- or 2nd-degree heart block
  - Ca-blockers (non-dihydropyridine): Low cardiac output, heart block
  - Aldosterone antagonists: Oliguria, anuria, renal dysfunction
  - Loop diuretics: Hypokalemia, hypomagnesemia
  - ACE inhibitors: Pregnancy, angioedema
- Precautions:
  - In patients with chronic kidney disease, digoxin dosage should be 0.125 mg/d or less, and drug levels followed carefully to avoid toxicity.
  - Closely monitor electrolytes.
  - ACE inhibitors: Initiate with care if BP is low. Begin with low-dose captopril, such as 6.25 mg t.i.d.
  - β-blockers: Avoid in patients with evidence of poor tissue perfusion; they may further depress systolic function.
  - Milrinone, amrinone: Contraindicated for long-term use due to increased mortality

Second Line

- Combination hydralazine/isosorbide dinitrate is recommended in addition to standard treatment in African American patients with class III–IV symptoms (1)[A], and for all patients with reduced EF and symptoms incompletely responsive to ACE inhibitor and beta blocker (3)
- Angiotensin receptor blockers as an alternative to, or in addition to, ACE inhibitors
- Inotropic therapy (e.g., dobutamine or milrinone) for support prior to surgery or cardiac transplantation

ADDITIONAL TREATMENT

General Measures

- Reduction of filling pressures
- Treatment of electrolyte disturbances

Issues for Referral

Management by a heart failure team improves outcomes and facilitates early transplant referral.

Additional Therapies

- Prophylactic implantable cardioverter defibrillator (ICD) should be considered for patients with an LVEF <30% (1)[A].
- Biventricular pacing should be considered for patients with QRS interval >120 ms, LVEF <35%, and class III CHF despite medical therapy (1)[A]. MADIT-CRT data suggests patients with class II and possibly class I may also benefit (4)[A].
- Patients with severe, refractory HF with no reasonable expectation of improvement should not be considered for an ICD (1)[C].
- Consideration of an LV assist device as "permanent" or destination therapy is reasonable in selected stage D patients.

ONGOING CARE

DIET

Low fat, low salt, fluid restriction

PROGNOSIS

20–40% of patients in NYHA functional class IV die within 1 year. With a transplant, a 1-year survival is as high as 94%.

COMPLICATIONS

Worsening CHF, syncope, renal failure, arrhythmias, or sudden death

REFERENCES

1. Richardson P, McKenna W, Bristow M, et al. Report of the 1995 World Health Organization/International Society and Federation of Cardiology Task Force on the Definition and Classification of cardiomyopathies. *Circulation*. 1996;93:841–2.
2. Nohria A, Lewis E, Stevenson LW. Medical management of advanced heart failure. *JAMA*. 2002;287:628–40.
3. 2009 Focused update: ACCF/AHA guidelines for the diagnosis and management of heart failure in adults: a report of the American College of Cardiology Foundation/American Heart Association Task Force on Practice Guidelines. *Circulation*. 2009;119:1977–2016.
4. Moss AJ, Hall WJ, Cannom DS, et al. Cardiac-Resynchronization Therapy for the Prevention of Heart-Failure Events. *N Engl J Med*. 2009.

ADDITIONAL READING

Hunt SA, et al. ACC/AHA 2005 guideline update for the diagnosis and management of chronic heart failure in adults. *J Am Coll Cardiol*. 2005;46:1116–43.

See Also (Topic, Algorithm, Electronic Media Element)

Alcohol Withdrawal; Alcohol Abuse and Dependence; Amyloidosis; Congestive Heart Failure; Diabetes Mellitus, Type 1; Diabetes Mellitus, Type 2; Hypertension; Hypothyroidism, Adult; Idiopathic Hypertrophic Subaortic Stenosis; Malnutrition, Protein-Calorie; Rheumatic Fever; Sarcoidosis

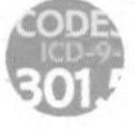

CODES

ICD9

- 425.4 Other primary cardiomyopathies
- 425.5 Alcoholic cardiomyopathy
- 425.8 Cardiomyopathy in other diseases classified elsewhere

CARIOTID SINUS SYNDROME

George E. Kikano, MD

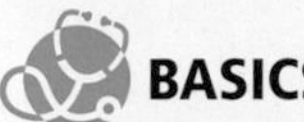

BASICS

DESCRIPTION

- Baroreceptors in the carotid sinus and aortic arch normally influence blood pressure (BP) and heart rate. An endogenous increase in BP or external pressure on the carotid sinus increases the baroreceptor firing rate and activates vagal efferents, resulting in a bradycardia and/or drop in BP.
- In carotid sinus syndrome, stimulation of 1 or both hypersensitive carotid sinuses may produce brief episodes of faintness or loss of consciousness.
- Carotid sinus syndrome is defined as an asystole of ≥3 seconds and/or a drop in systolic BP of ≥50 mm Hg elicited by cardiac sinus pressure.
- 4 types are described:
  - Cardioinhibitory: Vagally mediated, causing bradycardia, sinus arrest, or atrioventricular block for >3 seconds
  - Vasodepressor: A sudden drop of peripheral vascular resistance leads to a >50 mm Hg decrease in systolic BP without change in heart rate, or to a >30 mm Hg symptomatic drop in systolic BP.
  - Mixed: Combined cardioinhibitory and vasodepressor changes
  - Cerebral: Extremely rare; carotid sinus hypersensitivity occurs without bradycardia or hypotension.
- System(s) affected: Cardiovascular; Nervous
- Synonym(s): Carotid sinus syncope; Carotid sinus hypersensitivity

EPIDEMIOLOGY

- Predominant age: Elderly
- Predominant sex: Male > Female (2:1)

Geriatric Considerations

- More likely to occur in elderly
- Can be a cause of unexplained frequent falls

Incidence

- 35 million cases are reported every year.
- Incidence increases with age

Prevalence

- In 2 large studies of patients with syncope, 6–14% had carotid sinus hypersensitivity.
- In patients >80 years of age with unexplained syncope, prevalence of carotid sinus syndrome may be as high as 40%.

RISK FACTORS

- Diffuse atherosclerosis
- Age

ETIOLOGY

- Idiopathic
- Carotid body tumors
- Inflammatory and malignant lymph nodes in the neck
- Metastatic cancer

COMMONLY ASSOCIATED CONDITIONS

- Sick sinus syndrome
- Atrioventricular block
- Coronary artery disease

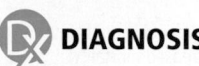

DIAGNOSIS

HISTORY

- Syncope
- Unexplained falls
- Abnormal gait and balance
- Absence of postictal symptoms

PHYSICAL EXAM

- Bradycardia
- Hypotension
- Pallor
- Abnormal visual acuity
- Diaphoresis
- Orthostatic vital signs (exclude orthostatic hypotension)

DIAGNOSTIC TESTS & INTERPRETATION

Electrocardiogram (ECG)

Imaging

Carotid duplex scan

Diagnostic Procedures/Surgery

- Special test: Unilateral carotid sinus pressure "massage" for 5–10 seconds:
  - With the patient in the supine position and while the BP and ECG are monitored, manual pressure on the carotid sinus causes asystole or reproduce the symptoms (commonly but somewhat erroneously termed "massage")
  - Diagnostic yield may be increased by combining with tilt-table testing.
  - Contraindications to this test include:
    - Carotid bruit
    - History of stroke or transient ischemic attack
    - Recent myocardial infarction
    - History of ventricular tachycardia or fibrillation
- The test can be falsely positive in elderly patients.

Pathological Findings

Pressure on the carotid sinus causes asystole of >3 seconds (cardioinhibitory) and/or a drop in systol BP ≥50 mm Hg.

DIFFERENTIAL DIAGNOSIS

- Neurocardiogenic syncope
- Postural hypotension
- Primary autonomic insufficiency
- Hypovolemia
- Dysrhythmias
- Sick sinus syndrome
- Cerebrovascular insufficiency
- Other causes of syncope

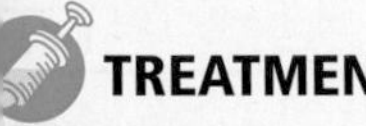

TREATMENT

MEDICATION

First Line

- Anticholinergics: Atropine (acutely) for cardioinhibitory type
- α-Sympathomimetics: Ephedrine, midodrine
- Precautions: Concomitant usage of digitalis, β-blockers, clonidine, and α-methyldopa may accentuate response to carotid sinus massage.

Second Line

Fludrocortisone can be used to improve orthostatic symptoms in patients with vasodepressor response.

ADDITIONAL TREATMENT

General Measures

- No treatment is required for asymptomatic individuals.
- Support hose may help with vasodepressor symptoms.
- Dietary high-salt intake may be helpful.

Issues for Referral

Symptomatic patients need to be referred for further evaluation.

SURGERY/OTHER PROCEDURES

- Carotid sinus denervation by surgery or radiation therapy for selected patients
- Adventitial stripping is a surgical technique that is effective and relatively safe in many patients.
- Permanent pacing may help prevent recurrent symptoms in patients with cardioinhibitory component.
- Carotid endarterectomy for patients with atheroma

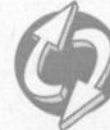

ONGOING CARE

PATIENT EDUCATION

- Avoid pressure on the neck, tight collars, and neckties.
- Restrictions on driving or other potentially hazardous activities until cleared by the physician
- Take medications as prescribed.
- Avoid medications that might cause hypotension.

PROGNOSIS

- May be serious if syncope is associated with atheromatous narrowing of sinus artery or basilar artery
- Recurrence rate is difficult to quantify.

COMPLICATIONS

- Frequent falls, leading to injuries and fractures
- Rarely, sudden death from asystole

ADDITIONAL READING

- ACC/AHA/NASPE 2002 Guideline update for implantation of cardiac pacemakers and antiarrhythmia devices: Summary article. A report of the American College of Cardiology/American Heart Association task force on practice guidelines (ACC/AHA/NASPE committee to update the 1998 pacemaker guidelines).
- Alboni P, Brignole M, Menozzi C, et al. Diagnostic value of history in patients with syncope with or without heart disease. *J Am Coll Cardiol*. 2001;37: 1921–8.
- Bartoletti A, Fabiani P, Bagnoli L, et al. Physical injuries caused by a transient loss of consciousness: main clinical characteristics of patients and diagnostic contribution of carotid sinus massage. *Eur Heart J*. 2008;29:618–24.
- Davies AJ, Kenny RA. Frequency of neurologic complications following carotid sinus massage. *Am J Cardiol*. 1998;81:1256–7.
- Humm AM, Mathias CJ. Unexplained syncope–is screening for carotid sinus hypersensitivity indicated in all patients aged >40 years? *J Neurol Neurosurg Psychiatry*. 2006;77:1267–70.
- Kenny RA, Richardson DA, Steen N, et al. Carotid sinus syndrome: a modifiable risk factor for nonaccidental falls in older adults (SAFE PACE). *J Am Coll Cardiol*. 2001;38:1491–6.
- Kerr SR, Pearce MS, Brayne C, et al. Carotid sinus hypersensitivity in asymptomatic older persons: implications for diagnosis of syncope and falls. *Arch Intern Med*. 2006;166:515–20.
- Mathias CJ, Deguchi K, Schatz I. Observations on recurrent syncope and presyncope in 641 patients. *Lancet*. 2001;357:348–53.

See Also (Topic, Algorithm, Electronic Media Element)

Syncope

CODES

ICD9

337.01 Carotid sinus syndrome

CLINICAL PEARLS

- Pressure on the carotid sinus causes asystole of >3 seconds (cardioinhibitory) and/or a drop in systolic BP ≥50 mm Hg, reproducing symptoms.
- It is clinically important to distinguish carotid sinus syndrome from sick sinus syndrome.
- The finding of carotid sinus hypersensitivity does not exclude other causes of syncope.

CAROTID STENOSIS

Charles Strom, MD
Jeremy Golding, MD

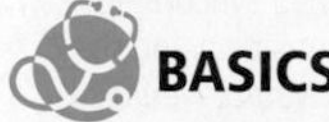

BASICS

DESCRIPTION

- Narrowing of carotid artery lumen, typically due to atherosclerotic changes in the vessel wall. Atherosclerotic plaques are responsible for 90% of extracranial carotid lesions and up to 30% of all ischemic strokes.
- Carotid lesions classified by:
  - Symptom status
    - Asymptomatic: Tend to be homogenous and stable
    - Symptomatic (stroke, transient cerebral ischemic event): Tend to be heterogeneous and unstable
  - Degree of stenosis
    - High grade: 80–99% stenosis
    - Moderate grade: 50–79% stenosis
    - Low grade: <50% stenosis

EPIDEMIOLOGY

More common in men and with increasing age (see Risk Factors)

Incidence

Unclear (asymptomatic patients often go undiagnosed)

Prevalence

- Of patients aged >50 years, 4.8% of men and 2.2% of women have moderate (≥50%) stenosis (1).
- Of patients aged >70 years, moderate stenosis affects 12.5% of men and 6.9% of women (1).

RISK FACTORS

- Nonmodifiable factors: Advanced age, hypercoagulable states, male sex, family history, carotid bruit, cardiac disease, race (African American, Latino)
- Modifiable factors: Smoking, hyperlipidemia, sedentary lifestyle, elevated body mass index, use of oral contraceptive pills, hypertension (HTN), diabetes mellitus, history of transient ischemic attack (TIA) or stroke, EtOH/drug abuse, low serum folate levels, elevated anticardiolipin antibodies, fibrinogen, or homocysteine levels

Genetics

Increased incidence among family members:

- Direct genetic factors (increased carotid artery stenosis/plaque formation seen in homozygotes):
  - apoE lipoprotein [varepsilon]4 polymorphism
  - TT Leu554Phe E-selectin variant
  - Apolipoprotein 5 (APOA5) 56C >G variant
- Genetically linked factors:
  - Hypercoagulability, diabetes mellitus, race, HTN, family history, obesity

GENERAL PREVENTION

- Antihypertensive therapy
- Statin therapy in appropriate candidates

PATHOPHYSIOLOGY

Atherosclerosis formation begins during adolescence, consistently at carotid bifurcation. The carotid bulb has unique blood-flow dynamics. Hemodynamic disturbances cause endothelial injury and dysfunction. Plaque formation in vessel wall results, and stenosis then ensues.

ETIOLOGY

Initial cause not well understood, but certain risk factors are frequently present (see Risk Factors). Tensile stress on the vessel wall, turbulence, and arterial wall shear stress seem to be involved.

COMMONLY ASSOCIATED CONDITIONS

- TIA/stroke
- Coronary artery disease (CAD)/myocardial infarction (MI)
- Peripheral vascular disease (PVD)
- HTN
- Diabetes mellitus
- Hyperlipidemia
- Hypercoagulable states

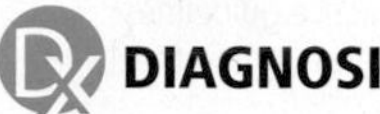

DIAGNOSIS

Screening for carotid stenosis is not recommended. However, in the setting of symptoms suggestive of stroke or TIA, workup for this condition may be indicated.

HISTORY

- Identification of modifiable and nonmodifiable comorbidities (see Risk Factors)
- History of cerebral ischemic event
- Stroke, TIA, amaurosis fugax (monocular blindness), aphasia
- CAD/MI
- PVD
- Full review of systems, with focus on risk factors for:
  - Cardiovascular disease
  - Stroke (HTN and arrhythmia)

PHYSICAL EXAM

- Lateralizing neurologic deficits:
  - Contralateral motor and/or sensory deficit
- Monocular blindness (amaurosis fugax):
  - Hollenhorst plaques on retinal examination
- Cerebellar abnormalities:
  - Binocular vision loss, falls without syncope, vertigo, loss of coordination
- Carotid bruit (low sensitivity and specificity)

DIAGNOSTIC TESTS & INTERPRETATION

Lab

Initial lab tests

- Complete blood count with differential
- Basic metabolic panel
- ESR (if temporal arteritis a consideration)
- Glucose/HbA1c
- Fasting lipid profile
- Hypercoagulable workup if (+) risk factors

Follow-Up & Special Considerations

Proceed to imaging if suggestion of stenosis from history or physical examination.

Imaging

Initial approach

Duplex ultrasound identifies ≥50% stenosis with 98% sensitivity and 88% specificity (2)[A]. Doppler ultrasound determines degree of stenosis by assessin velocity of blood flow through stenotic vessel. Although findings should be confirmed by angiogram (magnetic resonance [MR], computed tomography [CT], or contrast), ultrasound is increasingly used to screen prior to surgical assessment.

Follow-Up & Special Considerations

Other noninvasive imaging techniques can add detail to duplex results:

- CT angiography:
  - 88% sensitivity and 100% specificity
  - Requires contrast load with risk for subsequent renal morbidity
- MR angiography:
  - 95% sensitivity and 90% specificity (3)[A]
  - Evaluates cerebral circulation (extracranial and intracranial) as well as aortic arch and common carotid artery
  - Tends to overestimate degree of stenosis

Diagnostic Procedures/Surgery

Contrast angiography is the traditional gold standard for diagnosis:

- Delineates anatomy pertaining to aortic arch and proximal vessels
- However, procedure is invasive and has multiple risks:
  - Dye allergy and renal toxicity
  - Stroke
  - Should be used only when other tests are not conclusive

Pathological Findings

- Stenosis consistently occurs at carotid bifurcation, with plaque formation most often at proximal internal carotid artery:
  - Plaque thickest at carotid bifurcation
  - Plaque occupies intima and inner media, avoids outer media and adventitia

Plaque histology:
- Homogenous (stable) plaques, seldom hemorrhage or ulcerate:
  - Fatty streak and fibrous tissue deposition
  - Diffuse intimal thickening
- Heterogenous (unstable) plaques, may hemorrhage or ulcerate:
  - Presence of lipid-laden macrophages, necrotic debris, cholesterol crystals
  - Ulcerated plaques
- Soft and gelatinous clots with platelets, fibrin, and red and white blood cells

DIFFERENTIAL DIAGNOSIS

Aortic valve stenosis
Aortic arch atherosclerosis
Arrhythmia with cardiogenic embolization
Migraine
Brain tumor
Metabolic disturbances
Functional/psychologic deficit
Seizure

TREATMENT

Smoking cessation, good control of blood pressure, and use of antiplatelet medication and statin medication is the primary treatment for both asymptomatic and symptomatic carotid stenosis (4).

MEDICATION

Antihypertensives:
- Thiazide diuretic ± angiotensin-converting enzyme inhibitor (5)[A]

Statins (5)[A]
Antiplatelet (5)[A] agents:
- Aspirin 81–325 mg daily
- Clopidogrel 75 mg daily
- Aspirin/dipyridamole

ADDITIONAL TREATMENT

General Measures

Lifestyle modifications
Control of HTN, generally with target <140/90
Avoidance of cigarettes
Dietary control and weight loss

Issues for Referral

For acute symptomatic stroke, order imaging and contact neurology.
For known carotid stenosis, some suggest duplex imaging every 6 months if stenosis is >50% and patient is a surgical candidate.

SURGERY/OTHER PROCEDURES

Goal: Prevention of stroke:

Carotid endarterectomy (CEA) may be indicated in:
- Asymptomatic patients with >60–70% stenosis, but the absolute reduction in stroke risk is small, and long-term benefit is critically dependent upon low perioperative stroke rate (≤3% morbidity and mortality). CEA for asymptomatic carotid disease remains controversial.
- Symptomatic patients: Number needed to treat (NNT) to prevent 1 disabling stroke or death over 2–6 years is 15 for patients with severe stenosis (stenosis >70–80%) and 21 for patients with less severe stenosis (50–70%). Good outcomes depend upon surgeons and centers with <6% perioperative stroke risk.

- Regional anesthesia may be preferable to general (fewer strokes, arrhythmias, and MIs).
- Carotid angioplasty with stent placement is an alternative option in symptomatic high-risk patients with >80% stenosis.

IN-PATIENT CONSIDERATIONS

Initial Stabilization

Rapid evaluation for symptoms compatible with TIA should be obtained in the emergency department or inpatient setting.

Admission Criteria

Any patient with presentation of acute symptomatic carotid stenosis should be hospitalized for further diagnostic workup and appropriate therapy.

IV Fluids

Not necessary

Discharge Criteria

24–48 hours post-CEA, if ambulating, taking adequate p.o. intake, and neurologically intact

ONGOING CARE

FOLLOW-UP RECOMMENDATIONS

Patient Monitoring

After CEA, overnight in postanesthesia care unit or step-down:
- Duplex at 2–6 weeks postop
- Duplex every 6–12 months

DIET

- NPO postop (in case return to operating room)
- Low fat, low cholesterol, low salt at discharge

PATIENT EDUCATION

- Signs and symptoms of TIA/stroke:
  - Lateralizing neurologic deficits, monocular blindness, aphasia
- Diet and lifestyle modification

PROGNOSIS

Risk proportional to degree of stenosis

COMPLICATIONS

- Untreated:
  - TIA/stroke
- Postoperative (s/p CEA):
  - Perioperative (within 30 days):
    - Stroke/death, cranial nerve injury, hemorrhage, hemodynamic instability, MI (because of comorbid CAD)
  - Late (>30 days postop):
    - Recurrent stenosis, false aneurysm at surgical site

REFERENCES

1. de Weerd M, Greving JP, de Jong AW, et al. Prevalence of Asymptomatic Carotid Artery Stenosis According to Age and Sex. Systematic Review and Metaregression Analysis. *Stroke*. 2009.
2. Jahromi AS, Cinà CS, Liu Y, et al. Sensitivity and specificity of color duplex ultrasound measurement in the estimation of internal carotid artery stenosis: a systematic review and meta-analysis. *J Vasc Surg*. 2005;41:962–72.
3. Nederkoorn PJ, van der Graaf Y, Hunink MG. Duplex ultrasound and magnetic resonance angiography compared with digital subtraction angiography in carotid artery stenosis: a systematic review. *Stroke*. 2003;34:1324–32.
4. *Cochrane Database Syst Rev*. 2010;(2):CD005953.
5. Sacco RL, Adams R, Albers G, et al. Guidelines for prevention of stroke in patients with ischemic stroke or transient ischemic attack: a statement for healthcare professionals from the American Heart Association/American Stroke Association Council on Stroke: co-sponsored by the Council on Cardiovascular Radiology and Intervention: the American Academy of Neurology affirms the value of this guideline. *Stroke*. 2006;37:577–617.

ADDITIONAL READING

Barnett HJ, Taylor DW, Eliasziw M, et al. Benefit of carotid endarterectomy in patients with symptomatic moderate or severe stenosis. North American Symptomatic Carotid Endarterectomy Trial Collaborators. *N Engl J Med*. 1998;339:1415–25.

See Also (Topic, Algorithm, Electronic Media Element)

Algorithms: Transient Ischemic Attack; Stroke; Hypercholesterolemia

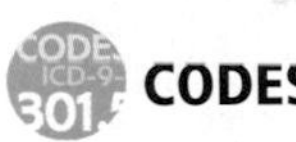

CODES

ICD9

433.10 Occlusion and stenosis of carotid artery without mention of cerebral infarction

CLINICAL PEARLS

- Atherosclerosis is responsible for 90% of all cases of carotid artery stenosis.
- The greater the degree of stenosis, the greater the risk of embolism and stroke.
- Amaurosis fugax (monocular blindness) is often described as "curtain pulled over eye" and is concerning for further ischemic events.
- Duplex is the best initial imaging modality.
- Medical management is the cornerstone of treatment, with surgical management in carefully selected cases and situations

CARPAL TUNNEL SYNDROME

Jay U. Howington, MD

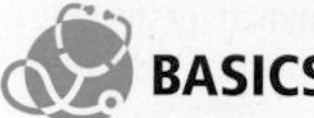

BASICS

DESCRIPTION

- Carpal tunnel syndrome is the most common cause of peripheral nerve compression.
- The median nerve is compressed as it traverses the carpal tunnel in the wrist and hand.
- The tunnel is composed of the carpal bones dorsally and the transverse carpal ligament ventrally. It contains flexor tendons and the median nerve.
- Symptoms tend to affect the dominant hand, but >50% of patients experience bilateral symptoms.
- System(s) affected: Musculoskeletal; Nervous

Pregnancy Considerations

Not uncommon during pregnancy

EPIDEMIOLOGY

- Predominant age: 40–60
- Predominant sex: Female > Male (3:1–10:1) (1)

Incidence

- Two peaks: Late 50s in women and late 70s when the sex ratio is more equal
- Older patients tend to have more severe carpal tunnel syndrome (59% >65 have thenar atrophy) (2).

Prevalence

Most common entrapment neuropathy. Most recent estimates of prevalence indicate that the disorder occurs in 346/100,000 population.

RISK FACTORS

- No clear evidence that repetitive flexion and extension of the wrist may influence the development of carpal tunnel syndrome.
- Occupation as a seamstress or computer operator may exacerbate carpal tunnel syndrome. There is, however, no universal agreement that carpal tunnel syndrome is job-related.
- Obesity is a risk factor in younger patients.

Genetics

Unknown; however, a familial type has been reported.

GENERAL PREVENTION

Take a break once an hour when doing repetitive work involving hands.

ETIOLOGY

- Disorders affecting the musculoskeletal system in the region of the wrist, including:
  - Trauma or Colles fracture
  - Degenerative joint disease
  - Rheumatoid arthritis
  - Ganglion cyst
  - Scleroderma
- Hypothyroidism and diabetes are frequently associated with this condition, which also occurs with increased frequency during pregnancy.
- Other miscellaneous causes include:
  - Acromegaly
  - Lupus erythematosus
  - Leukemia
  - Pyogenic infections
  - Sarcoidosis
  - Primary amyloidosis
  - Paget disease
- Hyperparathyroidism, hypocalcemia

COMMONLY ASSOCIATED CONDITIONS

- Diabetes
- Obesity
- Pregnancy

DIAGNOSIS

HISTORY

- Burning pain and/or tingling in the fingers, particularly at night (acroparesthesias):
  - The altered sensation (tingling or prickling) is characteristically confined to the thumb and the index and middle fingers, but many patients do not distinguish this localization and feel the entire hand is affected.
- Arm pain
- Symptoms characteristically are relieved by shaking or rubbing the hands.
- During waking hours, symptoms occur when driving the car, reading the newspaper, and occasionally when using the hands for repetitive maneuvers.

PHYSICAL EXAM

- Positive Tinel sign: Tapping of the wrist proximal to the carpal tunnel may produce electric sensation perceived by the patient, a sign of nerve compression (50% sensitivity and 77% specificity) (3)[A].
- Positive Phalen sign: Holding the wrist flexed for 60 seconds may precipitate the paresthesias experienced by the patient (68% sensitivity and 73% specificity) (3)[A].
- Finger sensory loss
- Wasting of the thenar and hypothenar muscles is a late sign.
- Weakness of the hand, however, for such tasks as opening jars is often noted by the patient early in the disorder.

DIAGNOSTIC TESTS & INTERPRETATION

Lab

- No laboratory test is diagnostic.
- Normal serum TSH and normal serum glucose may be helpful in excluding conditions associated with carpal tunnel syndrome.

Initial lab tests

- Special tests:
  - Electromyography:
    - Will be abnormal in >85% of cases
    - Prolonged distal latency of the median motor nerves may be seen.
    - The most sensitive indicator is the median sensory distal latency, which is prolonged. Further, the sensory nerve action potential may be reduced or unobtainable.
    - Not required as a diagnostic test where clinical symptoms are well defined or to predict surgical outcome (3)[A]
- Stimulation of the ulnar nerve should be done as well to exclude generalized polyneuropathy.

Imaging

Initial approach

- Special radiographic views of the carpal tunnel may be obtained. These are of limited usefulness unless heterotopic calcification can be identified.
- Magnetic resonance neurography may be used to confirm compression of the median nerve in the carpal tunnel and to assess the success of surgical decompression.

Diagnostic Procedures/Surgery

A BP tourniquet to cut off circulation to the arm may precipitate symptoms promptly.

DIFFERENTIAL DIAGNOSIS

- Cervical spondylosis
- Generalized peripheral neuropathy
- Brachial plexus lesion
- Pronator syndrome
- Anterior interosseous syndrome

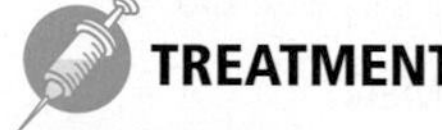

TREATMENT

MEDICATION

First Line

NSAIDs such as ibuprofen, 800 mg b.i.d. or t.i.d., or naproxen sodium, 500 mg b.i.d., may provide significant relief of symptoms in many patients:

- Contraindications: GI intolerance
- Precautions: GI side effects of NSAIDs may preclude their use in selected patients.

Second Line

Oral steroid

DDITIONAL TREATMENT

eneral Measures

Splinting of the wrist in extension while sleeping may provide significant relief of symptoms.

Prolonged use of splinting, if possible, may allow some symptoms to resolve.

Injection of the carpal tunnel with steroid may provide significant temporary relief. This is particularly useful during pregnancy. Can be expected to provide relief for up to 1 month or longer.

The combination of splinting and steroid injections provides long-term relief in only 10% of cases and is not better than either treatment in isolation (4,5)[A].

OMPLEMENTARY AND ALTERNATIVE EDICINE

espite studies, no data exists to support use of amin B_6 in the prevention or treatment of carpal nnel syndrome.

URGERY/OTHER PROCEDURES

Surgical decompression of the carpal tunnel by dividing the transverse carpal ligament completely provides almost total relief of symptoms in >95% of patients.

Surgical decompression is usually done as an outpatient procedure under local anesthesia.

Healing of the incision generally takes 2 weeks; an additional 2 weeks of recuperation may be required before the hand can be fully used for tasks requiring strength.

Recent randomized, controlled studies indicate that surgery is more effective than splinting at 18 months (6,7)[A].

Open vs endoscopic procedures produce similar outcomes at 1 year and approach should be driven based upon surgeon and patient preference (8)[A].

N-PATIENT CONSIDERATIONS

nitial Stabilization

Outpatient

Outpatient surgery

ONGOING CARE

FOLLOW-UP RECOMMENDATIONS

Patient Monitoring

- Patients treated with wrist splints or other palliative measures such as cortisone injections will require follow-up in the ensuing 4–12 weeks to assess the success of treatment modalities.
- Patients treated surgically rarely experience recurrence of the disorder. Routine follow-up once healing of the incision has occurred is not necessary.

PATIENT EDUCATION

Carpal Tunnel Syndrome Foundation. For patient education materials favorably reviewed on this topic, contact: American Academy of Family Physicians Foundation, P.O. Box 8418, Kansas City, MO 64114, (800) 274-2237, Ext. 4400.

PROGNOSIS

Untreated, more severe cases of the condition can be expected to lead to numbness and weakness in the hand, with atrophy of hand muscles and permanent loss of function of the extremity.

COMPLICATIONS

- Postoperative infection (rare)
- Injury to recurrent branch of the nerve

REFERENCES

1. Nordstrom DL, DeStefano F, Vierkant RA, et al. Incidence of diagnosed carpal tunnel syndrome in a general population. *Epidemiology.* 1998;9:342–5.
2. Blumenthal S, Herskovitz S, Verghese J. Carpal tunnel syndrome in older adults. *Muscle Nerve.* 2006;34:78–83.
3. Jordan R, Carter T, Cummins C. A systematic review of the utility of electrodiagnostic testing in carpal tunnel syndrome. *Br J Gen Pract.* 2002;52:670–3.
4. Graham RG, et al. A prospective study to assess the outcome of steroid injections and wrist splinting for the treatment of carpal tunnel syndrome. *Plas Reconst Surg.* 2004;113:550–6.
5. Marshall S, Tardif G, Ashworth N et al. Local corticosteroid injection for carpal tunnel syndrome. *Cochrane Database Syst Rev.* 2007;CD001554.
6. Verdugo RJ, Salinas RA, Castillo JL, et al. Surgical versus non-surgical treatment for carpal tunnel syndrome. *Cochrane Database Syst Rev.* 2008:CD001552.
7. Gerritsen AA, de Vet HC, Scholten RJ, et al. Splinting vs surgery in the treatment of carpal tunnel syndrome: a randomized controlled trial. *JAMA.* 2002;288:1245–51.
8. Scholten RJ, Mink van der Molen A, Uitdehaag BM, Bouter LM, de Vet HC et al. Surgical treatment options for carpal tunnel syndrome. *Cochrane Database Syst Rev.* 2007;CD003905.

ADDITIONAL READING

Cudlip SA, Howe FA, Clifton A, et al. Magnetic resonance neurography studies of the median nerve before and after carpal tunnel decompression. *J Neurosurg.* 2002;96:1046–51.

See Also (Topic, Algorithm, Electronic Media Element)

Arthritis, Rheumatoid; Hypoparathyroidism; Scleroderma; Systemic Lupus Erythematosus (SLE)

Algorithms: Carpal Tunnel Syndrome; Pain in Upper Extremity

CODES

ICD9

354.0 Carpal tunnel syndrome

CLINICAL PEARLS

- The altered sensation (tingling or prickling) in carpal tunnel syndrome is characteristically confined to the thumb and the index and middle fingers, but many patients do not distinguish this localization and feel the entire hand is affected.
- Tinel and Phalen signs have poor sensitivity and specificity.
- Normal serum TSH and normal serum glucose may be helpful in excluding conditions associated with carpal tunnel syndrome.
- Strongly consider surgical treatment for moderate and severe cases. Atrophy is a late finding indicating severe disease.

C

CATARACT

Christopher Gudas, MD
John W. Gittinger, Jr., MD

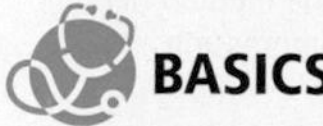

BASICS

DESCRIPTION

A *cataract* is any opacity or discoloration of the lens, localized or generalized; the term is usually reserved for changes that affect visual acuity:

- Etymology: From Latin *catarractes*, for "waterfall"; named after foamy appearance of opacity
- Leading cause of blindness worldwide, an estimated 20 million people
- Types include:
  - Age-related ("senile"): 90% of total
  - Congenital (1/250 newborns; 10–38% of childhood blindness)
  - Systemic disease associated (myotonic dystrophy, atopic dermatitis)
  - Metabolic (diabetes via accelerated sorbitol pathway, hypocalcemia, Wilson disease)
  - Secondary to associated eye disease, so-called complicated (e.g., uveitis associated with juvenile rheumatoid arthritis or sarcoid, tumor such as melanoma or retinoblastoma)
  - Traumatic (e.g., heat, electric shock, radiation, concussion, perforating eye injuries, intraocular foreign body)
  - Toxic/nutritional (e.g., corticosteroids, medications)
- Morphologic classification:
  - Nuclear: Exaggeration of normal aging changes of *central* lens nucleus, often associated with myopia due to increased refractive index of lens (some elderly patients consequently may be able to read again *without spectacles,* so-called second sight of the aged)
  - Cortical: Outer portion of lens; may involve anterior, posterior, or equatorial cortex; radial, spokelike opacities
  - Subcapsular: Posterior subcapsular cataract has more profound effect on vision than nuclear or cortical cataract; patients particularly troubled under conditions of miosis; near vision frequently impaired more than distance vision
- System(s) affected: Nervous

Geriatric Considerations

Some degree of cataract formation is expected in all people >70 years of age.

Pediatric Considerations

See Congenital Cataracts; may present as leukocoria.

Pregnancy Considerations

See Congenital Cataracts (i.e., medications, metabolic dysfunction, intrauterine infection, and malnutrition).

EPIDEMIOLOGY

Incidence

- Nearly 48% of the 37 million cases of blindness worldwide result from cataracts.
- Leading cause of treatable blindness and vision loss in developing countries
- Predominant age: Depends on type of cataract
- Predominant sex: Male Female (perhaps *slight* female predominance of cortical cataract)

Prevalence

- Cataract type and prevalence highly variable based on population demographic
- It is estimated that 50% of people 65–74 years of age and 70% of people >75 years of age have age-related cataract change.

RISK FACTORS

- Aging
- Cigarette smoking
- Ultraviolet B (UVB) sunlight exposure
- Diabetes
- Prolonged high-dose steroids
- Positive family history (see Genetics)
- Alcohol

Genetics

- Congenital sometimes associated (e.g., heredofamilial systemic disorders [Laurence-Moon-Biedl syndrome], chromosomal disorders [Down syndrome]) (1)[A]
- Genetics of age-related cataract not yet established, but likely multifactorial contribution (2)

GENERAL PREVENTION

- Use of UVB protective glasses (2,3)[A]
- Avoidance of tobacco products (2,3)[A]
- Effective control of diabetes (2,3)[A]
- Care with high-dose, long-term steroid use (systemic therapy > inhaled treatment) (2)[B]
- Protective methods using pharmaceutical intervention (e.g., antioxidants, ASA, hormone replacement therapy [HRT]) show no proven benefit to date (2,3)[C].

ETIOLOGY

- Age-related cataract:
  - Continual addition of layers of lens fibers throughout life creates hard, dehydrated lens nucleus that impairs vision (nuclear cataract).
  - Aging alters biochemical and osmotic balance required for lens clarity; outer lens layers hydrate and become opaque, adversely affecting vision.
- Congenital:
  - Usually obscure cause
  - Drugs (corticosteroids in 1st trimester, sulfonamides)
  - Metabolic diabetes in mother, galactosemia in fetus
  - Intrauterine infection during 1st trimester (e.g., rubella, herpes, mumps)
  - Maternal malnutrition
- Other cataract types:
  - Common feature is a biochemical/osmotic imbalance that disrupts lens clarity
  - Local changes in lens protein distribution lead to light scattering (lens opacity).

COMMONLY ASSOCIATED CONDITIONS

- Diabetes (especially with poor control)
- Myotonic dystrophy (90% of patients develop visually innocuous change in 3rd decade; becomes disabling in 5th decade)
- Atopic dermatitis: 10% of patients with severe AD develop cataracts in 2nd–4th decades, often bilateral.
- Neurofibromatosis type 2
- Associated ocular disease or "secondary cataract" (e.g., chronic anterior uveitis, acute [or repetitive] angle-closure glaucoma or high myopia)
- Drug-induced (e.g., steroids, chlorpromazine)
- Trauma

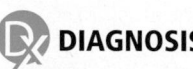

DIAGNOSIS

HISTORY

- Age-related cataract:
  - Blurred vision, distortion, or "ghosting" of image
  - Problems with visual acuity in bright light or night driving (glare)
  - Falls or accidents; injuries (e.g., hip fracture)
- Congenital: Often asymptomatic, or parents notice child's visual inattention or strabismus
- Other types of cataract:
  - May present with decreased visual acuity
  - Appropriate history or signs to help in diagnosis

HYSICAL EXAM

Age-related cataract: Lens opacity on eye examination

Congenital:
- Lens opacity present at birth or within 3 months of birth
- Leukocoria (white pupil), strabismus, nystagmus, signs of associated syndrome (as with Down or rubella syndrome)
- *Note:* Always must rule out ocular tumor; early diagnosis and treatment of retinoblastoma may be lifesaving.

Other types of cataract: May present with decreased visual acuity

IAGNOSTIC TESTS & INTERPRETATION

Visual quality assessment: Glare testing, contrast sensitivity sometimes indicated

Retinal/macular function assessment: Potential acuity meter testing

ab

iabetic control: HbA1c; hyperglycemic state creates n osmotic change within the lens and may alter sual acuity and refractive measurement.

athological Findings

onsistent with lens changes found in the type of ataract; however, diagnosis is made by clinical xamination.

IFFERENTIAL DIAGNOSIS

n opaque-appearing eye may be due to opacities of e cornea (e.g., scarring, edema, calcification), lens pacities, tumor, or retinal detachment.

iomicroscopic examination (slit lamp) or careful phthalmoscopic exam should provide diagnosis:

In the elderly, visual impairment is often due to multiple factors, such as cataract and macular degeneration, both contributing to visual loss.

Age-related cataract is significant if symptoms and ophthalmic exam support cataract as a major cause of vision impairment.

Congenital lens opacity in the absence of other ocular pathology may cause severe amblyopia.

Note: Cataract *does not* produce a relative afferent pupillary reaction defect. Abnormal pupillary reactions mandate further evaluation for other pathology.

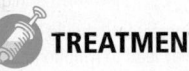

TREATMENT

Outpatient (usually) or inpatient surgery

~1.64 million cataract extractions in US yearly

MEDICATION

here is currently no medication to prevent or slow the rogression of cataracts.

ADDITIONAL TREATMENT

ssues for Referral

patient has cataract and symptoms do not seem to upport recommended surgery, a 2nd opinion by nother ophthalmologist may be indicated.

SURGERY/OTHER PROCEDURES

- Age-related cataract:
  - Surgical removal is indicated if visual impairment–producing symptoms are distressing to the patient, interfering with lifestyle or occupation, or posing a risk for fall or injury.
  - Because significant cataract may develop gradually, the patient may not be aware of how it has changed his or her lifestyle. Physician may note a significant cataract, and patient reports "no problems." Thus, evaluation requires effective physician–patient exchange of information.
  - Surgical technique: Cataract extraction via small incisions, followed by implantation of a prosthetic intraocular lens; lenses have power calculated based on size of the eye and curvature of cornea usually to correct for distance vision; surgery performed on 1 (worse) eye, with contralateral surgery only after recovery and if deemed necessary; generally takes less than an hour depending on surgical technique
  - Anesthesia: Usually local with sedation and monitoring of vital signs
  - Preoperative evaluation: By the primary-care physician; patients on anticoagulants may need to be temporarily discontinued 1–2 weeks before surgery if possible (but not always necessary; thus, need to discuss with ophthalmologist); patients who have ever taken an α-blocker should alert their ophthalmologist (risk of intraoperative floppy iris syndrome)
  - Postoperative care: Usually protective eye shield as directed, topical antibiotic, and steroid ophthalmic medications; avoid lifting or bending over for a few weeks.
- Congenital cataract:
  - Treatment is surgical removal of cataract. Newborn may require surgery within days to reduce risk of severe amblyopia. Use of lens implants is controversial.
  - Postoperative care: Long-term patching program for good eye to combat amblyopia; refractive correction of operative eye, with multiple repeat examinations; challenging for physician and parents

ONGOING CARE

FOLLOW-UP RECOMMENDATIONS

Patient Monitoring

- As cataract progresses, an ophthalmologist may change spectacle correction to maintain vision. When this is no longer successful and *interferes with patient's activities of daily living* (ADLs), surgery is indicated.
- Following surgery, spectacle correction may be required to maximize near and/or far visual acuity. Refraction is usually prescribed several weeks after surgery.

PATIENT EDUCATION

See Surgery.

PROGNOSIS

- Ocular prognosis good after cataract removal if no prior ocular disease: 95% of otherwise healthy eyes achieve best corrected visual acuity of 20/40 or better (90% when all eyes are considered, including comorbidity such as diabetes and glaucoma).
- In congenital cataracts, prognosis often is poorer because of the high risk of amblyopia.

COMPLICATIONS

- Vary widely from delay in visual recovery or protracted visual discomfort to blindness and loss of eye
- Nearly all reported complications occur rarely (<2% of eyes) except for posterior capsule opacification (~25% of eyes, usually treated with Nd-YAG laser capsulotomy in office).

REFERENCES

1. Tasman W, ed. *Duane's Ophthalmology.* Philadelphia: JB Lippincott Co, 2002.
2. Abraham AG, Condon NG, West Gower E. The new epidemiology of cataract. *Ophthalmol Clin North Am.* 2006;19:415–25.
3. Asbell PA, Dualan I, Mindel J, et al. Age-related cataract. *Lancet.* 2005;365:599–609.

ADDITIONAL READING

Bradford CA, ed. *Basic Ophthalmology* 8th ed. San Francisco: American Academy of Ophthalmology; 2004.

See Also (Topic, Algorithm, Electronic Media Element)

Algorithm: Cataracts

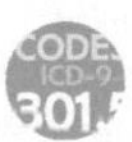

CODES

ICD9

- 366.9 Unspecified cataract
- 366.10 Senile cataract, unspecified
- 743.30 Congenital cataract, unspecified

CELIAC DISEASE

Brandi Kelly, PharmD
Gary Mark McWilliams, MD

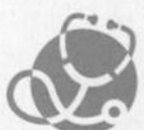

BASICS

DESCRIPTION
- Classically, a chronic diarrheal disease characterized by intestinal malabsorption of virtually all nutrients and precipitated by eating gluten-containing foods. Multiple forms exist.
- Nondiarrheal form may actually be more common (intestinal villous atrophy produces vitamin and mineral malabsorption)
- System(s) affected: Gastrointestinal
- Synonym(s): Sprue; Gluten enteropathy; Celiac sprue

EPIDEMIOLOGY
Incidence
- Disease primarily of individuals of Northern European ancestry
- Predominant sex: Female > Male (3:2)

Prevalence
~1 in 133 persons in US

RISK FACTORS
- 1st-degree relatives: 10% incidence
- 71% in monozygotic twins

Genetics
HLA-DQ2 and/or DQ8 closely associated (testing may be indicated if indeterminate small bowel pathology)

GENERAL PREVENTION
Avoid all gluten-containing products (wheat, barley, rye, and possibly oat products).

ETIOLOGY
Sensitivity to gluten, specifically gliadin fraction

COMMONLY ASSOCIATED CONDITIONS
- May have secondary lactase deficiency
- Extraintestinal manifestation may include marked decrease in bone density
- Dermatitis herpetiformis common
- Autoimmune thyroiditis
- Diabetes, type 1 (prevalence of celiac disease in type 1 diabetes is 3–8%)
- Elevated AST and ALT
- Recurrent fetal loss or infertility
- IBS (irritable bowel syndrome) (1)[A]
- Restless legs syndrome (2)

Pregnancy Considerations
- Celiac disease may be an underappreciated cause of male and female infertility. Consider celiac disease in pregnant women with severe anemia.

DIAGNOSIS

HISTORY
- Diarrhea
- Steatorrhea
- Muscle cramps
- Iron-deficiency anemia
- Nervousness
- Weight loss
- Failure to thrive (slowing velocity of weight gain)
- Weakness
- Lassitude
- Fatigue
- Large appetite
- Explosive flatulence
- Abdominal pain, nausea, vomiting rare
- Recurrent aphthous stomatitis
- Abdominal distention

Pediatric Considerations
- Failure to thrive and delayed growth with short stature may be early manifestations. A few children may outgrow intolerance to wheat after prolonged gluten-free diets, but should be cautioned to watch for signs of recurrence in middle age.

DIAGNOSTIC TESTS & INTERPRETATION
Lab
Initial lab tests

Positive IgA antiendomysial antibodies and IgA tissue transglutaminase (sensitivity 90–98%, specificity 98%) when on normal (nongluten-free) diet

Follow-Up & Special Considerations
- IgA-deficient patients have false-negative IgA antiendomysial and IgA antitransglutaminase antibodies
- tTG (the tissue transglutaminase antibody test) is the preferred test (over the deamidated gliadin peptide [DGP] antibody) (3,4)[A].
- 72-hour fecal fat showing >7% fat malabsorption
- Elevated liver function tests
- d-Xylose test showing malabsorption
- Decreased calcium
- Increased prothrombin time (PT)
- Decreased neutral fats
- Decreased cholesterol
- Decreased vitamin A
- Decreased vitamin B_{12} (rare)
- Decreased vitamin D
- Decreased vitamin C
- Decreased folic acid
- Decreased iron (common)
- Decreased total protein
- Decreased hemoglobin (common)

Imaging
Initial approach

Upper GI series showing flocculation of barium, edema, and flattening of mucosal folds

Follow-Up & Special Considerations

Evaluate for osteoporosis

Diagnostic Procedures/Surgery
- Endoscopy with diagnostic biopsy of the duodenal mucosa with repeat endoscopy and normal biopsy on a gluten-free diet is necessary before a firm diagnosis can be made.
- In general, diagnosis should not be made based on serology alone.

Pathological Findings
Small bowel biopsy:
- Flattened villi, hyperplasia and lengthening of crypts, infiltration of plasma cells, and lymphocytes in lamina propria

DIFFERENTIAL DIAGNOSIS
- Short bowel syndrome
- Pancreatic insufficiency
- Crohn disease
- Whipple disease
- Hypogammaglobulinemia
- Tropical sprue
- Lymphoma
- AIDS
- Acute enteritis
- Giardiasis
- Eosinophilic gastroenteritis
- Pancreatic disease

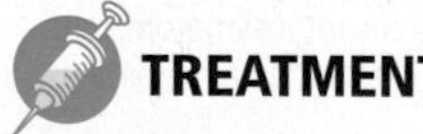

TREATMENT

MEDICATION
First Line
Usually none: Gluten-free diet is treatment

Second Line
- In refractory disease, consider:
  - Steroids (prednisone, 40–60 mg/d p.o. in cases of refractory sprue)
  - Azathioprine (immunosuppressants should be used with caution; use may lead to lymphoma in celiac disease)
  - Cyclosporine
  - Infliximab
  - Cladribine
- Patients may require supplemental calcium, calcium carbonate, 500 mg p.o. b.i.d., and vitamin D (ergocalciferol) 10–100 g/d; in severe malabsorption, up to 2.5 mg/d may be required.

ADDITIONAL TREATMENT

General Measures

- Removal of gluten from the diet. Rice, corn, and soybean flour are safe, palatable substitutes.
- Levels of IgA antigliadin normalize with gluten abstinence.

Issues for Referral

- Additional nutritional support
- Refractory disease

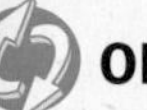

ONGOING CARE

FOLLOW-UP RECOMMENDATIONS

- Consultation with dietitian
- Screening for osteoporosis

Patient Monitoring

- Repeat endoscopy after 6–8 weeks on a gluten-free diet (in selected cases).
- IgA antigliadin assay may be used to monitor response to gluten-free diet.

DIET

Removal of gluten: Wheat, rye, barley, and those with gluten additives. This can be a challenging diet (especially learning sources of "hidden" gluten) and should be coordinated with a skilled dietitian.

PATIENT EDUCATION

- Discuss importance of recognizing gluten in various products.
- Highlight potential complications and outcomes of failing to follow a gluten-free diet.

PROGNOSIS

- Good with correct diagnosis and adherence to gluten-free diet
- Patient should feel better in 7 days.
- All symptoms usually disappear in 4–6 weeks.
- It is unknown whether strict dietary adherence decreases cancer risk.

COMPLICATIONS

- Malignancy: <10% of patients (50% of whom have small bowel lymphoma)
- Refractory sprue:
  - May respond to prednisone 40–60 mg/d p.o.
  - Refractory sprue unresponsive to corticosteroid therapy raises the specter of adult-onset autoimmune enteropathy or cryptic T-cell lymphoma. In this circumstance, screening for antienterocyte autoantibodies and careful scrutiny of the small intestine, including retroperitoneal lymph node biopsy with full-thickness small bowel biopsy, may be needed.
- Chronic ulcerative jejunoileitis:
  - Associated with multiple ulcers, intestinal bleeding, strictures, perforation, obstruction, and peritonitis
  - 7% mortality
- Osteoporosis secondary to decreased vitamin D and calcium absorption
- Dehydration
- Electrolyte depletion
- Refractory cases may need total parenteral nutrition.

REFERENCES

1. Ford AC, Chey WD, Talley NJ, et al. Yield of diagnostic tests for celiac disease in individuals with symptoms suggestive of irritable bowel syndrome: systematic review and meta-analysis. *Arch Intern Med*. 2009;169:651–8.
2. Weinstock L, Walters A, Mullin G, et al. Celiac disease is associated with restless legs syndrome. *Dig Dis Sci*. 2010;55:1667–73.
3. Lewis NR, Scott BB et al. Meta-analysis: deamidated gliadin peptide antibody and tissue transglutaminase antibody compared as screening tests for coeliac disease. *Aliment Pharmacol Ther*. 2010;31:73–81.
4. van der Windt DA, Jellema P, Mulder CJ, Kneepkens CM, van der Horst HE et al. Diagnostic testing for celiac disease among patients with abdominal symptoms: a systematic review. *JAMA*. 2010;303:1738–46.

ADDITIONAL READING

- AGA Institute. AGA Institute Medical Position Statement on the Diagnosis and Management of Celiac Disease. *Gastroenterology*. 2006;131: 1977–80.
- Celiac Disease: A Hidden Epidemic by Peter Green.
- Celiac Sprue Association (CSA) http://www.csaceliacs.org.
- *Guidelines for a Gluten-free Lifestyle*, 3rd. ed. Celiac Disease Foundation. http://www.celiac.org.
- Quick Start Diet Guide: Celiac Disease Foundation (CDF) & Gluten Intolerance Group (GIG). http://www.celiac.org,http://www.gluten.net.

C

See Also (Topic, Algorithm, Electronic Media Element)

Algorithms: Diarrhea, Chronic; Malabsorption Syndrome

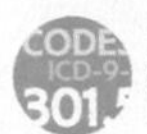

CODES

ICD9

579.0 Celiac disease

CLINICAL PEARLS

- Common condition (1 in 133)
- Characterized by mucosal inflammation and villous atrophy
- Associated with malabsorption of nutrients
- Treatment is gluten free diet.
- Test for celiac disease in patients with IBS.

CELLULITIS

Laura Sullivan Eurich, MD
Frank J. Domino, MD

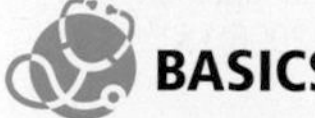

BASICS

DESCRIPTION

- A diffuse and nonpurulent infection of the skin and subcutaneous tissue. It initially affects the epidermis and dermis layers of the skin, and may subsequently spread within the superficial fascia.
- Several entities are recognized:
  - Cellulitis of the extremities
  - Recurrent cellulitis of the leg after saphenous vein removal
  - Dissecting cellulitis of the scalp
  - Facial cellulitis
  - Perianal cellulitis
  - *Pseudomonas* cellulitis
- System(s) affected: Skin/Exocrine

EPIDEMIOLOGY

- Cellulitis can affect any part of body, but commonly affects the extremities or head.
- Predominant age:
  - Perianal cellulitis: Principally in children
  - Facial cellulitis: In adults, usually <45 years; in children, <3 years
- Predominant sex: Male = Female (perianal cellulitis more common in boys)

Incidence

24.6 cases per 1,000 person-years

Prevalence

Unknown

RISK FACTORS

- Previous trauma (e.g., laceration, puncture, human or animal bite)
- Surgical procedures (saphenous vein removal, breast cancer axillary node dissection, or lymph node dissection for pelvic malignancy)
- Lower extremity lymphedema secondary to radical pelvic surgery, radiation therapy, chronic venous insufficiency
- Preexisting skin infections: Impetigo, ulceration, intertrigo, tinea pedis
- Immunocompromised patients, diabetics, IV drug users, cirrhotics, chronic renal disease, neutropenics

Geriatric Considerations

In cellulitis of lower extremities, older patients are more prone to develop thrombophlebitis.

GENERAL PREVENTION

- Avoid trauma, swimming with skin abrasions, and human or animal bites.
- Wear support stockings to decrease peripheral edema.
- Maintain good skin hygiene, especially with minor cuts.
- Maintain tight glycemic control and proper foot care for diabetics.

PATHOPHYSIOLOGY

Cellulitis is caused by bacterial penetration through a break in the skin integrity. Hyaluronidase mediates subcutaneous spread.

ETIOLOGY

- According to site (*S. aureus* most common overall):
  - Cellulitis of the extremities: Group A streptococcus, *Staphylococcus aureus*
  - Recurrent cellulitis of the leg: Non–group A β-hemolytic streptococci (groups C, G, and B)
  - Dissecting cellulitis of the scalp: *S. aureus*
  - Facial cellulitis in adults: *Haemophilus influenzae* type B
  - Facial cellulitis in children: *H. influenzae* type B, patients >3 years with portal of entry: Staphylococcal and streptococcal
  - Synergystic necrotizing cellulitis: Mixed aerobic-anaerobic flora
  - Intravenous drug use: MRSA, streptococci, Enterobacteriaceae, *Pseudomonas*, fungi
- Specific diseases:
  - Diabetes mellitus: *S. aureus*, streptococci, gram-negative bacilli, anaerobes
  - Human bites: *Eikenella corrodens*
  - Animal bites (e.g., cat, dog): *Pasteurella multocida, Capnocytophaga canimorsus*
- Patient groups:
  - Neonates: Group B streptococcus
  - Immunocompromised:
    - Bacteria (e.g., *Serratia*, *Proteus*, and other Enterobacteriaceae)
    - Fungi (e.g., *Cryptococcus neoformans*)
    - Atypical mycobacterium
  - Cirrhotics:
    - *Campylobacter fetus, Coliforms, Vibrio vulnificus*
  - Environmental and occupational exposures:
    - *Erysipelothrix rhusiopathiae* in patients handling fish, shellfish, meat, and poultry
    - *Vibrio* sp: Saltwater exposure
    - *Aeromonas hydrophila*: Freshwater exposure
    - *Pseudomonas aeruginosa:* Hot-tub exposure

COMMONLY ASSOCIATED CONDITIONS

- Facial cellulitis in children:
  - Upper respiratory tract infection
  - Unilateral or bilateral otitis media
  - Meningitis
- Perianal cellulitis:
  - Pharyngitis may precede infection.

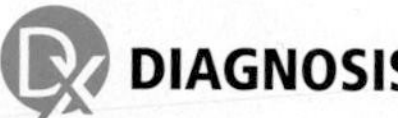

DIAGNOSIS

HISTORY

- Previous trauma, surgery, or animal/human bites
- High-risk comorbidities, trauma, surgery, bites

PHYSICAL EXAM

- Localized pain and tenderness (1)[A]
- Erythema
- Fever
- Chills
- Malaise
- Regional lymphadenopathy: Face, periorbital region, neck, or extremities
- Decreased visual activity and compromised extraocular movements
- Purulent drainage from burrowing interconnecting abscesses
- Itching
- Burning
- Irritability
- Intense perianal erythema or itching
- Pain on defecation
- Blood-streaked stools
- Area of local inflammation with redness, warmth, edema, tenderness, itchiness, poorly demarcated margins, regional lymphadenopathy.

DIAGNOSTIC TESTS & INTERPRETATION

Diagnosis based primarily on skin appearance and clinical setting, but laboratory, pathology, and imaging modalities can confirm diagnosis.

Lab

Initial lab tests

- Aspirates from point of maximum inflammation yield a 45% positive culture rate compared with a 5% rate from leading-edge culture; recommended in patients with systemic toxicity, immunocompromised, recurrent cellulitis, comorbidities, or special exposures (1)[B].
- Blood cultures: Potential pathogens isolated in <5% of patients. Better yield in patients with systemic symptoms (i.e., fever, tachycardia, hypotension, etc.). Blood cultures in children are more likely to show a contaminant than a true positive (2)[C].
- Mild leukocytosis with a left shift (1)[C]
- Mildly elevated erythrocyte sedimentation rate or C-reactive protein

Imaging

Initial approach

- Plain radiographs or computed tomography useful if a subjacent osteomyelitis, fracture, or early necrotizing fasciitis is suspected.
- Magnetic resonance imaging is helpful in differentiating cellulitis from necrotizing fasciitis.
- Ultrasonography is helpful in detecting subcutaneous accumulation of pus, and aids in guiding aspiration.
- Gallium^{67} scintillography is helpful for detecting cellulitis superimposed on recently increasing chronic lymphedema of a limb.

Diagnostic Procedures/Surgery

- Skin biopsy is not indicated in immunocompetent mild cellulitis.
- Lumbar puncture should be considered for all children with *H. influenzae* type B cellulitis or patients with meningeal signs associated with facial cellulitis.
- Gram stain of cellulitis aspirate may be useful for making preliminary microbial diagnosis to direct specific antibiotic therapy.

Pathological Findings

Biopsy of skin shows marked infiltration of the dermis with eosinophils and inflammatory changes.

DIFFERENTIAL DIAGNOSIS

- Toxic shock syndrome
- Bursitis
- Acute dermatitis
- Herpes zoster
- Deep vein thrombosis
- Insect stings
- Acute gout, pseudogout
- Necrotizing fasciitis or myositis
- Gas gangrene
- Deep venous thrombophlebitis
- Herpetic whitlow
- Osteomyelitis
- Cutaneous diphtheria
- Erythema chronicum migrans

C

TREATMENT

EDICATION

rst Line

- at 5–15 days or longer, depending on clinical sponse, and guided by culture results whenever ssible. Use IV therapy for rapidly spreading infection significant comorbidities:
- Empiric therapy or mild cellulitis infection (activity against β-hemolytic streptococci and methicillin-susceptible *S. aureus*): Oral dicloxacillin, cephalexin, clindamycin, or IV cefazolin, oxacillin, or nafcillin
- Parenteral therapy if severely ill or unable to tolerate oral therapy: Include penicillinase-resistant penicillins, a 1st-generation cephalosporin; if penicillin-allergic, use clindamycin or vancomycin
- Necrotizing fasciitis and gas gangrene: Use parenteral clindamycin and penicillin
- Recurrent infection underlying predisposing conditions, previous episode of proven methicillin-resistant *Staphylococcus aureus* (MRSA) infection, or systemic toxicity:
  - Use agents with activity against MRSA: Parenteral vancomycin or oral trimethoprim-sulfamethoxazole (TMP/SMX), doxycycline or minocycline, or clindamycin
- Mild early-suspected streptococcal etiology: Aqueous penicillin G, 600,000 U, then IM procaine penicillin at 600,000 U q8h–q12h.
- Freshwater exposure: Penicillinase-resistant: Penicillin plus gentamicin or fluoroquinolone
- Saltwater exposure: Doxycycline 200 mg IV in divided doses
- Human or animal bites: Oral amoxicillin-clavulanate or IV ampicillin-sulbactam or ertapenem in patients. If mildly allergic to penicillin, use cefoxitin or carbapenems. For severe penicillin reactions, use doxycycline, TMP/SMX, or a fluoroquinolone plus clindamycin.
- Facial cellulitis in adults and children (*H. influenza* B): Cefotaxime IV (1)[B]
- Diabetic foot infection: Ampicillin/sulbactam 3 g IV q6h or imipenem/cilastatin, or meropenem. Alternative: Combinations targeting anaerobes as well as gram-positive and gram-negative aerobes
- Severe infection, toxicity, immunocompromised patients, or worsening infection despite empirical therapy: Consider agents effective against MRSA (i.e., vancomycin, linezolid, tigecycline, quinupristin/dalfopristin, or daptomycin). Switch to oral dicloxacillin, cephradine, cephalexin, or cefadroxil when symptoms begin to resolve (3)[A].
- Recurrent streptococcal cellulitis: Penicillin IV 250 mg b.i.d., or if penicillin-allergic, use erythromycin 250 mg once or twice daily

ALERT

f community-acquired MRSA is a concern, reatment options (7–14 days) include:

- Trimethoprim/sulfamethoxazole: DS (160 mg TMP and 800 mg of SMX) 1–2 PO b.i.d. daily; doxycycline: 100 mg PO b.i.d., *or*
- Clindamycin: 300–600 mg PO t.i.d.

ediatric Considerations

- Review contraindications, including patient allergies to antibiotics as well as organ failure.
- Avoid doxycycline in children ≤8 years old and during pregnancy.
- Now that children are HIB-vaccinated, the most common predisposing conditions are conjunctivitis or an infected wound near the eye, rather than bacteremia (4)[A].

Second Line

Mild infection:

- Penicillin allergy: Erythromycin 500 mg PO q6h
- Cephalexin remains a cost-effective therapy for outpatient management of cellulitis at current estimated MRSA levels.

ADDITIONAL TREATMENT

General Measures

- Immobilization and elevation of the involved limb to reduce swelling
- Sterile saline dressings to decrease local pain
- Cool aluminum acetate compresses for pain relief
- Edema: Compression stocking, pneumatic pumps, and diuretic therapy
- Adjuvant corticosteroids (prednisone 0.5 mg/kg/d for 5–8 days) if partial response to parenteral antibiotics and hemorrhagic or bullous cellulitis
- Treat intertrigo with topical antifungals (miconazole, clotrimazole, or terbinafine).

Issues for Referral

Consider consulting Infectious Disease if patient is immunocompromised, not responding to treatment, or infection is severe.

SURGERY/OTHER PROCEDURES

- Debridement for gas and purulent matter collections
- Intubation or tracheotomy may be needed for cellulitis of the head or neck.

IN-PATIENT CONSIDERATIONS

Admission Criteria

- Severe infection, suspicion of deeper or rapidly spreading infection, tissue necrosis, or severe pain
- Marked systemic toxicity or worsening symptoms that do not resolve after 24–48 hours of therapy
- Patients with underlying risk factors or severe comorbidities

Nursing

- Ambulate patient in mild infection
- Bed rest in severe infection
- Elevate extremity to reduce swelling

ONGOING CARE

FOLLOW-UP RECOMMENDATIONS

Patient Monitoring

- Repeat needle aspirate culture.
- Repeat blood count if patient was toxic.
- Repeat lumbar puncture in case of meningitis.
- Consider prophylaxis of deep vein thrombosis.
- Symptomatic improvement usually occurs within 24–48 hours of therapy; however, visible improvement may take up to 72 hours.
- Cutaneous inflammation may worsen in first 24 hours due to inflammatory response from release of bacterial antigens.

PATIENT EDUCATION

- Practice good skin hygiene, especially with minor cuts.
- Report early skin changes to physician.

PROGNOSIS

With adequate antibiotic treatment, outlook is good.

COMPLICATIONS

- Bacteremia
- Local abscesses
- Superinfection with gram-negative organisms
- Lymphangitis, especially in recurrent cellulitis
- Thrombophlebitis or venous thrombosis of lower extremities in older patients
- Bacterial meningitis
- Gangrenous disorder

REFERENCES

1. Swartz MN. Clinical practice. Cellulitis. *N Engl J Med*. 2004;350:904–12.
2. Sadow KB, Chamberlain JM. Blood Cultures in the Evaluation of Children with Cellulitis. *Pediatrics*. 1998;101;e4.
3. Daum RS. Clinical practice. Skin and soft-tissue infections caused by methicillin-resistant Staphylococcus aureus. *N Engl J Med*. 2007;357: 380–90.
4. Rimon A, Hoffer V, Prais D, et al. Periorbital cellulitis in the era of Haemophilus influenzae type B vaccine: predisposing factors and etiologic agents in hospitalized children. *J Pediatr Ophthalmol Strabismus*. 2008;45:300–4.

ADDITIONAL READING

- Chira S, Miller LG et al. Staphylococcus aureus is the most common identified cause of cellulitis: a systematic review. *Epidemiol Infect*. 2010;138: 313–7.
- Wells RD, Mason P, Roarty J, et al. Comparison of initial antibiotic choice and treatment of cellulitis in the pre- and post-community-acquired methicillin resistant Staphylococcus aureus eras. *Am J Emerg Med*. 2009;27:436–9.

CODES

ICD9

- 682.0 Cellulitis and abscess of face
- 682.1 Cellulitis and abscess of neck
- 682.9 Cellulitis and abscess of unspecified sites

CLINICAL PEARLS

- Most common overall causes of cellulitis are *Staphylococcus aureus* and group A Streptococcus.
- Consider MRSA if cellulitis is not responding to antibiotics in the 1st 48 hours.
- Rapid expansion of infected area with red/purple discoloration and severe pain may suggest necrotizing fasciitis requiring urgent surgical evaluation.

CELLULITIS, ORBITAL

Congjun Yao, MD

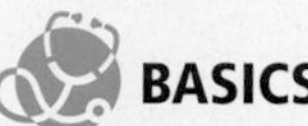

BASICS

DESCRIPTION
- Acute, spreading infection involving the fat and/or muscle within the bony orbit posterior to the orbital septum
- Synonym(s): Postseptal cellulitis

ALERT
Prompt diagnosis and intervention are critical, since delayed treatment can result in sustained or permanent vision loss, intracranial complications, and even death.

EPIDEMIOLOGY
- Occurs more commonly in the winter because of increased incidence of sinusitis (12)[C]
- No racial predilection or difference in frequency between the sexes in adults
- More common in children. Male > Female (2:1).
- The median age of children hospitalized with orbital cellulitis is 7–12 years.

RISK FACTORS
- Continuous sinusitis is the most common risk factor, accounting for up to 80–90% of cases (1,3)[C].
- Orbital trauma
- Dental or intracranial infection
- Retained orbital foreign body
- Preorbital or facial cellulitis
- Facial skin infection (i.e., impetigo, infected insect bite, acne, eczema)
- Acute dacryocystitis
- Acute dacryoadenitis
- Orbital mucopyocele
- Ophthalmologic surgery (for strabismus or detached retina, blepharoplasty, radial keratotomy, peribulbar anesthesia)

Genetics
No known genetic predisposition

GENERAL PREVENTION
- Appropriate treatment of bacterial sinusitis
- Proper postoperative wound care

PATHOPHYSIOLOGY
Orbital cellulitis often develops as a complication of acute sinusitis, as the sinuses are major components of the walls of the orbit.

ETIOLOGY
- Most common organisms (2,3)[C]:
  - *Staphylococcus aureus*
  - *Streptococcus pneumoniae*
- Less common organisms:
  - *Moraxella catarrhalis*
  - *Haemophilus influenza*
  - Nonspore–forming anaerobes
  - Group A β-hemolytic streptococcus
  - *Pseudomonas aeruginosa*
  - Fungal pathogens
  - *Mycobacterium tuberculosis*
  - *Mycobacterium avium* complex
- Since the introduction of routine vaccination in 1990, *Haemophilus influenzae* B is no longer a leading cause of orbital cellulitis (2,3)[B].

COMMONLY ASSOCIATED CONDITIONS
- More than 80% of orbital cellulitis cases result from contiguous sinusitis.
- Some cases are related to trauma, dental diseases, or hematogenous infection dissemination.

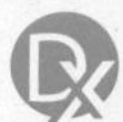

DIAGNOSIS

Chandler staging of orbital cellulitis is still widely used today (1,3)[C]:
- Stage I: Preorbital cellulitis (considered a different entity) (1,3)[B]
- Stage II: Edema of orbital lining, chemosis, proptosis, limitation of extraocular movement, fever
- Stage III: Include stage II with a subperiosteal abscess. Occasional vision loss.
- Stage IV: Orbital abscess. Ophthalmoplegia with visual loss.
- Stage V: Extension of the infection to the cavernous sinus, subdural space, meninges, or brain

HISTORY
- Malaise and fever
- Most patients with history of sinusitis, dental infection, or history of eye surgery or trauma
- Diffuse unilateral periorbital edema and erythema
- Chemosis (conjunctival swelling)
- Pain with eye movement
- Restricted extraocular mobility
- Diplopia
- Proptosis and globe displacement
- Blurred vision or loss of vision

ALERT
Ophthalmoplegia, mental status changes, contralateral cranial nerve palsy, or bilateral orbital cellulitis may herald intracranial involvement.

PHYSICAL EXAM
- Thorough inspection of the eye and surrounding structures
- Inspection of nasal vaults and sinus palpation for evidence of acute sinusitis
- Ocular motility testing
- Visual acuity testing

DIAGNOSTIC TESTS & INTERPRETATION

Lab
- Complete blood count with differential, C-reactive protein, and erythrocyte sedimentation rate
- Cultures can be obtained from sinus aspirates and abscesses.
- Cultures of eye secretions or nasopharyngeal aspirates are likely to be contaminated by normal flora, but may be helpful in identifying antibiotic-resistant organisms.
- Cultures from orbital and sinus abscesses are more likely to yield positive results, although these should be limited to cases where invasive procedures are clinically indicated.
- Blood cultures should be obtained prior to initiation of antibiotic therapy (more likely to be positive in children <5 years old) (3)[C].

Follow-Up & Special Considerations
A full septic evaluation, including lumbar puncture, should be considered before antibiotic administration in any toxic-appearing patient, or in the presence of any signs or symptoms suggestive of meningitis (3)[C].

Imaging
- Stage I: Preorbital cellulitis. Computed tomography (CT) scan normal.
- Stage II: CT scan shows no subperiosteal abscess. Might see mucosal edema or swelling.
- Stage III: CT scan shows subperiosteal abscess, globe displacement, and intraconal involvement of extraocular muscles.
- Stage IV: CT scan shows proptosis, abscess formation involving the extraocular muscles and orbital fat, and periosteal rupture (2,3,4)[C].

Initial approach
- Contrast CT is the most widely used modality for evaluating orbital cellulitis (5)[B]:
  - Consider CT imaging if concern for stage III or IV disease (5)[C]
  - Thin sections (2 mm) CT, coronal and axial views with bone windows
  - Differentiate preorbital from orbital cellulitis.
  - Confirm extension of inflammation into orbit, detect coexisting sinus disease, and identify orbital or subperiosteal abscesses.
  - Deviation of medial rectus on the affected side indicates intraorbital involvement.
- Magnetic resonance imaging offers superior resolution of soft tissue infections and is the modality of choice for identification of cavernous sinus thrombosis.
- Ultrasonography can be useful in ruling out orbital myositis, locating foreign bodies or abscesses, and following the progression of a drained abscess.

DIFFERENTIAL DIAGNOSIS
- Periorbital cellulitis:
  - Stage I orbital cellulitis in Chandler classification. Now it is mostly considered to be a different entity (1)[B].
  - Induration, erythema, warmth, and tenderness of the periorbital soft tissues
  - Extraocular motion is not affected and should be full.
  - Mostly caused by trauma (1)[C]
  - The inflammation does not extend into the bony orbit (1)[B].
- Idiopathic orbital inflammatory disease (3)[C]:
  - Usually no prodromal symptoms such as fever or malaise
- Atopic dermatitis
- Contact dermatitis
- Rosacea
- Trauma, including insect bites
- Conjunctivitis
- Blepharitis
- Hordeolum
- Herpes or varicella lesions
- Rapidly progressive tumors:
  - Rhabdomyosarcoma
  - Lymphoma
  - Leukemia
- Ruptured dermoid cyst

TREATMENT

Once diagnosed with orbital cellulitis, the patient should be admitted to a hospital for treatment and careful monitoring of ocular status.

Stage II: Intravenous antibiotics

Stage III: Intravenous antibiotics first; surgical intervention if no improvement within 24–48 hours of medical treatment or worsening signs discovered (impaired vision, complete ophthalmoplegia, or well-defined periosteal abscess)

Stage IV: Intravenous antibiotics and surgical drainage (2,4)[C]

MEDICATION

Empiric antibiotic therapy at all ages should provide coverage for pathogens associated with acute sinusitis (*S. pneumoniae*, *H. influenzae*, *M. catarrhalis*, *S. pyogenes*), as well as for *S. aureus* and anaerobes.

IV antibiotic treatment should be modified accordingly when microbiological sensitivities return. Duration of IV therapy is usually a week, based on clinical picture.

Oral antibiotic therapy should continue for 2–3 weeks. Longer duration (3–6 weeks) is recommended for patients with severe sinusitis and bony destruction.

First Line

Mainstay of therapy is broad-spectrum IV antibiotics: Ampicillin/sulbactam (Unasyn) or cefuroxime plus metronidazole or clindamycin if concurrent anaerobic infection is suspected (2)[C]:

- Ampicillin/sulbactam 1.5 to 3 g IV q6h for adult; 200-300 mg/kg/d divided q6h for children
- Cefuroxime 150 mg/kg/d divided q8h
- Clindamycin, 600–900 mg IV q8h for adults; 25–40 mg/kg/d IV q6–8h for children
- Metronidazole 30–35 mg/kg/d divided q8h

In severe, culture-proven methicillin-resistant *Staphylococcus aureus* infection, vancomycin remains parenteral drug of choice (2)[C]:

- Vancomycin 1g IV q12h for adults; 40 mg/kg/d IV divided q8–12h, max daily dose 2 g for children

Nafcillin or oxacillin plus cefotaxime or ceftriaxone can also be considered as initial IV treatment:

- Nafcillin or oxacillin 2 g IV q4h for adults; 200 mg/kg/d divided q6–8h for children, max daily dose 12 g

Second Line

f the patient is penicillin-allergic, clindamycin with a uoroquinolone (ciprofloxacin or levofloxacin) (>18 years only) may be used; or vancomycin and a uoroquinolone can be used. In children, consider lindamycin with cefazolin or clindamycin with ancomycin:

- Ceftriaxone 2 g IV q12h for adults; 80–100 mg/kg/g divided q12h for children, max daily dose 4 g
- Cefotaxime 2 g IV q4h for adults; 150–200 mg/kg/d divided q6–8h, max daily dose 12 g for children
- Ciprofloxacin or levofloxacin 500 mg q12h (>18 years only)

ADDITIONAL TREATMENT

Steroid use is still controversial. Short-term systemic steroid may be recommended for use in orbital cellulitis secondary to sinusitis (3)[C].

Issues for Referral

- Ophthalmology and otolaryngology should be consulted early when orbital cellulitis is suspected.
- Infectious disease consultation should be considered if available.
- Neurology or neurosurgery should be consulted if intracranial spread is suspected (3,4)[B].

SURGERY/OTHER PROCEDURES

- IV antibiotic therapy is still the best initial therapy. Surgical intervention is warranted when a patient has visual impairment, complete ophthalmoplegia, or well-defined large abscess (>10 mm) on presentation or no clinical improvement after 24 hours of antibiotic therapy.
- Treatment of choice for brain abscess is surgical excision or drainage with 4–8 weeks of antibiotics.
- Surgical interventions include external ethmoidectomy, endoscopic ethmoidectomy, uncinectomy, antrostomy, and subperiosteal drainage (1)[C].

IN-PATIENT CONSIDERATIONS

Patients with orbital cellulitis should be admitted for IV antibiotics and repeated eye examination to evaluate progression of infection or involvement of optic nerve (1,2,3)[A].

ONGOING CARE

FOLLOW-UP RECOMMENDATIONS

Patient Monitoring

- Visual acuity testing at least daily
- Pupillary light reflex monitored at least daily

ALERT

Close monitoring is indicated, as complications can develop rapidly.

PATIENT EDUCATION

- Maintain good skin hygiene.
- Avoid skin trauma.
- Promptly report periorbital swelling and/or erythema to health care professional.

COMPLICATIONS

- Complications can develop rapidly and include permanent vision loss, central nervous system involvement, and even death.
- Permanent vision loss:
  - Corneal opacification
  - Endophthalmitis
  - Septic uveitis or retinitis
  - Exudative retinal detachment
  - Globe rupture due to significantly increased intraocular pressure
  - Orbital compartment syndrome, compression of orbital soft tissues and optic nerve
  - Optic neuritis
  - Thrombophlebitis of ocular veins
  - Central retinal artery occlusion
  - Acute infarction of retina and choroids
- Central nervous system complications:
  - Intracranial abscess
  - Meningitis
  - Cavernous sinus thrombosis (2,3,4)[B]

REFERENCES

1. Botting AM, McIntosh D, Mahadevan M. Paediatric pre- and post-septal peri-orbital infections are different diseases A retrospective review of 262 cases. *Int J Pediatr Otorhinolaryngol*. 2008.
2. Hauser A, Fogarasi S et al. Periorbital and orbital cellulitis. *Pediatr Rev*. 2010;31:242–9.
3. Kloek CE, Rubin PA. Role of inflammation in orbital cellulitis. *Int Ophthalmol Clin*. 2006;46:57–68.
4. Brook I et al. Microbiology and antimicrobial treatment of orbital and intracranial complications of sinusitis in children and their management. *Int J Pediatr Otorhinolaryngol*. 2009;73:1183–6.
5. Rudloe TF, Harper MB, Prabhu SP, Rahbar R, Vanderveen D, Kimia AA et al. Acute periorbital infections: who needs emergent imaging? *Pediatrics*. 2010;125:e719–26.

ADDITIONAL READING

- Cannon PS, Mc Keag D, Radford R, Ataullah S, Leatherbarrow B et al. Our experience using primary oral antibiotics in the management of orbital cellulitis in a tertiary referral centre. *Eye (Lond)*. 2009;23:612–5.
- Ryan JT, Preciado DA, Bauman N, et al. Management of pediatric orbital cellulitis in patients with radiographic findings of subperiosteal abscess. *Otolaryngol Head Neck Surg*. 2009;140:907–11.
- Yang M, Quah BL, Seah LL, Looi A et al. Orbital cellulitis in children-medical treatment versus surgical management. *Orbit*. 2009;28:124–36.

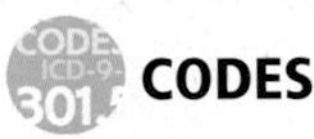

CODES

ICD9

376.01 Orbital cellulitis

CLINICAL PEARLS

- Most of orbital cellulitis cases result from contiguous sinusitis.
- Patients should be admitted to the hospital for monitoring and IV antibiotic treatment if orbital cellulitis is diagnosed.
- Ophthalmoplegia, mental status changes, contralateral cranial nerve palsy, or bilateral orbital cellulitis may herald intracranial involvement.
- Ophthalmology and otolaryngology should be consulted early when orbital cellulitis is suspected.

CELLULITIS, PERIORBITAL

Fozia A. Ali, MD

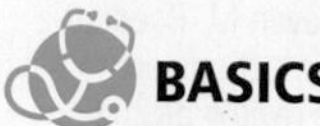

BASICS

DESCRIPTION

- An acute, spreading infection of the skin and subcutaneous tissue of the area surrounding the eye, usually secondary to external inoculation, but the inflammation does not extend into the bony orbit
- Synonym(s): Preseptal cellulitis

ALERT

It is important to distinguish periorbital cellulitis from orbital cellulitis (restricted extraocular mobility, diplopia, proptosis, and globe displacement vision loss), which is a potentially life-threatening condition.

EPIDEMIOLOGY

Occurs more commonly in children, with mean age 21 months

Incidence

Increased incidence in the winter months (due to increased number of cases of sinusitis)

RISK FACTORS

- Contiguous spread from upper respiratory infection
- Sinusitis
- Local skin trauma
- Insect bite
- Puncture wound
- Bacteremia

Genetics

No known genetic predisposition

GENERAL PREVENTION

- Avoid dermatologic trauma.
- Avoid swimming in fresh or salt water with skin abrasion.

PATHOPHYSIOLOGY

- An understanding of the anatomy of the eyelid is important in distinguishing preseptal from orbital cellulitis. The orbital septum is a sheet of connective tissue that extends from the orbital bones to the margins of the upper and lower eyelids, and it acts as a barrier to infection deep in the orbital structures. Infection of the tissues superficial to the orbital septum is called preseptal cellulitis, whereas infection deep in the orbital septum is termed orbital cellulitis.
- Periorbital cellulitis classically arises from a contiguous infection of soft tissues of the face, secondary to:
  - Sinusitis (via lamina papyracea)
  - Local trauma
  - Insect or animal bites
  - Foreign bodies

ETIOLOGY

- Common organisms:
  - *Streptococcus pneumoniae*
  - *Staphylococcus aureus*
  - *Streptococcus pyogenes*
- Atypical organisms:
  - *Acinetobacter sp.*
  - *Nocardia brasiliensis*
  - *Bacillus anthracis*
  - *Pseudomonas aeruginosa*
  - *Neisseria gonorrhoeae*
  - *Proteus sp.*
  - *Pasteurella multocida*
  - *Mycobacterium tuberculosis*
  - *Trichophyton sp.* (ringworm)
- Since the introduction of routine vaccination in 1990, *Haemophilus influenzae* B is no longer a leading cause of orbital cellulitis.

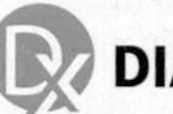

DIAGNOSIS

HISTORY

- Induration, erythema, warmth, and/or tenderness of periorbital soft tissues
- Chemosis (conjunctival swelling), proptosis, pain with extraocular eye movements
- Fever (although not necessary for diagnosis)

ALERT

Pain with eye movement and conjunctival swelling can occur, although both should raise the suspicion for orbital cellulitis.

PHYSICAL EXAM

- Thorough inspection of the eye and surrounding structures is key part in physical exam.
- Erythema, swelling, and tenderness of lids without orbital congestion. Violaceous discoloration of eyelid is more commonly associated with *Haemophilus influenza*.
- Also look for any break in skin if history of trauma causing periorbital cellulitis. Look for vesicle to rule out herpetic infection.
- Inspection of nasal vaults and sinus palpation for signs of acute sinusitis
- Ocular motility and visual acuity testing to rule out orbital cellulitis

DIAGNOSTIC TESTS & INTERPRETATION

Lab

- Complete blood count with differential
- Blood cultures

Follow-Up & Special Considerations

Children with periorbital or orbital cellulitis often have underlying sinusitis. If the child is febrile and appears toxic, blood cultures should be performed and lumbar puncture considered.

Imaging

If suspicious for orbital involvement, computed tomography (CT) scan can be used to evaluate the extent of infection and detect orbital inflammation or abscess (1)[B]. The classic sign of orbital cellulitis on CT scan is bulging of the medial rectus. CT should be performed with contrast, thin sections (2 mm), coronal and axial views with bone windows.

DIFFERENTIAL DIAGNOSIS

- Orbital cellulitis: Orbital cellulitis may have the same signs and symptoms in the periorbital tissue, but also results in proptosis, edema of the conjunctiva, ophthalmoplegia, or decreased visual acuity.
- Abscess
- Dacryocystitis
- Hordeolum
- Allergic inflammation
- Orbital or periorbital trauma
- Idiopathic orbital inflammatory syndrome
- Rapidly progressive tumors:
  - Rhabdomyosarcoma
  - Retinoblastoma
  - Lymphoma
- Leukemia

TREATMENT

MEDICATION

Empiric antibiotic treatment regimens are based on coverage of the most likely organisms, paying attention to local resistance patterns and the pathogens usually associated with sinusitis.

Uncomplicated post-traumatic:
- Usually due to skin flora, including *Staphylococcus* and *Streptococcus*
- Cephalexin, dicloxacillin, clindamycin

Extension from sinusitis:
- Amoxicillin, clavulanate, 3rd-generation cephalosporin

Bacteremic cellulitis:
- May be associated with meningitis
- Ceftriaxone plus vancomycin to cover methicillin-resistant *Staphylococcus aureus*

Duration of therapy should be 7–10 days:
- If symptoms do not improve within 24 hours, IV antibiotic therapy is indicated (2)[B].

ADDITIONAL TREATMENT

Issues for Referral

Although treatment may consist of intravenous antibiotics alone, management should be in consultation with otolaryngologists and ophthalmologists, especially when there is concern of orbital cellulitis.

SURGERY/OTHER PROCEDURES

Orbital surgery is indicated if the patient:
- Fails to respond
- No improvement by 24–48 hours
- Visual impairment
- Complete ophthalmoplegia
- Well-defined periosteal abscess (1,2)
- Deteriorates clinically despite treatment
- Has worsening visual acuity or pupillary changes
- Develops an abscess, except in selected pediatric cases of medial subperiosteal abscess, which may be successfully treated medically. Abscess formation necessitates incision and drainage.
- Endoscopic and transcaruncular surgery has been successfully employed to treat subperiosteal and intraorbital abscesses.

IN-PATIENT CONSIDERATIONS

- Mild cases in adults and children >1 year can be managed on an outpatient basis, provided the patient is stable and without systemic signs of toxicity.
- Preseptal cellulitis in children <4 years may warrant hospitalization and the use of intravenous antibiotics.

Admission Criteria

Consider hospitalization and IV antibiotics:
- For children <1 year
- Patients who have not been immunized for *S. pneumoniae* or *H. influenza*
- If no signs of clinical improvement are apparent after 24 hours of oral antibiotics

Discharge Criteria

- There are no strict guidelines to indicate when to switch therapy from parenteral to oral agents.
- Generally, we switch to oral therapy after the patient is afebrile and the skin findings have begun to resolve, which usually takes 3–5 days. Once we switch to oral therapy, it should be continued for 2–3 weeks. The longer duration is recommended for those patients with severe ethmoid sinusitis associated with bony destruction.

ONGOING CARE

FOLLOW-UP RECOMMENDATIONS

Patient Monitoring

The patient should be monitored for signs of orbital involvement, including decreased visual acuity or painful/limited ocular motility.

PATIENT EDUCATION

- Maintain good skin hygiene.
- Avoid skin trauma.
- Report early skin changes to health care professional.

PROGNOSIS

With adequate antibiotic treatment, outlook is good. Response to antibiotics in children with periorbital cellulitis usually is rapid, and a 10-day course of treatment generally is sufficient.

COMPLICATIONS

- Orbital cellulitis
- Abscess formation
- Scarring
- Delay in diagnosis and adequate treatment may result in serious complications, including blindness.

REFERENCES

1. Beech T, Robinson A, McDermott AL, et al. Paediatric periorbital cellulitis and its management. *Rhinology*. 2007;45:47–9.
2. Hennemann S, et al. Clinical inquiries. What is the best initial treatment for orbital cellulitis in children? *J Fam Prac*. 2007;56(8):662–4.
3. Georgakopoulos CD, Eliopoulou MI, Stasinos S, Exarchou A, Pharmakakis N, Varvarigou A et al. Periorbital and orbital cellulitis: a 10-year review of hospitalized children. *European journal of ophthalmology*. 2010.

ADDITIONAL READING

- *Br J Ophthalmol*. 2008;92:1337–41 doi:10.1136/bjo.2007.128975.
- Goldstein SM, Shelsta HN. Community-acquired Methicillin-resistant Staphylococcus aureus Periorbital Cellulitis: A Problem Here to Stay. *Ophthal Plast Reconstr Surg*. 2009;25:77.
- http://emedicine.medscape.com/article/798397-overview.

CODES

ICD9

682.0 Cellulitis and abscess of face

CLINICAL PEARLS

- Preseptal and orbital cellulitis occur most commonly in children.
- A multidisciplinary approach is needed in managing children with this condition, and CT scan of the patient's sinuses is essential to differentiate from orbital cellulitis.
- Early detection of periorbital cellulitis is important to prevent complications.
- The 2 most important factors for periorbital cellulitis are upper respiratory infection and eyelid trauma; sinusitis is more associated with orbital cellulitis (3)[C].

C

CEREBRAL PALSY

Jessica Hahn, MD
Beverly L. Nazarian, MD

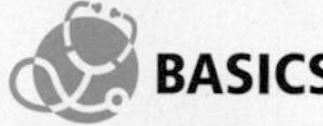

BASICS

DESCRIPTION

Cerebral palsy (CP): A group of chronic disorders of movement and posture caused by *nonprogressive* lesions in the developing brain. Some *activity limitation* must result from the motor impairment, and this motor dysfunction may be accompanied by impairment in other areas.

EPIDEMIOLOGY

Incidence

- Overall, 1.5–2.5 per 1,000 live births
- Incidence increases as gestational age (GA) at birth decreases (1):
  - 146/1,000 for GA of 22–27 weeks
  - 62/1,000 for GA of 28–31 weeks
  - 7/1,000 for GA of 32–36 weeks
  - 1/1,000 for GA of 37+ weeks

Prevalence

3–4/1,000 of the population

RISK FACTORS

- Prenatal:
  - Congenital anomalies
  - Multiple gestation
  - In utero stroke
  - Intrauterine infection (chorioamnionitis, TORCH)
  - Antepartum bleeding
  - Maternal factors (cognitive impairment, seizure disorders, hyperthyroidism)
  - Abnormal fetal position (e.g., breech)
- Perinatal:
  - Preterm birth
  - Low birth weight
  - Periventricular leukomalacia
  - Perinatal hypoxia/asphyxia
  - Intracranial hemorrhage/intraventricular hemorrhage
  - Neonatal seizure or stroke
  - Hyperbilirubinemia
- Postnatal:
  - Traumatic brain injury or stroke
  - Sepsis, meningitis, encephalitis
  - Asphyxia

Genetics

There are emerging reports of associations between cerebral palsy and candidate genes:

- Thrombophilic, cytokines, and apolipoprotein E

GENERAL PREVENTION

- Magnesium sulfate administration to mothers at risk for preterm delivery has a neuroprotective effect and reduces CP risk (2).
- Improved management of hyperbilirubinemia with decrease in kernicterus has greatly reduced dyskinetic CP.
- Prevention or reduction of chorioamnionitis and premature births (3)

PATHOPHYSIOLOGY

- Multifactorial; CP results from static injury or lesions in the developing brain, occurring prenatally, perinatally, or postnatally.
- Cytokines and free radicals and inflammatory response are likely contributing factors.

ETIOLOGY

- 50% of cases: Etiology is not established; most likely multifactorial.
- Spastic CP is most common, usually related to premature birth, with either periventricular leukomalacia or germinal matrix hemorrhage.
- Dyskinetic CP, often resulting from kernicterus, is now rare due to improved management of hyperbilirubinemia.

COMMONLY ASSOCIATED CONDITIONS

- Seizure disorder (22–40%)
- Cognitive impairment (23–44%)
- Behavior difficulties
- Speech and language disorders (42–81%)
- Sensory impairments:
  - Hearing deficits
  - Visual (62–71%):
    - Poor visual acuity, strabismus (50%), or hemianopsia
- Feeding impairment, swallowing dysfunction, and aspiration
- Poor dentition, excessive drooling
- Gastrointestinal conditions:
  - Constipation (59%), vomiting (22%), or gastroesophageal reflux
- Decreased linear growth or osteopenia
- Weight abnormalities (under- and overweight)
- Bowel and bladder incontinence
- Orthopedic: Contractures, hip subluxation/dislocation, or scoliosis

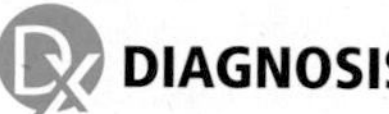

DIAGNOSIS

- A clinical diagnosis including:
  - Delayed motor milestones
  - Abnormal tone
  - Abnormal neurological exam suggesting a cerebral etiology
  - Absence of regression
  - Absence of underlying syndromes or alternative explanation for etiology
- Although the pathological lesion is static, clinical presentation may change as the infant grows and matures.
- Accurate early diagnosis remains difficult. Neurologic abnormalities observed in the first 1–2 years of life may resolve. Caution against diagnosis of CP before age 2.

HISTORY

- Presentation: Parental concerns over movements or motor development
- Ask about:
  - Prenatal, perinatal, and postnatal risk factors
  - Neurobehavioral signs:
    - Poor feeding/frequent vomiting
    - Irritability
  - Timing of motor milestones:
    - Delay in milestones is not sensitive or specific until after 6 months of age.
  - Abnormal spontaneous general movements
  - Asymmetry of movements, such as early hand preference
  - Symptoms of other conditions
- Regression of motor skills *does not* occur with cerebral palsy.

PHYSICAL EXAM

- Assess for 1 or more type of neurological impairment:
  - Spasticity: Increased tone/reflexes/clonus
  - Dyskinesia: Abnormal movements
  - Hypotonia: Decreased tone
  - Ataxia: Abnormal balance/coordination
- Areas of exam:
  - Tone: May be increased or decreased.
  - Trunk and head control: Often poor, but may be advanced due to high tone
  - Persistence of primitive reflexes
  - Asymmetry of movement or reflexes
  - Brisk DTRs
  - Clonus
  - Delayed motor milestones:
    - Serial exams most effective
  - Gait and stance:
    - Scissoring gait
    - Toe-walking
- Specific subtypes best diagnosed after 5 years of age:
  - Spastic hemiplegic CP:
    - Unilateral spasticity
  - Spastic diplegic CP:
    - Bilateral spasticity with leg > arm involvement
  - Spastic quadriplegic CP:
    - Bilateral spasticity with arm > or = leg involvement
  - Dyskinetic CP:
    - Dystonia-hypertonia and reduced movement
    - Choreoathetosis: Irregular spasmodic involuntary movements of the limbs or facial muscles
  - Ataxic CP:
    - Loss of orderly muscular coordination
  - Mixed

DIAGNOSTIC TESTS & INTERPRETATION

Cerebral palsy is a clinical diagnosis based on history, physical, and risk factors. Diagnostic tests rule out other conditions.

Lab

- Laboratory testing is not needed to make diagnosis, but can sometimes help to exclude other etiologies.
- Testing for metabolic and genetic syndromes (4):
  - Not routinely obtained in the evaluation for CP
  - If no specific etiology is identified by neuroimaging, or if there are atypical features in clinical presentation, genetic or metabolic testing may be useful.
  - Detection of certain brain malformations may warrant genetic or metabolic testing to identify syndromes.
- Screening for coagulopathies:
  - Diagnostic testing for coagulopathies should be considered in children with hemiplegic CP with cerebral infarction identified on neuroimaging (4)[C].

Imaging

- Neuroimaging is not essential, but recommended in children with CP for whom the etiology has not been established (4)[C].

Magnetic resonance imaging (MRI) is preferred to computed tomography (CT) scanning (4)[C].

Abnormalities in 80–90% of patients (5)[A]:
– Brain malformation, cerebral infarction, intraventricular or other intracranial hemorrhage, periventricular leukomalacia, ventricular enlargement, or other cerebrospinal fluid (CSF) space abnormalities

Diagnostic Procedures/Surgery

Assessing the functional impact of cerebral palsy can help to determine appropriate services and prognosis:
– The Gross Motor Function Classification System is commonly used
– A score of II or higher is considered significant. A score of IV or V indicates more severe involvement.

Screening for comorbid conditions: Developmental delay/cognitive impairment, basion/hearing impairments, speech and language disorders, or feeding/swallowing dysfunction

Pathological Findings

Perinatal brain injury may include:

White matter damage:
– Most common in premature infants
– Periventricular leukomalacia:
  ○ Gliosis with or without focal necrosis with resulting cysts and scarring
  ○ May be multiple lesions of various ages
  ○ Necrosis can lead to cysts/scarring.
– Germinal matrix hemorrhage:
  ○ May lead to intraventricular hemorrhage

Grey matter damage:
– More common in term infants
– Cortical infarcts, focal neuronal damage, myelination abnormalities

DIFFERENTIAL DIAGNOSIS

Benign congenital hypotonia, Brachial plexus injury, Familial spastic paraplegia, Dopa-responsive dystonia, Transient toe-walking, Muscular dystrophy, Metabolic disorders (e.g., glutaric aciduria type 1), Mitochondrial disorders, Genetic disorders (e.g., Rett syndrome)

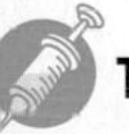

TREATMENT

Focuses on control of symptoms: Spasticity, management of comorbid conditions, improvement in functioning, and quality of life

MEDICATION

First Line

• Baclofen (6)[C]:
  – γ-aminobutyric acid B ($GABA_B$) agonist, facilitates presynaptic inhibition of mono- and polysynaptic reflexes
  – Adults: Initial dose is 5 mg t.i.d. and increase dosage every 3 days to an average maintenance dose of 20 mg t.i.d. 80 mg/24-hr maximum
  – Pediatric dose (>2 y/o): Initial 10–15 mg/24 hrs. Titrate to effective dose. <8 y/o = 40 mg/24 hrs. maximum. >8 y/o 60 mg/24 hrs. maximum
• Intrathecal Baclofen (Baclofen Pump):
  – Continuous intrathecal route allows greater maximal response with smaller dosage
  – Significantly reduces spasticity in children with cerebral palsy
  – Multiple adverse effects due to catheter placement and medication side effects
• Diazepam (6)[C]:
  – A $GABA_A$ agonist, facilitating CNS inhibition at spinal and supraspinal levels to reduce spasticity
  – Adult dose: 2–12 mg/dose p.o. q6–12 hrs.
  – Pediatric dose (<12 yrs): 0.12–0.8 mg/kg/24 h. p.o., divided q6–8h.
• Botulinum toxin type A:
  – Injected directly into muscles of interest
  – Acts at neuromuscular junction to inhibit the release of acetylcholine
  – Chemically denervates muscles, reducing tone
  – Lasts for 12–16 weeks following injection

Second Line

The following medications are used far less frequently:
• Dantrolene:
  – Limits calcium release from muscles, reducing spasticity
  – Adult dosing: 25 mg p.o. daily titrated to effective dose, maximum 100 mg p.o. q.i.d.
  – Pediatric dosing: 0.5 mg/kg p.o. daily titrated to effective dose, maximum 12 mg/kg/24 hrs.
• Tizanidine and other α-adrenergic agents:
  – α-adrenergic agonist, presynaptically inhibits motor activation, reducing spasticity
  – Adult dosing: 4 mg/day p.o., titrate to effective dose, up to 8 mg p.o. q4–6h, 36 mg/24 hrs. maximum
• Gabapentin:
  – Anticonvulsant structurally similar to GABA, increases levels of GABA in brain and reduces spasticity
  – Adult dosing: Titrate to starting dose 100 mg t.i.d. starting dosage, maximum dose 3600 mg/day in divided dosing

ADDITIONAL TREATMENT

• Care needs to be multidisciplinary, usually including specialists from orthopedics, neurology, ophthalmology, and physiatry, as well as physical, occupational, and speech therapists.
• "Medical home" with PCP (7) which requires:
  – Identification of patient's and family's needs for support, respite, and community resources
  – Care coordination among medical providers and with community agencies
  – Collaboration with schools and transition to adult care

General Measures

• Referral to early intervention for children ages 0–3 is essential.
• Various therapy modalities enhance functioning:
  – Physical therapy: Posture stability and gait, motor strength and control, contracture prevention
  – Occupational therapy: Functional activities of daily living and other fine motor skills
  – Speech therapy: Verbal and nonverbal speech and aid in feeding
• Equipment optimizes participation in activities:
  – Orthotic splinting: Maintains functional positioning and prevents contractures
    ○ AFOs (ankle-foot orthosis)
    ○ DAFOs (dynamic ankle-foot orthosis)
  – Spinal bracing (body jacket) may slow scoliosis.
  – Augmentative communication: Pictures, switches, or computer systems for nonverbal individuals
  – Electrical stimulation: Therapeutic and functional
  – Use of adaptive equipment such as standers to allow weight bearing
  – Mobility: Crutches, walkers, wheelchairs

COMPLEMENTARY AND ALTERNATIVE MEDICINE

• Hyperbaric oxygen: Conflicting results
• Hippotherapy: Therapeutic horse riding
• Aquatic therapy

SURGERY/OTHER PROCEDURES

• Dorsal root rhizotomy: Selectively cutting dorsal rootlets from L1–S2:
  – Best for patients with normal intelligence with spastic diplegia
  – Minimizes spasticity in lower limbs, but associated with adverse effects
• Surgical treatment of joint dislocations/subluxation, scoliosis management, tendon lengthening, etc.

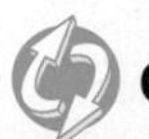

ONGOING CARE

PROGNOSIS

Reduced lifespan only in most severely affected.

REFERENCES

1. Himpens E, Van den Broeck C, Oostra A et al. Prevalence, type, distribution, and severity of cerebral palsy in relation to gestational age: a meta-analytic review. *Dev Med Child Neurol*. 2008;50:334–40.
2. Doyle LW, Crowther CA, Middleton P, et al. Magnesium sulphate for women at risk of preterm birth for neuroprotection of the fetus. *Cochrane Database Syst Rev*. 2009:CD004661.
3. Shatrov JG, Birch SC, Lam LT et al. Chorloamnionitis and cerebral palsy: a meta-analysis. *Obstet Gynecol*. 2010;116:387–92.
4. Ashwal S, Russman BS, Blasco PA et al., Practice parameter: diagnostic assessment of the child with cerebral palsy: report of the Quality Standards Subcommittee of the American Academy of Neurology and the Practice Committee of the Child Neurology Society. *Neurology*. 2004; 62:851–63.
5. Korzeniewski SJ, Birbeck G, Delano MC et al., A systematic review of neuroimaging for cerebral palsy. *J Child Neurol*. 2008;23:216–27.
6. Montané E, Vallano A, Laporte JR. Oral antispastic drugs in nonprogressive neurologic diseases: a systematic review. *Neurology*. 2004;63:1357–63.
7. Cooley WC, American Academy of Pediatrics Committee on Children With Disabilities. Providing a primary care medical home for children and youth with cerebral palsy. *Pediatrics*. 2004;114:1106–13.

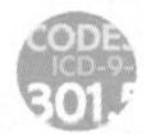

CODES

ICD9

• 343.0 Congenital diplegia
• 343.1 Congenital hemiplegia
• 343.2 Congenital quadriplegia

CLINICAL PEARLS

• Management should focus on maximizing functioning and quality of life with multidisciplinary team approach.
• Regression of motor skills *does not* occur with cerebral palsy.

CERVICAL HYPEREXTENSION INJURIES

Francesca L. Beaudoin, MS, MD
Stephanie Carreiro, MD

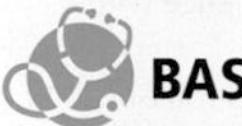

BASICS

DESCRIPTION

- Group of injuries involving the neck that result from a rapid, forceful, backwards motion
- May involve:
  - Injury to vertebral and paravertebral structures: Fractures, dislocations, ligamentous tears, and disc disruption/subluxation
  - Spinal cord injury: Traumatic central cord syndrome (CCS) secondary to cord compression or vascular insult
  - Vascular injury: Vertebral artery or carotid artery dissection
  - Soft tissue injury around cervical spine: Cervical strain/sprain
- System(s) affected: Musculoskeletal; Nervous; Vascular
- Synonym(s): Cervical acceleration-deceleration injury

EPIDEMIOLOGY

- Predominant age: Trauma and sports injuries more common in young adults (average age 29.4 years); however, CCS mostly seen in older population (average age 53 years)
- Predominant sex: Male > Female
- 25% spinal injuries caused by hyperextension

Incidence

In the US:

- Cervical fractures: 2–5/100 blunt trauma patients
- Central cord syndrome: 3.6/100,000 people/year
- Cervical artery dissection: 3 /100,000 people/year
- Cervical strain: 3 /1,000 people/year

RISK FACTORS

- Pre-existing spinal stenosis is present in >50% of cases of CCS, which may be:
  - Acquired: Prior trauma, spondylosis
  - Congenital: Klippel-Feil syndrome (congenital fusion of any 2 cervical vertebra) with cervical stenosis
- Conditions predisposing to spinal rigidity, such as ankylosing spondylitis, increase risk of vertebral fractures.

GENERAL PREVENTION

Wear seat belts and use proper safety equipment in sports activities.

ETIOLOGY

Trauma due to motor vehicle accidents, sports injuries, falls, and assaults.

COMMONLY ASSOCIATED CONDITIONS

Closed head injuries (concussion, cerebral contusions, intracranial bleeding), facial fractures, thoracic/lumbar spinal injury

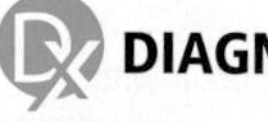

DIAGNOSIS

HISTORY

Usually acute presentation with mechanism of cervical hyperextension (see Etiology) and complaints of neck pain, stiffness or headaches, +/− neurologic symptoms

PHYSICAL EXAM

- External signs of trauma on the head and neck such as abrasions, lacerations, hematomas, or contusions
- Presence, severity, and location of neck tenderness:
  - Posterior midline, bony point tenderness concerning for bony injury
  - Paraspinal or lateral soft tissue tenderness suggestive of muscular/ligamentous injury.
  - Anterior tenderness concerning for carotid injury
- Range-of-motion (ROM) limitation
- Neurologic exam: Paresthesias/numbness, weakness
- CCS:
  - Typical symptom distribution: Distal > proximal, upper extremity > lower extremity
  - Extremity weakness/paralysis
  - Variable sensory changes below level of lesion (including paresthesias and dysesthesia)
  - Bladder/bowel dysfunction

DIAGNOSTIC TESTS & INTERPRETATION

Imaging

Initial approach

- Low-risk patients can be cleared clinically (without radiographic evaluation) using either the Canadian C-Spine Rule (CCR) or the National Emergency X-ray Utilization Study (NEXUS) Criteria:
  - CCR: Clinically clear a stable, adult patient with no history of cervical spine disease/surgery if all of the following conditions are met:
    - GCS = 15
    - Nonintoxicated patients without a distracting injury
    - No dangerous mechanism or extremity paresthesias
    - At least 1 "low-risk factor" (i.e., simple rear-end MVA, ambulation at the accident scene, no midline cervical tenderness, delayed onset of neck pain or sitting position at the time of exam)
  - NEXUS: Clinically clear if all of the following are met:
    - No alteration of mental status or intoxication
    - No focal neurodeficits
    - No distracting injury
    - No posterior, midline c-spine tenderness
  - Reported sensitivity/specificity: CCR (99.4%/45.1%), NEXUS (90.7%/36.8%) (1)[A]
- If imaging is required, choose from the following options based on the suspected injury and level of clinical suspicion:
  - Plain radiographs: Recommended by some in patients who cannot be cleared clinically but still are in low-suspicion category: Sensitivity for c-spine injury as low as 52% (2)[B]:
    - Static: Lateral, anterior-posterior (A-P) and odontoid views; in addition to bony abnormalities, may show prevertebral soft tissue swelling
    - Dynamic: Flexion/extension, only if asymptomatic and no neurologic deficits or mental impairment. Evaluates spine stability and union by amount of movement in fractures during or after treatment. Of limited utility in the acute setting given that technically adequate films are difficult to obtain in patients with restricted ROM (3)[C].
  - CT: Axial CT from occiput to T1 with coronal and sagittal reconstructions: Rapidly replacing plain radiography as the test of choice for cases with moderate to high clinical suspicion of c-spine injury given high sensitivity (95–99%) (2,4)[B]
  - MRI: Diagnostic test of choice in CCS with direct visualization of traumatic cord lesions (edema or hematomyelia), soft tissue compressing cord, and/or stenosis of canal. Also detects ligamentous injury and abnormalities of intervertebral discs and soft tissues, but modality is poor with fractures and is prone to false-positive results due to nonspecific findings.
  - CTA/MRA: Visualization of cervical and cerebral vascular structures to detect carotid or vertebral artery dissections

Follow-Up & Special Considerations

Cervical strain: May repeat flexion/extension lateral cervical spine views to confirm stability once muscula spasms have resolved

Pathological Findings

- Vertebral fractures: See General Measures.
- CCS: Currently thought to be due to axonal disruption within the white matter of the lateral column, particularly the corticospinal tracts
- Vascular dissection: Intimal disruption, leading to thrombosis and embolization
- Models of acute cervical strain/sprain based on animal, cadaver, and postmortem studies show myofascial tearing, edema, and inflammation; facet joint capsular pain may also play a role.
- Stretching or rupture of spinal ligaments
- Injuries to intervertebral discs

DIFFERENTIAL DIAGNOSIS

- Acute or chronic disc pathology (including herniation or internal disruption)
- Osteoarthritis
- Cervical radiculopathy
- For CCS:
  - Bell cruciate palsy
  - Bilateral brachial plexus injuries
  - Carotid or vertebral artery dissection

Geriatric Considerations

- Degenerative disease of c-spine may be confused with acute traumatic change on imaging; CT imaging more helpful to distinguish the 2
- Osteoporosis increases risk of fracture.

Pediatric Considerations

Consider SCI without radiographic abnormality, which has a high incidence at <9 years and accounts for up to 50% of all pediatric cervical spine injuries. MRI may help detect the injury.

TREATMENT

MEDICATION

- CCS: Methylprednisolone IV 30 mg/kg over 15 minutes, then 45 minutes later; start continuous infusion by IV 5.4 mg/kg/h for 24 hours. Further improvement in motor function recovery may be seen if infusion is given for 48 hours, especially if bolus dose is given 3–8 hours after injury (5)[A].
- Carotid/vertebral dissection: Anticoagulation with IV heparin, followed by warfarin therapy for 3–6 months, then long term antiplatelet therapy is currently recommended. However, an antiplatelet agent is recommended as the sole initial therapy in patients with contraindications to anticoagulation.

Cervical strain: Muscle relaxants, acetaminophen/nonsteroidal anti-inflammatory agents +/– opiate analgesics are commonly used

ADDITIONAL TREATMENT

General Measures

Fractures:
- Stability determined by imaging; decompression and stabilization are indicated in:
  - Incomplete SCIs with spinal canal compromise
  - Clinical deterioration or failure to improve despite conservative management
- Hangman fracture: Traumatic spondylolisthesis of C2 (the "axis") with bilateral fractures through C2 pedicles, often with anterior subluxation of C2 over C3: Can be unstable:
  - Managed with halo vest immobilization for 12 weeks until repeated flexion/extension films normalize
  - Unstable if C2 subluxation over C3; >50% of vertebral body of C3 in anteroposterior diameter, or if excessive angulation of C2 over C3
- Odontoid fracture: Treated according to type:
  - I: Through apex; usually stable; external immobilization with a cervical collar or halo vest for up to 12 weeks
  - II: Most common, at base of dens, usually unstable; nonunion rates of up to 67% with halo immobilization alone, especially with dens displacement >6 mm or age >50 years
  - III: Through C2 body, usually stable; initially immobilized in halo or cervical collar for 12–20 weeks (6)[B]
- Hyperextension teardrop fractures:
  - If stable, rigid collar or cervicothoracic brace for 8–14 weeks
  - If unstable, halo brace for up to 3 months

CCS: Neck immobilization with cervical collar, PT/OT

Cervical strain: Treatment depends on severity:
- No evidence that immobilization is beneficial; may use soft cervical collar for up to 10 days for symptomatic relief; otherwise, early mobilization and activity as tolerated

Issues for Referral

When cervical spine injury is suspected, the patient should be immobilized and sent to the emergency department for evaluation.

Emergent consultation from a spinal surgeon (neurosurgery and/or orthopedics) is indicated if there is any concern for unstable fracture or spinal cord injury.

COMPLEMENTARY AND ALTERNATIVE MEDICINE

Acupuncture for chronic neck pain resulting from cervical strain

SURGERY/OTHER PROCEDURES

Hangman's fracture: Consider surgical fixation in cases of excessive angulation or subluxation, disruption of intervertebral disc space or failure to obtain alignment with external orthosis (6)[B].

Odontoid fractures:
- Type II: Early surgical stabilization recommended in setting of age >50 years old, dens displacement >5 mm and in certain fracture patterns
- Type III: Surgical intervention often reserved for cases of nonunion/malunion after trial of external immobilization

- Hyperextension teardrop fractures: Consider surgical repair if unstable with neurologic deficit
- CCS:
  - If occurs in setting of unstable injury and/or herniated disc, surgical decompression/fixation is indicated
  - Otherwise, surgery considered when neurologic function plateaus or deteriorates (7)[B]

IN-PATIENT CONSIDERATIONS

Initial Stabilization

Advanced Trauma Life Support (ATLS) protocol with backboard and collar

Admission Criteria

Varies by injury; clinical judgment, radiographic findings, and need for operative intervention influence decision

ONGOING CARE

FOLLOW-UP RECOMMENDATIONS

Follow-up depends on the severity of injury, but all patients with hyperextension injuries should receive follow-up care.

Patient Monitoring

Patients with known injuries will often be followed with serial radiographs under the care of a specialist.

PATIENT EDUCATION

For patient instruction on prevention: THINK FIRST Foundation at: http://www.thinkfirst.org.

PROGNOSIS

- Overall, the most important prognostic factor is the initial neurologic status.
- Fracture dislocation:
  - Hangman fracture: 93–100% fusion rate after 8–14 weeks external immobilization
  - Odontoid fracture, fusion rate by type: Type I approximately 100% with external immobilization alone; Type III, 85% with external immobilization, 100% with surgical fixation (6)
- CCS:
  - Spontaneous recovery of motor function in >50% of cases over several weeks
  - Younger patients (<50 years old) are more likely to regain function.
  - Leg, bowel, and bladder functions return first; upper extremities follow, but recovery is often incomplete, especially manual dexterity (7)
- Cervical strain: 50% of patients continue to have neck pain at 1 year:
  - Greater initial disability, symptom severity, and psychological factors also predict slower recovery.
  - Prognostic factors for development of late whiplash syndrome (>6 months of symptoms affecting normal activity) include increased initial pain intensity, pain-related disability, and cold hyperalgesia.

COMPLICATIONS

- Nonunion/malunion of fractures
- Persistent instability requiring 2nd procedure
- Reactions and infection related to orthosis
- Embolic ischemic events and pseudoaneurysm formation after vascular dissection
- Persistent symptoms and pain/late whiplash syndrome

REFERENCES

1. Stiell IG, Clement CM, McKnight RD, Brison R, Schull MJ, Rowe BH, Worthington JR, Eisenhauer MA, Cass D, Greenberg G, MacPhail I, Dreyer J, Lee JS, Bandiera G, Reardon M, Holroyd B, Lesiuk H, Wells GA et al. The Canadian C-spine rule versus the NEXUS low-risk criteria in patients with trauma. *N Engl J Med*. 2003;349:2510–8.
2. Holmes JF, Akkinepalli R et al. Computed tomography versus plain radiography to screen for cervical spine injury: a meta-analysis. *J Trauma*. 2005;58:902–5.
3. Insko EK, Gracias VH, Gupta R, Goettler CE, Gaieski DF, Dalinka MK et al. Utility of flexion and extension radiographs of the cervical spine in the acute evaluation of blunt trauma. *J Trauma*. 2002;53:426–9.
4. Como JJ, Diaz JJ, Dunham CM, Chiu WC, Duane TM, Capella JM, Holevar MR, Khwaja KA, Mayglothling JA, Shapiro MB, Winston ES et al. Practice management guidelines for identification of cervical spine injuries following trauma: update from the eastern association for the surgery of trauma practice management guidelines committee. *J Trauma*. 2009;67:651–9.
5. Bracken MB. Steroids for acute spinal cord injury. Cochrane injuries group. *Cochrane Database Syst Rev*. 2008;3.
6. Pryputniewicz DM, Hadley MN et al. Axis fractures. *Neurosurgery*. 2010;66:68–82.
7. Aarabi B, Koltz M, Ibrahimi D et al. Hyperextension cervical spine injuries and traumatic central cord syndrome. *Neurosurg Focus*. 2008;25:E9.

See Also (Topic, Algorithm, Electronic Media Element)

Cervical Spinal Injury

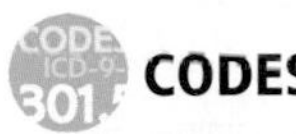

CODES

ICD9

- 847.0 Neck sprain
- 952.00 C1-c4 level spinal cord injury, unspecified
- 952.03 C1-c4 level with central cord syndrome

CLINICAL PEARLS

- Suspect SCI until exam and imaging suggest otherwise.
- Follow NEXUS or Canadian Cervical Spine rules on every patient with potential neck injury to determine imaging needs, but use clinical judgement!
- Inquire about preexisting cervical spine injuries or conditions, especially in the elderly, as they may increase risk of injury or alter radiographic interpretation.
- Consider vascular dissection when neurologic deficits are inconsistent with level of known injury.

CERVICAL MALIGNANCY

Amos O. Adelowo, MD, MPH
Antonella M. Leary, MD

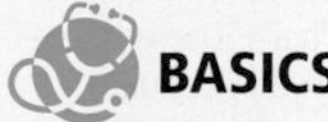

BASICS

DESCRIPTION
- Invasive cancer of the uterine cervix
- Commonly involves the vagina, parametria, and pelvic side walls
- Invasion of bladder, rectum, and other pelvic sites in advanced disease
- Disease prognosis differs with tumor stage.

EPIDEMIOLOGY
Incidence
- Worldwide, cervical cancer ranks 2nd among all malignancies for women (1).
- Higher incidence of cervical cancer in developing countries, contributing up to 83% of reported cases annually
- In the US, it is the 3rd most common gynecologic cancer and the 6th most common solid malignant neoplasm among women.
- Median age at diagnosis is bimodal: 35–50 years and >65 years

Prevalence
- In 2007, the American Cancer Society (ACS) estimated 11,150 new cases with 3,670 deaths from the malignancy.
- In 2008, the number of new cases decreased to 11,070 and the number of deaths increased to 3,870.
- African Americans and women in lower socioeconomic groups have the highest age-standardized cervical cancer death rates.
- Hispanic and Latino women have the highest incidence rate of the malignancy.

RISK FACTORS
- Strong association with sexually transmitted HPV infection
- Other risk factors include:
  - Early coitarche
  - Multiple sexual partners
  - Unprotected sex
  - A history of STDs
  - Nonbarrier methods of birth control
  - Low socioeconomic status
  - High parity
  - Cigarette smoking
  - Immunosuppression
  - DES exposure in utero
  - Lack of regular Pap smears

Genetics
Not an inherited disease

GENERAL PREVENTION
- Patient education regarding safer sex, condom use, decreasing number of sexual partners (2)[A]
- Smoking cessation
- Gardasil vaccine (3): Quadrivalent vaccine containing proteins from HPV strains 6, 11, 16, and 18. Recommended age of vaccination is 11–12 years, but can be given from age 9–26:
  - Vaccine is a series of 3 IM injections, with the 2nd and 3rd following 3 and 6 months after the 1st (4)[B].
- Regular screening: Pap smears and pelvic exams at appropriate intervals according to American College of Obstetricians and Gynecologists and the American Cancer Society
- Despite HPV vaccination, cervical cancer screening will remain the main preventive measure for both vaccinated and nonvaccinated women, but the nature of screening and management of women with cervical disease is being adapted to the new technologies (5).

PATHOPHYSIOLOGY
- Arise from preexisting dysplastic lesions usually following HPV infection
- Pattern of local growth may be exophytic or endophytic.
- Lymphatic spread typically through cervical lymphatic drainage
- Local tumor extension involving the bladder, ureters, rectum, and distant metastasis from hematogenous spread

ETIOLOGY
- Epidemiologic and experimental evidence supports oncogenic strains of HPV 16 and 18 as etiologic agents in cervical carcinogenesis.
- Association with the E6 and E7 oncogenic proteins responsible for malignant cell transformation by inactivation of the p53 and Rb tumor suppressor genes
- Slow progression from dysplasia to invasive cancer

COMMONLY ASSOCIATED CONDITIONS
- Condyloma acuminata
- Preinvasive/invasive lesions of the vulva and vagina

DIAGNOSIS

HISTORY
- May be asymptomatic
- Most common symptom is vaginal bleeding, often postcoital.
- Other gynecological symptoms include intermenstrual or postmenopausal bleeding and vaginal discharge.
- Other less common symptoms include low back pain with radiation down posterior leg, lower extremity edema, vesicovaginal and rectovaginal fistula, and urinary symptoms.

PHYSICAL EXAM
- Most patients have a normal physical exam.
- Thorough external genitalia and internal vaginal exam is needed to look for lesions:
  - Cervix may appear grossly normal with microinvasive disease.
  - Lesions may be exophytic, endophytic, polypoid, papillary, ulcerative, or necrotic.
  - Watery, purulent, or bloody discharge.
- Bimanual and rectovaginal examination for uterine size, vaginal wall, rectovaginal septum, parametrial, uterosacral, and pelvic sidewall involvement.
- Enlarged supraclavicular or inguinal lymphadenopathy, lower extremity edema, ascites, or decreased breath sounds with lung auscultation may indicate metastases.
- Examination under anesthesia for extent of pelvic tumor spread

DIAGNOSTIC TESTS & INTERPRETATION
Lab
Initial lab tests
- Pap smear
- CBC may show anemia.
- LFTs
- BUN and creatinine
- Urinalysis may show hematuria.

Follow-Up & Special Considerations
Prompt follow-up for test results and treatment plans

Imaging
Initial approach
CXR, IV pyelogram (IVP), CT scan of abdomen and pelvis, MRI, and PET scan:
- Evaluation of lung, lymph node, and distal organ metastasis; hydronephrosis; local extracervical invasion

Follow-Up & Special Considerations
Prompt multidisciplinary plan of care

Diagnostic Procedures/Surgery
- Biopsy of gross lesion
- Colposcopy with biopsy of abnormal blood vessels, irregular surface contour with loss of surface epithelium as indicated
- Endocervical curettage and cervical conization as indicated to determine depth of invasion and presence of lymphovascular involvement
- Cystoscopy to evaluate bladder invasion
- Proctoscopy for invasion into rectum

Pathological Findings
- Majority of cases (80%) are invasive squamous cell types usually arising from the ectocervix.
- Adenocarcinoma comprise 10–15% of cervical cancer arising from endocervical mucus-producing glandular cells.
- Other cell types that may be present include:
  - Rare mixed cell types
  - Neuroendocrine tumors
  - Sarcomas, lymphomas, melanomas

DIFFERENTIAL DIAGNOSIS
- Marked cervicitis and erosion
- Glandular hyperplasia
- STD
- Herpetic ulcer or chancre
- Cervical condyloma
- Cervical leiomyoma
- Cervical polyps
- Metastasis from endometrial carcinoma or gestational trophoblastic disease

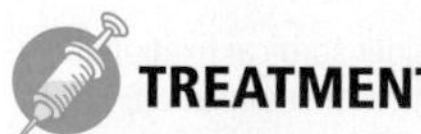

TREATMENT

MEDICATION
- Cisplatin, hydroxyurea, and fluorouracil have been used as adjuvant sensitizer to radiation therapy, but standard of care remains cisplatin as a radiosensitizer.
- Cisplatin/carboplatin, etoposide (VP-16), ifosfamide and bleomycin have been used as adjuvant therapy for recurrent, metastatic disease.

ADDITIONAL TREATMENT

General Measures

mprove nutritional state, correct any anemia, and eat any vaginal and/or pelvic infections.

Issues for Referral

Multidisciplinary management of patients as needed nd in a timely fashion

Additional Therapies

Radiation therapy forms the cornerstone of advanced-stage cervical cancer.

Combination of external beam pelvic radiation and brachytherapy is usually employed.

If para-aortic nodal metastases are evident, then extended-field radiation can be added to treat affected lymph nodes.

Chemoradiation with cisplatin-containing regimen has been associated with superior survival rates compared with pelvic and extended-field radiation alone.

SURGERY/OTHER PROCEDURES

Removal of precursor lesions (CIN) by LEEP, cold knife conization, laser ablation, or cryotherapy (6)[A]

Stage IA1 (lesions with <3 mm invasion from basement membrane): Cervical conization with total hysterectomy later when child-bearing is completed; otherwise, total hysterectomy

Stage IA2 (lesions with >3 mm but <5 mm invasion from the basement membrane) and stages IB1, IB2, IIA: Option of radical hysterectomy, bilateral pelvic lymphadenectomy, and para-aortic node sampling or primary radiation with brachytherapy and teletherapy

- Stage IVA (lesions limited to central metastasis to the bladder and/or rectum): Pelvic exenteration may be feasible.
- Radiotherapy:
  - For stage IB2 or higher:
    - Brachytherapy with intracavitary radium or cesium or interstitial cesium needles to treat the central tumor sites
    - Teletherapy with external radiation to treat tumor metastasis in the pelvic walls
  - For localized persistent or recurrent disease, radiation therapy or pelvic exenteration as appropriate
- Stage IVB disease has poor prognosis and is treated with goal of palliation.

IN-PATIENT CONSIDERATIONS

Initial Stabilization

- Active vaginal bleeding can be controlled with timely vaginal packing and radiation therapy.
- Recognition of ureteral blockage, hydronephrosis, urosepsis, and timely intervention

Admission Criteria

- Signs of active bleeding
- Urinary symptoms
- Dehydration
- Complications from surgery, chemotherapy, or radiation

IV Fluids

Adequate hydration and electrolyte repletion as needed

Nursing

Routine perioperative and postoperative care; pre- and postchemoradiation care

Discharge Criteria

Discharge criteria based on multidisciplinary assessment, including physicians, physical therapists, long- or short-term rehabilitation, home nursing care, or hospice.

Pregnancy Considerations

- Generally, the choice of treatment depends on the severity of the abnormal Pap smear, the length of gestation, the patient's wish to continue pregnancy to attainment of fetal lung maturity, and the treating physician's comfort level in delaying definitive therapy.
- Clinical stage at diagnosis is the single most important prognostic factor during pregnancy.
- If treatment is delayed, the patient must receive close follow-up care, with its frequency dependent on the severity of the disease.

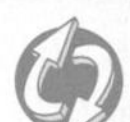

ONGOING CARE

FOLLOW-UP RECOMMENDATIONS

Patient Monitoring

- With completion of definitive therapy, each patient is evaluated with physical/pelvic examinations and Pap smears:
  - Every 3 months for 1–2 years
  - Every 6 months until the 5th year
  - Yearly thereafter
- Signs of cancer recurrence are unexplained weight loss, leg edema, and pelvic or thigh pain.

DIET

As appropriate

PATIENT EDUCATION

Patient education material available through the American Cancer Society at www.cancer.org

PROGNOSIS

After commonly accepted surgical and radiation treatments, 5-year survival:

Stage	5-yr Survival (%)
1	80
2	65
3	30
4	15

COMPLICATIONS

- Loss of ovarian function from radiotherapy or indication for bilateral oophorectomy
- Hemorrhage
- Pelvic infection
- Genitourinary fistula
- Bladder dysfunction
- Ureteral obstruction with renal failure
- Bowel obstruction
- Pulmonary embolism

REFERENCES

1. Scarinci IC, Garcia FA, Kobetz E, Partridge EE, Brandt HM, Bell MC, Dignan M, Ma GX, Daye JL, Castle PE et al. Cervical cancer prevention: new tools and old barriers. *Cancer*. 2010;116:2531–42.
2. Martin-Hirsch PL, et al. Surgery for cervical intraepithelial neoplasia. Cochrane Gynaecological Cancer Group. *Cochrane Database of Syst Rev*. 2007:3.
3. Kinney W, Stoler MH, Castle PE et al. Special commentary: patient safety and the next generation of HPV DNA tests. *Am J Clin Pathol*. 2010;134:193–9.
4. Markowitz LE, Dunne EF, Saraiya M, et al. Quadrivalent Human Papillomavirus Vaccine: Recommendations of the Advisory Committee on Immunization Practices (ACIP). *MMWR Recomm Rep*. 2007;56:1–24.
5. Grce M, Matovina M, Milutin-Gasperov N, Sabol I et al. Advances in cervical cancer control and future perspectives. *Coll Antropol*. 2010;34:731–6.
6. http://www.cancer.gov.

ADDITIONAL READING

- American Cancer Society: Cancer Facts and Figures 2007. Atlanta: American Cancer Society, 2007.
- Herrero R, Hildesheim A, Bratti C, et al. Population-based study of human papillomavirus infection and cervical neoplasia in rural Costa Rica. *J Natl Cancer Inst*. 2000;92:464–74.
- Jemal A, Siegel R, Ward E, et al. Cancer statistics, 2008. *CA Cancer J Clin*. 2008;58:71–96.
- Morris M, Eifel PJ, Lu J, et al. Pelvic radiation with concurrent chemotherapy compared with pelvic and para-aortic radiation for high-risk cervical cancer. *N Engl J Med*. 1999;340:1137–43.

See Also (Topic, Algorithm, Electronic Media Element)

Abnormal Pap and Cervical Dysplasia

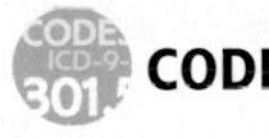

CODES

ICD9

- 180.0 Malignant neoplasm of endocervix
- 180.1 Malignant neoplasm of exocervix
- 180.8 Malignant neoplasm of other specified sites of cervix

CLINICAL PEARLS

- Worldwide, cervical cancer ranks 2nd among all malignancies for women.
- Women with cervical cancer may be asymptomatic and have a normal physical exam.
- Cervical carcinoma is clinically staged.
- Radiation therapy forms the cornerstone of advanced-stage cervical cancer.

CERVICAL POLYPS

Nicole D. Pilevsky, MD

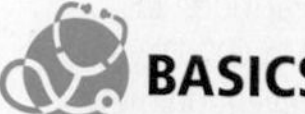

BASICS

DESCRIPTION

- Pedunculated masses, usually single, that vary in size from a few millimeters to 3 cm, that protrude from the cervix and may bleed
- System(s) affected: Reproductive

Geriatric Considerations

Rare

Pediatric Considerations

Rare

Pregnancy Considerations

Delay removal of polyps until postpartum unless bleeding or cervical dilation is found.

EPIDEMIOLOGY

- Predominant age: 40–60 years
- Predominant sex: Female only

Incidence

Common

RISK FACTORS

None

GENERAL PREVENTION

None known

PATHOPHYSIOLOGY

Hyperplastic proliferation of cervical or endometrial cells

ETIOLOGY

- Unknown for most cases
- Secondary reaction to cervical inflammatory or hormonal stimulation
- Extremely rare incidence of dysplasia or malignancy

COMMONLY ASSOCIATED CONDITIONS

There is some possibility of coexisting endometrial polyps.

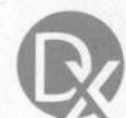

DIAGNOSIS

Cervical polyps are typically painless.

HISTORY

- The majority of cervical polyps are asymptomatic.
- Some cause abnormal vaginal bleeding or discharge:
  - Intermenstrual bleeding
  - Postcoital or postmenopausal bleeding
  - Leukorrhea

PHYSICAL EXAM

- Polyp may be an incidental finding on routine speculum exam.
- Document its location and size.

DIAGNOSTIC TESTS & INTERPRETATION

Lab

Send polyp for pathologic analysis.

Imaging

Sonohysterography may be helpful if there is suspicion of multiple polyps or to determine if polyp is originating from the endometrium.

Diagnostic Procedures/Surgery

Perform Pap smear before treatment if the patient is due for screening.

Pathological Findings

- Benign hyperplastic endocervical epithelium, often with a large number of blood vessels involved
- Extremely rare incidence of dysplasia or malignancy
  - Most atypia is found in the teens and 20s.
  - Most cancers are found in women >48 years.
- Case reports of lymphoma and sarcoma botryoides

DIFFERENTIAL DIAGNOSIS

- Prolapsed submucous myoma or endometrial polyp
- Other causes of intermenstrual bleeding
- Decidualized endometrium

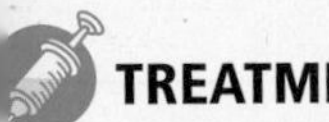

TREATMENT

There is no absolute need to remove a polyp unless there is a suspicion of malignancy, but removal may stop bleeding.

Smaller polyps may be removed in the office as long as hemostatic agents are available. The polyp is grasped with a ring forceps and twisted on its stalk until it detaches. Local anesthetic is not generally necessary. Silver nitrate or Monsel solution may be applied if cautery is needed. Sessile polyps may be removed using an electrosurgical loop (with local anesthetic).

Larger polyps may require removal in an operating room.

SURGERY/OTHER PROCEDURES

Outpatient management usually. If polyps are treated in the operating room, hysteroscopy may be a useful adjunct (1).

IN-PATIENT CONSIDERATIONS

Admission Criteria

Uncontrolled hemorrhage

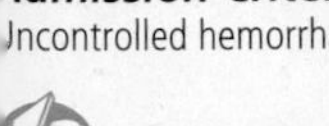

ONGOING CARE

FOLLOW-UP RECOMMENDATIONS

Following removal, avoid sexual intercourse, tampons, and douching for 2 weeks.

Patient Monitoring

Recheck at routine appointments or as needed.

PATIENT EDUCATION

Given the possibility of incomplete excision, patients should be educated about symptoms.

PROGNOSIS

Recurrence not likely with complete excision

COMPLICATIONS

Bleeding and mild pain with removal

REFERENCE

1. Stamatellos I, Stamatopoulos P, Bontis J. The role of hysteroscopy in the current management of the cervical polyps. *Arch Gynecol Obstet*. 2007.

ADDITIONAL READING

Schnatz PF, Ricci S, O'Sullivan DM. Cervical polyps in postmenopausal women: is there a difference in risk? *Menopause*. 2009.

CODES

ICD9

622.7 Mucous polyp of cervix

CLINICAL PEARLS

- There is no absolute need to remove a polyp unless there is a suspicion of malignancy, but removal may stop bleeding.
- Cervical polyps are extremely rarely cancerous.
- Smaller polyps may be removed in the office as long as hemostatic agents are available. Larger polyps may be removed in the operating room.

CERVICAL SPINE INJURY

Caroline Tschibelu, MD
Otis Warren, MD

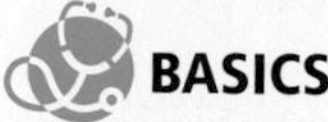

BASICS

DESCRIPTION

- Cervical spine injuries can result in vertebral fracture, ligamentous injury, or spinal cord injury.
- Vertebral and ligamentous injuries can cause cervical spine instability leading to cord injury.

EPIDEMIOLOGY

Incidence

- There are an estimated 12,000 new cases of spinal cord injury per year in the United States, with over half involving the cervical spine.
- Primarily affects young adults with active lifestyles, but the elderly are also affected due to prevalence of degenerative joint disease and increased risk of falls.
- Average age at time of injury: 39.5
- Male-to-female ratio: 4:1

RISK FACTORS

Anatomic irregularities:

- Degenerative joint disease (particularly the elderly)
- Osteoporosis
- Spinal canal stenosis
- Spina bifida

Genetics

Inherited connective tissue disorders (e.g., familial cervical spondylosis, a spondylitis)

GENERAL PREVENTION

- Use seat belts and child safety seats.
- Avoidance of high-risk activities such as driving while intoxicated
- Treatment of osteoporosis (e.g., calcium and vitamin D supplement, HRT, bisphosphonates)
- Fall prevention for the elderly

PATHOPHYSIOLOGY

4 major vertebral and ligamentous injuries are classified by mechanism:

- Flexion:
  - Simple wedge compression fracture:
    - Anterior compression fracture of vertebrae
    - Nuchal ligament stretch but not disruption
    - Diminished vertebral body height on x-ray
    - Stable fracture
  - Flexion teardrop fracture:
    - Anteroinferior vertebral body fracture
    - Displaced anterior fragment ("teardrop")
    - Posterior and anterior ligamentous disruption
    - Extremely unstable, high risk of cord injury
  - Anterior subluxation:
    - Posterior ligament rupture without fracture
    - Rarely associated with neurologic deficit
    - Seen on flexion-extension views
    - Treated as unstable due to risk while in flexion, but not unstable by definition
  - Bilateral facet dislocation:
    - More severe anterior subluxation
    - Includes disruption of annulus, anterior, and posterior ligaments
    - Inferior facets move superior and anterior to the superior facets, causing displacement.
    - Neurologic injury related to disk herniation
  - Clay shoveler fracture:
    - Oblique fracture at base of spinous process
    - Occurs with abrupt flexion with simultaneous contraction of lower neck and upper body
    - Also occurs with blunt trauma
    - Avulsed fragment seen on lateral views
    - Stable fracture, low risk for neurologic deficit
- Flexion–rotation:
  - Unilateral facet dislocation:
    - Less anterior displacement than bilateral
  - Rotary atlantoaxial dislocation (C1–C2):
    - Specific type of unilateral facet dislocation
    - Asymmetry of the lateral masses of C1 seen
    - Considered unstable due to location
- Extension:
  - Hangman fracture:
    - Traumatic spondylolisthesis of C2
    - Bilateral fractures through C2 pedicles
    - Unstable fracture, but cord injury rare
  - Extension teardrop fracture:
    - Avulsion fracture from stretch on anterior longitudinal ligament, causing anteroinferior bony fragment
    - Commonly found at lower cervical levels
    - Cord injury possible due to ligamenta flava encroaching into spinal canal
    - Unstable fracture in extension
  - Fracture of C1 posterior arch:
    - Stable fracture
  - Posterior atlantoaxial dislocation (C1–C2):
    - Cord injury possible
- Vertical compression (from axial load):
  - Jefferson fracture:
    - Burst fracture of C1 ring
    - Instability determined by severity of transverse ligamentous disruption
    - Unstable if more than 25% loss of height
  - Occipital condyle fracture:
    - Can be avulsion or compression fracture
    - Associated with cranial nerve deficits
- Unclear mechanisms:
  - Odontoid (dens) fracture, part of C2 (axis):
    - Type I: Involving tip of dens
    - Type II: Involving base of dens
    - Type III: Extends into body of axis
    - Types II and III can become unstable.
  - Atlanto-occipital dislocation:
    - Brainstem stretch may cause immediate respiratory arrest and death.
- Spinal cord injury (SCI):
  - Complete cord injury: Characterized by complete loss of sensory and motor functions below injury through S4–S5. Can also present with priapism, urinary retention, and bladder distention.
  - Incomplete deficits: Sensory and motor functions partially preserved below injury. Sensory preserved to a greater degree because sensory tracts peripherally located. Incidence of incomplete cord injury has increased compared to complete injury with implementation of ATLS protocols for all trauma patients (1). Most SCI are mixed injuries but there are some specific syndromes:
    - Central cord syndrome: Most common incomplete injury; motor deficits greater in upper than lower extremities. Sensory loss in the distribution of a "cape" and due to watershed injury affecting long fiber tracts; may be due to hyperextension.
    - Anterior cord syndrome: Posterior columns spared; affects spinothalamic, corticospinal, anterior, and lateral columns; loss of pain, temperature, motor with preserved vibration and position sense below the lesion
    - Posterior cord syndrome: Sensory deficits more pronounced than motor, due to contusion of posterior columns
    - Brown-Sequard syndrome: Ipsilateral motor los and vibration sensation deficits with contralateral loss of pain and temperature sensation; hemisection of cord most often due to penetrating trauma

ETIOLOGY

Traumatic injury to the head or neck from:

- Motor vehicle accidents or falls
- Violence, commonly gunshot wounds
- High-risk or high-impact sports

COMMONLY ASSOCIATED CONDITIONS

- Intracranial hemorrhage
- Skull and facial fractures
- Thoracolumbar spine injury
- Other: Visceral/extremities injuries in polytrauma

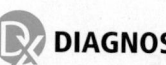

DIAGNOSIS

HISTORY

- History of traumatic injury to head or neck
- Neck pain or neurologic symptoms
- Past medical history, including medications
- Substance abuse or intoxication

PHYSICAL EXAM

- Midline cervical tenderness on palpation
- Limited or painful cervical range of motion
- Weakness, paresthesias, or numbness on complete neurological exam
- Abnormal rectal tone

DIAGNOSTIC TESTS & INTERPRETATION

Lab

Initial lab tests

- Complete blood count, basic metabolic panel
- Urine toxicology, blood alcohol level

Imaging

Initial approach

- Standard trauma series includes 5 x-ray views. However, if high suspicion for c-spine injury, consider CT as 1st-line imaging.
- Use Canadian C-spine Rules (CCR) or NEXUS Low-Risk Criteria (LRC) to decide when not to radiograph:
  - CCR, no imaging needed if (2)[A]:
    - Patient is alert (GCS = 15) and stable
    - No high-risk factors, no dangerous mechanism, no paresthesias, age <65
    - A low-risk factor (simple rear-end MVA, ambulatory, delayed pain, absence of midline tenderness) in a patient who can rotate neck 45 degrees left and right
  - NEXUS LRC, no imaging needed if (3)[A]:
    - No posterior midline cervical tenderness
    - Alert, without evidence of intoxication
    - No focal neurologic deficit
    - No painful distracting injury
- 2003 prospective cohort of 8,283 patients found CCR superior to NEXUS LRC.
- CT is superior to radiography in higher risk patients with decreased mentation.
- If C7–T1 cannot be visualized, consider CT.

Geriatric Considerations

In the geriatric population, avoid sedating medications. Strongly consider CT of cervical spine due to degenerative disease.

Pediatric Considerations

- Subluxation more likely than fracture
- Larger head size increases risk of cord injury
- C1–C3 more likely affected in children under 8
- Some sources support CT scan as 1st-line in children under 14, but risk of radiation outweighs the benefits in asymptomatic children (4)[B].
- Spinal Cord Injury Without Radiographic Abnormality (SCIWORA): Neurologic deficits without signs of bony or ligamentous injury on adequate radiographs or CT. SCIWORA primarily seen in children due to ligamentous laxity and incomplete ossification of the spine. Consider MRI to better visualize ligamentous injury in this population.

Follow-Up & Special Considerations

- If negative cervical spine CT with persistent midline tenderness, consider MRI in 72 hours.
- Flexion–extension radiographs were considered if the patient was alert and cooperative with persistent concern for ligamentous cervical spine injury not seen on standard x-rays. They are falling out of favor due to MRI ability to detect those injuries and because they may worsen spinal injury.
- MRI has NPV of 100% for noninjury, including injuries not seen on x-rays or CT (5)[A].

Diagnostic Procedures/Surgery

CT angiography of carotid or vertebral arteries if concerned for associated vascular injury

Pathological Findings

- Vertebral fractures on x-rays or CT
- Ligamentous tear or soft tissue edema on MRI
- Spinal cord entrapment on MRI

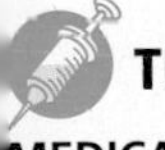

TREATMENT

MEDICATION

- Pain control
- Steroid treatment controversial for cord injury because effectiveness uncertain:
  - Methylprednisolone: Bolus: 30 mg/kg, then 5.4 mg/kg/h for the next 23 hours if within 3 hours of injury; if within 3–8 hours of injury, treat for total of 48 hours (6)[A]
- Increased risk of infection, GI bleeding, and steroid myopathy with steroid use (7)[C]

ADDITIONAL TREATMENT

General Measures

Long-term cervical collar or halo-style orthosis if evidence of vertebral, ligamentous, or cord injury

Issues for Referral

Orthopedics and/or neurosurgery

COMPLEMENTARY AND ALTERNATIVE MEDICINE

Massage therapy for residual muscular pain or spasm

SURGERY/OTHER PROCEDURES

Surgical stabilization used for a minority of cases

IN-PATIENT CONSIDERATIONS

Initial Stabilization

Follow the Advanced Trauma Life Support (ATLS) algorithm.

ALERT

- Immediately place patient in cervical collar if:
  - High-impact accident
  - Facial trauma, head injury, or direct cervical injury
  - Altered consciousness
- Presents from home after recent injury, despite functional status or time elapsed
- If transporting, use a backboard with stabilizing blocks to maintain neutral position.
- Keep oxygen saturation normal to prevent further cord injury from hypoxia.

Admission Criteria

- Respiratory: Oxygen requirements
- Cardiovascular: Hemodynamic instability
- Neurologic: Focal neurological findings, limited independent function, or concern for delayed intracranial bleed
- Surgical: Awaiting surgical stabilization

IV Fluids

Volume resuscitation or pressors as needed

Nursing

Frequent neurologic checks and use of appropriate, well-fitted collar

Discharge Criteria

Patient can be discharged if:

- Cleared according to NEXUS or CCR criteria or after neurology/orthopedic consults
- Ligamentous injury is present or suspected and sent home in cervical orthosis
- Stable vertebral fracture present and sent home in a cervical orthosis
- In permanent halo device and placed in a rehabilitation facility

ONGOING CARE

FOLLOW-UP RECOMMENDATIONS

Follow-up required if discharged with a collar

Patient Monitoring

If spinal cord injury, high cervical fracture, respiratory failure, or hemodynamic instability, critical care monitoring required

DIET

- n.p.o. until alert and protecting airway
- Early nutrition due to hypermetabolic state related to trauma and injury

PATIENT EDUCATION

- The national spinal cord injury association: http://www.spinalcord.org 1-800-962-9629
- NINDS spinal cord injury information page: http://www.ninds.nih.gov/disorders/sci/sci.htm

PROGNOSIS

Function after 1 year postinjury indicates long-term function.

COMPLICATIONS

- Common complications of cervical trauma:
  - Chronic musculoskeletal pain
  - Herniated discs
  - Chronic radiculopathy
- Common complications of spinal cord injury:
  - Pneumonia
  - Deep vein thrombosis
  - Pulmonary embolus
  - Pressure ulcers
  - Wound infections
  - Urinary tract infections
  - Chronic pain
  - Depression
  - Renal failure
- Death in cord injury patients usually related to pneumonia, pulmonary embolus, or sepsis.

REFERENCES

1. O'Dowd JK et al. Basic principles of management for cervical spine trauma. *Eur Spine J*. 2010;19 Suppl 1:S18–22.
2. Stiell IG, Wells GA, Vandemheen KL, et al. The Canadian C-spine rule for radiography in alert and stable trauma patients. *JAMA*. 2001;286:1841–8.
3. Hoffman JR, Mower WR, Wolfson AB, et al. Validity of a set of clinical criteria to rule out injury to the cervical spine in patients with blunt trauma. National Emergency X-Radiography Utilization Study Group. *N Engl J Med*. 2000;343(2):94–9.
4. Jimenez RR, DeGuzman MA, Shiran S, et al. CT versus plain radiographs for evaluation of c-spine injury in young children: do benefits outweigh risks? *Pediatr Radiol*. 2008;38:635–44.
5. Muchow RD, Resnick DK, Abdel MP. Magnetic resonance imaging (MRI) in the clearance of the cervical spine in blunt trauma: a meta-analysis. *J Trauma*. 2008;64(1):179–89.
6. Bracken MB. Steroids for acute spinal cord injury. *Cochrane Database Syst Rev*. 2002:CD001046.
7. Wuermser L, Ho CH, Chiodo AE, et al. Spinal Cord Injury Medicine: Acute Care Management of Traumatic and Nontraumatic Injury. *Arch Phys Med Rehabil*. 2007;88(1):S55–S61.

CODES

ICD9

- 805.00 Closed fracture of cervical vertebra, unspecified level
- 952.00 C1-c4 level spinal cord injury, unspecified
- 952.05 C5-c7 level spinal cord injury, unspecified

CLINICAL PEARLS

- Suspect cervical injury in any patient with facial or head trauma, especially if obtunded or intoxicated.
- Perform a comprehensive neurologic exam.
- Follow clear imaging guidelines, such as the Canadian C-spine Rules.
- Although controversial, consider early steroids if spinal cord injury suspected.

CERVICAL SPONDYLOSIS

Eric J. Kujawski, DO
Kenneth M. Bielak, MD
Brian K. Linn, MD

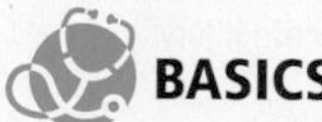

BASICS

DESCRIPTION

Considered the most common progressive disorder of the cervical spine due to the process of noninflammatory degeneration of the facet joints and intervertebral discs and osteophyte formation:

- Seen as a natural process of aging, most people remain asymptomatic.
- Symptomatic patients fall into three groups: Axial neck pain, cervical radiculopathy, and cervical myelopathy.
- System(s) affected: Musculoskeletal; Neurological
- Synonym(s): Cervical arthritis; Cervical myelopathy; Cervical osteophyte; Cervicalgia

Geriatric Considerations

- Patients <55 usually present due to a herniated disc.
- Patients >55 usually have osteophyte formation with canal or foraminal stenosis.
- Rule out myelopathy before considering conservative treatment.

Pediatric Considerations

Symptoms are less common, but radiographic changes can be seen as early as skeletal maturity.

EPIDEMIOLOGY

Incidence

Predominant sex: Male > Female (3:2)

Prevalence

- 10% by age 25
- 95% by age 65

RISK FACTORS

- Aging
- Smoking
- Laborers
- Congenital spinal canal narrowing

PATHOPHYSIOLOGY

- Loss of disc height:
  - Desiccation leads the nucleus pulposus to lose elasticity and become smaller and more fibrous.
  - The annulus fibrosus takes on more weight and can bulge into the spinal canal.
  - Loss of height begins ventrally, leading to loss of cervical lordosis and a resulting focal kyphosis.
- Osteophyte formation:
  - Bare edges of the vertebral bodies
  - Uncovertebral joints
  - Facet joints (C5–C7 most common)
- Thickened laminae
- Thickened or ossified posterior longitudinal ligament
- Thickened or buckling ligamentum flavum
- Vertebral artery involvement

COMMONLY ASSOCIATED CONDITIONS

See Etiology

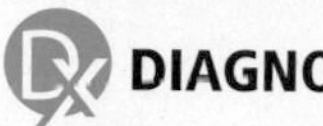

DIAGNOSIS

HISTORY

- Gradual chronic onset is more common than acute presentation. Radiculopathy can be acute, subacute, or chronic.
- Generally worse with movement. Common complaint of neck being "stiff."
- Pain in the posterior neck and trapezius muscle associated at times with radiation into the arms
- Scapular pain
- Arm pain usually on the outer aspect of the arm at least to the elbow (coronary heart pain is almost always on the inner aspect of the arm)
- Radicular pain may be present without neck pain.
- Loss of neck extension
- Lateral flexion is limited while erect but improves while lying down.
- Tenderness of biceps and pectoralis major in C5–C6 segment disease
- Tenderness of triceps in C6–C7 disease
- Long tract signs and positive Babinski may develop in severe cases with myelopathy.

PHYSICAL EXAM

- Tenderness over the affected segments
- Palpation occasionally reproduces radicular pain.
- Coughing, sneezing, Valsalva, and certain cervical movements can increase radicular pain.
- The "shoulder abduction sign" relieves pain in some patients. The patient holds the arm over their head and rests the wrist or forearm on top of the head.

DIAGNOSTIC TESTS & INTERPRETATION

Lab

Initial lab tests

Only if diagnosis is in question:

- Erythrocyte sedimentation rate
- Rheumatoid factor
- Complete blood count with differential

Imaging

Initial approach

X-rays of cervical spine, anteroposterior (AP), lateral, open-mouth odontoid, and obliques. Osteophytes and/or joint space narrowing will be evident (1)[C].

Follow-Up & Special Considerations

- CT or MRI scans are valuable in cases where surger is contemplated or the diagnosis is in doubt.
- Degenerative changes and disc herniations are commonly seen in asymptomatic patients, so correlation with neurological exam is needed.
- MRI better depicts cord changes, enlargement, compression, or atrophy.
- CT shows bony changes better, especially foraminal stenosis (2)[B].
- CT myelography in place of MRI in patients with metal hardware or pacemaker (3)[C]

Diagnostic Procedures/Surgery

Electromyogram (EMG) and nerve conduction studies may be needed to rule out other neurological causes. These studies are usually not needed in most patients with well-defined radiculopathy and correlating radiology findings.

DIFFERENTIAL DIAGNOSIS

- Cervical strain
- Rheumatoid arthritis
- Polymyalgia rheumatica
- Bone metastases
- Thoracic outlet syndrome
- With radiculopathy or myelopathy symptoms:
  - Multiple sclerosis
  - Syringomyelia
  - Tumor
  - Epidural abscess
  - Amyotrophic lateral sclerosis
  - Cervical herniated disc
  - Herpes zoster
  - Lyme radiculopathy
  - Diabetic polyradiculopathy

TREATMENT

MEDICATION

First Line

- NSAIDs (ibuprofen 800 mg t.i.d. 7–14 days or naproxen 500 b.i.d. 7–14 days) (4)[C]:
  - Contraindications: Gastrointestinal bleeding or ulcer
  - Precautions in patients with renal disease, hepatic disease, or coagulation disorders
- Acetaminophen 650 mg/dose 5 × per 24 hours or maximum of 3250 mg/day
- Muscle relaxants (up to 2 weeks) (4)[C]
- Topical pain relief cream (ketoprofen 20%, cyclobenzaprine 2%, lidocaine 10%; apply sparingly 2–3 × daily)
- Lidocaine or diclofenac patches
- Anticonvulsants for radiculopathy (gabapentin, pregabalin, tiagabine, or oxcarbazepine) (4)[C]

Second Line

- Short course of oral corticosteroids may benefit patients with acute radicular pain
- Facet joint steroid injections (3)[B]
- Opioids in patients who do not improve with other conservative treatments and are not surgical candidates.

ADDITIONAL TREATMENT

General Measures

- Avoidance of any provocative activities
- Physical therapy with exercise and gradual mobilization (5)[C]
- Return to normal activities as soon as possible.
- Conservative treatment for patients with only axial pain:
  - Oral analgesics (NSAIDS)
  - A short course of oral corticosteroids
  - Referral to physical therapy
  - Use of a cervical pillow
  - Soft cervical collar (up to 2 weeks)
  - Isometric exercises
- Patients with radicular pain with only paresthesia or numbness and no specific weakness:
  - Conservative treatment for 6–12 weeks
  - Facet joint injections if continued symptoms after conservative treatment
  - Epidural steroid injections (4)[C]
- Patients with myelopathy:
  - Surgical decompression is indicated (6)[B].

Issues for Referral

Immediate referral to an orthopedic surgeon for symptoms of myelopathy (gait disturbances, frequent falls, bowel or bladder dysfunction, loss of dexterity, Babinski sign, clonus, hyperreflexia)

Additional Therapies

- Cervical traction unit: 8–12 lbs at 24 degree angle of flexion for 15–20 minute intervals (3)[C]
- Avoid high-velocity manual manipulative therapy.

SURGERY/OTHER PROCEDURES

Surgical decompression for myelopathy can be beneficial in early cases. (5,6)[B]

ONGOING CARE

FOLLOW-UP RECOMMENDATIONS

Referral indicated for continued severe pain with conservative treatment, significant or progression of neurological deficits, or any sign/symptoms of myelopathy

Patient Monitoring

Follow-up visit in 3–4 weeks for evaluation of neurologic status. If no change, follow at intervals of 3–6 months, depending on severity of symptoms.

PATIENT EDUCATION

Patients should immediately report any weakness, eye symptoms, bladder or bowel incontinence, gait disturbance, loss of dexterity, or fine motor control.

PROGNOSIS

75% of patients have complete or significant relief of symptoms with nonoperative approach (4)[B].

REFERENCES

1. Pateder DB, Berg JH, Thal R et al. Neck and shoulder pain: differentiating cervical spine pathology from shoulder pathology. *J Surg Orthop Adv*. 2009;18:170–4.
2. Binder AI. Cervical spondylosis and neck pain. *BMJ*. 2007;334:527–31.
3. Eubanks JD. Cervical Radiculopathy: Nonoperative Management of Neck Pain and Radicular Symptoms. *American Family Physician*. 2010;81(1): 33–40.
4. Mazanec D, Reddy A. Medical management of cervical spondylosis. *Neurosurgery*. 2007;60: S43–50.
5. Rao RD, Currier BL, Albert TJ. , et al. Degenerative cervical spondylosis: clinical syndromes, pathogenesis, and management. *J Bone Joint Surg Am*. 2007;89:1360–78.
6. Hsu W, Dorsi MJ, Witham TF et al. Surgical Management of Cervical Spondylotic Myelopathy. *Neurosurgery quarterly*. 2009;19:302–307.

ADDITIONAL READING

- Robinson J, Kothari M. Treatment of Cervical Radiculopathy. Retrieved July 6, 2008, from http://www.utdol.com.
- Shedid D, Benzel EC. Cervical spondylosis anatomy: pathophysiology and biomechanics. *Neurosurgery*. 2007;60(1 Suppl 1 1):S7–13.
- Woiciechowsky C, et al. Degenerative spondylolisthesis of the cervical spine. *European Spine Journal*. 2004;13:680–4.
- Young WF. Cervical spondylotic myelopathy: a common cause of spinal cord dysfunction in older persons. *Am Fam Physician*. 2000;62:1064–70, 1073.

See Also (Topic, Algorithm, Electronic Media Element)

See videos: Neck Stretch with a Towel; Neck Extension in Prone; Neck Stretches - Chin Tucks; Neck Trigger Point Massage - Trapezius

CODES

ICD9

- 721.0 Cervical spondylosis without myelopathy
- 721.1 Cervical spondylosis with myelopathy

CLINICAL PEARLS

- Noninflammatory degeneration of the facet joints and intervertebral discs
- Considered a natural process of aging, most people remain asymptomatic:
  - Symptomatic patients fall into three groups: Axial neck pain, cervical radiculopathy, and cervical myelopathy.
- Patients <55 usually present due to herniated disc.
- Patients >55 usually present due to radicular symptoms related to osteophyte formation or foraminal stenosis.
- Diagnosis via X-rays of cervical spine, AP, lateral, open-mouth odontoid, and obliques
- Referral indicated for continued severe pain with conservative treatment, significant or progression of neurological deficits, or any sign/symptoms of myelopathy
- 75% of patients have complete or significant relief of symptoms with nonoperative approach.

CERVICITIS, ECTROPION AND TRUE EROSION

Jeremy Golding, MD
Barbara A. Majeroni, MD

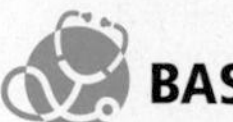

BASICS

DESCRIPTION

Cervicitis refers to inflammatory changes of the cervix.

- Ectropion: Presence of cervical columnar cells on the vaginal portion of the cervix (portio); often seen during adolescence and during pregnancy
- True erosion: Loss of overlying cervical epithelium owing to trauma (e.g., forceful insertion of vaginal speculum in patient with atrophic mucosa)
- System(s) affected: Reproductive

Geriatric Considerations

- Chronic cervicitis in postmenopausal women may be related to lack of estrogen.
- The possibility of infectious cervicitis should not be overlooked in geriatric patients because many remain sexually active.

Pregnancy Considerations

- Doxycycline should not be used during pregnancy.
- Screen all pregnant women for infectious cervicitis because of the risk of transmission to the fetus.

Pediatric Considerations

Infectious cervicitis in children should lead to an investigation for possible sexual abuse.

EPIDEMIOLOGY

Incidence

- Cervicitis: Cervicitis-specific data are not available. Based on CDC 2006 data:
  - Chlamydia incidence: Total actual cases reported to CDC were >1 million. CDC estimates 3 million new cases of chlamydia infection in both genders yearly.
  - Gonorrhea: Total actual cases reported to CDC approximately 358,000 both genders. CDC estimates actual incidence 700,000 new cases in both genders yearly.
  - Trichomoniasis: CDC estimates 7.4 million new cases in women and men yearly.
- Ectropion: Common with oral contraceptive use; very common in pregnant women
- True erosion: Occasionally seen in postmenopausal women
- Predominant age: 15–19 years
- Predominant sex: Women, especially sexually active women

RISK FACTORS

- Cervicitis:
  - Multiple sexual partners
  - Adolescence and young adulthood
  - Unprotected sex
  - History of STD
  - Smoking
  - Other reproductive tract infections: Vaginitis, PID
  - Foreign objects: Pessary, diaphragm, cervical cap, etc.
- Ectropion: Adolescence, pregnancy
- True erosion: Estrogen deficiency, trauma

GENERAL PREVENTION

- Sexually transmitted infection (gonorrhea, chlamydia, trichomoniasis):
  - Follow CDC-recommended screening measures: The US Preventive Services Task Force recommends screening for chlamydial infection in all sexually active nonpregnant young women ≤24 years and for older nonpregnant women who are at increased risk, but no routine screening for women >24 years not at increased risk (1)[C].
  - Treat sexual partners of infected women.
  - Advise use of condom during coitus.
- Estrogen deficiency: Estrogen replacement therapy

ETIOLOGY

- Cervicitis: *C. trachomatis, N. gonorrhoeae, T. vaginalis*, herpes simplex virus (HSV), mycoplasmas (e.g., *M. genitalium*), *Ureaplasma*, cytomegalovirus
- Non-sexually transmitted infectious cervicitis can be caused by β-hemolytic streptococcus or *E. coli*.
- Noninfectious causes include chemical irritation (e.g., from douching or latex exposure) and local trauma from vaginal foreign bodies such as diaphragms or cervical caps.
- Often no specific etiology is identified.
- Ectropion:
  - Hormonal changes with oral contraceptive use (especially with progesterone) or pregnancy
  - Resulting from cervical laceration during childbirth
- True erosion: Injury to atrophic epithelium owing to estrogen deficiency in menopause

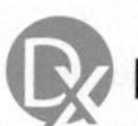

DIAGNOSIS

HISTORY

Patient may complain of vaginal discharge, dyspareunia, or bleeding/spotting following intercourse or may be asymptomatic.

PHYSICAL EXAM

- Cervicitis: Purulent vaginal discharge, cervical friability, erythema, ulceration (HSV); punctate hemorrhage causes "strawberry" cervix appearance in trichomoniasis.
- Ectropion: Cervix appears red, owing to the color of the columnar epithelium.
- True erosion: Vaginal bleeding, sharply defined ulcers of cervix
- Cervical motion tenderness may be appreciated on bimanual pelvic exam (suggests PID).

DIAGNOSTIC TESTS & INTERPRETATION

Lab

- Saline and KOH preparation of cervical and vaginal smears (endocervical sample with >10 WBC/hpf suggests cervicitis)
- Nucleic acid amplification tests: More sensitive and also may be used on urine, self-obtained vaginal swabs, and endocervical specimens (2)[A]. (Sensitivity and specificity between 95% and 99% for both gonorrhea and chlamydia.)
- Vaginal wet mount for *T. vaginalis*
- If ulcerations are present, culture for HSV.
- Pap smear of cervix

Diagnostic Procedures/Surgery

Colposcopy may be helpful in cases of chronic inflammation with a biopsy of suspicious areas.

Pathological Findings

- Cervicitis: Acute and chronic inflammatory changes, presence of infective organisms
- Ectropion: None/squamous metaplasia
- True erosion: Sharply defined ulcer borders, loss of epithelium

DIFFERENTIAL DIAGNOSIS

- Cervical dysplasia
- Carcinoma of the cervix
- Bacterial vaginosis (discharge is noninflammatory)

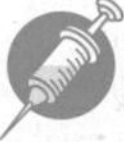

TREATMENT

Cervicitis increases HIV viral RNA present in vaginal secretions, so treatment of cervicitis therefore may reduce risk of HIV transmission in those with HIV and cervicitis (2).

MEDICATION

First Line

- If infectious cervicitis suspected, treat without awaiting culture results: Ceftriaxone (Rocephin) 125 mg single dose IM, followed by either doxycycline (Vibramycin) 100 mg PO b.i.d. × 7 days or azithromycin (Zithromax) 1 g single dose (3)[A]. Option of Rocephin and azithromycin removes patient-compliance factor because they are 1-time doses.
- Trichomoniasis: Metronidazole 2 g once or 500 mg b.i.d. × 7 days or 1 g b.i.d. × 2 doses
- Known or suspected chlamydial infection: For nonpregnant women, azithromycin 1 g PO once or doxycycline 100 mg b.i.d. PO × 7 days; for pregnant women, azithromycin 1 g once or erythromycin base 500 mg q.i.d. PO × 7 days or erythromycin ethylsuccinate 800 mg q.i.d. × 7 days

Ectropion: None, unless patient is extremely symptomatic with copious discharge. In that case, acid-buffered vaginal jelly can be used to decrease discharge. Cautery can be used but generally is considered overly invasive.
True erosion: Estrogen, conjugated vaginal cream daily for 1–2 weeks, followed by maintenance cream twice weekly or oral HRT
Contraindications:
- Metronidazole: Older references state that metronidazole is relatively contraindicated during 1st trimester of pregnancy. More recent meta-analyses suggest absence of teratogenicity. Treatment of trichomoniasis may be deferred until 2nd trimester if clinician remains concerned by product labeling.
- Doxycycline: Pregnancy or lactation
- Estrogen: See extended list of contraindications to estrogen use in standard texts.

Precautions:
- Metronidazole: See above; disulfiram reaction with ethanol ingestion
- Doxycycline: Possible fetal harm if used during pregnancy; staining of the infant's teeth if used during breast-feeding; allergy; photosensitization
- Erythromycin: Nausea or vomiting
- Estrogens: History of estrogen-dependent neoplasms; history of thromboembolic diseases. See extended list of contraindications to estrogen therapy in standard texts.

Significant possible interactions:
- Metronidazole: Ethanol
- Doxycycline: Dairy products, iron preparations, warfarin, and oral contraceptives (advise use of alternative contraceptive method)
Erythromycin: Theophylline (elevated theophylline level)
- Estrogen: N/A

Second Line
Cefixime 400 mg PO single dose is an acceptable alternative to ceftriaxone.

The rise of quinolone-resistant *N. gonorrhoea* has prompted a change in CDC recommendations concerning management of gonococcal disease (3)[A]. Quinolones are no longer recommended for primary management. The exception to this recommendation occurs only if the patient is penicillin-allergic and the organism is known to be sensitive to quinolones. The lack of availability of spectinomycin in the US creates a problem for patients with gonorrhea and true penicillin allergy. It seems reasonable to treat with a quinolone as below, with follow-up testing to ensure eradication in this case. Quinolones are contraindicated in pregnancy:
- Ofloxacin (Floxin) 400 mg PO single dose
- Ciprofloxacin (Cipro) 500 mg PO single dose
- Levofloxacin (Levaquin) 250 mg PO single dose

- Alternative to metronidazole for trichomoniasis: Tinidazole 2 g PO × 1 dose
- Estrogen deficiency: A number of estrogen vaginal preparations are available commercially.

SURGERY/OTHER PROCEDURES
Chronic cervicitis with negative cultures that does not respond to empirical medical treatment may be treated with cryosurgery, electrocautery, or loop excision.
- Adverse effects of cautery or cryosurgery can include cervical stenosis, which may affect fertility.

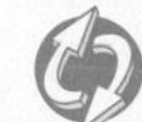

ONGOING CARE

FOLLOW-UP RECOMMENDATIONS
Patient Monitoring
- Follow-up assay is recommended in pregnant patients to document infection eradication.
- Estrogen deficiency: Re-examine in 1 month to confirm healing.

ALERT
Follow-up nucleic acid amplification tests should not be done <3 weeks after treatment because of false-positive results owing to dead organisms.

PATIENT EDUCATION
If the etiology of a patient's cervicitis is confirmed to be a sexually transmittable infection, educate patient on the necessity of treating her sexual partners to avoid reinfection.

PROGNOSIS
- Cervicitis: Excellent healing after infection is eradicated
- Ectropion: Spontaneous regression postpartum and with cessation of use of oral contraceptives
- True erosion: Spontaneous healing

COMPLICATIONS
Cervicitis owing to *C. trachomatis* or *N. gonorrhoeae* is associated with an 8–10% risk of developing subsequent PID. Adolescents are a high-risk group for reinfection with sexually transmitted organisms, and screening frequency should be once/twice yearly in this population.

REFERENCES

1. US Preventive Services Task Force. Screening for chlamydial infection: U.S. Preventive Services Task Force recommendation statement. *Ann Intern Med*. 2007;147:128–34.
2. Cook RL, Hutchison SL, Østergaard L, et al. Systematic review: noninvasive testing for Chlamydia trachomatis and Neisseria gonorrhoeae. *Ann Intern Med*. 2005;142:914–25.
3. Centers for Disease Control and Prevention. *Sexually transmitted diseases: Treatment guidelines 2006. MMWR*.

ADDITIONAL READING

- Arráiz R N, Colina Ch S, Marcucci J R, et al. Mycoplasma genitalium detection and correlation with clinical manifestations in population of the Zulia State, Venezuela. *Rev Chilena Infectol*. 2008;25:256–61.
- Brocklehurst P. Antibiotics for gonorrhea in pregnancy. *Cochrane Database Syst Rev*. 2006: 1. Accessed February 20, 2006.
- Johnson LF, Lewis DA. The Effect of Genital Tract Infections on HIV-1 Shedding in the Genital Tract: A Systematic Review and Meta-Analysis. *Sex Transm Dis*. 2008.
- Simpson T, Oh MK. Urethritis and cervicitis in adolescents. *Adolescent Med Clin*. 2004;15: 153–271.
- Wilson JF et al. In the clinic. Vaginitis and cervicitis. *Ann Intern Med*. 2009;151.

CODES

ICD9
- 616.0 Cervicitis and endocervicitis
- 622.0 Erosion and ectropion of cervix

CLINICAL PEARLS
- If infectious cervicitis is suspected, treatment of choice is ceftriaxone 125 mg IM plus azithromycin 1 g PO × 1 dose. Do not wait for test results.
- Encourage patient to have sexual partner(s) treated.
- Quinolones are no longer recommended to treat gonorrhea.
- Lubricants (e.g., KY Jelly) do not alter Pap smear results, so small quantities may be used when performing Pap smears.
- Positive results for *N. gonorrhoeae* or chlamydia should be reported to local or state health department.

CHANCROID

Jeffery T. Kirchner, DO

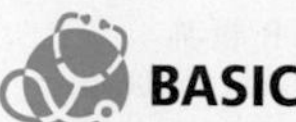

BASICS

DESCRIPTION

A sexually transmitted disease characterized by painful genital ulcerations and inflammatory inguinal adenopathy. Although uncommon in the US, it is found worldwide. Chancroid is endemic in developing countries, especially sub-Saharan Africa, and is a co-factor for HIV transmission.

EPIDEMIOLOGY

Incidence

- <50 cases reported to Centers for Disease Control (CDC) in 2004–2007 (from only 8 states)
- Actual numbers are considered higher due to lack of testing and thus underreporting.

Prevalence

- Endemic in developing countries, but actual prevalence is unknown due to lack of testing
- Thought to be extremely common in sub-Saharan Africa, southeast Asia, Latin America

RISK FACTORS

- Multiple sexual partners
- Uncircumcised men
- Prostitutes may be carriers.
- Patients presenting with other genital ulcerative diseases

GENERAL PREVENTION

Condom use

PATHOPHYSIOLOGY

Involves attachment of the bacteria to susceptible cells. Cytotoxin is secreted, which may play a role in epithelial injury and ulcer formation. Dendritic cells and natural killer cells respond to *H. ducreyi*, and this innate host response determines bacterial clearance versus disease progression.

ETIOLOGY

Haemophilus ducreyi (gram-negative rod)

COMMONLY ASSOCIATED CONDITIONS

- Syphilis: Concurrent in 10% of patients
- Herpes simplex virus or HIV infection

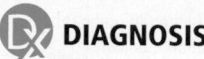

DIAGNOSIS

HISTORY

- Exposure to infected individual, but often not helpful or obtained
- Incubation period typically lasts 4–10 days.

PHYSICAL EXAM

- Tender erythematous genital papule that progresses into a pustule that erodes into an ulcer. Infected persons commonly have >1 ulcer.
- Typical ulcer is 1–2 cm, but size is variable.
- Ulcers are painful, with erythematous base and clearly demarcated borders, which are sometimes undermined.
- Common sites for ulcers in men include the penile shaft, glans, and meatus.
- Common sites for ulcers in women include labia, introitus, and perianal areas.
- Inguinal lymphadenitis with abscess (bubo) formation occurs in ~50% of men but less common in women.
- Buboes arise 1–2 weeks after ulceration, are typically painful
- Buboes may spontaneously rupture if the primary disease is untreated.
- Atypical presentations include folliculitis and foreskin abscess.

DIAGNOSTIC TESTS & INTERPRETATION

Lab

CDC criteria for presumptive diagnosis:

- Definite: Isolation of *H. ducreyi* from a lesion
- Probable: Clinical findings *plus* negative darkfield exam, negative serologic test for syphilis, negative cultures for herpes simplex virus (HSV), or a clinical presentation not typical for HSV.

Initial lab tests

- "School of fish" pattern on Gram stain with organisms clumped in long parallel strands
- Serologic testing for antibody to *H. ducreyi* with enzyme linked immunosorbent assay
- Culture of the organism on Mueller-Hinton agar with incorporated vancomycin but sensitivity is <80%.
- Multiplex polymerase chain reaction (PCR) has sensitivity of 95–98%, but no Food and Drug Administration-approved tests in the US; available from some commercial labs

Follow-Up & Special Considerations

All patients should also be tested for syphilis and HSV.

iagnostic Procedures/Surgery
ram stain and culture of exudate (1):
- Aspiration of inguinal bubo (lymph node)
- PCR testing of ulcer exudate for *H. ducreyi* DNA
- Darkfield examination of exudate to rule out *Treponema pallidum* infection
- Culture or PCR testing for HSV

IFFERENTIAL DIAGNOSIS
- Syphilis (*Treponema pallidum*)
- Genital herpes (HSV-1 and -2)
- Lymphogranuloma venereum (*Chlamydia trachomatis*)
- Granuloma inguinale (donovanosis)
- Drug eruption; Behçet disease

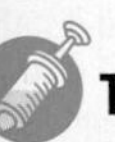

TREATMENT

IEDICATION
irst Line
zithromycin: 1 g p.o. single dose (2,3)[A]:
- Ceftriaxone 250 mg IM single dose

econd Line
- Ciprofloxacin 500 mg p.o. b.i.d. for 3 days (2,3)[A]
- Erythromycin base 500 mg q.i.d. for 7 days (2,3)[A]
- Contraindications:
  - Allergy to the medication
  - Ciprofloxacin during pregnancy and lactation and in patients <18 years

ADDITIONAL TREATMENT
ieneral Measures
- Outpatient treatment
- Saline or Burrow's solution to soak ulcers
- Aspiration of buboes if >5 cm; approached through adjacent skin. Also consider incision and drainage for larger lesions.

ALERT
HIV disease may affect treatment response.

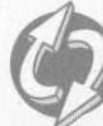

ONGOING CARE

FOLLOW-UP RECOMMENDATIONS
Patient Monitoring
- Avoid sexual activity until ulcers are resolved.
- Clinical improvement usually occurs within 48 hours.
- Patients should be reexamined 3–7 days after initiation of therapy and followed closely until all clinical signs of infection are resolved.
- Baseline syphilis serology and at 3 months
- Baseline HIV testing and at 3 months post-treatment

PATIENT EDUCATION
- Sexual counseling
- Use of condoms
- Local wound care
- Treatment of all sexual partners with same regimen as index
- HIV testing

PROGNOSIS
- Full clinical resolution with appropriate treatment
- Failure to respond may be due to incorrect diagnosis, coinfection with syphilis or HIV, medication nonadherence, or resistant *H. ducreyi*.
- 5% relapse after treatment.

COMPLICATIONS
- Phimosis
- Balanoposthitis
- Rupture of buboes with fistula formation and scarring

REFERENCES

1. Alfa M et al. The laboratory diagnosis of Haemophilus ducreyi. *Can J Infect Dis Med Microbiol*. 2005;16:31–4.
2. Lewis DA. Chancroid: Clinical manifestations, diagnosis, and management. *Sex Transm Inf*. 2003;79:68–71.
3. Centers for Disease Control and Prevention. Sexually transmitted diseases treatment guidelines—2006. *MMWR*. 2006;55:17–18.

ADDITIONAL READING

- Centers for Disease Control and Prevention. STD Surveillance. Division of STD Prevention—January 13, 2009.
- Janowicz DM, Li W, Bauer ME et al. Host-pathogen interplay of Haemophilus ducreyi. *Curr Opin Infect Dis*. 2010;23:64–9.
- Janowicz DM, Ofner S, Katz BP, et al. Experimental infection of human volunteers with Haemophilus ducreyi: fifteen years of clinical data and experience. *J Infect Dis*. 2009;199:1671–9.
- Montero JA. Chancroid: An update. *Infect Med*. 2002;191:174–8.
- Rosen T, Vandergriff T, Harting M. Antibiotic use in sexually transmissible diseases. *Dermatol Clin*. 2009;27:49–61.

CODES

ICD9
099.0 Chancroid

CLINICAL PEARLS
- Chancroid is a rare disorder in the US but more common elsewhere.
- Characterized by genital papules that progress to pustules that open, producing painful ulcers
- Treatment of choice is azithromycin 1 gm once.
- Treat sexual partners even in the absence of signs or symptoms of disease.

CHARCOT JOINT

Patrick W. Joyner, MD
Kristyn Fagerberg, MD

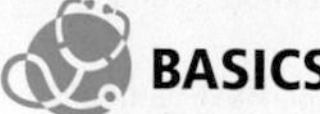

BASICS

In 1868, a French neurologist, Jean Martin Charcot, first described rapid joint deterioration in patients with tabes dorsalis. However, in 1703, Dr. William Musgrave first reported swollen, inflamed joints in a paralyzed patient. In 1936, Dr. William Jordan first described an association of diabetes mellitus with neuropathic changes in the foot and ankle.

DESCRIPTION

- A progressive destructive arthritis secondary to peripheral neuropathy and loss of pain sensation. The affected joints are subjected to repeated stress that is unrecognized by the patient, therefore causing continuous damage to the underlying bone and cartilage.
- Most often seen in tarsal and tarsometatarsal joints, less in metatarsophalangeal and talotibial joints. May also be seen in knee, hip, spine.
- Upper extremity joints rarely are involved.
- Diabetes mellitus (DM) is the most common cause in the US.
- 3 stages are identified:
  - Fragmentation/destruction
  - Coalescence
  - Consolidation/resolution
- Patients suspected to have a Charcot neuropathy should be referred to an orthopedic foot and ankle surgeon or podiatrist for follow-up and treatment.
- System(s) affected: Musculoskeletal; Endocrine; Neurologic
- Synonym(s): Neuropathic joint disease; Neuropathic arthropathy

EPIDEMIOLOGY

- Primarily seen in 5th and 6th decades
- Male = Female
- Bilateral involvement in 9–35% of cases

Incidence

- 0.1–0.4% in patients with DM
- 5–9% of patients with peripheral neuropathy

Prevalence

0.1% in all patients, up to 13% in high-risk diabetes foot clinics

RISK FACTORS

- >15-year history of diabetes
- Poor blood sugar control
- Poor foot hygiene; poor-fitting shoes, socks
- Diabetes mellitus is the most common cause in the United States.
- Globally, other medical conditions, such as syphilis and leprosy, are also risk factors.

Genetics

Family history of DM

GENERAL PREVENTION

- Excellent control of blood sugar
- Diabetic foot care
- Well-fitting footwear with adequate support
- Frequent exam of feet for signs of pressure sores or ulcerations
- Good foot hygiene

PATHOPHYSIOLOGY

Exact cause unknown, 3 major theories:

- Autonomic neuropathy: Autonomic neuropathy leads to local increase in blood flow, which leads to osteopenia secondary to increased osteoclastic activity.
- Neurotraumatic: Repetitive microtrauma not sensed by the patient leads to osseous destruction and progressive damage to ligaments, articular surfaces, and may lead to fractures and subluxation.
- Neurovascular: Underlying medical disorder creates hypervascularity; this in conjunction with increased osteoclastic resorption and osteoporosis. Both mechanisms in the setting of microfractures and subchondral collapse will lead to joint destruction.

ETIOLOGY

Many causes of peripheral neuropathy:

- Diabetes mellitus
- Multiple sclerosis
- Raynaud disease
- Any connective tissue disease (i.e., scleroderma, rheumatoid arthritis)
- Syphilis/tabes dorsalis
- Syringomyelia, upper extremity disease
- Meningomyelocele
- Frequent intra-articular steroid injections
- Alcoholism
- Pernicious anemia
- Charcot-Marie-Tooth disease
- Leprosy (Hansen disease)
- Renal dialysis
- Amyloidosis

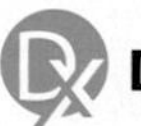

DIAGNOSIS

- Findings frequently confused with cellulitis
- Symptoms usually unilateral
- Significant swelling:
  - Early: Large effusion
  - Late: Swelling usually resolved
- Local increased warmth: 3–7°C higher than unaffected extremity
- Skin erythema:
  - Classically will resolve with elevation; helps to differentiate from infection (erythema from infection would not be affected by elevation)
- Effusion in joint
- Loss of distal sensation
- Skin intact
- Decreased pain, proprioception in affected limb
- Laxity/instability of joint:
  - May lead to calluses and/or ulcerations

HISTORY

- Long-standing diabetes
- May recall predisposing trauma, such as ankle twist/sprain, object dropped on foot
- May present with pain; however, proportionally less pain than expected by appearance
- Limited motion
- Diffuse swelling
- Erythema
- Can affect any number of joints. Charcot joint has been reported in the following anatomic locations: Spine, shoulder, elbow, wrist, hand, hip, knee, ankle and foot

PHYSICAL EXAM

- Localized warmth, swelling, erythema
- Brodsky test: Elevating the foot should resolve swelling.
- Neurologic exam:
  - Findings normally symmetric, sensory, and distal
  - Absent sensation on 4/10 sites using 5.07 g monofilament
  - Decreased or absent reflexes
  - Loss of pain, proprioception, and vibratory sensation
- Foot deformities:
  - Corns/calluses
  - Collapse of arch
  - Collapse of tarsal bones causing rocker-bottom foot
  - Protruding osteophytes
  - Plantar ulcer
- Peripheral circulation often normal

DIAGNOSTIC TESTS & INTERPRETATION

Resolution of erythema with elevation of affected extremity

Lab

- Blood sugar, hemoglobin A1c
- White blood cells may be elevated in osteomyelitis.
- Erythrocyte sedimentation rate: Elevated in osteomyelitis
- Basic metabolic panel: Blood urea nitrogen, creatinine to rule out renal disease
- B_{12}/folate, hematocrit, mean corpuscular volume
- Rapid plasma reagin, FTA-ABS to rule out syphilis
- Elevated alkaline phosphatase, calcium, parathyroid hormone, and low phosphate to rule out metabolic bone disease

Imaging

- Radiographs:
  - Early changes:
    - Slight fracture with joint subluxation
    - Joint effusion
    - Joint space narrowing
    - Sclerosis of subchondral bone
    - Bone fragmentation
  - Late changes:
    - Marked articular destruction
    - Fractures
    - Hypertrophic changes: Periarticular new bone, osteophytes, osseous debris, may look like severe arthritis
    - Bone resorption
    - Subluxation
    - Intra-articular loose bodies
    - Osteolysis
    - Large osteophytes
    - Atrophic changes: Massive bone resorption, joint disintegration, may look like chronic infection
- May be difficult to differentiate radiograph findings from those of osteomyelitis

- Magnetic resonance imaging (MRI): Assists in ruling out osteomyelitis, but can be difficult because joint will most likely have increased signal secondary to edema.
- Bone scan in conjunction with a tagged WBC scan: Assists in ruling out osteomyelitis:
  - Indium^{111} more specific than technetium^{99}

Initial approach
Rule out underlying neurologic disorder.

Diagnostic Procedures/Surgery
Arthrocentesis:
- Fluid for culture and sensitivity if osteomyelitis suspected
- Presence of WBC, calcium pyrophosphate dihydrate (CPPD) crystals
- Rule out malignancy of any cause for concern

DIFFERENTIAL DIAGNOSIS
- Cellulitis
- Osteomyelitis
- Osteonecrosis
- Advanced osteoarthritis
- Calcium pyrophosphate dihydrate crystal deposition disease
- Neoplasm

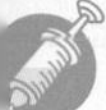

TREATMENT

- Early recognition of diabetic foot pathology
- No weight-bearing on affected extremity
- Total contact cast (gold standard)
- Reconstruction of foot to help prevent ulceration if conservative management fails. However, cannot be performed until erythema has resolved (i.e., late phase).

MEDICATION
Because pathophysiology is thought to involve increased osteoclastic activity, bisphosphonates have been used to halt progression of disease:

- Pamidronate, alendronate shown to give clinical improvement (1)[A]

- Bisphosphonates

ADDITIONAL TREATMENT
General Measures
- Goal of treatment is to restore joint stability and limit progression of disease.
- After casting, various braces are used to protect affected extremity:
  - Ankle-foot orthotic, rocker-bottom shoes, Charcot restraint orthotic walker, prefabricated pneumatic walking brace, custom prescription footwear
- Strict blood sugar control to limit progression of peripheral neuropathy

Additional Therapies
- Protective treatment with bracing, orthotics

- Radiotherapy does not appear to benefit healing of acute Charcot feet in people with diabetes (2)[B].

SURGERY/OTHER PROCEDURES
- Surgical treatment is reserved for severe cases and/or failure of conservative treatment.
- Surgery is indicated when a risk of skin ulceration, unstable fracture, or dislocation is present, or failure of medical therapy.
- Procedures performed vary, depending on joints involved and surgeon experience:
  - Exostosectomy of bony projections
  - Open reduction internal fixation
  - Osteotomy
  - Arthrodesis, with or without tendon lengthening
  - Amputation
  - Use of external fixation if poor skin quality or increase risk of postoperative healing complications
- Any surgical treatment should be delayed until after early fragmentation and inflammatory stages.
- Patients treated surgically often have long healing times.

IN-PATIENT CONSIDERATIONS
Initial Stabilization
- Immobilization of joint is initial treatment:
  - Casting:
    - Provides full immobilization
    - Casts must be checked weekly for correct fit, especially if underlying ulceration of skin.
    - Casts should be changed every 1–2 weeks.
    - Time in cast determined by clinical and radiographic measures
    - Total-contact cast better disperses pressure. Ensure pressure points are well padded, as these patients frequently have severely limited to no sensation and will likely not be aware of the development of pressure ulcer.
  - Brace/orthotic:
    - Alternative to casting
    - Removable
    - Patients may be noncompliant, and may not be able to sense a poor-fitting brace.
- Immobilization needed for minimum of 6 months; possibly 1 year or longer
- Also necessary to reduce stress on affected joint by limiting pressure:
  - Non-weight-bearing preferred, partial weight-bearing at minimum

Admission Criteria
Foot ulceration, suspicion of associated osteomyelitis, fractures

ONGOING CARE

FOLLOW-UP RECOMMENDATIONS
- Activity: Non- or partial weight-bearing initially
- Regular follow-up with podiatrist to maintain strict foot care

Patient Monitoring
- Regular monitoring of blood sugar, HbA1C
- After initial radiographs, repeat films should be obtained in 4–6 weeks.

Geriatric Considerations
Because most cases occur in patients >50, diabetic patients in this age group should be counseled about the symptoms and signs of neuropathic joint disease. The benefits of good blood sugar control should be discussed.

PATIENT EDUCATION
Multidisciplinary team approach

PROGNOSIS
- Patients often are immobilized for several months.
- Usually non-weight-bearing of extremity for an average of 6 months if surgery is required
- Total healing may take years to achieve.
- Patients must be vigilant about preventing further injury, receiving regular footcare, examining feet daily, and noting swelling and/or temperature of joints.
- Maintain strict diabetic control:
  - Especially critical if patient to undergo surgery. Increased likelihood of non-union, wound healing complications, and postoperative infection if diabetes not well controlled.

COMPLICATIONS
- Unidentified fractures can lead to debilitating joint deformities and skin ulcerations, increasing risk of infection.
- Collapse and inversion of arch into clubfoot or rocker-bottom foot
- Amputation

REFERENCES

1. Anderson JJ, et al. Bisphosphonates for the treatment of Charcot neuroarthropathy. *J Foot Ankle Surg*. 2004;43(5):285–9.
2. Chantelau E, et al. Palliative radiotherapy for acute osteoarthropathy of diabetic feet: A preliminary study. *Pract Diabetes Int*. 1997;14(6):154–6.

ADDITIONAL READING

Jude EB, et al. Medical treatment of Charcot's arthropathy. *J Am Podiatric Med Assoc*. 2002;92(7):381–3.

CODES

ICD9
- Neuropathic joint disease (Charcot's joints):
  - 094.0 Tabes dorsalis
  - 250.60 Diabetes mellitus with neurological manifestations, Type II or unspecified type, not stated as uncontrolled
- 713.5 Arthropathy associated with neurological disorders

CLINICAL PEARLS

- The most common presenting symptoms of Charcot joint are significant unilateral swelling, warmth, and erythema, usually in the feet. Patients may or may not recall minor preceding trauma.
- The goal of early prolonged immobilization is to prevent repetitive trauma and progression of arthropathy. Significant complications, such as severe foot deformities, ulcerations leading to infections, and amputation, can result if treatment is delayed.

CHICKENPOX (VARICELLA ZOSTER)

Kay A. Bauman, MD, MPH

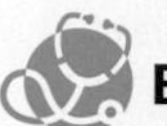

BASICS

DESCRIPTION

- Common, highly contagious generalized exanthem characterized by the development of crops of pruritic vesicles on the skin and mucous membranes.
- Fever in up to 70% of persons.
- Virus is spread by respiratory (airborne) droplets, direct contact with varicella vesicles, or rarely zoster lesions.
- Virus establishes latency in the dorsal root ganglia; reactivation results in herpes zoster or "shingles."
- Outbreaks tend to occur late winter to early spring in temperate climates.
- The usual incubation period is 14–16 days (range, 10–21). Patients are infectious from ~48 hours before appearance of the rash until the final lesions have crusted. Historically, most people acquire chickenpox during childhood and develop lifelong immunity. (1) Now it is an immunizable disease.
- System(s) affected: Nervous; Skin/Exocrine
- Synonym(s): Varicella

EPIDEMIOLOGY

- Predominant age: Peak incidence preschoolers to 9 years, but may occur at any age
- Predominant gender: Male = Female

Incidence

- Decreasing incidence since vaccine available: Estimated at 3.5 million cases annually prior to vaccine introduction with an incidence rate of 8–9% in children 1–9 years of age. Reported US varicella cases 1991: 147,076; reported for 2007: 40,146; reported for 2008: 30,386 (2,3).
- Prior to vaccine availability, ~100 deaths in the US/year were reported; for 2008, only 2 deaths were reported. (3,4,5)

RISK FACTORS

- No prior history of varicella infection
- Immunosuppressed patients (especially children with leukemia/lymphoma in remission or receiving high-dose corticosteroids)

Geriatric Considerations

- Infection more severe in adults than in children
- Latent varicella infection may reactivate and cause the exanthem known as shingles or zoster.
- Herpes zoster vaccine, a live attenuated vaccine licensed in 2006, is now recommended for persons ≥60 to prevent zoster (shingles):
  - 1-time dose. Recommended for those previously infected with varicella (chickenpox); those never infected should receive regular varicella vaccine (6). Dose: 0.65ml SQ, available as single dose vial.
- Most common cause of death: Primary viral pneumonia

Pediatric Considerations

- Neonates born to mothers who develop chickenpox from 5 days before to 2 days after delivery are at risk for serious disease. Must give varicella-zoster immune globulin
- Varicella bullosa seen mainly in children <2 years. Lesions appear as bullae instead of vesicles. The clinical course does not change.
- Most common cause of death: Septic complications and encephalitis
- Avoid aspirin/acetylsalicylic acid in children because of link to Reye syndrome.

Pregnancy Considerations

- Risk of transplacental infection after maternal infection is 25%.
- Congenital malformations are seen in 2% (1) of patients when the fetus is infected during the 1st or 2nd trimesters, characterized by limb atrophy and scarring of the skin of the extremities and occasional CNS and eye manifestations.
- Morbidity is increased in women infected during pregnancy (e.g., pneumonia).

GENERAL PREVENTION

- Exposed, susceptible people should be considered at risk and potentially infectious for 21 days.
- Isolate hospitalized patients.
- Passive immunization with IM varicella-zoster immune globulin given within 96 hours (preferably within 72 hours) of exposure to ensure efficacy (1):
  - Recommended for people exposed to chickenpox or shingles within 96 hours who are immunocompromised, ≥15 years old without prior history of chickenpox, newborns of mothers with onset of chickenpox <5 days before delivery or <2 days after delivery. Exposure criteria: Continued household contact, prolonged face-to-face contact (same room), or indoor playmate >1 hour
- Active immunization after exposure: Shown to prevent or reduce significantly the severity of varicella if given within 72 hours postexposure.
- Active immunization: Varicella virus vaccine (Varivax): Live attenuated vaccine approved by FDA in 1995 for pediatrics immunization and recommended by Advisory Committee on Immunization Practices for immunization of healthy patients ≥12 months who have not had chickenpox
- 12 months–12 years old: Initial dose 0.5 mL SC at age 12–15 months; 2nd dose age 4–6 years. Prelicensure studies showed efficacy rates: 70–90% against any disease and 95% against severe disease 7–10 years after vaccination. Other studies showed 100% efficacy at 1 year and 98% at 2 years after vaccination. More recent studies show rates of 85–94% effectiveness, the higher end for the prevention of severe disease. The 2-dose regimen is even more effective, with rates of 96–98% effectiveness. Breakthrough disease generally has <50 lesions, shorter duration of illness, and lower incidence of fever (7)[A].
- ≥13 years: 2 0.5 mL SC doses 4–8 weeks apart, seroconversion rates 78–82% after 1 dose, 99% after 2 doses (1). Adults have efficacy rates in the lower end of this range.
- Vaccine side effects are pain and redness at vaccine site.
- The newly approved MMRV vaccine which combines the measles, mumps, and rubella vaccine with varicella is equally effective. There are rare reports of an increased risk of febrile seizures 5–12 days after vaccination in 1/2300-2600 patients (8)[A].
- May be considered for a subset of HIV-positive children in CDC class I with CD4 >25% (1):
  - Vaccine recipients should avoid contact with immunocompromised people and pregnant women who have never had chickenpox and their newborns, for up to 6 weeks after vaccination.
  - Children needing catch-up vaccination need at least 3 months between doses 1 and 2.

PATHOPHYSIOLOGY

- Skin lesions identical histologically to those of herpes simplex virus.
- In fatal cases, intranuclear inclusions can be found in the endothelium of blood vessels and most organs.

ETIOLOGY

- Varicella-zoster virus is a member of the α-Herpesviridae subfamily; a double-stranded DNA virus.
- Reservoir is humans

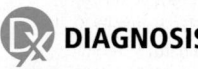

DIAGNOSIS

HISTORY

- Prodromal symptoms: Fever, malaise, anorexia, mild headache
- Malaise, muscle aches, arthralgias, and headache more common in adults (2)
- Subclinical in ~4% of cases

PHYSICAL EXAM

- Characteristic rash: Crops of "teardrop" vesicles on erythematous bases
- Lesions erupt in successive crops
- Progress from macule to papule to vesicle, then begin to crust
- Pruritic rash is present in various stages of development
- Lesions may be present on mucous membranes, both oral and vaginal

DIAGNOSTIC TESTS & INTERPRETATION

Generally used for complicated cases and epidemiologic studies

Lab

Initial lab tests

- Leukocyte count may be normal, low, or mildly increased.
- Marked leukocytosis suggests secondary infection.
- Multinucleated giant cells visible on Tzanck smear from scrapings of vesicles
- Isolated virus from human tissue culture

ollow-Up & Special Considerations

- Visualization of the virus by electron microscopy, tissue culture (costly), and various methods of acute and convalescent sera collection: Latex agglutination (most available), enzyme immunoassay, indirect immunofluorescence antibody, fluorescent antibody to membrane assay, or PCR assay, which can detect wild from vaccine viral strains (1)
- Vaccine-modified cases can be more difficult to diagnose; consider PCR testing of skin lesions (9)[B].

IFFERENTIAL DIAGNOSIS

- Herpes simplex virus infection
- Herpes zoster
- Impetigo
- Coxsackievirus infection
- Scabies
- Dermatitis herpetiformis
- Drug rash
- Rickettsial pox infection

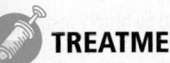

TREATMENT

utpatient except for complicating emergencies

MEDICATION

irst Line

- Supportive: Antipyretics for fever; avoid aspirin in children
- Local and/or systemic antipruritic agents for itching
- In immunocompromised patients: Varicella-zoster immune globulin available for passive immunization. Varicella-zoster immune globulin must be given within 96 hours after exposure to be beneficial. After 4th day postexposure, wait for rash to develop, then give acyclovir 500 mg/m^2/d q8 h for 7 days.
- Acyclovir: Decreases duration of fever and shortens time of viral shedding. Recommended for adolescents, adults, and high-risk patients. Most beneficial if initiated early in the disease (≤24 h).
  - 2–16-year-old patients: 20 mg/kg/dose (max. 800 mg/dose), q.i.d. for 5 days
  - Adults: 800 mg, 5 times daily.
- Contraindications.
  - Hypersensitivity to the drug
- Precautions
  - Possible renal insufficiency with acyclovir
  - Significant possible interactions
  - Concurrent administration of probenecid increases half-life; increased effects with zidovudine (e.g., drowsiness, lethargy)

Second Line

- Famciclovir: 500 mg t.i.d. for 7–10 days (adults)
- Valacyclovir: 1 g t.i.d. for 7–10 days (adults)

ADDITIONAL TREATMENT

General Measures

- Supportive/symptomatic treatment
- Antihistamines and/or Aveeno or oatmeal baths as needed for itch
- Acetaminophen and/or ibuprofen as needed
- Nail clipping in children to prevent scarring or secondary infection from itching

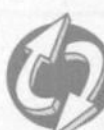

ONGOING CARE

FOLLOW-UP RECOMMENDATIONS

Patient Monitoring

- Usually none needed in mild cases. If complications occur, intensive supportive care may be required.
- Activity as tolerated. Children may return to school when lesions have scabbed.

DIET

No special diet

PATIENT EDUCATION

- In the healthy child, chickenpox is rarely serious and recovery is complete
- Confers lifelong immunity
- 2nd attack rare, but subclinical infection can occur; happens occasionally after vaccination in children
- Infection latent and may recur years later as herpes zoster in adults (and sometimes in children)
- Fatalities rarely occur from complications

COMPLICATIONS

- Although only 2% of cases are reported after 2nd decade, 35% of deaths occur in this age group (2)
- Secondary bacterial infection: Cellulitis, abscess, erysipelas, sepsis, septic arthritis/osteomyelitis, or staphylococcal pyomyositis
- Pneumonia: 20–30% of adults with chickenpox have lung involvement, 1/400 are hospitalized (2)
- Encephalitis (the most common CNS complication)
- Meningitis
- Reye syndrome
- Purpura
- Thrombocytopenia
- Glomerulonephritis
- Arthritis
- Hepatitis

REFERENCES

1. American Academy of Pediatrics. *Report of the Committee on Infectious Diseases (Red Book)*. Elk Grove Village, IL: American Academy of Pediatrics, 2003.
2. Goldman L, Bennett JC, ed. *Cecil Textbook of Medicine*, 21st ed. Philadelphia: WB Saunders, 2000.
3. Centers for Disease Control and Prevention. *MMWR* 2010;58:869.
4. Centers for Disease Control and Prevention. Summary of Notifiable Diseases, US, 1991. *MMWR*. 1992;40(No. 53).
5. Centers for Disease Control and Prevention (CDC). Varicella-related deaths–United States, January 2003-June 2004. *MMWR Morb Mortal Wkly Rep*. 2005;54:272–4.
6. *The Medical Letter*. 2006;48:73–4.
7. Marin M, Güris D, Chaves SS, Schmid S, Seward JF, Advisory Committee on Immunization Practices, Centers for Disease Control and Prevention (CDC) et al. Prevention of varicella: recommendations of the Advisory Committee on Immunization Practices (ACIP). *MMWR Recomm Rep*. 2007;56:1–40.
8. Marin M, Broder KR, Temte JL, Snider DE, Seward JF, Centers for Disease Control and Prevention (CDC) et al. Use of combination measles, mumps, rubella, and varicella vaccine: recommendations of the Advisory Committee on Immunization Practices (ACIP). *MMWR Recomm Rep*. 2010;59:1–12.
9. Leung J, Harpaz R, Baughman AL, Heath K, Loparev V, Vázquez M, Watson BM, Schmid DS et al. Evaluation of laboratory methods for diagnosis of varicella. *Clin Infect Dis*. 2010;51:23–32.

C

ADDITIONAL READING

- Campos-Outcalt D. Varicella vaccination: 2 doses now the standard. *J Fam Pract*. 2008;57:38–40.
- Galea SA, Sweet A, Beninger P, Steinberg SP, Larussa PS, Gershon AA, Sharrar RG et al. The safety profile of varicella vaccine: a 10-year review. *J Infect Dis*. 2008;197 (Suppl 2):S165–9.

See Also (Topic, Algorithm, Electronic Media Element)

Herpes Zoster

CODES

ICD9

052.9 Varicella without mention of complication

CLINICAL PEARLS

- Infection is more likely to produce serious illness in adults than in children.
- All people being immunized should receive two doses of vaccine, preferably at least 3 months but no fewer than 28 days apart.
- Herpes zoster vaccine (Zostavax) recommended for persons ≥60 years of age to prevent shingles (zoster).

CHILD ABUSE

Karen A. Hulbert, MD

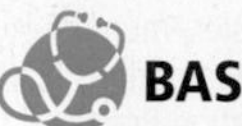

BASICS

DESCRIPTION

- Types of abuse: Neglect (most common and highest mortality), physical abuse, emotional/psychological abuse, sexual abuse—often in combination
- Child Abuse Hotline by state: http://www.childwelfare.gov/responding/reporting.cfm or call 800-4-A-Child (800-422-4453)
- System(s) affected: Gastrointestinal (GI); Endocrine/Metabolic; Musculoskeletal; Nervous; Renal; Reproductive; Skin/Exocrine; Psychiatric
- Synonym(s): Suspected nonaccidental trauma, child maltreatment, child neglect

EPIDEMIOLOGY

Prevalence

- An estimated 905,000 children in the US were victims of child abuse or neglect in 2006 out of approximately 3.6 million who received investigation (1).
- It is estimated that the actual number of victims is 3× greater than number reported
- Remains the 4th leading cause of childhood death in the US (2)

RISK FACTORS

- All ages; Male = Female:
  - Risk of physical abuse increases with age
  - Risk of fatal abuse more common <age 2
  - Physical abuse 2.1× higher among children with disabilities (3)
- Poverty, drug abuse, lower educational status, parental history of abuse, mentally ill parent/maternal depression, poor support network, and domestic violence:
  - Child abuse may be 4.9× more likely in family with spouse abuse (3)
  - Children in households with unrelated adults 50× more likely to die of inflicted injuries (3)
  - Adults who were abused as children are at much higher risk of becoming abusers than those not raised with abuse

GENERAL PREVENTION

- Know your patients and document their family situations; have increased suspicion to screen for risk factors at prenatal, postnatal, pediatric visit.
- Physicians can educate parents on range of normal behaviors to expect in infants and children:
  - Anticipatory guidance on ways to handle crying infants; methods of discipline for toddlers
- Train first responders—teachers, childcare workers—to look for signs of abuse
- Early childhood home visitation programs recommended to reduce maltreatment in high-risk families (4)[A]
- More research urgently needed to assess effectiveness of interventions such as parenting programs on ability to reduce abuse and neglect

COMMONLY ASSOCIATED CONDITIONS

- Failure to thrive
- Prematurity
- Developmental deficits
- Poor school performance
- Poor social skills
- Low self-esteem, depression

DIAGNOSIS

Documentation:

- Information in the medical record is an important piece of evidence for investigation and litigation (5)[C]
- Critical elements include (5)[C]:
  - Brief statement of child's disclosure or caregiver's explanation, including any alternate explanations offered
  - Time the incident occurred and date/time of disclosure
  - Whether witnesses were present
  - Developmental abilities of child
  - Objective medical findings
  - Interpretation of the findings
- DO NOT use terms such as "rule out," "R/O," and "alleged." They may cause ambiguity; clearly state physician opinion (5)[C].
- Documentation should include disposition of patient and record any report made to child protective services (5)[C].

HISTORY

- Use nonjudgmental, open-ended questions (ask: who, what, when, and where; NEVER why)
- Use quotes whenever possible
- Document past medical and developmental history, child's temperament, interactions among family members.
- Suggestive of intentional trauma:
  - No explanation or vague explanation (3)
  - Important detail of explanation changes dramatically (3)
  - Explanation is inconsistent with pattern, age, or severity (3)
  - Explanation is inconsistent with child's physical or developmental abilities (3)
  - Different witnesses provide markedly different history (3)
  - Considerable delay in seeking treatment
- Nonspecific symptoms of abuse:
  - Behavior changes; self-destructive behavior
  - Anxiety and/or depression
  - Sleep disturbances, night terrors
  - School problems

PHYSICAL EXAM

- General assessment for signs of physical abuse, neglect, self-injurious behaviors (6)[C]
- Thorough physical exam:
  - Skin, head, eyes, ears, nose, and mouth
  - Chest/abdomen
  - Genital (consider exam under sedation) or refer to ED
  - Extremities with focus on inner arms and legs
  - Growth data
- Maintain high index of suspicion for occult head, chest, and abdominal trauma
- Physical abuse:
  - Skin markings (e.g., lacerations, burns, ecchymoses, linear/shaped contusions, bites)
  - Immersion injuries with clearly distinguished outlines (e.g., from boiling water)
  - Oral trauma (e.g., torn frenulum, loose teeth)
  - Ear trauma (e.g., signs of ear pulling)
  - Eye trauma (e.g., hyphema, hemorrhage)
  - Head/abdominal blunt trauma
  - Fractures
- Sexual abuse:
  - Unexplained penile, vaginal, hymenal, perianal, or anal injuries/bleeding/discharge
  - Pregnancy or sexually transmitted infections (STIs)
  - Sperm is a definitive finding of child abuse
- Neglect:
  - Child may be undersized or unkempt
  - Rashes
  - Fearful or too trusting
  - Clinging to or avoiding caregiver
  - Flat or balding occiput
  - Abnormal development or growth parameters
- Measurements, photographs, careful descriptions are critical for accurate diagnosis
- Collaboration with specialist and child abuse assessment team (3)[C]

DIAGNOSTIC TESTS & INTERPRETATION

Lab

Initial lab tests

- Lab testing should be directed by history and physical exam:
  - Urinalysis (e.g., abdominal/flank/back/genital trauma)
  - Complete blood chemistry. Consideration of coagulation studies and platelet count (e.g., rule out bleeding disorder, abdominal trauma) as appropriate.
  - Electrolytes, creatinine, blood urea nitrogen, glucose
  - Liver and pancreatic function tests (e.g., abdominal trauma)
  - Guaiac stool (abdominal trauma)
- In cases of suspected neglect:
  - Stool exam, calorie count, purified protein derivative and anergy panel, sweat test, lead and zinc levels
- In cases of suspected sexual abuse:
  - STI testing: Gonorrhea, chlamydia, trichomonas; also consider HIV, HSV, hepatitis panel, syphilis (6)[C]
  - Serum pregnancy test (6)[C]

Follow-Up & Special Considerations

Bruising is a common presenting feature:

- Bruising in babies that are not independently mobile is very uncommon (<1%) (7)[A]
- Patterns suggestive of abuse (7)[A]:
  - Bruises seen away from bony prominences
  - Bruises to face, back, abdomen, arms, buttocks, ears, hands
  - Multiple bruises in clusters
  - Multiple bruises of uniform shape
  - Bruises that carry imprint of an implement

Imaging

Initial approach

Imaging should be directed by history and injury/condition:

- All children with fractures and children with suspicious injuries under age 2:
  - Skeletal survey (3)[B]: X-rays include 2 views of each extremity, skull: (AP) and lateral, spine: AP and lateral, chest x-ray, and/or rib (posterior), abdomen, pelvis, hands, and feet
  - Consider bone scan for acute rib fractures and subtle long bone fractures (3)[B]

Intracranial and extracranial injury:
- CT scan of head (3)[B]
- Consider MRI of head/neck for better dating of injuries, looking at subtle findings, intercerebral edema, or hemorrhage (3)[B]

Intra-abdominal injuries:
- CT scan of abdomen

Diagnostic Procedures/Surgery
Sexual abuse:
Consider photocolposcopy
<72 hours from time of abuse: Collect samples for the forensic laboratory (contact authorities for appropriate protocol) (6)[C]

Pathological Findings
Spiral fractures in nonambulatory patients (children that are not walking or cruising should not have bruising or fractures from "falls")
Chip or bucket-handle fractures
Epiphysial/metaphysial rib fractures in infants
Rupture of liver/spleen in abdominal blunt trauma
Retinal hemorrhages in shaken baby syndrome

DIFFERENTIAL DIAGNOSIS
Physical trauma (including but not limited to):
- Accidental injury; toxic ingestion
- Bleeding disorders (e.g., classic hemophilia)
- Metabolic diseases; congenital conditions
- Conditions with skin manifestations (e.g., mongolian spots, Henoch-Schönlein purpura, meningococcemia, erythema multiforme, hypersensitivity, car seat burns, staphylococcal scalded skin syndrome, chickenpox, impetigo)
- Cultural practices (e.g., cupping, coining)

Neglect (including but not limited to):
- Endocrinopathies (e.g., diabetes mellitus)
- Constitutional
- GI (clefts, malabsorption, irritable bowel)
- Seizure disorder
- Sudden infant death syndrome (SIDS)

Skeletal trauma (including but not limited to):
- Obstetrical trauma
- Nutritional (scurvy, rickets)
- Infection (congenital syphilis, osteomyelitis)
- Osteogenesis imperfecta

Neoplasm

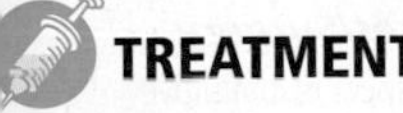

TREATMENT

MEDICATION
First Line
Antibiotics as indicated for treatment of documented STIs or infection

Second Line
Consider antidepressants if needed.

ALERT
Emergency contraception reduces rate of pregnancy after sexual assault if given within 5 days
- Levonorgestrel 1.5 mg as a single dose as effective as 2 split doses (0.75 mg each) 12 hours apart (8)[A]

ADDITIONAL TREATMENT
General Measures
- Always explain what the physical exam will involve and why certain procedures are necessary.
- Examine child in a comfortable setting.
- Allow child to choose who will be in the room.
- Use appropriate positions to examine the anal and genital areas of young children (6)[C].
- Test for STIs before treatment (6)[C].

Issues for Referral
- Consider managing in ER to collect forensic specimens and maintain chain of evidence.
- Mandatory reporting to child protective authorities

SURGERY/OTHER PROCEDURES
As clinically indicated

IN-PATIENT CONSIDERATIONS
Initial Stabilization
As clinically indicated

Admission Criteria
- Moderate-to-severe injuries or unstable
- Acute psychological trauma
- If safety of child outside the hospital cannot be guaranteed

IV Fluids
As clinically indicated

Nursing
As clinically indicated

Discharge Criteria
- Child should be sent to another relative or into foster care if the suspected abuser lives with the child.
- Counseling for individual and family
- After initial evaluation, consider referral to sexual assault center.

ONGOING CARE

FOLLOW-UP RECOMMENDATIONS
As clinically indicated

Patient Monitoring
- Refer to the state protective services
- Monitor injury healing over time
- Follow-up assessment for STIs that may not present acutely (e.g., HPV, herpes) (6)[C]

DIET
Routine

PATIENT EDUCATION
As clinically indicated

PROGNOSIS
Without intervention, child abuse is often a chronic and escalating phenomenon.

COMPLICATIONS
- Long-term physical and psychological damage
- Death

REFERENCES

1. Department of Health and Human Services, Administration on Children, Youth, and Families (ACF). Child Maltreatment 2006.
2. Deaths: Leading Causes for 2006. *Natl Vital Stat Rep*. 2010;58;14:1–100.
3. Kellogg ND, American Academy of Pediatrics Committee on Child Abuse and Neglect. Evaluation of suspected child physical abuse. *Pediatrics*. 2007; 119(6):1232–41.
4. Hahn RA, Bilukha OO, Crosby A et al. First reports evaluating the effectiveness of strategies for preventing violence: early childhood home visitation. Findings from the Task Force on Community Preventive Services. *MMWR Recomm Rep*. 2003;52(RR-14):1–9.
5. Jackson A, et al: Let the Record Speak: Medicolegal Documentation in Cases of Child Maltreatment. *Clin Ped Emerg Med*. 2006;7:181–5.
6. Nancy Kellogg and the Committee on Child Abuse and Neglect. The evaluation of sexual abuse in children. *Pediatrics*. 2005;116:506–12.
7. Maguire S, Mann MK, Sibert J, et al. Are there patterns of bruising in childhood which are diagnostic or suggestive of abuse? A systematic review. *Arch Dis Child*. 2005;90:182–6.
8. Cheng L, Gülmezoglu AM, Van Oel CJ, et al. Interventions for emergency contraception. *The Cochrane Database of Systematic Reviews*. 2004, Issue 3.

ADDITIONAL READING

Child Abuse Evaluation & Treatment for medical providers (http://www.ChildAbuseMD.com).

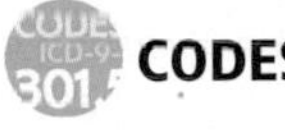

CODES

ICD9
- 995.50 Unspecified child abuse
- 995.51 Child emotional/psychological abuse
- 995.52 Child neglect (nutritional)

CLINICAL PEARLS

- High index of suspicion important for both prevention (knowing risk factors, ways to intervene) and recognition of abuse.
- Neglect is the most common and lethal form of abuse and should be aggressively reported.
- Detailed exam with documentation is key.
- Mandated reporting is required for suspected child abuse and neglect (reasonable suspicion); the physician does not have to prove abuse before reporting.
- Child Abuse Hotline by state: http://www.childwelfare.gov/responding/reporting.cfm or call 800-4-A-Child (800-422-4453).

CHLAMYDIA PNEUMONIAE

Lawrence M. Hwang, MD
Daniel T. Lee, MD

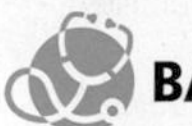

BASICS

DESCRIPTION
- *Chlamydia pneumoniae*, an obligate intracellular, gram-negative bacterium, has been established as an important cause of adult and pediatric respiratory disease and is capable of causing persistent latent infection.
- Humans are the only known reservoir.
- 1st recognized as a respiratory pathogen in 1989
- System(s) affected: Respiratory; Cardiovascular; Neurologic
- Synonym(s): Taiwan acute respiratory agent; *Chlamydophila pneumoniae*

EPIDEMIOLOGY
- Incubation period is approximately 30 days.
- Predominant age: More common in elderly; less common in children 2 months–5 years
- Serologic evidence of acute and chronic infection found in 1/3 of patients with acute chronic obstructive pulmonary disease (COPD) exacerbation, often together with other concurrent bacterial infection

Incidence
- Overall incidence rate of *C. pneumoniae* is unknown
- No particular seasonal variation
- Outbreaks have occurred among military recruits, university students, and nursing home residents.

Prevalence
- Accounts for 5–20% of community-acquired pneumonia in adults and children. Greatly varied rates exist between study locations.
- Most cases occur sporadically, although intrafamilial spread also occurs.

Pediatric Considerations
Uncommon in children 2 months–5 years of age

GENERAL PREVENTION
- As transmission is via contact with respiratory secretions, advise hand-washing and avoid exposure to infected persons.
- Flu and pneumococcal vaccines for high-risk groups

PATHOPHYSIOLOGY
Infection with *C. pneumoniae* and resultant host responses may lead to mucus production in the nasal passages, sinuses, bronchial tree, and alveoli, along with nasopharyngeal and airway inflammation and bronchospasm.

COMMONLY ASSOCIATED CONDITIONS
- COPD
- Asthma
- HIV infection
- Cystic fibrosis
- Diabetes mellitus
- Atherosclerosis
- Multiple sclerosis
- Alzheimer disease

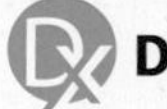

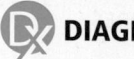

DIAGNOSIS

Geriatric Considerations
- Usually more severe disease in older adults, and more common in the elderly who also have concomitant medical problems.
- Elderly patients less likely to exhibit respiratory symptoms with pneumonia and may present with altered mental status or history of falls.

HISTORY
- Spectrum of illness may vary from mild and self-limited to severe pneumonia.
- Onset often gradual with delayed presentation
- Sore throat and hoarseness may precede cough by a week or more, giving biphasic appearance to illness (uncommon in *Legionella*, less common in *Mycoplasma, Streptococcus pneumoniae*, and *Haemophilus influenzae*).
- Dry cough
- Low grade fever (usually early in illness)
- Chills
- Rhinitis
- Headache
- Malaise
- Myalgias
- Sinus congestion
- Nausea
- Altered mental status

PHYSICAL EXAM
- General appearance usually nontoxic, unless extremely ill
- Fever
- Tachypnea
- Tachycardia
- Diminished breath sounds
- Crackles or wheezing
- Bronchial breath sounds
- Percussion dullness and egophony less sensitive but more specific for pneumonia
- Pharyngeal erythema (without exudates)
- Retropharyngeal lymphoid granulation

DIAGNOSTIC TESTS & INTERPRETATION

Lab
Initial lab tests
- Multiple unreliable laboratory methods for diagnos including culture, antigen detection, serology, PCR
- Leukocyte count usually normal or low, but may be mildly elevated
- Blood cultures recommended if toxic and requiring ICU admission; otherwise not likely to be helpful
- Culture has traditionally been the gold standard diagnostic method (1)[A]:
  - Many limitations include technical complexity, limited availability, and variable yield (1)[A]
  - Most easily cultured in HL or HEp2 cells (culture is 10–80% sensitive and >95% specific) (2)[A]
- Testing with microimmunofluorescence (MIF) is recommended by CDC, as enzyme immunoassay testing is less specific. However, MIF testing is not standardized for *C. pneumoniae* and may also lack specificity and sensitivity (2)[A].
  - 4-fold increase in IgG titer diagnostic of acute infection (10–100% sensitivity) (2)[A]
  - Presence of IgM antibody (≥1:16) (1)[A]
  - Single IgG titers are discouraged (1)[A]
- Complement fixation for *Chlamydia* is widely available but cannot distinguish *C. pneumonia* from *Chlamydophila psittaci*.
- PCR from pharyngeal swab or bronchioalveolar lavage specimen (30–95% sensitivity, >95% specificity) (2)[A]

Imaging
Initial approach
- Patients with suspected community-acquired pneumonia who are more than mildly ill should be evaluated with a chest x-ray (CXR) (2)[A].
  - CXR may be abnormal even in clinically mild disease.
- Variable radiographic abnormalities include unilateral and bilateral infiltrates and pleural effusions. Single, subsegmental funnel-shaped or circumscribed infiltrate is common.

Diagnostic Procedures/Surgery
Although serology is 95% specific, definitive diagnosis requires a positive culture or PCR testing (2)[A].

IFFERENTIAL DIAGNOSIS

Other causes of atypical pneumonia, including *M. pneumoniae* and *L. pneumophila*
Other bacterial causes of pneumonia, including *S. pneumoniae*. *H. influenzae*, *Moraxella catarrhalis*, and *Staphylococcus aureus*
Respiratory viruses: Adenovirus, influenza A, influenza B, parainfluenza virus, and respiratory syncytial virus
Endemic fungal pathogens: Blastomycosis, coccidioidomycosis, histoplasmosis
Bioterrorism agents: Anthrax, plague, tularemia
Conditions that mimic community-acquired pneumonia: Acute respiratory disease syndrome, atelectasis, idiopathic pulmonary fibrosis, neoplasm, pulmonary embolus, sarcoidosis, congestive heart failure

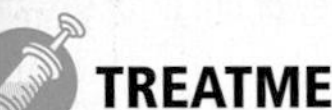

TREATMENT

IEDICATION

β-Lactam antibiotics and sulfasoxazole not effective for *C. pneumoniae*.

An advantage in clinical efficacy or mortality by empiric coverage of atypical pathogens in patients with community-acquired pneumonia has not been shown (3)[A].

The treatment course may be extended by several weeks in certain patients whose symptoms have not resolved.

irst Line

Azithromycin: 500 mg on day 1, then 250 mg on days 2–5 *OR*
Clarithromycin: 500 mg q12h for 10–14 days *OR*
Doxycycline, 100 mg q12h for at least 14 days (4)[C]:
- Tetracycline not for use during pregnancy or in children <8 years
- Tetracycline may cause photosensitivity; sunscreen is recommended.
  - Tetracyclines may increase the anticoagulant effect of warfarin.

econd Line

Alternative drugs: Erythromycin base, 250–500 mg q.i.d. for 14–21 days
Levofloxacin, 250–500 mg/d (PO or IV) or other respiratory fluoroquinolones have good bioavailability and the convenience of once-daily dosing, but are recommended for use only when patients have failed treatment with a 1st-line drug, or have had recent antibiotics, significant comorbidities, or allergies to alternatives.

regnancy Considerations

etracyclines and fluoroquinolones are ontraindicated.

COMPLEMENTARY AND ALTERNATIVE MEDICINE

In small studies, manipulative treatment was shown to reduce duration of intravenous antibiotic treatment and days in the hospital for hospitalized elderly patients with pneumonia (5)[C].

IN-PATIENT CONSIDERATIONS

- Usually outpatient care for most. Those with severe pneumonia or coexisting illness may require hospitalization.
- Pneumonia severity index or other validated prediction rule can assist in predicting those patients with community-acquired pneumonia with higher morbidity and those requiring hospitalization (6)[A].

Initial Stabilization

Infection in debilitated or hospitalized patients can be severe. Stabilize respiratory distress as per advanced cardiac life support protocol.

IV Fluids

Increased fluids generally recommended

Discharge Criteria

Reversal of any respiratory distress, with the patient tolerating oral medications, otherwise stable medically, and stable for discharge per the clinical judgment of the physician

ONGOING CARE

FOLLOW-UP RECOMMENDATIONS

Patient Monitoring

- Weekly patient monitoring until well
- Follow-up chest x-ray for resolution
- Reinfection is possible
- Some reports of individuals who are persistently culture-positive despite antibiotic treatment

PROGNOSIS

- Pneumonia is especially life-threatening in older adults and patients with other illnesses that affect the lungs (e.g., asthma, COPD) or the immune system (e.g., diabetes), with an overall 0.5–29% mortality rate.
- Estimated mortality rate from *C. pneumoniae* is 9%, but this may be an overestimate due to the number of subclinical cases.
- Death usually from secondary infection or underlying comorbidity

COMPLICATIONS

- Reactive airway disease
- Erythema nodosum
- Otitis media
- Endocarditis
- Pericarditis or myocarditis
- Meningoencephalitis
- Associated with atherosclerotic disease: *C. pneumoniae* has been cultured from atherosclerotic plaque in patients with coronary artery disease, but treatment has not been shown to affect mortality.

REFERENCES

1. Kumar S, Hammerschlag MR. Acute respiratory infection due to Chlamydia pneumoniae: current status of diagnostic methods. *Clin Infect Dis*. 2007;44:568–76.
2. Lutfiyya MN, et al. Diagnosis and treatment of community-acquired pneumonia. *AFP*. 2006;73:3: 442–50.
3. Shefet D, et al. Empiric antibiotic coverage of atypical pathogens for community acquired pneumonia in hospitalized adults. *Cochrane Database Syst Rev*. 2006;1:CD004418.
4. Kauppinen M, Saikku P. Pneumonia due to Chlamydia pneumoniae: prevalence, clinical features, diagnosis, and treatment. *Clin Infect Dis*. 1995;21(Suppl 3):S244–52.
5. Noll DR, Shores JH, Gamber RG, et al. Benefits of osteopathic manipulative treatment for hospitalized elderly patients with pneumonia. *J Am Osteopath Assoc*. 2000;100:776–82.
6. Fine MJ, Auble TE, Yealy DM, et al. A prediction rule to identify low risk patients with community-acquired pneumonia. *N Engl J Med*. 1997;336:243–50.

ADDITIONAL READING

- Blasi F, Tarsia P, Aliberti S. Chlamydophila pneumoniae. *Clin Microbiol Infect*. 2009;15:29–35.
- Miyashita N, et al. Clinical presentation of community-acquired *Chlamydia pneumonia* in adults. *Chest*. 2002;121:1176–81.
- Thibodeau KP, et al. Atypical pathogens and challenges in community-acquired pneumonia. *AFP*. 2004;69:7:1701–6.

See Also (Topic, Algorithm, Electronic Media Element)

Algorithm: Cough, Chronic

CODES

ICD9

483.1 Pneumonia due to chlamydia

CLINICAL PEARLS

- *C. pneumoniae* is a significant cause of adult and pediatric pneumonias.
- Formal and accurate diagnosis of *C. pneumoniae* is difficult due to lack of standardized diagnostic tests. Culture remains the gold standard.
- Initial treatment should include tetracyclines, macrolides, and quinolones.

CHLAMYDIAL SEXUALLY TRANSMITTED DISEASES

Autumn Davidson, MD
Jeremy Golding, MD

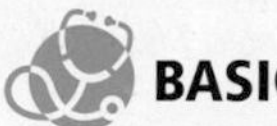

BASICS

DESCRIPTION

- An obligate intracellular membrane-bound prokaryotic organism, *C. trachomatis* is the most common bacterial sexually transmitted infection in the US.
- Transmitted through vaginal, anal, or oral sex. May also occur vertically from mother to infant during vaginal birth.
- Screening has increased over the last 20 years, but remains suboptimal with annual screening rates of only 42% among sexually active females ages 16–25 in 2007.
- Majority of cases are asymptomatic (75–90% females, 50–75% males)
- If untreated, may lead to pelvic inflammatory disease, ectopic pregnancies, and infertility.
- System(s) affected: Reproductive

Pregnancy Considerations

Perinatal acquisition may result in neonatal pneumonia and/or conjunctivitis.

EPIDEMIOLOGY

Incidence

- Mandatory reporting started in 1985 with national data showing steady increase in incidence since.
- 1.2 million *reported* cases in 2008, with >3 million estimated cases yearly in the US. Increasing incidence reflects greater screening and improved testing modalities.

Prevalence

- 401.3 per 100,000 people in the US in 2008. This was a 9.2% increase from 2007.
- Populations most affected: Young females, particularly those of ethnic minority groups
- Peak incidence: Late teens, early 20s
- Predominant sex: Females have higher reported incidence and prevalence than males, but this likely reflects increased testing in females.
- Minorities bear the highest burden, with infection rates among blacks in 2008, 8× that of whites. Rates among American Indian/Alaska natives and Hispanics were 4.9 and 2.9 times higher than whites, respectively. Rates higher in US southern states as compared with the Northeast.

RISK FACTORS

Risk correlates with:

- Number of lifetime sexual partners
- Number of concurrent sexual partners
- Use of oral contraceptives (due to resulting cervical ectopy)
- Younger age (highest in females 15–19 years, males 20–24 years)
- Black/Hispanic/American Indian and Alaskan native ethnicity (1)

GENERAL PREVENTION

- Populations with prevalence >5% should be screened at least annually (2). Screen if: New or >1 sex partner in past 6 months, attending an adolescent or family-planning clinic or an STD or abortion clinic, attending a jail or other detention-center clinic, rectal pain, discharge or tenesmus, testicular pain, testing of any individual with urethral or cervical discharge.
- All sexually active women <25 years of age should be screened at least yearly, and repeat testing in approximately 3 months is recommended for those who screen positive, not as test of cure but because reinfection rate is high regardless of whether the sexual partner is treated (2)[A].
- Screening sexually active men <25 years is controversial but should be strongly considered in high-risk populations (3,4)[A].

ETIOLOGY

C. trachomatis serotypes D–K

COMMONLY ASSOCIATED CONDITIONS

- Females:
  - PID: As many as 40% of untreated women will develop PID
  - Infertility
  - Ectopic pregnancies
  - Chronic pelvic pain
  - Mucopurulent cervicitis with cervical edema and propensity to bleed during speculum
  - Urethral syndrome (common in women with dysuria, frequency and pyuria in the absence of infection with uropathogen)
- Males:
  - Epididymitis
  - Nongonococcal urethritis
  - Reiter's syndrome (HLA-B27)
  - Proctitis (Men who have sex with men)
- Neonates:
  - Inclusion conjunctivitis
  - Otitis media
  - Pneumonia
- Diseases caused by other chlamydial species:
  - Lymphogranuloma venereum: *C. trachomatis* serotypes L1–L3
  - Trachoma: *C. trachomatis* serotypes A–C

DIAGNOSIS

- Majority of patients are asymptomatic. Of those with symptoms, the most common are as follows:
  - In females: Mucopurulent vaginal discharge, dysuria (urethral syndrome), bartholinitis, abdominopelvic pain (endometritis, salpingitis/PID), right upper quadrant pain (Fitz-Hugh-Curtis perihepatitis syndrome)
  - In males: Dysuria, urethral discharge (urethritis), scrotal pain (epididymitis), rectal pain or discharge (proctitis), acute arthritis (Reiter syndrome)
  - In infants: Conjunctivitis, pneumonitis, carriage in pharynx/gastrointestinal tract
- Lymphogranuloma venereum (LVG) (*C. trachomatis* serovars L1, L2, or L3): Primary lesion is a small genital or rectal papule that may ulcerate at the site of transmission after an incubation period of 3–30 days. Most common manifestation in heterosexuals is unilateral tender lymphadenopathy. With rectal transmission, LGV causes an invasive proctocolitis, which may be scarring and cause strictures.

HISTORY

- Complete sexual history, including number of sex partners lifetime and past year, prior history of sexually transmitted infections, use of barrier protection, exchange of money or drugs for sex, or or anal receptive intercourse
- Symptom history, with onset date for each symptom

PHYSICAL EXAM

- Men and women:
  - External genitalia (rash? lesions?)
  - Urethra (discharge?)
  - Inguinal lymph nodes
  - Pharynx and perianal area, if history indicates
- In addition, for women:
  - Cervix (discharge? motion tenderness?)
  - Uterus, ovaries, adnexae

DIAGNOSTIC TESTS & INTERPRETATION

Lab

- Test of choice: Nucleic acid amplification tests (NAAT)
  - Amplified molecular testing (e.g., PCR, ligase chain reaction, specific dynamic action, human chorionic somatotropin, thyroid microsomal antigen): Sensitivity >95%; specificity >99%. Urine equally as sensitive as cervical swab. Patient self-collected vaginal swabs have also been shown to be effective. Lab tests may remain positive for as long as 3 weeks after successful treatment
- Chlamydial cell culture: Sensitivity 50–90%; specificity >99%
- Enzyme immunoassay: Sensitivity 40-60%; specificity >99%
- Direct fluorescent antibody detection: Sensitivity 50–70%; specificity >99%
- Specimens should contain cell scrapings rather than inflammatory discharge because the organism lives only inside the epithelial cells.

Imaging

Imaging not indicated for initial screening; consider pelvic ultrasound/CT if high clinical suspicion for PID or tubo-ovarian abscess.

Initial approach

Offer testing for other STDs including gonorrhea, HIV, syphilis, and for HPV

Follow-Up & Special Considerations

Test of cure not routinely recommended with exceptions for the following patients: Those in whom symptoms persist, those in whom adherence to medication regimens may not be complete, and pregnant females.

DIFFERENTIAL DIAGNOSIS

- *N. gonorrhoeae:* Urethritis, proctitis, epididymitis, cervicitis, PID, Bartholin abscess, perihepatitis
- *Mycoplasma* or *U. urealyticum*: Urethritis, epididymitis, Reiter disease, PID
- *C. trachomatis* (serotypes L1–L3): LGV, Proctitis

TREATMENT

EDICATION

rst Line

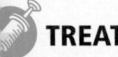

atment of chlamydial urethritis, cervicitis (including xual partners of infected persons):

- Azithromycin 1 g PO single dose, *or*
- Doxycycline: 100 mg PO b.i.d. × 7 days

egnancy Considerations

- In pregnant women: Tetracycline and ofloxacin are contraindicated during pregnancy; consider azithromycin or amoxicillin
  - Azithromycin as above, *or*
  - Amoxicillin 500 mg PO t.i.d. × 7 days
- 1st-line PID treatment (outpatient):
  - Ceftriaxone 250 mg IM × 1 PLUS Doxycycline 100 mg PO × 14 days with or without Metronidazole 500 mg PO b.i.d. × 14 days, *or*
  - Cefoxitin 2g IM × 1 with Probenecid 1 g PO × 1 PLUS doxycycline 100 mg PO × 14 days with or without Metronidazole 500 mg PO b.i.d. × 14 days
- 1st-line PID treatment parenteral therapy: See "Pelvic Inflammatory Disease"
- 1st-line treatment of LGV: Doxycycline 100 mg b.i.d. × 21 days *or* erythromycin base 500 mg orally q.i.d. × 21 days
- Tetracyclines may cause photosensitivity; sunscreen is recommended. Avoid concurrent administration of tetracyclines with antacids, dairy products, or iron.
- Practitioners may elect to give azithromycin and ceftriaxone together to the patient in the office to reduce patient noncompliance.

egnancy Considerations

tracyclines (e.g., doxycycline) and quinolones (e.g., loxacin, levofloxacin) are contraindicated in egnant women.

ediatric Considerations

tracyclines and quinolones are contraindicated in ildren.

econd Line

2nd-line therapy for chlamydial urethritis/cervicitis

- Erythromycin base: 500 mg PO q.i.d. × 7 days
- Erythromycin ethylsuccinate: 800 mg PO q.i.d. × 7 days
- Ofloxacin: 300 mg PO b.i.d. × 7 days
- Levofloxacin: 500 mg PO daily × 7 days

DDITIONAL TREATMENT

pedited partner therapy (EPT) is the practice of ysicians delivering medications or prescriptions to xual partners of persons infected with STIs without nical assessment of the partners.

- Treatment of sexual partners is a key component to STI control. EPT has been shown to be more effective than traditional partner referral in reducing recurrence rates.
- EPT is currently legal is 23 states, "potentially allowable" in 19 states, and illegal in 8. The logistics of this practice differ from state to state and continue to evolve.
- For an updated review on the legal status of EPT, please refer to the CDC website on this subject: http://www.cdc.gov/std/ept/legal/default.htm.

General Measures

- All patients with known or suspected chlamydia should be tested for gonorrhea, syphilis, and HIV (the latter requires individual counseling and consent) (2)[C].
- Ensure females are up to date with pap smears.
- Some experts recommend that all patients treated for chlamydia should be treated empirically for gonorrhea simultaneously, unless they are known to be negative for gonorrhea by sensitive lab testing.
- All partners of patients treated for chlamydia should be tested, if possible. They should be treated empirically rather than waiting for test results. They should also be treated empirically even if they were not tested.

IN-PATIENT CONSIDERATIONS

Treatment of PID: Trend toward outpatient treatment. However, decision to hospitalize made on case-by-case basis. Those falling into the following categories recommended for inpatient treatment: Pregnancy, lack of response or intolerance to oral meds, suspicion of poor compliance/nonadherence to therapy, severe clinical illness (fevers, severe vomiting, or abdominal pain), pelvic abscess, possible need for surgical intervention.

Initial Stabilization

Outpatient treatment, unless patient is moderately or severely ill with PID or other complications

Admission Criteria

As outlined above

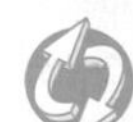

ONGOING CARE

FOLLOW-UP RECOMMENDATIONS

Abstinence from sexual contact until diagnosis and treatment complete for patient and all partners

Patient Monitoring

- It is not routine to test the patient to see if a cure has been obtained, except in pregnancy. However, retesting of infected women at 3 months is indicated because of high risk of reinfection (2,5)[A].
- Sexual partners must be evaluated and treated empirically, if necessary, to prevent passing the disease back and forth between partners. Partnerships with local public health departments should be fostered to assist with partner tracing.
- Lack of resolution or recurrence of symptoms must be reported immediately to the physician, and severe cases of urethritis/cervicitis, as well as the chlamydial syndromes, should be seen in follow-up after completion of therapy.
- Up to 25% of asymptomatic patients screened for chlamydia may not return for treatment after chlamydia culture results. Strategies must be developed to ensure treatment can be instituted.

PATIENT EDUCATION

- Suggest risk-reduction counseling and encourage delay of initiation of sexual activity, especially in younger adolescents.
- Encourage safe-sex practices, such as barrier protection (condoms particularly).
- Inform about serious sequelae of chlamydial disease, such as tubal infertility or chronic pelvic pain.
- Stress the need to finish entire course of antibiotics.

PROGNOSIS

Prognosis is good with early and compliant therapy; however, because of the asymptomatic nature of the early disease and the population affected, symptomatic PID still accounts annually for 2.5 million outpatient visits and >250,000 hospitalizations.

COMPLICATIONS

- Both sexes: Enhancement of transmission of and susceptibility to HIV
- Males: Transient oligospermia and postepididymitis urethral stricture (rare)
- Females: Tubal infertility (most common cause of acquired infertility), tubal (ectopic) pregnancy, chronic pelvic pain

REFERENCES

1. http://www.cdc.gov/std/chlamydia/default.htm#stat.
2. Centers for Disease Control and Prevention. Sexually transmitted disease treatment guidelines 2006. *MMWR*. 2006;55:No. RR-11.
3. Turner CF, Rogers SM, Miller HG, et al. Untreated gonococcal and chlamydial infection in a probability sample of adults. *JAMA*. 2002;287:726–33.
4. http://www.cdc.gov/std/chlamydia/ChlamydiaScreening-males.pdf.
5. Hosenfeld CB, Workowski KA, Berman S, Zaidi A, Dyson J, Mosure D, Bolan G, Bauer HM et al. Repeat infection with Chlamydia and gonorrhea among females: a systematic review of the literature. *Sex Transm Dis*. 2009;36:478–89.

See Also (Topic, Algorithm, Electronic Media Element)

Cervicitis; Epididymitis' Gonococcal Infections; HIV Infection and AIDS; Pelvic Inflammatory Disease; Syphilis; Urethritis

CODES

ICD9

- 099.55 Other venereal diseases due to chlamydia trachomatis, unspecified genitourinary site
- 616.11 Vaginitis and vulvovaginitis in diseases classified elsewhere

CLINICAL PEARLS

- *C. trachomatis* infection is common (but usually asymptomatic) in sexually active teens and young adults.
- Chlamydia infection is the most common cause of acquired infertility in the US.
- To prevent recurrence, treat patients and their partners concurrently.
- ACOG estimates that 40% of untreated chlamydial infections progress to PID, and 1 in 5 cases of PID lead to infertility.
- 2006 was the 1st year that new reported chlamydial cases in the US exceeded 1 million, and this is with only half the eligible sexually active women being screened.
- If all eligible women were screened, we would *annually* prevent an estimated 60,000 cases of PID, 8,000 cases of chronic pelvic pain, and over 7,000 cases of infertility.

CHOLANGITIS, ACUTE

Mallika Mundkur, MD
John M. Levey, MD

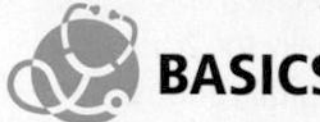

BASICS

DESCRIPTION

- An ascending bacterial infection of the bile duct system occurring in the context of a partial or complete obstruction of the biliary tree, most commonly caused by gallstones.
- Classically, presents with the clinical triad of fever, jaundice, and right upper quadrant (RUQ) pain (Charcot triad) or the pentad of fever, jaundice, RUQ pain, mental status changes and hypotension (Reynold pentad)
- Severity of the syndrome may range from mild to life-threatening
- Management includes medical and/or surgical interventions.
- System(s) affected: GI; Hepatobiliary

EPIDEMIOLOGY

- Predominant age: 55–70 years; rare in children, more common in adults
- The data on gender distribution is inconsistent; some studies note that though gallstones are more frequent in females than males, the frequency of cholangitis is equivalent between sexes.

RISK FACTORS

- As cholangitis often occurs secondary to gallstone obstruction, many of the risk factors for developing cholangitis are the same as those for developing gallstones: Populations such as Native Americans and African Americans with sickle cell disease
- Any condition that predisposes to bile stasis increases risk for cholangitis, including biliary strictures, biliary malignancies causing narrowing of the duct, or pancreatic tumors compressing the ductal system extrinsically.
- Endoscopic or surgical manipulation
- Parasitic infections of the Hepatobiliary system (*Ascaris lumbricoides, Clonorchis sinensis, Opisthorchis viverrini*)
- Biliary stents

GENERAL PREVENTION

Ensure surgical clearance of retained choledocholithiasis (CBD) stones at time of cholecystectomy with endoscopic or radiographic cholangiography or provide adequate drainage of the biliary tree

PATHOPHYSIOLOGY

- The composition of bile includes antibacterial components, such as immunoglobulins.
- The flow of bile from the liver to the GI tract via the ampulla enhances the maintenance of the bile as a sterile fluid.
- Obstruction to the flow of bile predisposes the system to an infection that festers in the biliary system and may ascend higher in the biliary tree.
- If the infection ascends unopposed to penetrate the hepatic circulation, the patient may present with generalized infection, severe sepsis, and a poor outcome.

ETIOLOGY

- *Escherichia coli, Klebsiella pneumoniae,* and *Streptococcus faecalis* are the most commonly cultured organisms from the bile of patients with cholangitis.
- *Bacteroides fragilis, Enterococcus, Enterobacter,* and *Pseudomonas* are also reported to have been frequently isolated from the bile of affected patients.

COMMONLY ASSOCIATED CONDITIONS

- Choledocholithiasis
- Malignant tumors
- Benign strictures
- Biliary-enteric anastomosis
- Invasive procedures
- Foreign bodies
- Parasites
- Secondary sclerosing cholangitis
- Immunosuppression

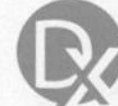

DIAGNOSIS

HISTORY

- Although the classic presentation, as per Charcot triad, includes fever, jaundice, and RUQ abdomina pain, the full triad is present in only approximately 2/3 of patients.
- More atypical presentations often occur in the elderly, who may present later in the evolution of t disease with sudden decompensation from sepsis.
- Reynold pentad includes the 3 symptoms of Charc triad (fever, jaundice, RUQ abdominal pain) as wel as the additional features of disorientation and hypotension. The presence of the pentad suggests much more severe manifestation of the disease.

PHYSICAL EXAM

Patient may have only 1 or 2 of the following symptoms, and the abdominal exam may be unrevealing:

- RUQ pain, not severe; abdominal exam may be similar or identical to that with acute cholecystitis
- Jaundice
- Chills and fever
- Shock
- CNS depression

DIAGNOSTIC TESTS & INTERPRETATION

Lab

- Complete blood count: Elevated white blood cell count (WBC), neutrophil predominant
- Liver function tests: Elevated bilirubin, GGT, alkalir phosphatase, transaminases
- Serum amylase and lipase (stone impacted at level of the ampulla)
- Blood cultures: Occasionally positive for growth, depending on severity of infection
- WBC $\geq$20,000, and *T. Bili* $\geq$10 mg/dl are selectiv predictors of adverse outcomes (1)[B].

naging
- See Diagnostic Procedures.
- CT may be helpful to distinguish suppurative from nonsuppurative cholangitis (2)[C].

iagnostic Procedures/Surgery
- Ultrasound (US) will rapidly diagnose gallstones and CBD dilatation
  - However, cholangiography is the definitive diagnostic test.
- Percutaneous transhepatic cholangiography or endoscopic retrograde cholangiopancreatography (ERCP) allow for both diagnostic confirmation and therapeutic intervention.
- ERCP allows for procedures such as stone extraction, stent-placement and sphincterotomy.
- MRCP is a newer noninvasive method of imaging the bile duct using magnetic resonance technology; may be useful in confirming biliary pathology prior to ERCP, and has high sensitivity and specificity for primary sclerosing cholangitis (3)[A].

IFFERENTIAL DIAGNOSIS
- Acute cholecystitis
- Mirizzi syndrome
- Biliary leaks
- Oriental cholangiohepatitis
- Pyogenic liver abscess
- Hepatitis
- Infected choledochal cysts
- Acute pancreatitis
- Perforated duodenal ulcer
- Pelvic inflammatory disease with peritonitis
- Kidney stones
- Pancreatitis
- Right lower-lobe pneumonia

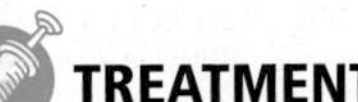

TREATMENT

- Monitor airway, breathing, and circulation, resuscitate as needed; intravenous crystalloid
- Make patient NPO, and if vomiting, place nasogastric tube

IEDICATION
- anagement consists of intravenous antibiotics, fluid suscitation, and biliary drainage.
- The initial empiric antibiotic therapy should be broad-spectrum until results of blood cultures are obtained, at which time the regimen should be modified according to the organism isolated
- Little data is available on the best initial antibiotic regimen, but sample initial broad-spectrum regimens are listed below in no particular order:
  - Monotherapy with a beta-lactam/beta-lactamase inhibitor, such as ampicillin-sulbactam (3 g every 6 hours) OR piperacillin/tazobactam (4.5 g every 6 hours) OR ticarcillin-clavulanate (3.1 g every 4 hours)
  - Metronidazole (500 mg IV every eight hours) PLUS a 3rd-generation cephalosporin, such as ceftriaxone (1 g IV every 24 hours)
  - Metronidazole (500 mg IV every eight hours) PLUS a fluoroquinolone (ciprofloxacin 400 mg IV every 12 hours or levofloxacin 500 mg IV daily)
  - Monotherapy with a carbapenem, such as imipenem (500 mg every six hours) OR meropenem (1 g every 8 hours) OR ertapenem (1 g daily)

ADDITIONAL TREATMENT
- The majority of patients will respond to antibiotics and conservative management and will be able to undergo elective biliary drainage.
- Approximately 1/5 of patients will require urgent biliary decompression, requiring invasive procedures that include ERCP with sphincterotomy, percutaneous transhepatic decompression, open surgical decompression, or T-tube placement
- Indications for urgent decompression include: Prolonged persistence of abdominal pain, mental status changes, fever >39C (102 F), hypotension not adequately responsive to fluid resuscitation

SURGERY/OTHER PROCEDURES
- Patients who do not respond to antibiotics and supportive care require emergency decompression of the biliary duct system. This may be accomplished by surgery, endoscopy, or transhepatic cholangiography.
- In case of obstruction secondary to stones, endoscopic papillotomy and stone extraction will drain the duct, may be definitive treatment of the underlying cause, and are shown to reduce mortality.

IN-PATIENT CONSIDERATIONS
See Treatment.

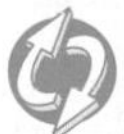

ONGOING CARE

FOLLOW-UP RECOMMENDATIONS
Some patients with recurrent symptoms of cholangitis may require maintenance antibiotics and imaging to exclude liver abscess.

DIET
NPO until acute phase is terminated.

PATIENT EDUCATION
For patient education materials favorably reviewed on this topic, contact National Digestive Diseases Information Clearinghouse, Box NDDIC, Bethesda, MD 20892, (301) 468-6344.

PROGNOSIS
- Historically the mortality rate was 100%.
- With current medical and surgical interventions, mortality from acute cholangitis has now decreased to approximately 5%.
- Coexistent cardiac or kidney impairment, malignancies, and hepatic abscesses worsen the prognosis of affected individuals.

COMPLICATIONS
- Hepatic abscess
- Sepsis
- Hepatic dysfunction
- Acute renal failure

REFERENCES

1. Rosing DK, De Virgilio C, Nguyen AT, et al. Cholangitis: analysis of admission prognostic indicators and outcomes. *Am Surg*. 2007;73: 949–54.
2. Lee NK, Kim S, Lee JW, et al. Discrimination of suppurative cholangitis from nonsuppurative cholangitis with computed tomography (CT). *Eur J Radiol*. 2008.
3. Dave M, Elmunzer BJ, Dwamena BA et al. Primary sclerosing cholangitis: meta-analysis of diagnostic performance of MR cholangiopancreatography. *Radiology*. 2010;256:387–96.

ADDITIONAL READING

Magnuson TH, Bender JS, Duncan MD., et al. Utility of magnetic resonance cholangiography in the evaluation of biliary obstruction. *J Am Coll Surg*. 1999;189: 63–71; discussion 71–2.

See Also (Topic, Algorithm, Electronic Media Element)
Cholelithiasis

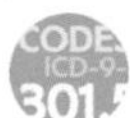

CODES

ICD9
576.1 Cholangitis

CLINICAL PEARLS

- The complete Charcot triad is present in only 2/3 of patients.
- Ultrasound helps with diagnosis, but ERCP is both diagnostic and therapeutic.

CHOLEDOCHOLITHIASIS

David Carne, MD

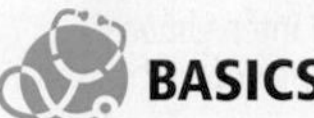

BASICS

DESCRIPTION
- Stones in common bile duct (CBD)
- 3 types: Cholesterol (majority), calcium bilirubinate or pigment, and mixed stones
- Pigment stones may form de novo in the CBD.
- System(s) affected: Gastrointestinal; Hepatobiliary
- Synonym(s): CBD stones; CBD calculi

EPIDEMIOLOGY
Incidence
- 700,000 cholecystectomies performed annually in US:
  - 4.6–20% of patients with gallstones have choledocholithiasis discovered at time of cholecystectomy, depending on whether routine cholangiography is used.
- Increases with age (30–50% of patients >60 years old with gallstones have CBD stones):
  - On average, present 10 years older than cholelithiasis patients
- Incidence of gallstones in US is 10–20%: Individuals >60 years old is up to 40%
- Internationally, incidence is increased due to parasitic infections such as *Ascaris lumbricoides*.
- Choledocholithiasis found with intraoperative cholangiography may be a false positive and may pass spontaneously without intervention.

Prevalence
Predominant sex: Female > Male

RISK FACTORS
- Cholelithiasis (most CBD stones migrate from the gallbladder [GB] into CBD)
- Pancreatitis (30%)
- Obesity
- Higher consumption of long-chain saturated fatty acids (1)[A]
- Chronic hemolysis
- Estrogen exposure
- Weight loss >25% of original weight after bariatric surgery (2)[A]
- Prior cholecystectomy:
  - <2 years prior: Considered a "retained" stone
  - >2 years prior: Considered "recurrent" stone

Genetics
- MDR3 defects may predispose to bile sludge formation, cholelithiasis, cholestasis of pregnancy, and subsequent choledocholithiasis.
- Increased prevalence in Hispanic population

GENERAL PREVENTION
- Maintain a normal weight.
- Avoid rapid weight loss.
- Regular exercise

PATHOPHYSIOLOGY
CBD stones may be primary or secondary:
- Primary stones form within the biliary tract: Caused by any condition leading to bile stasis or chronic bactibilia
- Secondary stones form within the gallbladder

ETIOLOGY
- Cholelithiasis: Majority of stones
- Chronic hemolytic states
- Formation of de novo pigment stones:
  - Dilated, sclerosed, or strictured ducts (e.g., from recurrent cholangitis)
  - Hepatobiliary parasitism (*Ascaris lumbricoides* or *Clonorchis sinensis*)

COMMONLY ASSOCIATED CONDITIONS
- Cholelithiasis, cholecystitis, cholangitis
- Gallstone pancreatitis
- Colorectal adenomas: Strong association between cholelithiasis and multiple (>/= 3) lesions [adjusted OR 2.39, 95% CI 1.21–4.72] and left-sided colorectal adenomas [adjusted OR 1.82, 95% CI 1.28–2.59] (3)[A]
- Cholangiocarcinoma [OR = 23.97, 95% CI 2.9–198.9] (4)[A]; cholecystectomy does not change risk.

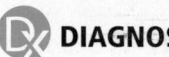

DIAGNOSIS

HISTORY
- Asymptomatic (30–50%)
- Right upper quadrant pain. Moderate/intense spasmodic pain, often intermittent, transient, recurrent:
  - May radiate to right shoulder/back
  - Worse after eating fatty or greasy foods
  - Occurs within minutes following meals
  - Pain not relieved by antacids
- Secondary effects of obstruction:
  - Clay-colored stool
  - Tea-colored urine
  - Jaundice
  - Nausea/vomiting
  - Pruritus
  - Pancreatitis (epigastric pain radiating to back, etc.)
  - Hepatomegaly
- Infection that may progress to cholangitis and septic shock:
  - Fever, chills
  - Hypotension, flushing
- History of CBD strictures, recurrent sclerosing cholangitis, sphincter of Oddi dysfunction, cystic dilation
- Weight loss

PHYSICAL EXAM
- Moderate right upper quadrant tenderness on palpation
- Jaundice
- Fever
- Anorexia
- Fever, RUQ pain, and jaundice (Charcot triad) strongly indicative of cholangitis:
  - With severe cholangitis: Shock and mental status changes possible (Reynolds pentad)
- Palpable gallbladder (less common)
- Rebound tenderness or guarding absent

DIAGNOSTIC TESTS & INTERPRETATION
Lab
Initial lab tests
- Lab tests may be entirely normal.
- Direct hyperbilirubinemia (with total serum bilirubin >3 mg/dL) indicates obstruction
- Leukocytosis
- Blood cultures positive in 30–60% of patients with cholangitis
- Alkaline phosphatase and gamma-glutamyl-transpeptidase elevated with CBD obstruction
- Combination of a dilated common bile duct, elevated alkaline phosphatase, and ALT has modest sensitivity and high specificity for patients with cholelithiasis and choledocholithiasis
- Possible elevation of pancreatic enzymes
- Increased liver transaminases

Imaging
Initial approach
- Imaging is the most effective method of confirming suspected choledocholithiasis.
- Transabdominal ultrasound:
  - Fastest modality
  - Poorly confirms/excludes CBD stones (sensitivity 15–50%, specificity 75%)
  - Can detect dilation of CBD, but difficult to identify stones
  - A dilated CBD is found in only half of those with choledocholithiasis.
- Endoscopic ultrasound:
  - Sensitivity 88–97% and specificity 96–100% improved over transabdominal U/S
  - More invasive and increased cost
- Magnetic resonance cholangiopancreatography (MRCP):
  - Sensitivity 92%, specificity 97%
  - Most accurate noninvasive test; no contrast required (5)[A]
  - Preferred by patients over endoscopic retrograde cholangiopancreatography (ERCP), no associated morbidity, and may be less costly than diagnostic ERCP (6)[A]
  - May miss calculi smaller than 5 mm
- Abdominal CT:
  - Less sensitive than MRCP, but faster
  - Good at detecting CBD dilation, complications, and delineating surrounding structures (e.g., pancreas)
- Cholescintigraphy (HIDA/DISIDA scan): CBD radionuclide imaging. Isotope derivatives taken up by hepatocytes and excreted into biliary tree. Can be used to assess for bile duct obstruction, cystic duct obstruction, or bile leakage:
  - May be combined with CCK to observe GB function and estimate GB "ejection fraction"

Diagnostic Procedures/Surgery
- Cholangiography is the gold standard for determining the presence of CBD stones:
  - ERCP (sensitivity 90–95%, specificity 95%): Most common diagnostic modality. Allows for papillotomy/stone extraction at time of diagnosis
  - Percutaneous transhepatic cholangiography (PTC): Puncture of hepatic duct by needle, injection of radiopaque dye, and subsequent radiograph imaging of abdomen. Used in place of ERCP in patients with extensive bile duct stone disease or in whom ERCP would be difficult.
  - Intraoperative cholangiography (IOC): Contrast inserted via opening in cystic duct during cholecystectomy. Ongoing debate if IOC should be routinely performed during cholecystectomy.
- Endoscopic ultrasound: More likely to detect stones than transabdominal route (sensitivity 85–97%, specificity 96–100%)
- Intraoperative intraluminal ultrasonography:
  - Can be performed during laparoscopic or open procedures
  - May be indicated in patients with contrast dye allergy
- Postoperative studies:
  - MRI (MRCP) can be commonly used postoperatively to diagnose CBD stone.

- T-tube cholangiography

Choledochoscopy can be used to extract stones intraoperatively or via t-tube tract.

IFFERENTIAL DIAGNOSIS

Biliary stricture
Narrowed biliary–enteric anastomosis
Cholangitis (acute or primary sclerosing)
Cholangiocarcinoma
Sphincter of Oddi dysfunction
Biliary parasites
Papillary stenosis
Blood clots

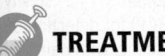

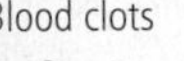
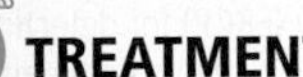

TREATMENT

IEDICATION

The obstruction needs to be removed. If not symptomatic and small, stones may pass spontaneously.

Antibiotics are used if infection is suspected (cholangitis) and need to cover enteric flora.

Broad-coverage antibiotics (substitute fluoroquinolones for penicillin-allergic patients).

Routinely prescribed for prophylaxis, although a 2003 study suggests prophylactic antibiotics did not prevent cholangitis in those with choledocholithiasis:
- Piperacillin-tazobactam (Zosyn) 3.375 g IV q6h
- Ampicillin-sulbactam (Unasyn) 1.5–3.0 g (1–2 g ampicillin + 0.5–1 g sulbactam) IV/IM q6–8h; not to exceed 8 g/d ampicillin or 4 g/d sulbactam

Fluoroquinolones have good biliary penetration:
- Levofloxacin 250–500 mg IV or p.o. once daily
- Ciprofloxacin 200 mg IV/p.o. b.i.d

Duration of therapy depends on rapidity of response, subsequent surgery, and presence of bacteremia, as well as correction of biliary obstruction.

Addition of metronidazole for anaerobic coverage in sepsis/infection, elderly patients, and patients with previous biliary manipulation (not necessary with newer broad-spectrum penicillins):
- Metronidazole 500 mg IV q8h

Consider stress ulcer prophylaxis.

DVT prophylaxis

SURGERY/OTHER PROCEDURES

Endoscopic CBD stone removal: Often performed following endoscopic cholangiography or following stone identification by other modalities:
- Relatively low complication rate (mortality 0.5%, pancreatitis 1–8%, perforation 0.4%, bleeding from sphincterotomy 1–2%, cholangitis 1%)
- Up to 90% success rate

Surgical CBD stone removal: High success rate (75–95%) and few complications:
- Laparoscopic: Often performed at the time of cholecystectomy. May be preferable to pre-/postoperative ERCP once laparoscopy has been initiated (7)[A],(8)[B].
- 1-stage management of symptomatic CBD stones with laparoscopic cholecystectomy + laparoscopic common bile duct exploration is associated with less morbidity and mortality (7% and 0.19%, respectively) than 2-stage management utilizing ERCP/ES (endoscopic sphincterotomy) followed by laparoscopic cholecystectomy (13.5% and 0.5%) (9)[A].
- Using a CBD lumen catheter may be considered if laparoscopic common bile duct exploration is not feasible and the chance of a CBD stone is less than 65% (9)[A].
- Open choledochotomy: Rarely used. Only for complex cases where laparoscopic and endoscopic techniques fail unless patient already undergoing an open procedure.

- Lithotripsy through a cholangioscope passed via duodenoscope to crush stones with a basket or fracture them with a laser or electrohydraulic method
- Surgical drainage via external catheter or by papillotomy through ampulla of Vater
- Indications for drainage: Sphincter of Oddi sclerosis or dysfunction, multiple or primary CBD stones, or previous stone
- Laparoscopic cholecystectomy with IOC is definitive treatment, unless patient unable to tolerate surgery
- New emerging techniques such as single port cholecystectomy and natural orifice transluminal endoscopic surgery (NOTES) cholecystectomy may offer advantages: Reduced abdominal pain, lower rates of wound infections, and reduced incidence of hernia formation (10)[B]

IN-PATIENT CONSIDERATIONS

Initial Stabilization

n.p.o. and antibiotics if infection suspected or with biliary manipulation

Admission Criteria

To control serious infection and urgently decompress common bile duct

Nursing

Early ambulation

Discharge Criteria

When stable

ONGOING CARE

FOLLOW-UP RECOMMENDATIONS

Retained stone extraction 6 weeks after placement of biliary drain

Patient Monitoring

- Liver function tests and bilirubin levels
- WBC and pancreatic enzymes
- Patients with weight loss >25% from original weight after bariatric surgery may benefit from U/S surveillance and subsequent cholecystectomy if gallstones are identified (2)[A].

PROGNOSIS

- With endoscopic or surgical treatment, prognosis is good.
- Untreated, 55% of patients experience complications.
- Filling defects found on intraoperative cholangiograms: 25% are false positives; 25% will pass spontaneously by 6 wks

COMPLICATIONS

- Cholangitis: Most frequent (60%)
- Retained CBD stones (2–10%)
- Pancreatitis
- Biliary enteric fistula
- Hemobilia
- Liver dysfunction/failure
- Bile duct injury

REFERENCES

1. Tsai CJ, Leitzmann MF, Willett WC, et al. Long-chain saturated fatty acids consumption and risk of gallstone disease among men. *Ann Surg*. 2008;247:95–103.
2. Li VK, Pulido N, Fajnwaks P, et al. Predictors of gallstone formation after bariatric surgery: a multivariate analysis of risk factors comparing gastric bypass, gastric banding, and sleeve gastrectomy. *Surg Endosc*. 2009.
3. Yamaji Y, Okamoto M, Yoshida H, et al. Cholelithiasis Is a Risk Factor for Colorectal Adenoma. *Am J Gastroenterol*. 2008.
4. Welzel TM, Mellemkjaer L, Gloria G, et al. Risk factors for intrahepatic cholangiocarcinoma in a low-risk population: A nationwide case-control study. *Int J Cancer*. 2006.
5. Romagnuolo J, Bardou M, Rahme E, et al. Magnetic resonance cholangiopancreatography: a meta-analysis of test performance in suspected biliary disease. *Ann Intern Med*. 2003;139:547–57.
6. Kaltenthaler E, Vergel YB, et al. A systematic review and economic evaluation of magnetic resonance cholangiopancreatography compared with diagnostic endoscopic retrograde cholangiopancreatography. *Health Technol Assess*. 2004;8(10):iii, 1–89.
7. Tranter SE, Thompson MH. Comparison of endoscopic sphincterotomy and laparoscopic exploration of the common bile duct. *Br J Surg*. 2002;89:1495–504.
8. Nathanson LK, O'Rourke NA, Martin IJ, et al. Postoperative ERCP versus laparoscopic choledochotomy for clearance of selected bile duct calculi: a randomized trial. *Ann Surg*. 2005;242:188–92.
9. Kharbutli B, Velanovich V. Management of Preoperatively Suspected Choledocholithiasis: A Decision Analysis. *J Gastrointest Surg*. 2008.
10. Auyang ED, Hungness ES, Vaziri K, et al. Natural orifice translumenal endoscopic surgery (NOTES): dissection for the critical view of safety during transcolonic cholecystectomy. *Surg Endosc*. 2009.

ADDITIONAL READING

Padda MS, Singh S, Tang SJ, et al. Liver test patterns in patients with acute calculous cholecystitis and/or choledocholithiasis. *Aliment Pharmacol Ther*. 2009.

See Also (Topic, Algorithm, Electronic Media Element)

Cholangitis (acute); Cholecystitis; Cholelithiasis; Jaundice

CODES

ICD9

- 574.30 Calculus of bile duct with acute cholecystitis without mention of obstruction
- 574.40 Calculus of bile duct with other cholecystitis, without mention of obstruction
- 574.50 Calculus of bile duct without mention of cholecystitis, without mention of obstruction

CLINICAL PEARLS

- Stones in the common bile duct may originate there (primary) or in the gallbladder (secondary) and then migrate to CBD.
- Cholangiography is "gold standard" for diagnosis.
- ERCP offers both diagnostic and therapeutic options.
- Cholangitis is most frequent complication.

CHOLELITHIASIS

Hongyi Cui, MD, PhD
John J. Kelly, MD

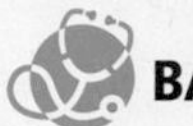

BASICS

DESCRIPTION

Cholelithiasis manifests in cholesterol, pigment, or mixed stones formed and contained in the gallbladder:

- Synonym(s): Gallstones

Pediatric Considerations

- Uncommon at <10 years of age
- Associated with blood dyscrasia
- Most gallstones in pediatric population are pigment stones.

EPIDEMIOLOGY

Incidence

- Increased in Native Americans and Hispanics
- Increases with age by 1–3% per year; peaks at 7th decade
- 2% of the US population develops gallstones annually.

Prevalence

- Population: 8–10% of US
- Predominant sex: Female > Male (2–3:1)

RISK FACTORS

- Age (peak in 60–70s)
- Female gender
- Caucasian, Hispanic, or Native American descent
- Hereditary (such as patients carrying the p.D19H variant for the hepatocanalicular cholesterol transporter ABCG5/ABG8 have an increased risk for gallstones)
- Metabolic syndrome (i.e., obesity, dyslipidemia, hypertension, and type 2 diabetes)
- Pregnancy and multiparity
- Cholestasis in association with prolonged fasting and long-term total parenteral nutrition
- Rapid weight loss following bariatric surgery
- Metabolic changes in association with short gut syndrome, terminal ileal resection, and inflammatory bowel disease
- Hemolytic disorders (e.g., hereditary spherocytosis and sickle cell anemia) and cirrhosis (for black or pigment stones)
- Medications (such as early use of birth control pills; estrogen replacement therapy at high doses)
- Biliary tract infection (such as liver flukes) and stricture (for intraductal formation of brown pigment stones)

Genetics

Animal studies indicate that gallstone formation is a dominant trait determined by at least 2 genes; susceptible strains fail to downregulate cholesterol synthesis during cholesterol feeding.

GENERAL PREVENTION

- Ursodiol (Actigall) taken during rapid weight loss prevents gallstone formation (1)[A]
- Regular exercise and dietary modification may reduce the incidence of gallstone formation.

PATHOPHYSIOLOGY

Gallstone formation is a complex process mediated by genetic, metabolic, immune, and environmental factors.

ETIOLOGY

- Production of bile supersaturated with cholesterol (cholesterol stones)
- Decrease in bile content of either phospholipid (lecithin) or bile salts
- Biliary stasis or impaired gallbladder motility
- Generation of excess unconjugated bilirubin in patients with hemolytic diseases; passage of excess bile salt into the colon with subsequent absorption of excess unconjugated bilirubin in patients with inflammatory bowel disease or after distal ileal resection (black or pigment stones)
- Hydrolysis of conjugated bilirubin or phospholipid by bacteria in patients with biliary tract infection or stricture (brown stones or primary bile duct stones; rare in the Western world and common in Asia)

COMMONLY ASSOCIATED CONDITIONS

90% of people with gallbladder carcinoma have gallstones.

DIAGNOSIS

HISTORY

- Mostly asymptomatic (80%):
  - 5–10% become symptomatic each year.
  - Over their lifetime, <1/2 of the patients with gallstones develop symptoms.
- Episodic right upper quadrant or epigastric pain lasting longer than 15 minutes and sometimes radiating to the back (biliary colic), usually postprandially; the majority of patients will develop recurrent symptoms after the 1st episode.
- Nausea
- Vomiting
- Fatty food intolerance (not proven)
- Indigestion or bloating sensation

PHYSICAL EXAM

- Physical exam is usually normal in patients with cholelithiasis.
- Epigastric and/or right upper quadrant tenderness (Murphy's sign) when in association with cholecystitis
- Fever and jaundice in patients with choledocholithiasis and cholangitis; jaundice can also be caused by extrinsic compression of the bile duct by a stone in the gallbladder or cystic duct (Mirizzi syndrome)
- Flank and periumbilical ecchymoses (Cullen sign and Grey-Turner sign) in patients with acute hemorrhagic pancreatitis
- In patients with concomitant acute calculus cholecystitis and gallbladder cancer, a mass in the right upper quadrant may be palpated.

DIAGNOSTIC TESTS & INTERPRETATION

Lab

- No lab study is specific for cholelithiasis.
- Leukocytosis and elevated C-reactive protein level are associated with acute calculus cholecystitis.

Imaging

- Ultrasound (best technique to diagnose gallstones and differentiate from cholecystitis). Ultrasound can detect gallstones in 97–98% of patients. Thickening of the gallbladder wall (5 mm or greater), pericholecystic fluid, and direct tenderness when the probe is pushed against the gallbladder (sonographic Murphy sign) are all radiographic sign of acute calculus cholecystitis.
- Computed tomography scan (no advantage over ultrasound except in detecting distal common bile duct stones)
- Magnetic resonance cholangiopancreatography is reserved for cases of suspected common bile duct stones due to high cost.
- Endoscopic ultrasound has been shown to be as sensitive as endoscopic retrograde cholangiopancreatography (ERCP) for detection of common bile duct stones in patients with gallstone pancreatitis.
- Hepatobiliary iminodiacetic acid (HIDA) scan is useful in differentiating acalculous cholecystitis from other causes of abdominal pain. False-positive results can arise from fasting status or insufficient resistance of the sphincter of Oddi. CCK-HIDA is specifically used to diagnose gallbladder dysmotility disorder (i.e., biliary dyskinesia).
- 10–30% of gallstones are radiopaque calcium or pigment-containing gallstones and are more likely to be visible on plain x-ray. A "porcelain gallbladder" is a calcified gallbladder, visible by x-ray; associated with gallbladder cancer (25%).

Pathological Findings

- Pure cholesterol stones have a white or slightly yellow color.
- Pigment stones may be black or brown. Black stones contain polymerized calcium bilirubinate, most often secondary to cirrhosis or hemolysis, and almost always form in the gallbladder. Brown stones are associated with biliary tract infection, caused by bile stasis, and as such may form either in the bile ducts or gallbladder.

DIFFERENTIAL DIAGNOSIS

- Peptic ulcer diseases
- Gastritis
- Hepatitis
- Pancreatitis
- Cholangitis
- Gallbladder cancer
- Gallbladder polyps
- Acalculous cholecystitis
- Biliary dyskinesia
- Biliary tree stricture
- Choledocholithiasis
- Choledochocyst
- Coronary artery disease
- Esophageal motility disorders
- Appendicitis
- Pneumonia
- Renal stones

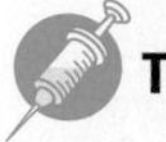

TREATMENT

Geriatric Considerations

Age alone should not alter the therapy plan.

MEDICATION

First Line

- Analgesics for pain relief
- Oral dissolution therapy is rarely used today.
- Antibiotics are indicated in patients with signs of acute cholecystitis.

Prophylactic antibiotics in low-risk patients do not prevent infections for laparoscopic cholecystectomies (2)[A].

Second Line

Nonsteroidal anti-inflammatory drugs (NSAIDs) may have a role in pain relief, given that prostaglandins are important in the development of pain.

ADDITIONAL TREATMENT

General Measures

- Treat only symptomatic gallstones and observe asymptomatic stones.
- Attempt conservative therapy during pregnancy. If necessary, perform surgery preferentially in the 2nd trimester.
- Prophylactic cholecystectomy for patients with calcified (porcelain) gallbladder (risk for gallbladder cancer), and patients with recurrent pancreatitis due to microlithiasis
- In morbidly obese patients, simultaneous cholecystectomy may be performed in combination with bariatric procedures in an effort to reduce later stone-related complications.

Issues for Referral

Patients with retained or recurrent bile duct stones following cholecystectomy should be referred to gastroenterology for ERCP.

SURGERY/OTHER PROCEDURES

- Surgical intervention should be considered for patients who have symptomatic cholelithiasis or gallstone-related complications such as cholecystitis (3)[B].
- Laparoscopic cholecystectomy is currently the standard of care for most cases (4)[B]. In well-selected patients, single incision/port laparoscopic cholecystectomy is a novel method for the treatment of symptomatic cholelithiasis. Natural orifice transluminal endoscopic surgery (NOTES) is still at an experimental stage, and NOTES cholecystectomy is only available in a limited number of specialized centers:
  - Surgery related complications include common bile duct injury (0.5%), right hepatic duct/artery injury, retained stones, cystic duct or duct of Luschka leak, biloma formation, or bile duct stricture in the long term.
  - Conversion to open procedure based on the judgment of the operating surgeon
  - Intraoperative cholangiogram (IOC) may help delineate bile duct anatomy when dissection proves difficult. Selective or routine use of IOC is a topic of debate, but may be associated with earlier recognition and decreased incidence of bile duct injury (5)[B].
- Open cholecystectomy is indicated for gallbladder cancer diagnosed preoperatively.
- Percutaneous cholecystostomy (PC) in high-risk patients with cholecystitis or gallbladder empyema. PC may also be used in patients with symptoms of cholecystitis for >72 hrs in which altered anatomy might significantly increase the surgical risk. Interval cholecystectomy is usually advisable after the resolution of cholecystitis and optimization of associated medical conditions to prevent recurrent cholecystitis.

IN-PATIENT CONSIDERATIONS

For patients with symptomatic cholelithiasis, laparoscopic cholecystectomy has become an outpatient procedure; for patients who developed gallstone-related complications (i.e., cholecystitis, cholangitis, and pancreatitis), inpatient care is necessary.

Initial Stabilization

- Patients are treated during the acute phase with nothing by mouth (n.p.o.), intravenous fluids, and antibiotics.
- Adequate pain control with narcotics and/or NSAIDs is also needed.

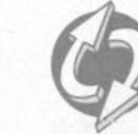

ONGOING CARE

FOLLOW-UP RECOMMENDATIONS

Patient Monitoring

- Medical attention if asymptomatic stones become symptomatic
- Patients on oral dissolution agents should be followed up with liver enzyme, serum cholesterol, and imaging studies.

DIET

A low-fat diet may be helpful.

PATIENT EDUCATION

- Change in lifestyle (e.g., regular exercise) and dietary modification (low-fat diet and reduction of total calorie intake) may reduce gallstone-related hospitalizations.
- Patients with asymptomatic gallstones should be educated about the typical symptoms of biliary colic and gallstone-related complications.

PROGNOSIS

- <1/2 of patients with gallstones become symptomatic.
- Cholecystectomy: Mortality <0.5% elective, 3–5% emergency; morbidity <10% elective, 30–40% emergency
- ~10–15% of the patients will have associated choledocholithiasis.
- After cholecystectomy, stones may recur in the bile duct.

COMPLICATIONS

- Acute cholecystitis (90–95% secondary to gallstones)
- Gallbladder empyema
- Gallstone pancreatitis
- Acute cholangitis
- Common bile duct stones with obstructive jaundice
- Biliary-enteric fistula
- Gallstone ileus
- Gallbladder perforation
- Peritonitis and sepsis
- Liver abscess
- Gallbladder cancer
- Mirizzi syndrome (bile duct obstruction caused by gallstones lodged in gallbladder or cystic duct)

REFERENCES

1. Uy MC, Talingdan-Te MC, Espinosa WZ, et al. Ursodeoxycholic Acid in the Prevention of Gallstone Formation after Bariatric Surgery: A Meta-analysis. *Obes Surg*. 2008.
2. Zhou H, Zhang J, Wang Q, et al. Meta-analysis: Antibiotic prophylaxis in elective laparoscopic cholecystectomy. *Aliment Pharmacol Ther*. 2009; 29:1086–95.
3. Bellows CF, Berger DH, Crass RA. Management of gallstones. *Am Fam Phys*. 2005;72:637–42.
4. Shamiyeh A, Wayand W. Current status of laparoscopic therapy of cholecystolithiasis and common bile duct stones. *Dig Dis*. 2005;23: 119–26.
5. Connor S, Garden OJ. Bile duct injury in the era of laparoscopic cholecystectomy. *Br J Surg*. 2006;93: 158–68.

ADDITIONAL READING

- Bogue CO, Murphy AJ, Gerstle JT, et al. Risk factors, complications, and outcomes of gallstones in children: a single-center review. *J Pediatr Gastroenterol Nutr*. 2010;50:303–8.
- Gurusamy KS, Samraj K, et al. Cholecystectomy versus no cholecystectomy in patients with silent gallstones. *Cochrane Database Syst Rev*. 2007; CD006230.
- Keus F, Gooszen HG, van Laarhoven CJ, et al. Open, small-incision, or laparoscopic cholecystectomy for patients with symptomatic cholecystolithiasis. An overview of Cochrane Hepato-Biliary Group reviews. *Cochrane Database Syst Rev*. 2010;:CD008318.
- Lammert F, Miquel JF. Gallstone disease: From genes to evidence-based therapy. *J Hepatol*. 2008.
- Sakorafas GH, Milingos D, Peros G, et al. Asymptomatic cholelithiasis: is cholecystectomy really needed? A critical reappraisal 15 years after the introduction of laparoscopic cholecystectomy. *Dig Dis Sci*. 2007;52:1313–25.

See Also (Topic, Algorithm, Electronic Media Element)

Cholangitis (acute); Cholecystitis; Choledocholithiasis

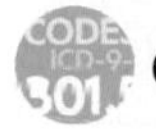

CODES

ICD9

- 574.00 Calculus of gallbladder with acute cholecystitis, without mention of obstruction
- 574.10 Calculus of gallbladder with other cholecystitis, without mention of obstruction
- 574.20 Calculus of gallbladder without mention of cholecystitis, without mention of obstruction

CLINICAL PEARLS

- Laparoscopic cholecystectomy has become the most frequently used procedure; lithotripsy and oral dissolution therapy may be considered in rare circumstances.
- Acute acalculous cholecystitis is associated with bile stasis and gallbladder ischemia.
- Prophylactic cholecystectomy is not indicated in patients with diabetes and asymptomatic gallstones. There is no evidence that asymptomatic diabetics are at increased risk of developing complications of gallstone disease.
- The best imaging modality for the diagnosis of gallstones is transabdominal ultrasound (sensitivity of 97% and specificity of 95%); not sensitive for occult gallstones or microlithiasis (stones smaller than 5 mm).
- Think of gallstones in the post-bariatric surgery patient complaining of "gas pains" as they are adjusting to their new diet.

CHOLERA

Abdulrazak Abyad, MD, PhD, MBA, MPH, AGSF, AFCHSE

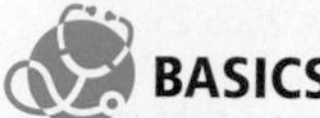

BASICS

DESCRIPTION

An acute infectious disease caused by *Vibrio cholerae* (El Tor type is responsible for the most recent epidemic; the other type, classic, is found only in Bangladesh). Characteristics include severe diarrhea with extreme fluid and electrolyte depletion, vomiting, muscle cramps, and prostration. (New serotype now in Bangladesh, India [0139]. Important because of lack of efficacy of standard vaccine.):

- Usual course: Acute, chronic, and relapsing
- Clinical course is 3–5 days; in the early stages, a severely affected patient can lose 1 L/h.
- Endemic areas: India, Southeast Asia, Africa, Middle East, southern Europe, Oceania, South and Central America
- System(s) affected: Gastrointestinal
- Synonym(s): Asiatic cholera; Epidemic cholera; Rice-water diarrhea; Cholera gravis

Pediatric Considerations

- Breastfeeding protects against cholera.
- Vaccine not recommended for children <6 months

EPIDEMIOLOGY

- Predominant age: All ages
- Predominant sex: Male = Female

Incidence

Since 1817, 7 cholera epidemics bave occurred.

Prevalence

About 0.01 cases/100,000. The few cases in the US have been found in returning travelers or are associated with food brought into this country illegally.

RISK FACTORS

- Traveling or living in epidemic/endemic areas
- Exposure to contaminated food or water
- Person-to-person transmission (rare)
- In endemic areas, children <5 years
- Attack more severe in patients with blood group O compared with AB
- People with low gastric acid secretion
- Gastrectomy
- Patients on acid-suppressing medications

GENERAL PREVENTION

- Water purification
- Careful food selection (e.g., no unpeeled raw fruits or vegetables, no raw or undercooked seafood)
- Enteric precautions
- Tetracycline for social contacts of an index case
- Natural infection confers long-lasting immunity.
- Prophylactic vaccine:
  - 50% effective for 3–6 months
  - Not recommended unless required by destination country and, if so, a single dose is sufficient.
  - Concomitant administration with yellow fever vaccine may result in reduced vaccine response to yellow fever.
  - Invariably associated with local side effects
  - Systemic side effects of fever and malaise
  - Newer oral killed-whole-cell vaccines provide longer immunity in adults, often up to 2 years from a single dose, and up to 3 or 4 years with annual boosters (1)[A].
  - There are a number of vaccines being developed, including:
    - Wyeth-Ayerst parenteral whole vaccine directed at *V. cholerae* O1 not effective
    - CVD 103-HgR highly protective against moderate and severe cholera
    - The WC/rBS stimulate both antibacterial and antitoxic antibodies.

ETIOLOGY

- Enterotoxin elaborated by gram-negative bacteria
- *Cholerae* (O-group 1)
- Human host
- Contaminated food
- Contaminated water
- Contaminated shellfish

COMMONLY ASSOCIATED CONDITIONS

Increased risk of disease with gastric achlorhydria

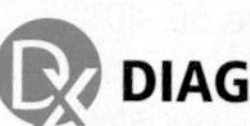

DIAGNOSIS

PHYSICAL EXAM

- Abdominal discomfort
- Anorexia
- Anuria
- Apathy
- Cyanosis
- Decreased skin turgor
- Dehydration
- Diarrhea, painless
- Distant heart sounds
- Diuresis, sudden
- Dysrhythmias
- Fever
- Hypotension
- Hypothermia
- Hypovolemic shock
- Increased or decreased bowel sounds
- Lethargy
- Listlessness
- Malaise
- Oliguria
- Rice-water diarrhea
- Seizures
- Sunken eyes
- Tachycardia
- Thirst
- Vomiting
- Washerwoman's fingers
- Weak peripheral pulses
- Weakness

DIAGNOSTIC TESTS & INTERPRETATION

Lab

- Stool culture: On selective media (thiosulfate citrate bile salts sucrose [TCBS])
- Typed antisera-specific agglutination
- Dark-field microscopy: Characteristic vibrio motility in stool
- Increased vibriocidal antibodies in nonimmunized patient
- Laboratory abnormalities of severe dehydration:
  - Acidemia
  - Acidosis
  - Hypokalemia
  - Hyponatremia
  - Hypochloremia
  - Hypoglycemia
  - Increased specific gravity
  - Polycythemia
  - Mild neutrophilic leukocytosis

Imaging

- Abdominal film: Ileus
- Chest radiograph: Microcardia

Diagnostic Procedures/Surgery

Physical examination and medical history that includes recent travel

Pathological Findings

- Electron microscopy: Organism adheres to mucosa.
- Intact mucosa
- Increased cellularity of lamina propria
- Increased cellularity of mucosa
- Vascular congestion
- Lymphoid hyperplasia of Peyer patches
- Lymphoid hyperplasia of mesenteric lymph nodes
- Lymphoid hyperplasia of spleen
- Cerebral edema
- Acute tubular necrosis
- Vacuolar hypokalemic nephropathy
- Pulmonary edema
- Hyaline membranes
- Bronchopneumonia
- Focal myocardial damage
- Lipid-depleted adrenals
- Tubularization of zona fasciculata

DIFFERENTIAL DIAGNOSIS

Other causes of severe diarrhea and dehydration (e.g., infection with Shigella, *Escherichia coli*, venous viruses)

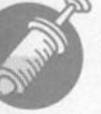

TREATMENT

Primary goal is to replenish fluid losses
Rehydration in 2 phases: Rehydration and maintenance
Practical guidelines for the treatment of cholera are as follows:
- Evaluate the degree of dehydration upon arrival.
- Rehydrate the patient in 2 phases. These include rehydration (for 2–4 h) and maintenance (until diarrhea abates).
- Register output and intake volumes on predesigned charts, and periodically review these data.
- Only use the intravenous route:
  - During the rehydration phase for severely dehydrated patients for whom an infusion rate of 50–100 mL/kg/h is advised
  - For moderately dehydrated patients who do not tolerate the oral route
  - During the maintenance phase in patients considered high stool purgers (i.e., >10 mL/kg/h)
- During the maintenance phase, use ORS at a rate of 800–1000 mL/h. Match ongoing losses with ORS administration.
- Reduced osmolarity ORS may cause low blood sodium levels with cholera (2)[A].
- Discharge patients to the treatment center if oral tolerance is greater than or equal to 1,000 mL/h, urine volume is greater than or equal to 40 mL/h, and stool volume is less than or equal to 400 mL/h.

MEDICATION

First Line

- Oral rehydration therapy for mild disease:
  - Oral rehydration solution (ORS) commercial brands available (Pedialyte, Rehydralyte, Resol, Rice-Lyte) or
  - Oral rehydration solution formula from World Health Organization, per liter:
    - Sodium chloride 3.5 g
    - Potassium chloride 1.5 g
    - Glucose 20 g
    - Trisodium citrate 2.9 g
    - Parenteral rehydration
- Rehydration for severely dehydrated patients:
  - IV rehydration (Ringer lactate) is followed by oral or nasogastric administration of glucose or sucrose-electrolyte solution.
  - Antibiotics:
    - For older children and adults: Doxycycline (Vibramycin): 300 mg once or 100 mg b.i.d. for 3 days or tetracycline 50 mg/kg/d for 3 days
    - For young children: Trimethoprim-sulfamethoxazole (SMX-TMP, Bactrim, Septra) 8 mg/kg trimethoprim plus 40 mg/kg sulfamethoxazole per day, divided q.12 h. This dosage is equivalent to 1 mL/kg of trimethoprim-sulfamethoxazole suspension.
    - In pregnant patients: Furazolidone 100 mg q.i.d. for 7–10 days
  - Contraindications:
    - Tetracycline: Not for use in pregnant patients or children <8 years old
    - Furazolidone and alcohol in combination may cause disulfiram-like reaction
  - Precautions:
    - Tetracycline: May cause photosensitivity; sunscreen recommended
  - Significant possible interactions:
    - Tetracycline: Avoid concurrent administration with antacids, dairy products, or iron.

Second Line

In young children: Furazolidone (Furoxone) 5–10 mg/kg/d divided q.6 h for 3 days

ADDITIONAL TREATMENT

General Measures

- Determination of the amount of fluid loss (may compare patient's previous with current weight)
- Rehydration therapy: Oral for mild-to-moderate cases. Patients with severe dehydration may require IV fluid replacement.

IN-PATIENT CONSIDERATIONS

Initial Stabilization

Outpatient for mild cases, inpatient for moderate-to-severe cases

ONGOING CARE

FOLLOW-UP RECOMMENDATIONS

Bed rest until symptoms resolve and strength returns

Patient Monitoring

Observe patient until symptoms are resolved.

DIET

Small, frequent meals when vomiting stops and appetite returns

PATIENT EDUCATION

- Centers for Disease Control and Prevention. Traveler's Information Hotline: (404) 332-4559 (available 24 hours via a touch-tone telephone)
- International Association for Medical Assistance to Travelers, 417 Center St., Lewiston, NY 14092; (716) 754-4883
- U.S. Centers for Disease Control and Prevention does not expect a major outbreak of cholera in the US, but has issued a "Cholera Preparedness Plan" outlining steps for proper surveillance, treatment, laboratory diagnosis, investigation of outbreaks, and public education.

PROGNOSIS

- Prompt p.o. or IV treatment can save lives.
- Appropriate disposal of human waste
- Antibiotic treatment reduces duration and infectivity of disease.
- Mortality <1% with appropriate supportive care
- Mortality higher with untreated hypovolemic shock

COMPLICATIONS

- Hypovolemic shock
- Chronic biliary infection
- Up to 50% mortality with untreated shock
- Intermittent stool shedding

REFERENCES

1. Shears P. Recent developments in cholera. *Curr Opin Infect Dis*. 2001;14:553–8.
2. Graves PM, Deeks JJ, Demicheli V et al. Vaccines for preventing cholera. *Cochrane Infectious Diseases Group Cochrane Database of Systematic Reviews*. 1, 2009.

ADDITIONAL READING

- Murphy C, Hahn S, Volmink J. Reduced osmolarity oral rehydration solution for treating cholera. *Cochrane Database of Systematic Reviews*. 2004, Issue 4. Art. No.: CD003754. DOI:10.1002/14651858.CD003754.pub2.
- Olsson L, Parment PA. Present and future cholera vaccines. *Expert Rev Vaccines*. 2006;5:751–2.

See Also (Topic, Algorithm, Electronic Media Element)

Diarrhea, Acute; Oral Rehydration

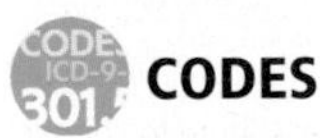

CODES

ICD9

001.9 Cholera, unspecified

CLINICAL PEARLS

- To avoid cholera while traveling, pay scrupulous attention to drinking only safe water and monitor personal hygiene.
- Currently available vaccine is of limited efficacy and should not be relied upon to prevent disease.
- During acute infection, patients may lose as much as 1 liter per hour in diarrhea and must be hydrated vigorously, then maintained on maintenance fluids until diarrhea abates.

CHRONIC COUGH

Jacqueline L. Olin, MS, PharmD, BCPS, CPP
Susan Ziglar, MD

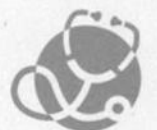

BASICS

DESCRIPTION

- Chronic cough persists >8 weeks in adults.
- Subacute cough describes cough lasting 3–8 weeks.
- In children, chronic cough is defined as cough for >4 weeks in duration.
- Patients present because of fear of the causative illness (e.g., cancer), as well as annoyance, self-consciousness, and hoarseness.
- Patients with stress urinary incontinence may find cough particularly troubling.
- At the primary care level, COPD and smoking-related cough are most common causes.
- System(s) affected: Gastrointestinal; Pulmonary

EPIDEMIOLOGY

- Predominant age: All age groups
- Predominant sex: Male = Female

Incidence

Recurrent cough has been reported at 3–40% by various population estimates.

Prevalence

Chronic cough is one of the most common reasons for primary care visits.

RISK FACTORS

Although various conditions may contribute to chronic cough, the main causes include smoking and pulmonary diseases.

PATHOPHYSIOLOGY

Varies with findings and disorders implicated

ETIOLOGY

- Often multiple etiologies, but most are related to bronchial irritation. Most frequent etiologies (account for >90% of cases) in nonsmokers include:
  - Upper airway cough syndrome (UACS) (postnasal drip syndrome)
  - Asthma
  - Nonasthmatic eosinophilic bronchitis (NAEB)
  - GERD
- Other causes:
  - Chronic smoking or exposure to smoke or pollutants
  - Aspiration
  - Bronchiectasis
  - ACE inhibitor therapy
  - Pertussis
  - Tuberculosis
  - Cystic fibrosis
  - Chronic interstitial lung disease
  - Restrictive lung disease
  - Neoplasms: lung or laryngeal cancer, other
  - Psychogenic (habit cough)

COMMONLY ASSOCIATED CONDITIONS

Patients with UACS, asthma, and GERD may present with chronic cough as the only symptom and not the usual symptoms associated with the diagnoses.

DIAGNOSIS

HISTORY

- The age of the patient, presence of associated signs/symptoms, medical history, medication history (ACE inhibitor), environmental exposures, potential for aspiration, and smoking history may make some causes more likely.
- The character of cough or description of sputum quality is rarely helpful in predicting the underlying cause.
- Cough diaries have not correlated well with objective measures.
- Various ambulatory systems for recording cough are under development.

PHYSICAL EXAM

- Signs and symptoms are variable and related to the underlying cause; usually a nonproductive cough with no other signs or symptoms.
- Possible signs and symptoms of UACS, sinusitis, GERD, congestive heart failure
- Absence of additional signs/symptoms of a particular condition not necessarily helpful (75% of GERD patients have no other signs or symptoms)

DIAGNOSTIC TESTS & INTERPRETATION

Extensive testing only if indicated by the history and physical. Simple testing (CXR, sinus CT) is followed by empiric therapy directed at likely underlying etiology.

Pediatric Considerations

Children with chronic cough should undergo, at a minimum, spirometry and chest radiograph (if age-appropriate).

Lab

Initial lab tests

As indicated by history and physical

Follow-Up & Special Considerations

If clinically indicated:

- Sweat chloride testing
- Sputum for eosinophils and cytology

Imaging

Initial approach

If clinically indicated: CXR

Follow-Up & Special Considerations

If clinically indicated:

- Chest CT
- Endoscopy

Diagnostic Procedures/Surgery

If diagnosis suspected and inadequate response to initial measures, procedures can be considered:

- Pulmonary function testing
- Purified protein derivative (PPD) skin testing
- 24-hour esophageal pH monitor
- Bronchoscopy if necessary
- Endoscopic or video fluoroscopic swallow evaluation or barium esophagram
- Sinus CT
- Ambulatory cough monitoring and cough challenge with citric acid or capsaicin (at specialized cough clinic)
- Echocardiogram

Pathological Findings

Specific to underlying cause

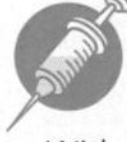

TREATMENT

- With chronic cough, empiric treatment should be directed at the most common causes (UACS, asthma, GERD, NAEB) (1)[C].
- Oral antihistamine/decongestant therapy with a 1st-generation antihistamine should be initial empiric treatment (1)[C].
- In patients with cough associated with the common cold, nonsedating antihistamines were not found to be effective in reducing cough (1)[C].
- In stable patients with chronic bronchitis, therapy with ipratropium bromide may reduce chronic cough (2)[C].
- Centrally-acting antitussive drugs (codeine, dextromethorphan) are recommended for short-term symptomatic relief of coughing in patients with chronic bronchitis (2)[C]:
  - These agents have limited efficacy in cough due to upper respiratory infections (2)[C].
- For cough associated with lung cancer, the use of narcotic cough suppressants is recommended (2)[C].

ediatric Considerations

In 2008, the FDA issued a public health advisory stating that OTC cough and cold medicines, including antitussives, expectorants, nasal decongestants, antihistamines, or combinations should not be given to children <2 years.

The American Academy of Pediatrics does not recommend central cough suppressants for treating any kind of cough (1)[B].

In children <14 years old, when pediatric recommendations are not available, adult recommendations should be used with caution (1)[C].

Some children with recurrent cough and no evidence of airway obstruction may benefit from an inhaled β-agonist (3)[C].

IEDICATION

eatments (antacids, bronchodilators, inhaled orticosteroids, proton pump inhibitors, antibiotics) hould be directed at the specific cause of cough.

irst Line

In adults, oral antihistamine/decongestant therapy should be empiric treatment. Multiple formulations are available OTC in combination with other ingredients. Advise patients to review labels carefully or consult pharmacist.

- Chlorpheniramine 2 mg/phenylephrine 5 mg/ Acetaminophen 325 mg (Tylenol Allergy Multi-Symptom) 2 caplets or gelcaps PO q12h (Maximum 12 caplets or gelcaps in 24 hours: Age >12 years.

Central cough suppressants for short-term symptomatic relief of nonproductive cough:

- Dextromethorphan 10–20 mg PO q4h. Age >12 years. Use 5–10 mg PO q4h for age 6–12 years.
- Narcotics: Codeine 15–30 mg PO q6h; hydrocodone (Vicodin) 5 mg PO q6h; hydrocodone (Tussionex Pennkinetic) 10 mg (5 mL) PO q12h for age 12 or over

econd Line

A peripherally acting antitussive agent has been used.

- Benzonatate (Tessalon Perles) 100–200 mg PO three times daily as needed (Maximum 600 mg daily): Age >10

Results from a small randomized placebo-controlled trial (n = 27) demonstrated subjective cough score improvement in patients using slow-release morphine sulfate. Patients had failed with other antitussive therapies. Side effects included constipation and drowsiness and there were no discontinuations due to adverse events (4)[C].

- Morphine was administered 5–10 mg PO twice daily.

For patients with cystic fibrosis, amiloride may increase cough clearance.

ADDITIONAL TREATMENT

General Measures

- In patients with chronic cough, considerations for potential etiology should include asthma (1)[B] or UACS (1)[C].
- With concomitant complaints of heartburn and regurgitation, GERD should be considered as a potential etiology (1)[C].
- 90% of patients will have resolution of cough after smoking cessation (1)[A].
- When indicated, ACE inhibitor therapy should be switched in patients in whom intolerable cough occurs (1)[A].
- Empiric treatment of postnasal drip and GERD.
- Consider nonpharmacological options such as warm fluids, hard candy, or nasal drops. In infants and children, can try clearing secretions with a bulb syringe.
- Attempt maximal therapy for single most likely cause for several weeks, then search for coexistent etiologies.

Issues for Referral

Refer based on specific diagnosis for cough.

SURGERY/OTHER PROCEDURES

Fundoplication may be effective for cough secondary to refractory GERD.

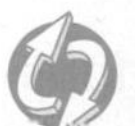

ONGOING CARE

FOLLOW-UP RECOMMENDATIONS

Consider stepwise withdrawal of medications after resolution of cough.

Patient Monitoring

Frequent follow-up is necessary to assess the effectiveness of the treatment and the addition of other medications as needed.

DIET

Patients with GERD may benefit by avoiding ethanol, caffeine, nicotine, citrus, tomatoes, chocolate, and fatty foods.

PATIENT EDUCATION

- Reassure patient that most cases do not have life-threatening causes and that the condition can usually be managed effectively.
- Counsel that several weeks to a month may be needed for significant reduction or total elimination of cough.
- Prepare the patient for the possibility of multiple diagnostic tests and therapeutic regimens, because the treatment is very often empiric.

PROGNOSIS

- >80% of patients can be effectively diagnosed and treated using a systematic approach.
- Cough from any cause may take weeks to months until resolution, and resolution depends greatly on efficacy of treatment directed at underlying etiology.

COMPLICATIONS

- Cardiovascular: Arrhythmias, syncope
- Stress urinary incontinence
- Abdominal and intercostal muscle strain
- GI: Emesis, hemorrhage, herniation
- Neurologic: Dizziness, headache, seizures
- Respiratory: Pneumothorax, laryngeal, or tracheobronchial trauma
- Skin: Petechiae, purpura, disruption of surgical wounds
- Medication side effects
- Other: Negative impact on quality of life

C

REFERENCES

1. Irwin RS, Baumann MH, Bolser DC, et al. Diagnosis and management of cough executive summary: ACCP evidence-based clinical practice guidelines. *Chest*. 2006;129:1S–23S.
2. Bolser DC. Cough suppressant and pharmacologic protussive therapy: ACCP evidence-based clinical practice guidelines. *Chest*. 2006;129:238S–249S.
3. Gupta A, et al. Management of chronic non-specific cough in childhood: An evidence-based review. *Arch Dis Child Educ Pract Ed*. 2007; 92:ep33–ep39.
4. Morice AH, Menon MS, Mulrennan SA et al. Opiate therapy in chronic cough. *Am J Respir Crit Care Med*. 2007;175:312–5.

ADDITIONAL READING

Pavord ID, Chung KF. Management of chronic cough. *Lancet*. 2008;371:1375–84.

See Also (Topic, Algorithm, Electronic Media Element)

Asthma; Bronchiectasis; Congestive Heart Failure; Eosinophilic Pneumonias; Gastroesophageal Reflux Disease (GERD); Laryngeal Cancer; Lung, Primary Malignancies; Pertussis; Pulmonary Edema; Rhinitis, Allergic; Sinusitis; Tuberculosis

Algorithm: Cough, Chronic

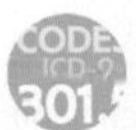

CODES

ICD9

786.2 Cough

CLINICAL PEARLS

- Chronic cough is defined as a cough that persists for >8 weeks in adults.
- In patients with chronic cough, most frequent etiologies include a history of smoking, asthma, UACS, and GERD.
- In 2008, the FDA issued a public health advisory stating that OTC cough and cold medicines should not be given to children <2 years.
- Consumer Healthcare Products Association (CHPA) members are voluntarily changing OTC product labels to state "do not use" in children <4 years old. New child-resistant packaging and measuring devices are being developed.

CHRONIC FATIGUE SYNDROME

Joan M. Stachnik, PharmD, BCPS
Anthony Valdini, MD

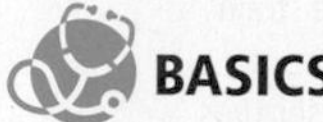

BASICS

DESCRIPTION

- A condition characterized by profound mental and physical exhaustion, with at least 6 months presence of multiple systemic and neuropsychiatric symptoms. At least 4 of 8 associated conditions are required per Centers for Disease Control and Prevention (CDC) definition:
  - Impaired memory
  - Sore throat
  - Tender lymph nodes
  - Persistent muscle or joint pain
  - New headaches
  - Unrefreshing sleep
  - Postexertion malaise
- Must have a new or definite onset (not lifelong). Fatigue is not relieved by rest and results in >50% reduction in previous activities (occupational, educational, social, and personal). Other potential medical causes must be ruled out.

EPIDEMIOLOGY

- Predominant age: 20–50 years
- Predominant sex: Male < Female
- All socioeconomic groups
- Because of cultural differences in presentation, doctors in less developed countries may not recognize the syndrome, making an accurate prevalence difficult to determine (1).
- Various associations between ethnicity and incidence have been reported. Higher rates found in ethnic minorities (Native Americans, Latinos, and African Americans) compared to white populations, based on population studies. Service-based studies (tertiary care) have reported higher rates among whites, or no association between incidence and ethnicity (2).

Incidence

Available studies have focused on prevalence of the disorder.

Prevalence

Estimates vary widely and depend upon case definition and population studied, but a reasonable estimate using a strict case definition is 100 cases per 100,000 population. Community-based studies have reported prevalence rates of 0.23% and 0.42%.

RISK FACTORS

Possible predisposing factors include (3,4):

- Personality characteristics (neuroticism and introversion)
- Lifestyle:
  - Childhood inactivity or overactivity
  - Inactivity in adulthood after infectious mononucleosis
  - Familial predisposition
  - Comorbid mood disorders of depression and anxiety
- Long-standing medical conditions in childhood
- Childhood trauma (emotional, physical, sexual abuse)

Genetics

- Higher concordance has been reported among monozygotic twins compared with dizygotic twins.
- Gender may be a significant predictor

ETIOLOGY

- Unknown and likely multifactorial:
  - Possible interaction between genetic predisposition, environmental factors, an initiating stressor, and perpetuating factors
- Physiologic or environmental stressor could be precipitant.
- Many patients with chronic fatigue recall significant stressors (e.g., major medical procedure, loss of a loved one, loss of employment) in months before symptoms began.
- Systems hypothesized to contribute to physiology include:
  - Neuroendocrine (e.g., diminished cortisol response to increased corticotropin concentrations)
  - Immune (e.g., increased C-reactive protein and beta-2 microglobulin) (5)
  - Neuromuscular (e.g., dysfunction of oxidative metabolism) (5)
- Serotonergic (e.g., hyperserotonergic mechanisms or upregulation of serotonin receptors).

COMMONLY ASSOCIATED CONDITIONS

- Common comorbidities include:
  - Fibromyalgia
  - Irritable bowel syndrome
  - Temporomandibular joint disorder
  - Anxiety disorders
  - Major depression
  - Post-traumatic stress disorder (including physical and/or sexual past abuse)
  - Domestic violence
- Exclusions:
  - Patients are excluded from chronic fatigue syndrome (CFS) definition until 2 years after resolution of substance/alcohol abuse and 5 years after resolution of anorexia nervosa or bulimia.

DIAGNOSIS

HISTORY

See "Description" for CFS historical features.

PHYSICAL EXAM

Complete physical examination to rule out other medical causes for symptoms. Note: Tender adenopathy is one of the defining criteria.

DIAGNOSTIC TESTS & INTERPRETATION

No single diagnostic test available

Lab

Standard laboratory tests are recommended to rule out other causes for symptoms (6):

- Chemistry panel
- Complete blood count (CBC)
- Urinalysis
- Thyroid-stimulating hormone (TSH)
- Erythrocyte sedimentation rate (ESR) or C-reactive protein
- Liver function
- Screen for drugs of abuse
- Age-/gender-appropriate cancer screening
- Additional studies, if clinical findings are suggestive (6):
  - Antinuclear antibodies (if +ESR)
  - Rheumatoid factor (if +ESR)
  - Creatine kinase
  - Tuberculin skin test
  - Serum cortisol
  - Human immunodeficiency virus (HIV)
  - Lyme serology
  - Gluten sensitivity (IgA tissue transglutaminase)

Follow-Up & Special Considerations

- Assessment for comorbid psychiatric disorders.
- Assessment for personality and psychosocial factor and maladaptive coping styles.
- In patients with sleep disturbance, polysomnograph may reveal a treatable comorbid disease.

Imaging

No applicable imaging tests available

DIFFERENTIAL DIAGNOSIS

- Insomnia: Primary (no clear etiology) vs. secondary (due to anxiety, depression, environmental factors, poor sleep hygiene, etc.)
- Idiopathic chronic fatigue (i.e., fatigue of unknown cause for >6 months without meeting criteria for CFS)
- Morbid obesity, body mass index (BMI) >40
- Malignancy
- Autoimmune disease
- Localized infection (e.g., occult abscess)
- Chronic or subacute bacterial disease (e.g., endocarditis)
- Lyme disease
- Fungal disease (e.g., histoplasmosis, coccidioidomycosis)
- Parasitic disease (e.g., amebiasis, giardiasis, helminth infestation)
- HIV-related disease
- Psychiatric disorders:
  - Major depression
  - Somatization disorder
- Chronic inflammatory disease (sarcoidosis, Wegene granulomatosis)
- Known chronic viral disease (HIV)
- Neuromuscular disease (multiple sclerosis, myasthenia gravis)
- Endocrine disorder (hypothyroidism, Addison disease, Cushing's syndrome, diabetes mellitus)
- Iatrogenic (e.g., medication side effects)
- Toxic agent exposure
- Other known or defined systemic disease (chronic pulmonary, cardiac, hepatic, renal, or hematologic disease)
- Pregnancy until 3 months post-partum
- Physiologic fatigue (inadequate or disrupted sleep, menopause)
- *Weakness* and *sleepiness* can indicate a different etiology.

TREATMENT

MEDICATION

- No established pharmacologic treatment recommendations
- Studies have been conducted with antidepressants, immunoglobulins, hydrocortisone, and modafinil. None have shown clear benefit (6).
- If insomnia present, use of non-addicting sleep aids (hydroxyzine, trazodone, doxepin, etc.) may improve outcomes.

ADDITIONAL TREATMENT

General Measures

Two treatments have been shown effective, often used in combination (7,8,9):
- Individual cognitive behavioral therapy (CBT): Challenge fatigue-related cognition. Plan social and occupational rehabilitation.
- Graded exercise therapy (GET): Track amount of exercise patient can do without exacerbating symptoms and gradually increase the intensity and duration. Both involve a carefully planned balance between activity and rest.

- Patients learn how to gradually increase activity in a way that will not exacerbate their illness. Vigorous exercise can trigger relapse, perhaps related to immune dysregulation; therefore, activity plan must be carefully monitored (8).
- Improves functional capacity and diminishes sense of fatigue (9).
- GET is more effective when delivered with educational interventions, explaining symptoms, and encouragement with telephone reminders (9).
- The duration of illness does not predict treatment outcome, so this approach can be applied to patients with chronic symptoms.

Issues for Referral

- Psychiatrist to assess for comorbid disorders if screening indicates need
- Rehabilitative medicine

COMPLEMENTARY AND ALTERNATIVE MEDICINE

- Although complementary and alternative medicines have been suggested, data are insufficient to recommend their use.
- Social support groups have not proven to be effective.

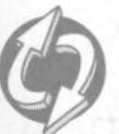

ONGOING CARE

FOLLOW-UP RECOMMENDATIONS

- Gradual increase in physical exercise with scheduled rest periods.
- Avoid extended periods of rest.

Patient Monitoring

Although no consensus exists, periodic re-evaluation is appropriate for support, relief of symptoms, and assessment for other possible causes of symptoms.

DIET

- No diet has been shown to be effective for treatment of CFS.
- A BMI of 40 has been associated with fatigue in general. Whether weight loss improves symptoms in such patients has yet to be tested.

PATIENT EDUCATION

- Patient education is an important part of treatment of CFS, such as education on the benefits of cognitive therapies, lifestyle changes, and pharmacologic therapy directed at specific associated symptoms.
- Chronic Fatigue and Immune Dysfunction Syndrome Association of America: www.cfids.org
- CDC Chronic Fatigue Syndrome: www.cdc.gov

PROGNOSIS

- Fluctuating course
- Generally, improvement is slow, with a course of months to years.
- An estimated 5% fully recover.

COMPLICATIONS

- Depression
- Unemployment. Although studies document improvement with treatment, fewer than 1/3 of patients in trials return to work (10).
- Polypharmacy

REFERENCES

1. Cho HJ, Menezes PR, Hotopf M et al. Comparative epidemiology of chronic fatigue syndrome in Brazilian and British primary care: prevalence and recognition. *Br J Psychiatry*. 2009;194:117–22.
2. Dinos S, Khoshaba B, Ashby D et al. A systematic review of chronic fatigue, its syndromes and ethnicity: prevalence, severity, co-morbidity and coping. *Int J Epidemiol*. 2009;38:1554–70.
3. Viner R, Hotopf M. Childhood predictors of self reported chronic fatigue syndrome/myalgic encephalomyelitis in adults: national birth cohort study. *BMJ*. 2004;329:941.
4. Heim C, Wagner D, Maloney E, et al. Early adverse experience and risk for chronic fatigue syndrome: results from a population-based study. *Arch Gen Psychiatry*. 2006;63:1258–66.
5. Fulle S, Pietrangelo T, Mancinelli R et al. Specific correlations between muscle oxidative stress and chronic fatigue syndrome: a working hypothesis. *J Muscle Res Cell Motil*. 2007;28:355–62.
6. Baker R, Shaw EJ. Diagnosis and management of chronic fatigue syndrome or myalgic encephalomyelitis (or encephalopathy): summary of NICE guidance. *BMJ*. 2007;335:446–8.
7. Margo KL, Margo GM. Two therapies lift mood in chronic fatigue syndrome. *Current Psychiatry*. 2006;5:91–100.
8. Nijs J, Paul L, Wallman K. Chronic fatigue syndrome: an approach combining self-management with graded exercise to avoid exacerbations. *J Rehabil Med*. 2008;40:241–7.
9. Price JR, Mitchell E, Tidy E, et al. Cognitive behaviour therapy for chronic fatigue syndrome in adults. *Cochrane Database Syst Rev*. 2008: CD001027.
10. Cairns R, Hotopf M. A systematic review describing the prognosis of chronic fatigue syndrome. *Occup Med-Oxford*. 2005;55:20–31.

ADDITIONAL READING

- Adams D, Wu T, Yang X et al. Traditional Chinese medicinal herbs for the treatment of idiopathic chronic fatigue and chronic fatigue syndrome. *Cochrane Database Syst Rev*. 2009;CD006348.
- Baker R, Shaw EJ et al. Diagnosis and management of chronic fatigue syndrome or myalgic encephalomyelitis (or encephalopathy): summary of NICE guidance. *BMJ*. 2007;335:446–8.
- Prins JB, van der Meer JW, Bleijenberg G et al. Chronic fatigue syndrome. *Lancet*. 2006;367: 346–55.
- Rimes KA, Chalder T et al. Treatments for chronic fatigue syndrome. *Occup Med (Lond)*. 2005;55: 32–9.

See Also (Topic, Algorithm, Electronic Media Element)

Algorithm: Fatigue

CODES

ICD9

780.71 Chronic fatigue syndrome

CLINICAL PEARLS

- CFS and depression can be comorbid. However, to differentiate between the two, sore throat, tender lymph nodes, and post-exercise fatigue are much more characteristic of CFS.
- Although a number randomized controlled trials on various pharmacologic agents (e.g., antidepressants, immune modulators) have been conducted, no single agent has been shown to be consistently effective.
- About 70% of patients show improvement with cognitive behavioral therapy, compared to 55% with graded exercise therapy; in many cases, these two treatments can be undertaken in combination.
- There are many more patients with idiopathic chronic fatigue than true CFS. To diagnose CFS, CDC criteria need to be met; standardized instruments (SF-36, Symptom Index) have been shown to be of use in the empirical diagnosis of CFS.

CHRONIC KIDNEY DISEASE

Lisa Pelunis-Messier, PharmD
Mhd Basheer Rahmoun, MD

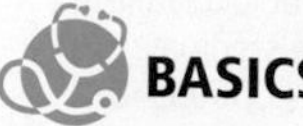

BASICS

Chronic kidney disease (CKD) is defined as:

- Kidney damage for ≥3 months, defined by structural or functional abnormalities of the kidney, with or without decrease in glomerular filtration rate (GFR), by either pathologic abnormalities or markers of damage, including abnormalities in blood or urine tests or imaging studies, *or*
- GFR <60 mL/min/1.73 m^2 for ≥3 months, with or without kidney damage (1)

DESCRIPTION

- CKD is classified into 5 stages by GFR estimated by Modification of Diet in Renal Disease (MDRD) equation:
  - Stage 1: Kidney damage with GFR >90 mL/min/1.73 m^2
  - Stage 2: Kidney damage with mild ↓ GFR 60–89 mL/min/1.73 m^2
  - Stage 3: Moderate ↓ GFR 30–59 mL/min/1.73 m^2
  - Stage 4: Severe ↓ GFR 15–29 mL/min/1.73 m^2
  - Stage 5: Kidney failure: GFR <15 mL/min/1.73 m^2 or dialysis
- System(s) affected: Renal/Urinary; Cardiovascular; Skeletal; Endocrine; Metabolic; Hematologic; Lymphatic; Immune; Neurologic
- Synonym(s): Chronic renal failure; Chronic renal insufficiency

Geriatric Considerations

GFR normally decreases with age, despite normal creatinine (Cr).

ALERT

- Adjust renally cleared drugs for GFR in elderly.
- Use nephrotoxic agents with caution in elderly.

Pediatric Considerations

- CKD definition is not applicable for children <6 years; lower GFR even when corrected for body surface area.
- Estimated GFR based on serum Cr can be compared with normative age-appropriate values to detect renal impairment.

Pregnancy Considerations

- Renal function in CKD may deteriorate during pregnancy.
- Cr >1.5 and hypertension are major risk factors for worsening renal function.
- Increased risk of premature labor, preeclampsia, and/or fetal loss
- Angiotensin-converting enzyme (ACE) inhibitors and angiotensin receptor blockers (ARBs) are contraindicated due to teratogenicity.
- Use diuretics with caution.

EPIDEMIOLOGY

- Majority of people with CKD in stages 1–3
- African Americans are 4 times more likely to develop chronic kidney failure than Caucasians.
- Predominant sex: For the CKD stages, was similar in both sexes; however, incidence rate of end-stage renal disease (ESRD) is males 409/million > females 276/million (USRDS 2004).

Incidence

- An estimated annual incidence of CKD was 1700/million population.
- Estimated ESRD patients by 2010: 129,200 ± 7742 new patients; 651,330 ± 15,874 long-term ESRD; 520,240 ± 25,609 dialysis; 178,806 ± 4349 with functioning transplants; and 95,550 ± 5478 patients on waiting lists

Prevalence

The unadjusted prevalence and incidence rates of ESRD (stage 5) are 1585 and 350.7/million, respectively. These numbers do not reflect the burden of earlier stages of CKD (1–40, which are estimated to affect 13.2% of population nationwide, or 26.3 million Americans (2).

RISK FACTORS

- Type 1 or 2 diabetes mellitus (most common)
- Age >60 years
- Cardiovascular disease (e.g., hypertension [HTN] [common])
- Acute kidney injury
- Urinary tract obstruction (e.g., benign prostatic hyperplasia)
- Autoimmune disease/vasculitis/connective tissue disorder
- Family history of CKD
- Nephrotoxic drugs (lithium, salicylate, high doses NSAIDs)
- Congenital anomalies; obstructive uropathy; renal aplasia/hypoplasia/dysplasia; reflux nephropathy
- Hyperlipidemia
- Low income/education/ethnic minority status
- Obesity/smoking
- Neoplasia

Genetics

- Alport syndrome, Fabry disease, sickle cell anemia, systemic lupus erythematosus (SLE), and autosomal-dominant polycystic kidney disease can lead to CKD
- Polymorphisms in gene that encodes for podocyte mom muscle myosin IIA are more common in African Americans than Caucasians and appear to increase risk for nondiabetic ESRD (3)

GENERAL PREVENTION

- Treat reversible causes: Hypovolemia, infections, diuretics, drugs (NSAIDS, aminoglycosides, IV contrast).
- Treat risk factors: diabetes mellitus, HTN, hyperlipidemia, smoking, and obesity.
- Adjust medication doses to prevent renal toxicity.

PATHOPHYSIOLOGY

Progressive destruction of kidney nephrons; GFR will drop gradually, and plasma Cr values will approximately double with 50% reduction in GFR and 75% loss of functioning nephrons mass.

ETIOLOGY

- Renal parenchymal/glomerular:
  - Nephritic: hematuria, red blood cell (RBC) casts, HTN, variable proteinuria:
    - Focal proliferative: IgA nephropathy, SLE, Henoch-Schöenlein purpura, Alport syndrome; proliferative glomerulonephritis; crescentic glomerulonephritis
    - Diffuse proliferative: Membranoproliferative glomerulonephritis, SLE, cryoglobulinemia, rapidly progressive glomerulonephritis (RPGN), Goodpasture syndrome.
  - Nephrotic: proteinuria (>3.5 g/day), hypoalbuminemia, hyperlipidemia and edema:
    - Minimal change disease, membranous nephropathy, focal segmental glomerulosclerosis
    - Amyloidosis, diabetic nephropathy
- Vascular: HTN, thrombotic microangiopathies, vasculitis (Wegener), scleroderma
- Interstitial-tubular: Infections, obstruction, toxins, allergic interstitial nephritis, multiple myeloma, connective tissue disease, cystic disease
- Postrenal: Obstruction (benign prostatic hyperplasia), neoplasm, neurogenic bladder

COMMONLY ASSOCIATED CONDITIONS

- HTN, Diabetes mellitus, Cardiovascular disease

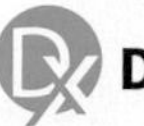

DIAGNOSIS

HISTORY

- Oliguria, nocturia, polyuria, hematouria, change in urinary frequency
- Bone disease
- Fatigue, depression, weakness
- Pruritus
- Metallic taste in mouth, anorexia, nausea, vomiting
- Dyspnea
- Hypertension
- Poorly controlled diabetes with retinopathy, neuropathy
- Hyperlipidemia
- Claudication, restless legs

PHYSICAL EXAM

- Volume status (pallor, blood pressure/orthostatics; edema; jugular venous distention; weight)
- Skin: Sallow complexion, uremic frost
- Ammonialike odor (uremic fetor)
- Cardiovascular: Assess for murmurs, bruits, pericarditis
- Chest: Pleural effusion
- Rectal: Enlarged prostate
- Central nervous system: (Asterixis, confusion, seizures, coma), peripheral neuropathy

DIAGNOSTIC TESTS & INTERPRETATION

Lab

Initial lab tests

- GFR can be estimated by MDRD equation:
  - GFR(mL/min/1.73 m^2) = 186 × {[serum Cr μmol/1/88.4] − 1.154} × {age (years) − 0.203} × 0.742 for females, or 1.21 for males
- Cr clearance (CrCl) can be calculated using Cockroft-Gault formula :
  - CrCl (male) = ([140-age] × weight(kg)/(serum Cr X72)
  - CrCl (female) = CrCl (male) × 0.82
- Urine analysis:
  - Urine microscopy: White blood cell/RBC casts, dysmorphic RBCs
  - Urine electrolytes: Sodium, Cr, urea (if on loop diuretics)

- Proteinuria/albuminuria
  - 24-hour urine collection: >20–200 μg/min
  - Spot urine sample: >30–300mg/L
  - Albumin/Cr ratio (ACR): ≥3.5 mg/mmol (Females); 2.5 mg/mmol (males)

Hematology:
- Normochromic, normocytic anemia, increased bleeding time

Chemistry:
- Elevated BUN, Cr, Hyperkalemia
- Increased parathyroid hormone, decreased 25-(OH) Vitamin D
- Hypocalcemia, Hyperphosphatemia
- Hyperlipidemia
- Metabolic acidosis
- Decreased albumin

ALERT

Drugs that may alter lab result:
- Cimetidine: Inhibits Cr secretion
- Trimethoprim: Inhibits Cr secretion
- Cefoxitin and flucytosine: Increases serum Cr
- Diltiazem and verapamil: Have significant antiproteinuric effects in patients with >300 mg/day of proteinuria

Follow-Up & Special Considerations

- Serology: ANA; antineutrophil cyplasmic antibody; complements (C3, C4, CH50); anti-GBM antibodies; hepatitis B, C; and HIV screening
- If proteinuria in patient >45 years, serum and urine immunoelectrophoresis

Imaging

- Ultrasound: Small, echogenic kidneys; may see obstruction (e.g., hydronephrosis); cysts; kidneys may be enlarged with HIV and diabetic nephropathy.
- Doppler ultrasound to assess for renovascular disease, thrombosis
- Noncontrast CAT scan: Obstruction; calculi; cysts; neoplasm; renal artery stenosis
- MRI/MRA; avoid gadolinium because of the risk of nephrogenic systemic fibrosis.
- Renal arteriogram for renal artery stenosis can be therapeutic (angioplasty or stenting).
- Renal scan to screen for differential function between kidneys

Diagnostic Procedures/Surgery

Biopsy: Hematuria, proteinuria, acute/progressive renal failure, nephritic or nephrotic syndrome

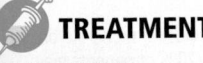

TREATMENT

MEDICATION

- Hypertension: Goal is blood pressure <130/80:
  - ACE inhibitors or ARBs for blood pressure control and antiproteinuric effect
    - Potential for hyperkalemia
    - Can tolerate up to 30% rise in serum Cr unless hyperkalemia develops
    - If goal not reached, add diuretic (thiazides, then loop diuretic), followed by diltiazem or verapamil or a β-blocker
    - Aldosterone antagonists for antiproteinuric effect; hyperkalemia potential.
- Secondary hyperparathyroidism:
  - Cinacalcet, paricalcitol (decrease PTH levels)
  - Recommended serum phosphate maintenance Levels for CKD patients (4)

Stage	mg/dL	mmol/L
Normal Range *may vary by institution*	2.5–4.5	0.81–1.45
Stage 3 and 4 CKD (not on dialysis)	2.7–4.6	0.87–1.49
Stage 5 and ALL stages on dialysis	3.0–5.0	1.13–1.78

  - Stages 3–5 CKD (not on dialysis): Restrict dietary phosphate to 900 mg/day
    - Calcium-containing phosphate binders (with meals): Calcium carbonate, calcium acetate—risk of hypercalcemia
    - Non-calcium phosphate binders (to be taken with meals): sevelamer, lanthanum
    - Vitamin D: Inactive vitamin D 25 (ergocalciferol or cholecalciferol), calcitriol (active vitamin D 1,25 [OH])
      - Vitamin D may increase absorption of phosphate by intestines and should not be started until serum phosphate concentration is controlled
- Anemia: Ferrous sulfate, erythropoietin:
  - Indication: Start when Hgb <10 g/dL; goal range 11–12 g/dL—not to exceed 13 g/dL
- Hyperlipidemia: Statins
- Glycemic control: Goal HbA1c <7; avoid metformin owing to the risk of metabolic acidosis.
- Metabolic acidosis: Start treatment when bicarb <20 mEq/L; goal >23 mEq/L.
  - Sodium bicarbonate: Daily dose of 0.5 to 1 mEq/kg per day
  - Sodium citrate: Should be avoided in patients taking aluminum-containing antacid

ADDITIONAL TREATMENT

General Measures

- Minimize radiocontrast exposure; prehydrate; N-acetylcysteine use is controversial.
- Renal replacement: Prepare for dialysis or transplant when GFR <30 mL/min/1.73 m^2.
- Vaccines: Pneumococcal; influenza
- Encourage smoking cessation.

Issues for Referral

- Nephrology consultation early to slow progression
- If GFR <15 immediate referral; 15<GFR<29 urgent referral; 30<GFR<59 routine referral in presence of risk factors; 60<GFR<89 no referral required unless other problem present

SURGERY/OTHER PROCEDURES

Placement of dialysis access or transplantation for ESRD

IN-PATIENT CONSIDERATIONS

Admission Criteria

Uremia: nausea/vomiting, fluid overload, pericarditis, uremic encephalopathy, resistant hypertension, hyperkalemia, metabolic acidosis, hyperphosphatemia (consider dialysis)

ONGOING CARE

DIET

Nutrition consult for CKD diet:
- For GFR <60 mL/min/1.73 m^2, assess protein and energy intake; important to maintain adequate nutrition.
- Restricted intake of phosphates
- Sodium restriction
- Potassium restriction if hyperkalemic

PATIENT EDUCATION

National Kidney Federation patient Web site at: http://www.kidney.org/patients

PROGNOSIS

Patients with CKD gradually progress to ESRD

COMPLICATIONS

HTN, anemia, 2° hyperparathyroidism, renal osteodystrophy, sleep disturbances, infections, malnutrition, increased magnesium, platelet dysfunction/bleeding, pseudogout, gout, metabolic calcification, sexual dysfunction

REFERENCES

1. K/DOQI clinical practice guidelines for chronic kidney disease: evaluation, classification, and stratification. *Am J Kidney Dis*. 2002;39(2 Suppl 1):S1–266.
2. Coresh J, Selvin E, Stevens LA, Manzi J, Kusek JW, Eggers P, Van Lente F, Levey AS et al. Prevalence of chronic kidney disease in the United States. *JAMA*. 2007;298:2038–47.
3. MYH9 is associated with nondiabetic end-stage renal disease in African Americans. *Nat Genet*. 2008;40(10):1185–92. Epub 2008 Sep 14
4. KDIGO Clinical Practice guidelines for the diagnosis, evaluation, and treatment of chronic kidney disease-mineral and bone disorder (CKD-MBD). *Kidney Int* 2009;76(Suppl 113):S1.

See Also (Topic, Algorithm, Electronic Media Element)

Proteinuria; Hydronephrosis; Nephrotic Syndrome; Polycystic Kidney Disease
Algorithm: Anuria or Oliguria

CODES

ICD9

- 585.1 Chronic kidney disease, stage i
- 585.2 Chronic kidney disease, stage ii (mild)
- 585.3 Chronic kidney disease, stage iii (moderate)

CLINICAL PEARLS

- Patient education is important in slowing the progression of CKD.
- Maintaining blood pressure <130/80 is crucial.
- Prevent and treat reversible causes of renal dysfunction.

CHRONIC OBSTRUCTIVE PULMONARY DISEASE AND EMPHYSEMA

Alan J. Cropp, MD

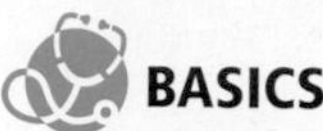

BASICS

DESCRIPTION

- Chronic obstructive pulmonary disease (COPD) encompasses several diffuse pulmonary diseases, including chronic bronchitis, asthma, cystic fibrosis, bronchiectasis, and emphysema:
  - The term usually describes a mixture of chronic bronchitis and emphysema.
  - Characterized by airflow limitation that is not fully reversible, is progressive, and inflammation is present (1,2,3)
- Chronic bronchitis is defined clinically by increased mucus production and recurrent cough present on most days for at least 3 months during at least 2 consecutive years.
- Emphysema is the destruction of interalveolar septa; it occurs in the distal or terminal airways and involves both airways and lung parenchyma.

EPIDEMIOLOGY

Incidence

Affects ~10–20% of adults; >100,000 deaths/year in US

Prevalence

- 14 million people have chronic bronchitis; 2 million people have emphysema.
- 4th leading cause of death in US

RISK FACTORS

- Smoking
- Passive smoking, especially adults whose parents smoked
- Severe viral pneumonia early in life
- Aging
- Alcohol consumption
- Airway hyperactivity

Genetics

- Chronic bronchitis is not a genetic disorder.
- Antiprotease deficiency (due to α_1 antitrypsin deficiency) is an inherited, rare disorder due to 2 autosomal-codominant alleles.

GENERAL PREVENTION

- Avoidance of smoking is the most important preventive measure.
- Passive smoke also has been shown to be harmful.
- Early detection through pulmonary function tests (PFTs) in high-risk patients may be useful in preserving remaining lung function.

PATHOPHYSIOLOGY

- Impaired gas (CO_2 and O_2) exchange
- Airway obstruction by mucus in chronic bronchitis (1)
- Destruction of lung parenchyma in emphysema

ETIOLOGY

Cigarette smoking, air pollution, antiprotease deficiency (α_1 antitrypsin), occupational exposure (firefighters), infection possibly (viral), occupational pollutants (cadmium, silica)

COMMONLY ASSOCIATED CONDITIONS

- Lung cancer
- Coronary artery disease
- Chronic sinusitis
- Malnutrition
- Laryngeal carcinoma
- Acute bronchitis
- Sleep apnea
- Chronic respiratory failure
- Osteoporosis

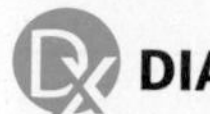

DIAGNOSIS

HISTORY

- Patient's habits with regard to tobacco should be discussed. Also review possible causes of exacerbation (e.g., recent infection) and history of cough, sputum, and dyspnea (1).
- Chronic bronchitis: Cough, sputum production, frequent infections, intermittent dyspnea, wheeze, hemoptysis, morning headache, pedal edema
- Emphysema: Minimal cough, scant sputum, dyspnea, weight loss, occasional infections

PHYSICAL EXAM

- Rarely diagnostic for COPD (3)
- Chronic bronchitis: Cyanosis, wheezing, weight gain, diminished breath sounds, distant heart sounds
- Emphysema: Barrel chest, minimal wheezing, accessory muscles used, pursed lip breathing, cyanosis slight or absent, breath sounds diminished

DIAGNOSTIC TESTS & INTERPRETATION

Lab

Initial lab tests

- Chronic bronchitis:
  - Arterial blood gases (ABGs) may show hypercapnia and hypoxia.
  - Hemoglobin may be increased.
- Emphysema:
  - Normal serum hemoglobin or polycythemia
  - Normal $PaCO_2$ on ABGs unless forced expiratory volume in 1 second (FEV1) <1 L, in which case it can be elevated.
  - Mild hypoxia

Follow-Up & Special Considerations

- Consider checking continuous overnight oximetry in selected patients.
- α_1-antitrypsin screening for those with COPD <45 years old or a blood relative with this disease

Imaging

Initial approach

- Chronic bronchitis chest x-ray (CXR): Increased bronchovascular markings and cardiomegaly
- Emphysema CXR: Small heart, hyperinflation, flat diaphragms, and possibly bullous changes

Follow-Up & Special Considerations

Chest computed tomography may show diffuse bullous changes or upper lobe predominance.

Diagnostic Procedures/Surgery

- PFTs:
  - Not indicated during acute exacerbation
  - Decreased FEV_1 and resulting reduction in FEV_1/FVC (forced vital capacity) ratio
  - Poor or absent reversibility to bronchodilator
  - Normal or reduced FVC
  - Normal or increased total lung capacity
  - Increased residual volume and functional residual capacity
  - Diffusing capacity is normal or reduced.
- Nocturnal oximetry

Pathological Findings

- Chronic bronchitis:
  - Bronchial mucous gland enlargement
  - Increased number of secretory cells in surface epithelium
  - Thickened small airways from edema and inflammation
  - Smooth muscle hyperplasia
  - Mucus plugging
  - Bacterial colonization of airways
- Emphysema:
  - Entire lung affected
  - Bronchi usually clear of secretions
  - Anthracotic pigment
  - Alveoli enlarged with loss of septa
  - Cartilage atrophy
  - Bullae

DIFFERENTIAL DIAGNOSIS

- Asthma
- Bronchiectasis
- Lung cancer
- Acute viral infection
- Normal aging of lungs
- Occupational asthma
- Chronic pulmonary embolism
- Sleep apnea
- Primary alveolar hypoventilation
- Chronic sinusitis
- Reactive airways dysfunction syndrome
- Congestive heart failure (CHF)
- Bronchiolitis obliterans
- Gastroesophageal reflux disease

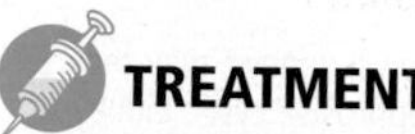

TREATMENT

MEDICATION

Medications help to reduce symptoms and exacerbations (3) and may prevent progression of disease (4,5)[A].

First Line

- Anticholinergics (2)[A]:
  - Ipratropium (Atrovent), tiotropium (Spiriva): 1 inhalation daily (6)[A]

  AND/OR
- Long-acting β-agonists:
  - Salmeterol (Serevent), formoterol (Foradil) 1 inhalation q12h or arformoterol (Brovana), formoterol (Perforomist) nebulized q12h (6)[A]

Second Line

- Trial of inhaled corticosteroids for moderate or severe disease (4)[A]. 10–20% of patients may have salutary response. Discontinue if no benefit in symptoms or objective measures in 6–8 weeks:
  - May initiate earlier if suggestion of asthmatic component to disease
  - Systemic corticosteroids; prednisone (Deltasone) can be given orally 7.5–15 mg/d
  - Consider pulse dosing (40 mg/d) with taper depending on length of therapy. Most useful in bronchitis with some reversibility (1)[A].
  - Among patients with COPD, inhaled corticosteroid use for at least 24 weeks is associated with a significantly increased risk of serious pneumonia, without a significantly increased risk of death (7)[A].
- Theophylline (1)[A]: 400 mg/d; increase by 100–200 mg in 1–2 weeks, if necessary:

- Reduce dosage in patients with impaired renal or liver function, age >55, or CHF.
- Monitor serum level. Therapeutic range is 8–13 μg/mL (1)[A].

Combination of inhaled corticosteroid, long-acting β-agonist, and anticholinergic indicated for severe disease (6)[A]

Mucolytic agents may improve secretions but do not improve outcomes.

Low-dose macrolides (clarithromycin or erythromycin) to decrease inflammation (8)[A]

α1-antitrypsin, if deficient: 60 mg/kg weekly to maintain level exceeding 80 mg/dL

Low-dose macrolides (clarithromycin, zithromycin, or erythromycin) to decrease inflammation

Precautions:
- Sympathomimetics: Excessive use may be dangerous. May need to reduce dosage or use levalbuterol (Xopenex) in patients with cardiovascular disease, hypertension (HTN), hyperthyroidism, diabetes, or convulsive disorders.
- Anticholinergics: Narrow-angle glaucoma, benign prostatic hyperplasia, bladder-neck obstruction
- Corticosteroids may mask infection or predispose to infection, especially fungal; subcapsular cataracts; glaucoma; adrenocortical insufficiency; psychic derangements; gastrointestinal bleeding; diabetes mellitus, reactivation of tuberculosis

Sympathomimetics may be aerosolized.

Anticholinergics: Ipratropium (Atrovent) may be aerosolized or combined with albuterol (Combivent).

ADDITIONAL TREATMENT

General Measures

Smoking cessation: This is the most important intervention to decrease risk (3).

Mucolytic agents

Aggressive treatment of infections (3)[A]

Treat any reversible bronchospasm.

Home oxygen: May improve survival in hypoxemia and cor pulmonale, and should be initiated early in these conditions if oxygen <89% (8)[A]

Influenza and pneumococcal immunizations

Issues for Referral

Severe exacerbation, frequent hospitalizations, age <40, rapid progression, weight loss, severe disease, or surgical evaluation

Additional Therapies

- Adequate hydration and pulmonary hygiene
- Consider postural drainage, flutter valve, or other devices to assist mucus clearance.
- Pulmonary rehabilitation may be of benefit (9).
- Occasionally, intermittent noninvasive ventilation may be of benefit with severe chronic respiratory failure (4)[A].

SURGERY/OTHER PROCEDURES

- Lung reduction surgery (selected cases)
- Lung transplantation (selected cases)

IN-PATIENT CONSIDERATIONS

Initial Stabilization

- Outpatient treatment is usually adequate.
- Supplemental oxygen and short-acting bronchodilators should be given in the emergency room (3)[A].
- Acute respiratory failure may require intensive care unit and mechanical ventilation.

Admission Criteria

- Exacerbation with acute decompensation (hypoxemia, hypercarbia) due to infection
- Need for mechanical ventilation
- Serious comorbidities, such as decompensated congestive heart failure (CHF)

Nursing

- Teach proper inhaler use.
- Monitor fluid balance.

Discharge Criteria

- Not waking at night due to dyspnea (3)
- Ability to ambulate
- Patient should have adequate gas exchange.
- Hypoxia can be treated with home O_2 (may only be temporary) (2)[A].
- Inhaled β-agonist therapy no more frequently than q4h (3).

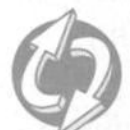

ONGOING CARE

FOLLOW-UP RECOMMENDATIONS

- May taper oral steroids as outpatient
- If pneumonia caused exacerbation, need to follow CXR until clear.

Patient Monitoring

- Severe or unstable patients should be seen monthly. When stable, see every 6 months.
- Check theophylline level with dose adjustment, then check every 6–12 months.
- With home O_2, check ABGs yearly or with change in condition. Monitor O_2 saturation (pulse oximetry) more frequently.
- Some patients only desaturate at night, thus only need nocturnal O_2.
- Avoid travel at high altitude.
- Discuss advance directive and health care proxy.
- Yearly PFTs

DIET

A high-protein diet is suggested. Decreased carbohydrates may benefit those with hypercarbia.

PATIENT EDUCATION

Printed material available from National Jewish Hospital in Denver, CO. Local branch of American Lung Association also has informational material.

PROGNOSIS

- Patient's age and postbronchodilator FEV_1 are the most important predictors of prognosis. Young age and FEV_1 >50% predicted to have a good prognosis. Older patients do worse.
- Supplemental O_2, when indicated, is shown to increase survival (may only need at night).
- Smoking cessation improves prognosis.
- Malnutrition, cor pulmonale, hypercapnia, and pulse >100 indicate a poor prognosis.

COMPLICATIONS

- Infections
- Cor pulmonale
- Secondary polycythemia
- Bullous lung disease
- Acute or chronic respiratory failure
- Pulmonary HTN
- Malnutrition
- Pneumothorax
- Poor sleep quality
- Arrhythmias

REFERENCES

1. Braman SS. Chronic cough due to chronic bronchitis: ACCP evidence-based clinical practice guidelines. *Chest*. 2006;129:104S–115S.
2. Celli BR. Update on the management of COPD. *Chest*. 2008;133:1451–62.
3. Wilt TJ, Niewoehner D, MacDonald R, et al. Management of stable chronic obstructive pulmonary disease: a systematic review for a clinical practice guideline. *Ann Intern Med*. 2007;147:639–53.
4. Maclay JD, Rabinovich RA, MacNee W. Update in chronic obstructive pulmonary disease 2008. *Am J Respir Crit Care Med*. 2009;179:533–41.
5. Rubins JB, Raci E, Kunisaki KM. Managing stable COPD in 2009: incorporating results from recent clinical studies into a goal-directed approach for clinicians. *Postgrad Med*. 2009;121:104–12.
6. Rabe KF, Hurd S, Anzueto A, et al. Global strategy for the diagnosis, management, and prevention of chronic obstructive pulmonary disease: GOLD executive summary. *Am J Respir Crit Care Med*. 2007;176:532–55.
7. Singh S, Amin AV, Loke YK. Long-term use of inhaled corticosteroids and the risk of pneumonia in chronic obstructive pulmonary disease: a meta-analysis. *Arch Intern Med*. 2009;169:219–29.
8. Cosio BG, Agusti A et al. Update in chronic obstructive pulmonary disease 2009. *Am J Respir Crit Care Med*. 2010;181:655–60.
9. Casaburi R, ZuWallack R. Pulmonary rehabilitation for management of chronic obstructive pulmonary disease. *N Engl J Med*. 2009;360:1329–35.

See Also (Topic, Algorithm, Electronic Media Element)

Bronchitis, Acute
Algorithms: Clubbing; Cyanosis

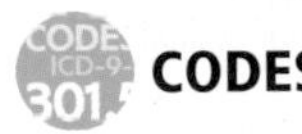

CODES

ICD9

- 492.8 Other emphysema
- 493.20 Chronic obstructive asthma, unspecified
- 496 Chronic airway obstruction, not elsewhere classified

CLINICAL PEARLS

- Screening PFTs should be done on all high-risk patients.
- Check overnight oximetry when daytime saturation is borderline.
- Influenza and pneumococcal vaccines should be kept up to date.
- Smoking cessation counseling, if applicable, is a critical component of care.

CHRONIC PAIN MANAGEMENT: AN EVIDENCE BASED APPROACH

Irene C. Coletsos, MD
Gail Gazelle, MD

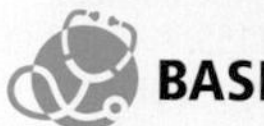

BASICS

- Defined as pain that extends beyond time of tissue healing or pain that cannot be explained by levels of pathology observed
- Because of changes in CNS, chronic pain becomes a disease state itself, continuing well beyond the initial event.
- Patients who experience chronic pain fall into three categories:
  - Those with known physical illnesses or traumas as the etiology of the chronic pain.
  - No identified physical etiology known to cause chronic pain, >50% of patients.
  - Those with psychiatric comorbidities.

EPIDEMIOLOGY

In the US, an estimated 35.5% of the residents suffer from chronic pain, the majority of which manage without use of chronic narcotics.

Prevalence

In the US, pain is the most common reason patients seek medical care. An estimated 50 million Americans suffer from chronic pain, and it is the major cause of adult disability.

RISK FACTORS

- Traumatic: Amputations, falls, motor vehicle accidents, repetitive motion injuries, sports injuries, work related injuries
- Postsurgical: e.g., failed back surgery, incisional pain, phantom limb pain, postthoracotomy syndrome.
- Medical conditions: Arthritis, back disease, cancer, fibromyalgia; neuropathies (diabetes, HIV, multiple sclerosis, shingles, past chemotherapy), radiculopathies; poststroke syndrome, spinal cord injuries
- Cancer
- Psychiatric comorbidities: Anxiety, borderline personality disorders, depression, dysthymia, post-traumatic stress disorder (PTSD), schizoaffective disorders, somatic disorders, the sequela of childhood sexual abuse
- Aging: Increased incidence with age, but should not be considered a "normal" part of aging
- Idiopathic: No pathological cause found despite repeated testing
- Secondary gain: Factitious disorder, malingering, Münchhausen's

GENERAL PREVENTION

- Avoidance of work-related injuries through the use of ergonomically correct workplace design
- Exercise and physical therapy to help prevent work-related low back pain
- Varicella vaccine and rapid treatment of shingles to lower risk of postherpetic neuralgia
- Tight glycemic control for diabetic patients, alcohol cessation for alcoholics, smoking cessation to avoid neuropathies

PATHOPHYSIOLOGY

With intense, repeated, or prolonged stimulation of damaged or inflamed tissues, the threshold for activating primary afferent pain fibers is lowered, the frequency of firing is higher, and there is increased response to noxious stimuli. The amygdala is thought to help modulate the relationship between pain and the emotions that may accompany it, such as anxiety and depression.

DIAGNOSIS

Chronic pain can be divided into 3 general categories:

- Nociceptive pain (2 types):
  - Somatic: Incisional, bone, soft-tissue disease. Well localized, dull, aching, throbbing, or gnawing
  - Visceral: Affecting viscera; poorly localized; described as deep, dull, and aching; may refer to sites remote from lesion
- Neuropathic pain: See "Neuropathic Pain."
- Sympathetically maintained pain: Peripheral nerve injury can cause severe burning pain associated with swelling of the affected limb, focal change in sweat production, and skin texture. Example: Complex regional pain syndrome.

HISTORY

- Use standardized tools to document baseline experience: Pain—Brief Pain Inventory (short form); Mood—Patient Health Questionnaire-9 (PHQ-9); Alcohol use—Alcohol Use Disorders Identification Test (AUDIT).
- Issues with substance abuse ("How many times in the last 12 months did you use an illegal drug or a prescription drug for nonmedical reasons?"); personal trauma; how patients have treated their pain in the past; and their current goals for pain relief (1)
  - Pain initiation, character and intensity (scale of 0–10, 10 being the worst)
  - Modifying factors (what lessens it and what makes it worse)
  - Questions about functioning—how the pain affects the patient's ability to carry on his/her life and job
  - Mood and sensory experience accompanying the pain
  - Past medical history, including arthritis, neoplasm, surgery, trauma, childhood or current abuse, psychiatric illness, substance abuse

PHYSICAL EXAM

- Physical exam begins in the waiting room. Note movement from chair to standing, ambulation. Does the patient change gait, grimace, express pain?
- Muscle wasting, localized tenderness, swelling, erythema, or increased warmth, muscle weakness. For joint pain, check passive and active range of motion.
- Neurological exam: Motor strength, reflexes, and sensation to light touch, noxious touch, and vibration; deep palpation of trigger points
- In chronic regional pain syndrome: Pain, swelling, limited range of motion, vasomotor instability, and skin changes (cyanosis, mottling, increased sweating, abnormal hair growth) in the affected area. Relief of the pain with a sympathetic block is diagnostic.

DIAGNOSTIC TESTS & INTERPRETATION

Lab

Testing should be directed at the differential diagnos regarding the area/body system involved.

Initial lab tests

- Complete blood count, erythrocyte sedimentation rate
- Urine drug screen (Urine Qualitative analysis for drugs of abuse and quantitative analysis of medication patient is reported to be using) and serum toxicology
- If abdominal: Liver function tests, amylase, lipase
- If pelvic: Ultrasound and possibly further imaging studies to rule out ovarian cancer
- If joint pain: RF, ANA, studies for Lyme disease, gonorrhea, septic arthritis

Follow-Up & Special Considerations

- Complex regional pain syndrome is possible, a ganglion block or sympathetic block can be diagnostic and possibly prevent the development o a chronic pain syndrome.
- If using opioids, order random urine drug screens: Qualitative analysis for drugs of abuse, quantitative analysis of the drug you are prescribing and urinalysis to confirm the specimen is in fact urine.

Diagnostic Procedures/Surgery

Consider referral to a pain center for interventional diagnostics such as facet joint blocks (to help diagnose facet joint disease); a nerve root block (to evaluate level of radicular pain); sacroiliac joint injection (to evaluate sacroiliac joint pain) (2).

DIFFERENTIAL DIAGNOSIS

- Abdominal adhesions, migraines, arthritis, bipolar disorder/depression, bursitis, chronic fatigue, drug abuse, endometriosis, fibromyalgia, lumbar degenerative disc disease, malignancy, neuromas, tendinitis
- Domestic abuse and violence, malingering, somatic disorders; Münchhausen syndrome and Münchhausen by proxy (in older children who are protecting the care provider who has been abusing the child)
- Diversion: Unintended use of a prescription medication for a nonmedical reason; for narcotics, i would include drug seeking to resell

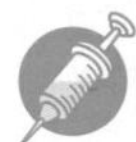

TREATMENT

- Trust between health care provider and patient
- Maintain clear boundaries: call frequency, amount of phone time, behavior toward staff
- Team approach: Involve family members, primary care doctor, substance abuse specialist, counselor, physical and occupational therapist, psychiatrist; relaxation training, spiritual counseling, complementary medicine. Patients cared for by multidisciplinary teams report a reduction in the intensity of their pain a year after these interventions (2).

MEDICATION

Sequential time-limited trials of medications, starting at low doses and gradually increasing until either effect or dose-limiting side effects are reached.

- For mild to moderate chronic pain:
  - Acetaminophen: Daily dose not to exceed total 4 grams in healthy adults and 2 grams in the elderly or those with hepatic disease or active or past history of alcohol use.
  - Nonsteroidal anti-inflammatory drugs (NSAIDS): Patients taking aspirin for cardiovascular protection should avoid the added gastrointestinal toxicity of NSAIDs. Cox-2 selective inhibitors should be used with caution because of cardiac risks.
  - "Weak" opioids, including codeine, hydrocodone, and tramadol. Avoid tramadol in elderly or patients at risk for seizures.
- For neuropathic pain (chronic low back pain, fibromyalgia, etc:
  - See "Neuropathic Pain" topic.
  - Classes of medications for neuropathic pain: (1) tricyclic, selective serotonin reuptake inhibitor (SSRIs), and selective serotonin-norepinephrine reuptake inhibitor (SSNRI) antidepressants; (2) anticonvulsants; (3) antiarrthymics; (4) opioids, particularly methadone.
  - Example: Combination of amitriptyline or duloxetine + gabapentin.
- For moderate-to-severe nonneuropathic chronic pain:
  - Strong opioids: Bind to central nervous system opioid receptors. Includes morphine, oxycodone, oral hydromorphone, oral morphine, Fentanyl. Check coanalgesic tables for differential dosing. Note no evidence supports any of these strong opioids as superior or having Improved side-effect profile. Morphine should be avoided in patients with significant renal insufficiency. Methadone: Only opioid that acts as N-methyl-D-aspartate receptor antagonist; is uniquely effective in neuropathic pain. Methadone has many drug interactions, and is easy to cause overdose. Methadone can contribute to potentially fatal cardiac arrhythmias.
  - Buprenorphine: A mixed opioid agonist and antagonist
  - Once stable dose of opioids is established, change to sustained-release formulations. Short-acting formulations only for break-through pain.
  - Common side effects: Constipation: senna and bisacodyl should be prescribed at time opioids are started. Also: nausea, sedation, mental status changes, pruritus.
  - Miscellaneous agents:
    - Capsaicin, found in hot chili peppers, depletes substance P in nociceptors.
    - Topical NSAIDS
    - Cannabinoids where legal

ALERT

All patients on chronic opioids should be managed with a "pain contract," random urine drug screening, and a "zero tolerance" approach when diversion is suspected.

ADDITIONAL TREATMENT

General Measures

Keep a "pain diary" to record pain, better or worse, and how much medication is taken.

COMPLEMENTARY AND ALTERNATIVE MEDICINE

- Acupuncture: Efficacy in chronic neck, back pain, and fibromyalgia
- Exercise: Efficacy in low back pain and fibromyalgia
- Improved mood and coping skills with behavioral and cognitive behavioral therapies (CBT). CBT may also decrease disability from chronic pain.
- Mind-body interventions: Yoga, tai chi, hypnosis, progressive muscle relaxation
- Children with chronic headaches, abdominal pain, etc: biofeedback, cognitive behavioral therapy, hypnosis, and relaxation exercises.

IN-PATIENT CONSIDERATIONS

Discharge Criteria

Discharge should include planning for:

- Chronic medication management (adding a stool regimen for opioids, adding liver and kidney function tests for chronic acetaminophen and NSAID use).
- Education and prescriptions for "rescue" medication doses for breakthrough pain.
- PT/OT, psychiatry, acupuncture, group/individual counseling, addiction counseling, stress-reduction techniques.

ONGOING CARE

FOLLOW-UP RECOMMENDATIONS

Patient Monitoring

- Contract between care provider and patient for all patients taking opioids. It should include:
  - 1 prescribing clinician (or designee)
  - No after-hours prescriptions or early refills
  - Mandatory police reports for medication thefts
  - Pain contracts (e.g., http://www.ohsu.edu/ahec/pain/med_contractlt.pdf)
- Random urine drug tests to reduce diversion and confirm no other illicit substances
- Taper and discontinue medications if patient does not benefit or side effects outweigh benefits, or if medications are abused or suspect diversion (1).
- Scheduled follow-up where patient's pain, function, and engagement in treatment (ex. physical therapy, occupational therapy, psychology therapies) (1)
- Scheduled follow-up appointments in which patient's mood is evaluated. Poorly controlled chronic pain is a risk factor for suicidality.

PATIENT EDUCATION

American Chronic Pain Association: http://www.theacpa.org

COMPLICATIONS

Substance abuse:

- Addiction: Includes 1 or more of following: Impaired control over drug use, compulsive use, and continued use despite harm. Taking drug for non-prescribed reasons.
- Physical dependence: Withdrawal syndrome produced by abrupt cessation or rapid dose reduction. Is a physiologic phenomenon
- Tolerance: A state of adaptation in which exposure to a drug induces changes that result in a diminution of 1 or more of the drug's effects over time.
- Addiction is common, but "problematic drug seeking behavior," due to other difficulties, including homelessness (loss of medications, improper dosing), genetic predispositions, and use of pain medications to self-treat anxiety or depressive disorder.
- Diversion: Selling drugs or giving them to persons other than for whom they are prescribed.

ALERT

Death: The rate of unintentional death due to opioid toxicity doubled between 1999 and 2005, accounting for more than 10,000 deaths. Narcotic overdose is the leading cause of accidental death of adults 25–55 (surpassing motor vehicle accidents) CDC/HVSS.

REFERENCES

1. Chou R, Fanciullo GJ, Fine PG, Adler JA, Ballantyne JC, Davies P, Donovan MI, Fishbain DA, Foley KM, Fudin J, Gilson AM, Kelter A, Mauskop A, O'Connor PG, Passik SD, Pasternak GW, Portenoy RK, Rich BA, Roberts RG, Todd KH, Miaskowski C, American Pain Society-American Academy of Pain Medicine Opioids Guidelines Panel et al. Clinical guidelines for the use of chronic opioid therapy in chronic noncancer pain. *J Pain*. 2009;10:113–30.
2. American Society of Anesthesiologists Task Force on Chronic Pain Management, American Society of Regional Anesthesia and Pain Medicine et al. Practice guidelines for chronic pain management: an updated report by the American Society of Anesthesiologists Task Force on Chronic Pain Management and the American Society of Regional Anesthesia and Pain Medicine. *Anesthesiology*. 2010;112:810–33.

See Also (Topic, Algorithm, Electronic Media Element)

Federation of State Medical Boards of the United States, Inc. Model Policy for the Use of Controlled Substances for the Treatment of Pain: www.painpolicy.wisc.edu/domestic/model04.pdf

CODES

ICD9

- 338.4 Chronic pain syndrome
- 338.21 Chronic pain due to trauma
- 338.22 Chronic post-thoracotomy pain

CLINICAL PEARLS

- Start with the presumption the patient's pain is *real*, even if pathophysiological evidence for it cannot be found.
- In taking the history, keep in mind that past/active sexual/domestic abuse can present as chronic physical pain.
- Have the patient keep a "pain diary."
- Emphasize that being pain free may not be possible, but that better function and quality-of-life can be shared goals.
- Written contracts and random urine testing for patients prescribed chronic opioids

CIRRHOSIS OF THE LIVER

Anne M. Walsh, PA-C, MMSc
Jill A. Grimes, MD

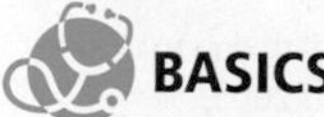

BASICS

DESCRIPTION

A chronic disease in which liver cell injury causes inflammation, necrosis, and stellate cell activation. Fibrosis replaces normal liver tissue and destroys the liver's vascular and lobular architecture, progressively diminishing blood flow and decreasing function. End result is liver failure and/or cancer.

Geriatric Considerations

- Jaundice and encephalopathy more common

Pediatric Considerations

- Inborn errors of metabolism (e.g., tyrosinemia), congenital anomalies (e.g., biliary atresia)

EPIDEMIOLOGY

- Predominant age: 40–50 years old
- Predominant sex: Male > female; but more females get cirrhosis from alcohol abuse.
- 12th leading cause of death in all US adults

RISK FACTORS

- Alcohol abuse
- IV drug abuse
- Obesity

Genetics

Hemochromatosis, Wilson disease, and Alpha-1-antitrypsin deficiency in adults

GENERAL PREVENTION

- Counsel patients to prevent risk factors for chronic liver disease (e.g., alcohol abuse); over 80% of chronic liver disease is preventable.
- Limit alcohol consumption to <2 drinks/day and advise weight loss for obesity
  - Raised BMI and alcohol consumption are both linked to liver disease, with evidence of a supra-additive interaction between the two. (1)[A]

ETIOLOGY

- Alcohol abuse (~60%)
- Chronic hepatitis B and/or C (~10%)
- Nonalcoholic steatohepatitis/obesity (~10%)
- Biliary obstruction (~10%)
- Hemochromatosis (~5%)
- Rare metabolic, genetic, toxic, infectious disorders (~5%)

COMMONLY ASSOCIATED CONDITIONS

- Diabetes
- Alcoholism
- Drug abuse
- Depression
- Obesity

DIAGNOSIS

HISTORY

- Review risk factors (alcohol abuse, viral hepatitis; family history of primary liver cancer, other liver disease, or autoimmune disease)
- Symptoms:
  - Fatigue, malaise, weakness
  - Anorexia, weight loss (gain if ascites/edema)
  - Right upper abdominal pain
  - Absent/irregular menses
  - Diminished libido, erectile dysfunction
  - Tea-colored urine, clay-colored stools
  - Edema, abdominal swelling/bloating
  - Bruising, bleeding, hematemesis, hematochezia, melena
  - Pruritus
  - Night blindness

PHYSICAL EXAM

Physical exam may be normal until end-stage disease develops.

- Skin changes:
  - Spider angiomata
  - Palmar erythema
  - Jaundice, scleral icterus
  - Ecchymoses
  - Caput medusa
  - Hyperpigmentation
- Hepatomegaly (small liver in end-stage disease)
- Splenomegaly if portal hypertension
- Central obesity
- Abdominal fluid wave, shifting dullness if ascites present
- Gynecomastia
- Dupuytren contractures
- Pretibial, presacral pitting edema
- Asterixis
- Mental status changes
- Muscle wasting, weakness

DIAGNOSTIC TESTS & INTERPRETATION

Lab

- ALT and AST mildly elevated; typically AST > ALT. Enzymes normalize as cirrhosis progresses.
- Elevated alkaline phosphatase (ALP), gamma-glutamyl transpeptidase (GGT), and total/direct bilirubin, indicates cholestasis
- Decreased platelet count from portal hypertension with splenomegaly
- Impaired synthetic liver function:
  - Low albumin and cholesterol
  - Prolonged prothrombin (PT), international normalized ratio (INR), partial thromboplastin time (PTT)
- Progressive cirrhosis:
  - Elevated ammonia level; decreased blood urea nitrogen (BUN), sodium, and potassium
- Alpha-fetoprotein level at diagnosis to screen for hepatocellular carcinoma (HCC)

Follow-Up & Special Considerations

To determine specific etiology consider:

- Hepatitis B surface antigen (HBsAg), core antibody (HBcAb), and surface antibody (HBsAb)
- Hepatitis C antibody
- Serum ethanol and GGT if suspected ongoing alcohol abuse
- Antimitochondrial antibody to screen for primary biliary cirrhosis
- Anti–smooth muscle and antinuclear antibodies to screen for chronic active (autoimmune) hepatitis
- Iron saturation (>50%) and ferritin (markedly increased) to screen for hemochromatosis; if abnormal, check hemochromatosis (HFE) genetics/mutation analysis
- Alpha-1-antitrypsin phenotype to screen for deficiency
- Ceruloplasmin level to screen for Wilson disease; if low, check copper excretion (serum copper plus 24-hour urine copper)

Imaging

- Abdominal ultrasound (US) every 6–12 months to screen for hepatocellular carcinoma
- Doppler US of hepatic/portal veins
- MRI to clarify patency of blood vessels and collaterals; best follow-up test for HCC if alpha-fetoprotein elevated and/or liver mass found on US

Diagnostic Procedures/Surgery

- Liver biopsy: percutaneous if INR <1.5 and no ascites; otherwise, transjugular biopsy
- Liver-spleen scan to diagnose portal hypertension if patient cannot be biopsied
- Endoscopy if portal hypertension, R/O esophageal varices/portal hypertensive gastropathy (2)[C]

Pathological Findings

- Fibrosis and regenerative nodules are general features of cirrhosis on biopsy
- Other histologic findings vary with etiology:
  - Alcoholic liver disease: Steatosis, polymorphonuclear leukocyte (PMN) infiltrate, ballooning degeneration of hepatocytes, Mallory bodies, giant mitochondria
  - Chronic hepatitis B and C: Periportal lymphocytic inflammation
  - Nonalcoholic steatohepatitis: Identical to alcoholic liver disease, confirmed by history. Steatosis may be absent in advanced disease ("burned-out NASH")
  - Biliary cirrhosis: PMN infiltrate in wall of bile ducts, inflammation increased in portal spaces, progressive loss of bile ducts in portal spaces
  - Hemochromatosis: Intrahepatic iron stores increased (iron stain or weighted biopsy tissue)
  - Alpha-1-antitrypsin deficiency: Positive Periodic Acid-Schiff (PAS) bodies in hepatocytes

DIFFERENTIAL DIAGNOSIS

- Diffuse hepatic parenchymal disease (e.g., fatty liver)
- Other causes of portal hypertension (e.g., portal vein thrombosis, lymphoma)
- Metastatic or multifocal cancer in the liver
- Vascular congestion (e.g., cardiac cirrhosis)
- Reversible (e.g., acute alcoholic hepatitis)

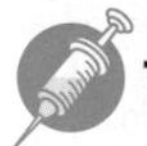

TREATMENT

Outpatient care except for major gastrointestinal bleeding, altered mental status, sepsis/infection, rapidly progressing hepatic decompensation, renal failure

MEDICATION

As indicated to treat the underlying cause (*Note prescribing precautions in decompensated cirrhosis*):

- Hepatitis C: Combination therapy with pegylated-interferon alpha 2a or 2b SC once weekly plus ribavirin 200 mg 2–3 pills PO b.i.d. for 6–12+ months eradicates virus permanently ("sustained viral response" or SVR) in ~50% of patients overall and in 80–90% of genotypes 2/3
- Hepatitis B: lamivudine 100 mg PO daily; adefovir, 10 mg PO daily; entecavir, 0.5–1 mg PO daily; or telbivudine, 600 mg PO daily until resistance develops; alternatively peginterferon alpha 2a SC weekly for 48 weeks. Due to high rates of resistance, combination recommended (3)[C].

Biliary cirrhosis: ursodeoxycholic acid (Ursodiol) 10–15 mg/kg PO daily, indefinitely (2)[A]

Wilson disease: penicillamine 1–3 g/d or tetrathiomolybdate, 100–400 mg/d. After 1 year, zinc acetate 250 mg b.i.d. for maintenance

Autoimmune (chronic active) hepatitis: prednisone 5–20 mg/d with or without azathioprine (Imuran) 0.5–1 mg/kg; adjust to keep transaminase levels normal.

Esophageal varices: propranolol 40–160 mg, or nadolol 10 mg daily, to lower portal pressure by 20 mm Hg, systolic pressure to 90–100 mm Hg, and pulse rate by 25% (2)[A]

Ascites/edema: Low-sodium (<2 g/day) diet and spironolactone, 100–400 mg daily with or without furosemide, 40–160 mg PO daily; torsemide may substitute for furosemide.

Encephalopathy: lactulose 15 mL b.i.d., titrate to induce 3 loose bowel movements daily. Neomycin or rifaximin may be combined with lactulose (4).

Pruritus: Ursodiol and antihistamines (e.g., hydroxyzine).

Renal insufficiency: Stop diuretics, nephrotoxic drugs; normalize electrolytes; hospitalize for plasma expansion or dialysis.

Prophylactic antibiotics for invasive procedures, GI bleeding, or history of spontaneous bacterial peritonitis (2)[A]

- Proton pump inhibitor for esophageal varices requiring banding or portal hypertensive gastropathy (5)[C]
- Recombinant factor VIIa to correct bleeding shows no survival benefit (4).

ADDITIONAL TREATMENT

General Measures

- Patients *must* abstain from alcohol, drugs, liver toxic medications, and herbs.
- Immunize for pneumococcal disease, hepatitis A and B, influenza.
- Nonalcoholic steatohepatitis (NASH): Weight reduction, exercise, optimal control of lipids/glucose.

Issues for Referral

Liver transplant evaluation at first onset complications (ascites, variceal bleed, encephalopathy), jaundice, or liver lesion suggestive of hepatocellular carcinoma, and/or when evidence of hepatic dysfunction develops (Child-Turcotte-Pugh >7 and MELD >10) (6)[C].

COMPLEMENTARY AND ALTERNATIVE MEDICINE

- Milk thistle (silymarin) may lower transaminases and improve symptoms; likely safe but offers no effect on overall mortality (7)[C]. *Caution*: Some preparations may contain hepatoxins and may interfere with INR and transaminase monitoring.
- Many herbal medications are liver toxic.

SURGERY/OTHER PROCEDURES

- Varices: Endoscopic ligation; 4–6 treatments typical (if acute bleed, use pre-esophagogastroduodenoscopy [EGD] octreotide as vasoconstrictor); transjugular intrahepatic shunt (TIPS) second-line or salvage therapy for acute bleed (8)
- Ascites: If tense, therapeutic paracentesis every 2 weeks PRN; caution if pedal edema absent.
- Fulminant hepatic failure: Liver transplantation
- Hepatocellular carcinoma: Curable if small with radiofrequency ablation or resection and transplant

IN-PATIENT CONSIDERATIONS

Admission Criteria

Major gastrointestinal (GI) bleeding, altered mental status, sepsis/infection, rapidly progressing hepatic decompensation, renal failure

ONGOING CARE

FOLLOW-UP RECOMMENDATIONS

Regular conditioning may help fatigue.

Patient Monitoring

- Once stable, monitor liver enzymes, platelets, and PT every 6–12 months.
- Patients >55 years old, with chronic hepatitis B or C, elevated INR, or low platelets are highest risk for HCC. Check alpha-fetoprotein and liver ultrasound every 6–12 months for screening in cirrhotics (4)[A].
- Endoscopy at diagnosis and every 2 years to screen for varices.

DIET

Protein 1–1.5 g/kg of body weight, high fiber, daily multivitamin (without iron), and <2 g/d sodium (essential if ascites/edema). A high-protein diet may precipitate encephalopathy, but protein restriction is no longer recommended (4). Coffee consumption has a graded and inverse association with liver cancer (9)[B].

PATIENT EDUCATION

- Educate caregivers on when to seek emergency care (e.g., hematemesis, altered mental status).
- Maintain sobriety/recovery/smoking cessation (includes no cannabis).
- Hepatitis A/B immunization and hepatitis C transmission precautions

PROGNOSIS

- At diagnosis of cirrhosis, expect 5–20 years of asymptomatic disease.
- At onset of complications, expect death within 5 years without transplant:
  - 5% per year develop HCC
  - 50% of cirrhotics develop ascites over 10 years; 50% 5-year survival if ascites develop
  - Acute variceal bleed most common fatal complication; carries 30% mortality
  - Median survival at onset decompensation (ascites, variceal bleed, encephalopathy) is 1.5 years (4).
  - With transplant, 85% survive 1 year; posttransplant deaths ~5% per year
- Fewer than 25% of eligible patients are transplanted due to donor organ shortage.

COMPLICATIONS

- Ascites
- Edema
- Infections
- Encephalopathy
- GI bleed: Esophageal varices, gastropathy, colopathy
- Hepatorenal syndrome
- Hepatopulmonary syndrome
- Hepatocellular carcinoma
- Fulminant hepatic failure
- Complications posttransplant (e.g., surgical, rejection, infections)

REFERENCES

1. Hart CL, Morrison DS, Batty GD, Mitchell RJ, Davey Smith G. Effect of body mass index and alcohol consumption on liver disease: analysis of data from two prospective cohort studies. *BMJ*. 2010;340:c1240.
2. Talwalkar JA, Kamath PS. Influence of recent advances in medical management on clinical outcomes of cirrhosis. *Mayo Clin Proc*. 2005;80: 1501–8.
3. Lok AS, McMahon BJ. Chronic hepatitis B. *Hepatology*. 2007;45:507–39.
4. Garcia-Tsao G. Managing the Complications of Cirrhosis, Hepatitis Annual Update 2008, Clinical Care Options Hepatitis, http://clinicaloptions.com/Hepatitis/Annual%20Updates/2008%20Annual%20Update.aspx
5. Nietsch HH. Management of portal hypertension. *J Clin Gastroenterol*. 2005;39:232–6.
6. Murray KF, Carithers RL, AASLD. AASLD practice guidelines: Evaluation of the patient for liver transplantation. *Hepatology*. 2005;41:1407–32.
7. Rambaldi A, Jacobs BP, Iaquinto G, et al. Milk thistle for alcoholic and/or hepatitis B or C virus liver diseases. Cochrane Hepato-Biliary Group *Cochrane Database Syst Rev*. 2006;Issue 4.
8. Garcia-Tsao G, Sanyal AJ, Grace ND. et al. Prevention and management of gastroesophageal varices and variceal hemorrhage in cirrhosis. *Hepatology*. 2007;46:922–38.
9. Hu G, Tuomilehto J, Pukkala E. et al. Joint effects of coffee consumption and serum gamma-glutamyltransferase on the risk of liver cancer. *Hepatology*. 2008.

ADDITIONAL READING

- Lebrec D, Thabut D, Oberti F et al. Pentoxifylline does not decrease short-term mortality but does reduce complications in patients with advanced cirrhosis. *Gastroenterology*. 2010;138:1755–62.
- Singal A, Volk ML, Waljee A, et al. Meta Analysis: Surveillance with Ultrasound for Early Stage Hepatocellular Carcinoma in Patients with Cirrhosis. *Aliment Pharmacol Ther*. 2009.

See Also (Topic, Algorithm, Electronic Media Element)

Algorithm: Cirrhosis

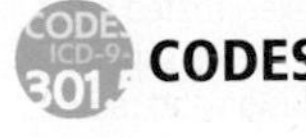

CODES

ICD9

- 571.2 Alcoholic cirrhosis of liver
- 571.5 Cirrhosis of liver without mention of alcohol

CLINICAL PEARLS

- 80% of chronic liver disease that leads to cirrhosis is preventable (primarily alcoholic).
- Check immunity to hepatitis A and B and vaccinate if not immune
- Check abdominal ultrasounds every 6 months for early detection of hepatocellular carcinoma

CLAUDICATION

William J. Knaus, II, MD
Arabinda Chatterjee, MD, FRCS, MS, D. Urology

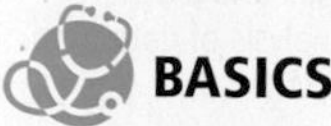

BASICS

DESCRIPTION

- Reproducible, exercise-induced muscle pain in the extremities associated with peripheral arterial disease:
  - Generally occurs in the lower extremities
- Intermittent claudication is the most common symptom of patients with peripheral arterial disease:
  - <20% of patients with peripheral arterial disease report typical symptoms.

EPIDEMIOLOGY

- 2/3 of patients with peripheral arterial disease are asymptomatic.
- Predominant sex: Male > Female (<2:1 ratio).

Incidence

- Incidence is related to age: 0.07% of men 35–44 years old and 1.4% of men > 65 years old develop the disease per year.
- Diabetic patients have an incidence 4–6 times greater than nondiabetic patients.

Prevalence

2–3% of men >60 years of age have symptomatic peripheral arterial disease compared to 1–2% of same-aged women.

RISK FACTORS

- Cigarette smoking:
  - 90% of all patients with claudication
- Diabetes mellitus
- Hypertension
- Hypercholesterolemia
- Family history
- Obesity
- Preexisting heart disease (15% of CHD patients have vascular disease in other beds)
- Advanced age

GENERAL PREVENTION

- Frequent walking exercises
- Smoking cessation
- Diet, lipid, and glucose control

PATHOPHYSIOLOGY

Atherosclerotic stenosis or occlusion of arterial flow diminishes blood pressure to the muscles of an extremity. Symptoms are generally exacerbated by exercise when blood-flow demand exceeds supply distal to the area of stenosis or occlusion and reduces tissue perfusion.

ETIOLOGY

- Sites affected depend upon the area of arterial supply involved.
- Symptoms occur distal to the area of arterial stenosis or occlusion.
- Superficial-femoral disease: Most common area associated with claudication. Pain may extend to the calf.
- Aortoiliac disease: Pain may extend from buttock to thigh.
- Femoropopliteal disease: Pain may extend from calf to foot.
- Subclavian, axillary, and brachial disease: Pain may extend to the upper extremity.

COMMONLY ASSOCIATED CONDITIONS

- Other manifestations of atherosclerosis:
  - Myocardial infarction
  - Carotid artery occlusive disease
  - Renovascular occlusive disease
  - Hypertension
- Of all patients with peripheral artery disease, 25–68% have concurrent coronary artery disease and 34–50% have a concomitant cerebrovascular disease (1)[B].

DIAGNOSIS

- Patients will limit their walking based on their symptoms:
  - Symptom continuum ranges from calf muscle fatigue to severe cramps and pain.
  - Pain occurring at rest is an ominous presentation.
- Cold feet are an early warning symptom.
- Paresthesias or numbness are later symptoms:
  - Diabetics less likely to report pain
- Rubor in dependent limb
- Leg color may darken to a dusky crimson when in lowered position.
- Lower extremities are hairless.
- Nonhealing ulcer is associated with poor circulation.
- Can lead to marked limitation of daily activities (1)

HISTORY

- Reproducible pain associated with restricted walking distance and relieved by rest.
- The Edinburgh is a questionnaire with the following criteria required for PVD diagnosis (sensitivity: 99%, specificity: 91%) (2):
  - Leg pain occurs with walking.
  - Pain does not have onset while standing or sitting.
  - Pain occurs while walking fast or uphill.
  - Pain resolves within 10 minutes of standing still.
- Modifiers:
  - Pain occurring even at normal pace on level ground suggests severe claudication.
  - Classic pain location is in the calf; thigh or buttock pain without calf pain is atypical.

PHYSICAL EXAM

- Signs of peripheral vascular disease: Abnormal skin coloration (pallor, rubor), cool feet, atrophy of nails, delayed capillary refill, loss of hair
- Diminished or absent femoral, popliteal, posterior tibial, or dorsalis pedis pulses (3)[B].

DIAGNOSTIC TESTS & INTERPRETATION

Lab

Initial lab tests

- Fasting lipid panel, fasting glucose
- Blood pressure readings in both arms
- ABI (arterial brachial index)
- Measuring fibrinogen and homocysteine and manipulation if elevated have not led to improved outcomes, so is not recommended.

Imaging

- Digital-subtraction angiography: The gold standard
- Contrast-enhanced magnetic resonance angiography: Highly accurate and reliable in identifying >50% stenosis (sensitivity 95%, specificity 97%)
- CT angiography (sensitivity 91%, specificity 91%)
- Duplex ultrasound (sensitivity 88%, specificity 96%) (4)

Diagnostic Procedures/Surgery

- The ankle–brachial index (ABI) is the systolic BP taken by a Doppler at the dorsalis pedis divided by the systolic pressure taken in the brachial artery. Sensitivity 95%, specificity 90%.
- Normal value is minimally ≥1. ABI <0.9 correlates with at ≥50% stenosis of at least 1 vessel (5)[B]:
  - ABI between 0.4 and 0.9 suggests stenosis and correlates with clinical claudication.
  - ABI <0.5 suggests multisegmental arterial stenoses.
  - ABI of <0.3 correlates with probable tissue death and/or rest pain.
- Photoplethysmography is another diagnostic option to evaluate blood pressure in the lower extremities.

DIFFERENTIAL DIAGNOSIS

- Osteoarthritis: Weight-bearing worsens pain.
- Pseudoclaudication: Attributed to spinal cord impingement or spinal stenosis. Relieved by sitting or squatting:
  - Neither pseudoclaudication nor osteoarthritis affects the arterial-brachial index.
- Thromboarterial occlusive disease (Buerger)
- Cystic adventitial disease
- Extraluminal compression (e.g., popliteal artery entrapment syndrome)
- Leriche syndrome: Lower extremity claudication, absence of femoral pulse, impotence, buttock muscle wasting
- Compartment syndrome
- Venous congestion

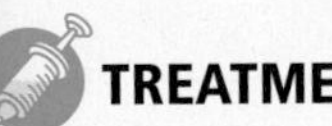

TREATMENT

Smoking cessation

Frequent exercise regimens are a mainstay of therapy:
- Supervised routines are more effective (6).
- Consider referral to physical therapy or supervised exercise program to develop structure to patient's exercise pattern

Recommended exercise regimen:
- Improve walking distance by 150% over 3–12 months.
- Recommend treadmill walking until pain elicited (7).
- Then, briefly rest until symptoms subside, then resume.
- Goal is 30–60 minutes per day, minimally 3 days per week for 3 months.

MEDICATION

First Line

- Antiplatelet therapy is recommended lifelong in patients with symptomatic disease (8):
  - Aspirin should be considered for all patients. It has no proven benefit for decreasing lower extremity claudication, but may be beneficial in reducing sequelae due to atherosclerotic disease:
    - Dose: Aspirin 80–325 mg PO/day
  - Clopidogrel (Plavix) can be used if aspirin is not tolerated. There is no evidence supporting dual antiplatelet therapy (8).
  - Ticlopidine (Ticlid) is effective in reducing mortality, but due to its side effect profile, is not preferred.
- Cilostazol (Pletal) improves maximal and pain-free walking distance (9).
- Recommended for moderate to severe disabling intermittent claudication that is unresponsive to exercise regimens in patients who are not candidates for surgical or percutaneous intervention (8):
  - Dose: 100 mg PO b.i.d.
  - Precautions: Headache occurs in >30% of patients taking cilostazol.
  - Contraindication: Patients with symptoms of congestive heart failure.
  - Significant possible drug-drug interactions: Use caution when combining with drugs metabolized by the cytochrome-P450 3A4 isoenzyme.
- HMG-CoA reductase inhibitor with a low-density lipoprotein goal of $\leq$100 mg/dL ($\leq$70 for high-risk patients) (7)
- Pentoxifylline 400 mg t.i.d. with meals; reduces symptoms by 25% but no more effectively than placebo, so is only used if exercise and other measures have failed.

Second Line

- Pentoxifylline (Trental): There is conflicting evidence regarding its efficacy in improving walking distance. 400mg PO t.i.d. (8)
- Arginine: 3g PO t.i.d.
- Propionyl levocarnitine: 1–2 g PO b.i.d.
- Ginkgo biloba: 120–160 mg PO b.i.d.
- Vitamin E: 50 mg PO per day (10)
- Naftidrofuryl (11)
- Prostaglandin analogues and stimulants continue to be investigated (12).

ADDITIONAL TREATMENT

General Measures

- Eliminate risk factors whenever possible.
- Smoking cessation is critical to success and is the single most important intervention.
- Optimize diet with low-fat and low-cholesterol regimen.
- Exercise is essential to management, significantly improving maximal walking time, distance to claudication, and calf blood flow.

COMPLEMENTARY AND ALTERNATIVE MEDICINE

Naftidrofuryl (unavailable in US; Cochrane review found clinical benefit to its use)

SURGERY/OTHER PROCEDURES

- Revascularization is reserved for a minority of patients:
  - Indications:
    - Severe claudication in which symptoms limit lifestyle or job performance
    - Unresponsive to exercise and medical management
- Angioplasty is preferred for patients with favorable anatomic features and younger patients ($\leq$50 years old).
- Arterial-bypass surgery is recommended for older patients ($\geq$50 years old) or with less certain anatomical features.
- Stenting modalities continue to be investigated (7).

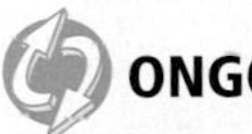

ONGOING CARE

FOLLOW-UP RECOMMENDATIONS

- Recommend continued, frequent exercise.
- Consider referral to vascular surgeon or cardiologist for follow-up of unresponsive or advanced cases.
- Peripheral noninvasive vascular studies every 6 months.
- If findings suggest condition of patient is worsening, this would be indication for surgery.

DIET

Cardiovascular diet (low-fat, low-cholesterol) is recommended.

PATIENT EDUCATION

- Encourage an exercise program, smoking cessation, healthy dietary choices, management of blood glucose levels in diabetic patients, and blood-pressure control.
- Reassurance that most patients improve walking distance over time and symptoms generally improve

PROGNOSIS

- Patients should experience gradual improvement with an intense walking program, appropriate medical therapy, as well as modification of risk factors.
- Disease progression may include rest pain, tissue loss, and gangrene.
- Select patients may require revascularization.

COMPLICATIONS

- Severe cases can result in tissue loss and gangrene, possibly requiring amputation of affected area.
- Largely affects patients with advanced, uncontrolled diabetes mellitus.
- Risk of venous thrombosis is increased due to the low-flow state indicated by claudication.

REFERENCES

1. Hiatt WR. The U.S. experience with cilostazol in treating intermittent claudication. *Atherosclerosis Suppl*. 2006;6:21–31.
2. Leng GC, Fowkes FG. The Edinburgh Claudication Questionnaire: an improved version of the WHO/Rose Questionnaire for use in epidemiological surveys. *J Clin Epidemiol*. 1992;45:1101–9.
3. Khan NA, Rahim SA, Anand SS et al. Does the clinical examination predict lower extremity peripheral arterial disease? *JAMA*. 2006;295:536–46.
4. Collins R, Burch J, Cranny G et al. Duplex ultrasonography, magnetic resonance angiography, and computed tomography angiography for diagnosis and assessment of symptomatic, lower limb peripheral arterial disease: systematic review. *BMJ*. 2007;334:1257.
5. Feringa HHH et al. The long-term prognostic value of the resting and postexercise ankle brachial index. *Arch Int Med*. 2006;166:529–35.
6. Watson L, Ellis B, Leng GC. Exercise for intermittent claudication. *Cochrane Database Syst Rev*. 2008:CD000990.
7. White C. Clinical practice. Intermittent claudication. *N Engl J Med*. 2007;356:1241–50.
8. Sobel M, Verhaeghe R. Antithrombotic therapy for peripheral artery occlusive disease: American College of Chest Physicians Evidence-Based Clinical Practice Guidelines (8th Edition). *Chest*. 2008;133:815S–843S.
9. Robless P, Mikhailidis DP, Stansby GP. Cilostazol for peripheral arterial disease. *Cochrane Database Syst Rev*. 2008:CD003748.
10. Kleijnen J, Mackerras D. Vitamin E for intermittent claudication. *Cochrane Database Syst Rev*. 2000: CD000987.
11. De Backer T, Vander Stichele R, Lehert P et al. Naftidrofuryl for intermittent claudication: meta-analysis based on individual patient data. *BMJ*. 2009;338:b603.
12. Reiter M, Bucek RA, Stümpflen A, et al. Prostanoids for intermittent claudication. *Cochrane Database Syst Rev*. 2004:CD000986.

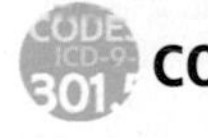

CODES

ICD9

- 440.21 Atherosclerosis of native arteries of the extremities with intermittent claudication
- 443.9 Peripheral vascular disease, unspecified

CLINICAL PEARLS

- Mainstay of treatment involves gradual increase in exercise in supervised setting and maximizing reduction of CHD risk factors: Smoking cessation, LDL reduction, glucose control in diabetes, etc.
- Available revascularization techniques include catheter-based balloon dilation with or without luminal stenting, endarterectomy, arterial reconstruction with an anatomically placed bypass graft, or with an extra-anatomically placed bypass prosthesis. Selection is based on patient risk, surgeon experience, and pattern of occlusions.
- Indications for revascularization are critical limb ischemia, patients with repeated atheroembolism, or severe lifestyle-limiting symptoms.

C

CLOSTRIDIUM DIFFICILE INFECTION

Aman D. Sabharwal, MD
Nathan T. Connell, MD

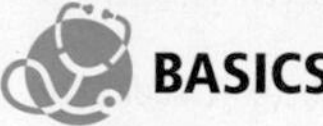

BASICS

DESCRIPTION

- *Clostridium difficile* is a gram-positive, spore-forming anaerobic bacillus.
- Infection caused by *C. difficile* is usually linked to broad-spectrum antibiotic use.
- Severity of infection can range from diarrhea to colitis to perforation to death.
- System(s) affected: GI
- Synonyms(s): *C. difficile*–associated disease or diarrhea (CDAD); antibiotic-associated diarrhea; *C. diff*

EPIDEMIOLOGY

Incidence

- Most cases of *C. difficile* infection occur in hospitals or long-term care facilities at a rate of 25–80 per 100,000 occupied bed-days (1).
- For outpatient setting, the rate is ~7.7 cases per 100,000 person-years.

Prevalence

- *C. difficile* causes ~25% of all cases of antibiotic-associated diarrhea.
- C. *difficile* infections account for ~25% of all nosocomial antibiotic associated infections (1).

RISK FACTORS

- Exposure to all antimicrobial agents (except aminoglycosides) is associated with *C. difficile* infection.
- Patients in health care settings have a higher risk of developing *C. difficile* infection.
- Age >65 years
- Duration of stay in the hospital
- Nasogastric intubation
- Previous *C. difficile* infection
- Severe primary illness
- Controversial: Use of anti-ulcer medications
- Chemotherapy
- Perioperative antibiotic prophylaxis:
  - Even if patients receive no other antibiotics other than perioperative prophylaxis, they are still at risk for developing *C. difficile* infection (2).

Geriatric Considerations

C. difficile is the most common cause of acute diarrheal illness in long-term care facilities. These patients are older and receive more antibiotics and antacids than the general public; thus, it is difficult to determine which factors contribute most to this increased risk.

Pediatric Considerations

Neonates have a higher rate of *C. difficile* colonization (25–80%), yet they are much less likely to be symptomatic than adults, possibly due to immature toxin receptors.

Genetics

No known genetic factors

GENERAL PREVENTION

- Implementation of a comprehensive infection-control program has resulted in a decrease in the incidence of *C. difficile* infection
- Disinfection with hypochlorite solution
- Handwashing with soap and water:
  - Alcohol-based hand gels do not kill spores.
- Reduction in the use of rectal thermometers
- Reduction of unnecessary broad-spectrum antibiotic use
- Isolation of infected patients and use of contact precautions
- Education of hospital personnel

PATHOPHYSIOLOGY

- *C. difficile* can thrive in the colon and cause infection if disruption of the normal flora and ingestion of *C. difficile* occur.
- *C. difficile* spores can survive for months.
- Host factors such as the presence of antibodies to *C. difficile* toxins can reduce the severity and prevent recurrences of infection.
- *C. difficile* produces toxins that are essential for disease to occur:
  - Toxins A (enterotoxin) and B (cytotoxin) attract neutrophils and monocytes, and degrade colonic epithelial cells, causing colitis, pseudomembrane colitis, and watery diarrhea.
  - BI/NAP1 strain of *C. difficile* has been shown to produce more virulent characteristics (3).
  - Binary toxin produces a virulent form of disease (different from toxin A or B); this may result in increased rates of colectomies and mortality.
  - Binary toxin has been identified in ~6% of clinical *C. difficile* isolates obtained in the US and Europe.

ETIOLOGY

- Altered colonic mucosa
- *C. difficile* spore ingestion
- Active toxin release

DIAGNOSIS

HISTORY

- Recent antibiotic use (especially broad-spectrum fluoroquinolones and cephalosporins)
- Diarrhea that is watery, foul-smelling
- Fever (typically <10%)
- Recent hospitalizations or stay at nursing facility

PHYSICAL EXAM

- Mild disease:
  - Mild lower abdominal cramping pain
- Moderate disease:
  - Fever
  - Nausea and vomiting
- Severe disease:
  - Peritonitis
  - Ileus
  - Hypovolemia
- Mild abdominal tenderness to peritonitis, depending on severity
- Hypovolemia

DIAGNOSTIC TESTS & INTERPRETATION

Markers of severe or fulminant infection include hypotension, sepsis, markedly elevated white blood cell count, and bandemia. Other signs include obstruction, perforation, toxic megacolon, colonic-wall thickening, or ascites.

Lab

- ELISA for toxins:
  - Available within several hours
  - Sensitivity 63–99%
  - Specificity 75–100%
  - Some labs only test for toxin A, others test for A and B.
- Tissue culture cytotoxicity assay:
  - Takes 24–48 hours for results; labor-intensive
  - Sensitivity 67–100%
  - Specificity 85–100%
- Microbiology culture:
  - Nontoxin-producing strains also detected
  - Mostly used to evaluate epidemiology studies
- PCR-based testing is currently research-based.
- Repeat testing during the same episode of diarrhea is discouraged (3).

Imaging

- Plain films may show thumbprinting and colonic distension.
- CT radiography may show mucosal wall thickening, thickened colonic wall, and pericolonic inflammation.

Diagnostic Procedures/Surgery

- Endoscopy can be used to evaluate for pseudomembranes and exclude other conditions.
- Flexible sigmoidoscopy may miss 15–20% of pseudomembranes that may be more proximal in the colon.
- Colonoscopy evaluates the entire colon: Used when diagnosis is in doubt or severity demands rapid diagnosis

Pathological Findings

Pseudomembranes consist of inflammatory and cellular debris that forms visible exudates that can obscure the underlying mucosa. These exudates have a yellow to grayish color.

DIFFERENTIAL DIAGNOSIS

- Food poisoning
- Enteric infections
- Antibiotic-associated diarrhea

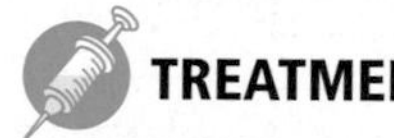

TREATMENT

MEDICATION

If clinically indicated (moderate-to-severe diarrhea, fever, significant leukocytosis, abdominal pain, etc.), consider antimicrobial against *C. difficile* (4)[A].

First Line

- Metronidazole is the drug of choice for mild-to-moderate *C. difficile* infection due to low cost and prevention of the emergence of vancomycin-resistant organisms (3)[A]:
  - 500 mg p.o. 3 times a day for 10–14 days
  - If patient is unable to take oral medications, then IV metronidazole or intraluminal vancomycin can be used.

Vancomycin is first-line therapy in patients with severe or fulminant *C. difficile* infection. Vancomycin is also first-line therapy for the 3rd and subsequent relapse in fewer than 6 months (3):
- 125 mg p.o. 4 times a day for 10–14 days
- Vancomycin retention enema if unable to take p.o. or there is evidence of poor GI motility.

For the first recurrence of *C. difficile* infection, the treatment is the same as the initial treatment, although current severity of illness should be taken into account. For subsequent relapses, use oral vancomycin as treatment in a pulse-taper format. Consultation with an infectious diseases specialist is recommended.

ALERT

When using vancomycin for treatment of *C. difficile* infection, oral or rectal formulations must be used since IV formulations are not excreted into the colonic lumen.

Second Line

- Vancomycin (4,5)[A]:
  - 125 mg p.o. 4 times a day for 10–14 days
  - Indicated for patients who cannot tolerate or have failed metronidazole therapy, and for those who are pregnant
- Immunoglobulin IV (IVIG) has been used in special cases.

ADDITIONAL TREATMENT

General Measures

- Avoid antimotility agents and opiates (4,6)[A].
- Avoid use of proton pump inhibitors (PPIs) unless absolutely necessary, as they have been associated with a 42% increased risk of recurrence if used concurrently with treatment for *C. difficile* colitis (7).

COMPLEMENTARY AND ALTERNATIVE MEDICINE

- Probiotics (*Lactobacilli* and *Saccharomyces)* have shown conflicting data, and have been associated with increased bacteremia (3):
  - Use oral *Lactobacilli* with caution if also using vancomycin, since the latter antibiotic is active against *Lactobacilli*.
- Fecal transplant in severe or relapsing disease

SURGERY/OTHER PROCEDURES

If *C. difficile* infection progresses to toxic megacolon, peritonitis, or sepsis after initiation of treatment, other therapeutic options should be explored, including a surgical consult (4,5)[A].

IN-PATIENT CONSIDERATIONS

Initial Stabilization

- Current nonessential antibiotic therapy should be discontinued if possible (3,4)[A].
- Institute supportive therapy with fluids and electrolytes if needed (3,4)[A].

Admission Criteria

- Hypovolemia
- Comorbid conditions
- Inability to keep up with enteric losses
- Hematochezia
- Electrolyte disturbances

IV Fluids

- Infuse to keep patient euvolemic
- Once over acute phase, patient can be weaned off IV fluids.

Nursing

See General Prevention.

Discharge Criteria

- Improved diarrhea severity and frequency
- Tolerating both medications and p.o.
- Afebrile

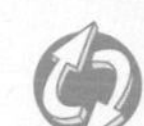

ONGOING CARE

FOLLOW-UP RECOMMENDATIONS

- Many patients can be treated as outpatients.
- Bed rest during acute phase

Patient Monitoring

- Relapses of colitis will occur in 15–30%.
- Relapses typically occur 2–10 days after discontinuation of antibiotics.
- Repeat treatment with 14-day course of antibiotics will result in 40% cure rate.
- The management of the first relapse following therapy for *C. difficile* diarrhea and colitis does not differ substantially from treatment of the initial episode.
- Administration of vancomycin or metronidazole every other day or every 3rd day allows spores to germinate on the off days and then be killed when the antibiotics are taken again.
- For multiple relapses, some success has been reported with the following oral vancomycin taper regimen:
  - Week 1: 125 mg q.i.d.
  - Week 2: 125 mg b.i.d.
  - Week 3: 125 mg daily
  - Week 4: 125 mg every other day
  - Weeks 5 and 6: 125 mg every 3 days
- If continued infection, consider pulse therapy with vancomycin in consultation with an infectious disease specialist.

DIET

No restrictions; as tolerated

PATIENT EDUCATION

Patients should be kept informed of the progress of disease and taught to practice good hygiene (i.e., handwashing).

PROGNOSIS

- Majority of patients will improve with conservative management and antibiotics
- 1–3% of patients will develop severe colitis requiring emergency colectomy.

REFERENCES

1. McDonald LC, Owings M, Jernigan DB. Clostridium difficile infection in patients discharged from US short-stay hospitals, 1996–2003. *Emerg Infect Dis*. 2006;12:409–15.
2. Carignan A, Allard C, Pépin J, et al. Risk of Clostridium difficile infection after perioperative antibacterial prophylaxis before and during an outbreak of infection due to a hypervirulent strain. *Clin Infect Dis*. 2008;46:1838–43.
3. Cohen SH, Gerding DN, Johnson S, Kelly CP, Loo VG, McDonald LC, Pepin J, Wilcox MH et al. Clinical practice guidelines for Clostridium difficile infection in adults: 2010 update by the society for healthcare epidemiology of America (SHEA) and the infectious diseases society of America (IDSA). *Infect Control Hosp Epidemiol*. 2010;31:431–55.
4. Bartlett JG. Narrative review: the new epidemic of Clostridium difficile-associated enteric disease. *Ann Intern Med*. 2006;145:758–64.
5. McFarland LV. Alternative treatments for *Clostridium difficile* disease: What really works? *J Med Micro*. 2005;54:101–11.
6. Koo HL, Koo DC, Musher DM, et al. Antimotility agents for the treatment of Clostridium difficile diarrhea and colitis. *Clin Infect Dis*. 2009;48:598–605.
7. Linsky A, Gupta K, Lawler EV, Fonda JR, Hermos JA et al. Proton pump inhibitors and risk for recurrent Clostridium difficile infection. *Arch Intern Med*. 2010;170:772–8.

ADDITIONAL READING

McFarland LV. Meta-analysis of probiotics for the prevention of antibiotic associated diarrhea and the treatment of Clostridium difficile disease. *Am J Gastroenterol*. 2006;101:812–22.

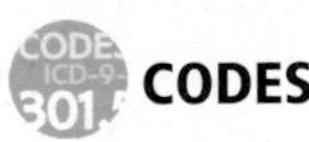

CODES

ICD9

008.45 Intestinal infection due to clostridium difficile

CLINICAL PEARLS

- Treatment of asymptomatic patients is not recommended.
- Therapeutic response should be based on clinical signs and symptoms. Patients may shed organism or toxin for weeks after treatment.

C

COLIC, INFANTILE

Daniel T. Lee, MD
Leanne Zakrzewski, MD

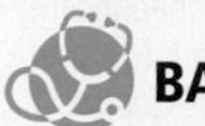

BASICS

DESCRIPTION

- Colic is defined as excessive crying in an otherwise healthy baby.
- A commonly used criteria is the Wessel criteria, or the "rule of 3": Crying lasts for >3 hours a day, >3 days a week, and persists >3 weeks.
- Many clinicians no longer use the criterion of persistence for >3 weeks because few parents or clinicians will wait that long before evaluation or intervention.
- Some clinicians feel that colic represents the extreme end of the spectrum of normal crying, whereas most feel that colic is a distinct clinical entity.

EPIDEMIOLOGY

Incidence

- Predominant age: Between 2 weeks and 4 months of age
- Predominant sex: Male = Female.

Prevalence

- Probably between 10% and 25% of infants
- Range is somewhere between 8% and 40% of infants

Pediatric Considerations

This is a problem during infancy.

RISK FACTORS

Physiologic predisposition in infant, but no definitive risk factors have been established.

GENERAL PREVENTION

Colic is generally not preventable.

ETIOLOGY

The cause is unknown. Factors that may play a role include

- Infant gastroesophageal reflux disease
- Allergy to cow's milk, soy milk, or breast milk protein
- Fruit juice intolerance
- Swallowing air during the process of crying, feeding, or sucking
- Overfeeding or feeding too quickly; underfeeding also has been proposed.
- Inadequate burping after feeding
- Family tension
- Parental anxiety, depression, and/or fatigue
- Parent-infant interaction mismatch
- Baby's inability to console itself when dealing with stimuli
- Increased gut hormone motilin, causing hyperperistalsis
- Tobacco smoke exposure
- Disorder of impaired synchronization between infant arousal and environment (1)[C]

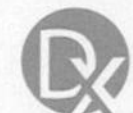

DIAGNOSIS

HISTORY

- Evaluation for Wessel criteria: Crying lasts for >3 hours per day, >3 days per week, and persists >3 weeks
- The colicky episodes may have a clear beginning and end.
- The crying is generally spontaneous, without preceding events triggering the episodes.
- The crying is typically different from normal crying. Colicky crying may be louder, more turbulent, variable in pitch, and appear more like screaming.
- The infant may be difficult to soothe or console regardless of how the parents try to help.
- The infant acts normally when not colicky.
- Assess the support system of caregivers and families, including coping skills.

PHYSICAL EXAM

- A comprehensive physical exam is normal.
- Since excessive crying may be a risk factor for shaken baby syndrome or other forms of child abuse (2)[B], be sure to examine the child carefully for signs of shaken baby syndrome or other forms of child abuse.

DIAGNOSTIC TESTS & INTERPRETATION

Diagnostic Procedures/Surgery

A thorough history and physical examination should be performed to rule out other causes. Otherwise, no diagnostic procedures or surgery is indicated.

DIFFERENTIAL DIAGNOSIS

Any organic cause for excessive or qualitatively different crying in infants such as

- Infections such as meningitis, sepsis, otitis media, or urinary tract infection
- GI issues such as gastroesophageal reflux, intussusception, lactose intolerance, constipation, anal fissure, or strangulated hernia
- Trauma such as foreign bodies, corneal abrasion, occult fracture, digit or penile hair tourniquet, or child abuse

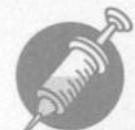

TREATMENT

MEDICATION

- Dicyclomine (Bentyl) has been proven beneficial, but the potential serious adverse effects such as apnea, seizures, and syncope have precluded its use. Further, the manufacturer has made the medication contraindicated for infants <6 months of age (3,4)[B].
- Simethicone has not been shown to be beneficial (3,4)[B].

ADDITIONAL TREATMENT

General Measures

- Soothe by holding and rocking the baby (3)[C].
- Use pacifier (3)[C].
- Use of gentle rhythmic motion (e.g., strollers, infant swings, car rides) (3)[C].
- Place near "white noise" (e.g., vacuum cleaner, clothes dryer, white noise machine) (3)[C].
- Crib vibrators or car-ride simulators have not proven to be helpful (3,5)[B].
- Increased carrying or use of infant carrier did not improve colic (3,5)[B].
- Employ the "5 S's" (need to be done concurrently):
  - Swaddling: Tight wrapping with blanket; may be especially beneficial in infants <8 weeks of age (6)[B]
  - Side/stomach: Laying baby on side or stomach
  - Shushing: Loud white noise
  - Swinging: Rhythmic, jiggly motion
  - Sucking: Sucking on anything (e.g., nipple, finger, pacifier) (3)[C]

sues for Referral

cessive vomiting, poor weight gain, recurrent spiratory diseases, or bloody stools should prompt 'erral to a specialist.

OMPLEMENTARY AND ALTERNATIVE EDICINE

- Herbal teas and supplements may help but are not recommended because of limited, inconclusive evidence. For example,
  - One study concluded that herbal teas containing mixtures of chamomile, vervain, licorice, fennel, and balm-mint used up to t.i.d. may be beneficial (4)[B]. However, the study used dosages of up to 150 cc t.i.d., raising clinical concerns that this dosage may impair needed milk consumption in infants and may be impractical to administer. Additionally, preparations used in the study may not be commercially available in the US.
  - A second double-blind, randomized trial of 0.1% fennel seed oil emulsion versus placebo demonstrated a decrease in colic symptoms according to the Wessel criteria. However, this preparation of fennel seed oil is not commercially available in the US, and the long-term health effects are unknown (7).
- A home-based intervention focusing on reducing infant stimulation and synchronizing infant sleep-wake cycles with the environment, as well as parental support, was effective (1)[B].
- Use of music may help (8,9)[C].
- Chiropractic treatment has shown no benefit over placebo (3)[C].
- Infant massage has not been shown to be helpful (3)[B].

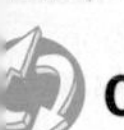

ONGOING CARE

OLLOW-UP RECOMMENDATIONS

equent outpatient visits as needed for parental assurance, education, and monitoring and to ensure e health of the infant and parents

atient Monitoring

ollow for proper feeding, growth, and development.

IET

- If breast-feeding:
  - Continue breast-feeding. Switching to formula probably will not help (3)[C].
  - Possible therapeutic benefit from eliminating milk products, eggs, wheat, and nuts from the diet of breast-feeding mothers (3,5)[B].
  - Along with eliminating the preceding foods from the maternal diet, removing soy, nuts, and fish may be beneficial (10)[C].
  - Probiotics (*Lactobacillus reuteri*) have been shown to be beneficial in a small study of breast-fed infants (11).
- If formula feeding:
  - Feeding the infant in a vertical position using a curved bottle or bottle with collapsible bag may help to reduce air swallowing.
  - Consider a 1-week trial of hypoallergenic formulas, such as whey hydrolysate (e.g., Good Start) or casein hydrolysate (e.g., Alimentum, Nutramigen, Pregestimil) (4,5)[B].
  - American Academy of Pediatrics concluded that there is no proven role for soy formula in the treatment of colic (12)[C].
  - Adding fiber to formula has not been shown to be helpful (5,8)[B].
- Supplementing with sucrose solution may be helpful, but the effect may be short-lived (<1 h) (4,5)[B].
- Use of lactase enzymes in formula or breast milk or given directly to the infant has no therapeutic benefit (5)[B].

PATIENT EDUCATION

- Reassure parents that colic is not the result of bad parenting, and advise parents about having proper rest breaks, adequate sleep, and help in caring for the infant.
- Explain spectrum of crying behavior.
- Avoid overfeeding or underfeeding.
- Instruct in better feeding techniques such as improved bottles (low air, curved) and sufficient burping after feeding.
- Colic: What You Should Know at www.aafp.org/afp/2004/0815/p741.html

PROGNOSIS

- Usually subsides by 3–6 months of age
- Despite apparent abdominal pain, colicky infants eat well and gain weight normally.
- A handful of studies indicate that temper tantrums may be more common among formerly colicky infants, as studied in toddlers up to 4 years of age (13,14).
- Colic has no bearing on the baby's intelligence or future development.

COMPLICATIONS

Colic is self-limiting and does not result in lasting effects to infant or maternal mental health (15)[C].

REFERENCES

1. Keefe MR, Lobo ML, Froese-Fretz A, et al. Effectiveness of an intervention for colic. *Clin Pediatr (Phila)*. 2006;45:123–33.
2. Reijneveld SA, van der Wal MF, Brugman E, et al. Infant crying and abuse. *Lancet*. 2004;364:1340–2.
3. Roberts DM, Ostapchuk M, O'Brien JG. Infantile colic. *Am Fam Physician*. 2004;70:735–40.
4. Wade S, Kilgour T. Extracts from "clinical evidence": Infantile colic. *BMJ*. 2001;323:437–40.
5. Garrison MM, Christakis DA. A systematic review of treatments for infant colic. *Pediatrics*. 2000;106:184–90.
6. van Sleuwen BE, L'hoir MP, Engelberts AC, et al. Comparison of behavior modification with and without swaddling as interventions for excessive crying. *J Pediatr*. 2006;149:512–7.
7. Alexandrovich I, Rakovitskaya O, Kolmo E, Sidorova T, Shushunov S et al. The effect of fennel (Foeniculum Vulgare) seed oil emulsion in infantile colic: a randomized, placebo-controlled study. *Altern Ther Health Med*. 58–61.
8. Clemons RM. Issues in newborn care. *Prim Care*. 2000;27:251–67.
9. McCollough M, Sharieff GQ. Common complaints in the first 30 days of life. *Emerg Med Clin North Am*. 2002;20:27–48, v.
10. Hill DJ, Roy N, Heine RG, et al. Effect of a low-allergen maternal diet on colic among breastfed infants: a randomized, controlled trial. *Pediatrics*. 2005;116:e709–15.
11. Savino F, Pelle E, Palumeri E, et al. Lactobacillus reuteri (American Type Culture Collection Strain 55730) versus simethicone in the treatment of infantile colic: a prospective randomized study. *Pediatrics*. 2007;119:e124–30.
12. O'Connor NR. Infant formula. *Am Fam Physician*. 2009;79:565–70.
13. Canivet C, Jakobsson I, Hagander B et al. Infantile colic. Follow-up at four years of age: still more "emotional". *Acta Paediatr*. 2000;89:13–7.
14. Rautava P, Lehtonen L, Helenius H, Sillanpää M et al. Infantile colic: child and family three years later. *Pediatrics*. 1995;96:43–7.
15. Clifford TJ, Campbell MK, Speechley KN, et al. Sequelae of infant colic: evidence of transient infant distress and absence of lasting effects on maternal mental health. *Arch Pediatr Adolesc Med*. 2002;156:1183–8.

CODES

ICD9

789.7 Colic

CLINICAL PEARLS

- Colic is defined as excessive crying in an otherwise healthy baby.
- Excessive crying may be a risk factor for shaken baby syndrome or other forms of child abuse.
- Provide advice, support, and reassurance to parents (3)[B].
- Prevent caregiver burnout by advising parents to get proper rest breaks, sleep, and help in caring for the infant.

COLONIC POLYPS

Macario C. Corpuz, Jr., MD
Pamela Lynn Grimaldi, DO

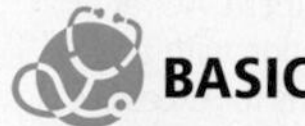

BASICS

DESCRIPTION

- A colonic polyp is an intraluminal outgrowth arising from the large intestinal epithelial lining, which is usually benign. The potential for malignant transformation necessitates close evaluation and monitoring. (See Colorectal Malignancy.)
- 3 types:
  - Adenomatous: May become malignant:
    - Villous: Polyps tend to be larger, most likely to become malignant (10%)
    - Tubular (75%)
    - Tubulovillous (15%)
  - Hyperplastic: Rarely become malignant
  - Inflammatory: No malignant potential

EPIDEMIOLOGY

- Varies considerably worldwide. Industrialized countries are generally at greater risk compared to the rest of the world.
- Age is an important determinant in the US and other high-risk countries.
- Adenomas more common in men than women

Incidence

- Estimated 5% of the US population
- ~20% of middle-aged and older adults
- 50% seen in ≥50 years

Prevalence

Average prevalence of 25% before age 40 to as high as 55% at age 80

RISK FACTORS

- Advancing age
- Male
- Obesity
- Family history of polyposis, polyps, or colorectal cancer (CRC)
- Inflammatory bowel disease
- Current cigarette smoking
- Excessive alcohol intake: >8 drinks of beer or spirits a week (1)
- Sedentary lifestyle

Genetics

May occur in the setting of genetic syndromes that are associated with gene mutations

GENERAL PREVENTION

- Diet: High-fiber diet has been a controversial risk. Two recent studies stressed that doubling fiber intake can significantly reduce colorectal cancer risk (2,3).
- Avoid smoking.
- Limit alcohol intake.
- Calcium supplement: Shown reduction of colorectal adenoma recurrence (4)
- Vitamin D, folic acid, vitamin B6
- Aspirin. Three randomized controlled trials (RCT) revealed that ASA caused significant reduction in the recurrence of sporadic adenomatous polyps after 1 to 3 years while short-term studies support regression of colorectal adenomas in FAP (5).

PATHOPHYSIOLOGY

- Adenomatous polyps: Formed from abnormal proliferation and from dysplasia
- Nonadenomatous polyps: Result from abnormal mucosal maturation, inflammation, or architecture

ETIOLOGY

Unknown. May be related to environmental and genetic factors.

COMMONLY ASSOCIATED CONDITIONS

Associated with several hereditary disorders:

- Familial adenomatous polyposis (FAP)
- Peutz-Jeghers syndrome
- Gardner syndrome
- Hereditary nonpolyposis colon cancer (HNPCC)

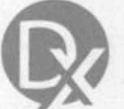

DIAGNOSIS

HISTORY

- Asymptomatic
- Hematochezia
- Melena
- Diarrhea or constipation
- Anemia
- Fatigue
- Abdominal pain

PHYSICAL EXAM

- Usually normal
- Rectal lesions may be felt by digital examination.

DIAGNOSTIC TESTS & INTERPRETATION

Lab

Initial lab tests

- Complete blood count (CBC): Anemia
- Electrolyte abnormalities: In villous adenoma

Diagnostic Procedures/Surgery

- Colonoscopy (6): Standard of goal. Most sensitive test available but its sensitivity is a concern. Chromoscopy enhances the detection of neoplastic lesions in the colon and the rectum (7).
- Chromoscopy: Studies are examining narrow-band imaging for histologic differentiation between adenomatous and hyperplastic polyps (7,8).
- CT colonography (formerly known "Virtual colonoscopy")
- Sigmoidoscopy
- Air-contrast barium enema: Misses small lesions
- Fecal occult blood test (FOBT): Many false positive results
- Fecal DNA testing
- Some polyps are more likely to become malignant, hence, they require histopathologic evaluation.

athological Findings
Villous adenoma:
– Gross: Velvety, multiple-frond projections
– Micro: Glands proliferate in fingerlike projections, malignant degenerations
Tubular adenoma:
– Gross: Smooth, firm, pink surface; microlobulated; fissures; pedunculated
– Glands proliferate in tubular fashion, nuclei elongated, hyperchromatic

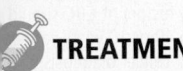

TREATMENT

URGERY/OTHER PROCEDURES
Endoscopic polypectomy: Major risks include perforation and bleeding
Colonic resection: For multiple intestinal polyps associated with FAP

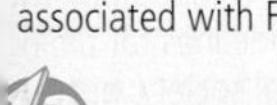

ONGOING CARE

OLLOW-UP RECOMMENDATIONS
enign polyps should have follow-up colonoscopy very 3–5 years.

atient Monitoring
ffer CRC screening for average risk patients eginning at age 50, earlier for at-risk patients. Most uidelines recommend to stop screening if life xpectancy is less than 10 years.

IET
alcium supplementation might contribute a noderate degree to the prevention of colorectal denomatous polyps (4).

ROGNOSIS
Curable with polypectomy
Projection estimates suggested that 50% of postpolypectomy patients will have a recurrence within 7.6 years; hence, need follow-up (9).

- Adenomatous polyps may undergo malignant transformation if not removed.
- Multiple polyps are particularly at increased risk of developing colorectal cancer.

COMPLICATIONS
Perforation with colonoscopy is rare.

REFERENCES

1. Anderson JC, Alpern Z, Sethi G, et al. Prevalence and risk of colorectal neoplasia in consumers of alcohol in a screening population. *Am J Gastroenterol*. 2005;100:2049–55.
2. Asano TK, McLeod RS. Dietary fibre for the prevention of colorectal adenomas and carcinomas. *Cochrane Database of Systematic Reviews*. 2002, Issue 1. Art. No.: CD003430. DOI:10.1002/14651858.CD003430.
3. Peters, Ulrike, et al. "Dietary fibre and colorectal adenoma in a colorectal cancer early detection programme." *Lancet*. 361.9368 (2003):1491–5.
4. Weingarten MA, Zalmanovici A, Yaphe J. Dietary calcium supplementation for preventing colorectal cancer and adenomatous polyps. *Cochrane Database Syst Rev*. 2008:CD003548.
5. Asano T, McLeod R. Non steroidal anti-inflammatory drugs (NSAID) and aspirin for preventing colorectal adenomas and carcinomas *Cochrane Database of Systematic Reviews*. 2010;2:CD004079.
6. Kim DH, Pickhardt PJ, Taylor AJ, et al. CT colonography versus colonoscopy for the detection of advanced neoplasia. *N Engl J Med*. 2007;357: 1403–12.
7. Brown SR, et al. Chromoscopy versus conventional endoscopy for the detection of polyps in the colon and rectum. *Cochrane Database Syst Rev*. 2007;4:CD006439. DOI:10.1002/14651858.CD006439.pub2.
8. Rastogi, Amit, et al. "Recognition of surface mucosal and vascular patterns of colon polyps by using narrow-band imaging: interobserver and intraobserver agreement and prediction of polyp histology." *Gastrointestinal endoscopy*. 2009;69(Suppl 3):716–22.
9. Yood,Marianne Ulcickas, et al. "Colon polyp recurrence in a managed care population." *Archives of internal medicine*.163.4 (2003):422–6.

C

ADDITIONAL READING

- Elwood PC, Gallagher AM, Duthie GG, et al. Aspirin, salicylates, and cancer. *Lancet*. 2009;373:1301–9.
- Kumar D, et al. *Pathologic Basis of Disease*, 7th ed. 2005;856–870.
- Larsen IK, Grotmol T, Almendingen K, et al. Lifestyle as a predictor for colonic neoplasia in asymptomatic individuals. *BMC Gastroenterol*. 2006;6:5.
- Seong-Eun K, et al. An association between obesity and the prevalence of colonic adenoma according to age and gender. *J Gastroenterol*. 2007;42(8).

See Also (Topic, Algorithm, Electronic Media Element)
Algorithm: Bleeding, GI

CODES

ICD9
211.3 Benign neoplasm of colon

CLINICAL PEARLS

- Villous adenomatous polyps are the "villains" (most likely to become malignant).
- Hyperplastic polyps rarely become cancer.
- Up to 50% of patients who have polyps removed have recurrent polyps.

COLORECTAL CANCER

Stephen M. Scott, MD, MPH

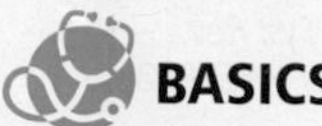

BASICS

DESCRIPTION

- Colorectal cancer (CRC) denotes a neoplasm that develops in the colon or rectum.
- CRC is the 3rd leading cause of cancer-related death in the US when men and women are considered separately; however, it is the 2nd leading cause when both sexes are combined.

EPIDEMIOLOGY

Incidence

In 2008, an estimated ~148,810 new cases of CRC were diagnosed, and 49,960 deaths occurred from CRC.

Prevalence

- The overall lifetime risk for developing CRC in the US is about 1 in 19 (5.4%).
- Death rates have been declining due to improved screening, prevention, and treatment.

RISK FACTORS

- Age: > 90% of people diagnosed with CRC are >50.
- Personal history of colorectal polyps:
  - Risks increase with multiple polyps, villous polyps, and larger polyps.
- Personal history of cancer:
  - Rectal cancer has a higher incidence of local recurrence than proximal cancers (20–30% vs. 2–4%)
- History of inflammatory bowel disease:
  - The prevalence of CRC in ulcerative colitis and Crohn disease is about 3%, with a cumulative risk of CRC of 2% at 10 years, 8% at 20 years, and 18% at 30 years (1,2).
- Family history of CRC (although most CRCs occur in people without a family history):
  - The risk doubles in those who have a single 1st-degree relative with a history of CRC.
  - The risk is > double for those who have a history of CRC or polyps in:
    - Any 1st-degree relative <60 years old
    - ≥2 1st-degree relatives, regardless of age
- Inherited syndromes:
  - Familial adenomatous polyposis (FAP):
    - Affected individuals develop hundreds to thousands of polyps in colon and rectum.
    - CRC usually present by age 40
    - Accounts for about 1% of CRCs
  - Hereditary nonpolyposis colon cancer (HNPCC, also called Lynch syndrome):
    - Often develops at a relatively young age
    - Lifetime risk of CRC 70–80%
    - Accounts for about 3–4% of all CRCs
  - Peutz-Jeghers syndrome:
    - Individuals may have freckles (mouth, hands, feet) and large polyps in gastrointestinal (GI) tract.
    - Greatly increased risk for CRC and cancers
- Race and ethnicity:
  - African Americans have highest CRC incidence and mortality rates in US.
  - Several different gene mutations have been identified among Ashkenazi Jews.
- Miscellaneous:
  - *Streptococcus bovis* bacteremia is associated with CRC.
  - Patients with acromegaly are at increased risk.

Genetics

- Most result from acquired DNA mutation
- There does not seem to be a single genetic pathway to CRC, although mutations are frequently seen in APC, K-Ras, p53, and SMAD4.
- A small percentage of colon cancers are known to be caused by inherited gene mutations:
  - APC, a tumor suppressor gene, is altered in FAP.
  - Genes encoding DNA repair enzymes implicated in HNPCC: MLH1, MSH2, MSH6, PMS1, PMS2, and others
  - STK11, a tumor suppressor gene, is altered in Peutz-Jeghers syndrome.

GENERAL PREVENTION

- Diets high in fruits and vegetables have been linked with decreased risk; those high in red and processed meats may increase CRC risk.
- People who are physically inactive are at higher risk for CRC.
- Long-term smokers are more likely than nonsmokers to develop and die from CRC.
- CRC has been linked to heavy alcohol consumption; may be related to low folic acid.
- Some studies suggest that vitamin D, calcium, and folate may lower CRC risk.
- NSAIDs may reduce risk in some groups; however, experts do not recommend NSAID use as a cancer prevention strategy in people at average risk for CRC.
- Colon cancer screening is one of the most powerful tools in preventing colon cancer:
  - The United States Preventive Services Task Force (USPSTF) strongly recommends that clinicians screen men and women between the ages of 50 and 75 for CRC (3)[A].
  - Current screening recommendations from the American Cancer Society include completing 1 of the following tests (1)[C]:
    - Fecal occult blood testing (FOBT) annually
    - Fecal immunochemical test (FIT) annually
    - Stool DNA test (sDNA), interval uncertain
    - Flexible sigmoidoscopy every 5 years
    - Double-contrast barium enema every 5 years
    - Colonoscopy every 10 years
    - Computed tomography (CT) colonography every 5 years (colonoscopy completed if positive)
  - The USPSTF does not recommend barium enema as a screening test and concludes that the evidence is insufficient to assess the benefits and harms of CT colonography and stool DNA testing as screening modalities for CRC (2)[A].
  - Digital rectal exam (DRE), alone or in combination with a 1-sample FOBT or FIT test, is not an acceptable method for CRC screening.
- Screening in high-risk groups:
  - People with a personal history of polyps need more frequent colonoscopy screening, depending on risk (i.e., 1 or 2 <1 cm polyps with low-grade dysplasia is deemed low-risk and may warrant repeat colonoscopy in 5–10 years; decision is influenced by family history, age, quality of initial colonoscopy, and patient comorbidities).
  - People who have a family history of CRC should begin colonoscopy at age 40 or 10 years younger than the age of relative at cancer diagnosis, whichever is earlier.
  - People with a family history of polyps should begin colonoscopy screening at age 40.
  - People with inflammatory bowel disease (IBD) should have regular surveillance colonoscopy with biopsies to detect dysplasia; guidelines for timing and location vary by professional society, but generally indicate starting surveillance by about 8 years of onset of disease followed by surveillance every 1–2 years.
  - Genetic testing may be appropriate for individuals with a strong family history of CRC or polyps:
    - Family members of a person affected by HNPCCC should start colonoscopy screening during their early 20s.
    - Individuals who test positive for the gene linked to FAP should start colonoscopy screening in their teens.

PATHOPHYSIOLOGY

The progression from the 1st abnormal cells to the appearance of CRC usually occurs over 10–15 years, a disease characteristic that contributes to the effectiveness of prevention.

ETIOLOGY

Multiple genetic and environmental factors have been linked to the development of CRC.

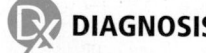

DIAGNOSIS

HISTORY

- Many patients with CRC are asymptomatic.
- Common presenting symptoms and signs in symptomatic patients include:
  - Abdominal pain or cramping
  - Change in bowel habits (constipation, diarrhea, narrowing of stool)
  - Rectal bleeding, dark stools, or blood in stool
  - Weakness or fatigue
  - Weight loss
  - Anemia
- Other presentations may include symptoms due to the presence of metastatic lesions (lymph nodes, liver, lung, peritoneum), fever of unknown origin, and *S. bovis* or *Clostridium septicum* sepsis.

PHYSICAL EXAM

- Weight loss
- Palpable abdominal mass
- Signs of anemia (i.e., conjunctival pallor)

DIAGNOSTIC TESTS & INTERPRETATION

Lab

Initial lab tests

- Complete blood count (CBC) (to evaluate anemia)
- Liver function (CRC may spread to the liver)

ɿaging

ɪtial approach

- CT scanning to evaluate the presence of metastatic disease
- Chest X-ray (CXR) may be used to evaluate the presence of chest metastases.
- Endoscopic ultrasound (EUS) may be used to evaluate the extent of rectal cancers; endorectal magnetic resonance imaging (MRI) may also provide further detail.
- Intraoperative ultrasound may be used to evaluate solid organs (such as the liver) after tumor resection.

ɪllow-Up & Special Considerations

- X-ray, CT, and/or MRI examinations may be used to monitor the presence or absence of CRC.
- Positron emission tomography (PET) may be used in some cases to detect metastatic disease.

iagnostic Procedures/Surgery

- Biopsy is usually performed (most often during colonoscopy) if CRC is suspected.
- CT needle-guided biopsy may be needed to evaluate a suspected tumor or metastasis.

athological Findings

- The American Joint Committee on Cancer (AJCC) TNM criteria and Duke's criteria are most often used for staging. TNM staging for CRC is:
  - Stage 0: Limited to the mucosa (*carcinoma in situ* or *intramucosal carcinoma*, Tis, N0, M0)
  - Stage I: Through the muscularis mucosa into the submucosa or muscularis propria; no invasion of lymph nodes or distant sites (T1, N0, M0 or T2, N0, M0)
  - Stage IIA: Invades serosa; no lymph nodes or distant sites (T3, N0, M0)
  - Stage IIB: Through the wall of the colon or rectum and into adjacent tissues or organs; no lymph nodes or distant sites (T4, N0, M0)
  - Stage IIIA: Through mucosa into submucosa or muscularis propria with spread to 1–3 lymph nodes; no distant sites (T1, N1, M0 or T2, N1, M0)
  - Stage IIIB: Through colon or rectum with or without invasion of adjacent tissues or organs plus spread to 1–3 lymph nodes; no distant sites (T3, N1, M0, or T4, N1, M0)
  - Stage IIIC: Through colon or rectum and spread to 4 or more nearby lymph nodes; no distant sites (any T, N2, M0)
  - Stage IV: Any level of invasion with spread to distant site (any T, any N, M1)
- CRCs are graded on a 4-point scale from G1–G4. G1–G2 may be called low-grade and G3–G4 high-grade.

ɪIFFERENTIAL DIAGNOSIS

- >95% of CRCs are adenocarcinomas.
- Other colonic tumors include carcinoid tumors, lymphomas, and Kaposi's sarcoma in HIV.
- Many conditions can mimic CRC, including other cancers, hemorrhoids, inflammatory bowel disease, infection, and extrinsic masses (i.e., cysts, abscesses).

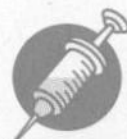

TREATMENT

MEDICATION

Surgical resection is the primary treatment for colorectal cancer. Chemotherapeutic regimens for metastatic disease may extend overall survival from 6 months to approximately 2 years. Adjuvant chemotherapy is most clearly beneficial for stage III (node-positive) disease, in which reductions of approximately 30% may be achieved in both disease recurrence and overall survival, compared with nontreated controls.

First Line

Chemotherapeutic agents include fluorouracil (5-FU), capecitabine (Xeloda, which is available in oral tablet form and is converted by body to 5-FU), irinotecan (Camptosar), and oxaliplatin (Eloxatin).

Geriatric Considerations

Elderly tend to tolerate CRC chemotherapy fairly well and should be considered when appropriate.

Second Line

Targeted therapies may be used alongside 1st-line agents or by themselves if 1st-line agents are ineffective:

- Bevacizumab (Avastin) is a monoclonal antibody that targets vascular endothelial growth factor (VEGF); inhibits angiogenesis.
- Cetuximab (Erbitux) and panitumumab (Vectibix) are monoclonal antibodies that target epidermal growth factor receptor (EGFR).

COMPLEMENTARY AND ALTERNATIVE MEDICINE

- May serve as an adjunct to treatment for CRC
- 70–75% of cancer survivors report using at least 1 type of complementary and alternative medicine (CAM), and almost all report that the alternative therapy improved their well-being.

SURGERY/OTHER PROCEDURES

- Surgery is the primary treatment for CRC:
  - May involve segmental resection, hemicolectomy, or colectomy, as well as resection of nodes, depending on size and invasion
  - Laparoscopic-assisted colectomy is an emerging option for earlier-stage tumors.
  - Surgery for rectal cancer may include local transanal, low anterior, or abdominoperineal resection, or pelvic exenteration.
- Radiation therapy is most often used for peritoneal or rectal cancers; it is rarely used for metastatic disease due to side effects.

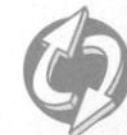

ONGOING CARE

FOLLOW-UP RECOMMENDATIONS

Patient Monitoring

- People with a personal history of proximal cancer (nonrectal) should have follow-up colonoscopy in 1 year, and if normal, in 3 and 5 years subsequently.
- Carcinoembryonic antigen (CEA) and/or CA 19-9 are used to detect recurrence in people treated for CRC. (Note: CEA levels may be elevated in ulcerative colitis, nonmalignant GI tumors, liver disease, lung disease, and in smokers.)

PATIENT EDUCATION

- NCI: What You Need to Know About Cancer of the Colon and Rectum: http://www.cancer.gov/cancertopics/wyntk/colon-and-rectal
- AAFP: Colorectal Cancer Screening (includes Spanish): http://familydoctor.org/online/famdocen/home/common/cancer/risk/556.html

PROGNOSIS

5-year relative survival rate is determined by stage (adjusted for patients dying of other diseases): Stage I: 92%; Stage II: 73%; Stage III: 56%; Stage IV: 8% (2)[A]

COMPLICATIONS

- Colorectal surgery: Pain, deep vein thrombosis (DVT), anastomotic leaks, infection, scarring, bowel obstruction
- Chemotherapy: Hair loss, nausea, vomiting, bruising, fatigue, increased risk for infections
- Radiation therapy: Skin irritation, nausea, rectal pain, incontinence, bladder irritation, fatigue, and sexual problems

REFERENCES

1. American cancer society guidelines for the early detection of cancer. Available at: http://www.cancer.org/docroot/PED/content/PED_2_3X_ACS_Cancer_Detection_Guidelines_36.asp?sitearea=PED. Accessed 9/30/2008.
2. O'Connell JB, Maggard MA, Ko CY. Colon cancer survival rates with the new American Joint Committee on Cancer sixth edition staging. *J Natl Cancer Inst*. 2004;96:1420–5.
3. Screening: Colorectal cancer. Available at: http://www.ahrq.gov/clinic/uspstf/uspscolo.htm. Accessed 9/30/2008.

ADDITIONAL READING

- Konda A, Duffy MC. Surveillance of patients at increased risk of colon cancer: Inflammatory bowel disease and other conditions. *Gastroenterol Clin North Am*. 2008;37:191–213, viii.
- National Cancer Institute. At: http://www.cancer.gov/cancertopics/types/colon-and-rectal.
- National Colorectal Cancer Roundtable. At: http://www.nccrt.org.

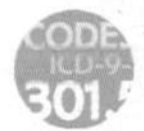

CODES

ICD9

- 153.9 Malignant neoplasm of colon, unspecified site
- 154.0 Malignant neoplasm of rectosigmoid junction
- 154.1 Malignant neoplasm of rectum

CLINICAL PEARLS

- The USPSTF recommends screening beginning at age 50, and notes that evidence supports several different screening regimens.
- 10% of cases of CRC occur in people younger than age 50. People who have a family history of CRC should begin colonoscopy at age 40, or 10 years younger than the age of relative at cancer diagnosis, whichever is earlier.
- Iron deficiency anemia in the elderly should prompt a search for CRC, and should not be attributed to normal aging.

COMPLEMENTARY AND ALTERNATIVE MEDICINE

Jennifer A. Caragol, MD
Anna Svircev, DO, MPH
Andrew Bentley, MS

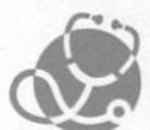

BASICS

Complementary and alternative medicine (CAM) are medical and health care systems, practices, and products that are not presently considered part of conventional medicine. The National Center for Health Statistics (NCHS) 2007 survey reports that 38% of adult Americans and 12% of children use some form of CAM, and this percentage is increasing as CAM healing practices and products become better known and more accessible. Medical professionals who incorporate CAM into their medical practice will often refer to their health care model as "integrative medicine."

DESCRIPTION

- Definitions and additional terms:
  - Complementary medicine is used with conventional medicine to address a health concern. For example, massage plus physical therapy to address low back pain, or medication plus osteopathic manipulation to address recurrent headaches.
  - Alternative medicine is used in place of conventional medicine to promote healing of conditions that cannot be explained by the conventional biomedical model or for which the effectiveness of therapy is not yet established by clinical research.
  - Integrative medicine is the combination of allopathic medicine with CAM, and may be provided to the patient by a single licensed medical professional versed in CAM or by a group of diverse health care providers. For example, a nurse on the oncology unit who integrates healing touch into the care of the patient.
  - Holistic is a descriptive term for a practitioner's approach to patient care. A holistic practitioner assesses the emotional, spiritual, mental, and physical state of wellness of the client and then works to provide comprehensive care. A holistic practice may include practitioners of different disciplines to best address all aspects of wellness or illness.
- Biologically based therapies: Diets, herbals, vitamins, supplements, flower essences
- Manipulative and body-based methods:
  - Massage therapy is the manipulation of the soft tissues of the body whereby the licensed practitioner uses knowledge of anatomy and physiology to restore function, promote relaxation, and relieve pain. There are several different types of massage.
  - Osteopathic manipulative medicine focuses on the musculoskeletal system. It includes indirect techniques, e.g., muscle energy, myofascial release, osteopathy in the cranial field, and strain-counterstrain approach, as well as direct action techniques (high-velocity thrusts).
  - Craniosacral therapy is a gentle manual treatment focusing on the release of bony and fascial restrictions in the craniosacral system, which includes the cranium, sacrum, spinal cord, meninges, and cerebrospinal fluid. Cranial osteopathy was developed in the early 1900s by American osteopath Dr. William Sutherland, who researched the subtle movements of the cranial bones and developed techniques to help release restrictions between sutures.
  - Chiropractic therapy is a discipline that focuses on the musculoskeletal and nervous systems and how imbalances in these systems can affect general health. It is most often used to treat back pain, neck pain, and joint pain. Doctors of chiropractic (DCs) complete 4–5 years of intensive training in anatomy, physiology, and manipulation.
- Mind-body medicine:
  - Meditation, traditionally a form of spiritual practice, is a practice of detachment in which a person sits quietly, generally focusing on the breath while releasing all thoughts from the mind with the intention to center the self, restore balance, and enhance well-being.
  - Spiritual practices/prayer
  - Yoga is an exercise of mindfulness, meditation, strength, and balance with the goal of achieving enlightenment. It is comprised of asanas (postures) and pranayamas (focused breathing). The discipline of yoga originated in India and has been practiced for thousands of years. Variations of yoga including Hatha, Raja, Jnana, Bhaki, and Tantra.
  - Aromatherapy utilizes highly concentrated plant extracts to stimulate physical, emotional, and energetic healing processes. These aromatic oils are rubbed on the skin, aerosolized, or used in compresses.
  - Tai chi and qigong are Chinese exercise systems that combine meditation, regulated breathing, and flowing dancelike movements to enhance and balance chi (qi), or life force energy.
- Alternative medical systems:
  - Traditional Chinese medicine incorporates Chinese herbs and acupuncture. Acupuncture is the practice of regulating chi by inserting hair-thin needles at specific points along meridian pathways of the body. Chi movement is responsible for animating and protecting the body; relieving pain; and regulating blood, oxygen, and nourishment to every cell.
  - Ayurvedic medicine originated in India and is one of the world's oldest medical systems. It utilizes healing modalities and herbs to integrate and balance the body, mind, and spirit.
  - Homeopathy is a system of therapy based on the concept that very dilute quantities of an offending agent can stimulate the body's own immune system to produce a reaction against this offense, thereby healing itself. In general, homeopathic remedies are considered safe and unlikely to cause serious adverse reactions.
  - Naturopathy is based on providing natural and minimally invasive options for prevention and treatment of disease. Treatment regimens can include herbs, vitamins, supplements, dietary counseling, homeopathic remedies, manipulative therapies, acupuncture, and hydrotherapy. 4-year doctoral training programs are available; however, because only 16 states have licensing laws for naturopathic physicians, patients are encouraged to research their prospective naturopath's credentials.
- Energy therapies:
  - Reiki, which means source energy, from Japan. Laying hands lightly on the patient or holding th hands just above the body, the Reiki practitioner facilitates spiritual and physical healing by replenishing and strengthening the patient's life force energy.
  - Healing touch designed by a registered nurse. Practitioners use their hands to clear, energize, and balance a patient's energy field to enhance well-being.
- Common reasons patients choose CAM:
  - Conventional medicine has been unsuccessful in fully addressing ailment.
  - Preventative health care
  - Desire for a holistic and natural approach to well-being
  - Preference for noninvasive treatment options
  - Concern about side effects of prescription medication
  - Desire for spiritual support to be incorporated in healing practice
  - Cultural or familial belief system may be more aligned with "natural" solutions not provided fo or supported by the standard allopathic model o health care.

EPIDEMIOLOGY

- All ages use CAM, but is most prevalent among adults aged 30–69 years
- Gender ratio: Female predominance
- College graduates and residents from Western states are more likely to use CAM.
- 10 most utilized CAM therapies based on the NCH 2007 survey; prayer is also reported. These 10 CAM therapies were used by the indicated percentage o survey participants:
  - Prayer/self (43%)
  - Prayer/others (24.4%)
  - Natural products (17.7%)
  - Deep breathing (12.7%)
  - Prayer group (9.6%)
  - Meditation (9.4%)
  - Chiropractic and osteopathic (8.6%)
  - Massage (8.3%)
  - Yoga (6.1%)
  - Diet-based therapies (3.6%)
  - Progressive relaxation (2.9%)
  - Guided imagery (2.2%)
  - Homeopathic treatment (1.8%)

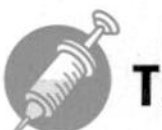

TREATMENT

- Evidence supports both safety and efficacy:
  - Meditation for lowering blood pressure (1)
  - Acupuncture for chronic low back pain (2)
  - Spinal manipulative therapy for prophylactic treatment of headaches
  - Manipulation, massage, and mobilization for acute low back and posterior neck pain
  - Massage therapy to promote weight gain in preterm infants
  - Acupuncture for nausea and vomiting
  - Tai chi for improving balance and decreasing the risk of and fear of falling in elderly (3)
  - Aromatherapy massage for temporary relief of anxiety or depression in cancer patients (4)

- Mind-body techniques for migraines, chronic pain, and insomnia
- Homeopathic remedy for the treatment of chemotherapy-induced stomatitis in children (5)
- Riboflavin for migraine prophylaxis (6)
- Horse chestnut seed extract to improve lower leg venous tone, pain, and edema
- Glucosamine and chondroitin sulfate for osteoarthritis and knee pain
- Yoga and meditation appear to improve endothelial function in patients with CAD.
- Yoga can have a potential beneficial effect on depressive disorders.

Evidence supports safety, but evidence regarding efficacy is inconclusive:
- Saw palmetto for benign prostatic hyperplasia
- Acupuncture for recurrent headache
- Homeopathy for induction and augmentation of labor
- Dietary fat reduction for certain types of cancer
- Mind-body techniques for metastatic cancer
- Copper and magnetic bracelets for pain

Evidence supports efficacy, but evidence regarding safety is inconclusive:
- St. John's wort extract for depression
- Ginkgo biloba for cognitive function in dementia

Evidence indicates serious risk:
- Delay in seeking medical care or replacement of curative conventional treatments
- Injections of unapproved substances
- Use of toxic herbs or substances
- Known herb-drug interactions

ONGOING CARE

PATIENT EDUCATION

National Library of Medicine: Alternative medicine (www.nlm.nih.gov)

The National Center for Complementary and Alternative Medicine (nccam.nih.gov)

COMPLICATIONS

Potentially toxic herbs:
- Serious adverse events from herbal remedies remain extremely rare.
- Some ethnic medicines, as those prescribed by practitioners of Ayurveda or traditional Chinese medicine, may intentionally contain heavy metals or other toxic substances. These are usually listed by their pharmacopial names, e.g., *qian dan* = lead oxide.
- Bitter orange (*Citrus sinensis*): Sympathomimetic; increases heart rate (HR), blood pressure (BP)
- California poppy (*Eschscholzia californica*): May cause respiratory depression, drowsiness; contains opioids
- Cascara sagrada (*Frangula purshiana*): Depletes serum potassium
- Chaparral (*Larrea tridentata*): Hepatotoxic
- Ephedra (*Ephedra* species): Sympathomimetic; increases HR, BP; insomnia, gastric distress
- Ginkgo (*Ginkgo biloba*): Extravasation, increased bleeding time
- Guarana (*Paullinia cupana*): Tachycardia, hypertension; contains caffeine
- Kava (*Piper methysticum*): Decreases utilization of niacin; possibly hepatotoxic
- Licorice (*Glycyrrhiza* species): Long-term use depletes serum potassium
- Lily of the valley (*Convallaria majalis*): Contains cardiac glycosides
- Poke root (*Phytolacca* species): Strong gastric irritant, may cause sedation
- Senna (*Cassia senna*): Depletes serum potassium
- Snakeroot (*Aristolochia* species): Nephrotoxic
- Wormwood (*Artemisia absinthum*): Elevates serotonin level, may raise BP
- Yohimbe (*Pausinystalia yohimbe*): Elevates BP

- Important herbal–medication interactions:
  - Ginkgo and St. John's wort account for most herb–drug interactions described in the medical literature.
  - Angelica, dong quai (*Angelica* species): Additive effect with calcium channel blockers
  - Bitter melon (*Momordicacharantia*): Additive effect with other hypoglycemic agents
  - Cascara sagrada (*Frangula purshiana*): Shortens transit time of intestinally absorbed drugs; Potential for causing hypokalemia may potentiate digoxin toxicity
  - Chamomile (*Anthemis, Matricaria* species): Antagonistic interaction with benzodiazepines
  - Echinacea (*Echinacea* species): May counteract immunosuppressants
  - Garlic (*Allium sativum*): Modest anticoagulant effect; decreases levels of saquinavir
  - Guarana (*Paullina cupana)*: Contains caffeine; may inhibit platelet aggregation
  - Ginkgo (*G. biloba*): Dangerous synergistic effect with anticoagulants (1)
  - Ginseng (*Panax* species): Potentiates dopaminergic drugs; counteracts phenothiazines
  - Kava (*Piper methysticum*): Additive effect with sedatives
  - Kelp (*Laminaria* species): May interfere with thyroxine and liothyronine
  - Lemon Balm (*Melissa officinalis*): Additive effect with sedatives; binds TSH and may interfere with thyroid testing and function
  - Licorice (*Glycyrrhiza* species): Increases potential for digoxin toxicity; depletes potassium
  - Lobelia (*Lobelia* species): Potentially counteracts β_2 adrenergic bronchodilators
  - Meadowsweet (*Filipendula ulmaria*): Increased anticoagulant effect; contains salicylates
  - Motherwort (*Leonurus cardiaca*): Can potentiate digoxin; contains cardiac glycosides
  - Milk thistle (*Silybum marianum*): Might accelerate clearance of liver-metabolized drugs
  - Pumpkin seed (*Cucurbita pepo*): Elevates levels of androgenic drugs
  - Red clover (*Trifolium pratense*): Partial agonistic/antagonistic interaction with estrogens
  - Saw palmetto (*Serenoa repens*): May potentiate or antagonize androgenic drugs
  - Soy isoflavones (*Glycine max*): Partial agonistic/antagonistic interaction with estrogens
  - St. John's wort (*Hypericum perforatum*): Induces CYP450 pathways, reducing levels of many drugs (2)
  - Tobacco (*Nicotiana tabacum*): May counteract β-blockers
  - Uva ursi (*Arctostaphylos uva-ursi*): Interferes with action of other diuretics; may cause faster clearance of kidney-metabolized drugs
  - Valerian (*Valeriana officinalis*): Potential for interference with valproic acid derivatives
  - Willow bark (*Salix alba*). Additive effect with anticoagulants; contains salicylates
- Vitamins and minerals with potential toxicity:
  - Iron is a leading cause of accidental poisoning in children under 6. Minerala (i.e., potassium, calcium, magnesium, zinc, copper, and selenium) may cause toxicity
  - Fat-soluble vitamins have the potential to cause hypervitaminosis
    - Vitamin A is most common cause of hypervitaminosis
    - β-carotene may have a limited potential for overdose.
  - Vitamin A: Pseudotumor cerebri, hepatic damage, loss of appetite, osteomalacia
  - Vitamin D: Constipation, hypercalcemia
  - Vitamin E: Coagulopathy, fatigue, pain in extremities

REFERENCES

1. Anderson JW, Liu C, Kryscio RJ. Blood pressure response to transcendental meditation: a meta-analysis. *Am J Hypertens*. 2008;21:310–6.
2. Manheimer E, White A, Berman B, et al. Meta-analysis: acupuncture for low back pain. *Ann Intern Med*. 2005;142:651–63.
3. Sattin RW, Easley KA, Wolf SL, et al. Reduction in fear of falling through intense tai chi exercise training in older, transitionally frail adults. *J Am Geriatr Soc*. 2005,53:1168–78.
4. Wilkinson SM, Love SB, Westcombe AM, et al. Effectiveness of aromatherapy massage in the management of anxiety and depression in patients with cancer: a multicenter randomized controlled trial. *J Clin Oncol*. 2007;25:532–9.
5. Oberbaum M, Yaniv I, Ben-Gal Y, et al. A randomized, controlled clinical trial of the homeopathic medication TRAUMEEL S in the treatment of chemotherapy-induced stomatitis in children undergoing stem cell transplantation. *Cancer*. 2001;92:684–90.
6. Schoenen J, Jacquy J, Lenaerts M. Effectiveness of high-dose riboflavin in migraine prophylaxis. A randomized controlled trial. *Neurology*. 1998;50: 466–70.

ADDITIONAL READING

- Bent S et al. Herbal medicine in the United States: review of efficacy, safety, and regulation: grand rounds at University of California, San Francisco Medical Center. *J Gen Intern Med*. 2008;23:854–9.
- Rakel D, Faas N. *Complementary Medicine in Clinical Practice*. Boston: Jones and Bartlett, 2006.

CLINICAL PEARLS

1/3 of adults and >10% of children use CAM; best evidence examples include:
- Meditation for lowering blood pressure (1)
- Acupuncture for chronic low back pain (2)
- Spinal manipulative therapy for prophylactic treatment of headaches

COMPLEX REGIONAL PAIN SYNDROME

Dennis E. Hughes, DO

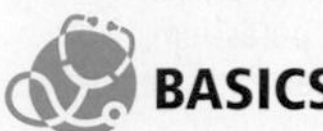

BASICS

Multidisciplinary approach with physical, occupational, and recreational therapy involvement

DESCRIPTION

- Pain syndrome after injury to bone and soft tissue; pathogenesis is obscure. Evidence suggests that these syndromes involve areas of the brain and nervous system.
  - Type I: No nerve injury [reflex sympathetic dystrophy (RSD)]
  - Type II: Associated with a demonstrable nerve injury (causalgia)
- System(s) affected: Nervous
- Synonym(s): Traumatic erythromelalgia, Weir Mitchell causalgia, causalgia, reflex sympathetic dystrophy, posttraumatic neuralgia, sympathetically maintained pain

EPIDEMIOLOGY

- Predominant age: Mean age 36–46 years (1)
- Predominant gender: Female > Male (3:1, 60–81%) (1)
- Extremely rare in children

Incidence

26.2/100,000 person-years, but may be higher owing to misdiagnosis initially

Prevalence

~6 million in the US

RISK FACTORS

- Minor or severe trauma (upper extremity fracture noted in 44%)
- Surgery
- Lacerations
- Burns
- Frostbite
- Casting
- Penetrating injury

Genetics

No known genetic pattern

GENERAL PREVENTION

- Early mobilization after fracture, stroke, and myocardial infarction has proven benefit in reducing incidence of complex regional pain syndrome (CRPS).
- 1 study of wrist fractures found that addition of 500 mg/d of vitamin C lowered rates of CRPS (2).

PATHOPHYSIOLOGY

Poorly understood activation of abnormal sympathetic reflex that lowers pain threshold

ETIOLOGY

Other than known nerve injury (type II or causalgia), no known definitive pathogenesis

COMMONLY ASSOCIATED CONDITIONS

- Serious injury to bone and soft tissue
- Herpes zoster
- Postherpetic neuralgia results from partial or complete damage to afferent nerve pathways.
- Pain occurs in dermatomes as a sequela of herpes zoster.

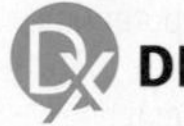

DIAGNOSIS

Unprovoked pain is the hallmark of the condition.

HISTORY

- Inciting injury ranges from minor sprains to major trauma
- Hyperhydrosis
- Thermal hypersensitivity
- Hair loss
- Burning paroxysms of pain
- Increased symptoms during emotional stress
- Muscle spasms
- Hypersensitivity to light touch
- Mottled skin
- Partial motor paralysis

PHYSICAL EXAM

- Smooth, glossy skin
- Guarding of extremity
- Diminished hair

DIAGNOSTIC TESTS & INTERPRETATION

Lab

Initial lab tests

- Complete blood count (CBC) (3)
- Erythrocyte sedimentation rate (ESR) (3)

Imaging

Initial approach

- Plain radiographs may show patchy demineralization within 3–6 weeks of onset of CRPS and more pronounced than one would see from disuse alone (3).
- 3-phase bone scanning has varying sensitivity but is most accurate for support of the diagnosis when there is diffuse activity (especially on phase 3) (1,3).
- Bone densometry (3)

Diagnostic Procedures/Surgery

- Electromyelography (EMG) shows nerve injury with type II CRPS (3).
- Sudomotor function testing (resting sweat testing, resting skin temperature, quantitative sudomotor axon reflex testing—all related to increased autonomic activity of the affected limb) (1)

Pathological Findings

- Partial or complete damage to afferent nerve pathways and probably reorganized central pain pathways
- Nerves most commonly involved are median and sciatic.
- Atrophy in affected muscles
- Incomplete nerve plexus lesion

DIFFERENTIAL DIAGNOSIS

- Infection
- Hypertrophic scar
- Bone fragments
- Neuroma
- CNS tumor or syrinx

TREATMENT

MEDICATION

First Line

- No single drug or combination of drugs has produced consistent results; early therapy is beneficial.
- α-Adrenergic blockers: Phenoxybenzamine: 40–120 mg/d PO in divided doses; the initial dose should not exceed 10 mg.
- Miscellaneous: Prednisone: 30 mg/d PO × 2–3 weeks, then tapered over 2–4 weeks (4)[B]
- Tricyclic antidepressants (response to each may be variable; therefore, several should be considered) (3,4)[C]:
  - Amitriptyline (Elavil): 25–100 mg/d at bedtime
  - Nortriptyline (Pamelor): 25–100 mg/d
- Anticonvulsants (serum drug level monitoring may be needed, except for clonazepam; individualize doses):
  - Carbamazepine (Tegretol): 200–1,000 mg/d PO
  - Phenytoin (Dilantin): 100–300 mg/d PO
  - Clonazepam (Klonopin): 1–10 mg/d PO
  - Valproic acid (Depakene): 750–2,250 mg/d PO, maximum of 60 mg/kg
  - Gabapentin: 100 mg/d at bedtime up to 600–1,200 mg t.i.d. (3,4)[B]

- Skeletal muscle relaxant: Baclofen: 10–40 mg/d PO; may act synergistically with carbamazepine and phenytoin (3)
- Contraindications: Refer to manufacturer's literature.
- Precautions: Refer to manufacturer's literature.
- Significant possible interactions: Many exist within this group of drugs. Refer to the manufacturer's literature for each drug.

econd Line

sphosphonates have the potential to reduce pain sociated with bone loss in patients with CRPS)[B].

DDITIONAL TREATMENT

eneral Measures

scourage maladaptive behaviors.

sues for Referral

- After 2 months of the illness, psychological evaluation generally is indicated to identify and treat any comorbid conditions (1)[C].
- Refer the patient to a specialty pain clinic in difficult cases (many advocate early referral to an expert in the management to reduce duration of symptoms).

dditional Therapies

- Available information about treatment is based on small studies or treatment reports; therefore, therapy remains largely empirical.
- Treatment response can be predicted by diagnosis (type I versus type II).
- Type I:
  - Physical therapy
  - Transcutaneous nerve stimulation
  - Psychotherapy

OMPLEMENTARY AND ALTERNATIVE IEDICINE

- Vitamin C (500 mg/d) may help to prevent CRPS in those with wrist fracture (2).
- Briskly rub the affected part several times per day.
- Acupuncture
- Hypnosis can be suggested.
- Relaxation training (alternate muscle relaxing and contracting)
- Biofeedback
- Mirror therapy (6)[A]

SURGERY/OTHER PROCEDURES

- Type II responds more favorably to nerve-directed treatment.
  - Sympathetic blocks
  - Sympathectomy (4)[C]
- Anesthetic blockade (chemical or surgical) of sympathetic nerve function:
  - Transient relief suggests that chemical or surgical sympathectomy will be helpful (1)[C].
  - Little in the way of quality clinical trials exist to support local sympathetic blockage as the "gold standard" of therapy (7).
- IV regional sympathetic block with guanethidine or reserpine by pain specialist or anesthetist
- Transcutaneous electric nerve stimulation (controversial)
- Inject myofascial painful trigger points
- Spinal cord stimulation (3)[C]
- Intrathecal analgesia (3)[C]

IN-PATIENT CONSIDERATIONS

Admission Criteria

Only for proposed surgical therapy

ONGOING CARE

FOLLOW-UP RECOMMENDATIONS

Weekly to monitor progress and initiate additional modalities as needed

PATIENT EDUCATION

- Stress need to remain active physically.
- Instruct carefully about any prescribed medications.
- Reflex Sympathetic Dystrophy Syndrome Association, www.rsds.org, (203) 877-3790 or American RSD Hope Group, www.rsdhope.org, (207) 583-4589

PROGNOSIS

Most improve with early treatment (1)

COMPLICATIONS

- Depression
- Disability
- Opioid dependence

REFERENCES

1. Rho RH, Brewer RP, Lamer TJ, et al. Complex regional pain syndrome. *Mayo Clin Proc.* 2002;77: 174–80.
2. Ghai B, Dureja GP. Complex regional pain syndrome: a review. *J Postgrad Med.* 2004;50: 300–7.
3. Cepeda MS, Carr DB, Lau J. Local anesthetic sympathetic blockade for complex regional pain syndrome. *Cochrane Database Syst Rev.* 2005:CD004598.
4. Malis A. Sympathetectomy for neuropathic pain. *The Cochrane Collaboration*, 2007.
5. Brunner F, Schmid A, Kissling R, et al. Biphosphonates for the therapy of complex regional pain syndrome I—Systematic review. *Eur J Pain.* 2008.
6. Ezendam D, Bongers RM, Jannink MJ et al. Systematic review of the effectiveness of mirror therapy in upper extremity function. *Disabil Rehabil.* 2009;31:2135–49.
7. Harden RN. Pharmacotherapy of complex regional pain syndrome. *Am J Phys Med Rehab.* 2005;84: s17–s28.

ADDITIONAL READING

Lang L, et al. *Living with RSDS. Your Guide to Coping with Reflex Sympathetic Dystrophy Syndrome.* Oakland CA: New Harbinger, 2003.

See Also (Topic, Algorithm, Electronic Media Element)

Algorithm: Pain in Upper Extremity

CODES

ICD9

- 337.20 Reflex sympathetic dystrophy, unspecified
- 337.21 Reflex sympathetic dystrophy of the upper limb
- 337.22 Reflex sympathetic dystrophy of the lower limb

CLINICAL PEARLS

- Pain control and early mobility are key to recovery.
- Regional sympathetic blocks may be useful.
- Use multidisciplinary approach.

CONCUSSION

J. Herbert Stevenson, MD

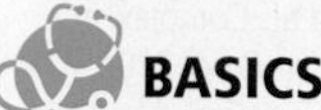

BASICS

DESCRIPTION

- A complex pathophysiologic process affecting brain function, induced by traumatic biomechanical forces that generally resolves over 7–10 days.
- Concussion severity can only be determined in retrospect.
- System(s) affected: Cardiovascular; Endocrine/Metabolic; Nervous; Psychiatric
- Synonym(s): Mild traumatic brain injury (TBI)

Pediatric Considerations

Children (ages 5–18) should not be allowed to return to training or play that same day and not until completely symptom-free. Resolution of symptoms and clinical findings often take longer in the pediatric athlete.

EPIDEMIOLOGY

- Predominant age: 12–24 years
- Predominant sex: Male > Female
- Usually related to accidents, sometimes sports related

Incidence

- 0.14–3.66 injuries/100 players each season at high school level
- 0.5–3.0 injuries/1,000 athlete exposures at college level (1)
- Average annual incidence 503:100,000.
- ~1.5 million cases of TBI in US annually, 85% of which are considered mild TBI.
- ~10% of TBIs are related to sports or cycling injuries.
- Among the 5–14 age group, 26.4% of mild TBI is related to sports or cycling (2).

RISK FACTORS

Contact sports, particularly football, and history of recent concussion.

GENERAL PREVENTION

- Educate athletes, coaches, parents, and officials on signs and symptoms of concussions.
- Rule enforcement in sports (e.g., penalties for spearing or head-to-head contact)
- Consideration of rule changes in sports to decrease dangerous plays
- Current protective headgear for contact sports decreases facial injuries, but has not been shown to decrease the overall concussion risk.
- Useful web site: www.thinkfirst.ca/default.asp

PATHOPHYSIOLOGY

Concussion represents a functional brain injury rather than a structural brain injury. The neurobiologic cascade has been shown to include excitatory amino acid release, ionic flux, hyperglycolysis, and reduced cerebral blood flow.

ETIOLOGY

- Falls
- Sports related
- Motor vehicle accidents

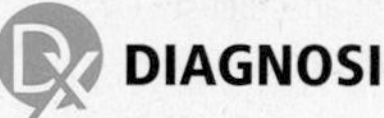

DIAGNOSIS

HISTORY

- Cognitive symptoms:
  - Confusion
  - Post-traumatic amnesia (PTA)
  - Retrograde amnesia (RGA)
  - Loss of consciousness (LOC)
  - Disorientation
  - Feeling "in a fog," "zoned out"
  - Inability to focus
  - Delayed verbal and motor responses
  - Slurred/incoherent speech
  - Excessive drowsiness
- Somatic:
  - Headache
  - Fatigue
  - Disequilibrium, dizziness
  - Visual disturbances
  - Phonophobia
- Affective:
  - Emotional lability
  - Irritability
- Sleep Disturbance

PHYSICAL EXAM

Variable and dependent on degree of injury:

- ABCs if seen acutely
- External evidence of major trauma
- Focal neurologic signs and symptoms
- Musculoskeletal: Evaluate for possible C-spine injury and stability.
- Detailed neurologic exam including:
  - State of alertness
  - Orientation
  - 3- or 5-word recall at 5 minutes
  - Concentration/attention (serial 3s or 7s)
  - Cerebellar function and postural stability assessment

DIAGNOSTIC TESTS & INTERPRETATION

- The sideline assessment of concussion (SAC) scale has been validated to drop from baseline after a concussion and return to baseline once symptoms clear.
- Serial cognitive evaluations should be done by an experienced health care provider using the neurologic exam listed above or by using other assessment tools such as the sport concussion assessment tool (SCAT) (3)[C].
- Computerized neurocognitive testing to date lacks sufficient evidence on validity, cost effectiveness, and improved management to warrant global usage (4)[B].
- Current gold standard is evaluation and treatment by a trained physician. Until improved outcomes, validity, and cost-effectiveness of computerized testing are established, use should be limited to experimental situations or possibly in management of complex concussions.

Lab

Generally not necessary.

Imaging

- Structural neuroimaging is usually normal in the setting of concussion.
- Consider MRI or CT with prolonged LOC, focal neurologic deficit, or overall worsening symptoms.
- Role of functional MRI is largely experimental and unvalidated at this time.
- Consider C-spine films.

Diagnostic Procedures/Surgery

Serial neurologic exams at least every 10–15 minute until symptoms are clearing and patient is stabilizing or patient has been transported to hospital for furthe evaluation.

DIFFERENTIAL DIAGNOSIS

- Concussion
- Subdural hematoma
- Epidural hematoma
- Cerebral contusion
- Facial or skull fracture

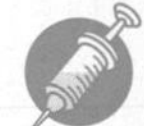

TREATMENT

MEDICATION

- Ibuprofen or acetaminophen may be used as adjun pain management for headache once structural brain injury ruled out.
- Prolonged symptoms such as sleep disturbance or anxiety, may benefit from appropriate pharmacologic treatment for symptom relief.

DDITIONAL TREATMENT

eneral Measures

Acute management depends on severity of injury. Most patients need only physical and cognitive rest, serial clinical evaluations to include neurologic checks, and a plan for follow-up evaluation (1)[C].

Prolonged LOC, abnormal neurologic exam, or deteriorating symptoms necessitate urgent or emergent referral to the hospital for further evaluation (1)[C].

ssues for Referral

Most concussions can be managed by primary care physicians using the standard guidelines for return to play; generally, referral to a specialist is not needed.

Patients with a complex or atypical concussion, or who have suffered recurrent concussions should be referred to a sports medicine physician or neurologist for management and clearance prior to returning to sports activities.

URGERY/OTHER PROCEDURES

enerally not indicated, unless signs of more severe BI present, with increased intracranial pressure or rge bleed.

N-PATIENT CONSIDERATIONS

nitial Stabilization

ABCs take priority over head injury and concussion.

C-spine immobilization should be considered in all head trauma.

dmission Criteria

Progressive neurologic symptoms, including deterioration of mental status, seizures, and focal neurologic signs

No competent adult at home

ischarge Criteria

Improving mental status at or near baseline

Competent adult at home for patient observation (see Patient Monitoring)

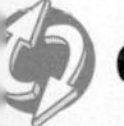

ONGOING CARE

OLLOW-UP RECOMMENDATIONS

Any athlete with a suspected concussion should be withheld that day from sports participation and not returned till a concussion has been ruled out or a diagnosed concussion has been appropriately treated as noted below (3).

Current recommendation on treatment involves an asymptomatic graduated return to play as follows (3)[C]:

- Complete rest until symptom-free, including cognitive rest (e.g., video games, and potentially scholastic activities)
- May then begin gradual reintroduction of activity as long as symptom free. Each step should be generally done 24 hours apart.
  - Light aerobic exercise
  - Sport-specific exercise
  - Noncontact training drills
  - Full contact training
  - Game play

- If postconcussive symptoms occur (exertional headache, visual disturbance, or disequilibrium), decrease level of activity until again asymptomatic, and progress again in 24 hours.
- High-risk athletes for more prolonged recovery include pediatric athletes, athletes with mood disorders, athletes with learning disabilities, and athletes with migraine headaches. These athletes should have a slower return to play progression and may require more intensive evaluation (formal neuropsychologic, balance, symptom testing).
- Athletes with multiple concussions should have slower return to play and may benefit from sports medicine consultation or neurology referral.

Patient Monitoring

- Written instructions regarding postconcussion management should be given to a competent adult describing signs to watch for and when to bring the patient back for further evaluation.
- Have a follow-up plan prior to discharge to home, ideally to be seen within a few days.
- Instruct patients and families regarding postconcussive symptoms, including the cognitive, somatic, and affective symptoms listed earlier.
- Ensure adequate rest and symptom-free return to both school and sports-related activities.

DIET

As tolerated.

COMPLICATIONS

- Delayed hematomas, including subdural hematomas, can present minutes to hours after initial injury, necessitating serial neurologic checks and close observation.
- Postconcussion syndrome occurs when symptoms of concussion, such as headache, fatigue, memory changes, or emotional lability, are persistent and last >1–3 months.
- Recurrent concussions can lead to second-impact syndrome or can occur with less and less impact force. Symptoms can persist longer than a 1st concussion, and progression to chronic cognitive and psychiatric symptoms is possible.
- Second-impact syndrome describes an additional insult or injury to the brain after a concussion and before the brain has had adequate time to completely recover. A rare, but life-threatening, cerebral edema after repeated head injury can occur. The etiology is thought to be due to loss of regulation of either cerebral circulation or glucose metabolism in the concussed brain.
- Chronic traumatic brain injury with chronic cognitive, mood, and potential Parkinson-type symptoms (5).

REFERENCES

1. Concussion (mild traumatic brain injury) and the team physician: a consensus statement. *Med Sci Sports Exerc*. 2006;38:395–9.
2. Bazarian JJ, McClung J, Shah MN et al. Mild traumatic brain injury in the United States, 1998–2000. *Brain Inj*. 2005;19:85–91.
3. McCrory P, Meeuwisse W, Johnston K, et al. Consensus Statement on Concussion in Sport: the 3rd International Conference on Concussion in Sport held in Zurich, November 2008. *Br J Sports Med* 2009;42(Suppl 1):i76–90.
4. Randolph C, McCrea M, Barr W. Is neuropsychological testing useful in the management of sport-related concussion? *J Athletic Train*. 2005;40(3):136–51.
5. Guskiewicz KM, Marshall SW, Bailes J et al. Association between recurrent concussion and late-life cognitive impairment in retired professional football players. *Neurosurgery*. 2005;57:.

C

ADDITIONAL READING

- Halstead ME, Walter KD. Council on Sports Medicine and Fitness et al. American Academy of Pediatrics. Clinical report- sport-related concussion in children and adolescents. *Pediatrics*. 2010;126:597–615.
- Mayers L. Return-to-play criteria after athletic concussion: a need for revision. *Arch Neurol*. 2008;65:1158–61.

See Also (Topic, Algorithm, Electronic Media Element)

Brain Injury, Traumatic; Brain Injury, Post Acute Care Issues; Postconcussive Syndrome; Seizure Disorders

CODES

ICD9

- 310.2 Postconcussion syndrome
- 850.9 Concussion, unspecified

CLINICAL PEARLS

- Most symptoms resolve completely within 7–10 days, but each person recovers at a different rate, and some symptoms may continue for weeks to months.
- Some athletes notice worsening symptoms, such as headache or nausea, while concentrating. If symptoms worsen while in class, they should stay home from school until their symptoms clear.
- Generally, patients who have been observed for at least 1–2 hours and are stable or improving do not need to be roused from sleep.
- When symptom-free at rest, the athlete may begin a gradual ramp-up of activity over 3–5 days, as listed above. If symptoms recur during any level of play, the athlete should postpone further activity for at least another 24 hours.

CONDYLOMATA ACUMINATA

Timothy R. McCurry, MD
Sujata Sharma, MD

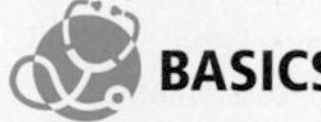

BASICS

DESCRIPTION

Condylomata acuminata are soft, skin-colored, fleshy warts that are caused by human papillomavirus (HPV):

- HPV types 6, 11, 16, 18, 31, 33, and 35 associated with condylomata acuminata
- Highly contagious; incubation period may be from 1–6 months.
- Warts appear singly or in groups, small or large; on the vagina, cervix, around the external genitalia and rectum, and in the urethra and anus. Reports of conjunctival, nasal, oral, and laryngeal warts and occasionally the throat.
- System(s) affected: Skin/Exocrine; Reproductive

Pediatric Considerations

Consider sexual abuse if seen in children, although they can be infected by other means (e.g., transfer from wart on another child's hand).

Pregnancy Considerations

- Warts often grow larger during pregnancy and regress spontaneously after delivery. Use cryotherapy.
- Virus does not cross the placenta. Treatment during pregnancy is somewhat controversial. Cesarean section is not absolutely indicated.
- Few documented cases of HPV transmission to infant at time of delivery have resulted in laryngeal papillomas, a rare and life-threatening condition.
- HPV vaccination is contraindicated in pregnancy.

EPIDEMIOLOGY

- Most common viral sexually transmitted infection (STI) in the US
- Predominant age: 15–30 years old
- Predominant sex: Male = Female

Incidence

- Venereal warts are increasing in an ever-younger population. A recent study of 487 college women showed an infection rate of 48%.
- Increased size and number in immunocompromised patients

Prevalence

- Peak prevalence in ages 17–33
- Minimum of 10–20% of sexually active women may be infected with HPV. Studies in men suggest a similar prevalence.
- Pregnancy and immunosuppression favor recurrence and increasing growth of lesions.

RISK FACTORS

- Young adults and adolescents
- Multiple sexual partners
- Not using condoms
- Possibly subclinical infection
- Young age of commencing sexual activity
- Cigarette smoking: Tobacco smoke has been shown to reduce cellular protection by decreasing cervical keratinocyte production.
- Poor hygiene
- History of genital warts

GENERAL PREVENTION

- Use of condoms (preventive effects not adequately evaluated; 40% of infected men have scrotal warts)
- Abstinence until treatment completed
- Circumcision may prevent recurrence in some men.
- Quadrivalent HPV vaccine available against genital warts and cervical cancer. This vaccination is targeted to adolescents before the period of their greatest risk for exposure to HPV. The vaccine does not treat previous infections:
  - Immunity has been documented to last at least 5 years after HPV vaccination.
  - The use of 4 HPV-specific virion protein capsids address the 2 most common HPV serotypes to be contracted in 6 and 11, and the 2 most cancer-promoting types in 16 and 18 (Gardasil) (1,2).
  - HPV quadrivalent vaccine protects against some types of condyloma-producing virus.
  - Quadrivalent vaccine, females and males (1) ages 9–26: Vaccine is administered IM; 3 doses to achieve optimal seroconversion.
  - Vaccination regimen: 0.5 mL IM injection first dose, and at months 2 and 6 after first dose to complete vaccination.
  - Observe recipients of vaccine for syncopal response.
- Bivalent HPV vaccine is available but does not cover the common viruses that cause condyloma lesions (Cervarix) (2).

ETIOLOGY

HPV is a circular double-stranded DNA molecule. There are >70 HPV subtypes. Types 6 and 11 cause common venereal warts. Cervical dysplasia and carcinoma in situ associates with types 16, 18, 31, 33, and 35.

COMMONLY ASSOCIATED CONDITIONS

- >90% of cervical cancer associated with HPV
- STIs (i.e., gonorrhea, syphilis, chlamydia); AIDS

DIAGNOSIS

HISTORY

Explore sexual history, contraception use, and other lifestyle issues.

- Pruritus
- Vaginal discharge
- Irritation (burning and redness)

PHYSICAL EXAM

- Multiple fingerlike projections; soft, sessile; smooth or rough
- Perianal condylomata acuminata usually rough and cauliflower-like
- Male sites include frenulum, corona, glans, prepuce, meatus, shaft, and scrotum.
  - Penile lesions often smooth and papular; occur in groups of 3 or 4
- Female sites include labia, clitoris, periurethral area, perineum, vagina, and cervix (flat lesions).
- Bleeding (result of trauma)
- Perianal area (both sexes)

DIAGNOSTIC TESTS & INTERPRETATION

Acetowhitening test: Subclinical lesions can be visualized by wrapping the penis with gauze soaked with 5% acetic acid for 5 minutes. Using a 10× hand lens or colposcope, warts appear as tiny white papules. A shiny white appearance of the skin represents foci of epithelial hyperplasia (subclinical infection); not highly specific, low positive predictive value.

Lab

- Serologic tests for syphilis negative
- Pap smear

Diagnostic Procedures/Surgery

Biopsy with highly specialized identification techniques rarely useful. HPV DNA detected through polymerase chain reaction

- Colposcopy
- Antroscopy, anoscopy, urethroscopy may be required

Pathological Findings

- Possible cervical dysplasia
- Sometimes difficult to differentiate from squamous cell carcinoma

DIFFERENTIAL DIAGNOSIS

- Condylomata lata (flat warts of syphilis)
- Lichen planus
- Normal sebaceous glands
- Seborrheic keratosis
- Molluscum contagiosum
- Keratomas, micropapillomatosis
- Scabies
- Crohn disease
- Skin tags
- Melanocytic nevi
- Vulvar intraepithelial neoplasia
- Buschke-Lowenstein tumor

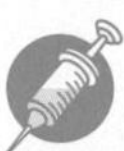

TREATMENT

MEDICATION

First Line

- Imiquimod (Aldara): self-treatment with a 5% cream applied overnight 3 times weekly until warts resolve for up to 16 weeks. The skin is then washed with soap and water 6 to 10 hours after application (3,4)
  - Precautions: Imiquimod has been noted to weaken condoms and diaphragms; therefore, patients should refrain from sexual contact while the cream is on the skin (3).
- Cryotherapy: Liquid nitrogen is applied to warts for 2 5- to 10-second bursts; usually requires 2–3 weekly sessions (3,5).
- Podophyllin in tincture of benzoin. Apply directly to warts. Leave on for 1–4 hours, then wash off. Repeat treatment every 7 days until gone (in-office procedure) *or* (3,6)
- Podofilox (Condylox): Apply to external warts (affected area) every 12 hours (allowing to dry) for 3 consecutive days. May repeat after 4 days (home application) (3,6).
- Trichloroacetic acid: 25–85%. Apply only to warts. Use powder/talc to remove unreacted acid. Repeat in office at weekly intervals.
- Trichloroacetic acid is ideal for isolated lesions in pregnant women.

Intralesion interferon has been shown to be effective in refractory cases and should be reserved for such cases (7,8).

Oral:
- Oral cimetidine: 30–40 mg/kg divided t.i.d. for 3 months in children with genital and perigenital condyloma. It is used as a primary and adjunctive therapy (9).

Contraindications:
- Podophyllin: Do not use in pregnant patients or on oral, cervical, urethral, or perianal warts. Can use on limited number of vaginal warts with careful drying after application. It is recommended that no more than 0.5 mL should be used.
- Cryotherapy: Cryoglobulinemia

Precautions:
- Podophyllin: To minimize local and systemic reactions, wash treated areas 1–4 hours after application and use ointments to protect surrounding skin from contact with podophyllin.
- Cryotherapy: None
- Electrocautery: Do not use in patients with pacemaker.

Second Line

External (penile and perianal):
- Podophyllin (3)
- Podofilox (Condylox) self-treatment (3)
- Intralesional interferon
- Small study of topical use of Calmette-Guérin bacillus for penile lesions (10)
- Cidovir 1% topical applied once daily for 5 contiguous days per week for 6 cycles (11)

Urethral meatus:
- Podophyllin (3)
- Cryrotherapy (3,5)
- Topical fluorouracil is no longer recommended due to severe side effects and teratogenicity. However, for refractory cases intralesional injection with fluorouracil/epinephrine/bovine collagen gel has been proven effective in phase clinical trials (12).

Anal:
- Trichloroacetic acid: Apply weekly (13).
- Topical fluorouracil is no longer recommended.

Uterine/cervix
- Trichloroacetic acid and Cryrotherapy are treatment options (3).
- Oral isotretinoins can be used for the treatment of recalcitrant condyloma acuminata of the cervix (note special prescription monitoring for this class of medications) (14).

ADDITIONAL TREATMENT

Pregnancy Considerations

- Podophyllin, podofilox, and fluorouracil should not be used in pregnancy due to the concern of possible teratogenicity (3).
- Surgical excision, trichloroacetic acid, Cryotherapy, and electrocautery are treatment options during pregnancy to minimize neonatal exposure to the virus (3).

General Measures

- May resolve spontaneously
- Change therapy if no improvement after 3 treatments, no complete clearance after 6 treatments, or therapy's duration or dosage exceeds manufacturer's recommendations.
- Appropriate screening/counseling of partners

SURGERY/OTHER PROCEDURES

- Larger warts require laser treatment or electrocoagulation including infrared therapy (15)
  - Precaution: Laser treatment may create smoke plumes that may contain HPV; therefore, it is recommended that physicians performing this procedure should wear appropriate masks.
- Surgical excision for large warts
- Intraurethral, external (penile and perianal), anal, and oral lesions can be treated with fulgurating CO_2 laser. Oral or external penile/perianal lesions can also be treated with electrocautery or surgery (3).

ONGOING CARE

FOLLOW-UP RECOMMENDATIONS

No restrictions, except for sexual contact

Patient Monitoring

- Patients seen every 2 weeks until lesions resolve and have annual Pap test
- Patients should also follow up 3 months after completion of treatment
- Persistent warts require biopsy.
- Sexual partners require monitoring.
- Treatment does not decrease transmissible infectivity.

PATIENT EDUCATION

- Provide pamphlets on HPV, STI prevention, and condom use.
- Emphasize the need for women to get regular Pap smears.

PROGNOSIS

- Warts will clear with treatment or resolve spontaneously, but recurrences are frequent and may necessitate repeated treatment.
- Some studies identified 3 independent risk factors for condylomatous relapse: Positive HIV status, male gender, and Langerhans cell level: Cell level per millimeter of anal tissue (15 vs. 30)
- Without treatment, may remain stable, worsen, or resolve completely
- Asymptomatic infection persists indefinitely.

COMPLICATIONS

- Cervical dysplasia
- Malignant change: Progression to cancer rarely, if ever, occurs.
- Male urethral obstruction
- The prevalence of high-grade dysplasia and cancer in anal canal is higher in HIV-positive than in HIV-negative patients, probably because of HPV activity.

REFERENCES

1. Centers for Disease Control and Prevention (CDC) et al. FDA licensure of quadrivalent human papillomavirus vaccine (HPV4, Gardasil) for use in males and guidance from the Advisory Committee on Immunization Practices (ACIP). *MMWR Morb Mortal Wkly Rep.* 2010;59:630–2.
2. Markowitz LE, Dunne EF, Saraiya M, et al. Quadrivalent human papillomavirus vaccine: Recommendations of the Advisory Committee on Immunization Practices (ACIP). *MMWR Recomm Rep.* 2007;56(RR-2):1–24.
3. Charles M, Kodner MD, Soraya Nasraty MD. University of Louisville School of Medicine, Louisville, Kentucky. *Am Fam Physician.* 2004; 70(12):2335–2342.
4. Edwards L. Imiquimod in clinical practice. *Aust J Dermatol.* 1998;39(Suppl 1):S14–S16.
5. Maw RD et al. Treatment of anogenital warts. *Dermatol Clin.* 1998;16:829–34, xv
6. Lacey CJ, et al. Randomised controlled trial and economic evaluation of podophyllotoxin solution, podophyllotoxin cream, and podophyllin in the treatment of genital warts. *Sex Transm Infect* 2003;79:270.
7. Welander CE, Homesley HD, Smiles KA, Peets EA et al. Intralesional interferon alfa-2b for the treatment of genital warts. *Am. J. Obstet. Gynecol.* 1990;162:348–54.
8. Klutke JJ, Bergman A. Interferon as an adjuvant treatment for genital condyloma acuminatum. *Int J Gynaecol Obstet.* 1995;49:171.
9. Franco I. Oral cimetidine for the management of genital and perigenital warts in children. *J Urol.* 2000;164:1074–5.
10. Böhle A, Büttner H, Jocham D. Primary treatment of condylomata acuminata with viable bacillus Calmette-Guerin. *J Urol.* 2001;165:834–6.
11. Snoeck R, Bossens M, Parent D, Delaere B, Degreef H, Van Ranst M, Noël JC, Wulfsohn MS, Rooney JF, Jaffe HS, De Clercq E et al. Phase II double-blind, placebo-controlled study of the safety and efficacy of cidofovir topical gel for the treatment of patients with human papillomavirus infection. *Clin Infect Dis.* 2001;33:597–602.
12. Swinehart JM, Sperling M, Phillips S, Kraus S, Gordon S, McCarty JM, Webster GF, Skinner R, Korey A, Orenberg EK. Intralesional fluorouracil/ epinephrine injectable gel for treatment of condylomata acuminata. A phase 3 clinical study. *Arch Dermatol.* 1997;133(1):67–73.
13. Sobhani I, Vuagnat A, Walker F, et al. Prevalence of high-grade dysplasia and cancer in the anal canal in human papillomavirus-infected individuals. *Gastroenterology.* 2001;120:857–66.
14. Georgala S, Katoulis AC, Georgala C, Bozi E, Mortakis A et al. Oral isotretinoin in the treatment of recalcitrant condylomata acuminata of the cervix: a randomised placebo controlled trial. *Sex Transm Infect.* 2004;80:216–8.
15. Bekassy Z, Weström L et al. Infrared coagulation in the treatment of condyloma acuminata in the female genital tract. *Sex Transm Dis.* 1987;14: 209–12.

ADDITIONAL READING

- Beutner KR, Spruance SL, Hougham AJ, et al. Treatment of genital warts. *J Am Acad Dermatol* 1998;38:230.
- Workowski KA, Berman SM. Sexually transmitted diseases treatment guidelines, 2006. *MMWR Recomm Rep.* 2006;55:1–94.

CODES

ICD9

078.11 Condyloma acuminatum

CONGESTIVE HEART FAILURE

Jeremy Golding, MD

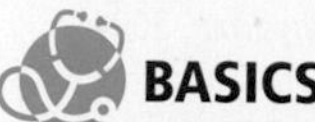

BASICS

DESCRIPTION

Congestive heart failure (CHF) (better term: heart failure [HF], because not all heart failure is *congestive*) affects both the cardiovascular and pulmonary systems. It is the principal complication of heart disease. The heart is unable to fill and/or pump blood sufficiently to meet tissue metabolic needs. Heart failure may involve the left heart, the right heart, or be biventricular. New York Heart Association (NYHA) Classification is a fundamental descriptive system used for classifying patients with HF: NYHA I—Asymptomatic; NYHA II—Symptomatic with moderate exertion; NYHA III—Symptomatic with mild exertion and may limit activities of daily living; NYHA IV—Symptomatic at rest.

EPIDEMIOLOGY

Medicare spends more to diagnose and treat heart failure than any other medical condition.

Incidence

- 500,000 new cases annually
- In 2002, the direct cost exceeded $15 billion.

Prevalence

- About 5 million people in the US have heart failure.
- <1% in those <50, increasing to 10% of those older than age 80
- Primarily a disease of the elderly; 75% of hospital admissions for HF are in persons >65.

RISK FACTORS

- For development of heart failure: Coronary artery disease (CAD) and myocardial infarction (MI), hypertension (HTN) (80% of cases of HF in the US caused by either CAD or HTN), valvular heart disease, diabetes mellitus, cardiotoxic medications
- For heart failure exacerbation: Sodium intake and/or fluid excess, nonadherence to medication regimen, arrhythmia (e.g., atrial fibrillation), ischemic ventricular dysfunction, negative inotropic drugs (e.g., calcium blocker, introduction of beta-blocker), excessive physical, emotional, or environmental stress, thyrotoxicosis, pregnancy, or increased metabolic demand

Genetics

Familial cardiomyopathy predisposes to development of heart failure (rare).

GENERAL PREVENTION

Control blood pressure (BP) and other risk factors. Thiazide diuretics and angiotensin-converting enzyme (ACE) inhibitors are superior to other agents in preventing development of heart failure.

PATHOPHYSIOLOGY

2 physiologic components explain most of the clinical findings of congestive heart failure:

- Systolic dysfunction: An *inotropic* abnormality, often due to MI or dilated or ischemic cardiomyopathy, resulting in diminished systolic emptying (ejection fraction <45%)
- Diastolic dysfunction: A *compliance* abnormality, often due to hypertensive cardiomyopathy, in which the ventricular relaxation is impaired (ejection fraction >45%)
- Patients with systolic dysfunction may also have diastolic dysfunction.

ETIOLOGY

- Coronary artery disease and ischemia, myocardial infarction
- Myocarditis and cardiomyopathy: Alcoholic, viral, longstanding HTN, drugs (e.g., chemotherapeutic agents), muscular dystrophy, amyloidosis (infiltrative), sarcoidosis (infiltrative), postpartum state, infectious (e.g., Chagas disease), HIV
- Valvular and vascular abnormalities: Aortic stenosis or regurgitation, rheumatic heart disease (mitral and aortic valvular disease). Renal artery stenosis, usually bilateral, may cause recurrent "flash" pulmonary edema, especially in setting of severe chronic hypertension.
- Chronic lung disease and pulmonary hypertension (right heart failure)
- Volume overload (requires extreme overload in patients with normal hearts and kidneys)
- Arrhythmias (atrial fibrillation and other tachyarrhythmias, high-grade heart block)
- Misc: High-output states: Hyperthyroidism, anemia, cardiac depressants (beta blocker overdose)

COMMONLY ASSOCIATED CONDITIONS

Dysrhythmia, followed by pump failure, are the leading causes of death in this condition.

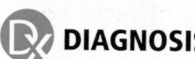

DIAGNOSIS

HISTORY

- Dyspnea on exertion: Cardinal sign of left heart failure. Deteriorating exercise capacity: Easy fatigue, generalized weakness.
- Nocturnal nonproductive cough, orthopnea, and paroxysmal nocturnal dyspnea; sometimes frothy or pink sputum
- Wheezing, especially nocturnal in absence of history of asthma or infection (cardiac asthma). Cheyne-Stokes breathing
- Anorexia/cachexia and/or fullness or dull pain in right upper quadrant (hepatic distension in right heart failure)
- Edema often with cool extremities due to peripheral vasoconstriction. Abdominal bloating (ascites) or anasarca. Cyanosis.

PHYSICAL EXAM

Rales (crackles) and sometimes wheezing, peripheral edema, S3 gallop, hepatomegaly, hepatojugular reflux, ascites, hypotension

DIAGNOSTIC TESTS & INTERPRETATION

Diagnosis of heart failure in patients with known heart failure and heart failure exacerbation should be primarily clinical, with laboratory data as adjunctive and indicative of complications.

Lab

Initial lab tests

- β-type natriuretic peptide (BNP) and N-type pro-BNP may be helpful in:
  - Emergency department (ED) setting to help differentiate the cause of dyspnea (BNP <100 essentially rules out HF as cause of dyspnea with NPV of ~99%. Most dyspneic patients with HF have BNP>400.)
  - Titrating treatment, because its value changes rapidly with LV functional status (unclear, however, that BNP-guided therapy improves outcomes) (1)
  - BNP values of 100–400 are most problematic, as they may indicate heart failure or may be due to conditions like pulmonary embolism, renal failure, acute coronary syndromes, and pulmonary hypertension.
  - Patients may have BNP elevation due to heart failure, but acute dyspnea may be from another cause (like pneumonia or pulmonary embolism).
- Lab findings in early and mild-to-moderately severe CHF include respiratory alkalosis, mild azotemia, decreased erythrocyte sedimentation rate (ESR), proteinuria (usually <1 g/24 h), elevated creatinine, dilutional hyponatremia (poor prognosis), and rarely hyperbilirubinemia.

Imaging

Initial approach

Chest x-ray (CXR) (changes lag clinical symptoms by up to 6 hours): Increased heart size, vascular redistribution/cephalization with "butterfly" pattern of pulmonary edema, interstitial and alveolar edema, Kerley B lines, pleural effusions

Diagnostic Procedures/Surgery

Determination of ejection fraction is critical to proper diagnosis and management of heart failure:

- Echocardiographic study is most useful single test to determine ejection fraction and valvular abnormalities. May be repeated if change suspected in underlying cardiac status.
- Nuclear imaging to estimate left and right ventricular size, perfusion and systolic function.

Pathological Findings

- Cardiac pathology depends upon underlying process (etiology) of heart failure.
- Noncardiac findings: Liver is engorged, firm, and fluid-filled. Microscopic analysis reveals dilated central hepatic veins and sinusoids. Late/chronic findings include hemosiderin deposits in lungs and "nutmeg" liver with centrilobular necrosis.

DIFFERENTIAL DIAGNOSIS

Simple dependent edema, pulmonary embolism, exertional asthma, cardiac ischemia with angina, chronic obstructive pulmonary disease (COPD), constrictive pericarditis, nephrotic syndrome, cirrhosis, venous occlusive disease with subsequent peripheral edema, High-output states: Anemia, sepsis, hyperthyroidism

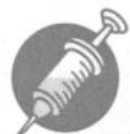

TREATMENT

MEDICATION

Diuretics are used initially in fluid-overload acute heart failure, with nitrates added if needed. Nitrates are primary therapy in ischemic acute heart failure (flash pulmonary edema), with diuretics secondary. Once acute HF is stabilized, an ACE inhibitor or beta-blocker should be started. Instruct patients not to use nonsteroidal anti-inflammatory drugs (NSAIDs), which markedly worsen HF. Avoid use of diltiazem and verapamil in patients with systolic dysfunction.

First Line

- ACE inhibitors:
  - Used to decrease afterload: Shown to increase survival, improve general symptomatology and overall exercise capacity in patients in all NYHA classifications; benefit greatest for patients with systolic dysfunction and post-MI. NNT approx 25/year for mortality (2).

- Angiotensin receptor blockers (ARBs) have fewer side effects than ACE inhibitors, but are less effective than ACE inhibitors and are therefore not 1st-line treatment.
- β-blockers used in systolic or diastolic HF (Note: Initiate in hospital or outpatient setting in hemodynamically stable patients at low dose and titrate upward slowly); NNT = 25 for mortality. Evidence mounting for titration to heart rate rather than specific dose:
  - Carvedilol: 3.125 mg b.i.d. to a maintenance of 25 mg b.i.d.; Metoprolol succinate extended release: 12.5 mg/d to a maximum of 200 mg/d (Note: Metoprolol tartrate may be equivalent but is taken b.i.d.) or bisoprolol 1.25–10 mg once daily
- Digoxin reduces symptoms, but has not shown any effect on mortality (2):
  - In patients with preserved renal function (creatinine clearance >50 mL/min), the recommended dose is 0.125 mg/d.
  - Levels lower than used for atrial fibrillation are effective and safer
- Diuretics helpful to manage volume overload:
  - Furosemide (Lasix): 20–320 mg IV/IM/p.o.
  - Metolazone (Zaroxolyn): 2.5–20 mg/d p.o.
  - Spironolactone (only diuretic to reduce mortality when added to standard therapy in NYHA Class III and IV, and probably Class II): 12.5–25 mg/d p.o.; maximum 50 mg/d p.o. Caution regarding hyperkalemia (2).
- Vasodilators:
  - IV nitroglycerin may be of short-term benefit to decrease preload, afterload, and systemic resistance, especially in acute heart failure.
  - The combination of hydralazine (75 mg/d divided b.i.d. or t.i.d.) and isosorbide dinitrate (40 mg q.i.d.) is effective for African Americans (2) or if unable to take ACE inhibitors or an ARB.
- Fish oil/omega-3 fatty acids: 1 gm daily of n-3 PUFA reduced mortality and time to hospitalization (NNT approx 170/year) (3)

Second Line

- Dobutamine in outpatient basis with intermittent infusions. Despite improving quality of life, it reduces short term survival.
- Nesiritide is approved for short-term use in decompensated heart failure. It is a recombinant form of human brain-type natriuretic peptide. Should not be used in ED. No better than nitroglycerine for most, and may increase mortality.

ADDITIONAL TREATMENT

Device therapy for heart failure increasingly successful, especially biventricular pacing for ventricular dyssynchrony and implantable cardiac defibrillators (AICDs):

- Biventricular pacing indicated for NYHA II, III (especially) or IV with low EF who are on optimal management for at least 6 months (2), with QRS >0.120 msec and who remain significantly symptomatic. Improves symptoms and may improve survival.
- AICD: Improve survival in dilated cardiomyopathy (4) and are recommended for: Primary prevention in patients with ischemic heart disease (HD) who are post-MI, LVEF<30%, Class 2 or 3 HF on optimal medical therapy, and >1 year estimated survival (2)[A], as well as for nonischemic HF EF<30%. Not indicated in Stage D (end-stage) HF.
- Treat anemia. Target minimum Hct at least 30 and possibly somewhat higher. Improves quality of life and may reduce mortality (5).

Additional Therapies

Home oxygen for pulse oximetry <89% (resting or with activity)

SURGERY/OTHER PROCEDURES

- Heart valve surgery if defective heart valve is responsible; mitral valve repair especially helpful if mitral regurgitation is aggravating condition.
- Cardiac transplantation to be considered in patients <55 and without other disqualifying medical problems who are developing CHF unresponsive to other therapeutic maneuvers, and who are considered to have a life expectancy of >1 year.

IN-PATIENT CONSIDERATIONS

Initial Stabilization

Sublingual nitroglycerin is rapid-onset and reduces both pre- and afterload. Bilevel positive airway pressure (BiPap) may help delay or avoid intubation, and often gives rapid symptomatic relief. Morphine titrated to reduce anxiety/air hunger.

Admission Criteria

Acute change in heart failure, with pulmonary edema accompanied by decreased oxygenation, change in mental status, with acute renal insufficiency, or significant hyponatremia

IV Fluids

Limit. Avoid sodium-containing fluids unless necessary to urgently correct hyponatremia. Fluid restriction is best for nonurgent correction of hyponatremia.

Discharge Criteria

Subjective improvement, resting heart rate (HR) <100, systolic BP >80 mm Hg, heart failure outpatient education performed

ONGOING CARE

FOLLOW-UP RECOMMENDATIONS

Critical patient education performed at all outpatient and inpatient physician visits "MAWDS":

- Medications: Take every day; don't skip.
- Activity: A little every day, don't overdo
- Weight: Daily. If gain >2 lb in a day or 5 lb above ideal, CALL!
- Diet: Eat less than 2,000 mg Na+ daily.
- Symptoms: Know the signs of worsening HF (cough, weight gain, worsening or rest dyspnea, swelling) and call the doctor early! Quit smoking, if a smoker!

Patient Monitoring

Rapid office follow-up after hospitalization and home health monitoring by specially trained nurses have both been shown to decrease frequency of hospitalizations.

DIET

Reduce sodium load (2 g).

PATIENT EDUCATION

- American Heart Association, 7320 Greenville Avenue, Dallas, TX 75231, (214) 373-6300
- American College of Cardiology, 911 Old Georgetown Road, Bethesda, MD 20814, (301) 897-5400

PROGNOSIS

After symptoms develop, 1-year mortality approximately 25% and 5-year mortality ~50%

COMPLICATIONS

- Sudden death (arrhythmic)
- Acute pulmonary edema and death

REFERENCES

1. Porapakkham P, Porapakkham P, Zimmet H, Billah B, Krum H et al. B-type natriuretic peptide-guided heart failure therapy: A meta-analysis. *Arch Intern Med*. 2010;170:507–14.
2. Hunt SA, Abraham WT, Chin MH, et al. 2009 Focused update incorporated into the ACC/AHA 2005 Guidelines for the Diagnosis and Management of Heart Failure in Adults A Report of the American College of Cardiology Foundation/American Heart Association Task Force on Practice Guidelines. *J Am Coll Cardiol*. 2009; 53:e1–e90.
3. Gissi-Hf Investigators. Effect of n-3 polyunsaturated fatty acids in patients with chronic heart failure (the GISSI-HF trial): a randomised, double-blind, placebo-controlled trial. *Lancet*. 2008.
4. Moss AJ, Hall WJ, Cannom DS, et al. Cardiac-Resynchronization Therapy for the Prevention of Heart-Failure Events. *N Engl J Med*. 2009.
5. Ngo K, Kotecha D, Walters JAE, Manzano L, Palazzuoli A, van Veldhuisen DJ, Flather M. Erythropoiesis-stimulating agents for anaemia in chronic heart failure patients. *Cochrane Database of Systematic Reviews* 2010, Issue 1. Art. No.: CD007613. DOI:10.1002/14651858. CD007613.pub2

ADDITIONAL READING

Hernandez AF, et al. Relationship between early physician follow-up and 30-day readmission among Medicare beneficiaries hospitalized for heart failure. *JAMA*. 2010;303:1716.

See Also (Topic, Algorithm, Electronic Media Element)

Algorithms: Congestive Heart Failure; Congestive Heart Failure, Treatment

CODES

ICD9

428.0 Congestive heart failure, unspecified

CLINICAL PEARLS

- Have patients weigh themselves daily and report weight gains of greater than 2 pounds in a day or 5 pounds above dry weight.
- An echocardiogram is the key test in initial workup of heart failure.
- Beta-blockers and ACE inhibitors are the core medications for management of this condition.
- Consider referral for biventricular pacing in patients with bundle branch block, and AICD in those with low EF.

CONJUNCTIVITIS, ACUTE

Frances Y. Wu, MD

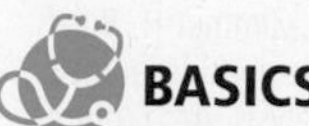

BASICS

DESCRIPTION

- Inflammation of the bulbar and/or palpebral conjunctiva <4 weeks duration
- System(s) affected: Nervous; Skin/Exocrine
- Synonym(s): Pink eye

Geriatric Considerations

Suspect autoimmune, systemic, or irritative conditions

Pediatric Considerations

- Neonatal conjunctivitis may be gonococcal, chlamydial, irritative, or related to dacryocystitis.
- Pediatric emergency room study; 78% positive bacterial cult, mostly *H. influenzae*; 13% no growth; other studies showed greater than 50% adenovirus
- Daycare regulations sometimes require any child with presumed conjunctivitis to be treated with a topical antibiotic despite the lack of evidence.

EPIDEMIOLOGY

- Predominant age:
  - Pediatric: Viral, bacterial
  - Adult: Viral, bacterial, allergic
- Predominant sex: Male = Female

Incidence

In the US: Variable, but accounts for 1–2% of all ambulatory office visits

RISK FACTORS

- History of contact with infected persons
- Sexually transmitted disease (STD) contact: Gonococcal, chlamydial, syphilis, or herpes
- Contact lenses: Pseudomonal or acanthamoeba keratitis
- Epidemic bacterial (streptococcal) conjunctivitis reported in school settings

GENERAL PREVENTION

- Wash hands frequently.
- Demonstrate eye dropper technique: Eye is closed and head back, several drops at nasal margin; open eyes to allow liquid to enter. Never touch tip of dropper to skin or eye.

ETIOLOGY

- Viral:
  - Adenovirus (common cold) or Coxsackie
  - Enterovirus (acute hemorrhagic conjunctivitis)
  - Herpes simplex
  - Herpes zoster or varicella
  - Measles, mumps, or influenza
- Bacterial:
  - *Staphylococcus aureus* or *epidermidis*
  - *Streptococcus pneumoniae*
  - *Haemophilus influenzae* (children)
  - Pseudomonas species or anaerobes (in contact lens users)
  - Acanthamoeba from contaminated contact lens solution may cause keratitis.
  - *Neisseria gonorrhoeae* and *meningitidis*
  - *Chlamydia trachomatis*: Gradual onset >4 weeks
- Allergic:
  - Hay fever, seasonal allergies, atopy
- Nonspecific:
  - Irritative: Topical medications, wind, dry eye, ultraviolet light exposure, smoke
  - Autoimmune: Sjögren, pemphigoid, Wegener granulomatosis
  - Rare: Rickettsial, fungal, parasitic, tuberculosis, syphilis, Kawasaki, chikungunya, Graves, gout, carcinoid, sarcoid, psoriasis, Stevens-Johnson, Reiter syndrome

COMMONLY ASSOCIATED CONDITIONS

- Viral infection (e.g., common cold)
- STD

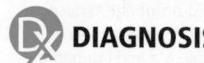

DIAGNOSIS

HISTORY

- RED FLAG: Any decrease in visual acuity is not consistent with conjunctivitis alone; must document normal vision for diagnosis of isolated conjunctivitis.
- Viral: Contact or travel:
  - May start with 1 eye, then both
  - If herpetic, recurrences or vesicles on skin
- Bacterial: Difficult to distinguish from viral, unless contact lens user. Assume bacterial in contact lens wearer unless cultures negative. If recent STD, suspect chlamydia or GC
- Allergic: Itching, atopy, seasonal, dander
- Irritative: Feels dry, exposure to wind, tear film deficit may persist 30 days after acute conjunctivitis, chemicals, or drug: Atropine, aminoglycosides, iodide, phenylephrine, antivirals, bisphosphonates, retinoids, topiramate, chamomile, COX-2 inhibitors
- Foreign body: Redness may persist 24 hours after removal.

PHYSICAL EXAM

- General: Common to all types of conjunctivitis:
  - Red eye, conjunctival injection
  - Foreign body sensation
  - Eyelid sticking or crusting, discharge
  - Normal visual acuity and pupillary reactivity
- Viral:
  - Palpable preauricular lymphadenopathy may be present.
  - Severe viral: Herpes simplex or zoster:
    - Burning sensation, rarely itching
    - Unilateral, herpetic skin vesicles in herpes zoster
    - Palpable preauricular node
- Bacterial (non-STD): May be epidemic:
  - Mild pruritus, discharge mild to heavy
  - Conjunctival chemosis/edema
  - If contact lens user, must rule out pseudomonal (or other bacterial) keratitis
- Bacterial: Gonococcal (or meningococcal) hyperacute infection:
  - Rapid onset 12–24 hours
  - Severe purulent discharge
  - Chemosis/conjunctival/lid edema
  - Rapid growth of superior corneal ulceration
  - Preauricular adenopathy
  - Signs of STDs (chlamydia, GC, HIV, etc.)
- Allergic:
  - Itching predominant
  - Seasonal or dander allergies
  - Chemosis/conjunctival/eyelid edema
- Nonspecific irritative:
  - Dry eyes, intermittent redness, chemical/drug exposure
  - Foreign body: May have redness and discharge 24 hours after removal
- Must document normal visual acuity
- Cornea should be clear and without fluorescein uptake. If cloudy or signs of keratitis, consult ophthalmologist.
- Recommend fluorescein exam:
  - Evert lid to inspect for foreign bodies.
- Skin: Look for herpetic vesicles, nits on lashes (lice), scaliness (seborrhea), or styes
- Limbal flush at corneal margin if uveitis
- If pupil is irregular (i.e., penetrating foreign body), emergent referral
- Discharge but no conjunctival injection: Blepharitis

DIAGNOSTIC TESTS & INTERPRETATION

Lab

- Usually not needed initially for the most common causes
- Culture swab if STD suspected, very severe symptoms, or patient is a contact lens user

Diagnostic Procedures/Surgery

- Fluorescein exam for ulcer or abrasion on cornea
- Small superficial foreign bodies may be removed with irrigation or moistened swab.

DIFFERENTIAL DIAGNOSIS

- Uveitis (iritis, iridocyclitis, choroiditis): Limbal flush (red band at corneal margin), hazy anterior chamber and decreased visual acuity
- Penetrating ocular trauma: Emergently hospitalize
- Acute glaucoma (emergency): Headache, corneal clouding, poor visual acuity
- Corneal ulcer(s) or foreign body: Lesions on fluorescein exam
- Dacryocystitis: Tenderness and swelling over tear sac (below medial canthus)
- Scleritis and episcleritis: Red injected vessels radially oriented, sectoral (pie wedge), nodularity of sclera
- Ophthalmia neonatorum: Neonates in 1st 2 days of life (gonococcal; 5–12 days of life): Chlamydial, HSV, very rare Neisseria meningitidis. Consider specialty consultation for required systemic therapy.
- Blepharitis: Lid margins inflamed and producing itching, scale, or discharge, but no conjunctival injection.

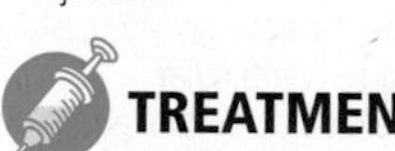

TREATMENT

MEDICATION

First Line

- Viral (nonherpetic):
  - Artificial tears for symptomatic relief
  - Vasoconstrictor/antihistamine (e.g., naphazoline/pheniramine) q.i.d. for severe itching
  - May consider topical antibiotic (see bacterial below) if return to daycare requires treatment (1)[C]
- Viral (herpetic) (by ophthalmologist):
  - Trifluridine: 1% drops 1 q2h (2)[C]
  - Acyclovir oral: 400 mg 5 × day for herpes simplex virus (HSV) (use 800 mg for zoster) × 7 days

Bacterial (non-STD) self-limited 5–7 days, so treatment is optional (and should take cost and bacterial resistance-production factors into consideration), although it may shorten the symptoms by half a day (3)[A]. Alternative strategy: Delay treatment until 3rd day (using simple warm moist towel cleansing of closed eye), same duration of symptoms (4)[B]. Contact lens wearers should be referred for evaluation of possible keratitis:

- Trimethoprim/polymyxin ophthalmic: 1 drop q4h (while awake) for 5 days *or*
- Erythromycin ophthalmic ointment: 1/2 inch b.i.d.–q.i.d. for 5 days *or*
- Sodium sulfacetamide (10% solution:) 2 drops q4h (while awake) for 5 days or
- Tobramycin 0.3% ophthalmic drops/ointment q4h (drops) to q8h (ointment)

Bacterial (gonococcal) hospitalize for IV ceftriaxone:

- If no corneal lesions, ceftriaxone 1 g IM as single dose and topical bacitracin ophthalmic ointment 1/2 inch q.i.d. Chlamydial in neonates requires oral erythromycin ethylsuccinate 30 mg/kg daily q6h p.o. × 14 d, max 3 g/d.

Allergic and atopic (by increasing approximate cost: All are efficacious, but evidence favoring one over another is inconclusive):

- Ketotifen 0.25% 1 drop b.i.d. (5)[A]
- Cromolyn (Opticrom) 4%, q.i.d. (4)[A]
- Epinastine (Elestat) 0.05% b.i.d. (5)[A]
- Ketorolac 0.1% 1 drop q.i.d. (5)[A]
- Emedastine 0.05% 1 drop q.i.d. (5)[A]
- Azelastine 0.05% 1 drop b.i.d. (4)[A]
- Olopatadine 0.1% 1 drop b.i.d. or 0.2% 1 drop daily (5)[A]
- Oral nonsedating antihistamines (Zyrtec [cetirizine] 10 mg/d, Allegra [fexofenadine] 60 mg b.i.d.), etc., to treat nasal and urticarial symptoms
- Oral antihistamine (e.g., diphenhydramine 25 mg t.i.d.) in severe cases

Contraindications: Avoid topical steroids unless able to monitor intraocular pressure. Also case report of HSV keratitis presenting without distinguishing findings from viral conjunctivitis would discourage initial use of steroids.

Precautions:

- Do not allow dropper to touch eye
- Vasoconstrictor/antihistamine: Rebound vasodilation after prolonged use

Second Line

Viral and allergic: Numerous over-the-counter products

Bacterial: Polymyxin-gramicidin, ciprofloxacin

ADDITIONAL TREATMENT

General Measures

Appropriate health care: Outpatient

Eyelid cleansing with wet cloth up to q.i.d.

Stop use of contact lenses while red

Patching of eye not beneficial

Avoid irritants such as smoke, wind, and sun

Issues for Referral

Any significantly decreased visual acuity, herpetic keratitis, or contact lens-related bacterial conjunctivitis: Ophthalmologic consultation

COMPLEMENTARY AND ALTERNATIVE MEDICINE

As it is usually benign and self-limited, saline flushes and other placebos would be expected to work.

SURGERY/OTHER PROCEDURES

No surgery for this condition. Other eye surgeries may be delayed until resolution of this condition.

IN-PATIENT CONSIDERATIONS

Acute gonococcal conjunctivitis (or very rare case of meningococcal conjunctivitis) would require inpatient treatment with ceftriaxone 50 mg/kg IV every day (pediatric), 1 gm IM x 1 (adult) along with ophthalmologic consultation.

Admission Criteria

Penetrating ocular trauma, GC

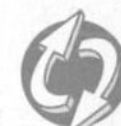

ONGOING CARE

FOLLOW-UP RECOMMENDATIONS

- If not resolved within 5–7 days, alternate diagnoses should be considered or consultation obtained.
- Children may be excluded from school until eye is no longer red if viral or bacterial, depending on school policy. Allergic conjunctivitis should be able to return to school with doctor's note.

Patient Monitoring

Referral if worse in 24 hours

PATIENT EDUCATION

- Patients should not wear contacts until their eyes are fully healed (typically 1 week).
- Patients should throw away current pair of contacts.
- Patients should throw away any eye makeup that they have been using, especially mascara.
- Cool, moist compresses can ease irritation and itch.

PROGNOSIS

- Viral: 5–10 days for pharyngitis with conjunctivitis, 2 weeks with adenovirus
- Herpes simplex: 2–3 weeks
- Bacterial: Self-limited, treated, 2–5 days; untreated, 5–7 days

COMPLICATIONS

- Corneal scars with herpes simplex
- Lid scars or entropion with varicella zoster
- Corneal ulcers or perforation, very rapid with gonococcal
- Hypopyon: Pus in anterior chamber
- Chlamydial neonatal ophthalmia: Could have concomitant pneumonia
- Otitis media may follow *H. influenzae* conjunctivitis.
- The very rare Neisseria meningitidis conjunctivitis may be followed by meningitis.

REFERENCES

1. David SP. Should we prescribe antibiotics for acute conjunctivitis? *Am Fam Physician*. 2002;66: 1649–50.
2. Greenberg MF, Pollard ZF. The red eye in childhood. *Pediatr Clin North Am*. 2003;50:105–24.
3. Sheikh A, Hurwitz B. Antibiotics vs. placebo for acute bacterial conjunctivitis. *Cochrane database of Systematic Reviews*. 2006, Issue 2. Art.No. CD001211.
4. Bielory L, Lien KW, Bigelsen S. Efficacy and tolerability of newer antihistamines in the treatment of allergic conjunctivitis. *Drugs*. 2005;65:215–28.
5. Chigbu DI et al. The management of allergic eye diseases in primary eye care. *Cont Lens Anterior Eye*. 2009;32:260–72.

ADDITIONAL READING

- Everitt HA, Little PS, Smith PW. A randomised controlled trial of management strategies for acute infective conjunctivitis in general practice. *BMJ*. 2006;333:321.
- Gupta R, Levent F, Healy CM, et al. Unusual soft tissue manifestations of Neisseria meningitidis infections. *Clin Pediatr (Phila)*. 2008;47:400–3.
- Hamerlynck JV, Rietveld RP, Hooft L. [From the Cochrane Library: Marginally higher chance of cure by antibiotic treatment in acute bacterial conjunctivitis] *Ned Tijdschr Geneeskd*. 2007;151: 594–6.
- Huang T, Wang Y, Liu Z, et al. Investigation of tear film change after recovery from acute conjunctivitis. *Cornea*. 2007;26:778–81.
- Rose PW, Harnden A, Brueggemann AB, et al. Chloramphenicol treatment for acute infective conjunctivitis in children in primary care: a randomised double-blind placebo-controlled trial. *Lancet*. 2005;366:37–43.

See Also (Topic, Algorithm, Electronic Media Element)

Rhinitis, Allergic

Algorithm: Eye Pain

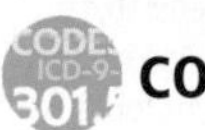

CODES

ICD9

- 077.99 Unspecified diseases of conjunctiva due to viruses
- 372.00 Acute conjunctivitis, unspecified
- 771.6 Neonatal conjunctivitis and dacryocystitis

CLINICAL PEARLS

- Conjunctivitis does not alter visual acuity; decreased acuity or photophobia should prompt consideration of more serious ophthalmic disorders.
- Culture discharge in all contact lens wearers, consider referral and remind patient to throw away current contacts and avoid contacts until eyes fully healed.
- Antibiotic therapy is of no value in viral conjunctivitis (most cases of infectious conjunctivitis), and does not significantly alter the course of most types of bacterial conjunctivitis (so is optional in these cases).

CONSTIPATION

Robert A. Baldor, MD
Abdulrazak Abyad, MD, PhD, MBA, MPH, AGSF, AFCHSE

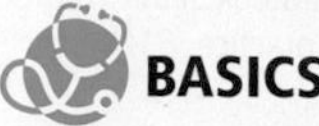

BASICS

A group of syndromes with similar findings that include unsatisfactory defecation characterized by infrequent stools, difficult stool passage, or both. Characteristics include fewer than 3 bowel movements a week, hard stools, excessive straining, prolonged time spent on the toilet, a sense of incomplete evacuation, and abdominal discomfort/bloating.

DESCRIPTION

- System(s) affected: Gastrointestinal (GI)
- Synonym(s): Obstipation

Geriatric Considerations

Increased incidence of colorectal neoplasms with age may be associated with constipation; thus, new onset of constipation after 50 years of age is considered a "red flag."

Pediatric Considerations

Consider Hirschsprung disease (absence of colonic ganglion cells): 25% of all newborn intestinal obstructions, milder cases diagnosed in older children with chronic constipation, abdominal distension, decreased growth. 5:1 male:female ratio. Associated with inherited conditions such as Down syndrome.

EPIDEMIOLOGY

- Predominant age: May affect all ages, but more pronounced in children and elderly
- Predominant sex: Female > Male (2:1)
- Non-whites > whites

Incidence

- 5 million office visits annually
- 100,000 hospitalizations

Prevalence

~15% of population effected

RISK FACTORS

- Extremes of life (very young and very old)
- Polypharmacy
- Sedentary lifestyle or condition
- Improper diet and inadequate fluid intake

Genetics

Unknown, but condition may be familial

GENERAL PREVENTION

High-fiber diet, adequate fluids, exercise, and bowel training to "obey the urge" to defecate are useful preventive strategies.

PATHOPHYSIOLOGY

- As food leaves the stomach, the ileocecal valve relaxes (gastroileal reflex) and chyme enters the colon (1–2 L/day). Peristaltic contractions move the chyme through the colon into the rectum. In the colon, sodium is actively absorbed in exchange for potassium and bicarb—water follows because of the generated osmotic gradient. The chyme is converted into feces (200–250 mL).
- Normal transit time for a meal to reach the cecum is 4 hours, and to the pelvic colon 8 hours later. Transit then slows to the anus. Rectal distention initiates the defecation reflex.
- Defecation follows as a reflex that can be inhibited by voluntarily contracting the external sphincter or facilitated by straining to contract the abdominal muscles while voluntarily relaxing the anal sphincter. The *urge to defecate* occurs as rectal pressures increase. Distention of the stomach by food also initiates rectal contractions and a desire to defecate.

ETIOLOGY

- Primary constipation:
  - Slow colonic transit time (13%)
  - Pelvic floor/anal sphincter dysfunction (25%)
  - Functional—normal transit time and sphincter function, yet problems (bloating, abdominal discomfort, perceived difficulty going, presence of hard stools) (69%)
- Secondary constipation:
  - Irritable bowel syndrome (IBS)
  - Endocrine dysfunction (diabetes mellitus, hypothyroid)
  - Metabolic disorder (increased calcium, decreased potassium)
  - Mechanical (obstruction, rectocele)
  - Pregnancy
  - Neurologic disorders (Hirschsprung, multiple sclerosis, spinal cord injuries)
- Medication effect:
  - Anticholinergic effects (antidepressants, narcotics, antipsychotics)
  - Antacids (calcium, aluminum)
  - Calcium channel blockers

COMMONLY ASSOCIATED CONDITIONS

- Debility, either general as in the aged or that imposed by specific underlying illness
- Dehydration
- Hypothyroidism
- Hypokalemia
- Hypercalcemia

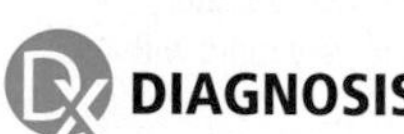

DIAGNOSIS

A group of syndromes with similar findings that include unsatisfactory defecation characterized by infrequent stools, difficult stool passage, or both.

ALERT

Red flags:
- New onset after age of 50
- Hematochezia/melena
- Unintentional weight loss
- Anemia
- Neurological defects

HISTORY

Ask about the Rome III criteria (1):
- At least 2 of the following, for 12 weeks, in the previous 6 months:
  - Fewer than 3 stools/week
  - Straining at least 1/4 of the time
  - Hard stools at least 1/4 of the time
  - Need for manual assist at least 1/4 of the time
  - Sense of incomplete evacuation at least 1/4 of the time
  - Sense of anorectal blockade at least 1/4 of the time
- Loose stools rarely seen without use of laxatives

PHYSICAL EXAM

- Digital rectal exam (masses, pain, stool, fissures, hemorrhoids, anal tone)
- Abdominal/gynecological exam (masses, pain)
- Neurological exam

DIAGNOSTIC TESTS & INTERPRETATION

For the most part, this is a clinical diagnosis, as evidence to support the use of routine labs/x-rays/scoping is lacking in the workup of constipation (2).

Lab

Initial lab tests

However, the American Gastroenterological Association guidelines suggest complete blood count BS, TSH, calcium, and creatinine routinely and sigmoid/colonoscopy if red flags are present (3).

Imaging

Initial approach

If condition is refractory to empiric approach, pursue further testing:
- Colonoscopy
- Barium enema to look for obstruction and/or megarectum, megacolon, or Hirschsprung disease

Follow-Up & Special Considerations

Measure colonic transit time by ingesting radiopaque (Sitz-Mark) markers:
- Plain abdominal film obtained 5 days later (120 hours): Retention >20% markers indicates slow transit
- Markers seen exclusively in distal colon/rectum suggests defecatory disorder.

Diagnostic Procedures/Surgery

Consider referral to evaluate defecation:
- Balloon expulsion
- Defecography using a barium paste
- Anorectal manometry with a rectal catheter

Pathological Findings

- None in common, functional constipation
- Paucity or absence of intramural enteric ganglia in certain cases of congenital or acquired megacolon
- Neuromuscular abnormalities in certain cases of pseudo-obstruction

DIFFERENTIAL DIAGNOSIS

- Congenital:
  - Hirschsprung disease/syndrome
  - Hypoganglionosis
  - Congenital dilation of the colon
  - Small left colon syndrome
- Meconium ileus
- Other causes of abdominal pain

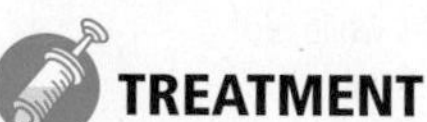

TREATMENT

Address immediate concerns:
- Bloating/discomfort/straining: Osmotic agents
- Post-op, childbirth, hemorrhoids, fissures: Stool softener to make defecation easier
- Stimulants and suppositories
- Manual disimpaction as needed, then approach the chronic condition

MEDICATION

In patients with no known secondary causes of constipation, conservative nonpharmacologic treatment measures generally are recommended, including:
- Regular exercise
- Increased fluid intake
- Bowel habit training

Other nonpharmacologic therapies include:
- Biofeedback therapy
- Behavior therapy
- Electric stimulation

First Line

Bulking agents (need to be accompanied by adequate amounts of liquid to be useful):

Hydrophilic colloids (bulk-forming agents):
- Psyllium (Konsyl, Metamucil, Perdiem Fiber): 1 rounded tsp in liquid p.o. daily up to t.i.d.
- Bran methylcellulose (Citrucel): 1 rounded tsp in 8 oz cold water p.o. daily up to t.i.d.
- Polycarbophil (Mitrolan, FiberCon): 1 g p.o. q.i.d.

Stool softeners:
- Docusate sodium (Colace): 100 mg b.i.d.

Osmotic laxatives:
- Polyethylene glycol (MiraLax) (0.8 mg/kg/d) 17 g daily (current evidence shows PEG to be superior to lactulose) (4)[A]
- Saccharines Lactulose (Chronulac) 15–60 ml q.h.s. (flatulence, bloating, cramping side effects)
- Sorbitol 15–60 ml q.h.s. (as effective as lactulose)
- Magnesium salts (Milk of Magnesia) avoid in renal insufficiency

Second Line

Stimulants (irritate bowel causing muscle contraction; usually combined with a softener; work in 8–12 hours)
- Senna/docusate (Senokot-S, ex-lax) 1–2 capsules or 15–30 mL at bedtime
- Bisacodyl/docusate (Dulcolax, Correctol) 2–3 tablets daily
- Casanthranol/docusate (Peri-Colace) lubricants (contain mineral oil, coating the stool)

ALERT

- Short-term use only. Can bind fat-soluble vitamins with the potential for deficiencies. May similarly decrease absorption of some drugs.
- Avoid in those at risk for aspiration (lipid pneumonia).
- Suppositories:
  - Osmotic: Sodium phosphate
  - Lubricant: Glycerin
  - Stimulatory: Bisacodyl
- Enemas:
  - Sodium phosphate (Fleet enema)
  - Lubiprostone (Amitiza): A selective chloride channel activator; 24 mcg b.i.d.

Pregnancy Considerations

- Avoid in pregnancy and breastfeeding
- Prokinetic agents (partial 5-HT4 agonists): Have been withdrawn due to cardiac side effects (tegaserod [Zelnorm], cisapride [Propulsid])
- Other agents not approved by the Food and Drug Administration:
  - Misoprostol (Cytotec) : A prostaglandin that increases colonic motility (5)
  - Colchicine: Neurogenic stimulation to increase colonic motility (6)

ADDITIONAL TREATMENT

General Measures

- Attempt to eliminate medications that may cause or worsen constipation
- Increase fluid intake
- Increase fiber in diet
- Enemas if other methods fail

Additional Therapies

Biofeedback with artificial silicon stool

SURGERY/OTHER PROCEDURES

Surgery rarely indicated

IN-PATIENT CONSIDERATIONS

Nursing

Manual disimpaction occasionally required in difficult chronic situations

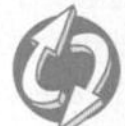

ONGOING CARE

FOLLOW-UP RECOMMENDATIONS

Encourage exercise and physical activity.

Patient Monitoring

If what seems to be simple, functional constipation persists, further investigate for a possible organic cause.

DIET

Increase fiber, but bloating and gas can be problematic:
- Gradually increase intake to 25 grams/day over a 6-week period.
- Insoluble, less fermentable fiber, like wheat bran, tends to be better tolerated.
- Bran (hard outer layer of cereal grains)
- Vegetables and fruits
- Whole grain foods
- Encourage liberal intake of fluids.

PATIENT EDUCATION

- Occasional mild constipation is normal.
- Instruction in consistent bowel training; the best time to move bowels is in the morning, after eating breakfast, when the normal bowel transit and defecation reflexes are typically functioning to move the bowels.

PROGNOSIS

- Constipation that is only occasional, brief, and responsive to simple measures is harmless.
- That which is habitual can be a lifelong nuisance.
- Those with neurologic compromise can suffer from ill effects such as obstipation and impaction to toxic megacolon.
- No evidence for dependence
- No evidence for harm from stimulant use; melanosis coli may develop, but it is a benign condition (7)

COMPLICATIONS

- Volvulus
- Toxic megacolon
- Acquired megacolon: In severe, long-standing cases
- Fluid and electrolyte depletion: Laxative abuse
- Rectal ulceration (stercoral ulcer) related to recurrent fecal impaction
- Anal fissures

REFERENCES

1. Longstreth GF, Thompson WG, Chey WD, et al. Functional bowel disorders. *Gastroenterology*. 2006;130:1480–91.
2. American College of Gastroenterology Chronic Constipation Task Force. An evidence-based approach to the management of chronic constipation in North America. *Am J Gastroenterol*. 2005;100 (Suppl 1):S1–4.
3. Locke GR, Pemberton JH, Phillips SF. American Gastroenterological Association Medical Position Statement: guidelines on constipation. *Gastroenterology*. 2000;119:1761–6.
4. Lee-Robichaud H, Thomas K, Morgan J et al. Lactulose versus Polyethylene Glycol for Chronic Constipation. *Cochrane Database Syst Rev*. 2010;7:CD007570–
5. Roarty TP, Weber F, Soykan I, et al. Misoprostol in the treatment of chronic refractory constipation: results of a long-term open label trial. *Aliment Pharmacol Ther*. 1997;11:1059–66.
6. Verne GN, Davis RH, Robinson ME, et al. Treatment of chronic constipation with colchicine: randomized, double-blind, placebo-controlled, crossover trial. *Am J Gastroenterol*. 2003;98: 1112–6.
7. Müller-Lissner SA, Kamm MA et al. Myths and misconceptions about chronic constipation. *Am J Gastroenterol*. 2005;100:232–42.

ADDITIONAL READING

- Spinzi G, Amato A, Imperiali G et al. Constipation in the elderly: management strategies. *Drugs Aging*. 2009;26:469–74.
- van Dijk M, Benninga MA, Grootenhuis MA, et al. Chronic childhood constipation: A review of the literature and the introduction of a protocolized behavioral intervention program. *Patient Educ Couns*. 2007.

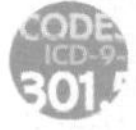

CODES

ICD9

564.00 Constipation, unspecified

CLINICAL PEARLS

- Constipation can be characterized as unsatisfactory defecation, with infrequent stools, difficult stool passage, or both, for 3 months.
- Functional constipation (normal transit time and sphincter function) seen most often
- Workup is necessary in the presence of red flags: Onset >50 yrs, hematochezia/melena, unintentional weight loss, anemia, neurological defects
- Best evidence for effectiveness is for osmotic agents (polyethylene glycol [PEG]).

CONTRACEPTION

Kristen Kelly, MD
Jeremy Golding, MD

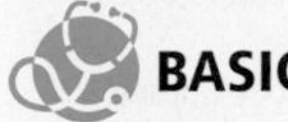

BASICS

DESCRIPTION

- Methods to prevent pregnancy
- Mechanisms include prevention/delay of ovulation, inhibition of sperm entry into the uterus, or interference with implantation of fertilized ovum.
- Natural family planning limits coitus to presumably nonfertile portions of the menstrual cycle.
- The most effective method of contraception is permanent sterilization. Reversal of sterilization may be difficult if not impossible.

Pediatric Considerations

Use of estrogen prior to pubertal growth spurt may reduce ultimate height due to epiphysial closure.

EPIDEMIOLOGY

Incidence

- ~98% of women of reproductive age have used some form of contraception, but 1/3–1/2 of pregnancies are unplanned or unwanted (1).
- OCs are leading method (31% of women) in the US, followed by tubal sterilization (1).
- Factors in choice of contraceptive method include efficacy, convenience, adverse effects, and affordability.

RISK FACTORS

Unintended pregnancy:

- Young adolescents
- Lower socioeconomic population
- Those with limited knowledge and access to reproductive service

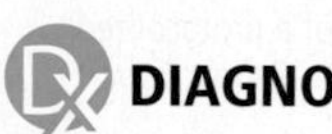

DIAGNOSIS

DIAGNOSTIC TESTS & INTERPRETATION

Lab

- No routine testing is needed prior to initiating contraception except reassurance that the patient is not pregnant (by history or laboratory).
- If family history of thrombophilia, consider testing for the specific defect (if known) or common disorders (factor V Leiden, prothrombin gene G20210A mutation) prior to initiation of hormonal contraception.

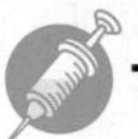

TREATMENT

CDC issued comprehensive guidelines in 2010 for use of contraceptive methods in patients with medical conditions (2).

MEDICATION

- Spermicides:
  - All contain nonoxynol-9; may alter vaginal flora and mucosal barrier
- Sponge:
  - 2-inch circular disk that contains nonoxynol-9. Moisten with water before insertion in vagina; effective for 24 hours.
- OCs:
  - Side effects minimized with pills having <50 μg estrogen. OCs with 35 μg of ethinyl estradiol provide the same blood hormone levels as 50 μg of mestranol.
  - Progestational agents vary. Newer progestogens are less androgenic and have less effect on lipoproteins (clinical significance unknown). Possible increased risk of thrombosis with desogestrel (3)[C].
  - Continuous pill (e.g., Seasonale with 84 active days and 7 inactive) used for endometriosis and premenstrual dysphoric disorder. Any monophasic may be used for continuous cycling: Skip the last 7 pills and begin new pack (off-label indication).
  - If adverse effects occur, pill may be changed based on nature of adverse reaction.
  - Progestin-only is the preferred OC for breast-feeding mothers, especially in the first few months of nursing because combined estrogen-progestin can suppress milk production.
- Weekly hormonal patch (Ortho-Evra):
  - Patch must be changed weekly; contains 20 μg ethinyl estradiol and 150 μg norelgestromin
  - Produces higher serum estrogen levels than oral 20 μg pill
  - Patch may cause local skin irritation.
  - Not as reliable in women >90 kg
- Vaginal contraceptive ring (NuvaRing):
  - Flexible polymer ring containing 15 μg ethinyl estradiol and 120 μg etonogestrel; inserted into vagina for 3 weeks per cycle (also may be used for continuous cycling for 4 weeks [off label])
- Medroxyprogesterone (Depo-Provera), also known as depot-medroxyprogesterone acetate (DMPA):
  - 150 mg IM *or* 104 mg/0.65 mL SC, both are given every 3 months
  - Contraceptive levels of hormone persist for up to 4 months (2–4-week margin of safety).
  - Potential for decreased bone mineral density if used for >2 years:
    - Recommend that women take 1300 mg of calcium and 400 IU of vitamin D when using DMPA (4).
- IUD:
  - ParaGard (Copper T): Interferes with sperm transport and ova fertilization; approved for up to 10 years, but likely remains effective for longer. May increase menstrual blood loss. Also effective as postcoital contraceptive up to 5 days from intercourse.
  - Mirena (Levonorgestrel intrauterine system):
    - T-shaped IUD that releases 20 μg of levonorgestrel per day (very low serum levels)
    - Approved for use up to 5 years; has been used off label for up to 7
    - Expect irregular menstrual spotting initially and then possibly amenorrhea after 6–9 months of use.
    - Ideally, insert during menses (ensures patient is not pregnant).
  - The literature on IUD use among adolescents is scant and obsolete. Nevertheless, published reports are generally reassuring (5), and both types of IUD are now commonly used in adolescents and other nulliparous women.
- Etonogestrel implant (Implanon):
  - Small, single, plastic rod that is implanted into the superficial subcutaneous tissue of the upper arm and provides continuous contraception via progestin hormone. This prevents ovulation and thickens cervical mucus to halt fertilization. Effective for up to 3 years.
  - The device may be inserted only by trained and certified providers, as improper placement may result in unintended pregnancy, pain, infection, and difficult removal.
  - Menstrual irregularities are common the 1st 6–12 months (and beyond); some will not have menses after 1 year, although others may have continuing irregular spotting for years.
- Emergency contraception: Start within 72 hours for maximum effectiveness, but evidence supports up to 120 hours:
  - Levonorgestrel: 1.5 mg taken as 2 0.75 mg tablets (Plan B), or 1 1.5 mg tablet (Plan B 1-Step). Less nausea and slightly more effective than the "Yuzpe regimen" (see below) (6):
    - Available over the counter, but may be less expensive for many women if prescribed
    - Prescription is needed for women under age 17
  - Estradiol/levonorgestrel (Preven, Ovral, Ogestrel): "Yuzpe regimen" 50 μg/0.25 mg, 2 tablets q12h (4 tablets total). Other OCs may be used as long as dose of estrogen component ≥100 μg/dose. *Note*: Antinausea medication (e.g., Phenergan) given 1–2 hours before the doses
  - Copper-bearing IUD (Paragard): Insert up to 5 days after intercourse; over 99% effective in preventing pregnancy and continues to provide contraception for up to 10 years.
  - Ulipristal acetate (Ella) 30 mg approved by FDA in 2010. Selective progesterone modulator, approved for use up to 5 days following unprotected intercourse
- Contraindications: Hormonal contraceptives, especially those containing estrogen (WHO Medical Eligibility Criteria for Contraceptive Use): History of coronary artery disease (CAD) or multiple risk factors (age >55, smoking, high blood pressure, diabetes mellitus); history of deep vein thrombosis (DVT)/pulmonary embolism (PE); history of cerebrovascular accident (CVA); history of migraines at age >35 or migraine at any age with aura; current or past breast cancer; active liver disease or hepatic tumor; pregnancy; unexplained abnormal uterine bleeding without further investigation. Relative contraindication: Smokers >35. Healthy nonsmokers may use oral contraceptives until menopause.

ALERT

Significant possible interactions due to increased metabolism of hormones (use higher estrogen dose and/or add barrier method):

ADDITIONAL TREATMENT

General Measures

Nondrug methods:

- Latex condom
- Diaphragm: Needs fitting
- IUD: Contraindications include pregnancy, undiagnosed genital bleeding, uterine anomalies, and large fibroids (3)[C].

Periodic abstinence:
- Calendar method: Track length of last 6 cycles; fertility period is calculated by subtracting 18 from the number of days of shortest cycle and 11 from number of days in longest cycle. Example: If shortest cycle is 28 days and longest cycle is 31 days, fertile period is from day 10–20.
- Symptothermal method: Calculate the 1st day of abstinence by subtracting 21 from the length of the shortest menstrual cycle in the previous 6 months, or the 1st day cervical mucus is detected, whichever comes first. End calculated as 3 days after body temperature rises 1°C.
- Withdrawal method: Male partner withdraws from vagina before ejaculation. Failure occurs if withdrawal is not timed accurately or if the pre-ejaculatory fluid contains sperm.

- Lactation delays resumption of ovulation postpartum due to prolactin-induced inhibition of gonadotropin-releasing hormone (GNRH) release. Breast-feeding is effective contraception only if (1) the infant is <6 months old, (2) the infant is exclusively breast-feeding, and (3) the mother has not resumed her regular menses (lactational amenorrhea method or LAM) (7).

SURGERY/OTHER PROCEDURES
Permanent sterilization:
- Tubal sterilization in the female
- Hysteroscopic sterilization via polyester fibers (Essure): Polyester fibers with a coiled spring are introduced into each fallopian tube by transcervical route. Requires another contraceptive to be used for 3 months after procedure (3)[C].
- Vasectomy in the male

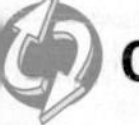

ONGOING CARE

FOLLOW-UP RECOMMENDATIONS
Patient Monitoring
- Pelvic exam and Pap smear per guidelines
- Sexually transmitted disease (STD) testing per guidelines
- Check for IUD 1 month after insertion. Spontaneous expulsion rate highest in first month. Pt should monitor presence of string monthly following menses.
- OC users: Monitor BP 3 months after starting, then annual follow up

DIET
Vitamin C and some herbals such as St. John's wort may alter estrogen levels, reducing efficacy or causing breakthrough bleeding.

PATIENT EDUCATION
- Condoms: Water-based lubricants (inside and outside) reduce the risk of breakage. Withdraw penis before it becomes flaccid.
- IUD: Check string periodically.
- Diaphragm:
  - Refit after childbirth or if weight changes by more than 10%.
  - Before inserting, 1 Tbs of water-soluble spermicidal jelly or cream should be placed in the dome.
  - Leave in at least 6 hours after coitus. If coitus is repeated before 6 hours, insert another teaspoon of spermicidal jelly into the vagina without removing the diaphragm.
- Female condom:
  - New condom required for each sex act
- OC:
  - Pill should be taken same time each day.
  - If a pill is missed, take 2 the following day, but use a barrier method until next period.
- Emergency contraception prevents pregnancy via several proposed mechanisms, including inhibition of sperm motility, alterations in tubal transport, unfavorable uterine receptivity, and/or fertilization inhibition. Emergency contraception does not affect an established pregnancy: 1-888-NOT-2-LATE or http://www.planbonestep.com/

COMPLICATIONS
- Hormonal contraceptives, serious:
  - Thromboembolism
  - Hypertension
  - Myocardial infarction, stroke
- OCs, minor:
  - Nausea and vomiting: Take after eating.
  - Breakthrough bleeding: Usually self-limiting after 3 months; if persists, change pill
  - Amenorrhea: Pregnancy must be ruled out.
  - Cyclic weight gain: Use smallest dose of estrogen available.
  - Breast tenderness: Rare with low-dose pill
  - Depression: Rare with low-dose pill
  - Chloasma: Stop pill or cover with makeup
  - Acne or hirsutism: Change to a less androgenic progesterone
  - Cholestatic jaundice: Stop pill; do not restart
  - Weight gain throughout cycle: Use triphasic pill to minimize dose of progesterone or use newer progesterone.
- Injectable contraceptive (Depo-Provera):
  - Irregular bleeding: No treatment needed; nonsteroidal anti-inflammatory drug (NSAID) may help
  - Weight gain
  - Amenorrhea: Common after 1 year of use
  - Possible ↑ bone resorption and ↓ bone mineral density (BMD), but rapid recovery following discontinuation. Food and Drug Administration (FDA) recommends BMD for use >2 years and to consider periodic estrogen.
- Sponge and diaphragm:
  - Associated with toxic shock syndrome
- IUD:
  - Pelvic inflammatory disease (PID) or salpingitis: Device removal is not necessary for mild PID treated as outpatient. For infections requiring hospitalization, most recommend that device be removed.
  - Heavy bleeding and cramps: Remove device.
  - Although absolute risk is no higher than without IUD, pregnancy, when it occurs, is more likely to be ectopic.

REFERENCES

1. CDC National Center for Health Statistics. *Use of Contraception and Use of Family Planning Services*: United States: 1992–2002. Hyattsville, MD; 2004.
2. Division of Reproductive Health, National Center for Chronic Disease Prevention and Health Promotion, Centers for Disease Control and Prevention (CDC), Farr S, Folger SG, Paulen M, Tepper N, Whiteman M, Zapata L, Culwell K, Kapp N, Cansino C et al. U S. Medical Eligibility Criteria for Contraceptive Use, 2010: adapted from the World Health Organization Medical Eligibility Criteria for Contraceptive Use, 4th edition. *MMWR Recomm Rep*. 2010;59:1–86.
3. Hatcher RA, Zietman M, Cwiak C, et al. *A Pocket Guide to Managing Contraception*. 8th ed. Tiger, GA: Bridging the Gap Foundation; 2005.
4. Schrager SB. DMPA's effect on bone mineral density: A particular concern for adolescents. *J Fam Pract*. 2009;58:E1–8.
5. Deans EI, Grimes DA. Intrauterine devices for adolescents: a systematic review. *Contraception*. 2009;79:418–23.
6. Cheng L, Gülmezoglu AM, Piaggio G, et al. Interventions for emergency contraception. *Cochrane Database Syst Rev*. 2008;CD001324.
7. Academy of Breastfeeding Medicine Clinical Protocol #13: Contraception during breastfeeding. 2005. Available at http://www.bfmed.org/Resources/Protocols.aspx

ADDITIONAL READING

- Hughes H. Postpartum contraception. *J Fam Health Care*. 2009;19:9–10, 12.
- Mestad RE, Kenerson J, Peipert JF. Reversible contraception update: the importance of long-acting reversible contraception. *Postgrad Med*. 2009; 121:18–25.
- Naz RK, Rowan S. Update on male contraception. *Curr Opin Obstet Gynecol*. 2009;21:265–9.

See Also (Topic, Algorithm, Electronic Media Element)
Thrombophilia, Factor V Leiden, Prothrombin Gene Mutation

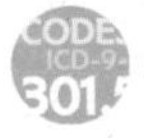

CODES

ICD9
- V25.01 General counseling on prescription of oral contraceptives
- V25.02 General counseling on initiation of other contraceptive measures
- V25.03 Encounter for emergency contraceptive counseling and prescription

CLINICAL PEARLS
- Hormonal and IUD contraceptives may be initiated immediately ("Quick-Start") as long as likelihood of established pregnancy is low.
- Quick-start may reduce risk of pregnancy occurring before next last menstrual period (LMP), and may improve long-term adherence.
- Clearly established benefits of OCs include reduction in ovarian cancer, endometrial cancer, ectopic pregnancies, and PID; less dysmenorrhea and anemia; reduced number of functional ovarian cysts, a regular menstrual cycle; improvement in acne.
- Barrier contraceptives lower the risk of STDs.

COR PULMONALE

Parag Goyal, MD
Oscar Starobin, MD

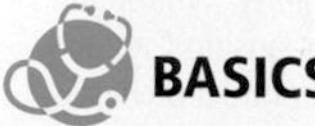

BASICS

DESCRIPTION
- Enlargement and subsequent dysfunction and failure of the right ventricle (RV) in the presence of pulmonary arterial hypertension secondary to abnormalities of the lungs, thorax, pulmonary ventilation or circulation
- May occur in acute or chronic setting:
  - Acute: Rapid increase of pulmonary arterial pressure causing RV overload and resulting dysfunction/failure
  - Chronic: Progressive hypertrophy and dilation of RV over months to years, with eventual dysfunction/failure

EPIDEMIOLOGY
- Approximately, 6–7% of all types of adult heart disease in US
- Between 10% and 30% of heart failure admissions in the US are the result of cor pulmonale (1).

Incidence
Difficult to assess. Best estimate is 1/10,000–3/10,000 per year (2).

Prevalence
Difficult to assess. Best estimate is 2/1,000–6/1,000 (2).

RISK FACTORS
- Acute cor pulmonale is most commonly caused by massive pulmonary embolism (PE):
  - Risk factors associated with PE include:
    - Vessel injury
    - Stasis
    - Hypercoagulable states
- Chronic cor pulmonale is most commonly caused by COPD and/or pulmonary arterial hypertension (PAH).
  - Risk factors associated with COPD and/or PAH include:
    - Tobacco use
    - Living at high altitudes
    - Industrial exposures such as asbestos
    - Alpha-1-antitrypsin deficiency
    - Connective tissue disease

GENERAL PREVENTION
- Prevention of pulmonary embolism via deep venous thrombosis prophylaxis when necessary
- Early detection and timely management of COPD to delay its progression
- Management of underlying disease, including aggressive correction of hypoxia and acidosis, that may contribute to worsening pulmonary hypertension

PATHOPHYSIOLOGY
- Acute: A sudden event, such as large pulmonary embolism, increases resistance to blood flow in the pulmonary vasculature, causing a quick and significant increase of pressure proximally. The RV is unable to overcome this pressure, leading to low cardiac output and RV failure.
- Chronic: PAH develops from many possible etiologies, although predominantly from alveolar hypoxia. The RV is initially able to compensate for this increased pressure through concentric hypertrophy. However, worsening pulmonary hypertension eventually overcomes the RV's accommodative abilities, leading to dilation of the RV. This results in both systolic and diastolic dysfunction, causing reduced cardiac output and right-sided heart failure.

ETIOLOGY
- Lung disease: COPD including emphysema and chronic bronchitis (80–90%) (3), cystic fibrosis, restrictive and interstitial lung disease, including scleroderma and sarcoidosis, pulmonary thromboembolism, tumor emboli, idiopathic pulmonary arterial hypertension
- Hematological abnormalities: Sickle cell anemia, polycythemia vera
- Neuromuscular disease: Amyotrophic lateral sclerosis, myasthenia gravis, Guillain-Barré syndrome, polio, spinal cord injuries
- Disorders of ventilator control: Primary central hypoventilation, sleep apnea syndromes
- Thoracic cage deformities: Kyphoscoliosis
- Collagen vascular disease
- Left ventricular failure is NOT considered a cause of cor pulmonale.

COMMONLY ASSOCIATED CONDITIONS
Pulmonary arterial hypertension (PAH): Classically defined as the presence of a resting mean pulmonary artery pressure (PAP) $>$20 mm Hg, though some sources define as $>$25 mm Hg at rest and $>$30 mm Hg with exercise

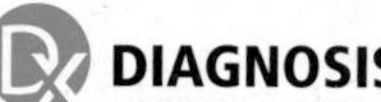

DIAGNOSIS

HISTORY
- Dyspnea, orthopnea
- Fatigue, lethargy, syncope
- Cyanosis, pallor, diaphoresis
- Pleuritic chest pain, cough, hemoptysis
- Exertional angina
- Hoarseness secondary to compression of the left recurrent laryngeal nerve by enlarged pulmonary vessels
- Anorexia and/or right upper quadrant discomfort from hepatic congestion
- Cardiovascular collapse, shock, and/or cardiac arrest may occur in acute setting or advanced chronic setting.

PHYSICAL EXAM
- Peripheral edema is the most common sign of right heart failure (RHF), though it is nonspecific.
- Tachypnea, wheeze
- Increased intensity of pulmonic component of 2nd heart sound (P2)
- Splitting of S2 over the cardiac apex with inspiration
- Audible S3 or S4
- Pansystolic murmur heard best at right midsternal border increasing with inspiration, consistent with tricuspid regurgitation (typically a late sign).
- Early diastolic murmur heard best at left upper sternal border, consistent with pulmonary regurgitation.
- Right ventricular heave
- Jugular venous distension with inspiration (Kussmaul sign)
- Prominent a and v waves on jugular venous pulse tracing
- Hepatomegaly
- Signs of DVT, such as tenderness or unilateral swelling, may or may not be present.

DIAGNOSTIC TESTS & INTERPRETATION
ECG (poor sensitivity; up to 67% patients will have normal findings) (1):
- Rightward P-wave axis deviation
- Peaked P waves anteriorly and in inferior leads (i.e., "P pulmonale")
- $S_1S_2S_3$ pattern, or $S_1Q_3T_3$, inverted pattern (McGinn-White pattern)
- RV hypertrophy (high specificity, low sensitivity)
- Right bundle-branch block
- Low-voltage QRS

Lab
Initial lab tests
- CBC and serum chemistries may be obtained to rule out other conditions:
  - Lab findings such as polycythemia and hypercapnia may be present due to COPD.
  - LFTs may be elevated due to hepatic congestion secondary to RV failure.
- Pulmonary function testing may show airflow obstruction with reduced PO_2, or other findings associated with COPD.
- Arterial blood gas, indicated for acute respiratory distress, may show hypercapnic acidosis and hypoxemia.
- BNP and cardiac troponins may be elevated secondary to RV stretch.

Imaging
- Chest x-ray:
  - Cardiomegaly
  - Increased width of right descending pulmonary artery
  - Left main pulmonary artery prominence below the aortic knob
- 2-dimensional echocardiogram:
  - RV mid-wall hypokinesis/akinesis plus normokinesis/hyperkinesis of RV apex (McConnell sign) are associated with acute cor pulmonale caused by acute pulmonary embolism.
  - RV dilatation and/or hypertrophy may be indicative of chronic cor pulmonale.
  - Doppler echocardiography with saline contrast to estimate tricuspid regurgitation is the most reliable noninvasive estimation of pulmonary artery pressure (PAP).
- Spiral CT scan of chest:
  - Most accurate modality for diagnosing emphysema and interstitial lung disease
  - Test of choice for assessment of acute pulmonary embolism
- V/Q scan may be used to assess for pulmonary embolism in acute cor pulmonale.
- MRI commonly used, as it can characterize right ventricular size, mass morphology, and gross function

Diagnostic Procedures/Surgery
- Right heart catheterization is the gold standard for quantitation of ventricular and pulmonary pressures, and exclusion of congenital heart disease as etiology. Right heart catheterization is also recommended to assess vasoreactivity prior to implementing calcium channel blocker therapy.

Pulmonary function tests should be performed in patients with a suggestive history of underlying lung disease and in those with normal cardiac function.

DIFFERENTIAL DIAGNOSIS

- Right-sided heart failure secondary to left-sided heart failure
- Right-sided cardiomyopathy, ischemic or nonischemic
- Tricuspid valvulopathy
- Severe congenital pulmonary hypertension secondary to congenital heart disease with left-to-right shunting, most frequently from unrepaired nonrestrictive ventricular septal defect (VSD)

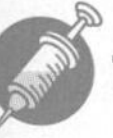

TREATMENT

Reduce disease burden via oxygenation, preservation of cardiac function, and attenuation of PAH (4).

MEDICATION

- Oxygenation:
  - Oxygen:
    - Long-term continuous oxygen therapy improves the survival of hypoxemic patients with COPD and cor pulmonale.
    - All patients with pulmonary hypertension whose PaO_2 is consistently <55 mm Hg or saturation ≤88% at rest, during sleep, or with ambulation should be prescribed oxygen to keep O_2 >90 mm Hg (5)[A].
- Preservation of cardiac function:
  - Diuretics: Decrease RV filling pressures; also improves peripheral edema secondary to right heart failure:
    - Furosemide: Starting at 20–80 mg p.o./IV, titrate and increase dose per diuresis.
    - Excessive volume depletion should be avoided.
    - Monitor closely for metabolic alkalosis, as this may suppress ventilatory drive and contribute to hypoxia.
  - Cardiac glycosides:
    - Impact of digoxin on cor pulmonale alone is unclear
    - Digoxin may be appropriate in the presence of co-existent left ventricular systolic failure.
    - Digoxin may also be appropriate in the presence of atrial fibrillation as adjunct for rate control.
- Amelioration of PAH:
  - Calcium channel blockers (CCB) (4):
    - May be used as adjunctive therapy in those with low-to-moderate disease
    - Vasodilator therapy to reduce pulmonary vascular resistance has been shown to be effective in a small subset of patients (10%).
    - Vasoreactivity trial should be attempted with short-acting vasodilator at cardiac catheterization to determine likelihood of response. Reduction of >20% PAP without reduction of cardiac output should prompt adding CCB such as nifedipine, diltiazem, amlodipine to treatment regimen.
    - Repeat vasoreactivity trial via cardiac catheterization is recommended at 3-6 months following initiation of CCB therapy to assess sustained response. For nonsustained response, discontinue CCB and pursue alternative medications (6).
  - For nonresponse or unsustained response to CCB, treatment with phosphodiesterase inhibitors, endothelin receptor antagonists, and/or prostanoids may be appropriate based on World Health Organization (WHO) classification (6):
    - WHO Class I: Supportive therapy.
    - WHO Class II: Monotherapy is recommended with either phosphodiesterase inhibitor or endothelin receptor antagonist.
    - WHO Class III: Combination therapy may be used with phosphodiesterase inhibitor, endothelin receptor antagonist, or prostanoids. There is currently little randomized data on which combination is most efficacious (7).
    - WHO Class IV: Epoprostenol IV is 1st-line therapy in critically ill patients; other classes of drugs may also be added for combination therapy.
    - Phosphodiesterase inhibitors: Vasodilates by increasing cAMP and therefore increasing nitric oxide, an endogenous vasodilator. Sildenafil, tadalafil: Endothelin receptor antagonists: Vasodilates by blocking the function of endothelin, a potent vasoconstrictor. Bosentan, Ambrisentan, Sitaxsentan.
    - Prostanoids: Vasodilates by mimicking endogenous vasodilators. Iloprost Inhaled. IV may also be used; evidence to date limited to expert opinion. Treprostinil SC. IV may also be used; evidence to date limited to expert opinion. Beraprost PO Epoprostenol IV: Currently recommended for WHO Class IV only.
  - Anticoagulation:
    - Recommended for patients with underlying thromboembolic disease
    - Recommended for patients with cor pulmonale in association with idiopathic pulmonary arterial hypertension (5)[B]
    - Use in secondary causes of PAH is widely accepted, though little supportive evidence to date (8)
    - In general, warfarin is recommended unless contraindications. Target international normalized ratio (INR) for prophylaxis is 2–3.

ADDITIONAL TREATMENT

General Measures

- Treat underlying disease.
- Supportive therapy as necessary:
  - Continuous positive airway pressure or bilevel positive airway pressure may be used for hypoxia/sleep disorders.
  - Ventilation using positive-pressure masks, negative-pressure body suits, or mechanical ventilation is suggested for patients with neuromuscular disease.
  - Phlebotomy may be indicated for severe polycythemia (hematocrit >55%).

Issues for Referral

Patients with cor pulmonale should be referred to a cardiologist or pulmonologist for expert consultation.

SURGERY/OTHER PROCEDURES

Moderate-to-severe disease refractory to medication may require atrioseptostomy and/or lung transplantation.

ONGOING CARE

Referral of patients with PAH to a specialized center with close follow-up is strongly recommended.

DIET

Salt and fluid restriction

PATIENT EDUCATION

- Smoking cessation and avoidance of exposure to secondary smoke is strongly recommended.
- Exertional activity should be limited.
- Pregnancy should be avoided in PAH.

PROGNOSIS

- Patients with cor pulmonale resulting from COPD have a greater likelihood of dying than do similar patients with COPD alone.
- The pulmonary artery pressure (PAP) is a reliable indicator of prognosis; higher pressure is associated with worse prognosis.
- In patients with COPD and mild disease (PAP 20–35 mm Hg), 5-year survival is 50%.

REFERENCES

1. Han MK, McLaughlin VV, Criner GJ, Martinez FJ et al. Pulmonary diseases and the heart. *Circulation*. 2007;116:2992–3005.
2. Naeije R et al. Pulmonary hypertension and right heart failure in chronic obstructive pulmonary disease. *Proc Am Thorac Soc*. 2005;2:20–2.
3. Weitzenblum E, Chaouat A et al. Cor pulmonale. *Chron Respir Dis*. 2009;6:177–85.
4. Hoeper MM et al. Drug treatment of pulmonary arterial hypertension: current and future agents. *Drugs*. 2005;65:1337–54.
5. Badesch DB, Abman SH, Simonneau G, et al. Medical therapy for pulmonary arterial hypertension: updated ACCP evidence-based clinical practice guidelines. *Chest*. 2007;131:1917–28.
6. Barst RJ, Gibbs JS, Ghofrani HA, Hoeper MM, McLaughlin VV, Rubin LJ, Sitbon O, Tapson VF, Galiè N et al. Updated evidence-based treatment algorithm in pulmonary arterial hypertension. *J Am Coll Cardiol*. 2009;54:S78–84.
7. Benedict N, Seybert A, Mathier MA et al. Evidence-based pharmacologic management of pulmonary arterial hypertension. *Clin Ther*. 2007;29:2134–53.
8. Alam S, Palevsky HI. Standard therapies for pulmonary arterial hypertension. *Clin Chest Med*. 2007;28:91–115, viii.

See Also (Topic, Algorithm, Electronic Media Element)

Pulmonary Embolism; Chronic Obstructive Pulmonary Disease and Emphysema; Pulmonary Arterial Hypertension, Idiopathic; Congestive Heart Failure

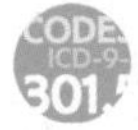

CODES

ICD9

- 415.0 Acute cor pulmonale
- 416.9 Chronic pulmonary heart disease, unspecified

CLINICAL PEARLS

- Continuous, long-term oxygen therapy improves life expectancy and quality of life in cor pulmonale.
- Referral of patients with PAH to a specialized center is strongly recommended.

CORNEAL ABRASION AND ULCERATION

Ken S. Ota, DO

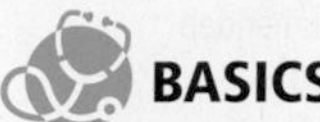

BASICS

DESCRIPTION

- Corneal abrasions result from scratching, denuding, abrading, or cutting of the outermost layer of the eye. They are usually due to trauma, but can occur spontaneously as well.
- Corneal ulcers usually represent an infection of the cornea by bacteria, viruses, or fungi as a result of breakdown in the protective epithelial barrier:
  - Both corneal abrasions and ulcerations can result in scarring, which may impair vision.
  - Both lesions can occur centrally or marginally.

EPIDEMIOLOGY

Incidence

- Corneal abrasion is the most common ophthalmologic visit to the emergency department and is commonly seen in urgent care as well.
- Ulceration is also common in the US.

RISK FACTORS

- Any abrasive injury
- Contact lenses (especially soft lenses)
- Blepharitis
- Dry eye syndrome
- Entropion (with lashes scratching cornea)
- Chronic topical steroid use
- Abuse of topical anesthetics
- Autoimmune disorders
- Vitamin A deficiency
- Chronic corneal exposure (Bell palsy, exophthalmos, etc.)
- Recent eye surgery
- Optic neuropathy

GENERAL PREVENTION

- Eye protection to avoid injury during work, crafts, and sport
- Proper contact lens handling
- Artificial tears for those with inability to blink or known dry eyes

ETIOLOGY

- Corneal abrasions typically result from accidental trauma (i.e., fingernail scratch).
- Corneal ulcers result from presence of an entryway to the external eye through dry eye, burns, abrasion, contact lenses, inappropriate use of topical anesthetics, antibiotics, or antiviral drops, immunosuppressant drugs, diabetes, or immunodeficiency.
- Causative agents of ulceration:
  - Gram-positive organisms (staphylococci, streptococci, and bacilli)
  - Anaerobes (cocci, bacilli)
  - Gram-negative organisms (*Pseudomonas*, diplococci, and rods)
  - Viruses, such as herpes
  - Fungal organisms (*Candida, Aspergillus, Fusarium, Acanthamoeba*) in agricultural workers or associated with ocular corticosteroid use
  - Peripheral ulcerative keratitis usually caused by autoimmune disorders such as rheumatoid arthritis (RA), systemic lupus erythematosus (SLE), scleroderma, etc.
  - Vitamin A deficiency may cause corneal necrosis or keratomalacia.

COMMONLY ASSOCIATED CONDITIONS

- Chronic ulcerations may be associated with neurotrophic keratitis due to lack of 5th nerve innervation of the cornea. Individuals with thyroid disease, diabetes, or immunosuppressive conditions are particularly at risk.
- Any cause of fat malabsorption may be associated with vitamin A deficiency.

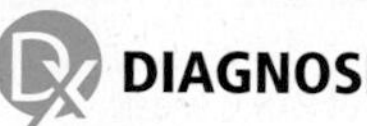

DIAGNOSIS

HISTORY

- History remarkable for contact lens use, dry eyes, rubbing eye, history of trauma from foreign body or chemical burn, or history of connective tissue disorder
- Signs and symptoms of abrasion or ulceration include sudden onset of eye pain, photophobia, tearing, foreign-body sensation, blurring of vision, and/or conjunctival injection.
- Abrasions and ulcerations are usually unilateral.

PHYSICAL EXAM

- Visual acuity may be decreased if abrasion of ulcer i centrally located.
- Conjunctival injection
- Increased lacrimation on affected side
- Photophobia
- Lesion seen on slit lamp exam and area of damage shows fluorescein uptake; staining seen using Wood lamp or cobalt blue slit lamp

DIAGNOSTIC TESTS & INTERPRETATION

Lab

Initial lab tests

- Culture ulcer and contact lens if applicable.
- *Note:* Pretreatment with topical antibiotics may alte culture results.

Diagnostic Procedures/Surgery

Scrapings of the corneal ulcer for culture and sensitivities ideally should be done before beginning local antibiotics. The sample should be plated directly onto the culture medium.

Pathological Findings

Scrapings for Gram and Giemsa stain may demonstrate bacteria, yeast, or intranuclear inclusions that may aid in the diagnosis.

DIFFERENTIAL DIAGNOSIS

- Foreign bodies
- Keratitis
- Herpes simplex or zoster
- Bilateral or true idiopathic lesions may suggest basement membrane dystrophy.

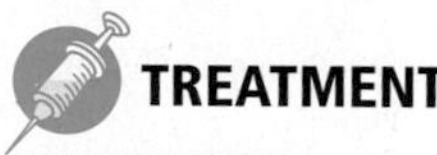

TREATMENT

MEDICATION

First Line

- Pain reduction can be achieved with ophthalmic NSAIDs (1)[A].
- Some ophthalmic NSAIDs include ketorolac 0.5% [Acular], diclofenac 0.1% [Voltaren], and bromfenac 0.09% [Xibrom].
- Ophthalmic antibiotics may help prevent further infection and ulceration of corneal abrasions (2)[C].
- Some ophthalmic antibiotics include chloramphenicol 1% [Chloroptic], ciprofloxacin 0.3% [Ciloxan], ofloxacin 0.3% [Ocuflox], gentamicin 0.3%, and erythromycin 0.5%. Note: ointment preparations may be more soothing to the eye than solutions.

Eye patching is not helpful and may be harmful; thus, it is not recommended (3)[A].

Consultation with an ophthalmologist is recommended for all ulcers to help determine appropriate therapy (4)[C].

Topical gentamicin and tobramycin are effective against *Pseudomonas, Enterobacter, Klebsiella*, and aerobic gram-negative organisms; cephalosporins (e.g., cefazolin 50 mg/mL) also may be used.

Fungal keratitis is treated with a protracted course of topical antifungal agents.

Herpetic keratitis should be treated initially with trifluridine. Vidarabine and acyclovir are alternatives (5)[A].

Second Line

Supplemental topical cycloplegia (i.e., homatropine 5% and cyclopentolate 1%) has not been found to be beneficial (6)[B].

Oral analgesic medication if topical analgesia not adequate

ADDITIONAL TREATMENT

General Measures

- Corneal abrasions can be managed by primary care physicians (7)[C]. See indications for referral below.
- All patients with corneal ulceration should be referred immediately to an ophthalmologist.
- For corneal ulcerations, appropriate antimicrobial therapy should be instituted after cultures have been obtained.
- Eye patching is not recommended (3)[A].
- Corneal abrasions should be evaluated regularly to determine if ophthalmology referral is necessary.

Issues for Referral

Refer to ophthalmologist if there is a history of significant ocular trauma, if corneal infection is suspected, or if a recurrent or nonhealing abrasion is encountered despite standard treatment (7)[C].

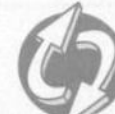

ONGOING CARE

FOLLOW-UP RECOMMENDATIONS

Patient Monitoring

The patient should be monitored every 1–3 days, depending on the depth/severity of the abrasion, until healed.

PATIENT EDUCATION

Prevention of abrasions and proper handling of contact lenses can prevent recurrence of corneal ulcers.

PROGNOSIS

Corneal abrasions and ulcerations should improve daily and heal with appropriate therapy. If healing does not occur or the lesion extends, obtain an ophthalmology consultation.

COMPLICATIONS

Recurrence, scarring of the cornea, loss of vision, and corneal perforation

REFERENCES

1. Weaver CS, Terrell KM et al. Evidence-based emergency medicine. Update: do ophthalmic nonsteroidal anti-inflammatory drugs reduce the pain associated with simple corneal abrasion without delaying healing? *Ann Emerg Med*. 2003;41:134–40.
2. Upadhyay MP, Karmacharya PC, Koirala S, Shah DN, Shakya S, Shrestha JK, Bajracharya H, Gurung CK, Whitcher JP et al. The Bhaktapur eye study: ocular trauma and antibiotic prophylaxis for the prevention of corneal ulceration in Nepal. *Br J Ophthalmol*. 2001;85:388–92.
3. Turner A, Rabiu M et al. Patching for corneal abrasion. *Cochrane Database Syst Rev*. 2006; CD004764.
4. Wirbelauer C. Management of the red eye for the primary care physician. *Am J Med*. 2006;119: 302–6.
5. Wilhelmus KR. Therapeutic interventions for herpes simplex virus epithelial keratitis. *Cochrane Database Syst Rev*. 2007;CD002898.
6. Carley F, Carley S et al. Towards evidence based emergency medicine: best BETs from the Manchester Royal Infirmary. Mydriatics in corneal abrasion. *Emerg Med J*. 2001;18:273.
7. Fraser S et al. Corneal abrasion. *Clin Ophthalmol*. 2010;4:387–90.

C

ADDITIONAL READING

- Ehler JP, Shah CP, Fenton GL. The Wills Eye Manual: Office and Emergency Room Diagnosis and Treatment of Eye Disease. Baltimore: Lippincott, Williams and Wilkins; 2008.
- Morden NE, Berke EM. Topical fluoroquinolones for eye and ear. *Am Fam Physician*. 2000;62:1870–6.
- Watson SL, Barker NH. Interventions for recurrent corneal erosions. *Cochrane Database Syst Rev*. 2007;CD001861.

CODES

ICD9

- 370.00 Corneal ulcer, unspecified
- 918.1 Superficial injury of cornea

CLINICAL PEARLS

- Contact lens use should be discontinued while corneal abrasion or ulcer is healing.
- Eye patching is not recommended.
- Prescribe topical and/or oral analgesic medication for symptom relief and consider ophthalmic antibiotics.
- Prompt referral to an ophthalmologist should be made for suspicion of an ulcer, recurrence of abrasion, retained foreign body, or lack of improvement despite therapy.
- Appropriate antimicrobial therapy should be instituted immediately when corneal infection is suspected.

CORNS AND CALLUSES

Neil J. Feldman, DPM

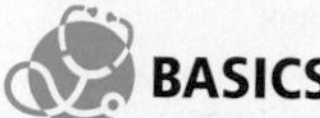

BASICS

DESCRIPTION

- A callus (tyloma) is a diffuse area of hyperkeratosis, usually without a distinct border.
- Typically the result of exposure to repetitive forces, including friction and mechanical pressure. Tend to occur on the palms of hands and soles of feet.
- A corn (heloma) is a circumscribed hyperkeratotic lesion with a central conical core of keratin that causes pain and inflammation. The conical core in a corn is a thickening of the stratum corneum.
- Hard corn or heloma durum (more common): More often on toe surfaces, especially 5th toe (PIP) joint
- Soft corn (heloma molle): Commonly in the interdigital space
- Digital corns are also known as clavi.
- Intractable plantar keratosis are usually located under a metatarsal head (1st and 5th most common), are typically more difficult to resolve, and resistant to usual conservative treatments.

EPIDEMIOLOGY

Corns and calluses have the largest prevalence of all foot disorders.

Incidence

Incidence of corns and calluses increases with age. Less common in pediatric patients. Women affected more often than men. Blacks report corns and calluses 30% more often than whites.

Prevalence

- 9.2 million Americans
- Nearly 38/1,000 people affected

RISK FACTORS

- Extrinsic factors producing pressure, friction, and local stress:
  - Ill-fitting shoes
  - Not using socks, gloves
  - Manual labor
  - Walking barefoot
  - Activities that increase stress applied to skin of hands or feet (running, walking, sports)
- Intrinsic factors:
  - Bony prominences: Bunions
- Enlarged bursa or abnormal foot function/structure: Hammertoe, claw toe, or mallet toe deformity

Genetics

No true genetic basis identified, since most corns and calluses are due to mechanical stressors on the foot/hands.

GENERAL PREVENTION

External irritation is by far the most common cause of calluses and corns. General measures to reduce friction on the skin are recommended to reduce incidence of callus formation. Examples include wearing shoes that fit well and using socks and gloves.

Geriatric Considerations

- In elderly patients, especially those with neurologic or vascular compromise, skin breakdown from calluses/corns may lead to increased risk of infection/ulceration. 30% of foot ulcers in the elderly arise from eroded hyperkeratosis. Regular foot exams are emphasized for these patients, as well as diabetic patients.

PATHOPHYSIOLOGY

Increased activity of keratinocytes in superficial layer of skin leading to hyperkeratosis. This is a normal response to excess friction, pressure, or stress.

ETIOLOGY

- Calluses typically arise from repetitive friction, motion, or pressure to skin.
- Soft corns arise from increased moisture from perspiration leading to maceration of the skin along with mechanical irritation, especially between toes.
- Hard corns are an extreme form of callus with a keratin-based core. Often found on the digital surfaces and commonly linked to bony protrusions causing skin to rub against shoe surfaces.

COMMONLY ASSOCIATED CONDITIONS

- Foot ulcers, especially in diabetic patients or patients with neuropathy or vascular compromise
- Infection; look for warning signs of:
  - Spreading or redness around sore
  - Pus-like drainage
  - Increased pain/swelling
  - Fever
  - Change in color of fingers or toes
- Signs of gangrene

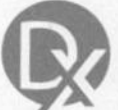

DIAGNOSIS

- Most commonly a clinical diagnosis based on visualization of the lesion.
- Examination of footwear may also provide clues

HISTORY

- Careful history can usually pinpoint cause.
- Ask about neurologic and vascular history and diabetes. These may be risk factors for progression of corns/calluses to frank ulcerations and infection.

PHYSICAL EXAM

- Calluses:
  - Thickening of skin without distinct borders
  - Often on feet, hands; especially over palms of hands, soles of feet
  - Colors from white to gray-yellow, brown, red
  - May be painless or tender
  - May throb or burn
- Corns:
  - Hard corns: Commonly on dorsum of toes or dorsum of 5th PIP joint:
    - Varied texture: Dry, waxy, transparent, to a hornlike mass
    - Distinct borders
    - More common to feet
    - Often painful
  - Soft corns:
    - Often between toes, especially between 4th and 5th digits at the base of the webspace
    - Often yellowed, macerated appearance
    - Often extremely painful

DIAGNOSTIC TESTS & INTERPRETATION

Imaging

Initial approach

- Radiographs may be warranted if no external cause found. Look for abnormalities in foot structure, bone spurs.
- Use of metallic radiographic marker and weight-bearing films often highlights the relationship between the callus and bony prominence.

Diagnostic Procedures/Surgery
Biopsy with microscopic evaluation in rare cases

Pathological Findings
Abnormal accumulation of keratin in epidermis, stratum corneum

DIFFERENTIAL DIAGNOSIS
- Plantar warts (typically a loss of skin lines within the wart)
- Porokeratoses (blocked sweat gland)

TREATMENT

MEDICATION
- Most therapy for corns and calluses can be done as self-care in the home.
- Use bandages, soft foam padding, or silicone sleeve over the affected area to decrease friction on the skin and promote healing with digital clavi.
- Use socks or gloves regularly.
- Use lotion/moisturizers for dry calluses and corns.
- Keratolytic agents such as urea or ammonium lactate can be applied safely.
- Use sandpaper discs or pumice stones over hard, thickened areas of skin.

Geriatric Considerations
- Use of salicylic acid corn plasters can cause skin breakdown and ulceration in patients with thin, atrophic skin; diabetes; and those with vascular compromise. The skin surrounding the callus will often turn white and can become quite painful.

ADDITIONAL TREATMENT

General Measures
- Debridement of affected tissue and use of protective padding
- Low-heeled shoes, soft upper with deep and wide toebox
- Extra-width shoes for 5th toe corns
- Avoidance of activities that contribute to painful lesions
- Prefabricated or custom orthotics

Issues for Referral
- May benefit from referral to podiatrist if use of topical agents and shoe changes are ineffective.
- Abnormalities in foot structure may require surgical treatment.
- Diabetic, vascular, and neuropathic patients may benefit from referral to podiatrist for regular foot exams to prevent infection, ulceration.

COMPLEMENTARY AND ALTERNATIVE MEDICINE
- Many OTC topical ointments and lotions available for calluses (Keralac, Callex, urea, Lac-Hydrin). Do not use on broken skin.
- Epsom salt soaks for 5–10 minutes at a time

SURGERY/OTHER PROCEDURES
- Surgical treatment of areas of protruding bone where corns and calluses form
- Rebalancing of foot pressure through functional foot orthotics
- Shaving or cutting off hardened area of skin using a chisel or 15-blade scalpel. For corns, remove keratin core and place pad over area during healing.

IN-PATIENT CONSIDERATIONS

Admission Criteria
- Admission usually not necessary, unless progression to ulcerated lesion with signs of severe infection, gangrene
- May require aggressive debridement in operating room should an abscess or deep-space infection be suspected.

Nursing
Wound care, dressing changes for infected lesions

ONGOING CARE

PATIENT EDUCATION
- General information available at: http://www.mayoclinic.com/health/corns-and-calluses/DS00033/DSECTION=9
- American Podiatric Medical Association. Available at: http://www.apma.org

PROGNOSIS
Complete cure is possible once factors causing injury are eliminated.

COMPLICATIONS
Ulceration, infection

ADDITIONAL READING

- Freeman DB. Corns and calluses resulting from mechanical hyperkeratosis. *Am Fam Physician*. 2002;65:2277–80.
- Pinzur MS, Slovenkai MP, Trepman E, et al. Guidelines for diabetic foot care: recommendations endorsed by the Diabetes Committee of the American Orthopaedic Foot and Ankle Society. *Foot Ankle Int*. 2005;26:113–9.
- Theodosat A. Skin diseases of the lower extremities in the elderly. *Dermatol Clin*. 2004;22:13–21.

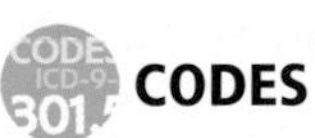

CODES

ICD9
700 Corns and callosities

CLINICAL PEARLS

Most therapy for corns and calluses can be done as self-care in the home using padding over the affected area to decrease friction.

C

COSTOCHONDRITIS

Scott A. Fields, MD

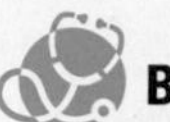

BASICS

DESCRIPTION

- Anterior chest wall pain associated with pain and tenderness of the costochondral and costosternal regions
- System(s) affected: Musculoskeletal
- Synonym(s): Costosternal syndrome; Parasternal chondrodynia; Anterior chest wall syndrome; Tietze disease and syndrome; Chondrocostal junction syndrome

Pediatric Considerations

Pay special attention to psychogenic chest pain in children who perceive family discord.

EPIDEMIOLOGY

- Predominant age: 20–40 years
- Predominant gender: Female

Incidence

~10% of chest pain complaints; 15–20% of teenagers with chest pain may have costochondritis.

RISK FACTORS

- Unusual physical activity or overuse
- Recent trauma (including motor vehicle accident, domestic violence, etc.) or new activity
- Recent upper respiratory infection (URI)

ETIOLOGY

- Not fully understood
- Trauma
- Overuse

COMMONLY ASSOCIATED CONDITIONS

URI

DIAGNOSIS

- Insidious onset
- Pain, usually sharp, sometimes pleuritic
- Pain involves multiple locations, the 2nd–5th costal cartilages are most often involved.
- Pain worsens with movement and breathing.
- Heat often relieves pain.
- Chest tightness is often associated with the pain.
- Pain sometimes radiates into arm.
- Nonsuppurative edema and tenderness at rib articulations
- Redness and warmth at sites of tenderness

HISTORY

A complete and thorough history is mandatory for the diagnosis, with special emphasis on cardiac risk factor evaluation.

PHYSICAL EXAM

A physical exam to exclude more serious conditions that may present with chest pain is necessary for the diagnosis. Tenderness elicited over the costochondral junctions is necessary to establish the diagnosis, but does not completely exclude other causes of chest pain.

Geriatric Considerations

- Often presents with multiple problems capable of causing chest pain, making a thorough history and physical exam imperative.

DIAGNOSTIC TESTS & INTERPRETATION

Lab

- The diagnosis of costochondritis is primarily based on a thorough history and physical exam.
- Laboratory exams should be used only if concern exists regarding other elements of the differential diagnosis.
- Erythrocyte sedimentation rate is inconsistently elevated.

Imaging

No imaging is indicated for the diagnosis of costochondritis; chest x-ray normal.

Diagnostic Procedures/Surgery

None indicated for the diagnosis of costochondritis

Pathological Findings

Costochondral joint inflammation

DIFFERENTIAL DIAGNOSIS

- Cardiac:
  - Coronary artery disease
  - Aortic aneurysm
  - Mitral valve prolapse
  - Pericarditis
  - Myocarditis
- Gastrointestinal:
  - Gastroesophageal reflux
  - Peptic esophagitis
  - Esophageal spasm
  - Gastritis
- Musculoskeletal:
  - Fibromyalgia
  - Slipping rib syndrome involves the lower ribs
  - Costovertebral arthritis
  - Painful xiphoid syndrome
  - Rib trauma with swelling
  - Thoracic disc compression
  - Ankylosing spondylitis
  - Epidemic myalgia
  - Precordial catch syndrome
- Psychogenic:
  - Anxiety disorder
  - Panic attacks
  - Hyperventilation
- Respiratory:
  - Asthma
  - Pulmonary embolism
  - Pneumonia
  - Chronic cough
  - Pneumothorax
- Other:
  - Domestic violence and abuse
  - Herpes zoster
  - Spinal tumor
  - Metastatic cancer
  - Substance abuse (cocaine)

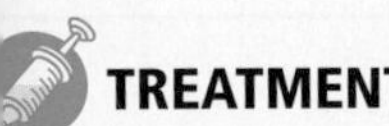

TREATMENT

eassurance of benign nature of condition

MEDICATION

irst Line

onsteroidal anti-inflammatory drugs (aspirin, uprofen, naproxen, or diclofenac). Narcotics rarely dicated (1,2)[C].

econd Line

cetaminophen (1,2)[C]

ADDITIONAL TREATMENT

General Measures

- Patient reassurance, rest, and heat (or ice massage)
- Stretching exercises

COMPLEMENTARY AND ALTERNATIVE MEDICINE

imited data on use of manipulation or ice massage, ut may be safely tried if patient interested

N-PATIENT CONSIDERATIONS

Admission Criteria

Only indicated if differential diagnosis is unclear and ardiac or other more serious etiology of chest pain is eing considered (3)[C]

Discharge Criteria

When diagnosis is established

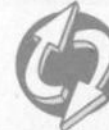

ONGOING CARE

FOLLOW-UP RECOMMENDATIONS

Follow-up within 1 week if diagnosis is unclear

DIET

Normal

PATIENT EDUCATION

Educate the patient in regard to the self-limited (although potentially recurrent) nature of the illness. Instruct patient on proper physical activity regimens to avoid overuse syndromes. Also stress importance of avoiding sudden, significant changes in activity.

PROGNOSIS

- Self-limited illness, although sometimes chronic
- Often recurs

COMPLICATIONS

Incomplete attention to differential diagnosis or inappropriate interventions in a desire to ensure that a more life-threatening diagnosis is not missed

REFERENCES

1. Freeston J, Karim Z, Lindsay K, et al. Can early diagnosis and management of costochondritis reduce acute chest pain admissions? *J Rheumatol*. 2004;31:2269–71.
2. Jensen S. Musculoskeletal causes of chest pain. *Aust Fam Physician*. 2001;30:834–9.
3. Mukamel M, Kornreich L, Horev G, et al. Tietze's syndrome in children and infants. *J Pediatr*. 1997;131:774–5.

ADDITIONAL READING

- Disla E, Rhim HR, Reddy A, et al. Costochondritis. A prospective analysis in an emergency department setting. *Arch Intern Med*. 1994;154:2466–9.
- Gregory PL, Biswas AC, Batt ME. Musculoskeletal problems of the chest wall in athletes. *Sports Med*. 2002;32:235–50.
- Rovetta G, Sessarego P, Monteforte P et al. Stretching exercises for costochondritis pain. *G Ital Med Lav Ergon*. 169–71.

See Also (Topic, Algorithm, Electronic Media Element)

Algorithm: Chest Pain

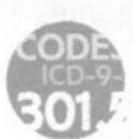

CODES

ICD9

733.6 Tietze's disease

CLINICAL PEARLS

- A very common disorder, accounting for perhaps 10% of all cases of chest pain, and a greater percentage in teenagers and young adults
- Educate the patient in regard to the self-limited (although potentially recurrent) nature of the illness. Instruct patient on proper physical activity regimens to avoid overuse syndromes. Also stress importance of avoiding sudden, significant changes in activity.
- Consider an anxiety disorder as a contributor to all cases of persistent chest pain, whether musculoskeletal or cardiac.

COUNSELING TYPES

William T. Garrison, PhD

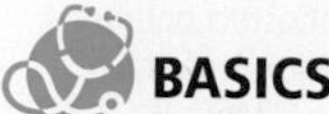

BASICS

DESCRIPTION

- Psychotherapeutic and counseling interventions play an important role in the management of chronic- and acute-onset diseases and disorders. They are typically the primary initial mode of evaluation and/or treatment for most mild-to-moderate psychiatric disorders that reach criteria using the DSM or ICD diagnostic classification systems. Treatment and successful control of either medical or psychological conditions require some form of professional counseling experience. Best outcomes occur when they are employed by a skilled practitioner. However, psychotherapy differs from generic counseling, which can take many forms and is delivered commonly in nonmedical settings with mixed results.
- Counseling approaches are usually tailored to the specific presenting problem or issue, and serve educational and emotional support functions. Typically, such counseling in medical settings will be time-limited and problem-focused, and is often not intended to lead to major medical symptom relief or major behavioral changes.
- The goals of psychotherapy range from increasing individual psychological insight and motivation for change, reduction of interpersonal conflict in the marriage or family, reduction of chronic or acute emotional suffering, and reversal of dysfunctional or habitual behaviors. There are several general types of psychotherapy, starting with individual, marital, or family approaches. In addition, a number of psychological theories guide various methods and treatment philosophies. The following is a brief overview of commonly used psychotherapeutic and counseling methods.
- Psychodynamic therapy: Unconscious conflict manifests as patient's symptoms/problem behaviors:
  - Short-term (4–6 mo) and long-term (1 yr+)
  - Focus is on increasing insight of underlying conflict to initiate symptomatic change.
  - Therapist actively helps patient identify patterns of behavior stemming from existence of an unconscious conflict.
- Cognitive behavioral therapy (CBT): Patterns of thoughts and behaviors can lead to development and/or maintenance of symptoms. Thought patterns may not accurately reflect reality and may lead to psychological distress:
  - Therapy aims at modifying thought patterns by increasing cognitive flexibility and changing dysfunctional behavioral patterns.
  - Encourages patient self-monitoring
  - Uses therapist-assisted challenges to patient's basic beliefs/assumptions
  - May utilize *exposure*, a procedure derived from basic learning theories
  - Can be offered in group or individual formats
  - Therapist role is suggestive and supportive.
- Dialectical behavior therapy (DBT): Techniques such as social skills training, mindfulness, and problem solving are used to modulate impulse control and affect management:
  - Derivative of CBT
  - Originally used in treatment of patients with self-destructive behaviors (e.g., cutting, suicide attempts)
  - Seeks to change rigid patterns of cognitions and behaviors that have been maladaptive
  - Utilizes both individual and group treatment modalities
  - Therapist takes an active role in interpretation and support.
- Interpersonal psychotherapy: Interpersonal relationships in a patient's life are linked to symptoms. Therapy seeks to alleviate symptoms and improve social adjustment through exploration of patients' relationships and experiences. Focus is on 1 of 4 potential problem areas:
  - Grief
  - Interpersonal role disputes
  - Role transitions
  - Interpersonal deficits: Therapist works with the patient in resolving the problematic interpersonal issues to facilitate change in symptoms
- Family therapy: Focuses on the family as a unit of intervention:
  - Uses psychoeducation to increase patient's and family's insight
  - Trains in communication and problem-solving skills
- Motivational interviewing: Focuses on motivation as a key to successful change process:
  - Short term
  - Focuses on identifying discrepancies between goals and behavior
  - "5 A's" model is a brief counseling framework developed specifically for physicians to effect behavioral change in patients:
    - Assess for a problem.
    - Advise making a change.
    - Agree on action to be taken.
    - Assist with self-care support to make the change.
    - Arrange follow-up to support the change.
- Counseling (heterogeneous treatment):
  - Often focuses on situational factors maintaining symptoms
  - Often encourages utilization of community resources
- Behavioral therapy: Relatively nontheoretical approach to behavioral change or symptom reduction/eradication through application of principles of stimulus and response

Pediatric Considerations

- Important distinctions are made between psychotherapy and counseling for children/teens compared to adults/couples.
- The focus of evaluation must include attention to parent and family processes and factors. Interventions typically include interactions and sessions with parents, as well as collateral work with teachers and other school personnel.
- Younger children will often be evaluated and diagnosed through behavioral descriptions provided by parents and other adults who know them well, as well as through direct observation and/or play techniques. Children of all ages should be screened using behavioral checklists that are norm-referenced for age.
- Any child or teenager who requests counseling should be interviewed initially by the primary care provider and referred appropriately. Most referrals will be in response to parental request, however.
- Psychotherapeutic interventions with the strongest empirical basis with children include behavior therapy/modification, CBT, and family/parenting therapy. Play therapy has the least empirical support, and insight-oriented therapies appear to be more effective with older children (>11 years).
- There is controversy regarding the efficacy of psychopharmacologic treatment in preadolescents, although clear benefits have been demonstrated in some studies. Treatment guidelines for mild-to-moderate depressed mood and/or anxiety disorders typically recommend pediatric CBT initially, and studies have supported this approach.

EPIDEMIOLOGY

- ~18.8 million adults suffer from clinical depression, and 20 million suffer from a diagnosable anxiety disorder.
- 1 in 4 Americans report seeking some form of mental health treatment in their adult life. This includes generic counseling in nonmedical settings such as work, clergy, or school settings, but also includes visits to primary care providers. It is estimated that between 3.5% and 5% of adults in the US actually participate in formal mental health psychotherapy annually.
- Public health experts report that the majority of those adults with diagnosable psychiatric disorders, however, do not receive professional mental health services. This is due to multiple factors, including failure to identify, noncompliance with psychiatric referral, regional shortages of providers, economic barriers, and excessive time duration from referral to available service.

A large study conducted between 1987 and 1997 concluded that the percentage of adults in psychotherapy remained relatively stable over that decade, the use of psychopharmacology doubled, and older adults (ages 55–64) increasingly sought psychotherapy services. In that same study, it was found that psychotherapy duration (number of sessions) decreased substantially and about 1/3 of psychotherapy patients only attended 1 or 2 sessions.

RISK FACTORS

The need for psychotherapy or counseling services is directly and indirectly associated with a host of socioeconomic and biogenetic factors, including the general effects of poverty, family or marital dysfunction, life stressors, medical diseases or conditions, and individual biologic predisposition to mental health disorders.

GENERAL PREVENTION

It is generally assumed that early identification and intervention of child and adolescent psychopathology increases the likelihood of reducing the risk for adult psychopathology, but this has not been sufficiently validated in all categories of psychological disorders. Data support such claims in disorders such as childhood attention deficit hyperactivity disorder, anxiety disorders, and habit disorders of childhood, however.

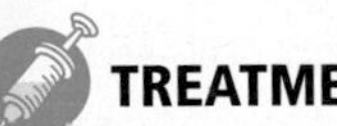

TREATMENT

MEDICATION

- Psychotherapy is most likely to be accompanied by use of pharmaceutical adjuncts in moderate-to-severe cases of psychological dysfunction that do not respond to other therapies, or in cases of extremely poor quality of life or high risk. The most common examples are in cases of clinical depression or anxiety that clearly incapacitates the patient or significantly reduces their quality of life. Patients at risk for suicide or who represent a danger to others are also candidates for acute psychopharmacotherapy. Studies suggest that verbal and behaviorally oriented therapies can add efficacy to medication treatment in both depression and anxiety.
- There is controversy in the research field regarding the efficacy of medication alone vs psychotherapy alone vs combined treatments. The most recent consensus has been that combined treatments in moderate-to-severe psychological dysfunction are most likely to render positive short-term results and increase the likelihood such effects can be sustained over time.

ADDITIONAL TREATMENT

General Measures

There is evidence of a "dose effect" in psychotherapy outcomes research, with some investigators suggesting that 6–8 sessions are necessary to yield positive initial effects, and upwards of 15–20 sessions for longer-term, sustainable therapeutic effects. This dose effect may not be applicable to counseling services with primarily informational or emotional/supportive functions.

Additional Therapies

- Anxiety disorders:
  - Panic disorder with and without agoraphobia (1)[A]: CBT, psychodynamic therapy
  - Generalized anxiety disorder: CBT (2)[A]
  - Obsessive-compulsive disorder: CBT (3)[A]
  - Post-traumatic stress disorder: CBT
  - Specific phobia: CBT
  - Social phobia: CBT (4)[A]
- Mood disorders:
  - Unipolar depression: CBT, interpersonal therapy, psychodynamic therapy (5)[A]
  - Bipolar disorder: Family therapy, interpersonal therapy, CBT
  - Schizophrenia: Psychodynamic therapy, family therapy, CBT
- Eating disorders:
  - Binge eating disorder: CBT, interpersonal therapy
  - Bulimia nervosa: CBT, interpersonal therapy
- Personality disorders:
  - Borderline: DBT, CBT
- Substance-use disorders:
  - Alcohol: Counseling, CBT, motivational interviewing
  - Cocaine: CBT, counseling
  - Heroin: CBT, counseling
  - Smoking: 5 A's
- Somatoform disorders:
  - Hypochondriasis: CBT
  - Body dysmorphic disorder: CBT

COMPLEMENTARY AND ALTERNATIVE MEDICINE

A host of nonempirically based psychological and nutritional therapies can be found outside of mainstream medicine and psychological science. Very little or no evidence exists to support such experimental therapies, but all have the considerable power of the placebo effect fueling their anecdotal supports or claims. Placebo effects are also thought to be further enhanced by the use of ingested or applied substances that create perceived or real physiologic changes in the patient.

REFERENCES

1. Furukawa TA, et al. Combined psychotherapy plus antidepressants for panic disorder with or without agoraphobia. *Cochrane Database Sys Rev.* 2007;2: CD004364.
2. Hunot V, et al. Psychological therapies for generalized anxiety disorder. *Cochrane Database Sys Rev.* 2007;2.
3. Eddy KT, Dutra L, Bradley R, et al. A multidimensional meta-analysis of psychotherapy and pharmacotherapy for obsessive-compulsive disorder. *Clin Psychol Rev.* 2004;24:1011–30.
4. Rodebaugh TL, Holaway RM, Heimberg RG. The treatment of social anxiety disorder. *Clin Psychol Rev.* 2004;24:883–908.
5. Bortolotti B, Menchetti M, Bellini F, et al. Psychological interventions for major depression in primary care: a meta-analytic review of randomized controlled trials. *Gen Hosp Psychiatry.* 2008;30: 293–302.

CODES

ICD9

- V65.49 Other specified counseling
- V65.8 Other reasons for seeking consultation

CLINICAL PEARLS

- Combined medication and psychotherapeutic treatments in moderate-to-severe psychological dysfunction are most likely to render positive short-term results and increase the likelihood such effects can be sustained over time. Relapse is common over time and/or as treatments are discontinued.
- There is evidence of a "dose effect" in psychotherapy outcomes research, with some investigators suggesting that 6–8 sessions are necessary to yield positive initial effects, and upwards of 15–20 sessions for longer-term, sustainable therapeutic effects. This dose effect may not be applicable to counseling services with primarily informational or emotional/supportive functions. Since many patients cease attendance to psychotherapy sessions after one or a few sessions, most interventions of this type cannot be accurately evaluated by the referring provider.

CROHN DISEASE

Gary I. Levine, MD

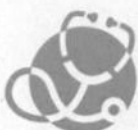

BASICS

DESCRIPTION
Idiopathic inflammatory disease of the alimentary tract that may present anywhere in the GI tract; most commonly found in the terminal ileum (60%), but may be limited to the colon in 15–20%, proximal small bowel 10%:
- Transmural disease
- May involve multiple regions of the intestine in between normal sections (skip lesions)

EPIDEMIOLOGY
Incidence
- Annual incidence of 3–7 cases per 100,000
- In US, more common in whites
- Predominant age: 15–25 years; 2nd, smaller peak in ages 55–65 years
- Female > Male
- 2–4 × increased risk in Ashkenazi Jewish ethnicity

Prevalence
20–100 per 100,000

RISK FACTORS
Cigarette smoking (2 × higher risk in smokers)

Genetics
- 15% of patients have 1st-degree relatives with inflammatory bowel disease, and develop the disease with similar patterns and age of onset.
- Chances of having a child with Crohn disease = 5% if mother has CD, 36% if both parents have CD

PATHOPHYSIOLOGY
- Segmental disease with patchy distribution and variable severity
- Strictures common; may prevent passage of the endoscope
- Aphthous ulcers found on mucosal surfaces
- Histologic features: Transmural inflammation, crypt abscesses, noncaseating granulomas

ETIOLOGY
- Combination of genetic factors, environmental factors, and immunologic abnormalities:
  - IBD locus on chromosome 16 - CARD15/NOD2; also on chromosomes 5q, 6p, and 19
- Idiopathic, immune-mediated Th-1 cells organize cell-mediated response, which involves tumor necrosis factor, interferon, and interleukin 12

COMMONLY ASSOCIATED CONDITIONS
- Arthritis, skin lesions, erythema nodosum, nonspecific rashes, pyoderma gangrenosum; gallstones; sclerosing cholangitis in ~10%
- Increased risk of both colorectal cancer and small bowel cancer: RR = 5–20 (1)

DIAGNOSIS

PHYSICAL EXAM
- Vary with area of intestinal involvement:
  - Diarrhea occurs in most patients.
  - Abdominal pain in 2/3; occasional mass
  - Weight loss, malaise
  - Growth failure in children
  - Low-grade fever
  - Fistula: Perirectal, bladder, skin, vagina
  - Extraluminal disease (25–35%): Skin, iritis, arthritis, sclerosing cholangitis, multifocal osteomyelitis
- Small-bowel disease only (15–30%):
  - Diarrhea prominent, including nocturnal
  - Vague abdominal pain frequent
  - Intestinal obstruction (1/3): Cramping abdominal pain precedes for months.
  - Bleeding in 20%, rarely massive
  - Perianal disease, including fistulae
- Colon disease only (25–30%):
  - Diarrhea prominent, including nocturnal
  - Hematochezia
  - Abdominal pain in 50%, relieved by stooling
  - Perianal disease in 40%, fistulae
  - Weight loss prominent
  - Megacolon in 10%
  - Intestinal obstruction occasional
- Colon and small-bowel disease (40–60%):
  - Intestinal obstruction much more common than in other types

DIAGNOSTIC TESTS & INTERPRETATION
Constellation of barium-identified distribution of lesions, endoscopic findings, and biopsies usually establish the diagnosis.

Lab
- Anemia (microcytic) is common.
- Albumin level decreased in severe cases
- Serum electrolytes imbalance
- Steatorrhea
- Elevated sedimentation rate, C-reactive protein
- Vitamin levels to evaluate specific nutrient deficiency (vitamin B_{12}, fat-soluble vitamins)
- Serologic biomarkers:
  - Used as adjuncts to other diagnostic modalities and clinical judgement
  - May predict disease behavior, but do not correlate with disease activity
  - ASCAs (anti-saccharomyces cerevisiae antibodies)
    - Elevated in Crohn disease (50–60% of patients) and ulcerative colitis (10–15%)
  - Atypical pANCA (perinuclear antineutrophil cytoplasmic antibody) titer:
    - Elevated in ulcerative colitis (40–80%) and Crohn disease (5–25%)
  - Antiglycan antibody titer
    - Highly specific, poor sensitivity for CD Dx
    - ALCA, ACCA, AMCA:
  - Anti-OmpC antibody
    - 55% CD, 10% UC
  - Anti-I2 IgA
    - 30–50% CD, 10% UC
  - Anti-pancreatic antibodies
    - 30% CD, 2–6% UC
  - Anti-CBir1 antibodies
    - 50% CD, 6% UC

Imaging
- Barium radiographs: Enema and small bowel:
  - Loss of smooth mucosa, undermined ulcers, narrowed lumen (string sign), fistulae, skip areas
- CT scans:
  - Thickening of bowel wall, strictures, and dilatation; abscess and fistulae; perirectal disease
  - CT enterography (CTE): Superior to plain CT
    - IV contrast and low-density oral contrast
- MR enteroscopy (MRE): Superior to CTE for pelvic soft tissue and perianal fistulae
  - Safer in pregnancy and renal insufficiency
- Ultrasound:
  - May identify bowel wall thickening, distinguish fibrosis from edema

Diagnostic Procedures/Surgery
- Colonoscopy; EGD; small bowel capsule endoscopy 40–70% diagnostic yield in CD (contraindicated if strictures)
- Double balloon endoscopy: Use when capsule endoscopy contraindicated or obstructive symptoms
- Biopsy of mucosa helpful but not diagnostic: Helps rule out other causes

Pathological Findings
- All layers of intestinal wall, with inflammation in at least focal areas in >95% of cases
- Skip areas; granuloma in up to 50% of resected specimen; fat hypertrophy

DIFFERENTIAL DIAGNOSIS
- Appendicitis; ulcerative, collagenous, lymphocytic, ischemic or drug-induced colitis; radiation enteritis
- PID, endometriosis, IBS, diverticulitis, infection, malignancy, or small bowel disease

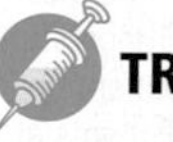

TREATMENT

General treatment goals include the reduction of abdominal pain, diarrhea, fatigue, anemia, nutritional deficiencies, extraintestinal manifestations, hospitalizations, surgeries, abcesses, fistulas, infections, and malignancies.

MEDICATION
First Line
- Traditional "step up" therapy. 5-ASA derivatives and adrenocorticosteroids are used to induce remission, and azathioprine and 6-MP are used to maintain remission. Treatment also includes appropriate symptomatic measures and supportive care (e.g., antispasmodic and antidiarrheals).
- "Top down" therapy. Anti-TNF alpha agents and immunomodulators as initial treatment if high risk of rapidly progressive disease.
- To induce remission in naive patient, relapse, or severe sx:
  - Sulfasalazine or mesalamine: 2–4 g/d
    - Useful in mild disease
    - Sulfasalazine more effective in CD colitis
    - Add folic acid 1–2 mg/day
  - Prednisone: 40–60 mg/d O:
    - For moderate disease, small bowel CD
    - 50% become steroid-dependent or resistant within 1 year
    - Not effective for maintaining remission

– Budesonide: 9 mg/day can be administered topically or orally; synthetic glucocorticoid with reduced bioavailability:
  ○ Alternative to prednisone in patients requiring long-term steroid use
  ○ Partially avoids steroid complications
– Antibiotics:
  ○ Ciprofloxacin 1 g/day
  ○ Rifaximin 800 mg b.i.d.: 50% achieve remission in 6–12 weeks
– Enteral nutritional therapy:
  ○ 60% remission rate, requires feeding tube

To achieve remission in patients who relapse with prednisone tapering or fail to respond, or to maintain remission:

– Add azathioprine (Imuran) 2–3 mg/kg/d or mercaptopurine (6-MP) 1–1.5 mg/kg/d. If good response, taper steroid, effective in maintaining remission:
  ○ Check TPMT levels prior to beginning therapy—predictive of development of leukopenia. Full level: Use normal dose; intermediate level: Use 1/2 normal dose; zero–low level: Do not use azathioprine or 6-MP
– Methotrexate 25 mg IM weekly to achieve remission, then 15 mg/week to maintain remission as an alternative to 6-MP or azathioprine
  ○ Add folic acid 1–2 mg/day, monitor LFTs.

- If inadequate response to achieve or maintain remission or for Rx of symptomatic nonresponsive fistulas or extraintestinal manifestations, maintain patient on immunosuppressant and start a course of anti-TNF monoclonal antibody:
  – Infliximab (Remicade)
    ○ Chimeric (75% human and 25% murine) IgG-1 monoclonal antibody vs TNF
    ○ 5 mg/kg infusion, repeat at 2 wks, 6 wks, then every 8 wks; can increase to 10 mg/kg if needed
    ○ Used with azathioprine, 6-MP, or methotrexate to reduce infliximab antibody formation
    ○ Increases risk of TB 7 ×, need to screen for latent TB prior to starting this medication
    ○ Active intra-abdominal abscess is a contraindication to use.
  – Adalimumab (Humira):
    ○ Recombinant human IgG-1 monoclonal antibody vs TNF
    ○ Given by subcutaneous injection
    ○ Used with infliximab failure or intolerance
  – Certolizumab pegol (Cimzia):
    ○ Pegylated 95% humanized Fab fragment of anti-TNF monoclonal antibody
    ○ Given by subcutaneous injection
    ○ Used with infliximab failure or intolerance
  – Natalizumab (Tysabri):
    ○ Humanized IgG4 monoclonal antibody vs alpha 4 integrin-mediated leukocyte migration
    ○ Used in CD patients with active inflammation not responsive to or unable to tolerate anti TNF alpha Rx
    ○ Increased risk of JC virus progressive multifocal leukoencephalopathy
- If tenesmus or bleeding prominent:
  – Mesalamine enema or hydrocortisone enema maintenance therapy
- Predominantly perirectal disease with fistulae:
  – Metronidazole (Flagyl) 250 mg t.i.d. for maximum of 8 weeks
- Patients with joint, eye, and skin extraintestinal manifestations:
  – Unresponsive to mesalamine, occasionally responsive to prednisone
  – Usually responsive to infliximab
- For all well-controlled patients:
  – Loperamide (Imodium) 2 mg to control diarrhea to avoid interference with daily life

Second Line

- Cyclosporine: Has assisted in closing fistulae when other measures fail; otherwise, not useful
- Tacrolimus: Reserved for nonresponders

ADDITIONAL TREATMENT

General Measures

- Attention to maintaining weight and nutrition
- Physical rest and relief of emotional stress
- Perirectal disease: Sitz baths, soap and water after stooling, surgical drainage of perirectal abscesses, surgical treatment of recurrent fistulae if medical management fails
- Folate supplementation may potentially decrease risk for malignancy (2)[B].

Additional Therapies

Vaccinations:

- Hepatitis B, HPV, pneumococcus, influenza, varicella; give at disease ONSET

COMPLEMENTARY AND ALTERNATIVE MEDICINE

Trichuris suis (porcine whipworm) ova administration has been effective in clinical trials in inducing and maintaining remission without significant side effects.

SURGERY/OTHER PROCEDURES

- Palliative, not curative: Laparoscopic or open
- Relapse rates after intestinal resection:
  – 5 years: 30–35%; 10 years: 50–55%; 15 years: 60–75%; 25 years: 95%
- Indications:
  – Failure of medical management
  – Total or recurrent intestinal obstruction or abscess
  – Perforation, hemorrhage, fistula, failure to thrive
  – Toxic megacolon, extensive disease, or cancer
  – Failure of ostomy to function after ≥1 year

ONGOING CARE

FOLLOW-UP RECOMMENDATIONS

Patient Monitoring

- Regular assessment (every 3–6 months if patient is stable), particularly status of weight, pain, diarrhea, hemoglobin, and sed rate
- Crohn Disease Activity Index (CDAI) score is an objective measure for recording disease activity that can be used to assess response to therapy:
  – <150 = remission, 150–220 = mild disease, 221–400 = moderate disease, >400 = severe disease
- Surveillance colonoscopy beginning 8 years after Crohn colitis diagnosis and every 1–3 years thereafter (1)[B]:
  – Biopsy any abnormal mucosa or stricture
  – 4-quadrant biopsy of normal mucosa every 10 cm
- Check liver tests yearly.
- Check vitamin B_{12} level in those with ileal disease or ileal resection.
- Check folate level in all on 5-aminosalicylate; use supplements in all.
- Follow CBC, LFTs, and consider monitoring 6-MMP and 6-TG levels in patients on AZA or 6-MP.
- Follow LFTs in patients on methotrexate.

DIET

- If fat malabsorption, diminish fat in diet.
- If strictures or recurrent obstruction, avoid highly fibrous substances.
- If diarrhea prominent, increase dietary fiber (sometimes recommended), decrease fat.
- Enteral nutrition preferred over parenteral

PATIENT EDUCATION

Crohn and Colitis Foundation of America, Inc., 11th floor, Park Ave. South, NY 10016, Phone (800) 343–3637.

PROGNOSIS

- Chronic condition with variable but nearly certain progression
- Average patient has surgery every 7 years: Short-bowel syndrome common after >4 surgeries:
  – 50–75% require surgery after 5 years, 70–90% after 10 years
- Most are able to maintain normal life.
- Fertility rate is the same as population at large.
- Pregnancy
  – Increased risk of spontaneous abortion/stillbirth; preterm birth and low birth weight infant; labor and delivery complications
  – No increased risk of congenital malformations
  – Risk of disease flare is same if pregnant or not pregnant.

COMPLICATIONS

- Fistulae (15%): Perirectal, cutaneous, enterovaginal, and enterovesicular
- Extraluminal disease (25%): Skin, uveal tract, joint, bone, and biliary tract
- Colon perforation, toxic megacolon, sepsis, hemorrhage, ischemia, gallstones in >25%, osteoporosis
- Depression and anxiety in 15%, 3 × normal population
- Colon cancer:
  – Extensive colon disease associated with 6 × increased risk of adenocarcinoma (3)

REFERENCES

1. Rubin DT, Kavitt RT. Surveillance for cancer and dysplasia in inflammatory bowel disease. *Gastroenterol Clin North Am*. 2006;35:581–604.
2. Chan EP, Lichtenstein GR. Chemoprevention: risk reduction with medical therapy of inflammatory bowel disease. *Gastroenterol Clin North Am*. 2006;35:675–712.
3. Jess T, Gamborg M, Matzen P, et al. Increased risk of intestinal cancer in Crohn's disease: a meta-analysis of population-based cohort studies. *Am J Gastroenterol*. 2005;100:2724–9.

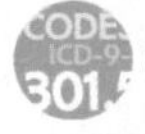

CODES

ICD9

- 555.0 Regional enteritis of small intestine
- 555.1 Regional enteritis of large intestine
- 555.2 Regional enteritis of small intestine with large intestine

CLINICAL PEARLS

- Crohn disease involves skip areas; ulcerative colitis extends continuously from rectum.
- Surgery is not curative; it is palliative. Recurrence is common after surgery.
- Cancer risk is greatest with Crohn colitis, and surveillance colonoscopy is strongly recommended.

CROUP (LARYNGOTRACHEOBRONCHITIS)

Garreth C. Biegun, MD

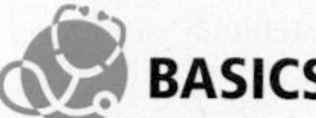

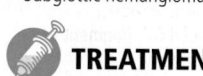

BASICS

DESCRIPTION

- Croup is a subacute viral illness characterized by upper-airway symptoms such as barking cough, stridor, and fever. "Croup" is used to refer to viral laryngotracheitis or laryngotracheobronchitis (LTB), though it is sometimes used for LTB with pneumonitis, bacterial tracheitis, or spasmodic croup.
- Most common cause of upper-airway obstruction or stridor in children
- System(s) affected: Pulmonary; Respiratory
- Synonym(s): Croup; Infectious croup; Viral croup; LTB
- Spasmodic croup: Noninfectious form with sudden resolution:
  - No fever or radiographic changes
  - Initially treated as croup
  - Usually self-limited and resolves with mist therapy at home
  - Often recurs on same night or in 2–3 nights

EPIDEMIOLOGY

- Predominant age (1):
  - Common, 7 months to 3 years
  - Most common in 2nd year of life
  - Rare >6 years
- Predominant sex: Male > Female (1.5:1) (1)
- Timing:
  - Any time of year possible, but most common in fall and winter (with parainfluenza 1 and respiratory syncytial virus [RSV])

Incidence

- 6 cases of croup per year per 100 children <6 years old
- 1.5–6% of cases require hospitalization.
- 2–6% of those require intubation.
- Decreasing incidence in the US and Canada

RISK FACTORS

- Past history of croup
- Recurrent upper respiratory infections
- Atopic disease increases risk of spasmodic croup.

PATHOPHYSIOLOGY

- Subglottic region/larynx is entirely encircled by the cricoid cartilage.
- Inflammatory edema and subglottic mucus production decrease airway radius.
- Small children have small airways with more compliant walls.
- Negative-pressure inspiration pulls airway walls closer together.
- Small decrease in airway radius causes significant increase in resistance (Poiseuille law: Resistance proportional to 1/radius^4).

ETIOLOGY

- Usually viruses that initially infect oropharyngeal mucosa and then migrate inferiorly
- Parainfluenza virus:
  - Most common pathogen: 75% of cases
  - Type 1 is most common, causing 18% of all cases of croup.
  - Types 2, 3, and 4 are also common.
  - Type 3 may cause a particularly severe illness.
- Other viruses:
  - RSV
  - Paramyxovirus
  - Influenza virus type A or B
  - Adenovirus
  - Rhinovirus
  - Enteroviruses (Coxsackie and Echo)
  - Reovirus
  - Measles virus where vaccination not common
- *Haemophilus influenzae* type B now rare with routine immunization (2)
- May have bacterial cause: *Mycoplasma pneumoniae* has been reported.

COMMONLY ASSOCIATED CONDITIONS

If recurrent (>2 episodes in a year) or in 1st 90 days of life, consider host factors:

- Underlying anatomic abnormality (e.g., subglottic stenosis)
- Paradoxical vocal cord dysfunction
- Gastroesophageal reflux disease
- Prolonged neonatal intubation

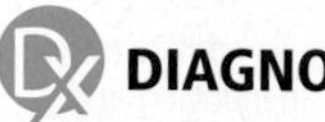

DIAGNOSIS

- Most children who present with acute onset of barky cough, stridor, and chest-wall indrawing have croup.
- Croup is a clinical diagnosis; labs and imaging serve only ancillary purposes (3).
- Classic "seal-like" barking, spasmodic cough
- May have biphasic stridor
- Low-grade to moderate fever
- Upper-respiratory infection prodrome lasting 1–7 days
- Severity usually determined by clinical observation for signs of respiratory effort: Nasal flaring, retractions, tripoding, sniffing position, abdominal breathing, tachypnea. Late: Hypoxia/cyanosis or fatigue.
- Westley Croup Scale (≤2 mild; 3–7 moderate; ≥8 severe):
  - Level of consciousness: Normal, including sleep = 0; disoriented = 5
  - Cyanosis: None = 0; with agitation = 4; at rest = 5
  - Stridor: None = 0; with agitation = 1; at rest = 2
  - Air entry: Normal = 0; decreased = 1; markedly decreased = 2
  - Retractions: None = 0; mild = 1; moderate = 2; severe = 3
- Nontoxic-appearing child: Normal voice, no drooling
- No change in stridor with positioning
- Nontender larynx
- Inflamed subglottic region with normal-appearing supraglottic region

HISTORY

- 2–3 days nonspecific prodromal syndrome with low-grade fever, coryza, rhinorrhea
- Onset and recurrence at night when child is sleeping
- Symptoms often resolve en route to hospital as child is exposed to cool night air.
- Lack of prodrome indicates spasmodic croup.

PHYSICAL EXAM

- Pulse oximetry often is normal because there is no disturbance of alveolar gas exchange.
- Overall appearance: Child comfortable or struggling?
- Work of breathing: Labored or comfortable?
- Sound of breathing and voice: Hoarse, stridor, inspiratory wheezing, short sentences?
- Observed/subjective tidal volume: Sufficient for child size?

DIAGNOSTIC TESTS & INTERPRETATION

Lab

- No laboratory abnormality is diagnostic.
- White blood cells may be low, normal, or elevated.
- Lymphocytosis expected but not required
- Rapid antigen or viral culture tests are available in some centers:
  - Guide isolation precautions not management

Imaging

- Posteroanterior and lateral neck films show funnel-shaped subglottic region with normal epiglottis: "Steeple," "hour glass," or "pencil point" sign (present in 40–60% of children with laryngotracheobronchitis).
- CT may be more sensitive for defining etiology of obstruction in a confusing clinical picture.
- Patient should be monitored during imaging; progression of airway obstruction may be rapid.

Pathological Findings

- Inflammatory reaction of respiratory mucosa
- Loss of epithelial cells
- Thick mucoid secretions

DIFFERENTIAL DIAGNOSIS

- Epiglottitis: Currently rare
- Foreign-body aspiration
- Subglottic stenosis (congenital or acquired)
- Bacterial tracheitis
- Simple upper-respiratory infection
- Retropharyngeal or peritonsillar abscess
- Trauma
- Allergic reaction (acute angioneurotic edema)
- Airway anomalies (e.g., tracheo/laryngomalacia)
- Subglottic hemangioma

TREATMENT

MEDICATION

First Line

- Well established in literature; cornerstones of treatment are immediate nebulized epinephrine and dexamethasone (4)[A].
- Racemic or L-epinephrine (equal efficacy and side-effect profiles; L-epinephrine is used for most other hospital purposes and is less expensive):
  - Racemic epinephrine: 0.05 mL/kg/dose (max, 0.5 mL) of 2.25% solution nebulized in normal saline total volume 3 mL (5)[A](6)[B]
  - L-epinephrine: 0.5 mL/kg per dose (max of 5 mL) of a 1:1000 dilution
  - Onset in 1–5 minutes, duration 2 hours
  - Repeat as necessary if side effects tolerated
  - Must observe child for 3–4 hours

Corticosteroids: (7)[A]:
- Dexamethasone (cheapest, most literature, easiest), 0.15–0.6 mg/kg; higher doses have been traditional care, but studies have proven 0.15 mg/kg has equal efficacy (8). Single dose, IV/IM/PO have proven equal efficacy (9)[A]
- Nebulized budesonide also proven effective (10)[B]
- Onset by 6 hours

Heli-Ox: A helium-oxygen mixture:
- Smaller, lower-mass helium molecule (compared to nitrogen) theoretically maintains laminar flow in narrower airways, serves as bridge therapy to steroids.
- Minimum 60% helium must be used; 70% preferable; 79% if patient has no O_2 requirement
- There is limited data. Anecdotal reports and 1 case series support its use, but 2 prospective studies showed no benefit (11,12). Also, a Cochrane review found insufficient evidence to support the use of Heliox in croup (13).

Antibiotics not indicated in this viral illness:
- Antecedent or subsequent bacterial infection is possible but uncommon.

Oxygen as needed

Contraindications, precautions, and significant possible interactions: Refer to the manufacturer's literature.

Second Line

Amantadine for influenza A: 100 mg PO b.i.d. for 3–5 days

ADDITIONAL TREATMENT

General Measures

- Minimize labs, imaging, and other procedures that upset the child; agitation that worsens tachypnea is more detrimental than accepting a clinical diagnosis.
- Electrocardiogram monitoring and pulse oximetry:
  - Frequent checks are more sensitive to worsening disease than is pulse-oximetry.

COMPLEMENTARY AND ALTERNATIVE MEDICINE

- Mist therapy often helps with symptoms. Do not use high-temperature misters (e.g., tea kettles) due to risk of burns. Sitting with child in bathroom with hot shower running is a good steam generator.
- Some children respond well to cold, dry air.

SURGERY/OTHER PROCEDURES

- Intubation rarely required; tube 0.5–1 mm smaller than normal:
  - After trial of medical management, intubation is for fatigue due to work of breathing or beginning total obstruction; not secondary to low oxygen saturation.
  - Extubate in 3–5 days when there is an appropriate air-leak around the endotracheal tube.
- Tracheotomy: Rarely, maintenance 3–7 days

IN-PATIENT CONSIDERATIONS

Initial Stabilization

- Outpatient care in mild cases
- Admission for patients who do not respond to therapy, or who have O_2 requirement, pneumonia, or congestive heart failure
- In most cases, emergency department observation after medical management is sufficient.

Admission Criteria

Minor cases need no visit to hospital or primary care physician (PCP):
- No stridor at rest, no difficulty breathing
- Child able to tolerate PO liquids
- No underlying medical condition
- Caretakers able to assess changes to clinical picture and reassess medical care

Discharge Criteria

Patients who maintain a good response to medical therapy for 3–4 hours (after epinephrine dose) may be safely discharged as long as they have reliable caretakers and good access to medical services if symptoms return (14)[C].

ONGOING CARE

FOLLOW-UP RECOMMENDATIONS

Patient Monitoring

Most patients will be seen in ED or PCP office setting. Some will be overnight by telephone.

DIET

- NPO and IV fluids for severe cases
- Frequent small feedings with increased fluids for mild cases

PATIENT EDUCATION

- Must keep patient quiet; crying may exacerbate symptoms.
- Educate parents about when to seek emergency care if mild cases progress.
- Emotional support and reassurance for the patient

PROGNOSIS

- Up to 1/3 of patients will have recurrence.
- Recovery is usually full and without lasting effects.

COMPLICATIONS

- Rare
- Subglottic stenosis in intubated patients
- Bacterial tracheitis
- Cardiopulmonary arrest
- Pneumonia

REFERENCES

1. Cherry JD. Clinical practice. Croup. *N Engl J Med*. 2008;358:384–91.
2. Sobol SE, Zapata S. Epiglottitis and croup. *Otolaryngol Clin North Am*. 2008;41:551–66, ix.
3. Everard ML. Acute bronchiolitis and croup. *Pediatr Clin North Am*. 2009;56:119–33, x–xi.
4. Johnson DW, Jacobson S, Edney PC, et al. A comparison of nebulized budesonide, intramuscular dexamethasone, and placebo for moderately severe croup. *N Engl J Med*. 1998; 339:498–503.
5. Westley CR, Cotton EK, Brooks JG. Nebulized racemic epinephrine by IPPB for the treatment of croup: a double-blind study. *Am J Dis Child*. 1978;132:484–7.
6. Waisman Y, Klein BL, Boenning DA, et al. Prospective randomized double-blind study comparing L-epinephrine and racemic epinephrine aerosols in the treatment of laryngotracheitis (croup). *Pediatrics*. 1992;89:302–6.
7. Russell K, Wiebe N, Saenz A, et al. Glucocorticoids for croup. *Cochrane Database Syst Rev*. 2004;CD001955.
8. Dobrovoljac M, Geelhoed GC et al. 27 years of croup: an update highlighting the effectiveness of 0.15 mg/kg of dexamethasone. *Emerg Med Australas*. 2009;21:309–14.
9. Geelhoed GC, Turner J, MacDonald WB. Efficacy of a small single dose of oral dexamethasone for outpatient croup: A double-blind placebo controlled clinical trial. *Br Med J*. 1996; 313(7050):140–2.
10. Cetinkaya F, Tüfekçi BS, Kutluk G. A comparison of nebulized budesonide, and intramuscular, and oral dexamethasone for treatment of croup. *Int J Pediatr Otorhinolaryngol*. 2004;68:453–6.
11. Vorwerk C, Coats TJ. Use of helium-oxygen mixtures in the treatment of croup: a systematic review. *Emerg Med J*. 2008;25:547–50.
12. Gupta VK, Cheifetz IM. Heliox administration in the pediatric intensive care unit: an evidence-based review. *Pediatr Crit Care Med*. 2005;6:204–11.
13. Vorwerk C, Coats T et al. Heliox for croup in children. *Cochrane Database Syst Rev*. 2010; 2:CD006822-
14. Klassen TP. Croup. A current perspective. *Pediatr Clin North Am*. 1999;46:1167–78.

ADDITIONAL READING

Bjornson CL, Johnson DW. Croup. *Lancet*. 2008;371: 329–39.

See Also (Topic, Algorithm, Electronic Media Element)

Bronchiolitis; Epiglottitis; Tracheitis, Bacterial

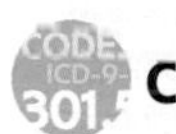

CODES

ICD9

464.4 Croup

CLINICAL PEARLS

- Parainfluenza virus is the most common pathogen.
- Also caused by RSV, paramyxovirus, influenza virus type A or B, adenovirus, rhinovirus, enteroviruses (Coxsackie and Echo)
- Established efficacy of inhaled epinephrine and corticosteroids
- Lateral neck films show funnel-shaped subglottic region with normal epiglottis: "Steeple," "hour glass," or "pencil point" sign (present in 40–60% of children with laryngotracheobronchitis).

CRYOGLOBULINEMIA

Luke Godwin, MD
Fred Schiffman, MD

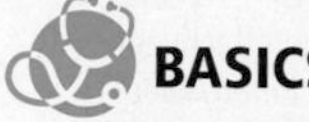

BASICS

DESCRIPTION

- Cryoglobulinemia is a state characterized by the presence of cryoglobulins in a patient's serum.
- Cryoglobulins are circulating immunoglobulins that precipitate at cold temperatures (below 37°C) and dissolve on rewarming.
- Clinical symptoms are often secondary to either small vessel occlusion and a hyperviscosity syndrome in Type I cryoglobulins, or the formation of cryoglobulin-containing immune complexes leading to vasculitis in Type II and Type III cryoglobulins (i.e., "mixed cryoglobulinemia"):
  - Type I
    - Monoclonal immunoglobulin (Ig); IgM is most common
    - 10–15% of all cryoglobulinemia
    - Less frequently IgG, IgA, free Ig light chains
  - Type II
    - Monoclonal IgM with rheumatoid factor activity (anti-IgG), which forms an immune complex with polyclonal IgG
    - 50–60% of all cryoglobulinemia
    - Monoclonal fraction rarely IgG or IgA
  - Type III:
    - Polyclonal IgM with rheumatoid factor activity (anti-IgG), which forms an immune complex with polyclonal IgG
    - 25–30% of cryoglobulinemia

EPIDEMIOLOGY

- No adequate epidemiological studies regarding overall prevalence
- Healthy patients may have low concentrations of cryoglobulins present in the serum (<0.06 g/L)
- Clinically relevant cryoglobulinemia is far more common in patients with chronic infections and/or inflammation

RISK FACTORS

- Type I: Associated with lymphoproliferative disorders:
  - Multiple myeloma
  - Waldenström's macroglobulinemia
  - Chronic lymphocytic leukemia (CLL)
  - Monoclonal gammopathy of unknown significance (MGUS)
  - B-cell lymphoma
- Type II (mixed cryoglobulinemia):
  - Main association with hepatitis C
  - 40–90% of patients with mixed cryoglobulinemia are hepatitis C positive
  - Higher association with hepatitis C compared to type III cryoglobulinemia
  - Also associated with Sjögren's syndrome, HIV, and other autoimmune/connective tissue disease
- Type III (mixed cryoglobulinemia):
  - Like Type II, also associated with chronic infection and inflammatory states:
    - Autoimmune disease: SLE, RA, IBD
    - Infection: EBV, CMV, TB, HIV, subacute endocarditis
  - Significant hepatitis C virus association, just less than type II

PATHOPHYSIOLOGY

- Exact mechanism of cold insolubility in these cryoproteins is unknown. Hypotheses include reduced concentrations of sialic acid and galactose in the Fc region of Ig, as well as steric conformation changes due to temperature variation.
- Type I:
  - An underlying lymphoproliferative disorder causes monoclonal B cell proliferation.
  - B cells produce cryoglobulin, which precipitates, causing hyperviscosity and vessel damage.
- Types II and III:
  - B cell hyperactivation (from hepatitis C virus or another chronic inflammatory state) produces immunoglobulin with rheumatoid factor activity, which leads to immune complex formation.
  - Immune complex deposition and subsequent complement activation causes small-vessel damage.

ETIOLOGY

Hepatitis C correlation:

- Hepatitis C virus displays lymphotropism. The E2 capsid protein of HCV binds site to CD81, a site present on hepatocytes, T lymphocytes, and B lymphocytes.
- Patients infected with HCV who have mixed cryoglobulinemia (MC) have been found to have higher viral loads than patients with HCV and no MC.

COMMONLY ASSOCIATED CONDITIONS

- NOTE: See above for specific association by cryoglobulinemia type classification
- Infections:
  - Viral: Hepatitis C, hepatitis B, hepatitis A, HIV, Epstein-Barr virus, VZV, cytomegalovirus, HTLV-1, adenovirus, influenza virus, parvovirus B19, rubella virus
  - Bacterial: Lyme disease, syphilis, Q fever, poststreptococcal nephritis, subacute bacterial endocarditis, leprosy, TB, brucella
  - Fungal: Coccidiomycosis
  - Parasitic: Kala-azar toxoplasmosis, echinococcosis, malaria, schistosomiasis, trypanosomiasis
- Hematologic disease:
  - Non-Hodgkin lymphoma
  - Chronic lymphocytic leukemia
  - Multiple myeloma
  - Waldenström's macroglobulinemia
  - Hodgkin lymphoma
  - Chronic myeloid leukemia
  - Castleman disease
  - Thrombocytopenic thrombotic purpura
  - Cold agglutinin disease
- Autoimmune diseases:
  - Sjögren syndrome
  - Systemic lupus erythematosus
  - Polyarteritis nodosa
  - Systemic sclerosis
  - Rheumatoid arthritis
  - Autoimmune thyroiditis
  - Temporal arteritis
  - Dermatomyositis/polymyositis
  - Henoch-Schönlein disease
  - Sarcoidosis
  - Inflammatory bowel disease
  - Pemphigus vulgaris

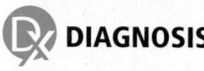

DIAGNOSIS

- Type I:
  - Commonly asymptomatic
  - More frequent association with signs of peripheral vessel occlusion, less with signs of vasculitis. Think of Raynaud's phenomenon, acrocyanosis, livedo reticularis, purpura, ulcers, gangrene.
- Types II and III: Mixed cryoglobulinemia syndrome
  - Caused by immune complex-mediated vasculitis
  - Characterized by Meltzer's triad:
    - Purpura
    - Weakness
    - Arthralgias
  - Multiple organ involvement is common:
    - Cutaneous vasculitis, purpura
    - Membranoproliferative glomerulonephritis (nephropathy)
    - Peripheral neuropathy

HISTORY

- Constitutional/nonspecific: Fever, myalgias, arthralgia, malaise, generalized weakness, sensory changes
- Hyperviscosity: Blurring of vision, headache, vertigo, dizziness, diplopia, ataxia, confusion, dementia, stroke
- Past medical history: Risk factors for hepatitis C, lymphoproliferative disorders

HYSICAL EXAM

- Skin: Purpura (intermittent, palpable, beginning in legs), ulcers, Raynaud phenomenon, livedo reticularis, acrocyanosis
- Gastrointestinal: Hepatomegaly, splenomegaly
- Endocrine: Lymphadenopathy
- Extremities: Synovitis, signs of peripheral vascular occlusion
- Neurological: Peripheral neuropathy

IAGNOSTIC TESTS & INTERPRETATION

nportant to rule out other small-vessel vasculitis (see ection Differential Diagnosis) (1)

ab

itial lab tests

- General:
  - Complete blood count (CBC), with peripheral smear
  - Electrolytes
  - Liver function tests (LFTs)
  - Blood urea nitrogen (BUN), creatinine
  - Urinalysis
  - Rheumatoid factor
- Specific:
  - Serological test for cryoglobulins (blood collection and initial storage needs to be at 37°C); following detection of cryoglobulins, further testing including electrophoresis and immunofixation should be completed.
  - Serum complement levels (low C4, normal or slightly decreased C3)
  - Serologic tests for hepatitis B and C
  - Rheumatologic (e.g., antinuclear antibody, ANCA)

iagnostic Procedures/Surgery

heck main organ systems involved:

- Kidneys: Proteinuria, microscopic hematuria, arterial hypertension common at diagnosis
- Nervous system: Peripheral neuropathy in types II and III cryoglobulinemia
- Liver: Normal or increased liver enzymes, steatosis, chronic hepatitis, cirrhosis

athological Findings

- Renal biopsy: Most common type of nephropathy is membranoproliferative glomerulonephritis
- Bone marrow: May be indicated for type I cryoglobulinemia; examination often reveals underlying hematological condition
- Liver biopsy: Inflammation is graded; fibrosis is staged

IFFERENTIAL DIAGNOSIS

- Possible causes of small-vessel vasculitis: Henoch-Schönlein purpura, lupus vasculitis, rheumatoid vasculitis, Sjögren syndrome vasculitis, hypocomplementemic urticarial vasculitis, Behçet syndrome, Goodpasture syndrome, serum sickness vasculitis, drug-induced immune complex vasculitis, infection-induced immune complex vasculitis, ANCA-associated vasculitis, paraneoplastic syndrome-associated vasculitis, inflammatory bowel disease-associated vasculitis
- Possible causes of hyperviscosity: Waldenstrom macroglobulinemia, polycythemia, sickle cell anemia, malaria, babesiosis

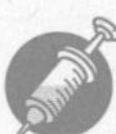

TREATMENT

- Most important to treat underlying disease
- Treat according to individual patient and severity of symptoms
- Mild disease treated with cold avoidance, analgesics, nonsteroidal anti-inflammatory drugs
- Intensive therapy with steroids, plasmapheresis, or cytotoxic agents only for organ-threatening or recalcitrant disease
- Type I:
  - Cytotoxic treatment of lymphoproliferative disease as appropriate
- Types II and III:
  - Antiviral hepatitis C treatment as appropriate

MEDICATION

- Hepatitis C-associated:
  - Antiviral therapy: Combination therapy of pegylated interferon (PEG-INF)α and ribavirin
- Non-hepatitis C-associated:
  - Immunosuppression, low-dose corticosteroids
- Rituximab: this chimeric monoclonal antibody directed against CD20 has shown some efficacy in treating both type I and mixed cryoglobulinemias, and should be considered in severely symptomatic patients.

ADDITIONAL TREATMENT

Plasmapheresis:

- For severe clinical manifestations of disease
- Used alongside immunosuppressive treatment to avoid rebound phenomena

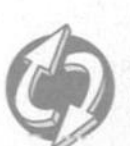

ONGOING CARE

DIET

At least one small study has suggested that a low antigen content (LAC) diet can be helpful in improving the symptoms of cryoglobulinemia. The hypothesized mechanism is a reduction in antigen input load for the reticuloendothelial system that allows that system to more efficiently process circulating immune complexes.

PATIENT EDUCATION

http://www.vasculitisfoundation.org/

PROGNOSIS

There seems to be no increased morbidity or mortality risk with cryoglobulinemia over the associated underlying conditions.

REFERENCES

1. Sargur R, White P, Egner W et al. Cryoglobulin evaluation: best practice? *Ann. Clin. Biochem.* 2010;47:8–16.

ADDITIONAL READING

- Alpers CE, Smith KD et al. Cryoglobulinemia and renal disease. *Curr Opin Nephrol Hypertens.* 2008;17:243–9.
- Dammacco F, Sansonno D, Piccoli C. , et al. The cryoglobulins: an overview. *Eur J Clin Invest.* 2001;31:628–38.
- Dispenzieri A et al. Symptomatic cryoglobulinemia. *Curr Treat Options Oncol.* 2000;1:105–18.
- Ferri C, Antonelli A, Mascia MT et al. B-cells and mixed cryoglobulinemia. *Autoimmun Rev.* 2007;7: 114–20.
- Sansonno D, Carbone A, De Re V et al. Hepatitis C virus infection, cryoglobulinaemia, and beyond. *Rheumatology (Oxford).* 2007.
- Tedeschi A, Baratè C, Minola E, et al. Cryoglobulinemia. *Blood Rev.* 2007.

CODES

ICD9

- 273.1 Monoclonal paraproteinemia
- 273.2 Other paraproteinemias

CLINICAL PEARLS

- Cryoglobulins are circulating immunoglobulins that precipitate at cold temperatures (below 37°F) and dissolve on rewarming.
- Type I: Associated with lymphoproliferative disorders (e.g., multiple myeloma, Waldenstrom macroglobulinemia, MGUS, CLL)
- Type II (mixed cryoglobulinemia): Main association with hepatitis C (40–90% are hepatitis C positive)
- Type III (mixed cryoglobulinemia): High association with chronic infection and inflammatory states
- Initial laboratory evaluation: CBC with peripheral smear, electrolytes, LFTs, BUN, creatinine, urinalysis, rheumatoid factor
- Specific:
  - Serological test for cryoglobulins (blood collection and initial storage needs to be at 37°C); electrophoresis and immunofixation if cryoglobulins present
  - Serum complement levels (low C4, normal or slightly decreased C3)
  - Serologic tests for hepatitis B and C
  - Rheumatologic (ANA, ANCA)

C

CRYPTORCHIDISM

Pamela I. Ellsworth, MD

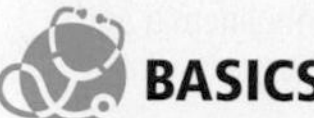

BASICS

DESCRIPTION

- Incomplete or improper descent of 1 or both testicles; normally, descent is in the 7th–8th month of gestation. The cryptorchid testis may be palpable or nonpalpable.
- Types of cryptorchidism:
  - Abdominal: Located inside the internal ring
  - Canalicular: Located between the internal and external rings
  - Ectopic: Located outside the normal path of testicular descent from abdominal cavity to scrotum; may be ectopic to perineum, femoral canal, superficial inguinal pouch (most common), suprapubic area, or opposite hemiscrotum
  - Retractile: Fully descended testis that moves freely between the scrotum and the groin
  - Iatrogenic: Previously descended testis becomes undescended secondary to scar tissue after inguinal surgery, such as an inguinal hernia repair or hydrocelectomy.
  - Also may be referred to as *palpable* versus *nonpalpable*
- System(s) affected: Reproductive
- Synonym(s): Undescended testes (UDT)

Pediatric Considerations

- This problem is usually detectable at birth or soon thereafter.
- If surgery is to be the treatment, it should be performed during the 1st 6–9 months of life (1).
- Puberty: If unilateral cryptorchidism is discovered at or after puberty, the usual treatment is orchiectomy.

EPIDEMIOLOGY

Incidence

- Predominant age: Premature newborns
- Predominant sex: Male only

Prevalence

- In the US, cryptorchidism occurs in 3% of full-term and 33% of premature newborn males.
- Spontaneous testicular descent occurs by age 1–3 months in 50–70% of full-term males with cryptorchidism.
- Descent at 6–9 months of age is rare.

RISK FACTORS

- Family history of cryptorchidism: Boys with UDTs: 4% of their fathers and 6.2–9.8% of their brothers have UDTs (23,).
- Low birth weight, prematurity, and small for gestational age are associated with a substantial increase in incidence of cryptorchidism, which may reach 20–25% in infants with birth weight less than 2.5 kg (4).

Genetics

Occurrence of UDT in siblings as well as fathers suggests a genetic etiology.

ETIOLOGY

- Not fully known
- May involve alterations in
  - Mechanical factors (gubernaculum, length of vas deferens and testicular vessels, groin anatomy, epididymis, cremasteric muscles, and abdominal pressure), hormonal factors (gonadotropin, testosterone, dihydrotestosterone, and müllerian inhibiting substance) and neural factors (ilioinguinal nerve and genitofemoral nerve)
  - Major regulators of testicular descent from intraabdominal location into the bottom of the scrotum are the Leydig cell–derived hormones testosterone and insulin-like growth factor 3 (IGF-3).
  - Mutations in the gene for IGF-3 and in the androgen receptor gene have been recognized as causes of cryptorchidism as well as chromosomal alterations.
  - Environmental factors acting as endocrine disruptors of testicular descent also may contribute to the etiology of cryptorchidism (5).

COMMONLY ASSOCIATED CONDITIONS

- Inguinal hernia/hydrocele
- Abnormalities of vas deferens and epididymis
- Intersex abnormalities
- Hypogonadotropic hypogonadism
- Germinal cell aplasia
- Prune-belly syndrome
- Meningomyelocele
- Hypospadias
- Wilms tumor
- Prader-Willi syndrome
- Kallman syndrome
- Cystic fibrosis

DIAGNOSIS

HISTORY

$\geq$1 testicles in a site other than the scrotum; may be an isolated defect or associated with other congenital anomalies

PHYSICAL EXAM

- Performed with warm hands, with child in sitting, standing, and squatting position
- A Valsalva maneuver and applied pressure to lower abdomen may help to identify the testes, especially a gliding testis.
- Failure to palpate a testis after repeated exams suggests an intraabdominal or atrophic testis.
- An enlarged contralateral testis in the presence of a nonpalpable testis suggests testicular atrophy/absence.

DIAGNOSTIC TESTS & INTERPRETATION

Lab

Initial lab tests

- In boys $\leq$3 months of age with bilateral nonpalpable UDTs, luteinizing hormone, follicle-stimulating hormone, and testosterone levels are helpful to determine whether the testes are present.
- $>$3 months of age, a human chorionic gonadotropin (hCG) stimulation test to determine presence/absence of testicular tissue (hCG 2,000 IU/d $\times$ 3 days, and check testosterone before and after stimulation)

Follow-Up & Special Considerations

In newborns and children $<$6–12 months of age, periodic examination to determine if testis is palpable and descended prior to considering further intervention

Imaging

Initial approach

- Ultrasonography has a sensitivity of 76%, a specificity of 100%, and an accuracy of 84% in the diagnosis on nonpalpable UDT, whereas MRI has a sensitivity of 86%, a specificity of 79%, and an accuracy of 85% (6)[C].
- CT scan findings in children are inconsistent.

Diagnostic Procedures/Surgery

Laparoscopy is useful in a child with nonpalpable cryptorchidism to accurately confirm testicular absence or presence and to determine the feasibility of performing a standard orchiopexy (7)[C].

Pathological Findings

- Higher incidence of carcinoma in UDT and alterations in spermatogenesis
- Histologic changes occur by 1.5 years of age and include smaller seminiferous tubules, fewer spermatogonia, and more peritubular tissue.

DIFFERENTIAL DIAGNOSIS

- Retractile testis (hypermobile testis): A normally descended testis that ascends into the inguinal canal because of an active cremasteric reflex (more common in males 4–6 years of age)
- Atrophic testis: May occur as a result of neonatal torsion
- Vanished testis may be the result of a lack of development or in utero torsion.

TREATMENT

EDICATION

The International Health Foundation recommends biweekly hCG injections for 5 weeks: 250 (IU) for infants, 500 IU for children ≤6 years of age, and 1,000 IU for children ≥6 years of age.

Success rates for descent into the scrotum range from 0–55% (8)[B].
- The more distal the testis, the more likely the descent.
- A systematic review with a meta-analysis of randomized clinical trials concluded that the evidence for the use of hCG versus gonadotropin-releasing hormone (GnRH) shows advantages for hCG but noted that the evidence was based on few trials (9)[B].

Contraindications: hCG therapy is contraindicated in patients with a clinically apparent inguinal hernia, those with a history of previous ipsilateral groin surgery, or those with ectopic testicles. Also refer to manufacturer's literature.

Precautions: (1) May induce precocious puberty; discontinue drug; effects should reverse in 4 weeks; (2) premature epiphyseal closure

Significant possible interactions: Refer to manufacturer's literature.

GnRH is approved for use in Europe, and neoadjuvant GnRH therapy may improve fertility index in UDT (10)[C].

DDITIONAL TREATMENT

eneral Measures

Rule out retractile testis.

Appropriate health care: Outpatient until surgery performed

Administration of chorionic gonadotropin may cause testicular descent in some boys. Reports of efficacy are inconsistent.

sues for Referral

Bilateral nonpalpable UDTs

≥1 testes not descended by 6 months to 1 year of age

URGERY/OTHER PROCEDURES

Reasons to consider: Avoids torsion, averts trauma, decreases but does not eliminate risk of malignancy, and prevents further alterations in spermatogenesis

Orchiopexy should be performed by age 1.

Alterations in germ cell count in the cryptorchid testis have been identified by age 2.

Laparoscopy is performed first if testis is nonpalpable.

If palpable, an inguinal approach is usually performed. Prepubertal approach is considered in select situations, but may increase the risk of hernia (11)[C].

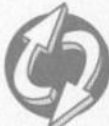

ONGOING CARE

FOLLOW-UP RECOMMENDATIONS

Initial follow-up within 1 month of surgery and periodically thereafter to assess testicular size/growth

Patient Monitoring

- Patients should be followed after surgery to evaluate testicular growth.
- Testicular tumors occur mainly during or after puberty; thus these children should be taught self-examination when they are older.

DIET

No restrictions

PATIENT EDUCATION

Discuss with parents about causes, available treatments, and possible effects on patient's reproductive potential; also increased risk for testicular cancer and need for regular self-examination.

PROGNOSIS

- Disorder is usually corrected with medical or surgical therapy; however, possible lifelong consequences.
- If testicle is absent or orchiectomy is required, may consider placement of testicular prosthesis.
- Early orchidopexy may decrease risk of testicular damage and risk of malignancy.

COMPLICATIONS

- Progressive failure of spermatogenesis, if left untreated; even with orchiopexy, the fertility rate is still reduced, especially with bilateral UDTs.
- Spermatogenesis is related to the duration of cryptorchidism and the location of the testis.
- Formerly bilaterally cryptorchid men have a greater decrease in fertility compared with unilateral cryptorchid male and the general male population.
- Abnormalities also have been identified in the contralateral descended testis, although less severe.

ALERT
- There is a 4–7× higher risk of developing testicular cancer in a male with a history of UDT (2)[C], but early orchidopexy appears to decrease the risk of cancer.
- Hernia development (25%)

REFERENCES

1. Lee PA. Fertility after cryptorchidism: epidemiology and other outcome studies. *Urology.* 2005;66: 427–31.
2. Cortes D. Cryptorchidism: Aspects of pathogenesis, histology and treatment. *Scan J Nephrol*. 1998;9:54.
3. Scorer CG, Farrington HG. *Congenital Deformities of the Testes and Epididymis*. London: Butterworths, 1971.
4. Cryptorchidism: a prospective study of 7500 consecutive male births, 1984–8. John Radcliffe Hospital Cryptorchidism Study Group. *Arch Dis Child*. 1992;67(7):892–9.
5. Foresta C, Zuccarello D, Garolla A, Ferlin A et al. Role of hormones, genes, and environment in human cryptorchidism. *Endocr Rev*. 2008;29: 560–80.
6. Kanemoto K, Hayashi Y, Kojima Y, et al. Accuracy of ultrasonography and magnetic resonance imaging in the diagnosis of non-palpable testis. *Int J Urol*. 2005;12:668–72.
7. Patil KK, et al. Laparoscopy for impalpable testis. *Br J Urol*. 2005;95:704–8.
8. Henna MR, Del Nero RG, Sampaio CZ, et al. Hormonal cryptorchidism therapy: systematic review with metanalysis of randomized clinical trials. *Pediatr Surg Int*. 2004;20:357–9.
9. Henna MR, Del Nero RG, Sampaio CZ, Atallah AN, Schettini ST, Castro AA, Soares BG et al. Hormonal cryptorchidism therapy: systematic review with metanalysis of randomized clinical trials. *Pediatr Surg Int*. 2004;20:357–9.
10. Schwentner C, Oswald J, Kreczy A, et al. Neoadjuvant gonadotropin-releasing hormone therapy before surgery may improve the fertility index in undescended testes: a prospective randomized trial. *J Urol*. 2005;173:974–7.
11. Al-Mandil M, Khoury AE, El-Hout Y, Kogon M, Dave S, Farhat WA et al. Potential complications with the prescrotal approach for the palpable undescended testis? A comparison of single prescrotal incision to the traditional inguinal approach. *J Urol*. 2008;180:686 9.

ADDITIONAL READING

Berkowitz GS, Lapinski RH, Dolgin SE, et al. Prevalence and natural history of cryptorchidism. *Pediatrics*. 1993;92:44–9.

CODES

ICD9

752.51 Undescended testis

CLINICAL PEARLS

- If testicular descent does not occur by 6–9 months of age, it is unlikely to occur. Therefore, refer patients to a urologist if a testes has not descended by 6 months to 1 year of age.
- Children with bilateral nonpalpable UDTs require laboratory evaluation to determine if viable testicular tissue is present.
- The risk of infertility is increased with bilateral UDTs.

CUBITAL TUNNEL SYNDROME

Joseph Blazuk, MD
Mark Kaplan, MD

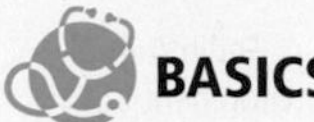

BASICS

DESCRIPTION

- Compression of the ulnar nerve on the medial aspect of the elbow where it enters the cubital tunnel. Often resulting in elbow pain and paresthesias of the forearm, wrist, 4th and 5th fingers.
- Synonym(s): Ulnar neuropathy

EPIDEMIOLOGY

- Predominant sex: Male > Female (3–8 times more common)
- Elbow is most common site of compression of ulnar nerve. Less common sites of entrapment include the arcade of Struthers, the medial intermuscular septum, the medial epicondyle, and the deep flexor pronator aponeurosis.
- 2nd most common nerve compression of upper extremity (behind median nerve compression in carpal tunnel) (1)

RISK FACTORS

- Patients who sleep or position themselves with their elbows bent, their arms overhead, or both
- Athletes in throwing sports, racquet sports, weightlifting, and skiing
- Preexisting polyneuropathy
- Patients with end-stage renal disease on hemodialysis
- Patients placed in dependent positioning (surgery, ICU)

GENERAL PREVENTION

- Avoid long periods with elbows bent or pressure on elbows.
- Sleep with elbows straight and avoid sleeping with arms overhead.
- Keep proper posture when working at a desk.

PATHOPHYSIOLOGY

- The ulnar nerve is the terminal branch of the medial cord of the brachial plexus and is composed from the C8 and T1 nerve roots.
- The ulnar nerve becomes more superficial as it enters the ulnar sulcus ~3.5 cm proximal to the medial epicondyle. The nerve courses posterior to the medial epicondyle and medial to the olecranon, then enters the cubital tunnel (2).
- The cubital tunnel is a fibro-osseous canal. The roof is defined by the arcuate ligament of Osbourne. The floor consists of the medial collateral ligament of the elbow, the joint capsule, and the olecranon.
- Elbow flexion increases distance from medial epicondyle to olecranon 5 mm for every 45°.
- Elbow flexion places stress on medial collateral ligament, overlying retinaculum, and ulnar nerve.
- Shape of cubital tunnel changes from a circle to an oval, with a 2.5-mm loss of height with elbow flexion.
- Loss of height of cubital tunnel with elbow flexion decreases tunnel volume by 55%, which doubles intraneural pressure on the ulnar nerve from 7–14 mm Hg.
- Maximal pressure on the ulnar nerve in cubital tunnel is created by shoulder abduction, elbow flexion, and wrist extension.

ETIOLOGY

- Elbow flexion decreases volume of cubital tunnel, causing compression of ulnar nerve.
- Compression of ulnar nerve causes pain at medial aspect of elbow and symptoms at forearm and hand.
- Caused by constricting fascial bands, subluxation of ulnar nerve over medial epicondyle, cubitus valgus, bony spurs, hypertrophied synovium, tumors, ganglia, or direct compression of ulnar nerve as it crosses cubital tunnel

COMMONLY ASSOCIATED CONDITIONS

- Ulnar nerve subluxation
- Osteoarthritis of elbow joint

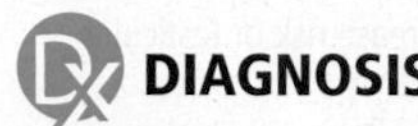

DIAGNOSIS

HISTORY

- Nocturnal elbow pain
- Medial elbow pain
- Paresthesias along lateral forearm, wrist, and 4th and 5th digits
- Paresthesias may be intermittent at first and then become more constant.
- History of trauma over the area
- Repetitive elbow flexion and extension activities (such as in hammering)
- Overhead throwing athlete with repetitive elbow motion
- Chronic symptoms: Loss of grip strength and loss of fine motor skills in hand

PHYSICAL EXAM

- Inspect carrying angle of both elbows.
- Palpate medial epicondyle and cubital tunnel for areas of tenderness or ulnar nerve subluxation.
- Check elbow range of motion.
- Positive Hoffman-Tinel test (tapping over ulnar nerve) (3)
- Pain on palpating over ulnar nerve
- Atrophy of intrinsic muscles
- Loss of sensation at ulnar side of 5th digit
- Wasting of hypothenar muscles and flexion contracture of 4th and 5th digits (ulnar claw)
- Wartenberg sign is clawing or abduction of the 5th digit with extension.
- Assess ability to cross 2nd and 3rd digits.
- Evaluate grip and pinch strength for weakness.
- Check vibration and light touch sensation.
- Recently, the "scratch-collapse test" has been described. The patient faces the examiner with arm adducted, elbows flexed, hands outstretched, and wrists at neutral. The patient resists bilateral shoulder adduction and internal rotation as examiner applies these forces to the forearm. The examiner "scratches" or swipes fingertips over course of compressed ulnar nerve. The force is then reapplied to the forearm. A positive result occurs when the patient has a temporary loss of external rotation resistance tone.
- Sensitivity for the scratch collapse was 69% compared with 54% and 46% for Tinel test and elbow flexion-compression test, respectively. Tinel test, however, had the highest negative predictive value (98%) of all tests for cubital tunnel (4).

DIAGNOSTIC TESTS & INTERPRETATION

McGowan grades quantify the degree of physical exam findings and are specific for cubital tunnel syndrome:

- McGowan Grade I: No wasting or weakness of intrinsic muscles, feeling of clumsiness in affected hand, mild paresthesias in ulnar nerve distribution
- McGowan Grade II: Intermediate lesions with weak interossei and muscle wasting
- McGowan Grade III: Severe lesions with paralysis of interossei and a marked weakness of the hand

Imaging

Initial approach

- X-rays may reveal osteophytes impinging on the area. Include anterior posterior (AP) lateral, and cubital tunnel views (3). Radiographs may also show signs of instability, deformity from old trauma, or presence of a supracondylar process (which can cause median nerve compression).
- Cubital tunnel view: Elbow is maximally flexed and x-ray beam is shot as an AP view of the distal humerus.

Follow-Up & Special Considerations

- Chest x-ray if patient has history of smoking and ulnar nerve symptoms (to exclude Pancoast tumor apical lung)
- Magnetic resonance imaging shows inflammation and irritation of ulnar nerve.
- High-resolution ultrasound

Diagnostic Procedures/Surgery

- Corticosteroid injection into ulnar groove
- Electromyogram (EMG) is not essential when diagnosis is obvious on clinical exam. Use to determine the efficacy of conservative treatment or when the diagnosis is unclear.
- EMG is considered positive if motor conduction delay across the elbow is <50 m/s or difference between motor velocity across elbow and below the elbow is >10 m/s.
- Nerve conduction studies

athological Findings
flammation and swelling of ulnar nerve

IFFERENTIAL DIAGNOSIS
- Cervical disc lesion
- Thoracic outlet syndrome
- Carpal tunnel syndrome
- Medial epicondylitis
- Thoracic outlet syndrome
- Pancoast syndrome
- Metabolic disorders creating peripheral neuropathies
- Multiple sclerosis and other myelopathies

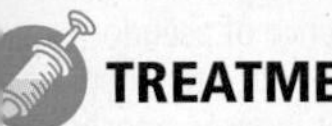

TREATMENT

ild cubital tunnel syndrome can often be treated ithout surgery. If provocative causes can be identified nd avoided, there is tendency for spontaneous covery. Patients with constant symptoms and/or uscle atrophy typically require surgical intervention.

IEDICATION

irst Line
onsteroidal anti-inflammatory drugs or other nalgesic

econd Line
orticosteroid (injection)

DDITIONAL TREATMENT

ieneral Measures
- Rest
- Avoidance of aggravating activities
- Conservative treatment is initial approach if no motor weakness.
- Instruct patient to avoid periods of prolonged elbow flexion.
- Instruct patient to avoid long periods of pressure and compression on ulnar nerve at elbow.
- Ice/heat for symptom relief
- Splint or brace while sleeping to keep affected elbow in extension and take pressure off cubital tunnel (e.g., wrap towel around elbow and hold in place with tape; use a small size soft knee splint but wear it on the elbow, tie a scarf around waist then around wrist)
- Physical therapy (nerve mobilization techniques)
- Workplace modifications (e.g., correct posture, avoid long periods with elbows bent)
- Avoid any activities that bring about symptoms. Otherwise activity as tolerated

ssues for Referral
ailure of conservative treatment, loss of grip strength, exion contracture of 4th and 5th digits, positive EMG or motor conduction delay

Additional Therapies
- Corticosteroid injection into ulnar groove
- Use 1 mL lidocaine and 20–40 mg methylprednisolone injected into ulnar groove, parallel to ulnar nerve (3).
- Hand therapy and custom splint prescription

COMPLEMENTARY AND ALTERNATIVE MEDICINE
Vitamin B_6 (100 mg/d) not found to be effective in randomized trials

SURGERY/OTHER PROCEDURES
- Goal of surgery is to create more space for ulnar nerve (5).
- Many surgical treatments exist for the treatment of cubital tunnel syndrome. *In situ* decompression, transposition of the ulnar nerve into the subcutaneous, intramuscular, or submuscular plane, or medial epicondylectomy have all been shown to be effective in the treatment of this disease process. Comparative studies have shown some short–term advantages to one or another technique, but overall results between the treatments have essentially been equivocal. The choice of surgical treatment is based on multiple factors, and a single surgical approach cannot be applied to all clinical situations (2).

ONGOING CARE

FOLLOW-UP RECOMMENDATIONS

Patient Monitoring
- In severe cases, the nerve damage may be permanent and the patient may not recover.
- The longer the nerve has been irritated, the more difficult it is to recover fully.

DIET
No restrictions

PATIENT EDUCATION
- Use correct posture; avoid putting pressure on your elbows, and place padding under your elbows.
- Inability to straighten fingers is often a sign of severe ulnar nerve damage. Patients with this level of irritation usually do not recover, even with surgery.

PROGNOSIS
- Both conservative and surgical methods result in 85–90% good-to-excellent results.
- For McGowan Grade III: Anterior intramuscular transposition has best outcome (6)[C].

COMPLICATIONS
Anterior transposition may have recurrent subluxation of the ulnar nerve.

REFERENCES

1. Fernandez E, Pallini R, Lauretti L, et al. Neurosurgery of the peripheral nervous system: cubital tunnel syndrome. *Surg Neurol*. 1998;50: 83–5.
2. Palmer BA, Hughes TB et al. Cubital tunnel syndrome. *J Hand Surg Am*. 2010;35:153–63.
3. Chumbley EM, O'Connor FG, Nirschl RP. Evaluation of overuse elbow injuries. *Am Fam Physician*. 2000; 61:691–700.
4. Cheng CJ, Mackinnon-Patterson B, Beck JL, Mackinnon SE et al. Scratch collapse test for evaluation of carpal and cubital tunnel syndrome. *J Hand Surg Am*. 2008;33:1518–24.
5. Mowlavi A, Andrews K, Lille S, et al. The management of cubital tunnel syndrome: a meta-analysis of clinical studies. *Plast Reconstr Surg*. 2000;106:327–34.
6. Bartels RH, Menovsky T, Van Overbeeke JJ, et al. Surgical management of ulnar nerve compression at the elbow: an analysis of the literature. *J Neurosurg*. 1998;89:722–7.

ADDITIONAL READING

Cutts S. Cubital tunnel syndrome. *Postgrad Med J*. 2007;83:28–31.

See Also (Topic, Algorithm, Electronic Media Element)
Ulnar Collateral Ligament Injury; Medial Epicondylitis; Lateral Epicondylitis

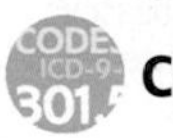

CODES

ICD9
354.2 Lesion of ulnar nerve

CLINICAL PEARLS
- Elbow flexion decreases depth of cubital tunnel, thus putting pressure on ulnar nerve.
- Sleeping with elbow bent and arm overhead can cause symptoms.
- Improper posture when working at a desk can cause symptoms.
- Conservative treatment consists of ice, rest, hand therapy, splint fabrication, and activity modifications.
- Both conservative and surgical methods result in good to excellent results 85–90% of the time.

CUSHING DISEASE AND CUSHING SYNDROME

David M. Barclay, III, MD, MPH, FAAFP
Colleen Veloski, MD

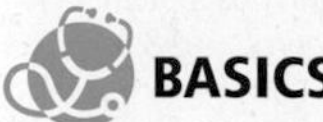

BASICS

DESCRIPTION
- Clinical abnormalities associated with chronic exposure to excessive amounts of cortisol (the major adrenocorticoid)
- Cushing disease is defined as glucocorticoid excess due to excessive adrenocorticotropic hormone (ACTH) secretion from a pituitary tumor. This is the most common cause of primary Cushing syndrome.
- Cushing syndrome is defined as excessive corticosteroid exposure from exogenous sources (medications) or endogenous sources (pituitary, adrenal, pulmonary, etc., or tumor)
- System(s) affected: Endocrine/Metabolic; Musculoskeletal; Skin/Exocrine; Cardiovascular; Neuropsychiatric

Pediatric Considerations
- Rare in infancy and childhood
- Most cases in children <8 years are a result of malignant adrenal tumors.

Pregnancy Considerations
Pregnancy may exacerbate disease.

EPIDEMIOLOGY

Incidence
Uncommon: 0.7–2.4 per million per year

Prevalence
In difficult-to-control diabetic patients with obesity and hypertension, prevalence has been reported at 2–5%.

RISK FACTORS
- Predominant sex: Female > Male (slightly). Cushing syndrome is equally prevalent in both sexes.
- Pituitary tumor
- Adrenal mass
- Neuroendocrine tumor (e.g., bronchial carcinoid)
- Prolonged use of corticosteroids

Genetics
- Multiple endocrine neoplasia type I
- Carney complex (an inherited multiple neoplasia syndrome)
- McCune-Albright syndrome (mutation of GNAS1 gene)

GENERAL PREVENTION
Avoid corticosteroid exposure when possible.

PATHOPHYSIOLOGY
- Disease: Pituitary tumor causing excess ACTH (corticotropin)
- Syndrome: Excessive corticosteroid exposure from exogenous sources (medications) or endogenous sources (pituitary, adrenal, pulmonary, etc., or tumor)

ETIOLOGY
- Exogenous glucocorticoids or ACTH
- Endogenous ACTH-dependent hypercortisolism (80–85%):
  - ACTH-secreting pituitary tumor: 70%
  - Ectopic ACTH production (e.g., small-cell carcinoma of lung, bronchial carcinoid): 20%
- Endogenous ACTH-independent hypercortisolism: 15–20%:
  - Adrenal adenoma
  - Adrenal carcinoma
  - Macronodular or micronodular hyperplasia

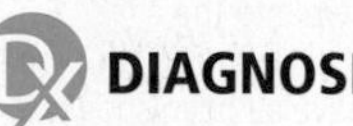

DIAGNOSIS

HISTORY
- Weight gain: 95% (1)[B]
- Decreased libido: 90%
- Menstrual irregularity: 80%
- Hirsutism: 75%
- Depression/emotional lability: 50–80%
- Easy bruising: 65%
- Proximal muscle weakness: 60%
- Diabetes or glucose intolerance: 60%

PHYSICAL EXAM
- Obesity: 95%
- Facial plethora: 90%
- Moon face (facial adiposity): 90%
- Thin skin: 85%
- Hypertension: 75%
- Skeletal growth retardation in children (epiphyseal plates remain open): 70–80%
- Purple striae on the skin
- Increased adipose tissue in neck and trunk
- Acne

DIAGNOSTIC TESTS & INTERPRETATION

Lab

Initial lab tests
- For initial evaluation, order either late-night salivary cortisol or 24-hour urinary-free cortisol. In normal circadian rhythm, cortisol secretion is highest in the morning and lowest between 11 PM and midnight. The nadir of serum cortisol is maintained in pseudo-Cushing (e.g., obesity, alcoholism, depression), but not in Cushing syndrome.
- Elevated late-night salivary cortisol provides sensitivity and specificity >90–95% (2,3)[B]. (Contact local lab for instructions to obtain this test.)
- 24-hour urinary-free cortisol level: Obtain ≥3 samples to rule out intermittent hypercortisolism if results are normal and suspicion is high. Also measure 24-hour urinary creatinine excretion to verify adequacy of collection. Results may be falsely low if glomerular filtration rate <30 mL/min. Overall sensitivity and specificity varies, but has been reported to be 90–97% and 85–96%, respectively (2)[B].
- Midnight plasma cortisol: Try to obtain samples on 3 consecutive nights. A late evening serum cortisol >7.5 μg/dL has a sensitivity of 96% and a specificity of 100% (4)[B].
- Persistently elevated serum cortisol implies Cushing syndrome; nadir of serum cortisol is maintained in obese patients, but not in those with Cushing.
- Low-dose dexamethasone suppression testing is no longer used as 1st-line testing. Dexamethasone 1 mg is given between 11 PM and midnight, and fasting plasma cortisol is measured between 8 and 9 AM the following morning. A serum cortisol leve below 1.8 μg/dL excludes Cushing syndrome, but specificity is limited. The presence of pseudo-Cushing states (depression, obesity, etc.), hepatic c renal disease, or any drug that induces cytochrome P-450 enzymes may cause a false result.
- High-dose dexamethasone suppression testing: Thi test is used to distinguish between an ACTH-secreting pituitary tumor and an ectopic ACTH-secreting tumor. 0.5 mg dexamethasone is given q.6h for 8 doses, with serum cortisol measured at 2 and 6 hours after last dose. Sensitivity 79%, specificity 74%.

ALERT
- Antiepileptic drugs, progesterone, oral contraceptives, rifampin, and spironolactone may cause a false-positive dexamethasone suppressior test.
- Corticotropin-releasing hormone (CRH) after dexamethasone: This test is used to distinguish Cushing syndrome from pseudo-Cushing syndrome. Dexamethasone 0.5 mg is given q.6h for 48 hours starting at noon. CRH (1 μg/Kg) is given 2 hours after the last dose of dexamethasone. Plasma cortisol is >1.4 μg/dL 15 minutes after CRH in patients with Cushing syndrome but not in those with pseudo-Cushing (5)[B].

Imaging

Initial approach
- Chest radiograph
- Lumbar spine radiograph:
  - Osteoporosis is common
- Pituitary MRI scan if pituitary tumor suspected
- Abdominal CT scan if adrenal disease suspected
- Chest CT scan if ectopic ACTH secretion is suspecte and inferior petrosal sinus sampling rules out pituitary source (6)[C]
- Octreotide scintigraphy to look for occult ACTH-secreting tumor

Diagnostic Procedures/Surgery
- Diagnostic procedure depends on circumstances an clinical judgment
- Inferior petrosal sinus sampling with CRH stimulation if ACTH-dependent tumor suspected (6)[C]

C

athological Findings

- Thyroid function suppressed
- Hypertension
- Dyslipidemia
- Polycystic ovarian syndrome/hyperandrogenism
- Oligomenorrhea/hypogonadism
- Myopathy/cutaneous wasting
- Neuropsychiatric problems
- Nodular adrenal disease
- Hypercoagulable state
- Osteoporosis
- Nephrolithiasis
- Growth hormone reduced

IFFERENTIAL DIAGNOSIS

- Obesity
- Diabetes mellitus
- Hypertension
- Metabolic syndrome X
- Polycystic ovarian disease
- Hypercortisolism secondary to alcoholism (pseudo-Cushing)

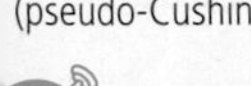

TREATMENT

MEDICATION

- Drugs are not usually effective as the primary long-term treatment, and are used primarily either in preparation for surgery or as adjunctive treatment after surgery, pituitary radiotherapy, or both.
- Metyrapone, ketoconazole, and mitotane can all be used to lower cortisol by directly inhibiting synthesis and secretion in the adrenal gland. As initial treatment, remission rates up to 85% (6,7)[C].

URGERY/OTHER PROCEDURES

- Tumor-specific surgery:
  - Trans-sphenoidal surgery for Cushing disease offers selective microadenectomy of the ACTH-producing adenoma, leaving the remaining pituitary intact (remission rate 60–80%).
  - For Cushing syndrome, resection of the ACTH-producing tumor is optimal treatment.
- Adrenal surgery:
  - For unilateral adrenal adenomas, laparoscopic surgery is treatment of choice.
  - For patients with Cushing disease, bilateral laparoscopic adrenalectomy is used more often, especially when the disease is severe or because of patient preference.
  - Pituitary radiotherapy can be used to treat persistent hypercortisolism after trans-sphenoidal surgery.

ONGOING CARE

PATIENT EDUCATION

- Comprehensive teaching to help patient cope with lifelong treatment may be needed, including:
  - Diet and monitoring weight daily
  - Early treatment of infections
  - Emotional lability prevention
- Refer to National Adrenal Disease Foundation: NADF 505 Northern Blvd. Great Neck, NY 11021; (516) 407-4992

PROGNOSIS

- Generally chronic course with cyclic exacerbations and rare remissions
- Guardedly favorable prognosis with surgery
- 20% long-term recurrence rate after surgery; more frequent following surgery for benign adrenal tumors:
  - Poor with small cell carcinoma of the lung producing ectopic hormone; neuroendocrine tumors (bronchial carcinoid) have much better prognosis (4)[C]

COMPLICATIONS

- Osteoporosis
- Increased susceptibility to infections
- Metastases of malignant tumors
- Increased cardiovascular risk even after treatment
- Lifelong glucocorticoid dependence following treatment with bilateral adrenalectomy
- Nelson syndrome (pituitary tumor) after treatment with bilateral adrenalectomy

REFERENCES

1. Newell Price J, Bertagna X, Grossman AB, et al. Cushing's syndrome. *Lancet*. 2006;367:1605–17.
2. Putignano P, et al. Midnight salivary cortisol versus urinary free and midnight serum cortisol as screening tests for Cushing's syndrome. *J Clin Endocrinol Metabol*. 88(9):4153–7.
3. Yaneva M, Mosnier-Pudar H, Dugué MA et al. Midnight salivary cortisol for the initial diagnosis of Cushing's syndrome of various causes. *J Clin Endocrinol Metab*. 2004;89:3345–51.
4. Isidori AM, et al. The ectopic adrenocorticotropin syndrome: Clinical features, diagnosis, management and long term follow up. *J Clin Endocrinol Metabol*. 2006;91(2):371–7.
5. Yanovski JA, Cutler GB, Chrousos GP et al. Corticotropin-releasing hormone stimulation following low-dose dexamethasone administration. A new test to distinguish Cushing's syndrome from pseudo-Cushing's states. *JAMA*. 1993; 269:2232–8.
6. Findling JF, et al. Cushing's syndrome: Important issues in diagnosis and management. *J Clin Endocrinol Metabol*. 2006;10:3746–53.
7. Nieman LK, Ilias I. Evaluation and treatment of Cushing's syndrome. *Am J Med*. 2005;118: 1340–6.

See Also (Topic, Algorithm, Electronic Media Element)

Algorithm: Cushing Syndrome

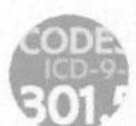

CODES

ICD9

255.0 Cushing's syndrome

CLINICAL PEARLS

- Cushing disease is due to excessive ACTH secretion from a pituitary tumor, resulting in corticosteroid excess.
- Cushing syndrome is due to excessive corticosteroid exposure from exogenous sources (medications) or endogenous sources (pituitary, adrenal, pulmonary, etc. or tumor).

CUTANEOUS DRUG REACTIONS

Nikki D.Y. Tang, MD
Nathaniel J. Jellinek, MD

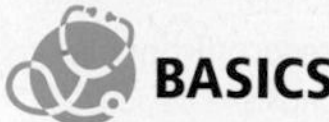

BASICS

DESCRIPTION

- An adverse cutaneous reaction in response to administration of a drug
- Cutaneous eruptions are the most common negative reactions to medications.
- Reactions are divided into immunologic and nonimmunologic reaction types.
- Morbilliform and urticarial eruptions are most common, but multiple morphologic types may occur.
- System(s) affected: Skin/Mucosa/Exocrine; Hematologic/Lymphatic/Immunologic
- Synonym(s): Drug eruptions; Drug rash; Dermatologic drug reactions' Dermatitis medicamentosa; Fixed drug eruption

Geriatric Considerations

- Possibly more likely in this age group due to greater number of medications
- Severe systemic reactions with greater morbidity

Pediatric Considerations

May occur in this age group

EPIDEMIOLOGY

- Predominant age: Geriatric, but all ages affected
- Predominant sex: Female > Male

Incidence

- In the US: 2–5% of inpatients, 0–8% overall, highest for antibiotic use (1–8%)
- Most are mild and resolve after removal of the offending agent, but severe and potentially fatal reactions may affect 1 in 1,000 inpatients.
- Likelihood of developing a cutaneous reaction is 10-fold greater in immunocompromised state

RISK FACTORS

Concurrent infections, immunocompromise (e.g., HIV, cancer, chemotherapy), metabolic disorders, large number of medications

GENERAL PREVENTION

- Always question patients about prior adverse drug events.
- Be aware of any potential cross-reactions.

PATHOPHYSIOLOGY

- Most drug reactions are nonimmunologic. Mechanisms include drug accumulation, idiosyncratic reactions (e.g., amoxicillin in infectious mononucleosis), direct release of mast-cell mediators (NSAID shift in leukotriene production causing histamine release), Jarisch-Herxheimer phenomenon, overdosage, phototoxic dermatitis, intolerance, or adverse effects.
- Reactions may be immunologically mediated, IgE-dependent, immune complex–dependent, cytotoxic, or most commonly delayed-type (type 4 hypersensitivity).

ETIOLOGY

- More than 700 drugs are known to cause a dermatologic reaction. Temporal relationship and type of reaction may elucidate the causative agent:
  - Acneform: OCPs, corticosteroids, iodinated compounds, hydantoins, lithium
  - Erythema multiforme: Sulfonamides, penicillins, barbiturates, hydantoins, NSAIDs, tetracycline, Cefaclor, Terbinafine
  - Erythema nodosum: OCPs, sulfonamides, penicillins
  - Fixed drug eruptions: OCPs, barbiturates, salicylates, tetracycline, sulfonamides
  - Lichenoid: Sildenafil, gold, antimalarials, thiazides, captopril
  - Photosensitivity: Doxycycline, thiazides, sulfonylureas, quinolones
  - Vasculitis: Thiazides, gold, sulfonamides, NSAIDs, tetracycline
  - Bullous: NSAIDs, thiazides, barbiturates, captopril
  - Skin necrosis: Warfarin, heparin
- Particularly common offenders: Antibiotics, NSAIDs, phenytoin, allopurinol, warfarin, gold, lithium

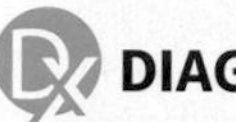

DIAGNOSIS

HISTORY

- Medications within past month: All oral, parenteral, and topical agents; all OTC drugs; vitamins, homeopathic, and herbal remedies
- Inquire about previous adverse reactions to medications.
- Ask about multiple courses of therapy or long-term use of a drug that can induce allergic sensitization.
- Consider other etiologies, including bacterial infections and viral exanthems.

PHYSICAL EXAM

May present as a number of different eruption types, including but not limited to:

- Morbilliform eruptions (exanthems):
  - Most frequent cutaneous reaction (28–95%) (1)[A]
  - May be indistinguishable from viral exanthem
  - Erythematous macules and papules; confluent, symmetric, and pruritic
  - Most common on trunk and in dependent areas
  - Onset 7–21 days after initiation
- Urticaria:
  - Also very common reaction
  - Pruritic erythematous wheals distributed anywhere on the body, including mucous membranes
  - 40% progress to angioedema, appearing as nonpitting edema without erythema or margins (2)[C]
  - May be annular in pediatric patient
  - Individual lesions fade within 24 hours, but new urticaria may develop.
- Fixed drug eruptions:
  - Single or multiple, round, sharply defined, dark violaceous plaques with gray center that leave residual macular hyperpigmentation
  - Appear shortly after drug exposure and reappear in the same location after drug ingestion; lesions can occur anywhere: Favored sites include mouth, genitalia, and acral areas
  - Onset usually 2 hours after ingestion of drug
  - Some patients have a refractory period during which the drug fails to activate lesions.
- Eczematous reactions:
  - Pruritic scalelike erythematous lesions typically on flexor surfaces of arms or legs
- Erythema multiforme (EM):
  - EM minor:
    - Target and bullous lesions predominantly on the extremities
    - Association with herpes simplex virus much more commonly than any drug
  - EM major:
    - Stevens-Johnson syndrome (SJS): Widespread skin and mucous membrane involvement with large atypical targetoid lesions with <10% skin sloughing; 5%-15% mortality (3)[C]
    - Toxic epidermal necrolysis (TEN): More extensive lesions with sloughing >30% of body surface, often with confluent areas of necrosis; 30% mortality (4)[C] with secondary infection and sepsis major concerns
  - Typical onset 1–3 weeks after starting offending agent
- Exfoliative erythroderma/dermatitis:
  - Erythema or eczema and scaling of over 50% of body surface
  - Lymphadenopathy, hepatosplenomegaly, leukocytosis, eosinophilia, or anemia may be present.
  - Potentially life-threatening
  - Difficult to distinguish between drug etiology, inflammatory etiology, cutaneous lymphoma etiology
- Acral erythema (erythrodysesthesia):
  - Common reaction to chemotherapeutic agents
  - Erythema, edema, and tenderness of palms and soles
  - Resolves in 2–4 weeks
- Lichen planuslike eruptions:
  - Violaceous, pruritic papules on extensor surfaces
  - Reticular pattern, buccal mucosa
- Photosensitivity reaction:
  - Phototoxic reactions within 24 hours of light exposure with exaggerated sun burn reaction
  - Photoallergic reactions; less common, more pruritic than painful, caused by UVA exposure
- Acneform eruptions:
  - Pustular lesions, but unlike true acne (no comedones)
- Vasculitis:
  - Petechiae or purpura concentrated on lower legs
  - Fever, myalgias, arthritis, and abdominal pain may also be present.
- Hypersensitivity syndrome (e.g., drug rash with eosinophilia and systemic symptoms—DRESS):
  - Related to anticonvulsants, sulfonamides, dapsone, minocycline, allopurinol
  - Classic triad of fever, exanthem, and internal organ involvement. May also present with pharyngitis and lymphadenopathy.
  - Internal organ involvement: 80% hepatic, 40% renal, 33% pulmonary (5)[C]
  - Atypical lymphocytosis with prominent eosinophilia (6)[C]
  - Onset 2–8 weeks, but may develop 3 months or later into therapy
- Acute generalized exanthematous pustulosis (AGEP):
  - Fever with multiple small, sterile, nonfollicular pustules on erythematous background with desquamation after 7–10 days
  - Appears similar to pustular psoriasis, but AGEP has more marked leukocytosis with neutrophilia and eosinophilia
  - Short time to onset (24 h to 2 weeks)

Serum sicknesslike reaction:
- Fever, nonspecific cutaneous eruption, arthralgias
- Onset 7–14 days
- Related to antibiotics, minocycline (6)[C]:
  - Detailed observation and morphologic description of all lesions facilitates diagnosis.
  - Nikolsky sign (epidermis sloughs with lateral pressure; may constitute medical emergency)

Sweet syndrome (acute febrile neutrophilic dermatosis):
- Fever, neutrophilia, tender reddish-blue or violet papules, plaques, or nodules, with or without pustules or vesicles that spontaneously resolve
- May have oral ulcers or ocular manifestations such as conjunctivitis
- Classically seen in young women after a mild respiratory illness, but 7–56% associated with malignancy (7)[C]
- Also associated with G-CSF, GM-CSF administration

Dermatomyositislike:
- Similar cutaneous findings (e.g., Gottron papules), but lack muscle involvement and antinuclear antibodies

DIAGNOSTIC TESTS & INTERPRETATION

Lab

Initial lab tests

- Routine laboratory tests generally are nonspecific and not helpful.
- Significant eosinophilia may be related to more severe disease in allergic reactions (4)[C].
- Special tests dependent on suspected mechanism (8)[C]:
  - Type I: Skin testing, RAST, serum tryptase
  - Type II: Direct or indirect Coombs test
  - Type III: ESR, C-reactive protein, ANA, antihistone antibody, tissue biopsy for immunofluorescence studies
  - Type IV: Patch testing, lymphocyte proliferation assay (investigational)
- Cultures may be useful to exclude infectious causes.

Imaging

For vasculitic eruptions, chest radiography and urinalysis

Diagnostic Procedures/Surgery

- Withdrawal of suspected offending agent and observation for resolution
- Punch biopsy sometimes helpful for fixed drug eruptions

Pathological Findings

Nonspecific histologic findings are superficial infiltrates composed variably of lymphocytes, neutrophils, and eosinophils (9).

DIFFERENTIAL DIAGNOSIS

- Viral exanthem: Presence of fever, lymphocytosis, and other systemic findings may help differentiate
- Primary dermatosis: Correlation of drug withdrawal to rash resolution may clarify diagnosis; skin biopsy may be helpful.

TREATMENT

MEDICATION

- Depends on the type of eruption; symptomatic treatment may be useful; most require no specific therapy except withdrawal of offending drug.
- Anaphylaxis or widespread urticaria: Epinephrine 1:1,000, 0.01 mL/kg (0.3 mL maximum) SC
- Acute urticaria (<6 weeks): First- or second-generation H1 antihistamines are mainstay of therapy (2)[A].
- Chronic urticaria (>6 weeks): Antihistamines, doxepin in increasing doses and antileukotriene medications are options (2)[A]. H4 receptor antagonists may be more beneficial than H1 receptor antagonists (8)[C].
- Anaphylaxis, severe urticaria, or erythema multiforme: Corticosteroids parenterally as indicated by condition; or prednisone p.o. 1 mg/kg in tapering doses (2)[A]
- Chronic erythema multiforme associated with herpes simplex: Prophylactic acyclovir (10)[A]
- Topical lubricants, emollients for eczematous reactions
- Topical corticosteroids (Groups I–III) for limited eczematous-type eruptions or lichenoid eruptions
- Contraindications, precautions, and significant possible interactions: Refer to manufacturer's information.

ADDITIONAL TREATMENT

General Measures

- Appropriate health care, monitor for signs of impending cardiovascular collapse:
  - Urticaria or bullous lesions, angioedema, and generalized erythroderma are all potentially more serious than other types of reactions; therefore, possible offending medications should be discontinued immediately, medical evaluation as soon as possible
  - Anaphylactic reactions, Stevens-Johnson syndrome, extensive bullous reactions, or TEN: Consider inpatient treatment.
- In patients on multiple medications, the decision to discontinue each medication should be based on the likelihood of each individual medication causing the reaction (e.g., 7% for penicillins, sulfonamides) and the risk/benefit ratio of continuing each medication.
- Do not rechallenge with drugs causing urticaria, bullae, angioedema, anaphylaxis, or erythema multiforme.
- Consider continuation of medications through morbilliform eruptions unless severe.

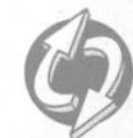

ONGOING CARE

FOLLOW-UP RECOMMENDATIONS

Patient Monitoring

- For urticarial, bullous, or erythema multiformelike lesions, close patient follow-up needed
- Patients with serious reactions (anaphylaxis, angioedema) should be given EpiPen for secondary prevention
- Label the patient's chart with the suspected agent and type of reaction.

PATIENT EDUCATION

American Academy of Dermatology, (708) 330-0230

PROGNOSIS

- Eruptions generally fade within days after removing offending agent
- Anaphylaxis, angioedema, and bullous reactions are potentially fatal.

COMPLICATIONS

- Anaphylaxis
- Bone marrow suppression
- Hepatitis (dapsone, hydantoin)
- Cross-reaction to chemically similar agents in future

REFERENCES

1. Bigby M. Rates of cutaneous reactions to drugs. *Arch Dermatol*. 2001;137:765–70.
2. Amar SM & Dreskin SC. Urticaria. *Prim Care Clin Office Pract*. 2008;(35):141–57.
3. Hazin R, Ibrahimi OA, Hazin MI, Kimyai-Asadi A et al. Stevens-Johnson syndrome: pathogenesis, diagnosis, and management. *Ann. Med*. 2008;40:129–38.
4. Granowitz EV & Brown RB. Antibiotic adverse reactions and drug interactions. *Crti Care Clin*. 2008:412–42.
5. Chen YC, Chiu HC, Chu CY et al. Drug Reaction With Eosinophilia and Systemic Symptoms: A Retrospective Study of 60 Cases. *Archives of dermatology*. 2010;
6. Knowles SR & Shear NH. Recognition and management of severe cutaneous drug reactions. *Dermatol Clin*. 2007;25:245–53.
7. Cohen PR, Kurzrock R et al. Sweet's syndrome: a neutrophilic dermatosis classically associated with acute onset and fever. *Clin. Dermatol*. 2000;18: 265–82.
8. Sicherer SH, et al. Advances in allergic skin disease, anaphylaxis and hypersensitivity reactions to foods, drugs and insects in 2007. *J All Clin Immunol*. 2008:1351–7.
9. Gerson D et al. Cutaneous drug eruptions: A 5-year experience. *J Am Acad Dermatol*. 2008;59;6:995–9.
10. Tatnall FM, Schofield JK, Leigh IM et al. A double-blind, placebo-controlled trial of continuous acyclovir therapy in recurrent erythema multiforme. *Br J Dermatol*. 1995;132:267–70.

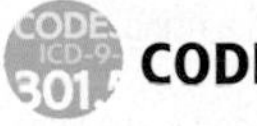

CODES

ICD9

- 693.0 Dermatitis due to drugs and medicines taken internally
- 708.0 Allergic urticaria

CLINICAL PEARLS

- Virtually any drug can cause any rash; antibiotics are the most common culprits causing cutaneous drug reactions.
- Focus on drug history with new suspicious skin eruptions.
- Morbilliform rashes are the most frequent.
- Usually self-limited after withdrawal of offending agent.
- Symptoms such as tongue swelling/angioedema, skin necrosis, blisters, high fever, dyspnea, and mucous membrane erosions signify more severe drug reactions.

CUTANEOUS SQUAMOUS CELL CARCINOMA

Herbert P. Goodheart, MD

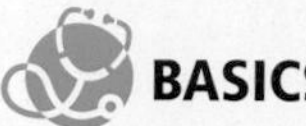

BASICS

- Squamous cell carcinoma (SCC) is a malignant epithelial tumor arising from keratinocytes of the epidermis. Cutaneous (nonmucous membrane) SCC is the second most common form of skin cancer. Lesions most frequently occur on sun-exposed sites of elderly, fair-skinned individuals. The majority of SCCs arise in solar keratoses *(actinic keratoses)*. Such actinically derived SCCs that develop from solar keratoses are slow-growing, minimally invasive, unaggressive; and the prognosis is usually excellent because distant metastases that arise from these lesions are extremely rare. An SCC may appear de novo without a preceding solar keratosis. SCCs may also develop from causes other than sun exposure. For example, an SCC may arise in an old burn scar or from sites previously exposed to ionizing radiation. An SCC may also emerge from preexisting human papilloma virus infection *(verrucous carcinoma)*. An SCC is capable of locally infiltrative growth, spread to regional lymph nodes, and distant metastasis, most often to the lungs. When metastases from SCC do occur, they are more likely to result from lesions that appear on the ears or on the vermilion border of the lips or from tumors >2 cm in diameter. Other risks for metastasis include lesions that arise on mucous membranes, from sites that received ionizing radiation, on the skin of organ transplant recipients, in chronic inflammatory lesions (e.g., discoid lupus erythematosus), or in long-standing scars or cutaneous ulcers (e.g., venous stasis ulcers) or other nonhealing wounds.
- System(s) affected: Skin/Exocrine
- Synonym(s): Squamous cell carcinoma of the skin; Epidermoid carcinoma; Prickle cell carcinoma

EPIDEMIOLOGY

- Predominant age: Elderly population
- Predominant sex: Males > Females
- More common in geographic areas that have a high frequency of sun exposure

Incidence

- The dramatic escalating incidence in the US due to an increase in sun exposure in the general population, aging of the population, earlier and more frequent diagnosis of SCC, and a rising number of immunosuppressed patients
- The incidence is highest in Australia and in the Sun Belt of the US.

ALERT

Bowen disease and frank squamous cell carcinoma are 2 of the few skin cancers that should be considered in blacks. These non-sun–related skin cancers tend to arise on the extremities de novo or in an old scar or in a lesion of discoid lupus erythematosus.

RISK FACTORS

- Older age
- Male sex: However, incidence is increasing in females due to lifestyle changes (e.g., suntan parlors, shorter dresses, etc.)
- Chronic sun exposure: SCC is noted more frequently in those with a greater degree of outdoor activity (e.g., farmers, sailors, gardeners).
- Patients with multiple solar keratoses are at increased risk.
- Personal or family history of skin cancer
- Northern European descent
- Fair complexion, fair hair, light eyes
- Poor tanning ability, with tendency to burn
- Organ transplant recipients, chronic immunosuppression
- Exposure to chemical carcinogens (e.g., arsenic, tar) or ionizing radiation
- Therapeutic UV and ionizing radiation exposure
- Defects in cell-mediated immunity related to lymphoproliferative disorders (CLL, lymphoma)
- Human papillomavirus (HPV) infection (certain subtypes)
- Chronic scarring and inflammatory conditions
- Specific genodermatoses (e.g., xeroderma pigmentosum)

Genetics

- Persons of Irish or Scottish ancestry have the highest prevalence of SCC.
- SCC is relatively rare in people of African and Asian descent, although it is the most common form of skin cancer in these populations.
- Patients with oculocutaneous albinism are at greater risk.

GENERAL PREVENTION

Sun-avoidance measures: Sunscreens, hats, etc. Sunglasses with UV protection. Tinted windshields and side windows in cars. Sun-protective garments.

ETIOLOGY

- Exact mechanisms are not established; however, it is well known that ultraviolet radiation damages skin cell nucleic acids (DNA) resulting in a mutant clone of the gene p53. This leads to uncontrolled growth of skin cells. Ultraviolet radiation also suppresses the immune response preventing recovery from this damage.
- Epidemiologic and experimental evidence suggests the following as causative agents: Sunlight (solar radiation), radiation exposure, tanning parlors, PUVA phototherapy exposure, inorganic arsenic exposure, coal tar and other oil derivatives
- Immunosuppression by medications or disease such as HIV

COMMONLY ASSOCIATED CONDITIONS

- Solar keratosis (some investigators consider a solar keratosis to be an early squamous cell carcinoma, although relatively few ultimately are found to develop into an SCC)
- Keratoacanthoma
- Cutaneous horn
- Actinic cheilitis (solar keratoses of the mucous membranes of the lips) and leukoplakia of lip
- Xeroderma pigmentosum, albinism, and vitiligo
- Immunosuppression
- Chronic skin ulcers and chronic thermal burns

DIAGNOSIS

HISTORY

Often a family or personal history of skin cancer

PHYSICAL EXAM

- Lesions occur chiefly on chronically sun-exposed areas:
  - The face and the backs of the forearms and hands
  - Bald areas of the scalp and top of ears in men
  - The sun-exposed "V" of the neck, as well as the posterior neck below the occipital hairline
  - In elderly females, lesions tend to occur on the legs and other sun-exposed locations.
  - In blacks: Equal frequency in sun-exposed and unexposed areas
- Clinical appearance:
  - Generally slow-growing, firm, hyperkeratotic papules, nodules, or plaques
  - Most SCCs are asymptomatic, although bleeding pain, and tenderness (all of which are unusual) may be noted.
  - Lesions may have a smooth, verrucous, or papillomatous surface.
  - Varying degrees of ulceration, erosion, crust, or scale
  - Color is often red to brown, tan, or pearly, and may be indistinguishable from basal cell carcinom

DIAGNOSTIC TESTS & INTERPRETATION

Diagnostic Procedures/Surgery

- Surgical biopsy to ensure diagnosis: Shave biopsy, punch biopsy, excisional biopsy, incisional biopsy
- Sentinel lymph node biopsy has been used to identi micrometastases in a small number of patients wit high-risk SCC and clinically negative nodes. Complete lymphadenectomy of the draining nodal basin has also been suggested for high-risk tumors

Pathological Findings

- Noninvasive SCC is characterized by an intraepidermal proliferation of atypical keratinocyte Hyperkeratosis, acanthosis, and confluent parakeratosis are seen within the epidermis. Cellula atypia, including pleomorphism, hyperchromatic nuclei, and mitoses, are prominent. Atypical keratinocytes may be found in the basal layer and often extend deeply down hair follicles, but they do not invade the dermis.
- In the in situ type of SCC (*Bowen disease*), only the full thickness of the epidermis is involved. The basement membrane remains intact.
- An invasive squamous cell carcinoma penetrates through the basement membrane into the dermis. I has various levels of anaplasia and may manifest relatively few to multiple mitoses and display varyin degrees of differentiation, such as keratinization.
- Poorly differentiated tumors are clinically more aggressive. SCCs proliferate 1st by local invasion. Metastases, when they do occur, spread via local lymph ducts to local lymph nodes.

DIFFERENTIAL DIAGNOSIS

- Solar keratosis *(actinic keratosis)*. Early SCC lesions may be clinically difficult, if not impossible, to distinguish from a precursor solar keratosis.
- Basal cell carcinoma may be also indistinguishable from an SCC, particularly if the lesion is ulcerated.
- Verruca vulgaris

ALERT

- The appearance of common warts is often similar to that of SCC lesions.
- A subungual SCC can easily be mistaken for a verruca.
- Seborrheic keratosis: "Stuck on" appearance
- Keratoacanthoma: This lesion also may be clinically impossible to differentiate from an SCC:
  - Occurs in the elderly >60 years
  - Fast growing
  - A nodular lesion that usually has a characteristic central crater

- If ignored, lesions may involute spontaneously.
- Resembles an SCC histologically and is considered by some dermatologists and dermatopathologists to be a low-grade variant of an SCC. (Some investigators feel that it should be treated as an SCC.)

- Melanoma:
  - Amelanotic melanoma and ulcerated melanoma may also be impossible to distinguish from an SCC.
- Clinical variants of SCC:
  - Bowen disease (*squamous cell carcinoma in situ)*: This is a solitary lesion that resembles a scaly psoriatic or eczematous plaque. By definition, the atypia of SCC in situ involves the full thickness of the epidermis without invasion into the dermis.
  - Cutaneous horn: SCC with an overlying cutaneous horn. A cutaneous horn represents a fingernail platelike keratinization produced by the SCC. Bowen disease may also produce a cutaneous horn on its surface.
  - HPV-associated SCC: Virally induced SCC most commonly manifests as a new or enlarging warty growth on the penis, vulva, perianal area, or periungual region.
  - Erythroplasia of Queyrat refers to Bowen disease of the glans penis, which manifests as 1 or more velvety red plaques.
  - Subungual SCC: Such lesions typically mimic a wart and are misdiagnosed prior to biopsy.
  - Anogenital SCC: SCC in the anogenital region may manifest as a moist, red plaque on the glans penis or perianal area; indurated or ulcerated lesions may be seen on the vulva, external anus, or scrotum.
  - Verrucous carcinoma, a subtype of SCC, can be locally destructive but rarely metastasizes. Lesions are "cauliflowerlike" verrucous nodules or plaques.

TREATMENT

MEDICATION

First Line

- Immunotherapy:
  - Imiquimod (Aldara) (1,2) 5% cream is approved for the treatment of solar keratoses, genital warts, and for superficial basal cell carcinomas. It is now being used "off-label" for SCC in situ (Bowen disease), and may have some utility in treating selected patients who have highly differentiated SCCs.
- In patients with multiple or recurrent SCCs, chemoprevention with systemic retinoids (3,4) such as acetrecin may be effective for reducing the number of new SCCs; shown to be beneficial in treating existing SCCs or at reducing the risk of recurrence after treatment.

Second Line

- Photodynamic therapy (PDT): Treatment with PDT involves the application of a photosensitizer (given topically or systemically) followed by exposure to a light source. PDT is used primarily to treat large numbers of solar keratoses and is not recommended for treatment of invasive SCC.
- Radiotherapy is a primary treatment option that is generally restricted to older patients who are physically debilitated or are unable to undergo, or refuse to undergo, excisional surgery.
- Topical chemotherapy: Topical formulations of 5-fluorouracil (5-FU) are available for the treatment of Bowen disease and solar keratoses.
- Intralesional 5-FU has also been used to successfully treat keratoacanthomas.

SURGERY/OTHER PROCEDURES

- Electrocautery (electrodesiccation) and curettage (ED&C):
  - For small lesions (generally <1 cm) on flat surfaces (e.g., forehead, cheek) and SCC in situ (Bowen disease). ED&C may be used to treat superficially invasive SCCs without high-risk characteristics, but it is not appropriate for certain high-risk anatomic locations (see below).
  - Cryosurgery with LN_2 in selected lesions, such as Bowen disease
- Total excision, which is the preferred method of therapy for SCC, permitting histologic diagnosis of the tumor margins
- Micrographic (Mohs) surgery is a microscopically controlled method of removing skin cancers that allows for controlled excision and maximum preservation of normal tissue. It has the highest cure rate of all surgical treatments. Mohs surgery may be indicated for:
  - Large or invasive carcinomas
  - Recurrent SCCs
  - Lesions with a poorly delineated clinical border
  - An SCC within an orifice (e.g., ear canals or nostrils)
  - Locations where preservation of normal tissue is extremely important (e.g., tip of the nose, eyelids, ala nasi, ears, lips, and glans penis)
  - Bone or cartilage invasion
  - A lesion in an area of late radiation change
  - Micrographic (Mohs) surgery provides the best available cure rates (94–99%) for SCC.
- Metastatic disease requires aggressive management by a multidisciplinary team involving plastic, ENT/maxillofacial, a general surgeon, or a surgical oncologist.

ONGOING CARE

FOLLOW-UP RECOMMENDATIONS

Patient Monitoring

After therapy, periodic skin exam every month for 3 months, 6 months after treatment, and then yearly

ALERT

- SCCs that arise in areas of non-sun–exposed skin or those that originate de novo on areas of sun-exposed skin have a greater tendency to metastasize.
- An SCC arising on a mucous membrane, one arising from a chronic ulcer, or one arising in an immunocompromised patient should be regarded as potentially metastatic.

PATIENT EDUCATION

Skin self-exam, encourage sun avoidance techniques, sunscreens, etc. Artificial tanning devices should be avoided.

PROGNOSIS

- 90–95% cure rate with appropriate treatment
- Head and neck lesions have better prognosis (5).
- The ability to produce scale (*keratinization)* indicates a tendency for a lesion to be more differentiated and less likely to metastasize.
- Softer, nonkeratinizing lesions are not as well differentiated and thus are more likely to spread.
- Lesions ≥2 cm more prone to recur
- SCCs that are deeply invasive in subcutaneous fat or deeper, or those that have perineural involvement, are more likely to metastasize.
- When SCC does metastasize, it usually occurs within several years from the time of diagnosis and involves draining lymph nodes.
- Once nodal metastasis of cutaneous SCC has occurred, the overall 5-year survival rate has historically been in the range of 25–35%.

ALERT

An SCC that is histopathologically described as being "poorly differentiated" should be treated more aggressively.

COMPLICATIONS

Untreated, SCC becomes indurated, with a tendency to ooze, ulcerate, or bleed. Local recurrence. Metastatic disease.

REFERENCES

1. Patel GK, Goodwin R. Imiquimod 5% cream monotherapy for cutaneous *squamous cell carcinoma in situ* (Bowen's disease): A randomized, double blind, placebo-controlled trial. *J Am Acad Dermatol*. 2006;54(1):25–32.
2. Hengge UR, Schaller J. Successful treatment of invasive squamous cell carcinoma using topical imiquimod. *Arch Dermatol*. 2004;140:404–6.
3. Harwood CA, Leedham-Green M, Leigh IM, et al. Low-dose retinoids in the prevention of cutaneous squamous cell carcinomas in organ transplant recipients: a 16-year retrospective study. *Arch Dermatol*. 2005;141:456–64.
4. Chen K, Craig JC, Shumack S. Oral retinoids for the prevention of skin cancers in solid organ transplant recipients: a systematic review of randomized controlled trials. *Br J Dermatol*. 2005;152:518–23.
5. Clayman GL, Lee JJ, Holsinger FC, et al. Mortality risk from squamous cell skin cancer. *J Clin Oncol*. 2005;23:759–65.

ADDITIONAL READING

Schmults CD. High-risk cutaneous squamous cell carcinoma: identification and management. *Adv Dermatol*. 2005;21:133–52.

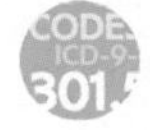

CODES

ICD9

- 173.0 Other malignant neoplasm of skin of lip
- 173.1 Other malignant neoplasm of skin of eyelid, including canthus
- 173.2 Other malignant neoplasm of skin of ear and external auditory canal

CLINICAL PEARLS

- An early lesion of SCC is difficult to distinguish from a solar keratosis.
- SCCs that develop from solar keratoses are generally unaggressive.
- An SCC arising on a mucous membrane such as the glans penis, lip, or from a chronic ulcer, or one arising in an immunocompromised patient, is potentially metastatic.

CUTANEOUS T-CELL LYMPHOMA

Sandra Cuellar, PharmD, BCOP
Paul G. Rubinstein, MD

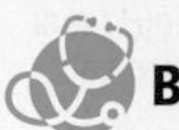

BASICS

Cutaneous T-cell lymphomas are a rare group of mature T-cell lymphomas presenting primarily in the skin. These diseases involve overlap of the disciplines of dermatology, medical oncology, and radiation oncology. Other than allogeneic stem cell transplant, there are no curative therapies for this disease (1,2,3,4).

DESCRIPTION

- A heterogeneous group of relatively uncommon extranodal non-Hodgkin lymphomas
- This section focuses on mycosis fungoides (MF), the most common type of cutaneous lymphoma. For other subtypes, please consult the reference section.

EPIDEMIOLOGY

- Median age at diagnosis is 55–60; however, it can occur in children and young adults (2).
- Male:Female = 2:1 (2)
- African American incidence greater compared to whites (2)

Incidence

0.4 cases per 100,000 per year

RISK FACTORS

No compelling evidence that mycosis fungoides is caused by viral infection or chemical exposure

Genetics

- Clonal T-cell receptor gene rearrangements are detected in most cases (4).
- No recurrent, mycosis fungoides-specific chromosomal translocations have been identified (2).
- Loss at chromosome 10q and abnormalities in the tumor suppressor genes p15, p16, and p53 are common (2,4).

PATHOPHYSIOLOGY

- Malignancy of $CD4^+$ helper T cells
- Malignant cells have a high affinity to the epidermis.
- Malignant T cells are also activated T cells ($CD45RO^+$) and produce cytokines, such as IL-4 and IL-5, which can lead to eosinophilia and atopylike symptoms.

ETIOLOGY

Unknown

DIAGNOSIS

- Diagnostic algorithm for MF is a point-based system. Points are scored for clinical, histopathologic, molecular biological, and immunopathological categories. A diagnosis of MF is made when a total of 4 points or more are determined (5).
- Clinical criteria: Patient has persistent and/or progressive patches and plaques plus lesions in a non-sun-exposed location, size/shape variation of lesions, poikiloderma (5)
- Histopathologic criteria: Superficial lymphoid infiltrate present plus epidermotropism without spongiosis, lymphoid atypia (5)
- Molecular biological criteria: Clonal TCR gene rearrangement is present (5).
- Immunopathologic criteria: <50% of T cells express CD2, CD3, CD5; <10% of T cells express CD 7; there is discordance of the epidermal and dermal cells with regard to expression of CD2, CD3, CD5, or CD7 (5)

PHYSICAL EXAM

- Examination of the entire skin, with assessment of percent of involved body surface area (%BSA), and lesions found, is critical.
- Pink scaly patches and plaques, typically in sun-protected areas such as the buttocks, thighs, and breasts
- Cutaneous tumors and ulcerations
- Exfoliative erythroderma
- Palmoplantar keratoderma (thickened scaly skin on palms and soles)
- Lymphadenopathy can be present in later stages.
- Hepatosplenomegaly can be present at late stages.

DIAGNOSTIC TESTS & INTERPRETATION

Lab

- Complete blood count (CBC) with differential and platelets and Sézary screen
- Polymerase chain reaction (PCR) of peripheral blood to detect clonal rearrangement of the T-cell receptor
- Flow cytometric studies to establish the presence of Sézary cells. Markers for CD3,4,7,8,26 need to be analyzed.
- If the CD4:CD8 ratio of >10, a circulating clonal T-cell population is identified, a positive Sézary cell count of over 1000 cells/mm^3 is found, this is consistent with Sézary syndrome; see below.
- Comprehensive metabolic profile
- LDH

Imaging

- Computed tomography (CT) of the neck, chest, abdomen for T2 disease or greater (see staging system described below)
- Chest x-ray should be used in limited disease without any palpable lymphadenopathy.

Diagnostic Procedures/Surgery

- Skin biopsy: Diagnostic procedure of choice
- Lymph node biopsy if there is clinical adenopathy o advanced disease
- Bone marrow biopsy for unexplained hematologic abnormality: Not normally done

Pathological Findings

- Skin biopsy shows superficial bandlike infiltrate, epidermotropism of lymphocytes, Pautrier microabscesses, and dermal infiltrates of atypical cells in tumors (5).
- Cells are usually CD3+, CD4+, CD45RO+, CD8–.
- Loss of T-cell antigens such as CD2, CD3, CD5, and CD7 is often seen.
- Sézary syndrome is diagnosed when Sézary cells are found in the peripheral circulation. Sézary cells are defined as atypical lymphocytes with cerebriform nuclei. Generalized erythroderma and lymphadenopathy usually accompanies this blood finding to complete the syndrome (2):
  - Sézary syndrome (leukemic phase of cutaneous T-cell lymphoma) is defined by the following: If th CD4:CD8 ratio >10, a circulating clonal T-cell population is identified, a positive Sézary cell count of over 1,000 cells/mm^3, a CD4/CD26- greater than or equal to 30% of all of the lymphocytes in the presence of a clonal T-cell population (2)
- Large cell transformation of cutaneous T-cell lymphoma is a rare and lethal event. If 25% of larg cells are found on a biopsy taken from an MF lesion this represents a transformation from an indolent lymphoma, MF, to a very aggressive form of cutaneous T-cell lymphoma. It is refractory to most chemotherapies, and overall survival is limited to just months (1,3,6).
- The treatment of the disease and prognosis (see prognosis section below) is determined by the stage (6):
  - Staging is done based on physical exam and pathology. Bone marrow biopsy is not needed for staging of the disease. The TNMB staging system ([T]umor, [N]ode, [M]Visceral, and [B]lood involvement with Sézary cells):
    - T1: Patches or plaques involving <10% of total body surface area
    - T2: Patches, papules, and/or plaques involving ≥10% of total body surface area
    - T3: 1 or more cutaneous tumors (≥1 cm in diameter)
    - T4: Erythroderma (>80% of total body surface area)

- N0: Lymph nodes clinically uninvolved
- N1: Lymph nodes clinically enlarged but not histologically involved
- N2: Lymph nodes clinically normal but histologically involved
- N3: Lymph nodes clinically enlarged and histologically involved
- M0: No visceral organ involvement
- M1: Visceral involvement with pathological confirmation
- B0: Absence of significant blood involvement (<5% of peripheral blood lymphocytes are Sézary cells)
- B1: Low blood tumor burden (>5% of the peripheral blood lymphocytes are Sézary cells)
- B2: High blood tumor burden: >1000/microliter Sézary cells

Stage groups:
- IA: T1N0M0B0-1
- IB: T2N0M0B0-1
- II: T1-2N1-2M0B0-1
- IIB: T3N0-2M0B0-1
- III: T4N0-2M0B0-1
- IIIA: T4N0-2M0B0
- IIIB: T4N0-2M0B1
- IVA1: T1-4N0-2M0B2
- IVA2: T1-4N3M0B0-2
- IVB: T1-4N0-3M1B0-2

DIFFERENTIAL DIAGNOSIS
- Patches and plaques seen in MF resemble lesions of:
  - Eczema
  - Parapsoriasis
  - Atopic dermatitis
  - Photodermatitis
  - Drug eruptions
  - Psoriasis
  - Contact dermatitis
- Cutaneous tumors:
  - Similar to other cutaneous lymphomas
- Erythroderma, though rare, can present like:
  - Atopic dermatitis
  - Contact dermatitis
  - Drug eruptions
  - Erythrodermic psoriasis

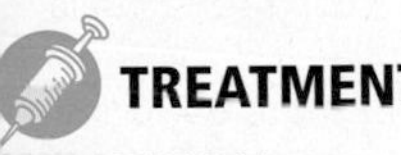

TREATMENT

MEDICATION
- Therapy must be individualized. No universally accepted standard approach exists to treat this disease. The stage of disease dictates the aggressiveness and type of therapy (13):
- T1 and T2 disease:
  - Topical potent corticosteroids
  - Topical mechlorethamine (nitrogen mustard)
  - Topical bis-chlor-nitrosourea
  - Topical bexarotene
  - Phototherapy: Psoralen and ultraviolet A light (PUVA) or narrow-band UVB
  - Oral retinoids (bexarotene)
  - Oral methotrexate
  - Radiation therapy (See Issues for Referral section below)
- T3 disease:
  - Oral retinoids (bexarotene)
  - Interferon α-2b
  - Denileukin diftitox
  - Chemotherapy: If the disease progresses on the above therapies, gemcitabine or pegylated doxorubicin is usually used first-line. If the disease continues to progress, low-dose methotrexate, bortezomib, cyclophosphamide, and fludarabine are used as second-line therapy. Stem cell transplantation can also be used in certain cases; see below.
- T4 disease and Sézary syndrome:
  - Oral retinoids (bexarotene)
  - Interferon α-2b
  - Denileukin diftitox
  - Phototherapy
  - Vorinostat (an oral deacetylase inhibitor)
  - Romidepsin (an injectable deacetylase inhibitor)
  - Extracorporeal photopheresis
  - Chemotherapy: If the disease progresses on the above therapies, gemcitabine or pegylated doxorubicin is usually used first-line. If the disease continues to progress, low-dose methotrexate, bortezomib, cyclophosphamide, and fludarabine are used as second-line therapy. Stem cell transplantation can also be used in certain cases; see below.
  - Stem cell transplantation (reserved for extensive and/or refractory disease)

ADDITIONAL TREATMENT

General Measures
- Most patients are managed on an outpatient basis
- Treatment should be individualized for each patient, based on their extent of disease and side effects of possible therapies (1,3).
- Skin lesions commonly become infected, and treatment with antibiotic may be necessary.

Issues for Referral
- Dermatology manages early disease.
- Hematology-oncology is involved for later-stage diseases.
- Radiation oncology can be referred for limited disease or to treat extensive or painful skin lesions when refractory to chemotherapy.

Additional Therapies
Localized or total skin electron-beam therapy can be used in most stages of disease, either as monotherapy or in combination with other agents.

ONGOING CARE

FOLLOW-UP RECOMMENDATIONS

Patient Monitoring
Must be individualized

PATIENT EDUCATION
Patient information can be found at:
- American Academy of Dermatology Web site: http://www.aad.org
- Cutaneous Lymphoma Foundation Web site: http://www.clfoundation.org

PROGNOSIS
- MF is a chronic disease, though early-stage disease is curable.
- Survival by stage:
  - Stage 1A: Survival similar to age-/sex-matched individuals without disease
  - Stage IB and IIA: 11 years
  - Stage IIB: 3.2 years
  - Stage III: 4.6 years
  - Stage IVA or B: 13 months

COMPLICATIONS
- Immunosuppression from the disease and treatments can lead to infections.
- Skin lesions commonly become infected and can lead to sepsis.

REFERENCES

1. Horwitz SM, Olsen EA, Duvic M, et al. Review of the treatment of mycosis fungoides and Sézary syndrome: a stage-based approach. *J Natl Compr Canc Netw*. 2008;6:436–42.
2. Hwang ST, Janik JE, Jaffe ES, et al. Mycosis fungoides and Sézary syndrome. *Lancet*. 2008;371: 945–57.
3. Prince HM, Whittaker S, Hoppe RT et al. How I treat mycosis fungoides and Sézary syndrome. *Blood*. 2009;114:4337–53.
4. Girardi M, Heald PW, Wilson LD. The pathogenesis of mycosis fungoides. *N Engl J Med*. 2004;350: 1978–88.
5. Pimpinelli N, Olsen EA, Santucci M, et al. Defining early mycosis fungoides *J Am Acad Dermatol*. 2005;53(6):1053–63.
6. Willemze R, Jaffe ES, Burg G, et al. WHO-EORTC classification for cutaneous lymphomas. *Blood*. 2005;105:3768–85.

CODES

ICD9

202.10 Mycosis fungoides, unspecified site

CYCLIC VOMITING SYNDROME

Salwa Khan, MD, MHS

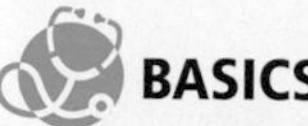

BASICS

DESCRIPTION

An idiopathic chronic functional GI disorder characterized by discrete, recurrent, stereotypical episodes of high-intensity nausea and vomiting lasting hours to days, separated by symptom-free intervals Cyclic vomiting syndrome (CVS) has a phasic pattern with four distinct phases.

- Interepisodic: Symptom-free period
- Prodromal: Often marked by nausea ± abdominal pain; able to take oral medications
- Vomiting: Nausea, vomiting, and retching
- Recovery: Nausea remits and patient has recovered appetite, strength, and energy.

EPIDEMIOLOGY

Incidence

Unknown

Prevalence

- 0.04–1.9%
- Whites more affected than other races
- Predominant sex: Female > Male (55:45).

RISK FACTORS

- Family history of migraine headaches
- Depression
- Anxiety
- Chronic cannabis use

Genetics

- Possible matrilineal inheritance
- A3243G mitochondrial DNA mutation
- Ion-channel mutations

GENERAL PREVENTION

- Handwashing to prevent upper respiratory infection (URI)
- Adequate sleep
- Avoiding triggers
- Psychological testing and stress-reduction techniques

PATHOPHYSIOLOGY

- Unknown
- Strong link between CVS and migraine, with similar symptoms, common coexistence in patients, and effectiveness of antimigraine therapy
- Proposed mechanism:
  - Heightened neuronal excitability owing to enhanced ion permeability, mitochondrial deficits, or hormonal state → increased susceptibility to physical or psychological trigger → release of corticotropin-releasing-factor (CRF) → vomiting
  - Vomiting perpetuated by altered brain stem regulation → sustained vomiting

ETIOLOGY

- Unknown
- Possible maternal inheritence
- Multiple theories:
  - GI motility dysfunction
  - Autonomic dysfunction
  - Mitochondrial enzymopathies
  - Food allergy or intolerance

COMMONLY ASSOCIATED CONDITIONS

- Irritable bowel syndrome (67%)
- Headaches (52%)
- Motion sickness (46%)
- Migraines (11–40%)
- Seizure disorder (5.6%)

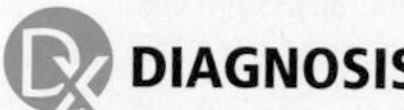

DIAGNOSIS

HISTORY

- Children with CVS often present with bilious emesis (83%), severe abdominal pain (80%) and/or hematemesis.
- The North American Society for Pediatric Gastroenterology, Hepatology, and Nutrition consensus statement recommends the following criteria to be fulfilled to diagnose CVS:
  - At least 5 attacks in any interval or a minimum of 3 attacks during a 6-month period
  - Episodic attacks of intense nausea and vomiting lasting 1 h to 10 days and occurring at least 1 week apart
  - Stereotypical pattern and symptoms in the individual patient
  - Vomiting during attacks occurs at least 4 times/h for at least 1 h
  - Return to baseline health between episodes
  - Not attributed to another disorder

PHYSICAL EXAM

Dehydration evaluation (seen in 30%):

- Orthostatic hypotension
- Tachycardia
- Skin turgor, decreased
- Mucous membranes, dry

DIAGNOSTIC TESTS & INTERPRETATION

Lab

There are no specific laboratory findings to diagnose CVS. Initial tests are mainly for screening purposes and to exclude other diagnoses.

Initial lab tests

- Electrolytes: Hypokalemia (Addison disease would show hyponatremia and hypoglycemia.)
- Complete blood count (CBC): Hemoconcentration and leukocytosis
- Amylase and lipase to check for pancreatitis
- Erythrocyte sedimentation rate (ESR)
- Hepatic transaminases: To exclude hepatitis or gallbladder disease
- Urinalysis: Granular casts, ketosis
- Urine pregnancy test
- Lactate, ammonia, amino acids, urine organic acids during an acute episode for young children to exclude metabolic diseases

Follow-Up & Special Considerations

Counseling:

- Anxiety and depression management
- Cannabis cessation (if applicable)

Imaging

Initial approach

- Upper GI series to exclude malrotation
- Small bowel follow-through
- Abdominal ultrasound to exclude transient hydronephrosis, gallstones, and ureteropelvic junction obstruction

Follow-Up & Special Considerations

CT scan of head, abdomen, and pelvis to evaluate biliary and urinary tracts and exclude structural reason

Diagnostic Procedures/Surgery

- Esophagogastroduodenoscopy (EGD): To evaluate for clinical suspicion of peptic ulcer disease or sign of hematemesis
- Electroencephalogram (EEG): Seizure disorder evaluation
- Gastric emptying studies
- Autonomic testing
- Neuropsychiatric testing

DIFFERENTIAL DIAGNOSIS

- Evaluate for causes of vomiting:
  - GI: Surgical and nonsurgical
  - Urologic
  - Renal
  - Gynecologic
  - Neurologic
  - Endocrinologic
  - Ear/nose/throat (ENT)
  - Psychiatric, including Münchausen by proxy
  - Metabolic
- Any child with suspected CVS should be evaluated for a possible metabolic or neurologic etiology of their symptoms if:
  - Child is <2 years of age.
  - Vomiting episodes are associated with other concurrent illnesses, prior fasting, or increased protein uptake.
  - Any focal findings on neurologic exam
  - Hypoglycemia, anion-gap metabolic acidosis, hyperammonia, or other findings suggestive of metabolic disorders

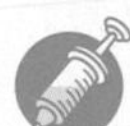

TREATMENT

MEDICATION

First Line

Lifestyle changes including avoidance of sleep deprivation, triggering foods, and motion sickness may reduce episode frequency. Prophylactic pharmacotherapy can be considered if the child is having repeated episodes requiring frequent hospitalization and school absences.

- Prophylactic: Decreases frequency or severity by >50%:
  - Amitriptyline (67–73%): Children >5 years: 0.3–0.5 mg/kg/d; adults: 50–75 mg/kg/d (1,2,3)[C]
  - Propranolol (57%): Children: 0.5 mg/kg/d divided b.i.d.–t.i.d.; adults: 10–20 mg/d b.i.d.–t.i.d.) (4)[C]
  - Cyproheptadine (39–66%): Children <5 years: 0.3 mg/kg/d divided b.i.d.–t.i.d.; appetite stimulant (1)[C]

Abortive:
- Ondansetron: Children: 0.3–0.4 mg/kg/dose q6h; adults: 4 mg IV/PO q6–8h (5)[C]
- Lorazepam: Children: 0.05–0.1 mg/kg/dose IV (not to exceed 4 mg/dose); adults: 1–2 mg IM/IV q4–6h p.r.n.) (5)[C]
- Sumatriptan: >40 kg/20 mg intranasal p.r.n. (5)[C]

Second Line

- Prophylactic: Decreases frequency or severity by >50%:
  - Phenobarbital (79%): 2–3 mg/kg/d (4)[C]
  - Erythromycin (75%): 20 mg/kg/d divided b.i.d.–t.i.d. (4)[C]
- Abortive:
  - Hydromorphone: Children: 0.015 mg/kg/dose IV for 1 dose; adults: 3 mg p.r.n. or 0.5–2 mg IM/SC × 1 dose (4,5)[C]
  - Diphenhydramine: Children: 1.25 mg/kg/dose q6h, not to exceed 300 mg/d; adults: 25–50 mg q4–6h p.r.n. (4,5)[C]

ADDITIONAL TREATMENT

General Measures

- Patient reassurance
- Nonstimulating environment
- Relaxation techniques
- Avoid recreational drugs

Issues for Referral

Mental health, weekly appointments

Additional Therapies

Relaxation techniques:
- Deep breathing
- Biofeedback
- Guided imagery

COMPLEMENTARY AND ALTERNATIVE MEDICINE

Coenzyme Q may play a role in helping CVS (6)[A].

IN-PATIENT CONSIDERATIONS

Initial Stabilization

- IV fluids
- IV ondansetron and lorazepam
- Analgesia for pain

Admission Criteria

- Dehydration requiring >2 L of IV fluids
- Failure of outpatient management
- Increased anion gap that reflects severe dehydration or metabolic decompensation

IV Fluids

Replacement of ongoing losses; may consider 10% dextrose-containing fluids to attenuate any metabolic crisis

Nursing

- Decrease stimulation; avoid noise and bright light.
- Supportive care
- Encourage relaxation techniques
- Avoid unnecessary interruptions during sleep

Discharge Criteria

- Resolution of vomiting phase
- Pain managed with oral analgesia
- Euvolemia
- Appropriate oral intake

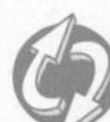

ONGOING CARE

FOLLOW-UP RECOMMENDATIONS

Patient Monitoring

- Weekly appointments for severe cases
- Monitoring of emesis-associated laboratory values: Hypokalemia, acid–base disturbances, ketosis
- Regular outpatient visits for support

DIET

- Foods rich in carbohydrates, proteins, vitamins, and minerals
- Limit fats and spicy foods.
- Avoid trigger foods: Chocolate, cheese, and monosodium glutamate (MSG).
- Regular meal schedules
- Maintenance of good hydration

PATIENT EDUCATION

- Information and explanation about CVS may greatly alleviate the burden of illness among older patients.
- Maintain vomiting diary to note patterns, which helps to identify potentially avoidable triggers in 75% of children.
- Stress management techniques
- Good sleep hygiene
- Regular, moderate exercise
- Online resources such as the Cyclic Vomiting Syndrome Association Web site at www.cvsaonline.org

PROGNOSIS

- Usually lasts 2.5–5.5 years
- Vomiting resolves in 60% of children with CVS.
- However, many children will continue to have somatic symptoms, including headache and abdominal pain
- 37% develop recurrent/migraine headaches.
- 50–75% with prophylactic treatment are asymptomatic at 1 year.

COMPLICATIONS

Occur during vomiting phase:
- Dehydration
- Electrolyte derangement, including the syndrome of inappropriate antidiuretic hormone (SIADH)
- Hematemesis
- Peptic esophagitis
- Mallory-Weiss tear
- Weight loss
- Hypovolemic shock

REFERENCES

1. Andersen JM, Sugerman KS, Lockhart JR, et al. Effective prophylactic therapy for cyclic vomiting syndrome in children using amitriptyline or cyproheptadine. *Pediatrics*. 1997;100:977–81.
2. Prakash C, Clouse RE. Cyclic vomiting syndrome in adults: clinical features and response to tricyclic antidepressants. *Am J Gastroenterol*. 1999;94: 2855–60.
3. Hejazi RA, Reddymasu SC, Namin F, Lavenbarg T, Foran P, McCallum RW et al. Efficacy of tricyclic antidepressant therapy in adults with cyclic vomiting syndrome: a two-year follow-up study. *J Clin Gastroenterol*. 2010;44:18–21.
4. Pareek N, et al. Cyclic vomiting syndrome: What a gastroenterologist needs to know. *Am J Gastroenterology*. 2007;102(12):2832–40.
5. Li BU. Cyclic Vomiting Syndrome. *Curr Treat Options Gastroenterol*. 2000;3:395–402.
6. Boles RG, Lovett-Barr MR, Preston A, Li BU, Adams K et al. Treatment of cyclic vomiting syndrome with co-enzyme Q10 and amitriptyline, a retrospective study. *BMC Neurol*. 2010;10:10.

C

ADDITIONAL READING

- Cyclic Vomiting Syndrome Association: Website: http://www.cvsaonline.org/
- Fitzpatrick E, Bourke B, Drumm B, Rowland M et al. Outcome for children with cyclical vomiting syndrome. *Arch. Dis. Child*. 2007;92:1001–4.
- Fleisher DR. Empiric guidelines for the management of cyclic vomiting syndrome. Available at: http://www.ch.missouri.edu/fleisher.
- Li BU, Balint JP. Cyclic vomiting syndrome: evolution in our understanding of a brain-gut disorder. *Adv Pediatr*. 2000;47:117–60.
- Li BU, Lefevre F, Chelimsky GG, et al. North American Society for Pediatric Gastroenterology, Hepatology, and Nutrition consensus statement on the diagnosis and management of cyclic vomiting syndrome. *J Pediatr Gastroenterol Nutr*. 2008;47:379–93.
- National digestive diseases information clearinghouse: http://www.digestive.niddk.nih.gov.

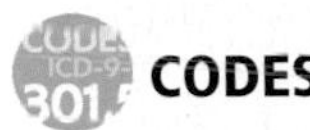

CODES

ICD9

536.2 Persistent vomiting

CLINICAL PEARLS

- Identify patterns and triggers for cycles.
- Encourage sleep hygiene, stress management, and appropriate diet.
- Treatment in the vomiting phase requires pharmacologic and psychosocial interventions.
- Educating families about CVS can help to reduce the burden of illness among patients.

CYSTIC FIBROSIS

Michael S. Stalvey, MD
Christian Müller, PhD
Terence R. Flotte, MD

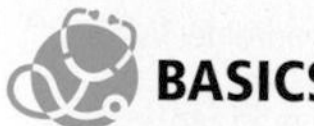

BASICS

DESCRIPTION

- Cystic fibrosis (CF) is an autosomal-recessive genetic condition that most prominently affects the lungs and pancreas.
- The intestinal tract, liver, endocrine system, reproductive organs, and skin can all be involved.
- Initially a pediatric disease, CF has become a chronic pediatric and adult medical condition as improvements in medical care have led to a dramatic increase in long-term survival.

EPIDEMIOLOGY

CF is the most common lethal inherited disease in Caucasians and is found in every racial group.

Incidence

- Prevalence varies according to country and ethnic background.
- Number of infants born with CF in relation to the total number of live births in the US:
  - 1 in 2,270 Ashkenazi Jewish Caucasian
  - 1 in 3,000 Caucasians
  - 1 in 10,000 Hispanics
  - 1 in 15,000 African Americans
  - 1 in 35,000 Asian Americans (reported frequency in Japan of 1 in 35,000) (1,2)[A]

Prevalence

- As per the 2008 CF Foundation Patient Registry, there are 30,000 patients with CF living in the US (3).
- ~1,000 new diagnoses are made annually (3).

RISK FACTORS

CF is a single-gene disorder. The severity of the phenotype can be affected by the specific CFTR mutation (most predictive of pancreatic disease), other modifier genes (CFTM1 for meconium ileus), and environmental factors, such as environmental tobacco smoke exposure, gastroesophageal reflux, and severe respiratory virus infections.

Genetics

CFTR gene (cystic fibrosis transmembrane conductance regulator). More than 1,500 mutations exist that can cause phenotypic CF, all of which are recessively inherited. Most common is loss of the phenylalanine residue at 508th position (deltaF508), which accounts for ~2/3 of affected alleles in the CF population in the US (2)[A].

GENERAL PREVENTION

- ACOG recommends genetic analysis for all North American couples planning a pregnancy, with appropriate counseling to identified carriers. Genetic analysis of siblings of known CF patients is highly recommended.
- Newborn screening for CF is offered throughout the United States. Identification of an affected newborn in a family has resulted in a reduction in the incidence of new cases, allowing genetic counseling prior to the birth of subsequent siblings.
- Prevention or amelioration of complications of CF can be accomplished through early diagnosis (by newborn screening or otherwise) followed by referral to an accredited regional CF center.

PATHOPHYSIOLOGY

- Abnormal CFTR function leads to abnormally viscous secretions that alter organ function.
- The lungs; obstruction, infection, and inflammation negatively affect lung growth, structure, and function:
  - Decreased mucociliary clearance
  - Infection is accompanied by an intense neutrophilic response.
  - Degradation of supporting tissues causes bronchiectasis and eventual failure.

COMMONLY ASSOCIATED CONDITIONS

- The GI tract:
  - Pancreatic exocrine insufficiency (85–90%):
    - Malabsorption of fat, protein, and fat-soluble vitamins (A, D, E, and K)
  - Hepatobiliary disease (11%) (3)[A]:
    - Focal biliary cirrhosis
    - Cholelithiasis
  - Meconium ileus at birth (10–15%)
  - Distal intestinal obstruction syndrome (DIOS): Intestinal blockage that typically occurs in older children and adults
- Endocrine:
  - CF-related diabetes (CFRD) (3)[A]:
    - May present as steady decline in weight, lung function, or increased frequency of exacerbation
    - Leading comorbid complication (21.5%)
    - Result of progressive insulin deficiency
    - Early screening and treatment may improve reduced survival found in CFRD (4).
  - Bone mineral disease (11.1%) (3)[A]
  - Hypogonadism:
    - Frequent low testosterone levels in men
    - Menstrual irregularities are common.
- Reproductive organs:
  - Congenital absence of the vas deferens: Obstructive azoospermia in 98% of males

Pregnancy Considerations

- Originally considered too dangerous for women with CF, successful pregnancies are occurring more frequently (3)[A].
- Pulmonary disease may worsen during pregnancy.

DIAGNOSIS

- General (any age):
  - Family history
  - Chronic/recurrent respiratory symptoms, including airway obstruction and infections
  - Persistent infiltrates on chest x-rays
  - Hypochloremic metabolic acidosis
- Neonatal:
  - Meconium ileus
  - Prolonged jaundice
- Infancy:
  - Failure to thrive
  - Chronic diarrhea
  - Anasarca/hypoproteinemia
  - Pseudotumor cerebri (vitamin A deficiency)
  - Hemolytic anemia (vitamin E deficiency)
- Childhood:
  - Recurrent endobronchial infection
  - Bronchiectasis
  - Recurrent sinusitis
  - Steatorrhea
  - Rectal prolapse
  - DIOS (distal intestinal obstruction syndrome)
  - Poor growth
  - Allergic bronchopulmonary aspergillosis
- Adolescence and adulthood:
  - Recurrent endobronchial infection
  - Bronchiectasis
  - Allergic bronchopulmonary aspergillosis
  - Chronic sinusitis
  - Hemoptysis
  - Pancreatitis
  - Portal hypertension
  - Azoospermia
  - Delayed puberty

HISTORY

Suspected in any child with failure to thrive, steatorrhea, and recurrent respiratory problems

PHYSICAL EXAM

- Respiratory:
  - Rhonchi and/or crackles
  - Hyper-resonance on percussion
  - Nasal polyps
- Gastrointestinal: Hepatosplenomegaly when cirrhosis present
- Other: Digital clubbing, growth retardation, and pubertal delay

DIAGNOSTIC TESTS & INTERPRETATION

Lab

Initial lab tests

- Newborn screening (42.8% of new cases) (3)[A]
- Sweat test (gold standard):
  - Sweat chloride:
    - >60 mmol/L is positive for CF.
    - <40 mmol/L is normal.
- CFTR mutation analysis:
  - Limited panel testing: Allele-specific PCR identifies >90% of mutations; finite chance of false-negative. Full sequence testing more costly and time-consuming. Greater sensitivity than PCR in patients of non-European descent.

Follow-Up & Special Considerations

- Sputum culture (common CF organisms)
- Pulmonary function tests (PFTs)
- 72-hour fecal fat
- Stool elastase
- Oral glucose tolerance test (OGTT)

Imaging

Initial approach

Chest x-ray:

- Hyperinflation early in disease
- Bronchial thickening and plugging
- Nodular densities, patchy atelectasis, and confluent infiltrates
- Bronchiectasis

Follow-Up & Special Considerations

Head CT: Abnormal sinus CT findings are nearly universal in CF and may include mucosal thickening, intraluminal sinus polyps, and sinus effusions. Many children with CF never develop aerated frontal sinuses.

Chest CT (not routine): Useful when unusual findings noted on CXR

Diagnostic Procedures/Surgery

Flexible bronchoscopy

Bronchoalveolar lavage

DIFFERENTIAL DIAGNOSIS

Pulmonary:
- Difficult-to-manage asthma
- Chronic bronchitis
- Recurrent pneumonia
- Chronic/recurrent sinusitis

GI:
- Celiac disease
- Protein-losing enteropathy
- Pancreatitis of unknown etiology
- Shwachman-Diamond syndrome

TREATMENT

MEDICATION

- Pulmonary:
  - Antibiotics, oral:
    - *S. aureus*: Bactrim or cephalexin
    - *P. aeruginosa*: Fluoroquinolones
    - Azithromycin (anti-inflammatory properties) (5)[A]
  - Antibiotics, inhaled:
    - TOBI (tobramycin 300 mg/dose via nebulizer)
    - Colistin (more commonly used in Europe)
    - Cayston (aerosolized aztreonam) 75 mg t.i.d. following bronchodilator use for 28 days (6)
  - Antibiotics, IV:
    - *S. aureus*: Zosyn or nafcillin
    - MRSA: Vancomycin or linezolid
    - *P. aeruginosa*: Zosyn or ceftazidime plus aminoglycoside (tobramycin)
    - *B. cepacia*: >3 drugs based on synergy studies
  - Inhalation therapy:
    - β-agonist in conjunction with chest physiotherapy
    - Recombinant human DNAse (7)[A]
    - Hypertonic saline (8)[A]
  - Anti-inflammatory agents:
    - Oral steroids (useful in setting of ABPA)
    - Ibuprofen (high dose)
- GI:
  - Pancreatic enzymes:
    - Use in pancreatic-insufficient patients.
  - Vitamin supplementation:
    - Fat-soluble vitamins (A, D, E, and K)
  - Liver disease (cholestasis):
    - Ursodeoxycholic acid

ADDITIONAL TREATMENT

General Measures

- Yearly influenza vaccination for all CF patients >6 months of age (3)
- Avoidance of smoke

Issues for Referral

All patients should be followed in a CF center (accredited sites are listed at www.cff.org).

Additional Therapies

- Airway clearance techniques (9)[A]
- Routine chest physiotherapy with postural drainage is critical in prevention of pulmonary exacerbations:
  - VEST (airway clearance system)
  - Flutter valve or acapella
- Endocrine:
  - CFRD: Dietary restrictions should be avoided.
  - CF-related bone disease: Consider bisphosphonate therapy.

SURGERY/OTHER PROCEDURES

- Lung transplantation reserved for patients with limited life expectancy (FEV_1 <30% predicted):
  - 158 patients with CF underwent lung transplantation during 2008 (3)[A].
  - 5-year post-transplant survival is 32.9–62% (10,11)[A].
- Liver transplantation is reserved for progressive liver failure and/or portal hypertension with GI bleeding.

IN-PATIENT CONSIDERATIONS

Initial Stabilization

Nasal cannula oxygen when the patient is hypoxic (SaO_2 <90%)

Admission Criteria

- Pulmonary exacerbation (most common reason for admission):
  - Increased cough, sputum production, and decreased pulmonary function
  - Change in lung examination (rales, retractions, tachypnea)
  - New abnormalities on CXR
  - Decreased energy level, appetite, and weight loss
  - Fever, leukocytosis, elevation of acute-phase reactants
- Bowel obstruction (due to distal intestinal obstruction syndrome, or DIOS, previously known as meconium ileus equivalent or MIE)
- Pancreatitis (in pancreatic-sufficient patients)

IV Fluids

- Increased salt loss increases risk of hyponatremic hypochloremic dehydration.
- Cautious use of IV fluids with worsening lung disease

Nursing

Nursing assignments should involve only one CF patient per nurse for isolation purposes.

ONGOING CARE

FOLLOW-UP RECOMMENDATIONS

- Upon discharge for a pulmonary exacerbation, follow up with their CF provider within 2–4 weeks
- Routine clinic visits every 3 months, with airway cultures and pulmonary function testing
- Annual comprehensive nutritional evaluation with morphometric analysis
- Yearly OGTT after 10 years of age (3)
- Bone densitometry every 1–4 years after age 18

DIET

High-calorie, high-fat diet with added salt

PATIENT EDUCATION

Cystic Fibrosis Foundation: www.cff.org

PROGNOSIS

- Most recent median survival is 37.4 years, as of 2008 CF Foundation Patient Registry (3)[A]
- Progression of lung disease usually determines length of survival.

REFERENCES

1. Palomaki GE, FitzSimmons SC, Haddow JE. Clinical sensitivity of prenatal screening for cystic fibrosis via CFTR carrier testing in a United States panethnic population. *Genet Med*. 2004;6: 405–14.
2. O'Sullivan BP, Freedman SD et al. Cystic fibrosis. *Lancet*. 2009;373:1891–904.
3. Cystic Fibrosis Foundation Patient Registry, 2008 Annual Data Report. Bethesda, Maryland, 2009.
4. Moran A, Dunitz J, Nathan B, Saeed A, Holme B, Thomas W et al. Cystic fibrosis-related diabetes: current trends in prevalence, incidence, and mortality. *Diabetes Care*. 2009;32:1626–31.
5. Saiman L, Marshall BC, Mayer-Hamblett N, et al. Azithromycin in patients with cystic fibrosis chronically infected with Pseudomonas aeruginosa: a randomized controlled trial. *JAMA*. 2003;290:1749–56.
6. O'Sullivan BP, Yasothan U, Kirkpatrick P, et al. Inhaled aztreonam. *Nat Rev Drug Discov*. 2010;9: 357–8.
7. Jones AP et al. Recombinant human deoxyribonuclease for cystic fibrosis. *Cochrane Database Sys Rev*. 2003;(3):CD001127.
8. Donaldson SH, Bennett WD, Zeman KL, et al. Mucus clearance and lung function in cystic fibrosis with hypertonic saline. *N Engl J Med*. 2006;354:241–50.
9. Main E et al. Conventional chest physiotherapy compared to other airway clearance techniques for cystic fibrosis. *Cochrane Database Sys Rev*. 2005;(1):CD002011.
10. Allen J, Visner G. Lung transplantation in cystic fibrosis–primum non nocere? *N Engl J Med*. 2007;357:2186–8.
11. Meachery G, De Soyza A, Nicholson A, et al. Outcomes of Lung transplantation for Cystic Fibrosis in a large United Kingdom cohort. *Thorax*. 2008.

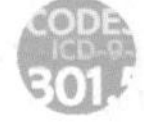

CODES

ICD9

- 277.00 Cystic fibrosis without mention of meconium ileus
- 277.01 Cystic fibrosis with meconium ileus
- 277.02 Cystic fibrosis with pulmonary manifestations

CLINICAL PEARLS

- CF must be considered in ANY child with chronic diarrhea, especially if associated with poor growth or failure to thrive.
- All children with nasal polyps should be evaluated.
- Children with CF may present with generalized edema due to protein/calorie malnutrition.
- The presence of digital clubbing or bronchiectasis should always trigger consideration of CF.
- A rapid decline in pulmonary function suggests the acquisition of resistant organisms (such as *B. cepacia*), CF-related diabetes, ABPA, or GE reflux disease.

CYTOMEGALOVIRUS INCLUSION DISEASE

Bonnie W. Lau, MD, PhD
Penelope Dennehy, MD

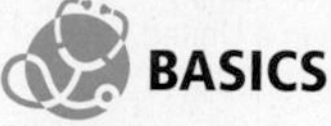

BASICS

Cytomegalovirus (CMV) infection is highly prevalent as illustrated by seroprevalence in 40–100% of the population (1). Serious disease can result in the perinatal period and in immunocompromised patients. Immunocompetent patients may become symptomatic with reinfection with different CMV strains. Prompt treatment and prophylaxis are the current mainstays of infection control.

DESCRIPTION

- β-infection from cytomegalovirus (CMV), a DNA virus in the *Herpesvirus* family
- Primary infection: Often asymptomatic; may remain latent throughout a person's life if no immunocompromise
- Severe disease can result from primary infection of newborns or reactivation in setting of immunocompromise or organ transplantation.
- Name derives from the infected cells, which are large and contain intranuclear inclusions, described as "owl's eye" inclusions
- Not highly contagious:
  - Spread via close contact with persons shedding virus from saliva, urine, blood, breast milk, or semen.
  - Also acquired via infected transplant organs.
  - Any organ can be affected.
- Categories of CMV infections:
  - Congenital: Vary greatly from mild viremia in a normal infant to the cause of abortion, stillbirth, postnatal morbidity and death from hemorrhage, anemia, or liver or central nervous system damage (including hearing loss, developmental delay and mental retardation) (2)
  - Acute infection in a normal host: Symptomatic infection commonly presents with acute mononucleosis syndrome (3).
  - Latent infection: Higher IgG titers may contribute to development of atherosclerotic disease (4).
  - Infection in bone marrow and solid organ transplant patients:
    - Bone marrow transplant: Usually interstitial pneumonia
    - Liver transplant: Hepatitis
    - Kidney transplant: CMV syndrome
  - Infection in patients with AIDS: Most commonly retinitis, 2nd most common is colitis, followed by esophagitis and neurologic disease (5)
  - Infections in other immunocompromised patients: Pulmonary, gastrointestinal (GI), or renal disease
- System(s) affected: Ophthalmic; Pulmonary; GI; Neurologic; Renal; Skin/Exocrine
- Synonym(s): Giant cell inclusion disease; CID CMV

Pregnancy Considerations

- CMV infection during pregnancy can be hazardous to the fetus.
- May lead to stillbirth, brain damage, birth defects, or to severe neonatal illness.

Pediatric Considerations

- May occur congenitally or postnatally.
- Breastfeeding can transmit virus to high-risk preterm infants. However there is low risk of symptomatic disease and no evidence of long-term sequelae from transmission from breastfeeding. Currently there are no recommendations for avoidance or treated breast milk (6).

EPIDEMIOLOGY

Incidence

- Common, but frequently asymptomatic
- <2–3 cases of end-organ disease per 100 person-years in HIV patients
- CMV infection is even more prevalent in populations at higher risk for HIV infection (IV drug users 75%, homosexual males 90%).
- Predominant age: All ages, peaks at <3 months, 16–40 years, and 40–75 years
- Predominant sex: Male > Female

Prevalence

- Occurs worldwide
- 40–100% of the general US population is seropositive from prior exposure during childhood or early adulthood (1).
- 20% of children in the US are seropositive before reaching puberty (1).
- Most common perinatally transmitted infection: 0.2–2.2% of births in the US (7)

RISK FACTORS

- HIV infection with specific risks, including:
  - CD4 count <50 cells/μL (5)[B]
  - Absence of treatment with or failure to respond to ART (5)[B]
  - Previous opportunistic infections (5)[B]
  - HIV viral load >100,000 (5)[B]
- Organ transplantation
- Blood transfusion
- Immunocompromise
- Living in closed population
- Corticosteroid therapy
- Day care environment, infant or geriatric (8)[B]
- For congenital infection, maternal infection during pregnancy
- Low socioeconomic status (7)[C]
- Critically ill immunocompetent adults in intensive care unit settings (up to 1/3 develop CMV, primarily between days 4–12 after admission) (9)[A]

GENERAL PREVENTION

- Handwashing/basic hygiene (8)[A]
- Avoid immunosuppression
- Highly active antiretroviral therapy (HAART) is the best method for high-risk HIV patients (1)[A].
- Chronic maintenance therapy for life in HIV patients with CMV end-organ disease unless successfully treated with ART (3)[A]
- Options include:
  - Parenteral or oral ganciclovir (3)[A]
  - Parenteral foscarnet (3)[A]
  - Combined parenteral ganciclovir and foscarnet (3)[A]
  - Parenteral cidofovir (3)[A]
  - Ganciclovir administration via intraocular implant or repetitive intravitreous injection of fomivirsen (3)[A]
- CMV antibody+, HIV+ children who are severely immunosuppressed require oral ganciclovir 30 mg/kg t.i.d. (8)[C]
- Antiviral suppression of CMV reactivation in CMV+ transplant recipients or recipients of CMV+ organs
  - Solid organ transplant: Prophylactic or preemptive treatment with oral ganciclovir, valganciclovir (10)[A]
  - Bone marrow transplant: IV ganciclovir
- CMV immunoglobulins decrease rate of severe disease after liver transplant (11)[A] and decrease incidence of disease after renal transplant.

ETIOLOGY

- Primary infection
- Reinfection with different CMV strains
- Reactivation of latent virus in patients who are immunosuppressed

COMMONLY ASSOCIATED CONDITIONS

- AIDS
- Corticosteroid therapy
- Leukemia
- Lymphoma

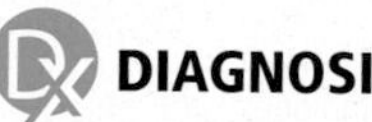

DIAGNOSIS

- Congenital:
  - Asymptomatic cytomegaloviremia
  - Symptomatic: Small for gestational age, purpura/petechiae, jaundice, hepatosplenomegaly, chorioretinitis, microcephaly, intracranial calcifications, hearing impairment
  - 90% have late complications: Sensorineural hearing loss occurs in 14%; 3–5% moderate to severe (11)[A]
  - Mental retardation, chorioretinitis, optic atrophy, seizures, learning disabilities (7)
- Acquired: Acute infection in a normal host:
  - Usually asymptomatic
  - Mononucleosis syndrome: Fever, malaise, sore throat, headache, antibiotic rash (3)
  - Less common: Exudative pharyngitis, splenomegaly, cervical adenopathy, rash (3)
- Infections in AIDS patients:
  - Retinitis: Usually unilateral, floaters, scotomata, peripheral field defects. Diagnosis made when characteristic retinal changes noted by ophthalmologist on funduscopic exam (5)
  - Colitis: Fever, weight loss, anorexia, abdominal pain, diarrhea, malaise; hemorrhage or perforation rare but serious (5)
  - Esophagitis: Fever, odynophagia, nausea, abdominal discomfort (5)
  - Pneumonitis: Dyspnea with or without exertion, nonproductive cough, hypoxemia (5)
  - Neurologic disease: Dementia, lethargy, confusion, fever, focal neurologic signs (5)
- Infections in transplant recipients:
  - Persistent fever (most common) (8)
  - Bone marrow transplant: Interstitial pneumonia (10)
  - Liver transplant: Hepatitis (10)
  - Kidney transplant: CMV syndrome (fever, leucopenia, atypical lymphocytes, hepatomegaly, myalgia, arthralgia) (10)

DIAGNOSTIC TESTS & INTERPRETATION

Lab

Acute infection in a normal host:
- Elevated liver transaminases in 92%, although transaminases rarely increase to >5 times normal ranges (3)
- Anemia (3)
- Thrombocytopenia (3)
- Positive cold agglutinins (3)
- Lymphocytosis with >10% atypical (3)
- Negative heterophil antibody test (rules out Epstein Barr virus mononucleosis) (3)
- Positive CMV IgM antibodies; may not peak until 4–7 weeks after acute infection (3)
- CMV IgG should increase 4–fold during acute infection (3)

Congenital/infant:
- <12 months: Positive CMV antibody indicates maternal infection, but not necessarily child infection (8)
- >12 months: Positive CMV antibody assay or culture indicates previous infection, but not necessarily active disease (8)
- Recovery of virus from tissue in symptomatic patient (GI or pulmonary tissue) indicates infection, although 1–6 weeks are required for distinctive cytopathic events to occur (8)
- Quantitative DNA polymerase chain reaction (PCR) evidences disease and can be used to monitor therapy (8)
- Direct hyperbilirubinemia >3 mg/dL (8)
- Thrombocytopenia (<75,000/mL) (7)
- Elevated liver transaminases (7)

- Immunocompromised:
  - Viremia: PCR, antigen assays (pp65 lower-matrix protein in leukocytes), blood culture, although viremia can be present without CMV disease (5)[A]
  - Serum CMV antibodies not useful; can be falsely negative due to immunosuppression (5)[C]
  - Neurologic disease: CMV detected in cerebrospinal fluid or brain tissue clinches diagnosis. Enhanced by PCR analysis (5)[A].

Imaging
- Head computed tomography or magnetic resonance imaging: Periventricular enhancement (CMV neurologic disease)
- Chest X-ray: Interstitial infiltrates (CMV pneumonitis)

Diagnostic Procedures/Surgery
- Bronchoscopy: Identification of CMV inclusion bodies in lung tissue in context of pulmonary infiltrates (pneumonitis)
- Endoscopic exam of GI tract: Mucosal ulcerations and colonoscopic, rectal, or esophageal biopsy (colitis, esophagitis) (5)[B]

Pathological Findings
Giant cells with basophilic inclusion bodies (owl's eye)

DIFFERENTIAL DIAGNOSIS
- Congenital: Toxoplasmosis, rubella, herpes, syphilis
- Acquired in immunocompetent: Epstein-Barr virus (EBV) mononucleosis, viral hepatitis
- Acquired immunocompromised: Other viral, bacterial, fungal opportunistic infections

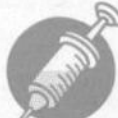

TREATMENT

MEDICATION

First Line
- Congenital disease: Ganciclovir 12 mg/kg IV q12h for 6 weeks (7)[B]
- Pediatric disseminated disease: IV ganciclovir (3)[A]
- CMV mononucleosis/asymptomatic viremia: No treatment (5)
- Retinitis: Effective treatments include the following and should be chosen in consultation with a specialist:
  - Oral valganciclovir (for peripheral lesions) (5)[A]
  - IV ganciclovir followed by oral valganciclovir (5)[A]
  - IV foscarnet (5)[A]
  - IV cidofovir (5)[A]
  - Ganciclovir intraocular implant with oral or IV valganciclovir (5)[A]
  - Treat until CD4 >100 for 3–6 months (5)[A]
- Colitis or esophagitis: IV ganciclovir or foscarnet for 21–28 days or until symptom resolution (5)[B]
- Neurologic disease: Prompt treatment with ganciclovir and foscarnet (5)[B]
- CMV disease in transplant patients: IV ganciclovir for 2–4 weeks (10)[B]

Second Line
- Adult CMV retinitis: Fomivirsen (7)[A]
- Pediatric disseminated disease: Foscarnet 60 mg/kg q8h for 14–21 days (7)[A], combination ganciclovir and foscarnet (7)[B]
- CMV disease in transplant patients: Valganciclovir (10)[C]
- CMV in bone marrow transplant patients:
  - Prophylaxis: Valacyclovir (10)[B]
  - Preemptive: Foscarnet (10)[B]

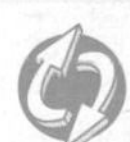

ONGOING CARE

FOLLOW-UP RECOMMENDATIONS
Bed rest

Patient Monitoring
- CMV urine culture at birth for all HIV-infected or -exposed (8)[C] and annual testing for CMV seronegative/HIV+ children (8)[C]
- Patients with CD4 counts <50 should have ophthalmologic screening every 3–6 months (8)[C].
- Patients on therapy should be followed for neutropenia, anemia, and thrombocytopenia.

DIET
Normal

PROGNOSIS
Severe disease with primary infection in newborns and reactivation in immunocompromised

COMPLICATIONS
- Congenital: Hearing loss, mental retardation, optic atrophy, seizures, learning disabilities
- Colitis: Hemorrhage and perforation

REFERENCES

1. Salzberger B, Hartmann P, Hanses F, et al. Incidence and prognosis of CMV disease in HIV-infected patients before and after introduction of combination antiretroviral therapy. *Infection*. 2005;33:345–9.
2. Yinon Y, Farine D, Yudin MH et al. Cytomegalovirus infection in pregnancy. *J Obstet Gynaecol Can*. 2010;32:348–54.
3. Taylor GH. Cytomegalovirus. *Am Fam Phys*. 2003;67(3):519–24.
4. Crumpacker CS. Invited commentary: human cytomegalovirus, inflammation, cardiovascular disease, and mortality. *Am J Epidemiol*. 2010;172(4):372–4.
5. Benson CA, Kaplan JE, Masur H, et al. Treating opportunistic infections among HIV-infected adults and adolescents: recommendations from CDC, the National Institutes of Health, and the HIV Medicine Association/Infectious Diseases Society of America. *MMWR Recomm Rep*. 2004;53:1–112.
6. Kurath S, Halwachs-Baumann G, Müller W et al. Transmission of cytomegalovirus via breast milk to the prematurely born infant: a systematic review. *Clin Microbiol Infect*. 2010;16:1172–8.
7. Mofenson LM, Oleske J, Serchuck L et al. Treating opportunistic infections among HIV-exposed and infected children: recommendations from CDC, the National Institutes of Health, and the Infectious Diseases Society of America. *MMWR Recomm Rep*. 2004;53:1–92.
8. Cohen J, et al. *Infectious diseases*, 2nd ed. New York: Elsevier, 2004.
9. Osawa R, Singh N. Cytomegalovirus infection in critically ill patients: a systematic review. *Crit Care*. 2009;13:R68.
10. Razonable RR, Emery VC, 11th Annual Meeting of the IHMF (International Herpes Management Forum). Management of CMV infection and disease in transplant patients. 27–29 February 2004. *Herpes*. 2004;11:77–86.
11. Grosse SD, Ross DS, Dollard SC. Congenital cytomegalovirus (CMV) infection as a cause of permanent bilateral hearing loss: a quantitative assessment. *J Clin Virol*. 2008;41:57–62.

ADDITIONAL READING

- Patel R, Paya CV. Infections in solid-organ transplant recipients. *Clin Microbiol Rev*. 1997;10:86–124.
- Sun HY, Wagener MM, Singh N. Prevention of posttransplant cytomegalovirus disease and related outcomes with valganciclovir: a systematic review. *Am J Transplant*. 2008;8:2111–8.

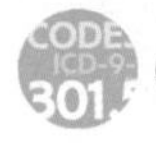

CODES

ICD9
- 078.5 Cytomegaloviral disease
- 771.1 Congenital cytomegalovirus infection

CLINICAL PEARLS
- CMV mono has much less cervical adenopathy and/or splenomegaly than EBV mono in adults.
- CMV is a major cause of sensorineural hearing loss in young children.

DE QUERVAIN TENOSYNOVITIS

J. Herbert Stevenson, MD

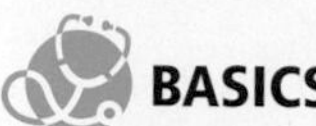

BASICS

DESCRIPTION

De Quervain tenosynovitis is a stenosis of the 1st dorsal compartment of the wrist including the extensor pollicis brevis (EPB) and abductor pollicis longus (APL). It is an inflammation or thickening of the tendon sheath that surrounds EPB and the APL, which leads to pain with certain movements of the thumb.

EPIDEMIOLOGY

- Predominant age: 30–50 years old
- Predominant sex: Female < Male (women 6–10× more likely than men)

Incidence

Common condition

RISK FACTORS

- Women age 30–50
- Pregnancy (primarily 3rd trimester and postpartum)
- Individuals participating in golf, fly fishing, and racquet sports
- Repetitive motions with the hand/thumb requiring forceful grasping or wrist ulna/radial deviation; often seen in carpenters and machine operators

GENERAL PREVENTION

Avoidance of repetitive actions of the thumb associated with forceful grasping or repetitive wrist ulna/radial deviation (e.g., hammering)

PATHOPHYSIOLOGY

Repetitive actions of the wrist and the thumb results in microtrauma and thickening of the surrounding tendon and tendon sheath (EPB, APL). This thickening causes inflammation and pain with movements of the thumb and wrist and may elicit pain over the radial styloid as they rub over the prominence.

ETIOLOGY

- Repetitive movements of the wrist and thumb and activities that require forceful grasping
- Trauma
- Systemic diseases (e.g., rheumatoid arthritis)

DIAGNOSIS

HISTORY

- Patients may complain of gradual worsening pain along their thumb and radial aspect of their wrist with certain movements, including ulnar deviation of the wrist.
- Usually insidious in onset
- Usually no associated trauma

PHYSICAL EXAM

- Pain and swelling is present over the radial styloid, which may be exacerbated when patients move their thumb or make a fist.
- Crepitus with movement of the thumb may be felt or heard.
- Occasionally, slight swelling at the base of the thumb and wrist is noted.
- Decreased range of motion of the thumb
- Swelling and tenderness may be appreciated over the distal radius.
- Pain over the 1st extensor compartment on resisted thumb abduction or extension
- Crepitus may be associated with movement of the thumb.

DIAGNOSTIC TESTS & INTERPRETATION

Finkelstein test is pathognomonic for De Quervain tenosynovitis. This test involves patient flexing thumb in palm, while the examiner ulnar deviates the wrist. The test is positive if patient's symptoms are reproduced.

Lab

No labs are indicated.

Imaging

This disease is primarily a clinical diagnosis, but if the diagnosis is questionable, then radiographs of the wrist may be indicated to rule out other pathology. Radiographs may rule out CMC arthritis, which can be misdiagnosed as De Quervain. MRI is the test of choice to rule out coexisting soft tissue injury or wrist joint pathology.

Pathological Findings

Inflamed and thickened retinacular sheath of the tendon

DIFFERENTIAL DIAGNOSIS

- Fracture of the scaphoid
- Dorsal wrist ganglion
- Osteoarthritis of the 1st carpometacarpal joint
- Flexor carpi radialis tendonitis
- Infectious tenosynovitis
- Tendonitis of the wrist extensors
- Intersection syndrome
- Trigger thumb

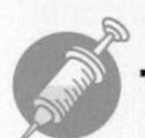

TREATMENT

- Rest and immobilization may be helpful early in the disease process. This is achieved with the use of a thumb spica splint.
- NSAIDs may help along with the splint to decrease the inflammation.

MEDICATION

First Line

Immobilization and NSAIDs

Second Line

Corticosteroid injection of the tendon sheath has shown significant cure rates. An 83% success rate after single injection has been reported (1)[B]. Additional injections are sometimes required.

ADDITIONAL TREATMENT

General Measures

- If full relief is not being achieved, a corticosteroid injection of the tendon sheath has been shown to result in 83% cure rate (1)[B].
- Anatomic variants may complicate treatment, including 2 tendon sheaths in the 1st compartment or the EPB tendon may travel in a separate compartment.
- Surgery is indicated for cases not responding to 3–6 months of conservative treatment. Surgery has been found to result in 91% cure rate (2)[B].

Issues for Referral

Referral to a hand surgeon is indicated if no improvement is noted after conservative treatments.

Additional Therapies

- Hand therapy along with iontophoresis/phonophoresis may help improve outcomes for moderate cases.
- Patients may incorporate thumb-stretching exercises into their rehabilitation.

SURGERY/OTHER PROCEDURES

Only indicated for patients who have failed conservative treatment. Surgical release has shown cure rates of up to 91% (2)[B].

IN-PATIENT CONSIDERATIONS

Initial Stabilization

- Splinting of the thumb (thumb spica splint or dorsal hood splint)
- Rest
- Ice (15–20 minutes 5–6× a day)
- Anti-inflammatory medications

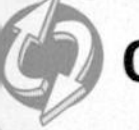

ONGOING CARE

FOLLOW-UP RECOMMENDATIONS

- Additional corticosteroid injection may be performed at 4–6 weeks if symptoms are not significantly reduced.
- Avoid repetitive activities and motions that aggravate the pain.

DIET

As tolerated

PATIENT EDUCATION

Modification of activities eliciting pain, such as repetitive movement of the wrist and thumb, and forceful grasping.

PROGNOSIS

Prognosis is extremely good with conservative treatments. 95% success rates have been shown with conservative therapy over 1 year, although up to 1/3 of patients will have recurrence (3)[A]. Surgery has shown success in 91% of patients who did not improve with conservative therapy.

COMPLICATIONS

- Most complications are secondary to the treatment modalities. This includes gastrointestinal, renal, and hepatic injury secondary to NSAIDs.
- Nerve damage may occur during surgery.
- Hypopigmentation, fat atrophy, bleeding, and infection are potential adverse events from corticosteroid injections.
- If not treated correctly, loss of flexibility of the thumb due to fibrosis may occur.

REFERENCES

1. Richie CA, Briner WW. Corticosteroid injection for treatment of de Quervain's tenosynovitis: a pooled quantitative literature evaluation. *J Am Board Fam Pract*. 2003;16:102–6.
2. Ta KT, Eidelman D, Thomson JG. Patient satisfaction and outcomes of surgery for de Quervain's tenosynovitis. *J Hand Surg [Am]*. 1999;24:1071–7.
3. Jirarattanaphochai K, Saengnipanthkul S, Vipulakorn K, et al. Treatment of de Quervain disease with triamcinolone injection with or without nimesulide. A randomized, double-blind, placebo-controlled trial. *J Bone Joint Surg Am*. 2004;86-A:2700–6.

ADDITIONAL READING

- Rettig AC. Athletic injuries of the wrist and hand. Part II overuse injuries of the wrist and traumatic injuries of the hand. *Am J Sport Med*. 2004;32: 262–73.
- Rossi R, et al. De Quervain Disease in volleyball players. *Am J Sport Med*. 2005;33:424–7.
- Tallia AF, Cardone DA. Diagnostic and therapeutic injection of the wrist and hand region. *Am Fam Physician*. 2003;67:745–50.

See Also (Topic, Algorithm, Electronic Media Element)

Algorithm: Pain in upper extremity

CODES

ICD9

727.04 Radial styloid tenosynovitis

CLINICAL PEARLS

- Repetitive movements of the wrist and thumb and activities that require forceful grasping are the most common causes of De Quervain tenosynovitis.
- De Quervain tenosynovitis is a stenosis of the 1st dorsal compartment of the wrist including the EPB and APL. It is an inflammation or thickening of the tendon sheath that surrounds EPB and the APL, which leads to pain with certain movements of the thumb.
- It is diagnosed via the Finkelstein test, which is pathognomonic for De Quervain tenosynovitis. This test involves patient flexing thumb in palm, while the examiner ulnar deviates the wrist. The test is positive if patient's symptoms are reproduced.
- Activity can be as-tolerated, using pain as a threshold; however, most people require modification of their activities to assist with rehabilitation and improvement.

D

DECOMPRESSION SICKNESS

Elise R. Bender, MD

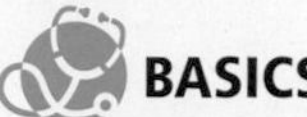

BASICS

DESCRIPTION

- Also known as "caisson disease" or "the bends"
- Occurs most often in SCUBA diving, free diving, high altitude flying, and aerospace events
- Rapid decrease in environmental pressure causing inert gases (usually nitrogen) to form bubbles in tissues or to obstruct small blood vessels, causing symptoms
- Type I (mild):
  - Musculoskeletal (70–85%): Mild joint pain that increases with time; most commonly shoulder or elbow pain
  - Cutaneous (10–15%): Rash, pruritus, edema
- Type II (serious):
  - Neurologic (10–15%): Headache, visual disturbance, paresthesias, paresis, paralysis, bladder or bowel incontinence, vertigo, memory loss, ataxia, seizures
  - Pulmonary (2–5%): Nonproductive cough, wheezing, pharyngeal irritation, chest discomfort on inspiration, respiratory distress
  - Death

Pregnancy Considerations

- A pregnant patient with decompression sickness is a priority, because the fetus may be affected and at greater risk for arterial gas emboli.
- No contraindication to recompression therapy during pregnancy

EPIDEMIOLOGY

- Predominant age: 20–29 years (although there is a trend toward increased susceptibility with increase in age, especially over age 42)
- Predominant sex: Male (although no evidence suggests increased male susceptibility)

Incidence

3.1/10,000 dives

Prevalence

<1% even in high-density diving areas and areas of caisson work

RISK FACTORS

- Large pressure reduction (i.e., flying after diving)
- Multiple repetitive SCUBA dives or ascents to altitudes above 18,000 feet
- High rate of ascent or decompression
- Previous decompression injury
- Obesity
- Cold-water diving
- Poor physical conditioning
- Vigorous physical activity
- Dehydration
- Local injury
- Patent foramen ovale or any intracardiac right-to-left shunt (increased risk of neurologic symptoms)

Genetics

No known genetic predisposition

GENERAL PREVENTION

- Travel by air after SCUBA diving should be restricted for 12 hours (after 1 dive per day) or 48 hours (after multiple dives or decompression).
- Chronic obstructive lung disease, cystic fibrosis, bronchiectasis, interstitial lung disease, or a history of thoracic surgery or prior pneumothorax should be absolute contraindications to diving.
- Intracardiac right-to-left shunts (e.g., patent foramen ovale, atrial septal defect, ventricular septal defect, patent ductus arteriosus, etc.) may be contraindications to diving.
- Follow decompression tables (Navy, National Association for Underwater Instructors [NAUI], Professional Association for Diving Instructors [PADI]) for diving to depth (>33 feet).
- Use dive computers that calculate nitrogen content of various tissues to estimate decompression limit.
- Breathing pure oxygen before exposure to a low barometric pressure environment (prebreathing) may decrease the risk of developing altitude decompression syndrome (1).
- Pre-dive oral hydration may also reduce bubble formation (2).
- Repeated dives and physical activity may have a protective effect (3).

PATHOPHYSIOLOGY

- As divers descend to increased pressures, the solubility of nitrogen in tissues increases.
- As the diver ascends, this dissolved gas may come out of solution and form bubbles, which can cause symptoms by blocking vessels, compressing tissue, or activating inflammatory cascades.
- Excess gas can be eliminated via respiration, so allowing for adequate breathing time is essential in disease prevention.

ETIOLOGY

- Rapid ascent from diving (depth >33 feet)
- Rapid ascent/decompression in an airplane
- Tunnel work (caisson disease)
- Inadequate pressurization/denitrogenation when flying
- Flying to high altitude too soon after diving

COMMONLY ASSOCIATED CONDITIONS

- Pulmonary barotrauma (pulmonary edema and hemorrhage; pneumomediastinum; pneumothorax; arterial gas embolism)
- Ear, sinus, or dental barotraumas
- Nitrogen narcosis
- Dysbaric osteonecrosis

DIAGNOSIS

HISTORY

- Recent history of diving or high-altitude flying, or occupational exposures to pressurized environments (e.g., miners, construction workers, divers, pilots)
- 75% present within 1 hour; 90% present within 12 hours; but can present >24 hours after diving
- Localized joint pain (e.g., elbow, shoulder, knee, hip wrist, ankle) ranges from dull ache to severe.
- Localized pruritus, which usually resolves without treatment, but may be painful (cutis marmorata)
- Painful lymphedema
- Headache, visual field deficits
- Confusion, memory loss, unexplained fatigue
- Seizures, dizziness/vertigo, nausea/vomiting
- Urinary and rectal incontinence
- Rapidly ascending paraplegia
- Substernal chest pain
- Coughing paroxysms (Behnken sign)
- Hemoptysis
- Coma, death

PHYSICAL EXAM

- Complete neurological exam required to rule out serious disease
- May see increased joint pain with active and passive motion
- Cutaneous and lymphatic signs:
  - Localized edema (mainly on chest and torso), lymphadenopathy
  - Localized erythema
  - Sharply defined area of pallor on tongue (Liebermeister sign)
  - Skin lesions:
    - Painful, pruritic, blotchy, red rash on torso
    - Burning blebs on skin
  - Joints:
    - Erythema and edema on periarticular surfaces
- Ataxia, nystagmus
- Arrhythmia, bradycardia, or tachycardia
- Hypotension
- Tachypnea

DIAGNOSTIC TESTS & INTERPRETATION

Lab

Initial lab tests

- Arterial blood gases:
  - May show decreased Po_2, decreased Pco_2, and metabolic acidosis
- Electrolytes, creatinine, BUN
- CBC:
  - Thrombocytopenia, increased hematocrit in severe cases due to dehydration
- Coagulation tests:
  - May see increased fibrin split products, increased prothrombin time
- Carboxyhemoglobin
- EEG:
  - Irregular slowing with cerebral bends

Imaging

Initial approach

- Chest X-ray:
  - Pneumothorax, mediastinal emphysema, right-sided heart enlargement
- Plain radiograph or ultrasound:
  - Gas bubbles in joints, tendons, bursae, muscles
- CT scan all patients with history of trauma or neurologic signs.
- MRI not very helpful in initial DCS:
  - Consider in spinal cord evaluation for continued symptoms

Diagnostic Procedures/Surgery

Test of pressure to ascertain response:

- Trial of recompression to 2.8 atmosphere absolute (ata)/100% oxygen for 10 minutes

DIFFERENTIAL DIAGNOSIS

- Arterial gas embolism
- Traumatic injury to extremity
- Cerebrovascular accident
- Musculoskeletal strains
- Urticaria
- Malingering
- Carbon monoxide poisoning

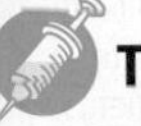

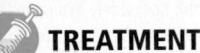

TREATMENT

MEDICATION

First Line

- 100% oxygen via tight nonrebreathing mask
- Isotonic fluid resuscitation:
  - Avoid D5W, hypotonic solutions in cord injury
  - No experimental or clinical studies support use of volume expanders (dextran, albumin).
- Steroids:
  - Advocated by some for the assumed vasogenic edema seen in decompression sickness
  - Controversial and not proven in controlled clinical trials
  - If prescribed, do not use for >4 days
- Diazepam: 5–15 mg IV (IM absorption unpredictable) for inner ear decompression sickness:
  - Relieves vertigo, nausea, and vomiting
  - Contraindications: Hypersensitivity to benzodiazepines, acute narrow-angle glaucoma
  - Precautions:
    - Monitor respiratory status, BP, and heart rate.
    - Reduce dose in elderly and patients with hepatic dysfunction.
  - Significant possible interactions: Benzodiazepines potentiate the effects of other CNS depressants.

Second Line

Adjunctive therapy:

- NSAIDs (tenoxicam) or use of heliox may reduce the number of recompressions required (although neither improves the odds of recovery).
- Digitalization for CHF/tachycardia
- Aminophylline *not* useful for decompression sickness
- Roles of steroids and heparin not determined

ADDITIONAL TREATMENT

General Measures

- Rapid referral to hyperbaric chamber facility
- Position in left lateral decubitus position (Durant maneuver)
- Trendelenburg is no longer recommended

Issues for Referral

- Prehospital: Referral through Divers' Alert Network (DAN; 919-684-8111) to nearest hyperbaric facility for recompression test
- Although recompression therapy is best administered as early as possible, some patients may still benefit even 6–9 days after the incident.

Additional Therapies

- Hyperbaric decompression (hyperbaric therapy for at least 4 hours)
- Transport via ground, low-altitude airplane, or aircraft pressurized to sea level

IN-PATIENT CONSIDERATIONS

IV Fluids

Isotonic fluid resuscitation

Nursing

Bed rest when neurologic involvement present

Discharge Criteria

Patients may be sent home when only cutaneous symptoms are present or if the appropriate response to therapy is observed in the emergency department.

ONGOING CARE

FOLLOW-UP RECOMMENDATIONS

Patient Monitoring

Symptomatic assessment

DIET

Normal

PATIENT EDUCATION

- SCUBA divers should be certified by an appropriate diving agency: NAUI, PADI, SSI, or YMCA.
- Sport divers who have not been diving for >6 months should review diving principles/skills via a refresher course.

PROGNOSIS

- Excellent for early symptomatic presentation, referral, and treatment
- Related to duration and severity of symptoms prior to treatment
- 16% of patients have residual symptoms for up to 3 months.

COMPLICATIONS

- Oxygen toxicity with seizures (infrequent and unpredictable)
- Neurologic sequelae for nonresponders
- Long-term risk of aseptic necrosis

REFERENCES

1. Castagna O, Gempp E, Blatteau JE. Pre-dive normobaric oxygen reduces bubble formation in scuba divers. *Eur J Appl Physiol*. 2009.
2. Gempp E, Blatteau JE, Pontier JM, et al. Preventive Effect Of Pre-Dive Hydration On Bubble Formation In Divers. *Br J Sports Med*. 2008.
3. Pontier JM, Guerrero F, Castagna O. Bubble formation and endothelial function before and after 3 months of dive training. *Aviat Space Environ Med*. 2009;80:15–9.

ADDITIONAL READING

- Barratt DM, Harch PG, Van Meter K. Decompression illness in divers: a review of the literature. *Neurologist*. 2002;8:186–202.
- Bennett MH, Lehm JP, Mitchell SJ, et al. Recompression and adjunctive therapy for decompression illness. *Cochrane Database Syst Rev*. 2007;CD005277.
- British Thoracic Society Fitness to Dive Group, Subgroup of the British Thoracic Society Standards of Care Committee. British Thoracic Society guidelines on respiratory aspects of fitness for diving. *Thorax*. 2003;58:3–13.
- DAN Annual Diving Report: 2007 Edition.
- DAN Scuba Diving Medical Services: http://www.diversalertnetwork.org/medical.
- Information from your family doctor: Medical problems of recreational scuba diving. *Am Fam Physician*. 2001;63(11):2225–6.
- Newton, HB. Neurologic complications of scuba diving. *Am Fam Physician*. 2001;63(11): 2211–8.
- Sheffield PJ. Flying after diving guidelines: a review. *Aviat Space Environ Med*. 1990;61:1130–8.
- Sulaiman ZM, Pilmanis AA, O'Connor RB. Relationship between age and susceptibility to altitude decompression sickness. *Aviat Space Environ Med*. 1997;68(8):695–8.
- Tetzlaff K, Shank ES, Muth CM. Evaluation and management of decompression illness–an intensivist's perspective. *Intensive Care Med*. 2003;29:2128–36.

CODES

ICD9

993.3 Caisson disease

CLINICAL PEARLS

- If the patient only has musculoskeletal and skin complaints, you should still worry about neurologic or pulmonary issues as well. 71% of nervous system decompression sickness presents with skin/limb bends.
- 75% of patients present within 1 hour; 90% present within 12 hours; but some patients may still present >24 hours after diving.
- If recompression therapy is delayed several days, you should still proceed. Early administration is best, but patients may benefit even 6–9 days after the incident.
- Travel by air after SCUBA diving should be restricted for 12 hours (after 1 dive per day) or 48 hours (after multiple dives or decompression).

DEEP VEIN THROMBOPHLEBITIS (DVT)

Alfonso J. Tafur, MD
Denisse Tafur Chang, MD

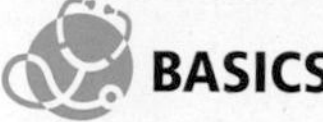

BASICS

DESCRIPTION

- Development of blood clot within the deep veins, usually accompanied by inflammation of the vessel wall.
- The major clinical consequences are embolization, usually to the lung, and postphlebitic syndrome.
- System(s) affected: Cardiovascular

EPIDEMIOLOGY

- The age- and gender-adjusted incidence of VTE is 100 times higher in the hospital than in the community (1).
- 1/3 of VTE cases die within 30 days, 1/5 will have sudden death due to PE. The 28-day DVT fatality rate is 9%.

Incidence

- In the US, VTE occurs for the 1st time in 100 persons per 100,000 per year.
- Approximately 2/3 of the new VTE cases are DVT alone.
- Higher incidence among Caucasians and African Americans relative to Hispanics and Asians
- Complicates approximately 1 in 1,000 pregnancies.

Prevalence

Variable; dependent on medical condition or procedure:

- 22–52% of the patients with PE have DVT.
- 25% of patients with superficial venous thrombosis (2)
- Present in 11% of patients with acquired brain injury entering to neurorehabilitation

RISK FACTORS

- Acquired: Age, previous thrombosis, iImmobilization, major surgery, orthopedic surgery, malignancy, oral contraceptives, hormonal replacement therapy, antiphospholipid syndrome, polycythemia vera, paroxysmal nocturnal hemoglobinuria, prolonged travel, pregnancy/puerperium
- Inherited: Antithrombin deficiency, protein C deficiency, protein S deficiency, factor V Leiden R506Q, prothrombin G20210A, dysfibrinogenemia
- Mixed/unknown: Hyperhomocysteinemia, high levels of factor VIII, activated protein C resistance not factor V Leiden, high levels of factor IX, high levels of thrombin activatable fibrinolysis inhibitor (TAFI), high levels of factor XI

Genetics

- Factor V Leiden is found in 5% of the population and in 20% of all VTE events. It is the most common thrombophilia. Homozygosity is found in 1 per 5,000 persons. It increases the risk of VTE 3- to 8-fold in heterozygous carriers and 50- to 80-fold in homozygous.
- PT20210A is found in 3% of Caucasians. Increases the risk of thrombosis about 3-fold.

GENERAL PREVENTION

- Mechanical thromboprophylaxis is recommended in patients with high bleeding risk and as an adjunct to anticoagulant based thromboprophylaxis. Mechanical measures include early ambulation, graduated compression stockings, venous foot pump, intermittent pneumatic compression.
- Level of risk
  - With minor surgery in mobile patient or fully mobile medical patients, risk of VTE <10%; early ambulation recommended
  - With medical patients on bed rest, general, and gynecologic or urologic surgeries, risk of VTE 10-40%; prophylactic LMWH, low-dose UFH or Fondaparinux recommended
- Hip or knee arthroplasty, major trauma, spinal cord injury, or hip fracture surgery, risk of VTE is 40–80%; LMWH, Fondaparinux, or oral vitamin K antagonist [INR 2-3] recommended

ETIOLOGY

Factors involved may include venous stasis, endothelial injury, and abnormalities of coagulation.

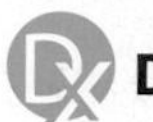

DIAGNOSIS

Wells criteria

- Active cancer within 6 months +1
- Paralysis or immobilization of lower extremity +1; Recent bedridden >3 days or major surgery within 4 weeks +1
- Tenderness/cord along vein +1
- Entire leg swollen +1
- Calf circumference >3 cm vs other leg +1
- Alternative diagnosis likely −2
- Interpretation
  - High probability +3
  - Moderate probability +3
  - Low probability 0

HISTORY

- Establish pretest probability based on Wells criteria.
- Classify as "Provoked" or "Idiopathic." Determine the presence of risk factors including family history.
- Clinical assessment of bleeding risk: bleeding with previous history of anticoagulation, history of liver disease, recent interventions, history of gastrointestinal bleed.

PHYSICAL EXAM

Physical exam is only 30% accurate for DVT. Resistance to dorsiflexion of the foot (Homan sign) is unreliable. Palpable tender cords are helpful if present but are often not present. Erythema over area of thrombosis (often not present). Fever is occasionally present. Swelling of collateral veins. Massive edema with cyanosis is a medical emergency (phlegmasia cerulea dolens, rare). Pain on medial tibia percussion (Lisker sign). Pain on compression of calf against tibia in the anteroposterior plane (Bancroft or Moses sign).Thoracic outlet maneuvers in Upper extremity DVT. Attention to signs of possible malignancy.

DIAGNOSTIC TESTS & INTERPRETATION

Lab

- D-dimer (sensitive but not specific; has a high NPV); most protocols are used to rule out DVT in low pretest probability cases: If D-dimer negative, DVT is ruled out with low pretest probability cases. Do not order D-dimer if pretest probability is moderate or high.
- CBC, platelet count, activated partial thromboplastin time (aPTT), prothrombin time (PT)/international normalized ratio (INR)
- In young patients with idiopathic or recurrent VTE consider:
  - Factor V Leiden, G20210A prothrombin, serum homocysteine, factor VIII level, and lupus anticoagulant
  - Protein C and S levels, antithrombin activity, anticardiolipin antibodies.
- Testing for genetic polymorphisms CYP2C9 and VKORC1 (www.warfarindosing.org for current recommendations)
- Thrombosis lowers antithrombin III; workup for deficiency performed after therapy completed. Secondary antithrombin deficiency is more common than primary.

Imaging

- Compression ultrasound (US): Noninvasive; sensitive and specific for popliteal, femoral thrombi, but has poor ability to detect calf vein thrombi
- Contrast venography: Gold standard, is technically difficult, risk of morbidity
- Impedance plethysmography: As accurate as duplex ultrasound, less operator dependency, but poor at detecting calf vein thrombi; not widely available
- Magnetic resonance venography: As accurate as contrast venography; may be useful for patients with contraindications to IV contrast
- ^{125}I-fibrinogen scan: Detects only active clot formation; very good at detecting ongoing calf thrombi; takes 4 hours for results

DIFFERENTIAL DIAGNOSIS

Cellulitis, fracture, ruptured synovial cyst (Baker cyst), lymphedema, muscle strain/tear, extrinsic compression of vein (for example, by tumor or enlarged lymph nodes), compartment syndrome, localized allergic reaction, filariasis (in developing countries)

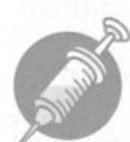

TREATMENT

MEDICATION

- All DVTs should receive treatment. Consider starting therapy even before confirmation in patients with high pre-test probability.
- 2008 American College of Chest Physicians Guidelines recommend low molecular weight heparin [LMWH], unfractionated heparin [UFH] (either IV, or fixed-dose or adjusted-dose subcutaneous heparin), or fondaparinux and warfarin for at least 5 days until the INR is 2–3 for 24 hours (3)[A].

First Line

- Unfractionated heparin (UFH):
  - IV drip: Initial dose of 80 units/kg or 5,000 Units followed by continuous infusion of 18 units/kg/hour. Target an APTT ratio >1.5. The APTT prolongation shall correspond to a 0.3 to 0.7 anti Xa level.
  - SC UFH: Monitored: 17,500 units or 250 units/kg b.i.d. with APTT adjustment to an equivalent to 0.3–0.7 anti Xa. Alternatively, fixed dose: 333 units/kg followed by b.i.d. dose 250 units/kg.
- Enoxaparin (Lovenox): 1 mg/kg/dose subcutaneously every 12 hours or 1.5 mg/kg/dose per day
- Dalteparin (Fragmin): 200 IU/kg subcutaneously every 24 hours

Fondaparinux (Arixtra): 5 mg (body weight <50 kg), 7.5 mg (body weight = 50–100 kg), or 10 mg (body weight >100 kg) subcutaneously once daily.
- Maintenance therapy:
  - Warfarin (Coumadin): 5 mg/d for 3 days, then adjust to a target INR of 2–3.
- Adverse effects:
  - Heparin or LMWH: Bleeding, edema, injection site irritation, skin eruptions, hematoma, thrombocytopenia
  - Fondaparinux: Bleeding, injection site irritation, rash, fever, anemia
  - Warfarin: Bleeding, skin necrosis, teratogenicity
- Contraindications:
  - Heparin or LMWH: Bleeding, heparin hypersensitivity, heparin-induced thrombocytopenia (HIT), ITP, infants/neonates
  - Fondaparinux: Bleeding, endocarditis, renal failure, thrombocytopenia
  - Warfarin: Current bleeding, alcoholism, preeclampsia, pregnancy, surgery, high fall risk

Second Line

f warfarin is contraindicated, heparin can be given by ntermittent subcutaneous self-injection.

Pregnancy Considerations

- Warfarin (Coumadin) is a teratogen; treat with full-dose heparin initially, followed by subcutaneous heparin starting at 15,000 units every 12 hours.
- Warfarin is safe with breast-feeding.
- LMWH, dalteparin, and fondaparinux are pregnancy category B.

ADDITIONAL TREATMENT

Additional Therapies

- Discharge with compression stockings 30–40 mm Hg. Stress use to prevent post-phlebitic syndrome. Continue compression therapy for 2 years.
- Intermittent pneumatic compression may be tried in patients with significant edema.

SURGERY/OTHER PROCEDURES

- In selected patients with proximal DVT (Iliofemoral DVT, <2 weeks of symptoms, good functional status, >1 year of life expectancy), catheter directed thrombolysis or open thrombectomy may be considered.
- When anticoagulants have failed or are contraindicated, filtering devices are recommended.

IN-PATIENT CONSIDERATIONS

Admission Criteria

Admission for: Respiratory distress, proximal VTE, candidates for thrombolysis, active bleeding, renal failure, phlegmasia cerulea dolens, history of heparin-induced thrombocytopenia

Nursing

Limb elevation

Discharge Criteria

Medically stable and properly anticoagulated; overlap of anticoagulation and warfarin monitoring may be done as an outpatient

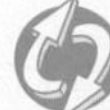

ONGOING CARE

FOLLOW-UP RECOMMENDATIONS

- Gradual resumption of normal activity, with avoidance of prolonged immobility.
- Duration of warfarin treatment after DVT:
  - 3 months for treatment of a DVT secondary to a reversible risk factor
  - Patients with unprovoked DVT shall be considered for prolonged secondary prophylaxis:
    - In patients who have completed 3 months of anticoagulation after an unprovoked VTE, a positive D Dimer 1 month after discontinuation of therapy correlates with the risk of VTE recurrence (4).
    - Tailoring the anticoagulation duration base on recanalization ultrasound evidence, may reduce the rate of recurrent VTE (5).
  - Consider prolonged secondary prophylaxis (1 year or indefinitely): Recurrent DVT; PE; active cancer (LMWH preferred over warfarin); life-threatening event (large pulmonary embolism, limb-threatening DVT); cerebral or visceral vein thrombosis; antithrombin deficiency with event; homozygous for factor V Leiden; combined clotting disorders (e.g., combined heterozygous factor V Leiden and PT20210A); antiphospholipid syndrome

Patient Monitoring

- Monitor platelet count while on heparin.
- Monitoring with LMWH and fondaparinux: Periodic platelet count. An anti-factor Xa activity level may help guide titration of therapy.
- Investigate significant bleeding (e.g., hematuria or GI hemorrhage) because anticoagulant therapy may unmask a preexisting lesion (e.g., cancer, peptic ulcer disease, or arteriovenous malformation).

DIET

Patients taking warfarin must be aware that foods high in vitamin K can affect INR.

PATIENT EDUCATION

- Patients should wear compression stockings post-DVT; these can be cumbersome and uncomfortable; however, they can reduce the risk of DVT recurrence and post-phlebitic syndrome.
- Dietary habits should be discussed when warfarin is initiated to ensure that intake of vitamin K-rich foods are identified.

PROGNOSIS

- 20% of untreated proximal (e.g., above the calf) DVTs progress to pulmonary emboli, and 10–20% of those are fatal; with anticoagulant therapy, mortality is decreased 5–10-fold.
- DVT confined to the infrapopliteal veins has a small risk of embolization, but can propagate into the proximal system. Best treatment uncertain, but most recommend 6–12 weeks of anticoagulation.

COMPLICATIONS

- Pulmonary embolism (fatal in 10–20%)
- Arterial embolism (paradoxical embolization) with AV shunting
- Chronic venous insufficiency
- Postphlebitic syndrome (pain and swelling in affected limb without new clot formation)
- Treatment-induced hemorrhage
- Soft tissue ischemia associated with massive clot and high venous pressures: phlegmasia cerulea dolens (rare, but a surgical emergency)

REFERENCES

1. Heit JA, Melton LJ, Lohse CM, et al. Incidence of venous thromboembolism in hospitalized patients vs community residents. *Mayo Clin. Proc.* 2001;76:1102–10.
2. Decousus H, Quéré I, Presles E, et al. Superficial venous thrombosis and venous thromboembolism: a large, prospective epidemiologic study. *Ann Intern Med*. 2010;152:218–24.
3. Kearon C, Kahn SR, Agnelli G, et al. Antithrombotic therapy for venous thromboembolic disease: American College of Chest Physicians Evidence-Based Clinical Practice Guidelines (8th Edition). *Chest*. 2008;133:454S–545S.
4. Palareti G, Cosmi B, Legnani C, et al. D-dimer testing to determine the duration of anticoagulation therapy. *N Engl J Med*. 2006; 355:1780–9.
5. Prandoni P, Prins MH, Lensing AW, et al. Residual thrombosis on ultrasonography to guide the duration of anticoagulation in patients with deep venous thrombosis: a randomized trial. *Ann Intern Med*. 2009;150:577–85.

See Also (Topic, Algorithm, Electronic Media Element)

Antithrombin Deficiency; Factor V Leiden; Protein C Deficiency; Protein S Deficiency; Prothrombin 20210 (Mutation); Pulmonary Embolism

CODES

ICD9

- 453.40 Acute venous embolism and thrombosis of unspecified deep vessels of lower extremity
- 453.41 Acute venous embolism and thrombosis of deep vessels of proximal lower extremity
- 453.42 Acute venous embolism and thrombosis of deep vessels of distal lower extremity

CLINICAL PEARLS

- Many cases are asymptomatic and are diagnosed after embolization.
- 25% of the patients with superficial thrombophlebitis will have DVT at presentation.
- Heparin and warfarin should overlap for a minimum of 5 days or longer to achieve target INR.
- Consider thoracic outlet syndrome in upper extremity DVT .
- Do a cancer-oriented review of systems and age- and gender-appropriate cancer screening in: Recurrent VTE, Not catheter associated Upper extremity DVT, bilateral lower extremity DVT, intra-abdominal DVT.

D

DEHYDRATION

Nitin Aggarwal, MD
Julie Scott Taylor, MD, MSc

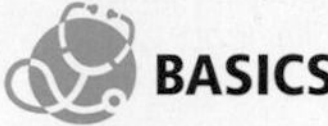

BASICS

DESCRIPTION

- Dehydration is a state of negative fluid balance.
- There are 2 types of dehydration:
  - Water loss dehydration (hyperosmolar, associated with either increased sodium or glucose)
  - Salt and water loss dehydration (hyponatremia)

EPIDEMIOLOGY

- Dehydration is the cause of 10% of all pediatric hospitalizations in the US.
- Gastroenteritis, one of the leading causes of dehydration, leads to hospital admission in 13 out of 1,000 children <5 years each year in the US (1).

Incidence

- There are more than a half million hospital admissions annually in the US for dehydration (2).
- 7.8% of hospitalized older persons have the diagnosis of dehydration (3).
- Worldwide, ~3–5 billion cases of acute gastroenteritis occur each year in children <5 years, resulting in nearly 2 million deaths (1).

RISK FACTORS

- Children <5 years old at highest risk
- Elderly
- Decreased cognition

Genetics

Some underlying causes of dehydration have a genetic component (diabetes), while others do not (gastroenteritis).

PATHOPHYSIOLOGY

- Negative fluid balance occurs when ongoing fluid losses exceed fluid intake.
- Fluid losses can be insensible (sweat, respiration), obligate (urine, stool), or abnormal (diarrhea, vomiting, osmotic diuresis in diabetic ketoacidosis).
- Negative fluid balance can ultimately lead to severe intravascular volume depletion and ultimately end-organ damage from inadequate perfusion.
- The elderly are at increased risk as kidney function, urine concentration, thirst sensation, aldosterone secretion, release of vasopressin, and renin activity are all significantly lowered with age. (4)

ETIOLOGY

- Decreased intake
- Increased output: Vomiting, diarrheal illnesses, sweating, frequent urination
- 3rd-spacing of fluids: Effusions, ascites, capillary leaks from burns or sepsis

COMMONLY ASSOCIATED CONDITIONS

- Hypo-/hypernatremia
- Hyperkalemia
- Hyperglycemia
- Hypovolemic shock
- Renal failure

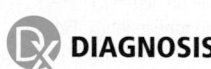

DIAGNOSIS

Calculate % dehydration = (preillness weight − illness weight)/preillness weight × 100:

Clinical Finding (5)	Mild Dehydration	Moderate Dehydration	Severe Dehydration
% Dehydration: Children	5–10%	10–15%	>15%
% Dehydration: Adults	3–5%	5–10%	>10%
General Condition: Infants	Thirsty, alert, restless	Lethargic or drowsy	Limp, cold, cyanotic extremities, may be comatose
General Condition: Older Children	Thirsty, alert, restless	Alert, postural dizziness	Apprehensive, cold, cyanotic extremities, muscle cramps
Quality of radial pulse	Normal	Thready or weak	Feeble or impalpable
Quality of respiration	Normal	Deep	Deep and rapid/tachypnea
Blood Pressure	Normal	Normal to Low	Low (shock)
Skin Turgor	Normal skin turgor	Reduced skin turgor, cool skin	Skin tenting, cool, mottled, acrocyanotic skin
Eyes	Normal	Sunken	Very sunken
Tears	Present	Absent	Absent
Mucous Membranes	Moist	Dry	Very dry
Urine Output	Normal	Reduced	None passed in many hours
Anterior Fontanelle	Normal	Sunken	Markedly sunken

GENERAL PREVENTION

- Patient/parent education on the early signs of dehydration
- Regular hand washing decreases the spread of contagious viral gastroenteritis.

Geriatric Considerations

A systematic approach in assessing risk factors is necessary for early prevention and management of dehydration in the elderly, especially those in long-term care facilities.

HISTORY

- Fever
- Intake (including description and amount)
- Diarrhea (including duration, frequency, consistency, +/− mucus or blood)
- Vomiting (including duration, frequency, consistency, +/− bilious/nonbilious)
- Urination pattern
- Sick contacts
- Medication history (e.g., diuretics, laxatives)

PHYSICAL EXAM

- Vitals: Pulse, BP, temperature
- Weight loss: <5%, 10%, or >15%
- Mental status
- Head: Sunken anterior fontanelle (for infants)
- Eyes: Sunken, +/− tear production
- Mucous membranes: Tacky, dry, or parched
- Capillary refill: Ranges from brisk to >3 sec

DIAGNOSTIC TESTS & INTERPRETATION

Lab

- For mild dehydration: Generally not necessary
- For moderate to severe dehydration:
  - Blood work including electrolytes, blood urea nitrogen (BUN), creatinine, and glucose
  - Urinalysis (specific gravity, hematuria, glucosuria)

Pediatric Considerations

Infants and the elderly may not concentrate urine maximally, so a nonelevated specific gravity should no be reassuring.

Imaging

Imaging does not play a role in diagnosis of dehydration, unless diagnosis of the specific medical condition causing the dehydration requires imaging.

DIFFERENTIAL DIAGNOSIS

- Decreased intake:
  - Ineffective breast-feeding
  - Inadequate thirst response
  - Anorexia
  - Malabsorption
  - Metabolic disorder
  - Obtunded state
- Excessive losses:
  - Gastroenteritis
  - Diarrhea
  - Febrile Illness
  - Diabetes/diabetic ketoacidosis (DKA)/ hyperosmolar hyperglycemic state (HHS)
  - Diabetes insipidus
  - Intestinal obstruction
  - Inadequate intravascular volume
  - Sepsis

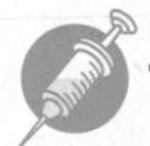

TREATMENT

MEDICATION

First Line

- If the patient is experiencing excessive vomiting, consider using an antiemetic.
- Antiemetic medications that are currently available include ondansetron, granisetron, tropisetron, dolasetron, ramosetron, promethazine, dimenhydrinate, metoclopramide, domperidone, droperidol, prochlorperazine, and trimethobenzamide.
- One randomized controlled trial (RCT) showed that a single oral dose of ondansetron reduced gastroenteritis-related vomiting and facilitated oral rehydration therapy (ORT) without significant adverse events (6)[B].

Second Line

- 2 RCTs found that in children with mild to moderate dehydration, loperamide reduced the duration of diarrhea compared with placebo. Another RCT found no significant difference. There is insufficient evidence to assess the risk of adverse effects (6)[B].
- In children ages 3–12 with mild diarrhea and minimal dehydration, loperamide improves diarrhea duration and frequency when used with oral rehydration (7)[A].

Pediatric Considerations

Given a higher risk for serious adverse events, loperamide is not indicated for children <3 years old with acute diarrhea (7)[A].

ADDITIONAL TREATMENT

Issues for Referral

- If dehydration is severe, or depending on underlying etiology, critical care referral and intensive care unit (ICU)-level care may be warranted.
- Consider surgical consultation for acute abdominal issues.

SURGERY/OTHER PROCEDURES

For specific underlying causes of dehydration, such as intestinal obstruction or appendicitis

IN-PATIENT CONSIDERATIONS

Initial Stabilization

- Stabilize ABCs.
- If mild dehydration, try oral rehydration therapy (ORT): See Oral Rehydration.
- If excessive vomiting or severe dehydration with shock, start IV access and IV fluids immediately.

Admission Criteria

- Intractable vomiting or diarrhea
- Electrolyte abnormalities
- Hemodynamic instability
- Inability to tolerate ORT

IV Fluids

- Stage I:
  - For moderate to severe dehydration in children: Isotonic saline or Ringer's lactate solution bolus of 10–20 mL/kg. May repeat up to 60 mL/kg; if still hemodynamically unstable, consider colloid replacement (blood, albumin, fresh frozen plasma) and address other causes for shock.
  - For moderate to severe dehydration in adults: Isotonic saline or Ringer's lactate 20 mL/kg/hour until normal state of consciousness returns or vital signs stabilize. Also consider colloid replacement if continued fluids required beyond 3L.
- Stage II: Replace fluid deficit along with maintenance over 48 hours. Fluid deficit = preillness weight – illness weight.
- An alternative IVF treatment option for moderate (10%) dehydration in children: (8)
  - Bolus with NS/LR at 20 mL/kg for 1 hour
  - Replete fluid deficit with D5 1/2NS + 20 mEq KCl/L at 10 mL/kg for 8 hours (hours 2–9)
  - Replete 1.5× maintenance fluids with D5 1/4NS + 20 mEq/L of KCl for 16 hours (hours 10–24)
- An alternative to IV fluids is hypodermoclysis, the subcutaneous infusion of fluids into the body.
  - Hypodermoclysis is indicated for the hydration of patients with mild to moderate dehydration who do not tolerate oral intake because of cognitive impairment, severe dysphagia, advanced terminal illness or intractable vomiting. It is also indicated to prevent dehydration, especially in frail elderly residents living in long-term care settings who reject the oral route for any reason.
  - It can also be a useful technique in rehydration for patients in whom IV access is difficult to obtain.
  - Hypodermoclysis is not indicated in patients with severe dehydration or shock, patients with coagulopathy or receiving full anticoagulation, patients with severe generalized edema (anasarca) or congestive heart failure, and those with fluid overload (9).

Nursing

- Strict I & Os.
- Document all oral and IV intake carefully.
- Document output of urine and stool, which may include weighing wet diapers.

Discharge Criteria

- Intake > output
- Underlying etiology treated and improving

ONGOING CARE

FOLLOW-UP RECOMMENDATIONS

Activity as tolerated

- If mild to moderate dehydration, the patient may be mobile without restrictions, although watch for orthostasis/falls.
- If moderate to severe dehydration, bed rest.

Patient Monitoring

Ongoing surveillance for recurrence

DIET

- Bland food such as a BRAT diet (bananas, rice, apples, toast)
- If diarrhea, avoid dairy for 48 hours after symptoms resolve. 1 systematic review of weak RCTs and 3 of 5 subsequent RCTs found that lactose-free feeds reduced the duration of diarrhea in children with mild to severe dehydration, compared with lactose-containing feeds. However, 2 subsequent RCTs found no difference between lactose-free and lactose-containing feeds in duration of diarrhea. (1)[A]
- Small frequent sips of room-temperature liquids
- For children, Pedialyte (liquid or Popsicles)
- Continue breast-feeding ad lib.

PATIENT EDUCATION

- Patients should go to the nearest emergency facility or call 911 if they or their child feels faint or dizzy when rising from a sitting or lying position, becomes lethargic and/or confused, or complains of a rapid heart rate.
- Patients should call their physician if they are unable to keep down any fluids, vomiting has been going on >24 hours in an adult or >12 hours in a child, diarrhea has lasted >2 days in an adult or child, an infant or child is much less active than usual or is very irritable, or if adult or child has excessive urination, especially if there is a history or family history of diabetes or diuretics administration.
- Patient information on dehydration at: http://www.mayoclinic.com/health/dehydration/DS00561
- Additional patient information at: http://familydoctor.org/online/famdocen/home/children/parents/common/stomach/196.html
- Treating gastroenteritis and dehydration in children at: http://www.aafp.org/afp/991201ap/991201a.html

PROGNOSIS

Self-limited if treated early. Potentially fatal.

COMPLICATIONS

- Seizures
- Renal failure
- Cardiovascular arrest

REFERENCES

1. Dalby-Payne J, et al. Clinical evidence concise: Gastroenteritis in children. *Am Fam Physician.* 2008;77(3):353. Available at: http://www.aafp.org/afp/20080201/bmj.html.
2. Xiao H, Barber J, Campbell ES et al. Economic burden of dehydration among hospitalized elderly patients. *Am J Health Syst Pharm.* 2004;61:2534–40.
3. Thomas DR, Cote TR, Lawhorne L, Levenson SA, Rubenstein LZ, Smith DA, Stefanacci RG, Tangalos EG, Morley JE, Dehydration Council et al. Understanding clinical dehydration and its treatment. *J Am Med Dir Assoc.* 2008;9:292–301.
4. Wotton K, Crannitch K, Munt R et al. Prevalence, risk factors and strategies to prevent dehydration in older adults. *Contemp Nurse.* 2008;31:44–56.
5. Gorelick MH, Shaw KN, Murphy KO et al. Validity and reliability of clinical signs in the diagnosis of dehydration in children. *Pediatrics.* 1997;99:E6-
6. Leung AK, Robson WL. Acute gastroenteritis in children: role of anti-emetic medication for gastroenteritis-related vomiting. *Paediatr Drugs.* 2007;9:175–84.
7. Barclay L, et al. Adjunctive loperamide therapy reduces acute diarrhea in children. Available at: http://www.medscape.com/viewarticle/554475.
8. Holliday MA, Ray PE, Friedman AL. Fluid therapy for children: facts, fashions and questions. *Arch Dis Child.* 2007;92:546–50.
9. Lopez JH, Reyes-Ortiz CA. Subcutaneous hydration by hypodermoclysis. *Reviews in Clinical Gerontology.* 2010;20(02):105–113.

See Also (Topic, Algorithm, Electronic Media Element)

Oral Rehydration

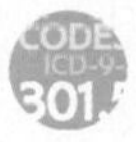

CODES

ICD9

- 276.1 Hyposmolality and/or hyponatremia
- 276.51 Dehydration

CLINICAL PEARLS

- Dehydration is the result of a negative fluid balance, when ongoing fluid losses exceed fluid intake for a variety of reasons.
- Dehydration is a common cause of hospitalization in both children and the elderly.
- Begin by assessing level of dehydration and determining the underlying cause.
- Treatment is directed at restoring fluid balance via oral rehydration therapy or IV fluids and treating underlying causes.

DELIRIUM

Jonathan M. Flacker, MD

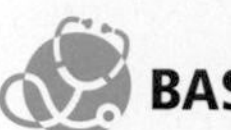

BASICS

DESCRIPTION

- A neurologic complication of illness and/or medication(s) especially common in older patients
- A medical emergency requiring immediate evaluation to decrease morbidity and mortality
- System(s) affected: Nervous
- Synonym(s): Acute confusional state; Altered mental status; Organic brain syndrome; Acute mental status change

EPIDEMIOLOGY

- Predominant age: Older persons
- Predominant sex: Male = Female

Incidence

>50% in high-risk older patients

Prevalence

- 10% in older emergency room patients
- 10–40% in hospitalized older patients
- 25% in older post–acute care patients
- Highest rates (>50%) in intensive care unit (ICU), post-hip fracture repair, post-cardiothoracic surgery

RISK FACTORS

- Predisposing risk factors:
  - Advanced age
  - Prior cognitive impairment
  - Functional impairment
  - High blood urea nitrogen: Creatinine ratio
  - Dehydration
  - Malnutrition
  - Hearing or vision impairment
  - Frailty
- Precipitating risk factors:
  - Severe illness in any organ system(s)
  - Need for a urinary catheter
  - >3 medications
  - Specific medications, especially long-acting sedative hypnotics (e.g., diazepam and flurazepam), narcotics (especially meperidine), and anticholinergics (especially diphenhydramine)
  - Pain
  - Any adverse iatrogenic event

GENERAL PREVENTION

Follow treatment approach.

PATHOPHYSIOLOGY

- Neuropathophysiology is not clearly defined; cholinergic deficiency is a leading hypothesis.
- Multicomponent approach addressing contributing factors can reduce incidence and complications.

ETIOLOGY

- Usually multifactorial
- Often interaction between predisposing and precipitating risk factors
- With more predisposing factors (i.e., frail patients), fewer precipitating factors needed to produce delirium
- If few predisposing factors (e.g., very robust patients), more precipitating factors needed to manifest delirium

COMMONLY ASSOCIATED CONDITIONS

Multiple, but most common are:

- New medicine or medicine changes
- Infections (especially lung and urine, but meningitis needs consideration as well)
- Toxic-metabolic (especially low sodium, elevated calcium, renal failure, and hepatic failure)
- Heart attack
- Stroke
- Alcohol or drug withdrawal
- Preexisting cognitive impairment increases risk.

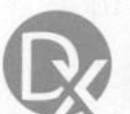

DIAGNOSIS

- The Confusion Assessment Method (CAM) may be used either pre- or post-hospital, or in hospital, and has been adapted for ICU setting (CAM-ICU).

ALERT

- Key diagnostic features of the CAM (1):
  - Acute change in mental status that fluctuates
  - Abnormal attention and **either** disorganized thinking **or** altered level of consciousness
- Any of the following nondiagnostic symptoms may be present:
  - Short- and long-term memory problems
  - Sleep-wake cycle disturbances
  - Hallucinations and/or delusions
  - Emotional lability
  - Tremors and asterixis
- Subtypes based on level of consciousness:
  - Hyperactive delirium (15%): Patients are loud, rambunctious, and disruptive.
  - Hypoactive delirium (20%): Quietly confused; may sit and not eat, drink, or move
  - Mixed delirium (50%): Features of both hyperactive and hypoactive delirium
  - Normal consciousness delirium (15%): Still display disorganized thinking, along with acute onset, inattention, and fluctuation

HISTORY

- Time course of mental status changes
- Recent medication changes
- Symptoms of infection
- New neurologic signs

PHYSICAL EXAM

- Comprehensive cardiorespiratory exam is essential.
- Focal neurologic signs usually absent
- Formal mini mental state exam is not diagnostic, but is helpful as structured interview and followed serially over time.

DIAGNOSTIC TESTS & INTERPRETATION

Electrocardiogram as necessary

Lab

Guided by history and physical exam

Initial lab tests

- Complete blood count
- Electrolytes, blood urea nitrogen, and creatinine
- Urinalysis, urine culture
- Medication levels (digoxin, theophylline where applicable)

Follow-Up & Special Considerations

If the above does not indicate a precipator of delirium, consider:

- Arterial blood gases
- Troponin
- Toxicology screen
- Liver panel
- Thyroid-stimulating hormone

Imaging

Guided by history and physical exam

Initial approach

- Chest radiograph for most
- Other if indicated by history and exam

Follow-Up & Special Considerations

Non-contrast-enhanced head computed tomography scan if:

- Unclear diagnosis
- Recent fall
- Receiving anticoagulants
- New focal neurologic signs
- Need to rule out increased intracranial pressure before lumbar puncture

Diagnostic Procedures/Surgery

- Lumbar puncture:
  - Rarely necessary
  - Perform if clinical suspicion of a central nervous system (CNS) bleed or infection is high
- Electroencephalogram:
  - Rarely necessary; consider after above evaluation if:
    - Diagnosis remains unclear
    - Suspicion of seizure activity

DIFFERENTIAL DIAGNOSIS

- Depression (slow onset, disturbance of mood, normal level of consciousness, and fluctuates over weeks to months)
- Dementia (insidious onset, memory problems, normal level of consciousness, and fluctuates over days to weeks)
- Psychosis (rarely sudden onset in older adults)

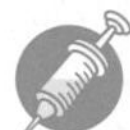

TREATMENT

- Stabilize vitals if needed.
- Ensure immediate evaluation. Addressing 6 risk factors (i.e., cognitive impairment, sleep deprivation dehydration, immobility, vision impairment, and hearing impairment) in at-risk hospitalized patients can reduce the incidence of delirium by 33%.

MEDICATION

- Nonpharmacologic approaches are preferred for initial treatment.
- Medications often treat only the symptoms and do not address the underlying cause.

First Line

- Neuroleptics:
  - Haloperidol (Haldol): Initially, 0.25–0.5 mg p.o./IM/IV unless urgent sedation needed; reevaluate and potentially redose hourly
  - Quetiapine (Seroquel): 25 mg/d to b.i.d.
  - Risperidone (Risperdal): 0.25–0.5 mg/d p.o.
- Short-acting benzodiazepines if neuroleptics do not work or should be avoided:
  - Lorazepam (Ativan): Initially, 0.25–0.5 mg p.o./IM/IV q6–8h; may need to adjust to effect (caution in patients with impaired liver function)
- Contraindications: Avoid neuroleptics in patients with parkinsonism or Parkinson disease
- Precautions: Neuroleptics may cause extrapyramidal effects, and benzodiazepines may lead to sedation. Both increase the risk of falls.

Second Line

Olanzapine (Zyprexa): 2.5–5.0 mg/d p.o.

Despite multiple trials there is no evidence to support the use of cholinesterase inhibitors in the prevention or treatment of delirium,

ADDITIONAL TREATMENT

General Measures

Postoperative patients should be monitored and treated for the following:
- Myocardial infarction/ischemia
- Pulmonary complications/pneumonia
- Pulmonary embolism
- Urinary or stool retention (attempt catheter removal by postoperative day 2)

Anesthesia route (general epidural) does not affect the risk of delirium.

Multifactorial treatment: Identify contributing factors and provide preemptive care to avoid iatrogenic problems (1,2)[A] with special attention to:
- CNS oxygen delivery (attempt to attain the following):
  - $SaO_2 > 90\%$ with goal of $SaO_2 > 95\%$
  - Systolic blood pressure <2/3 of baseline or >90 mm Hg
  - Hematocrit >30%

Fluid/electrolyte balance:
- Sodium, potassium, and glucose normal (glucose <300 mg/dL in diabetics)
- Treat fluid overload or dehydration.

Treat pain:
- Schedule acetaminophen (1 g q.i.d.) if daily pain
- Morphine or oxycodone for breakthrough pain if acetaminophen ineffective

ALERT
- Avoid meperidine (Demerol) (2)[A].
- Eliminate unnecessary medications:
  - Investigate new symptoms as potential medication side effects.
- Regulate bowel/bladder function:
  - Bowel movement at least every 48 hours
  - Screen for urinary retention or incontinence, especially after catheter removal.
- Prevent major hospital-acquired problems:
  - 6-inch-thick foam mattress overlay or a pressure-reducing mattress
  - Avoid urinary catheter.
  - Incentive spirometry, if bed-bound
  - SC heparin 5,000 U b.i.d., if bed-fast
  - Environmental stimulation:
    - Glasses and hearing aids
    - Clock and calendar
    - Soft lighting
    - Radio, tapes, and television, if desired
  - Sleep:
    - Quiet environment
    - Soft music
    - Therapeutic massage
- Restraints do not reduce risk of falls/injury:
  - Use only in the most difficult-to-manage patients, as briefly as possible

Issues for Referral

Psychiatric and/or neurologic assessment helpful if delirium not easily explainable after full evaluation

Additional Therapies

Early mobilization critical:
- Out of bed on hospital day 2 (or postoperative day 1) if no contraindications
- Out of bed several hours daily if able
- Daily therapy if not ambulating independently
- Daily therapy if not functionally independent

IN-PATIENT CONSIDERATIONS

General measures described above are also applicable to delirium prevention.

Admission Criteria

New delirium is a medical emergency and requires admission, except in the setting of palliative home care.

IV Fluids

As needed for dehydration

Nursing

- Institute skin care program for patients with established incontinence.
- Turning regimen if at risk of pressure ulcers
- Soft restraints are acceptable for a short time only if needed for protection of patient and others.

Discharge Criteria

- Resolution of precipitating factor(s)
- Safe discharge site if still delirious

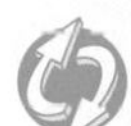

ONGOING CARE

FOLLOW-UP RECOMMENDATIONS

- If delirium at discharge, will usually be followed in post-acute facility
- If no delirium at discharge, follow up with primary care physician in 1–2 weeks.
- As tolerated
- Early physical therapy consultation to prevent deconditioning

Patient Monitoring

- Evaluate and assess mental status daily.
- Depends on specific conditions present

DIET

- Dentures used properly
- Proper positioning for meals
- Assistance with meals when necessary
- Nutritional supplements (1–3 cans daily) if intake is poor
- Temporary nasogastric tube if unable to eat and bowels working

PROGNOSIS

- Usually improves with treatment of underlying condition, but may become chronic
- Delirium complicating medical illness significantly increases a person's chance of dying from that illness

COMPLICATIONS

- Falls
- Pressure ulcers
- Malnutrition
- Functional decline
- Oversedation
- Polypharmacy

REFERENCES

1. Fong TG, Tulebave SR, Inouye SK. Delirium in elderly adults: Diagnosis, prevention, and treatment. Nature Reviews Neurology 2009;5: 210–220.
2. Hopkins RO, Jackson JC. Assessing neurocognitive outcomes after critical illness: are delirium and long-term cognitive impairments related? *Curr Opin Crit Care*. 2006;12:388–94.

ADDITIONAL READING

- Hshieh TT, Fong TG, Marcantonio ER, Inouye SK et al. Cholinergic deficiency hypothesis in delirium: a synthesis of current evidence. *J Gerontol A Biol Sci Med Sci*. 2008;63:764–72.
- van Eijk MM, van Marum RJ, Klijn IA, de Wit N, Kesecioglu J, Slooter AJ et al. Comparison of delirium assessment tools in a mixed intensive care unit. *Crit Care Med*. 2009;37:1881–5.
- Yang FM, Marcantonio ER, Inouye SK, Kiely DK, Rudolph JL, Fearing MA, Jones RN et al. Phenomenological subtypes of delirium in older persons: patterns, prevalence, and prognosis. *Psychosomatics*. 2009;50:248–54.

See Also (Topic, Algorithm, Electronic Media Element)

Substance Use Disorders; Dementia, Depression
Algorithm: Delirium

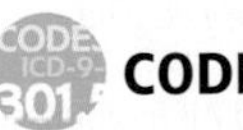

CODES

ICD9

- 293.0 Delirium due to conditions classified elsewhere
- 293.1 Subacute delirium
- 293.9 Unspecified transient mental disorder in conditions classified elsewhere

CLINICAL PEARLS

- The Confusion Assessment Method (CAM) criteria for delirium are acute onset of fluctuating mental status, inattention, disorganized thinking, AND EITHER disorganized thinking or altered level of consciousness.
- In the absence of active monitoring, the hypoactive subtype of delirium can easily be missed.
- Addressing 6 risk factors (i.e., cognitive impairment, sleep deprivation, dehydration, immobility, vision impairment, and hearing impairment) in at-risk hospitalized patients can reduce the incidence of delirium by 33%.
- Delirium may not resolve as soon as the treatable contributors are fixed; resolution may take weeks or months. Rarely will become chronic.
- Avoid diphenhydramine in older patients. Nonpharmacologic measures are preferable as a sleep aid, but if needed, zolpidem (5 mg hs) or trazodone (25 mg hs) are reasonable alternatives.

DEMENTIA

Alicia R. Desilets, PharmD
Karen Bryant, MD

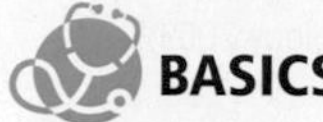

BASICS

DESCRIPTION

Dementia is a decline in cognitive function potentially caused by a number of disorders:

- Alzheimer dementia (AD):
  - Progressive deterioration of higher cortical functioning
- Vascular dementia (VaD):
  - Usually correlated with a cerebrovascular event and/or cerebrovascular disease
  - Stepwise deterioration with periods of clinical plateaus
- Lewy body dementia:
  - Fluctuating cognition associated with parkinsonism, hallucinations and delusions, gait difficulties, and falls
- Frontotemporal dementia:
  - Language difficulties, personality changes, and behavioral disturbances

EPIDEMIOLOGY

Prevalence

- In patients ≥71 years old:
  - AD: 70%
  - VaD: 17%
  - Other: 13%
- AD 60–64 years: <1%, approximately doubles every 5 years after age 60
- Estimated 5.2 million Americans had AD in 2008:
  - 5 million >65 years old; 200,000 <65 years

RISK FACTORS

- Increasing age
- Women > Men
- Lower educational status
- Genetic predisposition
- Head injury early in life
- Sedentary lifestyle
- Hypertension: AD; VaD
- Hypercholesterolemia: AD; VaD
- Diabetes: VaD
- Cigarette smoking: VaD

Genetics

- Heterogenous: Sporadic AD, ApoE4 allele on chromosome 19
- Familial: <0.1% AD, autosomal dominant

GENERAL PREVENTION

Data supporting specific preventative measures are limited and not conclusive:

- Smoking cessation
- Physical and mental activity
- Treatment of hypertension, hypercholesterolemia, and diabetes

ETIOLOGY

- AD:
  - Several mechanisms have been investigated.
  - Neurofibrillary tangles: Unable to support microtubules
  - Neuritic plaques (amyloid β-peptide):
    - Accumulation may lead to impaired cognitive function.
  - Other: Inflammatory mechanisms, oxidative:
    - Stress, mitochondrial dysfunction, apoptosis
- VaD:
  - Cerebral atherosclerosis or emboli with clinical or subclinical infarcts

COMMONLY ASSOCIATED CONDITIONS

- Anxiety and depression
- Delirium
- Behavioral disturbances (agitation, aggression)
- Sleep disturbances
- Caregiver stress

DIAGNOSIS

HISTORY

Probable diagnosis AD (1)[A]:

- Age between 40 and 90 (usually >65)
- Progressive cognitive decline of insidious onset
- No disturbances of consciousness
- Deficits in >2 areas of cognition
- No other explainable cause of symptoms
- Specifically, rule out thyroid disease, vitamin deficiency (B_{12}), grief reaction
- Supportive factors: Family history

PHYSICAL EXAM

- No disturbances of consciousness
- Cognitive decline demonstrated by standardized instruments, including:
  - Mini-Mental Status Exam
  - ADAS-Cog
  - Clock draw test
  - Change test
- Deficits in >2 areas of cognition

DIAGNOSTIC TESTS & INTERPRETATION

Lab

Initial lab tests

- Used to rule out other causes (1)[A]:
  - Comprehensive metabolic profile
  - Complete blood count
  - Thyroid stimulating hormone
  - Vitamin B_{12} level
  - Neuroimaging (preferably magnetic resonance imaging [MRI] of brain)
- Select patients:
  - HIV
  - Rapid plasma reagin
  - Erythrocyte sedimentation rate
  - Folate
  - Heavy metal screen
  - Toxicology screen

Imaging

Tests that support the diagnosis:

- Cerebral atrophy on neuroimaging
- Normal lumbar puncture

Initial approach

- Early age of onset (<65 years old), rapid progression, focal neurologic deficits, cerebrovascular disease risk, or atypical symptoms: Neuroimaging (MRI or computed tomography) to rule out other causes (1)[A]
- Important findings:
  - AD: Diffuse cerebral atrophy starting in association areas, hippocampus, amygdala
  - VaD: Old infarcts, including lacunes

Diagnostic Procedures/Surgery

Positron emission tomography scan not routinely recommended; has been approved to differentiate between Alzheimer disease and frontotemporal dementia (2)[A]

Pathological Findings

AD:

- Neurofibrillary tangles: Abnormally phosphorylated tau protein
- Senile plaques: Amyloid precursor protein derivative
- Microvascular amyloid

DIFFERENTIAL DIAGNOSIS

- Mild cognitive impairment
- Major depression
- Medication side effect
- Chronic alcohol use
- Delirium
- Subdural hematoma
- Normal pressure hydrocephalus
- Brain tumor
- Thyroid disease
- Parkinson disease
- Vitamin B_{12} deficiency
- Toxins (aromatic hydrocarbons, solvents, heavy metals, marijuana, opiates, sedative-hypnotics)

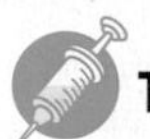

TREATMENT

MEDICATION

First Line

- Cognitive dysfunction, mild (2)[A]:
  - Cholinesterase inhibitors: Donepezil (Aricept), 5–10 mg/d; rivastigmine (Exelon), 1.5–6 mg b.i.d., transdermal system 4.6 mg/24 hours and 9.5 mg/24 hours; galantamine (Razadyne), 4–12 mg b.i.d., extended release 8–24 mg/d:
    - Adverse events: Nausea, vomiting, diarrhea, anorexia, nightmares
    - Galantamine warning: Associated with mortalit in patients with mild cognitive impairment in clinical trial
- Cognitive dysfunction, moderate to severe (2)[A]:
  - Cholinesterase inhibitors OR
  - Memantine (Namenda) 5–20 mg/d:
    - Adverse events: Dizziness, confusion, headache constipation
  - OR combination cholinesterase inhibitor and memantine
- Commonly associated conditions:
  - Psychosis and agitation/aggressive behavior:
    - Antipsychotics: Initiate low doses, haloperidol 0.25–0.5 mg/d; risperidone 0.25–1 mg/d; clozapine 12.5 mg/d; olanzapine 1.25–5 mg/d; quetiapine 12.5–50 mg/d; aripiprazole 5 mg/d; ziprasidone 20 mg/d (2)[A]
    - Atypical antipsychotics associated with a better side effect profile; quetiapine and aripiprazole often 1st-line due to decreased extrapyramidal side effects

ALERT
- Black box warning on atypical antipsychotics due to increased mortality found when used in elderly patients with dementia
- Depression:
  - Selective serotonin reuptake inhibitors (SSRIs): Initiate low doses, citalopram (Celexa) 10 mg/d; escitalopram (Lexapro) 5 mg/d; sertraline (Zoloft) 25 mg/d (2)[A]
  - Adverse events: Nausea, vomiting, agitation, parkinsonian effects, sexual dysfunction, hyponatremia
  - Fluoxetine (Prozac) and paroxetine (Paxil) should be avoided in elderly patients.
- Sleep disturbances:
  - Mirtazapine (7.5–60 mg) or trazodone (25–100 mg) at bedtime if also has depression (2)[A]
  - Atypical antipsychotics if psychotic symptoms present (2)[A]
  - Zolpidem (5–10 mg); zaleplon (5–10 mg) (2)[A]
  - Benzodiazepines only for short term if anxiety or as needed: Lorazepam 0.5–1.0 mg; oxazepam 7.5–15 mg (2)[A]

Second Line
Associated conditions:
- Depression: Venlafaxine, mirtazapine and bupropion (2)[A]
- Psychosis and agitation/aggressive behavior:
  - Some data for SSRIs (2)[A]
  - Benzodiazepines if agitation with anxiety; in elderly, use as needed (2)[A]

Geriatric Considerations
- Initiate pharmacotherapy at low doses and titrate slowly up if necessary.
- If benzodiazepines indicated for anxiety, choose drug with short half-life
- Watch decreased renal function and hepatic metabolism.

ADDITIONAL TREATMENT
Behavioral modification:
- Socialization such as adult day care to prevent isolation and depression
- Sleep hygiene program as alternative to pharmaceuticals for sleep disturbance
- Scheduled toileting to prevent incontinence

General Measures
- Daily schedules and written directions
- Emphasis on nutrition, personal hygiene, accident-proofing the home, safety issues, sleep hygiene and supervision
- Socialization (adult day care)
- Sensory stimulation (display of clocks and calendars) in the early to mid stages
- Discussion with the family concerning support and advance directives

Issues for Referral
- Neuropsychiatric evaluation particularly helpful in early stages or mild cognitive impairment
- Assessment and management of:
  - Cognitive problems
  - Mood disorders (e.g., depression, anxiety)
  - Psychosis
  - Behavioral problems (e.g., agitation, aggression)

COMPLEMENTARY AND ALTERNATIVE MEDICINE
- Vitamin E is no longer recommended due to lack of evidence and possible association with an increase in mortality (2)[A].
- Ginkgo biloba should not be recommended due to lack of evidence (2)[A].
- Huperzine-A appears to have potential in small trials; however, until clinical evidence can firmly establish its role, it should not be recommended.
- Use of nonsteroidal anti-inflammatory drugs, selegiline, and estrogen should not be recommended due to lack of efficacy and safety data (2)[A].

IN-PATIENT CONSIDERATIONS
Admission Criteria
- Patients who cannot be treated in an outpatient setting
- Patients who may require geripsychiatric admission for aggressive behaviors

ONGOING CARE

FOLLOW-UP RECOMMENDATIONS
Patient Monitoring
- Progression of cognitive impairment by use of standardized tool (e.g., MMSE, ADAS Cog)
- Development of behavioral problems
- Adverse events of pharmacotherapy
- Nutritional status
- Caregiver evaluation of stress
- Evaluate issues that may affect quality of life.

PATIENT EDUCATION
- Safety concerns
- Long-term issues: Management of finances, medical decision making, possible placement when appropriate
- Advance directives

PROGNOSIS
- AD: Progressive disease (variable rates) leading to profound cognitive impairment:
  - Without treatment average decline on MMSE of 2 points per year
- VaD: Less likely to be progressive, but cognitive improvement is unlikely
- Secondary dementias: Treatment of the underlying condition may lead to improvement.

COMPLICATIONS
- Wandering
- Falls with injury:
  - Hip fracture
  - Head trauma
  - Subdural hematoma
- Aspiration pneumonia in end stage
- Caregiver burnout

REFERENCES

1. Blass DM, Rabins PV. In the clinic. Dementia. *Ann Intern Med*. 2008;148:ITC4–1-ITC4-16.
2. APA Work Group on Alzheimer's Disease and other Dementias, Rabins PV, Blacker D, et al. American Psychiatric Association practice guideline for the treatment of patients with Alzheimer's disease and other dementias. Second edition. *Am J Psychiatry*. 2007;164:5–56.

ADDITIONAL READING

- Birks J. Cholinesterase inhibitors for Alzheimer's disease. *Cochrane Database Syst Rev*. 2006; CD005593.
- Blennow K, de Leon MJ, Zetterberg H. Alzheimer's disease. *Lancet*. 2006;368:387–403.
- Burns A, Iliffe S. Alzheimer's disease. *BMJ*. 2009;338:b158.
- Lleó A, Greenberg SM, Growdon JH. Current pharmacotherapy for Alzheimer's disease. *Annu Rev Med*. 2006;57:513–33.
- Lyketsos CG, Colenda CC, Beck C, et al. Position statement of the American Association for Geriatric Psychiatry regarding principles of care for patients with dementia resulting from Alzheimer disease. *Am J Geriatr Psychiatry*. 2006;14:561–72.

See Also (Topic, Algorithm, Electronic Media Element)
Algorithm: Dementia

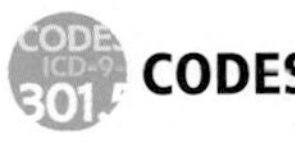

CODES

ICD9
- 290.0 Senile dementia, uncomplicated
- 290.40 Vascular dementia, uncomplicated
- 331.0 Alzheimer's disease
- 331.82 Dementia with Lewy bodies

CLINICAL PEARLS
- Dementia is loss of cognitive function in multiple areas.
- Time is diagnostic; AD is a progressive disease that will manifest with continual decline over time.
- Medications for AD show a small, statistically significant improvement in some cognitive measures, but it remains unclear if the improvement is clinically significant.

DENTAL INFECTION

Sheila O. Stille, DMD, MAGD
John J. Gentile, DMD

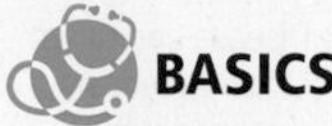

BASICS

DESCRIPTION

- Very painful area ± swelling in the head and neck region arising from the teeth and supporting structures. If left untreated, can lead to serious and potentially life-threatening illnesses.
- Assume any head and neck infection or swelling to be odontogenic in origin until proven otherwise.

EPIDEMIOLOGY

Incidence

- Caries is a contagious bacterial infection that is transmitted vertically from caregivers.
- The introduction of fluoride has dramatically decreased dental caries.

Prevalence

25% of children between ages of 5 and 17 years account for 80% of caries in the US (1).

RISK FACTORS

- Low socioeconomic status
- Poor access to care
- Fear of dentist
- Poor oral hygiene
- Poor nutrition
- Prior trauma to the teeth or jaws
- Heavily restored dentition
- Inadequate fluoride
- Gingival recession (increased risk of root caries)
- Physical and mental disabilities
- Decreased salivary flow
- Use of anticholinergic medications

GENERAL PREVENTION

- Preventable, contagious bacterial infection (*S. mutans*)
- Majority of dental problems can be avoided through flossing, brushing with fluoride toothpaste, and biannual cleaning (2)[B]
- Avoid smoking; linked to severe periodontal disease
- Good control of systemic diseases, i.e., diabetes

PATHOPHYSIOLOGY

Caries or trauma can lead to pulpal death, which in turn, leads to infection of pulp and/or abscess of adjacent tissues via direct or hematogenous bacterial colonization.

ETIOLOGY

- *Streptococcus mutans* vertically transmitted to newly dentate infants from caregivers
- Acidic secretions from *Streptococcus mutans* are implicated in early caries.
- Often polymicrobial
- Anaerobes, including *Pepto streptococci*, *Bacteroides*, *Prevotella*, and *Fusobacterium*, have been implicated. *Lactobacilli* may subsequently be involved.

COMMONLY ASSOCIATED CONDITIONS

- Rampant caries throughout dentition; multiple missing teeth
- Periodontal abscess
- Soft tissue cellulitis
- Pericoronitis
- Periodontitis

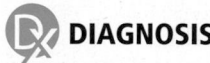

DIAGNOSIS

HISTORY

- Pain at infected site or referred to ears, jaw, cheek, or sinuses
- Sensitivity to hot or cold stimuli
- Unprovoked, intermittent, or constant throb along nerve pathway
- Pain on biting
- Bleeding or purulent drainage from gingival tissues
- When severe infection (systemic):
  - Fever
  - Difficulty breathing or swallowing
  - Death
- Children <4 years with stiff neck, sore throat, and dysphagia should be worked up for retropharyngeal abscess secondary to molar infection.

PHYSICAL EXAM

- Gingival edema and erythema
- Cheek or intraoral swelling
- Presence of fluctuant mass
- Suppuration of gingival margin or tooth
- Lymphadenopathy
- Severe infection may present with dysphagia, fever, and signs of airway compromise.

DIAGNOSTIC TESTS & INTERPRETATION

Lab

Initial lab tests

- No initial labs needed, unless patient looks acutely ill
- If acutely ill:
  - Consider complete blood count with differential.
  - Culture and sensitivity; if abscess present, aspirate pus. Test for aerobes and anaerobes.
  - Note: Multiple organisms involved; most likely anaerobic gram-negative rods and anaerobic gram-positive cocci (2).

Imaging

Initial approach

- Individual dental films of suspected teeth
- Panoramic film of the teeth and jaw for evaluation of the extent of infection

Follow-Up & Special Considerations

Computed tomography scan can be used to determine the extent and density of the swelling, locating the abscess within the soft tissue and bone. This aids in determining treatment course.

DIFFERENTIAL DIAGNOSIS

- Bacterial or viral throat infection
- Otitis media
- Sinusitis
- Viral or aphthous stomatitis
- Temporomandibular joint (TMJ) dysfunction (myofascial pain)
- Parotitis
- Cyst
- Jaw pain can be anginal equivalent, especially in women, and especially lower-left portion of the jaw.

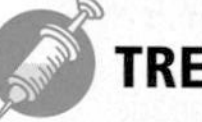

TREATMENT

- Place patient on appropriate antibiotic, if indicated.
- Tend to appropriate pain control: Anti-inflammatory agents
- Refer to dentist as soon as possible for definitive treatment: Root canal or extraction
- If infection is severe, consider hospitalization with IV antibiotics until stabilized. Patient may need incision and drainage of abscess.

MEDICATION

First Line

- Penicillin VK loading dose of 1,000 mg, followed by 500 mg q.i.d. for 7–10 days. In children, 40–60 mg/kg/d divided q.i.d.
- Amoxicillin loading dose of 1,000 mg, followed by 500 mg t.i.d. for 7–10 days. In children, 40–60 mg/kg/d divided t.i.d.
- If penicillin-allergic, use clindamycin

Second Line

long-standing infection or previously treated fection that does not respond to 1st-line eatment:

- Oral clindamycin 300 mg t.i.d. for 7–10 days
- If severe infection, load with clindamycin 600 mg, 900 mg IV, then 300 mg q6h; consider double coverage with metronidazole

ADDITIONAL TREATMENT

General Measures

- Ibuprofen 600–800 mg (or 10 mg/kg) q6h, or acetaminophen 650–1,000 mg (10–15 mg/kg) q4–6h
- For more severe pain, consider acetaminophen or ibuprofen + opioids.
- Can consider local anesthetic nerve block with long-acting anesthetic (bupivacaine) as adjunct; avoid penetrating infection with needle to avoid tracking infection

Issues for Referral

dentist should be consulted and follow-up definitive are appointment should be secured prior to discharge om medical office, emergency room, or hospital nit.

SURGERY/OTHER PROCEDURES

- Incision and drainage of abscess should be performed if abscess is large and fluctuant.
- Root canal or extraction should be performed as definitive treatment.

IN-PATIENT CONSIDERATIONS

Initial Stabilization

- Secure airway, if compromised, with either endotracheal intubation or tracheotomy.
- IV fluid resuscitation with normal saline may be indicated in acutely ill patients.

Admission Criteria

Criteria for hospital admission include swelling nvolving deep spaces of the neck, unstable vital signs, ever, chills, confusion or delirium, or evidence of nvasive infection.

Nursing

- Ensure good oral hygiene.
- Rinse mouth with chlorhexidine gluconate 2 times per day.
- Use warm salt water rinses several times per day to encourage drainage, especially after incision and drainage.

Discharge Criteria

Discharge patient if:

- Airway not compromised
- Abscess and sepsis eliminated
- Able to take p.o. intake and ambulate

ONGOING CARE

Educate patient in need for proper oral hygiene, need for follow-up dental care, need for routine dental care, and stress medical complications that can and have occurred due to lack of dental care.

FOLLOW-UP RECOMMENDATIONS

- Follow-up with dentist within 24 hours.
- Ensure adequate p.o. intake, including protein.

DIET

- Maintain a healthy diet. Bacteria thrive on refined sugar and starch.
- Avoid sugary foods that stick between the teeth.

Pediatric Considerations

In children, limit the frequency of sugary drinks, and advise against sleeping with a bottle to decrease the chance of dental caries.

PATIENT EDUCATION

- Biannual dental visits
- Nutritional education
- Limit the frequency of sugar/carbonated drinks and sugary or sticky foods.
- In young children, avoid sleeping with a bottle to decrease the chance of dental caries.
- Brush and floss daily.
- Caretakers should tend to their personal oral hygiene, +/− chlorhexidine rinses in 1st 3 years of the child's life to decrease the risk of transmission of the caries causing microorganisms.

PROGNOSIS

Prognosis is excellent with proper treatment.

COMPLICATIONS

- Ludwig angina
- Retropharyngeal and mediastinal infection
- Osteomyelitis
- Endocarditis
- Submental infection
- Submandibular infection
- Can cause unstable diabetes in diabetics/worsen preexisting heart disease
- Possible link to preterm labor
- Brain abscess/death

REFERENCES

1. Kaste LM, Selwitz RH, Oldakowski RJ, et al. Coronal caries in the primary and permanent dentition of children and adolescents 1-17 years of age: United States, 1988–1991. *J Dent Res.* 1996;75 Spec No:631–41.
2. Lockhart PB, ed. *Dental Care of the Medically Complex Patient*, 5th ed. New York: Elsevier, 2004.

ADDITIONAL READING

- Cliff K, et al. An evidence-based update of the use of analgesics in dentistry. *Periodontology.* 2008; 46(1):143–164.
- Marinho VCC, et al. Topical fluoride (toothpastes, mouthrinses, gels or varnishes) for preventing dental caries in children and adolescents. Cochrane Oral Health Group. *Cochrane Database Syst Rev.* 2007;(4):CD002781.
- Matijevi S, Lazi Z, Kulji-Kapulica N, et al. Empirical antimicrobial therapy of acute dentoalveolar abscess. *Vojnosanit Pregl.* 2009;66:544–50.
- Stefanopoulos PK, Kolokotronis AE. Controversies in antibiotic choices for odontogenic infections. *Oral Surg Oral Med Oral Pathol Oral Radiol Endod.* 2006;101:697–8.
- Stefanopoulos PK, Kolokotronis AE. The clinical significance of anaerobic bacteria in acute orofacial odontogenic infections. *Oral Surg Oral Med Oral Pathol Oral Radiol Endod.* 2004;98:398–408.
- Vargas CM, Crall JJ, Schneider DA. Sociodemographic distribution of pediatric dental caries: NHANES III, 1988–1994. *J Am Dent Assoc.* 1998;129:1229–38.
- Vellappally S, Fiala Z, Smejkalová J, et al. Smoking related systemic and oral diseases. *Acta Medica (Hradec Kralove).* 2007;50:161–6.

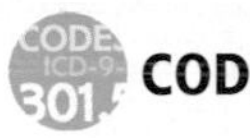

CODES

ICD9

- 521.00 Dental caries, unspecified
- 522.5 Periapical abscess without sinus
- 528.3 Cellulitis and abscess of oral soft tissues

CLINICAL PEARLS

- Do not ignore toothache pain.
- Treat patients with facial swelling aggressively, as infections can spread quickly.

DENTAL TRAUMA

Sheila O. Stille, DMD, MAGD
John J. Gentile, DMD

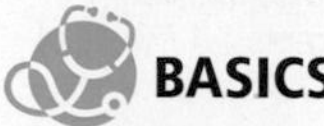

BASICS

DESCRIPTION

Loss or fracture of a tooth and/or supporting bone due to trauma. Trauma can result in shifting of remaining teeth, loss of teeth, loss of alveolar bone, displaced or nonunion of maxilla and/or mandible, resulting in functional and aesthetic deformities that may become difficult to correct.

EPIDEMIOLOGY

- Dental injuries of the teeth, supporting bone, and surrounding soft tissue constitute 7% of all physical injuries.
- Causes: Falls/sports, 63%; assault, 17%; auto or motorcycle accidents, 2%
- Male > Female (2–3:1)

Prevalence

- Prevalence: 5% of all school-age children; 7–13% in primary dentition, 1–16% in permanent dentition
- Affects 13% of population <12 years

RISK FACTORS

- Physical and mental disabilities
- Contact sports without wearing proper protective equipment, i.e., helmets, mouth guards
- Age: Youth <12 years
- Tongue rings
- Prior dental trauma
- Male gender

GENERAL PREVENTION

- Mouth guards and helmets may prevent traumatic dental injuries during sport exercises like football, soccer, baseball, hockey, bicycling, or skateboarding.
- Avoid tongue piercings.
- Wear seat belts while in the car.
- Monitor home for slippery areas.
- Childproof house gates and pad sharp table edges.

PATHOPHYSIOLOGY

Direct force sufficient to overcome the bond between the tooth and periodontal ligament within the alveolar socket or disruption of enamel and dentin. Force against maxilla or mandibular arch great enough to cause fracture.

COMMONLY ASSOCIATED CONDITIONS

- Tooth loss can cause loss of space in dental arch.
- Malocclusion causing functional problems
- Trauma to dentition resulting in pulpitis, which causes necrosis of the pulp
- Child abuse: Be alert for history inconsistent with injuries.

DIAGNOSIS

HISTORY

- Assess ABCs.
- Determine nature, time of injury; associated injuries
- Dental fractures:
  – Ask patient if they have possession of missing tooth pieces or swallowed/aspirated teeth.
  – Assess extent of fracture: Enamel only; enamel and dentin; enamel, dentin, and pulp; root fracture
- Concussion of teeth; subluxed; intruded; extruded
- Tooth avulsion:
  – Time out of socket (critical to management and prognosis)
  – Location of tooth when recovered
  – Type of tooth transfer media (milk, water, towel, etc.)
- Maxilla or mandibular fracture
- Consider child abuse in patients with dental fractures.

PHYSICAL EXAM

- Inspect the surrounding tissue for laceration, ecchymosis, embedded tooth fragments, or foreign bodies.
- Classify fracture by Ellis classification:
  – Ellis I fracture involves only the enamel.
  – Ellis II fracture includes enamel and dentin (pale yellow material underlying the enamel).
  – Ellis III fracture involves enamel, dentin, and pulp (red material under dentin).
- Check for sensitivity to hot/cold/percussion.
- Check if the tooth is mobile: Palpate tooth and surrounding bone.
- Check for mandibular fracture: Percuss/twist with tongue blade to evaluate.
- Bimanual palpation for maxilla fracture/alveolar fracture
- If tooth missing, investigate for intrusion of tooth or root fragment in socket.

DIAGNOSTIC TESTS & INTERPRETATION

Lab

Initial lab tests

No initial labs needed, unless patient appears acutely ill.

Imaging

Initial approach

Panoramic radiograph of the teeth and jaw for evaluation of the extent of injury; computed tomography (CT) scan only needed if other associated head trauma.

Follow-Up & Special Considerations

Chest x-ray may be needed for lost avulsed teeth: May be in trachea, lungs, esophagus, or stomach

DIFFERENTIAL DIAGNOSIS

- Crown fracture
- Root fracture
- Subluxation of tooth
- Extrusion/intrusion of tooth
- Trismus

TREATMENT

Assess ABCs for other problems associated with the traumatic injury.

MEDICATION

First Line

- Pain management:
  – Ibuprofen 600–800 mg (or 10 mg/kg) q6h, or acetaminophen 650–1,000 mg (10–15 mg/kg) q4–6h
  – For more severe pain, consider acetaminophen o ibuprofen + opioids.
  – Can consider local anesthetic nerve block with long-acting anesthetic (bupivacaine) as adjunct
- Antibiotics for fractures or avulsions to prevent complications:
  – Penicillin VK 500 mg q.i.d. for 7 days in adults. Fc children, 10 mg/kg/dose q.i.d.
  – Clindamycin 150–300 mg t.i.d. (or 5–7.5 mg/kg/ dose) in penicillin-allergic patients

Second Line

- Phenoxymethyl penicillin 200–500 mg p.o. q6h for children <12 years
- Clindamycin 150–300 mg t.i.d. (or 5–7.5 mg/kg/ dose) in penicillin-allergic patients

ADDITIONAL TREATMENT

General Measures

- Fractured teeth:
  – Ellis I: Smooth edges with emery board or dental drill; cosmetic repair can be done by dentist in follow-up.
  – Ellis II and III: Cover exposed area with calcium hydroxide paste (Dycal). Tooth must be dry befor adding Dycal. If not available, Coe-Pak (zinc oxid preparation) can be used. Wrap preparation around fractured tooth edge. Follow up with dentist within 24 hours, if other injuries permit.
- Primary goal of reimplantation/repositioning is to protect periodontal ligament; tooth pulp may die, but tooth can be saved by root canal.
- Subluxation (abnormal mobility) of teeth:
  – Patient should be referred to dentist as soon as possible to evaluate for possible repositioning an splinting.
  – Nonrigid splint should be placed ASAP.
- Intrusion (apical displacement of tooth into the alveolar bone):
  – Primary teeth should be left alone to allow for spontaneous eruption after dental follow-up.
  – For permanent teeth, do not reposition; refer to oral surgeon ASAP. Attempts to reposition may cause compromise of blood supply to supporting bone and nerve. Alveolar bone may have necrosi causing bony defect. Tooth usually needs to be extracted when bone heals.

Avulsed teeth: Dental emergency:
- Time is of the essence when reimplanting teeth.
- If primary tooth: Do not reimplant. If unsure, consult dentist.
- If permanent tooth: Avoid touching tooth root, handle only by the crown; rinse with normal saline. Minimize trauma to socket. If dirt or large clot in socket, perform gentle irrigation of the socket with normal saline and light aspiration of blood clot before implantation.
- If tooth is outside of socket <20 minutes, attempt implantation of tooth and stabilize with resin/metal splint, or, if not available, zinc oxide (Coe-Pak) splint.
- If tooth is outside of socket 20–60 minutes, soak tooth in Hanks solution for 30 minutes to preserve pH. If Hanks is not available, use saline. Attempt implantation and stabilization.
- If tooth is outside of socket >60 minutes, soak tooth in citric acid and fluoride for 30 minutes; attempt reimplantation and stabilization. If citric acid/fluoride not available, use Hanks or saline.
- Consult dentist for follow-up and for any questions.

Soft foods only for 10–14 days, depending on injury.

Jaw fracture:
- Assess for displacement.
- If nerve impingement, immediate surgery needed. Contact oral surgeon ASAP.
- If not displaced or no indication of nerve impingement, have patient see oral surgeon within 24 hours for fixation.

ssues for Referral

All patients should be referred to a dentist for follow-up.

Splints are typically maintained in place for 7–10 days for subluxed teeth and 2–8 weeks for avulsed teeth. Alveolar fractures should be splinted for 4–6 weeks and can take up to 6 months to heal.

Avulsed teeth continue to deteriorate up to 36 months after injury and typically require root canal therapy.

Oral surgeon should follow jaw fractures in consultation with general dentist.

\dditional Therapies

etanus booster should be considered if tetanus overage is uncertain or if tooth has been in contact vith soil or deep lacerations present.

COMPLEMENTARY AND ALTERNATIVE MEDICINE

Acupuncture (1)[C]

Clove oils (2)[C]

SURGERY/OTHER PROCEDURES

)ral surgeon referral within 1 hour if patient has lveolar bone fracture or jaw fracture. Reduction is asier before swelling.

N-PATIENT CONSIDERATIONS

nitial Stabilization

ecure airway if compromised with either ndotracheal intubation or tracheotomy.

Admission Criteria

Criteria for hospital admission include swelling ompromising airway, mental status change due to oncussion or hypoxia, after aspiration of teeth, or instable vital signs.

V Fluids

V fluid resuscitation with normal saline may be ndicated in septic patients.

Nursing

Ensure excellent oral hygiene. Rinse mouth with chlorhexidine gluconate to minimize bacterial load in oral cavity.

Discharge Criteria

Discharge patient when:
- Abscess and sepsis have been eliminated
- Patient able to take in adequate p.o. and ambulation
- Cleared from concussion

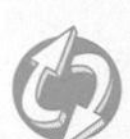

ONGOING CARE

FOLLOW-UP RECOMMENDATIONS

Follow-up with dentist or oral surgeon within 24 hours after any dental trauma:
- Restrict use of pacifiers if dental injuries are involved.
- Ellis III fractures in children <12 years are likely to get infected; clinicians should consider antibiotic coverage.

Patient Monitoring

Biannual cleaning and follow-up. First 36 months most critical to long-term prognosis.

DIET

Avoid any solid food before following up with dentist, and maintain diet as directed by dentist.

PATIENT EDUCATION

- Use a soft toothbrush and soft diet for 10–14 days after dental trauma. Rinse with chlorhexidine 0.1% twice a day for 1 week to prevent plaque and debris accumulation (3)[A].
- If tooth avulsion occurs, handle tooth only by the crown.
- Cold milk is the best transportation medium before coming to the emergency room, as it maintains the periodontal ligament for about 3 hours and has pH and osmolarity to maintain vitality of the cells. Saline or saliva is a good substitute. Water is the least desirable transport medium because it is a hypotonic solution that can lyse the cells.

PROGNOSIS

- <20 minutes of tooth separation from socket: Good prognosis
- >60 minutes of tooth separation: Poor prognosis for tooth reattachment
- Alveolar fracture: Poor prognosis for teeth involved
- Jaw fracture: Good prognosis with proper reduction/fixation

COMPLICATIONS

- Tooth loss
- Infection
- Cosmetic and/or functional deformity
- Anesthesia/paraesthesia of nerve entrapment with fractured jaw, especially mandibular fracture

REFERENCES

1. NIH Consensus Conference. Acupuncture. *JAMA*. 1998;280:1518–24.
2. Alan S. Marathon Man lessons for dental pain. *Emerg Med News*. 2005;27(9):20–21.
3. Flores MT, Andersson L, Andreasen JO, et al. Guidelines for the management of traumatic dental injuries. II. Avulsion of permanent teeth. *Dent Traumatol*. 2007;23:130–6.

ADDITIONAL READING

- Andreasen JO, Lauridsen E, Christensen SS. Development of an interactive dental trauma guide. *Pediatr Dent*. 2009;31:133–6.
- Celenk S, Sezgin B, Ayna B, et al. Causes of dental fractures in the early permanent dentition: a retrospective study. *J Endod*. 2002;28:208–10.
- Evidence-based review of clinical studies on trauma. *J Endod*. 2009;35:1160–2.
- Flores MT, Andersson L, Andreasen JO, et al. Guidelines for the management of traumatic dental injuries. I. Fractures and luxations of permanent teeth. *Dent Traumatol*. 2007;23:66–71.
- Flores MT, Andreasen JO, Bakland LK, et al. Guidelines for the evaluation and management of traumatic dental injuries. *Dent Traumatol*. 2001;17:193–8.
- Ong CKS, et al. An evidence-based update of the use of analgesics in dentistry. *Periodontology*. 2008;46(1):143–164.
- Vellappally S, Fiala Z, Smejkalová J, et al. Smoking related systemic and oral diseases. *Acta Medica (Hradec Kralove)*. 2007;50:161–6.
- Wilson S, et al. Epidemiology of dental trauma treated in an urban pediatric emergency department. *Pediatr Emerg Care*. l997;13:12–15.

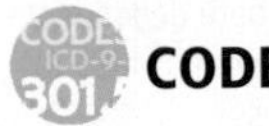

CODES

ICD9

- 802.20 Closed fracture of unspecified site of mandible
- 873.63 Open wound of internal structures of mouth, tooth (broken) (fractured) (due to trauma), uncomplicated
- 873.73 Open wound of internal structures of mouth, tooth (broken) (fractured) (due to trauma), complicated

CLINICAL PEARLS

- Do not reimplant primary teeth. Reimplant permanent teeth ASAP.
- Milk is the best transportation medium before coming to emergency room (ER), as it maintains the periodontal ligament for about 3 hours and has protective pH and osmolarity. Saline or saliva is a good substitute. Water is the least desirable transport medium because it is a hypotonic solution.
- Consider child abuse in younger patients.
- Young children are more likely to get infection after Ellis fractures; consider antibiotic coverage.
- Ensure tetanus vaccination is updated.

DEPENDENT PERSONALITY DISORDER

Heath A. Grames, PhD
W. Jeff Hinton, PhD

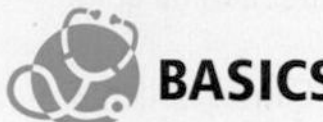

BASICS

DESCRIPTION

Beginning no later than adolescence or early adulthood, a consistent and pervasive pattern of dependency on others to make even the most trivial decisions, feelings of incompetence, and an excessive need for care by others (1):

- Common behaviors and variations:
  - Can be very clingy to caregivers
  - May isolate contact they have with other people to interactions with caregivers
  - May be very agreeable or submissive with others (even when they don't agree) out of fear of losing support/approval
  - May experience large amounts of distress when faced with decisions
  - May experience fear when alone
  - Lack of independence/fear of independence
  - Above behaviors are in excess of cultural norms
- Patients with this disorder typically display little insight into their behavior.

Geriatric Considerations

Illness (acute and chronic) may exacerbate dependent personality disorder (DPD) behaviors and may lead to intense feelings of fear and helplessness.

Pediatric Considerations

Diagnosis is rarely made for children/adolescents (may not be appropriate due to dependency needs of children/adolescents). Axis I disorders must be ruled out, as well as behavior related to a general medical condition or to the developmental cycle of the child. For diagnosis, baseline behaviors must be representative of DPD for a duration of at least 1 year.

Pregnancy Considerations

Physical and social changes may induce stress or increase fears, which may result in increased dependent behaviors. Distinguish this disorder from increased dependency due to pregnancy (i.e., when there is no, or poor, support system).

EPIDEMIOLOGY

- Predominant age: Onset no later than adolescence or early adulthood (may go undiagnosed for years)
- Predominant sex: Female > Male

Prevalence

- DPD accounts for 20–30% of all personality disorders in primary care outpatient settings (2).
- DPD is among the most common personality disorder in mental health clinics.

RISK FACTORS

- Chronic or severe illness or disability in children
- Childhood/adolescent separation anxiety
- Parenting style that does not encourage age-appropriate independence

GENERAL PREVENTION

Children with chronic illness or handicap may be more susceptible to DPD. When possible, foster appropriate independence in the face of disability.

ETIOLOGY

Undetermined; however, generally accepted that it is due to a combination of the following:

- Hereditary temperamental traits
- Environment (e.g., not allowed independence; age-appropriate)
- Developmental traits

COMMONLY ASSOCIATED CONDITIONS

- Co-occurring personality disorders: Frequent
- Increased risk with mood anxiety and adjustment disorders

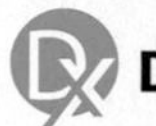

DIAGNOSIS

Due to high co-occurrence with other Axis II disorders, assess suicide ideation and self-harm behavior.

HISTORY

- Difficulty making decisions (even trivial decisions) without a great deal of reassurance and coaxing (1)
- Dramatic/urgent demands for medical attention (even when symptoms are not painful or life-threatening)
- May actively attempt to prolong illness or seek unnecessary medical procedures (3)
- Perception that he or she needs to be taken care of
- Clingy/demanding
- Seeks primary care provider and other caregivers to make decisions
- Once physician is in role of caregiver, may become submissive, agreeable (fear of losing relationship)
- Important to obtain collateral information (i.e., from family, partner) about patient behaviors
- Ask about substance abuse.

DIAGNOSTIC TESTS & INTERPRETATION

- Consider age of onset. To meet criteria for DPD, dependent pattern will be present from early adulthood.
- If symptoms begin later than early adulthood or are related to trauma (e.g., after a head injury), a general medical condition (GMC), or substance, consider other diagnoses.
- Rule out personality change due to a GMC:
  - Traits may emerge due to the effect of a GMC on the central nervous system (1).
- Rule out symptoms related to chronic substance abuse.
- Consider referring patient for formal psychological testing.
- Diagnostic accuracy may be improved through the utilization of the Structured Clinical Interview for DSM-IV Axis II Disorders (SCID-II) (4).

Diagnostic Procedures/Surgery

Must meet at least 5 of the following criteria for diagnosis (1):

- Indecisive: Needs support/reassurance from others to make decisions
- Defers personal responsibility (decision making, life choices) to others
- Does not voice disagreement with others without difficulty out of fear of losing relationship
- Not including realistic fears of abuse/retribution
- Difficulty starting/doing projects independently
- Seeks nurturance/support from others, even at great personal costs
- Experiences discomfort with solitude; fears having to care for self

DIFFERENTIAL DIAGNOSIS

Other psychiatric conditions, such as:

- Mood disorders:
  - Consider baseline behaviors when considering DPD vs mood disorder.
- Anxiety disorders:
  - With DPD, chronic baseline behaviors will suggest personality disorder (does not only occur at moments of stress or with Axis I disorders).

Adjustment disorder:
- Differentiate in that dependence from stressor is not chronic and is related to stressor

Other personality disorder:
- Consider patient's thoughts, feelings, and behavior to differentiate dependence from other personality disorders.
- High co-occurrence of DPD and other personality disorders, especially borderline, histrionic, and avoidant

General medical condition:
- Traits may emerge due to the effect of a GMC on the central nervous system.

Chronic substance abuse

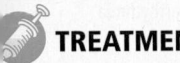

TREATMENT

Inpatient hospitalization is relatively ineffective in changing Axis II disorder behaviors.

Inpatient hospital services for conditions related to dependent personality disorder should be limited and of short duration to decrease dependence (decreasing likelihood of behavior change).

Hospitalization should be considered for the following:
- Adjust medications.
- Implement psychotherapy for crisis intervention.
- Stabilize patient (psychosocial stressors).

If suicidal, may need suicide watch and receive appropriate psychiatric care.

MEDICATION

No medications treat DPD.

Treat symptoms and Axis I disorders (2)[C].

Depression/anxiety (2)[C]:
- Serotonin reuptake inhibitors
- Benzodiazepines (short-term) if needed for anxiety symptom relief

ADDITIONAL TREATMENT

General Measures

Focus on patient management rather than fixing or curing behaviors (2)[C].

Schedule follow-up to relieve patient stress.

Meet with and rely on treatment team to avoid burnout and to provide opportunity for team to discuss issues with patient.

As necessary, refer patient to mental health therapist.

Issues for Referral

Treatment for Axis II disorder should include psychotherapy and/or psychiatry.

Additional Therapies

- Consider referring patient for specialty mental health services.
- Cognitive behavioral therapy has demonstrated some success with Axis II disorders in general.

IN-PATIENT CONSIDERATIONS

Admission Criteria

Refer to inpatient or outpatient psychiatry services if harm to self or others is expressed by the patient and/or suspected by the primary care provider.

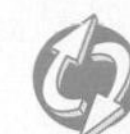

ONGOING CARE

FOLLOW-UP RECOMMENDATIONS

- Schedule routine follow-up with patient (relieves patient anxiety about medical care relationship with physician).
- Nurses can be helpful in managing the patient and calling the patient as needed (contact with the patient helps relieve patient stress).
- Focus should be on medical conditions and comorbid Axis I disorders.

PROGNOSIS

- Medical focus is on patient management and caring for medical and Axis I disorders (3).
- With appropriate treatment, including mental health services, patient is viewed as treatment-responsive (5).

REFERENCES

1. American Psychiatric Association. *Diagnostic and Statistical Manual of Mental Disorders*. 4th ed., text revision. Washington, DC: American Psychiatric Association; 2000.
2. Ward RK. Assessment and management of personality disorders. *Am Fam Physician*. 2004;70:1505–12.
3. Feder A, Robbins SW, Ostermeyer B. Personality disorders. In: Feldman, Christensen JF, eds. *Behavioral Medicine in Primary Care: A Practical Guide*. 2nd ed. New York: McGraw-Hill, 2003;231–52.
4. First MB, Gibbon M, Spitzer RL, Williams JBW, Benjamin LS. *Structured clinical interview for DSM-IV Axis II personality disorders, (SCID-II)*. Washington, DC: American Psychiatric Press, Inc., 1997.
5. Eskedal GA, Demetri JM. Etiology and treatment of cluster C personality disorders. *J Mental Health Counsel*. 2006;28:1–17.

CODES

ICD9

301.6 Dependent personality disorder

CLINICAL PEARLS

- To determine whether a patient has a DPD vs dependent behavior from an Axis I or substance-related disorder or from a general medical condition, note that personality disorders are chronic, so look at baseline behavior. Patients with DPD must have developed the personality disorder traits during adolescence or early adulthood rather than after a medical or Axis I change.
- In the outpatient setting, frequent, short visits help patients with DPD to calm their fears of losing support and help providers with time management. When possible, always have an appointment scheduled so patients can look forward to their next visit.
- To feel less overwhelmed when you are seeing a DPD patient, have an agenda ready for the visit. Be cordial—they deserve the same professionalism any patient gets. Address 1–2 issues per clinic visit.
- Many patients will benefit from additional psychotherapy treatments that target thoughts and behaviors associated with clients' underlying dependency needs.

DEPRESSION

Deborah S. Clements, MD

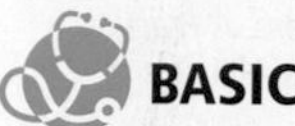

BASICS

DESCRIPTION

Depression is a primary mood disorder characterized by a depressed mood and/or decreased interest in things that used to give pleasure (anhedonia) during the same 2-week period, and representing a change from previous functioning:

- Synonym(s): Unipolar affective disorder
- System(s) affected: Nervous

EPIDEMIOLOGY

Incidence

Affects >78 million in the US

Prevalence

- 15% lifetime risk of having major depressive disorder (MDD)
- 4th most common reason to visit a physician

RISK FACTORS

- Female > Male (2:1)
- Predominant age: 1st onset usually in late 20s (earlier in women than men)
- Elderly (≥65)
- History of behavioral disorders
- Presence of chronic disease(s)
- Recent myocardial infarction/stroke
- Peptic ulcer disease
- Strong family history (depression, bipolar, suicide, alcoholism, other substance abuse)
- Domestic abuse or violence
- Substance abuse and dependence
- Losses and stressors
- Single, divorced, or unhappily married

Genetics

Multiple gene loci place a person at increased risk when faced with environmental stressors.

PATHOPHYSIOLOGY

- Changes in receptor–neurotransmitter relationship in the limbic system:
  - Serotonin and norepinephrine are the primary neurotransmitters involved; dopamine, acetylcholine, and γ-aminobutyric acid have also been involved.
- As action potential is passed on, the neurotransmitter is:
  - Reabsorbed into the neuron, where it is either destroyed by an enzyme or actively removed by a reuptake pump and stored until needed or
  - Destroyed by monoamine oxidase in the mitochondria
- Symptoms related to decreased levels of norepinephrine (dullness and lethargy) and serotonin (irritability, hostility, and suicidal ideation)

ETIOLOGY

- Impaired synthesis of neurotransmitters
- Increased metabolism of neurotransmitters
- Environmental factors and learned behavior may affect neurotransmitters and/or have an independent influence on depression.

COMMONLY ASSOCIATED CONDITIONS

- Manic depression (bipolar disorder)
- Cyclothymic and grief reactions
- Anxiety disorders
- Schizophrenia/schizoaffective disorders
- Psychophysiologic disorders
- Physical disorders
- Substance abuse

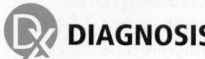

DIAGNOSIS

HISTORY

- Depressed mood most of the day, nearly every day
- Anhedonia
- Depression is probable when at least 4 of the following exist in addition to depressed mood or anhedonia:
  - Appetite: Significant weight gain or loss when not dieting (change of >5% of body weight in 1 month)
  - Sleep disturbance: Insomnia or hypersomnia nearly every day
  - Fatigue: Out of proportion to the amount of energy expended
  - Psychomotor retardation or agitation: Restlessness, irritability, or withdrawal
  - Poor self-image: Worthlessness, excessive or inappropriate guilt
  - Concentration: Diminished thinking or concentration, poor memory, indecisiveness
  - Suicidal ideation: Recurrent thoughts of death; sometimes, as patients begin to recover, they gain enough energy to think about and sometimes attempt suicide.

Geriatric Considerations

- Can present with pseudodementia
- More common in elderly and difficult to precisely diagnose due to medical comorbidities (highest rates of depression are associated with stroke, coronary artery disease, cancer, Parkinson disease, and Alzheimer disease)

Pediatric Considerations

Depression occurs in children and can present with somatic complaints, irritability (versus depressed mood), and social withdrawal.

PHYSICAL EXAM

Vital signs and complete physical exam with special attention paid to:

- Thyroid
- Cardiac exam, listening for arrhythmias
- Mental status, including affect

DIAGNOSTIC TESTS & INTERPRETATION

Lab

Initial lab tests

Labs may not be necessary, but are sometimes used to rule out other diagnoses:

- Thyroid-stimulating hormone
- Complete blood count
- Chem 7, including blood sugar
- Calcium
- Liver function tests

Follow-Up & Special Considerations

Electrocardiogram to rule out arrhythmia

Imaging

Initial approach

Electroencephalogram, computed tomography, or magnetic resonance imaging of brain to rule out organic brain disease if suspected

Diagnostic Procedures/Surgery

- Depression is primarily a clinical diagnosis made by eliciting personal, family, social, and psychosocial factors.
- Validated standard rating scales can assist:
  - Clinical Global Impressions Scale
  - Montgomery-Asberg Depression Rating Scale
  - Hamilton Rating Scale for Depression
  - Beck Depression Inventory

DIFFERENTIAL DIAGNOSIS

- Dysthymic disorder
- Bipolar disorder
- Organic brain diseases
- Endocrine/thyroid disorders, diabetes
- Metabolic abnormalities (hypercalcemia)
- Adrenal disease (Cushing)
- Liver/renal failure
- Malignancy
- Chronic fatigue syndrome
- Lupus
- Nutritional: Pernicious anemia, pellagra
- Medications: Abuse, side effects, overdose
- Substances: Abuse, dependence, withdrawal

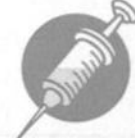

TREATMENT

MEDICATION

First Line

- Selective serotonin reuptake inhibitors (SSRIs):
  - Fluoxetine (Prozac): 20–80 mg/d
  - Sertraline (Zoloft): 50–200 mg/d
  - Paroxetine (Paxil): 10–50 mg/d
  - Paroxetine CR (Paxil CR): 12.5–62.5 mg/d
  - Citalopram (Celexa): 20–60 mg/d
  - Escitalopram (Lexapro): 10–20 mg/d
- Others:
  - Venlafaxine (Effexor): 75–375 mg/d (divided doses)
  - Venlafaxine XR(Effexor XR): 75–225 mg/d
  - Bupropion (Wellbutrin): 100–450 mg/d (divided doses, t.i.d.)
  - Bupropion SR (Wellbutrin SR): 100–450 mg/d (divided doses, b.i.d.)
  - Bupropion XL (Wellbutrin XL): 150–300 mg/d
  - Duloxetine (Cymbalta): 30–60 mg/d

ˈecond Line

Tricyclic antidepressants (TCAs) with sedating properties *condensed list*:
- Amitriptyline (Elavil): 50–150 mg/QHS, max 300
- Nortriptyline (Pamelor): 75–150 mg QHS
- Doxepin (Prudoxin, Zonalon): 75–150 mg QHS

TCAs with activating properties *condensed list*:
- Imipramine (Tofranil, Tofranil-PM): 150–200 mg QHS
- Desipramine (Norpramin): 150–300 mg/d

α_2-antagonists (sedating):
- Mirtazapine (Remeron): 15–45 mg QHS

SSRI/antagonists:
- Trazodone: 150 mg/d (divided doses), maximum 600 mg/d (divided doses)

Precautions:
- Bupropion: Increased risk of seizures
- TCAs: Advanced age, glaucoma, benign prostate hypertrophy, hyperthyroidism, cardiovascular disease, liver disease, urinary retention, MAOI treatment, potential for fatal overdose
- SSRIs: Abrupt discontinuation may result in withdrawal symptoms (i.e., dizziness), may raise serum levels of other drugs

Significant potential interactions:
- TCAs: Amphetamines, barbiturates, clonidine, epinephrine, ethanol, norepinephrine, MAOIs: Allow 14-day washout period before starting MAOIs, propoxyphene
- SSRIs and MAOIs: 14-day washout before instituting therapy
- Venlafaxine may cause fatal serotonin syndrome
- MAOIs: Significant drug and food interactions limit use, but can be useful in refractory cases.

ALERT

Black-box warning: Increased risk of suicidality in children, adolescents, and young adults up to age 25 treated with SSRI antidepressant medications. Although this has not been extended to adults, suicide risk assessments are warranted for all patients.

ˈeriatric Considerations

ˈeduce dosage of medications (1/2 usual starting ˈose); may need to treat longer than younger adults.

ˈediatric Considerations

ˈeduce dosage of medications in adolescents; also see ˈlert.

ˈregnancy Considerations

ˈSRIs: If possible, taper and discontinue. (Paroxetine is ˈategory D; the rest of SSRIs are Category C.)

ˈADDITIONAL TREATMENT

ˈeneral Measures

ˈsychotherapeutic interventions act synergistically ˈvith pharmacologic therapy.

ˈAdditional Therapies

ˈlectroconvulsive therapy for refractory cases

ˈCOMPLEMENTARY AND ALTERNATIVE ˈMEDICINE

ˈJse in mild depression; evidence is inconsistent:

Hypericum perforatum (St. John's wort) (1)[A]: Be aware of multiple drug interactions.

SAM-e (S-adenosyl methionine): 400–1,600 mg/d (2)[A]

IN-PATIENT CONSIDERATIONS

Admission Criteria

Inpatient care is indicated for severely depressed, psychotic, or suicidal patients.

Discharge Criteria

Depressive symptoms improving, no longer suicidal

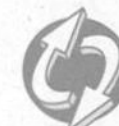

ONGOING CARE

FOLLOW-UP RECOMMENDATIONS

Patient Monitoring

- See within 2 weeks after starting medication.
- During follow-up, evaluate the side effects, dosage, and effectiveness of the medication.
- Follow up every 2 weeks until improvement.
- Follow up every 3 months thereafter.
- Explain treatment must continue for at least 6 months to 2 years; longer with family history, severe depression, and in the very young.

PATIENT EDUCATION

- Depression is a medical illness, not a character defect.
- Stress need for long-term treatment and follow-up, which includes lifestyle changes.
- 30 minutes of moderate-intensity exercise, 3–5 days per week for healthy adults (3)[A]

PROGNOSIS

- 70% significant improvement
- It has been shown that of patients with a single depressive episode, 50% develop a recurrent episode.

COMPLICATIONS

- Suicide
- Lower quality-of-life

REFERENCES

1. Keller MB. Issues in treatment-resistant depression. *J Clin Psychiatry*. 2005;66(Suppl 8):5–12.
2. Institute for Clinical Systems Improvement. *Major Depression in Adults in Primary Care*. Bloomington, MN: Institute for Clinical Systems Improvement; 2006.
3. American Psychiatric Association. *Diagnostic and Statistical Manual of Mental Disorders DSM-IV-TR*. 4th ed. [text revision]. Washington, DC: American Psychiatric Publishing, 2000.

ADDITIONAL READING

- Adams SM, Miller KE, Zylstra RG. Pharmacologic management of adult depression. *Am Fam Physician*. 2008;77:785–92.
- Fochtmann LJ, et al. *Guideline Watch: Practice Guideline for the Treatment of Patients with Major Depressive Disorder*, 2nd ed. Accessed June 1, 2008 at: http://www.psych.org/psych_pract/treatg/pg/prac_guide.cfm.
- Halfin A. Depression: the benefits of early and appropriate treatment. *Am J Manag Care*. 2007;13:S92–7.
- Kessler RC, Berglund P, Demler O, et al. The epidemiology of major depressive disorder: results from the National Comorbidity Survey Replication (NCS-R). *JAMA*. 2003;289:3095–105.
- Kocsis JH, et al. Prevention of recurrent episodes of depression with venlafaxine ER in a 1-year maintenance phase from the PREVENT Study. *J Clin Psychiatry*. 2007;68:1012–23.
- Kornstein SG, Bose A, Li D, et al. Escitalopram maintenance treatment for prevention of recurrent depression: a randomized, placebo-controlled trial. *J Clin Psychiatry*. 2006;67:1767–75.
- Maurer D, Colt R. An evidence-based approach to the management of depression. *Prim Care*. 2006;33:923–41.
- Roose SP, Sackeim HA, Krishnan KR, et al. Antidepressant pharmacotherapy in the treatment of depression in the very old: a randomized, placebo-controlled trial. *Am J Psychiatry*. 2004;161:2050–9.
- Skultety KM, Rodriguez RL. Treating geriatric depression in primary care. *Curr Psychiatry Rep*. 2008;10:44–50.
- Thase ME. Treatment of severe depression. *J Clin Psychiatry*. 2000;61(Suppl 1):17–25.

See Also (Topic, Algorithm, Electronic Media Element)

Algorithms: Depressive Episode, Major; Depressed Mood Resulting from Medical Illness

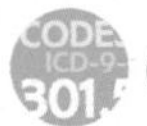

CODES

ICD9

- 296.20 Major depressive affective disorder, single episode, unspecified degree
- 296.30 Major depressive affective disorder, recurrent episode, unspecified degree
- 311 Depressive disorder, not elsewhere classified

CLINICAL PEARLS

- The relationship (therapeutic alliance) between the patient and health care provider is important to the success of treatment.
- Depression management has 2 main goals:
  - Remission: Absence of depressive symptoms with return to full functioning
  - Recovery: No longer meets MDD criteria for at least 8 weeks
- Given the high recurrence rates, long-term treatment is often necessary.

DEPRESSION, ADOLESCENT

Alyssa H. Tran, DO

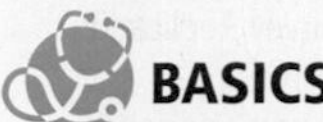

BASICS

DESCRIPTION

- Primary mood disorder characterized by sadness or irritability and a loss of self-worth and interest in typically pleasurable activities
- Depression in adolescents is undertreated, as an estimated 70–80% of these patients do not receive appropriate care.
- Dysthymic disorder is differentiated from major depression by less intense symptoms that are more persistent, lasting at least 1 year.
- Depressive disorder NOS is diagnosed when an adolescent presents with depressive symptoms but does not meet the criteria for other diagnoses.
- Treatment-resistant depression is a failure of treatment with 2 antidepressants administered in adequate dosage for at least 6 weeks.
- Depression is more likely to present as irritability or somatic complaints in adolescents (vs acutely depressed mood in adults). Adolescents may present with symptoms primarily when alone or with family, often "fine with friends." Symptoms may include declining grades, change in friends, or experimentation with drugs.

EPIDEMIOLOGY

Incidence

15–20% during adolescence

Prevalence

0.4–8.3% of adolescents. At least twice as common in females.

RISK FACTORS

- Female gender
- Prior depressive episodes
- History of anxiety disorders, ADHD, and/or learning disabilities
- Chronic illness
- Hormonal changes during puberty
- Use of certain medications (e.g., isotretinoin [Accutane]) (1)
- Family history: Risk is increased 3–6 times if 1st-degree relative has a major affective disorder.
- General stressors, such as socioeconomic deprivations, adverse life events/experiences, difficulties with peers, loss of a loved one, academic difficulties
- Childhood neglect or abuse
- Cigarette smoking
- Presence of specific serotonin-transporter gene variants (2)

Genetics

Studies have shown a 76% concordance rate in monozygotic twins reared together and a 67% concordance rate among those reared apart, along with a 19% concordance rate in dizygotic twins reared together.

GENERAL PREVENTION

Insufficient evidence supports the universal implementation of depression prevention programs (psychological and social) (3)[B]. May be a small benefit to regular exercise in preventing episodes of depression (4)[B]

PATHOPHYSIOLOGY

Still fairly unclear, but low functional levels of neurotransmitters may produce symptoms. Decreased norepinephrine may cause dullness and lethargy. Decreased serotonin may cause irritability, hostility, and suicidal ideation.

ETIOLOGY

External factors may affect neurotransmitters or independently affect depression

COMMONLY ASSOCIATED CONDITIONS

- Eating disorders (especially bulimia)
- Substance abuse
- Anxiety disorders
- Behavioral disorders (i.e., ADHD, oppositional defiant disorder, conduct disorder)
- Learning disorders
- Somatization disorders
- Depression in the adolescent population typically emerges after the comorbid disorder (except for substance abuse and conduct disorders).

DIAGNOSIS

HISTORY

- According to the DSM-IV, adolescents must display EITHER (3) depressed or irritable mood OR (4) loss of interest or pleasure (anhedonia) for most of the day, nearly every day, for at least 2 weeks, causing significant distress or functional impairment.
- In addition, 4 or more of the following symptoms must be present during the same 2-week period:
  - Change in appetite with weight loss or gain (change of >5% of body weight in 1 month)
  - Insomnia or hypersomnia nearly every day
  - Psychomotor agitation or retardation:
    - Adolescents will commonly talk or move more slowly and produce less speech with longer response latencies, and may display a flat affect.
    - Conversely, they may present with restlessness, excessive movements, and verbal outbursts.
  - Fatigue or loss of energy
  - Feelings of excessive guilt or worthlessness: Adolescents may be extremely self-critical, unable to identify positive self-attributes, or feel they deserve to be punished for things that are not their fault.
  - Indecisiveness or impaired thinking or concentration: School performance may decline significantly.
  - Recurring thoughts of death or suicide or actual attempts at suicide
- Symptoms must not: Meet the criteria for a mixed manic episode (suggestive of bipolar disorder); be due to the effects of a drug or other condition; be secondary to bereavement

PHYSICAL EXAM

Psychomotor retardation or agitation may be present.

ALERT

Clinicians should carefully assess patients for signs of self-injury (wrist lacerations) or abuse.

DIAGNOSTIC TESTS & INTERPRETATION

Lab

Initial lab tests

May be used to rule out other diagnoses (i.e., CBC, TSH, glucose, mono spot)

Imaging

Initial approach

CT or MRI of brain only if brain disease is suspected

Diagnostic Procedures/Surgery

- Depression is primarily diagnosed after conducting formal clinical interview with the adolescent, combined with supporting information obtained from caregivers and teachers.
- The following standardized tests can be useful as screening tools and to monitor response to treatment, but should not be used as the sole basis for diagnosis:
  - Beck Depression Inventory (BDI): All ages
  - Child Depression Inventory (CDI): Ages 7–17
  - Reynolds Adolescent Depression Scale (RADS): Teenagers in grades 7–12
  - Guidelines for Adolescent Preventive Services (GAPS): To be delivered to parents, younger and older adolescents during their 11–17-year-old annual health visits
- Suicide risk assessment should be performed.
- Office-based screening/case finding questionnaires have minimal impact on the detection, management or outcome of depression by clinicians (5)[A].

DIFFERENTIAL DIAGNOSIS

- Normal bereavement
- Substance-induced mood disorder
- Bipolar disorder
- Mood disorder secondary to a medical condition
- Endocrine diseases (hypo- or hyperthyroidism)
- Organic CNS diseases
- Malignancy
- Infectious mononucleosis
- Anemia
- Medication side effects (isotretinoin)
- Chronic diseases (diabetes)

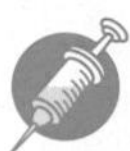

TREATMENT

Pediatric depression is often managed by primary care providers rather than psychiatrists (6).

MEDICATION

First Line

- Fluoxetine (Prozac): Starting dose 10 mg/day. Effective dose 20–60 mg/day: Fluoxetine is the only SSRI approved by the FDA for the treatment of depression in adolescence (7)[B].
- Careful monitoring of the patient for suicidal thoughts and behavior is required, given the possible increased risk while taking any antidepressant. However, completed suicide rates are higher in areas where SSRIs are not prescribed to adolescents (7)[C].

Second Line

- The following SSRIs are NOT approved by the FDA for treatment of adolescent depression, but may be tried as 2nd-line agents at the clinician's discretion (7)[B]:
  - Citalopram (Celexa): Starting dose 10 mg/day. Effective dose 20–60 mg/day.
  - Escitalopram (Lexapro): Starting dose 5 mg/day. Effective dose 10–20 mg/day.

- Fluvoxamine (Luvox): Starting dose 50 mg/day. Effective dose 150–300 mg/day.
- Paroxetine (Paxil) : Starting dose 10 mg/day. Effective dose 20–60 mg/day.
- Sertraline (Zoloft): Starting dose 25 mg/day. Effective dose 50–200 mg/day.

Venlafaxine (Effexor), nefazodone, mirtazapine, and bupropion may be tried in adolescents who have failed SSRIs, but no evidence supports the use of these atypical antidepressants in this population.

Tricyclic antidepressants have not been proven to be effective in adolescents and should NOT be used (7,8)[A].

ADDITIONAL TREATMENT

General Measures

Cognitive behavioral therapy (CBT) is effective in the treatment of mild-to-moderate adolescent depression (7)[A]:
- Goal is to alter a patient's negative thoughts and behaviors to improve his or her mood by encouraging pleasurable activities (behavioral activation), reducing negative thoughts (cognitive restructuring), and improving assertiveness and problem-solving skills to reduce feelings of hopelessness.
- Interpersonal psychotherapy (IPT) and family therapy may also be helpful: Treatment targets a patient's interpersonal problems to improve both interpersonal functioning and his or her mood.

Regular exercise may help reduce depressive symptoms (4)[B].

Issues for Referral

Referral to a child psychiatrist is recommended for adolescents with severe, recurrent, or treatment-resistant depression. Referrals are also recommended if the patient has comorbidities or if the clinician is uncomfortable prescribing complex therapies.

COMPLEMENTARY AND ALTERNATIVE MEDICINE

No evidence supports the use of St. John's wort or acupuncture.

IN-PATIENT CONSIDERATIONS

Admission Criteria

Indicated if an adolescent is severely depressed, psychotic, suicidal, or homicidal

Nursing

Patient may need one-on-one supervision or routine checks for safety if suicidal ideation is present.

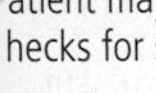

ONGOING CARE

Treatment for at least 6 months reduced the likelihood of suicide attempts compared with treatment for less than 8 weeks (9).

FOLLOW-UP RECOMMENDATIONS

Systematic and regular tracking of goals and outcomes from treatment should be performed, including assessment of depressive symptoms and functioning in home, school, and peer settings (9).

Recommendations from National Guideline Clearinghouse: Treatment (9):
- After initial diagnosis of mild depression, clinicians should consider a period of active support and monitoring before starting other evidence-based treatment.
- If a primary care provider (PCP) identifies an adolescent with moderate or severe depression or complicating factors/conditions such as coexisting substance abuse or psychosis, consultation with a mental health specialist should be considered. Appropriate roles and responsibilities for ongoing management by the PCP and mental health clinicians should be communicated and agreed upon. The patient and family should be consulted and approve the roles of the PC and mental health professionals.
- PCPs should recommend scientifically tested and proven treatments (i.e., psychotherapies such as cognitive behavioral therapy [CBT] or interpersonal therapy [IPT] and/or antidepressant treatment such as selective serotonin reuptake inhibitors [SSRIs]) whenever possible and appropriate to achieve the goals of the treatment plan.
- PCPs should monitor for the emergence of adverse events during antidepressant treatment.

- Recommendations from National Guideline Clearinghouse: Outgoing management (9):
  - Systematic and regular tracking of goals and outcomes from treatment should be performed, including assessment of depressive symptoms and functioning in several key domains: home, school, and peer settings.
  - Diagnosis and initial treatment should be reassessed if no improvement is noted after 6–8 weeks of treatment. Mental health consultation should be considered.
  - For patients who achieve only partial improvement after diagnostic and therapeutic approaches have been exhausted (including exploration of poor adherence, comorbid disorders, and ongoing conflicts or abuse), a mental health consultation should be considered.
  - PCPs should actively support depressed adolescents who are referred to mental health to ensure adequate management. PCPs may also consider sharing care with mental health agencies/professionals when possible. Appropriate roles and responsibilities regarding the provision and coordination of care should be communicated and agreed upon by the PCP and the mental health specialist.

Patient Monitoring

- Once started on antidepressants, patients should be seen weekly for the 1st month, biweekly for the 2nd month, and at least monthly thereafter: Careful monitoring for suicidal thoughts or behavior is required, particularly in the 1st 2 months after initiation or dose increase.
- Length of medication treatment:
  - First episode: Minimum 6 months followed by a slow taper over 6–8 weeks
  - Second episode: At least 1 year
  - Third episode: 1–3 years
  - >3 episodes: Lifelong
- Adverse effects (i.e., nausea, headaches, behavioral activation, etc.) occur in up to 93% of patients treated with SSRIs. Therefore, routine monitoring and discussion of possible medication side effects is critical for depressed youth who are treated with antidepressants.

PATIENT EDUCATION

Educate patients and parents about mental health and the fact that depression is a medical illness, not a character defect.

PROGNOSIS

- If left untreated, major depressive episode in adolescents typically lasts 7–9 months, with 90% resolving within 2 years.
- CBT alone is effective treatment in 40–50%.
- Combination therapy of CBT with fluoxetine results in improvement in 71% of patients.
- Recurrence is 40% by 2 years and 70% by 5 years.

COMPLICATIONS

- Lack of improvement in symptoms
- School failure or refusal
- Suicide

D

REFERENCES

1. Wysowski DK, Pitts M, Beitz J. An analysis of reports of depression and suicide in patients treated with isotretinoin. *J Am Acad Dermatol*. 2001;45:515–9.
2. Hariri AR, Mattay VS, Tessitore A, Kolachana B, Fera F, Goldman D, et al. Serotonin transporter genetic variation and the response of the human amygdala. *Science*. 2002;297:400–3.
3. Merry S, et al. Psychological and/or educational interventions for the prevention of depression in children and adolescents. Cochrane Depression, Anxiety and Neurosis Group. *Cochrane Database Syst Rev*. 2007:4.
4. Larun L, et al. Exercise in prevention and treatment of anxiety and depression among children and young people. Cochrane Depression, Anxiety and Neurosis Group. *Cochrane Database Syst Rev*. 2007:4.
5. Gilbody S, et al. Screening and case finding instruments for depression. Cochrane Depression, Anxiety and Neurosis Group. *Cochrane Database Syst Rev*. 2007:4.
6. Cheung AH, Dewa CS, Levitt AJ, et al. Pediatric depressive disorders: management priorities in primary care. *Curr Opin Pediatr*. 2008;20:551–9.
7. Bhatia SK, Bhatia SC. Childhood and adolescent depression. *Am Fam Physician*. 2007;75:73–80.
8. Hazell P, et al. Tricyclic drugs for depression in children and adolescents. Cochrane Depression, Anxiety and Neurosis Group. *Cochrane Database Syst Rev*. 2007:4.
9. Cheung AH, Zuckerbrot RA, Jensen PS, et al. Guidelines for Adolescent Depression in Primary Care (GLAD-PC): II. Treatment and ongoing management. *Pediatrics*. 2007;120:e1313–26.

CODES

ICD9

- 296.20 Major depressive affective disorder, single episode, unspecified degree
- 296.30 Major depressive affective disorder, recurrent episode, unspecified degree
- 311 Depressive disorder, not elsewhere classified

CLINICAL PEARLS

- Adolescent depression is underdiagnosed and often presents with irritability and anhedonia.
- CBT combined with fluoxetine is most efficacious for adolescents with major depression.
- Referral to a child psychiatrist is appropriate for complex cases.

DEPRESSION, GERIATRIC

Anna Mirk, MD
Frederick Wu, MD

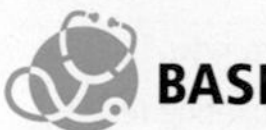

BASICS

DESCRIPTION

Depression is a primary mood disorder characterized by a depressed mood and/or a markedly decreased interest or pleasure in normally enjoyable activities for at least 2 weeks and causing significant distress or impairment in daily functioning.

EPIDEMIOLOGY

Prevalence rates among the elderly vary, largely depending on the specific diagnostic instruments used and their current health and/or home environment:

- 1–3% of community-dwelling elderly
- 7.5% seen in primary care clinics
- 10–21% of hospitalized elderly patients
- 12–27% of nursing home residents

RISK FACTORS

- General:
  - Chronic physical health condition(s)
  - History of mental health problems
  - Death of a loved one
  - Caregiving
  - Social isolation
  - Lack or loss of social support
  - Significant loss of independence
  - Uncontrolled pain
  - Insomnia/sleep disturbance
- Prevalence of depression in medical illness:
  - Stroke (22–50%)
  - Cancer (18–50%)
  - Myocardial infarction (15–45%)
  - Parkinson disease (10–39%)
  - Rheumatoid arthritis (13%)
  - Diabetes mellitus (5–11%)
  - Alzheimer's dementia (5-15%)
- Suicide:
  - Suicide is the 11th leading cause of death in the US for all ages.
  - Suicide rates are higher for Americans age >65 compared to the general population (approximately 15 per 100,000 people).
  - Suicide rates are highest for males aged >75 (rate 38.5 per 100,000).

PATHOPHYSIOLOGY

- There are still significant gaps in the understanding of the underlying pathophyisiology.
- Ongoing research has identified several possible mechanisms, including:
  - Monoamine transmission and associated transcriptional and translational activity
  - Epigenetic mechanisms and resilience factors
  - Neurotrophins, neurogenesis, neuroimmune systems, and neuroendocrine systems

ETIOLOGY

Depression appears to be a complex interaction between heritable and environmental factors.

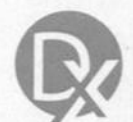

DIAGNOSIS

HISTORY

- Depressed mood most of the day, nearly every day, and/or loss of interest or pleasure in life
- Other common symptoms include:
  - Feeling hopeless, helpless, or worthless
  - Insomnia and loss of appetite/weight (alternatively, hypersomnia with increased appetite/weight in atypical depression)
  - Fatigue and loss of energy
  - Somatic symptoms (headaches, chronic pain)
  - Neglect of personal responsibility or care
  - Psychomotor retardation or agitation
  - Diminished concentration, indecisiveness
  - Thoughts of death or suicide

Screening with **SIGECAPS**:

- **S**LEEP: Changes in sleep habits from baseline, including excessive sleep, early waking, or inability to fall asleep
- **I**NTEREST: Loss of interest in previously enjoyable activities
- **G**UILT: Guilt that may or may not focus on a specific problem or circumstance
- **E**NERGY: Perceived lack of energy
- **C**ONCENTRATION: Inability to concentrate on specific tasks
- **A**PPETITE: Increase or decrease in appetite
- **P**SYCHOMOTOR: Restlessness and agitation, or the perception that everyday activities are too strenuous to manage
- **S**UICIDALITY: Desire to end life or hurt oneself, harmful thoughts directed internally, or thoughts of homicidality

DIAGNOSTIC TESTS & INTERPRETATION

Lab

Initial laboratory evaluation is done primarily to rule out potential medical factors that could be causing symptoms.

Initial lab tests

- Thyroid-stimulating hormone (TSH)
- Complete blood count with differential
- Comprehensive metabolic panel, including liver function
- Urine drug screen
- Vitamin B_{12}

Follow-Up & Special Considerations

Additional testing for possible confounding medical and cognitive disorders as warranted

Diagnostic Procedures/Surgery

Validated screening tools and rating scales:

- Geriatric Depression Scale: 15- or 30-point scales
- Patient Health Questionnaire (PHQ-2 or PHQ-9)
- The Hamilton Depression Rating Scale
- The Beck Depression Inventory

DIFFERENTIAL DIAGNOSIS

Concurrent medical conditions, cognitive disorders, and medications may produce neurovegetative symptoms that may mimic depression:

- Medical conditions: e.g., hypothyroidism, B_{12} deficiency, liver or renal failure, cancers, stroke
- Medication induced: e.g., interferon-α, β-blockers, isotretinoin
- Dementia and neurodegenerative disorders
- Delirium
- Psychiatric disorders: e.g., bipolar disorder, dysthymic disorder, anxiety disorders, substance abuse-related mood disorders, psychotic disorders

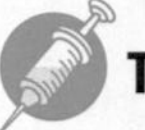

TREATMENT

Although response alone, usually interpreted as a 50% reduction in symptoms, can be clinically meaningful, the goal is to treat patients to the point of remission (i.e., essentially the absence of depressive symptoms)

MEDICATION

- Typically more conservative initial dosing and titration of antidepressants in the elderly, starting with 1/2 of the usual initiation dose and increasing within a couple of weeks if tolerated
- Continue titrating dose every 3–4 weeks as appropriate. It is important to reach an adequate treatment dose.

First Line

- Selective serotonin reuptake inhibitors (SSRIs) have been found to be effective in treating depression in the elderly (1,2)[A].
- No single SSRI clearly outperforms others in the class; choice of medication often reflects side effect profile or practitioner familiarity:
  - Citalopram: Start at 10 mg/day. Treatment range 20–60 mg/day.
  - Sertraline: Start at 25 mg/day. Treatment range 50–200 mg/day.
  - Escitalopram: Start at 5–10 mg/day. Treatment range 10-20 mg/day.
  - Fluoxetine: Start at 10 mg/day. Treatment range 20–60 mg/day.
  - Paroxetine: Start at 10 mg/day. Treatment range 20–60 mg/day.
- SSRIs should not be used concomitantly with monoamine oxidase inhibitors (MAOIs).

Second Line

- Atypical antidepressants: More effective than placebo in treatment of depression in the elderly, although additional studies are needed to better delineate patient factors that determine response (3)[A]:
  - Bupropion (immediate, sustained/twice a day, and extended/once daily available): Start at 100 mg/day. Increase dose in 3 days. Treatment range 200-300 mg/day. Avoid in patients with elevated seizure risk.
  - Venlafaxine (immediate and sustained release available): Start at 37.5 mg and titrate weekly. Treatment range 75–300 mg/day. May be associated with elevated blood pressure at higher doses.

- Duloxetine: Start at 30 mg/day. Treatment range 30–60 mg/day. Also may be associated with elevated blood pressure.
- Mirtazapine: Start at 7.5–15 mg/nightly. Treatment range 15–45 mg/day. Can produce problems with weight gain, sedation, and cognitive dysfunction.

For patients who have not responded to initial SSRI trial:

- Switch to a different SSRI medication, switch to an atypical antidepressant, or augment initial antidepressant with bupropion (4,5,6)[B].

ADDITIONAL TREATMENT

Tricyclic antidepressants (TCAs) have been shown to be effective in treating depression in the elderly (1,2)[A]. However, they are difficult for elderly patients to tolerate due to side effect profile and are potentially lethal in overdose, limiting their use as initial treatment agents.

Although not FDA approved, buspirone, lithium, or triiodothyronine are sometimes used off-label to augment a primary antidepressant (6)[B].

Monoamine oxidase inhibitors (MAOIs) also appear more effective than placebo in the treatment of depression in the elderly (1)[A]. They are not used frequently in clinical practice due to potential side effects and necessary dietary restrictions.

General Measures

Psychotherapy: Studies do show some benefit in depressed elderly patients (7)[B]:

- Cognitive behavioral therapy
- Problem-solving therapy
- Interpersonal therapy
- Psychodynamic psychotherapy

Issues for Referral

Depression with suicidal ideation, psychotic depression, bipolar disorder, co-morbid substance abuse issues, severe or refractory illness

Additional Therapies

- Electroconvulsive therapy (ECT): Has been shown to produce remission of depressive symptoms in the elderly (8)[B]. It should be considered as initial option for patients with severe or psychotic depression.
- Exercise: May be beneficial for depression in the elderly population (9,10)[B].

COMPLEMENTARY AND ALTERNATIVE MEDICINE

- St. John's wort may have minimal benefit (11)[A].
- Tryptophan and hydroxytryptophan: 150–300 mg/d; possible efficacy, additional investigation required (12)[B],(13)

IN-PATIENT CONSIDERATIONS

Inpatient care indicated for imminent safety risk (e.g., acutely suicidal patients) or for those patients unable to care adequately for themselves due to depression.

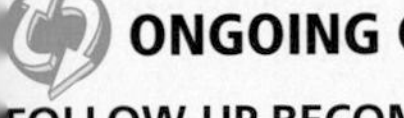

ONGOING CARE

FOLLOW-UP RECOMMENDATIONS

Due to the delay of benefit following initiation of antidepressant therapy (2–4 weeks), it is necessary to ensure open communication with the patient to prevent premature discontinuation of therapy. An adequate explanation of potential side effects with instructions to call the office before discontinuing therapy is imperative.

Patient Monitoring

- A patient with severe depression who exhibits suicidality may require admission to an appropriate facility.
- Monitor for worsening anxiety symptoms or increase in suicidality.

DIET

No dietary restrictions are necessary, except for patients taking MAOIs, which necessitate dietary restriction of foods high in tyramine.

PATIENT EDUCATION

- Depression is a treatable illness.
- Medications may need to be taken for at least 2–4 weeks before any beneficial effect is noted.
- Depression is often a recurring illness.
- National Suicide Prevention Lifeline at 1-800-273-TALK (8255) is a free, 24-hour hotline available to anyone in suicidal crisis or emotional distress. Calls will be routed to the nearest crisis center.

PROGNOSIS

- Treatment outcomes in the elderly may be worse than in the general population, possibly mediated by physical comorbidities and other factors.
- Depending on the population studied and specific clinical measures used, estimates vary for initial clinical response and remission (between 30% and 70%).

COMPLICATIONS

- Impairment in social, occupational, or interpersonal functioning
- Difficulty performing activities of daily living (ADLs) and self-care
- Increase in medical services utilization and increased costs of care
- Suicide

REFERENCES

1. Wilson K, Mottram PG, Sivananthan A, et al. Antidepressants versus placebo for the depressed elderly. *Cochrane Database of Systematic Reviews* 2001, Issue 1. Edited (no change to conclusions), published in Issue 1, 2009.
2. Mottram PG, Wilson K, Strobl JJ. Antidepressants for depressed elderly. *Cochrane Database of Systematic Reviews* 2006, Issue 1. Edited (no change to conclusions), published in Issue 1, 2009.
3. Nelson JC, Delucchi K, Schneider LS, et al. Efficacy of second generation antidepressants in late-life depression: a meta-analysis of the evidence. *Am J Geriatr Psychiatry*. 2008;16:558–67.
4. Ruhe HG, Huyser J, et al. Switching antidepressants after a first selective serotonin reuptake inhibitor in major depressive disorder: a systematic review. *J Clin Psychiatry* 2006;67(12): 1836–1855.
5. Rush AJ, Trivedi MH, et al. Bupropion-SR, sertraline, or venlafaxine-XR after failure of SSRIs for depression. *N Engl J Med*. 2006;354(12): 1231–1242.
6. Trivedi MH, Fava M, et al. Medication Augmentation after the Failure of SSRIs for Depression. *New England Journal of Medicine*. 2006;354(12):1243–1252.
7. Wilson KC, Mottram PG, Vassilas CA, et al. Psychotherapeutic treatments for older depressed people. *Cochrane Database Syst Rev*. 2008; CD004853.
8. Van der Wurff FB, et al. Electroconvulsive therapy for the depressed elderly. *Cochrane Database Sys Rev*. 2003;CD003593. DOI:10.1002/14651858. CD003593.
9. Blake H, Mo P, Malik S, et al. How effective are physical activity interventions for alleviating depressive symptoms in older people? A systematic review. *Clin Rehabil*. 2009.
10. Sjösten N, Kivelä SL et al. The effects of physical exercise on depressive symptoms among the aged: a systematic review. *Int J Geriatr Psychiatry*. 2006;21:410–8.
11. Linde K, et al. St. John's wort for depression. *Cochrane Database Sys Rev*. 2005;CD000448. DOI:10.1002/14651858.CD000448.pub2.
12. Shaw K, Turner J, DelMar C. Tryptophan and 5-hydroxytryptophan for depression. *Cochrane Database Sys Rev*. 2002;CD003198. DOI:10.1002/14651858.CD003198.
13. Sarris J, Schoendorfer N, Kavanagh DJ. Major depressive disorder and nutritional medicine: a review of monotherapies and adjuvant treatments. *Nutr Rev*. 2009;67:125–31.

See Also (Topic, Algorithm, Electronic Media Element)

Algorithms: Depressive Episode, Major; Depressed Mood Resulting from Medical Illness

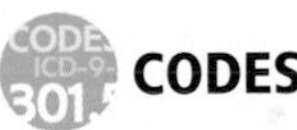

CODES

ICD9

- 290.21 Senile dementia with depressive features
- 311 Depressive disorder, not elsewhere classified

CLINICAL PEARLS

- Depression is not a normal part of aging.
- Depression in the elderly may be difficult to precisely diagnose due to medical and cognitive comorbidities.
- Depression may present primarily with cognitive dysfunction. Cognitive function may improve with treatment of the depression.
- A multidisciplinary approach to the treatment of depression is often most efficacious.
- SSRIs are considered first-line therapy for safety and tolerability. A full remission may take upwards of 12 weeks of treatment. Long-term treatment may be needed to prevent recurrence.

DEPRESSION, POSTPARTUM

Karla M. Rodriguez, MD
Nancy Byatt, DO, MBA

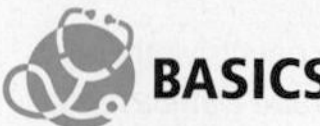

BASICS

DESCRIPTION

Major depressive disorder (MDD) that recurs or has its onset in the postpartum period. May also occur in mothers adopting a baby or in fathers (1).

EPIDEMIOLOGY

Incidence

10–15% of mothers within 1st year of giving birth (2)

Prevalence

- Controversial; assessments range from 10–20% during the early postpartum weeks
- Investigators have reported elevated depressive symptoms in 30–50% of women during the early postpartum period with continued symptoms throughout the 1st postpartum year (3).

RISK FACTORS

- Previous episodes of postpartum depression
- History of MDD
- MDD during pregnancy
- Anxiety during pregnancy (4)
- History of premenstrual dysphoria
- Family history of depression (5)
- Unwanted pregnancy
- Socioeconomic stress
- Low self-esteem
- Young maternal age
- Alcohol abuse
- Marital conflict
- Multiple births (6)
- Lack of social and family support system (7)
- Postpartum pain, sleep disturbance, and fatigue
- Assisted reproductive technology pregnancy (8)
- Recent immigrant status
- Increased stressful life events
- History of childhood sexual abuse
- Decision to decrease antidepressants during pregnancy

GENERAL PREVENTION

- Universal screening during the 3rd trimester to diagnose depression and risk factors for depression and to allow initiation of treatment before or immediately after delivery (9)[A]
- Postpartum screening using Edinburgh Postnatal Depression Scale within 4-6 weeks post-delivery (9)[A]
- Continuation of antidepressants in high-risk women during pregnancy may prevent postnatal depression.
- Provide postnatal visits and psychotherapy and/or education for high-risk women.
- Use of depression care manager who provides education, routine telephone contact, and follow-up in order to engage women in treatment

PATHOPHYSIOLOGY

May be related to sensitivity in hormonal fluctuations, including estrogen, progesterone, and other gonadal hormones, as well as neuroactive steroids; cytokines; HPA axis hormones; and altered fatty acid, oxytocin, and arginine vasopressin levels (4)

ETIOLOGY

Multifactorial, including biologic–genetic predisposition in terms of neurobiologic deficit, destabilizing effects of hormone withdrawal at birth, inflammation, and psychosocial stressors (2)

COMMONLY ASSOCIATED CONDITIONS

- Bipolar mood disorder
- Depressive disorder not otherwise specified
- Dysthymic disorder
- Cyclothymic disorder
- Major depressive disorder (10)

DIAGNOSIS

HISTORY

- Increased/decreased sleep
- Decreased interest in formerly compelling or pleasurable activities
- Guilt, low self-esteem
- Decreased energy
- Decreased concentration
- Increased/decreased appetite
- Psychomotor agitation or retardation
- Suicidal ideation

DIAGNOSTIC TESTS & INTERPRETATION

Lab

Initial lab tests

Thyroid-stimulating hormone (TSH) (11)[A]

Diagnostic Procedures/Surgery

- Edinburgh Postnatal Depression Scale is the primary screening tool.
- Beck, Hamilton, and Zung depression inventories may provide information about the severity of the depression and suicidal risks.
- Edinburgh Postnatal Depression Scale (Partner Version). To be completed by mother's partner to obtain his/her view of mother's depression.

DIFFERENTIAL DIAGNOSIS

- Baby blues: Not a psychiatric disorder, mood lability, resolves within days
- Postpartum psychosis: A psychiatric emergency
- Postpartum anxiety/panic disorder
- Postpartum obsessive-compulsive disorder
- Hypothyroidism
- Postpartum thyroiditis: Can occur in up to 7.5% of patients and can present as depression (12)[A]
- Sleep apnea

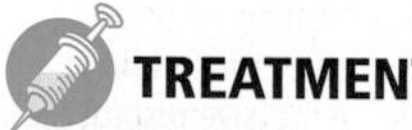

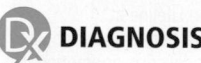

TREATMENT

MEDICATION

First Line

- Selective serotonin reuptake inhibitors (SSRIs) are generally effective and safe:
  - Fluoxetine (Prozac): 20–80 mg/d p.o. (most activating of all SSRIs); less expensive
  - Sertraline (Zoloft): 50–200 mg/d p.o. (sedating)
  - Paroxetine (Paxil): 20–60 mg/d p.o. (sedating)
  - Citalopram (Celexa): 20–60 mg/d p.o.
- Tricyclic antidepressants (TCAs) effective and less expensive, yet are lethal in overdose and have unfavorable side effects:
  - Avoid TCAs in mothers with a history of suicide attempts.
- Bupropion (Wellbutrin): 150–450 mg/d p.o. in patients with depression plus psychomotor retardation, hypersomnia, and with weight gain. Bupropion is less likely to cause weight gain or sexual dysfunction and is highly activating.
- Mirtazapine (Remeron): 15–45 mg/d p.o. q.h.s. Ma[y] assist with sleep restoration and weight gain; no sexual dysfunction
- Venlafaxine (Effexor XR): A dual-action antidepressant that blocks the reuptake of serotoni[n] in doses of up to 150 mg/d and then blocks the reuptake of norepinephrine in doses of 150–450 mg/d p.o.
- Bipolar disorder requires treatment with mood stabilizer.
- Among breastfeeding mothers:
  - Weigh potential efficacy of treatment with antidepressant, risks of exposure to infant, and known negative effects of not treating on child development.
  - All antidepressants are excreted in breast milk, but are generally compatible with lactation.
  - Paroxetine and sertraline offer best safety profile during lactation.
  - Start with low doses and increase slowly. Monitor infant for adverse side effects.
  - Minimize infant exposure to medication by avoiding breastfeeding at time of peak concentration.
  - Consider continuing medication that is efficacious while monitoring infant carefully, rather than switching antidepressants (4,13)[B].
  - For further information: *Medications and Mother's Milk* by Thomas Hale, PhD

Second Line

Electroconvulsive therapy (ECT): May be indicated in patients who cannot tolerate antidepressant medication, are actively engaged in suicidal self-destructive behaviors, or have a previous history of response to ECT (14)[C]

ADDITIONAL TREATMENT

General Measures

- Most patients respond to outpatient individual psychotherapy in combination with pharmacotherapy.
- Support/therapy groups may be helpful.
- Assess suicidal ideation.
- Assess homicidal ideation and thoughts of harming baby. Thoughts of harming baby require immediate hospitalization.
- Visiting nurse services can provide direct observations of the mother about safety issues and mother–child bonding (10)[A].

Issues for Referral

- Obtain psychiatric consultation for patients with psychotic symptoms.
- Immediate hospitalization is mandatory if delusions or hallucinations are present.
- Hospitalization is indicated if mother's ability to care for self and/or infant is significantly compromised.

ıdditional Therapies

Psychoeducation, including providing reading material for the patient and family (10)[C]

Psychotherapy: Interpersonal psychotherapy, cognitive behavioral therapy, and psychodynamic psychotherapy shown to be effective (4)[C]

:OMPLEMENTARY AND ALTERNATIVE ⁄IEDICINE

Breastfeeding is effective in reducing stress and protecting maternal mood (11)[A].

Infant massage, infant sleep intervention, exercise, and bright light therapy may be beneficial (4)[B],(15)[A].

N-PATIENT CONSIDERATIONS

ALERT

Obtain psychiatric consultation for patients with psychotic symptoms. If delusions or hallucinations are present, immediate hospitalization is mandatory. The psychotic mother should *not* be left alone with the baby.

ıdmission Criteria

ʼresence of suicidal or homicidal ideation and/or ısychotic symptoms and/or thoughts of harming baby ınd/or inability to care for self or infant, severe weight ɔss

Ͻischarge Criteria

- Absence of suicidal or homicidal ideation and/or psychotic symptoms and/or thoughts of harming baby
- Mother must be able to care for self and infant.

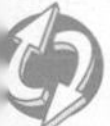

ONGOING CARE

FOLLOW-UP RECOMMENDATIONS

ʼatient Monitoring

- Collaborative care approach, including primary care visits and case manager follow-ups
- Consultation with the infant's doctor, particularly if mother is breastfeeding while taking psychotropic medications

DIET

- Good nutrition and hydration, especially when breastfeeding
- The addition of a multivitamin with minerals and Ω-3 fatty acids may be helpful.

PATIENT EDUCATION

- *This Isn't What I Expected: Overcoming Postpartum Depression*, by Karen R. Kleinman and Valerie Davis Radkin
- *Down Came the Rain: My Journey Through Postpartum Depression*, by Brooke Shields, 2005
- *Behind the Smile: My Journey Out of Postpartum Depression*, by Marie Osmond, Marcie Wilkie, and Judith Morre, 2001
- *A Medication Guide for Breastfeeding Moms*, by Thomas Hale and Ghia Mcafee, 2008
- Web resources:
  - Postpartum support international: http://www.postpartum.net
  - http://www.4women.gov
  - La Leche League: http://www.lalecheleague.org
  - http://toxnet.nlm.nih.gov
  - www.mededppd.org
  - www.womensmentalhealth.org
  - www.motherrisk.org

PROGNOSIS

- Treatment of maternal depression to remission has been shown to have a positive impact on children's mental health (13)[B].
- Some patients, particularly those with undertreated or undiagnosed depression, may develop chronic depression requiring long-term treatment (16)[A].
- Untreated maternal depression is linked to impaired child development, including poor cognitive functioning and emotional maladjustment in infants and children (4,13)[B].
- Postpartum psychosis associated with tragic outcomes, such as maternal suicide and infanticide (2,16)[C]

COMPLICATIONS

- Suicide
- Self-injurious behavior
- Psychosis
- Neglect of baby
- Harm to the baby (12)[A]

REFERENCES

1. Paulson JF, Dauber S, Leiferman JA. Individual and combined effects of postpartum depression in mothers and fathers on parenting behavior. *Pediatrics*. 2006;118:659–68.
2. Brett K, et al. Prevalence of self-reported postpartum depressive symptoms: 17 Sate, 2004–2005. *MMWR Weekly*. 2008;361–6.
3. Mayberry J, et al. Depression symptom prevalence and demographic risk factors among U.S. women during the 1st 2 years postpartum. *J Obstet Gynecol Neo Nurs*. 2007:542–9.
4. Pearlstein T, Howard M, Salisbury A, et al. Postpartum depression. *Am J Obstet Gynecol*. 2009;200:357–64.
5. Davey HL, Tough SC, Adair CE, et al. Risk Factors for Sub-Clinical and Major Postpartum Depression Among a Community Cohort of Canadian Women. *Matern Child Health J*. 2008.
6. Choi Y, Bishai D, Minkovitz CS. Multiple births are a risk factor for postpartum maternal depressive symptoms. *Pediatrics*. 2009;123:1147–54.
7. Lee AM, et al. Prevalence, course, risk factors for antenatal anxiety and depression. *Obstet Gyn*. 2007;5:1102–12.
8. Monti F, et al. Depressive symptoms during late pregnancy and early adulthood following assisted reproductive technology. *Fertility Sterility*. 2008;1–7.
9. Jomeen J, et al. Replicability and stability of the multidimensional model of the Edinburgh Postnatal Depression Scale I late pregnancy. *J Psychiatr Mental Health Nurs*. 2007;14:319–24.
10. Howard LM, et al. Antidepressant prevention of postnatal depression. *PLoS Medicine*. 2006;3:1741–2.
11. Kendall-Tackett K. A new paradigm for depression in new mothers: The central role of inflammation and how breastfeeding and anti-inflammatory treatments protect maternal health. *Intl Breastfeeding J*. 2007;2:6.
12. Harrington AR, Greene-Harrington CC. Healthy Start screens for depression among urban pregnant, postpartum and interconceptional women. *J Natl Med Assoc*. 2007;99:226–31.
13. Freeman MP. Breastfeeding and antidepressants: clinical dilemmas and expert perspectives. *J Clin Psychiatry*. 2009;70:291–2.
14. Forray A, Ostroff RB. The use of electroconvulsive therapy in postpartum affective disorders. *J ECT*. 2007;23:188–93.
15. Daley AJ, Macarthur C, Winter H. The role of exercise in treating postpartum depression: a review of the literature. *J Midwifery Womens Health*. 2007;52:56–62.
16. Tammentie T, Tarkka MT, Astedt-Kurki P, et al. Family dynamics and postnatal depression. *J Psychiatr Ment Health Nurs*. 2004;11:141–9.
17. Musters C, McDonald E, Jones I. Management of postnatal depression. *BMJ*. 2008;337:a736.

ADDITIONAL READING

- Gjerdingen D, et al. Stepped care treatment of postpartum depression. *Women's Health Issues*. 2007;18:44–52.
- Sit DK, Wisner KL et al. Identification of postpartum depression. *Clin Obstet Gynecol*. 2009;52:456–68.

CODES

ICD9

- 296.20 Major depressive affective disorder, single episode, unspecified degree
- 296.30 Major depressive affective disorder, recurrent episode, unspecified degree
- 648.44 Postpartum mental disorders of mother

CLINICAL PEARLS

- PPD is a common, debilitating medical condition that impairs a mother's ability to function and interact with her infant and family.
- Universal screening for PPD is recommended during the 3rd trimester and at regular intervals during the postpartum period.
- Early diagnosis and treatment are vital, as untreated PPD can lead to developmental difficulties for the infant and prolonged disability and suffering for the mother (4,17)[B].
- Breastfeeding is recommended for maternal and child health. There are several medication options for treating depression in mothers that are safe for breastfeeding infants.

DERMATITIS, ATOPIC

Dennis E. Hughes, DO

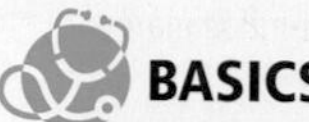

BASICS

DESCRIPTION

- Chronic, relapsing, pruritic eczematous condition affecting characteristic sites
- System(s) affected: Skin/Exocrine
- Synonym(s): Eczema; Atopic eczema; Atopic neurodermatitis; Constitutional dermatitis; Besnier prurigo

EPIDEMIOLOGY

Environmentally triggered in susceptible individuals

Incidence

- 45% of all cases begin in the 1st 6 months of life.
- 70% of affected children will have a spontaneous remission before adolescence.

Prevalence

- Mainly childhood disease; affects 10% of all children
- Also may have late-onset dermatitis in adults
- Visits for the condition have been rising over the last 10 years.
- Asians and blacks affected more often than whites
- 60% for one affected parent; rises to 80% if both parents affected

RISK FACTORS

- "Itch-scratch cycle"
- Skin infections
- Emotional stress
- Irritating clothes and chemicals
- Excessively hot or cold climate
- Food allergy in children (in some cases)
- Exposure to tobacco smoke
- Family history of atopy:
  - Asthma
  - Allergic rhinitis

Genetics

- Arises from gene-gene and gene-environment interactions
- Both epidermal and immune coding likely involved

PATHOPHYSIOLOGY

- Alteration in stratum corneum results in transepidermal water loss.
- Epidermal adhesion is reduced either as a result of genetic mutation or as a result of inflammatory response.
- Interleukin 31 (IL-31) upregulation is thought to be a major factor in pruritus rather than histamine excess.

COMMONLY ASSOCIATED CONDITIONS

- Food sensitivity/allergy in many cases
- Asthma
- Allergic rhinitis
- Hyper-IgE syndrome (Job syndrome):
  - Atopic dermatitis
  - Elevated IgE
  - Recurrent pyodermas
  - Decreased chemotaxis of mononuclear cells

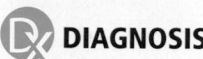

DIAGNOSIS

HISTORY

Pruritus is the most common symptom.

PHYSICAL EXAM

- Distribution of lesions:
  - Infants: Trunk, face, and flexural surfaces; diaper-sparing
  - Children: Antecubital and popliteal fossae
  - Adults: Hands, feet, face, neck, upper chest, and genital areas
- Morphology of lesions:
  - Infants: Erythema and papules; may develop oozing, crusting vesicles
  - Children and adults: Lichenification and scaling are typical with chronic eczema as a result of persistent scratching and rubbing (lichenification rare in infants).
- Associated signs:
  - Facial erythema, mild to moderate
  - Perioral pallor
  - Infraorbital fold (Dennie sign/Morgan line)
  - Dry skin
  - Increased palmar linear markings
  - Pityriasis alba (hypopigmented asymptomatic areas on face and shoulders)
  - Keratosis pilaris

DIAGNOSTIC TESTS & INTERPRETATION

Lab

Initial lab tests

- No test is diagnostic.
- Serum IgE levels are elevated in as many as 80% of affected individuals.
- Eosinophilia tends to correlate with disease severity.

Pathological Findings

- Epidermis thickened and hyperkeratotic
- Perivascular inflammation of dermis

DIFFERENTIAL DIAGNOSIS

- Photosensitivity rashes
- Contact dermatitis (especially if only the face is involved)
- Scabies
- Seborrheic dermatitis (especially in infants)
- Psoriasis or lichen simplex chronicus if only localized disease is present in adults
- Rare conditions of infancy:
  - Histiocytosis X
  - Wiskott-Aldrich syndrome
  - Ataxia-telangiectasia syndrome
- Ichthyosis vulgaris

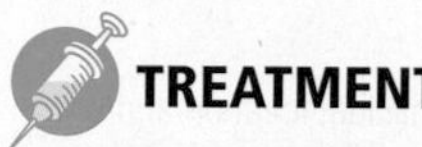

TREATMENT

Pediatric Considerations

Chronic potent fluorinated corticosteroid use may cause striae, hypopigmentation, or atrophy, especially in children.

MEDICATION

First Line

- Frequent systemic lubrication with thick emollient creams (e.g., Eucerin, Vaseline) over moist skin is the mainstay of treatment before any other intervention is considered.
- Infants and children: 0.5–1% topical hydrocortisone creams or ointments (1)[C]
- Adults: Higher-potency topical corticosteroids in areas other than face and skin folds
- Short-course higher-potency corticosteroids for flares; then return to the lowest potency (creams preferred) that will control dermatitis (2)[C]. Hypopigmentation can occur even with short-term use.
- Antihistamines for pruritus (e.g., Hydroxyzine 10–25 mg at bedtime and as needed)

Second Line

- Topical immunomodulators (tacrolimus or pimecrolimus) for episodic use for children >2 years of age. There is a black box warning from the Food and Drug Administration regarding potential cancer risk (3).
- Plastic occlusion in combination with topical medication to promote absorption
- For severe atopic dermatitis, consider systemic steroids × 1–2 weeks [e.g., Prednisone 2 mg/kg/d PO (maximum 80 mg/d) initially, tapered over 7–14 days].
- Topical tricyclic doxepin as a 5% cream may decrease pruritus.
- Modified Goeckerman regimen (tar and ultraviolet light)
- Immune modifiers (methotrexate, azathioprine, cyclosporine)

ADDITIONAL TREATMENT

General Measures

- Decrease stress if possible.
- Avoid agents that may cause irritation (e.g., wool, perfumes).
- Minimize sweating.
- Lukewarm (not hot) baths
- Minimize use of soap (superfatted soaps best).
- Frequent systemic lubrication with thick emollient creams (e.g., Eucerin) over moist skin
- Sun exposure may be helpful.
- Humidify the house.
- Avoid excessive contact with water.
- Avoid lotions that contain alcohol.
- If very resistant to treatment, search for a coexisting contact dermatitis.

Issues for Referral

- Ophthalmology evaluation for persistent vernal conjunctivitis
- If using topical steroids around eyes for extended periods, ophthalmology follow-up for cataract evaluation

Additional Therapies

- Methods to reduce house mite allergens (micropore filters on heating, ventilation, and air-conditioning systems, impermeable mattress covers) (4)[C]
- Behavioral relaxation therapy to reduce scratching (4)[B]

COMPLEMENTARY AND ALTERNATIVE MEDICINE

- Evening primrose oil (includes high content of fatty acids):
  - May decrease prostaglandin synthesis
  - May promote conversion of linoleic acid to omega-6 fatty acid
- Probiotics may reduce the severity of the condition, reducing medication use (4)[C].

ONGOING CARE

FOLLOW-UP RECOMMENDATIONS

Patient Monitoring

Evaluate to ensure that secondary bacterial or fungal infection does not develop as a result of disruption of the skin barrier.

DIET

- Trials of elimination may find certain "triggers" in some patients.
- Breast-feeding in conjunction with maternal hypoallergenic diets may decrease the severity in some infants.

PATIENT EDUCATION

- http://www.add.org/public/publications/pamplets/eczemaatopicdermatitis.htm
- National Eczema Association: www.nationaleczema.org

PROGNOSIS

- Chronic disease
- Declines with increasing age
- 90% of patients have spontaneous resolution by puberty.
- Localized eczema (e.g., chronic hand or foot dermatitis, eyelid dermatitis, or lichen simplex chronicus) may continue in some adults.

COMPLICATIONS

- Cataracts are more common in patients with atopic dermatitis.
- Skin infections (usually *Staphylococcus aureus*); sometimes subclinical
- Eczema herpeticum:
  - Generalized vesiculopustular eruption caused by infection with herpes simplex or vaccinia virus
  - Causes acute illness requiring hospitalization
- Atrophy and/or striae if fluorinated corticosteroids are used on face or skin folds
- Systemic absorption may occur if large areas of skin are treated, particularly if high-potency medications and occlusion are combined.

REFERENCES

1. Bieber T. Atopic dermatitis. *N Engl J Med*. 2008;358:1483–94.
2. Williams HC. Clinical practice. Atopic dermatitis. *N Engl J Med*. 2005;352:2314–24.
3. Trammell S, Shakil A, Wilder L, et al. Clinical inquiries. What is the role of tacrolimus and pimecrolimus in atopic dermatitis? *J Fam Pract*. 2005;54:714–6.
4. Weston S, et al. Effects of probiotics on atopic dermatitis: A randomized controlled trial. *Arch Disease Child*. 2005;90:892–897.

ADDITIONAL READING

Hill DJ, Hosking CS, Food Allergy and Atopic Dermatitis in Infancy: An Epidemiological Study. *Padiatr Allergy Immunol*. 2004;15(5):421–7.

See Also (Topic, Algorithm, Electronic Media Element)

Algorithm: Rash, focal

CODES

ICD9

691.8 Other atopic dermatitis and related conditions

CLINICAL PEARLS

- Institute early and proactive treatment to reduce inflammation.
- Monitor for secondary bacterial infection.
- Frequent systemic lubrication with thick emollient creams (e.g., Eucerin, Vaseline) over moist skin is the mainstay of treatment before any other intervention is considered.
- Use the lowest-potency topical steroid that controls symptoms.

DERMATITIS, CONTACT

Aamir Siddiqi, MD

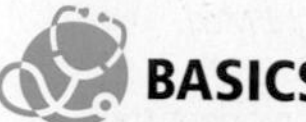

BASICS

DESCRIPTION

- The cutaneous reaction to an external substance
- Primary irritant dermatitis is due to direct injury of the skin. It affects individuals exposed to specific irritants and generally produces discomfort immediately after exposure.
- Allergic contact dermatitis (ACD) affects only individuals previously sensitized to the substance. It represents a delayed hypersensitivity reaction, requiring several hours for the cascade of cellular immunity to be completed to manifest itself.
- System(s) affected: Skin/Exocrine
- Synonym(s): Dermatitis venenata

EPIDEMIOLOGY

Common

Incidence

Occupational contact dermatitis: 20.5/100,000 workers

Prevalence

- Contact dermatitis represents >90% of all occupational skin disorders.
- Predominant sex: Male = Female:
  - Variations due to differences in exposure to offending agents as well as normal cutaneous variations between male and female (eccrine and sebaceous gland function and hair distribution)

Geriatric Considerations

Increased incidence of irritant dermatitis secondary to skin dryness

Pediatric Considerations

Increased incidence of positive patch testing due to better delayed hypersensitivity reactions

RISK FACTORS

- Occupation
- Hobbies
- Travel
- Cosmetics
- Jewelry

Genetics

Increased frequency of ACD in families with allergies

GENERAL PREVENTION

- Avoid causative agents.
- Use of protective gloves (with cotton lining) may be helpful (1)[A].

PATHOPHYSIOLOGY

Hypersensitivity reaction to a substance generating cellular immunity response

ETIOLOGY

- Plants:
  - Rhus-urushiol: Poison ivy, oak, sumac
  - Primary contact: Plant (roots/stems/leaves)
  - Secondary contact: Clothes/fingernails (not blister fluid)
- Chemicals:
  - Nickel: Jewelry, zippers, hooks, and watches
  - Potassium dichromate: Tanning agent in leather
  - Paraphenylenediamine: Hair dyes, fur dyes, and industrial chemicals
  - Turpentine: Cleaning agents, polishes, and waxes
  - Soaps and detergents
- Topical medicines:
  - Neomycin: Topical antibiotics
  - Thimerosal (Merthiolate): Preservative in topical medications
  - Anesthetics: Benzocaine
  - Parabens: Preservative in topical medications
  - Formalin: Cosmetics, shampoos, and nail enamel

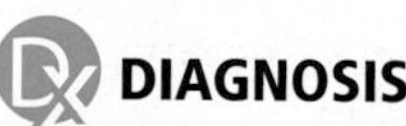

DIAGNOSIS

HISTORY

- Itchy rash
- Assess for prior exposure to irritating substance

PHYSICAL EXAM

- Acute:
  - Papules, vesicles, bullae with surrounding erythema
  - Crusting and oozing
  - Pruritus
- Chronic:
  - Erythematous base
  - Thickening with lichenification
  - Scaling
  - Fissuring
- Distribution:
  - Where epidermis is thinner (eyelids, genitalia)
  - Areas of contact with offending agent (e.g., nail polish)
  - Palms and soles more resistant
  - Deeper skin folds spared
  - Linear arrays of lesions
  - Lesions with sharp borders and sharp angles are pathognomonic.
- Well-demarcated area with a papulovesicular rash

DIAGNOSTIC TESTS & INTERPRETATION

Diagnostic Procedures/Surgery

Consider patch tests for suspected allergic trigger (systemic corticosteroids or recent, aggressive use of topical steroids may alter results) (2)[B]

Pathological Findings

- Intercellular edema
- Bullae

DIFFERENTIAL DIAGNOSIS

- Based on clinical impression:
  - Appearance, periodicity, and localization
- Groups of vesicles:
  - Herpes simplex
- Diffuse bullous or vesicular lesions:
  - Bullous pemphigoid
- Photodistribution:
  - Phototoxic/allergic reaction to systemic allergen
- Eyelids:
  - Seborrheic dermatitis
- Scaly eczematous lesions:
  - Atopic dermatitis
  - Nummular eczema
  - Lichen simplex chronicus
  - Stasis dermatitis
  - Xerosis

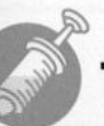

TREATMENT

MEDICATION

First Line

- Topical medications:
  - Lotion of zinc oxide, talc, menthol 0.25%, phenol 0.5% (Gold Bond, others)
  - Corticosteroids for allergic contact dermatitis as well as irritant dermatitis (1)[A]:
    - High-potency steroids: Fluocinonide (Lidex) 0.05% ointment t.i.d.–q.i.d.
    - Use high-potency steroids only for a short time and then switch to low- or medium-potency steroid cream or ointment.
    - Caution regarding face/skin folds: Use lower-potency steroids and avoid prolonged usage. Switch to lower-potency topical steroid once the acute phase is resolved.
- Calamine lotion for symptomatic relief
- Topical antibiotics for secondary infection (bacitracin, erythromycin)
- Systemic:
  - Antihistamine:
    - Hydroxyzine: 25–50 mg p.o. q.i.d., especially useful for itching
    - Diphenhydramine: 25–50 mg p.o. q.i.d.
  - Corticosteroids:
    - Prednisone: Taper starting at 60–80 mg/d p.o., over 10–14 days
    - Used for moderate-to-severe cases
    - May use burst dose of steroids for up to 5 days
  - Antibiotics for secondary skin infections:
    - Dicloxacillin: 250 mg p.o. q.i.d. for 7–10 days
    - Amoxicillin-clavulanate (Augmentin): 500 mg p.o. b.i.d. for 7–10 days
    - Erythromycin: 250 mg p.o. q.i.d. in penicillin-allergic patients
- Precautions:
  - Antihistamines may cause drowsiness.
  - Prolonged use of potent topical steroids may cause local skin effects (atrophy, stria, telangiectasia).
  - Use tapering dose of oral steroids if using more than 5 days.

Second Line

Other topical or systemic antibiotics, depending on organisms and sensitivity

Pregnancy Considerations

Usual cautions with medications

ADDITIONAL TREATMENT

General Measures

- Removal of offending agent:
  - Avoidance
  - Work modification
  - Protective clothing
  - Barrier creams, especially high-lipid content moisturizing creams (e.g., Keri lotion, petrolatum, coconut oil) (3)[A]
- Topical soaks with cool tap water, Burow solution (1:40 dilution), saline (1 tsp/pint water), or silver nitrate solution (25.5%)
- Lukewarm water baths
- Aveeno oatmeal baths
- Emollients (white petrolatum, Eucerin)

Issues for Referral

May need referral to a dermatologist or allergist if refractory to conventional treatment

COMPLEMENTARY AND ALTERNATIVE MEDICINE

The use of complementary and alternative treatment is a supplement and not an alternative to conventional treatment (4).

IN-PATIENT CONSIDERATIONS

Admission Criteria

Rarely will need hospital admission

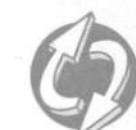

ONGOING CARE

FOLLOW-UP RECOMMENDATIONS

Stay active, but avoid overheating.

Patient Monitoring

- As necessary for recurrence
- Patch testing for etiology after resolved

DIET

No special diet

PATIENT EDUCATION

- Avoidance of irritating substance
- Cleaning of secondary sources (nails, clothes)
- Fallacy of blister fluid spreading disease

PROGNOSIS

- Self-limited
- Benign

COMPLICATIONS

- Generalized eruption secondary to autosensitization
- Secondary bacterial infection

REFERENCES

1. Saary J, Qureshi R, Palda V, et al. A systematic review of contact dermatitis treatment and prevention. *J Am Acad Dermatol*. 2005;53:845.
2. Saripalli YV, Achen F, Belsito DV. The detection of clinically relevant contact allergens using a standard screening tray of twenty-three allergens. *J Am Acad Dermatol*. 2003;49:65–9.
3. Hachem JP, De Paepe K, Vanpée E, et al. Efficacy of topical corticosteroids in nickel-induced contact allergy. *Clin Exp Dermatol*. 2002;27:47–50.
4. Noiesen E, Munk MD, Larsen K, et al. Use of complementary and alternative treatment for allergic contact dermatitis. *Br J Dermatol*. 2007.

See Also (Topic, Algorithm, Electronic Media Element)

Algorithm: Rash, Focal

CODES

ICD9

- 692.0 Contact dermatitis and other eczema due to detergents
- 692.3 Contact dermatitis and other eczema due to drugs and medicines in contact with skin
- 692.4 Contact dermatitis and other eczema due to other chemical products

CLINICAL PEARLS

- Anyone exposed to irritants or allergic substances is predisposed to contact dermatitis, especially in occupations that have high exposure to chemicals.
- The most common allergens causing contact dermatitis are plants of the *Toxicodendron* genus (poison ivy, poison oak, poison sumac).
- The usual treatment for contact dermatitis is avoidance of the allergen or irritating substance and temporary use of topical steroids.
- A contact dermatitis rash presents in a nondermatomal geographic fashion, due to the skin being in contact with an external source.

D

DERMATITIS, DIAPER

Dennis E. Hughes, DO

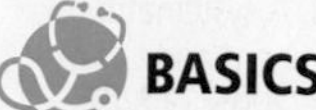

BASICS

DESCRIPTION

- Diaper dermatitis is a rash occurring under the covered area of a diaper. The rash may be a direct result of wearing the diaper, aggravated by the diaper, or coincidental with a rash that appears elsewhere on the body.
- System(s) affected: Skin/Exocrine
- Synonym(s): Diaper rash

Geriatric Considerations

Incontinence is a significant cofactor.

EPIDEMIOLOGY

Incidence

- The most common dermatitis found in infancy
- Peak incidence: 7–12 months of age, then decreases

Prevalence

Prevalence has been variably reported from 4–35% in the 1st 2 years of life.

RISK FACTORS

- Infrequent diaper changes
- Waterproof diapers
- Improper laundering
- Family history of dermatitis
- Hot, humid weather
- Recent treatment with oral antibiotics
- Diarrhea (>3 stools per day increases risk)
- Dye allergy
- Prior history of eczema may increase risk.

GENERAL PREVENTION

Attention to hygiene during bouts of diarrhea

PATHOPHYSIOLOGY

- Fecal proteases and lipases are irritants.
- Superhydrase urease enzyme found in the stratum cornium liberates ammonia from cutaneous bacteria.
- Fecal lipase and protease activity is increased by acceleration of GI transit; thus a higher incidence of irritant diaper dermatitis is observed in babies who have had diarrhea in the previous 48 h.
- Once the skin is compromised, secondary infection by *Candida albicans* is common. 40–75% of diaper rashes that last >3 days are colonized with *C. albicans*.
- Bacteria may play a role in diaper dermatitis through reduction of fecal pH and resulting activation of enzymes.
- Allergy is exceedingly rare as a cause in infants.

ETIOLOGY

- Wet skin from prolonged contact with urine or feces resulting in susceptibility to chemical, enzymatic, and physical injury; wet skin is also penetrated more easily.
- Some have raised the possibility of contact allergy from the dye in disposable diapers.

COMMONLY ASSOCIATED CONDITIONS

- Contact (allergic or irritant) dermatitis
- Seborrheic dermatitis
- Psoriasis
- Candidiasis
- Atopic dermatitis

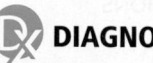

DIAGNOSIS

HISTORY

- Onset, duration, and change in the nature of the rash
- Presence of rashes outside the diaper area
- Associated scratching or crying
- Contact with infants with a similar rash
- Recent illness, diarrhea, or antibiotic use
- Fever
- Pustular drainage
- Lymphangitis

PHYSICAL EXAM

- Mild forms consist of shiny erythema ± scale.
- Margins are not always evident.
- Moderate cases have areas of papules, vesicles, and small superficial erosions.
- It can progress to well-demarcated ulcerated nodules that measure 1 cm or more in diameter.
- It is found on the prominent parts of the buttocks, medial thighs, mons pubis, and scrotum.
- Skin folds are spared or involved last.
- *Tidemark dermatitis* refers to the bandlike form of erythema of irritated diaper margins.
- Diaper dermatitis can cause an id (autoeczematous) reaction outside the diaper area.

DIAGNOSTIC TESTS & INTERPRETATION

Lab

Initial lab tests

- Rarely needed
- Consider a culture of lesions or a KOH preparation.

Follow-Up & Special Considerations

- The finding of anemia in association with hepatosplenomegaly and the appropriate rash may suggest a diagnosis of Langerhans cell histiocytosis or congenital syphilis.
- Finding mites, ova, or feces on a mineral oil preparation of a burrow scraping can confirm the diagnosis of scabies.

Pathological Findings

- Biopsy is rare.
- Histology may reveal acute, subacute, or chronic spongiotic dermatitis.

DIFFERENTIAL DIAGNOSIS

- Contact dermatitis
- Seborrheic dermatitis
- Candidiasis
- Atopic dermatitis
- Scabies
- Acrodermatitis enteropathica
- Letterer-Siwe disease
- Congenital syphilis
- Child abuse
- Streptococcal infection
- Kawasaki disease
- Biotin deficiency
- Psoriasis
- HIV infection

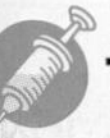

TREATMENT

ee "General-Measures" for 1st-line approach.

MEDICATION

First Line

For a pure contact dermatitis, a low-potency topical steroid (hydrocortisone 0.5–1% t.i.d.) and removal of the offending agent should suffice.

- If candidiasis is suspected or diaper rash persists, use an antifungal such as miconazole nitrate 2% cream, miconazole powder, econazole (Spectazole), clotrimazole (Lotrimin), or ketoconazole (Nizoral) cream at each diaper change (1)[B].
- If inflammation is prominent, consider a very low-potency steroid cream such as hydrocortisone 0.5–1% t.i.d. along with an antifungal cream ± a combination product such as clioquinol-hydrocortisone (Vioform–hydrocortisone) cream (1)[B].
- If a secondary bacterial infection is suspected, use an antistaphylococcal oral antibiotic or mupirocin (Bactroban) ointment topically.
- Precautions: Avoid high- or moderate-potency steroids often found in combination steroid antifungal mixtures (1)[B].

Second Line

Sucralfate paste for resistant cases

ADDITIONAL TREATMENT

General Measures

- Expose the buttocks to air as much as possible (1).
- Avoid waterproof pants during treatment (day or night); they keep the skin wet and subject to rash or infection.
- Change diapers frequently, even at night, if the rash is extensive (2).
- Superabsorbable diapers are beneficial (1,2)[B].
- Discontinue using baby lotion, powder, ointment, or baby oil (except zinc oxide).
- Disposable baby wipes contain substances that induce contact or irritant dermatitis, such as fragrance, benzalkonium chloride, and isothiazolinone or alcohol.
- Apply zinc oxide ointment or other barrier cream to the rash at the earliest sign and b.i.d. or t.i.d. (e.g., Desitin or Balmex). Thereafter, apply to clean, thoroughly dry skin (1).
- Use mild soap, and pat dry.
- Cornstarch can reduce friction. Talc powders that do not enhance the growth of yeast can provide protection against frictional injury in diaper dermatitis but do not form a continuous lipid barrier layer over the skin and obstruct the skin pores. These treatments are not recommended.

Issues for Referral

Consider if a systemic disease such as Langerhans cell histiocytosis, acrodermatitis enteropathica, or HIV infection is suspected.

IN-PATIENT CONSIDERATIONS

Admission Criteria

- Febrile neonates
- Recalcitrant rash suggestive of immunodeficiency
- Toxic-appearing infants

Nursing

Assist 1st-time parents with hygiene education.

ONGOING CARE

FOLLOW-UP RECOMMENDATIONS

Patient Monitoring

Recheck weekly until clear; then at times of recurrence.

PATIENT EDUCATION

Patient education is vital to the treatment and prevention of recurrent cases.

PROGNOSIS

- Quick, complete clearing with appropriate treatment
- Secondary candidal infections may last a few weeks after treatment is begun.

COMPLICATIONS

- Secondary bacterial infection [consider community-acquired methicillin-resistant *Staphylococcus aureus* (MRSA) in pustular dermatitis that does not respond to normal therapy]
- Rare complication is inoculation with group A β-hemolytic *Streptococcus* resulting in necrotizing fascitis.
- Secondary yeast infection

REFERENCES

1. Scheinfeld N. Diaper dermatitis: A review and brief survey of eruptions of the diaper area. *Am J Clin Derm*. 2005;6:273–81.
2. Janniger CK, Thomas I. Diaper dermatitis: an approach to prevention employing effective diaper care. *Cutis*. 1993;52:153–5.

ADDITIONAL READING

- Alberta L, et al. Diaper dye dermatitis. *Pediatrics*. 2005;116(3):450–2.
- Kazaks EL, et al. Diaper dermatitis. *Pediatr Clin North Am*. 2000;47(4):909–19.

See Also (Topic, Algorithm, Electronic Media Element)

Algorithm: Rash, Focal

CODES

ICD9

- 112.3 Candidiasis of skin and nails
- 691.0 Diaper or napkin rash

CLINICAL PEARLS

- Hygiene is the main preventative measure.
- Look for secondary infection in persistent cases.

DERMATITIS, EXFOLIATIVE

Herbert P. Goodheart, MD

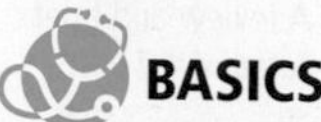

BASICS

DESCRIPTION

- Exfoliative dermatitis (ED), or *erythroderma*, is a rare disorder characterized by a generalized (often >90% of body) scaling eruption of most, if not all, of the skin.
- It may appear suddenly or gradually, occasionally accompanied by fever, chills, and lymphadenopathy.
- It arises idiopathically or secondary to an underlying cutaneous or systemic disease or as a reaction to medications.
- Cutaneous involvement consists of redness and/or scaling of most of the skin.
- When fulminant, this reaction is potentially life-threatening.
- System(s) affected: Skin/Exocrine
- Synonym(s): Erythroderma; Exfoliative erythroderm; Red man syndrome (*homme rouge*); Pityriasis rubra

EPIDEMIOLOGY

The vast majority of patients are older than 40 years of age and are mostly males.

Incidence

- In the US: Rare; estimated 1% of hospitalizations for skin disease
- Predominant age: >40 years, except when it results from atopic dermatitis, seborrheic dermatitis, staphylococcal scalded-skin syndrome, or hereditary ichthyosis, all of which are most common in the pediatric age group.
- Predominant sex: Male > Female (2–4:1)

RISK FACTORS

- Underlying diseases as noted below
- Male sex
- Age >40 years

PATHOPHYSIOLOGY

Arises idiopathically or secondary to an underlying cutaneous or systemic disease, or as a reaction to medications

COMMONLY ASSOCIATED CONDITIONS

- The most common associated conditions or diseases that have been reported to present with or develop into exfoliative dermatitis include:
  - In adults, psoriasis most frequently
  - In children, most often secondary to severe atopic dermatitis
  - Drug reactions
  - Idiopathic in up to 20–30% of cases
- Less commonly, ED has been noted as a finding in the following skin disorders:
  - Allergic contact dermatitis
  - Stasis dermatitis with secondary autoeczematization
  - Pityriasis rubra pilaris (a rare disorder of keratinization)
  - Graft-versus-host disease
  - Seborrheic dermatitis (Leiner disease) in infants
  - Ichthyosiform dermatoses
  - Pemphigus foliaceus
  - Papulosquamous dermatitis of AIDS
  - Fungal disease with id reaction
- Other rare reported associations include:
  - Reiter syndrome
  - SLE
  - Hailey-Hailey disease
  - Norwegian scabies
  - Sarcoidosis
  - Lichen planus
  - Dermatomyositis
- Medications: May occur as a reaction to the following drugs: Allopurinol, antimalarials, aspirin, barbiturates, captopril, codeine, cefoxitin, cimetidine, dapsone, gold salts, hydantoin, isoniazid, lithium, NSAIDs, omeprazole, para-aminosalicylic acid, penicillin, phenylbutazone, phenothiazine, St. John's wort, sulfonamide, sulfonylurea, thalidomide, and vancomycin
- May occur as a complication or presenting symptom of the following malignancies:
  - Mycosis fungoides (cutaneous T-cell lymphoma)
  - Sézary syndrome (leukemic variant of mycosis fungoides)
  - Hodgkin disease
  - Non-Hodgkin lymphoma and leukemia

DIAGNOSIS

- Diagnosis is made on a clinical basis.
- Determination of the cause is often elusive, but history is the most important aid in finding the underlying etiology of ED.

PHYSICAL EXAM

- Nail dystrophy in 40%
- Fever in 40–50%
- Chills
- Malaise/weakness
- Eosinophilia (30%)
- Hepatomegaly (20%)
- Splenomegaly when underlying lymphoma/leukemia is present
- Alopecia
- Hypoproteinemia
- Dehydration
- High-output cardiac failure
- Tachycardia (40%)
- In time, lichenification may occur.
- Postinflammatory dyspigmentation (hyper- or hypopigmented areas of the skin)
- Eliciting a history of drug ingestion or a preexisting dermatosis or disease may be valuable.
- Infrequently, the characteristic lichenification of atopic dermatitis or the nail pitting that suggests psoriasis or islands of sparing in pityriasis rubra pilaris may be found.
- There is marked generalized erythema followed by scaling.
- Pruritus may be severe.
- Edema and increased warmth of the skin
- Pedal or pretibial edema
- Lymphadenopathy, usually a reactive type (*dermatopathic lymphadenopathy*) is often present.
- Most often, primary lesions that might offer clues to making an etiologic diagnosis are obscured or lacking.

DIAGNOSTIC TESTS & INTERPRETATION

Lab

None are diagnostic; however, may have elevated WBC count with eosinophilia, anemia, elevated ESR, decreased albumin, and electrolyte abnormalities

Imaging

CXR and other imaging procedures as indicated to investigate any underlying disease process

Diagnostic Procedures/Surgery

- Laboratory testing can provide serologic evidence of Sézary syndrome or leukemia.
- Patch testing during a period of remission may uncover a contact allergen.
- Skin biopsy (lymph node or bone marrow) as indicated to investigate an underlying disease process
- Further tests are performed if suggested by the review of systems and physical examination.

Pathological Findings

- May have characteristics of an underlying cutaneous disease; however, findings are most often nonspecific and consist of hyperkeratosis, parakeratosis, and acanthosis in the epidermis and edema, vasodilation, and perivascular infiltrates with lymphocytes, histiocytes, and eosinophils in the dermis
- Repeated or multiple biopsies are sometimes helpful in finding an underlying cause.

DIFFERENTIAL DIAGNOSIS
- Extensive acute eczematous dermatoses, such as contact dermatitis and drug eruptions
- Toxic epidermal necrolysis
- Staphylococcal scalded-skin syndrome
- Erythema multiforme major

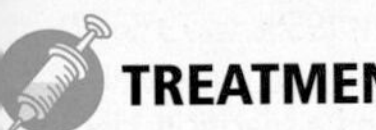

TREATMENT
- Cool tap water dressings
- Application of intermediate-strength topical steroids (e.g., triamcinolone cream 0.025–0.1%) beneath wet dressings
- Cool colloid baths with oatmeal (e.g., Aveeno)
- Local bland moisturizing ointments/lotions
- Systemic antibiotics if signs of secondary infection are observed
- Antihistamines act primarily as sedatives.

ALERT

Systemic steroids may be helpful in some cases, but should be avoided in suspected cases of psoriasis.

MEDICATION
First Line
- Midpotency topical steroids
- In addition, treatment specific to any underlying infection or disease should be provided.
- Systemic steroids: Initial dosage equivalent to prednisone 40 mg/d with increases in dosage by 20 mg/d if there is no response after 3–4 days. Subsequently, dosage should be tapered as symptoms are controlled.
- Oral retinoids: If psoriasis is determined to be the underlying cause of the ED, an oral retinoid such as isotretinoin probably is a better choice than systemic steroids, which may exacerbate psoriasis.

Second Line
- When psoriasis is the underlying cause, cyclosporine, methotrexate, etretinate, phototherapy, photopheresis, photochemotherapy, as well as monoclonal antibodies such as infliximab and alemtuzumab may be effective.
- Photochemotherapy also may be useful therapy for treating ED associated with mycosis fungoides.
- Oral acitretin and isotretinoin have been used when pityriasis rubra pilaris is the underlying cause.
- Antimetabolites/cytotoxic drugs
- Bexarotene
- Infliximab (1)
- Etanercept (2)

ADDITIONAL TREATMENT
General Measures
- Outpatient care except in patients with complications of secondary infection, dehydration, or heart failure
- Withdrawal of any implicated medications or treatment of any identified underlying infection/disease
- Protection from development of hypothermia
- When ED evolves rapidly, the patient frequently requires hospitalization, where measures such as fluid replacement, temperature control, and expert topical skin care are available.

IN-PATIENT CONSIDERATIONS
Admission Criteria
- Impending or actual heart failure
- Inability to control ED on an outpatient basis

Nursing
Bed rest, cool compresses, lubrication with emollients, antipruritic therapy with oral antihistamines, and low- to intermediate-strength topical steroids

ONGOING CARE

DIET
- Increased fluid intake
- Ensure adequate nutrition with emphasis on sufficient protein intake.

PROGNOSIS
- The prognosis of ED depends largely on underlying etiology.
- In patients with an identified underlying cause, the course and prognosis generally will parallel those of the primary disease. For example, in patients who have underlying psoriasis or atopic dermatitis, the progression of disease generally is gradual.
- ED due to a drug eruption usually clears after the drug is discontinued.
- A study of erythrodermic pediatric patients indicated that age <3 years, fever, ill appearance, hypotension, and elevated creatinine levels are poor prognostic signs, and the possibility of toxic shock syndrome should be considered.
- Acute, severe episodes, particularly in elderly persons or in persons with preexisting heart disease, also have a more guarded prognosis.
- In patients with idiopathic ED, the prognosis is poor, and recurrences are not uncommon.

COMPLICATIONS
- Secondary infection, sepsis
- A marked loss of exfoliated scales (uncontrolled mitosis and desquamation) and an increase in cutaneous blood perfusion may contribute to:
  - Dehydration/electrolyte disturbances
  - Hypoalbuminemia
  - Edema
  - Heat loss and hypothermia
  - Possible high-output cardiac failure and death
- Depending on the underlying cause and possible complications, the overall mortality ranges from 20–40%.

REFERENCES

1. Rongioletti F, Borenstein M, Kirsner R, et al. Erythrodermic, recalcitrant psoriasis: clinical resolution with infliximab. *J Dermatolog Treat.* 2003;14:222–5.
2. Querfeld C, Guitart J, et al. Successful treatment of recalcitrant, erythroderma-associated pruritus with etanercept. *Arch Dermatol.* 2004;140(12): 1539–40.

ADDITIONAL READING

- Byer RL, Bachur RG. Clinical deterioration among patients with fever and erythroderma. *Pediatrics.* 2006;118:2450–60.
- Heald P. The treatment of cutaneous T-cell lymphoma with a novel retinoid. *Clin Lymphoma.* 2000:1S45–1S49.
- Okoduwa C, Lambert WC, Schwartz RA, et al. Erythroderma: review of a potentailly life-threatening dermatosis. *Indian J Dermatol.* 2009;54(1):1–6.
- Ott H, Hütten M, Baron JM, et al. Neonatal and infantile erythrodermas. *J Dtsch Dermatol Ges.* 2008;6:1070–85; quiz 1086.
- Pruszkowski A, Bodemer C, Fraitag S, et al. Neonatal and infantile erythrodermas: a retrospective study of 51 patients. *Arch Dermatol.* 2000;136:875–80.
- Tomi NS, Kränke B, Aberer E. Staphylococcal toxins in patients with psoriasis, atopic dermatitis, and erythroderma, and in healthy control subjects. *J Am Acad Dermatol.* 2005;53:67–72.

See Also (Topic, Algorithm, Electronic Media Element)
Algorithm: Rash, Focal

CODES

ICD9
695.89 Other specified erythematous conditions

CLINICAL PEARLS
- In its more severe manifestations, ED is a medical and dermatologic emergency.
- In many cases, the underlying cause is never established.

DERMATITIS HERPETIFORMIS

Anne M. Mahoney, MD
Amit Garg, MD

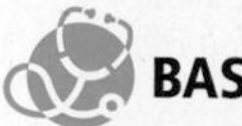

BASICS

DESCRIPTION

- Dermatitis herpetiformis (DH) is a chronic, intensely pruritic papulovesicular eruption involving primarily extensor skin surfaces (elbows, knees, buttocks, back) and the scalp.
- DH is distinguished from other bullous diseases by characteristic histologic and immunologic findings, as well as associated gluten-sensitive enteropathy (1).
- Within the spectrum of gluten-sensitive disorders, which include celiac disease (CD), some forms of IgA nephropathy, and gluten-sensitive ataxia (2)
- System(s) affected: Skin
- Synonym(s): Duhring disease

EPIDEMIOLOGY

- Occurs most frequently in those of Northern European origin
- Rare in persons of Asian or African-American origin
- Predominant age: Most common between the ages of 30 and 40 years but may occur in children
- Predominant sex: Male > Female (1.4:1 in the US, 2:1 worldwide)

Incidence

0.98/100,000 persons per year in US

Prevalence

11/100,000 persons in US population; as high as 39/100,000 persons worldwide

RISK FACTORS

- Gluten-sensitive enteropathy (GSE): >90% of those with DH will have GSE, which may be asymptomatic.
- Family history of DH or CD

Genetics

- High incidence of human leukocyte antigen A1, B8, DR3, and DQ2 (1)
- Strong association with combination of alleles DQA1*0501 and DQB1*02 OR DQA1*03 and DQB1*0302 (3)

GENERAL PREVENTION

Gluten-free diet (GFD) results in improvement of DH and reduces dependence on medical therapy. GFD also may prevent complications associated with DH.

PATHOPHYSIOLOGY

- Evidence suggests that epidermal transglutaminase (eTG) 3, a keratinocyte enzyme involved in cell envelope formation, is the autoantigen in DH (4).
- eTG is highly homologous with tissue transglutaminase (tTG), which is the antigenic target in celiac disease (3).
- The initiating event for DH is presumed to be the interaction of wheat peptides with TTGs, which results in activation of T cells and the humoral immune system.
- IgA antibodies against tTGs cross-react with eTG and result in IgA-eTG immune complexes that are deposited in the papillary dermis. Subsequent activation of complement and recruitment of neutrophils to the area result in inflammation and blistering.
- Skin eruption may be delayed 5–6 weeks after exposure to gluten.
- Gluten applied directly to the skin does not result in the eruption, whereas gluten taken by mouth or rectum does. This implies necessary processing by the GI system (2).

ETIOLOGY

Thought to be autoimmune or immune complex–mediated (3)

COMMONLY ASSOCIATED CONDITIONS

- Gluten-sensitive enteropathy
- Gastric atrophy, hypochlorhydria, pernicious anemia
- Gastrointestinal lymphoma, non-Hodgkin lymphoma
- Hyperthyroidism, hypothyroidism, thyroid nodules, thyroid cancer
- Down syndrome
- Glomerulopathy
- Autoimmune disorders, including systemic lupus erythematosus, dermatomyositis, Sjögren syndrome, rheumatoid arthritis, Raynaud phenomenon, insulin-dependent diabetes mellitus, myasthenia gravis, Addison disease, vitiligo, alopecia, and psoriasis

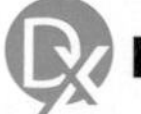

DIAGNOSIS

Diagnosis of DH involves a clinicopathologic correlation among clinical presentation, histologic and direct immunofluorescence evaluation, serology, and response to therapy or diet restriction.

HISTORY

- Waxing and waning, intensely pruritic eruption with papules and tiny vesicles
- Eruption may worsen with gluten intake.
- GI symptoms may be absent or may not be reported until prompted.

PHYSICAL EXAM

- Symmetric, grouped, erythematous papules and vesicles
- Only erosions, excoriations, and hyperpigmentation secondary to scratching may be apparent on presentation (5).
- Areas involved include extensor surfaces of elbows (90%), knees (30%), shoulders, buttocks, and sacrum. The scalp is also frequently affected. Oral lesions are rare. Palms and soles are spared (5).
- The eruption in children is similar to that in adults (2).
- Adults with associated enteropathy are most often asymptomatic, with <10% complaining of bloating, diarrhea, or steatorrhea.
- Children with associated enteropathy may present with abdominal pain, diarrhea, iron deficiency, and reduced growth rate (5).

DIAGNOSTIC TESTS & INTERPRETATION

The "gold standard" for diagnosing DH is direct immunofluorescence on skin, which demonstrates that granular IgA is deposited in the dermal papillae (5)[A].

Lab

Initial lab tests

- IgA TTG antibodies: Detection of tTG antibodies was noted to be 94.4% sensitive and 92.3% specific for DH in patients on unrestricted diets (6).
- IgA eTG antibodies: Antibodies to eTG, the primary autoantigen in DH, were shown to be more sensitive than antibodies to tTG in the diagnosis of patients with DH on unrestricted diets (95% vs 79%) (7).
- IgA endomysial antibodies: Have a sensitivity between 50% and 100% and a specificity close to 100% in patients on unrestricted diets (5)

Follow-Up & Special Considerations

Serologic assessment of anti-tTG and anti-endomysial antibodies (EMA) may be useful in monitoring major deviations from GFD (5).

Diagnostic Procedures/Surgery

Skin biopsy for hematoxylin and eosin stain and for direct immunofluorescence on skin

Pathological Findings

- Direct immunofluorescence of skin reveals a granular pattern of IgA deposition in the dermal papillae (5).
- Histopathology with routine staining reveals neutrophilic microabscesses in dermal papillae and also may show subepidermal blistering (2).

DIFFERENTIAL DIAGNOSIS

- In adults (5):
  - Bullous pemphigoid: Linear deposition of C3 and IgG at the basement membrane zone
  - Linear IgA disease: Homogeneous and linear deposition of IgA at the basement membrane zone, absence of GSE
  - Transient acantholytic dermatosis
  - Urticaria: Wheals, angioedema, dermal edema
  - Erythema multiforme
- In children (5):
  - Atopic dermatitis: Face and flexural areas
  - Scabies: Interdigital areas, axillae, genital region
  - Papular urticaria: Dermal edema
  - Impetigo

TREATMENT

MEDICATION

- Disease control is achieved with dietary modification, medication, or both.
- Medication is useful for immediate symptom management.
- A GFD is necessary for long-term management of underlying gluten sensitivity.
- Interdisciplinary treatment involves outpatient care with a dermatologist as well as consultations with a gastroenterologist and a registered dietician.

First Line

- Dapsone is the most widely used medication for DH (2)[A].
- It is the only medication approved by the Food and Drug Administration for use in this disease. Adult doses range from 25–400 mg/d, which result in improvement of symptoms within 24–48 h. Use of a minimum effective dose is recommended. Average maintenance dose is 1 mg/kg/d. Minor outbreaks on the face and scalp are common even with treatment.
- Dapsone works by inhibiting neutrophil recruitment, inhibiting the respiratory burst of neutrophils, and protecting cells from neutrophil-mediated injury, thereby suppressing the skin reaction. It has no role in preventing IgA deposition or mitigating the immune reaction in the gut (2).

Precautions:
- Common side effects include nausea, vomiting, headache, dizziness, and weakness
- A drop in hemoglobin of 1–2 g is characteristic with dapsone 100 mg/d.
- G6PD deficiency increases severity of hemolytic stress. Dapsone should be avoided if possible in those who are G6PD-deficient.
- Dose-related methemoglobinemia may occur, typically with doses >100 mg/d.
- Other adverse events include toxic hepatitis, cholestatic jaundice, hypoalbuminemia, sensory and motor neuropathy, psychosis, infectious mononucleosis syndrome with fever and lymphadenopathy, agranulocytosis, aplastic anemia, leukopenia, exfoliative dermatitis, erythema multiforme, erythema nodosum, and urticaria.
- The drug is secreted in breast milk and will produce hemolytic anemia in infants.

ALERT

- Monitor for potentially fatal sulfone syndrome: Fever, jaundice and hepatic necrosis, exfoliative dermatitis, lymphadenopathy, methemoglobinemia, and hemolytic anemia.
- Can occur 48 h or 6 months after treatment, most often 5 weeks after initiation

Pediatric Considerations

- <2 years: Dosing not established
- >2 years: 0.5–1.0 mg/kg/d

Pregnancy Considerations

- Category C: Safety during pregnancy is not established.
- Adherence to a strict GFD 6–12 months before conception should be considered with the hope of eliminating need for dapsone during pregnancy.

Second Line

Sulfasalazine (1–2 g/d), sulphamethoxypyridazine (0.25–1.5 g/d): Side effects include nausea, vomiting, anorexia, hypersensitivity reactions, hemolytic anemia, proteinuria, and crystalluria (5).

ALERT

- Prior to treatment, monthly for the first 3 months of treatment and biannually thereafter, complete blood count (CBC) with differential and urinalysis with urine microscopy should be done (5).
- Colchicine, prednisone, tetracycline plus nicotinamide, minocycline, cyclosporine, and topical steroids are 3rd-line medications.

ADDITIONAL TREATMENT

GFD:
- Average of 2 years is often necessary for diet to completely eliminate skin eruptions, and lesions usually recur within 12 weeks of gluten reintroduction (5).
- Fundamentals of the GFD (8):
  - Grains that should be avoided:
    - Wheat (includes spelt, kamut, semolina, and triticale)
    - Rye
    - Barley (including malt)
  - Safe grains (gluten-free):
    - Rice
    - Amaranth
    - Buckwheat
    - Corn
    - Millet
    - Quinoa
    - Sorghum
    - Teff (an Ethiopian cereal grain)
    - Oats
  - Sources of gluten-free starches that can be used as flour alternatives:
    - Cereal grains: Amaranth, buckwheat, corn, millet, quinoa, sorghum, teff, rice (white, brown, wild, basmati, jasmine), and montina
    - Tubers: Arrowroot, jicama, taro, potato, and tapioca
    - Legumes: Chickpeas, lentils, kidney beans, navy beans, pea beans, peanuts, and soybeans
    - Nuts: Almonds, walnuts, chestnuts, hazelnuts, and cashews
    - Seeds: Sunflower, flax, and pumpkin

ONGOING CARE

FOLLOW-UP RECOMMENDATIONS

Patient Monitoring

If treating with dapsone:
- Obtain baseline CBC and liver function tests.
- Quantify G6PD prior to initiating treatment in Asians, African Americans, and those of southern Mediterranean origin.
- Check CBC weekly for 1st month, monthly for the next 5 months, and semiannually thereafter.
- Check chemistry profile every 6 months.
- Patient should be made aware of potential hemolytic anemia and the signs associated with methemoglobinemia.

DIET

- 87% of patients showed complete remission of skin manifestations after 18 months of a GFD (9)[C]
- Improvement in cutaneous disease and normalization of small bowel mucosa result from strict compliance with a GFD in most patients (5)[C].

PATIENT EDUCATION

- American Academy of Dermatology, 930 N. Meacham Road., P.O. Box 4014, Schaumberg, IL 60168-4014; (708) 330-0230
- Gluten Intolerance Group of North America, 31214–124 Ave. SE, Auburn, WA 98092; phone (206) 246-6652; fax (206) 246-6531; www.gluten.net
- The Celiac Disease Foundation, 13251 Ventura Blvd., #1, Studio City, CA 9160; phone (818) 990-2354; fax (818) 990-2379

PROGNOSIS

- Lifelong disease
- Remission in 10–20%
- Skin disease responds readily to dapsone.
- Strict adherence to a GFD improves clinical symptoms and decreases dapsone requirement. GFD is the only sustainable method of eliminating cutaneous and GI disease. Dapsone does not alter GI mucosal pathology.
- Occasional new lesions (2–3 per week) are to be expected and are not an indication for altering daily dosage.
- Risk of lymphoma may be decreased in those who maintain a GFD.

COMPLICATIONS

- Malnutrition, weight loss
- Abdominal pain, dyspepsia
- Nutritional deficiencies (folate, B_{12}, iron)
- Osteoporosis
- Chronic fatigue
- Autoimmune diseases
- Lymphomas

REFERENCES

1. Patrício P, Ferreira C, Gomes MM, Filipe P et al. Autoimmune bullous dermatoses: a review. *Ann N Y Acad Sci*. 2009;1173:203–10.
2. Nicolas ME, Krause PK, Gibson LE, et al. Dermatitis herpetiformis. *Int J Dermatol*. 2003;42:588–600.
3. Kárpáti S et al. Dermatitis herpetiformis: close to unravelling a disease. *J Dermatol Sci*. 2004;34: 83–90.
4. Sárdy M, Kárpáti S, Merkl B, et al. Epidermal transglutaminase (TGase 3) is the autoantigen of dermatitis herpetiformis. *J Exp Med*. 2002;195: 747–57.
5. Caproni M, Antiga E, Melani L, et al. Guidelines for the diagnosis and treatment of dermatitis herpetiformis. *J Eur Acad Dermatol Venereol*. 2009.
6. Caproni M, Cardinali C, Renzi D, et al. Tissue transglutaminase antibody assessment in dermatitis herpetiformis. *Br J Dermatol*. 2001;144:196–7.
7. Rose C, Armbruster FP, Ruppert J, Igl BW, Zillikens D, Shimanovich I et al. Autoantibodies against epidermal transglutaminase are a sensitive diagnostic marker in patients with dermatitis herpetiformis on a normal or gluten-free diet. *J Am Acad Dermatol*. 2009;61:39–43.
8. Green PH, Cellier C. Celiac disease. *N Engl J Med*. 2007;357:1731–43.
9. Nino M, Ciacci C, Delfino M. A long-term gluten-free diet as an alternative treatment in severe forms of dermatitis herpetiformis. *J Dermatolog Treat*. 2007;18:10–2.

ADDITIONAL READING

Desai AM, Krishnan RS, Hsu S. Medical pearl: Using tissue transglutaminase antibodies to diagnose dermatitis herpetiformis. *J Am Acad Dermatol*. 2005;53:867–8.

See Also (Topic, Algorithm, Electronic Media Element)

Celiac Disease
Algorithm: Rash, Focal

CODES

ICD9

694.0 Dermatitis herpetiformis

CLINICAL PEARLS

- DH is a chronic, intensely pruritic papulovesicular eruption involving primarily extensor skin surfaces symmetrically as well as the scalp.
- Strong association with gluten-sensitive enteropathy
- Diagnosed by skin biopsy with direct immunofluorescence
- 1st-line treatment: Dapsone

D

DERMATITIS, SEBORRHEIC

Juan Qiu, MD, PhD

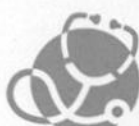

BASICS

DESCRIPTION

Chronic, superficial, recurrent inflammatory rash affecting sebum-rich, hairy regions of the body, especially scalp, eyebrows, and face

EPIDEMIOLOGY

Incidence

- Predominant age: Infancy, adolescence, and adulthood
- Predominant sex: Male > Female

Prevalence

Seborrheic dermatitis: 3–5%

RISK FACTORS

- Parkinson disease
- AIDS (disease severity correlated with progression of immune deficiency)
- Emotional stress
- Medications may flare or induce seborrheic dermatitis: Auranofin, aurothioglucose, buspirone, chlorpromazine, cimetidine, ethionamide, gold, griseofulvin, haloperidol, interferon alfa, lithium, methoxsalen, methyldopa, phenothiazine, psoralen, stanozolol, thiothixene, trioxsalen

Genetics

Positive family history; no genetic marker identified to date

GENERAL PREVENTION

Seborrheic skin should be washed more often than usual.

PATHOPHYSIOLOGY

Helper T cells, phytohemagglutinin and concanavalin stimulation, and antibody titers are depressed compared with those of control subjects.

ETIOLOGY

- Skin surface yeasts *Malassezia* (formerly *P. ovale*) may be a contributing factor (1).
- *Malassezia* spp. may have a role in T-cell suppression and complement activation.
- The mite *D. folliculorum* may have a direct or indirect role.
- Genetic and environmental factors: Flares are common with stress or illness.
- Parallels increased sebaceous gland activity in infancy and adolescence or as a result of some acnegenic drugs

COMMONLY ASSOCIATED CONDITIONS

- Parkinson disease
- AIDS

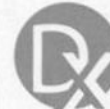

DIAGNOSIS

The diagnosis of seborrheic dermatitis usually can be made by history and physical examination.

HISTORY

- Intermittent active phases manifest with burning, scaling, and itching alternating with inactive periods; activity is increased in winter and early spring, with remissions commonly occurring in summer.
- Infants:
  - Cradle cap: Greasy scaling of scalp, sometimes with associated mild erythema
  - Diaper and/or axillary rash
  - Age at onset typically ~1 month
  - Usually resolves by 8–12 months
- Adults:
  - Red, greasy, scaling rash in most locations consisting of patches and plaques with indistinct margins
  - Red, smooth, glazed appearance in skin folds
  - Minimal pruritus
  - Chronic waxing and waning course
  - Bilateral and symmetric
  - Most commonly located in hairy skin areas: Scalp and scalp margins, eyebrows and eyelid margins, nasolabial folds, ears and retroauricular folds, presternal area, and middle to upper back, buttock crease, inguinal area, genitals, and armpits

PHYSICAL EXAM

- Scalp appearance varies from mild, patchy scaling to widespread, thick, adherent crusts. Plaques are rare.
- Seborrheic dermatitis can spread onto the forehead, the posterior part of the neck, and the postauricular skin, as in psoriasis.
- Skin lesions manifest as branny or greasy scaling over red, inflamed skin.
- Hypopigmentation is seen in blacks.
- Infectious eczematoid dermatitis, with oozing and crusting, suggests secondary infection.
- Seborrheic blepharitis may occur independently.

DIAGNOSTIC TESTS & INTERPRETATION

Diagnostic Procedures/Surgery

Consider biopsy if:

- Usual therapies fail
- Petechiae noted
- Histiocytosis X suspected
- Fungal cultures in refractory cases or when pustules and alopecia are present

Pathological Findings

Nonspecific changes:

- Hyperkeratosis, acanthosis, accentuated rete ridges, focal spongiosis, and parakeratosis are characteristic.
- Parakeratotic scale around hair follicles and mild superficial inflammatory lymphocytic infiltrate

DIFFERENTIAL DIAGNOSIS

- Atopic dermatitis: Distinction may be difficult in infants.
- Psoriasis:
  - Usually knees, elbows, and nails are involved.
  - Scalp psoriasis will be more sharply demarcated than seborrhea, with crusted, infiltrated plaques rather than mild scaling and erythema.
- *Candida*
- Tinea cruris or capitis: Suspect these when usual medications fail or if hair loss occurs.
- Eczema of auricle or otitis externa
- Rosacea
- Discoid lupus erythematosus: Skin biopsy will be beneficial.
- Histiocytosis X: May appear as seborrheic-type eruption
- Dandruff: Scalp only, noninflammatory

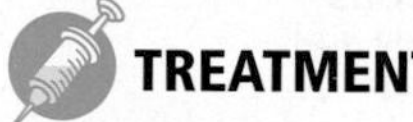

TREATMENT

MEDICATION

First Line

- Cradle cap: Use a coal tar shampoo or ketoconazole (Nizoral) shampoo if the nonmedicated shampoo is ineffective (2).
- Adults:
  - Topical antifungal agents:
    - Ketoconazole 2% foam or shampoo twice a week for clearance, then once a week or every other week for maintenance
    - Ketoconazole (Nizoral) cream may be used to clear scales in other areas.
    - Ciclopirox 1% shampoo twice weekly (1)[B]
  - Topical corticosteroids:
    - Begin with 1% hydrocortisone, and advance to more potent (fluorinated) steroid preparations as needed.

- Avoid continuous use of the more potent steroids to reduce the risk of skin atrophy, hypopigmentation, or systemic absorption (especially in infants and children).
- Precautions: Fluorinated corticosteroids and higher concentrations of hydrocortisone (e.g., 2.5%) may cause atrophy or striae if used on the face or on skin folds.
- Other topical agents:
  - Coal tar1% shampoo twice a week
  - Selenium sulfide 2.5% shampoo twice a week
  - Zinc pyrithione shampoo twice a week
  - Lithium succinate ointment twice a week
- Once controlled, washing with zinc soaps or selenium lotion with periodic use of steroid cream may help to maintain remission.

Second Line

- Calcineurin inhibitors:
  - Pimercolimus 1% cream twice daily
  - Tacrolimus 0.1% ointment twice daily
- Systemic antifungal therapy:
  - Data are limited.
  - For moderate to severe seborrheic dermatitis:
    - Ketoconazole 200 mg/d
    - Itraconazole 200 mg/d
    - Daily regimen for 1–2 months followed by twice-weekly dosing for chronic treatment
    - Monitor potential hepatotoxic effects.

ADDITIONAL TREATMENT

General Measures

- Increase frequency of shampooing.
- Sunlight in moderate doses may be helpful.
- Cradle cap:
  - Frequent shampooing with a mild, nonmedicated shampoo
  - Remove thick scale by applying warm mineral oil, and then wash off an hour later with a mild soap and a soft-bristle toothbrush or terrycloth washcloth (2).
- Adults: Wash all affected areas with antiseborrheic shampoos. Start with over-the-counter brands (Tegrin, Selsun Blue), and increase to more potent preparations (containing coal tar, sulfur, selenium, or salicylic acid) if no improvement is noted (2).
- For dense scalp scaling, 10% liquor carbonic detergens in Nivea oil may be used at bedtime, covering the head with a shower cap. This should be done nightly for 1–3 weeks.

Issues for Referral

No response to 1st-line therapy and concerns regarding systemic illness (HIV, etc.)

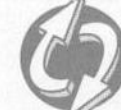

ONGOING CARE

FOLLOW-UP RECOMMENDATIONS

Patient Monitoring

Every 2–12 weeks as necessary depending on disease severity and degree of patient sophistication

PATIENT EDUCATION

http://familydoctor.org/online/famdocen/home/common/skin/disorders/157.html

PROGNOSIS

- In infants, seborrheic dermatitis usually remits after 6–8 months.
- In adults, seborrheic dermatitis is usually chronic and unpredictable, with exacerbations and remissions. Disease is usually easily controlled with shampoos and topical steroids.

COMPLICATIONS

- Skin atrophy or striae are possible from fluorinated corticosteroids, especially if used on the face.
- Glaucoma can result from use of fluorinated steroids around the eyes.
- Photosensitivity is caused occasionally by tars.
- Herpes keratitis is a rare complication of herpes simplex: Instruct patient to stop eyelid steroids if herpes simplex develops.

REFERENCES

1. Shuster S, Meynadier J, Kerl H, et al. Treatment and prophylaxis of seborrheic dermatitis of the scalp with antipityrosporal 1% ciclopirox shampoo. *Arch Dermatol*. 2005;141:47–52.
2. Johnson BA, Nunley JR. Treatment of seborrheic dermatitis. *Am Fam Physician*. 2000;61:2703–10, 2713–4.

ADDITIONAL READING

- Darabi K, Hostetler SG, Bechtel MA, et al. The role of Malassezia in atopic dermatitis affecting the head and neck of adults. *J Am Acad Dermatol*. 2008.
- Karincaoglu Y, Tepe B, Kalayci B, et al. Is Demodex folliculorum an aetiological factor in seborrhoeic dermatitis? *Clin Exp Dermatol*. 2009.
- Naldi L, Rebora A. Clinical practice. Seborrheic dermatitis. *N Engl J Med*. 2009;360:387–96.
- Shemer A, Kaplan B, Nathansohn N, et al. Treatment of moderate to severe facial seborrheic dermatitis with itraconazole: an open non-comparative study. *Isr Med Assoc J*. 2008;10:417–8.
- Shin H, Kwon OS, Won CH, et al. Clinical efficacies of topical agents for the treatment of seborrheic dermatitis of the scalp: A comparative study. *J Dermatol*. 2009;36:131–7.

See Also (Topic, Algorithm, Electronic Media Element)

Algorithm: Rash, Focal

CODES

ICD9

- 690.10 Seborrheic dermatitis, unspecified
- 690.11 Seborrhea capitis
- 690.12 Seborrheic infantile dermatitis

CLINICAL PEARLS

Search for an underlying systemic disease in a patient who is unresponsive to usual therapy.

DERMATITIS, STASIS

Joseph A. Florence, MD

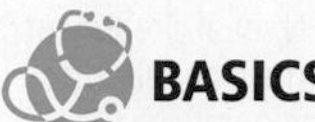

BASICS

DESCRIPTION

- Chronic, eczematous, erythremic, scaling, and noninflammatory edema of the lower extremities accompanied by cycle of scratching, excoriations, weeping, crusting, and inflammation in patients with chronic venous insufficiency, due to impaired circulation and other factors (nutritional edema)
- Clinical skin manifestation of chronic venous insufficiency usually appears late in the disease
- May present as a solitary lesion
- System(s) affected: Skin/Exocrine
- Synonym(s): Gravitational eczema; Varicose eczema; Venous dermatitis

EPIDEMIOLOGY

Incidence

- In the US: Common in patients >50 (6–7%)
- Predominant age: Adult, geriatric
- Predominant sex: Female > Male

Geriatric Considerations

- Common in this age group
- Estimated to affect 15–20 million patients >50 years in the US

RISK FACTORS

- Atopy
- Superimposition of itch–scratch cycle
- Trauma
- Previous deep vein thrombosis (DVT)
- Previous pregnancy
- Prolonged medical illness
- Obesity
- Secondary infection
- Low-protein diet
- Old age
- Deposition of fibrin around capillaries
- Microvascular abnormalities
- Ischemia
- Genetic propensity
- Edema
- Tight garments that constrict the thigh
- Vein stripping
- Vein harvesting for coronary artery bypass graft surgery
- Previous cellulitis

Genetics

Familial link probable

GENERAL PREVENTION

- Use compression stockings to avoid recurrence of edema and to mobilize the interstitial lymphatic fluid from the region of stasis dermatitis.
- Topical lubricants twice a day to prevent fissuring and itching

ETIOLOGY

- Incompetence of perforating veins causing blood to backflow to the superficial venous system leading to venous hypertension (HTN) and cutaneous inflammation
- Continuous presence of edema in ankles, usually present because of venous valve incompetency (varicose veins)
- Weakness of venous walls in lower extremities
- Trauma to edematous, eczematized skin
- Itch may be caused by inflammatory mediators (from mast cells, monocytes, macrophages, or neutrophils) liberated in the microcirculation and endothelium
- Abnormal leukocyte-endothelium interaction is proposed to be a major factor.
- A cascade of biochemical events leads to ulceration.
- Is associated with amlodipine therapy
- Elevated homocysteine has been noted in patients with stasis dermatitis.

COMMONLY ASSOCIATED CONDITIONS

- Varicose veins
- Venous insufficiency
- Other eczematous disease

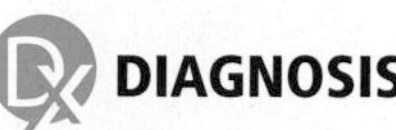

DIAGNOSIS

HISTORY

- Erythema, scaling, edema of lower extremities
- Pruritus
- Excoriations
- Weeping, crusting, inflammation of the skin
- Noninflammatory edema precedes the skin eruption and ulceration.
- Edema initially develops around the ankle.
- Itching, pain, and burning may precede skin signs, which are aggravated during evening hours (1)[B].
- Insidious onset
- Usually bilateral
- Description may include aching/heavy legs

PHYSICAL EXAM

- Evaluation of the lower extremities characteristically reveals:
  - Bilateral scaly, eczematous patches, papules, and/or plaques
  - Violaceous (sometimes brown), erythematous-colored lesions due to deoxygenation of venous blood (postinflammatory hyperpigmentation and hemosiderin deposition within the cutaneous tissue)
- Distribution: Medial aspect of ankle with frequent extension onto the foot and lower leg
- Brawny induration
- Stasis ulcers (frequently accompany stasis dermatitis) secondary to cuts, bruises, and excoriations to the weakened skin around the ankle
- Mild pruritus, pain (if ulcer present)
- Varicosities are often associated with ulcers.
- Clinical inspection reveals erythematous color with increased pigmentation, swelling, and warmth.
- Skin changes are more common in the lower 3rd of the extremity and medially.
- Early signs include prominent superficial veins and pitting ankle edema.
- May present as a solitary lesion (2)[C]

DIAGNOSTIC TESTS & INTERPRETATION

Lab

Initial lab tests

Culture stasis ulcers if bacterial infection is suspected.

Imaging

Initial approach

Duplex ultrasound imaging is helpful in diagnosis (3)[C].

Diagnostic Procedures/Surgery

Rule out arterial insufficiency (check peripheral pulses, leg blood pressures).

Pathological Findings

Chronic inflammation, characterized histologically by proliferation of small blood vessels in the papillary dermis

DIFFERENTIAL DIAGNOSIS

- Other eczematous diseases:
  - Atopic dermatitis
  - Uremic dermatitis
  - Contact dermatitis (due to topical agents used to self-treat)
  - Neurodermatitis
  - Arterial insufficiency
  - Sickle cell disease causing skin ulceration
  - Cellulitis
  - Erysipelas
- Tinea dermatophyte infection
- Pretibial myxedema
- Nummular eczema
- Lichen simplex chronicus
- Xerosis
- Asteatotic eczema
- Amyopathic dermatomyositis

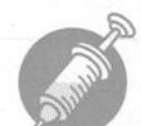

TREATMENT

MEDICATION

First Line

- Use of antibiotics topically or systemically is controversial, as stasis ulcer may not be infected.
- Antibiotics are indicated if bacterial infection is present, or may be used empirically if bacterial infection is suspected.
- If ulcer is present, local povidone-iodine treatment is as effective as systemic antibiotics (4)[B].
- If secondary infection, treat with oral antibiotics for *Staphylococcus* or *Streptococcus* organisms (e.g., dicloxacillin 250 mg q.i.d., cephalexin 250 mg q.i.d. or 500 mg b.i.d., or levofloxacin 250 mg q.i.d.).

Gram-negative colonization: Treat with topical antimicrobial agents (e.g., benzoyl peroxide, acetic acid, silver nitrate, or Hibiclens) or broad-spectrum topical antibiotics (e.g., neomycin or bacitracin-polymyxin B [Polysporin]).

5% Aluminum acetate (Burow solution) wet dressings and cooling pastes

Topical triamcinolone 0.1% (Kenalog, Aristocort) cream/ointment t.i.d. or topical betamethasone

Betamethasone valerate (Valisone) 0.1% cream/ointment/solution t.i.d. (5)[A]

Topical antipruritic: Pramoxine, camphor, menthol, and doxepin

Systemic steroids for severe cases

Calcium dobesilate has been shown to be an effective adjuvant therapy (6)[B].

Vitamin supplementation in patients with hyperhomocysteinemia (7)[C]

Evidenced-based treatment options for associated venous ulcers include aspirin and pentoxifylline (8)[B].

Second Line

Consider antibiotics on basis of culture results of exudate from ulcer craters.

Lubricants when dermatitis is quiescent

Chronic stasis dermatitis can be treated with topical emollients (e.g., white petroleum, lanolin, Eucerln).

Antipruritic medications (e.g., diphenhydramine, cetirizine hydrochloride, desloratadine)

ADDITIONAL TREATMENT

If the patient is on amlodipine therapy consider discontinuing amlodipine (9)[B].

General Measures

Primary role of treatment is to reverse effects of venous HTN. Appropriate health care:

Outpatient:

- Reduce edema (8)[B]:
  - Leg elevation: Heels higher than knees, knees higher than hips
  - Compression therapy: Elastic bandage wraps: Ace bandages or Unna paste boot (zinc gelatin) if lesions are dry or compression stockings (Jobst or nonfitted type) (10,11)[A]
  - Pneumatic compression devices
  - Diuretic therapy
- Treat infection:
  - Débride the ulcer base of necrotic tissue.
  - Improvement of lipodermatosclerosis
- Activity:
  - Avoid standing still.
  - Stay active and exercise regularly.
  - Elevate foot of bed unless contraindicated.

Inpatient for vein stripping, sclerotherapy, or skin grafts:

- Venous ulcer treatment includes autolytic, biologic, chemical, mechanical, and surgical:
  - Autolytic: Hydrogels, alginates, hydrocolloids, foams, and films
  - Biologic: Topical application of granulocyte macrophage colony-stimulating factor promotes healing of ulcers.
  - Chemical: Enzyme débriding agents
  - Mechanical: Wet to dry dressings, hydrotherapy, and irrigation
  - Surgical modifying cause of venous HTN, treat ulcer by graft

SURGERY/OTHER PROCEDURES

Sclerotherapy and surgery may be required.

ONGOING CARE

FOLLOW-UP RECOMMENDATIONS

Patient Monitoring

If Unna boot compression is used: Cut off and reapply boot once a week (restricts edema and prevents scratching).

DIET

- No special diet
- Lose weight, if overweight

PATIENT EDUCATION

- Stress staying active to keep circulation and leg muscles in good condition. Walking is ideal.
- Keep legs elevated while sitting or lying.
- Don't wear girdles, garters, or pantyhose with tight elastic tops.
- Don't scratch.
- Elevate foot of bed with 2–4-inch blocks.

PROGNOSIS

- Chronic course with intermittent exacerbations and remissions
- The healing process for ulceration is often prolonged and may take months.

COMPLICATIONS

- Sensations of itching, pain, and burning have negative impact on the quality of life
- Secondary bacterial infection
- DVT
- Bleeding at dermatitis sites
- Squamous cell carcinoma in edges of long-standing stasis ulcers
- Scarring, which in turn leads to further compromise to blood flow and increased likelihood of minor trauma

REFERENCES

1. Duque MI, Yosipovitch G, Chan YH, et al. Itch, pain, and burning sensation are common symptoms in mild to moderate chronic venous insufficiency with an impact on quality of life. *J Am Acad Dermatol*. 2005;53:504–8.
2. Weaver J, Billings SD et al. Initial presentation of stasis dermatitis mimicking solitary lesions: a previously unrecognized clinical scenario. *J Am Acad Dermatol*. 2009;61:1028–32.
3. Coleridge-Smith P, Labropoulos N, Partsch H, et al. Duplex ultrasound investigation of the veins in chronic venous disease of the lower limbs–UIP consensus document. Part I. Basic principles. *Eur J Vasc Endovasc Surg*. 2006;31:83–92.
4. Daróczy J. Quality control in chronic wound management: the role of local povidone-iodine (Betadine) therapy. *Dermatology*. 2006;212 (Suppl 1):82–7.
5. Weiss SC, Nguyen J, Chon S, et al. A randomized controlled clinical trial assessing the effect of betamethasone valerate 0.12% foam on the short-term treatment of stasis dermatitis. *J Drugs Dermatol*. 2005;4:339–45.
6. Kaur C, Sarkar R, Kanwar AJ, et al. An open trial of calcium dobesilate in patients with venous ulcers and stasis dermatitis. *Int J Dermatol*. 2003;42: 147–52.
7. Kartal Durmazlar SP, Akgul A, Eskioglu F et al. Hyperhomocysteinemia in patients with stasis dermatitis and ulcer: A novel finding with important therapeutic implications. *J Dermatolog Treat*. 2009;1–4.
8. Collins L, Seraj S et al. Diagnosis and treatment of venous ulcers. *Am Fam Physician*. 2010;81: 989–96.
9. Gosnell AL, Nedorost ST et al. Stasis dermatitis as a complication of amlodipine therapy. *J Drugs Dermatol*. 2009;8:135–7.
10. Partsch H, Flour M, Coleridge Smith P. Indications for compression therapy in venous and lymphatic disease Consensus based on experimental data and scientific evidence. Under the auspices of the IUP. *Int Angiol*. 2008;27:193–219.
11. Coleridge-Smith PD. Leg ulcer treatment. *J Vasc Surg*. 2009;49:804–8.

ADDITIONAL READING

- Antignani PL. Classification of chronic venous insufficiency: a review. *Angiology*. 2001; 52 (Suppl 1):S17–26.
- Durmazlar SPK, Akgul A, Eskioglu F. Hyperhomocysteinemia in patients with stasis dermatitis and ulcer: A novel finding with important therapeutic implications. *J Dermatolog Treat*. 2009;20:3;1–4.

See Also (Topic, Algorithm, Electronic Media Element)

Varicose Veins

Algorithm: Rash, focal

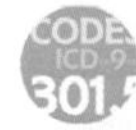

CODES

ICD9

- 454.1 Varicose veins of lower extremities with inflammation
- 459.81 Venous (peripheral) insufficiency, unspecified

CLINICAL PEARLS

Treatment of edema associated with stasis dermatitis via elevation and/or compression stockings is essential for optimal results.

DIABETES INSIPIDUS

Kristine Willett, PharmD
Susan White, MD

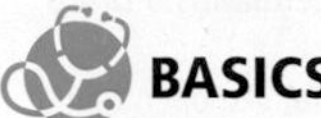

BASICS

DESCRIPTION

- A condition of intense thirst (polydipsia) and excessive urination (polyuria) owing to the kidneys' inability to conserve water as they filter blood.
- Most commonly, this results from decreased pituitary secretion of vasopressin [central diabetes insipidus (DI)] or failure of response to vasopressin (nephrogenic DI).
- Rarely, DI can be induced by pregnancy (gestational DI)
- System(s) affected: Endocrine/Metabolic

EPIDEMIOLOGY

Incidence

- 1/25,000 persons
- May occur in 18.3% following transsphenoidal microsurgery
- Causes of DI:
  - 30% idiopathic
  - 25% brain tumors (malignant or benign)
  - 16% head trauma
  - 20% after cranial surgery

Prevalence

- Vasopressin deficiency may occur at any age.
- Nephrogenic DI is usually manifest in infancy.
- Nephrogenic DI is encountered in males more commonly, reflecting its X-linked mode of inheritance.

RISK FACTORS

- Intracranial neoplasm
- Infection
- Following surgery
- Drug-induced (amphotericin B, colchicine, demeclocycline, foscarnet, gentamicin, lithium, loop diuretics, methoxyflurane)
- Head trauma
- Genetic predisposition

Genetics

- Central DI: Familial cases of vasopressin deficiency have been reported (commonly autosomal dominant; >20 mutations have been identified), but the disease usually is isolated and often secondary to other disorders.
- Nephrogenic DI:
  - Most common is an X-linked defect in the V_2 receptor that binds antidiuretic hormone (ADH).
  - Autosomal dominant or recessive defects in the aquaporin-2 gene that encodes an ADH-responsive water channel

PATHOPHYSIOLOGY

- Central DI:
  - Inadequate secretion of vasopressin may be due to loss or malfunction of the neurosecretory neurons that make up the neurohypophysis (posterior pituitary) and the pituitary stalk.
  - Posterior pituitary lesions rarely cause DI because ADH is produced in the hypothalamus and therefore still would be secreted.
- Nephrogenic DI:
  - Inadequate response of kidney to vasopressin
  - A disorder of renal tubular function resulting in inability to respond to vasopressin in absorption of water

ETIOLOGY

- Central DI (inadequate secretion of vasopressin; may be idiopathic or familial):
  - Idiopathic
  - Trauma/head injury: A study of 89 patients with traumatic brain injury found that primary hormonal dysfunction (including DI) occurred in 21% of patients and tended to occur in patients with the lowest Glasgow Outcome Scale scores (1).
  - Neurosurgery
  - Tumors (e.g., craniopharyngioma, lymphoma, metastasis)
  - Infections (e.g., meningitis, encephalitis)
  - Granulomas (e.g., sarcoid, histiocytosis)
  - Hypoxic encephopathy
  - Vascular disorders
  - Inheritable defects (rare, occurs in 1–2%)
- Nephrogenic DI (inadequate response of kidneys to vasopressin):
  - Familial genetic defect in resorption of water in renal collecting ducts, including X-linked V_2 receptor mutation and autosomal recessive aquaporin-2 mutation
  - Drug induced (amphotericin B, colchicine, demeclocycline, foscarnet, gentamicin, lithium, loop diuretics, methoxyflurane)

COMMONLY ASSOCIATED CONDITIONS

- Potassium depletion
- Chronic hypercalcemia
- Tumors
- Infection:
  - Encephalitis
  - Tuberculosis
  - Syphilis
- Xanthomatosis
- Pyelonephritis
- Renal amyloidosis
- Sjögren syndrome
- Sickle-cell anemia
- Multiple myeloma
- Wolfram syndrome (DIDMOAD: *DI*, *d*iabetes *m*ellitus, *o*ptic *a*trophy, *d*eafness)

DIAGNOSIS

The diagnosis of DI may be difficult to make because the clinical presentation depends on the cause, severity, and other medical conditions that may or ma not be present. The course of DI not associated with brain injury tends to be indolent and, as long as wate is available, may be hard to detect. Polyuria is highly variable, as is tolerance for dehydration.

HISTORY

- Thirst/polydipsia (with a particular preference for cold or iced drinks)
- Polyuria (3–20 L/d)
- Nocturia, bed wetting
- Dehydration
- Headache
- Visual disturbances
- Rate of onset of polydipsia is more rapid in central DI than in nephrogenic DI.
- Family history of polyuria
- In children, enuresis, anorexia, linear growth defects, and frequent fatigue may be found.
- In infants, crying, irritability, poor growth, hyperthermia, and weight loss are often found.

PHYSICAL EXAM

Signs of dehydration and an enlarged bladder may be present, but otherwise the exam is usually unremarkable.

DIAGNOSTIC TESTS & INTERPRETATION

Lab

- Low urine specific gravity and osmolality are indicative of DI.
- Urine/plasma osmolality ratio and plasma vasopressin concentration results may be difficult to interpret; low ratios may be found in patients with primary polydipsia.
- Water deprivation test (Miller-Moses test) to evaluate the ability to concentrate urine; aids in determining etiology.
  - Water is withheld, and urine and plasma osmolality are measured at hourly intervals.
  - A rise in urine osmolality indicates an intact ADH response.
  - A rise in plasma osmolality or stable urine osmolality indicates poor ADH response.
  - Perform the test during the day, not overnight, to avoid serious volume depletion or hypernatremia.
  - If the results support the diagnosis, desmopressin should be administered to test renal concentrating ability.

Initial lab tests

- Serum electrolyte levels
- Serum glucose to rule out diabetes mellitus
- Urine osmolality
- Urine specific gravity
- Urine electrolytes; hypokalemia and hypercalcemia alter the ability to concentrate urine.

- Plasma vasopressin or urinary vasopressin following osmotic stimulus, such as fluid restriction or administration of hypertonic saline
- Drugs that may alter lab results: Lithium, demeclocycline, and methoxyflurane may induce vasopressin insensitivity.

ɱaging

- ead MRI

ıitial approach

- the diagnosis of DI is made, appropriate studies ɔr cause, including MRI of the brain, must be erformed.

'athological Findings

- egeneration of neurosecretory neurons in the eurohypophysis

IFFERENTIAL DIAGNOSIS

- Diabetes mellitus and other causes of polydipsia and polyuria
- Increased solute load for excretion, as occurs with high salt intake; osmotic diuresis
- Psychogenic polydipsia (ultimately impairs vasopressin secretion)

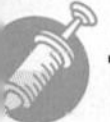

TREATMENT

ΛEDICATION

- Therapy depends on type of DI.
- Central DI (23):
  - Desmopressin (DDAVP), a derivative of vasopressin, may be given orally, parenterally (IV, IM, SQ), or intranasally.
    - Intranasally (100 μg/mL solution), recommended initial dose is 10 μg at bedtime to relieve nocturia; may dose twice daily if symptoms persist in daytime.
    - Orally available as 0.1- to 0.2-mg tablets; recommended initial dose in children >4 years of age is 0.05 mg twice daily.
  - Thiazide diuretic dosed once or twice daily
- Nephrogenic DI (23):
  - Does not respond to desmopressin (DDAVP)
  - Remove offending agent(s).
  - Correct electrolyte imbalances (I.e., hypokalemia, hypocalcemia).
  - Pitressin has vasopressor and ADH activity, increasing water resorption at collecting ducts.
    - Adults: 5–10 units SC q3–6h; children: 2.5–10 units SC b.i.d. to q.i.d.
    - Major side effect is coronary artery constriction.
    - Contraindicated in patients with hypertension, angina, coronary heart disease
    - Pregnancy category B
  - Chlorpropamide (Diabinese) promotes renal response to ADH.
    - Adult 125–250 mg PO b.i.d.; not recommended for pediatric patients
    - Contraindicated in type I diabetes mellitus, severe renal or hepatic impairment, thyroid dysfunction
    - Pregnancy category C
    - Hypoglycemia may occur.
- Contraindications: Use desmopressin with caution in the immediate postoperative period for intracranial lesions because of possible cerebral edema.
- Precautions: An overdose of desmopressin may produce water intoxication and hyponatremia in patients with excessive water intake.

First Line

- Desmopressin is the treatment of choice in patients with central DI or gestational DI (pregnancy category B).

ADDITIONAL TREATMENT

General Measures

- Control fluid balance, and prevent dehydration.
- Careful follow-up and management of electrolytes
- Check weight daily.
- Provide good skin and mouth care.
- Nephrogenic DI: Correct hypercalcemia and hypokalemia, and discontinue causative medications (2)[A].

Issues for Referral

- Dilatation of urinary tract (may be secondary to large urine volumes)
- Complications of primary disease (tumor, histiocytosis, etc.)
- In congenital nephrogenic DI, an associated retardation of mental development may occur in some patients.
- Subnormal growth rate

ONGOING CARE

FOLLOW-UP RECOMMENDATIONS

Continuing care is provided on an outpatient basis with self-medication.

Patient Monitoring

- Regular follow-up at 2- to 3-week intervals initially and 3–4 months later
- Adjust treatment on the basis of urine and electrolyte concentrations.
- Following moderate to severe traumatic brain injury, testing should done 6 and 12 months after injury.

DIET

- Normal, with free access to fluids
- Young infants with nephrogenic DI may benefit from low-solute formula.
- A low-sodium, low-protein diet may reduce urine output in nephrogenic DI.

PATIENT EDUCATION

- Reassurance of good prognosis
- Monitor medications/urinary pattern.
- Special precautions during travel, hot weather, exertion, and times of vomiting or diarrhea to avoid dehydration

PROGNOSIS

- Most reversible cases of nephrogenic DI are caused by medications, and patient symptoms improve with removal of the offending agent (4)[A]. Lithium may cause irreversible DI (4)[A].
- Generally good prognosis depending on underlying disorder

COMPLICATIONS

- Dilatation of the urinary tract has been observed (probably secondary to large volume of urine).
- Complications of the primary disease (tumor histiocytosis, etc.) should be anticipated. In congenital nephrogenic DI, an associated retardation of mental development may occur in some patients (cause undetermined).
- Without treatment, dehydration can lead to confusion, stupor, and coma.
- Subnormal growth rate

REFERENCES

1. Karhulik D, Zapletalova J, Frysak Z, et al. Dysfunction of hypothalamic-hypophysial axis after traumatic brain injury in adcults. *J Neurosurg*. 2009;0:1–4. Posted online November 20, 2009.
2. Makaryus AN, McFarlane SI. Diabetes insipidus: diagnosis and treatment of a complex disease. *Cleve Clin J Med*. 2006;73:65–71.
3. www.diabetesinsipidus.org
4. Garofeanu CG, Weir M, Rosas-Arellano MP, et al. Causes of reversible nephrogenic diabetes insipidus: a systematic review. *Am J Kidney Dis*. 2005;45:626–37.

ADDITIONAL READING

- Fukuda I, Hizuka N, Takano K. Oral DDAVP is a good alternative therapy for patients with central diabetes insipidus: experience of five-year treatment. *Endocr J*. 2003;50:437–43.
- Nemergut EC, Zuo Z, Jane JA, et al. Predictors of diabetes insipidus after transsphenoidal surgery: a review of 881 patients. *J Neurosurg*. 2005;103: 448–54.

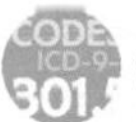

CODES

ICD9

253.5 Diabetes insipidus

CLINICAL PEARLS

- To distinguish primary polydipsia from DI in a patient with polyuria, a patient with primary polydipsia will have a normal response to a water restriction test and normal levels of plasma ADH.
- Vasopressin (IM) had been used previously but has been replaced by desmopressin, which provides the antidiuretic but not the vasoconstrictive activity of vasopressin for the treatment of central DI.
- The goal in adult patients with congenital nephrogenic DI is to prevent dehydration by ensuring proper fluid intake. Genetic testing should be recommended for access to genetic counseling and to facilitate newborn screening.

DIABETES MELLITUS, TYPE 1

Alfred Chege Gitu, MD

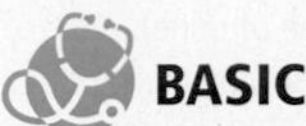

BASICS

DESCRIPTION

- Chronic disease caused by pancreatic insufficiency (deficiency) of insulin production
- Results in hyperglycemia and end-organ complications (e.g., accelerated atherosclerosis, neuropathy, nephropathy, and retinopathy)
- Features include:
  - Patients are insulinopenic and require insulin.
  - Ketosis
  - Usually rapid onset
  - Nutritional status: Normal or thin physique
- System(s) affected: Endocrine/Metabolic

Pregnancy Considerations

- During embryogenesis, hyperglycemia increases the incidence of congenital malformations. Tight control of blood sugar prior to conception is important.
- Women with microalbuminuria during the 1st trimester are at increased risk for preeclampsia and preterm delivery.
- A safe pregnancy is possible with vaginal delivery of a term baby. Close monitoring of blood sugar during labor is important.

EPIDEMIOLOGY

- Mean age of onset 8–12 years, peaking in adolescence
- Onset 1.5 years earlier in girls than boys
- Rapid decline in incidence after adolescence
- Overall incidence increasing worldwide
- Age of presentation has a bimodal distribution, being highest at ages 4–6 and 10–14 yrs.

Incidence

- 15/100,000 per year
- Racial predilection for whites
- African Americans have lowest overall incidence.

Pediatric Considerations

- Although onset is usually before the age of 19 yrs, true type 1 diabetes can occur for the first time in patients who are well into their 30s.
- Young children are more likely to present in diabetic ketoacidosis (DKA) due to atypical presentation, and because they may not express thirst or obtain fluids as readily as older children or adults.

RISK FACTORS

- Certain human leukocyte antigen (HLA) types
- Presence of a specific 64,000 mw protein may be responsible for antibody formation.
- Family history: Insulin-dependent or noninsulin-dependent diabetes in any 1st-degree relatives
- Dietary factors: Breastfeeding may provide a degree of protection against the disease, whereas exposure to cow's milk at an early age is associated with an increased risk of the disease.
- Maternal age at birth may play a role (1).
- Slightly greater risk for a child if the father has type 1 diabetes

Genetics

- Mode of genetic expression not clear
- Genes located on major histocompatibility complex on chromosome 6
- HLA DR3 and DR4 are individually associated with an increased risk; if a person is carrying both susceptibility genes, the relative risk is increased.
- HLA B8 and B15 associated with increased risk

PATHOPHYSIOLOGY

- Alteration in immunologic integrity, placing the β cell at special risk for inflammatory damage, accounts for most cases
- Autoantibodies to islet cells, glutamic acid decarboxylase (GAD), tyrosine phosphatase antibodies, and insulin identified in certain cases (type 1A diabetes)
- Some idiopathic cases (type 1B) have no evidence of autoimmune or other reason for beta cell damage.

ETIOLOGY

- Inherited defect
- Associated environmental triggers: None have been verified:
  - Viruses (such as mumps, coxsackie, cytomegalovirus, and hepatitis viruses)
  - Diet high in nitrosamines
  - Environmental toxins
- Emotional and physical stress

COMMONLY ASSOCIATED CONDITIONS

- Autoimmune diseases, such as hypothyroidism and Addison disease:
  - Screening regularly for hypothyroidism is particularly important in females.
- Diabetes mellitus can also be seen as part of multiple endocrine adenomatosis.

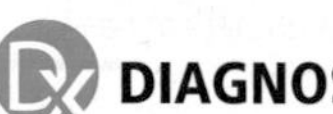

DIAGNOSIS

DIAGNOSTIC TESTS & INTERPRETATION

Lab

- Criteria for the diagnosis of diabetes:
  - Fasting glucose >126 mg/dL (7.0 mmol/L) OR
  - Random of >200 mg/dL (11.1 mmol/L) in a patient with classic symptoms of hyperglycemia OR
  - Oral glucose tolerance test; plasma glucose ≥200 mg/dL 2 hours after a glucose load of 1.75 g/kg (max. dose 75g) OR
  - Glycated hemoglobin (HbA1c) level ≥6.5% (2)[C]
- Other tests to consider:
  - Serum electrolytes, especially in sicker patients who may have ketoacidosis
  - Urinalysis for glucose and ketones and microalbuminuria
  - Pancreatic autoantibodies (to diagnose type 1A diabetes):
    - Islet cells, insulin, GAD, tyrosine phosphatase antibodies
  - Complete blood count (white blood cell count and hemoglobin may be elevated)
- C-peptide insulin level if needed to differentiate from type 2 diabetes

Pathological Findings

Inflammatory changes, lymphocytic infiltration around the islets of Langerhans, or islet cell loss

HISTORY

- Polyuria and polydipsia:
  - Polyuria may present as nocturia, bedwetting, or incontinence in a previously continent child.
  - Polyuria may be difficult to appreciate in diaper-clad children.
- Weight loss 10–30%:
  - Often almost devoid of body fat at diagnosis
  - Due to hypovolemia and increased catabolism
- Prolonged or recurrent candidal infection, usually in the diaper area
- Increased fatigue, lethargy, muscle cramps
- Irritability and emotional lability, headaches, abdominal discomfort, nausea
- Vision changes, such as blurriness
- Altered school or work performance
- Anxiety attacks

DIFFERENTIAL DIAGNOSIS

- Benign renal glycosuria
- Glucose intolerance
- Type 2 noninsulin-dependent diabetes:
  - Obese children might have maturity-onset diabetes of the young (MODY)
- Secondary diabetes:
  - Pancreatic disease (chronic pancreatitis, cystic fibrosis, hereditary hemochromatosis)
  - Hormonal disorders (pheochromocytoma, multiple endocrine adenomatosis)
  - Inborn errors of metabolism (glycogen storage disease, type 1)
  - Hereditary neuromuscular disease
  - Progeroid syndromes
  - Obesity (Prader-Willi syndrome)
  - Cytogenetic syndromes (trisomy 21, Klinefelter, and Turner syndromes)
  - Drug- or chemical-induced glucose intolerance: Glucocorticosteroids, HIV protease inhibitors, atypical antipsychotics, tacrolimus, cyclosporine
- Acute poisonings (salicylate poisoning can cause hyperglycemia and glycosuria, and may mimic diabetic ketoacidosis)

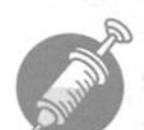

TREATMENT

MEDICATION

- All type 1 diabetes patients will require some form of insulin supplementation.
- Types of insulin:
  - Long-acting insulin analogues (insulin glargine [Lantus] and insulin detemir [Levemir]). These should not be mixed with other insulins in the same syringe.
  - Intermediate-acting insulin (NPH)—Humulin N or Novolin N—can be mixed with other insulins.
  - Short-acting (regular) insulin: Novolin R or Humulin R
  - Very rapid-acting insulin analogues (insulin lispro [Humalog], insulin aspart [Novolog], and insulin glulisine [Apidra])

First Line

- Flexible intensive insulin therapy is the gold standard.
- Frequent daily injections (FDI) or continuous subcutaneous insulin infusion (CSII) have equal efficacy.
- Total initial dose is 0.2–0.4 units per gg/day for insulin-naive patients.
- 40–60% of total dose given as basal insulin, and the rest as bolus insulin

FDI regime:
- Basal, long-acting insulin once or twice a day
- Prandial, short-acting insulin based on number of carbohydrate portions (e.g., 1:10, meaning 1 unit of insulin for every 10 g of carbohydrate to be eaten)
- Correctional short-acting mealtime insulin based on premeal blood glucose level (e.g., BS-100/50, meaning if the blood glucose is >150, subtract 100 from the BG level, and divide that number by 50)
- Administration of the mealtime insulin before a meal may be more efficacious than during or after the meal.

CSII regime:
- May use regular insulin or rapid-acting insulin analogues
- Basal insulin is infused continuously at a preset rate, and bolus doses are given with meals as above.

econd Line

Conventional insulin therapy

Once to twice daily injections with NPH mixed with regular or rapid-acting insulin in the same syringe

Not physiologic, but lower cost and fewer injections may improve compliance in the less motivated patient.

Premixed insulin available as NPH/regular (Novolin or Humulin 70/30) or NPH/rapid-acting insulin (e.g., Novolog 75/25 Mix or Humulin 75/25 Mix)

Pancreatic transplantation is usually reserved for patients with end-stage renal failure, who may receive kidney-pancreatic transplants at the same time.

Oral hypoglycemics not indicated in type 1 diabetes (except in obese patients, who may have MODY; or a combination of type 1 and type 2): Metformin (Glucophage)

DDITIONAL TREATMENT

eneral Measures

Overall control of carbohydrate metabolism for the very young child:
- Normoglycemia (adjusted for age): Strive for blood glucose levels in range of 80–150 mg/dl (4.4–8.3 mmol/L) all the time (80–120 in older patients)
- Very tight control might be dangerous in young children due to risk of repeated hypoglycemia.
- Hemoglobin A1c target levels:
  - Children <6 years: 7.5–8.5%
  - Children 6–12 years: <8.0%
  - Adolescents 13–19: <7.5% (<7.0% if achieved without excessive hypoglycemia)
  - Nonpediatric patients: <6.0%

Normal growth and development, and overall good health (asymptomatic):
- Reach optimal height for genetic potential
- Appropriate and timely pubertal maturation
- Coping psychosocial development: Normal school or work attendance and performance; normal goals/career plans. Screen adolescents annually for depression.

Prevent acute complications, including:
- Hypoglycemic insulin reactions
- Ketoacidosis

Delay or prevent chronic complications.

N-PATIENT CONSIDERATIONS

Jewly diagnosed type 1 diabetics may require ıospitalization during initiation of insulin therapy.

ONGOING CARE

FOLLOW-UP RECOMMENDATIONS

- Normal; full participation in sports activities
- Regular aerobic exercise is recommended.

Patient Monitoring

- Blood pressure (BP) monitoring at every office visit (3)[C]
- Monitor height, weight, and sexual maturation (in children).
- Daily home blood glucose monitoring with home blood glucose meter: Blood tests should be done at least 4–6 times daily (more frequently in pump patients) for optimal monitoring.
- Quarterly measurement of hemoglobin A1c
- Annual screenings after 5 years of diabetes, sooner if glycemic control is suboptimal:
  - Microalbuminuria for earliest signs of possible nephropathy
  - If elevated, depending on level, even if BP is normal, consider an angiotensin-converting enzyme inhibitor (such as Vasotec [enalapril])
  - Ophthalmology exam (after 3–5 years of diabetes, also depending on glycemic control); regularly thereafter
  - Yearly lipid profile, thyroid levels, blood chemistries, complete blood count
  - Annual influenza vaccine

DIET

- American Diabetic Association diet:http://www.diabetes.org/food-and-fitness/food/
- Carbohydrate counting using insulin-to-carbohydrate ratio with all meals and snacks. Allows patient flexibility of eating and ability to eat almost anything.

PROGNOSIS

- Initial remission or honeymoon phase with decreased insulin needs and easier control, usually 3–6 months and rarely beyond a year
- Progression to total diabetes when endogenous insulin is insignificant; usually is gradual, but stress or illness initiate it suddenly
- Current prognosis:
  - Increasing longevity and quality of life with careful blood glucose monitoring and improvement in insulin delivery regimens
- At this time, reduced life expectancy, but has improved greatly over the past 20 years

COMPLICATIONS

- Microvascular disease (retinopathy, nephropathy, neuropathy)
- Hyperlipidemia
- Macrovascular disease (coronary and cerebral artery disease)
- Chronic foot ulcers/amputations
- Hypoglycemia
- Diabetic ketoacidosis
- Excessive weight gain
- Increased risk for preeclampsia and preterm delivery (4)
- Driving mishaps (5)
- Psychologic problems of chronic disease

REFERENCES

1. Cardwell CR, Stene LC, Joner G, Bulsara MK, Cinek O, Rosenbauer J, Ludvigsson J, Jané M, Svensson J, Goldacre MJ, Waldhoer T, Jarosz-Chobot P, Gimeno SG, Chuang LM, Parslow RC, Wadsworth EJ, Chetwynd A, Pozzilli P, Brigis G, Urbonaite B, Sipetic S, Schober E, Devoti G, Ionescu-Tirgoviste C, de Beaufort CE, Stoyanov D, Buschard K, Patterson CC et al. Maternal age at birth and childhood type 1 diabetes: a pooled analysis of 30 observational studies. *Diabetes*. 2010;59:486–94.
2. THE INTERNATIONAL EXPERT COMMITTEE. International Expert Committee Report on the Role of the A1C Assay in the Diagnosis of Diabetes. *Diabetes Care*. 2009.
3. American Diabetes Association (ADA). Standards of medical care in diabetes. V. Diabetes care. *Diabetes Care*. 2006;29(Suppl 1):S8–17.
4. Jensen DM, Damm P, Ovesen P, Mølsted-Pedersen L, Beck-Nielsen H, Westergaard JG, Moeller M, Mathiesen ER et al. Microalbuminuria, preeclampsia, and preterm delivery in pregnant women with type 1 diabetes: results from a nationwide Danish study. *Diabetes Care*. 2010;33:90–4.
5. Cox DJ, Ford D, Gonder-Frederick L, Clarke W, Mazze R, Weinger K, Ritterband L et al. Driving mishaps among individuals with type 1 diabetes: a prospective study. *Diabetes Care*. 2009;32:2177–80.

ADDITIONAL READING

Silverstein J, Klingensmith G, Copeland K, et al. Care of children and adolescents with type 1 diabetes: a statement of the American Diabetes Association. *Diabetes Care*. 2005;28:186–212.

See Also (Topic, Algorithm, Electronic Media Element)

Diabetes Mellitus, Type 2; Diabetic Ketoacidosis (DKA)

CODES

ICD9

- 250.01 Diabetes mellitus without mention of complication, type I (juvenile type), not stated as uncontrolled
- 250.03 Diabetes mellitus without mention of complication, type I (juvenile type), uncontrolled

CLINICAL PEARLS

- Polyuria may present as nocturia, bedwetting, or incontinence in a previously continent child.
- Young children are more likely to present in DKA because they may not express thirst or obtain fluids as readily as older children or adults.
- Onset usually before the age of 19 yrs, but type 1 diabetes can present in patients who are well into their 30s.
- Obese children might have MODY.

D

DIABETES MELLITUS, TYPE 2

Ramothea L. Webster, MD, PhD

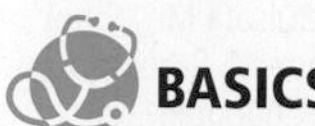

BASICS

DESCRIPTION
- Diabetes mellitus (DM) type 2 manifests in nonketotic hyperglycemia, insulin resistance, and relative impairment in insulin secretion.
- System(s) affected: Endocrine/Metabolic; Nervous; Renal/Urologic; Cardiovascular

Geriatric Considerations
- Significant contributing factor to blindness, renal failure, and lower limb amputations
- Dietary restrictions for elderly patients with DM in long-term facilities is not warranted; give regular diet.

Pediatric Considerations
Incidence is increasing dramatically, possibly related to increases in childhood obesity.

Pregnancy Considerations
First-line drug is insulin (class B), but may consider glyburide (class B) only after the 1st trimester or metformin (class B)

EPIDEMIOLOGY
Incidence
300/100,000; Male, 230/100,000; Female, 340/100,000

Prevalence
- 5,000/100,000; within race: 7.2% whites, 9% Hispanics, 11.2% blacks, and 35% Pima Indians
- If diagnosed <40, average reduction in life-years is 12 Yr (male) and 19 Yr (female).
- Lifetime risk of developing diabetes if born in 2000 is 33% (male) and 39% (female)

RISK FACTORS
- Family history: 1st-degree relative
- Gestational diabetes (GDM)
- Obesity: Induces resistance to insulin-mediated peripheral glucose uptake
- Ethnicity: African American, Latino, Native American, Asian American, and Pacific Islander
- Impaired fasting glucose (IFG) or impaired glucose tolerance (IGT)

Genetics
- Strong polygenic familial susceptibility
- Concordance nearly complete in identical twins

GENERAL PREVENTION
- Lose 5–10% body weight, exercise 150 min/week, and decrease fat and caloric intake
- Protein increases insulin response, but not to exceed 15% of caloric intake

PATHOPHYSIOLOGY
- Decrease in peripheral insulin effects ("insulin resistance") and resultant progressive loss of β-cell function and mass
- Cellular damage due to inability of cells to regulate uptake of glucose during hyperglycemic events via mitochondrial superoxide production to capillary endothelial cells in retina, mesangial cells in renal glomerulus, and to neurons and Schwann cells in peripheral nerves (1)[A].

ETIOLOGY
- Genetic factors (β-cell dysfunction, defects in insulin action, diseases of the exocrine pancreas, i.e., cystic fibrosis)
- Obesity, immune-mediated, infection, hemochromatosis
- Drug- or chemical-induced (e.g., medications used for psychosis, HIV, or transplant recipients)

COMMONLY ASSOCIATED CONDITIONS
- Hypertension
- Hyperlipidemia
- Impotence
- Stroke
- Peripheral neuropathy
- Syndrome X/metabolic syndrome
- Renal insufficiency/failure
- Cardiovascular disease
- Retinopathy
- Infertility
- Pancreatic cancer
- Polycystic ovary syndrome
- Acanthosis nigricans

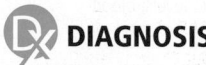

DIAGNOSIS

HISTORY
Polyuria, polydipsia, polyphagia, weight loss, weakness, fatigue, and frequent infections

PHYSICAL EXAM
Complications of hyperglycemia: Retinopathy, neuropathy, and poor wound healing

DIAGNOSTIC TESTS & INTERPRETATION
- According to the ADA, IFG 100–125mg/dL, and IGT 140–199 mg/dL 2 hours after ingestion of 75g of glucose are prediabetes categories (1)[A].
- Glucose tolerance test (GTT) is usually not necessary, except when diagnosing gestational diabetes.
- HbA_{1c} has advantages over fasting plasma glucose (FPG) for diagnosis and analysis (2)[A].
- HbA_{1c} approximately $\leq$8.5% is mostly due to postprandial hyperglycemia and less fasting hyperglycemia, whereas HbA_{1c} $\geq$8.5% is mostly due to fasting hyperglycemia and less by postprandial hyperglycemia (1)[A].

Lab
- Criteria for diagnosis:
  - HbA_{1c} $\geq$6.5% on 2 or more occasions is diagnostic; HbA_{1c}between 5.7–6.4% is prediabetes (2)[A].
  - Symptoms of diabetes plus random plasma glucose $\geq$200 mg/dL (11.1 mmol/L), *or*
  - FPG $\geq$126 mg/dL (7.0 mmol/L) on 2 occasions, *or*
  - 2-hour plasma glucose $\geq$200 mg/dL (11.1 mmol/L) during oral GTT with 75-g glucose load (3)[A]
- Drugs that may alter lab results: Atypical antipsychotics, pentamidine, nicotinic acid, glucocorticoids, thyroid hormone, diazoxide, beta-adrenergic agonists, thiazides, Dilantin, alpha-interferon, and some fluoroquinolones

DIFFERENTIAL DIAGNOSIS
- Type 1 DM
- GDM

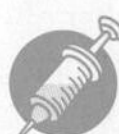

TREATMENT
- Goal FPG <110 mg/dL (5.5 mmol/L)
- Use drugs from different classes to achieve adequate control.
- Insulin might be the next best addition if uncontrolled by oral agents
- Goals remain unclear; some data suggest best A1C ~ 7.5%; ADA endorses <7.5%
- If HbA_{1c} >8%, consider starting 2 oral agents (3)[B].

MEDICATION
First Line
- Metformin: Preferred 1st medication because of its effects on weight loss and insulin resistance
- The following classes of agents may be used alone or in combination:
  - Biguanides
    - Metformin (Glucophage, Fortamet, Riomet, Glumetza): 500–1000 mg b.i.d.–t.i.d. or ER 1000–2000 mg qpm, max 2550 mg/d, except Glumetza, 2000 mg/d
    - Avoid situations that increase risk for lactic acidosis: Renal insufficiency, radiocontrast agents, surgery, or acute illnesses i.e., liver disease, cardiogenic shock, pancreatitis, or hypoxia
    - Caution with congestive heart failure (CHF), alcohol abuse, elderly, or with tetracycline
  - Sulfonylureas
    - Glipizide (Glucotrol): 2.5–40 mg/d; dosage >10 mg/d given b.i.d., take 30 minutes before meals
    - Glipizide extended-release: 5–20 mg/d
    - Glyburide (DiaBeta, Glynase, Micronase): 1.25–20 mg/d, Glynase 0.75–12 mg/d
    - Glimepiride (Amaryl): 1–8 mg/d
    - Caution with renal, liver, or thyroid disease, sulfa allergy, Cr CL <50, late pregnancy
    - Chlorpropamide (Diabinese): 100–500mg/d, max 750 mg/d
  - Thiazolidinediones
    - Pioglitazone (Actos): 15–45 mg/d
    - Monitor serum transaminase q2mo for the 1st year, contraindicated for liver disease and symptomatic heart failure patients; may cause or exacerbate CHF and myocardial infarction.
  - Alpha-glucosidase inhibitors
    - Acarbose (Precose): 25–100 mg t.i.d.
    - Miglitol (Glyset): 25–100 mg t.i.d.
    - Take at beginning of meals to decrease postprandial glucose peaks.
    - Poor patient compliance due to gastrointestinal symptoms
    - Avoid in renal insufficiency, inflammatory bowe disease, colonic ulceration, or partial bowel obstruction.
  - Dipeptidyl peptidase-4 inhibitor:
    - Sitagliptin (Januvia): 100 mg/d
    - Vildagliptin (Galvus): Awaiting FDA approval
    - Renally excreted; therefore, adjust dosage for renal patients.
- Precautions: Warn patients of signs of hypo- and hyperglycemia:
  - Combination of metformin and sulfonylurea can increase patient's relative risk of cardiovascular hospitalization or mortality

Significant possible interactions:
- Drugs that may potentiate sulfonylureas: Salicylates, clofibrate, warfarin (Coumadin), ethanol, and ACE inhibitors
- Thiazides can cause IGT.
- Gatifloxacin can cause either severe hypo- or hyperglycemia.
- TZD pioglitazone may decrease effectiveness of oral contraceptives.
- Drug binders, such as cholestyramine resin, should be taken at least 2 hours apart from alpha-glucosidase inhibitors

ALERT

Avandia: Associated with an increased risk of heart attack, stroke, and CHF. As of fall 2010, Avandia has been suspended in Europe; in U.S., is restricted to only when other diabetes medicine have failed and patients are aware of the drug's cardiovascular risks.

Second Line

Insulin: Rapid (Aspart, Lispro, Glulisine), short (regular insulin), intermediate (NPH), and long/peakless (Glargine) or long/peak (Detemir):
- Can be given up to t.i.d.
- May be used in combination with oral agents, or with an insulin of a different half-life
- Most often required in late stages of type 2 DM, when oral agents fail to control glucose levels
- Insulindetemir (Levemir) or insulin glargine (Lantus): 0.5–1 U/kg/d, onset 1 hour, no true peak, duration 6–23 hours, given QHS or b.i.d.; start with 10 U SC QHS, then increase by 1 Unit daily until FPG <100.
- Long-acting insulins have a lower risk of hypoglycemia and lower variability than other insulins

Amylinomimetic:
- Pramlintide (Symlin): 60–120 μg SC qAC:
- When used with insulin, may cause severe hypoglycemia
- Preprandial insulins, short-acting or rapid-acting, should be reduced by 50% at initiation of drug.
- Contraindicated in patients with gastroparesis
- Drug interactions: Anticholinergic drugs or agents that slow intestinal absorption of nutrients

GLP-1 (glucagonlike peptide-1) receptor agonist
- Exenatide (Byetta): 5–10 μg SC b.i.d. within 60 minutes before meals and at least 6 hours apart
- Liraglutide (Victoza): 0.6 mg SQ per day for 1 week, then increase to 1.2; max 1.8 mg/day; less expensive and better tolerated than exenatide; should not be used in patients with history or family history of medullary thyroid cancer or MEN type II (black box warning) (4)[A]

Promotes weight loss, increases high-density lipoprotein cholesterol, and decreases diastolic blood pressure (BP)

Sulfonylureas should be decreased to reduce the chance of hypoglycemia. Patients should be advised to take other oral medications 1 hour before injecting Exenatide.

Meglitinides:
- Repaglinide (Prandin): 0.5–4 mg before meals; may be useful in patients with sulfa allergy or renal impairment
- Nateglinide (Starlix): 60–120 mg before meals t.i.d.

ADDITIONAL TREATMENT

General Measures

- Foot exam every visit for neuropathy (monofilament), arterial insufficiency, and ulcers
- Nephropathy: Urine analysis to check microalbumin yearly
- Retinopathy: Yearly eye exams
- NCEP guidelines recommend a low-density lipoprotein cholesterol goal of <70 mg/dL in patients with existing cardiovascular disease (CVD) or risk factors for CVD.
- Strict control of hypertension (goal BP <130/80 mm Hg)
- Low-dose aspirin is recommended for all adults with diabetes, unless there is a contraindication.
- ACEI/ARB 1st-line hypertension drug (3)[A]; if contraindicated, consider a calcium channel blocker

COMPLEMENTARY AND ALTERNATIVE MEDICINE

- Cinnamon has no statistical significance with improving HbA_{1c} or lipid parameters, but has shown improvements with FBG in patients with DM types 1 or 2. Its role in preventing DM is unknown.
- Chromium studies have shown reduction in HbA_{1c} and FBG in patients with diabetes, although further studies are needed to fully understand its role in diabetes treatment and prevention.

ONGOING CARE

FOLLOW-UP RECOMMENDATIONS

Regular aerobic exercise about 150 min/week can improve glucose tolerance and decrease medication requirements (3)[A]. Lifestyle modifications with pharmacotherapy can delay progression from prediabetes to diabetes (1)[A].

Patient Monitoring

- Office visits every 2–4 months
- Monitor glucose, HbA_{1c}, lipids, BP, body weight, and renal function.
- HbA_{1c} twice a year for glycemic-controlled patients and quarterly for uncontrolled or change-in-therapy patients (3)[A]

DIET

ADA suggests mild caloric restriction to achieve mild to moderate weight loss. Carbohydrates should consist of <45%–65% of caloric consumption/day; fat <30%; protein <15%; and fiber 50 g/day (3)[A].

PATIENT EDUCATION

ADA patient education materials

PROGNOSIS

In susceptible individuals, complications begin to appear 10–15 years after onset, but can be present at time of diagnosis since disease may go undetected for years.

COMPLICATIONS

- Damage of macro- and microvascular arterial cell walls
- Peripheral neuropathy
- Proliferative retinopathy
- Nephropathy and chronic renal failure
- Atherosclerotic CVD and peripheral vascular disease
- Hyperosmolar coma
- Gangrene of extremities
- Blindness
- Glaucoma
- Cataracts
- Skin ulceration
- Charcot joints

REFERENCES

1. Blonde L et al. Current antihyperglycemic treatment guidelines and algorithms for patients with type 2 diabetes mellitus. *Am J Med*. 2010;123:S12–8.
2. The International Expert Committee. International Expert Committee Report on the Role of the A1C Assay in the Diagnosis of Diabetes. *Diabetes Care*. 2009.
3. American Diabetes Association. Standards of medical care in diabetes-2010. *Diabetes Care*. 2010;33(suppl 1)S11–S61.
4. Fakhoury WK, Lereun C, Wright D et al. A meta-analysis of placebo-controlled clinical trials assessing the efficacy and safety of incretin-based medications in patients with type 2 diabetes. *Pharmacology*. 2010;86:44–57.

See Also (Topic, Algorithm, Electronic Media Element)

Diabetes Mellitus, Type 1; Diabetic Ketoacidosis (DKA); Hypertension, Essential
Algorithm: Diabetes Mellitus, Type 2

CODES

ICD9

- 250.00 Diabetes mellitus without mention of complication, type ii or unspecified type, not stated as uncontrolled
- 250.02 Diabetes mellitus without mention of complication, type ii or unspecified type, uncontrolled

CLINICAL PEARLS

- Screening: ≥45 years with a body mass index (BMI) ≥25 kg/m^2 or <45 years, overweight (BMI > 25 kg/m^2), and other risk factors. Repeat every 3 years; if IFG or IGT, check every 1–2 years
- Criteria for testing children for DM II is: Overweight (BMI >85th percentile; weight for height >85th percentile or weight >120% of ideal height). Plus any 2 risk factors below:
  - Family history with 1st- or 2nd-degree relatives
  - Race/ethnicity
  - Signs of insulin resistance or conditions associated with insulin resistance (AN, hypertension, hyperlipidemia, or PCOS)
  - Maternal history of DM or GDM
  - Start at age 10 or at onset of puberty, whichever comes first
  - Frequency: every 2 years

D

DIABETIC KETOACIDOSIS (DKA)

Francesca L. Beaudoin, MS, MD
Nadine T. Himelfarb, MD

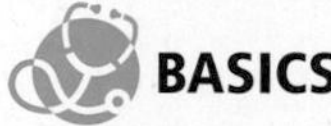

BASICS

DESCRIPTION
- A true medical emergency secondary to severe insulin deficiency and characterized by hyperglycemia, ketosis, and metabolic acidosis
- System(s) affected: Endocrine/Metabolic

EPIDEMIOLOGY
Incidence
- In US: 46 episodes/10,000 diabetic patients; 2/100 patient-years of type 1 diabetes mellitus (DM)
- Predominant age: 0–19 years
- Predominant sex: Male = Female.

RISK FACTORS
- Type 1 > type 2 DM
- Younger patients at higher risk

GENERAL PREVENTION
- Close monitoring of glucose during periods of stress, infection, and trauma
- Careful insulin control and monitoring of the blood glucose level
- "Sick day" management instructions

PATHOPHYSIOLOGY
A relative or absolute deficiency of insulin, exacerbated by an increase in counterregulatory hormones (e.g., catecholamines, cortisol, glucagon, and growth hormone) leading to a hyperglycemic crisis

ETIOLOGY
- Noncompliance/insufficient insulin: 25%
- Infection: 30–40%
- 1st presentation of DM: 10–20%
- Myocardial infarction (MI): 5–7%
- No cause identified: 10–30%
- Cerebrovascular accident (CVA)
- Medications (corticosteroids, thiazides)
- Drugs (cocaine)
- Trauma
- Surgery
- Emotional stress
- Pregnancy

COMMONLY ASSOCIATED CONDITIONS
Complications of chronic DM such as nephropathy, neuropathy, and retinopathy

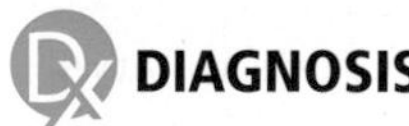

DIAGNOSIS

HISTORY
- Recent illness
- Changes in diet or medications
- Missed insulin doses
- Polyuria, nocturia
- Polydipsia
- Generalized weakness
- Malaise, lethargy
- Anorexia or increased appetite
- Nausea, vomiting
- Abdominal pain
- Decreased perspiration
- Fever
- Confusion
- Coma

PHYSICAL EXAM
- Hypotension
- Tachycardia
- Hypothermia or fever
- Tachypnea, Kussmaul respirations
- Fruity odor to breath (acetone smell)
- Decreased reflexes
- Abdominal tenderness
- Decreased bowel sounds
- Dry mucus membranes, poor skin turgor
- Decreased perspiration
- Confusion
- Coma
- Attempt to find precipitating cause (i.e., source of infection).

DIAGNOSTIC TESTS & INTERPRETATION
- Electrocardiogram (ECG):
  - Usually shows sinus tachycardia
  - Look for changes consistent with electrolyte abnormalities and ischemia/MI
- Urine and blood cultures
- Consider lumbar puncture (meningitis)

Lab

ALERT
- Hyponatremia: Hyperglycemia or hypertriglyceridemia may cause an artificially low or very low sodium concentration. The measured sodium is suppressed by 1.6 mg/dL for every 100 mg/dL of glucose over normal.
- Hyperglycemia (usually 250–800 mg/dL)
- Serum ketosis: Check β-hydroxybutyrate (β-HB) instead of ketones to evaluate ketosis (1)[B]. With concomitant lactic acidosis, acetoacetate production may be inhibited in the presence of high levels of β-HB. Nitroprusside reaction, which measures only acetoacetate, may not be strongly positive.
- Urine ketosis (may be falsely negative initially; urinalysis (UA) may only identify acetoacetate and not β-HB)
- Glycosuria
- Hyperamylasemia, hyperlipasemia
- Hypertriglyceridemia/hypercholesterolemia
- Increased creatinine and blood urea nitrogen (BUN): Markedly increased serum ketones may cross-react and cause a falsely high serum creatinine.
- HCO_3 (usually $\leq$15 mEq/L)
- Decreased calculated total-body K^+: Severe acidosis gives an artificially high K^+ level.
- Metabolic acidosis on arterial blood gases
- Increased serum osmolality
- Increased anion gap
- Elevated base deficit

Initial lab tests
- Complete blood count, electrolytes, BUN, creatinine
- Serum β-HB or ketones
- Arterial blood gases; venous blood gases (VBGs) also may be used (VBG pH 0.03 lower)

Imaging
- Chest X-ray to rule out pulmonary infection
- Head CT scan if suspected CVA or cerebral edema

Diagnostic Procedures/Surgery
Only if surgical problem is the underlying precipitant (e.g., appendicitis)

DIFFERENTIAL DIAGNOSIS
- Hyperosmolar nonketotic coma
- Alcoholic ketoacidosis
- Starvation ketosis
- Toxic ingestions (e.g., salicylates)
- Lactic acidosis
- Acute hypoglycemic coma
- Uremia/chronic renal failure

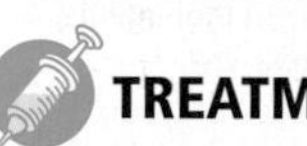

TREATMENT

- Oxygen and airway management as needed
- Establish IV access
- Cardiac monitoring
- Start isotonic crystalloid solution (0.9% saline)
- Fingerstick glucose testing
- Empirical naloxone if altered mental status

MEDICATION
First Line
- Insulin: IV infusion of regular insulin at 0.1 unit/kg/h; may use IM or SC route, but IV is recommended for moderate to severe DKA (1,2)[B].
- Potassium: Falsely elevated owing to acidosis; start replacement when $K^+ \leq 5.0$ mg/dL and urine output is adequate. Start 30–40 mEq/L IV fluids. Increase rate (up to 60 mEq/L) if $K^+ \leq 3.5$ mg/dL (2,1)[A].
  - Hold insulin if $K^+ \leq 2.5$ mg/dL; give IV potassium 1 mEq/kg over 1 h.
  - For each 0.1 unit of pH, serum K^+ will change by ~0.6 mEq in opposite direction.
- Phosphorus: Routine replacement may lead to hypocalcemia; if very low (<1.0), give 1/3 of K^+ replacement as KPhos.
- Sodium bicarbonate: No demonstrable benefit with a pH >7.0 (1,2)[B]; rehydration usually leads to resolution of acidosis. Consider its use in patients with arterial pH <6.9 or patients with life-threatening hyperkalemia.
- Magnesium: If Mg $\leq$1.8 mg/dL and the patient is symptomatic, consider replacement.
- Precautions:
  - If the patient is on an insulin pump, it should be stopped.
  - Double insulin if no response in serum glucose over 1st 2 h.
  - If blood glucose does not fall by ~75 mg every 2 h, increase insulin rate.
  - If using bicarbonate, add 50–100 mEq $NaHCO_3$ to 1 L 0.45% saline *or* 150 mEq $NaHCO_3$ to 1 L D_5W and give over 1 h. Once a pH of 7.1 has been reached, infusion should be stopped.

econd Line

sulin, SC or IM: Load with 0.3 unit/kg SC, followed y 0.1 unit/kg/h. Space dosing to q2h once glucose :250 mg/dL.

DDITIONAL TREATMENT

ieneral Measures

All but mild cases require inpatient management; severe DKA requires an ICU setting.

Goals:
- Fluid resuscitation
- Insulin therapy
- Resolution of anion-gap acidosis
- Correction of electrolytes

Laboratory testing during management:
- Serum glucose every 1–2 h until stable
- Electrolytes, phosphorous, and venous pH every 2–6 h as needed

ediatric Considerations

Children with moderate to severe DKA should be transferred to the nearest pediatric critical-care hospital.

In 0.3–1% of children/adolescents, fluid resuscitation and treatment may result in marked mental deterioration, including development of coma 4–6 h after therapy has begun; death is 21–24%.
- Think of cerebral edema secondary to rapid IV hydration.
- Diagnose by CT scan.
- Treat with IV bolus of mannitol 1 g/kg in 20% solution.
- If no response, hyperventilation to a pCO_2 of 28 mm Hg.

ieriatric Considerations

Aust be careful with impaired renal function or ongestive heart failure when correcting fluid and lectrolyte abnormalities.

regnancy Considerations

Pregnancy itself is diabetogenic. It also results in a compensated respiratory alkalosis (HCO_3 19–20 mEq/L) with theoretically reduced buffering capacity. Therefore, pregnant patients are more susceptible to DKA.

Euglycemic DKA

Increased risk of preeclampsia and fetal death

β-Tocolytics and corticosteroids can trigger DKA.

Perinatal death: 9–35%

N-PATIENT CONSIDERATIONS

Admission Criteria

ADA admission guidelines: Blood glucose >250 ng/dL; pH <7.3; HCO_3 ≤15 mEq/L; ketones in urine; CU setting for severe DKA (3)

IV Fluids

- 10–20 mL/kg over the 1st h, then 500 mL/h (~0.7 mL/kg/h) for 4 h or until hemodynamics improve; then 250 mL/h (3.5 mL/kg/h) until tolerating PO
- Switch to 5% dextrose in 0.45% saline at maintenance rate when serum glucose <250 mg/dL. Maintain blood glucose between 150 and 250 mg/dL. Too rapid correction of fluid balance may precipitate cerebral edema (1)[C]. If the blood glucose level is falling too rapidly, consider using a 10% dextrose solution instead.

Pediatric Considerations

Bolus 10–20 mL/kg initially; 4-h fluid total should be <50 mL/kg to reduce chance of cerebral edema.

Discharge Criteria

Discharge when DKA has resolved: glucose <200 mg/dL; pH >7.3; bicarbonate >18 mEq/L; additionally, patients must be tolerating PO intake and able to resume home medication regimen, and the underlying precipitant (e.g., infection) must be identified and treated.

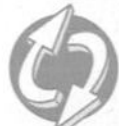

ONGOING CARE

FOLLOW-UP RECOMMENDATIONS

Bed rest

Patient Monitoring

- Monitor mental status, vital signs, and urine output q30–60min until improved, then q2–4h every 24 h.
- Monitor blood sugar q1h until <300 mg/dL, then q2–6h.
- Monitor electrolytes (Na, K, HCO_3) q2h.
- Monitor phosphate, calcium, and magnesium q4–6h.

DIET

- NPO initially
- Advance to preketotic diet when nausea and vomiting are controlled.
- Avoid foods with high glycemic index (e.g., soft drinks, white bread, etc.).

PROGNOSIS

- 16% of all diabetes-related fatalities
- Death 1–2%
- In children <10 years of age, DKA causes 70% of diabetes-related fatalities.

COMPLICATIONS

- Cerebral edema
- Pulmonary edema
- Vascular thrombosis
- Hypokalemia
- Cardica dysrhythmia
- MI
- Acute gastric dilatation
- Late hypoglycemia
- Erosive gastritis
- Infection, mucormycosis
- Respiratory distress

REFERENCES

1. Agus MS, Wolfsdorf JI. Diabetic ketoacidosis in children. *Pediatr Clin North Am*. 2005;52: 1147–63, ix.
2. Kitabchi AE, Umpierrez GE, Murphy MB, et al. Hyperglycemic crises in diabetes. *Diabetes Care*. 2004;27 (Suppl 1):S94–102.
3. American Diabetes Association. Hospital admission guidelines for diabetes. *Diabetes Care*. 2004;27 (Suppl 1):S103.

ADDITIONAL READING

- Carroll MA, Yeomans ER. Diabetic ketoacidosis in pregnancy. *Crit Care Med*. 2005;33:S347–53.
- Trachtenbarg DE. Diabetic ketoacidosis. *Am Fam Physician*. 2005;71:1705–14.

See Also (Topic, Algorithm, Electronic Media Element)

Diabetes Mellitus, Type 1

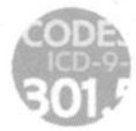

CODES

ICD9

- 250.12 Diabetes mellitus with ketoacidosis, type ii or unspecified type, uncontrolled
- 250.13 Diabetes mellitus with ketoacidosis, type I (juvenile type), uncontrolled

CLINICAL PEARLS

- Admit if blood glucose >250 mg/dL, pH <7.3, HCO_3 ≤15 mEq/L, and ketones in urine.
- Potassium is falsely elevated owing to acidosis; start replacement when K^+ ≤5.0 mg/dL and urine output is adequate.

DIABETIC POLYNEUROPATHY

Samir Malkani, MD

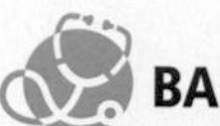

BASICS

DESCRIPTION

Peripheral nerve dysfunction seen in diabetes; several patterns described:

- Symmetric polyneuropathy:
  - Distal sensory or sensorimotor
  - Proximal lower extremity polyneuropathy
- Focal and multifocal neuropathy:
  - Cranial neuropathy
  - Focal limb neuropathy
  - Diabetic amyotrophy
  - Truncal neuropathy
- Autonomic neuropathies
- Chronic inflammatory demyelinating polyneuropathy (CIDP)

EPIDEMIOLOGY

Prevalence

- Prevalence increases with diabetes duration
- Generalized polyneuropathy:
  - 10% at diabetes diagnosis
  - 50% at 25 years
  - Cross-sectional prevalence: 15% by symptoms; 50% by nerve conduction
- Autonomic neuropathy: 16.7% in a UK study

RISK FACTORS

- Poor glycemic control
- Duration of diabetes
- Older age
- Presence of retinopathy

GENERAL PREVENTION

Maintenance of normal blood sugar

PATHOPHYSIOLOGY

- >1 pathogenetic factor may operate
- Metabolic derangement due to hyperglycemia:
  - Aldose reductase converts excess glucose to sorbitol, which causes nerve damage
  - Nonenzymatic glycation of neural proteins and lipids forms damaging advanced glycosylation end products
  - Protein kinase C activation causes vascular endothelial changes
  - Oxidative stress from excessive production of reactive oxygen species
- Vasculopathy causing nerve ischemia: Likely in mononeuropathies

ETIOLOGY

Diabetes mellitus (type 1 and 2)

DIAGNOSIS

HISTORY

- Most common form: Symmetric distal sensory or sensorimotor polyneuropathy:
  - Distressing numbness, tingling, pain of legs/feet, usually worse at night; allodynia; hyperalgesia
  - Sometimes silent and unnoticed by patient
  - Ataxia due to proprioceptive loss
  - Neuropathic foot ulcers due to analgesia and repetitive injury
  - Neuropathic degeneration of foot joints
  - Hands involved late
  - Distal muscle involvement, usually mild
- Symmetric proximal polyneuropathy:
  - Proximal leg weakness and wasting
  - Muscles of shoulder girdle rarely involved
  - Pain and sensory changes less prominent
- Focal cranial or limb mononeuropathy:
  - May involve 3rd, 4th, 6th, or 7th cranial nerve
  - Femoral, sciatic, or peroneal neuropathy: Weakness or pain in nerve distribution
  - Any major peripheral nerve can be involved
- Truncal neuropathies: Painful radiculopathy over dermatomes
- Diabetic amyotrophy (this term is used for a lumbar radiculoplexopathy):
  - Unilateral hip, thigh pain
  - Pelvic girdle, thigh weakness, atrophy
  - Recovery over months
- Diabetic autonomic neuropathy:
  - Gastrointestinal: Nocturnal diarrhea, sometimes alternating with constipation; gastroparesis with postprandial fullness; nausea and vomiting
  - Cardiovascular: Postural dizziness; increased risk for coronary event; exercise intolerance
  - Urogenital: Urinary hesitancy, overflow incontinence; erectile dysfunction; vaginal dryness; sexual dysfunction
  - Sudomotor: Anhidrosis or hyperhydrosis; gustatory sweating of head and upper body
- CIDP: Progressive, severe motor loss
- Diabetic cachexia: Weight loss and depression with polyneuropathy

PHYSICAL EXAM

- Symmetric distal polyneuropathy:
  - "Stocking-and-glove" distal sensory loss
  - Large-fiber neuropathy: Loss of vibratory perception and light touch (10-G monofilament)
  - Small-fiber involvement: Loss of temperature and pinprick
  - Absent ankle reflexes
  - Wasting, weakness of small muscles in foot; changes to arch of foot or clawing of toes
  - With small-fiber involvement, there may be lack of objective sensory deficit despite pain
- Symmetric proximal polyneuropathy:
  - Proximal leg, arm wasting and weakness
  - Loss of patellar reflexes
- Focal cranial or limb mononeuropathy:
  - 3rd cranial nerve palsy: Painful ophthalmoplegia and ptosis; preserved pupillary reflexes (in contrast to compressive palsies)
  - 6th cranial nerve: Lateral gaze palsy
  - Femoral neuropathy: Weakness of lower leg extension; hip flexion; quadriceps wasting; absent patellar reflex; sensory loss in anterior thigh
  - Sciatic neuropathy: Pain or sensory loss in back of thigh and leg; weakness of hamstrings, lower leg muscles
  - Peroneal neuropathy: Foot drop
- Truncal neuropathies: Sensory loss along dermatomes
- Lumbar radiculoplexopathy (amyotrophy):
  - Weakness and wasting pelvic girdle and thigh
  - Sensory loss in L2–L3
  - Absent patellar reflex
- Autonomic neuropathy:
  - Cardiovascular: Resting tachycardia; orthostatic hypotension
  - Gastroparesis: Postprandial distension; gastric splash
- CIDP: Motor weakness

DIAGNOSTIC TESTS & INTERPRETATION

Lab

Initial lab tests

- Fasting plasma glucose, 2-hr glucose tolerance test or hemoglobin A1c for diagnosis and to assess glycemic control
- Serum B_{12} levels
- Thyroid function
- Creatinine and blood urea nitrogen
- Syphilis testing
- Serum protein electrophoresis
- In mononeuropathy/mononeuritis multiplex, test for vasculitis, paraproteinemia, and sarcoid.

Imaging

Initial approach

In radiculopathy or mononeuropathy, imaging studies to exclude compressive lesions

Diagnostic Procedures/Surgery

- Quantitative sensory testing for vibratory and thermal thresholds:
  - Standardized measures for assessing severity and risk of foot ulceration
- Electromyogram nerve conduction velocity (1):
  - Useful to confirm mononeuropathy and entrapment syndromes
  - Sensitive but nonspecific index of presence and severity of diabetic polyneuropathy
  - In small unmyelinated fiber painful neuropathy, test may be normal
- Lumbar puncture:
  - In CIDP, elevation of spinal fluid protein
- Skin biopsy (1):
  - Enables direct study of small nerve fibers that are difficult to assess electrophysiologically
- Corneal confocal microscopy (2):
  - Noninvasive approach based on examination of corneal innervation

athological Findings

- In peripheral nerve, Wallerian degeneration, focal axonal swellings containing neurofilaments, axonal atrophy, and demyelination are seen.
- Thick neural capillary basement membrane
- Obliterative microvascular lesions and perivascular inflammation

IFFERENTIAL DIAGNOSIS

- Uremic polyneuropathy
- Drug-induced:
  - Antineoplastic drugs: Cisplatin, vincristine
  - Isoniazid
  - Amiodarone
- Toxic:
  - Chronic arsenic poisoning
  - n-Hexane, methyl-*n*-butyl ketone
- Nutritional deficiency:
  - Usually associated with alcoholism
- Paraneoplastic polyneuropathy
- Hypothyroidism

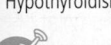

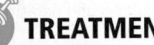

TREATMENT

MEDICATION

irst Line

- Management of pain and sensory neuropathy:
  - Tricyclic antidepressants (TCAs) (1,3,4)[A]:
    - Analgesia may be related to effects on sodium channels
    - Amitriptyline 25–150 mg at bedtime
    - Nortriptyline (25–150 mg); desipramine (25–200 mg) less sedating than amitriptyline
    - Anticholinergic side effects may occur.
  - Calcium channel modulators: Gabapentin (1,34)[A]:
    - Fewer side effects than TCAs
    - Act on subunits of voltage-gated calcium channels (same site as pregabalin)
    - Dose titration is from 300–1,200 mg t.i.d.
    - Reduce dose in renal insufficiency
    - Adverse effects: Dizziness, fatigue, edema
  - Calcium channel modulators: Pregabalin (34)[A]
    - Binds Ca^{2+} channel-associated protein α_2-δ, inhibits neurotransmitter release
    - Usual dose 150–600 mg
    - Adverse effects are dizziness and edema.
  - Duloxetine (3 ,4)[A]:
    - Selective serotonin and norepinephrine uptake inhibitor
    - Usual dose is 60–120 mg/d
    - Adverse effects are nausea and dizziness.
- Management of autonomic neuropathy (3):
  - Orthostatic hypotension:
    - Fludrocortisone
    - Midodrine
  - Gastroparesis:
    - Metoclopramide or domperidone
    - Erythromycin
  - Diabetic diarrhea:
    - Loperamide
    - Clonidine
    - Octreotide
    - Antibiotics for bacterial overgrowth
  - Erectile dysfunction:
    - Phosphodiesterase-5 inhibitors
    - Prostaglandin E_1 injection
    - Mechanical devices
  - Hyperhidrosis:
    - Propantheline

Geriatric Considerations

- Anticholinergic effects of TCAs may cause urinary retention, arrhythmias

Second Line

- Antidepressants:
  - Venlafaxine (75–225 mg daily) (4)[B]:
    - Serotonin norepinephrine reuptake inhibitor
  - Selective serotonin reuptake inhibitors (4)[B]:
    - Paroxetine and citalopram demonstrate some efficacy.
- Anticonvulsants:
  - Carbamazepine (1,3)[B]:
    - Alleviates pain by blocking sodium channels
    - Dose 400–1,200 mg/d
  - Lamotrigine/topiramate 200–600 mg (1,3)[B]
- Topical therapies:
  - Capsaicin 0.075% cream applied t.i.d. 3[B]:
    - Depletes C fibers in skin of substance P
  - Lidocaine 5% (700 mg) patches applied daily to feet (3)[B]:
    - Causes sodium channel blockade
- Opiate analgesia:
  - Tramadol 100–400 mg daily (1,3):
    - Nonnarcotic medication; binds opiate receptors; fewer opiate side effects
  - Oxycodone (1,3)[A]:
    - Controversial due to dependence potential
- α-Lipoic Acid (4)[B]:
  - Antioxidant properties may limit free radical-mediated damage
  - 600 mg oral daily dose; showed benefit in small studies

ADDITIONAL TREATMENT

General Measures

- Maintain blood glucose close to normal.
- Provide appropriate footwear to prevent pressure damage to insensate feet.

Issues for Referral

If CIDP suspected, refer to neurologist for investigation and treatment

Additional Therapies

- Transcutaneous electrical nerve stimulation
- Percutaneous nerve stimulation
- Electrical spinal cord stimulation

COMPLEMENTARY AND ALTERNATIVE MEDICINE

Acupuncture (1)[C]: Placebo response possible, as trials were unblinded

SURGERY/OTHER PROCEDURES

Electrical spinal cord stimulation (1)

ONGOING CARE

PROGNOSIS

- Generalized symmetric polyneuropathies:
  - Usually slow chronic progression
  - Insensitive but painless foot as pain lessens
- Focal neuropathies:
  - Recovery over months to years

COMPLICATIONS

- Claw foot deformity
- Neurotropic ulceration:
  - Painless ulcers on weightbearing area
  - Callus formation precursor to ulceration
- Neuropathic arthropathy:
  - Results in complete disorganization of joint structure in foot, Charcot joint

REFERENCES

1. Boulton AJ, Malik RA, Arezzo JC, et al. Diabetic somatic neuropathies. *Diabetes Care*. 2004;27: 1458–86.
2. Zochodne DW. Diabetic polyneuropathy: an update. *Curr Opin Neurol*. 2008;21:527–33.
3. Unger J, et al. Recognition and management of diabetic neuropathy. *Primary Care: Clin Office Pract*. 2007;34:887–913.
4. Ziegler D et al. Painful diabetic neuropathy: advantage of novel drugs over old drugs? *Diabetes Care*. 2009;32 (Suppl 2):S414–9.

ADDITIONAL READING

- Boulton AJ, Vinik AI, Arezzo JC, et al. Diabetic neuropathies: a statement by the American Diabetes Association. *Diabetes Care*. 2005;28:956–62.
- Casellini CM, Vinik AI et al. Clinical manifestations and current treatment options for diabetic neuropathies. *Endocr Pract*. 2007;13:550–66.
- Wong MC, Chung JW, Wong TK. Effects of treatments for symptoms of painful diabetic neuropathy: systematic review. *BMJ*. 2007;335:87.

See Also (Topic, Algorithm, Electronic Media Element)

Diabetes Mellitus, Type 1; Diabetes Mellitus, Type 2

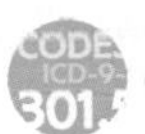

CODES

ICD9

- 250.60 Diabetes mellitus with neurological manifestations, type ii or unspecified type, not stated as uncontrolled
- 250.61 Diabetes mellitus with neurological manifestations, type I (juvenile type) not stated as uncontrolled
- 250.62 Diabetes mellitus with neurological manifestations, type ii or unspecified type, uncontrolled

CLINICAL PEARLS

- Occasionally, when glycemic control improves dramatically, as can occur when treatment for diabetes is initiated, there may be a worsening of neuropathy symptoms. Symptoms usually stabilize and gradually improve as glycemic control is maintained.
- It is common to combine agents with different mechanisms of action in the management of neuropathic pain. Topical therapies can also be combined with systemic therapies.

DIARRHEA, ACUTE

Cheryl Abel, PharmD
Jill A. Grimes, MD

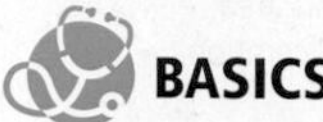

BASICS

DESCRIPTION

- Abnormal increase in stool frequency or liquidity in an otherwise healthy individual
- Often self-limiting; <14 days duration
- Acute viral diarrhea (50–70%):
  - Most common form; usually occurs for 1–3 days; self-limited
  - Causes changes in small intestinal cell morphology, such as villous shortening and an increase in the number of crypt cells
- Bacterial diarrhea (15–20%):
  - Develop 6–24 hours after infected food ingested
  - Suspect if simultaneous illness is present in others who have shared contaminated food
- Protozoal infections (10–15%):
  - Cause prolonged, watery diarrhea (travelers from areas with contaminated water supply)
- Traveler's diarrhea typically begins 3–7 days after arrival in foreign location; often quite acute.
- System(s) affected: Endocrine/Metabolic; Gastrointestinal

EPIDEMIOLOGY

Predominant age: All ages

Prevalence

- 11% of the general population
- Highest in children <5 years old

RISK FACTORS

- Individual from an industrialized country visiting a developing country
- Immunocompromised host
- Antibiotic use
- Day care attendance; nursing home residency

GENERAL PREVENTION

- Frequent handwashing; proper hygiene
- Rotavirus vaccine
- Strict food handling
- Care during foreign travel to avoid brushing teeth with contaminated water, ingesting ice cubes, or eating cold salads or meats
- Probiotics may be used to help prevent traveler's diarrhea (1)[A].

ETIOLOGY

- Bacterial:
  - *Escherichia coli*
  - *Salmonella*
  - *Shigella*
  - *Campylobacter jejuni*
  - *Vibrio parahaemolyticus*
  - *Vibrio cholerae*
  - *Yersinia enterocolitica*
  - *Clostridium difficile*
  - *Staphylococcus aureus*
  - *Bacillus cereus*
- Viral:
  - Rotavirus
  - Norwalklike virus (Norovirus)
- Protozoal:
  - *Giardia lamblia*
  - *Cryptosporidium*
  - *Entamoeba histolytica*
  - *Isospora belli*

Pediatric Considerations

- Rotavirus is a common cause of viral diarrhea in the winter months and is accompanied by vomiting.
- Other etiologies include overfeeding, medications, cystic fibrosis, and malabsorption.

COMMONLY ASSOCIATED CONDITIONS

- Diabetes mellitus
- Ileal resection
- Gastrectomy
- Hyperthyroidism

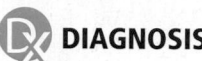

DIAGNOSIS

HISTORY

- Anorexia ± vomiting
- Malaise
- Headache
- Myalgia
- Assess stool characteristics: Frequency and quantity, presence of mucous or blood, consistency (2)[A]
- Travel history, day care attendance, ingestion of raw or undercooked meat, raw seafood, unpasteurized milk, sick contacts (2)[A]
- With *Giardia*: Cramping; pale, greasy stools; fatigue; weight loss; chronicity

PHYSICAL EXAM

- Loose liquid stools ± blood or mucus
- Fever
- Abdominal pain and distension
- Determine hydration status; look for decreased skin turgor, dry mucous membranes, hypotension, or decreased urination:
  - In children: Absence of tears, depressed fontanelles, dry diapers
- Abdominal exam to rule out potential surgical causes of diarrhea such as appendicitis or pelvic abscess

Geriatric Considerations

Watery diarrhea with chronic constipation may be caused by fecal impaction or obstructing neoplasm.

Pregnancy Considerations

Dehydration may lead to preterm labor.

DIAGNOSTIC TESTS & INTERPRETATION

Lab

Initial lab tests

- Consider testing if diarrhea is prolonged
- Complete blood count:
  - Increased white blood cells with a left shift may indicate an infectious process.
  - A decreased hemoglobin/hematocrit may indicate anemia from blood loss.
- Serum electrolytes:
  - Increased sodium from dehydration
  - Decreased potassium from diarrhea
- Blood urea nitrogen, creatinine: Elevated in dehydration
- pH: Hyperchloremic acidosis
- Stool sample:
  - Occult blood present in inflammatory bowel disease, bowel ischemia, bacterial infections
  - Fecal leukocytes present in diarrhea caused by *Salmonella, Campylobacter, Yersinia*
  - For community-acquired or traveler's diarrhea >1 day or accompanied by fever or bloody stools: Culture or test for *Salmonella, Shigella, Campylobacter*, *E. coli* O157:H7. If antibiotics or chemotherapy in recent weeks, *C. difficile* toxin A and B (2)[B].
  - For nosocomial diarrhea (onset ≥3 days in hospital): Test for *C. difficile* toxins A and B. Also consider bacterial cultures listed above in patients with bloody stools or infants (2)[B].
  - For diarrhea >7 days: Stool ova and parasites (O & P) plus bacterial cultures if immunocompromised (2)[B]
  - *Giardia* enzyme linked immunosorbent assay: >90% sensitive in at-risk population, consider prior to O & P

Imaging

Abdominal radiographs (flat plate and upright) indicated with abdominal pain or evidence of obstruction to rule out toxic megacolon and bowel ischemia

Diagnostic Procedures/Surgery

Sigmoidoscopy indicated with bloody diarrhea or suspected pseudomembranous or ulcerative colitis

Pathological Findings

- Viral diarrhea: Changes in small intestine cell morphology that include villous shortening, increased number of crypt cells, and increased cellularity of the lamina propria
- Bacterial diarrhea: Bacterial invasion of colonic wall leads to mucosal hyperemia, edema, and leukocytic infiltration.

DIFFERENTIAL DIAGNOSIS

- Inflammatory bowel disease
- Drugs (cholinergic agents, magnesium-containing antacids)
- Pseudomembranous colitis secondary to antibiotic use
- Diverticulitis
- Spastic (irritable) colon
- Fecal impaction
- Malabsorption
- Zollinger-Ellison syndrome
- Ischemic bowel
- Gastrinoma

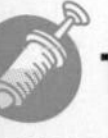

TREATMENT

MEDICATION

First Line

- Loperamide: 4 mg followed by 2-mg capsule after each unformed stool (see precautions below)
- Bismuth subsalicylate: 30 mL every 1/2 hour until 8 doses; may be helpful in mild diarrhea
- If diarrhea persists and a bacterial or parasitic organism is identified, antibiotic therapy should be started:
  - *Giardia*: Metronidazole 250 mg t.i.d. for 5 days
  - *E. histolytica*: Metronidazole 750 mg t.i.d. for 10 days
  - *Shigella*: Trimethoprim-sulfamethoxazole (Bactrim DS) 160 mg/800 mg b.i.d. for 5 days, or ciprofloxacin 500 mg b.i.d. for 3 days
  - *Campylobacter*: Erythromycin 500 mg q.i.d. for 5 days or ciprofloxacin 500 mg b.i.d. for 3 days
  - *C. difficile*: Discontinue antibiotics if possible. Consider metronidazole 500 mg t.i.d. for 10–14 days if diarrhea persists or worsens.
  - Traveler's diarrhea: Ciprofloxacin 750 mg 1 dose or, if severe, 500 mg divided p.o. twice a day for 3 days *or* TMP/SMX (Bactrim DS) 1 tab twice a day for 3 days
- Contraindications:
  - Antibiotics are contraindicated in *Salmonella* infections unless caused by *S. typhosa* or the patient is severely ill.
  - Avoid alcoholic beverages with metronidazole due to the possibility of a disulfiram reaction.
  - Antibiotics are not indicated in foodborne toxigenic diarrhea.
- Precautions:
  - Antiperistaltic agents (e.g., loperamide) should be used with caution in patients suspected of having infectious diarrhea (especially if *E. coli* 0157:H7 suspected) or antibiotic-associated colitis
  - Antiperistaltic agents may speed recovery from traveler's diarrhea when used in combination with antibiotics (3)[A].
  - Doxycycline, sulfamethoxazole-trimethoprim, and ciprofloxacin may cause photosensitivity; use sunscreen.
- Significant possible interactions:
  - Salicylate absorption from bismuth subsalicylate can cause toxicity in patients already taking aspirin-containing compounds and may alter anticoagulation control in patients taking Coumadin.
  - Ciprofloxacin and erythromycin increase theophylline levels.

Second Line

- Doxycycline: 100 mg b.i.d. for 3 days
- Diphenoxylate-atropine in nonpregnant adults
- Tinidazole or selnidazole for *E. histolytica*
- Oral vancomycin for *C. difficile* infections

ADDITIONAL TREATMENT

General Measures

Replace lost fluid and electrolytes (2)[A]:

- Clear liquids at room temperature, such as tea, broth, carbonated beverages (without caffeine), and rehydration fluids (e.g., Gatorade) to replace lost fluid.
- Packets of rehydration salts (1 packet to be diluted in 1 quart of water); drink until thirst is quenched (helps replace electrolytes); treatment of choice for pediatric patients
- ORS (oral rehydration solutions): Polymer-based ORS may be superior to glucose-based ORS in watery diarrhea (4)[A].
- IV fluids if patient cannot tolerate oral rehydration

COMPLEMENTARY AND ALTERNATIVE MEDICINE

- In children with acute infectious diarrhea, treatment with probiotics appears to be safe and effective for reducing the duration and frequency of diarrhea (5)[B].
- In patients being treated with antibiotics, administration of a probiotic at levels above 10^{10}/g may prevent diarrhea (6)[A].
- Zinc supplementation can decrease diarrhea-related morbidity and mortality (7)[A].

IN-PATIENT CONSIDERATIONS

Initial Stabilization

Outpatient health care except for complicating emergencies (dehydration)

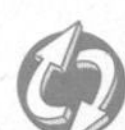

ONGOING CARE

DIET

- Early refeeding is encouraged.
- During periods of active diarrhea, avoid coffee, alcohol, dairy products, most fruits, vegetables, red meats, and heavily seasoned foods.
- Begin by eating clear soup with rice, salted crackers, dry toast or bread, and sherbet.
- As stooling rate decreases, slowly add to diet baked potato and chicken soup with noodles.
- As stool begins to retain shape, add to diet baked fish, poultry, applesauce, and bananas.
- The traditional bananas, rice, applesauce, toast diet has little evidence-based support despite heavy clinical use.

PATIENT EDUCATION

See guidelines in Prevention section.

PROGNOSIS

This common problem is rarely life-threatening if adequate hydration is maintained.

COMPLICATIONS

- Dehydration
- Sepsis
- Shock
- Anemia

REFERENCES

1. McFarland LV et al. Meta-analysis of probiotics for the prevention of traveler's diarrhea. *Travel Med Infect Dis*. 2007;5:97–105.
2. Guerrant RL, Van Gilder T, Steiner TS, et al. Practice guidelines for the management of infectious diarrhea. *Clin Infect Dis*. 2001;32:331–51.
3. Riddle MS, Arnold S, Tribble DR et al. Effect of adjunctive loperamide in combination with antibiotics on treatment outcomes in traveler's diarrhea: a systematic review and meta-analysis. *Clin Infect Dis*. 2008;47:1007–14.
4. Gregorio GV, Gonzales ML, Dans LF, et al. Polymer-based oral rehydration solution for treating acute watery diarrhoea. *Cochrane Database Syst Rev*. 2009;CD006519.
5. Chen CC, Kong MS, Lai MW, Chao HC, Chang KW, Chen SY, Huang YC, Chiu CH, Li WC, Lin PY, Chen CJ, Li TY et al. Probiotics have clinical, microbiologic, and immunologic efficacy in acute infectious diarrhea. *Pediatr Infect Dis J*. 2010;29:135–8.
6. McFarland LV et al. Evidence-based review of probiotics for antibiotic-associated diarrhea and Clostridium difficile infections. *Anaerobe*. 2009;15:274–80.
7. Walker CL, Black RE et al. Zinc for the treatment of diarrhoea: effect on diarrhoea morbidity, mortality and incidence of future episodes. *Int J Epidemiol*. 2010;39 (Suppl 1):i63–9.

ADDITIONAL READING

- Dupont HL. Systematic review: the epidemiology and clinical features of travellers' diarrhoea. *Aliment Pharmacol Ther*. 2009.
- Marcos LA, DuPont HL. Advances in defining etiology and new therapeutic approaches in acute diarrhea. *J Infect*. 2007;55:385–93.

See Also (Topic, Algorithm, Electronic Media Element)

Botulism; Cholera; Food Poisoning, Bacterial

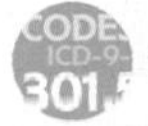

CODES

ICD9

- 005.9 Food poisoning, unspecified
- 008.5 Bacterial enteritis, unspecified
- 009.2 Infectious diarrhea

CLINICAL PEARLS

- Viruses, especially norovirus, are the most common causes of acute diarrheal illness in the US:
  - Antibiotics are not generally needed for routine bacterial causes of gastroenteritis.
- Early refeeding and use of probiotics is encouraged.
- Loperamide and bismuth are useful antidiarrheal medications.
- Bismuth can cause transient black tongues and stools.

D

DIARRHEA, CHRONIC

Cheryl Abel, PharmD
Jill A. Grimes, MD

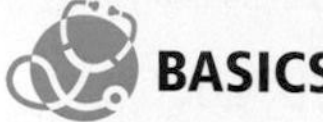

BASICS

DESCRIPTION

Chronic diarrhea refers to an increase in frequency or decrease in fecal consistency (typically >3 loose stools per day) for >4 weeks:

- Causes include inflammatory diarrhea, osmotic diarrhea (malabsorption), secretory diarrhea, and intestinal dysmotility.
- System(s) affected: Gastrointestinal

Geriatric Considerations

Patients with lifelong diarrhea may suffer increasing difficulty with advanced age.

EPIDEMIOLOGY

Prevalence

Depends on criterion used, but approximately 5% of US population is affected.

RISK FACTORS

- Female > Male
- Inflammatory:
  - AIDS
  - Infections
  - Radiation
  - Family history
- Osmotic:
  - Infectious
  - Abdominal surgery: Cholecystectomy, resection, vagotomy
  - Chronic alcohol abuse
  - Sorbitol, fructose, lactose, gluten
- Secretory: Distal ileal surgery
- Altered intestinal motility:
  - Diabetes
  - Fecal impaction
  - Neurologic diseases
- Factitious: Laxative use

Genetics

- Celiac sprue and inflammatory bowel disease may be familial.
- Lactose intolerance: Increased incidence in certain geographic regions

GENERAL PREVENTION

Refrain from dietary or pharmacologic agents that may precipitate a diarrhea event.

PATHOPHYSIOLOGY

Incomplete absorption of water from intestinal lumen

ETIOLOGY

- Inflammatory diarrhea:
  - Inflammatory bowel disease
  - Radiation enterocolitis
  - Eosinophilic gastroenteritis
  - Hypersensitivity (e.g., food allergy)
  - AIDS
- Infectious diarrhea:
  - Parasites (e.g., *Giardia lamblia, Isospora*)
  - Helminths (e.g., Strongyloides)
  - Bacterial (e.g., *Mycobacterium avium intracellulare, Clostridium difficile*)
- Osmotic diarrhea:
  - Celiac disease
  - Lactase deficiency
  - Pancreatic insufficiency
  - Bacterial overgrowth
  - Thyrotoxicosis
  - Whipple disease
  - Abetalipoproteinemia
  - Postsurgical (short gut, peptic ulcer disease [PUD] surgery)
  - Drugs: Osmotically active agents, antibiotics, nonsteroidal anti-inflammatory drugs (NSAIDs), prostaglandins, colchicine, metformin, digoxin, selective serotonin reuptake inhibitors (SSRIs), antineoplastic agents
  - Herbal products: St. John's wort, echinacea, feverfew, garlic, saw palmetto, ginseng, cranberry extract, pokeroot tea, aloe vera
- Secretory diarrhea:
  - Carcinoid syndrome
  - Zollinger-Ellison syndrome
  - Vasoactive intestinal peptide-secreting pancreatic adenomas
  - Medullary carcinoma of thyroid
  - Villous adenoma of rectum
  - Microscopic colitis (collagenous, lymphocytic)
  - Choleraic diarrhea: Excessive secretion of electrolytes
  - Diabetes mellitus
  - Laxatives (phenolphthalein, cascara, senna, aloe)
  - Toxins (arsenic, mushrooms, insecticides, alcohol)
- Altered intestinal motility (most common in clinical practice)
- Irritable bowel syndrome (most common in young females)
- Fecal impaction
- Neurologic diseases
- Diabetes: Increased transit and possible bacterial overgrowth
- In children: Secondary to dietary products (e.g., fructose and apple juice)

COMMONLY ASSOCIATED CONDITIONS

- Immune-complex-mediated extraintestinal complications of inflammatory bowel disease (IBD)
- Arthritis, uveitis, pyoderma gangrenosum, nephritis

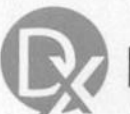

DIAGNOSIS

HISTORY

- Review the onset, pattern, duration, frequency of loose stools, and stool characteristics.
- Asses for fecal incontinence, aggravating factors (diet, stress), mitigating factors (diet, drugs), travel, or other exposures.
- Check for weight loss.
- Review previous evaluation.
- Appropriate review of systems for underlying causes hyperthyroidism, diabetes mellitus, collagen vascula diseases, tumor syndromes, AIDS, Ig deficiencies (review the Rome Criteria for IBS) (1)[C]:
  - ≥3 months of abdominal discomfort, relieved with defecation and associated with a change in frequency and consistency of stool
  - >2 of the following altered stools, at least 25% of the time:
    - Frequency
    - Form (e.g., loose or hard stools)
    - Stool passage (sensation of incomplete evacuation after bowel movements, straining, o urging)
    - Passing mucus

PHYSICAL EXAM

- General: Fluid balance, nutrition
- Skin: Flushing, rashes, dermatographism
- Thyroid: Mass
- Chest: Wheezing
- Heart: Murmur
- Abdomen: Hepatomegaly, mass, ascites, tenderness
- Anorectal: Sphincter competence, fecal occult blood test
- Extremities: Edema

DIAGNOSTIC TESTS & INTERPRETATION

Lab

Initial lab tests

- Complete blood count (CBC) with differential, electrolytes, total protein, albumin, thyroid-stimulating hormone (TSH), amylase/lipase (if weight loss)
- If celiac disease suspected: Antiendomysial antibody (AEA), transglutimase antibody (TGA), Ig A
- Initial stool analysis: WBCs, electrolytes, pH, fecal occult blood, fat output (Sudan stain), laxative screen
- Stool ova and parasites
- *C. difficile* toxin (if history of antibiotic use)
- Modified Ziehl-Neelson stain if immunocompromised (*Cryptosporidium*)

ollow-Up & Special Considerations
When tumor syndrome suspected: Gastrin, calcitonin, vasoactive intestinal peptide, somatostatin, urine excretion of 5-hydroxy acetic acid, metanephrine, histamine
24-hour stool collection: Weight (g/24 hours), pH, electrolytes, osmolality

maging
initial approach
Plain film abdomen
Flexible sigmoidoscopy with (if >45 years old) or without (if <45) barium enema (2)[B]
Computed tomography (CT) to rule out pancreatic cancer/chronic pancreatitis if abnormal pancreatic enzymes or evidence of malabsorption

Diagnostic Procedures/Surgery
Colonoscopy/sigmoidoscopy for inflammatory lesions; if occult blood in stool ± iron deficiency
- Barium enema with small bowel follow-through can help evaluate the small bowel.
- If barium enema is negative and diarrhea persists, biopsies are indicated.
- Esophagogastroduodenoscopy (EGD) with small bowel biopsies if malabsorption disorder suspected

Pathological Findings
- When present, the findings are those of the associated or underlying disease.
- None seen in functional disorder
- Melanosis coli suggests cathartic abuse.

DIFFERENTIAL DIAGNOSIS
- Functional disorder
- Inflammatory bowel disease: Look for systemic illness or extraintestinal manifestations (arthritis, pyoderma gangrenosum, erythema nodosum, uveitis, or vasculitis).
- Factitious: Psychiatric disease or past history
- Irritable bowel syndrome (IBS): Alternating diarrhea and constipation
- Tropical sprue
- Tuberculosis enteritis
- Chronic radiation enterocolitis
- Colonic neoplasm
- Diverticular disease
- Lactose intolerance (uncommon)

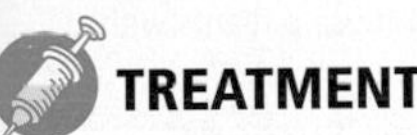

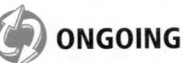

TREATMENT

MEDICATION
First Line
Opioid agonists are considered 1st-line symptomatic treatment relief of diarrhea:
- Diphenoxylate-atropine (Lomotil): 5–20 mg/d or loperamide (Imodium) 4–16 mg/d, doses calculated and timed according to patient's weight and individual needs
- Contraindicated in infectious diarrhea and ulcerative colitis toxic megacolon

Second Line
- Cholestyramine (Questran) for bile salt malabsorption, certain postsurgical patients (3)[C]:
  – 4–8 g t.i.d.
  – May interfere with absorption of fat-soluble vitamins and other medications
- Lactase (Lactaid, Lactrase) for lactose intolerance: Chew/swallow 3 original-strength tablets or 1 fast-acting tablet with 1st bite of food containing dairy products.
- Budesonide exhibits high clinical and histological response rates in collagenous colitis (pooled OR for clinical response 12.32 (95% CI 5.53-27.46) with NNT of 2 patients (4)[A]:
  – 9 mg p.o. daily for 6–8 weeks
- Steroids and sulfasalazine derivatives in inflammatory bowel disease
- Octreotide (Sandostatin): In carcinoid and other peptide-secreting tumors, dumping syndrome, chemotherapy-induced diarrhea:
  – 200–300 SC μg/d in 2–4 divided doses
  – Can be switched to IM depot form (Sandostatin LAR) 20 mg intragluteally q4wk. Revaluate after 2 months.

ADDITIONAL TREATMENT
There is little evidence to support treating children with antimicrobials for persistent diarrhea (5)[A].

General Measures
- Unless the patient is hypotensive or an electrolyte abnormality or deconditioning is present, outpatient therapy is adequate.
- Fluids with electrolyte supplementation

SURGERY/OTHER PROCEDURES
For villous adenomas, hormone-producing tumors, and refractory ulcerative colitis

ONGOING CARE

DIET
- Abstain from gluten products, sorbitol, lactose-containing products, and food allergens.
- In irritable bowel syndrome, add dietary fiber (e.g., 20–30 g/d supplemental fiber).

PATIENT EDUCATION
- Reassure that normal frequency varies widely.
- Restrict colon stimulants.
- Dietary consult when appropriate

PROGNOSIS
Variable, from a short (factitious and altered intestinal motility) and treatable course, to a chronic illness (e.g., Crohn disease, ulcerative colitis)

COMPLICATIONS
- Fluid and electrolyte abnormalities
- Malnutrition
- Anemia

REFERENCES

1. Longstreth GF, Thompson WG, Chey WD, et al. Functional bowel disorders. *Gastroenterology*. 2006;130:1480–91.
2. Thomas PD, Forbes A, Green J, et al. Guidelines for the investigation of chronic diarrhoea, 2nd edition. *Gut*. 2003;52 (Suppl 5):v1–15.
3. Ung KA, Gillberg R, Kilander A, et al. Role of bile acids and bile acid binding agents in patients with collagenous colitis. *Gut*. 2000;46:170–5.
4. Chande N, McDonald JWD, MacDonald JK. Interventions for treating collagenous colitis. *Cochrane Database of Systematic Reviews*. 2008, Issue 2. Art. No.: CD003575. DOI:10.1002/14651858.CD003575.pub5.
5. Abba K, Sinfield R, Hart CA, Garner P, et al. Antimicrobial drugs for persistent diarrhoea of unknown or non-specific cause in children under six in low and middle income countries: systematic review of randomized controlled trials. *BMC Infect. Dis*. 2009;9:24.

ADDITIONAL READING

- Baber KF, Anderson J, Puzanovova M, Walker LS, et al. Rome II versus Rome III classification of functional gastrointestinal disorders in pediatric chronic abdominal pain. *J. Pediatr. Gastroenterol. Nutr*. 2008;47:299–302.
- Fan X, Sellin JH. Review article: Small intestinal bacterial overgrowth, bile acid malabsorption and gluten intolerance as possible causes of chronic watery diarrhea. *Aliment Pharmacol Ther*. 2009.
- Nwachukwu CE, Okebe JU, et al. Antimotility agents for chronic diarrhoea in people with HIV/AIDS. *Cochrane Database Syst Rev*. 2008;CD005644.
- Saxena S, Mitton SG, Pollok R et al. Chronic diarrhoea in a teenager. *BMJ*. 2008;337:a430.

See Also (Topic, Algorithm, Electronic Media Element)
Algorithm: Diarrhea, Chronic

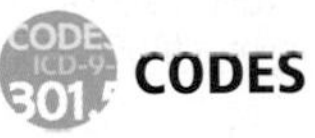

CODES

ICD9
787.91 Diarrhea

CLINICAL PEARLS

- The most common causes are functional disorders such as IBS, IBD, malabsorptive syndromes, chronic infections, and idiopathic secretory diarrhea.
- Opioids and opioid agonists (loperamide, diphenoxylate-atropine) should be considered as 1st-line for symptomatic relief of chronic, noninfectious diarrhea.
- The evaluation and treatment of diarrheal syndromes is often a multistep process that requires ruling out a wide variety of entities. However, most cases can be diagnosed through careful history and physical examination and select laboratory studies.

DIFFUSE INTERSTITIAL LUNG DISEASE

Jacqueline L. Olin, MS, PharmD, BCPS, CPP
Julie Scott Taylor, MD, MSc

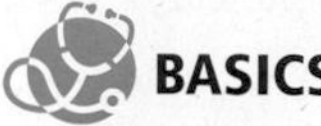

BASICS

DESCRIPTION

- Interstitial lung diseases (ILDs) represent a diverse group of chronic progressive lung diseases associated with alveolar inflammation and/or potentially irreversible pulmonary fibrosis.
- >200 individual diseases may present with similar characteristics, making ILD difficult to classify.
- A classification scheme proposed by the American Thoracic Society and European Respiratory Society includes these subtypes:
  - Known causes (environmental, occupational, or drug-associated disease)
  - Systemic disorders (sarcoidosis, Wegener granulomatosis, collagen vascular disease, etc.)
  - Rare lung diseases (pulmonary histiocytosis, lymphangioleiomyomatosis, etc.)
  - Idiopathic interstitial pneumonias (IIPs)
- Based on clinical, radiologic, and histologic features, IIPs are further subclassified into the following diagnoses:
  - Idiopathic pulmonary fibrosis (IPF), characterized by progressive dyspnea, cough, restrictive lung disease, and a specific histopathologic pattern
  - IIPs other than IPF (including nonspecific interstitial pneumonia [NSIP], respiratory bronchiolitis-associated ILD [RBILD], acute interstitial pneumonia [AIP], bronchiolitis obliterans with organizing pneumonia [BOOP], etc.)
- The classification of IIPs and relationships between the subtypes continues to be an area of controversy.

Pediatric Considerations

Interstitial lung disease (ILD) in infants and children represents a heterogeneous group of respiratory disorders that are mostly chronic and associated with high morbidity and mortality. In children, ILD is difficult to diagnose, as no classification scheme is entirely satisfactory (1). Classification can center around whether disease is primarily a pulmonary process or if symptoms occur as a result of a systemic disorder.

EPIDEMIOLOGY

Incidence

- Due to lack of consistency in disease presentation and definition, epidemiologic data are not well defined. Exact incidence has been difficult to determine because of differences in case definitions and procedures used in diagnosis.
- Ranges cited for incidence of IPF: 6.8–16.3 per 100,000 (2)
- According to the National Heart, Lung, and Blood Institute, about 50,000 new cases of IPF are diagnosed each year in the US.

Prevalence

- Exact prevalence has been difficult to determine because of differences in case definitions and procedures used in diagnosis.
- Ranges cited for prevalence of IPF: 14–42.7 per 100,000 (2) and above 175 per 100,000 in the older population (3)

RISK FACTORS

- Environmental or occupational exposure to inorganic or organic dusts
- 66–75% of patients with ILD have a history of smoking.
- Due to diversity of diseases, age is not a reliable predictor of pathology:
  - Most patients with connective tissue disease-related pathology and inherited subtypes present between ages 20 and 40.
  - Patients with IPF are typically age 50 or older.

Genetics

Some studies suggest that some subtypes of ILD may be associated with specific predisposing genes and environmental exposures; however, the role of genetic factors is unknown at this time; ~10% of IPF cases are inherited.

GENERAL PREVENTION

Avoiding environmental/occupational exposure to organic or inorganic dust and smoking cessation may reduce incidence or improve clinical course in patients with established ILD.

PATHOPHYSIOLOGY

- Alveolar inflammation may progress into irreversible fibrosis.
- Varying degrees of ventilatory dysfunction occur among the ILD subtypes.
- ILD associated with collagen vascular disease and systemic connective disorders can manifest involvement of skin, joints, muscular, and ocular systems.

ETIOLOGY

Some types of ILD are associated with specific exposures:

- Medications (amiodarone, antibiotics [especially nitrofurantoin], chemotherapy agents, gold, illicit drugs)
- Inorganic dusts (silicates, asbestos, talc, mica, coal dust, graphite)
- Organic dusts (moldy hay, inhalation of fungi, bacteria, animal proteins)
- Metals (tin, aluminum, cobalt, iron, barium)
- Gases, fumes, vapors, aerosols

COMMONLY ASSOCIATED CONDITIONS

- Many systemic disorders and primary diseases are associated with ILD.
- A partial list includes:
  - Collagen vascular disease
  - Sarcoidosis
  - Amyloidosis
  - Goodpasture syndrome
  - Churg-Strauss syndrome
  - Wegener granulomatosis

DIAGNOSIS

- Diagnosis should be based on clinical, radiologic, and histologic data.
- A multidisciplinary consensus is recommended for diagnosis since even among experts, diagnostic criteria are subject to interpretation.

HISTORY

- Symptoms may include progressive exertional dyspnea and nonproductive cough.
- Patients may also present with hemoptysis (due to idiopathic alveolar hemosiderosis) or fatigue.
- Obtaining a history of illness duration (acute vs chronic), potential environmental/occupational exposures, travel, and medical conditions (including systemic diseases) is important in assessing the cause of the ILD.
- Some cases of lung disease may occur weeks to years after discontinuation of an offending agent.

PHYSICAL EXAM

Physical findings are usually nonspecific. Some common features include:

- Rales
- Inspiratory "squeaks"
- Clubbing of the digits
- Cyanosis in advanced disease

DIAGNOSTIC TESTS & INTERPRETATION

Lab

Initial lab tests

- Arterial blood gas (ABG)
- If a systemic disorder is suspected, consider obtaining an antinuclear antibody (ANA), rheumatoid factor (RF), erythrocyte sedimentation rate (ESR), and antineutrophil cytoplasmic antibodies (ANCA).

Follow-Up & Special Considerations

If indicated, hypersensitivity pneumonitis panel, plasma angiotensin-converting enzyme (ACE) concentration (sarcoidosis)

Imaging

Patients may also present initially with an abnormal chest x-ray (CXR) as compared with previous imaging.

Initial approach

CXR

Follow-Up & Special Considerations

High-resolution computed tomography (HRCT) of the chest is the most useful tool for distinguishing among ILD subclasses, especially in those patients with normal CXRs.

Diagnostic Procedures/Surgery

- Pulmonary function testing (PFT; spirometry, lung volumes, carbon monoxide diffusing capacity):
  - Commonly demonstrates a restrictive defect (decreased vital capacity and total lung capacity)
- Bronchoscopy:
  - Bronchoalveolar lavage (BAL) cellular analysis studies may be useful in distinguishing some subtypes (including sarcoidosis, hypersensitivity pneumonitis, cancer), but its role in diagnosis, prognostication, and assessment of disease progression is not clear (4).
  - Bronchoscopic transbronchial lung biopsy may help diagnose sarcoidosis and, on occasion, is sufficiently supportive of other ILD diagnoses.
- Thoracoscopic surgery for lung biopsy has the greatest diagnostic specificity for ILDs, but is less frequently used given improved specificity of HRCT. It may be indicated if a specific diagnosis cannot be determined from transbronchial biopsy, HRCT, etc., or if deemed necessary prior to further treatment.

Pathological Findings

- The diagnostic classifications of IIPs are based on histopathologic patterns seen on lung biopsy.
- The major histologies include an inflammation and fibrotic and granulomatous patterns.
- Characteristic changes on HRCT may help to distinguish between subtypes:
  - Reticulonodular, ground-glass opacities, and, in later stages, honeycombing may be seen.
  - Associated hilar and mediastinal adenopathy are characteristic of stage I and II sarcoidosis.
- No specific test is the "gold standard," which emphasizes the importance of a multidisciplinary consensus for diagnosis with clinical, radiological, and pathological findings.

DIFFERENTIAL DIAGNOSIS

- Acute pulmonary edema
- Diffuse hemorrhage
- Atypical pneumonia
- Diffuse bronchoalveolar cell carcinoma or lymphatic spread of tumor

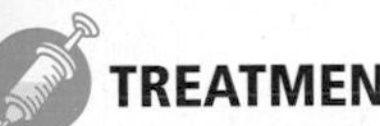

TREATMENT

- Evidence does not support the routine use of any specific therapy for ILD in general, and especially IPF.
- A single randomized-controlled trial did not demonstrate survival benefit of home oxygen use in ILD (5).
- There is no evidence that any pharmacologic therapies improve survival or quality of life (6)[B].
- Corticosteroids have a role in some ILD subtypes. (7)[A]
- Current evidence does not clearly support routine use of noncorticosteroid anti-inflammatory agents for IPF, including cyclosporine, azathioprine, colchicines, cyclophosphamide, cytokines, methotrexate, or interferon (8).
- Phase II studies of bosentan and etanercept had demonstrated trends towards improvement in some quality-of-life measures. A recent study showed limited effect of bosentan on health-related quality-of-life measures in a subset of patients who underwent lung biopsy (9).

MEDICATION

First Line

- In general, corticosteroids are most effective for certain ILDs, especially exacerbations of sarcoidosis, NSIP, BOOP, and hypersensitivity pneumonitis. However, response rates have been variable across and within subtypes. The optimal dose and duration of therapy is unknown.
- Common starting dose of prednisone is 0.5–1 mg/kg/d for 4–12 weeks, with potential up-titration to 0.5 mg/kg based on patient response.

Second Line

- 2nd-line agents have been used for IPF alone or in combination with steroids, with limited success rates:
  - Azathioprine was studied at 2–3 mg/kg/d (not to exceed 200 mg/d; adjusted to the nearest 25-mg dose increment) in combination with prednisone and ultimately as a steroid-sparing agent.
  - Cyclosporine has been studied in a limited number of patients.
  - The addition of acetylcysteine (1,800 mg/d for 12 months) to therapy with azathioprine and prednisone in IPF was studied in a double-blind, placebo-controlled trial. Improvements in vital capacity and carbon monoxide diffusing capacity were noted in the acetylcysteine-treated patients.
  - Pirfenidone, an orally active antifibroblast agent, currently submitted for Food and Drug Administration (FDA) approval, demonstrated potentially promising treatment effects in phase III trials of patients with IPF.
- Several 2nd-line agents have been used in Wegener granulomatosis:
  - Cyclophosphamide is commonly used in treatment of Wegener granulomatosis. It is given 1.5–2 mg/kg/d p.o. for 3–6 months.
  - Methotrexate has been used in treatment of mild Wegener granulomatosis in combination with corticosteroids. A studied dosing regimen consisted of an initial methotrexate dose of 0.3 mg/kg (maximum dose of 15 mg) once weekly, with 2.5 mg titration each week (maximum dose of 25 mg/wk).
  - Other 2nd-line agents that have been studied include mycophenolate mofetil and rituximab.

ADDITIONAL TREATMENT

General Measures

- Avoid/minimize offending environmental/occupational exposures.
- Smoking cessation
- Discontinue culprit medications.
- Supplemental oxygen, if indicated

Issues for Referral

Patients benefit from ongoing care by a pulmonary specialist.

SURGERY/OTHER PROCEDURES

Single- or double-lung transplantation may be a treatment of last resort in some patients. However, some ILDs associated with systemic disease may recur in the recipient lung.

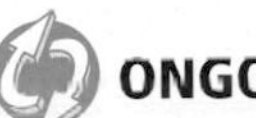

ONGOING CARE

FOLLOW-UP RECOMMENDATIONS

Follow-up testing should include PFTs, cardiopulmonary stress test, pulse oximetry, and CXR.

Patient Monitoring

Patients must be carefully monitored for objective response to treatments and adverse effects.

PATIENT EDUCATION

- Wide degree of prognostic variation occurs among ILD subtypes.
- National Heart, Lung, and Blood Institute at http://www.nhlbi.nih.gov/health/dci/Diseases/ipf/ipf_whatis.html

PROGNOSIS

Overall prognosis is varied among subtypes. IPF confers the worst prognosis (50–80% mortality in 5 years). Some entities, including hypersensitivity pneumonitis, nonspecific interstitial pneumonia, and cryptogenic organizing pneumonia, have a good prognosis.

COMPLICATIONS

- Cor pulmonale
- Pneumothorax
- Progressive respiratory failure

REFERENCES

1. Clement A, Eber E. Interstitial lung diseases in infants and children. *Eur Respir J*. 2008;31:658–66.
2. Raghu G, Weycker D, Edelsberg J, et al. Incidence and prevalence of idiopathic pulmonary fibrosis. *Am J Respir Crit Care Med*. 2006;174:810–6.
3. Rogliani P, Mura M, Assunta Porretta M, et al. New perspectives in the treatment of idiopathic pulmonary fibrosis. *Ther Adv Respir Dis*. 2008;2:75–93.
4. Reynolds HY et al. Present status of bronchoalveolar lavage in interstitial lung disease. *Curr Opin Pulm Med*. 2009;15:479–85.
5. Crockett AJ, Cranston JM, Antic N et al. Domiciliary oxygen for interstitial lung disease. *Cochrane Database Syst Rev*. 2001;CD002883.
6. King TE. Clinical advances in the diagnosis and therapy of the interstitial lung diseases. *Am J Respir Crit Care Med*. 2005;172:268–79.
7. Richeldi L, Davies HR, Ferrara G et al. Corticosteroids for idiopathic pulmonary fibrosis. *Cochrane Database Syst Rev*. 2003;CD002880.
8. Davies HR, et al. Immunomodulatory agents for idiopathic pulmonary fibrosis. *Cochrane Database Syst Rev*. 2006;(3).
9. Raghu G, King TE, Behr J et al. Quality of life and dyspnoea in patients treated with bosentan for idiopathic pulmonary fibrosis (BUILD-1). *Eur Respir J*. 2010;35:118–23.

ADDITIONAL READING

- Behr J, Thannickal VJ. Update in diffuse parenchymal lung disease 2008. *Am J Respir Crit Care Med*. 2009;179:439–44.
- Demedts M, Behr J, Buhl R, et al. High-dose acetylcysteine in idiopathic pulmonary fibrosis. *N Engl J Med*. 2005;353:2229–42.
- Dinwiddie R. Treatment of interstitial lung disease in children. *Paediatr Respir Rev*. 2004;5:108–15.
- King TE Jr, Behr J, Brown K et al. BUILD-1: a randomized placebo-controlled trial of bosentan in idiopathic pulmonary fibrosis. *Am J Respir Crit Care Med*. 2008;177:75–81.

CODES

ICD9

515 Postinflammatory pulmonary fibrosis

CLINICAL PEARLS

- ILD differs from COPD; anatomically, ILD involves the lung parenchyma (i.e., alveoli) and COPD involves both airways and alveoli.
- In some cases, for ILD due to organic or inorganic dust or drug-related ILD, avoiding or minimizing offending environmental/occupational exposures, medications, and smoking may alter the severity of disease, but other general preventative measures are not known at this time.
- A wide degree of prognostic variation occurs among different subtypes of ILD. For example, death is rare with cryptogenic organizing pneumonia, but acute interstitial pneumonia has 60% mortality in <6 months. Refer the patient to a pulmonologist for a thorough evaluation.

D

DIGITALIS TOXICITY

Katherine Boyle, MD
Kathryn W. Weibrecht, MD

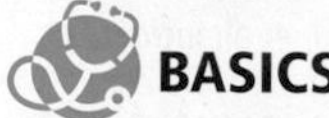

BASICS

DESCRIPTION

- A life-threatening condition resulting from intoxication by digitalis (digoxin) when used for chronic therapy, from accidental or intentional overdose, or from ingestion of naturally occurring compounds containing cardiac glycosides (e.g., foxglove, oleander)
- Can be acute or chronic
- System(s) affected: Cardiovascular; Gastrointestinal; Ocular; Central Nervous System

EPIDEMIOLOGY

Incidence

About 1.1% of outpatients on digitalis glycosides per year develop toxicity, with as many as 10–20% of nursing home residents annually experiencing some degree of digoxin-related toxicity.

Prevalence

In 2007, the American Association of Poison Control Centers' National Poison Data System reported more than 2,500 cases of cardiac glycoside overdose.

RISK FACTORS

- Advanced age
- Renal failure
- Hypoxemia
- Electrolyte disturbances:
  - Hypokalemia
  - Hypomagnesemia
  - Hypernatremia
  - Hypercalcemia
- Acid–base disturbances
- Decompensating congestive heart failure
- Myocardial infarction
- Myocarditis
- Recent cardiac surgery
- Hypothyroidism
- Cor pulmonale

GENERAL PREVENTION

- Use caution when prescribing digitalis if the patient is taking medications that interfere with digoxin metabolism or clearance.
- Adjust dosing when there are circumstances that increase total body levels of the drug (e.g., acute or chronic renal failure), increase cardiac sensitivity (e.g., ischemia, myocarditis), or increase bioavailability by altering gut flora (e.g., macrolides).
- Prescribe lower doses of digoxin (0.125 mg/day instead of 0.25 mg/day) (1). Digoxin is effective in heart failure at much lower levels than necessary for rate control in atrial fibrillation.

PATHOPHYSIOLOGY

- Digitalis inhibits Na^+-K^+-ATPase in myocytes, resulting in an increase in intracellular sodium and a decrease in the transmembrane sodium gradient.
- The loss of the sodium gradient decreases the drive of the Na^+-Ca^{2+} transporter, leading to increased intracellular calcium and thus increased inotropy.
- At high/toxic digoxin concentrations, elevated intracellular calcium generates small depolarizations, and the additive effects of these depolarizations produce dysrhythmias.
- Digitalis also acts on the parasympathetic system resulting in increased vagal tone and slowing AV node conduction.
- The combination of these effects can cause tachyarrhythmias and conduction block, which can present simultaneously.

ETIOLOGY

- Chronic therapy
- Intentional overdose (suicide attempt)
- Accidental overdose (children)
- Prescription/administration error
- Electrolyte disturbances
- Renal failure or any condition that decreases clearance of the drug
- Poisoning with plants containing cardiac glycosides (e.g., oleander, foxglove, lily of the valley)
- Concurrent use of medications:
  - Antibiotics: Rifampin, tetracycline, macrolides
  - Selective serotonin reuptake inhibitors (SSRIs)
  - Calcium channel blockers: Diltiazem, verapamil
  - Antiarrhythmics: Quinidine, amiodarone
  - Diuretics: Spironolactone
  - β-blockers

COMMONLY ASSOCIATED CONDITIONS

- Renal failure
- Congestive heart failure
- Dehydration
- Syncope

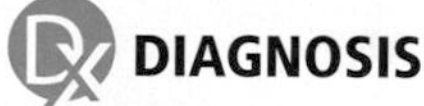

DIAGNOSIS

HISTORY

- For patients at risk for toxicity from chronic use, ask about new medications or new or worsened cardiac or renal disease.
- For suspected accidental overdose in children, a careful history of childproofing and available medications should be obtained.
- As with all suspected or confirmed intentional ingestions, ask about timing of ingestions and coingestions.
- Signs and symptoms generally nonspecific:
  - Anorexia
  - Nausea
  - Vomiting
  - Diarrhea
  - Visual disturbances (e.g., yellow halos)
  - Mydriasis
  - Confusion
  - Fatigue
  - Restlessness
  - Weakness
  - Headache
  - Depression
  - Hallucinations
  - Neuralgias
  - Vertigo

DIAGNOSTIC TESTS & INTERPRETATION

Lab

Initial lab tests

- Na^+, K^+, Cl^-, $HCO3^-$, Mg^+, Ca^+, blood urea nitrogen (BUN), Cr, and cardiac enzyme biomarkers
- Serum digoxin level: Total:
  - The accepted therapeutic range in serum is 0.8–2.0 ng/mL (for rate control in atrial fibrillation), with toxicity more common above 2.5 ng/mL (1)[B].
  - Toxicity may occur with plasma digoxin levels within therapeutic range, especially in chronic overdose (2)[C].
  - Digoxin level may be falsely high if measured <6 hours after acute ingestion or last dose (1)[C].
  - Non-digoxin cardiac glycoside (e.g., foxglove, oleander) may cross-react and generate a positive/elevated level; a negative level does not rule out exposure.
- Free serum digoxin level:
  - Free levels are useful for monitoring response to therapy after digoxin-specific Fab antibody fragments are given (Fab bound to digoxin increases the total digoxin level).
- Potassium:
  - In acute toxicity, hyperkalemia can be common, life-threatening, and predictive of lethality (1)[B].
  - Hypokalemia potentiates digoxin toxicity.

Diagnostic Procedures/Surgery

- Electrocardiogram (EKG):
  - Digoxin has been reported to cause a wide variety of rhythm disturbances, so consider the diagnosis with any sudden change in cardiac rhythm. Look for rhythms that suggest increased automaticity and/or delayed conduction (2)[C].
  - Characteristic EKG changes ("digitalis effect") can occur at therapeutic levels:
    - Prolonged PR segment
    - T-wave changes, prolonged QT interval, scooping of ST segment
  - EKG changes relatively specific for digitalis toxicity:
    - Accelerated junctional rhythm
    - Bidirectional ventricular tachycardia
    - New-onset Mobitz type I AV block
    - Nonparoxysmal atrial tachycardia with AV block
  - Other associated rhythms:
    - Ventricular ectopy, premature ventricular contractions
    - High-degree heart block
    - Sinus bradycardia
    - Sinus bradycardia with junctional tachycardia
    - Ventricular fibrillation or tachycardia
    - Atrial flutter
  - Digoxin toxicity is less likely to cause supraventricular tachycardia, rapid atrial fibrillation, or Mobitz Type II AV block.
- For suspected intoxication with naturally occurring cardiac glycosides, consider early consultation with a medical toxicologist or poison control center for help in identifying the toxic source and to guide treatment decisions.

DIFFERENTIAL DIAGNOSIS

- Conduction abnormalities:
  - Sick sinus syndrome
  - AV nodal dysfunction
- Medication effect
- Electrolyte disturbances
- Other causes of life-threatening arrhythmia

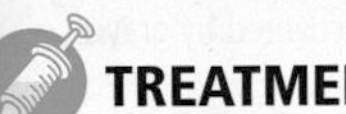

TREATMENT

MEDICATION

First Line

- Digoxin-specific Fab antibody fragments (Digibind) Indications:
  - Treatment of severe, life-threatening arrhythmias due to digitalis toxicity (3)[A]:
    - Sustained ventricular arrhythmias
    - Advanced AV block
    - Asystole
  - Hemodynamic instability
  - Plasma potassium concentration >5 mEq/L in the setting of acute overdose
  - Plasma digoxin concentration above 10 ng/mL (at steady state)
  - Acute ingestion of >10 mg digoxin in adults or >4 mg in children
- Dosage of Digibind:
  - If possible, obtain a total digoxin level before administration.
  - Use free levels to monitor treatment response.
  - To calculate Digibind dosage (1)[A]:
    - Number of vials = Ingested amount (mg) × 0.8/0.5
    - Number of vials = Digoxin level (ng/mL) × weight (kg)/100
  - Unknown acute ingestion or drug level:
    - Empiric dose is 10 vials (4)[C].
  - Dosing for children is the same as for adults.
  - Slow administration increases the efficiency and elimination of digoxin (5)[C].
  - Onset of action for reversal of digoxin toxicity is rapid (minutes) (1)[C].
- Adverse reactions:
  - Hypokalemia: Monitor potassium carefully, since rapid development of hypokalemia can occur after Digibind therapy (1)[A].
  - Exacerbation of heart failure, increased ventricular response in atrial fibrillation, and hypersensitivity reactions can occur (1)[A].

Second Line

- Activated charcoal (1)[C]:
  - Consider in acute or overdose settings
  - Increases GI elimination and systemic clearance
- Magnesium: 2 g IV initially, consider maintenance infusion (3)[C]
- Temporary pacing if no Digibind available (3)[C]
- Hemodialysis can be used to treat hyperkalemia, but is not effective for reversal of toxicity because of the extensive tissue distribution of digoxin (1)[C].

ADDITIONAL TREATMENT

General Measures

- Discontinue digoxin and other medications that interact with digoxin or exacerbate dysrhythmias.
- Correct electrolyte abnormalities and monitor potassium levels:
  - Maintain potassium in high–normal range.
  - Treat hyperkalemia with sodium bicarbonate, insulin, glucose, and Kayexalate.
  - Treat hypokalemia cautiously.
  - Do not use calcium salts, which can worsen ventricular arrhythmias by further increasing intracellular calcium (2)[C].
- For chronic toxicity, treat the underlying cause.

IN-PATIENT CONSIDERATIONS

Initial Stabilization

- Manage airway
- IV access/fluid resuscitation
- Supplemental oxygen
- Atropine for symptomatic bradycardia (1)[C]
- Temporary cutaneous pacing (1)[C]
- Hemodynamically unstable patients should receive Digibind as soon as possible (3)[A].

Admission Criteria

All patients with suspected digoxin toxicity who have cardiac dysrhythmias, toxic digoxin levels, or hyperkalemia should be admitted for continuous cardiac monitoring.

IV Fluids

Administration of appropriate IV fluids depends on underlying etiology for toxicity (e.g., decompensated congestive heart failure vs acute renal failure secondary to dehydration).

Discharge Criteria

Patients should remain in the hospital until the signs and symptoms have resolved and the serum digoxin level <2 ng/mL.

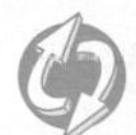

ONGOING CARE

FOLLOW-UP RECOMMENDATIONS

- Psychiatric referral is indicated for all intentional overdoses.
- In chronic toxicity, close follow-up by a primary care physician or cardiologist is recommended if digoxin therapy is continued after discharge.

Patient Monitoring

- Digoxin levels should be monitored in acute toxicity. However, Digibind administration can interfere with the assay and give unreliable results.
- Electrolytes, especially potassium, should be carefully monitored.
- Medications that may have precipitated or contributed to digoxin intoxication should be discontinued and restarted when clinical symptoms have resolved.
- EKG and cardiac monitoring should continue until resolution of dysrhythmias.

PROGNOSIS

Moderate/major morbidity or death has been reported from 20–25% of exposures treated in hospitals (6).

REFERENCES

1. Bauman JL, Didomenico RJ, Galanter WL. Mechanisms, manifestations, and management of digoxin toxicity in the modern era. *Am J Cardiovasc Drugs*. 2006;6:77–86.
2. Hauptman PJ, Kelly RA. Digitalis. *Circulation*. 1999;99:1265–70.
3. ACC/AHA/ESC 2006 guidelines for management of patients with ventricular arrhythmias and the prevention of sudden cardiac death-executive summary: A report of the American College of Cardiology/American Heart Association Task Force and the European Society of Cardiology Committee for Practice Guidelines. *Circulation*. 2006;114: 1088–1132.
4. Brubacher JR, Heller MB, Ravikumar PR, et al. Treatment of Toad Venom Poisoning with Digoxin-Specific Fab Fragments. *Chest*. 1996;110:1282–1288.
5. Lapostolle F, Borron S, Verdier C, et al. Digoxin-specific Fab fragments as single first-line therapy in digitalis poisoning. *Crit Care Med*. 2008;36(11):3014–3018.
6. Lapostolle F, Borron SW, Verdier C, et al. Assessment of digoxin antibody use in patients with elevated serum digoxin following chronic or acute exposure. *Intensive Care Med*. 2008;34: 1448–1453.

ADDITIONAL READING

- Rajapakse S. Management of yellow oleander poisoning. *Clinical Toxicology*. 2009;47(3): 206–212.
- Roberts DM, Buckley N. Antidotes for acute cardenolide (cardiac glycoside) poisoning (Review). *Cochrane Database of Systematic Reviews*. 2006; Issue 4.

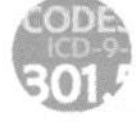

CODES

ICD9

972.1 Poisoning by cardiotonic glycosides and drugs of similar action

CLINICAL PEARLS

- The onset of vague symptoms accompanied by dysrhythmia should raise suspicion of toxicity by digitalis or other cardiac glycosides (e.g. foxglove, oleander).
- Toxicity may develop even when digoxin serum levels are within normal therapeutic range.
- Digoxin-specific Fab antibody fragments are the treatment of choice for severe, life-threatening arrhythmias due to digitalis toxicity.

D

DIPHTHERIA

Richard Kent Zimmerman, MD, MPH
Gregory A. Poland, MD

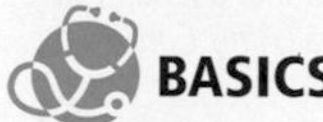

BASICS

DESCRIPTION

- Acute respiratory tract infection caused by *Corynebacterium diphtheriae*, usually producing a membranous pharyngitis
- Incubation period 2–5 days typically (range 1–10)
- Infection usually occurs during fall and winter in temperate regions. In the tropics, seasonal trends are less distinct.
- Transmission by respiratory route from infected person or carrier. Humans are the only reservoir.
- Several forms occur:
  - Membranous pharyngotonsillar diphtheria: The membrane is gray, adheres to the pharynx, and is surrounded by erythema. The underlying mucosa bleeds when the membrane is removed.
  - Nasal diphtheria: Unilateral discharge
  - Obstructive laryngotracheitis: Complication when membrane descends into larynx or bronchial tree. When it breaks up in young children, total obstruction of the airway may occur.
  - Cutaneous diphtheria: Punched-out ulcer covered by gray membrane (particularly in tropics and among homeless). Peaks August–October in southern US.
- System(s) affected: Cardiovascular; Nervous; Skin/Exocrine; Respiratory

EPIDEMIOLOGY

- Predominant age: Children <15 years old and poorly immunized adults
- Predominant sex: Male = Female

Incidence

In the US: For noncutaneous form, 1.6 in 100 million. Diphtheria is a rare condition in the US today. Fairly recent outbreaks have occurred in the independent states of the former Soviet Union.

RISK FACTORS

- Crowded living conditions
- Inadequate immunization
- Lower socioeconomic status
- Native Americans
- Alcoholism
- Travelers: Outbreaks have occurred in various countries; see CDC's travel Web site.

GENERAL PREVENTION

Prevention is by immunization:

- Children age 6 weeks up to 7 years of age should receive doses at 2, 4, 6, and 15–18 months and 4–6 years of age with 0.5 mL of DTaP vaccine IM. If the pertussis component is contraindicated, then pediatric diphtheria tetanus (DT) should be used. A booster dose of adult Tdap should be given at age 11–12 years.
- Unimmunized persons ≥7 years should receive 2 doses of adult Td 4–8 weeks apart with a 3rd dose 6–12 months later. 0.5 mL of Td should be given. Subsequently, booster doses with Td should be given every 10 years to all individuals without a contraindication. CDC currently recommends that Tdap substitute for 1 of the recommended decennial Td boosters.
- Immunized individuals may develop diphtheria, but their course is milder; immunization protects against the toxin, not infection or microbial carriage in the nose, pharynx, or skin. Disinfect all articles in contact with patient.
- Close contacts should be cultured and given antibiotic prophylaxis, regardless of immunization status.
- Contacts should receive an age-appropriate diphtheria toxoid-containing vaccine unless given a booster within the past 5 years.
- Contacts should receive a diphtheria toxoid-containing vaccine unless vaccinated within the past 5 years.

PATHOPHYSIOLOGY

Toxigenic strains produce an exotoxin that inhibits protein synthesis in all cell types.

ETIOLOGY

C. diphtheriae infection

DIAGNOSIS

- Membranous pharyngotonsillar diphtheria:
  - Initially, white-to-yellow membrane, which is easily removed
  - Adherent, whitish-gray, leathery membrane on tonsils or pharynx
  - Removing membrane causes bleeding of mucosa.
  - Injected pharynx
  - Membrane may become black due to hemorrhage.
  - Sore throat
  - Cervical adenopathy with swelling
  - Malaise and prostration
  - Enlarged, tender cervical and submandibular lymph nodes
  - May progress to edematous, swollen neck (bull neck)
  - Paralysis of soft palate
  - Low-grade fever of 37.8–38.8°C (100–100.9°F)
  - Thrombocytopenia and purpura
- Nasal diphtheria:
  - Serosanguineous or seropurulent discharge and excoriations
  - Often, discharge is unilateral.
  - Often chronic, mild course
- Obstructive laryngotracheitis:
  - Hoarseness
  - Croupy cough
  - Progresses to dyspnea and stridor
  - Labored breathing
  - Thick speech
- Cutaneous diphtheria:
  - On skin, conjunctiva, vulva, vagina, and penis
  - Primary cutaneous diphtheria: Starts as tender pustule on lower extremity and becomes deep, round, punched-out ulcer covered by grayish membrane
  - Secondary infection of preexisting wound, purulent exudate, partial membrane

DIAGNOSTIC TESTS & INTERPRETATION

Lab

- Gram-positive rods in the pathognomonic Chinese character configuration
- Moderate leukocytosis
- Thrombocytopenia
- Transient albuminuria
- In experienced hands, methylene-blue stains can assist in a presumptive diagnosis.
- Culture from nose and throat beneath membrane and plate on special media; inform lab that diphtheria is suspected.
- Should test for toxigenicity of strain
- Serial ECGs and cardiac enzymes to detect myocarditis
- Delayed peripheral nerve conduction velocities
- Culture on special media (cystine-tellurite blood agar or modified Tinsdale agar) is positive in 8–12 hours if not previously treated with an antibiotic. Laboratory must be alerted to use special media.
- Toxin production confirmed by modified Elek test.
- Polymerase chain reaction
- Drugs that may alter lab results:
  - If an antibiotic was used, then ≥5 days may be required for the culture to grow on medium.

Pathological Findings

- Pleomorphic gram-positive rods
- Necrotic epithelium
- Hyaline degeneration

DIFFERENTIAL DIAGNOSIS

- Bacterial pharyngitis including group A Streptococcus
- Viral pharyngitis
- Mononucleosis
- Oral syphilis
- Candidiasis
- Vincent angina
- Acute epiglottitis

TREATMENT

MEDICATION

First Line

- Both antitoxins and antibiotics are needed for noncutaneous diphtheria.
- Diphtheria antitoxin, equine: Use 20,000–40,000 U of antitoxin for laryngeal or pharyngeal disease of <48 hours' duration; 40,000–60,000 U for nasopharyngeal lesions; 80,000–120,000 U for extensive disease ≥3 days or swelling of the neck (bull neck) (1)[B].
- Some experts recommend treating cutaneous disease with 20,000–40,000 U of antitoxin, while others doubt its value when there are no signs of systemic disease.
- Antitoxin is obtained from the CDC under Investigation New Drug protocol at 770-488-7100.
- Erythromycin parenterally or p.o., 40–50 mg/kg/d; maximum of 2 g/d for 14 days (2)[B], or penicillin G IM or IV for 14 days, or penicillin G procaine IM for 14 days. For cutaneous diphtheria, 10 days of one of these antibiotics.
- Precautions:
  - Equine antitoxin: 7% of patients are sensitive to equine antitoxin and need desensitization. Always test for hypersensitivity to antitoxin prior to its administration:
    - 1st, a drop of 1:100 dilution of antitoxin is placed on a scratch on the forearm, read at 15–20 minutes. If negative, an intradermal skin test is done with 1:1,000 dilution (0.02 mL). A positive reaction is the development of urticaria within 20 minutes of injection.
    - If no reaction to 1st intradermal, then repeat test with a 1:100 dilution
    - If the person has a negative history for animal allergy, has not previously received animal serum, and had a negative scratch test, then 1:100 dilution may be used initially.

Second Line

DL-carnitine 100 mg/kg/d b.i.d. p.o. in children for 4 days in myocarditis is experimental

ADDITIONAL TREATMENT

Antibiotics recommended for close contacts (oral erythromycin for 10 days or single IM penicillin G benzathine). Contacts should receive an age-appropriate diphtheria toxoid-containing vaccine unless given a booster within the past 5 years. Contacts who are children <7 years and who lack their 4th dose of DTaP should be vaccinated. Antibiotics recommended for carriers.

General Measures

- Appropriate health care:
  - Inpatient, initially hospitalized in unit that can monitor cardiac and respiratory status (must act on presumptive diagnosis because therapy cannot wait for culture confirmation)
  - Droplet isolation for pharyngeal diphtheria until cultures on 2 consecutive days are negative. The 1st culture must be taken at least 24 hours after the cessation of antibiotic therapy.
  - Contact precautions for cutaneous diphtheria.
- Have intubation or tracheostomy readily available. For laryngeal disease, laryngoscopy is desirable. Intubation or tracheostomy should be considered early for laryngeal disease.
- Avoid hypnotics and sedatives while monitoring respiratory status.

Additional Therapies

Physical therapy in convalescence for range of motion exercises to prevent contractions

ONGOING CARE

FOLLOW-UP RECOMMENDATIONS

Rest for at least 3 weeks until risk of developing myocarditis has passed.

Patient Monitoring

- ECG, cardiac enzymes, and respiratory status. Serial ECG 2–3 times per week for 4–6 weeks to detect myocarditis
- Elimination of the organism should be documented by 2 negative cultures 24 hours apart. The 1st culture should 24 hours after the completion of antimicrobial therapy.
- During convalescence, patients should be immunized against diphtheria, because infection does not necessarily confer immunity.

DIET

Liquid to soft as tolerated

PATIENT EDUCATION

Explain aspects of illness and complications.

PROGNOSIS

- <5% mortality rate unless respiratory form for which case-fatality rate is 5–10%
- Prognosis guarded until recovery
- In convalescing patients, 5–10% persistence in nasopharynx
- Worse prognosis if myocarditis

COMPLICATIONS

- Myocarditis (10–25%) may occur early.
- Cranial and peripheral neuropathy (2–6 weeks after onset)
- ECG abnormalities in 2/3 of patients, including bundle branch block, tachycardia, atrial or ventricular fibrillation, and extrasystoles
- Right-sided heart failure
- Local paralysis of soft palate and posterior pharynx demonstrated by regurgitation of fluids through the nares
- Peripheral and cranial neuropathy affecting primarily motor nerve functions. Motor dysfunction starts proximally and extends distally. It usually resolves slowly.
- Syndrome resembling Guillain-Barré

REFERENCES

1. Hrobjartsson A, et al. The controlled clinical trial turns 100 years: Fibiger's trial of serum treatment of diphtheria. *Br Med J*. 1998;317:1243–5.
2. Kneen R, Pham NG, Solomon T, et al. Penicillin vs. erythromycin in the treatment of diphtheria. *Clin Infect Dis*. 1998;27:845–50.

ADDITIONAL READING

- American Academy of Pediatrics. Diphtheria. In Pickering LK: *Red Book: 2009 Report of the Committee on Infectious Diseases*. 28th Edition. Elk Grove Village, IL: American Academy of Pediatrics, 2009:280–3.
- Karam AG, Cherry JD. Hypotonic and Hyporesponsive Episodes After Diptheria-Tetanus-Acellular Pertussis Vaccination. *Pediatr Infect Dis J*. 2007;26:966–7.
- The original streptomycin trial paper: Fibiger J. Om Serumbehandling af Difteri. *Hospitalstidende*. 1898;6:309–25, 337–50

See Also (Topic, Algorithm, Electronic Media Element)

http://www.cdc.gov/vaccines/vpd-vac/diphtheria
http://wwwnc.cdc.gov/travel/yellowbook/2010/chapter-2/diphtheria.aspx

CODES

ICD9

- 032.0 Faucial diphtheria
- 032.2 Anterior nasal diphtheria
- 032.3 Laryngeal diphtheria

CLINICAL PEARLS

- Close contacts should be cultured, checked for immunization status, and considered for antimicrobial prophylaxis (penicillin or erythromycin).
- Past infection does not necessarily confer immunity.
- Alert lab if sending a culture because *C. diphtheriae* requires a special media to grow.

DISSEMINATED INTRAVASCULAR COAGULATION (DIC)

Jan Cerny, MD, PhD
Eva Medvedova, MD

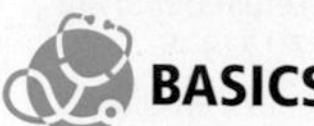

BASICS

DESCRIPTION

- Acquired syndrome characterized by diffuse activation of intravascular coagulation arising from different causes. It can originate from and cause damage to the microvasculature, which, if sufficiently severe, can produce organ dysfunction.
- Occurring in complications of obstetrics (eg, abruptio placentae, fetus retention, amniotic fluid embolism), infection (especially gram-negative), malignancy (uncontrolled, metastatic tumor or leukemia), trauma, and other severe illnesses
- System(s) affected: Hematologic/Lymphatic/Immunologic
- Synonym(s): Consumptive coagulopathy; DIC

EPIDEMIOLOGY

Incidence

Unknown

Prevalence

- Predominant age: None
- Predominant sex: Male = Female

RISK FACTORS

See Etiology

GENERAL PREVENTION

Aggressive interventions aimed at early treatment of the underlying clinical conditions

PATHOPHYSIOLOGY

- Systemic formation of fibrin is the result of the simultaneous coexistence of:
  - Increased thrombin generation via tissue factor/factor VII mediated pathway
  - Suppression of the physiologic anticoagulant pathways:
    - Antithrombin due to consumption, degradation, and impaired synthesis
    - Proteins C and S due to decreased levels of thrombomodulin
  - Impaired fibrinolysis (early on):
    - Sustained increase in plasminogen activator inhibitor, type 1
- Increased fibrinolysis (late during the process) leads to bleeding.

ETIOLOGY

Causes can be classified as acute or chronic, systemic or localized:

- Sepsis/severe infection (any microorganism)
- Trauma (polytrauma, neurotrauma)
- Obstetric complications (amniotic fluid embolism, abruptio placentae)
- Solid tumors and leukemias (especially acute promyelocytic leukemia)
- Vascular disorders, such as Kasabach-Merritt syndrome, large vascular aneurysms, and thrombosis
- Organ destruction (severe pancreatitis, severe liver failure)
- Severe toxic or immunologic reactions:
  - Snake bite
  - Recreational drugs
  - Transfusion reactions
  - Transplant rejection
  - Thermal injury
- Infant and adult respiratory distress syndrome
- Neonatal purpura fulminans

COMMONLY ASSOCIATED CONDITIONS

Thromboembolic phenomena are associated with venous thrombosis, thrombotic vegetations on the aortic heart valve, arterial emboli, and neonatal purpura fulminans (homozygous protein C or protein S deficiency).

Pediatric Considerations

Neonatal purpura fulminans is associated with DIC and protein C or protein S deficiency (homozygous).

DIAGNOSIS

Symptoms and signs are related to the underlying disease process and disseminated intravascular coagulation.

HISTORY

Symptoms of microvascular thrombosis (e.g., renal failure), as well as diffuse bleeding

PHYSICAL EXAM

- Bleeding manifestations:
  - Skin (petechiae, purpura, ecchymosis, generalized oozing from venipuncture sites and wounds)
  - Renal (hematuria)
  - Gastrointestinal (mucous membranes and intestinal bleeding)
  - Neurologic (hemorrhagic infarction, massive intracerebral bleeding)
  - Respiratory (epistaxis, pulmonary hemorrhage)
- Microvascular thrombosis:
  - Skin (skin infarction, digital gangrene)
  - Gastrointestinal (mucosal ulcerations, bowel infarction)
  - Renal (oliguria, anuria, uremia)
  - Pulmonary (hypoxemia, acute respiratory distress syndrome)
  - Neurologic (convulsions, delirium, coma, multifocal cortical infarction)

DIAGNOSTIC TESTS & INTERPRETATION

No single laboratory test is sensitive and specific enough to allow a definitive diagnosis of DIC.

Lab

- Thrombocytopenia
- Increased partial thromboplastin time (PTT)
- Increased prothrombin test (PT)
- Decreased fibrinogen (serial levels)
- Increased fibrin degradation product (FDP)
- Positive D-dimer
- Decreased antithrombin III, decreased protein C
- Microangiopathic hemolytic anemia (schistocytes, increased lactate dehydrogenase levels, low hemoglobin)
- Decreased factor VIII (can help differentiate DIC vs liver failure—normal in liver failure)

Initial lab tests

Diagnostic algorithm for overt DIC (International Society on Thrombosis and Haemostasis)

- Assess if underlying disease is known to be associated with DIC:
  - YES: Proceed with this algorithm.
  - NO: Do not use this algorithm.
- Order global coagulation tests (PT, PTT, fibrinogen, soluble fibrin monomers, or FDPs)
- Score global coagulation test results:
  - Platelet count ($>100 = 0$, $<100 = 1$, $<50 = 2$)
  - Elevated fibrin-related markers (no increase = 0, moderate increase = 1, strong increase = 3)
  - Prolonged PT (<3 seconds = 0, >3 but <6 seconds = 1, >6 seconds = 2)
  - Fibrinogen level (>1 g/l = 0, <1 g/l = 1)
- Calculate score:
  - If ≥ 5: Compatible with DIC, repeat scoring daily. If <5: Suggestive (not affirmative for nonovert DIC: Repeat in 1–2 days).

Follow-Up & Special Considerations

Frequent follow-up of initially abnormal laboratory tests to see effect of therapeutic interventions

DIFFERENTIAL DIAGNOSIS

- Fulminant liver failure or massive hepatic necrosis
- Vitamin K deficiency
- Thrombotic thrombocytopenic purpura
- Hemolytic–uremic syndrome
- Heparin-induced thrombocytopenia
- Primary fibrinolysis
- HELLP syndrome in pregnancy (hemolysis, elevated liver function, and low platelets)

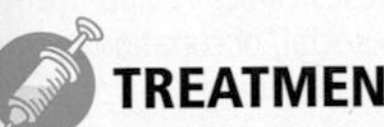

TREATMENT

Heterogeneity of the underlying disorders and the clinical presentations makes the therapeutic approach to DIC difficult:

- Appropriate health care: Inpatient and often intensive care unit (depending on underlying condition)
- Treat underlying condition (e.g., evacuation of uterus in abruptio placentae; broad-spectrum antibiotics for gram-negative sepsis)
- Supportive care with transfusions in patients who are bleeding, going for surgery, or at high risk of bleeding. Do not treat abnormal laboratory parameters:
  - Fresh frozen plasma
  - Platelet concentrates
  - Cryoprecipitate or fibrinogen concentrates
- Anticoagulants remain very controversial. Deep venous thrombosis prophylaxis is recommended in patients who are not bleeding.
- Restoration of anticoagulant pathways:
  - Recombinant human-activated protein C (benefit only in carefully selected patients at high risk of death from sepsis. The drug should only be administered in an Intensive Care Unit (ICU) when patient is monitored by trained personnel) (1)[A]
  - Activated factor VII use remains controversial.

MEDICATION

- Broad-spectrum antibiotics for sepsis
- Recombinant human-activated protein C in severe sepsis (1)

SURGERY/OTHER PROCEDURES

Surgical treatment or procedures should be considered, especially if they are treating the underlying condition (e.g., evacuation of uterus in abruptio placentae; some trauma or bleeding situations).

IN-PATIENT CONSIDERATIONS

Initial Stabilization

- Treat underlying disorder.
- Frequent monitoring of clinical and laboratory response

Admission Criteria

Usually dictated by severity of underlying condition. Some cases can be managed on a standard ward, but ICU care is typical.

Discharge Criteria

Once clinical and laboratory criteria are significantly improved and underlying reason for DIC is under control

ONGOING CARE

FOLLOW-UP RECOMMENDATIONS

Patient Monitoring

- Monitor closely until much improved
- Serial platelet count, coagulation tests, and fibrinogen levels to see effect of therapeutic interventions

PROGNOSIS

- Related to the severity of cause
- Decreased antithrombin level is a poor prognostic factor in DIC.

COMPLICATIONS

- Acute renal failure
- Shock
- Cardiac tamponade
- Hemothorax
- Intracerebral hematoma
- Various thrombotic complications, including myocardial infarction, stroke, gangrene, and loss of digits

REFERENCE

1. Vincent JL, Bernard GR, Beale R, et al. Drotrecogin alfa (activated) treatment in severe sepsis from the global open-label trial ENHANCE: further evidence for survival and safety and implications for early treatment. *Crit Care Med*. 2005;33:2266–77.

ADDITIONAL READING

- Franchini M, Lippi G, Manzato F. Recent acquisitions in the pathophysiology, diagnosis and treatment of disseminated intravascular coagulation. *Thromb J*. 2006;4:4.
- Levi M. Disseminated intravascular coagulation. *Crit Care Med*. 2007;35:2191–5.
- Levi M, Toh CH, Thachil J, Watson HG et al. Guidelines for the diagnosis and management of disseminated intravascular coagulation. British Committee for Standards in Haematology. *Br J Haematol*. 2009;145:24–33.
- Taylor FB, Toh CH, Hoots WK, et al. Towards definition, clinical and laboratory criteria, and a scoring system for disseminated intravascular coagulation. *Thromb Haemost*. 2001;86:1327–30.

CODES

ICD9

286.6 Defibrination syndrome

CLINICAL PEARLS

Treat underlying condition(s); transfusions represent supportive measures.

Transfusions are not indicated in patients with abnormal laboratory parameters without clinical bleeding.

DISSOCIATIVE DISORDERS

Moshe S. Torem, MD, DLFAPA

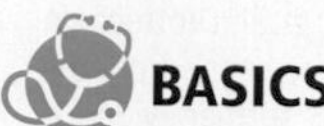

BASICS

DESCRIPTION

- Dissociative disorders bring about a sudden change in state of consciousness, identity, motor behavior, thoughts, feelings, and perception of reality so that these functions do not operate congruently.
- Numerous pathologic symptoms can be experienced, but all patients experience dysphoria, suffering, and maladaptive functioning.
- Disorders include dissociative amnesia, dissociative fugue, dissociative identity disorder, depersonalization disorder, and dissociative disorder not otherwise specified. Some authors may include somnambulism (sleepwalking disorder), conversion reactions, pseudo-epilepsy, and (in some cultures) a variety of possession syndromes.
- System(s) affected: Nervous
- Synonym(s): Hysterical neurosis, dissociative type; Ganser syndrome (1)

Geriatric Considerations

Decrease in frequency and intensity of dissociative symptoms; medication side effects are more likely

Pediatric Considerations

Suspect abuse or neglect.

EPIDEMIOLOGY

Incidence

- Predominant age: Adolescents and young to middle-age adults; rare as a new illness in the elderly. If untreated, it may linger from childhood into adulthood and old age.
- Predominant sex: Female > Male (2:1)

Prevalence

- Transient symptoms of depersonalization or derealization in the general population are common.
- Lifetime prevalence rate is 26–74%.
- 31–66% occurring at the time of a traumatic event
- Up to 70% of young adults report short periods of dissociative experiences that are self-limiting and resolve spontaneously without any treatment.
- Dissociative amnesia occurs in 2–7% of the general population.

RISK FACTORS

- Exposure to neglect, abuse, and trauma in childhood (2)
- Physical, emotional, verbal, or sexual abuse in childhood
- Sudden and severe trauma or threat to psychologic or physical integrity
- Sudden and unexpected exposure to watching others being killed or severely injured (as in an industrial or car accident)
- Tendency to cope with life's stresses by excessively using an escape mechanism of daydreaming and/or dissociation
- A preponderance of coping with trauma and internal or interpersonal conflicts by the use of dissociation
- Psychologic/social support to cope with the trauma/abuse was unavailable.
- Family history of dissociative disorders or posttraumatic stress disorder (PTSD)

GENERAL PREVENTION

- Child abuse prevention via parent education and community agency intervention
- Crisis intervention following individual trauma or disasters may prevent dissociative disorders.

PATHOPHYSIOLOGY

- All disorders share symptoms that:
  - Cause significant distress or impairment in social, occupational, or other important areas of functioning
  - Are not due to the direct physiologic effects of a substance (e.g., drug of abuse, a medication) or a general medical condition (e.g., temporal lobe epilepsy)
- Dissociative amnesia:
  - ≥1 episodes of inability to recall important personal information too extensive to be explained by ordinary forgetfulness
  - Not occurring during another psychiatric illness and not due to effects of chemical substance (e.g., drug abuse or medication)
  - Not due to a neurologic or other medical condition (e.g., epilepsy, head trauma)
- Dissociative fugue:
  - Sudden unexpected travel away from home or customary place of work with an inability to recall one's past
  - Confusion about personal identity or assumption of a new identity
  - Above symptoms do not occur during course of dissociative identity disorder.
  - Symptoms cause significant distress or impairment in social, occupational, or other activities of daily living (ADLs).
- Dissociative identity disorder:
  - Presence of ≥2 distinct identities or personality states (each with its own relatively enduring pattern of perceiving, relating to, and thinking about the environment and self)
  - At least 2 of these identities or personality states recurrently take control of the person's behavior.
  - Inability to recall important personal information that cannot be explained by ordinary forgetfulness
  - Reports of lost time, distortion, and lapses
  - Experiencing voices from inside one's head
  - Chronic headaches not due to other diagnoses
  - History of severe emotional or physical abuse as a child
  - Referring to self as he/she, we, they, us
  - Abnormal eating behaviors
  - Flashbacks
  - Feelings of derealization
  - Feelings of depersonalization
  - Amnesia about important childhood events
  - Personal objects and belongings that cannot be accounted for
  - Disowning unrecalled behaviors
  - Different handwriting styles
  - Different signatures and names
  - Sudden mood changes
  - Sudden behavioral changes (e.g., from adult to young child)
  - Episodes of déjà vu and déjà entendu
  - Feeling controlled by another person from within
  - Self-inflicted violence such as wrist cutting
- Depersonalization disorder:
  - Persistent or recurrent experiences of feeling detached from, and as if an outside observer of, mental processes or body (e.g., feeling like as if in a dream)
  - During the depersonalization experience, reality testing remains intact.
  - The depersonalization causes clinically significant distress or impairment in social, occupational, or other important areas of functioning.
  - The depersonalization experience does not occur exclusively during the course of another mental disorder, such as schizophrenia, panic disorder, acute stress disorder, or another dissociative disorder, and is not due to the direct physiological effects of a substance (e.g., a drug of abuse, a medication) or a general medical condition (e.g., temporal lobe epilepsy).
- Dissociative disorder not otherwise specified: Predominant feature is a dissociative symptom (e.g., a disruption in the usually integrated functions of consciousness, memory, identity, or perception of the environment) that does not meet the criteria for any other specific dissociative disorder. Examples:
  - Clinical presentations similar to dissociative identity disorder (DID) that fail to meet the full diagnostic criteria for DID
  - Derealization unaccompanied by depersonalization in adults
  - States of dissociation that occur in individuals who have been subjected to periods of prolonged and intense coercive persuasion (e.g., brainwashing, thought reform, or indoctrination while captive)
  - Dissociative trance disorder: Single or episodic disturbances in the state of consciousness, identity, or memory that are indigenous to particular locations and cultures. Dissociative trance involves narrowing of awareness, of immediate surroundings, or stereotyped behaviors or movements that are experienced as being beyond one's control.
  - Possession trance: Involves replacement of the customary sense of personal identity, attributed to the influence of a spirit, power, deity, or other person, and is associated with stereotyped involuntary movements or amnesia. This may be the most common dissociative disorder in Asia. Examples: *amok*, *bebainan* (Indonesia), *latah* (Malaysia), *pibloktoq* (Arctic). The dissociative or trance disorder is not a normal part of a broadly accepted collective cultural or religious practice.
  - Loss of consciousness, stupor, or coma not attributed to a general medical condition
- Ganser syndrome: Rare dissociative disorder characterized by nonsensical or wrong answers to questions or doing things incorrectly (e.g., 2 + 2 = 5) when not associated with dissociative amnesia or dissociative fugue

ETIOLOGY

Common link to a history of trauma

COMMONLY ASSOCIATED CONDITIONS

See Risk Factors.

DIAGNOSIS

HISTORY
Patient's personal history should be complemented with history obtained from a family member.

DIAGNOSTIC TESTS & INTERPRETATION
Lab
Initial lab tests
- Electroencephalogram to rule out epilepsy
- Polysomnogram to rule out sleep disorders

Follow-Up & Special Considerations
- Toxicology screening may be helpful.
- Computed tomography scan and magnetic resonance imaging of the head to rule out organic brain disorders

Imaging
Follow-Up & Special Considerations
- Avoid sleep deprivation.
- Avoid substance abuse.

Diagnostic Procedures/Surgery
- Neuropsychologic testing to rule out learning disabilities and cognitive deficits due to early dementia or borderline mental retardation
- Psychologic testing to identify specific disorders, personality structure, and dynamics
- Dissociation scales help assess the tendency to dissociate in daily living activities
- Amobarbital (Amytal) interviews (narcoanalysis) and interviews under hypnosis may be useful in selected cases.

DIFFERENTIAL DIAGNOSIS
- Other mental/central nervous system disorder: Schizophrenia, depression, anxiety disorder, bipolar, PTSD, obsessive-compulsive disorder, identity disorder, phobic disorders, and eating disorders
- Other: Extreme sensory deprivation, epilepsy, dementia, encephalitis, head trauma, migraine, cerebral vascular disease, brain tumors
- Endocrinopathy: Hypoglycemia, hypothyroidism, hyperthyroidism
- Miscellaneous: Huntington disease, carbon monoxide poisoning, mescaline intoxication, botulism, hyperventilation

TREATMENT

MEDICATION
First Line
- No medications are specifically curative. The following have been helpful:
  - Antidepressants for depression
  - Benzodiazepines for anxiety
  - Propranolol (80–400 mg/d) for flashbacks and other dissociative symptoms (off label)
  - Neuroleptics (low doses) for psychotic symptoms
  - Mood swings in dissociative disorders do not respond to the use of mood stabilizers.
- Precautions:
  - Potential abuse with short-acting benzodiazepines
  - Overdose/suicide potential with tricyclic antidepressants (TCAs)
  - Very low doses of neuroleptics can be used without producing tardive dyskinesia.
  - Atypical neuroleptics may be associated with hyperglycemia.
- Significant possible interactions:
  - Avoid monoamine oxidase inhibitors with TCAs or selective serotonin reuptake inhibitors.

Second Line
- Anxiety symptoms:
  - Buspirone (BuSpar), 30–80 mg/d for anxiety
- Obsessive-compulsive and/or depressive symptoms: Consider psychotropic medications.
- Atypical neuroleptics have recently been found useful for the control of self-inflicted violence or psychotic symptoms. Consider medications with the lowest effective dose.

ADDITIONAL TREATMENT
General Measures
- Individual psychotherapy plus behavior modification and in selective cases hypnotherapy (3)
- Adjuncts: Group therapy, expressive art therapy, occupational and recreational therapy when not associated with dissociative amnesia or dissociative fugue

Issues for Referral
Dissociative disorders are best treated by a well-trained mental health professional.

IN-PATIENT CONSIDERATIONS
Initial Stabilization
- Outpatient, individual psychotherapy
- At times of crisis: Intensive hospital-based treatment (as a protection for patients with suicidal or homicidal impulses)
- Use inpatient care to verify diagnosis with special tests and begin a treatment program.
- *Note*: Treatment emphasis should be on progress in the adaptive functions with daily living activities, symptom alleviation, ego strengthening, and preventing regressions.

ONGOING CARE

PATIENT EDUCATION
- Self-hypnosis, relaxation exercises, guided imagery, mindfulness meditation
- Encourage patients to get educated about their condition and be inspired by those who got better and recovered:
  - Benson, H. *The Relaxation Response*. New York: HarperCollins, 2000.
  - Kabat-Zinn J. *Coming to Our Senses*. New York: Hyperion, 2005.
  - Rossman, ML. *Guided Imagery for Self-Healing*. Novato, CA: New World Library, 2000.
  - Sizemore C. *A Mind of My Own*. New York: W. Morrow, 1989.
  - Tart TC. *Living the Mindful Life*. Boston: Shambhala Publications, 1994.
  - Steinberg, M & Schnall, M. *The Stranger in the Mirror*. New York: HarperCollins, 2001.

PROGNOSIS
- Ranges from spontaneous improvement in cases of dissociative amnesia, dissociative fugue, and depersonalization disorder to acute and chronic morbidity in others
- Without treatment, a dissociative identity disorder patient may have a healthy functioning facade, with episodes of depression, confusion, mood swings, etc. With age, the intensity and frequency of dissociative experiences may decrease and crystallize around 1–2 major personality states.
- Effective treatment produces partial or full recovery for many patients.

COMPLICATIONS
Self-inflicted violence, suicide attempts, substance abuse, chemical dependency

REFERENCES

1. American Psychiatric Association. *Diagnostic and Statistical Manual of Mental Disorders*. 4th ed. Washington, DC: American Psychiatric Association; 1994:477–91.
2. Savitz JB, van der Merwe L, Newman TK, et al. The relationship between childhood abuse and dissociation. Is it influenced by catechol-O-methyltransferase (COMT) activity? *Int J Neuropsychopharmacol*. 2008;11:149–61.
3. Maldonado JR, et al. Treatment for dissociative disorders. In: Natham P, *Gorman JM, eds. A guide to treatments that work*, 2nd ed. England: Oxford University; 2002:463–96.

ADDITIONAL READING

- Alvi T & Minhas FA. Type of Presentation of Dissociative Disorder and Frequency of Co-morbid Depressive Disorder. *J Coll Physicians Surg Pak*. 2009;19:113–16.
- Espirito-Santo H, Pio-Abreu JL. Psychiatric symptoms and dissociation in conversion, somatization and dissociative disorders. *Aust N Z J Psychiatry*. 2009;43:270–6.
- Foote B, Smolin Y, Neft DI, et al. Dissociative disorders and suicidality in psychiatric outpatients. *J Nerv Ment Dis*. 2008;196:29–36.
- Maaranen P, Tanskanen A, Hintikka J, et al. The course of dissociation in the general population: a 3-year follow-up study. *Compr Psychiatry*. 2008; 49:269–74.
- Ozturk E, Sar V. Somatization as a predictor of suicidal ideation in dissociative disorders. *Psychiatry Clin Neurosci*. 2008;62:662–8.
- Phillips KA, et al. Special DSM-V issues on anxiety, obsessive-compulsive spectrum, posttraumatic, and dissociative disorders. *Depress Anxiety*. 2010; 27:91–92.
- Ross CA. Borderline personality disorder and dissociation. *J Trauma Dissoc*. 2007;8:71–80.
- Simeon D, et al. Temporal disintegration in depersonalization disorder. *J Trauma Dissoc*. 2007;8:11–24.

CODES

ICD9
- 300.12 Dissociative amnesia
- 300.13 Dissociative fugue
- 300.14 Dissociative identity disorder

CLINICAL PEARLS

- Focus on improving and maintaining adaptive functioning with ADLs.
- Symptom stabilization and ego-strengthening come before exploration of past trauma.
- Regularly assess and reassess levels of functioning. Prevent unnecessary regressions.

DIVERTICULAR DISEASE

David M. Navel, MD
Justin M. Bailey, MD

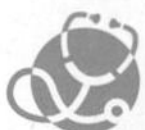

BASICS

DESCRIPTION

- Diverticular disease includes asymptomatic diverticula, symptomatic uncomplicated diverticular disease (recurrent pain, distention), diverticulitis, and diverticular hemorrhage
- Diverticula: Saclike protrusion of the mucosal and submucosal wall
  - Diverticulosis develops more commonly in countries where people eat a low-fiber diet.
  - In Western societies, 90–95% are found in the sigmoid colon, whereas Asian populations have more right-sided disease.
  - Diverticula number increase with age.
- Diverticular hemorrhage: Occurs in 3–5% of patients with diverticular disease:
  - Accounts for >40% of lower GI bleeds and 17–40% of cases of hematochezia in general
  - Bleeding is more common from right-sided diverticula.
- Diverticulitis: The most usual clinical complication, affects 10–25% of patients
- Complicated diverticulitis includes associated abscess, perforation, fistula, or stricture.
- System(s) affected: GI

EPIDEMIOLOGY

Incidence

- Diverticula in up to 20% general population, but increases progressively with age reaching up to 2/3 of people by the 8th decade
- Diverticulitis: 2,400–3,800/100,000
- Yearly mortality rate: 2.5/100,000

Prevalence

- Predominant age: <10% of people <40 years old, 2/3 of people in their 80s have diverticula
- Predominant sex: Male = Female overall, but more male <65 and female >65 years old

RISK FACTORS

- Age >40
- Low-fiber diet
- Sedentary lifestyle, obesity
- Previous diverticulitis and number of diverticula
- NSAID use may increase the risk of perforation.

Genetics

- No known genetic pattern
- Asian populations have a higher predominance of right-sided disease.

GENERAL PREVENTION

High-fiber diet; best with >30 g/day of fiber

ETIOLOGY

- Increased intraluminal pressure from dense, fiber-depleted stools and abnormal colonic motility
- Occur at areas of weakness from junctures of penetrating arteries in the muscular wall
- Bleeding is caused by medial thinning of the vasa recta and weakening of the artery.
- Diverticulitis occurs when increased pressures and fecal particles cause local inflammation and necrosis.

COMMONLY ASSOCIATED CONDITIONS

Connective tissue diseases, colon cancer, and inflammatory bowel disease

DIAGNOSIS

HISTORY

- Diverticulosis:
  - 80–85% of patients remain asymptomatic. Of the 15–20% with symptoms, 1–2% will need hospitalization and 0.5% will need surgery.
  - Pain: Dull, colicky, mostly in left lower quadrant, can be worse after eating, some relief following bowel movement or passage of flatus
  - Diarrhea or constipation
- Diverticulitis: Uncomplicated (75%) and complicated (25%):
  - Pain: Acute onset, mostly localized in left lower quadrant; prominently associated with tenderness in same region
  - Fever with chills as severity increases
  - Anorexia, nausea (20–62%), or vomiting
  - Constipation (50%) or diarrhea (25–35%)
  - Dysuria, frequency if bladder involved
  - Pneumaturia, fecaluria if colovesical fistula develops
- Diverticular hemorrhage:
  - Melena, hematochezia,
  - Painless rectal bleeding

PHYSICAL EXAM

- Diverticulosis:
  - Abdomen normal or distended and tympanitic
  - Absent signs of peritoneal inflammation
- Diverticulitis:
  - Rebound tenderness, involuntary guarding, or boardlike rigidity
  - Palpable mass (20%) that is tender, firm, or fixed
  - Abdomen distended and tympanitic
  - Bowel sounds depressed or could be exaggerated if obstruction ensues
  - Rectal exam may reveal tenderness, induration, or mass in the cul-de-sac.
  - Enterocutaneous, enterovaginal, and perirectal fistulae may be the initial manifestation.

DIAGNOSTIC TESTS & INTERPRETATION

Lab

Initial lab tests

- White blood cell count normal in diverticulosis; usually elevated with immature polymorphs in diverticulitis (normal in up to 45% of diverticulitis patients)
- Hemoglobin low, if bleeding present
- Erythrocyte sedimentation rate elevated in diverticulitis
- Urine analysis may be abnormal with microscopic pyuria, hematuria, pneumaturia, or fecaluria possibly suggesting fistula formation.
- Urine culture: Persistent infection in colovesical fistula
- Blood culture: Positive in diverticulitis with generalized peritonitis
- Drugs that may alter lab results:
  - Steroids
  - Other immunosuppressive drugs
- Disorders that may alter lab results:
  - Severe malnutrition

Imaging

Initial approach

- Diverticulosis:
  - Symptomatic uncomplicated disease: Consider a colonoscopy or a barium enema to rule out malignancy or colitis.
  - Recurrent uncomplicated diverticular disease: Evaluate by either a CT scan or a barium enema.
- Diverticulitis:
  - Plain film abdomen supine and upright; useful in peritonitis and perforation
  - Patients with suspected diverticulitis should have a CT scan with intravenous, oral, and rectal contrast to rule out complicated disease (1)[A].
  - CT may help in determining degree of acute perforation when present and assist in surgical planning.
  - Ultrasound has been shown to be effective in identifying diverticulitis in the acute setting (2)[B].
  - Avoid endoscopy or barium enemas due to risk of extravasation into the peritoneum.
- Diverticular hemorrhage/hematochezia:
  - Endoscopy is generally considered the test of choice for the evaluation of lower GI bleeding (3).
  - Angiography is used if massive bleeding obscures endoscopy or when endoscopy cannot visualize a source (3). It may also be used in some institutions as a primary evaluation tool for patients with acute lower GI bleeding.

Follow-Up & Special Considerations

- After resolution of an initial episode of acute diverticulitis, the colon should be evaluated with endoscopy to exclude any associated malignancies, strictures, or inflammatory bowel disease (1).
- After an episode of lower GI bleeding, colonoscopy should be performed to exclude neoplasia (2).

Diagnostic Procedures/Surgery

- For evaluation of hematochezia in suspected diverticular hemorrhage:
  - A nasogastric tube should be placed to exclude upper GI sources of bleeding (3).
  - 99mTc-pertechnetate–labeled red blood cell scans can be used before angiography to evaluate if angiography can be effective or not in revealing a source; however, this has not been studied in a comparison trial (3).
- For diverticulitis, gallium- or indium-labeled leukocytes to localize abscess (rarely used)

Pathological Findings

- Right-sided diverticula are true diverticula (all layers of the colonic wall).
- Left-sided diverticula are actually pseudodiverticula (outpouchings of the mucosa and submucosa).
- Surgical and autopsy studies show mycosis, a constellation of thickened circular muscle (pseudohypertrophy due to increased elastin in the taeniae), short taeniae, and luminal narrowing.
- Diverticulitis: Inflammation with lymphocytic infiltrate, ulceration, mucin depletion necrosis, Paneth cell metaplasia, and cryptitis.

DIFFERENTIAL DIAGNOSIS

rritable bowel syndrome, lactose intolerance, carcinoma, inflammatory bowel disease, fecal mpaction, incarcerated hernia, gallbladder disease, angiodysplasia, colitis, acute appendicitis, ectopic pregnancy

Pregnancy Considerations

- Rule out ectopic pregnancy.
- Carefully select antibiotic use in pregnant women due to teratogenicity of some medications.

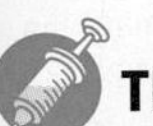

TREATMENT

MEDICATION

First Line

- Diverticulosis:
  - High fiber intake is recommended (preferably above 20–30 g/day).
- Symptomatic uncomplicated diverticular disease in the absence of a history of complicated disease can be treated with cyclical rifaximin or mesalamine continuously.
- Diverticulitis:
  - Oral antibiotics for outpatient treatment of mild disease: Cover for anaerobes and gram-negative rods with:
    - A quinolone (ciprofloxacin or levofloxacin) plus metronidazole (Flagyl) *OR*
    - Bactrim plus metronidazole
  - More severe cases in hospitals use intravenous antibiotics:
    - Mild/moderate disease: Zosyn or Unasyn or Ertapenem
    - Severe disease: Imipenem or Meropenem
  - Recurrences of acute diverticulitis may be decreased by using mesalamine ± rifaximin (4)[A] or probiotics
- Diverticular bleeding:
  - Consider Vasopressin 0.2–0.3 units/min through selective intra-arterial catheter
- Precautions:
  - Avoid morphine and other opiates that may increase intraluminal pressure or promote ileus.
  - Increased fiber intake is not recommended in the acute management of diverticulitis.

Second Line

- For outpatient therapy, Augmentin or Moxifloxacin
- For mild/moderate inpatient therapy:
  - Intravenous quinolone (ciprofloxacin or levofloxacin) + metronidazole or tigecycline
- For severely ill patients:
  - Ampicillin + metronidazole + a quinolone *OR*
  - Ampicillin + metronidazole + an aminoglycoside (if renal function allows)

ADDITIONAL TREATMENT

General Measures

- Diverticulosis: Outpatient with fiber supplements to soften stools
- Outpatient diverticulitis: Pain, tenderness, leukocytosis, but no toxicity or peritoneal signs; treat with oral antibiotics. 1–2% of subjects require hospitalization for toxicity, septicemia, peritonitis, or failure of symptoms to be resolved in a few days. Up to 30% of patients may require surgery at 1st episode of diverticulitis. Up to 50% of all patients with diverticulitis eventually may come to surgery.
- Toxic patients require hospitalization, bowel rest with clear liquids or nothing by mouth, and intravenous antibiotics at least until there is a positive response.
- Symptomatic improvement is expected within 2–3 days of initiating antibiotics, and antibiotics continued for 7–10 days (2).
- 80% of diverticular hemorrhages will resolve spontaneously (3).

Issues for Referral

Acutely suspected perforation, peritoneal signs, persistent lower GI bleeding requiring multiple transfusions

COMPLEMENTARY AND ALTERNATIVE MEDICINE

Probiotics may have benefit in symptomatic uncomplicated diverticular disease.

SURGERY/OTHER PROCEDURES

- Indication for emergent surgery: Peritonitis, uncontrolled sepsis, visceral perforation, colonic obstruction, or acute deterioration
- Surgery for nonemergent state controversial, sometimes even in complicated cases of diverticulitis (5)
- Elective surgery after acute diverticulitis: Decision for elective resection should be made on a case-by-case basis (1)[B].
  - After 1st episode, there is a 33% chance of a recurrence; if it does recur, there is a 66% chance of a 3rd bout.
  - Most complicated cases occur on the 1st presentation with subsequent presentations being uncomplicated (5).
  - Emergent surgery carries a 9-fold increase in mortality when compared to elective resection (6).
  - Elective resection is typically advised after recovery from a complicated diverticulitis treated nonoperatively (1)[B].
  - Age: Younger patients more likely to have recurrence; but should not determine the need for surgery.
  - Immunocompromised patients: More likely to present with acute complicated diverticulitis, fail medical management and have complications from elective surgery.
- Large abscesses (>4 cm) are usually drained radiologically and many of these patients can be acutely managed nonoperatively. As stated above, the ASCRS generally recommends elective resection after resolution of such a case (1)[B].
- In diverticular hemorrhage, patients requiring more than 4 units of red blood cells transfused have a 60% chance of requiring surgical intervention to stop bleeding. Patients requiring <4 units typically do not need surgery (3).

IN-PATIENT CONSIDERATIONS

Initial Stabilization

Intravenous fluids, analgesics, antibiotics, nasogastric suction

Admission Criteria

~1–2% of subjects require hospitalization for toxicity, septicemia, peritonitis

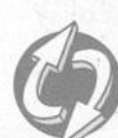

ONGOING CARE

DIET

- NPO during acute diverticulitis; progress to fluids, then high-fiber as bowel function returns
- Patients with known diverticulosis should eat a high-fiber diet (>30 g/day) to prevent recurrence.
- Nuts, corn, and popcorn do not increase risk for diverticulosis or diverticular complications (7).

PROGNOSIS

- Good with early detection and treatment of complications.
- Recurrence risk increases with each bout.
- If diverticular bleeding, rebleeding occurs in up to 6%.

COMPLICATIONS

Hemorrhage, perforation, peritonitis, obstruction, abscess, or fistula

REFERENCES

1. Standards Committee of The American Society of Colon and Rectal Surgeons, Rafferty J, Shellito P, et al. Practice Parameters for Sigmoid Diverticulitis. *Dis Colon Rectum*. 2006.
2. Stollman NH, Raskin JB. Diagnosis and management of diverticular disease of the colon in adults. Ad Hoc Practice Parameters Committee of the American College of Gastroenterology. *Am J Gastroenterol*. 1999;94:3110–21.
3. Zuccaro G. Management of the adult patient with acute lower gastrointestinal bleeding. American College of Gastroenterology. Practice Parameters Committee. *Am J Gastroenterol*. 1998;93:1202–8.
4. Gatta L, Vakil N, Vaira D, Pilotto A, Curlo M, Comparato G, Leandro G, Ferro U, Lera M, Milletti S, Di Mario F et al. Efficacy of 5-ASA in the treatment of colonic diverticular disease. *J Clin Gastroenterol*. 2010;44:113–9.
5. Nelson RS, Ewing BM, Wengert TJ, et al. Clinical outcomes of complicated diverticulitis managed nonoperatively. *Am J Surg*. 2008;196:969–72; discussion 973–4.
6. Novitsky YW, Sechrist C, Payton BL, et al. Do the risks of emergent colectomy justify nonoperative management strategies for recurrent diverticulitis? *Am J Surg*. 2008.
7. Strate LL, Liu YL, Syngal S, et al. Nut, corn, and popcorn consumption and the incidence of diverticular disease. *JAMA*. 2008;300:907–14.

CODES

ICD9

- 562.00 Diverticulosis of small intestine (without mention of hemorrhage)
- 562.01 Diverticulitis of small intestine (without mention of hemorrhage)
- 562.02 Diverticulosis of small intestine with hemorrhage

CLINICAL PEARLS

- Diverticula occur in up to 20% of general population, but increases progressively with age, reaching up to 2/3 of people by the 8th decade.
- Patients with known diverticulosis should eat a high-fiber diet to prevent recurrence, and nuts, corn, and popcorn do not increase risk for diverticular complications.
- WBC are not elevated in up to 45% of cases of diverticulitis

D

DOMESTIC VIOLENCE

Rhonda A. Faulkner, PhD
Meg Lekander, MD

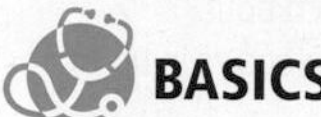

BASICS

DESCRIPTION

- Domestic violence (DV) is behavior in any relationship that is used to gain or maintain power and control over an intimate partner.
- May include physical, sexual, and/or emotional abuse, economical or psychological actions, or threats of actions that influence another person.
- Although women are at greater risk of experiencing DV, it occurs among patients of any race, age, sexual orientation, religion, gender, socioeconomic background, and education level.
- Synonym(s): Intimate partner violence (IPV); Spousal abuse; Family violence

EPIDEMIOLOGY

Incidence

Approximately 8%; women were more likely to report partner violence than men (1)[B]

Prevalence

- Domestic violence occurs in 1 in 4 American families. In the US, 2–4 million women are abused by an intimate partner each year. Nearly 5.3 million incidents of DV occur each year among US women ≥18 years, and 3.2 million incidents among men.
- DV results in nearly 2 million injuries and 2,000–4,000 deaths nationwide each year.
- Reportedly, 30% of women and 22% of men have experienced physical, sexual, or psychological IPV during their lifetime in the U.S.
- DV is estimated to affect at least 1/3 of patients cared for by primary care physicians, with 5% of women patients in current abusive relationship.

Geriatric Considerations

- ~4–6% of elderly are abused, with ~1–2 million elderly persons experiencing abuse and/or neglect each year. In 90% of cases, the perpetrator is a family member.
- Elder abuse is any form of mistreatment that results in harm or loss to an older person; may include physical, sexual, emotional, financial abuse, and/or neglect.

Pediatric Considerations

- >3 million children aged 3–17 years are at risk of witnessing acts of DV.
- Approximately 1 million abused children are identified in the US each year.
- Children living in violent homes are at increased risk of physical, sexual, and/or emotional abuse; anxiety and depression; decreased self-esteem; emotional, behavioral, social, and physical disturbances.

Pregnancy Considerations

DV occurs during 7–20% of pregnancies. Women with unintended pregnancy are at 3 times greater risk of DV compared with those whose pregnancy was planned. 25% of abused women report exacerbation of abuse during pregnancy.

RISK FACTORS

Patient/victim risk factors:

- Substance abuse
- Poverty/financial stressors/unemployment
- Recent loss of social support
- Family disruption and life cycle changes
- History of abusive relationships or witness to abuse as child
- Mental or physical disability in family
- Social isolation
- Pregnancy

Abuser risk factors:

- Substance abuse (e.g., heavy drinking)
- Young age
- Unemployment
- Low academic achievement
- Witnessing or experiencing violence as child
- Depression
- Personality disorders

Relational risk factors:

- Marital conflict
- Marital instability
- Economic stress
- Traditional gender role norms
- Poor family functioning

Geriatric Considerations

Factors associated with the abuse of older adults include increasing age, nonwhite race, low income status, functional impairment, cognitive disability, substance use, poor emotional state, low self-esteem, cohabitation, and lack of social support.

Pediatric Considerations

Factors associated with child abuse or neglect include low-income status, low maternal education, nonwhite race, large family size, young maternal age, single-parent household, parental psychiatric disturbances, and presence of a stepfather.

DIAGNOSIS

- DV is often underdiagnosed, with only 10–12% of physicians conducting routine screening.
- Although prevalence of DV in primary care settings is 7–50%, <15% are screened.
- Pregnancy increases risk.
- 15–20% of women in US emergency departments are there related to DV.
- Barriers to screening: Time constraints, discomfort with the subject, fear of offending the patient, and lack of perceived skills and resources to manage DV.
- Abused patients may refuse to disclose abuse for many reasons:
  - Not feeling emotionally ready to admit the reality of the situation
  - Shame and self-blame
  - Feelings of failure if abuse is admitted
  - Fear of rejection by the physician
  - Fear of retribution from abuser
  - Belief that abuse will not happen again
  - Believe that no alternatives or available resources exist
- Physicians should introduce the subject of DV in a general way (i.e., "I routinely ask all patients about domestic violence. Have you ever been in a relationship where you were afraid?").
- How to screen:
  - Screen patient alone, without partner or others present
  - Ask screening questions in patient's primary language; do not use children or other family members as interpreters
- Partner violence screening:
  - "Have you ever been hit, kicked, punched, or otherwise hurt by someone?"
  - "Have you ever been verbally threatened or abused by someone?
  - "Do you feel safe in your current relationship?"
  - "Is there a partner from a previous relationship who is making you feel unsafe now?"
  - "Has your child(ren) ever witnessed anything violent or frightening in your home, neighborhood, or school?"
- CDC-recommended RADAR system:
  - R: Routinely screen every patient; make screening a part of everyday practice in prenatal, postnatal, routine gynecologic visits, and annual health screenings.
  - A: Ask questions directly, kindly, and be nonjudgmental.
  - D: Document findings in the patient's chart using the patient's own words, with details. Use body maps and photographs as necessary.
  - A: Assess the patient's safety and see if the patient has a safety plan.
  - R: Review options for dealing with domestic violence with the patient and provide referrals.
- Additional DV screening tools:
  - SAFE Questions:
    - Stress/Safety: "Do you feel safe in your relationship?"
    - Afraid/Abused: "Have you ever been in a relationship where you were threatened, hurt, or afraid?"
    - Friends/Family: "Are your friends or family aware that you have been hurt? Could you tell them, and would they be able to give you support?"
    - Emergency Plan: "Do you have a safe place to go and the resources you need in an emergency?"
  - HITS screening tool (1-never, 2-rarely, 3-sometimes, 4-often, 5- frequently; Score >9 is considered abuse):
    - How often does your partner: Hurt you (physically)?; Insult you?; Threaten you with harm?; Scream or curse at you?

HISTORY

- Pregnancy difficulties such as poor/late prenatal care, low-birth-weight babies. and perinatal deaths
- Pelvic and abdominal pain, chronic without demonstrable pathology
- Headaches
- Back pain
- Gynecologic disorders
- Sexually transmitted infections including HIV/AIDS
- Central nervous system disorders
- Gastrointestinal disorders

- Depression
- Suicidal ideation
- Anxiety
- Fatigue
- Substance abuse
- Eating disorders
- Overuse of health services/frequent emergency room visits
- Noncompliance

PHYSICAL EXAM

- Psychological signs and symptoms:
  - Signs of Battered Woman Syndrome &/or PTSD (flat affect/avoidance of eye contact; evasiveness; heightened startle response; sleep disturbance; traumatic flashbacks)
  - Depression, anxiety, chronic fatigue, substance abuse
  - Suspicious partner accompaniment at appointment; overly solicitous partner and/or refusal to leave exam room
- Physical signs and symptoms:
  - Tympanic membrane rupture
  - Rectal or genital injury (centrally located injuries with bathing-suit pattern of distribution—concealable by clothing)
  - Head and neck injuries (site of 50% of abusive injuries)
  - Facial scrapes, loose or broken tooth, bruises, cuts, or fractures to face or body
  - Knife wounds, cigarette burns, bite marks, welts w/outline of weapon (such as belt buckle)
  - Broken bones
  - Defensive posture injuries
  - Injuries inconsistent with the explanation given
  - Injuries in various stages of healing

DIAGNOSTIC TESTS & INTERPRETATION

- The US Preventive Services Task Force (USPSTF) found insufficient evidence to recommend for/against routine screening of parents or guardians for the physical abuse or neglect of children, of women for intimate partner violence, or of older adults or their caregivers for elder abuse.
- Other recommendations:
  - American College of Physicians recommends routine screening for DV in primary care settings and when women present for emergency care with traumatic injuries.
  - US Surgeon General and American Association of Family Practitioners recommend that physicians consider the possibility of DV as a cause of illness and injury.

Pediatric Considerations

American Academy of Pediatrics (AAP) and American Medical Association (AMA) recommend that physicians remain alert for signs and symptoms of child physical and sexual abuse in the routine exam.

Pregnancy Considerations

ACOG and AMA guidelines on DV recommend that physicians should routinely assess all pregnant women for DV.

Lab

Initial lab tests

LFTs, amylase, lipase if abdominal trauma is suspected

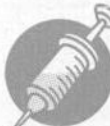

TREATMENT

- Treatment includes: Initial diagnosis; ongoing medical care; emotional support, counseling, and patient education regarding the DV cycle; referrals to community and supportive services as needed.
- Upon diagnosis, offer validation and emotionally supportive statements:
  - "You are not to blame. I am sorry this is happening to you. There is no excuse for DV."
  - Remind patient of your commitment to confidential communication.
- Listen and respond to safety issues for the patient:
  - "Are you afraid to go home?"
  - "Are there guns in the home?"
- Provide information about DV and help where needed:
  - "DV is a health issue for you (and your children)."
- Make referrals to local resources:
  - "Do you need or want to access a safety shelter or DV service agency?"
  - "Do you want police intervention and if so, would you like me to call the police so they can make a report with you?"
  - Offer numbers to local resources and National DV Hotline: 1.800.799.SAFE (open 24/7; can provide physicians in every state with information on local resources).
- Document findings:
  - Use patient's own words regarding injury and abuse.
  - Legibly document injuries: Use a body map.
  - If possible, take instant photographs of patient's injuries if given patient consent.
- Make patient safety plan.
- If patient is planning to leave:
  - Is there a friend or supportive family member nearby with whom the patient can stay?
  - Does patient want to go to a DV shelter or contact police; obtain an order of protection?
- If patient is not planning to leave:
  - Can she or he anticipate the escalation of violence and take precautions?
  - Are there weapons in the home?
- Preparing patient to get away in an emergency:
  - Encourage patient to keep the following items in a safe place: Keys (house and car); important papers (Social Security card, birth certificates, photo ID/driver's license, passport, green card); cash, food stamps, credit cards; medication for self and children; children's immunization records; important phone numbers/addresses (friends, family, local shelters); personal care items, extra glasses, etc.
  - Encourage patient to arrange a signal with someone to let that person know when she or he needs help.

ADDITIONAL TREATMENT

- National DV Hotline: 1.800.799.SAFE (7233)
- Post in all exam rooms posters in both English and Spanish; available at http://www.thehotline.org/resources/resource-download-center/

General Measures

- Reporting child and elder abuse to protective services is mandatory in most states. Several states have laws requiring mandatory reporting of IPV.
- Contact the local DV program to find out about laws and community resources before they are needed.
- Display resource materials (National DV Hotline: 1.800.799.SAFE) in the office, all exam rooms, and restrooms.

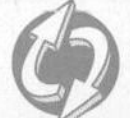

ONGOING CARE

FOLLOW-UP RECOMMENDATIONS

- Schedule prompt follow-up appointment.
- Inquire about what has happened since last visit.
- Review medical records and ask about past episodes to convey concern for the patient and a willingness to address this health issue openly.
- DV often requires multiple interventions over time before it is resolved.

PATIENT EDUCATION

- Counsel patients about nonviolent ways to resolve conflict.
- Educate patients about the cycle of violence.
- Counsel parents about developmentally appropriate ways to discipline their children.
- Educate parents about the negative consequences of arguments on children and each other.
- National Coalition Against Domestic Violence: www.ncadv.org
- CDC: www.cdc.gov/violenceprevention

PROGNOSIS

Most DV perpetrators do not voluntarily seek therapy unless pressured by partners or upon legal mandate. Current evidence is insufficient on effectiveness of therapy for perpetrators.

REFERENCE

1. Walton MA, Murray R, Cunningham RM, Chermack ST, Barry KL, Booth BM, Ilgen MA, Wojnar M, Blow FC et al. Correlates of intimate partner violence among men and women in an inner city emergency department. *J Addict Dis*. 2009;28:366–81.

ADDITIONAL READING

MacMillan HL, Wathen CN, Jamieson E, et al. Screening for intimate partner violence in health care settings: A randomized trial. *JAMA*. 2009;302:493–501.

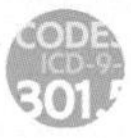

CODES

ICD9

- 995.50 Unspecified child abuse
- 995.51 Child emotional/psychological abuse
- 995.52 Child neglect (nutritional)

CLINICAL PEARLS

- Display resource materials in the office (e.g., posting Abuse Awareness posters/National DV Hotline, 1.800.799.SAFE, in both English and Spanish, in all exam rooms and restrooms).
- Despite lack of data, screen all women: "Have you ever been threatened, hit, kicked, or are you afraid of your partner?"
- For those who screen positive, offer resources, reassure confidentiality, and provide close follow-up.

D

DOWN SYNDROME

Michele Roberts, MD, PhD

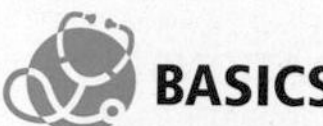

BASICS

DESCRIPTION

- Congenital condition associated with mental retardation and an increased risk of multisystem medical problems
- One of the most common identifiable causes of mental retardation
- System(s) affected: Neurologic (100%); Cardiac (40–50%); Gastrointestinal (GI) (8–12%)
- Etiology: The presence of all or part of an extra chromosome 21
- Synonym(s): Trisomy 21; DS

Pediatric Considerations

- Congenital heart disease is major cause of morbidity/mortality. Murmur may not be present at birth. Delay in recognition may lead to irreversible pulmonary hypertension.
- Early treatment of subclinical thyroid disease may improve growth and development (1)[B].

Geriatric Considerations

- Life expectancy has increased to 56 years in 2008 (2).
- Age-related health issues occur at earlier age than in general population.
- Communication difficulties may interfere with prompt recognition of:
  - Alzheimer disease, which is more prevalent and may occur at a younger age, and other psychiatric illness
  - Thyroid/autoimmune disorders
  - Cataracts/hearing loss

Pregnancy Considerations

- Most DS males are infertile:
- Females are subfertile but can conceive:
  - 36% of reported offspring have DS
  - Assess mental and physical fitness to carry pregnancy/care for child

EPIDEMIOLOGY

Incidence

In the US, 1 in 700 live births

Prevalence

350,000 persons in the US

RISK FACTORS

- DS occurs in all races with equal frequency.
- Risk increases dramatically with mother's age:
  - Age 20, 1 in 1,445
  - Age 35, 1 in 270
  - Age 37, 1 in 100
  - Age 45, 1 in 25
- With prenatal screening of older mothers, relatively more DS infants are born to younger mothers.

Genetics

- Online Mendelian Inheritance in Man (OMIM) #190685
- Inheritance: Most commonly sporadic nondisjunction resulting in trisomy 21
- Chance of having another child with DS is:
  - 1% (or age risk, whichever is greater) after conceiving a pregnancy with nondisjunction trisomy 21
  - 10–15% for mothers and 3–5% for fathers who carry a balanced translocation
  - 100% if the parental translocation is 21:21(45,t [21:21])
- Unclear after child with mosaic DS, but ~1%
- Chromosome 21 has been sequenced; it is the smallest human chromosome.
- The majority of identifiable phenotypic characteristics associated with DS map to a 37–44 Mb region of distal 21q. Broad susceptibility regions for 25 phenotypes have been identified, arguing against a single Down syndrome critical region (DSCR) (3).

GENERAL PREVENTION

- No prevention for nondisjunction
- The American College of Medical Genetics and the American College of Obstetrics and Gynecology recommend that all pregnant women be offered prenatal screening for DS.
- Preimplantation diagnosis with in vitro fertilization (IVF) or prenatal diagnosis and termination are current options.
- Maternal prenatal screening includes:
  - Pregnancy-associated plasma protein A (PAPP-A): 1st trimester
  - Quadruple test: 2nd trimester
  - Sequential/integrated screen combines both
  - Ultrasound (nuchal translucency or NT)
- Chorionic villi sampling or amniocentesis: if high a priori risk or positive screen

ETIOLOGY

- Trisomy 21: In 95% of patients, an extra chromosome 21 is found in all cells due to nondisjunction usually in maternal meiosis.
- Translocation DS: In 3% of patients, extra chromosome 21q material is translocated to another chromosome (usually 13, 14, or 21). For translocation trisomy 21, 2/3 are new, 1/3 have a parental carrier:
  - Translocation DS more likely if mother <30 years of age
- Mosaic trisomy 21: Found in 2% of patients with DS. Manifestations may be milder.

COMMONLY ASSOCIATED CONDITIONS

- Cardiac:
  - Congenital heart defects (40–50%):
  - Mostly endocardial cushion or ventricular septal defect (VSD)
- GI/growth:
  - Structural defects (12%):
    - Duodenal or anal atresia/stenosis
    - Hirschsprung disease, annular pancreas
  - Gastroesophageal reflux
  - Constipation
  - Celiac disease
- Pulmonary:
  - Tracheal stenosis/tracheoesophageal fistula
  - Pulmonary hypertension
  - Obstructive apnea
- Genitourinary:
  - Cryptorchidism, hypospadias
  - Renal anomaly
- Hematologic/neoplastic:
  - Macrocytosis (66%)
  - Transient leukemoid reaction (10%):
    - Generally resolves spontaneously, but can be preleukemic (AMKL) in 20–30%
  - Leukemia (0.5–1%):
  - Acute lymphoblastic leukemia (ALL) risk: 10–20 × that of ALL in non-DS
  - Decreased risk of most solid tumors; increased ris of germ cell tumors
- Endocrine:
  - Hypothyroidism: Congenital or acquired (20–40%
  - Diabetes
  - Hypogonadism
- Skeletal:
  - Altered growth pattern
  - Atlantoaxial instability (15%); 2% symptomatic
  - Ligamentous laxity
  - Scoliosis (some cases have adult onset)
  - Hip problems (8%)
- Immune/rheumatologic:
  - Abnormal immune function with increased rate of and mortality from infection, especially respiratory
  - Increased risk of autoimmune disorders including thyroid, celiac disease, lupus
- Neurologic:
  - Mental retardation ranging from near-normal to severe. Average is moderate retardation.
  - Seizures:
    - Infantile spasms (5–10%)
    - Increased risk child-/adult-onset seizures
  - Alzheimer disease: 100% develop neuropathologic changes, though not all develop symptoms
- Psychiatric:
  - Emotional/conduct disorders (25–33%)
  - Depression: Up to 10% of adults
- Sensory:
  - Hearing loss (60–90%):
    - Mostly conductive due to high frequency of asymptomatic middle ear effusion
  - Visual impairment (60–70%): Mostly strabismus, nystagmus, cataracts
- Dermatologic, worsens with increasing age:
  - Palmoplantar hyperkeratosis (>75%), atopic or seborrheic dermatitis (50%), onychomycosis (50%), syringomas (30%), furunculosis/folliculitis (15%)

DIAGNOSIS

- The mother should be informed of the diagnosis promptly by a physician (preferably the obstetrician and pediatrician, or family physician), on the basis of clinical observations and before the karyotype is available, but with consideration of extenuating circumstances (e.g., mother's medical condition).
- The spouse/partner and infant should be present unless this would cause undue delay. The meeting should be private.
- Refer to the baby by name.
- The physician should be knowledgeable on the subject of DS, and should conduct a discussion with content that is current, respectful, balanced, informative, and realistic but not overly pessimistic, concentrating on what is relevant to the first year of life.

HISTORY

85% of mothers of infants with DS learn of the diagnosis postnatally

PHYSICAL EXAM

- DS-specific growth curves should be used.
- Infants and children:
  - Brachycephaly (100%)
  - Hypotonia (80%)
  - Small ears, often low set and simplified
  - Upslanting palpebral fissure (90%)
  - Epicanthic folds (90%)
  - Brushfield spots
  - Depressed nasal bridge
  - Short neck, often with increased nuchal folds
  - Abnormal dermatoglyphics, including single palmar crease, single flexion crease on 5th finger
  - Increased space between toes 1–2; 5th finger clinodactyly; brachydactyly
- Adults: Features may become less obvious.

DIAGNOSTIC TESTS & INTERPRETATION

Lab

Initial lab tests

- A chromosome test is definitive and should always be done at the time of clinical suspicion.
- Parental chromosome study indicated only if translocation DS found in child.

Imaging

Initial approach

- Echocardiogram at the time of diagnosis. A ventricular septal defect (VSD)/endocardial cushion defect may not be apparent at birth.
- Radiographs of neck currently recommended for all children once between ages 3 and 5 years.

Follow-Up & Special Considerations

- Repeat neck films for minor trauma, neck pain, long-tract symptoms, or breathing problems.
- Cardiac follow-up as indicated

Pathological Findings

Upslanting palpebral fissures, epicanthic folds, 5th-finger clinodactyly, and single palmar crease individually may be a benign familial trait. Unilateral single palmar crease seen in 4% of general population; bilateral in 1%.

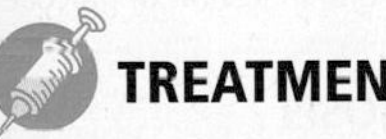

TREATMENT

ADDITIONAL TREATMENT

General Measures

Genetic evaluation and counseling

Issues for Referral

- Infant stimulation programs
- Physical/occupational/speech therapy
- Special needs educational support
  - Inclusion programs generally work well.

COMPLEMENTARY AND ALTERNATIVE MEDICINE

- Antioxidant therapy has theoretical basis for future benefits, although a 2008 randomized controlled trial provided no evidence to support the use of antioxidant or folinic acid supplements in children with Down syndrome (4).
- Vitamin E, selenium, and zinc may be beneficial (5)[C].
- Many unproven and dangerous procedures and therapies are offered to vulnerable parents:
  - Craniosacral manipulation is dangerous due to potential atlantoaxial instability.
  - Sicca is illegal in US, potentially dangerous, and without any evidence of benefit.
- Piracetam is much publicized, without scientific evidence of benefit.

SURGERY/OTHER PROCEDURES

Repair of congenital anomalies is appropriate. Plastic surgery for facial features generally not recommended.

IN-PATIENT CONSIDERATIONS

Discharge Criteria

If the social situation indicates adoption, there are families specifically seeking to adopt DS children.

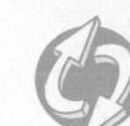

ONGOING CARE

FOLLOW-UP RECOMMENDATIONS

Patient Monitoring

Surveillance recommendations (6,7,8)[C] (repeat additionally for clinical suspicion):

- Vision: Assess for strabismus, cataracts, and nystagmus at birth and on each routine visit:
  - Should be seen by ophthalmologist by 6 months and every 2 years in early childhood, annually in later childhood and adulthood
- Hearing: Neonatal screen with ABR or OAE, then audiogram every 6 months until age 3 years, then annual hearing assessment
- Thyroid: Initial newborn screen. Repeat thyroid-stimulating hormone (TSH) at 6 months, 12 months, and then annually.
- Screening for celiac disease is controversial, but does not appear to be cost effective.
- C-spine flexion/extension films once at 3–5 years of age and as indicated clinically.
- Echocardiogram for all newborns, regardless of murmur. Monitor clinically for later cardiac complications throughout life.

DIET

- No special diet, but caloric needs are lower in adolescents/adults with DS than in their peers
- Obesity is prevalent at all ages.
- No scientific evidence to support megavitamin therapy and dietary supplements that are widely discussed in the lay press

PATIENT EDUCATION

- National Down Syndrome Congress (800) 232-NDSC http://www.ndsccenter.org
- National Down Syndrome Society (800) 221-4602 http://www.ndss.org
- Dr. Len Leshin, a pediatrician whose son has Down syndrome, has written an extensive collection of accurate and accessible articles about Down syndrome: http://www.ds-health.com/
- The Down Syndrome Research Foundation provides information on the latest research and educational programs for people with Down syndrome: http://dsrf.org/index.cfm?fuseaction=publications.dsq

PROGNOSIS

- Associated congenital anomalies are the immediate concern during the newborn period.
- Adults can often work in protected situations; a few are largely independent.
- Earlier onset of age-related health issues, shortened life expectancy.
- Clinical Alzheimer disease in at least 1/3 of patients after age 35 years

REFERENCES

1. van Trotsenburg AS, Vulsma T, van Rozenburg-Marres SL, et al. The effect of thyroxine treatment started in the neonatal period on development and growth of two-year-old Down syndrome children: a randomized clinical trial. *J Clin Endocrinol Metab*. 2005;90:3304–11.
2. http://www.ndss.org.
3. Lyle R, Béna F, Gagos S et al. Genotype-phenotype correlations in Down syndrome identified by array CGH in 30 cases of partial trisomy and partial monosomy chromosome 21. *Eur J Hum Genet*. 2009;17:454–66.
4. Ellis JM, Tan HK, Gilbert RE, et al. Supplementation with antioxidants and folinic acid for children with Down's syndrome: randomised controlled trial. *BMJ*. 2008;336:594–7.
5. Roizen NJ. Complementary and alternative therapies for Down syndrome. *MRDD Res Rev*. 2005;11:149–55.
6. American Academy of Pediatrics: Health supervision for children with Down syndrome *Pediatrics*. 2001;107:442–9.
7. Cohen WI. Current dilemmas in Down syndrome clinical care. *Am J Med Genet*. 2006;142C:141–8.
8. Smith DS. Health care management of adults with Down syndrome. *Am Fam Physician*. 2001;64: 1031–8.

ADDITIONAL READING

- Mégarbané A, Ravel A, Mircher C et al. The 50th anniversary of the discovery of trisomy 21: the past, present, and future of research and treatment of Down syndrome. *Genet Med*. 2009;11:611–6.
- Ranweiler R. Assessment and care of the newborn with down syndrome. *Adv Neonatal Care*. 2009;9:17–24.
- Reynolds T, Vranken G, Van Nueten J, et al. Down's syndrome screening: population statistic dependency of screening performance. *Clin Chem Lab Med*. 2008;46:639–47.
- Roizen NJ, Patterson D. Down's syndrome. *Lancet*. 2003;361:1281–9.
- Skotko BG, Capone GT, Kishnani PS, et al. Postnatal diagnosis of Down syndrome: synthesis of the evidence on how best to deliver the news. *Pediatrics*. 2009;124:e751–8.

See Also (Topic, Algorithm, Electronic Media Element)

Algorithm: Mental Retardation

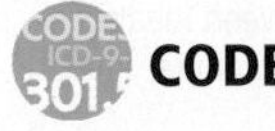

CODES

ICD9

758.0 Down's syndrome

CLINICAL PEARLS

- DS can affect all systems, including neurologic, cardiac, gastrointestinal, and endocrine.
- As life expectancy increases, regular health monitoring can improve outcomes.

DUMPING SYNDROME

Hongyi Cui, MD, PhD
John J. Kelly, MD

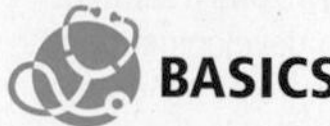

BASICS

DESCRIPTION

Gastrointestinal and vasomotor symptoms resulting from rapid gastric emptying and delivery of large amounts of hyperosmolar content into the small intestine. Usually occurs following gastric and esophageal surgery (gastrectomy, vagotomy, pyloroplasty, esophagectomy, Nissen fundoplication, or gastric bypass procedures).

EPIDEMIOLOGY

- Overall, about 10% of patients following gastric surgery and up to 50% of patients who undergo esophagectomy develop dumping symptoms.
- Predominant age: Middle age to elderly
- Predominant sex: Female > Male

Incidence

- In the US, 0.9% of proximal gastric vagotomy without any drainage procedure; 10–22% truncal vagotomy and drainage. After partial gastrectomy, 14–20% of patients develop symptoms of dumping.
- It is a prominent feature after bariatric surgery. Over 70% of patients that have undergone gastric bypass procedure experience varying degree of dumping symptoms. It is regarded as a beneficial feature of gastric bypass surgery since patients learn to avoid calorie-rich foods and eat small meals.

RISK FACTORS

Accelerated gastric emptying resulting from gastric surgery is a main risk factor for dumping syndrome. In fact, the severity of dumping syndrome is proportional to the rate of gastric emptying. The common gastric surgical procedures associated with dumping syndrome are:

- Bariatric surgery (i.e., Roux-en-Y gastric bypass)
- Gastric drainage procedures (e.g., pyloroplasty)
- Partial gastrectomy
- Total gastrectomy. Those with pouch formation have significantly less dumping and heartburn (1)[A].
- Esophagectomy
- Antiulcer surgery (e.g., vagotomy)
- Antireflux surgery (e.g., Nissen fundoplication, especially in pediatric patients)

GENERAL PREVENTION

- Dietary modifications (i.e., eating frequent, small, dry meals that contain limited amount of refined carbohydrates; restrict fluids to between meals; avoid milk products and increase protein/fat intake and supplement dietary fibers, etc.)
- Postural changes (i.e., lying supine for 30 minutes after meals)

ETIOLOGY

The pathogenesis of dumping syndrome is multifactorial. It includes at least the following interplaying factors:

- Alterations in the storage function of the stomach and/or the pyloric emptying mechanism, leading to rapid delivery of hyperosmolar material into the intestine. This results in fluid shifts from the intravascular compartment into the bowel lumen, leading to rapid small-bowel distention and an increase in the frequency of bowel contractions (early dumping).
- Supraphysiologic release of various GI peptides/vasoactive mediators, leading to paradoxical vasodilation in a relatively volume-contracted state.
- Reactive hypoglycemia secondary to hyperinsulinemia caused by high concentration of carbohydrates in the proximal small intestine and rapid absorption of glucose (late dumping).
- Pancreatic islet cell hyperplasia, rather than late dumping, is thought to be the underlying mechanism for hyperinsulinemic hypoglycemia with nesidioblastosis after gastric bypass.

COMMONLY ASSOCIATED CONDITIONS

- Peptic ulcer disease
- Reactive hypoglycemia
- Gastrectomy/vagotomy/pyloroplasty
- Esophagectomy
- After Nissen fundoplication for reflux disease in pediatric population
- After gastric bypass procedure for morbid obesity

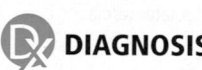

DIAGNOSIS

A suggestive symptom profile in a patient who has undergone gastric (including bariatric) or esophageal surgery warrants the investigation for dumping syndrome.

HISTORY

- History of gastric procedures
- GI symptoms (in early dumping):
  - Cramping abdominal pain
  - Diarrhea (postprandial)
  - Borborygmi
  - Bloating or epigastric fullness
  - Nausea/vomiting
- Systemic/vasomotor symptoms (both early and late dumping):
  - Palpitations
  - Diaphoresis
  - Faintness, fatigue, and headache
  - Flushing
  - Light-headedness and desire to lie down
  - Confusion and syncope
  - Malnutrition and weight loss
- Early dumping symptoms include gastrointestinal (abdominal pain, nausea, bloating, borborygmi and diarrhea, etc.) and vasomotor (perspiration and facial flushing, a desire to lie down, palpitations, weakness and syncope, etc.) symptoms; late dumping symptoms include perspiration, palpitations, hunger, weakness, confusion and syncope, etc.

PHYSICAL EXAM

- Diagnosis is mainly based on typical symptoms in patients with history of gastric procedures. A diagnostic scoring system has been developed by Sigstad based on various weighting factors allocated to the symptoms of dumping. A score index >7 is suggestive of dumping syndrome. The score index is very helpful in assessing a response to therapy.
- No physical signs are specific for dumping syndrome

DIAGNOSTIC TESTS & INTERPRETATION

Lab

- Postprandial hypoglycemia
- Anemia
- Hypoalbuminemia
- Drugs that may alter lab results: Insulin
- Disorders that may alter lab results: Diabetes mellitus

Imaging

- Upper gastrointestinal series: Barium rapidly emptying from stomach
- Nuclear medicine gastric emptying study
- Endoscopy (to define anatomy and exclude mechanical obstruction)

Diagnostic Procedures/Surgery

- Dumping syndrome is a clinical diagnosis based on typical symptoms in patients who have undergone gastric surgery.
- Oral glucose challenge test (i.e., oral intake of 50 grams of glucose following 10-hour fasting) can elicit typical signs and symptoms in patients with dumping syndrome. A rise in heart rate by 10 beats per minute or more in the first hour is diagnostic.
- Hydrogen breath test after oral ingestion of glucose is also a sensitive test.

DIFFERENTIAL DIAGNOSIS

- Mechanical obstruction
- Gastroenteric fistula
- Celiac sprue
- Crohn disease
- Pancreatic exocrine insufficiency
- Neuroendocrine tumors (e.g., carcinoid)
- Irritable bowel syndrome
- Lactose intolerance

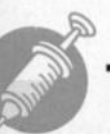

TREATMENT

Dietary modifications are the mainstay of treatment in patients with dumping syndrome. Medical therapy is effective in patients with incapacitating symptoms who fail dietary modifications. Remedial surgery is only considered in patients refractory to medical management.

MEDICATION

First Line

- Octreotide (Sandostatin) 100–500 μg SC b.i.d. Can be very expensive (2)[B]. Patients may have increased steatorrhea during octreotide treatment, and pancreatic enzyme supplement is effective in relieving this symptom.
- Late dumping symptoms can be ameliorated by the α-glucosidase inhibitor acarbose (100–200 mg, PO t.i.d.), which lowers blood glucose by delaying GI absorption of carbohydrates.
- Pectin/guar gum are effective by delaying glucose absorption and prolonging small bowel transit time.

Second Line

Anticholinergics: Results generally are disappointing.

ADDITIONAL TREATMENT

General Measures

Most patients can be managed conservatively with dietary modification and medical treatment. Only a small percentage of patients ultimately require surgical intervention.

Additional Therapies

Continuous trophic enteral feeding via a jejunostomy has been reported to be an effective approach in patients refractory to all other treatment measures.

SURGERY/OTHER PROCEDURES

- Remedial surgery only if dietary and medical management unsuccessful and symptoms debilitating; the results are variable and unpredictable. A proper selection of the surgical intervention is very important. Most patients with dumping syndrome as a result of gastric bypass will find that the effects ameliorate with time (>2 years).
- Options of surgery include Roux-en-Y conversion (from Billroth I and II), pyloric reconstruction (for patients who have severe dumping following pyloroplasty), reversed jejunal segment (for patients who failed Roux-en-Y reconstruction), and conversion of Billroth II to Billroth I anastomosis.
- Patients with refractory dumping symptoms after loop gastrojejunostomy may benefit from simple takedown of the anastomosis; conversion to Roux-en-Y gastrojejunostomy is a reasonable option for patients with disabling dumping after distal gastrectomy. Other procedures have been attempted with limited success.
- The syndrome of hyperinsulinemic hypoglycemia with nesidioblastosis (a hyperplasia of islet cells) after Roux-en-Y gastric bypass (>1–2 year post-op) can usually be managed with low-carbohydrate diet and alpha-glucosidase inhibitors. Subtotal or total pancreatectomy (as has been suggested in the literature) is usually unnecessary.

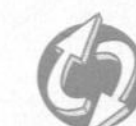

ONGOING CARE

FOLLOW-UP RECOMMENDATIONS

Lying supine for 30 minutes after eating or when symptoms occur may reduce the chance of syncope.

Patient Monitoring

Follow to be sure of adequate nutrition.

DIET

- Low-carbohydrate, high-protein diet
- Add dietary fiber.
- Milk or milk products should be avoided.
- Frequent small meals with minimal liquid
- Avoid hyperosmolar liquids.

PATIENT EDUCATION

National Digestive Diseases Information Clearinghouse, Box NDDIC, Bethesda, MD 20892, (301) 468-6344, digestive.niddk.nih.gov

PROGNOSIS

Favorable

COMPLICATIONS

- Hypoglycemia
- Malnutrition and weight loss
- Electrolyte disturbances, including hypokalemia

REFERENCES

1. Gertler R, Rosenberg R, Feith M, Schuster T, Friess H et al. Pouch vs. no pouch following total gastrectomy: meta-analysis and systematic review. *Am J Gastroenterol*. 2009;104:2838–51.
2. Ukleja A. Dumping syndrome: pathophysiology and treatment. *Nutr Clin Pract*. 2005;20:517–25.
3. Gonzalez-Sánchez JA, Corujo-Vázquez O, Sahai-Hernández M. Bariatric surgery patients: reasons to visit emergency department after surgery. *Bol Asoc Med P R*. 2007;99:279–83.
4. Penning C, Vecht J, Masclee AA. Efficacy of depot long-acting release octreotide therapy in severe dumping syndrome. *Aliment Pharmacol Ther*. 2005;22:963–9.
5. Bouras EP, Scolapio JS. Gastric motility disorders: management that optimizes nutritional status. *J Clin Gastroenterol*. 2004;38:549–57.

D

ADDITIONAL READING

Tack J, Arts J, Caenepeel P et al. Pathophysiology, diagnosis and management of postoperative dumping syndrome. *Nat Rev Gastroenterol Hepatol*. 2009;6: 583–90.

See Also (Topic, Algorithm, Electronic Media Element)

Diarrhea, Chronic; Hypoglycemia, Non-diabetic; Peptic Ulcer Disease

Algorithm: Diarrhea, Chronic

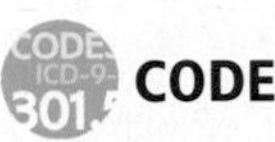

CODES

ICD9

564.2 Postgastric surgery syndromes

CLINICAL PEARLS

- Vagotomy affects gastric emptying through increased gastric tone and decreased receptive relaxation.
- Dumping syndrome is the most common cause for ER presentation after bariatric surgery (3)[B].
- An increase in heart rate of 10 BPM is noted after glucose challenge (50 g oral glucose) in patients with dumping syndrome.
- Depot octreotide has shown some promise as an alternative to standard SC octreotide (4)[B].
- Some side effects of octreotide are gallstones, steatorrhea, and diarrhea (5)[B].

DUPUYTREN CONTRACTURE

Jeffrey F. Minteer, MD

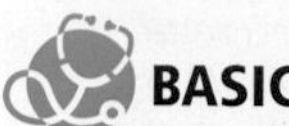

BASICS

DESCRIPTION

- Palmar fibromatosis; due to progressive fibrous proliferation and tightening of the fascia inside the palms, resulting in flexion deformities and loss of function
- Not the same as "trigger finger," which is caused by thickening of the distal flexor tendon
- Similar change may rarely occur in plantar fascia; it usually appears simultaneously.
- System(s) affected: Musculoskeletal

EPIDEMIOLOGY

Prevalence

- Unknown in United States
- Norway: 9% males and 3% females

RISK FACTORS

- Smoking (mean 16 pack-years, odds ratio 2.8)
- Increasing age
- Male/Caucasian
- Workers exposed to vibration
- Diabetes mellitus (1/3 affected, increases with time, usually mild; middle and ring finger involved)
- Epilepsy
- Chronic illness (e.g., pulmonary tuberculosis, liver disease, HIV)
- Hypercholesterolemia
- Alcohol consumption

Genetics

- Autosomal-dominant with variable penetrance
- 68% of male relatives of affected patients develop disease at some time

GENERAL PREVENTION

Avoid risk factors, especially with a strong family history.

ETIOLOGY

Unknown; possibly a T-cell–mediated autoimmune disorder

COMMONLY ASSOCIATED CONDITIONS

- Alcoholism
- Epilepsy
- Diabetes mellitus
- Chronic lung disease
- Occupational hand trauma (vibration white finger)
- Shoulder–hand syndrome
- Status postmyocardial infarction
- Hypercholesterolemia
- Carpal tunnel syndrome

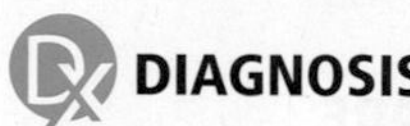

DIAGNOSIS

HISTORY

- Caucasian male aged 50–60 years
- Family history
- Mild pain early
- Unilateral or bilateral (50%)
- Right hand more frequent
- Ring finger more frequent
- Ulnar digits more affected than radial digits

PHYSICAL EXAM

- Painless plaques or nodules in palmar fascia
- Extends into a cordlike band in the palmar fascia
- Skin adheres to fascia and becomes puckered.
- Nodules can be palpated under the skin.
- Digital fascia becomes involved as disease progresses
- Reduced flexibility of metacarpophalangeal (MCP) and proximal interphalangeal (PIP) joints
- No sign of inflammation
- Web space contractures
- Dupuytren diathesis can involve plantar (Ledderhose—10%) and penile (Peyronie—2%) fascia
- Knuckle pads over PIP
- Disease stages:
  - Early: Skin pits (can also be seen in nevoid basal cell cancer and palmar keratosis)
  - Intermediate: Nodules and cords
  - Late: Contractures

DIAGNOSTIC TESTS & INTERPRETATION

Diagnostic Procedures/Surgery

Magnetic resonance imaging (MRI) can assess cellularity of lesions that correlate with higher recurrence after surgery.

Pathological Findings

- Myofibroblasts
- 1st stage (proliferative): Increased myofibroblasts
- 2nd stage (residual): Dense fibroblast network
- 3rd stage (involutional): Myofibroblasts disappear

DIFFERENTIAL DIAGNOSIS

- Early for callosity
- Tendon abnormalities
- Camptodactyly: Early teens; tight fascial bands on ulnar side of small finger
- Diabetic cheiroarthropathy: All 4 fingers
- Volkmann ischemic contracture

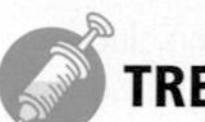

TREATMENT

MEDICATION

First Line

- Steroid injection for an acute tender nodule, painful knuckle pad
- Clostridial collagenase injections (FDA approved 2010):
  - Degrades collagen to allow manual rupture of diseased cord
  - Best for isolated cord of MCP joint
  - Recurrence rate at 8 years 67% in MCP joints but less severe than initial contracture (1)[B]

Second Line

- Topical high-potency steroids: Case report of improvement with clobetasol 0.1% b.i.d. and at bedtime for 2–4 weeks
- Surgery for contracture >30%

DDITIONAL TREATMENT

eneral Measures

Physiotherapy alone is ineffective:
- Intermittent splinting unlikely to be effective
- Continuous splinting may be helpful in pre- and postoperative

Isolated involvement of palmar fascia can be followed.

MCP joint involvement can be followed if flexion contracture is <30°.

sues for Referral

Any involvement of PIP joints

MCP joints contracted >30°

Positive Hueston test

dditional Therapies

Continuous elongation technique is useful to prepare a severely contracted PIP joint for surgery. The digit can frequently be completely extended; however, it will relapse if surgery is not performed.

Prophylactic external beam radiation: 87% either no progression or improvement at 12 months; concern about local effects in a benign disease

Intraoperative 5-fluorouracil ineffective

Percutaneous and needle fasciotomy:
- Best for MCP joint
- Recurrence common
- Not indicated in severe or recurrent disease

URGERY/OTHER PROCEDURES

Selective fascial ray release/partial fasciectomy (2)[B]

Indications:
- Any involvement of the PIP joints
- MCP joints are contracted at least 30°.
- Positive Hueston tabletop test: When the palm is placed on a flat surface, the digits cannot be simultaneously placed fully on the same surface as the palm because of flexion contractures.

- May require skin grafts for wound closure with severe cutaneous shrinkage. Reports of clinical regression with continuous passive skeletal traction in extension and under a skin graft.
- 80% have full range of movement if operated on early.
- Amputation of little finger if severe and deforming
- MCP joints respond better than PIP joints, especially if contracted >45°.

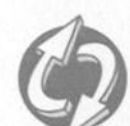

ONGOING CARE

FOLLOW-UP RECOMMENDATIONS

Patient Monitoring

Regular follow-up by physician every 6 months–1 year

PATIENT EDUCATION

- Avoid risk factors, especially with a strong family history.
- Mild disease: Passively stretch digits twice a day and avoid recurrent gripping of tools.

PROGNOSIS

- Unpredictable, but usually slowly progressive
- 10% may regress spontaneously.
- Patients likely to have aggressive disease if 1 or more of the following are present: Age <40 years at onset, knuckle pads, positive family history, bilateral disease involving radial side of hand
- Recurrence rate after surgery is high; more with aggressive features
- Prognosis better for MCP joint vs PIP joint after surgery and collagenase injection

COMPLICATIONS

- Postsurgery development of reflex sympathetic dystrophy
- Postoperative recurrence or extension in 46–80%
- Postoperative hand edema and skin necrosis
- Digital infarction

REFERENCES

1. Watt AJ, Curtin CM, Hentz VR et al. Collagenase injection as nonsurgical treatment of dupuytren's disease: 8-year follow-up. *J Hand Surg Am.* 2010;35:534–9, 539.e1.
2. van Rijssen AL, Werker PM et al. [Treatment of Dupuytren's contracture; an overview of options] *Ned Tijdschr Geneeskd*. 2009;153:A129.
3. Rayan GM. Clinical presentation and types of Dupuytren's disease. *Hand Clin*. 1999;15:87–96, vii.

ADDITIONAL READING

- Hunt TR. What is the appropriate treatment for Dupuytren contracture? *Cleve Clin J Med*. 2003;70: 96–7.
- Hurst LC, Badalamente MA, Hentz VR, Hotchkiss RN, Kaplan FT, Meals RA, Smith TM, Rodzvilla J, CORD I Study Group et al. Injectable collagenase clostridium histolyticum for Dupuytren's contracture. *N Engl J Med*. 2009;361:968–79.
- Rayan GM. Duypuytren Disease: Anatomy, Pathology, Presentation, and Treatment. *J of Bone & Joint Surgery*. 2007;89(1):189–98.

CODES

ICD9

- 728.6 Contracture of palmar fascia
- 728.71 Plantar fascial fibromatosis

CLINICAL PEARLS

- 90% of cases are progressive.
- Refer those with any involvement of the PIP joints or MCP involvement >30°.
- Neither surgical nor enzymatic fasciotomy offers a cure with high rate of recurrence (3)

DYSFUNCTIONAL UTERINE BLEEDING

Meaghan Delaney, MD
Debra Papa, MD
Ginger Allister, MD

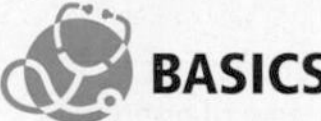

BASICS

DESCRIPTION

- Dysfunctional uterine bleeding (DUB) is irregular (usually heavy, prolonged, or frequent) bleeding that occurs in the absence of anatomic pathology
- Associated with anovulatory menstrual cycles
- Typically a diagnosis of exclusion: Need to exclude anatomic pathology and medical illnesses
- Systems affected: Endocrine/Metabolic, Reproductive

EPIDEMIOLOGY

- Predominant age: 12–50 years
- Predominant gender: Female only
- Adolescents and perimenopausal women are most often affected

Incidence

Accounts for 5–10% of outpatient gynecologic visits

Prevalence

Abnormal uterine bleeding occurs in:

- ~ 1 in 3 women of reproductive age
- ~1 in 10 post-menopausal women

RISK FACTORS

Risk factors for endometrial cancer (which can cause DUB):

- Age >40
- Obesity
- Diabetes Mellitus
- Nulliparity
- Early menarche or late menopause (>55 years)
- Hypertension
- Chronic anovulation or infertility
- Unopposed estrogen therapy
- History of breast cancer or endometrial hyperplasia
- Tamoxifen use
- Family history: Gynecologic, breast, or colon cancer

Genetics

Unclear

PATHOPHYSIOLOGY

- Disruption of normal hormonal sequence of ovulatory menstrual cycle
- Anovulation accounts for 90% of DUB:
  - Loss of cyclic endometrial stimulation
  - Elevated estrogen levels stimulate endometrial growth
  - Endometrium does not shed and eventually outgrows blood supply
  - Tissue breaks down and sloughs from uterus

ETIOLOGY

The diagnosis of DUB is made when pathologic causes of abnormal bleeding have been ruled out:

- Pregnancy
  - Ectopic pregnancy, threatened or incomplete abortion, or hydatidiform mole
- Reproductive pathology & structural disorders
  - Uterus: leiomyomas, endometritis, hyperplasia, polyps, trauma
  - Adnexa: Salpingitis, functional ovarian cysts
  - Cervix: Cervicitis, polyps, sexually transmitted diseases (STDs), trauma
  - Vagina: Trauma, foreign body
  - Vulva: Lichen sclerosis, STDs
- Malignancy of the vagina, cervix, uterus, & ovaries
- Systemic diseases
  - Inflammatory bowel disease
  - Hematologic disorders (Von Willebrand's disease, thrombocytopenia, etc.)
  - Advanced or fulminant liver disease
  - Chronic renal disease
- Diseases causing anovulation
  - Hyper/hypothyroidism
  - Adrenal disorders
  - Pituitary disease (prolactinoma)
  - Polycystic ovarian syndrome (PCOS)
  - Eating disorders
- Medications (iatrogenic causes)
  - Anticoagulants
  - Steroids
  - Tamoxifen
  - Hormonal medications: Intrauterine devices (IUDs)
  - Selective-serotonin reuptake inhibitors
  - Antipsychotic medications
- Other causes of abnormal uterine bleeding:
  - Excessive weight gain
  - Increased exercise
  - Stress

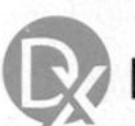

DIAGNOSIS

A thorough medical, surgical, social, and family history should be obtained.

HISTORY

- History of bleeding:
  - Onset, severity (quantified in pad/tampon use, presence & size of clots)
  - Association with other factors (i.e. coitus, contraception, weight loss/gain)
- Menstrual history:
  - Unpredictable or episodic, heavy or light bleeding
  - Menstrual symptoms do not typically precede bleeding
- Review of symptoms (exclude symptoms of pregnancy, symptoms of bleeding disorders, bleeding from other orifices, stress, exercise, recent weight change, visual changes, headaches, galactorrhea)
- Medication history (evaluate for use of aspirin, anticoagulants, hormones, herbal supplements)

ALERT

Postmenopausal bleeding is any bleeding that occurs >1 year after the last menstrual period; cancer must always be ruled out

PHYSICAL EXAM

Discover anatomic or organic causes of DUB:

- Assess hemodynamic stability
- Evaluate for:
  - Obesity (BMI)
  - Pallor
  - Visual field defects (pituitary lesion)
  - Hirsutism or acne (hyperandrogenism)
  - Goiter
  - Galactorrhea (hyperprolactinemia)
  - Purpura, ecchymosis (bleeding disorders)
- Pelvic exam:
  - Evaluate for uterine irregularities
  - Check for foreign bodies
  - Rule out rectal or urinary tract bleeding
  - Include Pap smear and tests for STDs

Pediatric Considerations

Premenarchal children with vaginal bleeding should be evaluated for foreign bodies, physical/sexual abuse, possible infections, and signs of precocious puberty.

DIAGNOSTIC TESTS & INTERPRETATION

Lab

Not always necessary

Initial lab tests

- Urine human chorionic gonadotropin (rule out pregnancy and/or hydatiform mole)
- Complete blood count (CBC)
- Thyroid-stimulating hormone (TSH) (1)[B]
- Prolactin level
- Consider other tests based on differential diagnosis:
  - Follicle-stimulating hormone (FSH) to evaluate for hypo/hypergonadotropism
  - Coagulation studies & factors (2)[A]
  - Liver function tests
  - 17-hydroxyprogestrone
  - Androgenic hormones
  - *Neisseria gonorrhea*, *Chlamydia trachomatis* tests

Imaging

Initial approach

- Transvaginal ultrasound (TVUS):
  - Indications: postmenopausal patients, suspicion of pregnancy or anatomic abnormalities, PCOS
  - High sensitivity for endometrial carcinoma in postmenopausal women (3)[A]. If ≤4 mm, endometrial cancer unlikely
  - If endometrial thickness >5 mm, proceed to endometrial biopsy (EMB)
- Saline infusion sonohistogram: Often superior to TVUS in screening for anatomic abnormalities (4). Can perform if TVUS suspicious for lesion.

Diagnostic Procedures/Surgery

- Pap smear to exclude cervical cancer
- Endometrial biopsy (EMB) should be performed in women:
  - Women >35 years of age with DUB to rule out cancer or premalignancy
  - Women with endometrial thickness >5 mm
  - Women aged 18–35 with DUB and risk factors for endometrial cancer (see Risk Factors)
  - Perform ≥day 18 of cycle if known; secretory endometrium confirms ovulation occurred
  - Does not diagnose leiomyosarcoma or fibroids because lesions are deep to endometrial lining
- Dilation & curettage:
  - Performed if bleeding is heavy, uncontrolled, and/or failed emergent medical management
  - If unable to perform EMB in office
- Hysteroscopy if lesion suspected (diagnostic and therapeutic)

Pathological Findings

Pap smear could reveal carcinoma or inflammation indicative of cervicitis. Most EMBs show proliferative or dyssynchronous endometrium (suggesting anovulation)

DIFFERENTIAL DIAGNOSIS

See Etiology

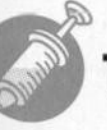

TREATMENT

Attempt to diagnose other causes of bleeding prior to instituting therapy.

MEDICATION

First Line

- Acute, emergent, nonovulatory bleeding: (5)
  - Conjugated equine estrogen (Premarin): 25 mg IV Q4H (maximum of 6 doses) or 2.5 mg PO Q6H should control bleeding in 12–24 hours (6)[A]
  - Then change to OCP or progestin for cycle regulation
- Acute, nonemergent, nonovulatory:
  - Combination OCP with ≥30 mcg estrogen given as a taper. An example of a tapered dose: 4 pills/d until bleeding stopped for 24 hours; 3 pills/d for 3 days; 2 pills/d for 3 days.
  - Then begin once-a-day regimen (7)[B]
- Nonacute, nonovulatory:
  - OCPs: 20–35 mcg estrogen plus progesterone (mono- or triphasic)
  - Progestins: Medroxyprogesterone acetate (Provera) 10 mg/d for 5–10 days each month. Daily progesterone for 21 days per cycle results in significantly less blood loss (8)[A].
  - Levonorgestrel intrauterine devices (Mirena) are most effective (9)[A].
- Do not use estrogen if contraindications are present
- Precautions:
  - Exclude endometrial hyperplasia & carcinoma before administering estrogen
  - Consider deep vein thrombosis prophylaxis when treating with high-dose estrogens
  - Failed medical treatment requires further workup
  - Smokers >35 years of age should be counselled on the risk of thromboembolic disease when using OCPs

Second Line

- Gonadotropin-releasing hormone (GnRH) agonists create a hypogonadotropic state, usually used as a bridge to definitive therapy.
- Danazol (Danocrine 200–400 mg/d) is more effective than nonsteroidal anti-inflammatory drugs (NSAIDs), but is limited by androgenic side effects & cost (10)[A]. It has been essentially replaced by GnRH agonists.
- Antifibrinolytics like tranexamic acid (Lysteda, 650mg, 2 tabs three times daily (max of 5 days during menstruation) (11)[A].

ADDITIONAL TREATMENT

General Measures

NSAIDs (naproxen sodium 500 mg BID, mefenamic acid 500 mg TID, ibuprofen 600–1,200 mg/d):

- Decreases amount of blood loss compared to placebo (10)[A]
- Diminishes pain

Issues for Referral

- If an obvious cause for vaginal bleeding is not found in a pediatric patient, refer to a pediatric endocrinologist.
- Patients with persistent bleeding despite medical treatment require reevaluation and referral to a gynecologist.

Additional Therapies

- Antiemetics if treating with high-dose estrogen
- Iron supplementation if anemia (usually iron deficiency) is identified

SURGERY/OTHER PROCEDURES

- Hysterectomy if endometrial cancer, if medical therapy fails, or uterine pathology
- Endometrial ablation is less expensive than hysterectomy with high satisfaction; medical treatment does not have to fail first (12)[A]

IN-PATIENT CONSIDERATIONS

Initial Stabilization

With acute bleeding, replace volume with crystalloid and blood as necessary

Admission Criteria

Significant hemorrhage causing acute anemia with signs of hemodynamic instability

Nursing

Pad counts and clot size can be helpful to determine and monitor amount of bleeding

Discharge Criteria

- Hemodynamic stability
- Control of vaginal bleeding

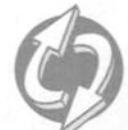

ONGOING CARE

FOLLOW-UP RECOMMENDATIONS

Routine follow-up with a primary care or ob/gyn provider

Patient Monitoring

Women treated with estrogen or OCPs should keep a menstrual diary to document bleeding patterns & their relation to therapy.

DIET

No restrictions

PATIENT EDUCATION

- Explain possible/likely etiologies
- Answer all questions, especially those related to cancer and fertility
- http://www.acog.org

PROGNOSIS

- Varies with pathophysiologic process
- Most anovulatory cycles can be treated with medical therapy and do not require surgical intervention.

COMPLICATIONS

- Iron-deficiency anemia
- Uterine cancer in cases of prolonged unopposed estrogen stimulation

REFERENCES

1. Albers J, et al. Abnormal uterine bleeding. *Am Fam Physician*. 2004;69:8.
2. Kouides PA, et al. Hemostasis and menstruation: Appropriate investigation for underlying disorders of hemostasis in women with extensive menstrual bleeding. *Fertil Steril*. 2005;84(5):1345–51.
3. Dijkhuizen FP, et al. The accuracy of transvaginal ultrasonography in the diagnosis of endometrial abnormalities. *Obstet Gynecol*. 1996;87(3):345–9.
4. Maness DL, Reddy A, Harraway-Smith CL, Mitchell G, Givens V et al. How best to manage dysfunctional uterine bleeding. *J Fam Pract*. 2010;59:449–58.
5. Casablanca Y. Management of dysfunctional uterine bleeding. *Obstet Gynecol Clin North Am*. 2008;35:219–34.
6. DeVore GR, et al. Use of intravenous Premarin in the treatment of dysfunctional uterine bleeding: A double-blind randomized control study. *Obstet Gynecol*. 1982;59(3):285–91.
7. Rimsza ME. Dysfunctional uterine bleeding. *Pediatr Rev*. 2002;23(7):227–33.
8. Lethaby A, et al. Cyclical progestogens for heavy menstrual bleeding. *Cochrane Database Syst Rev*. 2004.
9. Lethaby A, et al. Progesterone or progesterone-releasing intrauterine systems for heavy menstrual bleeding. *Cochrane Database Syst Rev*. 2005.
10. Lethaby A, et al. Nonsteroidal anti-inflammatory drugs for heavy menstrual bleeding. *Cochrane Database Syst Rev*. 2004.
11. Lethaby A, et al. Antifibrinolytics for heavy menstrual bleeding. *Cochrane Database Syst Rev*. 2004.
12. Lethaby A, et al. Endometrial resection and ablation versus hysterectomy for heavy menstrual bleeding. *Cochrane Database Syst Rev*. 2004.

D

ADDITIONAL READING

- Chen EC, Danis PG, Tweed E et al. Clinical inquiries. Menstrual disturbances in perimenopausal women: what's best? *J Fam Pract*. 2009;58:E3.
- LaCour DE, Long DN, Perlman SE et al. Dysfunctional uterine bleeding in adolescent females associated with endocrine causes and medical conditions. *J Pediatr Adolesc Gynecol*. 2010;23:62–70.

See Also (Topic, Algorithm, Electronic Media Element)

Menorrhagia; Dysmenorrhea
Algorithm: Menorrhagia

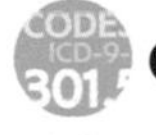

CODES

ICD9

626.8 Other disorders of menstruation and other abnormal bleeding from female genital tract

CLINICAL PEARLS

- Uterine bleeding in premenarchal & postmenopausal women is always abnormal and should prompt immediate evaluation.
- Dysfunctional uterine bleeding is irregular bleeding occurring in the absence of pathology, making it a diagnosis of exclusion.
- Anovulation accounts for 90% of DUB.
- An endometrial biopsy should be performed in all women >35 years of age with DUB to rule out cancer or premalignancy, and considered in women aged 18–35 with DUB and risk factors for endometrial cancer.

DYSHIDROSIS

Katherine A. Mansalis, MD
Rebecca A. Frye, DO

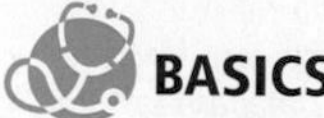

BASICS

DESCRIPTION

- A skin rash (dermatitis) of which there are several different classes within the family "dyshidrosis" and strict definitions are disputed.
- Dyshidrotic eczema:
  - Common, chronic, or recurrent, nonerythematous, vesicular eruption primarily of the palms, soles, and interdigital areas
  - Associated with burning, itching, and pain
- Pompholyx (from Greek, "bubble"):
  - Rare condition characterized by abrupt onset of large bullae, primarily on hands
  - Sometimes used interchangeably with dyshidrosis, although many believe them to be discrete entities
- Lamellar dyshidrosis:
  - Fine, spreading exfoliation of the superficial epidermis in the same distribution as described above
- System(s) affected: Dermatologic; Exocrine; Immunologic
- Synonym(s): Pompholyx; Cheiropompholyx; Keratolysis exfoliativa; Dyshidrotic eczema; Vesicular palmoplantar eczema; Desquamation of interdigital spaces; Palmar pompholyx reaction

EPIDEMIOLOGY

Incidence

- Incidence is 0.5%.
- Mean age of onset is <40 years.
- Male = Female
- Comprises 5–20% of hand eczema cases

Prevalence

20 cases per 100,000

RISK FACTORS

- Many risk factors are disputed in the literature, with none being consistently associated
- Atopy
- Other dermatologic conditions:
  - Atopic dermatitis (early in life)
  - Contact dermatitis (later in life)
  - Dermatophytosis
- Sensitivity to
  - Foods
  - Drugs: neomycin, quinolones, acetaminophen, and oral contraceptives
  - Nickel (seen in patients treated with disulfiram, which causes a high serum level of nickel)
  - Smoking in males

Genetics

- Atopy: 50% of patients with dyshidrotic eczema have atopic dermatitis.
- Rare autosomal dominant form of pompholyx found in Chinese population maps to chromosome 18q22.1–18q22.3

GENERAL PREVENTION

- Control emotional stress.
- Avoid excessive sweating.
- Avoid exposure to irritants.
- Avoid diet high in metal salts (chromium, cobalt, nickel).

PATHOPHYSIOLOGY

- Exact mechanism unknown; thought to be multifactorial
- On dermatopathology, vesicles are found in spongiotic dermatitis
- Thick stratum corneum of palmar and plantar skin keeps the vesicles intact

ETIOLOGY

- Exact cause not known
- Aggravating factors (debated):
  - Hyperhidrosis (in 40% of patients with the condition)
  - Climate: Hot or cold weather; humidity
  - Nickel sensitivity
  - Irritating compounds and solutions
  - Stress
  - Dermatophyte infection
  - Prolonged wear of occlusive gloves
  - Intravenous immunoglobulin therapy
  - Smoking

COMMONLY ASSOCIATED CONDITIONS

- Atopic dermatitis
- Allergic contact dermatitis
- Parkinson disease

DIAGNOSIS

HISTORY

- Episodes of pruritic rash alternating with periods that are symptom free
- Recent emotional stress
- Familial or personal history of atopy
- Exposure to allergens or irritants (1):
  - Occupational, dietary, or household
  - Cosmetic and personal hygiene products
- Costume jewelry use
- IV immunoglobulin therapy
- HIV
- Smoking

PHYSICAL EXAM

- Symmetric distribution on the palms and soles; also may affect the dorsal aspects of hands and feet
- Early findings:
  - 1–2 mm, clear nonerythematous deep-seated vesicles
- Late findings:
  - Unroofed vesicles with inflamed bases
  - Desquamation
  - Peeling, rings of scale, or lichenification common

DIAGNOSTIC TESTS & INTERPRETATION

Lab

Initial lab tests

Skin culture in suspected secondary infection (most commonly *staph aureus*) (2)

Follow-Up & Special Considerations

Consider antibiotics based on culture results and severity of symptoms.

Diagnostic Procedures/Surgery

- Diagnosis is based on clinical exam
- Patch test (to elicit allergic cause)
- KOH wet mount (if concerned about dermatophyte infection)

Pathological Findings

- Fine 1–2-mm spongiotic vesicles intraepidermally with little to no inflammatory changes
- No eccrine glandular involvement

DIFFERENTIAL DIAGNOSIS

- Vesicular tinea pedis/manus
- Vesicular id reaction
- Contact dermatitis (allergic or irritant)
- Chronic vesicular hand dermatitis
- Drug reaction
- Dermatophytid
- Bullous disorders: Dyshidrosiform bullous pemphigoid, pemphigous, bullous impetigo, epidermolysis bullosa
- Pustular psoriasis
- Acrodermatitis continua
- Erythema multiforme
- Herpes infection
- Pityriasis rubra pilaris
- Vesicular mycosis fungoides

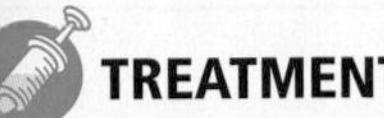

TREATMENT

entification and avoidance of aggravating factors.

MEDICATION

irst Line

- Mild cases: Topical steroids (high potency) (2)[B]
- Moderate to severe cases:
  - Ultrahigh-potency topical steroids with occlusion over treated area (3)[B]
  - Psoralens plus UV therapy (PUVA), either oral *or* immersion in psoralens (4)[B]:
    - Oral 8-methoxypsoralen (8-MOP) dose: 0.6 mg/kg taken 1 h prior to UVA irradiation
    - Immersion in 8-MOP: Solution of 5 mg/L of water × 15 minutes immediately preceding UVA irradiation
- Recurrent cases (3)[C]:
  - Systemic steroids at onset of itching prodrome
  - Single morning dose of 60 mg × 3–4 days every 2–4 months

econd Line

- Topical calcineurin inhibitors (mitigate the long term risks of topical steroid use):
  - Topical tacrolimus (5)[A]
  - Topical pimecrolimus (5)[A]
- Oral cyclosporine (2)[A]
- Injections of botulinum toxin type A (BTXA) (5)[A]
  - Newer topical forms of BTXA currently being developed and show promise
- Systemic alitretinoin (5)[A]
- Topical bexarotene (a retinoid X receptor agonist approved for use in cutaneous T-cell lymphoma) (5)[B]
- Methotrexate (5)[C]

ADDITIONAL TREATMENT

- Radiation therapy (6)[C]
- UV-free phototherapy (5)[C]

General Measures

- Avoid possible causative factors: Stress, chemical irritants, nickel, occlusive gloves, smoking, sweating
- Moisturizers/emollients for symptomatic relief
- Foot care:
  - Wear shoes with leather rather than rubber soles (e.g., sneakers).
  - Wear socks made of cotton instead of synthetic materials.
  - Remove shoes and socks whenever possible to allow sweat evaporation and to apply lubricants.

ssues for Referral

- Allergist (if allergen testing required)
- Psychologist (if stress modification needed)

COMPLEMENTARY AND ALTERNATIVE MEDICINE

- Topical treatments to minimize pruritus (not curative) (2)[C]: Burrow solution (aluminum acetate) or vinegar compress
- Exposure to sunlight as maintenance therapy (7)[C]
- Dandelion juice (avoid in atopic patients) (5)[C]

ONGOING CARE

FOLLOW-UP RECOMMENDATIONS

Patient Monitoring

- Dyshidrotic Eczema Area and Severity Index (DASI)
- Parameters used in the DASI score:
  - Number of vesicles per square centimeter
  - Erythema
  - Desquamation
  - Severity of itching
  - Surface area affected
- Grading: Mild (0–15), moderate (16–30), severe (31–60)
- Monitor BP and glucose in patients receiving systemic corticosteroids.
- Monitor for adverse effects of medications.

DIET

- Consider diet low in metal salts if there is history of nickel sensitivity (2)[A].
- Updated recommendations for low-cobalt diet are available (8).

PATIENT EDUCATION

- Instructions on self-care, complications, and avoidance of triggers/aggravating factors
- Suggested web site for patients: www.nlm.nih.gov

PROGNOSIS

- Condition is benign.
- Usually heals without scarring
- Lesions often resolve spontaneously but resolve more quickly with appropriate treatment (9).
- Recurrence is common.

COMPLICATIONS

- Secondary bacterial infections (*staphylococcus aureus* most common)
- Dystrophic nail changes
- Fissures
- Skin tightening/discomfort
- Psychological distress

REFERENCES

1. Guillet MH, Wierzbicka E, Guillet S, et al. A 3-year causative study of pompholyx in 120 patients. *Arch Dermatol.* 2007;143:1504–8.
2. Lofgren SM. Dyshidrosis: Epidemiology, clinical characteristics, and therapy. *Dermatitis.* 2006;17:165–81.
3. Chen J, et al. The gene for a rare autosomal dominant form of pompholyx maps to chromosome 18q22.1–18q22.3. *J Invest Dermatol.* 2006;126: 300–4.
4. Tzaneva S, Kittler H, Thallinger C, et al. Oral vs. bath PUVA using 8-methoxypsoralen for chronic palmoplantar eczema. *Photodermatol Photoimmunol Photomed.* 2009;25:101–5.
5. Wollina U. Pompholyx: what's new? *Expert Opinion in Investigational Drugs.* 2008;17:897–904.
6. Sumila M, Notter M, Itin P, et al. Long-term Results of Radiotherapy in Patients with Chronic Palmo-plantar Eczema or Psoriasis. *Strahlentherapie und Onkologie.* 2008;184:218–223.
7. Leti M. Exposure to sunlight as adjuvant therapy for dyshidrotic eczema. *Med Hypotheses.* 2009.
8. Stuckert J, Nedorost S. Low-cobalt diet for dyshidrotic eczema patients. *Contact Dermatitis.* 2008;59:361–5.
9. Rashid RD, Salah W, Keuer EJ. Vexing Vesicles. *Journal of Medicine.* 2007;120:589–590.

ADDITIONAL READING

- Thiers BH. What's new in dermatologic therapy. *Dermatol Ther.* 2008 Mar–Apr;21:142–9.
- Veien NK. Acute and Recurrent Vesicular Hand Dermatitis. *Dermatologic Clinics.* 2009;27:337–353.

See Also (Topic, Algorithm, Electronic Media Element)

Algorithm: Rash, Focal

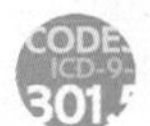

CODES

ICD9

705.81 Dyshidrosis

CLINICAL PEARLS

- Dyshidrosis is a transient, recurrent vesicular eruption most commonly of the palms, soles, and interdigital areas.
- The etiology and pathophysiology are unknown but are most likely related to a combination of genetic and environmental factors.
- The best prevention is limiting exposure to irritating agents.
- Treatments are based on severity of disease and include topical steroids, UV therapy, botulinum toxin A, and various immunosuppressants.
- The condition is benign and usually heals spontaneously and without scarring. Medical treatment decreases healing time and risk for progression to secondary bacterial infection.

DYSMENORRHEA

Janice E. Daugherty, MD

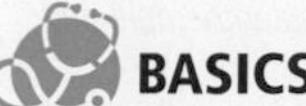

BASICS

DESCRIPTION

- Pelvic pain occurring at or around the time of menses; a leading cause of absenteeism for women <30 years
- Primary dysmenorrhea: Without pathologic physical findings
- Secondary dysmenorrhea: Often more severe than primary, having a secondary pathologic (structural) cause
- Classified by severity:
  - Mild: Pelvic discomfort, cramping, or heaviness on 1st day of bleeding with no associated symptoms
  - Moderate: Discomfort occurring on 1st 2–3 days of menses and accompanied by mild malaise, diarrhea, and headache
  - Severe: Intense, cramp-like pain lasting 2–7 days, often with nausea, diarrhea, back pain, thigh pain, and headache
- System(s) affected: Reproductive
- Synonym(s): Menstrual cramps

EPIDEMIOLOGY

- Predominant age:
  - Primary: Teens to early 20s
  - Secondary: 20s–30s
- Predominant sex: Female only

Prevalence

- >50% of adult females have menstrual pain.
- 10% are incapacitated for 1–3 days each cycle.

RISK FACTORS

- Primary:
  - Nulliparity
  - Obesity
  - Cigarette smoking
  - Positive family history
- Secondary:
  - Pelvic infection
  - Sexual transmitted diseases (STDs)
  - Endometriosis

Genetics

Not well studied

GENERAL PREVENTION

- Primary: Choose a diet low in animal fats, dairy products, and eggs. Increase vegetables, raw seeds, and nuts to increase production of beneficial prostaglandins. Consider supplementation with zinc 30 mg, taken 1–3 times daily for 1–4 days prior to the expected onset of menses [C].
- Secondary: Reduce risk of STDs

PATHOPHYSIOLOGY

See Etiology.

ETIOLOGY

- Primary: Elevated production (2–7 times normal) of prostaglandins and other mediators in the uterus that produce uterine ischemia through:
  - Platelet aggregation
  - Vasoconstriction
  - Uterine contractions generating pressures higher than the systemic blood pressure (BP)
- Secondary:
  - Congenital abnormalities of uterine or vaginal anatomy
  - Cervical stenosis
  - Pelvic infection
  - Adenomyosis
  - Endometriosis
  - Pelvic tumors, especially leiomyomata (fibroids)
  - Uterine polyps
  - Copper-containing intrauterine device (IUD)

Pediatric Considerations

Onset with first menses raises probability of genital tract anatomic abnormality, such as transverse vaginal septum, minimally perforate hymen, and uterine anomalies.

COMMONLY ASSOCIATED CONDITIONS

- Obesity
- Hyperestrogenic states
- Longer menstrual cycle length

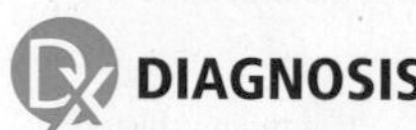

DIAGNOSIS

- Primary: History is characteristic.
- Based on characteristic history of cramping pain felt in suprapubic or low back
- Patients may have associated diarrhea, headache, or pain radiating into inner thighs.

HISTORY

- Onset of symptoms
- Recurrence at or just before the onset of the menstrual flow:
  - Pelvic pain occurring between menstrual periods is not likely to be dysmenorrhea.
- Relief associated with:
  - Continued bleeding for the usual duration
  - Use of analgesics, especially nonsteroidal anti-inflammatory drugs (NSAIDs)
  - Orgasm
  - Local heat application
- Response to dietary supplements or NSAIDs helps confirm diagnosis.

PHYSICAL EXAM

- Primary: Physical exam is typically normal.
- Secondary: Exam may show evidence of uterine enlargement, tenderness, irregularity, or fixation.

DIAGNOSTIC TESTS & INTERPRETATION

Lab

- Pregnancy test to rule out ectopic pregnancy
- Cervical cultures to rule out infection
- Drugs that may alter lab results:
  - Antibiotics

Follow-Up & Special Considerations

Counsel regarding appropriate preventive measures for sexually transmitted infection and pregnancy.

Imaging

Initial approach

- Primary: Consider pelvic ultrasound to rule out secondary abnormalities if history is not characteristic.
- Secondary: Ultrasound or laparoscopy to define anatomy

Diagnostic Procedures/Surgery

Laparoscopy is rarely needed.

Pathological Findings

- Primary:
  - None
- Secondary:
  - Uterine enlargement
  - Leiomyomata
  - Ligamentous thickening
  - Fixation of pelvic structures
  - Endometritis
  - Salpingitis
  - Adenomyosis

DIFFERENTIAL DIAGNOSIS

- Primary:
  - History is characteristic
- Secondary:
  - Pelvic or genital infection
  - Complication of pregnancy
  - Missed or incomplete abortion
  - Ectopic pregnancy
  - Uterine or ovarian neoplasm
  - Endometriosis
  - Urinary tract infection (UTI)
  - Complication of intrauterine device

Pregnancy Considerations

Consider ectopic pregnancy in differential diagnosis of pelvic pain with vaginal bleeding.

TREATMENT

- Reassure patient that treatment success is very likely with adherence to recommendations.
- Relief may require the use of several treatment modalities at the same time.

MEDICATION

First Line

- NSAIDs (1): All NSAIDs studied have been found equally effective in the relief of dysmenorrhea. As NSAIDs work by inhibiting prostaglandin synthesis, taking them at the very onset of menses (or whenever the cramping starts) provides the most relief.
  - Ibuprofen 400–600 mg q6h
  - Naproxen sodium 550 mg q12h
- Combination oral contraceptives in monthly and especially in 3–5-month cycles may improve or eliminate dysmenorrhea, although they may be associated with increased breakthrough menstrual spotting (2)[B]:
  - Combination oral contraceptives containing 20 mcg or less of ethinyl estradiol have not been found effective in reducing menstrual pain.
- Potential contraindications to NSAIDs and combination oral contraceptive (OC) methods:
  - Platelet disorders
  - Gastric ulceration or gastritis
  - Thromboembolic disorders
  - Vascular disease
  - Other contraindications to oral contraceptives
- Precautions:
  - Gastrointestinal irritation
  - Lactation
  - Coagulation disorders
  - Impaired renal function
  - Congestive heart failure (CHF)
  - Liver dysfunction
- Significant possible interactions:
  - Coumadin-type anticoagulants
  - Aspirin with other NSAIDs
  - Methotrexate
  - Furosemide
  - Lithium

econd Line

- Mefenamic acid 500 mg at once, then 250 mg q6h may be tried if other NSAIDs are ineffective, as it blocks production of prostaglandins as well as already-formed prostaglandins (1)[A].
- Progestin-containing IUD (Mirena) in suitable candidates

DDITIONAL TREATMENT

eneral Measures

- General physical conditioning, exercise to raise endorphins
- Transcutaneous electrical nerve stimulation (3)[B]
- Secondary dysmenorrhea: Treatment of infections; suppression of endometrium if endometriosis is suspected

OMPLEMENTARY AND ALTERNATIVE MEDICINE

- Because of low methodologic quality and small sample size in 30 different randomized controlled trials (RCTs), there is no convincing evidence for acupuncture in the treatment of primary dysmenorrhea (4)[A].
- However, in individual studies, acupuncture has been shown to be effective for both treatment and prevention. The lack of significant adverse effects of acupuncture, compared with common effects of NSAIDs including GI bleeding, blood pressure elevation, and potential renal impairment make acupuncture a choice to be considered early in the treatment plan (5,6,7).
  - Acupressure at Sanyinjiao (SP6) is quickly effective and can be taught to women for self-treatment.
  - Acupuncture at SP6, with or without 60 HZ, 2–3 mV electrical stimulation, was significantly more effective than ibuprofen.
  - Acupuncture at Hegu (LI4) and Taichong (LR3) was effective in decreasing menstrual pain.
  - Ear acupressure at appropriate points with vaccaria seeds was significantly more effective than indomethacin.
  - For endometriosis, acupuncture was more effective than oral danazol to decrease pain, irregular menstruation, back pain, and perineal swelling.
- Aromatherapy with lavender, clary sage, rose oils, and abdominal massage decreases intensity of pain (8)[B].
- Osteopathic manipulation, including pressure over the sacrum, can decrease the intensity of menstrual pain (9)[B].

URGERY/OTHER PROCEDURES

- Adenomyosis may require hysterectomy.
- Uterine artery embolization may be an alternative to hysterectomy for patients with leiomyomata (fibroid tumors) (10).

N-PATIENT CONSIDERATIONS

oth primary and secondary dysmenorrhea are usually ıanaged in the outpatient setting.

nitial Stabilization

- Primary: Outpatient care
- Secondary: Usually outpatient care

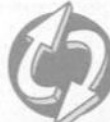

ONGOING CARE

FOLLOW-UP RECOMMENDATIONS

Normal

DIET

- Several dietary supplements have been found to be effective at treating dysmenorrhea:
  - Vitamin B1 100 mg daily
  - Fish oil 3,000–5,000 mg + vitamin E 1.5 mg daily (vitamin E is preservative)
  - Diosmin 450 mg + hesperidin 50 mg t.i.d. with onset of menses
  - Magnesium 400 mg daily (11)
- Several dietary supplements are possibly effective, although have not studied in large trials:
  - Vitamin E 200 mg b.i.d. beginning 2 days before expected menses and continuing for the 1st 3 days of bleeding (12)[B]
  - Vitamin B1 (thiamine) 100 mg/d p.o. for at least 90 days (13)[C]
  - Fish oil capsule 1,000 mg daily for 2 months (14)[B]
  - Zinc 30 mg 1–3 times daily for 1–4 days preceding expected menses has been found effective for prevention (15)[C].
- Low-fat vegetarian diet significantly decreases pain.

PATIENT EDUCATION

Reassure patient that primary dysmenorrhea is treatable with use of dietary supplements and/or NSAIDs prior to menses and/or oral contraceptives, and that it will usually abate with age and parity.

PROGNOSIS

- Primary: Improves with age and parity
- Secondary: Likely to require therapy based on underlying cause

COMPLICATIONS

- Primary: Anxiety and/or depression
- Secondary: Infertility from underlying pathology

REFERENCES

1. Marjoribanks J, Proctor ML, Farquhar CI. Nonsteroidal anti-inflammatory drugs for primary dysmenorrhoea (Cochrane Review). *The Cochrane Library*. 2003;4.
2. Proctor ML, Roberts H, Farquhar CM. Combined oral contraceptive pill (OCP) as treatment for primary dysmenorrhoea (Cochrane Review). In: *The Cochrane Library*. 2003;4.
3. Milsom I, Hedner N, Mannheimer C. A comparative study of the effect of high-intensity transcutaneous nerve stimulation and oral naproxen on intrauterine pressure and menstrual pain in patients with primary dysmenorrhea. *Am J Obstet Gynecol*. 1994;170:123–9.
4. Yang H, Liu CZ, Chen X, et al. Systematic review of clinical trials of acupuncture-related therapies for primary dysmenorrhea. *Acta Obstet Gynecol Scand*. 2008:1–9.
5. Proctor ML, Smith CA, Farquhar CM, et al. Transcutaneous electrical nerve stimulation and acupuncture for primary dysmenorrhoea (Cochrane Review). 2003;4.
6. Zhao L, Li P. A survey of acupuncture treatment for primary dysmenorrhea. *J Tradit Chin Med*. 2009;29:71–6.
7. Ziaei S, Zakeri M, Kazemnejad A, et al. A randomised controlled trial of vitamin E in the treatment of primary dysmenorrhoea. *BJOG*. 2005;112:466–9.
8. Han SH, Hur MH, Buckle J, Choi J, Lee MS, et al. Effect of aromatherapy on symptoms of dysmenorrhea in college students: A randomized placebo-controlled clinical trial. *J Altern Complement Med*. 2006;12:535–41.
9. Chadwick K and Morgan A. The efficacy of osteopathic treatment for primary dysmenorrhea in young women. *The AAO Journal: A Publication of the American Academy of Osteopathy*. 1996 Fall;6(3):15–17, 29–31.
10. Bradley LD et al. Uterine fibroid embolization: a viable alternative to hysterectomy. *Am J Obstet Gynecol*. 2009;201:127–35.
11. Guerrera MP, Volpe SL, Mao JJ et al. Therapeutic uses of magnesium. *Am Fam Physician*. 2009;80:157–62.
12. Transdermal nitroglycerine in the management of pain associated with primary dysmenorrhoea: a multinational pilot study. The Transdermal Nitroglycerine/Dysmenorrhoea Study Group. *J Int Med Res*. 1997;25:41–4.
13. French L. Dysmenorrhea. *Am Fam Physician*. 2005;71:285–91.
14. Harel Z, Biro FM, Kottenhahn RK et al. Supplementation with omega-3 polyunsaturated fatty acids in the management of dysmenorrhea in adolescents. *Am J Ob Gyn*. 1996;174:1335–8.
15. Eby G. Zinc treatment prevents dysmenorrhea. *Med Hypoth*. 2007;69.2:297–301.

ADDITIONAL READING

- Cho SH, Hwang EW et al. Acupuncture for primary dysmenorrhoea: a systematic review. *BJOG*. 2010;117:509–21.
- Giudice LC et al. Clinical practice. Endometriosis. *N Engl J Med*. 2010;362:2389–98.
- Sanfilippo J, Erb T. Evaluation and management of dysmenorrhea in adolescents. *Clin Obstet Gynecol*. 2008;51:257–67.
- Stones RW, Mountfield J. Interventions for treating chronic pelvic pain in women (Cochrane Review). *The Cochrane Library*. 2003;4.
- White AR. A review of controlled trials of acupuncture for women's reproductive health care. *J Fam Plan Reprod Health Care*. 2003;29:233–6.

See Also (Topic, Algorithm, Electronic Media Element)

- Endometriosis
- Algorithm: Pelvic Girdle Pain

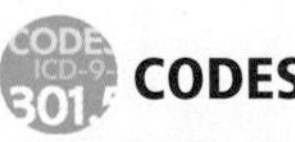

CODES

ICD9

- 625.3 Dysmenorrhea

CLINICAL PEARLS

- Dysmenorrhea is a leading cause of absenteeism for women <30 years old.
- Lifestyle and dietary supplement therapies are preferable for long-term treatment, as they have equal or greater efficacy and pose fewer health risks than NSAIDs or hormonal contraceptives.
- All NSAIDs studied have been found equally effective in the relief of dysmenorrhea.

D

DYSPAREUNIA

Scott T. Henderson, MD

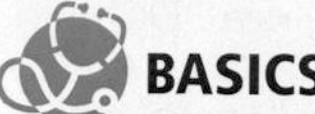

BASICS

DESCRIPTION

- Recurrent and persistent genital pain associated with sexual activity that is not exclusively due to lack of lubrication or vaginismus
- May be the result of organic, emotional, or psychogenic causes:
  - Primary: Present throughout one's sexual history
  - Secondary: Arising from some specific event or condition (e.g., menopause, drugs)
  - Superficial: Pain at or near the introitus or vaginal barrel associated with penetration
  - Deep: Pain after penetration located at the cervix or lower abdominal area
  - Complete: Present under all circumstances
  - Situational: Occurring selectively with specific situations
- System(s) affected: Reproductive

EPIDEMIOLOGY

- Predominant age: All ages
- Predominant sex: Female > Male.

Incidence

More than 50% of all sexually active women will report dyspareunia at some time.

Geriatric Considerations

Incidence increases dramatically in postmenopausal women primarily because of vaginal atrophy.

Prevalence

- Most sexually active women will experience dyspareunia at some time in their lives.
  - ~15% (4–40%) of adult women will have dyspareunia on a few occasions during a year.
  - ~1–2% of women will have painful intercourse on a more-than-occasional basis.
- Male prevalence is ~1%.

RISK FACTORS

- Fatigue
- Stress
- Diabetes
- Estrogen deficiency:
  - Menopause
  - Lactation
- Vaginal surgery
- Alcohol/marijuana consumption
- Medication side effects (antihistamines, tamoxifen, bromocriptine, low-estrogen oral contraceptives, depo-medroxyprogesterone, desipramine)

Pregnancy Considerations

Pregnancy is a potent influence on sexuality; dyspareunia is common.

PATHOPHYSIOLOGY

See Etiology section.

ETIOLOGY

- Disorders of vaginal outlet:
  - Adhesions
  - Clitoral irritation
  - Decreased lubrication
  - Episiotomy scars
  - Fissures
  - Hymenal ring abnormalities
  - Infections
  - Lichen planus
  - Lichen sclerosus
  - Postmenopausal atrophy
  - Trauma
  - Vulvar papillomatosis
  - Vulvar vestibulitis/vulvodynia
- Disorders of vagina:
  - Abnormality of vault owing to surgery or radiation
  - Congenital malformations
  - Decreased lubrication
  - Infections
  - Inflammatory or allergic response to foreign substance
  - Masses or tumors
  - Pelvic relaxation resulting in rectocele, uterine prolapse, or cystocele
- Disorders of pelvic structures:
  - Endometriosis
  - Levator ani myalgia
  - Malignant or benign tumors of the uterus
  - Ovarian pathology
  - Pelvic adhesions
  - Pelvic inflammatory disease
  - Pelvic venous congestion
  - Prior pelvic fracture
- Disorders of the GI tract:
  - Constipation
  - Crohn disease
  - Diverticular disease
  - Fistulas
  - Hemorrhoids
  - Inflammatory bowel disease
- Disorders of the urinary tract:
  - Interstitial cystitis
  - Ureteral or vesical lesions
- Male:
  - Cancer of penis
  - Genital muscle spasm
  - Infection or irritation of penile skin
  - Infection of seminal vesicles
  - Lichen sclerosus
  - Musculoskeletal disorders of pelvis and lower back
  - Penile anatomy disorders
  - Phimosis
  - Prostate infections and enlargement
  - Testicular disease
  - Torsion of spermatic cord
  - Urethritis
- Psychological disorders:
  - Anxiety
  - Conversion reactions
  - Depression
  - Fear
  - Hostility toward partner
  - Phobic reactions
  - Psychological trauma

COMMONLY ASSOCIATED CONDITIONS

Vaginismus

Pregnancy Considerations

- Episiotomies do not have a protective effect (1)[A].
- Mediolateral episiotomy increases the risk of dyspareunia compared with no episiotomy (2)[B].

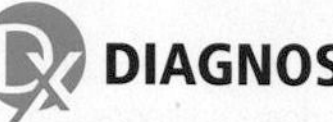

DIAGNOSIS

HISTORY

- Include menstrual, obstetric, reproductive, and sexual histories.
- Identify pain characteristics.
  - Onset and duration
  - Location
  - Intensity/quality: Varying degrees of pelvic/genital pressure, aching, tearing, and/or burning
  - Pattern (precipitating or aggravating factors): When pain occurs (at entry, during or after intercourse)
  - Relief measures (avoid intercourse, change positions, have intercourse only at certain times of the month)
- Question for history of domestic violence or history of rape.

PHYSICAL EXAM

- A complete exam, including a focused pelvic exam, to identify pathology and provide patient education
- Since exam often reproduces the pain, it must include inspection and palpation of vaginal area and urethral structures as well as palpation of the uterus

DIAGNOSTIC TESTS & INTERPRETATION

Lab

Initial lab tests

Based on history and exam findings:

- Wet mount
- Gonorrhea culture
- Chlamydia culture
- Herpes culture
- Urine analysis
- Urine culture
- Pap smear

naging

itial approach

mited and based on history and exam findings

ollow-Up & Special Considerations

Voiding cystourethrogram if urinary tract involvement

GI contrast studies if GI symptoms

Ultrasound and CT scan are of limited value; perform if clinically indicated.

iagnostic Procedures/Surgery

ased on history and exam findings:

Colposcopy and biopsy if vaginal/vulvar lesions

Laparoscopy if complex deep-penetration pain

Cystoscopy if urinary tract involvement

Endoscopy if GI involvement

athological Findings

epend on etiology

IFFERENTIAL DIAGNOSIS

aginismus

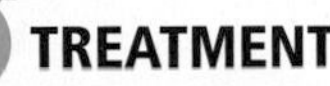

TREATMENT

Primary dyspareunia might be related to vaginismus, low libido, and/or arousal disorders.

Endocrine factors, such as primary amenorrhea, might reduce the biologic basis of sexual response.

If pain prevents penetration, severe vaginismus may be present.

IEDICATION

irst Line

epends on the etiology:

Antibiotics, antifungals, or antivirals as indicated for infection

Estrogen for vaginal and vulvar atrophy

Analgesics and topical anesthetics for pain

Lubricants for dryness

Vulvar vestibulitis/vulvodynia may respond to tricyclic antidepressants or gabapentin.

DDITIONAL TREATMENT

ieneral Measures

Educate the patient and partner as to the nature of the problem. Reassure them that the problem can be solved.

If an organic cause is identified during the initial evaluation, initiate specific treatment.

Once organic causes are ruled out, treatment is a multidimensional and multidisciplinary approach (2)[C].

- Individual behavioral therapy: Indicated to help the patient deal with intrapersonal issues and assess the role of the partner
- Couple behavioral therapy:
  - Indicated to help resolve interpersonal problems
  - May involve short-term structured intervention or sexual counseling
  - Designed to systemically desensitize uncomfortable sexual responses and intercourse through a series of interventions over a period of weeks
  - Interventions range from muscle relaxation and mutual body massage to sexual fantasies and erotic massage.

Issues for Referral

Referral for long-term therapy may be necessary.

Additional Therapies

No benefit of therapeutic ultrasound (3)[A]

COMPLEMENTARY AND ALTERNATIVE MEDICINE

- Sitz baths may relieve painful inflammation.
- Perineal massage

SURGERY/OTHER PROCEDURES

- Laparoscopic excision of endometriotic lesions has shown benefit (4)[B].
- Surgical vestibulectomy can be considered if conservative measures fail with vulvar vestibulitis.

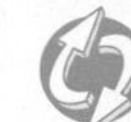

ONGOING CARE

FOLLOW-UP RECOMMENDATIONS

Patient Monitoring

- Outpatient follow-up depends on therapy.
- Every 6–12 months once resolved

DIET

A high-fiber diet may help if constipation is a contributing cause.

PATIENT EDUCATION

- Boston Women's Health Book Collective. *Our Bodies, Ourselves: A New Edition for a New Era*. New York: Simon & Schuster, 2005
- Kegel exercise information
- Provide couples with information about sexual arousal techniques.

PROGNOSIS

Most patients will respond to treatment.

REFERENCES

1. Carroli G, Mignini L. Episiotomy for vaginal birth. *Cochrane Database Syst Rev*. 2009;CD000081.
2. Crowley T, Richardson D, Goldmeier D, et al. Recommendations for the management of vaginismus: BASHH Special Interest Group for Sexual Dysfunction. *Int J STD AIDS*. 2006;17:14–8.
3. Sartore A, De Seta F, Maso G, et al. The effects of mediolateral episiotomy on pelvic floor function after vaginal delivery. *Obstet Gynecol*. 2004;103:669–73.
4. Ferrero S, Abbamonte LH, Giordano M, et al. Deep dyspareunia and sex life after laparoscopic excision of endometriosis. *Hum Reprod*. 2006.

ADDITIONAL READING

- Boardman LA, Stockdale CK et al. Sexual pain. *Clin Obstet Gynecol*. 2009;52:682–90.
- Frank JE, Mistretta P, Will J. Diagnosis and treatment of female sexual dysfunction. *Am Fam Physician*. 2008;77:635–42.
- Steege JF, Zolnoun DA. Evaluation and treatment of dyspareunia. *Obstet Gynecol*. 2009;113:1124–36.

See Also (Topic, Algorithm, Electronic Media Element)

Balanitis; Endometriosis; Pelvic Inflammatory Disease (PID); Sexual Dysfunction in Women; Vaginismus; Vulvovaginitis, Prepubescent; Vulvovaginitis, Estrogen Deficient

Algorithms: Dyspareunia; Discharge, Vaginal

CODES

ICD9

- 302.76 Dyspareunia, psychogenic
- 625.0 Dyspareunia

CLINICAL PEARLS

- Determine whether patient feels pain before, during, or after intercourse to help identify cause.
  - Pain before intercourse suggests a phobic attitude toward penetration and/or the presence of vestibulitis.
  - Pain during intercourse combined with the location of the pain is most predictive of the causes of pain.
  - Introital pain after intercourse suggests vestibulitis in women of childbearing age, hypertonic pelvic floor, or vulvovaginal dystrophia.
- Primary dyspareunia might be related to vaginismus, low libido, and/or arousal disorders.
- Episiotomy does not offer any benefit in the prevention of dyspareunia; a mediolateral episiotomy in fact may cause more future discomfort.

DYSPEPSIA, FUNCTIONAL

Anthony M. Zizza, III, MD
Randall S. Pellish, MD

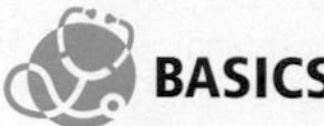

BASICS

DESCRIPTION

- A condition characterized by the presence of chronic intermittent symptoms for at least 3 months of epigastric pain, postprandial fullness, early satiety, or epigastric burning without mucosal lesions or other structural abnormalities of the gastrointestinal (GI) tract (1)[A]
- Analogous to irritable bowel syndrome (IBS) of the upper GI tract
- System(s) affected: GI
- Synonym(s): Nonulcer dyspepsia; Moynihan dyspepsia; Pseudo-ulcer dyspepsia; Phantom ulcer; Nonorganic dyspepsia; Nervous dyspepsia

EPIDEMIOLOGY

Incidence

- Common in US
- Affecting 15–20% of patients referred to gastroenterologists
- Accounts for 60% of patients with dyspepsia

Prevalence

- Predominant age: Adults, but can be seen in children
- Predominant gender: Females > Males

RISK FACTORS

- Other functional disorders
- Anxiety
- Depression

Genetics

Possible link to G-protein β-3 subunit 825 CC genotype and serotonin transport genes

GENERAL PREVENTION

Avoid foods and habits known to exacerbate symptoms (see Diet).

PATHOPHYSIOLOGY

- Not well understood
- Motility disorder
- Possible visceral hypersensitivity to gastric distention
- Psychosocial factors

ETIOLOGY

- Often unknown; may be of several different etiologies
- Evanescent ulcers (20–30% go on to develop ulcers)
- Gastric motility disorder (delayed or accelerated)
- Visceral hypersensitivity
- Impaired gastric accommodation
- Controversial relationship to *Helicobacter pylori*
- Adverse drug effects
- Carbohydrate malabsorption
- Food intolerance
- Psychosocial factors

COMMONLY ASSOCIATED CONDITIONS

Other functional bowel disorders

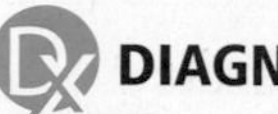

DIAGNOSIS

HISTORY

- Belching
- Aerophagia, gaseousness, abdominal distension
- Borborygmus
- Epigastric pain, gnawing or burning; eating may improve or worsen symptoms
- Substernal pain, gnawing, or burning
- Early satiety
- Anorexia, nausea, or vomiting
- Change in bowel habits
- Abdominal tenderness
- Stress, anxiety, depression
- Exclude (2)[A]:
  - IBS
  - Peptic ulcer disease
  - Malignancy
  - Biliary tract disease
  - Gastroesophageal reflux disease (GERD)
  - Medication-induced dyspepsia

Pediatric Considerations

Look for family system dysfunction.

Pregnancy Considerations

Pregnancy may exacerbate condition.

Geriatric Considerations

Cancer risk is higher.

PHYSICAL EXAM

To rule out other disorders

DIAGNOSTIC TESTS & INTERPRETATION

Lab

Initial lab tests

- Complete blood count
- Chemistry panel
- *H. pylori* serology
- Stool for occult blood

Imaging

Initial approach

- Extensive workup only in patients with *alarm symptoms*:
  - Onset of symptoms >45–55 years (3)[B]
  - Unexplained weight loss
  - Change in stool caliber
  - With symptoms and signs suggesting more serious disease
  - Who need added reassurance
  - Who are younger and do not respond rapidly to empiric treatment
- Usual:
  - Endoscopy (2)[A],(4)
  - Upper GI series
  - Test and treat for *H. pylori* (in areas of high prevalence) (3)[B]
- Sometimes:
  - Barium enema
  - Gallbladder studies for right upper quadrant pain (e.g., ultrasound or gallbladder cholecystokinin function testing)
  - Nuclear medicine gastric emptying study (in selected cases)

Diagnostic Procedures/Surgery

- Esophageal manometry (rarely needed)
- 24-hour intraesophageal pH monitoring (rarely needed unless dysphagia is present)

Pathological Findings

None (by definition)

DIFFERENTIAL DIAGNOSIS

- GERD
- Cholecystitis
- Peptic ulcer disease
- Gastric cancer
- Esophageal spasm
- Malabsorption syndromes
- Pancreatic disease
- IBS
- Aerophagia
- Ischemic heart disease
- Diabetes mellitus
- Thyroid disease
- Connective tissue disorders
- Conversion disorder

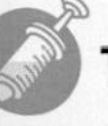

TREATMENT

MEDICATION

First Line

- 40% of patients improve with placebo.
- Acid reduction drugs:
  - H_2 antagonists: Ranitidine, others
  - Over-the-counter omeprazole (5)[A]
  - *H. pylori* eradication (often does not relieve symptoms, but may be worth trying)
- Contraindications:
  - Avoid magnesium-containing antacids in patients with significant renal dysfunction.
- Precautions:
  - Monitor H_2 antagonist dosages in patients with renal disease.
  - Calcium-containing antacids may precipitate the formation of kidney stones.
- Significant possible interactions:
  - H_2 blockers interact with drugs metabolized by and affecting the liver.

Second Line

- Gastric motility drugs (2)[A]:
  - Metoclopramide (Reglan); although neurologic side effects are significant
  - Erythromycin
- Amitriptyline: 50 mg q.h.s.
- Selective serotonin reuptake inhibitors
- Itopride (6)[C]:
  - Placebo-controlled trial showed symptom improvement.
  - Mechanism unknown, requires more studies

ADDITIONAL TREATMENT

General Measures

- Appropriate health care: Outpatient
- Supportive measures:
  - Reassurance
  - Do not investigate excessively.
  - Dietary changes (see Diet)
  - Elevate head of bed (where applicable).
  - Maintain ideal body weight.
  - Explore psychological issues.

Additional Therapies

- Stress reduction:
  - Relaxation techniques
  - Physical exercise
  - Reflux precautions where applicable
- Psychological therapy (1)[B]:
  - Cognitive behavioral therapy
  - Hypnotherapy
  - Psychotherapy

COMPLEMENTARY AND ALTERNATIVE MEDICINE

In combination with caraway oil, peppermint oil can be used for reducing symptoms of nonulcer dyspepsia (7).

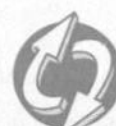

ONGOING CARE

FOLLOW-UP RECOMMENDATIONS

Patient Monitoring

- Usual duration of medication is 4 weeks, then 2 weeks intermittently for exacerbations. If chronic medication use is needed, endoscopy evaluation is indicated.
- Continue observation to provide support and reassurance.
- Minimize diagnostic studies unless disabling symptoms persist or new problems arise.

DIET

- Symptoms are frequently triggered or exacerbated by fatty foods (8).
- Eat frequent small meals.
- AVOID:
  - Foods known to exacerbate symptoms
  - Regular and decaffeinated coffee
  - Tea, cocoa, and chocolate
  - Heavy alcohol use
  - Cigarette smoking
  - Aspirin-containing compounds and NSAIDs

PATIENT EDUCATION

Prevention: Continue healthy habits listed under Treatment and Diet (i.e., avoid activities known to exacerbate problems, maintain healthy lifestyle, continue stress-reduction techniques).

PROGNOSIS

Long-term or chronic symptoms with symptom-free periods

COMPLICATIONS

Iatrogenic, from evaluation to rule out serious pathology

REFERENCES

1. Drossman DA. The functional gastrointestinal disorders and the Rome III process. *Gastroenterol*. 2006;130:1377–90.
2. Dickerson LM, et al. Evaluation and management of nonulcer dyspepsia. *Am Fam Phys*. 2004;70: 107–14.
3. Kandulski A, Venerito M, Malfertheiner P, et al. Therapeutic strategies for the treatment of dyspepsia. *Expert Opin Pharmacother*. 2010;11: 2517–25.
4. Delaney B, Ford AC, Forman D, et al. Initial management strategies for dyspepsia. *Cochrane Database Syst Rev*. 2005:CD001961.
5. Moayyedi P, et al. The efficacy of proton pump inhibitors in nonulcer dyspepsia: A systematic review and economic analysis. *Gastroenterol*. 2004;127:1329–37.
6. Holtmann G, Talley NJ, Liebregts T, et al. A placebo-controlled trial of itopride in functional dyspepsia. *N Engl J Med*. 2006;354:832–40.
7. Madisch A, Holtmann G, Mayr G, et al. Treatment of functional dyspepsia with a herbal preparation. A double-blind, randomized, placebo-controlled, multicenter trial. *Digestion*. 2004;69:45–52.
8. Pilichiewicz AN, Feltrin KL, Horowitz M, et al. Functional Dyspepsia Is Associated With a Greater Symptomatic Response to Fat But Not Carbohydrate, Increased Fasting and Postprandial CCK, and Diminished PYY. *Am J Gastroenterol*. 2008.

D

ADDITIONAL READING

- Choung RS, et al. Novel mechanisms in functional dyspepsia. *W J Gastroenterol*. 2006;12:673–7.
- Faure C, Patey N, Gauthier C, Brooks EM, Mawe GM et al. Serotonin signaling is altered in irritable bowel syndrome with diarrhea but not in functional dyspepsia in pediatric age patients. *Gastroenterology*. 2010;139:249–58.
- Keohane J, et al. Functional dyspepsia and nonerosive reflux disease: Clinical interactions and their implications. *Med Gen Med*. 2007;9:31.

See Also (Topic, Algorithm, Electronic Media Element)

Dyspepsia, Endoscopic-Negative Reflux Disease, Gastritis; Irritable Bowel Syndrome

Algorithms: Dyspepsia; Epigastric Pain; Esophageal Regurgitation

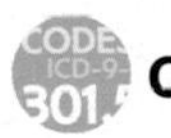

CODES

ICD9

536.8 Dyspepsia and other specified disorders of function of stomach

CLINICAL PEARLS

- When no organic cause for dyspepsia is found, it is considered functional or idiopathic.
- Extensive diagnostic testing is not recommended unless the patient presents with alarm symptoms (vomiting, early satiety, weight loss, or anemia).
- Consider empiric treatment with acid suppressants or *H. pylori* eradication if serology is positive.

DYSPHAGIA

Archit Sharma, MD
Mark D. Goodman, MD

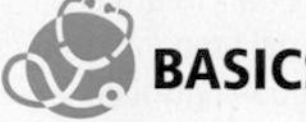

BASICS

Difficulty or discomfort during the progression of the alimentary bolus from the mouth to the stomach

DESCRIPTION

- Difficulty in swallowing
- A disorder of transferring the food bolus from oropharynx to esophagus or of impairment in transport of the bolus through the esophagus
- Commonly divided based on:
  - Anatomical standpoint: Oropharyngeal or esophageal dysfunction
  - Pathophysiological standpoint: Structure-related or functional causes
- Associated symptoms: *Odynophagia* (painful swallowing); *globus* (lump in throat)
- System(s) affected: GI; Nervous

EPIDEMIOLOGY

Incidence

- In US: 7% incidence lifetime
- Predominant age: All ages; increasing prevalence with age
- Predominant sex: Male = Female

Prevalence

- 16–22% of people >50 years
- Up to 60% of nursing home residents
- 25% of hospitalized patients

RISK FACTORS

- Children: Hereditary and/or congenital malformations
- Adults: Age >50 years (esophageal cancer, neurologic disorders) more likely
- Smoking, excess alcohol, obesity
- Long history of GERD
- Medications (quinine, potassium chloride, vitamin C, tetracycline, Bactrim, clindamycin, NSAIDs, and others)
- Neurologic events or diseases (CVA, neuromuscular disease, multiple sclerosis, Parkinson disease, ALS)
- Trauma or irradiation of head, neck, and chest

GENERAL PREVENTION

- Observe feeding of infants closely for aspiration; have suction available.
- Correct poorly fitting dentures in older patients.
- Avoid drinking alcohol with meals.
- Give consideration to positioning during meals, texture of foods being eaten
- In infants/children: Discuss underlying problem and therapy for recurrent aspiration.
- Positioning and texture in older adults, dentures, supervision to prevent aspiration

ETIOLOGY

- In children:
  - Malformations: Congenital (esophageal atresia, cleft palate, choanal atresia, TE fistula, Zenkers diverticulum)
  - Malformations: Acquired (corrosive or herpetic esophagitis)
  - Neuromuscular/neurologic: Delayed maturation, CP, MD, poliomyelitis
  - GERD
- In adults (esophageal):
  - Structural: Tumors (cancer or benign), strictures (peptic, chemical, trauma, radiation), lower esophageal rings (Schatzki rings), esophageal webs
  - Mechanical: Extrinsic compression from enlarged left atrium, aortic aneurysm, aberrant subclavian artery (termed dysphagia lusoria), substernal thyroid, cervical bony exostosis, and thoracic tumor
  - GERD
  - Neuromuscular: Achalasia, diffuse esophageal spasm, hypertensive lower esophageal sphincter, scleroderma, myasthenia gravis, nutcracker esophagus
- In adults (oropharyngeal):
  - CVA
  - Parkinson disease
  - Neurodegenerative diseases (MS, ALS, Huntington disease, pseudobulbar palsy)
  - Zenker diverticulum
  - Myasthenia gravis
  - Polio
  - Cricopharyngeal achalasia
  - Cervical spondylosis (cervical osteophytes)
  - Obstructive lesions (tumors, inflammatory masses)

Pediatric Considerations

- Congenital malformations
- Tonsillar hypertrophy, large tongue, dental problems (overbite)

Geriatric Considerations

- Poor dentition and/or dentures
- Drug-induced

COMMONLY ASSOCIATED CONDITIONS

- Esophageal carcinoma
- GERD-induced peptic stricture
- Dysphagia lusoria (extrinsic compression)
- Achalasia
- Symptomatic diffuse esophageal spasm
- Eosinophilic esophagitis
- Foreign body
- Scleroderma
- Myasthenia gravis
- CVA

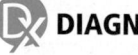

DIAGNOSIS

ALERT

Rapidly progressive symptoms and/or profound weight loss is indicative of malignant process; requires immediate attention; should undergo endoscopy with/without biopsy

HISTORY

- Is the dysphagia for solids, liquids, or both? Which started first?
- Does the food bolus feel stuck? If so, where?
- Are there symptoms of oropharyngeal dysfunction?
- Do you have any cough while swallowing? Is it early in swallowing or late?
- Is the dysphagia intermittent or progressive?
- Have you ever brought food back up or vomited?
- Is there a history of chronic heartburn?
- How much alcohol and/or tobacco do you use?
- Are there associated symptoms such as weight loss or chest pain?
- What medications are being taken?
- Is there odynophagia? (Does it hurt with just solid food or both solid and liquids?)
- Is there any halitosis?

PHYSICAL EXAM

- Oropharyngeal type:
  - Choking with swallowing
  - Coughing with swallowing
  - Nasal speech (wet voice)
  - Hoarseness of voice
  - Sialorrhea (drooling of saliva)
  - Frequent respiratory infections
  - Weight loss
  - Dysarthria
  - Nasopharyngeal regurgitation with swallowing
- Esophageal type:
  - Pressure sensation in midchest (localizing below suprasternal notch highly likely to be esophageal disorder); narrow the diagnostic possibilities by asking if this occurs for solids, liquids, or both.
  - Oral or pharyngeal regurgitation
  - Recurrent aspiration pneumonia
  - Weight loss
  - Symptoms of GERD
- Neck and oral cavity for lesions, masses, goiter
- Signs of collagen: Vascular disease
- Detailed neurologic exam, especially cranial nerves with gag reflex testing (CVA, neuromuscular disease, Parkinson)
- In infants:
  - Breastfeeding problems
  - Vomiting or spitting up during feeds
  - Lengthy feeding or eating times (>30 min)

DIAGNOSTIC TESTS & INTERPRETATION

- In infants/children:
  - Observe sucking/eating.
  - Attempt to pass NG tube to assess esophageal patency.
  - Radiography of neck and chest
  - Contrast radiography
  - Endoscopy
- In adults:
  - Barium swallow
  - Fiberoptic endoscopic examination of swallowing (FEES)
  - Gastroesophageal endoscopy
  - Barium cine/video esophagogram
  - Ambulatory 24-h pH testing
  - Esophageal manometry
  - Videofluoroscopic swallowing study (VFSS)

Lab

As suggested by specific differential diagnosis under consideration

Initial lab tests

- CBC to screen for infectious and inflammatory condition
- Serum protein and albumin levels for nutritional assessment
- Thyroid function studies to detect dysphagia associated with hypothyroidism or hyperthyroidism

Imaging

- Barium swallow
- CT scan of chest
- MRI of brain and cervical spine
- Videofluoroscopic swallowing study (VFSS)

Diagnostic Procedures/Surgery
- Endoscopy with biopsy
- Esophageal manometry
- Esophageal pH monitoring

Pathological Findings
- Squamous cell or adenocarcinoma
- Barrett metaplasia
- Fibrous tissue of a ring, web, or stricture
- Loss of smooth muscle (scleroderma)
- Acute or chronic inflammatory changes
- Oropharyngeal lesions

DIFFERENTIAL DIAGNOSIS
- Cardiac chest pain
- Globus hystericus
- Functional heartburn or dysphagia

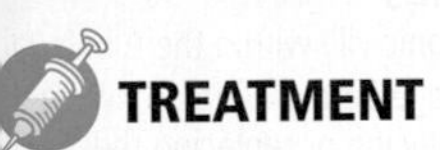

TREATMENT

MEDICATION
- For spasms: Calcium channel blockers: Nifedipine (Procardia) 10–30 mg t.i.d.; amitriptyline 0.5–2 mg/kg q.h.s.; dicyclomine (Bentyl) 20 mg q.i.d.
- For esophagitis:
  - Antacids: Tums, Mylanta, Maalox
  - H_2 blockers: Cimetidine (Tagamet), ranitidine (Zantac), nizatidine (Axid), famotidine (Pepcid)
  - Proton pump inhibitors: Omeprazole (Prilosec), lansoprazole (Prevacid), rabeprazole (AcipHex), esomeprazole (Nexium), pantoprazole (Protonix)
  - Prokinetic agents: Metoclopramide (Reglan), erythromycin (Ery-Tab)
- Contraindications:
  - Anticholinergics: Obstructive uropathy, glaucoma, myasthenia gravis, achalasia, dementia/delirium, advanced age
  - Nitrates: Early MI, severe anemia, increased ICP, HTN
- Investigational: Cilostazol for dysphagia in poststroke patients is under investigation; may improve swallowing and reduce risk of aspiration pneumonia; mechanism is not completely understood
- Precautions: May need to use liquid forms of medications, as patients might have difficulty swallowing pills

ADDITIONAL TREATMENT

General Measures
- Exclude cardiac disease.
- Ensure airway and pulmonary function.
- Assess nutritional status.
- Speech therapy evaluation is helpful.

Issues for Referral
- Need for endoscopy, refractory: Gastroenterology
- Failure of dilation or medications: Surgery for esophageal myotomy

Additional Therapies
Speech therapy for swallowing assessment, dietary and positioning recommendations, and muscle-strengthening exercise; no eating at bedtime; remaining upright after eating

SURGERY/OTHER PROCEDURES
- Esophageal dilatation (pneumatic or bougie)
- Esophageal stent; laser for cancer palliation
- Treatment for underlying problem (e.g., thyroid goiter, vascular ring, esophageal atresia)
- Nd: YAG laser incision of lower esophageal rings refractory to dilation
- Photodynamic therapy (cancer)
- Cricopharyngeal myotomy for oropharyngeal dysphagia
- Surgery for Zenker diverticulum, refractory strictures, or myotomy for achalasia
- Nissens fundoplication to prevent reflux

IN-PATIENT CONSIDERATIONS

Initial Stabilization
- Outpatient for conditions where patient is able to maintain nutrition and has little risk of complications
- Hospitalization may be required for either infants or adults when dysphagia is associated with total or near-total obstruction of esophageal lumen.
- Endoscopy and/or esophageal dilation may be needed for stenoses and strictures (often recur).
- Surgery may be required in either benign or malignant processes.

Admission Criteria
- Complete or partial esophageal obstruction with malnutrition or hypovolemia/dehydration
- Comorbid conditions complicating etiology of dysphagia
- Enteral feeding might be required in patients with:
  - Impaired level of consciousness
  - Massive aspiration or recurrent respiratory infections
  - Esophageal obstruction

IV Fluids
For dehydrated, hypovolemic patients and patients with impaired consciousness

Nursing
- Monitor for aspiration.
- Ensure correct posture of patient while feeding.
- Consider bedside screening tests using water swallowing and pulse oximetry to screen neurologic patients for dysphagia (1)[A].

Discharge Criteria
- Correction of dysphagia
- Tolerating adequate diet without nausea/pain
- Adequate nutritional intake
- Control of pain syndrome

ONGOING CARE

FOLLOW-UP RECOMMENDATIONS
- No restrictions
- Sit upright for meals, stay upright afterward; appropriately fitting dentures
- Follow speech therapy/swallow therapy recommendations.
- Strengthening exercises and rehab for post-CVA

Patient Monitoring
Related to specific etiology of the dysphagia

DIET
Depends on etiology and severity:
- Counsel the patient on avoiding irritating drugs.
- Counsel the patient on the importance of chewing food well.
- Speech therapy texture recommendations like mechanical soft diet or pureed diet

PATIENT EDUCATION
Dietary modification, no eating at bedtime, remaining upright after eating, pharmacologic therapy, smoking cessation

PROGNOSIS
Course and prognosis vary with specific diagnosis (cancer, poor; esophageal peptic stricture, good).

COMPLICATIONS
- Aspiration/aspiration pneumonia
- Esophageal "asthma"
- Upper respiratory tract infections
- Malnutrition
- Esophagitis: Reflux based or pill induced
- Death

REFERENCE

1. Bours GJ, Speyer R, Lemmens J, et al. Bedside screening tests vs. videofluoroscopy or fibreoptic endoscopic evaluation of swallowing to detect dysphagia in patients with neurological disorders: systematic review. *J Adv Nurs*. 2009;65:477–93.

ADDITIONAL READING

- Rofes L, Arreola V, Almirall J, Cabré M, Campins L, García-Peris P, Speyer R, Clavé P et al. Diagnosis and Management of Oropharyngeal Dysphagia and Its Nutritional and Respiratory Complications in the Elderly. *Gastroenterology research and practice*. 2011;2011.
- Speyer R, Baijens L, Heijnen M, Zwijnenberg I et al. Effects of therapy in oropharyngeal dysphagia by speech and language therapists: a systematic review. *Dysphagia*. 2010;25:40–65.
- White GN, O'Rourke F, Ong BS, Cordato DJ, Chan DK et al. Dysphagia: causes, assessment, treatment, and management. *Geriatrics*. 2008;63:15–20.

See Also (Topic, Algorithm, Electronic Media Element)
Esophageal Tumors; Gastroesophageal Reflux Disease

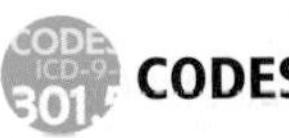

CODES

ICD9
- 530.3 Stricture and stenosis of esophagus
- 750.3 Congenital tracheoesophageal fistula, esophageal atresia and stenosis
- 787.20 Dysphagia, unspecified

CLINICAL PEARLS
- Careful history taking of types of food involved, progression, and associated symptoms will help to determine where the problem is.
- The alarm symptoms to look for are weight loss, chest pain, rapid progression, and risk factors such as chronic GERD and alcohol or tobacco use.
- A barium study (esophagram) is the first step in evaluating patients with dysphagia if you suspect obstruction or achalasia, and then endoscopy; or directly to endoscopy if achalasia is less likely.
- An EGD with esophageal biopsies should be considered in patients with intermittent solid-food dysphagia to rule out eosinophilic esophagitis even if they have normal endoscopic findings.

ECTOPIC PREGNANCY

Janelle M. Evans, MD
Shaila V. Chauhan, MD

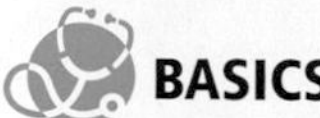

BASICS

DESCRIPTION

- Ectopic: Pregnancy occurs outside the confines of the uterine cavity
- Tubal: Pregnancy implanted in any portion of the fallopian tube
- Abdominal: Pregnancy implanted intra-abdominally, most commonly in the posterior cul-de-sac
- Heterotopic: Pregnancy implanted intrauterine and a separate pregnancy implanted outside uterine cavity
- Ovarian: Implantation of pregnancy in ovarian tissue
- Cervical: Implantation in cervix (associated with large blood loss)
- Intraligamentary: Implantation of pregnancy within the broad ligament

EPIDEMIOLOGY

Incidence

- 108,800 cases in 1992 in the US according to Centers for Disease Control census (most recent data available)
- 15.8 per 1,000 total reported pregnancies, or 9.5 per 10,000 women
- 28,000 hospitalizations reported in 2006 in the US for ectopic pregnancy
- Heterotopic pregnancy, although rare (1:30,000), occurs with greater frequency in women undergoing in vitro fertilization (IVF) (1–2/1,000)
- Leading cause of 1st-trimester maternal death and accounts for 9% of national pregnancy deaths

Prevalence

- Predominant age: >40% occur in women between ages 20 and 29
- 12–15% recurrence rate if prior ectopic pregnancy

RISK FACTORS

- History of tubal surgery (7:1,000 for tubal ligation)
- Previous ectopic pregnancy
- History of pelvic inflammatory disease (PID), endometritis, or current gonorrhea/chlamydia infection
- Pelvic adhesive disease (infection, prior surgery)
- Use of an intrauterine device: Reduction of the absolute risk of ectopic pregnancy overall, but increased likelihood of pregnancy being ectopic if pregnancy occurs
- Use of assisted reproductive technologies in up to 4% (e.g., IVF, embryo transfer)
- Diethylstilbestrol exposure in utero
- Cigarette smoking
- Some evidence that vaginal douching is a modifiable risk factor
- Patients with disorders that affect ciliary motility may be at increased risk.

GENERAL PREVENTION

- Reliable contraception or abstinence
- Screening and treatment of sexually transmitted diseases (gonorrhea, chlamydia) that can cause PID and tubal scarring

PATHOPHYSIOLOGY

- 98% of ectopic pregnancies occur in the fallopian tube, 70% in the ampullary portion of the tube, 12% in the isthmus, 11% in the fimbria, and 2% in the cornua.
- Abdominal pregnancies account for 1.3% of all ectopics; ovarian and cervical sites account for 0.2% each.

ETIOLOGY

- For a tubal pregnancy:
  - Damage or compromise to the integrity of the fallopian tubes leads to dysfunction of the tubal cilia, which are required for proper movement of the fertilized ovum to the uterine cavity.
  - Scarring or narrowing of the tube damages tubal integrity.
- Other locations are rare and may occur from reimplantation of an aborted tubal pregnancy or uterine structural abnormalities (mainly cervical pregnancy).

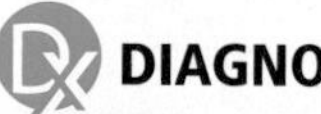

DIAGNOSIS

HISTORY

- In more than half of presenting cases, patients have sudden-onset abdominal pain coupled with cessation of menses or irregular menses.
- Nausea and/or vomiting
- Abdominal pain or mass
- Referred shoulder pain (secondary to hemoperitoneum)

PHYSICAL EXAM

- Abdominal tenderness
- Vaginal bleeding
- Palpable mass on pelvic exam
- Cervical motion tenderness may also be appreciated.
- In cervical cases, an hourglass-shaped cervix might be noted.
- In cases of rupture and intraperitoneal bleeding, signs of shock such as pallor, tachycardia, and hypotension may be present.

DIAGNOSTIC TESTS & INTERPRETATION

Lab

Initial lab tests

- Human chorionic gonadotropin (HCG): Serial quantitative serum levels normally increase by ~66% every 48 hours:
  - Abnormal rise should prompt workup for gestational abnormalities.
- Serial hematocrit and abdominal exams to quantify blood loss only if not immediately going to the operating room
- Serum progesterone level (>20 mg/mL associated with lower risk of ectopic pregnancy)

Imaging

Initial approach

- Transvaginal ultrasound (TVUS) is the gold standard for diagnosis (1)[A]:
  - Doppler flowmetry is usually coupled with ultrasound for more accurate diagnosis.
- Magnetic resonance imaging is also useful, but costly, and rarely used if ultrasound is available.

Follow-Up & Special Considerations

Consider TVUS in the 1st trimester of future pregnancies.

Pathological Findings

- Tubal pregnancy: Chorionic villi within the tubal wal
- Ovarian pregnancy (Spiegelberg criteria):
  - Pregnancy found displacing or replacing the ovarian tissue
  - Possible utero-ovarian ligament attachment
  - Ovarian tissue identified as part of gestational sac
- Abdominal pregnancy—primary form:
  - Both ovaries and tubes appear normal.
  - No uteroperitoneal fistula is present.
  - Limited to peritoneal attachment of conceptus
- Cervical pregnancy: Villi seen in the cervical canal
- Intraligamentary pregnancy: The products of conception (POCs) are within the confines of the broad ligament.

DIFFERENTIAL DIAGNOSIS

- Missed or threatened abortion
- Appendicitis
- Salpingitis, PID
- Ruptured corpus luteum or hemorrhagic cyst
- Ovarian tumor, benign or malignant
- Ovarian torsion
- Endometrioma
- Cervical cancer
- Cervical phase of uterine abortion

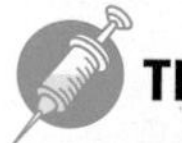

TREATMENT

MEDICATION

- Methotrexate: Primary treatment for unruptured tubal pregnancy or for remaining POCs after laparoscopic salpingotomy. It inhibits DNA synthesis via folic acid antagonism.
- Most effective when pregnancy is <3 cm diameter, HCG <5,000 mIU/mL, and no fetal heart rate is seen. Success rate is 85–90% with proper selection.
- Dosage:
  - Single: IM methotrexate: 50 mg/m^2 of body surface area; may repeat once (preferred method) if <15% decline in HCG by day 7
  - Multidose: Methotrexate 1 mg/kg IM/IV every other day, with leucovorin 0.1 mg/kg IM in between. Maximum 4 doses; course may be repeated 7 days after last dose if necessary.

- Contraindications:
  - Hemodynamic instability or any evidence of rupture
  - Fetal heart rate seen
  - Large gestational sac (>3 cm)
  - Noncompliance or limited access to hospital or transportation
- Precautions:
  - Immunologic, hematologic, renal, gastrointestinal, hepatic, and pulmonary disease, or interacting medications
- Pretreatment testing: serum HCG, complete blood count, liver and renal function tests, type and screen
- Patient counseling: During therapy, refrain from use of alcohol, aspirin, nonsteroidal anti-inflammatory drugs, or folate supplements (decreases efficacy of MTX), avoid excessive sun exposure

ADDITIONAL TREATMENT

- After evidence of repeat medical failure or rupture, surgery is necessary.
- Follow all patients treated medically to an HCG of 0 to prevent surgical intervention.
- Expectant management in asymptomatic patients with no evidence of rupture or hemodynamic instability coupled with an appropriately low BHCG, no evidence of fetal cardiac activity

Issues for Referral

- Co-manage with or refer to a gynecologist for medical treatment.
- Consult a gynecologist for surgical care.

COMPLEMENTARY AND ALTERNATIVE MEDICINE

Watchful waiting: If no clear adnexal mass and low HCG (usually 1,000–2,000), may follow with HCG/ultrasound. Rare cases of rupture have been described with low quants.

SURGERY/OTHER PROCEDURES

- Indications include ruptured ectopic, inability to comply with medical follow-up, previous tubal ligation, known tubal disease or current heterotopic pregnancy, desire for permanent sterilization at time of diagnosis
- Laparoscopy is 1st-line surgical management.
- Salpingostomy preferred in patients who wish to maintain fertility:
  - Slightly higher recurrence rate than with salpingectomy
  - Slightly higher rate of persistent trophoblastic tissue with laparoscopy vs open laparotomy (8% vs 3.4%)
- Salpingectomy indicated for uncontrolled bleeding, recurrent ectopic pregnancy, severely damaged tube, gestational sac >4 cm, or patient desire for sterilization

IN-PATIENT CONSIDERATIONS

Initial Stabilization

Surgical emergency:

- 2 IV access lines should be placed immediately if suspicion of rupture; aggressive resuscitation as needed
- Blood product transfusion and fluids if necessary en route to operating room
- In cases of shock, pressors and cardiac support may be necessary.

Admission Criteria

Fails criteria for methotrexate management, suspicion of rupture, orthostatic, shock, and severe abdominal pain requiring IV narcotics

Nursing

Strict input/output, hourly vitals, orthostatics if mobile, frequent abdominal exams, serial hematocrit, pad counts if heavy vaginal bleeding

Discharge Criteria

Afebrile; abdominal pain resolving or resolved

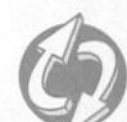

ONGOING CARE

FOLLOW-UP RECOMMENDATIONS

Patient Monitoring

- Serial serum quantitative HCG until level drops to negative
- Pelvic ultrasound for persistent or recurrent masses
- Pain control: Brief course of narcotics usually necessary
- Liver and renal function tests following methotrexate administration
- Delay of subsequent pregnancy for at least 3 months after treatment with methotrexate due to teratogenicity

DIET

- Avoid foods and vitamins high in folate due to interaction with methotrexate efficacy.
- Maintain excellent hydration.

PROGNOSIS

- Recurrence rate 12–15% for ectopic pregnancy
- Future fertility depends on fertility prior to ectopic, history of tubal compromise
- Referral to reproductive endocrinology appropriate if infertility persists beyond 12–18 months

COMPLICATIONS

- Hemorrhage and hypovolemic shock
- Persistent trophoblastic tissue after medical or surgical management
- Infection
- Infertility (more commonly with salpingectomy)
- Blood transfusions with associated infections/transfusion reaction
- Disseminated intravascular coagulation

REFERENCE

1. *Ann Emerg Med*. 2010;56(6):674–683.

ADDITIONAL READING

- ACOG practice bulletin. Medical management of tubal pregnancy. Number 3, December 1998. Clinical management guidelines for obstetrician-gynecologists. American College of Obstetricians and Gynecologists. *Int J Gynaecol Obstet*. 1999;65:97–103.
- Bisharah M, Tulandi T. Laparoscopic surgery in pregnancy. *Clin Obstet Gynecol*. 2003;46:92–7.
- Braude P, Rowell P. Assisted conception. III–problems with assisted conception. *BMJ*. 2003;327:920–3.
- Centers for Disease Control and Prevention. Sexually Transmitted Disease Surveillance 2007. Atlanta, GA: U.S. Department of Health and Human Services; December 2008.
- Centers for Disease Control and Prevention. Sexually Transmitted Disease Surveillance 2007. Atlanta, GA: U.S. Department of Health and Human Services; December 2008.
- Elson J, et al. Expectant management of tubal ectopic pregnancy: Prediction of successful outcome using decision tree analysis. *Ultrasound Obstet Gynaecol*. 2004;23:552–6.
- Hajenius PJ, Mol F, Mol BW, et al. Interventions for tubal ectopic pregnancy. *Cochrane Database Syst Rev*. 2007;CD000324.
- Lipscomb GH. Medical therapy for ectopic pregnancy. *Semin Reprod Med*. 2007;25:93–8.
- Mol F, Mol BW, Ankum WM, et al. Current evidence on surgery, systemic methotrexate and expectant management in the treatment of tubal ectopic pregnancy: a systematic review and meta-analysis. *Hum Reprod Update*. 2008.
- Murray H, et al. Diagnosis and treatment of ectopic pregnancy. *Can Med Assoc J*. 2005;173(8):905–912.
- Nama V, Manyonda I. Tubal ectopic pregnancy: diagnosis and management. *Arch Gynecol Obstet*. 2008.
- Ramakrishnan K, Scheid DC. Ectopic pregnancy: expectant management of immediate surgery? *J Fam Pract*. 2006;55:517–22.
- Tay JI, Moore J, Walker JJ. Ectopic pregnancy. *BMJ*. 2000;320.916–9.

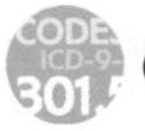

CODES

ICD9

- 633.00 Abdominal pregnancy without intrauterine pregnancy
- 633.10 Tubal pregnancy without intrauterine pregnancy
- 633.20 Ovarian pregnancy without intrauterine pregnancy

CLINICAL PEARLS

- Ectopic pregnancy is the leading cause of 1st-trimester maternal death and accounts for 9% of national pregnancy deaths.
- 98% of ectopic pregnancies occur in the fallopian tube.
- TVUS is the gold standard for diagnosis.
- When an ectopic pregnancy is <3 cm diameter, HCG <5,000 mIU/mL, and no fetal heart rate is seen, a single dose of methotrexate is the preferred medical treatment, with a success rate of 85–90%.
- Indications for surgery include ruptured ectopic, inability to comply with medical follow-up, previous tubal ligation, known tubal disease or current heterotopic pregnancy, or desire for permanent sterilization at time of diagnosis.

EJACULATORY DISORDERS

Andrew Leone, MD
Kyle D. Wood, MD

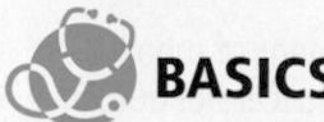

BASICS

DESCRIPTION

- Premature/rapid ejaculation: Inability to control the ejaculatory reflex is the most common type of sexual dysfunction affecting all age groups:
  - American Urological Association (AUA) 2003 Guidelines definition: "Ejaculation that occurs sooner than desired, either before or shortly after penetration, causing distress to either one or both partners." (1)
  - Natural biologic response is to ejaculate within 2–5 minutes after vaginal penetration.
  - Ejaculatory control is an acquired behavior that increases with experience.
- Delayed (retarded) ejaculation: Prolonged time to ejaculate despite desire, stimulation, and erection.
- Aspermia (lack of sperm in the ejaculate):
  - Anejaculation: Lack of emission or contractions of bulbospongiosus muscle
  - Retrograde ejaculation: Partial or complete ejaculation of semen into the bladder
  - Obstruction: Ejaculatory duct obstruction or urethral obstruction
- Painful ejaculation: Genital or perineal pain during or after ejaculation
- Ejaculatory anhedonia: Normal ejaculation lacking orgasm or pleasure
- Hematospermia: Presence of blood in the ejaculate
- Ejaculatory duct obstruction
- System(s) affected: Nervous; Reproductive
- Synonym(s): Premature ejaculation; rapid ejaculation; retarded ejaculation; retrograde ejaculation; anejaculation; inhibited orgasm in males; ejaculatory dysfunction

EPIDEMIOLOGY

- Premature ejaculation is common. Reported prevalence in US males ages 18–59: 21%
- Retarded ejaculation is reported in ~5–8% of men between 18 and 59, but <3% experience the problem for >6 months.
- Predominant age: All sexually mature age groups
- Predominant sex: Male only

Prevalence

20% of men affected

RISK FACTORS

See Etiology

PATHOPHYSIOLOGY

Male sexual response:

- Erection mediated by parasympathetic nervous system
- Ejaculation consists of 2 phases:
  - Emission phase: Semen is deposited into urethra by contraction of prostate, seminal vesicles, and vas deferens. Under autonomic sympathetic control.
  - Ejaculation phase: Semen is forcibly propelled out of urethra by rhythmic contractions of the bulbospongiosus and ischiocavernosus muscles. This is mediated by the somatic nervous system on the motor branches of the pudendal nerve.
- Bladder neck contracture occurs during the above process and is induced by alpha-adrenergic receptors to ensure anterograde ejaculation.
- Orgasm: The pleasurable sensation associated with ejaculation (cerebral cortex) (2)

ETIOLOGY

- Untreated erectile dysfunction is the most common treatable cause.
- Premature ejaculation (many potential causes but all without evidence base):
  - Penile hypersensitivity
  - 5-hydroxytryptamine (5-HT)-receptor sensitivity
  - Sexual inexperience
  - High level of sexual arousal and/or long interval since last ejaculation
  - Fear of sexual transmitted diseases (STDs)
  - Anxiety
  - Guilty feelings about sex
  - Lack of privacy
  - Interpersonal maladaptation (e.g., marital problems, unresponsiveness of partner)
- Retarded ejaculation:
  - Rarely may be caused by an underlying painful disorder (e.g., prostatitis, seminal vesiculitis)
  - May be psychogenic as part of erectile dysfunction
  - Sexual performance anxiety and other psychosocial factors
  - Some drugs may impair ejaculation (e.g., certain monoamine oxidase inhibitors [MAOIs], selective serotonin reuptake inhibitors [SSRIs], α- and β-blockers, thiazides, antipsychotics, tricyclic and quadricyclic antidepressants, nonsteroidal anti-inflammatory drugs [NSAIDs], opiates, or alcohol).
- Never any ejaculate:
  - Congenital structural disorder (Müllerian duct cyst, Wolffian abnormality)
  - Acquired (radical prostatectomy, postinfectious, post-traumatic, T10–12 neuropathy)
- Anejaculation:
  - Medications (α- and β-blockers, benzodiazepines, SSRIs, MAOIs, TCAs, antipsychotics, aminocaproic acid)
  - Diabetes mellitus (DM) (neuropathy)
  - Retroperitoneal lymph node dissection
  - Sympathetic nerve injury (spinal cord injury, intraoperative injury)
  - Radical prostatectomy
- Retrograde ejaculation:
  - Transurethral resection of the prostate (25%) or other prostate resection procedures
  - Surgery on the neck of the bladder
  - Extensive pelvic surgery
  - Retroperitoneal lymph node dissection for testicular cancer (also may produce failure of emission)
  - Neurologic disorders (multiple sclerosis, DM)
  - Medications (alpha-blockers, in particular tamsulosin, ganglion blockers, antipsychotics)
  - Urethral stricture
  - Trauma
- Painful ejaculation:
  - Infection or inflammation (orchitis, epididymitis, prostatitis, urethritis)
  - Ejaculatory duct obstruction
  - Seminal vesicle calculi
  - Obstruction of the vas deferens
  - Psychological
- Ejaculatory anhedonia:
  - Medications
  - Psychological
  - Hormonal imbalances
  - Decreased libido
- Hematospermia:
  - Inflammation/infection
  - Calculi: Bladder, seminal vesicle, prostate, urethra
  - Trauma to genital area, i.e., cycling or constipation
  - Obstruction
  - Cyst
  - Tumor (prostate cancer [1–3% present with hematospermia])
  - Arteriovenous malformations
  - Iatrogenic
  - Hypertension
- Endocrinopathies can result in ejaculatory dysfunction

COMMONLY ASSOCIATED CONDITIONS

- Neurologic disorders (e.g., multiple sclerosis)
- Diabetes mellitus
- Prostatitis
- Ejaculatory duct obstruction
- Urethral stricture
- Psychologic disorders
- Endocrinopathies
- Relationship/interpersonal difficulties

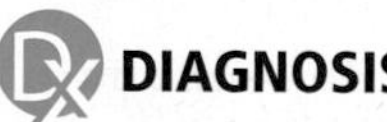

DIAGNOSIS

- Ejaculation occurs before individual wishes.
- Ejaculation does not occur following normal stimulation (including masturbation).

HISTORY

- Detailed sexual history, including:
  - Time frame of the problem
  - Evaluation of the quality of patient's sexual response
  - Sense of ejaculatory control and sexual distress
  - Overall assessment of the relationship
- Detailed history of recent and current medications
- History of past trauma or recent infections
- Past surgical history with particular attention to genitourinary surgeries
- Inquire about home remedies attempted.
- Many men do not distinguish initially between problems related to erection and ejaculation.
- Some men have unrealistic expectations of ejaculatory response and frequency.
- Include the sexual partner in the interview, especially if the patient expresses a belief that he is not meeting his partner's needs.
- In review of systems, elicit any evidence of testosterone deficiency or prolactin excess for diagnosis of anhedonia.

PHYSICAL EXAM

- Look for multiple sclerosis, spinal cord injury, and emotional disorders
- Thorough genitourinary (GU) exam, including (3):
  - Size and texture of testes and epididymis
  - Verification of the presence of the vas deferens
  - Location and patency of urethral meatus
  - Digital rectal examination to evaluate prostate consistency and size and possible midline lesions

DIAGNOSTIC TESTS & INTERPRETATION

Lab

- Laboratory test results may be normal.
- Fasting blood sugar to rule out diabetes
- Postorgasmic urinalysis will confirm retrograde ejaculation. Sperm, fructose level, and viscosity can be measured.
- Anejaculation will have fructose negative, sperm negative, nonviscous postorgasmic urinalysis.
- In painful ejaculation, urinalysis and urine culture
- If prostate cancer is considered, check prostate-specific antigen (PSA).
- In anhedonia, consider checking testosterone, prolactin, and thyroid levels.

Imaging

- In hematospermia, painful ejaculation, or if ejaculatory duct obstruction is considered, transrectal ultrasound (TRUS) may be helpful.
- TRUS-guided seminal vesicle aspiration; if ejaculatory duct obstruction is present, then the aspirate will contain sperm.
- If suspicious of anatomic abnormality, can use ultrasound and/or MRI

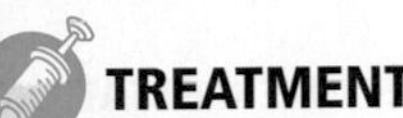

TREATMENT

MEDICATION

- Premature ejaculation:
  - Treating underlying erectile dysfunction (if identified) may allow for a decrease in the rapidity.
  - Behavioral/sex therapy is important when appropriate.
  - Topical anesthetic gel applied (2.5% prilocaine + 2.5 % lidocaine (EMLA)) 2.5 g under a condom for 30 minutes prior to intercourse
  - Experimental PSD502 topical aerosol preparation of lidocaine/prilocaine effective in phase III trials (4)
  - Clomipramine 20–50 mg/d or sertraline 25–200 mg/d, fluoxetine 5–20 mg/d, or paroxetine 10–40 mg/d have been shown to delay ejaculation.
  - Clomipramine shown to be the most effective, but has higher rate of side effects
  - On-demand use of clomipramine 20–40 mg 4–24 hours before intercourse or sertraline 50 mg 4–8 hours before intercourse or paroxetine 20 mg 3–4 hours before intercourse
  - Switching antidepressants to bupropion, nefazodone, mirtazapine, or possibly trazodone may eliminate drug-induced ejaculatory disturbance.
- Delayed (retarded) ejaculation:
  - Retarded orgasm and ejaculation in patients who must continue SSRIs may respond to bupropion, buspirone, cyproheptadine, or yohimbine supplementation before intercourse.
  - Some evidence that cyproheptadine and amantadine may be helpful (5)
- Anejaculation/retrograde ejaculation:
  - Alpha-agonists and antihistamines can be helpful but are not approved by Food and Drug Administration (FDA):
    - Pseudoephedrine 60 mg p.o. every day to q.i.d.
    - Imipramine 25 mg p.o. b.i.d.
    - Ephedrine sulfate 50 mg p.o. q.i.d.
- Painful ejaculation:
  - Treat underlying infection/inflammatory process
  - Alpha-blockers may have some benefit

ADDITIONAL TREATMENT

General Measures

- Identifying any medical cause (even if not reversible) helps patient accept condition.
- Improve partner communication.
- Psychological counseling may be beneficial for some patients.
- Reduce performance pressure through reassurance.
- Use of a variety of resources may be necessary (e.g., psychiatrist, psychologist, sex therapist, vascular surgeon, urologist, endocrinologist, neurologist).
- Premature ejaculation
  - Use sensate focus therapy (gradual progression of nonsexual contact to sexual contact)
  - Quiet vagina: Female partner stops moving just prior to ejaculation
  - Techniques to learn ejaculatory control (e.g., coronal squeeze technique [squeezing the glans penis until ejaculatory urge ceases] or start-and-stop technique [cessation of penile stimulation when ejaculation approaches and resumption of stimulation when ejaculatory feeling ends])
- Delayed ejaculation:
  - Change medications to an antidepressant that is less likely to cause delayed ejaculation (citalopram, fluvoxamine, nefazodone).
  - If patient has diabetes, better control of diabetes may improve ejaculation.
  - Penile vibratory stimulation (not frequently used)
- Anejaculation/retrograde ejaculation:
  - Discontinue offending medication(s).
  - Diabetic control
  - If urethral obstruction present, referral to urology for management
  - Retrograde ejaculation may be helped if intercourse occurs when bladder is full.
  - Consider penile vibratory stimulation (effective in spinal cord injuries greater than T10) or electroejaculation (place on monitor if lesions above T6 since autonomic dysreflexia may result) to collect sperm in anejaculation cases.
- Painful ejaculation:
  - Counseling may be beneficial.
  - If seminal vesicle stones possible, refer to urology.
- Hematospermia:
  - If persistent or high degree of suspicion for abnormality, refer to urologist for proper evaluation.

Issues for Referral

The following conditions, when suspected, should be referred to a urologist:

- Ejaculatory duct obstruction
- Seminal vesicle or prostatic stones
- Urethral obstruction
- Vas deferens obstruction
- Calculi
- Persistent or severe hematospermia

SURGERY/OTHER PROCEDURES

Surgical treatment of ejaculatory duct obstruction:

- Transurethral resection of the ejaculatory ducts

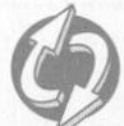

ONGOING CARE

PATIENT EDUCATION

See General Measures

PROGNOSIS

Often improves with therapy and counseling

COMPLICATIONS

Psychologic impact on some males: Signs of severe inadequacy, self-doubt, additional anxiety, and guilt

REFERENCES

1. Montague DK, Jarow J, Broderick GA, et al. AUA guideline on the pharmacologic management of premature ejaculation. *J Urol*. 2004;172:290–4.
2. Master VA, Turek PJ. Ejaculatory physiology and dysfunction. *Urol Clin North Am*. 2001;28: 363–75, x.
3. Schuster TG, Ohl DA. Diagnosis and treatment of ejaculatory dysfunction. *Urol Clin North Am*. 2002;29:939–48.
4. Dinsmore WW, Wyllie MG. PSD502 improves ejaculatory latency, control and sexual satisfaction when applied topically 5 min before intercourse in men with premature ejaculation: results of a phase III, multicentre, double-blind, placebo-controlled study. *BJU Int*. 2009.
5. McMahon CG, Abdo C, Incrocci L, et al. Disorders of orgasm and ejaculation in men. *J Sex Med*. 2004;1:58–65.

ADDITIONAL READING

- Mercer CH, et al. Sexual function problems and health seeking behaviour in Britain: Probability sample survey. *Br Med J*. 2003;327:426–7.
- Richardson D, Goldmeier D, BASHH Special Interest Group for Sexual Dysfunction. Recommendations for the management of retarded ejaculation: BASHH Special Interest Group for Sexual Dysfunction. *Int J STD AIDS*. 2006;17:7–13.
- Waldinger MD. Premature ejaculation: definition and drug treatment. *Drugs*. 2007;67:547–68.

CODES

ICD9

- 302.75 Premature ejaculation
- 608.87 Retrograde ejaculation

CLINICAL PEARLS

- If erectile dysfunction is contributing to ejaculatory difficulty, management of erectile dysfunction should precede attempted management of ejaculatory disorders.
- Medications should always be thoroughly reviewed, as they may be the primary cause of ejaculatory disorders.
- A multidisciplinary approach, including the primary care physician, urologists, psychologists, and other appropriate health care professionals, is essential to the proper treatment of ejaculatory disorders.

E

ELDER ABUSE

Thomas Price, MD

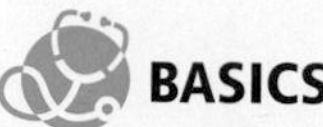

BASICS

DESCRIPTION

Elder abuse, or elder mistreatment, is a condition where the physical, psychological, or financial well-being of an older adult is infringed upon through intentional acts or lack of action, even if harm is not intended. 3 basic entities comprise this problem:

- Abuse: Includes physical, sexual, or psychological harm
- Neglect: Withholding of necessary treatments or services
- Exploitation: Use of an older adult's property counter to their needs or benefit

EPIDEMIOLOGY

Incidence

2–10% of persons worldwide over the age of 65 suffer abuse on an annual basis, as many as 1 new case every 8 hours (1)

Prevalence

1–2 million seniors affected in the US as of 2003 data (1)

RISK FACTORS

- 5 major risk factors (2):
  - Shared living situation (abuser/victim)
  - Dementia or other cognitive impairment
  - Social isolation (abuser or victim)
  - Mental illness/alcohol abuse (abuser)
  - Financial/material dependence (abuser) on the victim
- The presence of all of these risk factors does not convey increased diagnostic accuracy; likewise, the absence of all risk factors does not preclude abuse.

GENERAL PREVENTION

- Improve patient social contact and support.
- Monitor patients for self-neglect and functional decline.
- Recognition of caregiver stressors and burden
- Assist management of behavioral and functional changes that occur in dementia
- While several screening tools exist, screening questionnaires are not helpful in patients with cognitive impairment (3). Common screening questions include:
  - "Have you felt unsafe at home?"
  - "Has anyone hurt you, called you names, or taken things from you?"
  - " What happens when you disagree with [caregiver]?"

ETIOLOGY

The most common scenario of abuse is a caregiver with poor family/social support who is providing care for an older person with a degree of disability. These caregivers are often relatives of the possible victim. Abuse can occur in any setting (home, assisted living, nursing home), and any older person with an impaired ability to defend or care for themself can be at risk.

COMMONLY ASSOCIATED CONDITIONS

- Nearly 2/3 of patients diagnosed as suffering from elder abuse had dementia in an international study (4)[B].
- Older patients that are admitted with a geriatric syndrome of "failure to thrive" may be victims and should be screened for abuse.

DIAGNOSIS

As neglect and exploitation are more common forms of elder mistreatment than abuse, the history is extremely important and will allow the practitioner to develop their own suspicion threshold for an individual case.

HISTORY

- Interviewing the patient separate from the suspected abuser is helpful. The patient may give vague explanations of the causes of injury, or may refuse to answer questions.
- A history of dementia or functional decline can be associated with increased risk, as is an increase in physical and psychological aggression as is often seen in dementia.
- Observe interaction between patient and caregiver: Suspicion is raised if there is withdrawal of patient from caregiver, or caregiver interrupting the patient and providing answers for them. Caregivers with anxiety, depression, and reduced social support are more likely to mistreat their care recipients (3)[C].

PHYSICAL EXAM

- Documentation of abnormal findings on physical exam may be used as evidence in court cases and should not include subjective or editorial comments or conclusions.
- Context of the physical condition of the patient is important. If they are examined in their own bed, look for bedding or mattress soiled by bodily fluids. If found in sheets, copious flakes of skin or shedded hair can point to restricted mobility and care:
  - Appearance of poor personal hygiene
  - Bruises and soft tissue injury:
    - Common areas include surfaces of the upper back, upper arms, and lower legs
    - Lesions with shapes (such as buckles, snaps, or buttons) suggest prolonged immobility or blunt trauma
  - Pressure ulcers can indicate neglect but are equivocal outside of context.
  - Poor dentition or evidence of oral sores, candidiasis, etc.
  - Findings of lice, scabies, or saprophytes
- Fearful or withdrawn affect
- A genital exam is indicated if sexual abuse is suspected, but should be performed with a documented chaperone of the patient's gender. The use of a rape kit if trained personnel is available may be appropriate.

DIAGNOSTIC TESTS & INTERPRETATION

Lab

The following workup is recommended:

- Urine and blood screen for narcotics, intoxicants, and other psychoactive agents (extended panels may be necessary depending on your laboratory)
- Nutritional assessment, including appropriate serology (albumin, prealbumin, iron), blood count, and extended blood chemistry
- Additional labs to consider in patients with cognitive impairment: Thyroid stimulating hormone, syphilis serology, vitamin B_{12} level
- Assessment of infection (may include urinalysis and culture, chest radiograph, blood count, and cultures)
- If sexual abuse suspected, culture and microscopy of any present exudate or residue and viral serology (rape kit lab package)

Imaging

- Radiographic imaging of areas below soft tissue injury is indicated if there is evidence of infection (osteomyelitis) at a pressure ulcer site or bruising of a limb (fracture).
- If physical abuse is suspected and cognitive impairment present, then cranial imaging looking for hemorrhage (subdural, etc.) is indicated.

Diagnostic Procedures/Surgery

- Pulse test: Check blood pressure and pulse in presence and absence of suspected abuser. Elevation of either in the presence of the suspected abuser should raise suspicion. Useful in patients with dementia or other condition that makes history taking difficult.
- Documentation: Practitioners may make statements of "suspected mistreatment" but should avoid making definitive diagnosis of abuse in their initial assessment.

DIFFERENTIAL DIAGNOSIS

- Self-neglect is a condition where a patient fails to provide adequate self-care. It can occur in patients with cognitive impairment and may be a sign of early-stage dementia. It is also seen in patients with psychiatric disorders such as schizophrenia and depression. Many consider this a condition related to elder abuse and place it in the category of elder mistreatment.
- Alzheimer's disease alone can manifest with poor nutrition, withdrawal from society, and feelings of persecution.
- Delusions due to dementia, such as the Alzheimer's type, may manifest early with accusations of theft and deception.
- Parkinson's disease patients often fall and may exhibit fractures and bruises on a frequent basis that may mimic recurrent physical abuse.
- Coagulopathy such as due to use of antiplatelet or warfarin therapy can cause easy bruising of the forearms, but usually spares the upper arm.
- Adenocarcinoma of the lung, prostate, and colon can present with weight loss, apathy, and pressure ulcers.
- Pancreatic adenocarcinoma may present with severe weight loss, depression, and a failure-to-thrive picture.
- Hypothyroidism can present with apathy, weight loss, and confusion that may be confused for neglect.
- Chronic lung disease can present as weight loss, reduced functional reserve, and withdrawal.
- Acute psychosis can be due to infection, medications, or metabolic disturbances and may result in delusional accusations of harm and neglect.
- Impaired financial status often leads to a lack of access to appropriate food, clothing, shelter, and medical care.

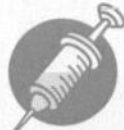

TREATMENT

In most states, the physician or allied health care worker is a mandated reporter of suspicion of elder abuse. This does not put a burden of charge on the physician.

IN-PATIENT CONSIDERATIONS

Initial Stabilization

Patient's living situation must be explored and determination of a safe alternative environment made. This is usually in conjunction with a social worker.

Admission Criteria

- Victims of elder abuse should be admitted to the hospital (observation status) if there are no safe discharge alternatives.
- Often, these victims will have acute or chronic medical illness that requires medical attention and possible conversion from observation to inpatient status.
- Cases of suspected abuse *must be reported* to the state's Adult Protective Services agency or a designated alternative (e.g., if patient resides in nursing home, then report to that state's regulatory entity). Social services may help. If physical harm has occurred, consider reporting to local law enforcement for investigation.
- Hospital security may need to be notified if restricted visitor access to a patient is required and the patient's name may be hidden from the public hospital census.

Discharge Criteria

Victims should not be discharged back to a potentially abusive environment without active investigation or protection (e.g., court order). Alternatives to discharge to the unsafe environment may include:

- Another friend or family member
- Nursing home
- Personal care home
- Assisted living facility
- Local victims rescue or sheltering program if available

ONGOING CARE

FOLLOW-UP RECOMMENDATIONS

Victims of abuse should not be discharged without adequate follow-up, including:

- Primary care physician visit in 1 week
- Follow up with Adult Protective Services or other agency
- Home Health Agency for assessment of safety (physical therapy)
- Follow up with appropriate psychiatric or psychological care.

Patient Monitoring

Frequent follow-up with appropriate state agency as discussed above

PATIENT EDUCATION

To locate Elder Abuse Hotline in your state, go to: http://www.nccafv.org/state_elder_abuse_hotlines.htm

PROGNOSIS

Patients with corroborated elder abuse have a 3-fold increase in mortality over 10 years when compared to controls (5)[B].

COMPLICATIONS

Victims of elder abuse who are seen by an Adult Protective Services caseworkers are 4 times more likely to be admitted to a nursing home (6)[B].

REFERENCES

1. National Center on Elder Abuse. *Elder Abuse Prevalence and Incidence*. Washinton, DC: American Public Human Services Association: 2005.
2. Lachs MS, Pillemer K et al. Elder abuse. *Lancet*. 2004;364:1263–72.
3. Wiglesworth A, Mosqueda L, Mulnard R, Liao S, Gibbs L, Fitzgerald W et al. Screening for abuse and neglect of people with dementia. *J Am Geriatr Soc*. 2010;58:493–500.
4. Cooper C, Katona C, Finne-Soveri H, Topinková E, Carpenter GI, Livingston G et al. Indicators of elder abuse: a crossnational comparison of psychiatric morbidity and other determinants in the Ad-HOC study. *Am J Geriatr Psychiatry*. 2006;14:489–97.
5. Lachs MS, Williams CS, O'Brien S, Pillemer KA, Charlson ME et al. The mortality of elder mistreatment. *JAMA*. 1998;280:428–32.
6. Lachs MS, Williams CS, O'Brien S, Pillemer KA, et al. Adult protective service use and nursing home placement. *Gerontologist*. 2002;42:734–9.

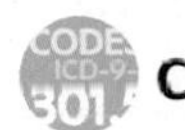

CODES

ICD9

- 995.80 Unspecified adult maltreatment
- 995.82 Adult emotional/psychological abuse
- 995.83 Adult sexual abuse

CLINICAL PEARLS

Patients with dementia or other psychiatric illness may accuse caregivers of physical harm or theft due to disease-induced elusions. Corroborating evidence may be needed to support suspicion of abuse, but these claims should not be summarily dismissed.

E

ENCEPHALITIS, VIRAL

Mary Cataletto, MD
Paul J. Lee, MD
Margaret McCormick, MS, RN

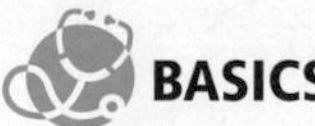

BASICS

DESCRIPTION

- Inflammatory process of the brain associated with clinical evidence of neurologic dysfunction
- System(s) affected: Nervous
- Synonym(s): Meningoencephalitis

EPIDEMIOLOGY

Incidence

3.5–7.4/100,000 persons/year

Prevalence

- Seasonal variation: (e.g., arboviruses, enteroviruses, mumps, varicella)
- Nonseasonal: Most others (e.g., herpes simplex virus [HSV])

RISK FACTORS

- Age: Increased incidence in infants and elderly
- Contact with animals or insect vectors
- Impaired immune status
- Ingestions (e.g., raw meat)
- Occupation (e.g., lab or animal-care workers)
- Recreational activities (e.g., camping, hunting)
- Transfusion and transplantation
- Travel to endemic areas
- Recent vaccinations or unvaccinated status

GENERAL PREVENTION

- Appropriate clothing to protect against mosquitos
- Use of mosquito repellants (DEET, Picaridin)
- Avoidance and removal of ticks
- Elimination of mosquito breeding sources
- Vaccines, when available

PATHOPHYSIOLOGY

- Most common entry site is through the blood.
- Specific cell lines may be infected and are associated with specific symptom complexes:
  - Neurons: Associated with seizures
  - Oligodendroglia: May cause demyelination alone, cortical infection, or reactive parenchymal swelling; changes in state of consciousness
  - Brainstem neurons: Coma, respiratory failure
  - Microglia, macrophages: Neurologic dysfunction
- Pathologic changes seen with postinfectious and postvaccinal encephalomyelitis include perivascular infiltration of mononuclear inflammatory cells.

ETIOLOGY

- Vaccines have changed epidemiology in US.
- Despite extensive evaluations, the etiologic agent is frequently not identified (32–75%).
- Most commonly identified etiologies in US: HSV, West Nile, enteroviruses

COMMONLY ASSOCIATED CONDITIONS

- Seizures
- Hyperthermia
- Increased intracranial pressure (ICP)
- Inappropriate ADH

DIAGNOSIS

- Seek epidemiologic clues and assess risk factors in all patients with encephalitis (1)[A].
- Consider acute disseminated encephalomyelitis (ADEM) with history of recent infectious illness or vaccination associated with clinical presentation of encephalitis (2)[B].
- Specific diagnostic studies should be done in the majority of patients (see testing section) (2)[A].

HISTORY

General and specific neurological findings may include headache, fever, nausea/vomiting, altered consciousness

PHYSICAL EXAM

- General signs:
  - Rash
  - Mucus membrane lesions
  - Concurrent or prodromal upper respiratory findings
  - Parotitis
  - Erythema nodosum
- Neurologic findings:
  - Altered level of consciousness
  - Acute cognitive dysfunction
  - Behavioral changes
  - Neck stiffness
  - Focal neurologic signs
  - Motor weakness
- Other:
  - Loss of temperature or vasomotor control
  - Diabetes insipidus
  - Syndrome of inappropriate secretion of antidiuretic hormone

DIAGNOSTIC TESTS & INTERPRETATION

Lab

- Recommended general diagnostic studies for all suspected encephalitis patients (diagnostic studies outside of the CNS):
  - Blood cultures (2)[B]
  - Serum samples: Should be obtained at time of initial presentation and stored for future studies
- Additional studies based on risk factors and clinical findings may include:
  - Cultures of stool, nasopharynx, sputum (2)[B]
  - Skin scrapings of active vesicles (DFA testing to identify viral antigen)
  - Biopsy of specific tissues with culture, antigen detection, nucleic acid amplification testing and histology (2)[A]
  - Serologic testing: IgM antibodies (2)[A], IgM and IgG capture ELISAs
  - Plaque reduction neutralization
  - Acute and convalescent-phase serum to show seroconversion: Not helpful to initiate therapy but may be helpful for the retrospective diagnosis of a specific pathogen (2)[B]
  - Serum IgG antibodies should be considered in patients where the encephalitis may be the result of reactivation of a previously acquired infection.
  - Nucleic acid amplification tests (such as PCR) (2)[B]

Initial lab tests

- Lumbar puncture is essential (unless specific contraindication) (2)[A]:
  - CSF shows pleocytosis (10–2,000 cells/mm^3). Mononuclear cells usually predominate. Finding of CSF eosinophils may suggest certain pathogens (e.g., highest with helminths but can also be seen with other pathogens).
  - CSF glucose normal or mildly depressed
  - CSF protein usually mild or moderately increased
  - Direct examination of CSF fluid with Gram stain for bacteria, acid fast stain for *Mycobacteria*, by India ink for *Cryptococcus*, wet preparation for free living amoeba, Giemsa stain for trypanosomes
  - CSF culture for bacteria, mycobacteria, fungi, amoeba, and viruses
  - CSF culture for viruses has limited value; not routinely recommended
  - CSF nucleic acid amplification tests (e.g., PCR) (2)[A]; herpes simplex PCR should be performed on all specimens (2)[A]; if negative, consider repeat in 3–7 days in those with compatible clinical syndrome or temporal lobe localization on neuroimaging (2)[B]
  - Viral-specific IgM (2)[A]
- In up to 10% of cases with viral encephalitis, CSF findings are normal.

Follow-Up & Special Considerations

- PCR may be negative early on; repeat in 48–72 hours; may be useful in detecting herpesvirus, enterovirus, seasonal and 2009 H1N1 influenza virus, and polyomavirus.
- Rapid Influenza Diagnostic Tests (RIDTs) may be helpful in diagnosing seasonal and 2009 H1N1 in a clinically useful time frame. However, their sensitivity ranges from 10–70% and the currently available RIDTs cannot distinguish between the different influenza A subtypes (seasonal H1N1 vs. 2009 H1N1 vs H3N2).

Imaging

Initial approach

- MRI: Most sensitive and most specific; however, in some cases it may be normal either initially or during clinical course (3)[A].
- Diffusion-weighted imaging is superior to conventional MRI in encephalitis caused by herpes simplex, enterovirus, and West Nile virus.
- FLAIR (fluid attenuated inversion recovery) imaging may be helpful with enterovirus 71 encephalitis, flaviviruses, and Eastern equine encephalitis.
- CT, with and without contrast enhancement, if MRI not an option (2)[B]
- FDG-PET not routinely recommended, but may be helpful as an adjunct diagnostic tool

Follow-Up & Special Considerations

Imaging studies (e.g., CT, MRI, brain scan) may be normal early; later, nonspecific abnormalities may be seen (exception: herpes simplex encephalitis).

Diagnostic Procedures/Surgery
- CXR may be helpful
- EEG is nondiagnostic but may be useful in early herpes simplex encephalitis and less commonly in other herpes viruses (VAV, EBV, HHV6). It is recommended for all patients with encephalitis (2)[A].
- Serologic testing
- Brain biopsy: Rarely used and not routinely recommended. Consider in patients with encephalitis of unknown etiology whose condition is deteriorating despite treatment with acyclovir (2)[B].

Pathological Findings
- Prominent inflammatory reaction in meninges and in a perivascular distribution
- Swelling and degenerative changes of neural elements

DIFFERENTIAL DIAGNOSIS
- Vasculitis
- Paraneoplastic syndromes
- Postinfectious encephalitis
- Postimmunization encephalitis
- ADEM
- Secondary encephalopathy

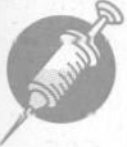

TREATMENT

- Most will require intensive care.
- Initial empiric therapy includes prompt administration of intravenous acyclovir (unless there is a contraindication).
- When appropriate, combine with appropriate therapy for bacterial, rickettsial, or ehrlichial infection.
- Once an etiologic agent has been identified, therapeutic intervention should be reevaluated, focusing on pathogen specific therapy and discontinuing therapy if there is no available therapy against the specific etiologic agent.

MEDICATION
- No specific drug therapy is available for most types of viral encephalitis.
- Antiviral agents are available for encephalitides caused by herpes viruses, especially HSV, and for both seasonal and 2009 H1N1 influenza viruses.
- Acyclovir is recommended as initial treatment for all patients with suspected encephalitis as soon as possible, pending results of diagnostic studies (2)[A].
- Appropriate antiviral therapy (i.e., Oseltamivir or Zanamivir) should be started as soon as possible for hospitalized patients with neurologic symptoms and suspected seasonal or 2009 H1N1 influenza infection (4)[C].
- Empiric antimicrobial therapy should be initiated if indicated by the clinical history or specific epidemiologic factors (2)[A].
- Doxycycline should be added to empiric regimen when clinical clues suggest rickettsial or ehrlichial infection (2)[A].
- Once etiology is determined, treat specifically.

ADDITIONAL TREATMENT
General Measures
- Supportive therapy
- Monitoring for drug-related toxicities

Issues for Referral
- Monitoring and management of ICP
- Evaluation and treatment of seizures
- Multidisciplinary teams often provide care.

Additional Therapies
Adjunctive agents: Limited data; consider risks and benefits; infectious disease consultation should be considered.
- IFN alpha: Tried with West Nile virus encephalitis; results inconclusive
- IFN alpha 2b (limited series): Reduce severity and duration of complications of St. Louis *encephalitis virus meningoencephalitis* (further studies are necessary).
- Intravenous immunoglobulin containing high anti–West Nile virus antibody titers in patients with West Nile virus nueroinvasive disease (in trial)

SURGERY/OTHER PROCEDURES
The following procedures may be required during stabilization and care:
- Intracranial pressure monitor
- Intubation
- Mechanical ventilation
- Central line for hemodynamic monitoring
- Arterial line
- Central line for total parenteral nutrition
- Nasogastric tube placement
- Foley catheter placement

IN-PATIENT CONSIDERATIONS
- Admit suspected cases of encephalitis to hospital for evaluation, supportive care, and treatment. Most will require intensive care services.
- Although standard isolation precautions are appropriate for most viral encephalitides, droplet precautions are necessary for patients with confirmed or suspected seasonal or 2009 H1N1 influenza infection.

Initial Stabilization
- Protect airway when appropriate.
- When indicated:
  - Supplemental oxygen
  - Intubation and mechanical ventilatory support
- Assessment and management of circulatory status, fluids, glucose, and electrolytes
- Precautions for seizure and altered mental status
- Consider isolation for immunosuppressed patients and those with exanthems.

Admission Criteria
- Suspicion of encephalitis
- Altered level of consciousness
- Need for intensive monitoring
- Need for airway protection, cardiopulmonary support

IV Fluids
- Monitor glucose, chemistries, and fluid balance
- Monitor for SIADH
- Monitor for drug-specific toxicities

Nursing
- Isolation should be considered for immunosuppressed patients and those with exanthems.
- Precautions for seizure and altered mental status
- Comfort measures to reduce headache
- Injury prevention and safety
- Monitor level of consciousness, neurologic signs, cardiorespiratory parameters, and fluid balance.
- Establish and maintain open lines of communication with patient and family.
- Educate families about the importance of vaccines when available and postexposure prophylaxis for seasonal or 2009 H1N1 influenza virus.
- Skin care to prevent decubitus ulcers

Discharge Criteria
Resolution of acute symptoms:
- No longer need hospital-level care
- Outpatient services in place if needed

ONGOING CARE

Patients with suspected or proven encephalitis are best cared for, at least initially, in an intensive care unit.

FOLLOW-UP RECOMMENDATIONS
- Postencephalitis sequelae are primarily neurologic, and follow-up should be guided by patient's condition (e.g., anticonvulsants for seizures).
- Physical therapy may be necessary.

Patient Monitoring
Postencephalitis patients should be followed carefully after discharge. Specialty services and follow-up may be required.

DIET
Guided by clinical condition

PATIENT EDUCATION
- DEET-containing mosquito repellants
- Avoidance of outdoor activities during periods of peak mosquito activity
- Use of protective clothing
- Adequate vector control and environmental sanitation
- Vaccines when available
- http://www.mayoclinic.com/health/encephalitis/DS00226

PROGNOSIS
Often difficult to predict; prognosis related to etiologic agent, age, and clinical course

COMPLICATIONS
Vary with age, etiologic agent, and clinical course

REFERENCES

1. Hinson VK, Tyor WR. Update on viral encephalitis. *Curr Opin Neurol*. 2001;14:369–74.
2. Mandell G, et al. *Principles & Practice of Infectious Diseases*, 6th ed. New York: Elsevier, 2005: 1143–7.
3. Chaudhuri A, Kennedy PG. Diagnosis and treatment of viral encephalitis. *Postgrad Med J*. 2002;78:575–83.
4. CDC. Neurologic Complications Associated with Novel Influenza A (H1N1) Virus Infection in Children — Dallas, Texas, May 2009. *MMWR* 2009;58:773–8.

CODES

ICD9
049.9 Unspecified non-arthropod-borne viral diseases of central nervous system

CLINICAL PEARLS

- Neurologic signs are unlikely to distinguish etiologies, but location and type of skin lesions may be helpful.
- Think of ADEM if there is a history of recent mild viral illness.

E

ENCOPRESIS

Jay Gar-Yee Fong, MD
William T. Garrison, PhD

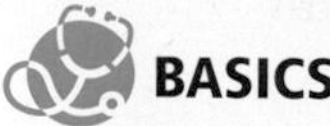

BASICS

DESCRIPTION

- The involuntary or intentional passage of feces into clothing or other inappropriate places by a child 4–18 years of age:
  Age may be chronologic or developmental.
  - Absence of underlying organic process explaining these symptoms
  - At least 1 event per month for 3 months
  - Classified into functional constipation (retentive encopresis) and functional nonretentive fecal incontinence (FNRFI): Both cause fecal incontinence, but no constipation in FNRFI. Functional constipation more common.
- System(s) affected: GI; Psychological
- Synonyms(s): Fecal incontinence

EPIDEMIOLOGY

Incidence

Predominant sex: Male > Female (3:1). Constipation accounts for 3% of general pediatric referrals; up to 84% of constipated children have fecal incontinence at some point.

Prevalence

1–3% of children >4 years of age

RISK FACTORS

- Male gender
- Constipation
- Very low birth weight
- Painful defecation
- Difficulty with bowel training, including pressure related to early daycare placement
- Organic/anatomic causes
- Anxiety and depression

Genetics

None known, although incidence may be higher in children with family history of constipation

GENERAL PREVENTION

Family education regarding constipation, avoid toilet training prior to readiness, optimal feeding, early detection of problems. Look for signs of relapse: Large-caliber stools, decrease in stool frequency, and soiling.

PATHOPHYSIOLOGY

- In 90% of cases, encopresis develops as a consequence of chronic constipation with resulting overflow incontinence, which typically is termed *retentive encopresis*. The other 10% are caused by specific organic etiologies.
- Chronic constipation due to irregular and incomplete evacuation results in progressive rectal distension and stretching of both the internal and external anal sphincters.
- As the child habituates to chronic rectal distension, he or she may no longer sense the normal urge to defecate. Eventually, soft or liquid stool begins to leak around the retained fecal mass, resulting in fecal soiling.
- Many children voluntarily withhold stool in response to the urge to defecate for fear of pain.

ETIOLOGY

- Psychological:
  - Stool withholding, fear, anxiety
  - Difficulty with toilet training, including unusual anxiety or conflict with parent
  - Resistance to using public toilet facilities, such as school bathrooms or outdoor toilets
  - Known association with sexual abuse in boys; likely similar association in girls as well
  - Developmental delay
- Anatomic:
  - Rectal distension and desensitization
  - Anal fissure or painful defecation
  - Muscle hypotonia
  - Slow intestinal motility
  - Hirschsprung disease
  - Cystic fibrosis
  - Spinal cord defects, e.g., spina bifida
  - Congenital anorectal malformations
  - Anal stenosis
  - Anterior displacement of the anus
  - Postoperative stricture of anus or rectum
  - Pelvic mass
  - Neurofibromatosis
- Dietary or metabolic:
  - Lack of fiber
  - Excessive protein or milk intake
  - Inadequate water intake
  - Hypothyroidism
  - Hypercalcemia
  - Hypokalemia
  - DI or DM
  - Food allergy
  - Gluten enteropathy
- Medication side effects

COMMONLY ASSOCIATED CONDITIONS

- Constipation (common)
- Developmental and behavioral diagnoses
- Cerebral palsy (intermediate)
- Cystic fibrosis (intermediate)
- Hirschsprung disease (common)
- Urinary incontinence

DIAGNOSIS

HISTORY

- Look for signs/symptoms of constipation:
  - Hard, large-caliber stools
  - <3 defecations/week
  - Pain or discomfort with stool passage, withholding of stool
  - Blood on stools
  - Decreased appetite
  - Abdominal pain improving with stool passage
  - Hiding while defecating before child is toilet trained; avoiding use of the toilet
  - Diet low in fiber or fluids, high in dairy
  - Passed stool within 1st 48 h of life
  - Pasty stool found on underclothes
  - Recurrent UTIs
- Abrupt onset after age 5 years more likely to be associated with psychological trauma
- Overlap with ADD common in children >5 years of age
- Medications such as opiates, phenobarbital, and TCAs
- Family history of constipation

PHYSICAL EXAM

- Detailed history and physical exam usually make the diagnosis without need for lab testing.
- Neurologic exam of lower extremities and perineal area with attention to S1–S4 distribution, perineal sensation, cremasteric reflex, and anal sphincter tone
- Genital area
- Digital rectal exam: Assess for anal fissures, sphincter tone, rectal distension/impaction, presence of occult or visible blood
- Abdominal exam: Mild abdominal distension; palpable stool in left lower quadrant.

DIAGNOSTIC TESTS & INTERPRETATION

Lab

Most cases of fecal incontinence do not require extensive lab work.

Initial lab tests

Done to rule out organic causes when conventional treatment fails: UA/urine culture: UTI/glucosuria; Thyroid function tests: Hypothyroidism; electrolyte panel including calcium may show hypokalemia, hypercalcemia, or hyperglycemia

Follow-Up & Special Considerations

Failure to pass meconium within 48 h of birth, failure to thrive, bloody diarrhea, or bilious vomiting in neonate is almost always associated with aganglionic megacolon, and that history would warrant a barium enema and/or rectal biopsy. Constipation and diarrhea, rash, failure to thrive, or recurrent pneumonia should prompt evaluation for cystic fibrosis. Celiac disease should also be a consideration. Patients with abdominal distension or ileus should be evaluated for possible obstruction.

Imaging

Abdominal plain films may be useful if an impaction is suspected but not detected by abdominal or rectal exam.

Initial approach

Comprehensive history and physical exam. Management includes education, disimpaction if necessary, prevention, and follow-up.

Diagnostic Procedures/Surgery

Manometric studies may be useful in patients who have constipation that does not respond to treatment.

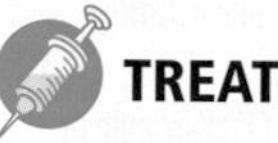

TREATMENT

A treatment approach that integrates both laxative treatment and behavioral therapy improves continence in children with fecal incontinence over laxative treatment alone (1).

MEDICATION

- Remove stool impaction, then start maintenance treatment program.
- No randomized, controlled studies have compared methods of disimpaction: Can use oral agents, enemas, and rectal suppositories; oral agents least traumatic. Glycerin suppositories best option for infants.

First Line

- Disimpaction with PEG has been shown to be more effective than lactulose in 1 study (2)[B]:

- Give 17 g (240 mL) water or juice: 1–1.5 g/kg/d × 3 days for disimpaction
- 0.26–0.084 g/kg/d for maintenance

- Disimpaction with mineral oil for child >1 year also effective; give 15–30 mL/year of age to maximum of 240 mL:
  - Maintenance: 1–3 mL/kg/d or divided b.i.d.
  - May mix with orange juice to make palatable; *avoid in infants to avoid aspiration and lipoid pneumonia*
- Other maintenance regimens include:
  - Milk of magnesia (MOM) 400 mg (5 mL): 103 mL/kg/d b.i.d. (3)[A]
  - Lactulose 10 g (15 mL) 1–3 mL/kg/d b.i.d.
  - Senna syrup 8.8 g sennoside (5 mL): Age 2–6 years: 2.5–7.5 mL/d b.i.d.; age 6–12 years: 5–15 mL/d b.i.d.
  - Bisacodyl suppository 10 mg: 0.5–1 suppository once or twice per day

Second Line
Another disimpaction protocol is as follows:
- Give 1 oz (28.4 g) of mineral oil the 1st day.
- On the next day, give 1–3 enemas until clear; this may be repeated over the next 1–2 days.
- Give an oil-retention enema.
- Follow the oil-retention enema with hypophosphate enemas (e.g., sodium phosphate [Fleet] 1 oz [28.4 g] per 20 lb [9.1 kg]) of body weight *or*
- Normal saline enemas: 2 tsp table salt/qt (946 mL) of warm water, and give 2 oz (60 mL)/year of age to a maximum of 16 oz (480 mL)

ADDITIONAL TREATMENT
General Measures
- Anticipatory guidance relative to toilet training beginning at 18 months, with special attention to when children should reduce reliance on diapers or pull-ups during the daytime hours
- Eliminate impaction prior to maintenance Rx.
- Avoid frequent and repeated rectal exams, enemas, and suppositories, especially in infants.
- Once stools seem regular in frequency, child should sit on toilet b.i.d. at the same time each day for 10–15 minutes and for 10–15 minutes after meals. Incorporate positive reinforcement for successfully produced bowel movements.

Issues for Referral
If symptoms do not improve after 6 months of good compliance with a multifactorial treatment model, refer to pediatric GI for further evaluation.

Additional Therapies
Behavioral treatment and counseling

COMPLEMENTARY AND ALTERNATIVE MEDICINE
- Behavioral treatment is recommended as an adjunct to medical therapy in children with functional constipation (4)[A].
- Children who receive behavioral treatment in addition to medications are more likely to have resolution of encopresis at 3 and 6 months than children who get medication alone.
- Biofeedback is not recommended because it does not improve outcomes when it is combined with medical therapy for functional constipation in children (1)[B].

SURGERY/OTHER PROCEDURES
Some children who have ongoing constipation that is refractory to a combination of medical and behavioral therapy should be considered for evaluation with anorectal manometry to evaluate for internal anal sphincter achalasia (or ultrashort-segment Hirschsprung's disease). If present, this condition can be treated successfully in the majority of patients with an internal sphincter myectomy.

IN-PATIENT CONSIDERATIONS
Initial Stabilization
Hospital admission and abdominal films may be necessary to ensure complete removal of impaction. This may include gastric administration of balanced electrolyte–polyethylene glycol solutions if the patient cannot tolerate the medication by mouth. Serial abdominal films as well as careful observation of the rectal effluent can help to determine when the patient is adequately treated.

Admission Criteria
Admission criteria should include:
- Continued soiling and recurrent impaction on outpatient medical therapy, whether from lack of medication efficacy or patient medication nonadherence
- Decreased p.o. intake for fluid and food
- Vomiting or obstructive-type symptoms

IV Fluids
IV fluids should be considered when the pediatric patient is heading toward dehydration while undergoing bowel cleanout.

Nursing
Nursing is essential to observing and documenting the stool consistency and clarity.

Discharge Criteria
Stools that are becoming more loose in consistency and clear in appearance would signify a successful inpatient endpoint for discharge consideration. In addition, an abdominal radiograph that shows much less fecal loading as compared with a pretreatment radiograph in combination with serial abdominal exams can provide additional evidence that the patient is ready for discharge.

ONGOING CARE

FOLLOW-UP RECOMMENDATIONS
Patient Monitoring
- Continue the maintenance treatment program for at least 6 months, possibly 1–2 years.
- Visits every 4–10 weeks for support and to ensure compliance; more often with oppositional or anxious children.
- Telephone availability to adjust doses and to provide continued encouragement to caregivers
- Treat redevelopment of impaction promptly.
- Chief target behaviors in a behavior plan for such children include compliance with medication, compliance with sits, and self-initiation of bathroom visits.
- Children who do not progress with a well-designed behavior plan should be referred for more in-depth mental health evaluation and counseling.

DIET
Hydration, high fiber, decrease or avoid cow's milk products if a trial shows this to be helpful. Avoid excessive bananas, rice, apples, and gelatin.

PATIENT EDUCATION
- Education and demystifying of the process
- Careful and full explanation of the treatment plan and dietary changes
- Avoid punishment for soiling.
- In children >4 years of age, explain to parents how overreliance on diapers and pull-ups, while convenient, can prolong the problem.
- Always attempt to use positive reinforcement 1st for successful toilet sits and medication compliance.
- If positive approach is unsuccessful, consider removing daily desired privileges (e.g., TV, video games, time with friends, etc.) for noncompliance with behavioral plan. Some children respond better to use of a token economy (chips or tickets to earn privileges the child desires).

PROGNOSIS
- Initial good response with a high relapse rate due to noncompliance by parents and/or child
- Depending on the study, anywhere from 30–50% of children still may have encopresis after 5 years of treatment.
- Children with psychosocial or emotional problems that preceded the encopresis are more recalcitrant to treatment.

COMPLICATIONS
- Colitis due to excessive enema/suppository
- Perianal dermatitis
- Anal fissure

E

REFERENCES

1. Brazzelli M, et al. Behavioural and cognitive interventions with or without other treatments for the management of faecal incontinence in children. *Cochrane Database Syst Rev*. 2008;3:CD002240.
2. Loening-Baucke V, Pashankar DS. A randomized, prospective, comparison study of polyethylene glycol 3350 without electrolytes and milk of magnesia for children with constipation and fecal incontinence. *Pediatrics*. 2006;118:528–35.
3. Baker S, et al. Evaluation and the treatment of constipation in infants and children: Recommendation of the north American Society for Pediatric Gastroenterology, Hepatology, and Nutrition. *J Pediatr Gastroenterol Nutr*. 2006; 43e1–13.
4. Borowitz SM, et al. Treatment of childhood encopresis: A randomized trial comparing 3 treatment protocols. *J Ped Gastroenterol Nutr*. 2002;34:378–84.

CODES

ICD9
- 307.7 Encopresis
- 787.60 Full incontinence of feces
- 787.62 Fecal smearing

CLINICAL PEARLS

Most children (84%) with constipation have some fecal incontinence, but diagnosis of encopresis requires at least 1 event per month for 3 months. 90% of encopresis results from chronic constipation. Address toddler constipation early (decrease excessive milk intake, increase fruits/vegetables) to avoid future issues.

ENDOCARDITIS, INFECTIVE

William L. Marshall, MD

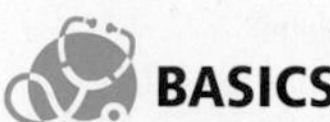

BASICS

DESCRIPTION

- An infection primarily of the valvular endocardium; and occasionally, the mural endocardium
- System(s) affected: Cardiovascular; Endocrine/Metabolic; Hematologic/Lymphatic; Immunologic; Pulmonary; Renal/Urologic; Skin/Exocrine; Neurologic
- Synonym(s): Bacterial endocarditis; Subacute bacterial endocarditis; Acute bacterial endocarditis

EPIDEMIOLOGY

Incidence

In the US: 1.5–6.2/100,000

Geriatric Considerations

- Incidence increased in the elderly
- Cumulative rate of endocarditis at 1 year after prosthetic valve replacement: 1.5–3.0%
- At 5 years: 3–6%
- Highest risk during 6-month period following valve replacement

RISK FACTORS

- Injection drug use
- IV catheterization
- Certain malignancies (colon cancer)
- High-risk cardiac conditions:
  - Prosthetic cardiac valve
  - Previous infective endocarditis (IE)
  - Congenital heart disease (CHD):
    - Unrepaired cyanotic CHD, including palliative shunts and conduits
    - Repaired CHD with prosthetic device during the prior 6 months
    - Repaired CHD with residual defects at or near the site of prosthetic material
    - Cardiac transplantation recipients who develop valvulopathy (1)[B]

GENERAL PREVENTION

- Maintain good oral hygiene.
- Antibiotic prophylaxis is now only recommended for people with cardiac conditions predicting the highest risk of adverse outcome from IE (1).
- Procedures requiring prophylaxis:
  - Oral/upper respiratory tract: Manipulation of gingival tissue or periapical region of teeth or perforation of the oral mucosa (1)[C], invasive respiratory procedures involving incision, or biopsy of the respiratory mucosa:
    - Prophylaxis for dental/oral procedures (1)[C]
  - Amoxicillin: 2 g PO (if penicillin-allergic, clindamycin 600 mg PO) 30–60 min before procedure
  - Alternative: Ampicillin 2 g IV/IM (penicillin-allergic patients, clindamycin 600 mg IV), *or*
  - Cephalexin 2 g PO, *or*
  - Azithromycin/clarithromycin 500 mg PO, *or*
  - Cefazolin/ceftriaxone 1 g IV/IM 30 minutes before procedure
  - Pediatric doses: Amoxicillin 50 mg/kg PO; cephalexin 50 mg/kg PO; clindamycin 20 mg/kg PO; and ampicillin or ceftriaxone 50 mg/kg IM/IV
  - GI/GU: Only consider coverage for enterococcus (with penicillin, ampicillin, piperacillin, or vancomycin) for patients with an established infection undergoing procedures (1)[B].
  - Cardiac valvular surgery or placement of prosthetic intracardiac/intravascular materials (1)[B], perioperative prophylaxis with cefazolin 1–2 g IV 30 min preop, or vancomycin 15 mg/kg 60 min preop in the penicillin-allergic patient
  - Skin: Incision and drainage of infected tissue; patients should receive treatment with agents active against skin pathogens, e.g., cefazolin 1–2 g IV q8h or vancomycin 15 mg/kg q12h in the penicillin-allergic patient or where MRSA is suspected.

ETIOLOGY

- Acute endocarditis:
  - Gram-positive: *Staphylococcus aureus; Streptococcus* groups A, B, C, G; *Streptococcus pneumoniae; Staphylococcus lugdunensis; Enterococcus* spp.
  - Gram-negative: *Haemophilus influenzae* or *parainfluenzae; Neisseria gonorrhoeae*
- Subacute endocarditis:
  - Gram-positive: α-Hemolytic streptococci (Viridans group strep), *Streptococcus bovis, Enterococcus* spp., *S. aureus, Staphylococcus epidermidis*
  - HACEK organisms: ***H****aemophilus aphrophilus* or *paraphrophilus,* ***A****ctinobacillus actinomycetemcomitans,* ***C****ardiobacterium hominis,* ***E****ikenella corrodens,* ***K****ingella kingae*
- Endocarditis in IV drug abusers (tricuspid valve):
  - Gram-positive: *S. aureus, Enterococcus* spp.
  - Gram-negative: *Pseudomonas aeruginosa, Burkholderia cepacia*, other bacilli
  - *Candida* spp.
- Early prosthetic-valve endocarditis (<60 days after valve implantation):
  - Gram-positive: *S. aureus, Staphylococcus epidermidis*
  - Gram-negative bacilli
  - Fungi: *Candida* spp., *Aspergillus* spp.
- Late prosthetic-valve endocarditis (>60 days after valve implantation):
  - Gram-positive: α-Hemolytic streptococci, *Enterococcus* spp., *S. epidermidis*
  - Fungi: *Candida* spp., *Aspergillus* spp.
- Culture-negative endocarditis:
  - *Bartonella quintana* (homeless people)
  - *Bartonella henselae* (cat owners)
  - Fastidious organism: *Brucella* spp., fungi, *Coxiella burnetii* (Q fever), *Chlamydia trachomatis, Chlamydia psittaci*, HACEK organisms
  - Use of antibiotics prior to blood cultures
  - Abiotrophia (formerly B_6 deficient streptococci)

DIAGNOSIS

- Modified Duke Criteria for Diagnosis of IE (2)[B] (definite: 2 major criteria, or 1 major and 3 minor criteria, or 5 minor criteria; possible: 1 major and 1 minor criteria, or 3 minor criteria)
- Major clinical criteria:
  - Positive blood culture:
    - Typical microorganism for infective endocarditis (viridans strep., *S. aureus*, or community-acquired *Enterococcus*) from 2 separate blood cultures, *or*
    - Persistently positive blood culture
  - Single positive blood culture for *C. burnetii* or anti–phase-1 IgG antibody titer >1:800
  - Positive transesophageal echocardiogram recommended with prosthetic valves and "possible IE," or with complicated IE):
    - Oscillating mass on valve or supporting structures, in the path of regurgitant jets, on implanted material, *or*
    - Periannular abscess, or
    - New partial dehiscence of prosthetic valve
  - New valvular regurgitation (change in preexisting murmur not sufficient)
- Minor criteria:
  - Predisposing heart condition or IV-drug use
  - Fever ≥38.0°C (100.4°F)
  - Vascular phenomena: Major arterial emboli, septic pulmonary infarcts, mycotic aneurysm, intracranial hemorrhage, conjunctival hemorrhage, Janeway lesions
  - Immunologic phenomena: Glomerulonephritis, Osler nodes, Roth spots, rheumatoid factor
  - Microbiologic evidence: Positive blood culture, but not of major criterion (excluding single positive cultures for coagulase-negative staphylococci and organisms that do not cause endocarditis) or serologic evidence of infection with an organism likely to cause infective endocarditis

DIAGNOSTIC TESTS & INTERPRETATION

Lab

- Positive blood cultures drawn >2 hours apart
- Leukocytosis in acute endocarditis
- Anemia in subacute endocarditis
- Elevated ESR, CRP
- Decreased C3, C4, CH50 in subacute endocarditis
- Hematuria, microscopic or macroscopic
- Rheumatoid factor in subacute endocarditis
- Consider serologies for *Chlamydia*, Q fever, and *Bartonella* in "culture-negative" endocarditis.

Imaging

- Transthoracic or transesophageal echocardiogram
- CT scan may be useful in locating abscesses (e.g., splenic abscess).

Pathological Findings

- Vegetations are composed of platelets, fibrin, and colonies of microorganisms. Destruction of valvular endocardium, perforation of valve leaflets, rupture of chordae tendineae, abscesses of myocardium, rupture of sinus of Valsalva, and pericarditis may occur.
- Emboli, infarction, abscesses, and/or infarction may be found in any organ.
- Immune-complex glomerulonephritis

DIFFERENTIAL DIAGNOSIS

- Marantic endocarditis; Connective tissue diseases; Fever of unknown origin
- Intra-abdominal infections; Rheumatic fever; Salmonellosis
- Malignancy; Tuberculosis; Atrial myxoma; Septic thrombophlebitis; Infected central venous catheter

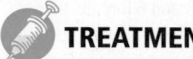

TREATMENT

MEDICATION

First Line

- PCN-susceptible Viridans group streptococci or *S. bovis*, native valve:
  - Pen G 12–18 million U/d IV either continuously or in 4–6 equally divided doses *or* ceftriaxone 2 g/d IV/IM in 1 dose, both for 4 weeks (3)[A]

– For prosthetic valve infection, Pen G 24 million units/d IV either continuously or 4–6 equally divided doses for 6 weeks *or* ceftriaxone 2 g/d IV/IM in 1 dose ± gentamicin 3 mg/kg IV/IM q24h for 2 weeks (peak gentamicin level 3 mcg/ml and trough <1 mcg/ml)

- PCN-resistant Viridans group streptococci or *S. bovis*, native valve:
  – Pen G 24 million U/d IV either continuously or in 6 equally divided doses *or*ceftriaxone 2 g/d IV/IM in 1 dose for 4 weeks plus gentamicin 3 mg/kg IV/IM q24h for 2 weeks (peak gentamicin level 3 mcg/ml and trough <1 mcg/ml) (3)[B]
  – Regimen for prosthetic valve infection is equivalent, but length of therapy is 6 weeks for all antibiotics.
- *Staphylococcus* on native valve:
  – Oxacillin-sensitive: Oxacillin or nafcillin 2 g IV q4h for 4–6 weeks. Use of gentamicin 1 mg/kg q8h IV/IM for the 1st 3–5 days does not improve survival and increases the chance of nephrotoxicity (4).
  – Oxacillin-resistant: Vancomycin 15 mg/kg/d IV q12h for 6 weeks for goal trough of 15–20 mcg/ml (3)[B]
- Daptomycin may also be considered for continued outpatient therapy (5).
- *Staphylococcus* of prosthetic valve:
  – Oxacillin-sensitive: Oxacillin or nafcillin 12 g/d IV in 6 equally divided doses plus rifampin 300 mg IV/PO q8h, for 6 weeks, plus gentamicin 1 mg/kg q8h IV/IM for the 1st 2 weeks (peak gentamicin level 3 mcg/ml and trough <1 mcg/ml) (3)[B]
  – Oxacillin-resistant: Vancomycin 15 mg/kg IV q12h, plus rifampin 300 mg IV/PO q8h, both for 6 weeks, plus gentamicin 3 mg/kg/d IV/IM in 2–3 doses for the 1st 2 weeks (peak gentamicin level 3 mcg/ml and trough <1 mcq/ml) (3)[B]
- Pan-sensitive *Enterococcus*, native or prosthetic valve: Ampicillin 2g IV q4h *OR*Pen G 18–30 million units/d IV either continuously or in 6 equally divided doses, plus gentamicin 1 mg/kg IV q8h for 4–6 weeks (peak gentamicin level 3 mcg/ml and trough <1 mcg/ml) (3)[A] Consider expert consultation for resistant enterococci.
- HACEK organisms: Ceftriaxone 2 g IM or IV q24h for 4 weeks (3)[B] *OR* ampicillin-sulbactam 2g IV q6h for 4 weeks (3)[B] *OR* Ciprofloxacin 1 g/d PO or 800 mg/d IV in 2 equally divided doses for 4 weeks (3)[C]
- Precautions:
  – In patients with renal impairment, dosage adjustment should be made for penicillin G, gentamicin, cefazolin, ampicillin, ampicillin/sulbactam, ciprofloxacin, and vancomycin.
  – Rapid infusion of vancomycin <1 hour may cause "red-man syndrome; due to histamine release, not an allergic reaction; will disappear when rate of infusion is reduced.
- Significant possible interactions:
  – Vancomycin plus gentamicin increases renal toxicity.
  – Rifampin increases the requirement for Coumadin and oral hypoglycemic agents.

Second Line

For patients allergic to penicillin:

- Penicillin-susceptible or resistant Viridans group streptococci or *S. bovis*: Vancomycin 30 mg/kg (not to exceed 2 g/d) IV for 4 weeks (6 weeks for prosthetic valve endocarditis) for goal trough of 10–15 mcg/ml (3)[B]
- *Enterococcus*, native or prosthetic valve: Desensitization to penicillin should be considered. Vancomycin15 mg/kg (usual dose, 1 g) IV q12h, plus gentamicin or streptomycin (peak gentamicin level 3 mcg/ml and trough <1 mcg/ml) for 4–6 weeks (6 weeks for prosthetic valve endocarditis) (3)[B].
- *Staphylococcus* of native valve: Cefazolin 2 g IV q8h (not to be used in patients with immediate-type hypersensitivity to penicillin) for 4–6 weeks (3)[B] *OR* vancomycin 30 mg/kg (usual dose, 1 g) IV q12h for a goal trough of 15–20 mcg/ml, for 6 weeks (3)[B]

SURGERY/OTHER PROCEDURES

Surgical therapy (i.e., valve replacement) should be considered for:

- CHF due to valve incompetence (3)[B]
- Embolic event in 1st 2 weeks of antibiotic therapy (3)[B] and stroke if hemorrhage has been excluded (6)[B]
- Persistent bacteremia after 1 week of antibiotic therapy or infection caused by resistant organisms (e.g., fungus, *Pseudomonasaeruginosa*, S. *marcescens*) (3)[B], *S. aureus* on a prosthetic valve, or most cases of relapsing IE (6)[B]
- Valve dehiscence, perforation, rupture or fistula, heart block, or large perivalvular abscess (3,7)[B]. Anterior mitral valve leaflet vegetation >10 mm in size, persistent vegetation after systemic embolization (3)[B], or increase in vegetation size despite antibiotic therapy (3,7)[C]
- Early prosthetic valve IE (6)[B]

ONGOING CARE

FOLLOW-UP RECOMMENDATIONS

Patient Monitoring

- Check gentamicin peak (~3 μg/mL) and trough (<1 μg/mL) levels if used for >5 days, and with renal dysfunction.
- Check vancomycin trough (15–20 μg/mL) levels in all patients (8)[B].
- Perform twice-weekly BUN and serum creatinine while on gentamicin.
- Consider audiometry baseline and follow-up during long-term aminoglycoside therapy.
- Baseline EKG, and monitor EKG for conduction disturbances/MI in initial weeks.
- TTE at the end of therapy
- Blood cultures q48h until negative

PROGNOSIS

Regardless of the mode of treatment, the mortality for IE remains high.

COMPLICATIONS

- Arterial emboli and infarcts (e.g., myocardial infarction, mesenteric, splenic, cerebral infarct)
- Infectious emboli (e.g., abscesses of heart, lung, brain, meninges, bone, pericardium)
- Inflammatory/immune disorders (e.g., arthritis, myositis, glomerulonephritis)
- Miscellaneous complications (e.g., CHF, ruptured valve cusp, sinus of Valsalva aneurysm, cardiac arrhythmia, intra- and extracranial mycotic aneurysms)

REFERENCES

1. Wilson W, et al. Prevention of infective endocarditis. Guidelines from the American Heart Association. A Guideline from the American Heart Association Rheumatic Fever, Endocarditis, and Kawasaki Disease Committee, Council on Cardiovascular Disease in the Young, and the Council on Cardiology, Council on Cardiovascular Surgery and Anesthesia, and the Quality of Care and Outcomes Research Interdisciplinary Working Group. *Circulation*. 2007; epub 19 Apr. 2007.
2. Li JS, Sexton DJ, Mick N, et al. Proposed modifications to the Duke criteria for the diagnosis of infective endocarditis. *Clin Infect Dis*. 2000;30:633–8.
3. Baddour LM, Wilson WR, Bayer AS, et al. Infective endocarditis: diagnosis, antimicrobial therapy, and management of complications: a statement for healthcare professionals from the Committee on Rheumatic Fever, Endocarditis, and Kawasaki Disease, Council on Cardiovascular Disease in the Young, and the Councils on Clinical Cardiology, Stroke, and Cardiovascular Surgery and Anesthesia, American Heart Association: endorsed by the Infectious Diseases Society of America. *Circulation*. 2005;111:e394–434.
4. Cosgrove SE, Vigliani GA, Campion M, et al. Initial Low-Dose Gentamicin for Staphylococcus aureus Bacteremia and Endocarditis Is Nephrotoxic. *Clin Infect Dis*. 2009.
5. Rehm S, Campion M, Katz DE, et al. Community-based outpatient parenteral antimicrobial therapy (CoPAT) for Staphylococcus aureus bacteraemia with or without infective endocarditis: analysis of the randomized trial comparing daptomycin with standard therapy. *J Antimicrob Chemother*. 2009.
6. Prendergast BD, Tornos P et al. Surgery for infective endocarditis: who and when? *Circulation*. 2010; 121:1141–52.
7. Paterick TE, Paterick TJ, Nishimura RA, et al. Complexity and subtlety of infective endocarditis. *Mayo Clin Proc*. 2007;82:615–21.
8. Rybak M, Lomaestro B, Rotschafer JC, et al. Therapeutic monitoring of vancomycin in adult patients: a consensus review of the American Society of Health-System Pharmacists, the Infectious Diseases Society of America, and the Society of Infectious Diseases Pharmacists. *Am J Health Syst Pharm*. 2009;66:82–98.

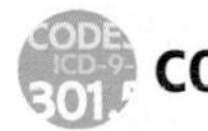

CODES

ICD9

421.0 Acute and subacute bacterial endocarditis

CLINICAL PEARLS

- Antibiotic prophylaxis is now only recommended for people with artificial heart valves, past history of IE, certain congenital heart diseases, and cardiac transplants with a heart-valve problem.
- Mitral valve prolapse by itself is no longer an indication for antibiotic prophylaxis.

E

ENDOMETRIAL CANCER AND UTERINE SARCOMA

Michael P. Hopkins, MD, MEd
Jonna M. Quinn, DO

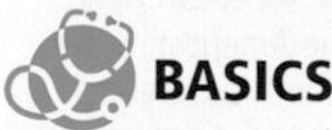

BASICS

DESCRIPTION

- Endometrial cancer: Malignancy of the endometrial lining of the uterus
  - Two types
    - I: estrogen dependent, lower grade, better prognosis
    - II: estrogen independent, higher grade, more aggressive
- Cell types: Adenocarcinoma, adenosquamous (malignant squamous elements), clear cell, and papillary serous
- Sarcomas: Malignancy of the uterine mesenchyme and mixed tumors:
  - Mixed müllerian sarcoma (carcinosarcoma): Heterologous sarcoma elements are not native to the müllerian system (e.g., cartilage or bone); homologous sarcoma elements are native to the müllerian system.
  - Endometrial stromal sarcoma develops from the stromal component of the endometrium.
  - Leiomyosarcoma develops in the myometrium or rarely in a myoma (fibroid).
  - Poorer prognosis
- Predominant age:
  - Endometrial cancer: The majority are postmenopausal
    - Median age: 66 years old
  - Sarcomas: Age 40–69 years old
- System(s): Reproductive
- Synonym(s): Uterine cancer; Endometrial cancer; Corpus cancer

Pregnancy Considerations

This malignancy is not associated with pregnancy.

EPIDEMIOLOGY

Incidence

- Most common gynecologic malignancy, 4th most common cancer in women, 8th leading cause of cancer-related death in women
- ~40,000 new cases per year and 7,000 deaths per year

Prevalence

500,000 women in the US

RISK FACTORS

- Early menarche/late menopause
- Nulliparity
- Personal or family history of colon or reproductive system cancer
- Obesity
- Diabetes mellitus
- Hypertension
- Polycystic ovarian syndrome
- Menstrual irregularities
- Endometrial hyperplasia
- Unopposed estrogens
- Tamoxifen
- Age
- Prior pelvic irradiation (sarcoma)

Genetics

- Endometrial: Lynch syndrome (hereditary nonpolyposis colorectal cancer)
- Sarcoma: African American

GENERAL PREVENTION

- In young women who are obese or anovulatory, the risk of endometrial cancer can be reduced by taking oral contraceptive pills, permanently losing weight, or taking cyclic progesterone to prevent unopposed estrogens effects on the uterus.
- Estrogen replacement therapy should always include progesterone unless the woman has undergone a hysterectomy.
- Cigarette smoking has been associated with a lower risk of endometrial cancer; however, it is not recommended secondary to its many health risks.

PATHOPHYSIOLOGY

Continuous estrogen stimulation unopposed by progesterone

ETIOLOGY

- Endometrial: Unopposed estrogen:
  - Estrogen replacement therapy without concomitant progesterone increases the risk. Addition of progesterone decreases risk to that of general population
- Sarcomas: Etiology unknown

COMMONLY ASSOCIATED CONDITIONS

- Endometrial Hyperplasia: 1–25% will progress to endometria adenocarcinoma
  - Simple without Atypia
  - Complex without Atypia
  - Simple with Atypia
  - Complex with Atypia
    - 43% with Complex Hyperplasia with Atypia have concurrent endometrial cancer
- Endometrial cancer patients should be screened regularly for breast and colon cancer because of an increased risk of these cancers.
- Patients who have breast or colon cancer are at increased risk for endometrial cancer.
- Granulosa cell tumors of the ovary produce estrogen; these patients will have an increased risk of endometrial cancer.

DIAGNOSIS

HISTORY

- Endometrial cancer:
  - Postmenopausal bleeding is the most frequent sign. Any spotting or abnormal discharge mandates evaluation.
- Sarcoma:
  - Mixed müllerian sarcoma: Bleeding and prolapsing tissue, pain
  - Leiomyosarcoma: Increasing size of presumed uterine myomas, pain

PHYSICAL EXAM

Pelvic exam: Enlarged uterus

DIAGNOSTIC TESTS & INTERPRETATION

Lab

Initial lab tests

- Liver and renal function tests
- Levels of cancer antigen 125 (CA-125) may be elevated when intra-abdominal disease is present.

Follow-Up & Special Considerations

- A biopsy of a pregnant uterus can produce tissue that looks hyperplastic or premalignant.
- Pap smear is rarely positive.

Imaging

Initial approach

- Transvaginal ultrasound usually shows increased endometrial thickness.
- CXR: Most common site of metastases is the lungs.
- Mammogram and colonoscopy: Endometrial cancer is associated with breast and colon cancer.

Follow-Up & Special Considerations

- CT scan, bone scan, liver spleen scan: Not part of the routine evaluation, but may be needed if suspected metastasis
- MRI has been reported to show the depth of myometrial penetration accurately but is not always cost effective.

Diagnostic Procedures/Surgery

- Office endometrial biopsy (90% accurate). If this is negative with high suspicion for cancer, a dilation and curettage is necessary. Endometrial stromal sarcoma and leiomyosarcoma are rarely diagnosed preoperatively.
- Fractional dilation and curettage is 99% accurate except in cases of sarcoma.
- Hysteroscopy may be associated with higher risk of positive washings/cytology – controversial

Pathological Findings

- Stage I (confined to corpus uteri):
  - A. No or less than half myometrial invasion
  - B. Invision equal to or more than half the myometrium
- Stage II: Tumor invades cervical stroma, but does not extend beyond the uterus
- Stage III: Local and/or regional spread
  - A. Uterine serosal and or adnexal invasion
  - B. Vaginal and/or parametrial involvement
  - C. Metastases to pelvic and/or para-aortic lymph nodes
    - IIIC1: +pelvic nodes
    - IIIC2: +para-aortic LN +/– positive pelvic lymph nodes
  - Stage IV: Tumor invades bladder and/or bowel mucosa, and or distant metastases
    - A. Tumor invades bladder and/or bowel mucosa,
    - B. Distant metastases, including intra-abdominal metastases and/or inguinal lymph nodes
- FIGO Staging System: revised 2009 (1)

DIFFERENTIAL DIAGNOSIS

- Atypical complex hyperplasia: A premalignant lesion of the endometrium
- Cervical cancer
- Ovarian cancer invading the uterus
- Endometriosis
- Adenomyosis

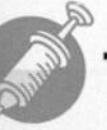

TREATMENT

MEDICATION

First Line

Endometrial:

- Chemotherapy for advanced or recurrent disease incurable with surgery and radiation (2,3)[A]:
  - Doxorubicin + Cisplatin + Paclitaxel
  - Paclitaxel + Carboplatin
- Hormonal therapy:
  - Medroxyprogesterone acetate: For recurrence or metastases (2)[A]
  - Megestrol (Megace) 160 mg/d for 3 months for women with premalignant lesions, atypical complex hyperplasia, or well-differentiated endometrial cancer patients desiring fertility. Follow with dilation and curettage to determine cancer resolution.
  - Levonorgestrel containing IUD: As above for patients desiring future fertility

- Sarcoma:
  - Chemotherapy:
    - Doxorubicin as single-agent or in combination (4)[A]
  - Hormonal:
    - Tamoxifen or aromatase inhibitors- not fully studied
    - Progesterones

Second Line

Ondansetron (Zofran), dronabinol (Marinol), metoclopramide (Reglan), and others to control nausea from chemotherapy

ADDITIONAL TREATMENT

General Measures

- Main treatment for uterine cancer is surgery
- Radiation is used to prevent tumor recurrence at the vaginal cuff.

Issues for Referral

Patients should be referred to gynecologic oncologist, radiation oncologist, and medical oncologist as indicated.

Additional Therapies

Radiation therapy:

- Nonoperative candidates: Radiation therapy alone (5)[A]
- Low-risk: No adjuvant radiation therapy (5)[A]
- Intermediate-risk: Consider adjuvant vaginal brachytherapy. Reduces local recurrences but has no effect on overall survival (5)[A].
- High-risk: Chemotherapy and radiation therapy in some cases.

SURGERY/OTHER PROCEDURES

Surgical staging:

- Extrafascial hysterectomy and bilateral salpingo-oophorectomy
- Cytologic washings
- Pelvic and para-aortic lymph node dissection
- Omental sampling as indicated
- Optimal tumor debulking

Geriatric Considerations

Older (especially obese) patients may be at high risk for surgery. Alternative radiation therapy can be considered.

IN-PATIENT CONSIDERATIONS

Admission Criteria

- Excessive vaginal bleeding
- Preoperative stabilization

Nursing

Routine; ensure postoperative pain is controlled.

Discharge Criteria

Postsurgical criteria: Pain controlled, tolerating diet, ambulating, and voiding

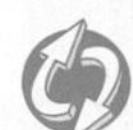

ONGOING CARE

FOLLOW-UP RECOMMENDATIONS

Speculum and rectovaginal exam every 3–4 months for 2–3 years then every 6 months for 3 years then annually for life

Patient Monitoring

CXR annually

DIET

As tolerated and according to comorbidities

PATIENT EDUCATION

Following surgery:

- No intercourse for ~6 weeks
- No lifting >10–15 lbs
- No driving until pain free
- Do not expect resumption of full activity for 6 weeks.

PROGNOSIS

5-year survival rates:

- Uterine Adenocarcinoma

Stage	Survival (%)
IA	88
IB	75
II	69
IIIA	58
IIIB	50
IIIC	47
IVA	17
IVB	15

- Uterine Sarcoma

Stage	Survival (%)
I	70
II	45
III	30
IV	15

COMPLICATIONS

- Surgical: Excessive bleeding, wound infection, lymphedema, DVT, and damage to the urinary or intestinal systems
- Radiation: Diarrhea, ileus, bowel obstruction or fistula, radiation cystitis, proctitis, vaginal stenosis, DVT
- Chemotherapy: Per the drug given

REFERENCES

1. Creasman W. Revised FIGO staging for carcinoma of the endometrium. *Int J Gynaecol Obstet*. 2009;105(2):109. Epub 2009 Apr 3. PubMed PMID: 19345353.
2. Polyzos NP, Pavlidis N, Paraskevaidis E, et al. Randomized evidence on chemotherapy and hormonal therapy regimens for advanced endometrial cancer: an overview of survival data. *Eur J Cancer*. 2006;42:319–26.
3. Fleming GF, Brunetto VL, Cella D, et al. Phase III trial of doxorubicin plus cisplatin with or without paclitaxel plus filgrastim in advanced endometrial carcinoma: a Gynecologic Oncology Group Study. *J Clin Oncol*. 2004;22:2159–66.
4. Bramwell VH, Anderson D, Charette ML, et al. Doxorubicin-based chemotherapy for the palliative treatment of adult patients with locally advanced or metastatic soft tissue sarcoma. *Cochrane Database Syst Rev*. 2003:CD003293.
5. Einhorn N, Tropé C, Ridderheim M., et al. A systematic overview of radiation therapy effects in uterine cancer (corpus uteri). *Acta Oncol*. 2003;42:557–61.

ADDITIONAL READING

- American Cancer Society, 2010 http://www.cancer.org.
- American College of Obstetricians & Gynecologists (ACOG), http://www.acog.com.
- American College of Obstetricians and Gynecologists. ACOG practice bulletin, clinical management guidelines for obstetrician-gynecologists, number 65, August 2005: management of endometrial cancer. *Obstet Gynecol*. 2005;106:413–25.
- Gadducci A, Cosio S, Romanini A, et al. et al. The management of patients with uterine sarcoma: A debated clinical challenge. *Crit Rev Oncol Hematol*. 2007.
- Humber C, et al. Chemotherapy for advanced, recurrent or metastatic endometrial carcinoma. *Cochrane Database Syst Rev*. 2005;(4):CD003915.

See Also (Topic, Algorithm, Electronic Media Element)

Cervical Malignancy
Algorithm: Pelvic Pain

CODES

ICD9

182.0 Malignant neoplasm of corpus uteri, except isthmus

CLINICAL PEARLS

- Most common presenting symptom is abnormal uterine bleeding.
- Primary cause is unopposed estrogen.
- Endometrial thickness on transvaginal ultrasound of less than 5 mm makes endometrial cancer very unlikely.
- Primary treatment is with surgery with possible chemotherapy ± radiation.

E

ENDOMETRIOSIS

Ginger Allister, MD
Julie Scott Taylor, MD, MSc

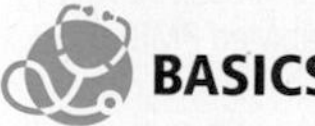

BASICS

DESCRIPTION

- Endometriosis is a common, recurring disease in females of reproductive age that may even persist into early menopause (1).
- Heterotopic islands of endometrial glands and stroma found outside the uterus:
  - Pelvic sites: Peritoneal surfaces (bladder, cul-de-sac, pelvic walls, ligaments, and fallopian tubes), vagina, cervix, lymph nodes, ovaries, bowel
  - Distant sites: Abdominal wall, spleen, gallbladder, stomach, nasal mucosa, spinal canal, lungs, breasts, diaphragm, pleura, pericardium
- Classified as peritoneal, ovarian, or deep endometriosis
- Staged according to the American Society for Reproductive Medicine surgical scoring system:
  - Based on disease severity: Extent and characteristics of endometrial implants and adhesions
  - Stage I (minimal) to IV (severe)
- System affected: Reproductive
- Synonym: Endometriosis externa

ALERT

Staging is useful in therapeutic planning but does not correlate with severity of pain or predict response to treatment for symptoms or infertility.

EPIDEMIOLOGY

Incidence

- Affects 0.5–5% of fertile women
- Found in 30-50% of infertile women (2)
- Found in 50-60% of women and adolescent females with pelvic pain (3)

Pediatric Considerations

Endometriosis may begin with puberty, causing debilitating pelvic pain and severe dysmenorrhea associated with missed school, social, and family activities.

Pregnancy Considerations

Pelvic endometriosis is generally ameliorated with pregnancy, but infertility is significantly associated with the disease itself.

Geriatric Considerations

Although menopause often results in resolution of symptoms, pelvic endometriosis may extend into menopause and is exacerbated by hormone replacement therapy (HRT).

Prevalence

- Predominant sex: Female only
- Affects 6-10% of reproductive-age women

RISK FACTORS

- Diethylstilbestrol (DES) exposure in utero
- Low birth weight
- Obstruction of menstrual flow (Müllerian anomalies)
- Prolonged exposure to endogenous estrogen
  - Early menarche
  - Short menstrual cycles
  - Late menopause
  - Delayed childbearing
  - Obesity
- Hereditary/genetic predisposition
- Exposure to endocrine-disrupting chemicals
- Increased dietary intake of red meat and trans fats

Genetics

Genetic predisposition is common.

GENERAL PREVENTION

- Prevention is not possible, but some factors are considered protective:
  - Fruits, green vegetables, n-3 long-chain fatty acids
  - Multiple pregnancies
  - Prolonged lactation
- Early diagnosis and treatment might help prevent the possible sequelae.

PATHOPHYSIOLOGY

- Not fully understood; tendency for abnormal endometrial tissue to implant and proliferate, causing chronic peritoneal inflammation
- Endometrial-associated infertility is multifactorial:
  - Pelvic inflammation
  - Anatomic disruption of pelvic structures (involvement of the fallopian tube may cause isthmic tubal obstruction)
  - Proliferation and activation of peritoneal macrophages (may predispose to gamete phagocytosis)
  - Alteration in eutopic endometrium

ETIOLOGY

Not fully understood. Theories:

- Sampson theory: Retrograde menstruation results in peritoneal implantation and disease
  - Affected women have an immune dysfunction that prevents clearing of implants
- Halban theory: Distant disease probably caused by hematogenous/lymphatic dissemination or metaplastic transformation
- Coelomic metaplasia: Coelomic epithelium undergoes metaplasia, forming functioning endometrium

COMMONLY ASSOCIATED CONDITIONS

Associated with increased risk of other autoimmune diseases (3). Increased risk of ovarian, endometrioid, and clear-cell cancers as well as other cancers (non-Hodgkin's lymphoma)

DIAGNOSIS

- Diagnosis can be challenging because symptoms overlap with many other gynecological and nongynecological conditions.
- A complete medical, surgical, social, and family history should be collected from patients.
- A complete physical exam, including a pelvic exam, should be performed.

HISTORY

- Dysmenorrhea (50–90% of cases)
- Dyspareunia
- Chronic pelvic pain (≥6 months) that worsens with time and activity
  - Intermittent or continuous
  - Dull, throbbing, or sharp
- Premenstrual spotting
- Dyschezia
- Cyclic nausea, abdominal distention, and early satiety
- Painful defecation
- Hematochezia
- Hematuria
- Infertility
- Spontaneous abortion (theoretical)
- History of pelvic pain, infertility, and hysterectomy in 1st- or 2nd-degree relative

PHYSICAL EXAM

- Focal pain/tenderness on pelvic exam (associated with endometriosis in 66% of patients) (3)
- Pelvic mass
- Immobile pelvic organs (frozen pelvis)
- Rectovaginal exam revealing uterosacral nodules, beading, or tenderness

DIAGNOSTIC TESTS & INTERPRETATION

Lab

Initial lab tests

No special labs; CA-125 levels are not recommended (poor sensitivity and specificity) and may be falsely elevated due to peritoneal irritation.

Imaging

Initial approach

- Routine imaging is not recommended.
- If history and physical exam reveal adnexal pain or tenderness with/without fullness on pelvic exam:
  - Transvaginal ultrasound (US) and MRI are equally effective in detecting ovarian endometriomas. Sensitivity 80–90% and specificity 60-98% for both (3)
  - US is preferred (less costly).
  - Both modalities are poor in detecting peritoneal implants and adhesions.

Diagnostic Procedures/Surgery

- Definitive diagnosis is made via visualization of lesions during surgery (laparoscopy or laparotomy).
- Hysterosalpingography for tubal occlusion (proximal or distal) and periadnexal adhesions

Pathological Findings

- Red and blue-black lesions, adhesions, and "chocolate cysts"
- Endometrial glands and stroma on histologic analysis of biopsied lesions

DIFFERENTIAL DIAGNOSIS

Differential diagnosis of pelvic pain includes all causes of acute abdomen, and:

- Complications of intrauterine or ectopic pregnancy
- Pelvic adhesions
- Acute salpingitis/Pelvic inflammatory disease
- Ruptured ovarian cyst
- Uterine leiomyomas
- Adenomyosis
- Irritable bowel syndrome
- Inflammatory bowel disease
- Intussusception
- Urinary tract infection (UTI)/Cystitis
- Interstitial cystitis
- Malignancies
- Depression
- History of sexual abuse
- Myofascial pain

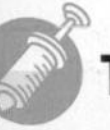

TREATMENT

MEDICATION

Medications may be helpful in treatment symptoms of pain and dysmenorrhea, but symptoms frequently recur.

First Line

Empirical medical treatment is indicated for symptom management, but has not been shown to improve fertility (4):

- Nonsteroidal anti-inflammatory drugs (NSAIDs) initiated at the beginning or just before menses
- Cyclic combined oral contraceptive pills (OCPs)

Second Line

- Continuous combined OCPs. Switch from cyclic to continuous OCPs for 3–6 months if symptoms persist or in chronic, noncyclic pelvic pain
- Progestogens
  - Levonorgestrel IUD (Mirena), especially for symptomatic rectovaginal endometriosis (although not FDA approved) or instead of continuous OCPs in pain that persists despite 1st-line treatment
  - Medroxyprogesterone acetate 150 mg IM or 104 mg SC every 3 months
- GnRH agonists inhibit pituitary gonadotropin synthesis and induce a hypoestrogenic state (3)[A]:
  - Leuprolide acetate (Depo-Lupron) 3.75 mg IM each month or 11.25 mg IM every 3 months (gluteal)
  - Nafarelin (Synarel) intranasal spray 400 μg/day divided into 2 inhalations per day, 1 in each nostril (start between days 2–4 of menstrual cycle)
  - Goserelin (Zoladex) implant 3.6 mg SC in upper abdominal wall every 28 days for 6 months
- GnRH agonists should be given with estrogen-progestogen add-back therapy to minimize effects of hypoestrogenism (most importantly reduced bone mineral density) (3)[A]:
  - Norethindrone acetate 5 mg p.o. once daily
  - Conjugated equine estrogen 0.635 mg p.o. once daily
- Danazol was an early treatment (now 2nd-3rd line). Use limited by androgenic side effects.

ADDITIONAL TREATMENT

General Measures

Calcium / vitamin D supplementation (1,000–1,500 mg/day) is recommended when using GnRH agonists to prevent calcium loss.

Issues for Referral

- Early referral to a board-certified reproductive endocrinologist or gynecologist with expertise in infertility if the patient has difficulty conceiving
- Other indications for referral to a gynecologist include:
  - Need for definitive diagnosis (failure to respond to a conservative 1st-line therapy)
  - Chronic pelvic pain
  - Adolescent with severe dysmenorrhea/dyspareunia

Additional Therapies

Regular exercise and counseling for pain-management strategies (avoidance of narcotics is ideal)

COMPLEMENTARY AND ALTERNATIVE MEDICINE

- Physical therapy (3)[C]
- Acupuncture (3)[C]

SURGERY/OTHER PROCEDURES

Surgery (laparoscopy or laparotomy) is both diagnostic and therapeutic (1st line or when conservative measures fail):

- Peritoneal endometriosis: Laser ablation, excision, or fulguration,
- Ovarian endometriosis (endometriomas) >3 cm: Ablation, excision, drainage

ALERT

- Surgery for endometriomas may decrease ovarian reserve in advanced disease.

- Lysis of adhesions (LOA)
- Hysterectomy with bilateral salpingo-oophorectomy for debilitating symptoms refractory to other medical or surgical treatments (3)[C]
  - Relieves pain in 80–90% but pain recurs in 10% within 1–2 years after surgery
  - Postoperative hormone replacement should include estrogen and progestogen (3)[C]
- Interruption of nerve pathways:
  - Laparoscopic ablations and presacral neurectomy improve dysmenorrhea (3)[A].

  Fertility procedures:
- Ablation of lesions with LOA is recommended to treat infertility in Stage I–II disease (3)[A]
  - Spontaneous conception should be attempted for 1 year prior to assisted reproduction techniques
- GnRH agonists 3–6 months before in vitro fertilization (IVF) significantly increases live birth rates (3)[A].
  - Disease does not endanger IVF pregnancies.

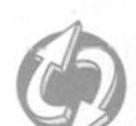

ONGOING CARE

FOLLOW-UP RECOMMENDATIONS

Routine gynecological care with Pap smears, mammograms, etc.

Patient Monitoring

- Symptomatic and asymptomatic pelvic masses <5 cm may be followed with serial US
- Patients on GnRH agonist therapy should have serum estradiol levels monitored to assess degree of hypoestrogenemia & efficacy of add-back therapy: Maintaining estradiol between 30–45 pg/mL (109–164 pmol/L) prevents bone loss without stimulating disease
- Endometriosis is likely an independent risk factor for the development of epithelial ovarian cancer.

DIET

No restrictions.

PATIENT EDUCATION

- American Congress of Obstetrics and Gynecology at www.acog.org
- American Academy of Family Physicians at www.familydoctor.org

PROGNOSIS

- Excellent, especially if diagnosis and treatment plans are initiated early in disease course
- Poor for recovery of fertility if the disease has progressed to stage III or IV

COMPLICATIONS

Possible sequelae include chronic pelvic pain, repetitive surgical intervention, costs, infertility, and the psychological manifestations thereof.

REFERENCES

1. Ozkan S, Murk W, Arici A. Endometriosis and infertility: epidemiology and evidence-based treatments. *Ann N Y Acad Sci*. 2008;1127:92–100.
2. Härkki P, Tiitinen A, Ylikorkala O et al. Endometriosis and assisted reproduction techniques. *Ann N Y Acad Sci*. 2010;1205: 207–13.
3. Giudice LC et al. Clinical practice. Endometriosis. *N Engl J Med*. 2010;362:2389–98.
4. Rodgers AK, et al. Treatment strategies for endometriosis. *Exp Opin Pharmacother*. 2008;9(2): 243–55.

ADDITIONAL READING

- Davis L, Kennedy SS, Moore J, et al. Modern combined oral contraceptives for pain associated with endometriosis. *Cochrane Database Syst Rev*. 2007:CD001019.
- de Ziegler D, Borghese B, Chapron C et al. Endometriosis and infertility: pathophysiology and management. *Lancet*. 2010;376:730–8.
- Ferrero S, Remorgida V, Venturini PL et al. Current pharmacotherapy for endometriosis. *Expert Opin Pharmacother*. 2010;11:1123–34.
- Harada T, Taniguchi F et al. Dienogest: a new therapeutic agent for the treatment of endometriosis. *Womens Health (Lond Engl)*. 2010;6:27–35.
- Hughes E, Brown J, Collins JJ, et al. Ovulation suppression for endometriosis. *Cochrane Database Syst Rev*. 2007:CD000155.
- Jacobson TZ, Duffy JM, Barlow D, Koninckx PR, Garry R et al. Laparoscopic surgery for pelvic pain associated with endometriosis. *Cochrane Database Syst Rev*. 2009;CD001300.
- Nothnick WB et al. Endometriosis: in search of optimal treatment. *Minerva Ginecol*. 2010;62: 17–31.
- Vercellini P, Somigliana E, Viganò P, et al. Endometriosis: current and future medical therapies. *Best Pract Res Clin Obstet Gynaecol*. 2008;22: 275–306.

See Also (Topic, Algorithm, Electronic Media Element)

Algorithm: Pelvic Pain

CODES

ICD9

- 617.0 Endometriosis of uterus
- 617.1 Endometriosis of ovary
- 617.2 Endometriosis of fallopian tube

CLINICAL PEARLS

- Severe dysmenorrhea and dyspareunia are never normal. Failure to respond to NSAIDs and/or OCPs warrants further investigation.
- In patients suspected of having endometriosis, always perform a rectovaginal exam looking for uterosacral tenderness, nodules, and beading.

E

ENDOMETRITIS AND OTHER POST-PARTUM INFECTIONS

Justin P. Lavin, Jr., MD
Allison Kreiner, MD

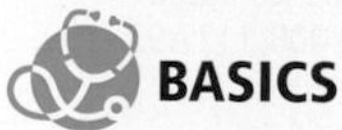

BASICS

DESCRIPTION

- Bacterial infection of the genital tract, usually within the 1st week after delivery, but can occur 1–6 weeks postpartum
- Endometritis (infection of the endometrium) is the most common postpartum infection.
- Less common are postpartum infections of the myometrium and parametrial tissues, vaginal and cervical infections, perineal cellulitis, pelvic cellulitis, septic pelvic vein thrombophlebitis, and parametrial phlegmon.
- System: Reproductive
- Synonym(s): Postpartum infection; endometritis; endoparametritis; endomyometritis; myometritis; endomyoparametritis; metritis; metritis with pelvic cellulitis

EPIDEMIOLOGY

Incidence

- Predominant age: Women of childbearing years
- Predominant sex: Female only

Prevalence

- Occurs in 1–3% of all births
- 10 times more likely with cesarean section:
  - 2–15% prior to labor
  - 30–35% after labor without prophylaxis
  - 2–15% after labor with prophylaxis
  - Accounts for 7% of maternal deaths
  - 4th leading cause of maternal mortality

RISK FACTORS

- Cesarean delivery is the most important risk factor
- Chorioamnionitis
- Bacterial vaginosis
- Group B streptococcal colonization of genital tract
- HIV infection
- Prolonged labor
- Prolonged rupture of membranes
- Multiple vaginal examinations
- Internal fetal monitoring during labor
- Operative vaginal delivery
- Manual extraction of the placenta
- Low socioeconomic status

GENERAL PREVENTION

- Avoid unnecessary vaginal examinations.
- Treat chorioamnionitis during labor.
- Spontaneous placental extraction
- Avoid retained placental fragments or membranes.
- Antibiotic prophylaxis for 3rd- and 4th-degree laceration (1)[B]
- Use of aseptic technique during operative vaginal delivery
- No data to support antibiotic prophylaxis for operative vaginal delivery (2)[A]
- Administering prophylactic antibiotics prior to skin incision in cesarean delivery (as opposed to the prior practice of waiting to cord clamping) is considered the standard of care. Antibiotics should be administered within 1 hour of the surgery start time. There is a 40% reduction in postpartum maternal infections without any increase in neonatal infectious outcomes or difficulty in evaluating the neonate (3)[B].
- Extending the spectrum of coverage to include not only a cephalosporin but also azithromycin decreases the incidence of infections (4)[A],(5)[B].

ETIOLOGY

- Endometritis commonly follows chorioamnionitis.
- Other infections follow trauma to the perineum, vagina, cervix, and uterus.
- Infection is nearly always polymicrobial and involves organisms that have ascended from the lower genital tract:
  - Aerobic isolates in 70%: *Streptococcus faecalis, S. agalactiae, S. viridans, Staphylococcus aureus, Escherichia coli*
  - Anaerobic isolates in 80%: *Peptococcus* sp., *Peptostreptococcus* sp., *Clostridium* sp., *Bacteroides bivius, B. fragilis, Fusobacterium* sp.
- Other genital mycoplasmata; role in endometritis unclear
- *Chlamydia trachomatis* responsible for some late (2–10 days) postpartum endometritis (see Medication, Second Line)
- Range of number of isolates is 1–8

COMMONLY ASSOCIATED CONDITIONS

- Chorioamnionitis
- Wound infection

DIAGNOSIS

HISTORY

- Fever, chills, malaise, headache, anorexia
- Abdominal pain

PHYSICAL EXAM

- Oral temperature >38.7°C (101.6°F) in 1st 24 hours postpartum or >38°C (100.4°F) in 2 of 1st 10 days postpartum (excluding 1st 24 hours)
- Tachycardia
- Uterine tenderness on exam
- Other localized tenderness on exam
- Purulent or malodorous lochia
- Heavy vaginal bleeding
- Ileus
- Group A or B streptococcal bacteremia may have no localizing signs.

DIAGNOSTIC TESTS & INTERPRETATION

Lab

Initial lab tests

- Complete blood count (CBC): Interpret with care, because *physiologic leukocytosis may be as high as 20,000 white blood cells (WBCs)*
- 2 sets of blood cultures (especially if sepsis is suspected)
- Note: Diagnosis is usually made clinically, but consider additional testing, including:
  - Genital tract cultures and rapid test for group B streptococci, which may be done while patient is in labor
  - Amniotic fluid Gram stain: Usually polymicrobial
  - Uterine tissue cultures: Prep the cervix with Betadine and use a shielded specimen collector or Pipelle. Difficult to obtain without contamination.

Imaging

Initial approach

If patient is not responsive to antibiotics in 24–48 hours:

- Ultrasound (US) for retained products of conception, pelvic abscess, or mass
- Computed tomography (CT) or magnetic resonance imaging (MRI) looking for pelvic vein thrombophlebitis, abscess, or deep-seated wound infection

Diagnostic Procedures/Surgery

Paracentesis or culdocentesis with culture rarely is necessary.

Pathological Findings

- Superficial layer of infected necrotic tissue in microscopic sections of uterine lining
- >5 neutrophils per HPF in superficial endometrium; ≥1 plasma cell in endometrial stroma
- Thrombosis of any of the pelvic veins, including the vena cava
- Phlegmon on leaves of the broad ligament
- Abscess

DIFFERENTIAL DIAGNOSIS

- Urinary tract infection
- Viral syndrome
- Dehydration
- Pneumonia
- Wound infection
- Thrombophlebitis
- Thyroid storm
- Mastitis

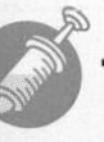

TREATMENT

MEDICATION

First Line

Clindamycin 900 mg IV every 8 hours plus gentamicin 5 mg/kg IV every 24 hours (6)[A]

Potential side effects include nephrotoxicity, ototoxicity, pseudomembranous colitis, or diarrhea (in up to 6%).

Second Line

Clindamycin 900 mg IV every 8 hours plus aztreonam 1–2 g every 8 hours (6)[A].

Metronidazole 500 mg every 12 hours plus penicillin 5 million units every 6 hours. *OR*

Ampicillin 2 g every 6 hours plus gentamicin 5 mg/kg every 24 hours (6)[A].

Cefoxitin 2 g IV every 6 hours. Add ampicillin 2 g IV every 6 hours, if clinical failure after 48 hours (6)[A]

Cefotetan 2 g IV every 12 hours. Add ampicillin 2 g IV every 6 hours, if clinical failure after 48 hours (6)[A].

Note: Base therapy on cultures, sensitivities, and clinical response

Contraindications:
- Drug allergy
- Renal failure (aminoglycosides)
- Avoid sulfa, tetracyclines, and fluoroquinolones before delivery and if breastfeeding. Metronidazole is relatively contraindicated if breastfeeding; however, clinical scenario should be considered.

Precautions:
- Clindamycin and other antibiotics occasionally cause pseudomembranous colitis.

Significant possible interactions: Refer to the manufacturer's literature for each drug.

Note: Consider adding a macrolide antibiotic (for chlamydia coverage) for infections occurring after 48 hours.

Note: Heparin may be indicated for septic pelvic vein thrombophlebitis; requires 10 days of full anticoagulation.

SURGERY/OTHER PROCEDURES

- Curettage of retained products of conception
- Surgery to drain an abscess
- Surgery to decompress the bowel
- Surgical drainage of a phlegmon is not advised unless it is suppurative.

IN-PATIENT CONSIDERATIONS

Initial Stabilization

- Inpatient care for severe infection
- Low-grade endometritis may respond to outpatient treatment with oral antibiotics (see "Medication, Second Line").
- Most infections (94%) occur after hospital discharge.
- IV antibiotics and close observation for severe infections
- Open and drain infected wounds.
- Normalize fluid status.
- Note: Amnioinfusion during labor may decrease infections when membranes have been ruptured for >6 hours (7)[B].

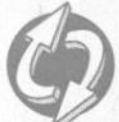

ONGOING CARE

FOLLOW-UP RECOMMENDATIONS

Patient Monitoring

- Individualize according to severity
- IV antibiotics can be stopped when the patient is afebrile for 24–48 hours.
- Oral antibiotics on discharge are not necessary, except in cases of bacteremia; then continue oral antibiotics to complete a 7-day course.

DIET

As tolerated, although may be limited by ileus

PATIENT EDUCATION

- Advise patient to call her doctor if she has fever >38°C (100.4°F) postpartum, heavy vaginal bleeding, foul-smelling lochia, or other symptoms of infection.
- Information available at: http://www.healthline.com/yodocontent/pregnancy/infections-postpartum-endometritis.html

PROGNOSIS

- With supportive therapy and appropriate antibiotics, most patients improve within a few days.
- If no improvement occurs on antibiotics, consider retained placental fragments or membranes, abscess, wound infection, hematoma, cellulitis, phlegmon, or septic pelvic vein thrombosis.

COMPLICATIONS

- Resistant organisms
- Peritonitis
- Pelvic abscess
- Septic pelvic thrombophlebitis
- Ovarian vein thrombosis
- Sepsis
- Death

REFERENCES

1. Duggal N, Mercado C, Daniels K, et al. Antibiotic prophylaxis for prevention of postpartum perineal wound complications: a randomized controlled trial. *Obstet Gynecol*. 2008;111:1268–73.
2. Liabsuetrakul T, et al. Antibiotic prophylaxis for operative vaginal delivery. *Cochrane Databse Sys Rev*. 2009;1:CD004455.
3. Owens SM, Brozanski BS, Meyn LA, Wiesenfeld HC et al. Antimicrobial prophylaxis for cesarean delivery before skin incision. *Obstet Gynecol*. 2009;114:573–9.
4. Costantine MM, Rahman M, Ghulmiyah L, et al. Timing of perioperative antibiotics for cesarean delivery: a metaanalysis. *Am J Obstet Gynecol*. 2008;199:301.e1–6.
5. Tita AT, Owen J, Stamm AM, et al. Impact of extended-spectrum antibiotic prophylaxis on incidence of postcesarean surgical wound infection. *Am J Obstet Gynecol*. 2008;199:303.e1–3.
6. French LM, Smaill F. Antibiotic regimens for endometritis after delivery. *Cochrane Database Sys Rev*. 2009;1:CD001067.
7. Parilla BV, McDermott TM. Prophylactic amnioinfusion in preganancies complicated by chorioamnionitis: a prospective randomized trial. *Am J Perinatol*. 1998;15:649–52.

ADDITIONAL READING

- Belfort MA, Clark SL, Saade GR, Kleja K, Dildy GA, Van Veen TR, Akhigbe E, Frye DR, Meyers JA, Kofford S et al. Hospital readmission after delivery: evidence for an increased incidence of nonurogenital infection in the immediate postpartum period. *Am J Obstet Gynecol*. 2010;202:35.e1–7.
- Maharaj D. Puerperal pyrexia: a review. Part I. *Obstet Gynecol Surv*. 2007;62:393–9.
- Maharaj D. Puerperal pyrexia: a review. Part II. *Obstet Gynecol Surv*. 2007;62:400–6.

See Also (Topic, Algorithm, Electronic Media Element)

Algorithm: Pelvic Pain

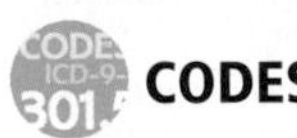

CODES

ICD9

- 615.9 Unspecified inflammatory disease of uterus
- 670.04 Major puerperal infection unspecified, postpartum

CLINICAL PEARLS

- Endometritis is a postpartum complication causing fever and uterine tenderness that occurs in 1–3% of all births.
- Infection is nearly always polymicrobial and involves organisms that have ascended from the lower genital tract.
- Evidence supports antibiotic prophylaxis prior to skin incision for all cesarean deliveries, but not for operative vaginal deliveries.
- Recommended treatment of endometritis is clindamycin 900 mg IV evert 8 hours and gentamicin 5 mg/kg every 24 hours until the patient is afebrile for 24–48 hours.
- Antibiotics can be stopped completely when the patient has been afebrile for 24–48 hours, except in cases of documented bacteremia, which require a 7-day course of therapy.

ENURESIS

Melanie J.S. Malec, MD

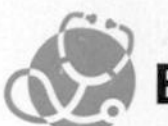

BASICS

DESCRIPTION

- Nocturnal enuresis (NE): Repeated spontaneous voiding of discrete amounts of urine during sleep after the anticipated age of bladder control (age 5)
- Daytime incontinence: Uncontrollable leakage of urine while awake
- Classification:
  - Primary NE: 1% of adult population; 80% of all cases; child/adult who has never established urinary continence on consecutive nights for a period of 6 months or more
  - Secondary NE: 20% of cases; resumption of enuresis after at least 6 months of urinary continence
- Also categorized as:
  - Monosymptomatic NE (uncomplicated): Bed wetting without lower urinary tract symptoms other than nocturia and no history of bladder dysfunction
  - Nonmonosymptomatic NE: Bed wetting with lower urinary tract symptoms such as frequency, urgency, daytime wetting, hesitancy, straining, weak or intermittent stream, posturination dribbling, lower abdominal or genital discomfort, sensation of incomplete emptying
- Adult-onset NE with absent daytime incontinence is a serious symptom; complete urologic evaluation and therapy are warranted; usually associated with diurnal symptoms, voiding dysfunction, and urinary incontinence (UI).
- System(s) affected: Nervous; Renal/Urologic
- Synonym(s): Bed wetting; Sleep enuresis; Nocturnal incontinence; Primary nocturnal enuresis

EPIDEMIOLOGY

Incidence

- Dependent upon family history
- Spontaneous resolution: 15% per year, 99% children are dry by age 15

Prevalence

- Very common. Affects 5–7 million children in the US
- 40% of 3 year olds; 10% of 6 year olds; 3% of 12 year olds; 1% of adults
- Predominant sex: Male > Female (3:1)
- Predominant timing: Nocturnal > Day (3:1)

Geriatric Considerations

Infrequent; often associated with daytime incontinence (formerly referred to as diurnal enuresis)

RISK FACTORS

- Family history
- Stressors (emotional, environmental) common in secondary enuresis (e.g., divorce, death)
- Constipation and encopresis
- Organic disease: 1% of monosymptomatic NE (e.g., urologic and nonurologic causes)
- Psychological disorders:
  - Comorbid disorders are highest with secondary NE: Depression, anxiety, social phobias, conduct disorder, hyperkinetic syndrome, internalizing disorders
  - Association with attention deficit hyperactivity disorder (ADHD; more pronounced in older children ages 9–12 years); 30% greater chance of enuretic events
  - Abuse; victims may present with NE; 11% sexually abused girls
- Altered mental status or impaired mobility

Genetics

Most commonly, NE is an autosomal dominant inheritance pattern with high penetrance (90%); more heritable in boys than in girls:

- 1/3 of all cases are sporadic.
- 4 loci associated with NE identified (chromosomes 8, 12, 13, and 22)
- Higher rates in monozygotic versus dizygotic twins (68% vs. 36%)
- 75% of children with enuresis have a 1st-degree relative with the condition.
- If both parents had NE, risk in child is 77%; 44% if 1 parent affected. Parental age of resolution often predicts when child's enuresis should resolve.

GENERAL PREVENTION

No known measures

PATHOPHYSIOLOGY

A disorder of sleep arousal, a low nocturnal bladder capacity, and nocturnal polyuria are the three factors that interrelate to cause nocturnal enuresis (1).

ETIOLOGY

- Both functional and organic causes; many theories, none absolutely confirmed
- Primary NE owing to disparity between bladder capacity, nocturnal urine production, and the child's failure to awaken in response to a full bladder
- Detrusor instability
- Deficiency of arginine vasopressin (AVP); owing to decreased inherent nocturnal AVP or decreased AVP stimulation secondary to an empty bladder (bladder distension stimulates AVP)
- Maturational delay of CNS
- Severe NE with some evidence of interaction between bladder overactivity and brain arousability: Association between children with severe NE and frequent cortical arousals in sleep
- Organic urologic causes in 1–4% of enuresis in children: Urinary tract infection (UTI), occult spina bifida, ectopic ureter, lazy bladder syndrome, irritable bladder with wide bladder neck, posterior urethral valves
- Organic nonurologic causes: Epilepsy, diabetes mellitus, food allergies, obstructive sleep apnea, chronic renal failure, hyperthyroidism, pinworm infection, sickle-cell disease
- No evidence of sleep disorder/altered sleep pattern; NE occurs in all stages of sleep.

COMMONLY ASSOCIATED CONDITIONS

- Obstructive sleep apnea syndrome; ↑ atrial natriuretic factor → inhibits renin-angiotensin-aldosterone pathway → ↑ diuresis
- Constipation (1/3 of NE patients)
- Behavioral problems

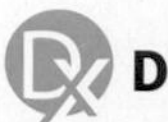

DIAGNOSIS

HISTORY

- Age of onset, duration, severity
- Lower urinary tract symptoms
- Constipation and encopresis (15% with comorbid encopresis)
- Daily intake patterns
- Voiding and elimination patterns
- Psychosocial history
- Family history of enuresis
- Investigation and previous treatment history

PHYSICAL EXAM

- ENT: Evaluation for adenotonsillar hypertrophy
- Abdomen: Enlarged bladder, kidneys, or fecal masses or impaction
- Look for dimpling or tufts of hair on sacrum
- Genital urinary exam:
  - Males: Meatal stenosis, hypospadias, epispadias, phimosis
  - Females: Vulvitis, vaginitis, labial adhesions, ureterocele at introitus; wide vaginal orifice with scar or healed laceration may be evidence of abuse.
- Rectal exam: Tone and constipation
- Neurologic exam

DIAGNOSTIC TESTS & INTERPRETATION

Lab

Initial lab tests

- Only obligatory test in children is urinalysis.
- Urinalysis and culture: UTI, pyuria, hematuria, proteinuria, glycosuria, and poor concentrating ability (low specific gravity) may suggest organic etiology, especially in adults.

Follow-Up & Special Considerations

Select tests for diagnosing causes of secondary enuresis: Serum glucose, blood urea nitrogen (BUN), creatinine, thyroid-stimulating hormone (TSH).

Imaging

Initial approach

- Urinary tract imaging is usually not necessary.
- If abnormal clinical findings or adult onset: Renal ultrasound (US) and bladder US IV pyelogram, voiding cystourethrogram, or retrograde pyelogram as indicated
- Spine radiographs for spina bifida occulta

Follow-Up & Special Considerations

In children, imaging and urodynamic studies are helpful for significant daytime symptoms, history of UTIs, suspected structural abnormalities, and refractory cases.

Diagnostic Procedures/Surgery

Urodynamic studies may be beneficial in adults and nonmonosymptomatic NE.

Pathological Findings

- Dysfunctional voiding
- Detrusor instability and/or reduced bladder capacity most common findings

DIFFERENTIAL DIAGNOSIS

- Primary NE:
  - Delayed physiologic urinary control
  - UTI (both)
  - Spina bifida occulta
  - Obstructive sleep apnea (both)
  - Idiopathic detrusor instability

- Previously unrecognized myelopathy or neuropathy (e.g., multiple sclerosis, tethered cord, epilepsy)
- Anatomic urinary tract abnormally (e.g., ectopic ureter)

Secondary NE:
- Bladder outlet obstruction
- Neurologic disease, neurogenic bladder (e.g., spinal cord injury)

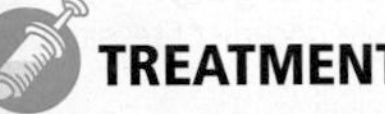

TREATMENT

Combined therapy (e.g., enuresis alarm, bladder training, motivational therapy, and pelvic floor muscle training) is more effective than each component alone or than pharmacotherapy (2)[A].

MEDICATION

First Line

- Desmopressin (DDAVP): Synthetic analogue of vasopressin that decreases nocturnal urine output (3)[A]:
  - Adults only: 20 μg intranasally at bedtime
  - As of 2007, USFDA recommends against use in children due to reports of severe hyponatremia resulting in seizures and deaths in children using intranasal formulations of desmopressin (45)[A].
  - Oral DDAVP: dose dependent: begin at 0.2 mg tablet taken at bedtime on empty stomach; may titrate to 0.6 mg
    - Maximally effective in 1 h; cleared within 9 h
    - Trial nightly for 6 months then stop for 2 weeks for test of dryness
    - Suspend dose in children who experience acute condition affecting fluid/electrolyte balances (fever, vomiting, diarrhea, vigorous exercise)
  - 10–60% success; safe even when used for >12 months; high relapse rate after discontinuation without a structured withdrawal program
- Anticholinergics:
  - Oxybutynin (Ditropan, Ditropan XL, Oxytrol patch): Anticholinergic; smooth muscle relaxant, antispasmodic; may increase functional bladder capacity and aids in timed voiding
    - Ditropan: Adults and children >5 years of age: 5 mg PO t.i.d.–q.i.d.; children 1–5 years of age: 0.02 mg/kg/dose b.i.d.–q.i.d. (syrup 5 mg/5 mL)
    - Ditropan XL: Adults: 5 mg/d PO; increase to 30 mg/d PO (5-, 10-mg tabs)
    - Oxytrol patch: 1 patch every 3–4 days (3.9 mg/patch) (periodic trials off the medication, i.e., weekends or weeks at a time, will help determine efficacy and resolution of primary disturbance)
    - Ditropan 5–10 mg at night; 30–50% success; 50% relapse after stopped
  - Tolterodine (Detrol, Detrol LA): Anticholinergic; fewer side effects than Ditropan:
    - Detrol: 1–2 mg PO b.i.d.
    - Detrol LA: 2–4 mg/d

Pediatric Considerations

USFDA recommends against using intranasal formulations of desmopressin in children due to reports of severe hyponatremia resulting in seizures and deaths (45)[A].

Second Line

- Imipramine (Tofranil): Tricyclic antidepressant, anticholinergic effects; increases bladder capacity, antispasmodic properties
  - Primarily in adults; use in children reserved for resistant cases
  - Dose: Adults, 25–75 mg and children >6 years, 10–25 mg PO at bedtime; increase by 10–25 mg at 1- to 2-week intervals; treat for 2–3 months; then taper;
  - 25–30% success when used >3 months
  - Pretreatment ECG recommended to identify underlying rhythm disorders
- Precautions:
  - Oxybutynin: Glaucoma, myasthenia gravis, GI or genitourinary obstruction, ulcerative colitis, megacolon; use a decreased dose in the elderly.
  - Tolterodine: Urinary retention, gastric retention, or uncontrolled narrow-angle glaucoma; significant drug interactions with CYP2D6, CYP3A3/4 substrates
  - DDAVP: Avoid in patients at risk for electrolyte changes or fluid retention (congestive heart failure [CHF], renal insufficiency).
  - Imipramine: Do not use with monoamine oxidase inhibitors (MAOIs), hypotension, and arrhythmias; low toxic therapeutic ratio.
- Combination therapy with DDAVP and oxybutynin has better results than individual use.
- Prostaglandin inhibitors (e.g., indomethacin) have been studied; may increase bladder capacity.

ADDITIONAL TREATMENT

General Measures

- Use non-pharmacologic approaches as 1st line before prescribing medications (6)[A].
- Simple behavioral interventions (e.g., scheduled wakening, positive reinforcement, bladder training, minimizing fluid/caffeine 2 hours prior to sleep, limiting dairy consumption to 4 hours prior to bedtime)
- Motivational therapy
- Enuresis alarms (bells or buzzers)
  - 66–70% success rate; must be used nightly for 3–4 months; offers cure; significant parental involvement; disruption of sleep for entire family

Issues for Referral

- Primary NE: Persistent enuresis despite nonpharmacologic and pharmacologic therapies
- Diurnal incontinence or nonmonosymptomatic enuresis with voiding dysfunction or underlying medical condition

Additional Therapies

Individual psychotherapy, crisis intervention, and family therapy

COMPLEMENTARY AND ALTERNATIVE MEDICINE

Acupuncture and hypnosis are other treatments offered; few data support their use (7,8)[B]

SURGERY/OTHER PROCEDURES

Only for surgically correctable causes (e.g., tethered cord, ectopic ureter, benign prostatitic hypertrophy, obstructive sleep apnea)

ONGOING CARE

FOLLOW-UP RECOMMENDATIONS

Patient Monitoring

Follow patient until condition resolved. Monitor therapy.

DIET

Limit fluid and caffeine intake prior 2 hours to bedtime. Limit dairy products 4 hours prior to bedtime (decrease osmotic diuresis).

PATIENT EDUCATION

Web resources for alarms and supplies:
- http://www.bedwettingstore.com/index.htm
- http://www.pottypager.com/

PROGNOSIS

In children, NE usually self-limiting; 1% will persist as adult; evaluate for organic causes.

COMPLICATIONS

UTI, perineal excoriation, psychological disturbance (especially in children)

E

REFERENCES

1. Robson WL. Current management of nocturnal enuresis. *Curr Opin Urol*. 2008;18:425–30.
2. Zaffanello M, Giacomello L, Brugnara M, et al. Therapeutic options in childhood nocturnal enuresis. *Minerva Urol Nefrol*. 2007;59:199–205.
3. Vande Walle J, Stockner M, Raes A, et al. Desmopressin 30 years in clinical use: a safety review. *Curr Drug Saf*. 2007;2:232–8.
4. Graham KM, Levy JB et al. Enuresis. *Pediatr Rev*. 2009;30:165–72; quiz 173.
5. http://www.fda.gov/Drugs/DrugSafety/PostmarketDrugSafetyInformationforPatientsandProviders/ucm107924.htm
6. Robson WL et al. Clinical practice. Evaluation and management of enuresis. *N Engl J Med*. 2009; 360:1429–36.
7. Neveus T, Eggert P, Evans J et al. Evaluation of and treatment for monosymptomatic enuresis: a standardization document from the International Children's Continence Society. *J Urol*. 2010;183: 441–7.
8. Libonate J, Evans S, Tsao JC et al. Efficacy of acupuncture for health conditions in children: a review. *Scientific World Journal*. 2008;8:670–82.

See Also (Topic, Algorithm, Electronic Media Element)

Incontinence, Urinary Adult Female; Incontinence, Urinary Adult Male
Algorithm: Enuresis

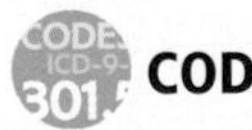

CODES

ICD9

- 307.6 Enuresis
- 788.30 Urinary incontinence, unspecified
- 788.36 Nocturnal enuresis

CLINICAL PEARLS

- Diagnosis is usually made based on history, physical examination, and urinalysis.
- If the condition is not distressing to child and caretakers, treatment is unnecessary.
- Dryness is possible for most children.

EPICONDYLITIS

Shawn M. Ferullo, MD

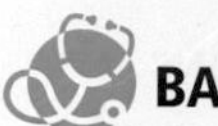

BASICS

DESCRIPTION

- Tendon injury characterized by pain and tenderness at the tendinous origins of the wrist flexors/extensors on the epicondyles of the humerus
- May be acute (traumatic) or chronic (overuse)
- 2 types:
  - Medial epicondylitis or "golfer's elbow":
    - Involvement of the wrist flexors and pronators on the medial epicondyle
  - Lateral epicondylitis or "tennis elbow":
    - Involvement of the wrist extensors and supinators on the lateral epicondyle
- May be caused by many different athletic or occupational activities
- Common in carpenters, plumbers, gardeners, and politicians
- Usually occurs unilaterally on the epicondyles of the dominant arm
- Lateral epicondyle involvement is more common than medial.

EPIDEMIOLOGY

- Predominant age: >40
- Predominant sex: Male = Female

Incidence

- Very common site of overuse injury
- Lateral > Medial

RISK FACTORS

Repetitive wrist motions:

- Flexion/pronation → medial
- Extension/supination → lateral

GENERAL PREVENTION

- Limit overuse of the wrist flexors, extensors, pronators, and supinators.
- Use proper techniques when working.
- Use lighter tools that have smaller grips.

PATHOPHYSIOLOGY

- Acute (tendonitis):
  - Inflammatory response to injury
- Chronic (tendonosis):
  - Overuse injury
  - Tendon degeneration, fibroblast proliferation, microvascular proliferation, lack of inflammatory response

ETIOLOGY

- Repetitive wrist motions
- Tool/racquet gripping
- Shaking hands
- Sudden maximal muscle contraction
- Direct blow

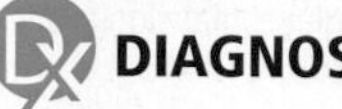

DIAGNOSIS

HISTORY

- Occupational activities
- Sport participation
- Direct trauma
- Duration of symptoms
- Treatments or medication use
- Pain with gripping
- Sensation of mild forearm weakness

PHYSICAL EXAM

- Localized pain just proximal to the affected epicondyle
- Increased pain with wrist flexion/pronation (medial)
- Increased pain with wrist extension/supination (lateral)
- Medial epicondylitis:
  - Tenderness at origin of wrist flexor tendons
  - Increased pain with resisted wrist flexion and pronation
  - Normal elbow range of motion
  - Increased pain with gripping
- Lateral epicondylitis:
  - Tenderness at origin of wrist extensors
  - Increased pain with resisted wrist extension/supination
  - Normal elbow range of motion
  - Increased pain with gripping

DIAGNOSTIC TESTS & INTERPRETATION

Imaging

- None required
- Anterior-posterior/lateral radiograph if decreased range of motion or trauma
- Magnetic resonance imaging for recalcitrant cases

Diagnostic Procedures/Surgery

Local injection of anesthetic to document resolution of symptoms

DIFFERENTIAL DIAGNOSIS

- Elbow osteoarthritis
- Fractures of the epicondyles
- Posterior interosseous nerve entrapment (lateral)
- Ulnar neuropathy (medial)
- Synovitis
- Medial collateral ligament injury
- Referred pain from shoulder or neck

TREATMENT

- May take weeks to months to resolve
- Majority of patients will improve with conservative treatment
- Relative rest with reduction of aggravating activities
- Changing technique of activities
- Ice to area for 10 minutes b.i.d.
- Elbow straps during activity (counterforce bracing) (1)[B]

MEDICATION

First Line

Nonsteroidal anti-inflammatory drugs (NSAIDs): Good for short-term relief. There are no data to support long-term usefulness (2)[B].

Second Line

Corticosteroid injections (3)[B] help relieve pain in acute setting; no effect in long-term outcome.

ADDITIONAL TREATMENT
Physical therapy:
Begin once acute pain resolved
Focus on eccentric strength training.
Grip exercises
Ultrasound (4)[B]
Corticosteroid iontophoresis

General Measures
Relative rest

Issues for Referral
Failure of conservative therapy

Additional Therapies
- Botulinum toxin injections (5)[B]
- Platelet-rich plasma injections (6)[C]:
  - Involves the injection of a concentrated portion of the patient's plasma. Specifically, the platelet-rich portion of plasma is used. The localized injection of the concentrate leads to a local inflammatory response causing the platelets to degranulate, releasing growth factors, which then stimulate the physiologic healing cascade.
- Prolotherapy:
  - Involves the injection of a dextrose solution into and around the tendon attachment. This stimulates a localized inflammatory response, leading to increased blood supply to the area, which increases the flow of nutrients and healing mediators to stimulate tendon healing.
  - Research is currently being performed to look at efficacy of use in epicondylitis.

COMPLEMENTARY AND ALTERNATIVE MEDICINE
Acupuncture (7)[A]

SURGERY/OTHER PROCEDURES
- May be indicated in refractory cases
- Involves debridement and release of the involved tendons
- Can be performed open or arthroscopically (1)[B]

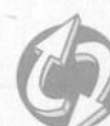

ONGOING CARE

PROGNOSIS
Good: Majority resolve with conservative care

REFERENCES

1. Dunkow PD, Jatti M, Muddu BN. A comparison of open and percutaneous techniques in the surgical treatment of tennis elbow. *J Bone Joint Surg.* 2004;86-B:701.
2. Green S, et al. Non-steroidal anti-inflamatory drugs for treating lateral elbow pain in adults. *Cochrane Database Syst Rev.* 2001;(4):CD002267.
3. Assendelft W, Green S, Buchbinder R, et al. Tennis elbow (lateral epicondylitis). *Clin Evid.* 2002: 1290–300.
4. Smidt N, van der Windt DA, Assendelft WJ, et al. Corticosteroid injections, physiotherapy, or a wait-and-see policy for lateral epicondylitis: a randomised controlled trial. *Lancet.* 2002;359: 657–62.
5. Wong SM, Hui AC, Tong PY, et al. Treatment of lateral epicondylitis with botulinum toxin: a randomized, double-blind, placebo-controlled trial. *Ann Intern Med.* 2005;143:793–7.
6. Mishra A, Pavelko T. Treatment of chronic elbow tendinosis with buffered platelet-rich plasma. *Am J Sports Med.* 2006;34:1774–8.
7. Trinh KV, Phillips SD, Ho E, et al. Acupuncture for the alleviation of lateral epicondyle pain: a systematic review. *Rheumatology (Oxford).* 2004;43:1085–90.

ADDITIONAL READING

Wilson JJ, Best TM. Common overuse tendon problems: A review and recommendations for treatment. *Am Fam Physician.* 2005;72:811–8.

See Also (Topic, Algorithm, Electronic Media Element)
Algorithm: Pain in Upper Extremity

CODES

ICD9
- 726.31 Medial epicondylitis
- 726.32 Lateral epicondylitis

CLINICAL PEARLS

- Tendon injury characterized by pain and tenderness at the tendinous origins of the wrist flexors/extensors on the epicondyles of the humerus
- 2 types:
  - Medial epicondylitis or "golfer's elbow":
    - Involvement of the wrist flexors and pronators on the medial epicondyle
  - Lateral epicondylitis or "tennis elbow":
    - Involvement of the wrist extensors and supinators on the lateral epicondyle
- May take weeks to months to resolve
- Majority of patients will improve with conservative treatment.
- NSAIDs 1st line; steroid injection 2nd line
- Ice to area for 10 minutes b.i.d.
- Elbow straps during activity (counterforce bracing)
- Physical therapy as symptoms improve

E

EPIDIDYMITIS

Andrew Leone, MD
Kyle D. Wood, MD

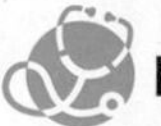

BASICS

- Acute epididymitis: Pain for <6 weeks
- Chronic epididymitis: Pain for >3 months

DESCRIPTION

Inflammation (infectious or noninfectious) of epididymis resulting in scrotal pain and swelling, induration of the posterior epididymis, and eventual scrotal wall edema, involvement of the adjacent testicle, and hydrocele formation:

- System(s) affected: Reproductive
- Synonym(s): Epididymo-orchitis
- Classification: Infectious (bacterial, viral, fungal, parasitic) versus sterile (chemical, traumatic, autoimmune, idiopathic, industrial, noninfectious, vasoepididymal reflux syndrome, vasal reflux syndrome); chronic versus acute

EPIDEMIOLOGY

- Predominant age: Usually younger, sexually active men or older men with urinary tract infections; in older men usually secondary to bladder outlet obstruction
- Predominant sex: Male only

Pediatric Considerations

Occurs in prepubertal boys: Epididymitis is found to be the most common cause of acute scrotum, more common than testicular torsion.

Incidence

- Common (600,000 cases annually in United States)
- 1 in 1,000 males per year

Prevalence

Common

RISK FACTORS

- Urinary tract infection (UTI), prostatitis
- Indwelling urethral catheter
- Urethral instrumentation or transurethral surgery
- Urethral or meatal stricture
- Transrectal prostate biopsy
- Prostate brachytherapy (seeds) for prostate cancer
- Anal intercourse
- High-risk sexual activity
- Strenuous physical activity
- Prolonged sedentary periods
- Bladder obstruction (benign prostatic hyperplasia, prostate cancer)
- HIV-immunosuppressed patient
- Severe Behçet disease
- Presence of foreskin (1)
- Constipation
- Sterile epididymitis:
  - Increased intra-abdominal pressure (occupation requiring frequent physical strain):
    - Military recruits, especially who begin their physically unprepared
    - Laborers; Restaurant kitchen workers
    - Full bladder during intense physical exertion

GENERAL PREVENTION

- Vasectomy or vasoligation during transurethral surgery
- Safer sexual practices
- Mumps vaccination
- Antibiotic prophylaxis for urethral manipulation
- Early treatment of prostatitis/benign prostatic hyperplasia
- Avoid vigorous rectal exam with acute prostatitis.
- Sterile epididymitis:
  - Emptying the bladder prior to physical exertion
  - Physically conditioning the body prior to engaging in regular intense physical exertion (2)
  - Treating constipation

PATHOPHYSIOLOGY

- Infectious epididymitis:
  - Retrograde spread of urine or urinary bacteria from the prostate or urethra via the ejaculatory ducts and the vas deferens into the epididymis; rarely, hematogenous spread
  - Causative organism is identified in 80% of patients, and varies according to patient age.
- Sterile epididymitis:
  - Urine in full bladder when exposed to increased intra-abdominal pressure is pushed through internal urethral sphincter (located at proximal end of prostatic urethra).
  - Reflux of urine through orifice of ejaculatory ducts at verumontanum may occur with history of urethritis/prostatitis, as inflammation may produce rigidity in musculature surrounding orifice to ejaculatory ducts, holding them open.
  - Exposure of epididymis to foreign fluid may produce inflammatory reaction within 24 hours

ETIOLOGY

- <35 years and sexually active:
  - Usually *Chlamydia trachomatis* or *Neisseria gonorrhoeae*
  - Look for serous urethral discharge (chlamydia) or purulent discharge (gonorrhea).
  - With anal intercourse, likely *Escherichia coli* or *Haemophilus influenzae*
- >35 years:
  - Coliform bacteria usually, but sometimes *Staphylococcus aureus* or *S. epidermidis*
  - In elderly men, often with distal urinary tract obstruction, BPH, UTI, or catheterization
  - Tuberculosis, if sterile pyuria and nodularity of vas deferens (hematogenous spread)
  - Sterile urine reflux after transurethral prostatectomy
  - Granulomatous reaction following BCG intravesical therapy for bladder cancer
- Prepubertal boys:
  - Usually coliform bacteria
  - Evaluate for underlying congenital abnormalities, such as vesicoureteral reflux, ectopic ureter, or anorectal malformation (rectourethral fistula).
- Amiodarone may cause noninfectious epididymitis; resolves with decreasing drug dosage.
- Syphilis, blastomycosis, coccidioidomycosis, and cryptococcosis are rare causes, but brucellosis can be a common cause in endemic areas (3).

COMMONLY ASSOCIATED CONDITIONS

- Prostatitis/Urethritis/Orchitis
- Hemospermia
- Constipation
- Urinary Tract Infection

DIAGNOSIS

- Scrotal pain, sometimes radiating to the groin region, may begin acutely over several hours.
- Urethral discharge or symptoms of UTI, such as frequency of urination, dysuria, cloudy urine, or hematuria (4)
- Initially, only the posterior-lying epididymis, usually the lowermost tail section, is very tender and indurated; will eventually progress to involvement of body and head of epididymis.
- Elevation of the testes/epididymis improves the discomfort (Prehn sign).
- Entire hemiscrotum becomes swollen and red, the testis becomes indistinguishable from the epididymis, the scrotal wall becomes thick and indurated, and reactive hydrocele may occur.
- Sterile epididymitis:
  - Unilateral scrotal pain and swelling preceded by intense physical exertion by several hours. Patient may recall full bladder prior to exertion.
  - No symptoms of infection

Pediatric Considerations

- In prepubertal patients, may be postinfectious inflammatory condition; treat with anti-inflammatories, analgesics, and usually no antibiotics (5)
- Bacteremia from *Haemophilus influenzae* infection may produce acute epididymitis.
- In adolescent males, particularly >13 years old, must rule out testicular torsion.
- History not helpful in distinguishing epididymitis from testicular torsion.

Geriatric Considerations

- Diabetics with sensory neuropathy may have pain despite severe infection/abscess.

PHYSICAL EXAM

- The tail of the epididymis is larger in comparison to the contralateral side.
- Epididymis is markedly tender to palpation.
- Cremasteric reflex should be present in epididymitis; if absent, suspect testicular torsion.

DIAGNOSTIC TESTS & INTERPRETATION

Lab

Initial lab tests

- Urinalysis (pyuria and bacteruria suggestive of infectious origin)
- Urine culture (negative does not rule out)
- GC/chlamydia testing (urethral swab or urine testing)
- Gram stain urethral discharge
- White blood cell count may be elevated.
- Urinalysis clear and culture-negative suggest sterile epididymitis

Imaging

- If testicular torsion cannot be excluded (especially in pediatrics), Doppler ultrasound test of choice (6)
- In adult men, Doppler ultrasound: Sensitivity and specificity of 100% in evaluation of acute scrotum, but usually not needed (7)

Follow-Up & Special Considerations

Pediatric Considerations

Further radiographic imaging in children should be done to rule out anatomic abnormalities:

Diagnostic Procedures/Surgery
This is a clinical diagnosis.

Pathological Findings
- Epididymis:
  - Surrounding tissue fibrosis and scarring
  - Interstitial nonspecific acute infiltration, edema, congestion, PMNs, and lymphocytes
  - Fine inflammatory adhesions
  - Can progress to abscess or necrosis (2)
- Vas deferens:
  - Possible fibrosis of this structure

DIFFERENTIAL DIAGNOSIS
- Epididymal congestion following vasectomy
- Testicular torsion
- Torsion of testicular appendages
- Orchitis
- Testicular malignancy
- Testicular trauma
- Epididymal cyst
- Inguinal hernia
- Urethritis
- Spermatocele
- Hydrocele
- Hematocele
- Varicocele
- Epididymal adenomatoid tumor
- Epididymal rhabdomyosarcoma
- Vasculitis (Henoch-Schönlein purpura)

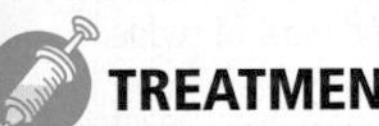

TREATMENT

- Bed rest or restriction on activity
- Athletic scrotal supporter
- Scrotal elevation
- Ice pack/warm compress
- If chemical epididymitis:
  - Cessation of strenuous physical activity for several weeks
  - Empty bladder prior to strenuous exercises.

MEDICATION
First Line
- <35 years, for chlamydia: Doxycycline 100 mg PO bid for 10 PO ceftriaxone 250 mg IM × 1. Treat sexual partner(s) (8).
- If penicillin-allergic or participates in insertive anal intercourse: Ciprofloxacin (Cipro) 500 mg PO bid or ofloxacin (Floxin) 200 mg PO bid for 10 days
- Older men with bacteriuria:
  - Levofloxacin (Levaquin) 500 mg PO every day for 7–10 days (8)
  - Ofloxacin 300 mg orally bid for 10 days (8)
  - Ciprofloxacin (Cipro) 500 mg PO bid or ciprofloxacin (Cipro XL) 1000 mg/day for 10–14 days
- Analgesia (infectious and chemical epididymitis):
  - Nonsteroidal anti-inflammatory drugs (NSAIDs) (e.g., naproxen or ibuprofen) for mild to moderate pain
  - Consider corticosteroid if patient cannot tolerate NSAID.
  - Acetaminophen-codeine or acetaminophen-oxycodone for moderate-to-severe pain
- Septic or toxic patient:
  - 3rd-generation cephalosporin or aminoglycoside
- For Beçhet, sarcoid, Henoch Schönlein purpura:
  - Corticosteroids such as methylprednisolone 40 mg/day recommended

Second Line
- Trimethoprim-sulfamethoxazole (Bactrim, Septra) double-strength PO bid for 10–14 days; increasing bacterial resistance may limit effectiveness.
- Add rifampin (rifampicin) or vancomycin as required.

ADDITIONAL TREATMENT
General Measures
Spermatic cord block with local anesthesia in severe cases

Issues for Referral
- If suspicion is high for testicular torsion or cancer, consult urologist.
- If failed medical management, should be referred to urologist to rule out anatomic abnormality or to diagnosis chemical epididymitis.

SURGERY/OTHER PROCEDURES
- Vasostomy to drain infected material if severe or refractory case
- Scrotal exploration if unable to clinically distinguish between epididymitis or testicular torsion
- Drainage of abscesses, epididymectomy (acute suppurative), or epididymo-orchiectomy in severe cases refractory to antibiotics
- Surgery to correct underlying anatomic abnormality or obstruction

IN-PATIENT CONSIDERATIONS
Initial Stabilization
- The majority of cases can be managed with outpatient care.
- Inpatient care needed if septic or if surgery is scheduled

Admission Criteria
- Intractable pain
- Sepsis
- Abscess
- Persistent vomiting
- Purulent drainage

ONGOING CARE

FOLLOW-UP RECOMMENDATIONS
Patient Monitoring
- Office visits until all signs of infection have cleared
- In chemical epididymitis, follow-up in 4 weeks to assess efficacy of NSAIDs and lifestyle changes

DIET
If constipation is contributing to chemical epididymitis, consider a high-fiber diet.

PATIENT EDUCATION
- Stress completing course of antibiotics, even when asymptomatic.
- Early recognition and treatment of UTI or prostatitis
- Safer sexual practices
- If chemical epididymitis, then educate on noninfectious etiology and proper lifestyle changes

PROGNOSIS
- Pain improves within 1–3 days, but induration may take several weeks/months to completely resolve.
- If bilateral involvement, sterility may result.
- In chemical epididymitis, symptoms resolve in usually <1 week

COMPLICATIONS
- Recurrent epididymitis
- Infertility
- Oligospermia
- Testicular necrosis or atrophy
- Secondary abscess formation
- Fournier gangrene (necrotizing synergistic infection)

REFERENCES

1. Bennett RT, Gill B, Kogan SJ. Epididymitis in children: the circumcision factor? *J Urol*. 1998;160:1842–4.
2. Wolin LH. On the etiology of epididymitis. *J Urol*. 1971;105:531–3.
3. Akinci E, Bodur H, Cevik MA, et al. A complication of brucellosis: epididymoorchitis. *Int J Infect Dis*. 2006;10:171–7.
4. Tracy CR, Steers WD, Costabile R. Diagnosis and management of epididymitis. *Urol Clin North Am*. 2008;35:101–8; vii.
5. Somekh E, Gorenstein A, Serour F. Acute epididymitis in boys: evidence of a post-infectious etiology. *J Urol*. 2004;171:391–4; discussion 394.
6. Trojian TH, Lishnak TS, Heiman D. Epididymitis and orchitis: an overview. *Am Fam Physician*. 2009;79:583–7.
7. Süzer O, Ozcan H, Küpeli S, et al. Color Doppler imaging in the diagnosis of the acute scrotum. *Eur Urol*. 1997;32:457–61.
8. Drugs for sexually transmitted infections. *Treat Guidel Med Lett*. 2007;5:81–8.

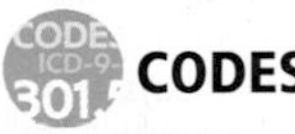

CODES

ICD9
- 604.90 Orchitis and epididymitis, unspecified
- 604.91 Orchitis and epididymitis in diseases classified elsewhere
- 604.99 Other orchitis, epididymitis, and epididymo-orchitis, without mention of abscess

CLINICAL PEARLS

- With epididymitis, the pain is more gradual in onset, and the tenderness is mostly posterior to the testis. With testicular torsion, the symptoms are quite rapid in onset, the testis will be higher in the scrotum and may have a transverse lie, and the cremasteric reflex will be absent. The absence of leukocytes on urine analysis and decreased blood flow on scrotal ultrasound with Doppler will suggest torsion.
- Prostatic massage is contraindicated in epididymitis because the risk for worsening local infection and potential for sepsis is increased with acute prostatitis.
- Chemical epididymitis is a clinical diagnosis of exclusion, and infectious causes are much more common, but certain occupations, such as soldiers and laborers, must be considered.

E

EPIGLOTTITIS

Vassiliki P. Syriopoulou, MD

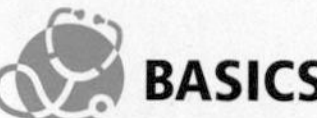

BASICS

DESCRIPTION
- An illness with acute onset characterized by inflammation and edema of the supraglottic structures, epiglottis, vallecula, arytenoepiglottic folds, and arytenoids
- System(s) affected: Pulmonary
- Synonym(s): Supraglottitis

EPIDEMIOLOGY
Incidence
- Has decreased dramatically since the introduction of the *Haemophilus influenzae* type b (Hib) vaccine in the mid-1980s (1,2)
- In adults: 1–3 per 100,000 per year
- In the pre-vaccine era, the most commonly affected group was children 2–4 years old.
- With use of Hib vaccine, the predominant age is shifting to older children (median age, 7 years) and adults (1,2).
- Predominant sex: Male > Female (1.8:1)

Prevalence
More prevalent in countries without universal immunization

RISK FACTORS
- Absence of immunization against Hib
- Immunocompromise

GENERAL PREVENTION
- *H. influenzae* type B vaccine is effective, although not 100% protective.
- Rifampin prophylaxis (20 mg/kg/d for 4 days, maximum daily dose 600 mg) for all household and daycare contacts of invasive Hib. Family and close contacts may be asymptomatic carriers of Hib.

Pediatric Considerations
Rare since introduction of Hib vaccine

Geriatric Considerations
Rare

PATHOPHYSIOLOGY
- In epiglottitis, usually a local invasion of the epiglottis occurs, followed by bacteremia.
- The epiglottis, aryepiglottic folds, false vocal cords, and supraglottic structures become inflamed and edematous, leading to narrowed airway and respiratory compromise.
- Inspiratory airway occlusion often occurs prior to total occlusion from supraglottic edema.

ETIOLOGY
- Bacterial:
  - Hib
  - *Streptococcus pyogenes*
  - *Streptococcus pneumoniae*
  - *Staphylococcus aureus*
  - Other bacteria
- Fungal
- Viral
- Traumatic: Caustic ingestion
- Allergic reactions

DIAGNOSIS

HISTORY
- Sudden onset of severe symptoms and a fulminant course over a period of hours, unless airway control and medical management are initiated promptly.
- Fever is the 1st symptom, followed by stridor and labored breathing.
- Dysphagia, refusal to eat, drooling, and sore throat are common.
- Muffled voice/cry (vs hoarseness in croup)
- Minimal cough (vs barking cough in croup)
- Usually no history of prodromal upper respiratory infection (vs positive history in croup)
- In adults, presentation is more indolent (sore throat and odynophagia are the predominant symptoms).

PHYSICAL EXAM
- Toxic appearance/shock (occasionally, due to associated septicemia)
- Marked restlessness, irritability, and anxiety are common.
- Airway obstruction resulting in respiratory distress
- Tripod position (sitting propped up on hands with head forward and tongue out)
- Stridor softer and less prominent than in croup
- Anterior neck exam may reveal tender adenopathy.
- Definitive diagnosis is established by visualizing a swollen and erythematous epiglottis during careful exam of the oropharynx, although this should not normally be attempted without specific training and equipment available to manage an obstructed airway, such as in an operating room.
- Cyanosis indicates a poor prognosis.

DIAGNOSTIC TESTS & INTERPRETATION
Lab
Initial lab tests
- Blood culture (positive in >75–90% of children with Hib-acute epiglottitis). *Do not* visualize/swab epiglottis except in controlled environment (e.g., operating room). Blood tests are also contraindicated until airway is secured.
- Epiglottic swab culture (positive in 70%)
- Complete blood count: Leukocytosis with left shift
- Hib antigen test in serum/urine useful in children with previous antibiotic treatment
- Hypoxia usually not present until airway obstructed

Imaging
Initial approach
- Lateral neck radiographs typically show an enlarged edematous epiglottis (the thumbprint sign) (1,3); however, radiographs are contraindicated because of danger of sudden complete airway obstruction with delay of important airway intervention.
- If radiographs are obtained, ensure adequate staff i case complete airway obstruction occurs.
- Chest x-rays after intubation to check position of endotracheal tube and to rule out pneumonia, which may occur as a complication.

Diagnostic Procedures/Surgery
- Visualization of epiglottis with tongue depressor is contraindicated because of danger of sudden complete airway obstruction.
- Controlled visualization of epiglottis at intubation i operating room is diagnostic (cherry red, edematou epiglottis).
- Lumbar puncture is indicated if there is clinical suspicion of meningitis.
- In an adult, indirect laryngoscopy is generally safe.

DIFFERENTIAL DIAGNOSIS
- Viral croup (laryngotracheobronchitis)
- Acute angioneurotic edema (no fever)
- Aspirated foreign body (history, no fever)
- Bacterial tracheitis (pseudomembranous croup)
- Retropharyngeal or peritonsillar abscess
- Diphtheria in an unimmunized patient (often an adult)
- Sepsis from other cause

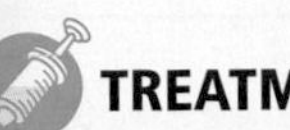

TREATMENT

ere are 2 key aspects to the treatment of acute iglottitis:

- Maintenance of an adequate airway should be the primary concern (1,2,3)[C].
- Administration of antimicrobial agents

EDICATION

irst Line

- Begin empiric antibiotic promptly after blood and epiglottic cultures are obtained. Use antibiotics guided by cultures thereafter. Duration of antimicrobial: 7–10 days (1,3)[C]
- Cefotaxime (Claforan) 100–200 mg/kg/d q8h IV (1,3)[C]
- Ceftriaxone (Rocephin) 50–100 mg/kg/d q12h IV (1,3)[C]

econd Line

- Other 3d- or 4th-generation cephalosporins IV or only ampicillin if Hib is sensitive (3)[C]
- Ampicillin-sulbactam (Unasyn) 150 mg/kg/d q6h, IV
- The role of steroids and racemic epinephrine remains controversial (1,3)[C].
- Antipyretics if necessary

DDITIONAL TREATMENT

eneral Measures

- Each institution should have an emergency protocol involving a team of emergency room physicians, pediatricians, anesthesiologists, surgeons, pediatric intensivists, and pediatric intensive care unit (ICU) nurses (principles are similar for pediatric and adult patients).
- Call anesthesiologist to bedside.
- Have equipment for intubation and needle cricothyrotomy or percutaneous tracheostomy at bedside.
- Notify operating room (OR).
- Notify pediatric surgeon or ear/nose/throat (ENT) specialist for standby in OR in case tracheostomy becomes necessary.
- Keep patient quiet, calm, sitting up (in parent's arms).
- Avoid venipuncture, blood gases, oxygen masks, IV lines, injections, monitors, and radiographs.
- Judicious use of sedation that does not depress respirations may be appropriate.
- Racemic epinephrine is without benefit.
- Avoid examining the pharynx.
- Transport patient and parent together to OR in a wheelchair.
- Intubate all patients, preferably in OR under controlled circumstances by experienced anesthesiologist, with surgeon or ENT specialist on standby for emergency tracheostomy.
- Tracheostomy is not indicated unless intubation is unsuccessful (1,2,3)[C].
- Tape airway securely in place, and use a bite block if indicated.
- Splint elbows and restrain arms to avoid self-extubation.
- Use humidity and avoid T-piece (traction increases risk of accidental extubation).
- Continuous positive airway pressure, mechanical ventilation, and sedation are usually unnecessary.
- Pay attention to supervision and pulmonary suctioning to minimize risk of endotracheal tube plugs.

SURGERY/OTHER PROCEDURES

Emergency tracheotomy may be necessary (1,2,3)[C].

IN-PATIENT CONSIDERATIONS

Initial Stabilization

Acute epiglottitis is a medical emergency. During acute illness, hospitalize patient in ICU (1,2,3)[C].

Admission Criteria

Whenever the diagnosis of epiglottitis is suspected, immediate hospitalization is required.

IV Fluids

Initially, while intubated

Nursing

Expert respiratory nursing care is essential.

Discharge Criteria

Extubated patients afebrile in good clinical condition

ONGOING CARE

FOLLOW-UP RECOMMENDATIONS

Immunization

Patient Monitoring

- Rule out secondary foci of infection.
- Observe swallowing ability and presence of an air leak around endotracheal/nasotracheal tube.
- Follow-up with laryngoscopy prior to extubation (advocated by some).
- Observe in ICU for 24 hours following extubation.

DIET

IV fluid initially, then nasogastric feedings while intubated

PATIENT EDUCATION

Reassurance about treatment and outcome

PROGNOSIS

- Most patients can be extubated after 24–48 hours.
- Morbidity and mortality are low with appropriate intervention.

COMPLICATIONS

- Pneumonia, meningitis, septic arthritis, cervical adenitis, and cellulitis (rare)
- Progression of infection to deep neck tissue
- Epiglottic abscess
- Septic shock (~1%)
- Pneumothorax (rare)
- Death from asphyxia

REFERENCES

1. Mayo-Smith MF, Spinale JW, Donskey CJ, et al. Acute epiglottitis. An 18-year experience in Rhode Island. *Chest*. 1995;108:1640–7.
2. Guldfred LA, Lyhne D, Becker BC. Acute epiglottitis: epidemiology, clinical presentation, management and outcome. *J Laryngol Otol*. 2008;122:818–23.
3. Glynn F, Fenton JE. Diagnosis and management of supraglottitis (epiglottitis). *Curr Infect Dis Rep*. 2008;10:200–4.

E

ADDITIONAL READING

- Cheung CS, Man SY, Graham CA, Mak PS, Cheung PS, Chan BC, Rainer TH et al. Adult epiglottitis: 6 years experience in a university teaching hospital in Hong Kong. *Eur J Emerg Med*. 2009;16:221–6.
- Sobol SE, Zapata S et al. Epiglottitis and croup. *Otolaryngol Clin North Am*. 2008;41:551–66, ix

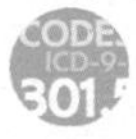

CODES

ICD9

- 464.30 Acute epiglottitis without mention of obstruction
- 464.31 Acute epiglottitis with obstruction
- 487.1 Influenza with other respiratory manifestations

CLINICAL PEARLS

- Acute epiglottitis is a medical emergency and requires immediate hospitalization. The airway must be secured before transport of all patients with suspected epiglottitis. Transport must be done by an experienced team.
- Evident respiratory distress, stridor, drooling, and shorter duration of symptoms are clinical features associated with a higher likelihood of airway obstruction in children with epiglottitis.
- Security of the airway is always of primary concern in acute epiglottitis; failure to intervene prior to loss of the airway associated with an increase in mortality. Avoid interventions that may upset the child, and proceed directly to operating room in parent's lap
- Avoid use of tongue blade, which may worsen obstruction. Direct laryngoscopy should be done in OR.

EPISTAXIS

Julie Yeh, MD, MPH

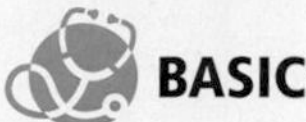

BASICS

DESCRIPTION
- Hemorrhage from the nose involving either the anterior or posterior mucosal surfaces
- Synonym(s): Nosebleed

EPIDEMIOLOGY
Incidence
- In the US: Common
- Estimated lifetime incidence approximately 60%
- Bimodal, with peaks in children up to 15 and in adults >50
- Rare in children under age 2

RISK FACTORS
- Local irritation from multiple causes (see Etiology)
- Medications/supplements, including aspirin and clopidogrel

GENERAL PREVENTION
- Humidification at night
- Cut fingernails to minimize picking.

PATHOPHYSIOLOGY
- Local vs systemic disease. Large majority are due to local causes.
- Anterior: 90–95% of all cases (Kiesselbach plexus)
- Posterior: Usually branches of sphenopalatine arteries: May be asymptomatic or may present with other symptoms

ETIOLOGY
- Idiopathic
- Local inflammation/irritation:
  - Infection
  - Irritant inhalation
  - Topical steroid use
  - Septal deviation (more air movement on 1 side)
  - Low humidity
- Trauma:
  - Epistaxis digitorum (nose picking)
  - Foreign bodies
  - Septal perforation
  - Sinus fracture

COMMONLY ASSOCIATED CONDITIONS
- Vascular malformation/telangiectasia
- Neoplasm (rare, but consider in persistent unilateral cases)
- Systemic:
  - Coagulopathy, primary or iatrogenic
  - Thrombocytopenia
  - Cirrhosis
  - Renal failure
  - Alcoholism
- No proven association with HTN, but may make control of bleeding more difficult.

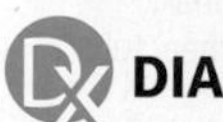

DIAGNOSIS

HISTORY
- Initial presentation, including detail on where bleeding started (which side?)
- Trauma, including nose picking
- Previous episodes
- Comorbid conditions
- Current medications, including over-the-counter and supplements

PHYSICAL EXAM
- Blood loss through 1 or both nostrils in the majority of cases is due to anterior nasal septal bleeding and can often be directly visualized.
- Examiner should wear protective gear, including gown, gloves, and goggles.
- Patient seated, head forward, to avoid blood going down the posterior pharynx.

DIAGNOSTIC TESTS & INTERPRETATION
Indicated only in complicated cases

Lab
Lab testing is not indicated in the majority of uncomplicated cases in which bleeding is reasonably easily controlled and is not truly hemorrhagic.

Initial lab tests
- For recurrent or intractable cases
- CBC, platelet count, prothrombin time
- Cross-match when appropriate
- Toxicology screen when nasal use of illicit drugs is suspected

Imaging
For most cases, imaging not indicated

Diagnostic Procedures/Surgery
Nasal endoscopy

DIFFERENTIAL DIAGNOSIS
- Diagnosis usually apparent; the differential for the etiology is key
- Posterior bleeding must be included in the differential for any chronic blood loss.

Pediatric Considerations
More likely anterior, idiopathic, and recurrent

Geriatric Considerations
More likely to be posterior bleed

TREATMENT

- Most cases managed as outpatient
- Patient applies direct pressure by pinching the lowe part of the nose for 5–20 minutes without a break. This will stop active bleeding in the majority of patients.
- An ice pack placed over the dorsum of the nose ma help with hemostasis.
- Inspect the nasal septum for the bleeding site.

MEDICATION
First Line
If general measures fail, affected naris may be spraye with topical vasoconstrictor such as phenylephrine or oxymetazoline.

Second Line
NosebleedQR: A nonprescription powder of hydrophilic polymer with potassium salt; induces formation of scab

ADDITIONAL TREATMENT

- Nasal packing: Either with ribbon gauze or preformed nasal tampons
- FloSeal: A biodegradable hemostatic sealant (a thrombin-type gel) in 1 study more effective and better tolerated than packing (1)[B]
- If an actively bleeding anterior septal site is visualized, this may be treated with gentle and specific silver nitrate cautery for ~10 seconds for definitive treatment.
- Limit to 1 side of septum, or wait 4–6 weeks in between treatments to reduce risk of perforation (2).
- Posterior: Posterior packing or tamponade with balloon devices (Foley catheter has been used)
- Recurrent epistaxis: Cochrane Review of issue in children shows no difference in effectiveness between antiseptic nasal cream, petroleum jelly, silver nitrate cautery, or no treatment (3)[A]:
  – Silver nitrate cautery followed by 4 weeks of antiseptic cream may be better than antiseptic cream alone (4)[B].

General Measures

Resuscitation as indicated. Use universal "ABC" approach.

Issues for Referral

- Posterior bleeding, frequently requires an otolaryngology consultation
- Intractable bleeding. May require more specialized measures:
  – Endoscopic laser or electrocauterization
  – Angiography with arteriolar embolization

SURGERY/OTHER PROCEDURES

- Packing:
  – Layering of Vaseline ribbon gauze:
    ◦ For gauze packing, be certain both ends of the ribbon gauze protrude from the nostril.
    ◦ The packing is layered from the floor upward.
    ◦ Secure packing with gauze across the outside of the nostril
  – Nasal tampon may be used after lubricating the tip with KY Jelly or antibiotic cream or ointment.
  – Additional saline may be needed to expand the tampon if the bleeding has slowed.
  – Merocel and Rapid Rhino packs are easier to use than gauze packing and are usually well tolerated.
- Posterior bleed:
  – In the emergent setting, this may be attempted utilizing a Foley catheter or a specific posterior packing balloon.
  – With both methods, the tubing is introduced through the nose similar to the passage of a nasogastric tube. Once it reaches the posterior oral pharynx, the balloon is inflated and the tubing is pulled back outward to tamponade the posterior bleeding source:
    ◦ If using a Foley catheter (10–14 French), the balloon can be inflated with 10 mL of saline.
    ◦ Traction is maintained with an umbilical cord clamp with adequate padding between the clip and the nose to avoid injury.

IN-PATIENT CONSIDERATIONS

Consider for elderly or for patients with posterior bleeding or coagulopathy. May also consider if significant comorbidities.

Initial Stabilization

Universal "Airway/Breathing/Circulation" (ABC) approach. Stop blood loss.

Admission Criteria

- Posterior bleed
- Hemodynamic changes
- Clotting dysfunction

ONGOING CARE

FOLLOW-UP RECOMMENDATIONS

Patient Monitoring

- When significant blood loss, hemodynamic monitoring
- With packing, 24-hour minimum; some authors recommend 3–5 days. The latter recommendation carries the risk of mucosal injury and toxic shock syndrome. The former has the risk of rebleed, which usually occurs between 24 and 48 hours.

PATIENT EDUCATION

- Demonstrate proper pinching pressure techniques.
- Avoidance of trauma or irritants is key.
- Management of systemic illness and proper use of medication

PROGNOSIS

- Most are self-limited.
- Good results with proper treatment

COMPLICATIONS

- Septal perforation
- Pressure-induced tissue necrosis of the nasal mucosa
- Toxic shock syndrome with packing
- Arrhythmias triggered by packing

REFERENCES

1. Mathiasen RA, Cruz RM. Prospective, randomized, controlled clinical trial of a novel matrix hemostatic sealant in patients with acute anterior epistaxis. *Laryngoscope*. 2005;115:899–902.
2. Hanif J, Tasca RA, Frosh A, et al. Silver nitrate: histological effects of cautery on epithelial surfaces with varying contact times. *Clin Otolaryngol Allied Sci*. 2003;28:368–70.
3. Burton MJ, Dorée CJ. Interventions for recurrent idiopathic epistaxis (nosebleeds) in children. *Cochrane Database Syst Rev*. 2004:CD004461.
4. Calder N, Kang S, Fraser L, Kunanandam T, Montgomery J, Kubba H et al. A double-blind randomized controlled trial of management of recurrent nosebleeds in children. *Otolaryngol Head Neck Surg*. 2009;140:670–4.

ADDITIONAL READING

- Douglas R, Wormald PJ. Update on epistaxis. *Curr Opin Otolaryngol Head Neck Surg*. 2007;15:180–3.
- Gifford TO, Orlandi RR. Epistaxis. *Otolaryngol Clin North Am*. 2008;41:525–36, viii.
- Kucik CJ, et al. Management of epistaxis. *Am Fam Physician*. 2005;7(2).
- Robertson S, Kubba H. Long-term effectiveness of antiseptic cream for recurrent epistaxis in childhood: five-year follow up of a randomised, controlled trial. *J Laryngol Otol*. 2008:1–4.
- Viehweg TL, Roberson JB, Hudson JW. Epistaxis: diagnosis and treatment. *J Oral Maxillofac Surg*. 2006;64:511–8.

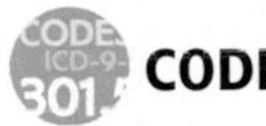

CODES

ICD9

784.7 Epistaxis

CLINICAL PEARLS

- Most episodes are anterior in etiology and respond to timed pressure over the anterior nares for 5–20 minutes.
- Most are idiopathic or as a result of nose picking.
- Posterior nosebleeds can be asymptomatic or present with nausea, hematemesis, or heme-positive stool.

EPSTEIN-BARR VIRUS INFECTIONS

Dennis E. Hughes, DO

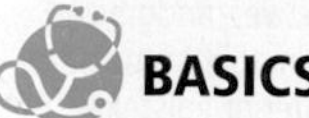

BASICS

DESCRIPTION

- Epstein-Barr virus (EBV) is the cause of heterophile-positive infectious mononucleosis.
- All seropositive persons actively shed the virus in the saliva.
- System(s) affected: Hemic/Lymphatic/Immunologic

EPIDEMIOLOGY

Incidence

Worldwide, infects >90% of people (antibody-positive) (1)

Prevalence

- Military and college student groups have the most active infection rate (0.1–0.48%) (2).
- Predominant age: 10–19 years (2)
- By young adult life, 60–90% of persons are antibody-positive to EBV; antibodies persist for lifetime (1).
- Predominant gender: Male = Female

RISK FACTORS

- Age
- Sociohygienic level
- Geographic location
- Close, intimate contact
- EBV may play a cofactor role in chronic inflammatory and autoimmune diseases such as multiple sclerosis (MS) (3)[C].

GENERAL PREVENTION

- Avoiding close physical contact with persons known to be currently symptomatic
- Good handwashing and hygiene
- EBV vaccine currently under development

PATHOPHYSIOLOGY

- A polyclonal B-cell proliferative response is characteristic of infectious mononucleosis. Relatively few circulating lymphocytes are infected by EBV and represent <0.1% of circulating mononuclear cells in the acute illness.
- EBV is tropic for B-lymphocytes, which are infected in the oropharynx through salivary exchange; infected B cells then circulate in the blood and are distributed to the bone marrow and lymphoreticular system.
- EBV can also be found in infected epithelial cells of the buccal mucosa, salivary glands, tongue, and endocervix; this suggests that chronic epithelial replication brings about continuous reinfection of B lymphoid cells.
- Immune T-cell responses to latently infected B cells account for the clinical findings.

ETIOLOGY

EBV, a member of the herpesvirus (DNA virus) group

COMMONLY ASSOCIATED CONDITIONS

- Infectious mononucleosis: The symptomatic primary EBV infection seen in otherwise healthy older children, adolescents, and young adults:
  - Clinical features vary in severity and duration: In children, generally mild; in adults, more severe and protracted.
  - Incubation period is 30–50 days.
- X-linked lymphoproliferative syndrome (Duncan disease)
- Lymphoproliferative syndromes due to EBV infections in transplant patients
- Lymphomas (B-cell lymphoblastic, T cell)
- Lymphocytic interstitial pneumonitis
- Hairy leukoplakia of the tongue and central nervous system (CNS) lymphomas in AIDS patients
- Burkitt lymphoma
- Nasopharyngeal carcinoma
- Parotid carcinoma
- Hodgkin lymphoma

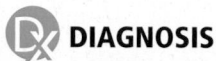

DIAGNOSIS

HISTORY

- May begin abruptly or insidiously
- Syndrome of fatigue, malaise, and sore throat
- In adults, temperature may rise to 103°F (39.4°C) and gradually fall over a variable period of 7–10 days; in severe cases, temperature elevations of 104–105°F (40.0–40.6°C) may persist for 2 weeks.
- Children usually have a low-grade fever or may be afebrile.
- Diffuse hyperemia and hyperplasia of oropharyngeal lymphoid tissue
- Gelatinous, grayish-white exudative tonsillitis persists for 7–10 days in 50%.
- Petechiae develop at border of hard and soft palates in 60%.
- Axillary, epitrochlear, popliteal, inguinal, mediastinal, and mesenteric nodes may also be affected (95% of patients) (2).
- Lymph node enlargement subsides over days or weeks.
- Chest pain (myocarditis and pericarditis)

PHYSICAL EXAM

- Fever, lymphadenopathy, pharyngitis in >50%, with palatal petechiae and hepatosplenomegaly ~10% (1,4)
- Tender lymphadenopathy (cervical nodes are most commonly enlarged)
- Splenomegaly in 50%
- Skin manifestations (3–16%):
  - Erythematous macular or maculopapular rash
  - Petechial and purpuric exanthems have been reported.
  - Rash location: Trunk and upper arms; occasionally the face and forearms involved

DIAGNOSTIC TESTS & INTERPRETATION

Lab

Initial lab tests

- Complete blood count (CBC) with differential
- Lymphocytes and atypical lymphocytes:
  - Increased numbers of lymphocytes (especially atypical lymphocytes; may be up to 70% of leukocytes) in peripheral blood
  - In 1st week after onset, white blood cell (WBC) count is normal or moderately decreased. By the 2nd week, lymphocytosis develops with >10% atypical lymphocytes (4).
  - During early illness, atypical lymphocytes are B cells transformed by the EBV; later, atypical cells are primarily T cells having an immunoregulatory function.
- Antibodies:
  - Heterophile antibodies in 80–90% of adults
  - Heterophile antibody is an IgM response, which appears during the 1st or 2nd week of illness and persists for 3–6 months.
  - In general, agglutinin titer is higher in infectious mononucleosis than in other disorders; an unabsorbed heterophile titer >1:128 and 1:40 or higher after absorption is significant.
- Specific antibodies to EBV-associated antigens:
  - Develop regularly in infectious mononucleosis
  - Viral capsid-specific IgM and IgG are present early in illness; viral capsid-IgM responses disappear after several months, whereas viral capsid-IgG antibodies persist for life.
- Liver function studies; AST and ALT elevations and hyperbilirubinemia are common; frank jaundice is rare.
- Disorders that may alter lab results: Atypical lymphocytes are not specific for EBV infections and may be present in other clinical conditions, including rubella, infectious hepatitis, allergic rhinitis, asthma, and primary atypical pneumonia:
  - In infectious mononucleosis, increased numbers of atypical forms are present in peripheral blood; in other disorders, quantitative percentage is usually less.

ollow-Up & Special Considerations

ıbnormal hepatic enzymes in 80% of patients for ›everal weeks after onset; hepatomegaly in 15–20%

maging

nitial approach

Abdominal ultrasound to monitor for splenic enlargement is not supported routinely (2).

Consider for those wishing to return to strenuous activity or contact sports at day 21 of illness to evaluate for resolution of splenomegaly.

Diagnostic Procedures/Surgery

Chest x-ray (CXR):

Hilar adenopathy may be observed in infectious mononucleosis cases with extensive lymphoid hyperplasia.

Pathological Findings

- Mononuclear infiltrations involve lymph nodes, tonsils, spleen, lungs, liver, heart, kidneys, adrenal glands, skin, and CNS.
- Bone marrow hyperplasia develops regularly, and small granulomas may be present; these are nonspecific and have no prognostic significance.

DIFFERENTIAL DIAGNOSIS

- Streptococcal pharyngitis and tonsillitis
- Diphtheria
- Blood dyscrasias
- Rubella
- Measles
- Viral hepatitis
- Cytomegalovirus
- Toxoplasmosis

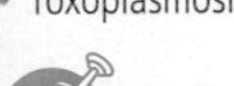

TREATMENT

MEDICATION

- Antimicrobial agents (usually a penicillin) if throat culture is positive for group A, beta-hemolytic streptococci (5)
- Warm saline gargles for the pain of pharyngeal involvement and enlarged lymph nodes
- Corticosteroids:
  - Support unclear; may provide some symptomatic relief, but no improvement in resolution of illness
  - Consider in severe pharyngotonsillitis with oropharyngeal edema and airway encroachment. Dexamethasone (0.3 mg/kg/day) may be used for 1–3 days (2,5,6)[B].
  - Also for patients with marked toxicity or major complications (e.g., hemolytic anemia, thrombocytopenic purpura, neurologic sequelae, myocarditis, pericarditis) (1)
- Precautions: Refer to the manufacturer's literature.

ADDITIONAL TREATMENT

General Measures

- The treatment is chiefly supportive.
- Nonsteroidal anti-inflammatory drugs
- During acute stage, limit activity for 4 weeks to reduce potential complications (splenic rupture, etc.) and aid in recovery.

SURGERY/OTHER PROCEDURES

With profound thrombocytopenia, refractory to corticosteroid therapy, splenectomy may be necessary.

IN-PATIENT CONSIDERATIONS

Admission Criteria

- Inability to eat food or drink fluids
- Splenic rupture

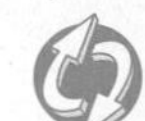

ONGOING CARE

FOLLOW-UP RECOMMENDATIONS

ALERT

Rupture of the spleen may be fatal if not recognized, and requires blood transfusions, treatment for shock, and splenectomy. Occurrence is estimated at 0.1% (2).

Patient Monitoring

- Avoid contact sports, heavy lifting, and excess exertion until spleen and liver have returned to normal size.
- Eliminate alcohol or exposure to other hepatotoxic drugs until liver function tests return to normal.
- Monitor patients closely during the 1st 2–3 weeks after the onset of symptoms. Thereafter, follow patients until their symptoms subside.
- Rarely, laboratory results resolve more slowly, and symptoms (malaise, fatigue, intermittent sore throat, lymphadenopathy) may persist for several months (4).

DIET

No restrictions. Hydration during acute phase is very important.

PATIENT EDUCATION

Mononucleosis on Familydoctor.org

PROGNOSIS

- Vast majority will be recovered by 4 weeks.
- Fatigue symptoms may persist for months (2).

COMPLICATIONS

- Neurologic (rare):
  - Aseptic meningitis
  - Bell palsy
  - Meningoencephalitis
  - Guillain-Barré syndrome
  - Transverse myelitis
  - Cerebellar ataxia
  - Acute psychosis
- Hematologic (rare):
  - Thrombocytopenia, slight to moderate, early in illness
  - Hemolytic anemia with marked neutropenia during early weeks
  - Aplastic anemia
  - Agammaglobulinemia
- Pneumonitis
- Splenic rupture:
  - Rare, but most often occurs in 1st 21 days of illness

REFERENCES

1. Cohen JI. Epstein-Barr virus infection. *N Engl J Med*. 2000;343:481–92.
2. Ebell MH. Epstein-Barr virus infectious mononucleosis. *Am Fam Physician*. 2006;70(7): 1279–88.
3. Pohl D. Epstein-Barr virus and multiple sclerosis. *J Neurol Sci*. 2009.
4. Rea TD, Russo JE, Katon W, et al. Prospective study of the natural history of infectious mononucleosis caused by Epstein-Barr virus. *J Am Board Fam Pract*. 2001;14:234–42.
5. Halstead ME, Bernhardt DT. Common infections in the young athlete. *Pediatr Ann*. 2002;31:42–8.
6. Thompson SK, Doerr TD, Hengerer AS. Infectious mononucleosis and corticosteroids: management practices and outcomes. *Arch Otolaryngol Head Neck Surg*. 2005;131:900–4.

ADDITIONAL READING

Roy M, Bailey B, Amre DK, et al. Dexamethasone for the treatment of sore throat in children with suspected infectious mononucleosis: a randomized, double-blind, placebo-controlled, clinical trial. *Arch Pediatr Adolesc Med*. 2004;158:250–4.

CODES

ICD9

075 Infectious mononucleosis

CLINICAL PEARLS

- False-negative monospot (heterophile antibody) in the 1st 10–14 days of illness
- 98% have fever, sore throat, cervical node enlargement, and tonsillar hypertrophy.
- Although splenic rupture is extremely rare, athletic activity should be curtailed for 3–4 weeks.
- Lab shows a lymphocytosis, not a monocytosis.

ERECTILE DYSFUNCTION

Michael C. Barros, PharmD, BCPS
Erica Tavares, PharmD, RPh
Frank J. Domino, MD

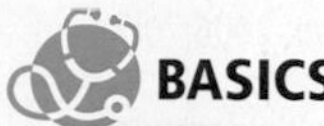

BASICS

DESCRIPTION

- Inability to achieve or maintain an erection sufficient for satisfactory sexual performance (1)[C]
- Erectile dysfunction is sometimes assumed to be a symptom of the aging process in men, but it can likely result from concurrent medical conditions of the patient or from medications that patients may be taking to treat those conditions.
- Normal penile erection requires full functioning of the vascular, nervous, and hormonal systems.
- System(s) affected: Cardiovascular; Nervous; Urologic; Reproductive
- Synonym: Impotence

EPIDEMIOLOGY

Prevalence

- Overall prevalence for erectile dysfunction per the Massachusetts Male Aging Study (2):
  - 52% in men age 40–70 years
  - Age-related increase ranging from 12.4% in men age 40–49 years up to 46.6% in men age 50–69 years
- A study of US health professionals found prevalence of sexual dysfunction 12% in men <59 years old, 22% age 60–69 years, and 30% >69 years old (3).

RISK FACTORS

- Age
- Cardiovascular disease
- Diabetes
- Metabolic syndrome
- Lower urinary tract systems of benign prostatic hyperplasia
- Medications that induce erectile dysfunction
- Urologic surgery or trauma/injury to pelvic area or spinal cord
- Central neurologic and endocrinologic conditions
- Substance abuse
- Psychological conditions: stress, anxiety, or depression
- Smoking

Genetics

Rarely related to chromosomal disorders

ETIOLOGY

- Erectile dysfunction may result from problems with systems required for normal penile erection:
  - Vascular: Diseases that compromise blood flow:
    - Peripheral vascular disease, arteriosclerosis, essential hypertension
  - Neurologic: Diseases that impair nerve conduction to brain or penile vasculature:
    - Spinal cord injury, trauma (bicycling accident), stroke, diabetes
  - Endocrine: Diseases associated with changes in testosterone, luteinizing hormone, prolactin levels
  - Psychological: Patients suffering from malaise, depression, performance anxiety, or Alzheimer's disease
- Social habits such as smoking or excessive alcohol intake
- Medications may cause erectile dysfunction.
- Structural injury or trauma

Geriatric Considerations

Aging alone is not a cause.

COMMONLY ASSOCIATED CONDITIONS

- Cardiovascular disease
  - Men with erectile dysfunction have a greater likelihood of having angina, myocardial infarction, stroke, transient ischemic attack, congestive heart failure, or cardiac arrhythmia compared to men without erectile dysfunction (3).
- Diabetes
- Psychiatric disorders

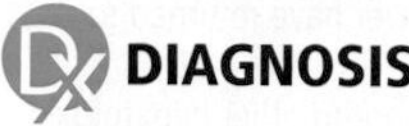

DIAGNOSIS

- Inability to maintain erection satisfactory for intercourse
- Inability to achieve erection
- Reduced body hair
- Thyromegaly
- Gynecomastia
- Testicular atrophy or absence
- Deformed penis
- Peripheral vascular disease
- Neuropathy

HISTORY

- Identify concurrent medical illnesses or surgical procedures
- Social history: Smoking, ethanol intake, recreational drug use
- List of prescription and nonprescription medications

PHYSICAL EXAM

- Assess vital signs (blood pressure and heart rate)
- Signs and symptoms of hypogonadism: Gynecomastia, small testicles, decreased body hair
- Abnormal penile curvature (Peyronie's disease)
- Assess for central obesity, thyroid goiter
- Detailed examination of the cardiovascular, neurologic, and genitourinary systems
  - Check femoral and lower extremity pulses to assess vascular supply to genitals
  - Check anal sphincter tone and genital reflexes for adequate nerve supply
  - Digital rectal exam for patients age >50 years to rule out benign prostatic hyperplasia (BPH)
- Screen for cardiovascular risk factors

DIAGNOSTIC TESTS & INTERPRETATION

- Nocturnal penile tumescence and rigidity assessment
- Consider the following only in rare circumstances, when indicated:
  - 24-hour urine zinc
  - Dorsal nerve somatosensory-evoked potentials
  - Sacral evoked response
  - Penile–brachial blood pressure (BP)
  - Aortogram
  - Selective pudendal angiogram
  - Dynamic cavernosography
  - Penile BP
- Optional diagnostic tests: psychological or psychiatric evaluation

Lab

Initial lab tests

- Fasting serum glucose
- Lipid profile
- Serum testosterone levels drawn in the morning (2 serial levels are needed to confirm hypogonadism)
- Thyroid-stimulating hormone
- Prolactin

Imaging

Doppler, angiogram, cavernosogram

Diagnostic Procedures/Surgery

International Index of Erectile Function (IIEF) Survey may be used to assess the severity of a patient's erectile dysfunction. The survey is also available in an abbreviated form (IIEF-5).

DIFFERENTIAL DIAGNOSIS

- Endocrine:
  - Thyroid dysfunction
  - Low testosterone
  - High prolactin
  - Diabetes
  - High estrogen effect
  - Renal failure
  - Zinc deficiency
- Neurologic: Central, Spinal, Peripheral
- Vascular: Arterial insufficiency, Cavernosal insufficiency, Venous insufficiency
- Medication: β-blockers, thiazides, antidepressants
- Psychological: Depression, Schizophrenia, Relationship disorders, Personality disorders, Anxiety
- Structural:
  - Microphallus, Chordee and Peyronie's disease, Cavernosal scarring
  - Phimosis, Hypospadias
- Postsurgical sequelae

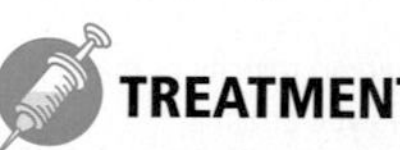

TREATMENT

Use least invasive therapy first; reserve more invasive therapies for nonresponders.

MEDICATION

First Line

Phosphodiesterase type 5 (PDE-5) inhibitors are effective in the treatment of erectile dysfunction associated with diabetes mellitus and spinal cord injury, and sexual dysfunction associated with antidepressants (3).

- Sildenafil (Viagra): Usual daily dose: 25–100 mg within 30–60 min of sexual intercourse on an empty stomach, at least 2 hours before meals. Duration up to 4 hours.

- Vardenafil (Levitra): Usual daily dose 5–20 mg within 30–60 minutes of sexual intercourse on an empty stomach, at least 2 hours before meals. Duration up to 4 hours.
- Tadalafil (Cialis): Usual daily dose 5–20 mg, 2 hours before intercourse. May take without regard to meals. Duration up to 36 hours.

Geriatric Considerations

- Use doses at the lower end of the dosing range for elderly patients:
  - Sildenafil 25 mg daily
  - Vardenafil 5 mg daily
- Adverse effects of PDE-5 inhibitors: Headache, facial flushing, dyspepsia, nasal congestion, dizziness, hypotension, increased sensitivity to light (sildenafil and vardenafil), vision changes, lower back pain (tadalafil), and priapism (with excessive doses)

Second Line

- Penile injectables:
  - Alprostadil, also known as prostaglandin E_1, causes smooth muscle relaxation of the arterial blood vessels and sinusoidal tissues in the corpora. Available in 2 formulations:
    - Alprostadil (Caverject): Usual dose: 10–20 mcg, with max dose of 60 mcg. Injection should be made at right angles into one of the lateral surfaces of the proximal third of the penis using a 0.5-inch 27- or 30-gauge needle. Do not use >3 times a week or > once in 24 hours. Patient to notify physician if erection lasts >4 hours for immediate attention. Apply manual pressure at site of injection to prevent hematoma formation. Use with caution in patients with sickle cell disease: Initial trial dose should be administered under supervision of a physician
    - Alprostadil may also be combined with papaverine (Bimix) plus phentolamine(Tri-Mix).
    - Alprostadil (Muse) urethral suppository: 125-, 250-, 500-, and 1,000-mcg pellets. Administer 5–50 minutes before intercourse. No more than 2 doses in 24 hours are recommended.
- Miscellaneous:
  - Testosterone replacement regimens for patients with primary or secondary hypogonadism as confirmed by decreased libido and low testosterone concentrations.
    - Testosterone patch (Testoderm) 4 mg/patch, 6 mg/patch: Apply 4–6 mg/day to scrotum
    - Testosterone patch (Testoderm TTS) 4 mg/patch, 6 mg/patch: Apply 4–6 mg/day to arm, buttock, back
    - Testosterone patch (Androderm) 2.5 mg/patch: Apply 2.5–5 mg/day to arm, back, abdomen, thigh
    - Testosterone gel (AndroGel 1%) 5 g/packet, 10 g/packet: Apply 5–10 g/day to shoulders, upper arms, abdomen
    - Testosterone cypionate (Depo-Testosterone) 100 mg/mL, 200 mg/mL
    - Testosterone enanthate (Delatestryl) 100 mg/mL, 200 mg/mL: Inject 200–400 mg intramuscularly every 2-4 weeks
  - Contraindications:
    - Avoid injections in patients with bleeding disorders, sickle cell disease or trait, and penile deformities.
    - Avoid use in patients with known allergies to constituents.
    - Nitroglycerin (or other nitrates) and phosphodiesterase inhibitors: Potential for severe, potentially fatal hypotension
  - Precautions:
    - Testosterone: Urinary retention, acne, sodium retention, and gynecomastia
    - Injection therapy: Priapism, fibrosis, hypotension, and nausea
    - Urethral suppositories: Penile pain and irritation, as well as testicular pain
    - Sildenafil: Hypotension (caution for patients on nitrates)
    - PDE-5 inhibitors: Use caution with congenital prolonged QT syndrome, class Ia or II antiarrhythmics, nitroglycerin, α-blockers (e.g., terazosin, tamsulosin), retinal disease, unstable cardiac disease, liver and renal failure
  - Significant possible interactions:
    - PDE-5 inhibitor concentration is affected by CYP3A4 inhibitors (e.g., erythromycin, indinavir, ketoconazole, ritonavir, amiodarone, cimetidine, clarithromycin, delavirdine, diltiazem, fluoxetine, fluvoxamine, grapefruit juice, itraconazole, nefazodone, nevirapine, ritonavir, saquinavir, and verapamil). Serum concentrations and/or toxicity may be increased. Lower starting doses should be used in these patients.
    - PDE-5 inhibitor concentration may be reduced by rifampin and phenytoin.

ADDITIONAL TREATMENT

General Measures

- Penile prosthesis should be reserved for patients who have failed 1st- or 2nd-line therapies.
- Psychotherapy alone or in combination with psychoactive drugs may be helpful in men whose erectile dysfunction is caused by depression or anxiety.
- Weight loss and increased physical activity for obese men with erectile dysfunction.
- Improve partner communication.
- Reduce performance pressure.
- Try vacuum erectile device or oral therapy (can be used in conjunction with intracavernous injections). Do not use vacuum devices in men with sickle cell anemia or blood dyscrasias, or those on anticoagulants.
- Use of psychiatrists, psychologists, sex therapists, vascular surgeons, urologists, endocrinologists, neurologists, or plastic surgeons is often necessary for refractory cases.

COMPLEMENTARY AND ALTERNATIVE MEDICINE

Yohimbine and herbal therapies are not recommended for the treatment of erectile dysfunction (1).

SURGERY/OTHER PROCEDURES

Penile prosthesis is the most invasive treatment of erectile dysfunction and is reserved for patients who do not respond or are not candidates for oral or injectable therapies. Penile arterial reconstructive surgery is controversial.

ONGOING CARE

FOLLOW-UP RECOMMENDATIONS

Patient Monitoring

Treatment should be assessed at baseline and after the patient has completed at least 1–3 weeks of a specific treatment: Monitor the quality and quantity of penile erections and Monitor the level of satisfaction patient achieves.

DIET

Diet and exercise recommended to achieve a normal body mass index; limit alcohol

PROGNOSIS

- All commercially available PDE-5 inhibitors are equally effective. In the presence of sexual stimulation, sildenafil produces satisfactory erections in 56–82% of patients. Similar results are seen in 65–80% of patients taking vardenafil and 62–77% in patients taking tadalafil:
  - Lower success rates with diabetes mellitus or who have postoperative nerve damage.
- Overall effectiveness is 70–90% for intracavernosal alprostadil and 43–60% for intraurethral alprostadil (4,5).
- Penile prostheses are associated with a 90% patient satisfaction rate, and the surgical success rate after insertion is 82–98% (4).

E

REFERENCES

1. Montague DK, Jarrow JP, Broderick GA, Dmochowski RR, Heaton JP, Lue TF, et al. *The Management of Erectile Dysfunction: An Update*. Linthicum, MD: American Urological Association, 2006.
2. Johannes CB, Aranjo AB, Feldman HA, et al. Incidence of erectile dysfunction in men 40-69 years old: Longitudinal results from the Massachusetts Male Aging Study. *J Urol*. 2000;163:460–3.
3. Heidelbaugh JJ et al. Management of erectile dysfunction. *Am Fam Physician*. 2010;81:305–12.
4. Lue TF. Erectile dysfunction. *N Engl J Med*. 2000;342:1802–13.
5. McVary KT. Clinical practice. Erectile dysfunction. *N Engl J Med*. 2007;357:2472–81.

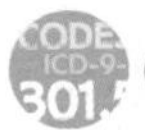

CODES

ICD9

- 302.72 Psychosexual dysfunction with inhibited sexual excitement
- 607.84 Impotence of organic origin

CLINICAL PEARLS

- Nitrates should be withheld for 24 hours after sildenafil or vardenafil administration and for 48 hours after use of tadalafil.
- Reserve surgical treatment for patients who do not respond to drug treatment.
- The use of PDE-5 inhibitors with alpha-adrenergic antagonists may increase the risk of hypotension. Tamsulosin is the least likely to cause orthostatic hypotension.
- Consult a cardiologist for use of PDE-5 inhibitors in patients with left ventricular dysfunction or NYHA class II. Do not use in patients with NYHA class III or IV.

ERYSIPELAS

James G. Anderson, MD
Richard A. Moriarty, MD

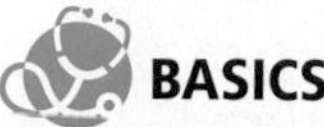

BASICS

DESCRIPTION

- Distinct form of cellulitis notable for acute, well-demarcated, superficial bacterial skin infection with lymphatic involvement almost always caused by *Streptococcus pyogenes*. Usually acute, but a chronic recurrent form also exists (1).
- System(s) affected: Skin/Exocrine
- Synonym(s): Saint Anthony's fire

EPIDEMIOLOGY

- Predominant age: Infants, children, and adults >40 years. Greatest in elderly (>75 years).
- Predominant sex: Male = Female
- Affects all races

Incidence

- Erysipelas occurs in about 1 person/1,000/year (2)
- Incidence on the rise since the 1980s (3)

Prevalence

Unknown

RISK FACTORS

- Toe-web intertrigo and lymphedema (2)
- Skin barrier disruption (surgical incisions, insect bites, eczematous lesions, local trauma, abrasions, dermatophytic infections)
- Fissured skin (especially at the nose and ears)
- Leg ulcers/stasis dermatitis
- Venous or lymphatic insufficiency (saphenectomy, varicose veins of leg, phlebitis, radiotherapy, mastectomy, lymphadenectomy)
- Chronic diseases (diabetes, malnutrition, nephrotic syndrome, heart failure)
- Immunocompromised (HIV) or debilitated
- Alcohol abuse
- Morbid obesity
- Recent streptococcal pharyngitis

GENERAL PREVENTION

- Good skin hygiene.
- Appropriate management of underlying medical condition that might predispose to the condition: Tinea pedis, stasis dermatitis, etc.
- Men who shave within 5 days of facial erysipelas are more likely to have a recurrence.
- With recurrences, search for other possible source of streptococcal infection (e.g., tonsils, sinuses).
- Compression stockings should be encouraged for patients with lower extremity edema.
- Consider suppressive prophylactic antibiotic therapy in patients with ≥2 episodes in a 12-month period.

PATHOPHYSIOLOGY

- Group A streptococci induce inflammation and activation of the contact system, releasing proteinases and pro-inflammatory cytokines.
- The generation of antibacterial peptides and the release of bradykinin, a proinflammatory peptide, increase vascular permeability and induce fever and pain.
- The M proteins from the group A streptococcal cell wall interact with neutrophils, leading to the secretion of heparin-binding protein, an inflammatory mediator that also induces vascular leakage.
- These cascades of reactions lead to the symptoms seen in erysipelas: Fever, pain, erythema, and edema

ETIOLOGY

- Group A β-hemolytic streptococci primarily; occasionally other streptococcus groups C or G
- Rarely, group B streptococci or *Staphylococcus aureus* may be involved.

Pediatric Considerations

- Group B streptococcus may be a cause in neonates/infants.

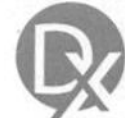

DIAGNOSIS

- Prodromal symptoms may include chills, malaise, moderate- to high-grade fever, headache, vomiting, and anorexia, usually in the 1st 48 hours.
- Arthralgias

ALERT

Important to differentiate erysipelas from MRSA infection, which usually has an indurated center, significant pain, and later evidence of abscess formation

PHYSICAL EXAM

- Vital signs: Moderate- to high-grade fever with resultant tachycardia. Hypotension may occur.
- Fever may be a differentiating factor among other skin infections.
- Headache and vomiting may be prominent.
- Acute onset of erythematous patch
- Sharply demarcated, raised border, fiery-red plaque that spreads circumferentially over hours/days
- Lesion characteristically hot, indurated, tender with marked swelling
- Peau d'orange appearance
- Vesicles and bullae may form, but are not uniformly present.
- Desquamation may occur later.
- Location:
  - Lower extremity 70–80% of cases
  - Face involvement is less common (5–20%), especially nose and ears
  - Chronic form usually recurs at site of the previous infection, and may recur years after initial episode.
- Patients on systemic steroids may be more difficult to diagnose because signs and symptoms of the infection may be masked by anti-inflammatory action of the steroids.
- Systemic toxicity resolves rapidly with treatment; skin lesions desquamate on days 5–10, but usually heal without scarring.

Pediatric Considerations

- Abdominal involvement more common in infants, especially around umbilical stump
- Face, scalp, and leg common in older children

Geriatric Considerations

- Fever may not be as prominent.
- More prone to complications
- High-output cardiac failure may occur in debilitated patients with underlying cardiac disease.
- Face and lower extremity are most common areas
- Integument: Hot, tender, erythematous, superficial plaque with sharply demarcated borders. Facial involvement presents in a butterfly pattern. Pustules characteristically absent.
- Lymphatics: Regional lymphadenopathy, lymphangitic streaking

DIAGNOSTIC TESTS & INTERPRETATION

Lab

- Classic erysipelas can be diagnosed and treated without laboratory workup. Reserve diagnostic for severely ill, toxic patients or those who are immunosuppressed.
- Leukocytosis
- Blood culture (<5% positive)
- Elevated erythrocyte sedimentation rate (ESR) and C-reactive protein (CRP)
- Streptococci may be cultured from exudate or noninvolved sites.
- Antistreptolysin, streptozyme, anti-DNase, and antihyaluronidase titers may not be helpful acutely.

Imaging

Usually not indicated

Pathological Findings

- Dermal and epidermal edema, extending into the subcutaneous tissues
- Peau d'orange appearance caused by edema in the superficial tissue surrounding the hair follicles
- Vasodilation and enlarged lymphatics
- Mixed interstitial infiltrate mainly consisting of neutrophils and mononuclear cells
- Endothelial cell swelling
- Gram-positive cocci in lymphatics and tissue with rare invasion of local blood vessels
- Fibrotic thickening of lymphatic vessel walls with possible luminal occlusion may be seen in recurrent erysipelas.

DIFFERENTIAL DIAGNOSIS

- Cellulitis (margins are less clear)
- Necrotizing fasciitis (systemic illness and more pain)
- Dermatophytes
- Impetigo (blistered or crusted appearance; superficial)
- Ecthyma (ulcerative impetigo)
- Herpes zoster (dermatomal distribution)
- Erythema annulare centrifugum (raised pink-red ring or bulls-eye marks)
- Contact dermatitis (no fever, pruritic)
- Giant cell urticaria (transient, wheal-appearance, severe itching)
- Angioneurotic edema (no fever)
- Scarlet fever (widespread rash with indistinct borders and without edema; rash is most common early in skin folds; develops generalized "sandpaper" feeling as it progresses)
- Toxic shock syndrome (diffuse erythema with evidence of multiorgan involvement)
- Lupus (of the face; less fever, positive antinuclear antibodies)
- Polychondritis (common site is the ear)

- Tuberculoid leprosy
- Inflammatory breast carcinoma
- Other bacterial infections to consider:
  - Meat, shellfish, fish, and poultry workers: *Erysipelothrix rhusiopathiae* (known as erysipeloid)
  - Human bite: *Eikenella corrodens*
  - Cat or dog bite: *Pasteurella multocida* or *Capnocytophaga canimorsus*
  - Salt water exposure: *Vibrio vulnificus*
  - Fresh or brackish water exposure: *Aeromonas hydrophilia*

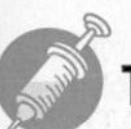

TREATMENT

Infectious Diseases Society of America guidelines for the diagnosis and management of skin and soft tissue infections recommends penicillin, either p.o. or parenterally, depending on clinical severity, as the treatment of choice for erysipelas (4).

MEDICATION

First Line

- Adults:
  - Mild: Penicillin VK 500 mg p.o. q6h for 10–14 days (improvement in 24–48 hours) or penicillin G procaine 0.6–1.2 million U IM b.i.d. for 10 days (4)[A]
  - Moderate-severe: Cefazolin 1–2 grams q8h IM/IV or ceftriaxone 1 gram q24h IM/IV
- Children:
  - Penicillin VK:
    - <12 years: 25–50 mg/kg/d p.o. div. q6–8h with max: 3 g/d
    - >12 years: Adult dose
  - Penicillin G procaine:
    - <30 kg: 300,000 U/d IM
    - >30 kg: Adult dose
- Nafcillin or oxacillin 2.0 g IV q4h or penicillin G parenterally is recommended for severe or complicated cases (1 million–2 million units q4–6h).
- No reported group A streptococci resistance to beta-lactam antibiotics
- In chronic recurrent infections, prophylactic treatment after the acute infection resolves:
  - Penicillin G benzathine 1.2 million U IM q month, or Penicillin VK 250 mg p.o. b.i.d.
- If staphylococcal infection is suspected or patient is acutely ill, a beta-lactamase-stable antibiotic should be considered.
- Consider community-acquired methicillin-resistant *Staphylococcus aureas* (MRSA) and, depending on regional sensitivity, may treat MRSA with trimethoprim-sulfamethoxazole, clindamycin, or tetracycline. If resistance is a concern or patient is clinically unstable, treat with vancomycin, daptomycin, or linezolid.

Second Line

- Cephalosporins:
  - Cephalexin:
    - Children: 25 mg/kg/d p.o. divided q6h
    - Adults: 500 mg p.o. q6h
  - Cefazolin:
    - Children: 50 mg/kg/d IV divided q8h
    - Adults: 1 g IV q8h
  - Contraindications: Allergy
  - Pregnancy Category B
- Clindamycin for penicillin-allergic patients in regions with high macrolide resistance:
  - Children: 10-25 mg/kg/d p.o. divided q6–8h or alternatively: 15–25 mg/kg/d IV/IM divided q6–8h
  - Adults: 150–450 mg p.o. q6h or alternatively: 600–2,700 mg/d IV/IM divided q6–12h
  - Use IV for severe infections.
- Macrolides in penicillin-allergic patients:
  - Azithromycin 500 mg on day 1, then 250 mg/d for 4 days or clarithromycin 500 mg b.i.d. for 10 days
  - Macrolide resistance among group A streptococci has increased regionally in the US, but there has never been penicillin or cephalosporin resistance reported.
- Recurrent erysipelas in adults:
  - Pen V 250 mg p.o. b.i.d.
  - Azithromycin 500 mg/d p.o.
  - Clarithromycin 500 mg/d p.o.

ADDITIONAL TREATMENT

Consider prednisolone 30 mg daily with taper over 8 days as optional adjunct for treatment of uncomplicated erysipelas in adults (5)[B].

General Measures

- Symptomatic treatment of myalgias and fever
- Adequate fluid intake
- Local treatment with cold compresses
- Elevation of affected extremity
- Appropriate therapy for any underlying predisposing condition

Issues for Referral

Recurrent infection, treatment failure

IN-PATIENT CONSIDERATIONS

Initial Stabilization

Outpatient care

Admission Criteria

- Patient with systemic toxicity
- Patient with high-risk factors (elderly, lymphedema, postsplenectomy, diabetes, etc.)

IV Fluids

IV therapy if systemic toxicity or unable to tolerate p.o.

Discharge Criteria

No evidence of systemic toxicity with improvement of erythema and swelling

ONGOING CARE

FOLLOW-UP RECOMMENDATIONS

Bed rest with elevation of extremity during acute infection, then activity as tolerated

Patient Monitoring

Patients should be treated until all symptoms and skin manifestations have resolved.

DIET

No special diet

PATIENT EDUCATION

Stress importance of completing medication regimen prescribed

PROGNOSIS

- Patients should recover fully if adequately treated.
- Mortality less than 1% in patients receiving appropriate treatment.
- Bullae formation suggests longer disease course, and often indicates a concomitant *Staphylococcus aureus* infection that may require antibiotic coverage for MRSA.
- Chronic edema/scarring may result from chronic recurrent cases.
- Rarely, obstructive lymphadenitis may result from chronic recurrent cases.

COMPLICATIONS

- Recurrent infection
- Abscess (suggests staphylococcal infection)
- Necrotizing fasciitis
- Lymphedema
- Bacteremia (which may lead to sepsis or involvement of other organ systems)
- Sepsis
- Pneumonia (due to sepsis or toxin-producing organism)
- Meningitis (due to sepsis or toxin-producing organism)
- Embolism
- Gangrene
- Bursitis
- Septic arthritis, tendinitis, or osteitis

REFERENCES

1. Gabillot-Carré M, Roujeau JC. Acute bacterial skin infections and cellulitis. *Curr Opin Infect Dis.* 2007;20:118–23.
2. Bernard P. Management of common bacterial infections of the skin. *Curr Opin Infect Dis.* 2008;21:122–8.
3. Celestin R, Brown J, Kihiczak G, et al. Erysipelas: a common potentially dangerous infection. *Acta Dermatovenerol Alp Panonica Adriat.* 2007;16: 123–7.
4. Stevens DL, et al. Practice guidelines for the diagnosis and management of skin and soft tissue infections. *Clin Infect Dis.* 2005;41:1973.
5. Bergkvist PI, Sjöbeck K et al. Antibiotic and prednisolone therapy of erysipelas: a randomized, double blind, placebo-controlled study. *Scand J Infect Dis.* 1997;29:377–82.

ADDITIONAL READING

Breen JO et al. Skin and soft tissue infections in immunocompetent patients. *Am Fam Physician.* 2010;81:893–9.

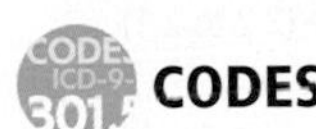

CODES

ICD9

035 Erysipelas

CLINICAL PEARLS

- Athlete's foot is the most common portal of entry for this superficial bacterial skin infection caused by *Streptococcus pyogenes*.
- Erysipelas is distinguished from cellulitis by its sharp, shiny, fiery-red, raised border.
- In recurrent cases, search for other possible source of streptococcal infection (e.g., tonsils, sinuses, intertrigo).
- Most erysipelas infections now occur on the legs, rather than the face.

ERYTHEMA MULTIFORME

Congjun Yao, MD

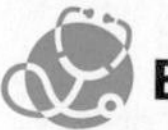

BASICS

- Erythema multiforme (EM) is an acute, self-limited hypersensitivity reaction:
  - Mostly triggered by infectious agents (more than 50% by herpes simplex virus [HSV]-1 or -2) or drugs (1,2)[B]
  - Involving the skin and sometimes the mucous membrane, most commonly the mouth
  - Skin lesions include typical target or "iris" lesions, flat or raised atypical lesions, macules with or without blisters.
- Currently, there are no universal diagnostic criteria for EM. It was previously considered to be a spectrum of disease, consisting of EM, EM major, Stevens-Johnson syndrome (SJS), and toxic epidermal necrolysis (TEN). However, it appears to be a growing consensus that EM is a distinct condition from SJS and TEN due to the differences in clinical presentation, histopathology manifestation, patient demographics, possible etiology and pathogenesis, and treatment plan (1,2,3,4)[C].

DESCRIPTION

- Two subtypes, erythema multiforme minor (EMm) and erythema multiforme major (EMM), with the former involving none or 1 mucous membrane, and the latter involving at least 2 mucous sites (1)[C]
- Recurrent EM has a mean number of 6 attacks (range 2–24) per year and a mean duration of 9.5 years (range 2–36) (1)[B].
- System(s) affected: Skin/Exocrine
- Synonym(s): Erythema polymorphe

EPIDEMIOLOGY

Incidence

The annual incidence in the US has been estimated at between 0.01 and 1% (4)[C].

Prevalence

- Predominant age: Peak incidence in 20s and 40s; rare <age 3 and >age 50
- Predominant sex: Male > Female (3:2 to 2:1) (1,2)[C]

RISK FACTORS

Previous history of erythema multiforme

Genetics

Strong association with HLA-DQ3 in herpes-related cases. Possible association in recurrent cases with HLA-B15, -B35, -A33, -DR53, DQB1*0301, and DQW3 (1)[C]

GENERAL PREVENTION

- Known or suspected etiologic agents should be avoided.
- Acyclovir may help prevent herpes-related erythema multiforme (1,2)[B].

PATHOPHYSIOLOGY

- The exact pathophysiology of EM is unknown.
- Possible immunologically mediated lymphocytic reaction to an infectious agent or a drug at the dermal-epithelial junction
- HSV-triggered EM seems to involve CD4+ T-cell infiltration and associated IFN-γ activation.
- Drug-triggered EM involves CD8+ T-cells and associated TNF-α activation (4)[C].

ETIOLOGY

- Most cases appear to be due to a preceding infection.
- Viral infections, particularly herpes simplex (accounting for more than 50% of cases); also Epstein-Barr, coxsackie, echovirus, varicella, mumps, poliovirus, hepatitis C, cytomegalovirus, HIV, molluscum contagiosum virus
- Bacterial infections, particularly *Mycoplasma pneumoniae;* other occasional reported bacterial infections include *Treponema Pallidum* and *Gardnerella vaginalis*
- Fungal infection, including *Histoplasma capsulatum* and *Coccidioides immitis*
- Medications, including sulfonamides, penicillins, barbiturates, hydantoins, nonsteroidal anti-inflammatory drugs (NSAIDs), phenothiazines. Other sparsely reported medications include candesartan, cilexetil, rofecoxib, metformin, bupropion, ciprofloxacin, sorafenib, gemfibrozil, risperidone, paclitaxel, metoprolol, adalimumab, etanercept, and infliximab.
- Vaccines: Tetanus/diphtheria, bacillus Calmette-Guérin, oral polio, hepatitis B, human papillomavirus
- Protozoan infections
- Radiation therapy
- Premenstrual hormone changes
- Sarcoidosis

COMMONLY ASSOCIATED CONDITIONS

Any of the infections or diseases listed under Etiology

DIAGNOSIS

Diagnose clinically by careful review of the history and detailed physical examination. No specific labs are required for the diagnosis.

HISTORY

- Absent or mild prodromal symptoms.
- Preceding HSV infection (over 50% of cases) 10–15 days before the skin eruptions (1,2)[B]
- Rash involving the skin and sometimes the mucous membrane, most commonly the mouth

PHYSICAL EXAM

- Skin pleomorphic eruption with a mixture of macules, papules of various sizes, and target lesions:
  - Typical target lesions: Raised and cyanotic center, edematous light intermediate ring and bright erythematous border (three zones)
  - Flat or raised atypical target lesions: 2 zones only (center and intermediate ring) with poorly defined border
  - Symmetrically distributed rash, mainly on the palms, soles, dorsum of the hands, and extensor surface of the extremities and the face
  - Lesions may coalesce and become generalized.
  - Body surface area with epidermal detachment <10% (1,2,3,4)[B]
- Mucosal involvement:
  - Minimal involvement in EM minor; if present, most commonly involves the mouth
  - At least 2 mucosal sites involved in EM major, including eyes (conjunctivitis, keratitis), mouth (stomatitis, cheilitis), and probable trachea, bronchi, gastrointestinal tract, or genital tract (balanitis and valvulitis)
  - Multiple papules and vesicles, superficial irregular erosions, shallow painful ulcers with erythematous margin (1)[C]

DIAGNOSTIC TESTS & INTERPRETATION

Lab

- No specific lab test is indicated to make the diagnosis of EM (1,2,3,4)[B].
- Skin biopsy of lesional and perilesional tissue in equivocal conditions (1,2,3,4)[C]
- Direct and indirect immunofluorescence to differentiate EM from other vesiculobullous diseases (1)[C]. Indirect immunofluorescence is detected on a biopsy of perilesional skin, and direct immunofluorescence is detected from a blood sample.
- HSV tests in recurrent EM (serologic tests, swab culture, or tests using skin biopsy sample to check HSV antigens or DNA in keratinocytes by immunofluorescence or polymerase chain reaction (PCR)) (4)[C]
- Antibody staining to IFN-γ and TNF-α to differentiate HSV-associated EM and drug-associated EM (4)[C]
- Elevated *M. pneumonia* antibody titer in *M. pneumonia* infection–associated EM (1)[C]

Imaging

Initial approach

No specific imaging studies are indicated in most cases.

Follow-Up & Special Considerations

Chest x-ray may be necessary if an underlying pulmonary infection (M. *pneumonia* infection) is suspected.

Pathological Findings

- A predominantly perivascular inflammatory infiltrate with CD4+ T lymphocytes and histocytes in papillary dermis and the epidermal-dermal junction
- Focal necrotic keratinocytes mainly in the basal layer
- Dermal edema (1,2,4)[C]

DIFFERENTIAL DIAGNOSIS

- Stevens-Johnson syndrome (3)[C]:
  - Different pattern and location of the skin lesions. No typical target lesion. Atypical flat target lesions or macules, generalized or mainly in the trunk
  - Blisters and skin detachment less than 10% of the total body surface area
  - Usually with systemic complications (i.e., Central Nervous System, lung, gastrointestinal system, kidney)
  - 1–5% mortality rate

Toxic epidermal necrolysis (1,3)[C]:
- Blisters and skin detachment more than 30% of the total body surface area
- 10–30% mortality rate

Urticaria
Necrotizing vasculitis
Drug eruptions
Contact dermatitis
Pityriasis rosea
Herpes simplex
Secondary syphilis
Ringworm
Pemphigus vulgaris
Pemphigoid
Dermatitis herpetiformis
Herpes gestationis
Septicemia
Serum sickness
Viral exanthems
Rocky Mountain spotted fever
Collagen vascular diseases
Mucocutaneous lymph node syndrome
Meningococcemia
Lichen planus
Behçet syndrome
Recurrent aphthous ulcers
Herpetic gingivostomatitis
Granuloma annulare

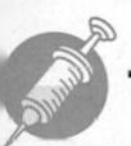

TREATMENT

MEDICATION

First Line

- Treatment of any underlying or causative disease (1,2)[B]
- Withdrawal of any drugs that might be the cause (1,2)[B]
- Symptomatic treatment with oral antihistamines and topical corticosteroids for mild cases (1,2)[B]
- Early treatment with acyclovir may lessen the number and duration of cutaneous lesions for patients with coexisting or recent HSV infection (2)[B]:
  - Acyclovir for adults: 200 mg, 5 times a day for 7–10 days in the onset of EM
  - For pediatric patients: 10 mg/kg or 500 mg/s^2, 3 times a day for 7–10 days
- Recurrent EM may be treated with oral acyclovir (400 mg 2 times per day) , even if HSV infection has not been confirmed (2)[B].
- Valacyclovir (Valtrex, 500–1,000 mg per day) and famciclovir (Famvir, 125–250 mg per day) may be tried in patients who are resistant to acyclovir (2)[C]:
  - Reduce the dosage once the patient is recurrence-free for 4 months, and eventually discontinue the drug.

Second Line

- Recurrent EM cases nonresponsive to antiviral therapy could also try dapsone (100–150 mg per day), azathioprine (Imuran, 100–150 mg per day), thalidomide (100–200 mg per day), mycophenolate mofetil (CellCept <2 g daily), hydroxychloroquine (<400 mg daily), colchicine (<1.2 mg daily) (25)[C].
- Cyclosporine given intermittently (4 mg/kg per day for a week) may also be used for recurrent EM (2)[C].
- Systemic steroid use is controversial, because it may decrease the patient's resistance to HSV and increase recurrent HSV infection (1,2)[C].
- Precautions: Refer to the manufacturer's profile of each drug.
- Significant possible interactions: Refer to the manufacturer's profile of each drug.

ADDITIONAL TREATMENT

General Measures

- Meticulous wound care and Burow's solution or Domeboro solution dressings for severe cases with epidermal detachment
- Mouth washes with warm saline or a solution of diphenhydramine, lidocaine (Xylocaine), and Kaopectate for oral lesions to provide symptomatic relief and oral hygiene, and to facilitate oral intake

IN-PATIENT CONSIDERATIONS

Admission Criteria

- Care at home
- Hospitalization needed for fluid, electrolyte management if patient with severe mucous membrane involvement, impaired oral intake and dehydration.
- IV antibiotics if secondary infection develops

ONGOING CARE

FOLLOW-UP RECOMMENDATIONS

Patient Monitoring

- The disease is self-limiting.
- Complications are rare, with no mortality.

DIET

As tolerated with increased fluid intake

PATIENT EDUCATION

- The disease is self-limiting. However, the recurrence risk may be 30%.
- Antiviral therapy with acyclovir may reduce the duration and frequency of outbreaks.
- Avoid any identified etiological agents.

PROGNOSIS

- Rash evolves over 1–2 weeks and subsequently resolves within 2–6 weeks, generally without scarring or sequelae.
- Following resolution, there may be some postinflammatory hyper- or hypopigmentation.

COMPLICATIONS

Secondary infection

REFERENCES

1. Al-Johani KA, Fedele S, Porter SR. Erythema multiforme and related disorders. *Oral Surg Oral Med Oral Pathol Oral Radiol Endod*. 2007.
2. Lamoreux MR, Sternbach MR, Hsu WT. Erythema multiforme. *Am Fam Physician*. 2006;74:1883–8.
3. Auquier-Dunant A, Mockenhaupt M, Naldi L, et al. Correlations between clinical patterns and causes of erythema multiforme majus, Stevens-Johnson syndrome, and toxic epidermal necrolysis: results of an international prospective study. *Arch Dermatol*. 2002;138:1019–24.
4. Aurelian L, Ono F, Burnett J. Herpes simplex virus (HSV)-associated erythema multiforme (HAEM): a viral disease with an autoimmune component. *Dermatol Online J*. 2003;9:1.
5. Wetter DA, Davis MD et al. Recurrent erythema multiforme: clinical characteristics, etiologic associations, and treatment in a series of 48 patients at Mayo Clinic, 2000 to 2007. *J Am Acad Dermatol*. 2010;62:45–53.

ADDITIONAL READING

- Chen M, Doherty SD, Hsu S et al. Innovative uses of thalidomide. *Dermatol Clin*. 2010;28:577–86.
- Nikkels AF, Pièrard GE. Treatment of mucocutaneous presentations of herpes simplex virus infections. *Am J Clin Dermatol*. 2002;3:475–87.
- Williams PM, Conklin RJ. Erythema multiforme: a review and contrast from Stevens-Johnson syndrome/toxic epidermal necrolysis. *Dent Clin North Am*. 2005;49:67–76, viii.

See Also (Topic, Algorithm, Electronic Media Element)

Cutaneous Drug Reactions; Dermatitis Herpetiformis; Herpes Gestationalis; Urticaria; Stevens-Johnson Syndrome; Toxic Epidermic Necrotisis

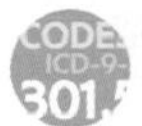

CODES

ICD9

695.10 Erythema multiforme, unspecified

CLINICAL PEARLS

- EM is diagnosed clinically by careful review of the history, through detailed physical examination, and by excluding other similar disorders. No lab tests are required for the diagnosis.
- Typical lesions are pleomorphic macules, papules, and characteristic target or "iris" lesions
- Lesions are symmetrically distributed on palms, soles, dorsum of the hands, and extensor surfaces of extremities and face. Mucosal involvement is minimal.
- Management of EM involves determining the etiology when possible. The first step is to treat the suspected infection or discontinue the causative drug.
- Complications are rare. Most cases are self-limited. However, the recurrence risk may be as high as 30%.
- Recurrent cases often are secondary to herpes simplex infection. Antiviral therapy may be beneficial.

ERYTHEMA NODOSUM

Sophia L. Delano, MD
Nikki Levin, MD, PhD

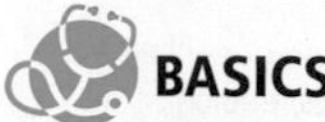

BASICS

DESCRIPTION

- A delayed-type hypersensitivity reaction to infectious agents, medications, or malignancies, or in the setting of autoimmune disorders, presenting as a subcutaneous panniculitis
- Clinical pattern of multiple, bilateral, erythematous, tender subcutaneous nodules that undergo a characteristic pattern of color changes, similar to that seen in bruises. Unlike erythema induratum, the lesions of erythema nodosum do not typically ulcerate.
- Occurs most commonly on the shins, less commonly on the thighs and forearms
- May be accompanied by fever and arthralgias
- Often idiopathic but may be associated with a number of clinical entities
- Usually remits spontaneously in weeks to months without scarring or atrophy
- Synonym(s): Dermatitis contusiformis

Pregnancy Considerations

May have repeat outbreaks during pregnancy

EPIDEMIOLOGY

Incidence

- 1-5/100,000
- Predominant age: 20–30 years
- Predominant sex: Female > Male (3:1).

Prevalence

Varies geographically depending on the prevalence of disorders associated with erythema nodosum

RISK FACTORS

See "Etiology."

ETIOLOGY

- Idiopathic: 37–60%
- Bacterial: Streptococcal infections (most common cause in children), tuberculosis, leprosy, tularemia, gonorrhea, *Yersinia enterocolitica*, *Campylobacter*, *Salmonella*, *Shigella*
- Sarcoid
- Drugs: Sulfonamides, amoxicillin, oral contraceptives, bromides
- Pregnancy
- Fungal: Dermatophytes, coccidioidomycosis, histoplasmosis, blastomycosis
- Viral/chlamydial: Infectious mononucleosis, lymphogranuloma venereum, paravaccinia
- Enteropathies: Ulcerative colitis, Crohn disease, Behçet disease (1), celiac disease (2)
- Malignancies: Lymphoma/leukemia, sarcoma, after radiation therapy

COMMONLY ASSOCIATED CONDITIONS

See "Etiology."

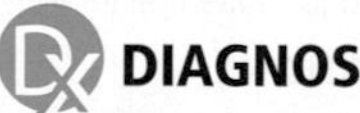

DIAGNOSIS

HISTORY

- Increasingly tender and aching nodules on the legs, usually over the shins.
- Fever, malaise, chills, fatigue
- Eruptions often preceded by symptoms of pharyngitis or upper respiratory infection
- Headache
- Arthralgias

PHYSICAL EXAM

- Initially warm, tender, brightly erythematous nodules, which may be raised, on anterior shins; lesions become bluish and fluctuant, gradually fading to yellowish, resembling a bruise.
- May occur on any area with subcutaneous fat
- Diameter usually 2–6 cm, but may rarely be larger

DIAGNOSTIC TESTS & INTERPRETATION

Diagnosis is usually clinical.

Lab

- Erythrocyte sedimentation rate (ESR). May be elevated or normal.
- Complete blood count (CBC): Mild leukocytosis
- Antistreptolysin titers may be elevated.
- Throat culture (usually negative because the infection typically resolves before lesions appear)
- Stool culture and leukocytes, if indicated
- Skin testing for mycobacteria, if indicated
- Drugs that may alter lab results: Antecedent antibiotics may affect cultures.

Imaging

CXR for hilar adenopathy or infiltrates related to sarcoidosis or tuberculosis

Diagnostic Procedures/Surgery

Deep incisional skin biopsy including subcutaneous fat; rarely necessary except in atypical cases with ulceration, duration greater than 12 weeks or a presentation that does not include skin lesions.

Pathological Findings

- Septal panniculitis without vasculitis.
- Neutrophilic infiltrate in septa of fat tissue early in course.
- Actinic radial (Miescher's) granulomas, consisting of collections of histocytes around a central stellate cleft, may be seen (3).
- Fibrosis, paraseptal granulation tissue, lymphocytes, and multinucleated giant cells predominate late in course.

DIFFERENTIAL DIAGNOSIS

- Nodular vasculitis or erythema induratum (warm ulcerating calf nodules)
- Superficial thrombophlebitis
- Cellulitis
- Septic emboli
- Weber-Christian disease (violaceous, scarring nodules)
- Lupus panniculitis
- Cutaneous polyarteritis nodosa
- Sarcoidal granulomas
- Cutaneous T-cell lymphoma
- Erythema nodosum leprosum (clinically similar to EN but shows vasculitis on histopathology)
- Vasculitis

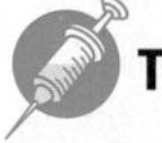

TREATMENT

All medications listed as treatment for erythema nodosum are off-label uses of the medications. There are no FDA-approved medications for erythema nodosum.

MEDICATION

First Line

- Medication usually more effective in acute than in chronic disease
- Condition often self-limited
- Nonsteroidal anti-inflammatory drugs (NSAIDs):
  - Ibuprofen: 400 mg po q4–6 hours (not to exceed 3200 mg per day)
  - Indomethacin: 25–50 mg po t.i.d.
  - Naproxen (Naprosyn): 250–500 mg po b.i.d.

- Aspirin: 325 mg 1–2 tablets po q4–6 hours (not to exceed 12 tablets a day); use enteric-coated tablets to decrease GI upset.
- Contraindications:
  – Active or recent peptic ulcer disease
  – History of hypersensitivity to NSAIDs
- Precautions:
  – GI upset/bleeding
  – Fluid retention
  – Dose reduction in elderly, especially those with renal disease, diabetes, or heart failure
  – May mask fever
  – NSAIDs may elevate liver function tests.
- Significant possible interactions:
  – May blunt antihypertensive effects of diuretics and β-blockers
  – NSAIDs can elevate plasma lithium levels.
  – Caution is advised with naproxen or any highly protein-bound drug because it may compete for albumin binding and elevate levels.
- NSAIDs can cause significant elevation and prolongation of methotrexate levels.

Second Line

- Potassium iodide 400–900 mg/d divided 2–3×/day × 3–4 weeks (for persistent lesions). Need to monitor for hypothyroidism with prolonged use. Pregnancy Class D.
- Corticosteroids for severe, refractory cases in which an infectious workup is negative. Prednisone 1mg/kg/d for 1–2 weeks often helps resolve the lesions (4). Potential side effects include hyperglycemia, hypertension, weight gain, mood changes, bone loss, osteonecrosis, myopathy.
- Recent reports of improvement with colchicine 0.6–1.2 mg b.i.d.
- Hydroxychloroquine, thalidomide and cyclosporine may also be used.

ADDITIONAL TREATMENT

General Measures

- Mild compression bandages and leg elevation may reduce pain. (Wet dressings, hot soaks, and topical medications are not useful.)
- Discontinue potentially causative drugs.
- Treat underlying disease.

COMPLEMENTARY AND ALTERNATIVE MEDICINE

Vitamin B12 replacement. A single case report of resolution of lesions with B12 replacement in a patient who had B12 deficiency and erythema nodosum (5).

IN-PATIENT CONSIDERATIONS

Admission Criteria

Occasionally, admission may be needed for the antecedent illness (e.g., tuberculosis).

ONGOING CARE

FOLLOW-UP RECOMMENDATIONS

- Keep legs elevated.
- Elastic wraps or support stockings may be helpful when patients are ambulating.

Patient Monitoring

Monthly follow-up or as dictated by underlying disorder

DIET

No restrictions

PATIENT EDUCATION

- Lesions will resolve over a few weeks to months.
- No scarring is anticipated.
- Joint aches and pains may persist.
- <20% recur.

PROGNOSIS

- Individual lesions resolve generally within 2 weeks.
- Total time course of 6–12 weeks but may vary with underlying disease.
- Joint aches and pains may persist for years.
- Lesions do not scar.
- Recurrences in 12–14% of patients: Occurs over variable periods, averaging several years; seen most often in sarcoid, streptococcal infection, pregnancy, and oral contraceptive use

COMPLICATIONS

- Vary according to underlying disease
- None expected from lesions of erythema nodosum

REFERENCES

1. Psychos DN, Voulgari PV, Skopouli FN, et al. Erythema nodosum: the underlying conditions. *Clin Rheumatol*. 2000;19:212–6.
2. Bartyik K, Várkonyi A, Kirschner A, et al. Erythema nodosum in association with celiac disease. *Pediatr Dermatol*. 2004;21:227–30.
3. Schwartz RA, Nervi SJ et al. Erythema nodosum: a sign of systemic disease. *Am Fam Physician*. 2007;75:695–700.
4. Requena L, Yus ES et al. Erythema nodosum. *Dermatol Clin*. 2008;26:425–38, v
5. Volkov I, et al. Successful treatment of chronic erythema nodosum with vitamin B12. *J Am Board Fam Pract*. 2005;18:6.

ADDITIONAL READING

- González-Gay MA, García-Porra C, Pujol RM, et al. Erythema nodosum: a clinical approach. *Clin Exp Rheumatol*. 2001;19:365–8.
- Habif T. *Clinical Dermatology*, 4th ed. St. Louis, MO: CV Mosby, 2004.
- Requena L, et al. Erythema nodosum. *Dermatol Online J*. 2002;8:4.
- Wolff K, et al., eds. *Fitzpatrick's Dermatology in General Medicine*, 7th ed. New York: McGraw-Hill Professional, 2007.

CODES

ICD9

695.2 Erythema nodosum

CLINICAL PEARLS

- Lesions of erythema nodosum appear to be erythematous patches, but when palpated, their underlying nodularity is appreciated.
- Erythema nodosum in the setting of hilar adenopathy may be seen with multiple etiologies and does not exclusively indicate sarcoidosis.
- In patients with a history of Hodgkin lymphoma, erythema nodosum may be a warning of impending recurrence.

ERYTHROBLASTOSIS FETALIS

Donald A.F. Nelson, MD

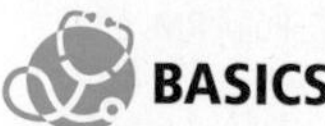

BASICS

DESCRIPTION

- Hemolytic anemia of the fetus or newborn caused by transplacental transmission of maternal antibody
- When severe, the anemia may result in extramedullary hematopoiesis, secondary organ dysfunction, heart failure, hydrops, and death.
- The term *erythroblastosis* refers to the presence of immature erythrocytes in the peripheral blood from accelerated hematopoiesis.
- System(s) affected: Cardiovascular; Hemic/Lymphatic/Immunologic; Nervous
- Synonym(s): Erythroblastosis neonatorum; Hemolytic disease of the fetus and newborn (HDFN); Congenital anemia of the newborn; Immune hydrops fetalis; Icterus gravis neonatorum

EPIDEMIOLOGY

- Predominant age: Affects fetus and newborn
- Predominant sex: Male = Female

Incidence

Universal screening for Rh sensitization and widespread use of RhIG in 3rd trimester and/or at birth have made this disease relatively rare.

RISK FACTORS

Prior transfusion with incompatible blood:

Pregnancy Considerations

- Any Rh-positive pregnancy in an Rh-negative woman (~9% of pregnancies have an Rh-negative mother with an Rh-positive fetus)
- Without prophylactic immunotherapy (RhIG), risk of Rh sensitization is up to 16% during or after term pregnancy, ~3% for spontaneous abortion, and 5–6% for surgical abortion.
- Sensitization by exposure to fetal blood may also occur with ectopic pregnancy, amniocentesis, chorionic villus sampling, placental trauma or manipulation, and placental abruption.
- Prophylaxis with Rho(D) immune globulin (RhIG) reduces risk of sensitization to <1% of susceptible pregnancies (1).
- Universal screening for Rh sensitization and widespread use of RhIG in 3rd trimester and/or at birth have made this disease relatively rare.

Genetics

- May occur when the fetus inherits a paternal blood group antigen lacking in the mother
- The Rh D antigen is most frequently implicated (for more on inheritance of Rh antigens, see Rh Incompatibility).
- In cases of a heterozygous paternal genotype, new DNA techniques now make it possible to diagnose the fetal blood type through free fetal DNA in maternal plasma (2).

GENERAL PREVENTION

- RhIG (RhoGAM, Rhophylac, HyperRHO) given prophylactically to unsensitized, Rh-negative pregnant women at risk. Usually at 28–32 weeks' gestation and at birth if infant is Rh-positive (see Rh Incompatibility).
- Artificial insemination with sperm from antigen-negative donor for isoimmunized woman whose partner is antigen-positive

ETIOLOGY

- Maternal isoimmunization to Rh antigen by transfusion of Rh-positive blood
- Maternal isoimmunization from exposure to fetal Rh antigens in prior or current pregnancy
- Maternal isoimmunization to other blood group antigens (e.g., Kell, Duffy, Kidd, M, Diego, S) is unusual, but may cause serious disease (3).

DIAGNOSIS

PHYSICAL EXAM

- Pallor
- Respiratory distress
- Jaundice
- Hepatomegaly
- Splenomegaly
- Ascites
- Purpura/bleeding problems
- Edema
- Anasarca (extreme generalized edema)
- Hydrops (fluid accumulation in ≥2 or more fetal compartments, including ascites, pericardial effusion, pleural effusion, and skin edema)
- Hypotension/shock
- Fetal death in utero

DIAGNOSTIC TESTS & INTERPRETATION

Lab

Initial lab tests

- Complete blood count:
  - Anemia
  - Thrombocytopenia
  - Nucleated red blood cells on differential count
- Reticulocytosis
- Hyperbilirubinemia (indirect bilirubin)
- Elevated amniotic fluid bilirubin (δ OD 450)
- Positive indirect Coombs test (antibody screen) during pregnancy
- Positive direct Coombs test
- If paternity is certain, paternal blood typing may exclude pregnancy from being at risk.

Follow-Up & Special Considerations

- Maternal antibody titer measured by 20 weeks and q.4wk. during pregnancy. A titer of 1:16 or greater, particularly if rising, indicates need for further testing (3)[C].
- Formerly, periodic amniocentesis for photometric determination of amniotic fluid bilirubin levels was the preferred method of monitoring in pregnancies with elevated antibody titers. Results estimated the extent of fetal hemolysis. High fluid bilirubin levels indicated the need for percutaneous umbilical blood sampling (cordocentesis) to determine the degree of fetal anemia (3)[C].
- Improvements in fetal ultrasonography now permit assessment of fetal anemia by Doppler measurement of flow velocity in the fetal middle cerebral artery. This noninvasive procedure is gradually replacing invasive methods for monitoring affected pregnancies (3)[C].
- Fetal heart rate testing/ultrasonography to assess fetal status (3)[C]
- Amniocentesis for fetal lung maturity at the point of pregnancy when early delivery is a management option, especially after 34 weeks (3)[C]
- Prior administration of Rho(D)IG during pregnancy may lead to weakly (false) positive indirect Coombs test in mother and direct Coombs test in infant.

Imaging

Initial approach

- Serial peak middle cerebral artery velocities by Doppler ultrasonography to detect/assess fetal anemia (2).
- Ultrasound may demonstrate hepatomegaly, abdominal enlargement, ascites, or signs of hydrops.
- When there is a history of an affected fetus or infant, maternal titers are no longer predictive of risk in subsequent pregnancies (2).

Follow-Up & Special Considerations

Fetus may be severely affected without hydrops; the presence or absence of hydrops on ultrasonography is poor at predicting the need for intervention.

Diagnostic Procedures/Surgery

- Amniocentesis
- Umbilical cord blood sampling

Pathological Findings

- Erythroid hyperplasia of bone marrow
- Extramedullary hematopoiesis
- Hepatomegaly
- Splenomegaly
- Cardiac enlargement
- Pulmonary hemorrhages
- Enlargement, edema of placenta

IFFERENTIAL DIAGNOSIS

Fetal blood loss anemia
Twin-to-twin transfusion
Arteriovenous or cardiac malformations
Hereditary hemolytic anemias
Drug-induced hemolytic anemia
Nonimmune fetal hydrops
Hemolysis from intrauterine infection (syphilis, toxoplasmosis, cytomegalovirus, others)

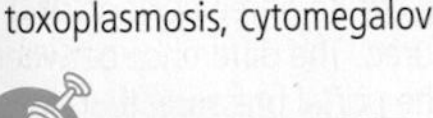

TREATMENT

MEDICATION

First Line

IG infusion has been used antenatally in combination with intrauterine transfusion to reduce the number of transfusions needed (4)B].

IG infusion in the newborn can reduce the number of exchange transfusions or the duration of phototherapy required for treatment (4)B].

Second Line

- Maternal plasmapheresis combined with IG infusion has been used successfully in some severe cases (5)C].
- Diuretics or inotropic agents may be used in addition to transfusion to manage heart failure in the newborn.

ADDITIONAL TREATMENT

General Measures

Depending on severity of involvement, treatment of nfant may include:

- Intrauterine transfusion: Intravascular approach via the umbilical vein is becoming preferred over the intraperitoneal approach and appears to be more effective.
- Early delivery
- Phototherapy
- Transfusion after delivery
- Exchange transfusion
- Diuretics and digoxin for hydrops

Issues for Referral

- Affected pregnancies are usually managed at the tertiary care level by perinatologists because of the specialized, somewhat hazardous, treatment measures involved.
- Delivery should occur in an institution capable of performing exchange transfusion, even if only mild involvement of the infant is expected.
- Infants with moderate or severe disease require neonatal intensive care.

ONGOING CARE

PROGNOSIS

- 50% of affected infants have mild disease and require no treatment (or treatment of anemia and jaundice only after delivery) and can be delivered at or near term.
- 30% have moderate disease with anemia and hepatomegaly. They require close follow-up of the pregnancy for signs of deterioration, which may require early delivery after 32–34 weeks or intrauterine transfusion prior to that age. After delivery, exchange transfusion is usually needed to treat anemia and hyperbilirubinemia.
- 20% have fetal hydrops, require intrauterine transfusion, and delivery as early as 32–34 weeks.
- Disease severity tends to worsen in successive affected pregnancies.
- Hydrops is associated with a poorer prognosis.
- Without treatment, overall perinatal mortality is ~50%.
- With appropriate monitoring and treatment, most infants do well, even those requiring intrauterine transfusion, and perinatal mortality has been reduced to 2–3% (1).
- Long-term studies have revealed normal neurologic outcomes in more than 90% of cases (2).

COMPLICATIONS

- Fetal distress requiring emergent delivery
- Fetal death in utero
- DIC
- Pregnancy loss from umbilical blood sampling
- Pregnancy loss from intrauterine transfusion
- Asphyxia
- Neonatal hemolytic anemia, mild to severe
- Neonatal anemia from hematopoietic suppression after intrauterine transfusion
- Pulmonary edema
- Congestive heart failure
- Shock
- Neonatal jaundice, mild to severe
- Kernicterus

REFERENCES

1. Bowman J. Thirty-five years of Rh prophylaxis. *Transfusion*. 2003;43:1661–6.
2. Moise KJ. Management of rhesus alloimmunization in pregnancy. *Obstet Gynecol*. 2008;112:164–76.
3. Management of alloimmunization during pregnancy. *ACOG Practice Bulletin 75*. Aug 2006.
4. Alcock GS, et al. Immunoglobulin infusion for isoimmune haemolytic jaundice in neonates. *Cochrane Database Sys Rev*. 2006;1.
5. Ruma MS, et al. Combined plasmapheresis and IV immune globulin for the treatment of severe maternal red cell alloimmunization. *Am J Obstet Gynecol*. 2007;196:138.e1–138.e6.

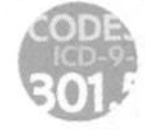

CODES

ICD9

- 773.0 Hemolytic disease of fetus or newborn due to Rh isoimmunization
- 773.1 Hemolytic disease of fetus or newborn due to abo isoimmunization
- 773.2 Hemolytic disease of fetus or newborn due to other and unspecified isoimmunization

CLINICAL PEARLS

- Prior administration of Rho(D)IG during pregnancy may lead to weakly (false) positive indirect Coombs test in mother and direct Coombs test in infant.
- Ultrasound is poor at predicting need for intervention.
- As for prognosis, 50% of affected infants have mild disease and require minimal treatment, 30% have moderate disease with anemia and hepatomegaly, and 20% have fetal hydrops.
- With appropriate monitoring and treatment, most infants do well, even those requiring intrauterine transfusion.
- Perinatal mortality has been reduced to 2–3% for this rare condition.

E

ESOPHAGEAL VARICES

James G. Nee, MD

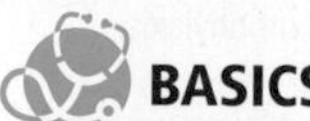

BASICS

DESCRIPTION

- Dilated collateral veins in the lamina propria of the distal esophagus connecting the portal and systemic circulations
- Results from chronic hypertension in the portal circulation due to increased resistance to blood flow.
- Increased pressure and turbulent flow within these vessels as well as their superficial location in the distal esophagus make them prone to rupture with significant morbidity and mortality.

EPIDEMIOLOGY

- Esophageal varices occur in ~50% of patients with cirrhosis.
- 50% of patients with esophageal varices bleed during their lifetime.
- Bleeding from esophageal varices is associated with 15–20% mortality.
- Predominant sex: Male > Female

RISK FACTORS

Cirrhosis of the liver

Genetics

No known pattern

GENERAL PREVENTION

- Endoscope esophagus annually in patients with cirrhosis
- Consider use of nonselective beta-blockers or obliteration of varices with esophageal banding for those intolerant of medication to prevent bleeding.

PATHOPHYSIOLOGY

Portal hypertension is caused by elevated portal pressure due to splanchnic arteriolar vasodilatation and increased resistance through dilated hepatic sinusoids.

ETIOLOGY

- Portal hypertension is defined as a pressure gradient >10 mm Hg.
- Cirrhosis accounts for >90% of cases. Alcohol and hepatitis C are the most common etiologies.
- Hemochromatosis, hepatitis B, nonalcoholic fatty liver disease, biliary cirrhosis, and autoimmune cirrhosis account for remainder. Extrahepatic portal vein thrombosis from umbilical vein infection, trauma, chronic pancreatitis, thrombotic conditions, and polycythemia.
- Malignant invasion of liver sinusoids or portal vein; seen in lymphoma, leukemia, hepatocellular carcinoma, and pancreatic carcinoma.
- Metabolic diseases altering liver sinusoids—amyloid, Gaucher disease, fatty liver
- Budd-Chiari syndrome
- Veno-occlusive disease

COMMONLY ASSOCIATED CONDITIONS

- Portal hypertensive gastropathy
- Hemorrhoids

DIAGNOSIS

- GI bleeding:
  - 75% of time, painless hematemesis and/or melena
  - Occult bleeding with anemia 25%
- Signs of cirrhosis

HISTORY

- Generally a history of cirrhosis or liver disease
- Painless hematemesis or melena

PHYSICAL EXAM

- Possible hypotension/tachycardia
- Small, hard liver
- Splenomegaly
- Ascites
- Visible abdominal periumbilical collateral circulation (Caput medusae)
- Spider angiomata on upper chest/back
- Palmar erythema

DIAGNOSTIC TESTS & INTERPRETATION

Lab

Initial lab tests

- Anemia related to blood loss
- Possibly abnormal liver function tests, thrombocytopenia, prolonged prothrombin time or low albumin-reflecting cirrhosis

Imaging

Initial approach

- Barium swallow:
  - Adequate for advanced varices, but is insensitive to small ones
  - Precludes possible urgent endoscopy
- Doppler sonography: Demonstrates patency, diameter, and flow in portal vein, and splenic vein, and large collaterals intra-abdominally.
- MRI:
  - Demonstrates large vascular channels intra-abdominally, and in the mediastinum.
  - Can demonstrate patency of the intrahepatic portal vein and splenic vein
- Venous phase celiac arteriography: Demonstrates portal vein and its collaterals, also can diagnose hepatic vein occlusion.

Diagnostic Procedures/Surgery

- Esophagoscopy as part of esophagogastroduodenoscopy:
  - Can identify and treat varices that appear as protruding submucosal veins in the distal 3rd of the esophagus.
  - Can identify actively bleeding varices as well as those with stigmata of recent hemorrhage.
  - Can treat actively bleeding vessels with sclerotherapy or esophageal band ligation or can obliterate vessels to prevent rebleeding. Can also identify associated conditions, including gastric varices and portal hypertensive gastropathy.
- Capsule endoscopy has acceptable sensitivity and specificity for detecting varices, and may be an alternative for those unwilling to undergo an EGD (1)[A].
- Endoscopic ultrasound is particularly sensitive to gastric varices.
- Portal pressure measurement:
  - Radiologist introduces a catheter retrograde into the hepatic vein in a wedged position to occlude flow.
  - The catheter is withdrawn to a free position and pressure again measured. The difference between wedged and free is the portal pressure. If <12 mm Hg, bleeding is less likely. Progressive increases above 12 correlate with the likelihood of hemorrhage
  - This is sometimes used to monitor successful treatment with beta-adrenergic blocking agent though it is not widely available.

Pathological Findings

- Extensive collateral circulation in the mediastinum and in the abdomen in addition to large vessels in the submucosa of the esophagus
- When bleeding occurs, these large veins explode into the submucosa of esophagus and rupture into the lumen.

DIFFERENTIAL DIAGNOSIS

- Upper GI bleeding:
  - Pulmonary bleeding; hemoptysis
  - Peptic ulcer disease
  - Gastric or esophageal malignancy
  - Arteriovenous malformation (AVM)
  - Nosebleed
- Lower GI bleeding:
  - Hemorrhoids
  - Colonic neoplasia
  - Diverticulosis
  - AVMs

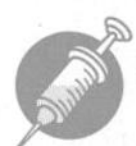

TREATMENT

MEDICATION

- For varices
  - β-Blockers: Decrease risk of first bleed by 45–50% in primary prophylaxis of variceal hemorrhage (2)[A]
  - Propranolol: 40 mg b.i.d. increase until heart rate decreased by 25% from baseline
  - Nadolol 80 mg daily, increase as above
  - Isosorbide mononitrate further reduces portal pressure. Begin at 20 mg b.i.d. No significant benefit in preventing first bleeds when given in combination with β-blockers. Should not be given as monotherapy (3)[B].
  - During banding or sclerotherapy: Proton pump inhibitor, such as lansoprazole 30 mg/d until varices obliterated
- During bleeding, consider antibiotic prophylaxis for spontaneous peritonitis and other infections with ciprofloxacin for 7–10 days.
- Contraindications: Severe asthma with β-blockers
- Precautions: Symptomatic hypotension

First Line

β-Blockers, proton pump inhibitors, antibiotics

Second Line

Isosorbide mononitrate

ADDITIONAL TREATMENT

General Measures

- Treat co-morbidities, generally related to cirrhosis.
- Hospital management of bleeding varices:
  - Appropriate resuscitation and maintenance of blood volume
  - Treat coagulopathy, if necessary.
  - IV somatostatin to lower portal venous pressure usually used as adjuvant to endoscopic management. Begin with IV bolus of 50 mg followed by drip of 50 mg/h (4)[A].
  - Urgent upper endoscopy for diagnosis and treatment. Variceal band ligation or sclerotherapy for bleeding varices or those not bleeding, which are medium to large in size, to decrease risk of bleeding. Variceal band ligation is preferred due to better bleeding cessation with fewer complications (5)[A].
  - Vasoactive drugs may be safe and effective whenever endoscopic therapy is not promptly available and seems to be associated with less adverse events than emergency sclerotherapy (6,7)[A].
  - Pharmacotherapy may be as effective as endoscopic therapy in reducing rebleeding rates and all-cause mortality (8)[A].
  - Pharmacotherapy plus endoscopic intervention is more effective than endoscopic intervention alone (8)[A].
  - Repeat ligation or sclerosant injection if bleeding recurs.
  - If endoscopic treatment fails to stop bleeding or cannot be accomplished, may need to use Sengstaken Blakemore or Minnesota tube to stabilize patient for a transjugular intrahepatic portosystemic shunt.
- Management of nonbleeding varices:
  - If ligation started, usually in medium to large varices (grade 2–4), repeat banding at 1- to 3-week intervals. 4–6 treatments are usually required to obliterate varices.
  - For those not treated endoscopically, begin nonselective β-blockers such as propranolol or nadolol. Increase dose for goal of heart rate reduction of 25% of baseline (SBP >90, HR >50). For those who do not tolerate the side effects of this regimen, proceed with endoscopic variceal band ligation as primary prophylaxis (9)[A].
  - If bleeding recurs, or portal pressure measurement shows portal pressure still >12 mm Hg, isosorbide mononitrate may be added, though endoscopic band ligation preferred if possible (10)[B].
  - Refractory bleeding may require use of transjugular intrahepatic portasystemic shunt (TIPS) or portocaval shunt (11)[B]
  - Refer for liver transplantation where appropriate.

Issues for Referral

Primarily those associated with liver transplantation

SURGERY/OTHER PROCEDURES

- Endoscopic variceal ligation: Preferred approach to those who cannot tolerate β-blockers.
- Endoscopic sclerotherapy
- Transjugular intrahepatic portasystemic shunt (TIPS)
- Portacaval shunt
- Esophageal transection
- Liver transplantation
- In patients with current or prior bleeding from esophageal varices, endoscopic variceal ligation is superior to endoscopic sclerotherapy (12)[A].

IN-PATIENT CONSIDERATIONS

Admission Criteria

Inpatient for acute bleeding

Discharge Criteria

Cessation of bleeding, stability of other comorbidities

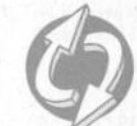

ONGOING CARE

FOLLOW-UP RECOMMENDATIONS

Patient Monitoring

- Close monitoring of vital signs if actively bleeding
- Endoscopic variceal ligation, repeated every 1–4 weeks until varices eradicated
- All patients with cirrhosis should undergo endoscopy to document the presence of varices and risk of hemorrhage (2)[B].
- If TIPS or other portacaval shunt, repeat endoscopy only if clinically bleeding
- If TIPS present, follow-up as recommended by radiologist; usually Doppler sonogram every 6 months

PATIENT EDUCATION

- Appropriate to cirrhosis
- National Digestive Information Clearinghouse, 2 Information Way, Bethesda, MD 20892 (digestive.niddk.nih.gov/) or American Liver Foundation, 1425 Pompton Way, Cedar Grove, NJ 07009 (www.liverfoundation.orq)

PROGNOSIS

- Depends heavily on ability to treat or reverse underlying condition
- In those with cirrhosis, 1 year survival for those who are alive 2 weeks after variceal bleed is ~50%.

COMPLICATIONS

- Bleeding
- Gastric or other uncommon varices may occur following successful eradication of esophageal varices.
- Esophageal varices can recur after obliteration.

REFERENCES

1. Lu Y, Gao R, Liao Z, et al. Meta-analysis of capsule endoscopy in patients diagnosed or suspected with esophageal varices. *World J Gastroenterol*. 2009;15:1254–8.
2. Groszmann RJ, Garcia-Tsao G, Bosch J, et al. Beta-blockers to prevent gastroesophageal varices in patients with cirrhosis. *N Engl J Med*. 2005;353: 2254–61.
3. D'Amico , et al. Pharmacological treatment of portal hypertension: an evidence based approach. *Semin Lever Dis*. 1999;19:475.
4. Zhou Y, Qiao L, Wu J, et al. Comparison of the efficacy of octreotide, vasopressin, and omeprazole in the control of acute bleeding in patients with portal hypertensive gastropathy: a controlled study. *J Gastroenterol Hepatol*. 2002;17:973–9.
5. Laine L, el-Newihi HM, Migikovsky B, et al. Endoscopic ligation compared with sclerotherapy for the treatment of bleeding esophageal varices. *Ann Intern Med*. 1993;119:1–7.
6. D'Amico G, Pagliaro L, Pietrosi G, Tarantino I et al. Emergency sclerotherapy versus vasoactive drugs for bleeding oesophageal varices in cirrhotic patients. *Cochrane Database Syst Rev*. 2010;3:CD002233.
7. Lo GH et al. Management of acute esophageal variceal hemorrhage. *Kaohsiung J Med Sci*. 2010;26:55–67.
8. Ravipati M, Katragadda S, Swaminathan PD et al. Pharmacotherapy plus endoscopic intervention is more effective than pharmacotherapy or endoscopy alone in the secondary prevention of esophageal variceal bleeding: a meta-analysis of randomized, controlled trials. *Gastrointest Endosc*. 2009;70:658–664.e5.
9. Boyer TD. Primary prophylaxis for variceal bleeding: are we there yet? *Gastroenterology*. 2005;128:1120–2.
10. Merkel C., et al. Randomised trial of nadolol alone or with isosorbide mononitrate for primary prophylaxis of variceal bleeding in cirrhosis. *Lanc*. 1996;348:1677.
11. Sanyal AJ, Freedman AM, Luketic VA, et al. Transjugular intrahepatic portosystemic shunts for patients with active variceal hemorrhage unresponsive to sclerotherapy. *Gastroenterology*. 1996;111:138–46.
12. Qureshi W, Adler DG, Davila R, et al. ASGE Guideline: the role of endoscopy in the management of variceal hemorrhage, updated July 2005. *Gastrointest Endosc*. 2005;62:651–5.

ADDITIONAL READING

Cheung J, Zeman M, van Zanten SV., et al. Systematic review: secondary prevention with band ligation, pharmacotherapy or combination therapy after bleeding from esophageal varices. *Aliment Pharmacol Ther*. 2009.

See Also (Topic, Algorithm, Electronic Media Element)

Cirrhosis of the Liver; Hemorrhoids; Portal Hypertension

CODES

ICD9

- 456.0 Esophageal varices with bleeding
- 456.1 Esophageal varices without mention of bleeding
- 456.20 Esophageal varices in diseases classified elsewhere, with bleeding

CLINICAL PEARLS

- Esophageal varices occur in ~50% of patients with cirrhosis.
- 50% of patients with esophageal varices bleed during their lifetime.
- Bleeding from esophageal varices is associated with 15–20% mortality.
- Endoscopy can identify and treat actively bleeding varices.

ESSENTIAL TREMOR SYNDROME

Jonathon M. Firnhaber, MD

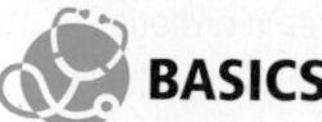

BASICS

DESCRIPTION

- A postural (occurring with voluntary maintenance of a position against gravity) or kinetic (occurring during voluntary movement) flexion–extension tremor that is slow and rhythmic and primarily affects the hands and forearms, head, and voice with a frequency of 4–12 Hz.
- Older patients tend to have lower frequency tremors, while younger patients exhibit frequencies in the higher range.
- May be familial, sporadic, or associated with other movement disorders
- Can begin at any age, but the incidence and prevalence increase with age
- The tremor can be exacerbated by emotional or physical stresses, fatigue, and caffeine.

EPIDEMIOLOGY

Essential tremor is the most common pathological tremor in humans.

Incidence

- Can occur at any age, but bimodal peaks exist in the 2nd and 6th decades
- Incidence rises significantly after age 49.
- System(s) affected: Neurologic; Musculoskeletal; ENT (voice)

Prevalence

0.4–5% of the general population

RISK FACTORS

Genetics

- Positive family history in 50–70% of patients; autosomal dominant inheritance is demonstrated in many families, but twin studies suggest that environmental factors are also involved.
- There is a link to genetic loci on chromosomes 2p22–25, 3q13, and 6p23. In addition, a Ser9Gly variant in the dopamine D_3 receptor gene on 3q13 has been suggested as a risk factor.

PATHOPHYSIOLOGY

Suspected to originate from an abnormal oscillation within thalamocortical and cerebello-olivary loops, as lesions in these areas tend to reduce essential tremor. Essential tremor is not a homogenous disorder; many patients have other motor manifestations and nonmotor features, including cognitive and psychiatric symptoms.

COMMONLY ASSOCIATED CONDITIONS

Can be present in 10% of patients with Parkinson disease (PD); characteristics of PD that distinguish it from essential tremor include 3- to 5-Hz resting tremor; accompanying rigidity, bradykinesia, or postural instability; and no change from alcohol consumption.

DIAGNOSIS

HISTORY

- Core criteria for diagnosis:
  - Bilateral action (postural or kinetic) tremor of the hands and forearms (but not rest tremor)
  - Absence of other neurologic signs, with the exception of cogwheel phenomenon
  - May have isolated head tremor with no signs of dystonia
- Secondary criteria include long duration (>3 years), positive family history, and beneficial response to alcohol (1)[C].

PHYSICAL EXAM

- Tremor can affect upper limbs (~95% of patients).
- Less commonly, the tremor affects head (~34%), lower limbs (~30%), voice (~12%), tongue (~7%), face (~5%), and trunk (~5%).

DIAGNOSTIC TESTS & INTERPRETATION

Lab

Initial lab tests

- Ceruloplasmin and serum copper to rule out Wilson disease
- Thyroid-stimulating hormone to rule out thyroid dysfunction
- Serum electrolytes, blood urea nitrogen, creatinine

Imaging

Initial approach

Brain magnetic resonance imaging (MRI) usually is not necessary or indicated unless Wilson disease is found or exam implies central lesion.

Diagnostic Procedures/Surgery

Electromyogram usually is not necessary.

Pathological Findings

Posture-related tremor

DIFFERENTIAL DIAGNOSIS

- Wilson disease
- Hyperthyroidism
- Multiple sclerosis
- Dystonic tremor
- Cerebellar tremor
- Asterixis
- Psychogenic tremor
- Drug-induced tremor [valproic acid, selection serotonin reuptake inhibitors, steroids, lithium, cyclosporine, β-adrenergic agonists, ephedrine, theophylline, tricyclic antidepressants (TCAs), antipsychotics]
- PD is manifested by a tremor at rest.

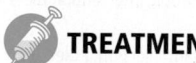

TREATMENT

MEDICATION

Pharmacologic treatment should be considered when tremor interferes with activities of daily living or causes psychological distress.

First Line

- Propranolol 60–320 mg/d in divided doses or in long-acting formulation reduces limb-tremor magnitude by ~50%, and almost 70% of patients experience improvement in clinical rating scales. There is insufficient evidence to recommend propranolol for vocal tremor. Single doses of propranolol, taken before social situations that are likely to exacerbate tremor, are useful for some patients.

- Primidone 25 mg q.h.s., gradually titrated to 150–300 mg q.h.s., improves tremor amplitude by 40–50%. Maximum dose is 750 mg/d, with doses greater than 250 mg/d typically divided to b.i.d. or t.i.d. Low-dose therapy (<250 mg/d) is just as effective as high-dose (750 mg/d) therapy.
- Propranolol and primidone have similar efficacy when used as initial therapy for limb tremor; both carry a level A recommendation.

Second Line

- Topiramate at a mean dose of 292 mg/d demonstrated significantly greater reduction in tremor rating scale (TRS) compared with placebo (7.7 vs 0.08; $p < .005$; baseline TRS = 37.0) in a small study combining results of 3 double-blind randomized controlled trials following a common protocol (2)[B]. Use is limited by dropout rates as high as 40% due to appetite suppression, weight loss, paresthesias, and concentration difficulties.
- Gabapentin up to 400 mg t.i.d.
- Sotalol, nadolol, and atenolol are alternative β-blockers; each has less evidence than propranolol to support use.
- Clonazepam and alprazolam should be used with caution because of abuse potential.
- Clozapine has shown efficacy at doses of 6–75 mg/d but is recommended only for refractory cases of limb tremor because of a 1% risk of agranulocytosis.
- Other medications that have been used to treat essential tremor include acetazolamide, flunarizine, levetiracetam, methazolamide, olanzapine, pregabalin, sodium oxybate, and zonisamide.
- Botulinum toxin A injections should be offered as a treatment option for cervical dystonia (Level A recommendation from American Association of Neurology), and may be offered for blepharospasm, focal upper extremity dystonia, adductor laryngeal dystonia and upper extremity essential tremor (3)[B]. Limited data support its use for head and voice tremor (4).

ADDITIONAL TREATMENT

Issues for Referral

Referral to a neurologist can help to differentiate those with dystonia, neuropathic tremor, PD, or drug-induced tremor.

SURGERY/OTHER PROCEDURES

- Deep brain stimulation may be used to treat medically refractory limb tremor and has fewer adverse effects than thalamotomy.
- Bilateral thalamic stimulation is effective in reducing tremor and functional disability; however, dysarthria is a possible complication.
- Unilateral thalamotomy may be used to treat limb tremor that is refractory to medical management.
- Bilateral thalamotomy is not recommended because of adverse side effects.

ONGOING CARE

DIET

Avoid caffeine.

PROGNOSIS

Tremor tends to worsen with age, increasing in amplitude.

REFERENCES

1. Bain P, Brin M, Deuschl G, et al. Criteria for the diagnosis of essential tremor. *Neurology*. 2000;54:S7.
2. Connor GS, Edwards K, Tarsy D. Topiramate in essential tremor: findings from double-blind, placebo-controlled, crossover trials. *Clin Neuropharmacol*. 2008;31:97–103.
3. Simpson DM, et al. Therapeutics and Technology Assessment Subcommittee of the American Academy of Neurology. Assessment: Botulinum neurotoxin for the treatment of movement disorders (an evidence-based review): report of the Therapeutics and Technology Assessment Subcommittee of the American Academy of Neurology. *Neurology*. 20086;70(19):1699–1706.
4. Zesiewicz TA, et al. Practice parameter: Therapies for essential tremor: Report of the Quality Standards Subcommittee of the American Academy of Neurology. 2005;28;64(12):2008–20.

ADDITIONAL READING

Sullivan KL, Hauser RA, Zesiewicz TA. Essential tremor. Epidemiology, diagnosis, and treatment. *Neurologist*. 2004;10:250–8.

CODES

ICD9

333.1 Essential and other specified forms of tremor

CLINICAL PEARLS

- Core criteria for diagnosis of essential tremor include bilateral action (intention) tremor of the hands, forearm, and/or head without resting component.
- Beneficial response to alcohol and positive family history help to differentiate essential tremor from PD; PD is characterized by tremor at rest.
- 10% of patients with PD will have both resting tremors of PD and essential (intention) tremors.
- Wilson disease, thyroid disease, and medication effect should be ruled out.
- Brain MRI is usually not necessary or indicated.
- 1st-line treatments include propranolol and primidone.

EUSTACHIAN TUBE DYSFUNCTION

Teresa V. Chan, MD

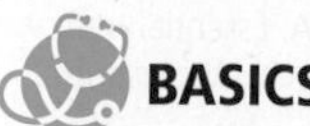

BASICS

DESCRIPTION

- Eustachian tube dysfunction (ETD) is classically described as a functional or structural obstruction of the eustachian tube. The eustachian tube does not open or close properly in response to pressure changes within the middle ear or outside the ear.
- Acute ETD may occur in the setting of pressure changes (e.g., plane travel) or acute upper airway inflammation (e.g., URI, sinusitis).
- Chronic ETD may lead to negative middle ear pressure, retracted tympanic membrane, serous effusions, otitis media, adhesive otitis media, or cholesteatoma.
- Patulous eustachian tube (PET), a distinct entity, is failure of the eustachian tube to close. It is often manifested as autophony, when an individual's own breathing and voice sounds excessively loud.
- System(s) affected: Auditory
- Synonym(s): Auditory tube dysfunction; Eustachian tube disorder; Blocked eustachian tube; Patulous eustachian tube

ALERT

- Sudden single-sided deafness (SSNHL) can be misdiagnosed as ETD.
- A simple 512-Hz tuning fork test lateralizes to the opposite ear in sudden sensorineural hearing loss and to the affected ear in ETD with conductive hearing loss.
- Any sudden sensorineural hearing loss is a medical emergency and should be referred to an otolaryngologist immediately.
- Treatment of SSNHL with high-dose steroids should begin ASAP, ideally within 14 days of onset.

EPIDEMIOLOGY

- Most common in children <5 years of age (1)
- Usually decreases with age but may persist into adulthood in some patients

Pediatric Considerations

Refer to an otolaryngologist if hearing loss or recurrent or chronic middle ear infections.

RISK FACTORS

- Adult and pediatric:
  - Tobacco and pollutant exposure, GERD, allergy, chronic sinusitis, sleep apnea with continuous positive airway pressure use, adenoid hypertrophy or nasopharyngeal mass, neuromuscular disease, altered immunity
  - Native American, Inuit, Australian Aborigine
- Pediatric:
  - 2nd-hand smoke, prematurity and low birth weight, young age, daycare, exposure to many other children, crowded living conditions, low socioeconomic status, prone sleeping position, prolonged bottle use
  - Craniofacial abnormalities (e.g., cleft palate, Down syndrome)

Pregnancy Considerations

- ETD may be exacerbated by rhinitis of pregnancy.
- Symptoms typically resolve postpartum.

Genetics

Twin studies show a genetic component (1). Specific genetic cause is still undefined.

GENERAL PREVENTION

- Control sources of upper airway inflammation: Allergens, GERD, URIs
- Autoinsufflation of middle ear (i.e., blow gently against pinched nostril and closed mouth)
- Avoid exposure to pressure changes (e.g., plane flight, scuba diving) in the setting of URI.
- Avoid exposure to environmental irritants: Smoking and 2nd-hand smoke

PATHOPHYSIOLOGY

- ETD is failure of the system at the proximal end (ET, palate, nasal cavities, and nasopharynx) to regulate the middle ear and mastoid gas cell system at its distal end.
- Eustachian tube functions:
  - Ventilation/regulation of middle ear pressure
  - Protection from nasopharyngeal secretions
  - Drainage of middle ear fluid
  - ET is closed at rest and opens with yawning, swallowing, and sneezing.
- Cycle of dysfunction: Structural or functional obstruction of the ET compromises 3 functions of this system:
  - Negative pressure develops in middle ear.
  - Serous exudate is drawn from the middle ear mucosa by negative pressure or refluxed into the middle ear if the ET opens momentarily.
  - Infection of static fluid causes edema and release of inflammatory mediators, which exacerbates cycle of inflammation and obstruction.
- Pathologic constriction of the ET in adults and children with chronic otitis media (COM) or in monkeys with a chemically or mechanically damaged tensor veli palatini (1)

ETIOLOGY

- In children, a horizontal ET predisposes to difficulties with ventilation and drainage (1).
- Shorter ET predisposes to reflux (1).
- Adenoid hypertrophy can block the torus tubarius (proximal opening of the ET) (1).
- In adults, paradoxical closing with swallowing has been noted in a majority of patients (1).

COMMONLY ASSOCIATED CONDITIONS

- Hearing loss
- Middle ear effusion
- Cholesteatoma
- Allergic rhinitis
- Chronic sinusitis
- URI
- Adenoid hypertrophy
- GERD
- Cleft palate
- Down syndrome
- Obesity
- Nasopharyngeal carcinoma or other tumor

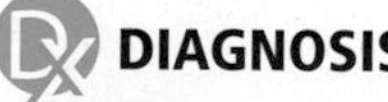

DIAGNOSIS

HISTORY

- Fullness, pressure, clogged feeling in the ear
- Otalgia or ear discomfort
- Relieved by "popping ears" (i.e., yawn or swallow tenses the tensor veli palatini, causing the ET to dilate)
- Hearing loss
- Symptoms: Unilateral or bilateral
- Tinnitus (usually popping, fluttering, clicking instead of high-pitched ringing)
- Dizziness or lightheadedness
- Recent onset vs chronic lifelong problem
- History of previous ear infections
- Previous ear surgeries, including tubes
- Constant vs waxing and waning symptoms
- Smoking history
- Antecedent URI
- Difficulty breathing through nose
- Allergic symptoms
- Trauma
- Voice change (hypo- or hypernasal voice, consider NP mass or palatal dysfunction)
- Recent flying or diving

ALERT

Unilateral symptoms and/or recent onset of symptoms in the absence of identifiable cause for ETD warrants workup for nasopharyngeal process such as tumor (1)[A].

PHYSICAL EXAM

- Pneumatic otoscopy: Retracted tympanic membrane, decreased movement, effusion
- Toynbee maneuver: View changes of the drum while patient autoinsufflates against closed lips and pinched nostrils. May show various degrees of retraction:
  - Entire drum may be retracted and "lateralize" with insufflation.
  - Posterosuperior quadrant (pars flaccida) may form a retraction pocket. Early on, this can be "lateralized" with autoinsufflation. If long-standing or severe, this pocket is well established and even may be scarred down to the middle ear mucosa or filled with cholesteatoma.
- Nasopharyngoscopy: Adenoid hypertrophy or nasopharyngeal mass
- Anterior rhinoscopy: Nasal obstruction, turbinate hypertrophy
- Tuning fork test: 512-Hz fork lateralizes to affected ear in setting of conductive hearing loss.

DIAGNOSTIC TESTS & INTERPRETATION

Imaging

- Radiologic studies are not performed routinely if clinical signs/symptoms suggest ETD.
- CT scan may show middle ear/mastoid opacification or other sequelae of chronic ETD and OM.
- Lateral neck film may help to confirm diagnosis of adenoid hypertrophy in an uncooperative pediatric patient.

Diagnostic Procedures/Surgery

- Tympanometry: Type B or C tympanograms indicate fluid or retraction, respectively. Negative middle ear peak pressures seen even with normal (type A) tympanograms.
- Audiogram may show conductive hearing loss.

Pathological Findings

- Blockage of the ET orifice by mucopurulent nasal discharge or edema
- Compression of the orifice by adenoid tissue
- Hypertrophy of the peritubal tonsil
- Paradoxical ET closure when swallowing
- Atrophy of the orifice
- In over 1/3 of patients, endoscopic findings were normal (2).

DIFFERENTIAL DIAGNOSIS

- SSNHL (a medical emergency)
- Tympanic membrane perforation
- Barotrauma
- TMJ disorder
- Ménière disease
- Superior semicircular canal dehiscence
- Skull base tumor

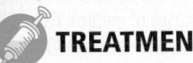

TREATMENT

- Reduce cycle of infection/inflammation.
- Tympanostomy tubes ± adenoidectomy when indicated for recurrent ear infections or severe progressive retractions

MEDICATION

- Few data exist demonstrating efficacy for ETD.
- Initiate treatment based on individual patient's symptoms and possible cause.
- Decongestants (1)[C]: There are common ingredients in many OTC brands; encourage patients to read labels. In general, avoid prolonged use of intranasal decongestants >3 days; use with caution in patients with hypertension or cardiac risk factors:
  - Phenylephrine (Neo-synephrine Nasal Spray, Sudafed PE oral) Adults: 1 (10 mg) tablet or 1 spray each nostril every 4 hours p.r.n., children (<4y) 1 tsp (2.5 mg) q4h p.r.n.
  - Pseudoephedrine (Sudafed), Adults: 2 (30 mg) tablets every 4–6 hours p.r.n., children <12 y: 1 tablet every 4–6 hours p.r.n.
  - Oxymetazoline (Afrin Nasal Spray), Adults: 1–2 sprays each nostril every 12 hours p.r.n.
  - Xylometazoline (Otrivin Nasal Spray), Adults 2 sprays of 0.1% solution each nostril every 8 hours p.r.n., children (2–12 y): 2 sprays of 0.05% solution each nostril every 8 hours p.r.n.
- Nasal steroids (may be beneficial for those with allergic rhinitis) (1)[B]:
  - Beclomethasone (Beconase, Vancenase), Adults and children >12 y: 1–2 sprays each nostril b.i.d., children 6-12 y, 1 spray each nostril b.i.d. Not recommended for children <6 y.
  - Budesonide (Rhinocort): Adults and children >6 y, 1 spray each nostril daily
  - Ciclesonide (Omnaris) (a prodrug that is activated on nasal mucosa): Adults and children >6 y: 2 sprays each nostril daily
  - Flunisolide (Nasarel, Nasalide): Adults and children >6 y: 2 sprays each nostril b.i.d.
  - Fluticasone furoate (Veramyst): Adults and children >12 y: 2 sprays each nostril daily; children 2–11 y: 1 spray each nostril daily
  - Fluticasonepropionate (Flonase): Adults 1–2 sprays each nostril daily; children >4 y: 1 spray each nostril daily
  - Triamcinolone (Nasocort): Adults and children >6 y: 1–2 sprays each nostril daily, children 2–5 y; 1 spray each nostril daily
- 2nd-generation H_1 antihistamines (may be beneficial for those with allergic rhinitis) (1)[B]:
  - Loratadine (Claritin) (tablets, redi-tabs and liquid available): Adults and children >6 y: 10 mg orally daily, children 2–6 y: 5 mg orally daily
  - Desloratadine (Clarinex) (tablets, redi-tabs and liquid available): Adults and children >12 y: 5 mg orally daily, children 6-11 y: 2.5 mg orally daily, children 12 m-5 y: 1.25 mg orally daily, children 6–11 m: 1 mg orally daily
  - Fexofenadine (Allegra) (tablets, redi-tabs and liquid available): Adults and children >12 y: 60 mg orally b.i.d. or 180 mg orally daily, children 6–11 y: 30 mg orally b.i.d.
  - Cetirizine (Zyrtec) (tablets, chewable tablets or liquid available): Adults and children >6 y: 5–10 mg orally daily, children 6 months-5 y: 2.5–5 mg orally daily or divided b.i.d.
  - Levocetirizine (Xyzal) (tablets and liquid available): Adults and children >12 y: 2.5–5 mg orally q.p.m., children 6–11 y: 2.5 mg orally q.p.m., children 6 m–5 y: 1.25 mg orally q.p.m.
- Antihistamine nasal sprays:
  - Olopatadine (Patanase) (antihistamine): Adults and Children >12y: 2 sprays each nostril BID, Children 6–11y: 1 spray each nostril BID
  - Azelastine (Astepro or Astelin) (antihistamine), Adults and children >12 y: 1–2 sprays each nostril b.i.d., children 6–11 y: 1 spray each nostril b.i.d.
- Antibiotics (not routinely used unless ETD is associated with acute OM):
  - Amoxicillin, 1st-line (1)[A]: Adults and children >3 months: 25 mg/kg/day in divided doses every 12 hours or 20 mg/kg/day in divided doses every 8 hours, children <12 weeks: 30 mg/kg/day divided q12h
  - Treatment for 10 days is most effective (1)[B].
- If ETD leads to OM associated with tympanic membrane perforation or if ventilation tube present, topical antibiotic drops are more efficacious than oral antibiotics (1)[A]:
  - Ciprofloxacin-dexamethasone (Ciprodex): 4–5 drops b.i.d. × 7 days
  - Ciprofloxacin–hydrocortisone suspension (Cipro HC) 3–5 drops b.i.d. × 7 days
  - Neomycin–polymyxin–hydrocortisone suspension (Cortisporin) 3–4 drops q.i.d. × 10 days
  - Ofloxacin (Floxin): 5 drops b.i.d. × 10 days
- Pain control, anti-inflammatory: Acetaminophen, NSAIDs

ADDITIONAL TREATMENT

General Measures

- Reduce cycle of inflammation with decongestants, antihistamines, topical steroids, antireflux medications, and antibiotics when indicated.
- Culture-directed antibiotics are 90% effective in treating sequela of ETD (chronic suppurative otitis media [CSOM] and mastoiditis) (1)[B].

Issues for Referral

Refer to an otolaryngologist if conservative 1st-line medications have provided no relief of symptoms or for surgical consideration.

SURGERY/OTHER PROCEDURES

- Myringotomy and pressure equalization tube placement to ventilate middle ear, relieve pressure, and prevent sequelae of chronically retracted drum (1)[A]
- Adenoidectomy if tissue is present:
  - In children, 1st set of tubes alone, then adenoidectomy in conjunction with second set of tubes if problems recur (1)[A]
  - Some advocate adenoidectomy even in absence of excess tissue; reduces frequency and number of subsequent tubes (3)[A].
- Direct nasopharyngoscopy and biopsy if mass
- Mastoidectomy for associated sequelae (e.g., chronic otomastoiditis, cholesteatoma)

ONGOING CARE

FOLLOW-UP RECOMMENDATIONS

- Monitor pressure equalization tubes every 6–8 months in children and every 6–12 months in adults.
- Monitor tympanic membrane retraction pocket for progression every 6–12 months to allow for early intervention for erosion or cholesteatoma.
- Avoid pressure changes (e.g., scuba diving, plane flights) with URI (1)[C].

DIET

- Generally no restrictions; avoid foods that would exacerbate reflux symptoms.
- In newborns, breastfeeding has been associated with a lower incidence of ETD and OM (1)[A].

PROGNOSIS

- May resolve with age in pediatric patients
- For some, it is a chronic disorder; current treatments provide symptomatic relief; usually require prolonged use.

COMPLICATIONS

Morbidity related to hearing compromise or associated chronic ear infections

REFERENCES

1. Bluestone CD. Studies in otitis media: Children's Hospital of Pittsburgh-University of Pittsburgh progress report–2004. *Laryngoscope*. 2004;114: 1–26.
2. Butler CC, Van Der Voort JH. Oral or topical nasal steroids for hearing loss associated with otitis media with effusion in children. *Cochrane Database Syst Rev*. 2002:CD001935.
3. Bluestone CD, Hebda PA, Alper CM, et al. Recent advances in otitis media. 2. Eustachian tube, middle ear, and mastoid anatomy; physiology, pathophysiology, and pathogenesis. *Ann Otol Rhinol Laryngol Suppl*. 2005;194:16–30.

See Also (Topic, Algorithm, Electronic Media Element)

Algorithm: Ear Pain

CODES

ICD9

381.81 Dysfunction of eustachian tube

CLINICAL PEARLS

- SSNHL can be missed diagnosed as ETD, and the optimal window to commence high-dose steroids is lost.
- A simple 512-Hz tuning fork test lateralizes to the opposite ear in sudden sensorineural hearing loss and to the affected ear in ETD with conductive hearing loss.
- Any sudden sensorineural hearing loss is a medical emergency and should be referred to an otolaryngologist immediately.
- Treatment of SSNHL with high-dose steroids should begin ASAP, ideally within 14 days of onset.

E

FACTITIOUS DISORDER/MÜNCHAUSEN SYNDROME

Irene C. Coletsos, MD
William G. Elder, Jr., PhD
Harold J. Bursztajn, MD

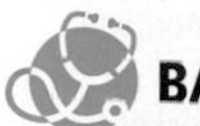

BASICS

DESCRIPTION

- Patients appear ill because they are feigning, exaggerating, or inducing symptoms.
- A mental disorder because the patient has an abnormal need for a sick role. Patients are aware of but will deny their deceit.
- Becomes apparent when there is a disease history stated in absence of symptoms, when symptom patterns are puzzling, or when there are nonhealing or unremitting symptoms despite adequate and correct treatment
- In factitious disorder by proxy, or Munchausen by proxy, an individual falsifies or induces illness in another person to vicariously accrue emotional payoffs, including sympathy, admiration, and/or feelings of power over care providers. Children are the usual victims and the mother is the usual perpetrator. The updated term for this activity is medical child abuse.
- Types of factitious disorder:
  - Factitious disorder with predominantly physical signs and symptoms:
    - Typically simulates 1 physical disease
  - Factitious disorder with predominantly psychological signs and symptoms:
    - These patients mimic the behavior of people with mental illnesses, claiming they are hearing voices or having visual hallucinations. In Ganser syndrome, patients may also give wrong answers to simple questions.
  - Münchausen syndrome is an extreme form usually with predominantly physical symptoms. Patients spend much of their lives seeking medical care from different providers and hospitals (changing hospitals when treatment is refused) and are willing to undergo painful procedures and surgeries to maintain their sick role. Named after an 18th-century nobleman who told tall tales.

EPIDEMIOLOGY

Incidence

Estimates vary on the incidence of medical child abuse. In the US, an estimated 200 new cases of serious abuse are expected to be uncovered yearly.

Prevalence

Factitious disorder with predominantly physical signs and symptoms: ~1–5% of people presenting with medical illness, according to some studies, but hard to estimate due to the secretive nature of the disorder. Identified as the probable cause of 3–9% of fevers of unknown origin in prospective studies.

RISK FACTORS

- Abuse/deprivation in childhood
- Childhood traumas, including hospitalizations
- Growing up with ill or emotionally unavailable caretakers
- Experience as health care professional
- Female gender 2:1 in factitious disorder
- Male gender 2:1 Münchausen syndrome
- Most by-proxy presentations involve a mother inducing symptoms in a child. Siblings of children known to have suffered this abuse are at grave risk.

ETIOLOGY

- The psychological basis is thought to be an unresolved sense of deprivation from childhood that, in a time of stress in adulthood, leads to a false claim of medical illness in order to get care. In Münchausen, this behavior is chronic.
- Personality predisposition and shaping may be factors, evident in the high degree of deceitfulness, lack of remorse, disregard for safety, inability to manage work and interpersonal situations, and failure to conform to social norms.

COMMONLY ASSOCIATED CONDITIONS

- History of many medical procedures
- Substance abuse
- Suicide attempts
- Psychiatric comorbidities, including adjustment disorder, borderline personality disorder, depression, somatoform disorder, eating disorders
- In medical child abuse, the siblings of the currently affected child may have been improperly diagnosed with a rare, intractable condition or may even have died.
- Delusional disorder

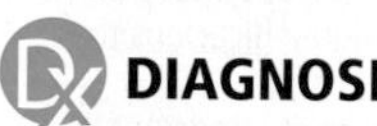

DIAGNOSIS

HISTORY

- A patient will relate a history of disease symptoms, often with "classic" textbook details, but has no signs of disease on examination. Or, if signs are noted, there may be evidence they were self-inflicted or are not medically caused.
- Careful elicitation of the developmental history may reveal early abuse or deprivations (1)[C].

PHYSICAL EXAM

- Normal, or evidence of self-inflicted wounds, such as scars
- Old wound with fresh bleeding (1)[C]
- Abscesses and rashes
- Tenderness on palpation with no tenderness noted by patient when the same areas are auscultated with pressure applied

DIAGNOSTIC TESTS & INTERPRETATION

Lab

- Abnormal urine studies not reproducible if the patient is directly observed. (Patients may surreptitiously heat their thermometers or contaminate urine specimens.)
- Skin infection (abscesses, IV sites, Foley sites): Culture may show infection via *E. coli*, presumably a patient's own fecal material.
- Repeated blood cultures showing uncommon pathogens in a patient who is immunocompetent and has no history of IV drug use (2)[C]
- Lab results fail to show the expected disease markers suggested by the reported symptoms.
- Agents taken to mimic disease states (insulin, to produce hypoglycemia; thyroxine or Cytomel to produce hyperthyroidism; laxative or diuretics, to produce hypokalemia; self-injection of epinephrine or isoproterenol hydrochloride, to mimic Cushing disease; warfarin, to produce bleeding; quinidine, to produce purpura; alkylating agents, to produce pancytopenia)

Diagnostic Procedures/Surgery

- Patients often undergo many diagnostic or surgery procedures before the psychological nature of their illness is discovered. Procedures are often welcome by the patient and, in the cases of medical child abuse, by the patient's caregiver. Avoid if possible.
- Psychological testing (3)[B]:
  - The Minnesota Multiphasic Personality Inventory, neuropsychological tests, and forensic tests are sensitive to faking and identify unusual profiles associated with factitious disorders.
- Cameras and other means of surveillance have frequently been used accidentally or purposely to detect patients or parents feigning or inflicting illness. Check with hospital attorney.

DIFFERENTIAL DIAGNOSIS

- Factious disorders are mental disorders where the patient has an abnormal need to maintain a sick role. Factitious disorders may be contrasted with other mental disorders where symptoms are beyond the patient's control, such as delusional disorders with bizarre somatic beliefs, and somatoform disorders such as hypochondriasis, conversion, and somatization disorders where the patient has and experiences symptoms for psychological reasons:
  - In hypochondriasis the person believes or fears that they have a disorder. Anxiety is marked.
  - Somatization disorder involves recurrent physical symptoms, such as gastrointestinal (GI), sexual, pain, and neurologic symptoms where these symptoms cannot be explained fully by physical disorder. Worsens in times of stress and begins in late adolescence.
  - Conversion disorder manifests in pseudoneurological symptoms classically originating from an unconscious psychological conflict.
- Factitious disorders may be contrasted with malingering where secondary gain is sought such as financial goal or avoiding responsibility and as a result of a conscious decision.
- Cultural differences in expressing pain and experiencing illness
- Occult medical illness (early stages of disease when blood tests may still show negative results)
- Unusual presentations of disease
- False-negative lab results
- For factitious disorder with predominantly psychological signs and symptoms, in addition to psychiatric illnesses that can have true psychotic symptoms, consider other medical etiologies:
  - Drugs, ingested as prescribed or abused (i.e., benzodiazepines, cocaine, PCP, steroids)
  - Poisoning (alcohol, lead, mercury)
  - Stroke or traumatic brain injury
  - Also consider:
    - Infection (especially sepsis)
    - Postsurgical anesthesia
    - Pneumonia (especially in older patients)
    - Urinary tract infection (especially in older patients)
    - Thiamine deficiency/Wernicke encephalopathy

ALERT

- Factitious disorder (or Münchausen syndrome) by proxy is a form of abuse.
- Parent may injure their child and then bring the child to care with a false history.
- Parents may appear overly involved and comfortable in the hospital setting, and not saddened or frightened by the child's illnesses.
- A child in this situation may become quite ill, can have frequent hospitalizations, and may die from injuries.
- Older children who are victims of Münchausen by proxy may collude with the care provider who is victimizing them in order to maintain their relationship with the care provider (4)[C].
- Take steps to protect the child and siblings. Medical providers are legally required to report this and other types of abuse. Most experts recommend a multisystem approach that includes separating children from the abuser; therapy for the abuser, the abuser's significant other, and children; court monitoring to determine when/if the abuser can be reunited with children; medical monitoring to make sure future medical care for the child is warranted (and not part of an on-going abuse). Visits between the abuser and child can be therapeutic, but all must be carefully monitored to prevent the abuser from giving the child any food/drinks or medicine (5).

TREATMENT

ADDITIONAL TREATMENT

General Measures

- When possible, review medical and mental health records and mental health history. Mental disorders may be initially denied (3)[B].
- In cases of known or suspected factitious disorder, emergency department providers protect the patients (and protect themselves legally) by proceeding with the necessary treatment (e.g., if the patient has swallowed a foreign object, consult GI), putting the patient under observation during the hospital stay (to avoid having the patient inflict further self-injury), and consulting psychiatry as part of the treatment plan (6)[C].
- Management may be limited to clinician recognition of the disorder and making sure patients are not offered unnecessary drugs, risky procedures, or surgeries (7).
- Directly confronting patients ("You did this to yourself!") is usually met with angry denial. The patients often leave and try to get the treatment they had wanted from other providers and hospitals. Face-saving techniques that allow patients to give up their symptoms without being humiliated are thought to be more effective (8)[C].
- For example:
  - Patients with factitious disorder may accept a frank but empathetic assessment that their actions themselves constitute the disorder (6).
  - The Inexact Interpretation method may eventually help the patient begin to understand that the self-harm is part of a pattern of trying to cope with (usually) unresolved childhood stresses, without directly accusing them of the self-harm. For example, if a patient with a history of childhood abuse at the hands of a parent is believed to be creating/reinfecting a skin wound, a provider can say: "I think your anger at your parent is making it more difficult for you to heal. It could also make it more difficult for you to work with your doctors." This type of interaction has been found to advance the therapy and can help lessen the inclination to self-harm (8)[C].
  - A double-blind diagnostic explanation may assist remission (8)[C]. The clinician should perform a thorough physical examination and go through a rapport-building interview. The diagnosis is then delivered in 2 parts:
    - Part 1: "Sometimes people do things to make themselves ill. We call doing that factitious disorder."
    - Part 2: "Your problem is unusual and I believe it will respond to 1 more attempt to treat it. If that doesn't improve it, it is likely that you have a factitious disorder." The *medical* therapy should be a benign one, such as biofeedback, self-hypnosis, or, in the case of a "nonhealing" skin wound (due to a patient's persistent reinfecting of it), a skin graft and antibiotics.
- In treating perpetrators of by proxy/medical child abuse: They must be able to admit what they have done, have an appropriate emotional response, have strategies in place to treat their own emotional issues without abusing those they care for, and can demonstrate, over time (6 months to a year), that they have put those strategies in place. One mode of therapy is "story construction," in which abusers can be helped to construct life narratives that explain why they were abusive, but then create alternative narratives that would prevent them from abusing in the future. The clinician advising the court on possible reunification of the abuser and child(ren) should be different from the one offering therapy. Despite therapy and intervention, relapse risk is high (9).
- In all clinical settings, be aware of the possibility of countertransference. Remain aware of personal responses and feelings toward these patients. Anger at these patients hinders the therapeutic alliance, and could lead to missed diagnoses. On the other hand, overidentification with these patients (who are often health care providers themselves) interferes with the timely identification of this syndrome and treatment (6)[C]. In all cases, consider consulting with a psychiatrist or psychologist (7)[B].

IN-PATIENT CONSIDERATIONS

Initial Stabilization

- Form an alliance with the patient, identifying their suffering.
- Seek a detailed history of childhood events. Health history of parents and siblings may reveal early traumas to the patient (3)[B].

Admission Criteria

- Patients whose behavior threatens their own lives should be considered for an emergency inpatient psychiatric commitment and evaluation (10)[C].
- In by proxy/medical child abuse cases, children may have to be hospitalized for monitored detoxification from the unneeded medications they had been given.

Nursing

IV and other in-room equipment should be monitored for tampering.

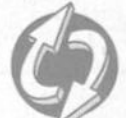

ONGOING CARE

PROGNOSIS

- Fair to poor especially if etiology underlying the disorder cannot be addressed
- The long-term outcomes of patients with untreated factitious disorder has been judged to be worse than those with other severe mental disorders such as schizophrenic, bipolar, and delusional disorders.

COMPLICATIONS

Patient illness or death from self-harm and unnecessary medical interventions

REFERENCES

1. Peebles R, Sabella C, Franco K, et al. Factitious disorder and malingering in adolescent girls: Case series and literature review. *Clin Pediatr.* 2005;44(3):237–43.
2. Galanos J, Perera S, Smith H, et al. Bacteremia due to three Bacillus species in a case of Munchausen's syndrome. *J Clin Microbiol.* 2003;41:2247–8.
3. Binder LM, Campbell KA. Medically unexplained symptoms and neuropsychological assessment. *J Clin Experiment Neuropsychol.* 2004;26(3): 369–92.
4. Awadallah N, Vaughan A, Franco K, et al. Munchausen by proxy: a case, chart series, and literature review of older victims. *Child Abuse Negl.* 2005;29:931–41.
5. Schreier H et al. On the importance of motivation in Munchausen by Proxy: the case of Kathy Bush. *Child Abuse Negl.* 2002;26:537–49.
6. Jagoda P. Factitious disorder in the emergency department. *Primary Psychiatry.* 2009;16(1): 61–66.
7. Krahn LE, Li H, O'Connor MK. Patients who strive to be ill: factitious disorder with physical symptoms. *Am J Psychiatry.* 2003;160(6):1163–8.
8. Eisendrath SJ. Factitious physical disorders. *West J Med.* 1994;160:177–9.
9. Sanders MJ, Bursch B et al. Forensic assessment of illness falsification, Munchausen by proxy, and factitious disorder, NOS. *Child Maltreat.* 2002;7:112–24.
10. Johnson BR, Harrison JA. Suspected Munchausen's syndrome and civil commitment. *J Am Acad Psychiatry Law.* 2000;28:74–6.

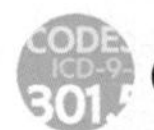

CODES

ICD9

- 300.16 Factitious disorder with predominantly psychological signs and symptoms
- 300.19 Other and unspecified factitious illness
- 301.51 Chronic factitious illness with physical symptoms

CLINICAL PEARLS

- Atypical emotional responses to illness are telling.
- Respond as you would to someone who cannot control self-harm rather than someone who wants to deceive you.
- In cases of by proxy disorders/medical child abuse, watch for children growing more ill after parental visits.

F

FACTOR V LEIDEN

Marc Jeffrey Kahn, MD
Rebecca Kruse-Jarres, MD, MPH

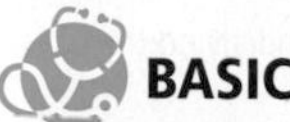

BASICS

DESCRIPTION

- Factor V Leiden is a genetic disease that is the most common hereditary cause of venous thrombosis. It leads to resistance to activated protein C.
- System(s) affected: Cardiovascular; Gastrointestinal; Hemic/Lymphatic/Immunologic; Nervous; Pulmonary; Reproductive
- Synonym(s): Factor V Leiden thrombophilia; factor V Leiden mutation

Pediatric Considerations

Increased thrombosis risk in patients with factor V Leiden

Pregnancy Considerations

Heterozygous patients are not at increased risk for thromboembolism or fetal loss.

EPIDEMIOLOGY

- Predominant age: Thrombosis typically occurs after the 2nd decade.
- Predominant sex: Male = Female

Prevalence

- ~3–12% of Caucasians are affected:
  - The mutation is rare in other ethnic groups.
- ~15–20% of patients who present with thrombosis have factor V Leiden.

RISK FACTORS

- Risk for venous embolism is 2.7-fold in heterozygous and 18-fold in homozygous factor V Leiden individuals, compared with individuals without the mutation.
- Oral contraceptives increase the risk of thrombosis:
  - In homozygotes, the risk increases 100-fold; in heterozygotes, 35-fold.
  - The increased risk is halved when the patient uses desogestrel-containing oral contraceptives.
- Hormone replacement therapy (HRT) and selective estrogen receptor modulators (SERMs) both increase the risk of thrombosis, and in patients with factor V Leiden, that risk is increased substantially.
- Pregnancy and homozygous factor V Leiden increase the risk of thrombosis 7–16-fold during pregnancy and the puerperium. Other complications of pregnancy may be increased in patients with factor V Leiden.
- Recurrence risk after an initial thrombosis is not increased in individuals who are heterozygous for factor V Leiden mutation. Data is conflicting in individuals who are homozygous, but it may not be increased (1).

Genetics

- Deep and superficial thrombosis of the venous system occurs with an odds ratio of 50–100 times greater for homozygotes.
- The odds ratio is closer to 2.5 times greater for heterozygotes.

GENERAL PREVENTION

Patients with factor V Leiden without thrombosis do not require prophylactic anticoagulation.

PATHOPHYSIOLOGY

- Point mutation causing substitution of arginine for glycine in residue 506 of factor V gene, rendering it less susceptible to inactivation by activated protein C
- Activated protein C is generated when protein C binds to its endothelial receptor, thrombomodulin.
- Activated protein C and its cofactor, protein S, lead to inactivation of factors V and VIII.
- Factor V Leiden is the most common cause of resistance to activated protein C.

ETIOLOGY

Genetic defect

COMMONLY ASSOCIATED CONDITIONS

Venous thrombosis

DIAGNOSIS

HISTORY

- Previous thrombosis
- Family history of thrombosis
- Family history of factor V Leiden mutation

PHYSICAL EXAM

- Arterial thrombosis is rare in adults with factor V Leiden.
- Thrombosis in unusual locations, such as the sagittal sinus, mesentery, and portal systems, is less common in patients with factor V Leiden than in patients with deficiency of protein C or S.
- Obstetric complications and venous thrombosis are increased in patients with factor V Leiden, and especially in those taking oral contraceptives.

DIAGNOSTIC TESTS & INTERPRETATION

Lab

Initial lab tests

- Genetic test: DNA-based test for factor V mutation; is reliable while on anticoagulation
- Functional test: Plasma-based coagulation assay using factor V–deficient plasma to which patient plasma is added along with purified activated protein C. The relative prolongation of the activated partial thromboplastin time (aPTT) is used to assay for the defect. May be unreliable while taking heparin products (2).

Imaging

Initial approach

- Extremity ultrasound for deep vein thrombosis (DVT)
- V/Q scan of spiral CT for pulmonary embolism (PE)

Follow-Up & Special Considerations

- Ultrasound may not show DVT acutely; repeat in 1–2 days if strong suspicion.
- V/Q scan may be difficult to interpret in patients with other lung disease.

Diagnostic Procedures/Surgery

Magnetic resonance angiography (MRA), venography, or arteriography to detect thrombosis

Pathological Findings

Venous thrombus

DIFFERENTIAL DIAGNOSIS

- Protein C deficiency
- Protein S deficiency
- Antithrombin deficiency
- Other causes of activated protein C resistance (e.g., antiphospholipid antibodies)
- Dysfibrinogenemia
- Dysplasminogenemia
- Homocystinemia
- Prothrombin 20210 mutation
- Elevated factor VIII levels

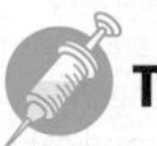

TREATMENT

Indicated for thrombosis

MEDICATION

First Line

- Low-molecular-weight heparin (LMWH) (2)[A]:
  - Enoxaparin (Lovenox): 1 mg/kg SC b.i.d., start warfarin simultaneously, continue Lovenox for at least 5 days and until international normalized ratio (INR) is >2.0, at which time it can be stopped
  - Fondaparinux (Arixtra): 7.5 mg SC daily
  - Tinzaparin (Innohep): 175 anti-Xa IU/kg SC daily for 6 days and patient is adequately anticoagulated with warfarin (INR of at least 2 for 2 consecutive days)
  - Dalteparin (Fragmin): 200 IU/kg SC daily
- Oral anticoagulant:
  - Warfarin (Coumadin) 5 mg daily p.o. initially and adjusted to an INR of 2–3
- Contraindications:
  - Active bleeding precludes anticoagulation (2)[A].
  - Risk of bleeding is a relative contraindication to long-term anticoagulation (2)[A].
  - Warfarin is contraindicated in patients with history of warfarin skin necrosis (2)[A].
  - Warfarin is contraindicated in pregnancy.
- Precautions:
  - Observe patient for signs of embolization, further thrombosis, or bleeding.
  - Avoid IM injections. Periodically check stool and urine for occult blood; monitor complete blood counts (CBCs), including platelets.
  - Heparin: Thrombocytopenia and/or paradoxic thrombosis with thrombocytopenia
  - Warfarin: Necrotic skin lesions (typically breasts, thighs, or buttocks)
  - LMWH: Adjust dosage in renal insufficiency. May also need dose adjustment in pregnancy (check anti-Xa level)

- Significant possible interactions:
  - Agents that intensify the response to oral anticoagulants: Alcohol, allopurinol, amiodarone, anabolic steroids, androgens, many antimicrobials, cimetidine, chloral hydrate, disulfiram, all nonsteroidal anti-inflammatory drugs (NSAIDs), sulfinpyrazone, tamoxifen, thyroid hormone, vitamin E, ranitidine, salicylates, acetaminophen
  - Agents that diminish the response to anticoagulants: Aminoglutethimide, antacids, barbiturates, carbamazepine, cholestyramine, diuretics, griseofulvin, rifampin, oral contraceptives

Second Line

- Heparin 80 mg/kg IV bolus followed by 18 g/kg/hour continuous infusion
- Adjust dose depending on aPTT.
- In patients requiring large daily doses of heparin, measure an anti-Xa level for dose guidance.
- Alternatively, unfractionated heparin can be given at 35,000 U per 24 hours SQ, with subsequent dosing to maintain a therapeutic aPTT (3)[C].

ADDITIONAL TREATMENT

General Measures

- Patients with factor V Leiden and a 1st thrombosis should be anticoagulated initially with heparin or LMWH (4)[A].
- Treatment with LMWH is recommended over unfractionated heparin, unless the patient has severe renal failure (3)[B].
- Treat as outpatient, if possible (3)[B].
- Initiate warfarin with heparin on the 1st treatment day, and discontinue heparin after 5 days and when INR >2.0 (3)[A].
- Patients should be maintained on warfarin with an INR of 2–3 for at least 6 months (3)[A].
- Recurrent thrombosis requires indefinite anticoagulation (4)[B].
- Compression stockings for prevention

Issues for Referral

- Recurrent thrombosis on anticoagulation
- Difficulty anticoagulating
- Genetic counseling

SURGERY/OTHER PROCEDURES

- Anticoagulation must be held for surgical interventions.
- For most patients with deep vein thrombosis (DVT), recommendations are against routine use of vena cava filter in addition to anticoagulation (3)[A].
- Thrombectomy may be necessary in some cases.

IN-PATIENT CONSIDERATIONS

Initial Stabilization

Heparin

Admission Criteria

Complicated thrombosis, such as pulmonary embolus

Nursing

- Teach LMWH and warfarin use.
- See above for drug interactions.

Discharge Criteria

Stable on anticoagulation

ONGOING CARE

FOLLOW-UP RECOMMENDATIONS

Patient Monitoring

Warfarin use requires periodic (~monthly after initial stabilization) INR measurements, with a goal of 2–3 (2)[A].

DIET

- No restrictions
- Foods rich in vitamin K may interfere with anticoagulation with warfarin.

PATIENT EDUCATION

- Patients should be educated about:
  - Use of oral anticoagulant therapy
  - Avoidance of NSAIDs while on warfarin
- The role of family screening is unclear, as most patients with this mutation do not have thrombosis. In a patient with a family history of factor V Leiden, consider screening during pregnancy or if considering oral contraceptive use.

PROGNOSIS

- Most patients heterozygous for factor V Leiden do not have thrombosis.
- Homozygotes have about a 50% lifetime incidence of thrombosis.
- Recurrence rates after a 1st thrombosis are not clear, with some investigators finding rates as high as 5% and others finding rates similar to the general population.
- Despite the increased risk for thrombosis, factor V Leiden does not increase overall mortality.

COMPLICATIONS

- Recurrent thrombosis
- Bleeding on anticoagulation

REFERENCES

1. Lijfering WM, Middeldorp S, Veeger NJ, Hamulyák K, Prins MH, Büller HR, van der Meer J et al. Risk of recurrent venous thrombosis in homozygous carriers and double heterozygous carriers of factor V Leiden and prothrombin G20210A. *Circulation*. 2010;121:1706–12.
2. Moll S. Thrombophilias–practical implications and testing caveats. *J Thromb Thrombolysis*. 2006; 21:7–15.
3. Büller HR, Agnelli G, Hull RD, et al. Antithrombotic therapy for venous thromboembolic disease: the Seventh ACCP Conference on Antithrombotic and Thrombolytic Therapy. *Chest*. 2004;126: 401S–428S.
4. Kim RJ, Becker RC. Association between factor V Leiden, prothrombin G20210A, and methylenetetrahydrofolate reductase C677T mutations and events of the arterial circulatory system: a meta-analysis of published studies. *Am Heart J*. 2003;146:948–57.

ADDITIONAL READING

Seligsohn U, Lubetsky A. Genetic susceptibility to venous thrombosis. *N Engl J Med*. 2001;344: 1222–31.

See Also (Topic, Algorithm, Electronic Media Element)

Thrombosis; Deep Vein Thrombophlebitis (DVT)

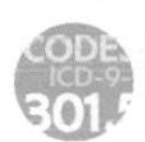

CODES

ICD9

289.81 Primary hypercoagulable state

CLINICAL PEARLS

- Extremely rare in Asian and African populations
- Asymptomatic patients with factor V Leiden do not need anticoagulation.

FAILURE TO THRIVE (FTT)

Jessica Davidson, MD

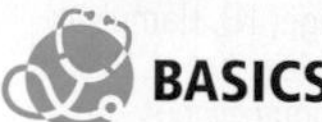

BASICS

DESCRIPTION

- Failure to thrive (FTT) is a general sign characterized by failure of physical growth, malnutrition, and potential retardation of development in children. The term is usually based on weight. In severe cases, it may lead to decreased length and/or head circumference.
- FTT describes a child with any of the following growth abnormalities:
  - Weight for age <5th percentile on >1 occasion
  - Weight that drops 2 or more major percentile lines on the standard growth charts
  - Weight <80% ideal body weight (IBW) based on National Center for Health Statistics' growth charts
  - Weight for height <10th percentile
  - Height for age <10th percentile
- Note that children with Down syndrome, intrauterine growth restriction (IUGR), premature infants, and infants with other syndromes follow different growth patterns.

EPIDEMIOLOGY

Incidence

- Predominant age: 6–12 months; most <3 years but can occur in older age groups
- Predominant sex: Male = Female

Prevalence

- Difficult to ascertain, as many studies do not exclude low birth weight (LBW) infants.
- As many as 10% of children seen in primary care have signs of growth failure.
- 1–5% of pediatric inpatient admissions are for evaluation of FTT.

RISK FACTORS

- Psychosocial risks:
  - Poverty is the leading risk factor.
  - Other risk factors include parent(s) with mental health disorder or limiting cognitive impairment, parent(s) with poor parenting skills or hypervigilant parents, families with unique health/nutritional beliefs, history of physical or emotional abuse, substance abuse, and social isolation
- Medical risks:
  - Intrauterine exposures, history of IUGR (symmetric or asymmetric), congenital abnormalities, premature or sick newborn, infant with physical deformity, acute or chronic medical conditions, developmental delay

Pregnancy Considerations

FTT is linked to intrauterine exposures, IUGR, and prematurity.

Genetics

No consistent genetic pattern but genetic disorders and inborn errors of metabolism can lead to FTT.

GENERAL PREVENTION

- Adequate parenting/caregiving skills
- Stable home life

PATHOPHYSIOLOGY

- Inadequate caloric intake (most frequent)
- Inadequate caloric absorption
- Excessive caloric expenditure
- Defective utilization

ETIOLOGY

- Traditional classifications of FTT have been listed as organic and nonorganic but most cases are a combination of these factors.
- Many cases of FTT begin with organic etiology. However, as the problem progresses, the caregivers and child begin to have interaction difficulties that also need to be addressed.
- Causes of FTT can be grouped by pathophysiology (including examples):
  - Inadequate intake: Breastfeeding difficulty, incorrect formula preparation, poor transition to food (6–12 months), poor feeding habits (e.g., excessive juice, avoidance of high calorie foods), mechanical problems (e.g., oropharyngeal dysfunction, congenital anomalies, GERD, CNS or PNS anomalies), poverty, neglect, poor parent-child interaction
  - Inadequate absorption: Necrotizing enterocolitis, short gut syndrome, biliary atresia, liver disease, cystic fibrosis, celiac disease, milk protein allergy, vitamin/mineral deficiency
  - Increased expenditure: Hyperthyroidism, congenital heart disease, chronic lung disease, HIV, congenital immunodeficiencies, malignancy, renal disease
  - Defective utilization: Metabolic disorders, congenital infections
- NOTE: Approximately 25% of children will decrease their weight or height by more than 25 percentile points in the first . years of life. These children are falling to their genetic potential or demonstrating constitutional growth delay (slow growth with a bone age less than chronologic age). After shifting down, these infants grow at a normal rate along their new percentile and do not have FTT.

DIAGNOSIS

HISTORY

- Prenatal history
- Developmental history
- Past medical history: Any acute or chronic disease that would affect caloric intake, digestion/absorption, cause increased energy need, or defective utilization
- Medication history, including complementary and alternative medications
- Family history: Stature of parents and growth trajectories of siblings; chronic diseases; genetic disorders; developmental delay
- Diet history from birth: Breast or formula feeding; timing and introduction of solids; who feeds the child, when, and how often; placement of child during feeds; amounts consumed; beverages consumed; snacking; vomiting or stooling associated with feeds
- Social history: Family composition, socioeconomic status, child-rearing beliefs, stressors, parental depression, parental substance abuse, caretaker personal history of abuse/neglect
- Review of systems: Anorexia, activity level, mental status, fevers, dysphagia, vomiting, gastro-esophageal reflux (GER), stooling pattern/consistency; dysuria; urinary frequency

PHYSICAL EXAM

- Accurate measurement of height, weight, and head circumference on National Center for Health Statistics (NCHS) growth charts (www.cdc.gov/growthcharts). Be sure that parameters are correctly plotted.
- Observe for signs of dehydration or severe malnutrition
  - Severity of malnutrition assessed via Gomez classification: Compare current weight for age with expected weight for age (50th percentile): Severe: <60% of expected; Moderate: 61–75%; Mild: 76–90%
- Medical disease that may be contributing to malnutrition
- Dysmorphic features
- Mental status (alert, responsive to stimuli)
- Any signs of physical abuse and/or neglect
- Observe interaction with caregivers and feeding techniques, specifically bonding and social/psychological cues

DIAGNOSTIC TESTS & INTERPRETATION

- Routine newborn screen in infants.
- Labs useful only in approximately 1.4% of cases.
- A period of re-nutrition is preferable prior to extensive lab workup.

Lab

Labs should be ordered based on history and physical exam findings and the age of the patient.

Initial lab tests

- CBC
- Electrolytes, serum BUN and creatinine
- Urinalysis and urine culture
- Erythrocyte sedimentation rate (ESR)
- Lead level
- If severe malnutrition is evident also include: Albumin, alkaline phosphatase, calcium, and phosphorus
- Other tests as dictated by the history and exam:
  - Thyroid-stimulating hormone (TSH), amylase and lipase, serum zinc level, iron studies, karyotype, genetic testing, sweat chloride test, stool for ova and parasite, guaiac, alpha-1-antitrypsin and elastase, RAST testing for IgE food allergies, tissue transglutaminase and total IgA (celiac sprue), P-ANCA and ASCA (anti-Saccharomyces cerevisiae antibodies for IBD), TB test, HIV ELISA, hepatitis A, B, other infections

Follow-Up & Special Considerations

- Evaluation by a multidisciplinary team including primary care physicians (PCPs), dietitians, occupational, physical and speech therapists, social workers, developmental specialists, psychiatrists, psychologists, visiting nurses, and/or child protection services.
- Evaluation should include a home visit by the child's PCP or visiting nurse for observation of infant, interaction with caretakers, and home environment
- Prospective food diary over 3–5 day
- Individual or family counseling for caregivers, parenting classes

Imaging

Not routine. Performed only as indicated by specific history or physical exam findings.

Initial approach

- Skeletal survey if suspicion or evidence of physical abuse
- Radiographs for bone age (wrist film)
- Swallowing studies, small bowel follow through
- Brain imaging if microcephalic and/or neurologic findings on examination.

DIFFERENTIAL DIAGNOSIS

Consider by system and disease process. Also consider psychosocial factors and abuse.

Differentiate based on growth patterns:

If low weight for age, normal linear growth, normocephalic OR low weight for age, followed by decreased linear growth OR low weight for age, leading to decreased linear growth and decreased head circumference (w/o neurological signs) = INADEQUATE NUTRITION (most common)

- Consider the following:
  - Inadequate food offered
  - Poor appetite
  - Oral aversion or food aversion
  - Oromotor dysfunction
  - Maldigestion/malabsorption
  - Hypermetabolic state

If low linear growth with normal weight for length OR low linear growth and proportionately low weight and decreased head circumference = short stature

- Consider the following:
  - Genetic potential
  - Genetic syndromes
  - Teratogens
  - Endocrine disorder

If microcephaly with prominent neurologic signs with poor growth secondary to presumed neurologic disorder

- Consider the following:
  - TORCHES
  - Genetic syndromes
  - Teratogens
  - Brain injury (i.e., hypoxic/ischemic)

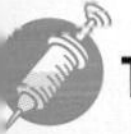

TREATMENT

MEDICATION

- Increase (and document) caloric intake.
- Consider multivitamin supplementation.

ADDITIONAL TREATMENT

General Measures

- Treatment is to improve nutrition to allow catch-up growth (weight gain 2–3 times greater than average for age).
- May use either of the following to calculate energy needs:
  - Increase intake 50% greater than the dietary reference intake (DRI) for age:
    - 0–6 months: 108 kcal/kg per day
    - 6–12 months: 98 kcal/kg per day
    - 1–3 years: 102 kcal/kg per day (1)[B]
  - General guideline for caloric requirements for infants with poor growth (for catch-up growth):
    - kcal/kg/d required = [RDA for age (kcal/kg) × Ideal wt. for ht.] / Actual wt., where ideal wt. for ht. is the median wt. for the patient's ht. (from NCHS curves)
- Rapid high-calorie intake can cause diarrhea, malabsorption, hypokalemia, hypophosphatemia. Therefore, increasing formulas above 24 kcal/oz is not recommended.
- The target energy intake should be slowly increased to goal over 5–7 days.
- Catch-up growth should be seen in 2–7 days.
- Accelerated growth should be continued for 4–9 months to restore weight and height:
  - Manage organic causes.
  - Establish appropriate nutritional intake.
  - Assist with social and family problems (WIC Program, food stamps, and other transitional assistance).

Issues for Referral

Multidisciplinary care is key. Referrals are dictated by the known or suspected cause of FTT.

Additional Therapies

- In severe cases, nasogastric (NG) tube feedings can be used to supplement oral feedings.
- Gastrostomy may also be considered.

IN-PATIENT CONSIDERATIONS

Most cases of FTT can be managed as outpatients.

Initial Stabilization

- During catch-up growth, some children will develop nutritional recovery syndrome.
  - Symptoms include sweating, increased body temperature, hepatomegaly (increase glycogen deposits), widening of cranial sutures (brain growth > bone growth), increased periods of sleep, fidgetiness and mild hyperactivity.
- There may also be an initial period of malabsorption with resultant diarrhea.

Admission Criteria

Consider hospitalization if outpatient management fails, severe malnutrition or dehydration exists, and/or psychosocial situation presents harm to child.

Discharge Criteria

Catch-up growth should be seen in 2–7 days. If this is not seen, reevaluation of causes is needed.

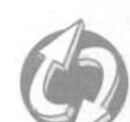

ONGOING CARE

FOLLOW-UP RECOMMENDATIONS

- When the etiology is organic, follow-up depends on the particular disease involved.
- Close long-term follow-up with frequent visits is important to create and maintain a healthy, supportive environment.
- If the family fails to comply, child protection authorities must be notified.

DIET

- Consider the presence of vegetarian or all-soy diets that may contribute to FTT. Safe vegetarian diets for children do exist, but must be chosen carefully.
- Nutritional requirements for a "normal" child:
  - Infant:
    - 110 kcal/kg, decreased to 100 kcal/kg at 6 months; if breastfed, ensure feeding occurs 8 times/day (minimum) w/ 5 minutes at each breast
    - Between 6 and 12 months, milk provides most of calories, but pureed foods should be consumed several times a day during this period
  - Toddler:
    - Minimum 5.5 oz/kg (110 kcal/kg) of formula; ensure proper formula mixing; if breastfed, ensure adequate supplemental foods
    - By middle of 2nd postnatal year, non-milk foods should provide at least 50% of caloric intake: 3 meals plus 2 nutritional snacks, 16–32 oz. milk/day, avoid juice and soda, and feed in a social environment
  - Rate of weight gain expected for age:
    - 0–3 months: 26–31 g/d
    - 3–6 months: 17–18 g/d
    - 6–9 months: 12–13 g/d
    - 9–12 months: 9 g/d
    - 1–3 years: 7–9 g/d

PATIENT EDUCATION

- Educate parents regarding infant social and physiological cues, formula/food preparation, proper feeding techniques, and importance of relaxed mealtimes
- When environmental deprivation is established, attempting to educate in a nonpunitive way is essential.
- Assist family with financial and nutritional assistance programs.
- Failure to Thrive: Why Is My Child Underweight? Available at http://www.aafp.org/afp/20030901/886ph.html
- The Women, Infants, and Children Program (WIC) provides Federal grants to states for supplemental foods, health care referrals, and nutrition education for low-income pregnant, breastfeeding, and non-breastfeeding postpartum women, and to infants and children up to age five who are found to be at nutritional risk. http://www.fns.usda.gov/wic/

PROGNOSIS

- Many children with FTT show adequate improvement in dietary intake with intervention.
- A significant proportion (1/3–1/2) will have long-term cognitive or behavioral abnormalities, the etiology of which is unclear.
- FTT may stunt neurologic development especially if head circumference is affected.
- Children with FTT are at increased risk for future undernutrition, overnutrition, and eating disorders.

REFERENCE

1. Krugman SD, Dubowitz H. Failure to thrive. *Am Fam Physician*. 2003;68:879–84.

See Also (Topic, Algorithm, Electronic Media Element)

Down Syndrome; Turner Syndrome; Irritable Bowel Syndrome

Algorithm: Failure to Thrive

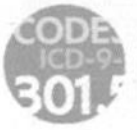

CODES

ICD9

783.41 Failure to thrive

CLINICAL PEARLS

- FTT is usually multifactorial. A multidisciplinary team approach to diagnosis and treatment is critical to help children with FTT and their families.
- Accurate weight and length and head circumference should be followed regularly.

F

FATTY LIVER SYNDROME

Dhvani Shah, MD
Edward Feller, MD

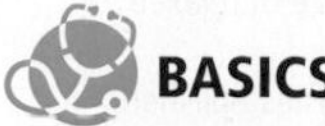

BASICS

Nonalcoholic fatty liver disease (NAFLD) describes a spectrum of fatty changes in the liver ranging from asymptomatic hepatic steatosis (fatty liver) to nonalcoholic steatohepatitis (NASH) and cirrhosis. NAFLD may be implicated to up to 90% of patients with asymptomatic, mild aminotransferase elevation not caused by alcohol, viral hepatitis, or medications.

DESCRIPTION

- Fatty liver:
  - Reversible condition where large vacuoles of triglyceride fat accumulate in hepatocytes; liver biopsy diagnosis usually shows fatty deposits in >30% of liver cells; No necrosis, no fibrosis
  - ALT and AST enzymes usually normal but may be elevated, rarely >3–4× the upper limit of normal
- NAFLD:
  - Fatty liver not due to excess alcohol consumption
  - Risk factors include associated obesity, metabolic syndrome, dyslipidemia, insulin resistance, and type 2 diabetes.
- NASH:
  - Progressive form of NAFLD; liver biopsy diagnosis of fatty deposits in >50% of liver cells associated with acute and chronic inflammation and fibrosis
  - Asymptomatic; ALT and AST elevated, generally <3–4× the upper limit of normal
  - Disease may progress to cirrhosis and/or hepatocellular cancer; incomplete data exists to assess natural history, although some evidence indicates that 30% with NASH have progression of fibrosis over 5 years.
- Both diseases usually identified in the 4th and 5th decade but may occur at any age,
- Synonym(s): Steatosis; Steatonecrosis; Nonalcoholic fatty liver disease (NAFLD); Steatohepatitis; Nonalcoholic steatohepatitis (NASH)

Pregnancy Considerations

- A severe complication of 3rd trimester is acute fatty liver of pregnancy. May be associated with signs of preeclampsia.
- Abrupt onset of confusion and restlessness with possible jaundice and right upper quadrant pain
- ALT and AST always elevated, usually <1000 IU/liter
- Emergency liver biopsy confirms diagnosis.
- Prompt delivery corrects the liver disease.
- Recurrence rare in subsequent pregnancies.

EPIDEMIOLOGY

NAFLD is the most common chronic liver disease globally, usually as benign, asymptomatic fatty liver (steatosis). NASH may be symptomatic with potential for progressive inflammation and fibrosis.

Incidence

- Present in up to 2/3 of obese (BMI >30) and in 90% of morbidly obese (BMI >39)
- Present in 5–10% type 2 DM patients
- Predominant age: 40s–50s; does occur in children
- Predominant sex: Male = Female

Prevalence

US prevalence is estimated at 6–24%

RISK FACTORS

- Obesity: BMI >30; DM; Hypertension; Hyperlipidemia (Metabolic syndrome)
- Protein–calorie malnutrition
- TPN >6 weeks
- Severe acute weight loss, including starvation and bariatric surgery
- Organic solvent (e.g., chlorinated hydrocarbons, toluene) exposure; vinyl chloride; hypoglycin A
- Gene for hemochromatosis or other conditions with increased iron stores
- Drugs: Tetracycline, glucocorticoids, tamoxifen, methotrexate, valproic acid, fialuridine, most chemotherapy regimes, and nucleoside analogues

Pediatric Considerations

- Reye syndrome: Fatty liver with encephalopathy characterized by
  - Vomiting with dehydration; usually postviral URI
  - Progressive CNS damage
  - Signs of hepatic injury: Liver morphologically shows extensive fatty vacuolization.
  - Hypoglycemia
- Etiology unknown; viral agents and drugs, especially salicylates, are implicated.
- Mortality rate 50%
- Tx: Mannitol, IV glucose, and FFP

Genetics

Largely unknown; carriers of hemochromatosis gene are more likely to be affected; possible genetic variants in the apolipoprotein C3 gene may play a role in fatty liver disease, insulin resistance, and hypertriglyceremia.

GENERAL PREVENTION

- Avoid excessive alcohol intake: >30 g/d for men, >20 g/d for women.
- Maintain or attain appropriate BMI.
- Avoid hepatotoxic medications
- Obtain HAV and HBV vaccination if not immune
- Obtain Pneumovax and yearly influenza vaccination.

PATHOPHYSIOLOGY

Primary pathophysiological derangement is *insulin resistance*, which leads to increased lipolysis, triglyceride synthesis, and increased hepatic uptake of fatty acids.

ETIOLOGY

- NAFLD: Most commonly an impaired ability of the liver to remove fatty acids
- NASH: "Two-hit" hypothesis involving macrovascular steatosis due to increased hepatic lipid synthesis, reduced transfer of lipids from the liver, and increasing insulin resistance with increased hepatic oxidative stress (1). Mitochondrial damage leading to impaired restoration of ADT stores, lipid peroxidation, and increased iron stores each have been found in 25–40% of the NASH patients.

COMMONLY ASSOCIATED CONDITIONS

Preeclampsia in pregnancy-related disease, central obesity, type 2 diabetes, insulin resistance, hyperlipidemia, hypertension

DIAGNOSIS

- Consider hepatic steatosis in any patient with asymptomatic aminotransferase elevation
- NAFLD can be present with normal or fluctuating AST and ALT.
- NASH has no distinguishing historical or laboratory features from other chronic liver disorders.
- Index of suspicion is higher in patients with associated risk factors such as metabolic syndrome, insulin resistance, or obesity.
- Noninvasive biomarkers of steatosis or fibrosis are not sufficiently reliable for diagnosis. Liver biopsy is the definitive diagnostic test. Biopsy should be considered when the results are likely to change management decisions.

HISTORY

Typically asymptomatic but some may experience fatigue and/or abdominal fullness

PHYSICAL EXAM

Hepatomegaly: Incidentally observed enlarged liver or spleen on physical exam or imaging.
Most common signs (each is infrequent):

- Liver pain or tenderness
- Mild to marked hepatomegaly
- Splenomegaly
- Limited to advanced cases: cutaneous stigmata of chronic liver disease or portal hypertension, variceal hemorrhage, ascites, hepatic encephalopathy, edema

DIAGNOSTIC TESTS & INTERPRETATION

Lab

- Liver function tests: Both ALT and AST may be elevated
  - Nonalcoholic, usually ALT:AST >1
  - If alcohol-induced, usually AST:ALT ≥2; serum alkaline phosphatase and direct bilirubin may be mildly elevated.
  - If advanced cirrhosis is present, marked, nonspecific enzyme abnormalities may exist.
- Level of enzyme elevation does not correlate with degree of fibrosis (2)[C].
- Severity in acute liver disease is marked by defects in ability to produce plasma proteins (serum albumin, prothrombin time), which are also clues to chronic hepatic disorders. Thrombocytopenia may be indicative of chronic liver disease and portal hypertension.
- Lipids almost always abnormal with elevated cholesterol, LDL, triglyceride, and decreased HDL
- Biomarkers of inflammation, increased oxidative stress or hepatocyte apoptosis such as ROS, leptin, adiponectin, CRP, serum caspase, and cytokeratin 18 remain investigational but may help differentiate NASH from NAFLD.

Initial lab tests

Serologic studies for viral hepatitis are vital: Serum ALT and AST, alkaline phosphatase, direct and total bilirubin, albumin and globulin, CBC, serum electrolytes, BUN, and creatinine

Follow-Up & Special Considerations

Patients with NAFLD have a 13% increase in carotid intima–media thickness; consider carotid ultrasound to assess (3)[A].

Imaging

- Fatty liver can be identified on ultrasound as hyperechoic liver and remains the 1st-line imaging modality for assessment of liver function test abnormalities; other imaging modalities such as MRI or CT may also be used; imaging modalities such as Fibroscan and magnetic resonance spectroscopy are currently being evaluated (4)[B].

No imaging modality can distinguish between simple steatosis from NASH.

Diagnostic Procedures/Surgery

- Liver biopsy is the only reliable diagnostic method; however it is not without risk, cost, and sampling error.
- Predictors associated with increased risk of fibrosis on biopsy are BMI >30, age >50, insulin resistance or diabetes mellitus, and elevated serum aminotransferases.

Pathological Findings

- Anatomic pathology liver biopsy is the gold standard to differentiate fatty liver with good prognosis from NASH (2)[B].
- In NASH, steatosis, ballooning, and lobular inflammation are considered common set of minimal criteria for diagnosis; other findings that are common but not necessary include mild-moderate portal inflammation, acidophil bodies, perisinusoidal zone 3 fibrosis, megamitochondria, and Mallory hyaline in hepatocytes (5)[B].
- Staging is based largely on the extent of fibrosis.

DIFFERENTIAL DIAGNOSIS

- Viral hepatitis
- Alcoholic fatty liver (history of alcoholism may be difficult to document or exclude)
- Drug- or toxin-induced hepatitis
- Occupational exposure
- Metabolic liver disease
- Autoimmune hepatitis
- Celiac disease
- Muscle disease if nonhepatic cause of elevated ALT and ALT are possible

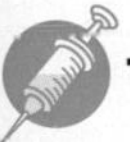

TREATMENT

Lifestyle modification through diet and exercise is the primary recommendation for patients with NAFLD and especially those with NASH. There have been a number of studies looking at the use of insulin-sensitizing and hepatoprotective agents; however currently there is no proven medication treatment regimen besides interventions that produce sustained weight loss, regular exercise, and diet composition modification.

MEDICATION

No specific therapy currently exists, but several promising agents are under investigation.

- There have been several studies that show drugs improving insulin resistance for patients with NAFLD may have a favorable role, but they are not definitive. These include metformin and pioglitazone (6)[A].
- Vitamins E and C have been shown to show mild improvement in hepatic steatosis and some improvement in inflammation (7)[B].
- Several other drugs have been studied in small pilot trials and animal studies. These include fibrates, gemfibrozil, statins, betaine, angiotensin-receptor blockers, and ursodeoxycholic acid. However, validation in larger randomized controlled studies have yet to be undertaken (7)[B].

ADDITIONAL TREATMENT

General Measures

- Aerobic exercise should occur 3× weekly for 20–45 minutes at the least.
- DM should be tightly regulated.
- Other components of metabolic syndrome such as hypertension, dyslipidemia, and obesity should be treated.
- All alcohol use should be discontinued permanently (2)[C].
- Avoid hepatotoxic medications.

Issues for Referral

Individuals with persistent elevation of liver enzymes 2–3 times above the upper limit of normal or with fibrosis on liver biopsy benefit from regular hepatologist follow-up.

COMPLEMENTARY AND ALTERNATIVE MEDICINE

Be wary of potential hepatotoxicity of complementary medications, which may also contain impurities.

SURGERY/OTHER PROCEDURES

Newer bariatric procedures have been found to have a positive impact on NASH (2)[B]. However careful case selection assessing risk-benefit ratio is vital since natural history is generally uncomplicated.

ONGOING CARE

FOLLOW-UP RECOMMENDATIONS

Patient Monitoring

- Repeat liver function tests yearly.
- Perform yearly US or CT scan to document diminution in fat.
- Changes toward normal provide major motivation to continue lifestyle changes.
- Routine repeat liver biopsy is not recommended (2)[C].

DIET

Diet low in fat; low in simple carbohydrates; low in high fructose corn syrup; devoid of industrial trans fats; and replete with vitamins, minerals, and natural antioxidants; avoidance of alcohol

PATIENT EDUCATION

Planning for lifelong change in eating, exercise, and alcohol use is required.

PROGNOSIS

Within the spectrum of NALFD, only NASH has been convincingly shown to have a progressive course, potentionally leading to cirrhosis, hepatocellular carcinoma, or liver failure.

- Cirrhosis develops in 25% of patients >20–30 years of age, with liver failure from cirrhosis occurring in 1–5%.
- Transplantation is effective, but NASH may recur after transplantation (2)[C].

COMPLICATIONS

Progressive disease may be complicated by features of decompensated cirrhosis and portal hypertension, such as ascites, encephalopathy, bleeding varices, hepato-renal or hepatopulmonary syndromes.

REFERENCES

1. Edmison J, McCullough AJ et al. Pathogenesis of non-alcoholic steatohepatitis: human data. *Clin Liver Dis*. 2007;11:75–104, ix
2. Ghali P, et al. The spectrum of nonalcoholic fatty liver disease. *J Clin Outcomes Managem*. 2005;12:585–93.
3. Sookoian S, Pirola CJ. Non-alcoholic fatty liver disease is strongly associated with carotid atherosclerosis: A systematic review. *J Hepatol*. 2008.
4. Rafiq N, Younossi ZM et al. Nonalcoholic fatty liver disease: a practical approach to evaluation and management. *Clin Liver Dis*. 2009;13:249–66.
5. Brunt EM et al. Nonalcoholic steatohepatitis. *Semin. Liver Dis*. 2004;24:3–20.
6. Angelico F, Burattin M, Alessandri C, Del Ben M, Lirussi F. Drugs improving insulin resistance for non-alcoholic fatty liver disease and/or non-alcoholic steatohepatitis. *Cochrane Database of Systematic Reviews*. 2007, Issue 1. Art. No.: CD005166. DOI:10.1002/14651858.CD005166.pub2.
7. Torres D, Harrison S. Diagnosis and Therapy of Nonalcoholic Steatohepatitis. *Gastroenterology*. 2008;134:1682–1698.
8. Schwimmer JB, Pardee PE, Lavine JE, et al. Cardiovascular risk factors and the metabolic syndrome in pediatric nonalcoholic fatty liver disease. *Circulation*. 2008;118:277–83.

See Also (Topic, Algorithm, Electronic Media Element)

Alcohol Abuse and Dependence; Cirrhosis of the Liver; Diabetes Mellitus, Type 2; Metabolic Syndrome

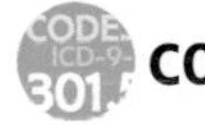

CODES

ICD9

- 571.0 Alcoholic fatty liver
- 571.8 Other chronic nonalcoholic liver disease

CLINICAL PEARLS

- NAFLD: Spectrum of liver damage ranging from simple steatosis to NASH, advanced fibrosis, and, rarely, progression to cirrhosis. Once thought to be benign, it is increasingly recognized as a major cause of liver-related morbidity and mortality.
- NAFLD: Most common cause of liver disease in children. Overweight children with NAFLD are more likely to have metabolic syndrome and central obesity; elevated levels of total cholesterol, LDL cholesterol and triglyceride; low HDL cholesterol levels; elevated blood pressure, and impaired fasting glucose (8)[B].
- NAFLD: A major cause of asymptomatic mild serum aminotransferase elevation.
- Benefit of statins in hypercholesterolemic patients generally outweighs risk of hepatoxicity. Continue statins and monitor hepatic enzymes.

FECAL IMPACTION

Benjamin Hilliker, MD
Eric Schmidt, MD

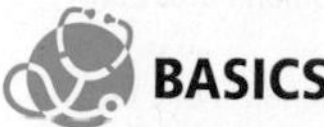

BASICS

DESCRIPTION

- Incomplete evacuation of feces, leading to formation of a large, firm, immovable mass of stool in the rectum (70%), sigmoid flexure (20%), or proximal colon (10%)
- System(s) affected: GI
- Synonym(s): Terminal reservoir syndrome

EPIDEMIOLOGY

Incidence

- General population: 1% (1,000/100,000)
- Children: 1.5%
- Nursing home residents: 30%
- Constipation more common in women, nonwhites, low income, <12 years of education (1)[C]
- Predominant age: >60 years
  Predominant sex:
- No sex preponderance in adults
- Among children, 75% are boys.

Geriatric Considerations

- Much more likely to occur in patients >80 years of age
- Megarectum may be present in physically and mentally impaired elderly.
- Constipation appears to correlate with decreased caloric intake in the elderly.

RISK FACTORS

- Institutionalization
- Psychogenic illness
- Immobility, inactivity
- Pica
- Excessive seed consumption (common in Middle East cultures), leading to rectal seed bezoars
- Chronic renal failure; renal transplant recipients
- Urinary incontinence
- Cognitive decline
- Constipation
- Heavy metal ingestion
- Poor toileting routines

Pediatric Considerations

- Habitual neglect of defecation urge, because of interference with play, may promote impaction.
- Fecal impaction has been reported to occur in >50% of all children with chronic constipation.

Genetics

Fecal impaction of the cecum may be seen in cystic fibrosis.

GENERAL PREVENTION

- Establish regular, consistent toilet time using gastrocolic reflex (2)[C]
- Maintain adequate hydration
- Maintain high-fiber diet (2)[C]
- Regular exercise (2)[B]
- Install user-friendly commodes.
- Psyllium 7–24 g PO daily (1)[B]
- Use periodic enemas, if indicated
- Periodic polyethylene glycol powder (MiraLax): 1 heaping tsp in 8 oz (240 mL) water daily × 2 weeks (1)[A]
- Lactulose 30–60 mL/d (1)[A]

PATHOPHYSIOLOGY

- The rectosigmoid colon dilates to accommodate mass, which, in turn, is not pliable enough to pass through the disproportionately small anal canal as a result of the patient's weak defecation effort.
- Impacted stool may exist as a single mass (stercolith) or as a composite of small, rounded fecal particles (scybalum).

ETIOLOGY

- Diet lacking in fiber
- Drug side effects (2)[C]:
  - Stimulant laxatives
  - Opiates
  - Benzodiazepines
  - Tricyclic antidepressants
  - Phenothiazines
  - Antihypertensives (calcium channel blockers)
  - Aluminum (sucralfate, antacids)
  - Iron
  - Antispasmodics
  - Vinca alkaloids
  - 5HT3 antagonist
- Painful rectal conditions inhibiting voluntary defecation (e.g., anal fissure, hemorrhoids, fistulas)
- Neoplastic or inflammatory obstructing lesions (e.g., rectal bezoars)
- Neurogenic disorders:
  - Hirschsprung disease
  - Chagas disease
  - DM
  - Autonomic neuropathy
  - Multiple sclerosis
  - Spinal cord injury
  - Cauda equine
  - Parkinson disease
- Nonneurogenic:
  - Hypothyroidism
  - Hypokalemia
  - Hypercalcemia
  - Anorexia nervosa
  - Systemic sclerosis
  - Myotonic dystrophy
- Excess of GI inhibitory hormones (e.g., prolactin, endorphins, glucagon, secretin)
- Severe idiopathic chronic constipation
- Irritable bowel syndrome
- Pelvic floor dysfunction
- Pelvic floor dyssynergia
- Encopresis

COMMONLY ASSOCIATED CONDITIONS

- Pulmonary aspiration
- Urinary tract obstruction
- Recurrent UTIs
- Intestinal obstruction
- Spontaneous perforation of colon
- Stercoral ulceration
- Hernia
- Volvulus
- Megacolon or megarectum
- Rectal prolapse
- Pneumothorax
- Hypoxia
- Hypovolemic shock
- Iliac occlusion

Pregnancy Considerations

Impaction can produce dysfunctional labor, dystocia.

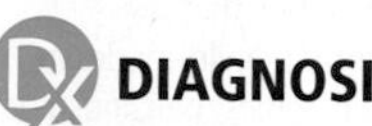

DIAGNOSIS

HISTORY

- Fecal incontinence, interpreted as diarrhea
- Postprandial abdominal pain
- Tenesmus
- Colic
- Nausea
- Vomiting
- Anorexia
- Weight loss
- Headache
- General malaise
- Agitation; confusion
- Urinary frequency
- Urinary incontinence

PHYSICAL EXAM

The general physical exam is not helpful in most patients.

- Weight loss
- Dehydration
- Agitation; confusion
- Fever to 39.4°C (103°F)
- Tachycardia
- Tachypnea
- Digital rectal exam:
  - Identify fissures or hemorrhoids.
  - Loss of sphincter tone: Neurologic disorders
- Large mass of stool palpable in lower left quadrant and rectal vault

DIAGNOSTIC TESTS & INTERPRETATION

Lab

Often normal

- Leukocytosis to 15,000 WBCs/mm^3
- Hyponatremia
- Hypokalemia
- Hypercalcemia
- TSH
- Stool may be positive for occult blood.
- Anemia, owing to chronic blood loss
- Pediatrics:
  - Antigliadin and antiendomysium antibodies
  - Lead

Geriatric Considerations

- Measure TSH, electrolyte activity, and BUN in elderly patients presenting with impaction.

Imaging
- Plain abdominal radiography may reveal stool or signs of obstruction if digital exam unrevealing.
- Stool retention is associated with megacolon.
- Barium enema can differentiate feces from tumor.

Diagnostic Procedures/Surgery
Sigmoidoscopy may be used to clarify the nature of a rectosigmoid mass.

DIFFERENTIAL DIAGNOSIS
- Irritable bowel syndrome
- Gastroenteritis, colitis
- Diverticulitis
- Appendicitis
- Carcinoma of the colon

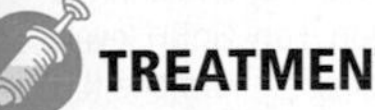

TREATMENT

MEDICATION
- A daily 1-L bolus of polyethylene glycol–electrolyte (GoLYTELY) solution given over 4–6 hours up to 3 days (2)[B]
- Polyethylene glycol-electrolyte (GoLYTELY) is better than lactulose in outcomes of frequency per week, form of stool, relief of abdominal pain, and the need for additional products (3)[A].
- Disimpaction in children; Consider combination:
  - Day 1: 1–2 phospho-soda enemas, 1 oz/10 kg; 4.5 oz maximum
  - Day 2: Bisacodyl suppository per rectum daily or b.i.d.
  - Day 3: Bisacodyl tablet PO every day or b.i.d.
  - Repeat 3-day cycle if needed once or twice.
- High-dose mineral oil: 15–30 mL PO per year of age per day to 8 oz maximum daily; b.i.d. for 3 days. Avoid if aspiration risk.
- Enemas: 1–2 oz/10 kg to 4.5 oz maximum, daily; b.i.d. for 1–2 days
- Children with constipation or fecal impaction who are treated with polyethylene glycol–electrolyte (GoLYTELY) have demonstrated consistently good outcomes. Dosages range from 0.3–0.7 g/kg/day (4)[A].
- Enemas and polyethylene glycol-electrolyte (GoLYTELY) were equally effective in treating fecal impaction in children. Polyethylene glycol-electrolyte (GoLYTELY) caused more fecal incontinence with comparable behavior scores (5)[B].
- Methylnaltrexone (Relistor) is approved for opioid-induced constipation by the FDA and can be considered in patients who do not have a reasonable response to a laxative regimen. Its use may be limited by cost (6)[B].
- Precautions:
  - Use magnesium citrate with caution in patients with renal insufficiency.
  - Be careful with lactulose; colonic distension can result from its bacterial fermentation.

ADDITIONAL TREATMENT

General Measures
- Manual fragmentation and extraction of fecal mass (after lubrication with lidocaine jelly) may be attempted.
- Larger masses can be disimpacted with water jet directed through fiberoptic sigmoidoscope.
- Enemas containing 20% water-soluble contrast material (Hypaque) may help.
- If incomplete fragmentation: Suppositories or enemas with mineral oil, tap water, or sodium phosphate
- Ensure minimum fluid intake of 1.5–2.0 L/d.

Issues for Referral
In the pediatric population, consultation with a pediatric gastroenterologist should be considered in children in whom oral or rectal medication is ineffective for disimpaction and in whom dietary changes and laxative therapy are ineffective.

COMPLEMENTARY AND ALTERNATIVE MEDICINE
Biofeedback improves constipation in patients with dyssynergic bowel function (7)[B].

SURGERY/OTHER PROCEDURES
- Laparotomy necessary only in extreme cases (2)[B]
- Electrohydraulic lithotripsy has been used to safely remove large, calcified fecaliths.

IN-PATIENT CONSIDERATIONS

Admission Criteria
- Disimpaction usually is performed in outpatient setting.
- Hospitalization is necessary if several attempts at outpatient management have failed.
- Presence of complications

ONGOING CARE

FOLLOW-UP RECOMMENDATIONS
Increased activity is important.

Patient Monitoring
<1 bowel movement every other day may lead to impaction.

DIET
- High fiber
- Home remedy: Mix 2 cups bran, 2 cups applesauce, and 1 cup unsweetened prune juice; refrigerate; take 2–3 tbs b.i.d.

PATIENT EDUCATION
- Avoid catharsis.
- Comprehensive program, including use of laxative, behavior changes, dietary changes
- Effective education of the parents and child with regard to constipation is crucial in changing chronic behavior patterns.
- No hot water, soap, or hydrogen peroxide enemas. They may burn or irritate rectal mucosa, causing bleeding.

PROGNOSIS
- Reimpaction is likely if program is not followed.
- Prognosis is poor for perforation with peritonitis.
- Mortality with impaction and obstruction is highest in the very young and the very old (up to 16%).

COMPLICATIONS
- Sepsis
- Hypotension
- Instrumental perforation
- Bleeding
- Postoperative obstruction

REFERENCES

1. Brandt LJ, Prather CM, Quigley EM, et al. Systematic review on the management of chronic constipation in North America. *Am J Gastroenterol*. 2005;100 (Suppl 1):S5–S21.
2. Hsieh C. Treatment of constipation in older adults. *Am Fam Physician*. 2005;72:2277–84.
3. Lee-Robichaud H, Thomas K, Morgan J, Nelson RL et al. Lactulose versus Polyethylene Glycol for Chronic Constipation. *Cochrane Database Syst Rev*. 2010;7:CD007570.
4. Candy D, Belsey J. Macrogol (polyethylene glycol) laxatives in children with functional constipation and faecal impaction: a systematic review. *Arch Dis Child*. 2009;94:156–60.
5. Bekkali N, van den Berg M, Dijkgraaf M, van wijk P, Bongers EJ, Liem O, Benninga M. Rectal Fecal Impaction Treatment in Childhood Constipation: Enemas versus High Doses Oral PEG. *Pediatrics* 2009;124;e1108–e1115.
6. Enck R. An Overview of Constipation and Newer Therapies. *American Journal of Hospice & Palliative Medicine*. 2009;26(3):157–158.
7. Rao SS, Seaton K, Miller M, et al. Randomized controlled trial of biofeedback, sham feedback, and standard therapy for dyssynergic defecation. *Clin Gastroenterol Hepatol*. 2007;5:331–8.

F

ADDITIONAL READING

- Constipation Guideline Committee of the North American Society for Pediatric Gastroenterology, Hepatology and Nutrition. Evaluation and treatment of constipation in infants and children: recommendations of the North American Society for Pediatric Gastroenterology, Hepatology and Nutrition. *J Pediatr Gastroenterol Nutr*. 2006;43: e1–13.
- Tariq SH. Geriatric fecal incontinence. *Clin Geriatr Med*. 2004;20:571–87, ix.

See Also (Topic, Algorithm, Electronic Media Element)
Constipation; Diarrhea, Chronic; Encopresis

CODES

ICD9
560.32 Fecal impaction

CLINICAL PEARLS
- Any elderly person with a fever of uncertain cause should be considered to have a fecal impaction until you can disprove it with a DRE.
- When treating chronic pain patients with opioid preparations, be sure to supplement with stool softeners or osmotic laxatives. Hydrophilic colloid (fiber) is not that helpful in frail, end-of-life, or nonmobile patients.

FEMALE ATHLETE TRIAD

Rahul Kapur, MD, CAQSM
Natasha Harrison, MD
Kristyn Newhall, MD

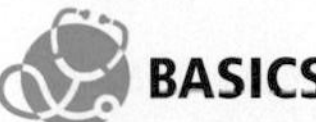

BASICS

Consisting of three interrelated spectrums of:
- Low energy availability
- Menstrual dysfunction
- Decreased bone health

DESCRIPTION
- First recognized in 1992.
- 2007 American College of Sports Medicine (ACSM) criteria recommends to consider each component of the triad as a continuous spectrum. The criterion of disordered eating has been replaced by "low energy availability with or without an eating disorder." Amenorrhea is considered within a spectrum from "eumenorrhea" to "functional hypothalamic amenorrhea." The endpoint diagnosis of osteoporosis has been replaced by a spectrum from "optimal bone health" to "osteoporosis." The ACSM 2007 revision underscores the importance of energy availability as the 1st step in the propagation of the triad, emphasizing that without correction of this triad component, full recovery is not possible (1).
- Energy availability: The dietary energy intake minus exercise energy expenditure, which represents the amount of dietary energy remaining for body functions after exercise training. When energy availability is low, the body compensates to restore energy balance by reducing mechanisms of cellular maintenance, thermoregulation, growth and reproduction. Athletes with low energy availability may develop an imbalance by increasing training disproportionately to energy intake, while others may reduce energy intake by restricting, fasting, bingeing and purging, or by using diet pills, laxatives, diuretics, or enemas. Only some of these athletes will meet the (DSM-IV) criteria for eating disorders including anorexia nervosa and bulimia nervosa.
- Menstrual dysfunction: A spectrum ranging from eumenorrhea to amenorrhea, allowing for the inclusion of athletes who have low estrogen levels but may still experience menstruation:
  - This spectrum includes luteal suppression (shortened luteal phase, prolonged follicular phase and decreased estradiol level), anovulation, oligomenorrhea (menstrual cycle greater than 35 days) and primary and secondary hypothalamic amenorrhea. Primary amenorrhea, though less common, can occur in young athletes. Secondary amenorrhea is defined as the absence of menstrual cycles for greater than three months after menarche has occurred.
  - Hypothalamic suppression is the most common cause of secondary amenorrhea in these athletes, although other causes must be ruled out prior to attributing the problem to low energy availability.
- Bone health: Bone health exists on a spectrum from optimal bone health to osteoporosis, a skeletal disorder characterized by compromised bone strength predisposing a person to an increased fracture risk. Bone health refers to bone strength, or bone mineral density (BMD), as well as bone quality. Current technology allows for the measurement of bone density but not quality, which helps to explain why 2 athletes with the same BMD may have very different bone fracture histories:
  - Athletes with a BMD Z-score that is 2 standard deviations (SD) below the mean are termed low bone density below the expected range for age for premenopausal women and low bone density for chronologic age for children.
  - Because most athletes have a higher BMD than nonathletes, the ACSM recommends physicians consider further workup for any athlete with a Z-score <-1.0, even in the absence of fracture (2).

EPIDEMIOLOGY
Unknown as often hidden by patients

Prevalence
- Prevalence unclear; data suggests between 3.4–4.3%. The 2 other triad studies, found all 3 components of triad in 2.7% of collegiate and 1.2% of high school athletes (1,3).
- Disordered eating: Prevalence of clinically diagnosed (DSM-IV) eating disorders in elite athletes 25–31% vs 5.5-9% in the general population.
- Menstrual dysfunction: Prevalence of secondary amenorrhea found to be as high as 69% in dancers and 65% in long-distance runners compared to 2–5% in the general population. Majority exhibit a luteal deficiency or anovulatory cycle in 1 in 3 menstrual cycles.
- Bone health: A systematic review of past studies using the World Health Organization (WHO) criteria for low BMD revealed prevalence of osteopenia (T-score between -1.0 and -2.5) from 22–50% in female athletes, compared to 12% in the normal population and of osteoporosis (T-score ≤ -2.5) as high as 13%, compared to 2.3% in the normal population.

RISK FACTORS
- Sports with an aesthetic component,e.g., ballet, figure skating, gymnastics, distance running, diving and swimming, or sports with weight classifications, e.g., martial arts and wrestling. Frequent weigh-ins, consequences for weight gain, domineering coaches or parents, and a win-at-all-cost attitude increase risk of developing the triad.
- A lack of family or social support, either secondary to intense training hours causing social isolation or entering a new environment (boarding school or college)
- Athlete with comorbid psychological conditions, e.g., anxiety, depression, and/or obsessive-compulsive disorder is more likely to develop the triad (3).

GENERAL PREVENTION
- Education of athletes, coaches, trainers, parents, and physicians about the triad is crucial. Young athletes are extremely impressionable and may turn negative comments and unhealthy advice from adults into maladaptive eating and exercising habits.
- Primary care physicians should screen all adolescents for disordered eating, menstrual dysfunction, and injury history.
- Athletes presenting with "red flag" conditions such as fractures, weight changes, fatigue, amenorrhea, bradycardia, orthostatic hypotension, syncope, arrhythmia, electrolyte abnormalities, or depression should also be screened for the triad.

PATHOPHYSIOLOGY
- Current theory is based on a baseline caloric defici[t] or low energy availability causing a disruption in th[e] hypothalamic-pituitary-ovarian axis, decreasing the pulsatile release of gonadotropin-releasing hormo[ne] (GnRH).
- Low energy availability alters the levels of various metabolic hormones including insulin, cortisol, growth hormone, insulin-like growth factor-1 (ILGF-1), 3.3.5-triiodothyronine (T3) and leptin, some of which are thought to play a role in the regulation of GnRH secretion. Low GnRH levels subsequently decrease luteinizing hormone (LH) an[d] follicle-stimulating hormone (FSH) levels causing a decrease in estrogen production, resulting in varyi[ng] degrees of menstrual dysfunction.
- Estrogen deficiency also negatively affects bone density and a chronic state of malnutrition reduces the rate of bone formation and increases the rate o[f] bone resorption. This change in increased bone resorption and declined rate of bone formation began within 5 days of energy availability reductio[n] (1,4).

COMMONLY ASSOCIATED CONDITIONS
- Anorexia nervosa or bulimia nervosa
- Psychological disorders including low self-esteem, depression, and anxiety. In one study, 5.4% of athletes with eating disorders reported suicide attempts (5).
- Low BMD predisposes athletes to stress fractures and may not be fully reversible. This may lead to an even higher rate of fractures as these athletes reac[h] postmenopausal status.

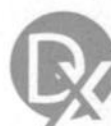

DIAGNOSIS

- The female athlete triad is a clinical diagnosis base[d] mainly on patient history.
- Screening for the female athlete triad should occur at annual sports physicals, routine exams, and acut[e] visits for any concerning complaints or components of the triad (1)[C].

HISTORY
- A 24-hour food recall diary may be helpful in this process. Athletes should be assessed for menstrual history (including oral contraceptive use), fracture history, and symptoms of depression (5)[C].
- Special dietary practices, eating behaviors, and weight changes should also be collected.
- Body image, fear of weight gain, fluctuations in weight, history of disordered eating, and use of laxatives, diet pills, or enemas are crucial to understanding the extent of the disease.

PHYSICAL EXAM
- Height, weight, and vital signs
- Common findings in patients with disordered eating include bradycardia, orthostatic hypotension, hypothermia, cold or cyanotic extremities, lanugo, hypercarotenemia, parotid gland enlargement or tenderness, epigastric tenderness, eroded tooth enamel, and knuckle or hand calluses (Russell sign) (5)[C].
- Patients with primary amenorrhea should undergo a pelvic exam to determine the presence of a uterus. A pelvic exam in patients with secondary amenorrhea

is warranted to rule out anomalies. Vaginal atrophy may be present in the hypoestrogen state (1)[C].

IAGNOSTIC TESTS & INTERPRETATION

ab

- Electrolytes and kidney function, complete blood count with differential, erythrocyte sedimentation rate, thyroid stimulating hormone (TSH), 25 vitamin D, and urinalysis.
- Primary evaluation for secondary amenorrhea includes a urine pregnancy test, follicle stimulating hormone, luteinizing hormone, prolactin and thyroid stimulating hormone (1)[B].

naging

- Electrocardiogram (EKG) to rule out a prolonged QT interval. The QT interval may be prolonged even in the absence of electrolyte abnormalities (5)[C].
- Evidence for bone mineral density testing by dual-energy x-ray absorptiometry (DXA) is controversial. Current guidelines recommend DXA studies for patients with disordered eating, eating disorders, amenorrhea, or oligomenorrhea for at least 6 months and/or patients with a history of stress fractures or fractures from minimal trauma. In patients with persistent components of the triad, reevaluation by the same DXA machine is recommended in 12 months from initial scan (1)[C].

IFFERENTIAL DIAGNOSIS

ne diagnosis of each component of the female hlete triad must be one of exclusion. Patients must e screened for anorexia nervosa and bulimia nervosa sing the DSM-IV criteria. Similarly, before presuming diagnosis of hypothalamic amenorrhea secondary to nergy deficit, the following groups of diagnoses must e ruled out:

- Pregnancy
- Hypothalamic dysfunction: Psychological stress induced amenorrhea, medication induced amenorrhea, Kallmann syndrome
- Pituitary dysfunction: Prolactinoma or other pituitary neoplasm, Sheehan syndrome, sarcoidosis, empty-sella syndrome
- Ovarian dysfunction: Polycystic ovarian syndrome, premature ovarian failure, menopause, gonadal dysgenesis, Turner syndrome, ovarian neoplasm, autoimmune disease
- Uterine dysfunction: Asherman syndrome, absence of uterus
- Endocrine abnormalities: Thyroid dysfunction, Cushing syndrome (3)[B]

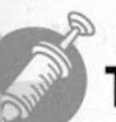

TREATMENT

The treatment goal is to optimize nutritional status by establishing healthy eating behaviors and treating any associated maladaptive thought processes or psychological disorders.

- A multidisciplinary team including a physician (or other health care provider), registered dietitian and a mental health provider is crucial for treatment (1)[C]. Diet and exercise behaviors must be modified by a combination of increasing dietary intake and reducing energy expenditure. Nutritional counseling by a registered dietitian is necessary for energy availability estimates as well as modification of eating behaviors. Individual, group and family psychotherapy may also be needed for the full treatment of the triad (5)[B]. Communication with team coaches, trainers, and family is also a critical intervention.
- Studies have shown a positive energy availability of more than 30 kcal/kg of fat-free muscle mass/day is sufficient to restore menstrual cycling, while an energy availability of more than 45 kcal/kg of fat-free muscle mass/day is likely needed for BMD improvement. Increases in body weight have been accompanied by improved BMD by up to 5% per year in previously amenorrheic athletes (1).

MEDICATION

The use of oral contraceptive pills (OCPs), hormone replacement therapy (HRT), and/or bisphosphonates has not been clearly shown to increase BMD or aid in the restoration of normal menstrual cycling. OCPs can be considered to minimize further bone loss in patients over age 16, who, despite adequate nutrition and body weight gain, continue to have decreasing BMD and functional hypothalamic amenorrhea (1)[C].

ADDITIONAL TREATMENT

Issues for Referral

Referrals to registered dietitians, mental health professionals who specialize in disordered eating behaviors, and sports medicine specialists for treatment of fractures often are needed (1)[C].

IN-PATIENT CONSIDERATIONS

Patients with disordered eating or clinically diagnosable eating disorders must be evaluated for potentially life-threatening conditions requiring hospital admission including bradycardia, severe orthostatic hypotension, significant electrolyte imbalances, hypothermia, arrhythmias, or prolonged QT interval on EKG (3,5)[C].

ONGOING CARE

- Patients with components of the triad should undergo frequent monitoring by all members of the multidisciplinary treatment team. In order to continue training and competing, athletes with disordered eating or clinically diagnosable eating disorders must agree to the following criteria:
  - To comply with all treatment strategies; to be closely monitored by heath care providers; to place treatment goals over training goals; and to modify the type, duration, and intensity of training or competition if necessary.
- Athletes with disordered eating behaviors who do not comply with this agreement may need to be restricted from training (1)[C].

PATIENT EDUCATION

All young female patients should be counseled on the importance of proper nutrition, calcium, and vitamin D intake and the benefits of regular weight-bearing exercise. Patients presenting with one or more components of the triad should be educated about the short-term and long-term effects of low BMD (6).

PROGNOSIS

- The short- and long-term prognosis for patients with female athlete triad is dependent on time to diagnosis and treatment. Assuming early intervention with a multidisciplinary team, prognosis is very good. With adequate treatment and an increase in energy availability, patients will regain normal menstrual cycling and fertility and begin to increase BMD.
- Because the triad often occurs within the age window of optimal bone strengthening, patients with a prolonged disease course may suffer from complications of decreased bone mineral density throughout their adolescent and adult life. In addition, patients with disordered eating behaviors may require long-term ongoing therapy to manage their disease (3).

REFERENCES

1. Otis CL, Drinkwater B, Johnson M, et al. American College of Sports Medicine position stand. The Female Athlete Triad. *Med Sci Sports Exerc.* 1997;29:i–ix.
2. International Society for Clinical Densitometry Writing Group for the ISCD Position Development Conference. Diagnosis of osteoporosis in men, women, and children. *J Clin Densitom.* 2004;7:17–26.
3. Hobart JA, Smucker DR. The female athlete triad. *Am Fam Physician.* 2000;61:3357–64, 3367.
4. The female athlete triad. *Med Sci Sports Exerc.* 2007;39:1867–82.
5. American Psychiatric Association Working Group on Eating Disorders. Treatment of patients with eating disorders, third edition. *Am J Psychiatry.* 2006;163.4–54.
6. American Academy of Pediatrics. Committee on Sports Medicine and Fitness. Medical concerns in the female athlete. *Pediatrics.* 2000;106:610–3.

See Also (Topic, Algorithm, Electronic Media Element)

Algorithms: Amenorrhea, Secondary; Amenorrhea, Primary; Weight Loss

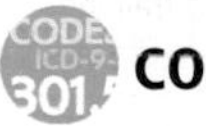

CODES

ICD9

- 307.50 Eating disorder, unspecified
- 626.0 Absence of menstruation
- 733.00 Osteoporosis, unspecified

CLINICAL PEARLS

- The female athlete triad consists of three related spectrums of energy availability, menstrual function, and BMD. Athletes may exhibit varying degrees of dysfunction along each of the 3 spectra.
- Regular screening of adolescent and adult females at all routine and relevant acute visits is critical to early diagnosis and intervention.
- Immediate intervention by a multidisciplinary team including physicians, registered dietitians, mental heath professionals, coaches, trainers, and parents is crucial to minimize further bone loss, recover bone mineral density, and regain menstrual cycling.

F

FEVER OF UNKNOWN ORIGIN (FUO)

Scott T. Henderson, MD

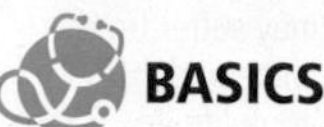

BASICS

DESCRIPTION

- Classic definition by Petersdorf and Beeson:
  - Fever over 38.3°C on several occasions
  - Fever duration at least 3 weeks
  - Uncertain diagnosis after 1 week of study in the hospital
- Modifications to the definition have been proposed, including eliminating the in-hospital evaluation and shortening the exam time.
- Some have suggested expansion of the definition to include nosocomial, neutropenic, and HIV-associated fevers that may not be prolonged.

EPIDEMIOLOGY

Incidence

No data on actual incidence

RISK FACTORS

- Recent travel
- Exposure to biologic or chemical agents
- HIV-infected patients with advanced disease
- Persons in AIDS risk group
- Elderly
- Drug abuse
- Immigrants
- Young female health care workers; consider factitious fever

ETIOLOGY

- >200 causes; each with prevalence 5% or less
- Infection:
  - Abdominal abscesses
  - Amebic hepatitis
  - Catheter infections
  - Cytomegalovirus
  - Endocarditis/pericarditis
  - HIV (late stage)
  - Mycobacterial infection (often with advanced HIV)
  - Osteomyelitis
  - Renal
  - Sinusitis
  - Wound infections
  - Other miscellaneous infections
- Neoplasms:
  - Atrial myxoma
  - Colon cancer
  - Hepatoma
  - Lymphoma
  - Leukemia
  - Solid tumors (hypernephroma)
- Collagen vascular disease:
  - Giant cell arteritis
  - Polyarteritis nodosa
  - Polymyalgia rheumatica
  - Systemic lupus erythematosus
  - Rheumatic fever
  - Rheumatoid arthritis
- Other causes:
  - Alcoholic hepatitis
  - Cerebrovascular accident
  - Cirrhosis
  - Drug fever/medication induced:
    - Allopurinol, captopril, carbamazepine, cephalosporins, cimetidine, clofibrate, erythromycin, heparin, hydralazine, hydrochlorothiazide, isoniazid, meperidine, methyldopa, nifedipine, nitrofurantoin, penicillin, phenytoin, procainamide, quinidine, sulfonamides
  - Endocrinologic diseases
  - Factitious/fraudulent fever
  - Granulomatous diseases
  - Occupational causes
  - Periodic fever
  - Pulmonary emboli/deep vein thrombosis
  - Thermoregulatory disorders
- In up to 20% of cases, the cause of the fever will not be identified despite thorough workup.

Geriatric Considerations

- Most common causes are acute leukemia, Hodgkin lymphoma, intra-abdominal infections, TB, and temporal arteritis

Pediatric Considerations

- Infections and collagen-vascular diseases are the most likely etiology.
- Inflammatory bowel disease is the common etiology in older children and adolescents.

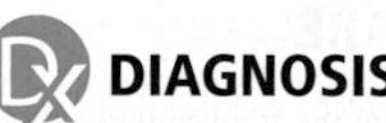

DIAGNOSIS

HISTORY

- History should focus on relevant symptoms:
  - Constitutional symptoms almost always accompany a fever:
    - Chills, night sweats, myalgias, weight loss with an intact appetite (infectious)
    - Arthralgias, myalgias, fatigue (inflammatory)
    - Fatigue, night sweats, weight loss with loss of appetite (neoplasms)
- Past medical history should include information about previously treated chronic infections and any prior diagnosis of cancer.
- Past surgical history should include specific information about type of surgery performed, postoperative complications, and any indwelling foreign materials.
- Obtain a comprehensive list of all medications, including over-the-counter and herbal remedies.
- Family history to identify prior illnesses in family members that may have a genetic link, such as periodic fever syndromes, and recent illnesses in family members to which the patient may have been exposed

ALERT

Special attention should be paid to travel, occupational, sexual, and drug exposure.

Geriatric Considerations

- Signs and symptoms in the elderly are much more nonspecific.
- Coexisting diseases and numerous medications ma cloud features.

PHYSICAL EXAM

- Physical exam should focus on areas that have hig diagnostic yield:
  - Fundoscopic exam for choroid tubercles or Roth spots; temporal artery palpation; gums and oral cavity; auscultation for bruits and murmurs; abdominal palpation for organomegaly; rectal examination; testicular examination; palpate for adenopathy; skin and nail bed exam for clubbing nodules, lesions, and rashes; focal neurologic signs; bony tenderness; and joint effusion
- Repeated exams are essential to determine cause.

DIAGNOSTIC TESTS & INTERPRETATION

Lab

Initial lab tests

- Complete blood count
- Peripheral blood smear
- Liver function tests
- C-reactive protein
- Erythrocyte sedimentation rate
- HIV antibody test
- Blood cultures (not to exceed 6 sets)
- Urinalysis and urine culture

Geriatric Considerations

- Residents of long-term care facilities have unique guidelines; review advanced directives first to determine if any testing should be done.
- Blood cultures are shown to have lower yield (1)[A

Follow-Up & Special Considerations

- Rheumatoid factor and antinuclear antibody test
- Serologic tests: Epstein-Barr, hepatitis, syphilis, Lym disease, Q fever, cytomegalovirus, amebiasis, coccidioidomycosis
- Serum ferritin
- Serum protein electrophoresis
- Sputum and urine cultures for TB
- Thyroid function tests
- Tuberculin skin test:
  - May not be helpful if anergic or acute infection
  - If test negative, repeat in 2 weeks

Imaging

Initial approach

- CXR
- CT scan or MRI of abdomen and pelvis (plus directe biopsy, if indicated) (2)[C]

Follow-Up & Special Considerations

- Technetium-based scan if infectious process or tumor suspected (2)[B]
- PET scan using the radiolabeled glucose analogue ^{18}F-fluorodeoxyglucose if infectious process, inflammatory process, or tumor suspected; PET scans have a high negative predictive value (3)[B]

- Ultrasound of abdomen and pelvis (plus directed biopsy, if indicated) if mass lesions, renal obstruction, or gallbladder/biliary tree pathology suspected
- ECG if cardiac valve lesions (endocarditis), atrial myxomas, or pericardial effusion suspected (transthoracic vs transesophageal)
- Leg Doppler if deep vein thrombosis/pulmonary embolism suspected
- CT scan of chest if pulmonary emboli suspected
- Indium-labeled leukocyte scanning if inflammatory process suspected
- Bone scan if osteomyelitis or metastatic disease suspected

›iagnostic Procedures/Surgery

- Liver biopsy if granulomatous disease suspected (2)[C]
- Temporal artery biopsy, particularly in the elderly (2)[B]
- Lymph node, muscle or skin biopsy if clinically indicated
- Bone marrow biopsy if clinically indicated
- Spinal tap if clinically indicated

’athological Findings

’epends on etiology

›IFFERENTIAL DIAGNOSIS

ee Etiology.

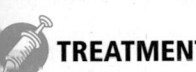

TREATMENT

⁄IEDICATION

‘irst Line

- 1st-line drugs are dependent on the diagnosis.
- Evidence does not support treatment of fever (4)[C].

’ediatric Considerations

Aspirin should be avoided in children because of the risk of Reye syndrome.

;econd Line

‘ the patient has symptoms with the fever or continues ɔ decline, a therapeutic trial may be indicated:

- Antibiotic trial based on patient's history
- Antituberculous therapy if there is a high risk for granulomatous disease pending culture results
- Steroid trial based on patient's history (once occult malignancy is ruled out)

ALERT

If a steroid trial is initiated, patient may have a relapse after treatment or if certain conditions (such as TB) have been undiagnosed.

‹DDITIONAL TREATMENT

;eneral Measures

- Attempt to determine the etiology before initiating the therapy.
- Avoid therapeutic trials unless as a last resort and only if therapy is reasonably specific.
- "Shotgun" approaches are condemned, as they obscure the clinical picture, have untoward effects, and do not solve the problem (2)[C].

Additional Therapies

With temperature elevations, patients will have increased caloric and fluid demands.

SURGERY/OTHER PROCEDURES

Need for exploratory laparotomy has been largely eliminated with the advent of more sophisticated tests and imaging modalities.

IN-PATIENT CONSIDERATIONS

Admission Criteria

- Reserved for the ill and debilitated
- Consider if factitious fever has been ruled out or an invasive procedure is indicated

ONGOING CARE

FOLLOW-UP RECOMMENDATIONS

Patient Monitoring

If the etiology of the fever remains unknown, repeat the history and physical exam along with screening lab studies.

DIET

With temperature elevations, patients will have increased caloric and fluid demands.

PATIENT EDUCATION

Maintain an open line of communication between physician and patient/family as the workup progresses:

- The extended time required in establishing a diagnosis can be frustrating.

PROGNOSIS

- Depends on etiology and age:
  - Patients with HIV have the highest mortality.
- 1-year survival rates reflecting deaths due to all causes

Age	Survival
<35	91%
35–64	82%
>64	67%

COMPLICATIONS

Dependent on etiology

Pregnancy Considerations

Fever is known to increase the risk of neural tube defects and trigger preterm labor.

REFERENCES

1. High KP, Bradley SF, Gravenstein S, et al. Clinical practice guideline for the evaluation of fever and infection in older adult residents of long-term care facilities: 2008 update by the Infectious Diseases Society of America. *J Am Geriatr Soc*. 2009;57: 375–94.
2. Mourad O, Palda V, Detsky AS. A comprehensive evidence-based approach to fever of unknown origin. *Arch Intern Med*. 2003;163:545–51.
3. Keidar Z, Gurman-Balbir A, Gaitini D, Israel O et al. Fever of unknown origin: the role of 18F-FDG PET/CT. *J Nucl Med*. 2008;49:1980–5.
4. Plaisance KI, Mackowiak PA. Antipyretic therapy: physiologic rationale, diagnostic implications, and clinical consequences. *Arch Intern Med*. 2000;160: 449–56.

ADDITIONAL READING

- Cunha BA. Fever of unknown origin: Clinical overview of classic and current concepts. *Infect Dis Clin N Am*. 2007;21:867–915.
- Cunha BA. Fever of unknown origin: Focused diagnostic approach based on clinical clues from the history, physical examination, and laboratory tests. *Infect Dis Clin N Am*. 2007;21:1137–87.
- Williams J, Bellamy R et al. Fever of unknown origin. *Clin Med*. 2008;8:526–30.

See Also (Topic, Algorithm, Electronic Media Element)

Arthritis, Juvenile Idiopathic; Colorectal Cancer; Cytomegalovirus Inclusion Disease; Endocarditis, Infective; Giant Cell Arteritis; Hepatoma; HIV Infection and AIDS; Leukemia; Osteomyelitis; Polyarteritis Nodosa; Polymyalgia Rheumatica; Pulmonary Embolism; Rheumatic Fever; Sinusitis; Stroke (Brain Attack); Lupus Erythematosus, Discoid;
Algorithms: Fever, Acute; Fever of Unknown Origin; Fever in the First 3 Months of Life

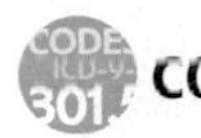

CODES

ICD9

780.60 Fever, unspecified

CLINICAL PEARLS

- The history, exam, and test should focus on the relevant causes of FUO:
  - A sequential approach leads to a rational sequentially diagnosis or rules out causes of FUO.
- A "shotgun" approach to treatment should be avoided; empiric therapy should be used only in carefully defined circumstances.
- FUO cases that defy precise diagnosis after intensive investigation and prolonged observation generally carry a favorable prognosis.
- In many cases, FUO in older persons may represent atypical, nonclassic presentations of common infectious and noninfectious diseases.

F

FIBROCYSTIC CHANGES OF THE BREAST

Katherine M. Callaghan, MD
Dawn S. Tasillo, MD

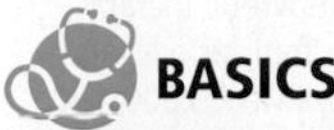

BASICS

DESCRIPTION

- Fibrocystic changes of the breast (FCC) is a generalized term for a heterogeneous group of changes affecting the stromal and glandular tissues of the breast.
- The most common of all benign breast conditions
- Commonly presents as mastalgia, engorgement, increased breast nodularity, and/or cysts:
  - Mastalgia (breast pain) is usually in upper outer quadrants of breast, bilateral, and may radiate to shoulders or upper arms.
  - Localized pain may occur with a rapidly enlarging cyst.
  - Nodules are usually small (2–10 mm), diffuse, and bilateral, with a rubbery consistency.
  - Cysts are more common in women in their 40s.
  - Larger cysts may have consistency of a water-filled balloon.
- Symptoms are most prominent in premenstrual (luteal) phase.
- System(s) affected: Endocrine/Metabolic; Reproductive
- Synonym(s): Fibrocystic breast disease; Mammary dysplasia; Chronic cystic mastitis

EPIDEMIOLOGY

Most common in women of reproductive years; occasionally seen after menopause with hormone replacement

Incidence

Unknown but very frequent

Prevalence

Present in up to 90% of women during their lifetime

RISK FACTORS

- The effect of consumption of methylxanthine-containing substances (e.g., coffee, tea, cola, and chocolate) has not been found to be a contributing factor (1)[A].
- Diet high in fruits and vegetables and high parity independently decrease risk of FCC (2)
- Diet high in saturated fats may increase risk of FCC

PATHOPHYSIOLOGY

May be the result of an exaggerated response of breast tissue to cycling hormones or a subtle imbalance in the ratio of estrogen to progesterone

ETIOLOGY

Estrogen likely a causative factor for many (3)[B]

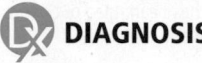

DIAGNOSIS

HISTORY

- May present in 3 overlapping, indistinct stages:
  - Mastoplagia and mastalgia, which may subside after menses; common in women in their 20s
  - Adenosis: Appearance of multiple small breast nodules; common in women in their 30s
  - Cystic phase: Tender cysts, usually small but up to 5 cm in diameter; common in women in their 40s
- Family history of breast disease (benign or malignant)

PHYSICAL EXAM

- With patient in supine position and rotated on contralateral hip, evaluate all breast tissue from sternum to midaxillary line, from clavicle to mammary ridge.
- Using fingertip, proceed in a linear fashion from top of sternum past breast tissue using 3 different depths of pressure at each palpation. Continue superiorly again to clavicle in a "lawnmower" fashion.
- Quantitate size, consistency, mobility, location, and skin changes.
- Findings in FCC may include:
  - Smooth, tense, or fluctuant masses
  - Bilateral masses
  - Breast thickening
  - Nipple discharge
- Palpate for axillary lymph nodes.

DIAGNOSTIC TESTS & INTERPRETATION

Evaluation should focus on excluding breast cancer. Testing may be conducted based on level of clinical suspicion.

Imaging

Initial approach

- Ultrasound (US): Signs of malignancy include irregular mass, clustered masses, calcifications, architectural distortion, dilated duct; US is useful fo[r] differentiating cystic from solid lesions.
- Mammography may reveal mass or dense tissue ± calcifications.

Follow-Up & Special Considerations

- Mammogram may be normal in presence of malignancy and difficult to interpret in women <35 years of age due to dense breast tissue; US may be helpful.
- Magnetic resonance imaging is indicated in patient[s] with *BRCA1* or *BRCA2* mutation or in any woman with 25% or greater lifetime risk for breast cancer (4).

Diagnostic Procedures/Surgery

- Fine-needle aspiration (FNA) and biopsy:
  - Allows differentiation of cystic and solid lesions
  - Aspirate may be straw-colored, dark brown, or green.
  - Cells sent for cytology can reveal cancer with hig[h] accuracy.
  - Low morbidity
- If mass disappears, no further evaluation is necessar[y] (including cytologic evaluation of aspirated fluid).

Pathological Findings

- Atypia: Relative risk of 4.24 for eventual breast cancer
- Proliferative changes without atypia: Relative risk o[f] 1.88 for eventual breast cancer
- Nonproliferative changes: Relative risk of 1.27 for eventual breast cancer (5)

DIFFERENTIAL DIAGNOSIS

Pain: Mastitis, costochondritis, pectoralis muscle strain, neuralgia, breast cancer, angina pectoris, gastroesophageal reflux, superficial phlebitis of the thoracoepigastric vein (Mondor disease)

Masses: Breast cancer, sebaceous cyst, fibroadenoma, lipoma, fat necrosis

Skin changes: Breast cancer (peau d'orange: Thickened skin similar to peel of an orange), eczema

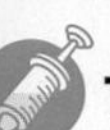

TREATMENT

After ruling out malignancy by means of imaging and diagnostic procedures, FCC may not require treatment and often resolves with time.

Cool compresses and a well-fitting, supportive bra (worn day and night) may be useful for symptom relief.

MEDICATION

First Line

For cyclic pain and swelling: Nonsteroidal anti-inflammatory drugs:

Ibuprofen 400 mg q.i.d./p.r.n.

Naproxen 500 mg b.i.d./p.r.n.

Second Line

Oral contraceptives may be useful in modulating symptoms or in preventing the development of new changes.

For severe pain, consider (6):

- Danazol (Danocrine) 100–400 mg/d divided in 2 doses × 4–6 months
- Bromocriptine 2.5 mg b.i.d. × 3 months
- Tamoxifen 10 mg/d × 3–6 months

ADDITIONAL TREATMENT

Issues for Referral

- If discrete lesion in a woman ≤35 years, US then refer to a surgeon
- If discrete lesion in a woman >35 years, diagnostic mammography ± US then refer to surgeon

COMPLEMENTARY AND ALTERNATIVE MEDICINE

Evidence supporting evening primrose oil, vitamin E, or pyridoxine as treatment for the discomforts of FCC is insufficient to draw conclusions about effectiveness (1).

SURGERY/OTHER PROCEDURES

Breast cyst aspiration can be both diagnostic and therapeutic.

ONGOING CARE

FOLLOW-UP RECOMMENDATIONS

Condition is benign, chronic, and recurrent.

Patient Monitoring

- Patient needs to be assessed with clinical examination, radiologic studies, and sometimes biopsy to be certain a lump is not malignant.
- Follow-up times are variable depending on the clinical situation.
- US is useful to differentiate cysts from solid lesions and in evaluating women <35 years of age for FCC but is not useful for screening.
- Screening mammograms should be obtained yearly after age 40.
- Aspiration cytology is useful for diagnosis of cysts and solid lesions. The false-positive rate ranges from 0–5.8%. The false-negative rate ranges from 1.7–22%.
- When physical examination, mammography, and FNA are used in combination, detection rates for breast cancer range from 93–100%.

PATIENT EDUCATION

- Patient info on fibrocystic breasts from the Mayo Foundation for Medical Education and Research: http://www.mayoclinic.com/health/fibrocystic-breasts/DS01070
- Info on breast cancer prevention from the National Cancer Institute: http://www.cancer.gov or 1-800-4-CANCER

REFERENCES

1. Horner NK, Lampe JW. Potential mechanisms of diet therapy for fibrocystic breast conditions show inadequate evidence of effectiveness. *J Am Diet Assoc*. 2000;100:1368–80.
2. Wu C, Ray RM, Lin MG, et al. A case-control study of risk factors for fibrocystic breast conditions: Shanghai Nutrition and Breast Disease Study, China, 1995-2000. *Am J Epidemiol*. 2004;160: 945–60.
3. Meisner AL, Fekrazad MH, Royce ME. Breast disease: benign and malignant. *Med Clin North Am*. 2008;92:1115–41, x.
4. Morris E. Diagnostic breast MR imaging: Current status and future directions. *Radio Clin N Am*. 2007;45(5).
5. Hartmann LC, Sellers TA, Frost MH, et al. Benign breast disease and the risk of breast cancer. *N Engl J Med*. 2005;353:229–37.
6. Srivastava A, Mansel RE, Arvind N, Prasad K, Dhar A, Chabra A et al. Evidence-based management of Mastalgia: a meta-analysis of randomised trials. *Breast*. 2007;16:503–12.

ADDITIONAL READING

- Kutson D, et al. Screening for breast cancer: current recommendations and future directions. *Am Fam Phys*. 2007;7(11):1660–6.
- Santen RJ, Mansel R. Benign breast disorders. *N Engl J Med*. 2005;353:275–85.
- Saslow D, et al. American Cancer Society guidelines for breast screening with MRI as an adjunct to mammography. *CA J Clin*. 2007;57(2):75–89.

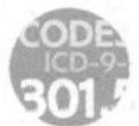

CODES

ICD9

- 610.0 Solitary cyst of breast
- 610.1 Diffuse cystic mastopathy
- 610.2 Fibroadenosis of breast

CLINICAL PEARLS

- Immediate office aspiration of breast cysts is a relatively easy procedure and often provides pain relief.
- If a mass is still present after cyst aspiration, patient may need surgery.

F

FIBROMYALGIA

Jhilam Biswas, MD
Robert E. Berry, Jr., MD

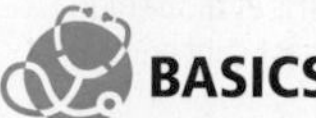

BASICS

DESCRIPTION

- Noninflammatory soft tissue pain disorder diagnosed by:
  - ≥3 months' duration
  - Widespread musculoskeletal pain
  - Excess tenderness in at least 11 of 18 defined anatomic sites
- Synonym(s): Fibrositis

EPIDEMIOLOGY

Incidence

- Predominant sex: Female > Male (6× more common in females)
- Predominant age: 30–60 years

Prevalence

- 2% of adult U.S. population
- Uncommon juvenile form with 1% prevalence
- Up to 8% of population >70 years of age may meet diagnostic criteria

RISK FACTORS

- Female gender
- Lower socioeconomic status
- Poor functional status
- Negative/stressful life events

Genetics

- Odds ratio may be as high as 8.5 for 1st-degree relatives, but shared environmental factors may play a role.
- Co-aggregates with mood disorders in families

GENERAL PREVENTION

No specific prevention known

ETIOLOGY

- Combination of:
  - Abnormal responsiveness or dysfunction of nervous system
  - Genetic/familial/environmental factors
  - Mood or anxiety disorder
- In 50% of patients, starts after a negative event or flulike illness

COMMONLY ASSOCIATED CONDITIONS

- Chronic fatigue syndrome
- Irritable bowel syndrome
- Headaches
- Mood disorders
- Anxiety disorders
- Unexplained pelvic pain
- Bladder dysfunction syndromes
- Multiple chemical sensitivities
- Temporomandibular joint (TMJ) syndrome

DIAGNOSIS

- Signs and symptoms are chronic in nature.
- Nonrestorative sleep with early morning awakening in an unrefreshed state
- Pain is increased with anxiety and/or stress.
- Pain improved by mild physical activity or vacations (stress-relieving situations)
- Generalized fatigue or tiredness
- Anxiety
- Chronic headache
- Alternating diarrhea, constipation, and tenesmus
- Subjective complaints of swelling or numbness
- Dizziness
- Depression
- Reduced physical endurance
- Decreased social interaction

HISTORY

- >3 months of symptoms of widespread musculoskeletal pain unexplained by other diagnoses (diagnosis of exclusion)
- Fatigue
- Sleep disturbances
- Female usually of age 20–65 years
- Impaired social/occupational functioning
- Depressed/anxiety symptoms
- Absence of identifiable contributing disease
- Adverse effect of medication excluded (eg, statins)

PHYSICAL EXAM

- Multiple painful sites may be present; patient may have general hyperalgesia. There will be an absence of features in the joints or skin of any inflammatory musculoskeletal disease.
- Neurological exam may show some abnormalities in hoarseness and gait.
  - 4 kg of pressure (whitens examiner's nail bed) manually applied to specific sites, referred to as *trigger points*, causes significant pain.
    - Insertion of suboccipital muscle
    - Middle upper trapezius muscle
    - Under the lower sternocleidomastoid muscle
    - Near the 2nd costochondral junction
    - Origin of the supraspinatus muscle
    - 2 cm distal to lateral epicondyle
    - Upper outer quadrant of the buttocks
    - At the prominence of the greater trochanter
    - At the medial fat pad of the knee

DIAGNOSTIC TESTS & INTERPRETATION

Lab

Initial lab tests

Testing done to exclude other diseases:

- Normal Westergren erythrocyte sedimentation rate and/or C-reactive protein
- Normal muscle enzymes (creatine kinase and aldolase)
- Normal thyroid-stimulating hormone
- Normal complete blood count with differential
- Normal renal and liver function
- 25 OH vitamin D
- Antinuclear antibodies not helpful if preceding tests are normal

Imaging

Not indicated except to exclude other diagnoses

Diagnostic Procedures/Surgery

- Sleep studies if indicated to rule out obstructive sleep apnea or narcolepsy as cause of fatigue
- Neuropsychiatric testing for vegetative symptoms (SIGECAPS, HAM-D)
  - Depression
  - Anxiety
  - Cognitive disturbance
  - Memory

DIFFERENTIAL DIAGNOSIS

- Overlap syndromes:
  - Chronic fatigue syndrome
  - Myofascial pain (more localized than fibromyalgia)
- Common coexisting disorders:
  - Connective tissue diseases
  - Psychiatric illness
  - Sleep disorders
  - TMJ syndrome

TREATMENT

- Multicomponent nonpharmacologic treatment along with medication shown to be effective in the short term in reducing key symptoms
- Essential nonpharmacologic elements include engaging in exercise, education on condition, and psychotherapy. Some weak data exists that short-term benefit may result from hydrotherapy (1,2)[A].
- Mainstay of therapy includes tricyclic antidepressants or cyclobenzaprine, daily aerobic exercise, sleep hygiene, and careful attention to mental status plus psychotherapy (cognitive behavioral therapy, etc.)
- Medications have shown to decrease pain, fatigue, depressed mood, sleep disturbance, and health-related quality of life.

MEDICATION

Nonsteroidal anti-inflammatory drugs are less likely to help because there is no identified inflammation, except as an additional pain measure.

ALERT

Avoid narcotics.

First Line

- Amitriptyline 25–50 mg p.o. at bedtime (1,2,3)[A]: Alternative: Desipramine (less sedating)
- Cyclobenzaprine 10–30 mg p.o. at bedtime (3)[A]
- Acetaminophen 325–1000 mg p.o. q.i.d. p.r.n.
- Tramadol 200–300 mg/d p.o. divided doses (3)[A]
- Combinations of acetaminophen and tramadol effective for pain control
- Gabapentin 1200–2400 mg/d p.o. b.i.d.–t.i.d.; start with lower doses (3)[A]. May be considered 1st line if exercise and TCAs are not sufficient at controlling pain scores.

Second Line
- Pregabalin 300–600 mg/day p.o. b.i.d.–t.i.d.; start with 150 mg/day and then advance as needed. Most improvement shown at 450 mg/day p.o. (4).
- Duloxetine 60 mg p.o. b.i.d.
- Milnacipran 100 mg/day or 200 mg/day p.o. (became available in 2009)
- Fluoxetine 20–80 mg/d p.o. (higher doses may be needed) (3)[A]
- Clonazepam 0.5 mg p.o. at bedtime may help sleep.
- Combinations of medicines such as amitriptyline and fluoxetine may be tried.

ADDITIONAL TREATMENT

General Measures
- Patient understanding of the illness and goals of therapy are key.
- Low-impact cardiovascular exercise is useful as long as the exercise program continues. Strength training has also shown improvement (4)[A].
- Cognitive behavioral therapy (3)[A]
- Stress management
- Patient education; consider group format (3)[A]
- Sleep hygiene
- Psychosocial support
- Consider job/workplace modifications.

Issues for Referral
Referrals for nonresponders may go to rheumatology, psychiatry, and pain management centers.

COMPLEMENTARY AND ALTERNATIVE MEDICINE
- Physical therapy may be helpful as part of conditioning program/fitness.
- Moderate efficacy shown in some studies for:
  - Hydrotherapy (5)[A]
  - Hypnotherapy
  - Biofeedback
- Weak evidence for efficacy:
  - Chiropractic
  - Acupuncture
  - Massage therapy
  - Electrotherapy
  - Ultrasonography

Pregnancy Considerations
May require therapy modification

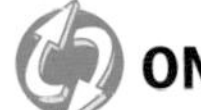

ONGOING CARE

FOLLOW-UP RECOMMENDATIONS
Encourage full activity as able, especially with fitness exercises.

Patient Monitoring
- For efficacy of therapy at 2–4 weeks
- For medication side effects every 3–6 months

DIET
No restrictions; no proven efficacy of any specific diet

PATIENT EDUCATION
It is very important that the patient understand the diagnosis and participate in developing and continuing a treatment program.

PROGNOSIS
- 50% with partial remission after 2–3 years of therapy
- Typically has fluctuating, chronic course
- Poorer outcome with:
  - Longer illness duration
  - More severe symptoms
  - Depression
  - Advanced age
  - Lack of social support

COMPLICATIONS
Chronic pain, chronic loss of work

REFERENCES

1. Hauser W, Bernhard M, Schiltenwolf M. Efficacy of multicomponent treatment in fibromyalgia syndrome: A meta-analysis of randomized controlled clinical trials. *Arth and Rheum.* 2009; 61(2):216–224.
2. Hauser W, Bernandy K, Uceyler N, Sommer C. Treatment of fibromyalgia syndrome with antidepressants: A meta-analysis. *JAMA.* 2009;301(2):198–209.
3. Goldenberg DL, Burckhardt C, Crofford L. Management of fibromyalgia syndrome. *JAMA.* 2004;292:2388–95.
4. Busch AJ, et al. Exercise for treating fibromyalgia. *Cochrane Database Syst Rev.* 2007:4CD003786.
5. McVeigh JG, McGaughey H, Hall M, Kane P. The effectiveness of hydrotherapy in the management of fibromyalgia syndrome: a systematic review. *Rheumatology International.* 2008;29(2):119–30.

ADDITIONAL READING

- Aaron LA, Burke MM, Buchwald D. Overlapping conditions among patients with chronic fatigue syndrome, fibromyalgia, and temporomandibular disorder. *Arch Intern Med.* 2000;160:221–7.
- Abeles AM, Pillinger MH, Solitar BM, et al. Narrative review: the pathophysiology of fibromyalgia. *Ann Intern Med.* 2007;146:726–34.
- American College of Rheumatology. Practice guidelines, patient education. At http://www.rheumatology.org.
- Arnold LM. Biology and therapy of fibromyalgia. New therapies in fibromyalgia. *Arthritis Res Ther.* 2006;8:212.
- Carville SF, Arendt-Nielsen S, Bliddal H, et al. EULAR evidence-based recommendations for the management of fibromyalgia syndrome. *Ann Rheum Dis.* 2008;67:536–41.
- National Fibromyalgia Association. At http://www.fmaware.org.
- Moore RA, Straube S, Wiffen PJ, Derry S, McQuay H. Pregabalin for acute and chronic pain in adults. *Chchrane Database of Syst Rev.* 2009;(3): CD007076.

See Also (Topic, Algorithm, Electronic Media Element)
Algorithm: Fatigue

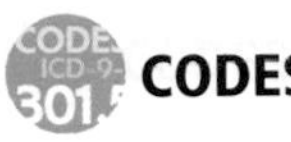

CODES

ICD9
729.1 Myalgia and myositis, unspecified

CLINICAL PEARLS
- Coexisting severe complaints of chronic pain, fatigue, multiple symptoms in the *absence* of laboratory or physical exam findings
- Biologic basis is still unclear, but the disease is considered a disorder of pain regulation termed *central sensitization*.
- Overlap with stress, depression, and anxiety must be recognized in treatment plan.
- Best outcomes occur in patients who understand their illness and are willing to engage in multimodal treatment, including medications, exercise, psychotherapy, and changing lifestyle habits.

FOOD ALLERGY

Stanley Fineman, MD

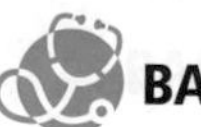

BASICS

DESCRIPTION

- Hypersensitivity reaction caused by certain foods
- System(s) affected: GI; Hemic/Lymphatic/Immunologic; Pulmonary; Skin/Exocrine
- Synonym(s): Allergic bowel disease; dietary protein-sensitivity syndrome

EPIDEMIOLOGY

- Predominant age: All ages, but more common in infants and children
- Predominant sex: Male > female (2:1)

Incidence

Prospective studies indicate that ~2.5% of infants experience hypersensitivity reactions to cow's milk in their 1st year of life (1)[B].

Prevalence

- The prevalence of IgE-mediated food allergy is likely between 1–2% in the US. (2,3)[A]
- In young children, the most common food allergies are cow's milk (2.5%), egg (1/3%), peanut (0.8%), and wheat (0.4%).
- Adults tend to have allergies to shellfish (2%), peanut (0.6%), tree nuts (0.5%), and fish (0.4%). (3)[B]
- In general, only 3–4% of children >4 years have persisting food allergy; therefore, it is frequently a transient phenomenon.
- 20% of children with peanut protein allergy outgrow their sensitivity by school age (4,3)[B].

RISK FACTORS

- Persons with allergic or atopic predisposition have increased risk of hypersensitivity reaction to food.
- Family history of food hypersensitivity

Genetics

In family members with a history of food hypersensitivity, the probability of food allergy in subsequent siblings may be as high as 50%.

GENERAL PREVENTION

Avoidance of offending food

PATHOPHYSIOLOGY

Allergic response owing to immunologic mechanisms, such as the classic IgE allergic response or nonimmunologic-mediated mechanisms

ETIOLOGY

- Any food or ingested substance can cause allergic reactions:
  - Most commonly implicated foods include cow's milk, egg whites, wheat, soy, peanuts, fish, tree nuts (walnut and pecan), shellfish, melons, sesame seeds, and sunflower seeds.
- Several food dyes and additives can elicit allergic-like reactions.

DIAGNOSIS

PHYSICAL EXAM

- GI (system usually affected):
  - More common: Nausea, vomiting, diarrhea, abdominal pain, occult bleeding, flatulence, and bloating
  - Less common: Malabsorption, protein-losing enteropathy, eosinophilic-enteritis, colitis
- Dermatologic:
  - More common: Urticaria/angioedema, atopic dermatitis, pallor, or flushing
  - Less common: Contact rashes
- Respiratory:
  - More common: Allergic rhinitis, asthma and bronchospasm, cough, serous otitis media
  - Less common: Pulmonary infiltrates (Heiner syndrome), pulmonary hemosiderosis
- Neurologic:
  - Less common: Migraine headaches
- Other symptoms:
  - Systemic anaphylaxis, vasculitis

DIAGNOSTIC TESTS & INTERPRETATION

Lab

- Eosinophilia in blood or tissue suggests atopy
- Epicutaneous (prick or puncture) allergy skin tests are used for documenting IgE-mediated immunologic hypersensitivity.
- Skin testing using the suspect food may be helpful. When fresh food skin testing is negative, an oral challenge may be completed to accurately determine the clinical hypersensitivity. The overall agreement between allergy skin testing and oral food challenge is 60% (i.e., a positive skin test showing a positive challenge reaction to a particular food) (5)[A].
- Food-specific IgE assays can also detect specific IgE antibodies to offending foods:
  - In certain laboratories, the ImmunoCap food-specific IgE was almost as accurate as a skin test in predicting positive oral challenges (6)[B].
- Periodic monitoring of the peanut-specific IgE levels every 2 years may be helpful. If the level of peanut-specific IgE falls below 0.5 kU/L, then a cautious oral challenge under the supervision of an allergist may be considered. A fresh food skin test with peanut protein should be considered prior to the oral challenge.
- Patch tests for foods are reported to be useful for determining delayed-sensitivity immunologic reactions, which are reported in patients with eosinophilic esophagitis and atopic dermatitis, although the addition of these is considered of marginal benefit (7)[B].
- Leukocyte histamine release and assays for circulating immune complexes are predominantly research procedures and are of limited use in clinica practices:
  - Assays for IgG and IgG 4 subclass antibodies are commercially available.
  - No convincing data suggest that these tests are reliable for the diagnosis of food allergy.
- The provocative injection and sublingual provocative tests are both highly controversial and have been proven to be useless for the diagnosis of food allergy.
- The leukocytotoxic assay is an unproven diagnostic procedure and is not useful for the diagnosis of allergy (8)[A]

Diagnostic Procedures/Surgery

Elimination and challenge test is the best procedure for confirming food allergy:

- The suspected food is eliminated from the diet for 1–2 weeks.
- The patient's symptoms are monitored. If the patient's symptoms disappear or substantially improve, an oral challenge with the suspected food should be performed under medical supervision.
- Optimally, this challenge should be performed in a double-blind, placebo-controlled manner.
- Patients with a history of anaphylaxis should not have an oral challenge unless lack of significant IgE sensitivity can be documented.
- Most allergic reactions will occur within 30 minutes–2 hours after the challenge, although late reactions have also been described, which may occur from 12–24 hours.

Pathological Findings

Pathologic findings are not common in food allergies; however, inflammatory changes can sometimes be seen in the GI tract.

DIFFERENTIAL DIAGNOSIS

- A careful history is necessary to document a temporal relationship with the manifestations of suspected food hypersensitivity.
- The GI, dermatologic, respiratory, neurologic, or other systemic manifestations may mimic a variety of clinical entities.

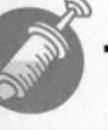

TREATMENT

MEDICATION

- Patients with significant type 1, IgE-mediated hypersensitivity should have epinephrine for auto-injection available in case of accidental ingestion and resulting severe anaphylactic reaction.
- Symptomatic treatment for milder reactions (e.g., antihistamine)
- The use of cromolyn has been suggested but is not practical for use in most patients with food allergy.

ADDITIONAL TREATMENT

General Measures

- Avoidance of the offending food is the most effective mode of treatment for patients with food allergies.
- Those patients with exquisite and severe allergy hypersensitivity to a food should be more cautious in their avoidance of that food. They should carry epinephrine for self-administration in the event that the offending food is ingested unknowingly and a subsequent immediate reaction develops.
- Immunotherapy or hyposensitization with food extracts by various routes, including subcutaneous immunotherapy or sublingual neutralization, are not recommended. Research studies are in progress, but immunotherapy with foods is considered experimental at this time.

COMPLEMENTARY AND ALTERNATIVE MEDICINE

There are reports of benefit using various Chinese herbal medicines in laboratory animals with induced food allergy. Benefits have not been reported in humans at this time.

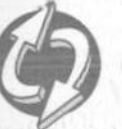

ONGOING CARE

FOLLOW-UP RECOMMENDATIONS

Patient Monitoring

As needed

DIET

- As determined by tests and clinical evaluation
- Strict avoidance of offending food

PATIENT EDUCATION

- Patients should be counseled by a dietitian to be sure that they maintain a nutritionally sound diet despite avoiding those foods to which the patient is sensitive.
- Patient support: Food Allergy and Anaphylaxis Network: 4744 Holly Ave., Fairfax, VA 22030-5647; 703-691-3179; Web site http://www.foodallergy.org
- Other information available at http://www.acaai.org and http://www.aaaai.org

PROGNOSIS

- Most infants will outgrow their food hypersensitivity by 2–4 years.
  - It may be possible to reintroduce the offending food cautiously into the diet (particularly helpful when the food is one that is difficult to avoid). It is critical that a specific IgE to the offending food is checked, optimally by fresh food allergy skin test, and is negative prior to an oral challenge.
  - 20% of young children with peanut allergy experience resolution by age of 5 years (4)[B].
- Adults with food hypersensitivity (particularly to milk, fish, shellfish, or nuts) tend to maintain their allergy for many years.

COMPLICATIONS

- Anaphylaxis
- Angioedema
- Bronchial asthma
- Enterocolitis
- Eosinophilic esophagitis
- Eczematoid lesions

REFERENCES

1. Høst A, Halken S. A prospective study of cow milk allergy in Danish infants during the first 3 years of life. Clinical course in relation to clinical and immunological type of hypersensitivity reaction. *Allergy*. 1990;45:587–96.
2. Chafen JJ, Newberry SJ, Riedl MA, Bravata DM, Maglione M, Suttorp MJ, Sundaram V, Paige NM, Towfigh A, Hulley BJ, Shekelle PG et al. Diagnosing and managing common food allergies: a systematic review. *JAMA*. 2010;303:1848–56.
3. Sicherer SH, Sampson HA et al. Food allergy. *J Allergy Clin Immunol*. 2010;125:S116–25.
4. Sicherer SH, Sampson HA et al. Peanut allergy: emerging concepts and approaches for an apparent epidemic. *J Allergy Clin. Immunol*. 2007;120.
5. Sampson HA. Utility of food-specific IgE concentrations in predicting symptomatic food allergy. *J Allergy Clin Immunol*. 2001;107:891–6.
6. Maloney JM, Rudengren M, Ahlstedt S, et al. The use of serum specific IgE measurements for the diagnosis of peanut, tree nut, and seed allergy. *J Allergy Clin Immunol*. 2008.
7. Spergel JM, Brown-Whitehorn T, Beausoleil JL, Shuker M, Liacouras CA et al. Predictive values for skin prick test and atopy patch test for eosinophilic esophagitis. *J Allergy Clin Immunol*. 2007;119:509–11.
8. Bernstein IL, Li JT, Bernstein DI, et al. Allergy diagnostic testing: an updated practice parameter. *Ann Allergy Asthma Immunol*. 2008;100:S1–148.
9. Chapman JA, Bernstein IL. Food Allergy: a practice parameter. *Ann Allergy Asthma Immunol*. 2006;96:S1–S68.
10. Greer FR, Sicherer SH, Burks AW, et al. Effects of early nutritional interventions on the development of atopic disease in infants and children: the role of maternal dietary restriction, breastfeeding, timing of introduction of complementary foods, and hydrolyzed formulas. *Pediatrics*. 2008;121:183–91.

See Also (Topic, Algorithm, Electronic Media Element)

Celiac Disease; Irritable Bowel Syndrome; Anaphylaxis

CODES

ICD9

- 708.0 Allergic urticaria
- 995.60 Anaphylactic shock due to unspecified food
- 995.7 Other adverse food reactions, not elsewhere classified

CLINICAL PEARLS

- Recent studies suggest that up to 20% of children with peanut allergy may outgrow their sensitivity.
  - Periodic monitoring of the peanut-specific IgE levels every 2 years may be helpful. If the level of peanut-specific IgE falls below 0.5 kU/L, then a cautious oral challenge under the supervision of an allergist may be considered. A fresh food skin test with peanut protein should be considered prior to the oral challenge.
- Oral itching following ingestion of fresh fruit may be a warning of risk for anaphylaxis, but may only represent oral allergy syndrome.
  - This syndrome is the result of cross-reacting proteins in pollens (example: Patients sensitive to birch tree pollen frequently have this cross-reactivity to fresh apples and pears. Cooked fruits are usually tolerated) (9)[B].
- Current evidence does not support a major role for maternal dietary restrictions during pregnancy or lactation in the prevention of atopic disease in infants. It is generally recommended to exclusively breast-feed for the first 6 months of life, particularly when there is a family history of atopy and food allergy. Although solid foods should not be introduced before 4–6 months of age, there is no convincing evidence that delaying their introduction beyond this period has a significant protective effect on the development of allergies (10)[B].

FOOD POISONING, BACTERIAL

Thomas J. Hansen, MD

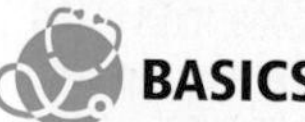

BASICS

DESCRIPTION

- Food poisoning, also called foodborne infection, is an illness resulting from the consumption of contaminated food.
- The illness may be produced by bacterial infection or by toxins produced by the bacteria.
- The most commonly recognized foodborne infections are those caused by the bacteria *Campylobacter*, *Salmonella*, and *E. coli* 0157:H7 (1).

EPIDEMIOLOGY

Incidence

In the US, it is estimated that there are more than 76 million cases of foodborne poisoning annually, resulting in 325,000 hospitalizations and 5,000 deaths (1).

RISK FACTORS

- Travel to developing countries
- Improper food storage or handling
- Cross-contamination during preparation of food
- Weakened immune system, pregnancy, very young age
- Underlying gastrointestinal disorders
- Patients taking antacids, H-2 blockers, and proton pump inhibitors (2)

GENERAL PREVENTION

- When preparing food at home (3):
  - Clean
    - Wash hands, cutting boards and surfaces before food preparation and after preparing each food item.
    - Wash fresh produce thoroughly before eating.
  - Separate
    - Keep raw meat, poultry, fish, and their juices away from other food.
  - Cook: Thoroughly cook meat to the following temperature:
    - Fresh beef, veal, and lamb: 145° F
    - Fresh pork: 160°F
    - Ground beef, pork, veal, lamb, egg dishes: 160°F
    - Poultry: 165° F. Cook chicken eggs thoroughly until the yolk is firm.
  - Chill
    - Refrigerate leftovers within 2 hours in clean, shallow, covered containers. If the temperature is above 90°F, refrigerate within 1 hour.
- When traveling to underdeveloped countries (4):
  - Eat only foods that are freshly prepared.
  - Avoid beverages diluted with nonpotable water, such as ice and milk.
  - Avoid food washed in nonpotable water, such as salads.
  - Other risky foods include raw or undercooked meat and seafood, unpeeled raw fruits and vegetables.
  - Bottled, carbonated, and boiled beverages are generally safe to drink.
- Bismuth subsalicylate (Pepto-Bismol), two 262-mg tablets four times daily has been shown to protect travelers to developing countries approximately 60% of the time. However, it is not recommended for persons taking anticoagulants or other salicylates (5).

ETIOLOGY

- Short incubation period (1–6 hours)
  - *Bacillus cereus* (preformed enterotoxin)
    - Food sources: Improperly cooked rice/fried rice and red meats.
    - Causes sudden onset of severe nausea and vomiting. Diarrhea may be present.
  - *Staphylococcus aureus*
    - Food sources: Unrefrigerated or improperly refrigerated meats, potato and egg salads.
    - Causes sudden onset of severe nausea and vomiting. Abdominal cramps and fever may be present.
- Medium incubation period (8–16 hours)
  - *Bacillus cereus* (toxin)
    - Food sources: Meat, stew gravy, vanilla sauce.
    - Causes watery diarrhea, abdominal cramps, nausea.
  - *Clostridium perfringens*
    - Food sources: Dry or precooked meats and poultry
    - Causes watery diarrhea, nausea, abdominal cramps.
- Long incubation period (>16 hours)
  - Toxin-producing organisms
    - *Clostridium botulinum*: Food source is home-canned or improperly canned commercial foods. Causes vomiting, diarrhea, blurred vision, diplopia, dysphagia, and descending muscle weakness.
    - *Enterohemorrhagic E. coli*: Food sources are undercooked beef, especially hamburger, unpasteurized milk, raw fruits and vegetables, and contaminated water. Causes severe diarrhea that is often bloody, abdominal pain, vomiting. More common in children <4 years of age.
    - *Enterotoxigenic E. coli*: Food sources are foods or water contaminated by human feces. Causes watery diarrhea, abdominal cramps, and vomiting.
    - *Vibrio cholerae*: Food sources are contaminated water, fish, and shellfish, especially food sold by street vendors. Causes profuse watery diarrhea and vomiting which can lead to severe dehydration and death within hours.
  - Invasive organisms
    - *Campylobacter jejuni*: Food sources are raw and undercooked poultry, unpasteurized milk, contaminated meats. Causes diarrhea (may be bloody), cramps, vomiting, and fever.
    - *Salmonella*: Food sources are contaminated eggs, poultry, unpasteurized milk or juice, cheese, contaminated raw fruits and vegetables. Causes diarrhea, fever, abdominal cramps, vomiting.
    - *Shigella*: Food sources are food or water contaminated by human fecal material. Causes abdominal cramps, fever, diarrhea.
    - *Vibrio parahaemolyticus*: Food source is raw shellfish. Causes nausea vomiting, diarrhea, and abdominal pain.
    - *Vibrio vulnificus:* Food source is undercooked and raw seafood; wounds exposed to sea water. Causes vomiting, diarrhea, abdominal pain, bacteremia, wound infections. Can be fatal in patients with liver disease or who are immunocompromised.
    - *Y. pentoerocolitica* and *Y. pseudotuberculosis*: Food sources are undercooked pork, unpasteurized milk, tofu, contaminated water. Causes appendicitis-like symptoms: abdominal pain, fever, diarrhea, and vomiting; occurs primarily in older children and younger adults (6).

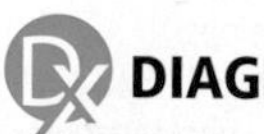

DIAGNOSIS

HISTORY

- Food poisoning most often presents as gastroenteritis (5).
- Most cases of gastroenteritis have a viral etiology. Suspect bacterial food poisoning when multiple persons become ill after eating the same meal, possibly with high fever and blood or mucus in stool.
- Suspect bacterial gastroenteritis if traveling in or recent travel to an underdeveloped country (5,7).
- Timing and presentation can aid in establishing an etiology (6).

PHYSICAL EXAM

- The physical exam should focus on signs of dehydration, including evaluating skin turgor and mucous membranes, and observing for hypotension or orthostatic changes.
- The abdominal exam should focus on abdominal distension with tenderness, suggestive of bowel obstruction. Auscultation may demonstrate increased bowel sound in obstruction or decreased bowel sounds with an ileus (7).

DIAGNOSTIC TESTS & INTERPRETATION

Lab

Initial lab tests

- Culture of stool and sensitivity, fecal leukocytes, and Hemoccult testing; consider ova and parasites if history of foreign travel or symptoms lasting longer than 2 weeks.
- BMP and white blood cell count if diarrhea is severe, temperature >101.5°F (38.5°C), persistently bloody stools, severe abdominal pain, or if patient is immunocompromised, elderly, or very young

Follow-Up & Special Considerations
Epidemiologic investigation may be warranted.

DIFFERENTIAL DIAGNOSIS

- Infectious gastroenteritis of any kind
- *C. difficile* colitis
- Inflammatory bowel disease
- Appendicitis and other acute abdominal surgical processes

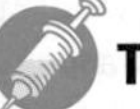

TREATMENT

- Most cases of food poisoning are self-limiting and do not require medication.
- A health care provider should be consulted for food poisoning if the following are present: High fever (≥101.5° F); blood in the stools; prolonged vomiting; signs of dehydration (decrease in urination, a dry mouth and throat, and feeling dizzy when standing up); diarrheal illness that lasts more than 3 days (4)[C].

First Line

Children, the elderly and pregnant patients with sign of mild diarrhea should be started on oral rehydration solution to prevent dehydration (2)[B].

Second Line

- For severe cases of food poisoning, the following medications are recommended:
- *Bacillus cereus:*
  - Supportive care only.
- *Campylobacter jejuni*:
  - Supportive care only.
- *Clostridium botulinum*:
  - Supportive care. Antitoxin can be helpful if administered early in the course of the illness.
- *Clostridium perfringens:*
  - Supportive care only.
- *Enterohemorrhagic E. coli*:
  - Supportive care only. Closely monitor renal function, hemoglobin and platelets. Infection associated with hemolytic uremic syndrome (HUS).
- *Enterotoxigenic E. coli* (common cause of traveler's diarrhea):
  - Generally self-limited. Antibiotics shorten course of illness.
  - Children: Azithromycin 10 mg/kg/day for 3 days or Ceftriaxone 50 mg/kg/day for 3 days
  - Adults: Ciprofloxacin 500 mg once a day for 3 days or SMX/TMP one DS tab twice daily for 3 days.
- *Salmonella*:
  - Children: Ceftriaxone: 100 mg/kg/day divided into two doses for 7–10 days or Azithromycin 20 mg/kg/day for 7 days.
  - Adults: Levofloxacin 500 mg a day for 7–10 days or azithromycin 500 mg daily for 7 days. Either can be given for 14 days for immunosuppressed patients.
- *Shigella*:
  - Children: Azithromycin 10 mg/kg/day for 3 days or Ceftriaxone 50 mg/kg/day for 3 days.
  - Adults: Metronidazole 500 mg three times a day for 10–14 days or Vancomycin 125 mg four times a day for 10–14 days or Rifaximin 400 mg four times a day for 10–14 days.
- *Staph. aureus*:
  - Supportive care only.
- *Vibrio cholerae*:
  - Children: Erythromycin 30 mg/kg/day given three times a day for 3 days or Azithromycin 10 mg/kg/day for three days.
  - Adults: Doxycycline 300 mg one time dose or Tetracycline 500 mg four times a day for 3 days or Erythromycin 250 mg three times a day for 3 days or Azithromycin 500 mg a day for three days.
- *Vibrio parahaemolyticus*:
  - Supportive care only.
- *Vibrio vulnificus:*
  - Adults: Minocycline or Doxycycline 100 mg twice daily plus either Cefotaxime 2 gm IV every eight hours or Ceftriaxone 1 g IV daily with doses appropriately adjusted for underlying renal or hepatic disease.
- *Yersinia*:
  - Supportive care only (6)[C]

ADDITIONAL TREATMENT

Loperamide 4 mg initially, then 2 mg after each loose stool to a maximum of 16 mg in a 24-hour period may be used unless high fever, bloody diarrhea, and/or severe abdominal pain are present (signs of enteroinvasion).

ONGOING CARE

DIET

- Avoid food while nausea is present but drink plenty of fluids.
- As the nausea subsides, drink adequate fluids, eat small, low-fat meals, and rest.
- Nursing infants should continue to be breastfed on demand, and infants and older children should be offered their usual food (5).

PROGNOSIS

Most infections are self-limited and will resolve over the course of 4–5 days.

COMPLICATIONS

- Dehydration
- Hemolytic uremic syndrome
- Guillain-Barré syndrome after Campylobacter enteritis
- Reiter syndrome
- *Clostridium difficile* colitis after antibiotic use
- Postinfectious irritable bowel (5)

REFERENCES

1. U.S. Food and Drug Administration, Foodborne Illness-Causing Organisms in the U.S.-What You Need to Know. October 2008, http://www.fda.gov/Food/ResourcesForYou/Consumers/ucm103263.htm
2. Ang JY, Mathur A. Traveler's Diarrhea: Updates for Pediatricians. *Pediatric Annals* 2008;37:814–820.
3. http://www.fsis.usda.gov/PDF/Kitchen_Companion.pdf
4. http://www.cdc.gov/ncidod/dbmd/diseaseinfo/foodborneinfections_g.htm#howtreated
5. Yates J. Traveler's diarrhea. *Am Fam Physician.* 2005;71:2095–100.
6. American Medical Association, Diagnosis and Management of Foodborne Illnesses: A Primer for Physicians and Other Health Care Professionals, February 2004, http://www.ama-assn.org/ama1/pub/upload/mm/36/2004_food_table_bact.pdf
7. Scorza K, Williams A, Phillips JD, Shaw J. Evaluation of Nausea and Vomiting. *Am Fam Physician.* 2007;76:76–84.

ADDITIONAL READING

- Diagnosis and management of foodborne illnesses: A primer for physicians. *MMWR Recomm Rep.* 2004;53(RR04):1–33.
- Reduced osmolarity oral rehydration solution. *Cochrane Database Syst Rev.* 2007, Issue 3.
- The Community Summary Report on Trends and Sources of Zoonoses and Zoonotic Agents in the European Union in 2007. *The European Food Safety Authority Journal.* 2009;223.

See Also (Topic, Algorithm, Electronic Media Element)

Appendicitis, Acute; Botulism; Brucellosis; Dehydration; Diarrhea, Acute; Guillain-Barré Syndrome; Hypokalemia; Intestinal Parasites; Salmonella Infection; Typhoid Fever

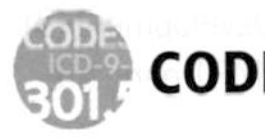

CODES

ICD9

- 003.9 Salmonella infection, unspecified
- 005.89 Other bacterial food poisoning
- 008.00 Intestinal infection due to e. coli, unspecified

CLINICAL PEARLS

- Consider bacterial food poisoning when multiple people present with symptoms after ingesting the same food and show fevers and blood or mucus in stool, or have recently returned from a developing nation.
- Consider antibiotics in a prolonged febrile state with blood/mucus in stool, septicemic states, and traveler's diarrhea.
- Reintroduce food as soon as tolerated; limit high-fat foods and foods high in simple sugars. Lactose limitation is controversial.

F

FROSTBITE

Alan M. Ehrlich, MD

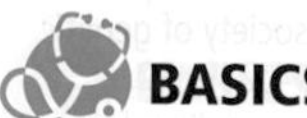

BASICS

DESCRIPTION

- A localized complication of exposure to cold, causing tissue to freeze, resulting in diminished blood flow to the affected part (especially hands, face, or feet)
- System(s) affected: Endocrine/Metabolic; Skin/Exocrine
- Synonym(s): Dermatitis congelationis; Frostnip; Environmental injuries

EPIDEMIOLOGY

- Predominant age: All ages
- Predominant sex: Male = Female

RISK FACTORS

- Previous cold-related injury
- Decreased caloric intake (<1,500 calories/day)
- Dehydration or hypovolemia
- Impaired cerebral function
- Under the effects of alcohol or drug abuse
- Underlying psychiatric disturbance
- Ambient temperature ≤−17.8°C (0°F)
- Smoker
- Elderly
- Lean body mass
- Low level of fitness
- Lack of proper clothing or shelter
- Raynaud phenomenon
- Constriction from excessively tight clothing (including too many layers of socks)
- Vehicular failure leading to prolonged cold exposure

GENERAL PREVENTION

- Dress in layers with appropriate cold-weather gear.
- Avoid clothing that is too constricting.
- Cover exposed areas and extremities appropriately.
- Prepare properly for trips to cold climates.
- Avoid alcohol.

PATHOPHYSIOLOGY

- Ice crystals form intracellularly.
- Dehydration, enzymatic destruction, and ultimately cell death occur.
- In severe cases, deep-tissue freezing may occur with damage to underlying blood vessels, muscles, and nerve tissue.

ETIOLOGY

- Prolonged exposure to cold
- Refreezing thawed extremities

COMMONLY ASSOCIATED CONDITIONS

Alcohol and/or drug abuse

DIAGNOSIS

HISTORY

- Throbbing pain
- Paresthesia
- Excessive sweating
- Joint pain

PHYSICAL EXAM

- Feet, hands, and face most commonly affected
- Injured area appears cold, hard, and white and is anesthetic to touch. It progresses to blotchy-red, swollen, and painful regions after rewarming.
- 1st degree: Redness and edema without blister formation
- 2nd degree: Redness, edema, and blister formation
- 3rd degree: Same as above with addition of hemorrhagic vesicles
- 4th degree: Necrosis and gangrene
- Pallor
- Loss of cutaneous sensation
- Numbness
- Limited movement of affected joints
- Subcutaneous edema
- Hyperemia
- Blistering
- Blue discoloration
- Skin necrosis
- Gangrene

DIAGNOSTIC TESTS & INTERPRETATION

ECG in hypothermia may show bradycardia, atrial fibrillation, atrial flutter, ventricular fibrillation, diffuse T-wave inversion, Osborn waves (upward-going "hump" following S wave in the RS–T segment)

Lab

- May show signs of hemoconcentration such as elevated hemoglobin or high BUN/creatinine ratio
- Liver function tests for decreased hepatic function

Imaging

- Triple-phase bone scan can identify tissue viability at early stage and facilitate early debridement.
- Other imaging techniques sometimes used include MRI/MRA, infrared thermography, angiography, digital plethysmography, and laser Doppler studies.

Pathological Findings

- Ice crystallization in the intravascular extracellular space
- Atrophy
- Fibroblastic proliferation
- Skin necrosis

DIFFERENTIAL DIAGNOSIS

- Frostnip, a superficial cold injury that does not cause permanent damage
- Chilblains (pernio), an inflammatory reaction to short-term cold, wet exposure without tissue freezing
- Immersion syndrome (trench foot), inflammatory reaction to prolonged cold, wet exposure, typically socks or footwear

TREATMENT

Geriatric Considerations

- Associated disease states increase mortality
- Periarticular osteoporosis complicates
- More prone to hypothermia

Pediatric Considerations

Loss of epithelial growth centers

ALERT

Acidosis

MEDICATION

First Line

- tPA administered within 24 hours of injury may prevent damage from thrombosis and may reduce amputation rate (1,2)[C].
- Tetanus toxoid
- Penicillin G 500,000 units every 6 hours for 48–72 hours prophylactically (3)[B]
- Ibuprofen 400 mg every 12 hours to inhibit prostaglandins (3)[C]
- NSAIDs for mild-moderate pain. For severe pain, narcotic analgesia.
- Precautions: tPA should not be used with history of recent bleeding, stroke, ulcer, etc.

Second Line

Vasodilators such as iloprost and pentoxifylline have been tried with some success (3)[C].

ADDITIONAL TREATMENT

General Measures

- If transport time will be short (1–2 hours at most), the risks posed by improper rewarming or refreezing outweigh the risks of delaying treatment for deep frostbite (4)[C].

If transport will be prolonged (more than 1–2 hours), frostbite will often thaw spontaneously. It is more important to prevent hypothermia than to rewarm frostbite rapidly in warm water. This does not mean that a frostbitten extremity should be kept in the cold to prevent spontaneous rewarming. Anticipate that frostbitten areas will rewarm as a consequence of keeping the patient warm and protect them from refreezing at all costs (4)[C].

Rapid rewarming (3)[B]:
- Immerse frozen body part in warm water (37–39°C [99–102°F]) for 15–30 minutes or until thawing is complete.
- Continue rewarming until a red/purple color appears and the affected part becomes pliable.
- It is critical not to allow refreezing after thawing has occurred.

After rewarming, injured parts should be covered with nonadhesive dressings, splinted, and elevated.
Remove jewelry and clothing, if present, from the affected area.
Application of aloe vera every 6 hours
Sterile cotton between fingers or toes, if applicable, to prevent maceration
- Keep the patient dry.
- If conscious, give the patient warm fluids with high sugar content.
- Prevent infection once treatment begins.
- Institute ongoing whirlpool therapy for cleansing and debridement.
- Prevent damage to other body parts.
- Prohibit use of nicotine-containing products (including cigarettes) or other vasoconstrictive agents.
- Maintenance: Gastric lavage, peritoneal dialysis, hemodialysis, and mediastinal lavage if needed (using warmed fluids)

Additional Therapies
- Heated oxygen
- Warm intravenous fluids via central venous pressure line

SURGERY/OTHER PROCEDURES
- Urgent surgery rarely needed except fasciotomy for compartment syndrome (suspect if tissue swollen and compartment pressures greater than 37–40 mm Hg)
- Surgical debridement as needed to remove necrotic tissue
- Amputation should not be considered until it is definite that tissues are dead: May take ~3 weeks to know whether the tissue is permanently injured

IN-PATIENT CONSIDERATIONS
Initial Stabilization
- Institute emergency measures for hypothermic patient without pulse or respiration. Such measures may include CPR and internal warming with warm intravenous fluids and warm oxygen (see topic Hypothermia).
- Prevent refreezing.
- It may be necessary to keep the frostbitten part frozen until the patient can be transported to a care facility. Prolonged freezing is preferable to warming and refreezing (5)[C].
- Remove nonadherent wet clothing.
- Treat for hypothermia.
- Treat for pain:
  - NSAIDs and/or narcotics if needed
- Do not rub areas to warm them; increased tissue damage may occur (1)[C].
- Do not allow patient with frostbitten feet to walk except when the life of the patient or rescuer is in danger (4)[C].

Admission Criteria
Hospitalization generally recommended (2)

ONGOING CARE

FOLLOW-UP RECOMMENDATIONS
Outpatient or inpatient, depending on severity:
- As tolerated; protect injured body parts
- Initiate physical therapy once healing progresses sufficiently.

Patient Monitoring
- Preferably electronic probe for temperature monitoring (rectal or vascular)
- Follow-up for physical therapy progress, infection, other complications

DIET
- As tolerated
- Warm oral fluids

PATIENT EDUCATION
- Refer to local library for information.
- Provide education on:
  - Exposure protection
  - Early signs and symptoms of frostbite

PROGNOSIS
- Anesthesia and bullae may occur.
- The affected areas will heal or mummify without surgery; the process may take 6–12 months for healing.
- Patient may be sensitive to cold and experience burning and tingling.
- Cyanotic nonblanching skin and blisters with dark fluid suggest worse prognosis (5)[C].

COMPLICATIONS
- Hyperglycemia
- Acidosis
- Refractory arrhythmias
- Tissue loss: Distal parts of an extremity may undergo spontaneous amputation
- Gangrene
- Death

REFERENCES

1. Bruen KJ, Ballard JR, Morris SE, et al. Reduction of the incidence of amputation in frostbite injury with thrombolytic therapy. *Arch Surg*. 2007;142: 546–51; discussion 551–3.
2. Jurkovich GJ. Environmental cold-induced injury. *Surg Clin North Am*. 2007;87:247–67, viii.
3. Imray C, Grieve A, Dhillon S, Caudwell Xtreme Everest Research Group et al. Cold damage to the extremities: frostbite and non-freezing cold injuries. *Postgrad Med J*. 2009;85:481–8.
4. State of Alaska Cold Injury Guideline: Alaska Multi-level 2003 Version. http://www.chems.alaska.gov/EMS/documents/AKColdInj2005.pdf.
5. Biem J, Koehncke N, Classen D, et al. Out of the cold: management of hypothermia and frostbite. *CMAJ*. 2003;168:305–11.

ADDITIONAL READING

- Cappaert TA, Stone JA, Castellani JW, et al. National Athletic Trainers' Association position statement: environmental cold injuries. *J Athl Train*. 2008;43: 640–58.
- Murphy JV, Banwell PE, Roberts AH, et al. Frostbite: pathogenesis and treatment. *J Trauma*. 2000;48: 171–8.
- Reamy BV. Frostbite: review and current concepts. *J Am Board Fam Pract*. 1998;11:34–40.
- Twomey JA, Peltier GL, Zera RT. An open-label study to evaluate the safety and efficacy of tissue plasminogen activator in treatment of severe frostbite. *J Trauma*. 2005;59:1350–4; discussion 1354–5.

See Also (Topic, Algorithm, Electronic Media Element)
Hypothermia
Algorithm: Hypothermia

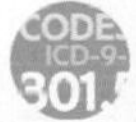

CODES

ICD9
- 991.0 Frostbite of face
- 991.1 Frostbite of hand
- 991.2 Frostbite of foot

CLINICAL PEARLS
- Frostbite is considered a tetanus-prone injury. Treat as any injury involving tissue destruction.
- Avoid rewarming en route to the hospital if there is a chance of refreezing. Avoid burns to affected areas, which may be numb and insensitive to heat.

FROZEN SHOULDER

J. Herbert Stevenson, MD
Jeffrey Manning, MD

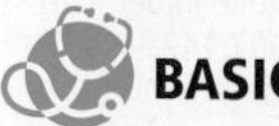

BASICS

DESCRIPTION

- Syndrome of painful restriction of active and passive range of motion (ROM) in 1 or both shoulders. Idiopathic adhesive capsulitis has 3 stages: Painful, adhesive, and recovery.
- System(s) affected: Musculoskeletal
- Synonym(s): Pericapsulitis; adherent bursitis; obliterative bursitis; adhesive capsulitis

EPIDEMIOLOGY

- Predominant age: 40–70 years
- Predominant sex: Female > Male

Geriatric Considerations

Common

Pediatric Considerations

Rare, but reported

Pregnancy Considerations

Primary (idiopathic): 2–3%

Prevalence

- General population is reported to be 2%.
- 11% in unselected individuals with diabetes

RISK FACTORS

- Systemic diseases (See Etiology. Diseases and conditions associated with secondary adhesive capsulitis) (1)[A]
- Prolonged immobilization
- Age (more common in elderly)
- Diabetes
- Thyroid disease

Genetics

Frequent trisomy 7 and trisomy 8 identified in fibroblasts

GENERAL PREVENTION

- Early ROM exercises after injury
- Stretching, frequent physical activity
- Avoid extended periods of immobilization.

PATHOPHYSIOLOGY

A chronic inflammatory response with fibroblastic proliferation, which may be immunomodulated (2)[B]

ETIOLOGY

Idiopathic (primary)

COMMONLY ASSOCIATED CONDITIONS

- Trauma
- Diabetes (most common)
- Postinflammatory
- After cerebrovascular accident or myocardial infarction (MI)
- After mastectomy (immobilization is the speculated cause)
- Hypothyroidism/hyperthyroidism
- Avascular necrosis
- Tuberculosis
- Scleroderma; rheumatoid arthritis
- Lung cancer or chronic lung disease

DIAGNOSIS

HISTORY

- Subacute onset of shoulder pain and decreased ROM without trauma
- Night pain often interrupting sleep
- Pain aggravated with movement and alleviated with rest
- Pain and tenderness to palpation:
  - May interrupt sleep
- Preceding injury, illness, or immobilization (secondary adhesive capsulitis)
- Loss of active and passive ROM in all planes
- Loss of natural arm swing with gait
- Because of compensatory scapular elevation (to lift the arm), muscles may be painful and spastic.
- Muscle atrophy and weakness with time
- Inability to reach into a back pocket or fasten the back of a garment
- Stages of adhesive capsulitis:
  - Painful stage (weeks to months):
    - Pain with movement
    - Generalized shoulder ache that is difficult to pinpoint
    - Muscle spasm
    - Increasing pain at night and at rest
  - Adhesive stage (up to 1 year):
    - Less pain
    - Increasing stiffness and restriction of movement
    - Decreasing pain at night and at rest
    - Discomfort felt at extreme ranges of movement
  - Recovery stage (weeks to months):
    - Decreased pain
    - Marked restriction with slow, gradual increase in range of motion
    - Recovery is spontaneous, frequently incomplete.

PHYSICAL EXAM

- Possible diffuse shoulder tenderness, but discrete point tenderness makes the diagnosis less likely.
- Marked limitation of passive and active shoulder abduction, flexion, internal and external rotation
- Normal 5/5 strength in all planes
- Hawkins, Neer, Yergason, and Speed testing can be positive.
- No neurovascular deficits

DIAGNOSTIC TESTS & INTERPRETATION

Lab

Initial lab tests

No lab is diagnostic for frozen shoulder, but may be required to rule out other disorders if suspected, such as systemic autoimmune disease.

Imaging

Initial approach

- Plain radiograph [anteroposterior (AP), axillary, supraspinatus outlet views] to rule out osteoarthritis, calcific tendinitis, avascular necrosis, osteomyelitis, fracture, dislocation, and tumor:
  - AP: Check osteopenia, fractures, dislocations, and superior migration of humeral head.
  - Axillary: Check subluxation or articular head damage (Bankart or Hills-Sachs lesions).
  - Supraspinatus outlet views: Check supraspinatus outlet narrowing to rule out acromial impingement.
- Arthrography:
  - Joint volume is reduced to 5–10 mL (normal, 20–30 mL).
  - Since this is invasive, arthrography is reserved for patients with uncertain diagnosis.
- Consider magnetic resonance imaging (MRI) to evaluate rotator cuff, evaluating for thickening of the shoulder capsule and to rule out other shoulder disorders.

Diagnostic Procedures/Surgery

- Joint aspiration if septic joint is suspected (rarely necessary)
- Arthroscopy to visualize fibrous bands in the joint space (rarely necessary)

Pathological Findings

- Active process of hyperplastic fibroplasia and excessive type III collagen secretion that lead to soft tissue contractures
- Fibrous bands traversing the glenohumeral joint space (occasional)
- Surgical findings of adherence of capsule to humeral head

DIFFERENTIAL DIAGNOSIS

- Rotator cuff strain/tear/impingement syndrome
- Bicipital/rotator/calcific tendinitis
- Septic arthritis
- Bursitis
- Polymyalgia rheumatica
- Glenohumeral or acromioclavicular joint osteoarthritis
- Cervical osteoarthritis/strain/disc disease
- Rheumatoid arthritis
- Bony neoplasm/metastases
- Dislocation
- Fracture (distal clavicle, proximal humerus)
- Avascular necrosis
- Fibromyalgia
- Myofascial pain syndrome
- Myelomeningocele
- Thoracic outlet syndrome
- Parkinson disease

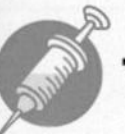

TREATMENT

Make patient aware of a 6–18-month recovery.

MEDICATION

First Line

- Nonsteroidal anti-inflammatory drugs (NSAIDs) during painful stage
- Acetaminophen if NSAIDs contraindicated
- Opioid analgesics (with physical therapy) if NSAIDs contraindicated and not responding
- Oral corticosteroids: 3–4-week taper (40 mg, 30 mg, 20 mg, 10 mg, then discontinue) (3)[A]
- Contraindications:
  - NSAIDs: Gastrointestinal (GI) ulcer disease/bleeding
  - Renal disease: See the manufacturer's literature.

Second Line

- Low-dose tricyclic antidepressants (e.g., amitriptyline) may help with pain and sleep.
- Subacromial bursa corticosteroid injection (4,5)[A]:
  - Increased ROM and decreased pain temporarily

ADDITIONAL TREATMENT

- Glenohumeral corticosteroid injection (e.g., triamcinolone, betamethasone) (4,5)[A]:
  - Does not shorten recovery, but may aid in decreasing discomfort with mobility exercises (controversial)
- Glenohumeral distention arthrography (controversial)
- Iontophoresis (electromotive drug administration) is generally not recommended in this condition.

General Measures

- Control of pain and preservation of mobility
- Avoid prolonged immobilization.
- Heat and/or ice
- Address underlying causes of secondary adhesive capsulitis (see Differential Diagnosis).
- Physical therapy

Issues for Referral

Not responding to conservative treatment within 3 months, but usually self-limiting

Additional Therapies

- Low-power laser therapy (6)[C]
- Physical therapy:
  - Avoid in the painful stage, as it will aggravate symptoms.
  - Focus on passive and active ROM exercises in the adhesive and recovery stages.

COMPLEMENTARY AND ALTERNATIVE MEDICINE

- Osteopathic manipulative technique may help decrease pain and increase shoulder ROM.
- Electroacupuncture or interferential electrotherapy may be of benefit (7)[C].

SURGERY/OTHER PROCEDURES

- Arthroscopic lysis of adhesions and manipulation under anesthesia are reserved for refractory cases.
- Arthroscopic capsular release with manipulation can offer good results to refractory cases (8,9,10)[A].

IN-PATIENT CONSIDERATIONS

Initial Stabilization

Outpatient care

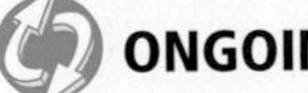

ONGOING CARE

FOLLOW-UP RECOMMENDATIONS

Monthly follow-up to determine ongoing treatment plan

Patient Monitoring

Close monitoring and frequent encouragement are usually needed for successful recovery.

DIET

No restrictions

PATIENT EDUCATION

- Long-term course of treatment until resolution of symptoms
- Stretching exercises daily or b.i.d. during and after improvement
- Codman exercises: Sit sideways in a straight chair; rest armpit on the back of the chair; swing the arm slowly in circles. Start with smaller circles and then bigger circles (clockwise and counterclockwise).
- Climbing the wall: Put the hand flat on a wall in front of you; use the fingers to "climb" the wall; pause 30 seconds every few inches.
- Reaching: Put everyday objects on a high shelf so that reaching is done more often.

PROGNOSIS

- Disorder is considered self-limiting (11)[A]
- Adhesive capsulitis may last from 6–9 months to as long as 1–3 years:
  - Painful stage: 2–6 months
  - Adhesive stage: 4–6 months
  - Recovery stage: 1–3 months

COMPLICATIONS

- Long-term loss of some mobility (7–30%) or function (rare)
- Residual pain and stiffness
- Long-term disability

REFERENCES

1. Milgrom C, Novack V, Weil Y, Jaber S, Radeva-Petrova DR, Finestone A. Risk factors for idiopathic frozenshoulder. *Israel Medical Association Journal: Imaj*. 2008;10(5):361–4.
2. Hand GC, Athanasou NA, Matthews T, Carr AJ. The pathology of frozenshoulder. *Journal of Bone & Joint Surgery - British Volume*. 2007;89(7): 928–32.
3. Buchbinder R, Green S, Youd JM, Johnston RV. Oral steroids for adhesive capsulitis. *Cochrane Database of Systematic Reviews*. 2006.
4. Arroll B, Goodyear-Smith F. Corticosteroid injections for painful shoulder: a meta-analysis. *Br J Gen Pract*. 2005;55(512):224–8. Review.
5. Arslon S, et al. Comparison of the efficacy of local corticosteroid injection and physical therapy for the treatment of adhesive capsulitis. *Rheumatol Int*. 2001;21:20–3.
6. Stergioulas A. Low-power laser treatment in patients with frozenshoulder: preliminary results. *Photomedicine and Laser Surgery*. 2008;26(2): 99–105.
7. Cheing GL, So EM, Chao CY. Effectiveness of electroacupuncture and interferential electrotherapy in the management of frozenshoulder. *Journal of Rehabilitation Medicine*. 2008;40(3):166–70.
8. Liem D, Meier F, Thorwesten L, Marquardt B, Steinbeck J, Poetzl W. The influence of arthroscopic subscapularis tendon and capsule release on internal rotation strength in treatment of frozenshoulder. *American Journal of Sports Medicine*. 2008;36(5):921–6.
9. Ozbaydar MU, Tonbul M, Altun M, et al. [Arthroscopic selective capsular release in the treatment of frozen shoulder] *Acta Orthop Traumatol Turc*. 2005;39:104–13.
10. Pearsall AW, Osbahr DC, Speer KP. An arthroscopic technique for treating patients with frozen shoulder. *Arthroscopy*. 1999;15:2–11.
11. Hand C, Clipsham K, Rees JL, Carr AJ. Long-term outcome of frozenshoulder. *Journal of Shoulder & Elbow Surgery*. 2008;17(2):231–6.

F

ADDITIONAL READING

- Daigneault J, et al. Shoulder pain in older people. *J Am Geriatr Soc*. 1998;46:1145–51.
- Siegel LB, et al. Adhesive capsulitis: A sticky issue. *Am Fam Physician*. 1999;59:1843–51.
- Woodward T, et al. The painful shoulder. II: Acute and chronic disorders. *Am Fam Physician*. 2000;61:3291–3300.

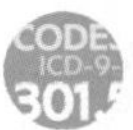

CODES

ICD9

726.0 Adhesive capsulitis of shoulder

CLINICAL PEARLS

- Syndrome of painful restriction of active and passive ROM commonly occurring in elderly
- Consider in symptomatic diabetic patients
- Primary cause is idiopathic.
- Treatment mainly consists of conservative measures: NSAIDs, corticosteroid injection, physical therapy.
- Prognosis is generally good, with self-limiting course over months to years.

FURUNCULOSIS

Zoltan Trizna, MD, PhD

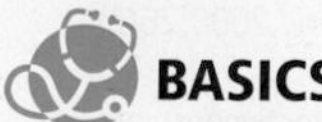

BASICS

DESCRIPTION

Acute bacterial abscess of a hair follicle (often *Staphylococcus aureus*):

- System(s) affected: Skin/Exocrine
- Synonym(s): Boils

EPIDEMIOLOGY

Incidence

- Predominant age:
  - Adolescents and young adults
  - Clusters have been reported in teenagers living in crowded quarters, within families, or in high school athletes.
- Predominant sex: Male = Female

Prevalence

Exact data are not available.

RISK FACTORS

- Carriage of pathogenic strain of *Staphylococcus* sp. in nares, skin, axilla, and perineum
- Rarely, polymorphonuclear leukocyte defect or hyperimmunoglobulin E–*Staphylococcus* sp. abscess syndrome
- Diabetes mellitus, malnutrition, alcoholism, obesity, atopic dermatitis
- Primary immunodeficiency disease and AIDS (common variable immunodeficiency, chronic granulomatous disease, Chediak-Higashi syndrome, C3 deficiency, C3 hypercatabolism, transient hypogammaglobulinemia of infancy, immunodeficiency with thymoma, Wiskott-Aldrich syndrome)
- Secondary immunodeficiency (e.g., leukemia, leukopenia, neutropenia, therapeutic immunosuppression)
- Medication impairing neutrophil function (e.g., omeprazole)

Genetics

Unknown

GENERAL PREVENTION

Patient education regarding self-care (see General Measures); treatment and prevention are interrelated.

PATHOPHYSIOLOGY

Infection spreads away from hair follicle into surrounding dermis.

ETIOLOGY

Pathogenic strain of *S. aureus* (usually); increasing incidence of community-acquired methicillin-resistant *S. aureus* (CA-MRSA)

COMMONLY ASSOCIATED CONDITIONS

- Usually normal immune system
- Diabetes mellitus
- Polymorphonuclear leukocyte defect (rare)
- Hyperimmunoglobulin E–*Staphylococcus* sp. abscess syndrome (rare)
- See Risk Factors.

DIAGNOSIS

HISTORY

- Located on hair-bearing sites, especially areas prone to friction or repeated minor traumas (e.g., underneath belt, anterior aspects of thighs, nape, buttocks)
- No initial fever or systemic symptoms
- The folliculocentric nodule may enlarge, become painful, and develop into an abscess (frequently with spontaneous drainage).

PHYSICAL EXAM

- Painful erythematous papules/nodules (1–5 cm) with central pustules
- Tender, red, perifollicular swelling, terminating in discharge of pus and necrotic plug
- The lesions may be solitary or clustered.

DIAGNOSTIC TESTS & INTERPRETATION

Lab

Initial lab tests

Culture of the purulent contents

Follow-Up & Special Considerations

- Immunoglobulin levels in rare (e.g., recurrent or otherwise inexplicable) cases
- If culture grows gram-negative bacteria or fungus, consider polymorphonuclear neutrophil leukocyte functional defect

Pathological Findings

Histopathology (though a biopsy is rarely needed):

- Perifollicular necrosis containing fibrinoid material and neutrophils
- At deep end of necrotic plug, in subcutaneous tissue, is a large abscess with a Gram stain positive for small collections of *S. aureus*.

DIFFERENTIAL DIAGNOSIS

- Folliculitis
- Pseudofolliculitis
- Carbuncles
- Ruptured epidermal cyst
- Myiasis (larva of botfly/tumbafly)
- Hidradenitis suppurativa
- Atypical bacterial or fungal infections

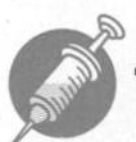

TREATMENT

MEDICATION

First Line

- If suspect CA-MRSA, see Second Line.
- If abscesses multiple, if lesions have marked surrounding inflammation, cellulitis, systemic symptoms such as fever, or if immunocompromised:
  - Obtain culture, and place on antibiotics directed at *S. aureus* × 10–14 days.
  - Dicloxacillin (Dynapen, Pathocil) 500 mg p.o. q.i.d. *or*
  - Cephalexin 250 mg p.o. q.i.d. *or*
  - Clindamycin 150 mg q.i.d. if penicillin-allergic
- Suppression of pathogenic strain (if topical treatment fails):
  - Dicloxacillin/cloxacillin 500 mg b.i.d. × 10–14 days
  - Cephalexin or clindamycin (if penicillin-allergic)
  - If preceding fails, dicloxacillin/cloxacillin 500 mg plus rifampin 600 mg p.o. daily × 7–10 days *or* clindamycin 150 mg/d × 3 months (1)[C]
- Contraindications: Allergy to the particular drug selected
- Precautions: Cloxacillin and dicloxacillin: Anaphylactic reaction

Second Line

- Resistant strains of *S. aureus* (MRSA): Clindamycin 300 mg q6h or doxycycline 100 mg q12h or TMP-SMX DS 1 tab q8h or minocycline 100 mg q12h (2)[C]
- If known or suspected impaired neutrophil function (e.g., impaired chemotaxis, phagocytosis, superoxide generation), add vitamin C 1,000 mg/d × 4–6 weeks (prevents oxidation of neutrophils)
- If fail with antibiotic regimens:
  - May try oral pentoxifylline 400 mg t.i.d. × 2–6 months (3)[C]
  - Contraindications: Recent cerebral and/or retinal hemorrhage; intolerance to methylxanthines (e.g., caffeine, theophylline); allergy to the particular drug selected
  - Precautions: Prolonged prothrombin time (PT) and/or bleeding; if on warfarin, frequent monitoring of PT

ADDITIONAL TREATMENT

General Measures

- Moist, warm compresses (provide comfort, encourage localization/pointing/drainage) 30 minutes q.i.d.
- If pointing or large, incise and drain
- Consider packing.
- Routine culture not necessary for localized abscess in nondiabetic patients with normal immune system
- Systemic antibiotics usually unnecessary, unless extensive surrounding cellulitis or fever
- If recurrent, usually related to chronic skin carriage of *Staphylococci* (nares or on skin). Treatment goals are to decrease or eliminate pathogenic strain *or* suppress pathogenic strain:
  - Culture nares, skin, axilla, and perineum (culture nares of family members).
  - Apply mupirocin ointment to anterior nares b.i.d. × 5 days (patient and family members/carriers).
  - Culture anterior nares every 3 months. If failure, retreat with mupirocin or consider oral antibiotics (4)[C].
  - See Medications, First Line, Suppression of Pathogenic Strain.
- Especially in recurrent cases, wash entire body and fingernails (with nailbrush) daily for 1–3 weeks with povidone–iodine (Betadine), hexachlorophene (Hibiclens), or pHisoHex soap (all can cause dry skin)
- Sanitary practices: Change towels, washcloths, and sheets daily; clean shaving instruments; avoid nose picking; change wound dressings frequently; do not share items of personal hygiene.

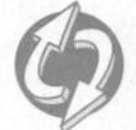

ONGOING CARE

FOLLOW-UP RECOMMENDATIONS

Patient Monitoring

Instruct patient to see physician if compresses unsuccessful

DIET

Unrestricted

PROGNOSIS

- Self-limited: Usually drains pus spontaneously and will heal with or without scarring within several days
- Recurrent/chronic: May last for months or years

COMPLICATIONS

- Scarring
- Bacteremia
- Seeding (e.g., septal/valve defect, arthritic joint)

REFERENCES

1. Klempner MS, Styrt B. Prevention of recurrent staphylococcal skin infections with low-dose oral clindamycin therapy. *JAMA*. 1988;260:2682–5.
2. *Up To Date 2007*. Impetigo, Folliculitis, Furunculosis, and Carbuncles.
3. Wahba-Yahav AV. Intractable chronic furunculosis: prevention of recurrences with pentoxifylline. *Acta Derm Venereol*. 1992;72:461–2.
4. Doebbeling BN, et al. Long Term Efficacy of Intranasal Mupirocin, A Prospective Cohort Study of Staphylococcal Aureus. *Arch Int Med*. 1994;154: 1505.
5. Winthropp KL, et al. An outbreak of mycobacterium furunculosis associated with footbaths at a nail salon. *N Engl J Med*. 2002;346(18):1366–71.

ADDITIONAL READING

Frazee BW, Lynn J, Charlebois ED, Lambert L, Lowery D, Perdreau-Remington F et al. High prevalence of methicillin-resistant Staphylococcus aureus in emergency department skin and soft tissue infections. *Ann Emerg Med*. 2005;45:311–20.

See Also (Topic, Algorithm, Electronic Media Element)

Folliculitis; Hidradenitis Suppurativa

CODES

ICD9

680.9 Carbuncle and furuncle of unspecified site

CLINICAL PEARLS

- The pathogens may be different in different localities. Keep up-to-date with the locality-specific epidemiology.
- If few, furuncles/furunculosis do not always need antibiotic treatment. If systemic symptoms (e.g., fever), cellulitis, or multiple lesions occur, oral antibiotic therapy is needed.
- Other treatments for MRSA include linezolid p.o. or IV and IV vancomycin.
- Folliculitis, furunculosis, and carbuncles are parts of a spectrum of pyodermas.
- Other causative organisms include anaerobic (e.g., *Escherichia coli*, *Pseudomonas aeruginosa*, and *Streptococcus faecalis*), anaerobic (e.g., *Bacteroides*, *Lactobacillus*, *Peptobacillius*), and *Peptostreptococcus*), and *Mycobacteria* (5).

GALACTORRHEA

Katherine M. Callaghan, MD
Dawn S. Tasillo, MD

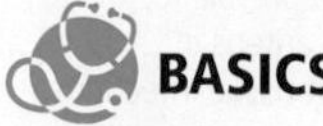

BASICS

DESCRIPTION
- Milky nipple discharge not associated with gestation. Galactorrhea does not include serous, purulent, or bloody nipple discharge.
- System(s) affected: Endocrine/Metabolic; Nervous; Reproductive
- Synonym(s): Disordered lactation; Nipple discharge

Pregnancy Considerations
- Most cases of galactorrhea during pregnancy are physiologic.
- Adenomas can grow rapidly during pregnancy.

EPIDEMIOLOGY
- Predominant age: 15–50 years
- Predominant sex: Female > Male (rare, 20% of patients with *MEN1* have prolactinomas)

Prevalence
1–50% of nonpregnant reproductive-age women

GENERAL PREVENTION
Keep medication causes in mind.

PATHOPHYSIOLOGY
Disorders of lactation are associated with hyperprolactinemia from overproduction or loss of inhibitory regulation by dopamine.

ETIOLOGY
- Nipple stimulation
- Pituitary gland overproduction:
  - Prolactinoma, acromegaly, empty sella, lymphocytic hypophysitis
- Hypothalamic region dysregulation:
  - Craniopharyngiomas, meningiomas, dysgerminomas, tumors, sarcoid, irradiation, vascular insult, stalk disruption, or dissection
- Medications that suppress dopamine:
  - Phenothiazines, atypical antipsychotics, selective serotonin reuptake inhibitors, tricyclic antidepressants, butyrophenones, cimetidine, ranitidine, reserpine, alpha methyl-dopa, verapamil, estrogens, isoniazid, opioids, stimulants, neuroleptics, metoclopramide, domperidone, protease inhibitors (1)
- Chest wall conditions:
  - Zoster, fibrocystic breast disease, or surgical or other trauma
- Postoperative condition, especially oophorectomy
- Other causes:
  - Primary hypothyroidism, cirrhosis, Cushing disease, ectopic prolactin secretion, renal failure, sarcoid, lupus, multiple sclerosis, polycystic ovary syndrome
- Physiologic with pregnancy or up to 6 months after stopping lactation
- Chiari-Frommel:
  - Galactorrhea >6 months postpartum
- Idiopathic:
  - Normal prolactin levels

COMMONLY ASSOCIATED CONDITIONS
See Etiology.

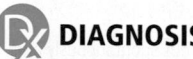

DIAGNOSIS

- Findings vary with causes
- Signs/symptoms of associated conditions:
  - Adrenal insufficiency, acromegaly, hypothyroidism, chest wall conditions

HISTORY
- Usually bilateral milky nipple discharge
- Hypogonadism from hyperprolactinemia:
  - Oligomenorrhea, amenorrhea
  - Inadequate luteal phase, anovulation, infertility
  - Decreased libido (especially in affected males)
- Mass effects from pituitary enlargement:
  - Headache, cranial neuropathies
  - Bitemporal hemianopsia, amaurosis, scotomata

PHYSICAL EXAM
Breast examination should be performed with attention to the presence of spontaneous or induced nipple discharge.

DIAGNOSTIC TESTS & INTERPRETATION
Formal visual field testing if pituitary adenoma suspected

Lab
- Check prolactin level and thyroid-stimulating hormone.
- Check pregnancy test, liver, and renal functions.
- Consider follicle-stimulating hormone and leuteinizing hormone if amenorrheic.
- Consider growth hormone levels if acromegaly suspected.
- Check adrenal steroids if signs of Cushing disease.
- Drugs that may alter lab results:
  - See medications that can cause hyperprolactinemia.
- Situations that may alter lab results:
  - See Etiology.
  - Lab evaluation of prolactin may be falsely elevated by a recent breast examination, vigorous exercise, sexual activity, or high-carbohydrate diet. Consider repeating the test under different circumstances if the value is borderline (30–40) elevated.

Follow-Up & Special Considerations
- Prolactin levels may fluctuate. Elevated prolactin levels should be confirmed with at least 1 additional level drawn in a fasting, nonexercised state, with no breast stimulation (2).
- Prolactin levels above 200 ng/mL are highly suggestive of a pituitary adenoma (2).

Imaging
Pituitary magnetic resonance imaging (MRI) with gadolinium enhancement if the serum prolactin level is significantly elevated (>200 ng/mL) or if a pituitary tumor is otherwise suspected

Diagnostic Procedures/Surgery
Confirm that microscopic evaluation of secretions is lipoid.

Pathological Findings
None unless pituitary resection required

DIFFERENTIAL DIAGNOSIS
- Primary hypothyroidism
- Nonmilky nipple discharge:
  - Intraductal papilloma
  - Fibrocystic disease
- Purulent breast discharge:
  - Mastitis
  - Breast abscess
  - Impetigo
  - Eczema
- Bloody breast discharge:
  - Consider malignancy

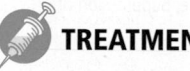

TREATMENT

- Treat underlying cause if possible.
- Idiopathic galactorrhea (normal prolactin levels) does not require treatment.
- Treat to manage symptoms, reduce patient anxiety, and restore fertility.
- Reduce tumor size or prevent progression to prevent neurologic sequelae.
- If microadenoma, watchful waiting can be appropriate, as 95% do not enlarge.
- Treat asymptomatic tumors if >10 mm.
- Discontinue offending medications.

MEDICATION

- The dopamine agonists work to reduce prolactin levels and shrink tumor size. Therapy is suppressive, not curative.
- Treatment is discontinued when tumor size has reduced or regressed completely or after pregnancy has been achieved.
- Contraindications are similar for all and include:
  - Uncontrolled hypertension
  - Sensitivity to ergot alkaloids
  - Preeclampsia
- Precautions:
  - Nausea, vomiting, and drowsiness are common.
  - Orthostasis, lightheadedness, or syncope
  - Hypertension, seizures, acute psychosis, and digital vasospasm are rare.
- Significant possible interactions:
  - Phenothiazines, butyrophenones, other drugs listed under "Etiology"
- Bromocriptine:
  - Start at 1.25 mg/d p.o. with food and increase weekly by 1.25 mg/d until therapeutic response achieved. (Usually 2.5–15 mg/d, divided once daily/3 times daily.)
  - More expensive and more frequent dosing; however, most providers have experience with this effective drug.
  - Long-term treatment can cause woody fibrosis of the pituitary gland.
- Cabergoline (Dostinex):
  - Start at 0.25 mg p.o. weekly and increase by 0.25 mg monthly until prolactin levels normalize. Usual dose ranges from 0.25 mg–1 mg p.o. once or twice weekly.
  - More effective and better tolerated than bromocriptine
  - Convenient dosing
  - Although cabergoline has been associated with valvular heart disease in patients treated for Parkinson disease, the lower doses used in treatment of prolactinomas have not been adequately studied (3).

SURGERY/OTHER PROCEDURES

- Surgery:
  - Macroadenomas need surgery if medical management does not halt growth, if neurologic symptoms persist, if size >10 mm, or if patient cannot tolerate medications. Also considered in young patients with microadenomas in order to avoid long-term medical therapy (4).
  - Trans-sphenoidal pituitary resection
  - 50% recurrence after surgery
- Radiotherapy:
  - Radiation is an alternate tumor therapy for macroprolactinomas not responsive to other modes of treatment:
    - 20–30% success rate
    - 50% risk of panhypopituitarism after radiation
    - Risk of optic nerve damage (5)
- Gamma knife is effective with high-volume surgeons (1)[B].

ONGOING CARE

FOLLOW-UP RECOMMENDATIONS

- Outpatient care unless pituitary resection required
- Bromocriptine patients need adequate hydration.

Patient Monitoring

- Varies with cause; check prolactin levels every 6 weeks until normalized, then every 6–12 months
- Monitor visual fields and/or MRI at least yearly until stable.

DIET

No restrictions

PATIENT EDUCATION

- Warn about symptoms of mass enlargement in pituitary.
- Discuss treatment rationale and risks of treating or not.
- Patient education material available from American Family Physician: http://www.aafp.org/afp/20040801/553ph.html

PROGNOSIS

- Depends on underlying cause
- Symptoms can recur after discontinuation of medication.
- Surgery can have 50% recurrence (6).
- Prolactinomas <10 mm can resolve spontaneously.

COMPLICATIONS

- Depends on underlying cause
- If enlarging pituitary adenoma, risk of permanent visual field loss
- Panhypopituitarism can complicate radiation or surgical therapy.
- Osteoporosis if amenorrhea persists without estrogen replacement

REFERENCES

1. Molitch M. Medication-induced hyperprolactinemia. *Mayo Clin Proc Rochester*. 2005;80(8):1050–8.
2. Leung AK, Pacaud D. Diagnosis and management of galactorrhea. *Am Fam Physician*. 2004;70:543–50.
3. Kars M, Pereira A, Bax J, et al. Cabergoline and cardiac valve disease in prolactinoma patients:Additional studies during long-term treatment are required. *Eur J Endocrinol*. 2008.
4. Mancini T, Casanueva FF, Giustina A. Hyperprolactinemia and prolactinomas. *Endocrinol Metab Clin North Am*. 2008;37:67–99.
5. Prabhakar VK, Davis JR. Hyperprolactinaemia. *Best Pract Res Clin Obstet Gynaecol*. 2007.
6. Schlechte JA. Long-term management of prolactinomas. *J Clin Endocrinol Metab*. 2007;92:2861–5.

See Also (Topic, Algorithm, Electronic Media Element)

Hyperprolactinemia

CODES

ICD9

- 611.6 Galactorrhea not associated with childbirth
- 676.60 Galactorrhea associated with childbirth, unspecified as to episode of care

CLINICAL PEARLS

- Galactorrhea is a common disorder, affecting between 1% and 50% of reproductive-age, nonlactating women.
- Lab evaluation of prolactin may be falsely elevated due to recent sexual activity, breast examination, exercise, or high-carbohydrate diet. Repeat any borderline elevation before continuing evaluation or initiating treatment.
- Most cases may be adequately evaluated by thyroid-stimulating hormone, prolactin, and human chorionic gonadotropin measurement, with additional testing as suggested by the presence of other symptoms or signs.
- Evaluate prolactin >200 ng/mL (or suspicion of pituitary macroadenoma) with a gadolinium-enhanced MRI.

GAMBLING ADDICTION

Amy Shah, MD
Christopher C. White, MD, JD

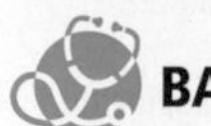

BASICS

DESCRIPTION

Gambling is the act of placing something of value at risk in the hopes of gaining something of greater value. Gambling addiction is an impulse-control disorder ranging in severity from problem gambling to the more severe pathologic gambling (PG). Disordered gambling is a dynamic behavior, and patients frequently move in both directions along the continuum of normal and PG behavior over relatively short time periods. Gambling addiction is further categorized into levels:

- Level 0: Nongamblers
- Level 1: Gambled without adverse consequences
- Level 2: Experienced negative consequences from gambling behavior but do not meet criteria for PG
- Level 3: Gambling meets *Diagnostic and Statistical Manual of Psychological Disorders*, Fourth Edition (DSM-IV), criteria for PG: Persistent and recurrent maladaptive gambling behavior indicated by ≥5 DSM-IV criteria.
- Level 4: Seeking help for gambling addiction regardless of degree of gambling addiction

EPIDEMIOLOGY

- Predominant sex: Male > Female
- The younger the person starts gambling, the more likely he or she is to become a pathologic gambler.
- A higher likelihood exists if parents have PG.
- Family history of substance abuse and mental disorders

Incidence

There are limited incidence studies, but some research states that the number of people affected by gambling addiction remains stable over time.

Prevalence

- According to the National Gambling Impact Study Commission, prevalence of problem and pathologic gambling was 1.7–7.3% of adults in the 17 states where surveys were done.
- 0.2–2.1% of the world's population meets diagnostic criteria for level 3 pathologic gamblers, with prevalence changing little over time.

GENERAL PREVENTION

Focus on treatment, patient education, and awareness of risk factors, associated conditions, and warning signs of pathologic or problematic gambling behaviors.

RISK FACTORS

- Some types of gambling present a greater risk to cause PG than other types: pull tabs, casino gambling, and bingo and cards outside a casino.
- Being involved with several gaming modalities is related to PG and suggests that the gambler is very captivated with risking money for excitement as opposed to risking money for social pleasure or for an interest in sports.
- Alcohol abuse and dependence are correlated with problem gambling.
- Lower socioeconomic status positively correlates with increased gambling pathology because these persons have few financial resources and cannot recover as easily from losses. Persons even may believe that gambling is a way to ease their financial burden.

Genetics

SLC6A4 serotonin transporter gene has been associated with PG in males but not females.

PATHOPHYSIOLOGY

- The brains of pathologic gamblers may have some predisposition to illness. Functional MRI studies indicate that the ventromedial prefrontal cortex is less activated when gambling stimuli are presented to pathologic gamblers.
- Abnormalities in the neurotransmitters serotonin, norepinephrine, dopamine, and glutamate may be implicated in PG.
  - Norepinephrine: Still unclear but plays a part in arousal or excitement
  - Serotonin: Involved in impulse control
  - Dopamine: May induce reversible PG in Parkinson patients who take dopamine agonists

COMMONLY ASSOCIATED CONDITIONS

- Poor nutrition
- Stress-related medical conditions (e.g., PUD, hypertension, migraine)
- Suicidal ideation and attempts
- Substance abuse disorder
- Attention deficit–hyperactivity disorder (ADHD)
- Bipolar disorder and other mood disorders
- Impulse-control disorders
- Personality disorders
- Incarceration
- Financial problems

DIAGNOSIS

DSM-IV criteria for PG:

- Persistent and recurrent maladaptive gambling behavior, as indicated by five or more of the following:
  - Preoccupation with gambling
  - Need to gamble with increasing amounts of money to achieve the desired excitement
  - Repeated unsuccessful efforts to control, cut back, or stop gambling
  - Restless or irritable when attempting to cut down or stop gambling
  - Gambles as a way of escaping from problems or of relieving a dysphoric mood
  - After losing money gambling, often returns another day to get even
  - Lies to family members, therapist, or others to conceal the extent of involvement with gambling
  - Has committed illegal acts such as forgery, fraud, theft, or embezzlement to finance gambling
  - Has jeopardized or lost a significant relationship, job, or educational or career opportunity because of gambling
  - Relies on others to provide money to relieve a desperate financial situation caused by gambling
- The gambling behavior is not better accounted for by a manic episode.

HISTORY

- Preoccupation with gambling
- Preoccupation with money
- Unexplained new financial problems
- New participation in illegal or dishonest money-making endeavors or activities
- Disruptions in personal life or career
- Patient may ask his or her family and friends to pay off his or her debts ("bailing them out").

DIAGNOSTIC TESTS & INTERPRETATION

- Lie/bet method: Have you ever had to lie to people important to you about how much you gambled? Have you ever felt a need to bet more money?
  - A patient who answers at least one question with a "Yes" screens positively for PG.
  - This test has been shown to have >85% specificity and >95% sensitivity (1).
- South Oaks Gambling Screen (SOGS):
  - 20-question screen for PG
  - Score of 3–4 suggests problem gambling.
  - Score of 5 or more indicates probable PG.
  - Criticized as overestimating the number of pathologic gamblers and being too lengthy to administer (2)[B].
- Gamblers Anonymous 20 questions:
  - Easily obtainable from Gamblers Anonymous Web site
  - Scores of >7 are indicative of problem/PG.

Imaging

- Neuroimaging research indicates that the neural structures of the mesolimbic pathway are involved in PG, including the orbitofrontal cortex, amygdala, and ventral striatum/nucleus accumbens.
- There are some data to suggest the idea that because there is lower activity in the ventral striatum when receiving a reward in PG, these patients have decreased sensitivity to reward.

DIFFERENTIAL DIAGNOSIS

- Social gambling
- Professional gambling
- Bipolar disorder, manic episode
- Substance use disorder
- Personality disorder

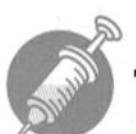

TREATMENT

In order to treat PG, treat the comorbidities first. The usual comorbid disorders are substance abuse, bipolar disorder, ADHD, and other impulse-control disorders. There is no Food and Drug Administration (FDA)–approved therapy for PG. Nonpharmacologic therapies are more effective than pharmacologic therapies. There are some data suggesting that gambling abstinence is not necessary for treatment; patients still can exhibit controlled gambling.

MEDICATION

- Selective serotonin reuptake inhibitors (SSRIs):
  - Beneficial for treating comorbid impulse-control disorders
  - Used to treat gambling addiction because of link with serotonergic dysfunction: Some studies show that low levels of serotonin cause a suppression of inhibitory responses.
  - Citalopram (Celexa) has shown significant improvement on all gambling measures, including number of days gambled, urge to gamble, and preoccupation with gambling. Celexa is also a low-cost medication with few drug interactions.
  - Fluvoxamine (Luvox) has been shown to be effective in a short-term acute trial as well.
  - Use of paroxetine (Paxil) in PG needs further studies.
- Modafinil helps pathologic gamblers with high impulsivity but increases gambling behavior in low-impulsivity pathologic gamblers. Modafinil shows decreases in motivation to gamble, risky decision making, and impulsivity in high-impulsivity pathologic gamblers (3)[B].
- Valproate and carbamazepine, as well as lithium carbonate, are effective treatments (3)[A].
- Opiate antagonists have the ability to decrease dopamine release in the dopamine reward pathway. Naltrexone and nalmefene are efficacious for PG and reduce urges to gamble. Positive family history of alcoholism predicted a positive response to opiate antagonist treatment (3).
- Selected antipsychotics have been shown to be ineffective in PG (i.e., olanzapine is not efficacious for the treatment of PG, and haloperidol may increase the desire to gamble in pathological gamblers) (3)[B].
- *N*-acetylcysteine (NAC), a glutamate-modulating agent, causes significant improvements in gambling thoughts and behaviors.

ADDITIONAL TREATMENT

- Patients are often forced to come in for treatment after an ultimatum, such as threat of divorce or prosecution.
- Patients' personal characteristics (i.e., pride, denial, or impatience) can hinder therapy.
- Additionally, pathologic gamblers may leave when therapy does not work fast enough.
- Mental health workers must avoid negative transference.
- Because of increased suicide rates, patients may need to be hospitalized acutely for safety and to prevent gambling.
- Since patients are at increased risk from mental and physical illness, they benefit from relaxation exercises to reduce stress, identify triggers, substitute gambling with other activities, and a complete physical and lab work with nutrition evaluation.

General Measures

- Get a sense of the patient's readiness for change.
- Provide intervention/patient education. While there are no FDA-approved drug treatments for PG, make clinically based medication recommendations.
- Screen for and treat comorbid conditions.
- Provide referrals:
  - Addiction psychiatrist/counselor
  - Gamblers Anonymous
  - Consumer credit organizations
  - Bankruptcy lawyers
  - Gam-Anon for family members

Additional Therapies

- Cognitive-behavioral therapy (CBT):
  - The main effective interventions for CBT are psychoeducation, cognitive restructuring, problem solving, social skills training, and relapse prevention. Studies indicated that CBT resulted in significant improvement for short-term therapy (4)[A].
  - CBT may be done in several formats: Individual, group, brief group, and dual diagnosis. All these formats have been shown to be effective. Group therapy is favored because patients are often extroverted. Couple or family therapy also may be used.
- Gamblers Anonymous:
  - A 12-step program similar to Alcoholics Anonymous for a person suffering from a gambling addiction
  - Dropout rate is high if this is the only means of therapy (1)[B].
  - Patients may deny need to attend in the 1st place, and for that reason, Gamblers Anonymous may not be appropriate for patients who are in the precontemplation stage.
- Motivational enhancement therapy (MET):
  - Provides nonargumentative exploration of patient's stage of change
  - Patient receives positive reinforcement from clinician.
  - Motivational enhancement strategies support self-efficacy.
  - Improves patient rapport; aids in removing barriers to treatment
  - In one study, MET alone did not show any improvement, but MET and CBT together improved outcome measures (3)[B].

ONGOING CARE

FOLLOW-UP RECOMMENDATIONS

Patients seeking treatment for gambling addiction should be followed routinely by physicians and counselors to monitor the response to treatment, tolerance to medications, and possibility of relapse.

PATIENT EDUCATION

- Gamblers Anonymous:
  - http://www.gamblersanonymous.org
  - National hotline 1-888-GA-HELPS (888-424-3577)
- Gam-Anon: Support group for spouses, family, or close friends of compulsive gamblers: http://www/gam-anon.org
- Responsible Gambling Council: http://www.responsiblegambling.org
- Humphrey H. This Must Be Hell: A Look at Pathological Gambling. IUniverse, 2000.
- Lee B. Born to Lose: Memoirs of a Compulsive Gambler. Hazelden, 2005.

PROGNOSIS

- Patients with gambling addiction can be treated, but many relapse.
- 36–39% of patients did not experience any gambling-related problems according to one study, and only 7–12% sought formal treatment or Gamblers Anonymous meetings.
- Roughly 1/3 of patients who have a gambling addiction recover without any intervention.

REFERENCES

1. Potenza MN, Fiellin DA, Heninger GR, et al. Gambling: an addictive behavior with health and primary care implications. *J Gen Intern Med*. 2002;17:721–32.
2. Rossow I and Molde H. Chasing the criteria: comparing SOGS-RA and the Lie/Bet screen to assess prevalence of problem gambling and "at-risk" gambling among adolescents. *Journal of Gambling Issues*. 2006;(18):57–71.
3. Leung KS, Cottler LB. Treatment of pathological gambling. *Curr Opin Psychiatry*. 2009;22:69–74.
4. Hodgins DC, Peden N. Cognitive-behavioral treatment for impulse control disorders. *Rev Bras Psiquiatr*. 2007.

ADDITIONAL READING

- Brewer JA, Potenza MN. The neurobiology and genetics of impulse control disorders: Relationships to drug addictions. *Biochem Pharmacol*. 2007.
- Potenza MN. Review. The neurobiology of pathological gambling and drug addiction: an overview and new findings. *Philos Trans R Soc Lond B Biol Sci*. 2008.

CODES

ICD9

- 312.31 Pathological gambling
- V69.3 Gambling and betting

CLINICAL PEARLS

- There are several brief screening strategies that can be used to identify PG, including the lie/bet method, the SOGS, and the Gamblers Anonymous 20 questions.
- To treat PG, 1st treat comorbidities such as substance abuse, bipolar disorder, ADHD, and other impulse-control disorders.
- Nonpharmacologic therapies are more effective than pharmacologic therapies. There is no FDA-approved therapy for PG.
- Patients seeking treatment for gambling addiction should be followed routinely by physicians and counselors to monitor the response to treatment, tolerance to medications, and possibility of relapse.

GANGLION CYST

Christopher Garofalo, MD

BASICS

- Ganglions are common benign tumors.
- Can be located throughout the body and usually located adjacent to joints and tendons, mostly on wrist, foot, ankle
- Average size is 3 cm.
- Most are not symptomatic except for changing size.

EPIDEMIOLOGY

- Can affect all age groups but unusual in children
- Most common in young adults
- Mucous cysts are usually seen in older patients.
- Hand and wrist ganglions are commonly seen in dorsal wrist, radial wrist, and dorsum of the DIP joint (which is referred to as a mucous cyst).
- 60–70% of hand and wrist ganglions are in dorsal wrist, 15–20% are at the volar wrist.

Prevalence

- Prevalence of wrist ganglia in patients presenting with wrist pain has been reported as 19%.
- Prevalence of ganglia in patients with a palpable mass in the wrist has been reported as 27%.

RISK FACTORS

- No specific risk factors
- No known occupational risk factors

PATHOPHYSIOLOGY

Pathogenesis is unclear. Several theories:

- Herniation of synovial lining creating a one-way valve; this is supported by dye studies that show communication of fluid from the wrist joint into the cyst but not from the cyst to the joint.
- Ganglions are benign tumors of synovium. However, pathologic analysis of surgical specimens from ganglion excision do not show a synovial lining, which brings these theories into question.
- A rent in the joint capsule or tendon sheath allows synovial fluid to leak, irritating surrounding tissue, which creates a pseudocapsule and ganglion and would explain why no lining is seen on pathology.
- Mucoid degeneration of collagen fibers in the joint with the collagen products forming a pool of hyaluronic acid and then a cyst
- Recurrent stress and microtrauma at the synovial-capsular interface may stimulate mucin production by mesenchymal cells or fibroblasts.

ETIOLOGY

- Etiology is unknown.
- May be associated with trauma but majority of patients cannot recall specific trauma

COMMONLY ASSOCIATED CONDITIONS

Mucous cysts are usually associated with some level of osteoarthritis of DIP joint.

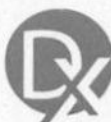

DIAGNOSIS

- Usually made on basis of history and physical examination
- Patients usually present when there is pain, increased size, interference with activities, or weakness.

HISTORY

- Patients usually present with asymptomatic mass present for months or years, decreasing and increasing in size.
- Mostly asymptomatic but can be associated with pain, limitations in activity.
- 1/3 of patients presenting with ganglion cyst elected for surgical intervention (1).

PHYSICAL EXAM

- Mass is compressible, subcutaneous, transilluminating, slightly mobile; no overlying skin changes.
- Extension of wrist often elicits pain at the site.
- Small ganglions may only be palpable in full wrist flexion.
- Occult ganglions are not palpable but can be quite painful.

DIAGNOSTIC TESTS & INTERPRETATION

Most ganglions do not require imaging to confirm diagnosis unless unclear wrist pain presents.

Imaging

- Several options:
  - Ultrasound
  - MRI
  - Bone scintigraphy, arthroscopy
- Ultrasound and MRI have similar rates of sensitivity and specificity.
- Scintigraphy is less specific.
- Ultrasound is less expensive than MRI but more operator-dependent.
- Arthroscopy is both diagnostic and therapeutic but should be considered when initial workup is nondiagnostic and conservative treatment effective.

Initial approach

Most are apparent clinically and do not need imaging

Pathological Findings

- Gross pathologic evaluation shows that cysts are often multilobulated.
- Microscopic exam reveals outer wall w/several layers of randomly oriented collagen fibers, relatively acellular with a few fibroblasts and mesenchymal cells in the collagen fibers.
- As pathology does not show an epithelial lining it is therefore not a true cyst.
- Fluid contains glucosamine, albumin, globulin, hyaluronic acid.
- Ganglions are histopathologically identical regardless of anatomic location.

DIFFERENTIAL DIAGNOSIS

- A mobile mass of extensor tendons of wrist may be a ganglion or tendon sheath, giant cell tumor, tenosynovitis from infection or inflammation.
- Other tumors include lipoma, sarcoma, hamartoma, interosseous neuroma.
- Firm mass may represent osteophyte.

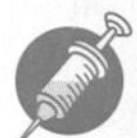

TREATMENT

3 primary treatment options (2):

- Reassurance that ganglia is not likely to be malignant or to cause damage, and observation; 33% dorsal ganglions and 45% volar ganglions resolve spontaneously by 6 years, up to 80% of ganglion in children resolve.
- Closed rupture, historically by hitting cyst with a book; results in initial decreased clinical symptoms by 22–66% but often leads to recurrence
- Aspiration can be done in an office under local anesthesia with 18-gauge or larger needle.
- Studies demonstrate mixed results on aspirations of a ganglion; evidence supporting injecting steroids is weak, and splinting after the procedure may help cure rate but recurrence may be as high as 80% after single aspiration. This can be reduced to 20% with multiple aspirations.
- Volar ganglion are not aspirated due to risk of neurovascular structures:
  - Mucous cysts can be aspirated but recurrence is over 50% and pain may not resolve if it is due to underlying osteoarthritis.
- Surgical excision

- Tricyclic antidepressants (TCAs):
  - Imipramine 75 mg PO daily; increase to maximum of 200 mg/d (NNT = 4.07). May start at 10–20 mg at night, and titrate up to 75–300 mg at night. Usual maintenance: 50–150 mg/d. Geriatric: 25–75 mg at night; maximum of 200 mg/d
- Benzodiazepines (should be tapered as the antidepressant dose is titrated to therapeutic levels after 6–8 weeks):
  - Clonazepam: 0.25–0.5 mg PO b.i.d., titrated up to 1 mg b.i.d. or t.i.d.
  - Lorazepam: 0.5–1.0 mg PO t.i.d., titrated up to 1 mg PO t.i.d. or q.i.d.
  - Diazepam: 2–10 mg PO 2–4 times daily as needed; geriatric: 2–2.5 mg PO once or twice daily; increase gradually
    - Have a rapid onset of action and are effective in GAD
    - Often recommended as adjunctive therapy to help patients in acute crisis or while waiting for a SSRI/SNRI to take effect.
    - Not recommended as monotherapy for depression, dysthymia, obsessive-compulsive disorder, and PTSD, which commonly occur with GAD.
    - Use for short-term treatment duration (up to 4 weeks) to avoid the risk of physical dependence and withdrawal (rebound anxiety).
    - Tapering usually takes months, with about 10% reduction per week.
    - If symptoms recur, it may be difficult to differentiate between benzodiazepine withdrawal or recurrence of GAD symptoms; symptoms that worsen within 2 weeks are most likely due to benzodiazepine withdrawal and suggest that the taper rate be decreased slightly.
    - Avoid in patients with polydrug or alcohol use, chronic pain disorders, and severe personality disorders owing to high risk of dependence.
- Antihistamines
  - Hydroxyzine: Should not be used as 1st therapy because of associated side effects (in particular, sedation and anticholinergic effects), slow onset of action, and lack of efficacy for comorbid disorders (3).
- Pregabalin
  - Approved in Europe for treatment of GAD
  - Improves both psychic and somatic symptoms in adults with GAD, including the elderly (4)
  - Discontinuation symptoms if abruptly stopped.
- Atypical antipsychotic
  - Quetiapine 50–150 mg daily
    - Could be considered after other classes of drugs have proved ineffective or when certain types of symptoms are present (5)
    - Most trials used this for augmentation; however, more trials are needed to validate the efficacy of this class of drug

Pregnancy Considerations

- Paroxetine (Paxil): Association with congenital heart (septal) defects in 1st-trimester exposure and with persistent pulmonary hypertension in 3rd-trimester exposure; Category D; fetal echocardiography should be considered for women who are exposed in early pregnancy.
- Venlafaxine (Effexor): Association with congenital heart defects in 1st-trimester exposure
- Benzodiazepines: 1st-trimester exposure is associated with craniofacial deformities. Maternal benzodiazepine use shortly before delivery is associated with floppy infant syndrome.

ADDITIONAL TREATMENT

Propranolol is not recommended for the treatment of GAD (no significant efficacy over placebo after 3 weeks in one randomized, controlled trial).

General Measures

Both psychological and medication therapies are effective and work well when used together.

Issues for Referral

Refer to a psychiatrist for comorbid depression, for prolonged use of benzodiazepines, and for patients with suicidal ideation.

Additional Therapies

- Patient surveys have shown a preference for psychological therapy to medications (6).
- Cognitive-behavioral therapy is frequently recommended as the 1st-line psychological treatment for GAD and has been shown to be superior to placebo in alleviating the symptoms of GAD.

COMPLEMENTARY AND ALTERNATIVE MEDICINE

- Kava is not recommended for the treatment of anxiety. Associated with fatal hepatotoxicity, and the FDA has issued a safety alert.
- Valerian is marketed principally for insomnia but also has been used as a mild sedative for anxiety disorders.
  - Clinical studies are inconclusive about effectiveness for treatment of insomnia; mild sedative effects in animals; no human studies available
  - Few adverse effects reported, but no data about long-term safety

IN-PATIENT CONSIDERATIONS

Initial Stabilization

Evaluate for suicidality, and begin pharmacologic treatment as soon as possible. Faster-acting medications (e.g., benzodiazepines) may be required for initial stabilization.

Admission Criteria

Inpatient admission is generally not necessary unless the patient expresses suicidal ideation.

Discharge Criteria

When suicidal ideation is no longer present and treatment has been started

ONGOING CARE

FOLLOW-UP RECOMMENDATIONS

- Efficacy, medication tolerance, symptoms, and side effects should be assessed within 2 weeks of starting any new treatment.
- Once the patient has begun to experience relief from symptoms, follow-up should be every 4 weeks.

DIET

Patients should discontinue or limit consumption of caffeine and other stimulant-type food/beverages.

PATIENT EDUCATION

- Patients should be presented with both medication and psychological treatment options.
- Patients treated with benzodiazepines should be made aware of the potential for dependence and the resulting short-term nature of this type of treatment.

PROGNOSIS

- GAD is a chronic disorder that rarely goes into remission, with long-term recovery achieved in only 1/3 of patients.
- Many patients will need chronic treatment with medication to prevent relapse; other patients may be treated with intermittent courses of acute treatment.
- Patients experience fluctuating levels of symptoms provoked by stressful life events. Augment treatment as needed.

REFERENCES

1. Davidson J, Feltner D, Dugar A. Management of Generalized Anxiety Disorder in Primary Care: Identifying the Challenges and Unmet Needs. *Prim Care Companion J Clin Psychiatry* 2010;12(2): e1–e13.
2. American Psychiatric Association. *Diagnostic and Statistical Manual of Mental Disorders*, 4th ed, Primary Care Version (DSM-IV-PC). American Psychiatric Association, Washington, DC, 1995.
3. Bandelow B, Zohar J, Hollander E, et al. World Federation of Societies of Biological Psychiatry (WFSBP) guidelines for the pharmacological treatment of anxiety, obsessive-compulsive and post-traumatic stress disorders-first revision. *World J Biol Psychiatry*. 2008;9:248–312.
4. Montgomery S, Chatamra K, Pauer L, Whalen E, Baldinetti F et al. Efficacy and safety of pregabalin in elderly people with generalised anxiety disorder. *Br J Psychiatry*. 2008;193:389–94.
5. Bandelow B, Chouinard G, Bobes J, Ahokas A, Eggens I, Liu S, Eriksson H et al. Extended-release quetiapine fumarate (quetiapine XR): a once-daily monotherapy effective in generalized anxiety disorder. Data from a randomized, double-blind, placebo- and active-controlled study. *Int J Neuropsychopharmacol*. 2010;13:305–20.
6. Hunot V, Churchill R, Teixeira V, et al. Psychological therapies for generalized anxiety disorder. *Cochrane Database of Systematic Reviews*. 2007, Issue 1. Art. No.: CD001848. DOI:10.1002/14651858.CD001848.pub4.

See Also (Topic, Algorithm, Electronic Media Element)

Depression

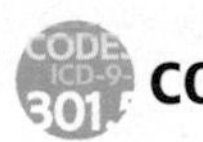

CODES

ICD9

300.02 Generalized anxiety disorder

CLINICAL PEARLS

- GAD is defined as excessive anxiety and worry more days than not for a period of 6 months or more, which the patient has a difficult time controlling and which causes significant impairment and distress.
- Patients should be evaluated for medical conditions that can cause hyperarousal and other anxiety disorders.

G

GIARDIASIS

Jill A. Grimes, MD

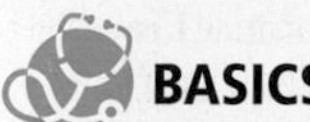

BASICS

DESCRIPTION

- Intestinal infection caused by the protozoan parasite *Giardia lamblia* (1)
  - *G. lamblia* is also called *G. duodenalis* and *G. intestinalis*.
- Infection results from ingestion of the cysts, which excyst into trophozoites. These colonize the small intestine and cause symptoms.
- Cycle is continued when the trophozoites encyst in the small intestine and water, food, or hands are contaminated by feces of the infected person.
- Most infections result from fecal–oral transmission or ingestion of contaminated water (such as while swimming) and are less commonly the result of contaminated food.

EPIDEMIOLOGY

- Predominant age: All ages, but most common in early childhood ages 1–9 and adults 35–44 (2)[A]
- Predominant gender: Male > Female (slightly)

Pediatric Considerations

Common in early childhood

Prevalence

- 5% of patients with stools submitted for ova and parasite exams
- >19,000 cases/year in the United States (although it is not reportable in Indiana, Kentucky, Mississippi, North Carolina, and Texas)

RISK FACTORS

- Daycare centers
- Anal intercourse
- Wilderness camping
- Travel to developing countries
- Children adopted from developing countries
- Public swimming pools

Genetics

No known genetic risk factors

GENERAL PREVENTION

- Good hand-washing when caring for diapered children
- Water purification when camping and when traveling to developing countries
- Cooking all foods

PATHOPHYSIOLOGY

Giardia trophozoites colonize the surface of the proximal small intestine. The mechanism by which they cause diarrhea is unknown.

ETIOLOGY

Protozoan parasite (*G. lamblia*) infection acquired through fecal–oral transmission or ingestion of contaminated water, less commonly from contaminated food

COMMONLY ASSOCIATED CONDITIONS

Hypogammaglobulinemia and possibly IgA deficiency; diarrhea more severe and prolonged in these patients

DIAGNOSIS

HISTORY

- ~25–50% of infected persons are symptomatic.
- Chronic diarrhea (lasting >5–7 days and frequently weeks)
- Abdominal bloating
- Flatulence
- Loose, greasy, foul-smelling stools
- Weight loss
- Nausea
- Lactose intolerance

PHYSICAL EXAM

Nonspecific; abdominal bloating and afebrile

DIAGNOSTIC TESTS & INTERPRETATION

Lab

Initial lab tests

- Stool for ova and parasites:
  - Repeated 3 times if necessary
  - Cysts are seen in fixed or fresh stools and, occasionally, trophozoites are found in fresh diarrheal stools.
- Fluorescent antibody (FA) and ELISA tests of fecal specimens are available. *A single FA or ELISA is at least as sensitive as 3 stools for ova and parasites.*
- Polymerase chain reaction (PCR) techniques have been found to be more sensitive than microscopy, but have not been widely adopted secondary to cost (3).

Follow-Up & Special Considerations

String test (Enterotest): A gelatin capsule on a string is swallowed and left in the duodenum for several hours or overnight. The end of the string is then visualized microscopically.

Diagnostic Procedures/Surgery

Esophagogastroduodenoscopy with biopsy and sample of small intestinal fluid

Pathological Findings

Intestinal biopsy shows flattened, mild lymphocytic infiltration and trophozoites on the surface.

DIFFERENTIAL DIAGNOSIS

- Includes other etiologies of small intestinal diarrhea
- Infectious causes include cryptosporidiosis, isosporiasis, and cyclosporiasis.
- Other causes of malabsorption include celiac sprue, tropical sprue, bacterial overgrowth syndromes, and Crohn ileitis.
- Irritable bowel is suspected when diarrhea is not accompanied by weight loss.

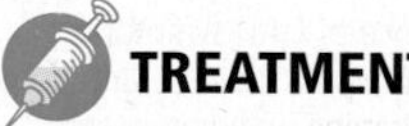

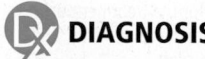

TREATMENT

Outpatient for mild cases, inpatient if symptoms are severe enough to cause dehydration

MEDICATION

First Line

- Metronidazole (Flagyl): 250 mg t.i.d. for 5–7 days (4)[B]
- Tinidazole 2 g single dose (50 mg/kg up to 2 g for children) (4)[B]
- Albendazole 400 mg once daily for 5 days:
  - Albendazole has comparable effectiveness to metronidazole with fewer side effects and low cost (5)[A].

- Precautions:
  - Theoretical risk of carcinogenesis with metronidazole
- Significant possible interactions: Occasional disulfiram reaction with metronidazole or tinidazole

Pregnancy Considerations

- Concern for potential teratogenicity of medications; consult infectious disease specialist or gastroenterologist for symptomatic disease
- Contraindications: Relatively contraindicated in pregnancy, especially 1st trimester

Second Line

- Furazolidone: 8 mg/kg/d t.i.d. for 10 days (slightly less effective, but commonly used in pediatrics because it is well tolerated)
- Paromomycin (Humatin): A nonabsorbable aminoglycoside that is probably less effective but commonly recommended in pregnancy because of theoretical risk of teratogenicity of other agents
- Quinacrine: 100 mg t.i.d. for 5–7 days; was the treatment of choice for giardiasis, but is withdrawn from the market in US
- Nitazoxanide suspension was approved by the FDA in 2003 for treatment of giardiasis in children ages 1–11. Children ages 1–4 receive 100 mg b.i.d. and ages 5–11 receive 200 mg b.i.d. for 3 days (1)[B].

ADDITIONAL TREATMENT

Lactose intolerance may follow Giardia infection and be a cause of persistent diarrhea post treatment.

General Measures

- Medical therapy for all infected individuals
- Fluid replacement if dehydrated

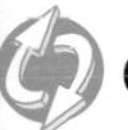

ONGOING CARE

FOLLOW-UP RECOMMENDATIONS

Patient Monitoring

Symptoms, weight, stool exams

DIET

Good nutrition, low lactose, low fat, monitor for dehydration

PATIENT EDUCATION

Hand washing may be more important than water purification to prevent transmission in outdoor recreationalists (6)[A].

PROGNOSIS

- Untreated giardiasis lasts for weeks.
- Patients usually (90%) respond to treatment within a few days:
  - Most nonresponders or relapses respond to a 2nd course with the same or a different agent.

COMPLICATIONS

Malabsorption and weight loss

REFERENCES

1. Yoder JS, Beach MJ, Centers for Disease Control and Prevention (CDC). Giardiasis surveillance–United States, 2003–2005. *MMWR Surveill Summ*. 2007;56:11–8.
2. Yoder JS, Harral C, Beach MJ, Centers for Disease Control and Prevention (CDC) et al. Giardiasis surveillance - United States, 2006-2008. *MMWR Surveill Summ*. 2010;59:15–25.
3. Haque R, Roy S, Siddique A, et al. Multiplex real-time PCR assay for detection of Entamoeba histolytica, Giardia intestinalis, and Cryptosporidium spp. *Am J Trop Med Hyg*. 2007;76:713–7.
4. Fallah M, Rabiee S, Moshtaghi AA. Comparison between efficacy of a single dose of tinidazole with a 7-day standard dose course of metronidazole in giardiasis. *Pakistan Journal of Medical Sciences*. 2007;23(1):43–6.
5. Solaymani-Mohammadi S, Genkinger JM, Loffredo CA, Singer SM et al. A meta-analysis of the effectiveness of albendazole compared with metronidazole as treatments for infections with Giardia duodenalis. *PLoS Negl Trop Dis*. 2010;4:e682.
6. Welch TP et al. Risk of giardiasis from consumption of wilderness water in North America: a systematic review of epidemiologic data. *Int J Infect Dis*. 2000;4:100–3.

ADDITIONAL READING

- Pawlowski SW, Warren CA, Guerrant R: Diagnosis and treatment of acute or persistent diarrhea. *Gastroenterology*. 2009;136(6):1874–86.
- Shields JM, Gleim ER, Beach MJ. Prevalence of Cryptosporidium spp. and Giardia intestinalis in Swimming Pools, Atlanta, Georgia. *Emerg Infect Dis*. 2008;14:948–50.

See Also (Topic, Algorithm, Electronic Media Element)

Algorithm: Diarrhea, Chronic

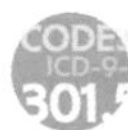

CODES

ICD9

007.1 Giardiasis

CLINICAL PEARLS

- Daycare facilities and public swimming pools are common sources of *Giardia* (don't assume camping or travel is required).
- Treatment with metronidazole is often poorly tolerated, but has higher cure rates.
- Most treatment failures respond to a second course of antibiotics (whether or not you switch drugs).

G

GINGIVITIS

Hugh J. Silk, MD
Sheila O. Stille, DMD, MAGD
Liang Zhao, MD

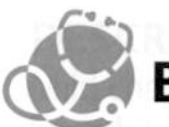

BASICS

DESCRIPTION

Gingivitis is a reversible form of inflammation of the gingiva. It is a mild form of periodontal disease. Classification includes:

- Plaque-induced
- Not plaque-induced (acute necrotizing gingivitis, Vincent disease, denture-related)
- Modified by systemic factors (e.g., pregnancy, HIV, diabetes, leukemia)
- Modified by medications (antihypertensives, antipsychotics, antiepileptics, hormones)
- Modified by malnutrition (vitamin deficiencies)
- System(s) affected: Gastrointestinal
- Synonym(s): Mild periodontal disease; Gum disease

Geriatric Considerations

More frequent in this age group (owing more to lifelong accumulation than to increased susceptibility)

Pediatric Considerations

Mild cases common in children (most common form of pediatric periodontal disease) and usually require no specific interventions

Pregnancy Considerations

- Very common in pregnant women; hormonal effect
- Hyperplasia
- Common; self-limited

EPIDEMIOLOGY

- Predominant age: >35 years old (but as young as 5)
- Predominant sex: Male = Female

Prevalence

- ~50% of children
- ~90% of adolescents and adult population
- ~30–75% of pregnant women

RISK FACTORS

- Poor dental hygiene/plaque formation
- Pregnancy
- Diabetes mellitus
- Malocclusion or dental crowding
- Smoking
- Mouth breathing
- Faulty dental restoration
- HIV-positive; AIDS
- Stress
- Vitamin C deficiency; coenzyme Q10 deficiency
- Dental appliances (dentures, braces)
- Eruption of primary or secondary teeth
- Necrotizing ulcerative gingivitis:
  - Stress
  - Lack of sleep
  - Malnutrition
  - Viral illness
  - Typically younger patients
- Bronchial asthma (1)
- Rheumatoid arthritis (2)

Genetics

Possible genetic link (up to 30% of population). Rare condition called hereditary gingival fibromatosis associated with hirsutism

GENERAL PREVENTION

- Good oral hygiene:
  - Adults
    - Regular twice daily brushing with fluoride toothpaste and increased benefit of using circular oscillating electric brush rather than regular brush (3)
    - Daily flossing
  - Pediatrics
    - Regular twice daily brushing with fluoride toothpaste with parental supervision until full manual dexterity (~age 8)
    - Regular flossing if no spaces between teeth
- Cleaning by a dentist or hygienist every 6 months or more frequently if indicated

PATHOPHYSIOLOGY

Inflammation of gingiva that may progress to deeper inflammation (see "Periodontitis")

ETIOLOGY

- Noncontagious
- Inadequate plaque removal
- Blood dyscrasias (pregnancy)
- Oral contraceptives
- Allergic reactions
- Nutritional deficiencies
- Vasoconstriction (nicotine)
- Endocrine/hormonal variations:
  - Pregnancy
  - Menses
  - Menarche
- Chronic debilitating disease
- Vincent disease:
  - Synergistic infection with fusiform bacillus (*Fusobacterium* spp.) and spirochete (*Borrelia vincentii*)

COMMONLY ASSOCIATED CONDITIONS

- Periodontitis
- Glossitis
- Pedunculated growths (pyogenic granulomata)

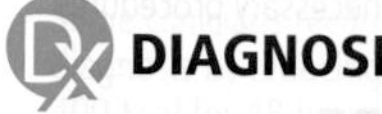

DIAGNOSIS

HISTORY

- Gum swelling and edema (usually painless)
- Gum erythema
- Bleeding of gums when brushing, flossing, or eating
- Inquire about HIV risk, pregnancy, nutritional deficiencies, diabetes, and other risk factors as indicated (See "Risk Factors").
- Smoking history
- Oral hygiene, dental visit history

PHYSICAL EXAM

- Normal gums should appear pink, firm, and shiny
- Gum swelling and edema (usually painless)
- Erythema
- Bleeding with manipulation of gums
- Change of normal gum contours
- Plaque and calculus (not easily removed)
- Edema of interdental papillae
- HIV gingivitis:
  - Also called linear gingival erythema
  - Narrow band of bright red inflamed gum surrounding neck of tooth
  - Painful
  - Bleeds easily
  - Rapid destruction of tissue
- Vincent disease:
  - Ulcers
  - Fever
  - Malaise
  - Regional lymphadenopathy
  - Pain
  - Mouth odor

DIAGNOSTIC TESTS & INTERPRETATION

Lab

Initial lab tests

- Possible smear or culture to identify causative agent (HIV gingivitis includes gram-negative anaerobes, enteric strains, and candida)
- Labs for contributing conditions (HIV, pregnancy, diabetes, nutritional deficiencies)

Imaging

Initial approach

No tests usually needed

Pathological Findings

- Acute or chronic inflammation
- Hyperemic capillaries
- Polymorphonuclear infiltration
- Papillary projections in subepithelial tissue
- Fibroblasts

DIFFERENTIAL DIAGNOSIS
- Periodontitis (deeper inflammation to connective tissue, ligaments, and alveolar bone)
- Glossitis
- Desquamative gingivitis (painful, persistent, usually middle-aged women)
- Pericoronitis (gum flap traps food and plaque over partially erupted molar), common in adolescence
- Gingival ulcers (aphthous, herpetic, malignancy, TB, syphilis)
- Specific forms of gingivitis: See "Description" including acute necrotizing ulcerative gingivitis (Vincent disease) and HIV gingivitis (linear gingival erythema)

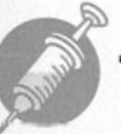

TREATMENT

MEDICATION
First Line
- Chlorhexidine rinses or varnishes may be used (4)
- Antibiotics indicated only for acute necrotizing ulcerative gingivitis (Vincent disease)
- Antibiotics:
  - Penicillin V: Pediatric dose, 25–50 mg/kg/d divided q6h; adult dose, 250–500 mg q6h, OR
  - Erythromycin: Pediatric dose 30–40 mg/kg/d divided q6h; adult dose, 250 mg q6h
- Topical corticosteroids:
  - Triamcinolone (0.147 mg/g) in Orabase (spray), applied locally t.i.d., q.i.d.
- Contraindications:
  - Allergy to specific medication
- Precautions:
  - Erythromycin frequently causes significant gastrointestinal issues.

Second Line
- Acetaminophen or ibuprofen for any pain (rare)
- Other antibiotics or antifungal rinses or systemics according to culture or smear
- Decapinol oral rinse (surfactant that acts as a physical barrier, making it harder for bacteria to stick to tooth surfaces) to reduce bacteria (not recommended for pregnant women or children under 12). Should be used in conjunction with other oral hygiene practices when those practices alone are not enough.

ADDITIONAL TREATMENT
General Measures
- Stop any contributing medications
- Remove irritating factors (plaque, calculus, faulty dentures)
- Good oral hygiene (see "General Prevention")
- Regular dental checkups (for scaling and polishing if plaque and/or tartar are present)
- No smoking
- Warm saline rinses b.i.d.

Issues for Referral
- Dental referral for cleanings and further treatment as needed
- If gingivitis becomes periodontitis, deep root scaling and planing may be indicated.

COMPLEMENTARY AND ALTERNATIVE MEDICINE
- Bilberry: Potentially helpful in reducing inflammation and stabilizing collagen tissue
- Coenzyme Q10: Topically, to restore coenzyme Q10 deficiency
- Replace any other deficiencies (e.g., vitamin C).

SURGERY/OTHER PROCEDURES
- Debridement for acute necrotizing gingivitis
- Minor surgery may be necessary to correct tissue overgrowth for gingivitis caused by medicines.

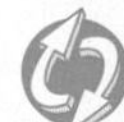

ONGOING CARE

FOLLOW-UP RECOMMENDATIONS
- Outpatient
- No restrictions

Patient Monitoring
Until clear; dental follow-up for continued cleanings and secondary prevention

DIET
- Well-balanced diet that includes fruits, vegetables, vitamin C; avoid sugary snacks and drinks, which contribute to plaque formation.
- Soft foods during flare if significant inflammation/bleeding for a few days

PATIENT EDUCATION
- Good oral hygiene including twice daily brushing with fluoridated toothpaste and daily flossing; regular dental visits
- Printable and viewable patient information available under "periodontal diseases" from the American Dental Association at http://www.ada.org; and the American Academy of Periodontology at http://www.perio.org

PROGNOSIS
- Usual course: Acute, relapsing, intermittent, chronic
- Prognosis: Generally favorable, responds well to appropriate treatment
- Left untreated may progress to periodontitis (controversial), which is a major cause of tooth loss

COMPLICATIONS
Severe periodontal disease (which is associated with heart disease, diabetes, and preterm birth)

REFERENCES

1. Mehta A, Sequeira PS, Sahoo RC, et al. Is bronchial asthma a risk factor for gingival diseases? A control study. *N Y State Dent J*. 2009;75:44–6.
2. Nilsson M, Kopp S. Gingivitis and periodontitis are related to repeated high levels of circulating tumor necrosis factor-alpha in patients with rheumatoid arthritis. *J Periodontol*. 2008;79:1689–96.
3. Deery C, Heanue M, Deacon S, et al. The effectiveness of manual versus powered toothbrushes for dental health: a systematic review. *J Dent*. 2004;32:197–211.
4. Puig-Silla M, Montiel-Company JM, Almerich-Silla JM. Use of chlorhexidine varnishes in preventing and treating periodontal disease. A review of the literature. *Med Oral Patol Oral Cir Bucal*. 2008;13:E257–60.

ADDITIONAL READING

- Armitage GC. Development of a classification system for periodontal diseases and conditions. *Ann Periodont*. 1999;4:1.
- Coventry J, Griffiths G, Scully C et al. Periodontal disease: ABC of oral health. *Br Med J*. 2000;321:36–9.
- Genco RJ. Current view of risk factors for periodontal diseases. *J Periodontol*. 1996;67:1041–9.
- Loesche WJ, Grossman NS. Periodontal disease as a specific, albeit chronic, infection: diagnosis and treatment. *Clin Microbiol Rev*. 2001;14:727–52.
- New Oral Rinse Helps Treat Gingivitis. FDA Consumer [serial on the Internet]. (2005, July), [cited July 22, 2008]; 39(4):5–6. Available from: Alt HealthWatch.
- Oliver RC, Brown LJ, Loer H. Peridontal disease in the United States population. *J Peridontol*. 1998; 69(2):269–78.

See Also (Topic, Algorithm, Electronic Media Element)
Glossitis, Dental Infection

Algorithm: Bleeding Gums

CODES

ICD9
- 523.00 Acute gingivitis, plaque induced
- 523.01 Acute gingivitis, non-plaque induced
- 523.10 Chronic gingivitis, plaque induced

CLINICAL PEARLS
- Gingivitis may be treated with regular dental cleanings, good oral hygiene, and use of chlorhexidine rinses.
- Untreated, gingivitis may progress to periodontitis, a possible contributor to systemic inflammation and its consequences (such as coronary artery disease and preterm labor).
- New onset or difficult to treat gingivitis, consider differential of etiology - pregnancy, HIV, diabetes, medications, vitamin deficiencies .

GLAUCOMA, PRIMARY CLOSED-ANGLE

Samantha R. Llanos, PharmD, RPh
Mark Iverson, MD

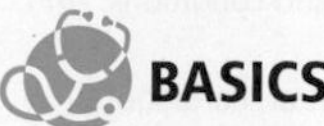

BASICS

DESCRIPTION

- Acute-angle closure (the term *glaucoma* is added when glaucomatous optic neuropathy is present):
  - At least 2 of the following symptoms: Ocular pain; N/V; intermittent blurred vision with halos, *plus*
  - At least 3 of the following signs: Intraocular pressure (IOP) >21 mm Hg; conjunctival injection; corneal epithelial edema; mid-dilated nonreactive pupil; shallower chamber in the presence of occlusion
- Primary-angle closure (the term *glaucoma* is added when glaucomatous optic neuropathy is present):
  - Occludable drainage angle *plus* signs that the peripheral iris has obstructed the trabecular meshwork (e.g., elevated IOP, lens opacities)
- Chronic angle-closure glaucoma: Refers to an eye with permanent closure of areas of the anterior chamber angle by peripheral anterior synechiae

Geriatric Considerations

Increased risk with age and prior history of cataract, hyperopia, and/or uveitis

Pediatric Considerations

Rare

Pregnancy Considerations

Medications used may cross the placenta and be excreted into breast milk.

EPIDEMIOLOGY

- 6th and 7th decades of life
- Female > Male
- Inuit and Asian > African and European
- Most common form of glaucoma worldwide, but only 10% of glaucoma in the US

Prevalence

Acute-angle closure glaucoma occurs in 1 in 1,000 Caucasians; 1 in 100 Asians; 2–4 in 100 Eskimos (lifetime)

RISK FACTORS

- Hyperopia
- Age >40–50 years old
- Shallow anterior chamber
- Female gender
- Family history of angle closure
- Asian or Inuit descent
- Pseudoexfoliation
- Medications that may induce angle-closure glaucoma:
  - Angiotensin-converting enzyme inhibitors (rare)
  - Adrenergic agonists (albuterol)
  - Anticholinergics
  - Antihistamines
  - Antidepressants: Selective serotonin reuptake inhibitors, TCAs
  - Cholinergic agents (pilocarpine)
  - Noncatecholamine adrenergic agonists
  - Sulfa-based drugs
  - Topiramate
  - Warfarin (rare)

Genetics

Polygenic inheritance: 1st-degree relatives have a 2–5% lifetime risk.

GENERAL PREVENTION

- Routine eye exam with gonioscopy for high-risk populations
- United States Preventive Services Task Force: Insufficient evidence to recommend for or against screening adults for glaucoma

PATHOPHYSIOLOGY

- Peripheral iris apposition to the trabecular meshwork obstructs the outflow of aqueous humor through the trabecular meshwork, which causes elevation in IOP.
- The underlying mechanism is anterior lens displacement or other anatomic abnormality, leading to pupillary block in which aqueous humor egress through the pupil is limited. This causes pressure to build posterior to the iris, leading to anterior iris displacement.

ETIOLOGY

Predisposing ocular anatomy

COMMONLY ASSOCIATED CONDITIONS

- Cataract
- Hyperopia
- Microphthalmos
- Systemic hypertension

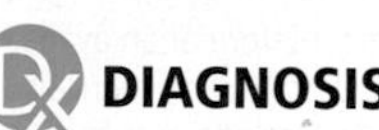

DIAGNOSIS

HISTORY

- Patient's previous medical and ophthalmologic history
- Family history of glaucoma
- Obtain history of prescription and over-the-counter medications
- Precipitating factors (dim light, meds)
- Review of symptoms
- Acute:
  - Severe unilateral ocular pain
  - Blurred vision
  - Lacrimation
  - Photophobia
  - Halos around lights/objects
  - Frontal, ipsilateral, headache
  - Nausea and vomiting
- Chronic:
  - May have subacute symptoms (intermittent subacute attacks)
  - Compromised peripheral, then central vision
  - May be asymptomatic

PHYSICAL EXAM

- Includes, but is not limited to, the following in the undilated eye (1)[C]:
  - Visual acuity
  - Visual field testing and ocular motility
  - Pupil size and reactivity (mid-dilated, minimally reactive)
  - External examination
  - Undilated fundus exam (congestion, cupping, atrophy of optic nerve)
  - Slit-lamp biomicroscopy (anterior segments)
  - Tonometry (determination of IOP)
  - Gonioscopy (visualization of the angle)
- Acute:
  - Elevated intraocular pressure (usually 40–80 mm Hg)
  - Corneal microcystic edema (haze)
  - Lid edema, conjunctival hyperemia, and circumcorneal injection (ciliary flush)
  - Fixed mid-dilated pupil (often oval) and firm globe
  - Shallow anterior chamber, often with inflammatory reaction (cell and flare)
  - Blepharospasm (severe cases)
  - Pain with eye movement
  - Closed angle by gonioscopy
- Chronic:
  - Multiple peripheral anterior synechiae
  - Normal or elevated intraocular pressure
  - Increased cup-to-disc ratio or excavation of disc
  - Glaucoma flecks (lens) and iris atrophy (previous acute attacks)

DIAGNOSTIC TESTS & INTERPRETATION

Imaging

Ultrasound biomicroscopy

Diagnostic Procedures/Surgery

Careful ophthalmic examination, including gonioscopy and tonometry (1,2,3)[C]

Pathological Findings

- Corneal stromal and epithelial edema
- Endothelial cell loss (guttata)
- Iris stromal necrosis
- Anterior subcapsular cataract (*glaukomflecken*)
- Optic disc congestion, cupping, excavation
- Optic nerve atrophy

DIFFERENTIAL DIAGNOSIS

- Acute orbital compartment syndrome
- Traumatic hyphema
- Conjunctivitis, episcleritis
- Corneal abrasion
- Glaucoma, malignant or neovascular
- Herpes zoster ophthalmicus
- Iritis and uveitis
- Orbital/periorbital infection
- Plateau iris syndrome
- Vitreous or subconjunctival hemorrhage
- Tight necktie, causing increased IOP

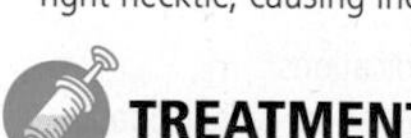

TREATMENT

Goals of Treatment

- Reduce acutely increased IOP.
- Remove anything causing pupillary block .
- Treat residual increased IOP caused by permanent trabecular meshwork dysfunction.

MEDICATION

- Practically speaking, acute angle glaucoma is managed with oral mannitol **or** glycerin for a rapid decrease in IOP, and then, once the cornea clears, a peripheral iridotomy is done.
- Initiate medical therapy first, using some or all of the following (1)[C],(4)[B]:

- Topical/systemic carbonic anhydrase inhibitor
  - Acetazolamide (Diamox) 500 mg IV *plus/or* 500 mg PO; dorzolamide 2% eyedrops or brinzolamide (Azopt) 1% suspension; 1 drop in affected eye q8h.
  - Contraindications/precautions: Sulfa-allergy (risk of cross-sensitivity), bitter taste, eyelid reactions
- β-Blockers:
  - Timolol (Timoptic) 0.5% solution, levobunolol (Betagan) 0.5% solution *or* betaxolol (Betoptic) 0.5% solution; also carteolol (generic) 1% solution or metipranolol (OptiPranolol) 0.3% solution, 1 drop in affected eye q12h.
  - Contraindications/precautions: Decompensated heart failure, sinus bradycardia $\geq$2nd-degree heart block, severe COPD/asthma; increased risk of bradycardia or heart block with digoxin, verapamil, diltiazem, or clonidine; effect on IOP may be lessened in patients taking oral β-blockers
- α-Agonists:
  - Apraclonidine (Iopidine) 0.5–1% solution, 1 drop in affected eye q8h; brimonidine 1 drop 2–3 times daily
  - Prostaglandin analogs: latanoprost (Xalatan), travoprost (Travatan), bimatoprost (Lumigan) 1 drop daily. Precautions: Irreversible changes to iris, eyelid and eyelash pigmentation, eyelash growth, itching, redness, edema
- Topical steroid: (Prednisolone 1% solution) 1–2 drops 2–4+ times daily
- Miotics:
  - Pilocarpine (2–4% solution, 1 drop in affected eye q6–8h); do not use unless directed by ophthalmologist .
  - Carbachol 3% solution, 1 drop 4 times daily or echothiophate iodide (phospholine iodide) 0.125% solution, 1 drop twice daily
  - Precautions: May worsen the condition due to anterior rotation of the lens-iris diaphragm, impaired night vision,
- Hyperosmotic agents:
  - Glycerin, 1–2 g/kg PO, repeat q5h p.r.n.; isosorbide, 1.5 g/kg PO; mannitol 20% solution, 1.5–2 g/kg over 30 minutes
  - Precautions: Glycerin-caution in patients with congestive heart failure or diabetes; mannitol-caution in patients with congestive heart failure or renal failure

ADDITIONAL TREATMENT

General Measures

- For acute form:
  - Manage extraocular symptoms, such as nausea and pain.
  - Obtain immediate ophthalmology consult.
- Ocular goals of therapy through medical and surgical treatment:
  - Reduce IOP to <35 mm Hg or by >25% of presenting IOP (4)[B].
  - Prevent damage to the optic nerve.
  - Prevent central retinal artery occlusion.
  - Prevent or reverse angle closure.

Additional Therapies

- Initiate immediate emergency ophthalmologic treatment.
- Keep patient supine.

SURGERY/OTHER PROCEDURES

- Acute (1,5)[B]:
  - Laser peripheral iridotomy per ophthalmology (1,5)[B]
  - Perform surgical iridectomy if laser is not possible.
- Chronic:
  - Goniosynechialysis
  - Phacoemulsification

IN-PATIENT CONSIDERATIONS

Admission Criteria

- Patient requires metabolic $\pm$ electrolyte and volume status monitoring (with osmotic agents)
- Maintain ophthalmology follow-up.

IV Fluids

IV access

Nursing

Implement emergency ophthalmic plan of care.

Discharge Criteria

Patient is stable for outpatient follow-up.

ONGOING CARE

FOLLOW-UP RECOMMENDATIONS

- Schedule immediate ophthalmologic follow-up.
- Hospital admission if clinically warranted

Patient Monitoring

- Postsurgical follow-up
- Fellow eye evaluation
- Chronic monitoring post acute attack per ophthalmology

DIET

Regular as tolerated

PATIENT EDUCATION

- Advise patient to seek emergency medical attention if experiencing a change in visual acuity, blurred vision, eye pain, or headache.
- New medication counseling
- If narrow angles but no peripheral iridotomy performed: Avoid decongestants, motion sickness medications, adrenergic agents, antipsychotics, antidepressants, and anticholinergic agents.
- Proper eyedrop administration technique
- Patients with significant visual impairment should be referred to vision rehab and social services
- Patient education materials:
  - Glaucoma Research Foundation at: http://www.glaucoma.org
  - National Eye Institute at: http://www.nei.nih.gov
  - Glaucoma handout from American Academy of Family Physicians
  - Handout on using glaucoma eyedrops in Am Fam Physician 1999;59(7):1882

PROGNOSIS

- With timely treatment, most patients do not have permanent vision loss.
- Depends on:
  - Time to treatment
  - Underlying eye disease
  - Ethnicity

COMPLICATIONS

- Chronic corneal edema
- Corneal fibrosis and vascularization
- Iris atrophy
- Cataract
- Optic atrophy
- Malignant glaucoma
- Central retinal artery/vein occlusion
- Permanent decrease in visual acuity
- Repeat episode
- Fellow eye attack

REFERENCES

1. American Academy of Ophthalmology. *Primary angle closure preferred practice pattern*. San Francisco: American Academy of Ophthalmology, 2005. Available at: http://www.aao.org.
2. Asrani S, Sarunic M, Santiago C, et al. Detailed visualization of the anterior segment using fourier-domain optical coherence tomography. *Arch Ophthalmol*. 2008;126:765–71.
3. Barkana Y, Dorairaj SK, Gerber Y, et al. Agreement between gonioscopy and ultrasound biomicroscopy in detecting iridotrabecular apposition. *Arch Ophthalmol*. 2007;125:1331–5.
4. Choong YF, Irfan S, Menage MJ. Acute angle closure glaucoma: an evaluation of a protocol for acute treatment. *Eye*. 1999;13(Pt 5):613–6.
5. Saw SM, Gazzard G, Friedman DS. Interventions for angle-closure glaucoma: an evidence-based update. *Ophthalmology*. 2003;110:1869–78; quiz 1878-9, 1930.

ADDITIONAL READING

Tripathi RC, Tripathi BJ, Haggerty C. Drug-induced glaucomas: mechanism and management. *Drug Saf*. 2003;26:749–67.

See Also (Topic, Algorithm, Electronic Media Element)

Glaucoma, Primary Open-Angle

CODES

ICD9

- 365.20 Primary angle-closure glaucoma, unspecified
- 365.22 Acute angle-closure glaucoma
- 365.23 Chronic angle-closure glaucoma

CLINICAL PEARLS

- Examiner can determine if patient is hyperopic by observing the *magnification* of the patient's face through their glasses (myopic lenses minify).
- A careful history may reveal similar episodes of angle closure that resolved spontaneously.
- Miotics are ineffective in the setting of high IOP (due to iris sphincter ischemia) and can potentially worsen angle closure by causing anterior rotation of the lens–iris diaphragm.

GLAUCOMA, PRIMARY OPEN-ANGLE

Richard W. Allinson, MD

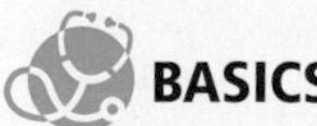

BASICS

DESCRIPTION

- Primary open-angle glaucoma (POAG) is an optic neuropathy resulting in visual field loss frequently associated with increased intraocular pressure (IOP).
- Normal IOP is 10–22 mm Hg. However, glaucomatous optic nerve damage also can occur with normal IOP and as a secondary manifestation of other disorders, such as corticosteroid-induced glaucoma.
- System(s) affected: Nervous
- Synonym(s): Chronic open-angle glaucoma

Pregnancy Considerations

Prostaglandins should be avoided during pregnancy in the treatment of POAG.

EPIDEMIOLOGY

Incidence

- Predominant age: Usually >40 years
- Increases with age
- Predominant gender: Male = Female

Prevalence

Prevalence of POAG in persons >40 years of age is ~1.8%.

Geriatric Considerations

Increasing prevalence with increasing age

RISK FACTORS

- Increased IOP
- Myopia
- DM
- African American
- Elderly
- Positive family history
- Central corneal thickness <550 μm
- Larger vertical cup-to-disc ratio
- Larger horizontal cup-to-disc ratio
- Disc hemorrhage
- Prolonged use of topical, periocular, inhaled, or systemic corticosteroids

Genetics

A family history of glaucoma increases the risk for developing glaucoma.

GENERAL PREVENTION

- Genetic testing may help to screen for POAG.
- Possible reduced risk of open-angle glaucoma with long-term use of oral statins

PATHOPHYSIOLOGY

- Abnormal aqueous outflow resulting in increased IOP
- Normally, aqueous is produced by the ciliary epithelium of the ciliary body and is secreted into the posterior chamber of the eye.
- Aqueous then flows through the pupil and enters the anterior chamber to be drained by the trabecular meshwork in the iridocorneal angle of the eye into the Schlemm canal and into the venous system of the episclera.
- 5–10% of the total aqueous outflow leaves via the uveoscleral pathway.

ETIOLOGY

- Impaired aqueous outflow through the trabecular meshwork
- Increased resistance within the aqueous drainage system

COMMONLY ASSOCIATED CONDITIONS

DM

DIAGNOSIS

HISTORY

Painless, slowly progressive visual loss; patients are generally unaware of the visual loss until late in the disease. Central visual acuity remains unaffected until late in the disease.

PHYSICAL EXAM

- Increased IOP
- Cup-to-disc ratio (C:D) >0.5: Normal eyes show a characteristic configuration for disc rim thickness of inferior ≥ superior ≥ nasal ≥ temporal (ISNT rule).
- Earliest visual field defects are paracentral scotomas and peripheral nasal steps.

DIAGNOSTIC TESTS & INTERPRETATION

Imaging

Initial approach

- Optical coherence tomography can be useful in the detection of glaucoma by measuring the thickness of the retinal nerve fiber layer (RNFL).
- RNFL is thinner in patients with glaucoma.
- RNFL thickness is affected by age, ethnicity, axial length, and optic disc area. RNFL tends to be thinner with older age, Caucasians, greater axial length, and smaller optic disc area.
- Factors associated with variability in RNFL thickness measurements include signal-strength variability, low analysis confidence, and low RNFL thickness.

Diagnostic Procedures/Surgery

- Visual field testing: Perimetry
- Tonometry to measure IOP
- Ophthalmoscopy to assess optic nerve for glaucomatous damage

Pathological Findings

- Atrophy and cupping of optic nerve
- Loss of retinal ganglion cells and their axons produces defects in the retinal nerve fiber layer.

DIFFERENTIAL DIAGNOSIS

- Normal-tension glaucoma
- Optic nerve pits
- Anterior ischemic optic neuropathy
- Compressive lesions of the optic nerve or chiasm
- Posthemorrhagic (shock optic neuropathy)

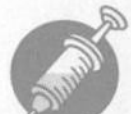

TREATMENT

MEDICATION

- >1 medication, with different mechanisms of action, may be needed.
- When ≥3 medications are required, compliance is difficult, and surgery may be needed. Ocular hypotensive agent categories:
  - β-Adrenergic antagonists (nonselective and selective): Decrease aqueous formation: Timolol 0.5% 1 drop in affected eye q12h
  - Parasympathomimetics (miotic), including cholinergic (direct-acting) and anticholinesterase agents (indirect-acting parasympathomimetic): Increase aqueous outflow:
    - Pilocarpine 1–4% 1 drop in affected eye b.i.d.–q.i.d. (cholinergic)
    - Demecarium bromide 0.125% 1 drop in affected eye b.i.d. (anticholinesterase)
- Carbonic anhydrase inhibitors (oral, topical): Decrease aqueous formation:
  - Acetazolamide 250 mg p.o. q.i.d.
  - Dorzolamide 2% 1 drop t.i.d.
- Adrenergic agonists (nonselective and selective α_2-adrenergic agonists):
  - Epinephrine 0.5–2% 1 drop b.i.d. and dipivefrin 0.1% 1 drop b.i.d. (nonselective agents) increase aqueous outflow through the trabecular meshwork and increase uveoscleral outflow.
  - Brimonidine tartrate 0.1% 1 drop t.i.d. (α_2-adrenergic agonist) decreases aqueous formation and increases uveoscleral outflow.
- Prostaglandin analogues: Enhance uveoscleral outflow: Latanoprost 0.005% 1 drop at bedtime
- Hyperosmotic agents: Increase blood osmolality, drawing water from the vitreous cavity:
  - Mannitol 20% solution administered IV at 2 g/kg of body weight
  - Glycerin 50% solution administered orally; dosage is usually 4–7 oz
- Contraindications:
  - Nonselective β-adrenergic antagonists: Avoid in asthma, COPD, 2nd- and 3rd-degree A-V block, and decompensated heart failure. Betaxolol is a selective β-adrenergic antagonist and is safer in pulmonary disease.
  - Parasympathomimetics (miotic): Indirect-acting parasympathomimetic agents increase risk of ocular and systemic side effects and are used rarely.
  - Carbonic anhydrase inhibitors:
    - Do not use with sulfa drug allergies.
    - Do not use with cirrhosis because of the risk of hepatic encephalopathy.
  - Adrenergic agonists: Caution recommended when using brimonidine and MAO inhibitor or TCA and in patients with vascular insufficiency. Brimonidine can cause excessive sleepiness and lethargy in children.
  - Prostaglandin analogues: Caution with uveitis and avoided during pregnancy
  - Hyperosmotic agents:
    - Glycerin can produce hyperglycemia or ketoacidosis in diabetic patients.
    - Can cause congestive heart failure
    - Do not use in patients with anuria.

- Precautions:
  - β-Adrenergic antagonists: Caution with obstructive pulmonary disease, heart failure, and DM
  - Parasympathomimetics (miotic): Cause pupillary constriction and may cause decreased vision in patients with a cataract, and may cause an eye ache or myopia due to increased accommodation. All miotics break down the blood–aqueous barrier and may induce chronic iridocyclitis.
  - Adrenergic agonists (e.g., brimonidine): Caution with vascular insufficiency
  - Prostaglandin analogues may cause increased pigmentation of the iris and periorbital tissue (eyelid):
    - Increased pigmentation and growth of eyelashes
    - Should be used with caution in active intraocular inflammation (iritis/uveitis)
    - Caution is also advised in eyes with risk factors for herpes simplex, iritis, and cystoid macular edema.
    - Macular edema may be a complication associated with treatment.
  - Hyperosmotic agents: Caution in diabetics, dehydrated patients, and those with cardiac, renal, and hepatic disease
- Significant possible interactions: β-Adrenergic antagonists: Caution in patients taking calcium antagonists because of possible A-V conduction disturbances, left ventricular failure, or hypotension
- Parasympathomimetics (miotic): Indirect-acting parasympathomimetic agents, anticholinesterase eye drops, can reduce serum pseudocholinesterase levels. If succinylcholine is used for induction of general anesthesia, prolonged apnea may result.

ADDITIONAL TREATMENT

General Measures

- Early Manifest Glaucoma Trial:
  - Early treatment delays progression.
  - The magnitude of initial IOP reduction influences disease progression (1)[A].
- Ocular Hypertension Treatment Study:
  - Patients who only had increased IOP in the range of 24–32 mm Hg were treated with topical ocular hypotensive medication.
  - Treatment produced ~20% reduction in IOP.
  - At 5 years, treatment reduced the incidence of POAG by >50%: 9.5% in the observation group vs 4.4% in the medication-treated group (2)[A]
- The Collaborative Normal-Tension Glaucoma Study Group:
  - Therapeutic intervention that resulted in a 30% decrease in IOP and helped to prevent progression of visual field loss (3)[A]
- The Advanced Glaucoma Intervention Study:
  - Eyes were randomized to laser trabeculoplasty or filtering surgery when medical therapy failed.
  - In follow-up, if the IOP was always <18 mm Hg, the visual fields tended to stabilize. When IOP was >17 mm Hg more than 1/2 of the time, patients tended to have worsening of their visual fields (4)[A].
  - Whites did better with trabeculectomy first, whereas African Americans did better with argon laser trabeculoplasty as the initial procedure.
- Collaborative Initial Glaucoma Treatment Study:
  - Both initial medical and surgical treatment achieved significant IOP reduction, and both had little visual field loss over time (5)[A].

SURGERY/OTHER PROCEDURES

- Argon laser trabeculoplasty (ALT):
  - Applied to 180 degrees of the trabecular meshwork
  - Improves aqueous outflow
  - The Glaucoma Laser Trial Research Group showed in newly diagnosed, previously untreated patients with POAG that ALT was as effective as topical glaucoma medication within the 1st 2 years of follow-up.
  - Usually reserved for patients needing better IOP control while taking topical glaucoma drops
- Trabeculectomy (glaucoma filtering surgery):
  - Usually reserved for patients needing better IOP control after maximal medical therapy and who may have previously undergone an ALT
  - Mitomycin C can be applied at the time of surgery to increase the chances of a surgical success.
  - Subconjunctival bevacizumab may be a beneficial adjunctive therapy for reducing late surgical failure after trabeculectomy.
- Shunt (tube) surgery:
  - For example, Molteno and Ahmed devices
  - Generally reserved for difficult glaucoma cases in which conventional filtering surgery has failed or is likely to fail
- Tube Versus Trabeculectomy (TVT) Study.
  - After 3 years of follow-up, both procedures were associated with similar intraocular pressure reduction and the number of glaucoma medications needed (6)[A].
- Ciliary body ablation: Indicated to lower IOP in patients with poor visual potential or those who are poor candidates for filtering or shunt procedures

ONGOING CARE

FOLLOW-UP RECOMMENDATIONS

Patient Monitoring

- Monitor vision and IOP every 3–6 months.
- Visual field testing every 6–18 months
- Optic nerve evaluation every 3–18 months depending on POAG control
- A worsening of the mean deviation by 2 dB on the Humphrey field analyzer and confirmed by a single test after 6 months had a 72% probability of progression.
- The IOP response to ocular hypotensive agents tends to be reduced in persons with thicker corneas.

PATIENT EDUCATION

POAG is a silent robber of vision, and patients may not appreciate the significance of their disease until much of their visual field is lost.

PROGNOSIS

- With standard glaucoma therapy, the rate of visual field loss in POAG is slow.
- Patients still may lose vision and develop blindness, even when treated appropriately.
- The rate of legal blindness from POAG over a follow-up of 22 years is 19%.

COMPLICATIONS

Blindness

REFERENCES

1. Heijl A, Leske MC, Bengtsson B, et al. Reduction of intraocular pressure and glaucoma progression: results from the Early Manifest Glaucoma Trial. *Arch Ophthalmol*. 2002;120:1268–79.
2. Kass MA, Heuer DK, Higginbotham EJ, et al. The Ocular Hypertension Treatment Study: a randomized trial determines that topical ocular hypotensive medication delays or prevents the onset of primary open-angle glaucoma. *Arch Ophthalmol*. 2002;120:701–13; discussion 829–30.
3. Comparison of glaucomatous progression between untreated patients with normal-tension glaucoma and patients with therapeutically reduced intraocular pressures. Collaborative Normal-Tension Glaucoma Study Group. *Am J Ophthalmol*. 1998;126:487–97.
4. The Advanced Glaucoma Intervention Study (AGIS): 7. The relationship between control of intraocular pressure and visual field deterioration.The AGIS Investigators. *Am J Ophthalmol*. 2000;130: 429–40.
5. Lichter PR, et al. CIGTS Study Group. Interim clinical outcomes in the Collaborative Initial Glaucoma Treatment Study comparing initial treatment randomized to medications or surgery. *Ophthalmol*. 2001;108:1943–53.
6. Gedde SJ, Schiffman JC, et al. Three-Year Follow-up of the Tube Versus Trabeculectomy Study. *Am J Ophthalmol*. 2009;148:670–684.

CODES

ICD9

365.11 Primary open angle glaucoma

CLINICAL PEARLS

- Topical or systemic steroids can cause the IOP to increase.
- Pain is not a frequent symptom of POAG.
- Painless, slowly progressive visual loss; patients generally are unaware of the visual loss until late in the disease. Central visual acuity remains unaffected until late in the disease.
- Patients still may lose vision and develop blindness, even when treated appropriately.

GLOMERULONEPHRITIS, ACUTE

Carla M. Nester, MD

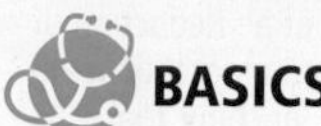

BASICS

DESCRIPTION

- Acute glomerulonephritis (GN) is an inflammatory process involving the glomerulus of the kidney, resulting in a clinical syndrome consisting of hematuria, proteinuria, hypertension, and renal insufficiency.
- Acute glomerulonephritis may be one of many primary diseases, or it may present as part of a systemic disease:
  - Postinfectious GN
  - IgA nephropathy–Henoch Schönlein purpura
  - Antiglomerular basement membrane disease (anti-GBM disease)
  - Antineutrophil cytoplasmic antibody (ANCA)-associated GN
  - Membranoproliferative GN (MPGN)
  - Lupus nephritis
  - Cryoglobulin-associated GN
- Clinical severity ranges from asymptomatic microscopic or gross hematuria to a rapid loss of kidney function (rapidly progressive glomerulonephritis: RPGN).

ALERT

Urgent investigation and treatment are required to avoid irreversible loss of kidney function.

EPIDEMIOLOGY

- Postinfectious GN:
  - Most commonly follows group A beta-hemolytic *Streptococcus* infection, but can occur as a result of other infections.
  - Onset occurs 1–3 weeks after an infectious process (throat or skin).
  - Accounts for 80% of acute GN in children
- IgA nephropathy:
  - Most common form of primary acute GN
  - Occurs mainly in the 2nd and 3rd decades
  - Male:Female: 3:1
  - Incidence differs geographically: Asia > US
- Anti-GBM disease:
  - Also known as Goodpasture disease
  - A noted cause of the pulmonary–renal syndrome
  - Occurs most commonly in the 2nd or 3rd decade
  - Male:Female: 6:1
- ANCA-associated GN:
  - Uncommon: Often has a relapsing and remitting course
  - 3 disease presentations:
    - Wegener granulomatosis
    - Churg-Strauss disease
    - Microscopic polyangiitis
  - Older patients are more commonly affected, though this GN can affect any age group.
- MPGN:
  - May be primary or secondary
  - May present in the setting of a systemic viral or rheumatic illness
- Lupus nephritis:
  - 30–70% of systemic lupus patients will have renal involvement.
- Cryoglobulin-associated vasculitis:
  - 80% of cases are associated with hepatitis C infection.

RISK FACTORS

- Epidemics of nephritogenic strains of streptococci are triggers for postinfectious GN.
- Hepatic cirrhosis and celiac disease place patients at risk for IgA nephropathy.
- Anti-GBM disease has been associated with influenza A infection and inhaled hydrocarbon solvent exposure.
- ANCA-associated GN is increased in settings where there is increased silica exposure (i.e., earthquakes and farming).
- Complement factor abnormalities and infection with hepatitis B and/or C are known to be associated with MPGN.
- Infection with hepatitis C is a risk factor for developing cryoglobulinemic GN.
- Mutations in alternate complement pathway genes are associated with membranoproliferative glomerulonephritis.

Genetics

There are likely to be genetic factors that play a role in susceptibility to many of the acute GNs, though these have not been sufficiently defined to be useful clinically.

GENERAL PREVENTION

Early detection is paramount.

ETIOLOGY

- In general, an immunologic mechanism triggers inflammation and proliferation of glomerular tissue.
- Postinfectious GN:
  - Host immune reaction to nephritogenic strains of streptococci are triggers.
- IgA nephropathy:
  - Relates to an abnormal glycosylation of IgA
- Anti-GBM disease:
  - Caused by autoantibodies that target type IV collagen of basement membranes
- ANCA-associated GN:
  - Autoantibodies against neutrophil granules are involved in the pathogenesis.
- MPGN:
  - An immune or genetic etiology is presumed, which triggers renal deposits and inflammation.
- Lupus nephritis:
  - An immune complex-mediated glomerular disease
- Cryoglobulin-associated GN:
  - An immune etiology is presumed, but not clearly defined.

DIAGNOSIS

HISTORY

- Patients may complain of cola- or tea-colored urine and decreased urine volume.
- Edema occurs in many patients, typically face and lower extremities
- Shortness of breath may occur with significant fluid overload.
- Generalized malaise
- Patients may also present with complaints more specific to the associated disease:
  - Joint pain or rash in lupus nephritis
  - Hemoptysis in anti-GBM disease
  - Sinusitis and pulmonary infiltrates in ANCA-associated GN
  - Abdominal pain and purpura in IgA-Henoch Schönlein purpura
  - Purpura and skin vasculitis in cryoglobulinemia-associated GN

PHYSICAL EXAM

- A complete physical exam may discover clues to systemic disease as a potential cause.
- Sinus disease: ANCA-associated GN
- Pharyngitis or impetigo: Postinfectious GN
- Pulmonary abnormality: Anti-GBM disease or lupus nephritis
- Hepatomegaly or liver tenderness could point to cryoglobulinemia-associated GN or IgA nephropathy.
- Purpura may point to ANCA-associated GN or Henoch Schönlein purpura GN.

DIAGNOSTIC TESTS & INTERPRETATION

Lab

- Urinalysis with examination of sediment:
  - Dysmorphic red blood cells (RBCs) or RBC casts on urine microscopy indicate glomerular hematuria and suggest the diagnosis of an acute glomerulonephritis.
- Electrolytes, blood urea nitrogen, creatinine, complete blood count
- Antistreptolysin O titer
- Streptozyme
- Complement levels (C3 and C4):
  - C3 complement levels are abnormal in postinfectious GN; C3 and C4 are abnormal in lupus nephritis and MPGN; C4 can be low in cryoglobulinemia.
- Proteinuria:
  - 24-hour collection or random urine protein/creatinine ratio
- Antinuclear antibody to rule out lupus nephritis
- ANCA antibody screen:
  - MPO and PR3 antibodies
- Anti-GBM antibody
- Hepatitis B antigen
- Hepatitis C antibody

Imaging

A chest x-ray may be useful to define the significance of hemoptysis or a suspected infiltrate on exam.

Pathological Findings

Renal biopsy:

- If clinical picture is consistent with postinfectious GN in a child, a biopsy may not be needed.
- If there is clinical suspicion for other causes of acute GN, renal biopsy should be done.
- Light microscopy:
  - Diffuse hypercellularity suggests a proliferative disease such as IgA nephropathy, lupus nephritis, or postinfectious GN.

- Immunofluorescence:
  - IgA staining is pathognomonic for IgA nephropathy, with the absence of staining suggesting ANCA-associated GN.
- Electron microscopy:
  - The location of immunoglobulin deposits is useful in pointing to a particular diagnosis.

DIFFERENTIAL DIAGNOSIS

- The differential for hematuria (without clear indication that it is from a glomerular origin) should include trauma, prostate diseases, urologic cancer, or renal stone disease.
- If the urine blood is felt to be of glomerular origin, the differential should include each of the glomerular diseases that can present as an acute glomerulonephritis.

TREATMENT

Supportive in post infectious

MEDICATION

First Line

- Hypertension:
  - Diuretics are useful, given that salt retention and edema are often present.
  - Calcium channel blockers
  - Avoid angiotensin-converting enzyme inhibitors if significant renal dysfunction is present.
- Peripheral edema:
  - Loop diuretics are often required due to the degree of edema.
- Pulmonary edema:
  - Oxygen and diuretic
- Hyperkalemia:
  - Sodium polystyrene sulfonate (Kayexalate) resin: 15 g p.o. every day to q.i.d. in 10% sorbitol
- Acidosis: Sodium bicarbonate 1–2 mEq/kg per dose (1–2 mmol/kg per dose) IV or p.o.

Second Line

- Each of the glomerular diseases often requires a specific treatment plan based on renal biopsy results; therefore, a nephrologist is often guiding care at this point.
- Pulse methylprednisolone has been reported to be useful in rapidly progressive forms of glomerulonephritis (1,2)[A].
- Crescents noted on renal biopsy are treated with the alkylating agent known as cyclophosphamide (1,2)[A].
- ANCA-associated renal disease, anti-GBM disease, and proliferative forms of lupus are treated with steroids plus either cyclophosphamide or mycophenolate (1,2,3,4,5)[A].
- Plasmapheresis has been shown to be effective in cases of pulmonary hemorrhage and in some patients who present in renal failure (2)[A].
- Dialysis may be needed for uremia, hyperkalemia refractory to medical management, intractable acidosis, and diuretic-resistant pulmonary edema.

ADDITIONAL TREATMENT

Issues for Referral

Consultation with a nephrologist is often required in order to assist with renal biopsy to confirm diagnosis and to assist with management.

IN-PATIENT CONSIDERATIONS

Admission Criteria

Consider admission for patients with no urine output, significant hypertension, and suspicion of pulmonary hemorrhage or fluid overload that is compromising heart or respiratory function.

Discharge Criteria

Hemodynamically stable patients without complications may be managed as outpatients.

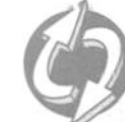

ONGOING CARE

FOLLOW-UP RECOMMENDATIONS

Patient Monitoring

Depends on type of glomerulonephritis:

- Regular blood pressure checks and urinalysis to detect recurrence; assessment of renal function to detect acute or follow chronic renal disease as a result of the primary event; and regular clinical assessment to detect suspicious symptoms that may herald a recurrence (i.e., rash, joint complaint, hemoptysis)
- Periodic reassessment of serology tests to detect asymptomatic individuals

DIET

- No-added-salt diet and fluid restriction until edema and hypertension clear
- Avoid high-potassium foods if significant renal dysfunction is present.

PATIENT EDUCATION

- National Kidney Foundation, 30 E. 33rd Street, Suite 1100, New York, NY 10016; (212) 889-2210
- Web site: http://vsearch.nlm.nih.gov/vivisimo/cgi-bin/query-meta?v%3Aproject=medlineplus&query=glomerulonephritis&x=48&y=10 - then search under the individual disease

PROGNOSIS

- In general, the prognosis depends on the cause of the glomerulonephritis.
- The GN may be self-limited (i.e., postinfectious GN) or part of a chronic disease that makes the possibility of recurrence likely.

COMPLICATIONS

- Hypertensive retinopathy and encephalopathy
- Rapidly progressive glomerulonephritis
- Microscopic hematuria may persist for years.
- Chronic kidney disease
- Nephrotic syndrome (~10%)

REFERENCES

1. Flanc RS, Roberts MA, Strippoli GF, et al. Treatment for lupus nephritis. *Cochrane Database Syst Rev.* 2004;CD002922.
2. Walters G, Willis NS, Craig JC. Interventions for renal vasculitis in adults. *Cochrane Database Syst Rev.* 2008;CD003232.
3. Hu W, Liu C, Xie H, et al. Mycophenolate Mofetil Versus Cyclophosphamide for Inducing Remission of ANCA Vasculitis with Moderate Renal Involvement. *Nephrol Dial Transplant.* 2007.
4. Walsh M, James M, Jayne D, et al. Mycophenolate Mofetil for Induction Therapy of Lupus Nephritis: A Systematic Review and Meta-Analysis. *Clin J Am Soc Nephrol.* 2007.
5. Isenberg D, Appel GB, Contreras G, Dooley MA, Ginzler EM, Jayne D, Sánchez-Guerrero J, Wofsy D, Yu X, Solomons N et al. Influence of race/ethnicity on response to lupus nephritis treatment: the ALMS study. *Rheumatology (Oxford).* 2010;49:128–40.

ADDITIONAL READING

Kaplan AA et al. The use of apheresis in immune renal disorders. *Ther Apher Dial.* 2003;7:165–72.

See Also (Topic, Algorithm, Electronic Media Element)

Hyperkalemia; Hypertensive Emergencies; Renal Failure, Acute

Algorithm: Hematuria

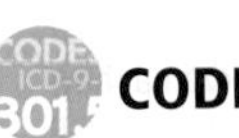

CODES

ICD9

580.9 Acute glomerulonephritis with unspecified pathological lesion in kidney

CLINICAL PEARLS

- Dysmorphic RBCs and RBC casts are a key component of the urinalysis in glomerulonephritis.
- Postinfectious GN in children is typically a self-limited disease.
- Searching for other organ involvement is useful in establishing a definitive diagnosis.
- With discovery of a GN, monitor the initial renal function labs frequently to identify a rapidly progressive GN.

GONOCOCCAL INFECTIONS

Paul E. Lyons, MD

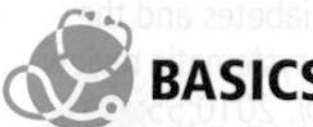

BASICS

DESCRIPTION

Gonorrhea is a sexually or vertically transmitted bacterial infection that has a predilection for epithelial cells.

- Caused by the gram-negative intracellular diplococci, *Neisseria gonorrhoeae*; virtually any mucosal membrane can be infected.
- Infection commonly manifests itself as urethritis, salpingitis, cervicitis, pelvic inflammatory disease (PID), epididymitis, or proctitis.
- Hematogenous dissemination may also occur and lead to fever, skin lesions, arthralgias, purulent arthritis, tenosynovitis, endocarditis or, rarely, meningitis.
- Asymptomatic carrier state can occur in both sexes.
- In newborns, gonococcal ophthalmia neonatorum, a purulent conjunctivitis, may occur after vaginal delivery by an infected mother and may lead to blindness if not treated promptly.
- System(s) affected: Cardiovascular; Musculoskeletal; Nervous; Reproductive; Skin/Exocrine
- Synonym(s): GC; Clap

EPIDEMIOLOGY

- Predominant age: 15–24 years
- Predominant sex: Prior to 1996, rates of gonorrhea among men were higher than rates among women. However, gonorrhea rates in women are now slightly higher than in men.

Incidence

- In 2008, 336,742 cases were reported to the Centers for Disease Control (CDC), resulting in rate of 111.6/100,000 US population.
- Highest rates are among black women aged 15–19 (2,934.6 /100,000)
- Blacks (625/100,000) have 20.2 times greater rate than whites (31/100,000)

Prevalence

As a treatable disease, incidence and prevalence of diagnosed disease are approximately equal. The asymptomatic nature of the disease (especially among women) would suggest that the prevalence is higher than the reported incidence.

RISK FACTORS

- History of previous gonorrhea infection
- Sexual exposure to an infected individual without barrier protection (condom)
- Other sexually transmitted infections
- New or multiple sexual partners
- Inconsistent condom use
- Sex work
- Drug use
- Infants: Passage through infected birth canal of mother
- Children: Sexual abuse by infected individual
- Autoinoculation (finger to eye)
- For PID: Use of intrauterine devices

Genetics

Individuals with congenital deficiency of late components of complement cascade (C7,8,9) are prone to develop dissemination of local gonococcal infections.

GENERAL PREVENTION

- Condoms offer partial protection, but must be used for oral, anal, and vaginal intercourse to be effective.
- Sexual contacts should be treated.

PATHOPHYSIOLOGY

Infection requires 4 steps:

- Mucosal attachment
- Local penetration/invasion
- Local proliferation
- Inflammatory response or dissemination

ETIOLOGY

N. gonorrhoeae (gonococcus)

COMMONLY ASSOCIATED CONDITIONS

Other sexually transmitted infections:

- Chlamydia
- Syphilis
- HIV
- Hepatitis B
- Herpes

DIAGNOSIS

HISTORY

- For all patients: Sexual history including number of partners and age of onset of sexual activity, new/recent change in sexual partner, contact with sex workers, condom use, history of STIs, menses, and possibility of pregnancy
- Patients should be screened for additional STIs, including HIV
- For patients with symptoms: Onset, context, duration, timing, severity, associated symptoms, and modifying factors of symptoms
- Remember 10% males and 20–40% of women are asymptomatic.
- Patients with symptoms should also be asked about symptomatic partner(s).
- Signs and symptoms may include:
  - General: Urinary symptoms: Urinary frequency, urgency, dysuria
  - Urethral symptoms: Copious urethral discharge, meatus and anterior urethral inflammation
  - Ocular symptoms: Purulent discharge, conjunctivitis, chemosis, eyelid edema, corneal ulceration
  - Pharyngeal symptoms:
    - Pharyngeal infection: Asymptomatic infection (98%), sore throat, exudative pharyngitis (<1%)
  - GI symptoms: Acute diarrhea
  - Males: Scant to copious purulent urethral discharge (82%); dysuria (53%); testicular pain (1%); asymptomatic infection (10%), proctitis
  - Females: Asymptomatic cervical infection (20%), endocervical discharge (96%), vaginal discharge, Bartholin gland abscess, dysmenorrhea, menometrorrhagia, abdominal pain/tenderness, cervical motion tenderness, rebound, infertility, chronic pelvic pain
  - Either sex, for receptive anal intercourse: Rectal discharge, tenesmus, rectal burning, asymptomatic
  - Disseminated syndromes:
    - Fever, chills, malaise, tenosynovitis, dermatitis, polyarthralgia, purulent arthritis
    - Endocarditis: Rapid cardiac valve destruction, high fevers
    - Meningitis: Meningeal signs, headache, skin lesions, fever, altered mental status

PHYSICAL EXAM

A full physical exam with an emphasis on vital signs, throat, abdomen, pelvic/rectal, genital, skin, and joints

DIAGNOSTIC TESTS & INTERPRETATION

Lab

Initial lab tests

CDC recommends nucleic acid amplification as the most sensitive and specific test for *N. gonorrhoeae*. Other options include:

- Genital culture
- Consider adding pharyngeal culture in adolescents (1)[A]
- Gram stain (recommended for urethritis)
- Urethral smear, sensitivity in symptomatic male: ≥95%. Sensitivity of endocervical smear in infected woman: 40–60%. Specificity: 100%
- DNA probes and PCR sensitivity: 92–99% dependent on population. Specificity: >97%; can replace culture
- Sensitivity of blood culture in disseminated disease: 50%. Sensitivity of joint fluid culture in septic arthritis: 50%
- If a clinical consideration, order with chlamydia, rapid plasma reagin (RPR), and HIV testing

Follow-Up & Special Considerations

- Test-of-cure testing is not generally recommended.
- Follow-up testing may be considered in cases of recurrent infection and/or in areas where significant antibiotic resistance exists.

Imaging

Initial approach

Imaging is not generally recommended for initial evaluation of uncomplicated gonococcal urethritis or clinically apparent PID.

Follow-Up & Special Considerations

Pelvic ultrasound or CT scan may demonstrate thick, dilated fallopian tubes or abscess formation.

Diagnostic Procedures/Surgery

Culdocentesis may demonstrate free purulent exudate and provide material for gram staining and culture. Gram staining material from unroofed skin lesions may show typical organisms.

Pathological Findings

- Exudate of polymorphonuclear leukocytes is typical.
- Gram-negative intracellular *diplococci*
- Nonpathologic gram-negative *diplococci* may be found in extragenital locations. For this reason, gram stain of pharyngeal or rectal swabs is not recommended.

DIFFERENTIAL DIAGNOSIS

- *Chlamydia trachomatis*
- Urinary tract infections
- Nongonococcal vaginitis
- Nongonococcal urethritis

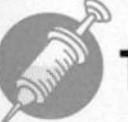

TREATMENT

MEDICATION

Because of the public health importance of untreated gonococcal infection, only antibiotics with a demonstrated success rate of 95% or higher should be used.

First Line

- Uncomplicated gonorrheal infection of the cervix, urethra, or rectum:
  - Ceftriaxone, 125 mg IM in a single dose or Cefixime, 400 mg PO in a single dose plus treatment for chlamydia
  - Note: During pregnancy, ceftriaxone is treatment of choice.
  - Pharyngitis: Ceftriaxone, 125 mg IM once
  - Conjunctivitis: Ceftriaxone, 1 g IM
  - PID: Outpatient regimens (for inpatient regimens, see citations):
    - Ceftriaxone, 250 mg IM once *plus* Doxycycline, 100 mg PO b.i.d. for 14 days *with or without* Metronidazole, 500 mg PO b.i.d. for 14 days
- Disseminated infection in adults:
  - Ceftriaxone, 1 g IM or IV q24h for 24–48 hours, also treat for chlamydial infection. Then for 1 week:
    - Cefixime, 400 mg PO b.i.d.
- Meningitis and endocarditis:
  - Ceftriaxone, 1–2 g IV q12h 10–14 days for meningitis; 4 weeks for endocarditis
- Treatment of infants and children: <45 kg (patients >45 kg should receive full adult dose)
- Uncomplicated genital, pharyngeal, rectal, or conjunctival infection, and infants born to mothers with untreated gonorrhea:
  - Ceftriaxone, 125 mg IM in single dose
  - Disseminated infections: Ceftriaxone, 25–50 mg/kg IV or IM daily, or cefotaxime, 25 mg/kg IV or IM q12h; bacteremia: 7 days; meningitis: 10–14 days; endocarditis: 4 weeks
- Ophthalmic neonatorum prophylaxis: Single application of:
  - Erythromycin (0.5%) ophthalmic ointment *or* tetracycline ophthalmic ointment (1%)
- Contraindications: Tetracyclines such as doxycycline are contraindicated in pregnancy and young children.
- Precautions: Refer to the manufacturer's profile of each drug.
- Significant possible interactions: Refer to the manufacturer's profile of each drug.
- Note: All medication recommendations from source

Second Line

- No 2nd-line agent available in the US for gonococcal infections:
  - Recent gonococcal isolates within the US have demonstrated significant rates of resistance to both azithromycin and quinolones. Neither is currently recommended for treatment.
  - Progressive resistance to sulfonamides, penicillins, tetracyclines, fluoroquinolones and now developing resistance in Asia, Australia, and elsewhere to 3rd-generation cephalosporins makes prevention critically important (2)[B].
- PID can be treated with clindamycin and gentamicin.
- For treatment options other than those listed in previous section, please see CDC report on sexually transmitted diseases treatment guidelines at: http://www.cdc.gov/std/treatment/2006/updated regimens.htm

ADDITIONAL TREATMENT

General Measures

Counseling concerning risk reduction and condom use

IN-PATIENT CONSIDERATIONS

Initial Stabilization

In rare cases, individual may be hemodynamically unstable from sepsis; stabilize with IV fluids if necessary.

Admission Criteria

- Hematogenously disseminated infection
- Pneumonia or eye infection in infants
- PID: If unable to take oral medications, significant tubo-ovarian abscess, or patient is pregnant

IV Fluids

Indicated for patients whose presenting complaints include significant nausea/vomiting with clinical evidence of dehydration

ONGOING CARE

FOLLOW-UP RECOMMENDATIONS

Patient Monitoring

US Preventive Services Task Force (USPSTF) recommends:

- Screen all sexually active women if they are at increased risk of infection (which includes having a new partner).
- Insufficient evidence to recommend screening men at increased risk of infection
- No screening for men or women not at increased risk of infection
- Strongly recommend prophylactic ocular topical medication for all newborns (3)[C].

PATIENT EDUCATION

- Counseling concerning risk reduction and condom use
- Counseling concerning future fertility
- Encourage patient and partner HIV testing.
- This is a reportable disease:
  - Reportable diseases are diseases considered to be of great public health importance. Local, state, and national agencies require that such diseases be reported when they are diagnosed. All states have a reportable diseases list. Most of these lists are similar. Gonorrhea is generally a mandatory written-report disease. A provider must contact both the state health department and the CDC.

PROGNOSIS

With adequate, early therapy, complete cure with return to normal function is the rule.

COMPLICATIONS

- Infertility
- Urethral stricture
- Corneal scarring
- Destruction of joint articular surfaces
- Cardiac valves

Pediatric Considerations

Vertical transmission to newborn infants is a significant risk among patients with gonococcal infection at the time of delivery.

Pregnancy Considerations

USPSTF found insufficient evidence to recommend for or against routine screening for gonorrheal infection in pregnant women who are not at increased risk for infection (3)[C].

REFERENCES

1. Giannini CM, Kim HK, Mortensen J, Mortensen J, Marsolo K, Huppert J et al. Culture of non-genital sites increases the detection of gonorrhea in women. *J Pediatr Adolesc Gynecol*. 2010;23: 246–52.
2. Barry PM, Klausner JD. The use of cephalosporins for gonorrhea: the impending problem of resistance. *Expert Opin Pharmacother*. 2009; 10:555–77.
3. US Preventive Services Task Force. Screening for Gonorrhea: Recommendation Statement. AHRQ Publication No. 05-0579-A. Rockville MD: Agency for Healthcare Research and Quality, May 2005. Available at: http://www.ahrq.gov/clinic/uspstf05/gonorrhea/gonrs.htm.

ADDITIONAL READING

- Centers for Disease Control and Prevention (CDC). Increases in fluoroquinolone-resistant Neisseria gonorrhoeae among men who have sex with men–United States, 2003, and revised recommendations for gonorrhea treatment, 2004. *MMWR Morb Mortal Wkly Rep*. 2004;53:335–8.
- *MMWR Morb Mortal Wkly Rep*. Update to CDC's sexually transmitted diseases treatment guidelines, 2006: fluoroquinolones no longer recommended for treatment of gonococcal infections. 2007;56(14): 332–6.

See Also (Topic, Algorithm, Electronic Media Element)

Chlamydial Sexually Transmitted Diseases; Pelvic Inflammatory Disease (PID); Syphilis; HIV Infection and AIDS

CODES

ICD9

- 098.0 Gonococcal infection (acute) of lower genitourinary tract
- 098.10 Gonococcal infection (acute) of upper genitourinary tract, site unspecified
- 098.11 Gonococcal cystitis (acute)

CLINICAL PEARLS

- The USPSTF recommends screening sexually active women at high risk of infection. High risk of infection is defined as <35 years of age, history of previous gonorrhea infection or other STD, NEW or multiple sexual partners, inconsistent condom use, sex work, and drug use.
- The USPSTF does not recommend routine screening of men at high risk or anyone at low risk.
- Patients testing positive for gonorrhea should also be considered for additional STI testing including chlamydia, syphilis, HIV, and hepatitis.
- Treat also for chlamydia, unless chlamydia infection ruled out.

G

GOUT

Janice A. Litza, MD
Jacob L. Bidwell, MD

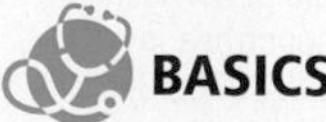

BASICS

DESCRIPTION

- Gout refers to a group of disorders related to hyperuricemia. Although hyperuricemia is necessary for the development of gout, it is not the only determining factor.
- Characterized by deposition of monosodium urate (MSU) crystals in tissue, resulting in acute and chronic arthritis, soft tissue masses called tophi, urate nephropathy, and uric acid nephrolithiasis
- Natural history involves 4 stages:
  - Asymptomatic hyperuricemia
  - Acute arthritis
  - Intercritical gout
  - Chronic tophaceous gout
- Acute gouty arthritis can affect ≥1 joints. The 1st metatarsophalangeal joint is most commonly involved at presentation (podagra).
- Other common sites include midtarsal, ankle, and knee joints.
- After an initial attack, patients can be attack-free for months or even years. Some patients will develop more frequent attacks or go on to develop chronic tophaceous gout.
- Management involves treating acute attacks and preventing recurrent disease by long-term reduction of serum uric acid levels through pharmacology and lifestyle adjustments.

Geriatric Considerations

- Presentation may lack acute pain, swelling, and inflammation
- More common in women >80
- Can present with tophi and finger joint pain
- Commonly triggered by diuretic use, especially in women

Pediatric Considerations

Often due to an inborn error of metabolism or other disease

EPIDEMIOLOGY

Incidence

Increases with age, especially in women

Prevalence

6 per 1,000 population for men; 1 per 1,000 population for women

RISK FACTORS

- Hyperuricemia
- Male gender (age <65)
- Increasing age
- Ethanol ingestion (beer and liquor > wine)
- Obesity (50%)
- Hypertension (50%)
- Diabetes
- Medications: Diuretics induce 20% of secondary gout
- Diet: High-purine animal-origin foods (e.g., meats and seafood)
- Family history
- Keto- and lactic acidosis
- Surgery or trauma
- Renal impairment
- Hypothyroidism
- Parathyroid disease
- Hyperlipidemia types II, IV, V
- Paget disease
- Hyperproliferative skin disorders (psoriasis)
- Lymphoproliferative disorders, hemolytic anemia, hemoglobinopathies, pernicious anemia
- Glycogen storage diseases

Genetics

- Primary gout runs in families and follows multifactorial inheritance.
- Phosphoribosyl pyrophosphate (PRPP) deficiency and hypoxanthine-guanine-phosphoribosyltransferase (HGPRT) deficiency are inherited enzyme defects associated with a primary overproduction of uric acid.
- URAT1 (urate transporter) deficiency is also a hereditary enzyme defect resulting in primary underexcretion of uric acid.

GENERAL PREVENTION

- Treat underlying cardiovascular risk factors.
- Maintain weight at optimal BMI of <26.
- Regular exercise
- Diet modification
- Reduce alcohol consumption (beer and liquor).
- Maintain fluid intake and avoid dehydration.

PATHOPHYSIOLOGY

- Humans have a narrow window for urate to remain soluble before crystal precipitation due to lack of uricase enzyme.
- Precipitation of MSU crystals can occur in the synovium, joint cartilage, kidneys, and soft tissue.
- MSU crystals can initiate and sustain an inflammatory response, leading to an acute gout attack.
- Chronic and untreated hyperuricemia lead to tophi formation in and around the joint space.
- Tophi contribute to chronic synovitis, often resulting in joint damage.

ETIOLOGY

- Increased uric acid production
- Impaired renal excretion of uric acid
- Enzyme defects
- Increased purine turnover
- Dehydration or starvation

COMMONLY ASSOCIATED CONDITIONS

- Metabolic syndrome (obesity, hyperglycemia, hyperlipidemia, hypertension [HTN])
- Myeloproliferative disorders
- Lymphoproliferative disorders
- Alcoholism
- Endocrinopathies
- Lesch-Nyhan syndrome

DIAGNOSIS

HISTORY

- Rapid onset of severe pain, usually beginning in early morning with 1 or 2 joints (75% are monoarticular) +/− fever
- Soft tissue redness, swelling, warmth
- Exquisite tenderness
- 1st metatarsophalangeal joint in 50% of initial attacks
- Acute untreated attacks last 2–21 days.
- Recurrent attacks last longer and occur more frequently with each recurrence.
- Between attacks, absence of inflammation (until the chronic or tophaceous phase occurs)
- Rarely polyarticular
- Migratory polyarthritis is a rare presentation.
- 50% untreated develop chronic arthritis
- Subcutaneous or intraosseous nodules (20%), referred to as tophi, may affect ears (antihelix), extensor aspects of peripheral joints (e.g., olecranon), cornea, aorta, spine, even intracranial space (1).
- Pain with urination secondary to uric acid renal stones

PHYSICAL EXAM

- Examine suspected joint(s) for tenderness, swelling, and range of motion (ROM).
- Assess for presence of firm nodules known as tophi.

DIAGNOSTIC TESTS & INTERPRETATION

Lab

Initial lab tests

- Synovial fluid analysis: Urate crystals, (negatively birefringent under polarizing microscopy), cell count (white blood count [WBC] usually 5,000–50,000/mm^3; predominantly neutrophils); culture to rule out infection
- Blood studies: Elevated serum uric acid level, complete blood count (can show elevated WBC during acute attack)
- Urine studies: Urine analysis, 24-hour urine testing for uric acid and creatinine (urate excretion will likely not be accurate during an acute attack)

Imaging

Initial approach

- Radiograph is usually normal early in disease.
- Radiograph in chronic gout reveals "punched-out" erosions (lytic areas), often with periosteum overgrowing the erosion ("overhanging edge").
- Urate kidney stones are radiolucent, and thus invisible on radiograph.

Diagnostic Procedures/Surgery

- Arthrocentesis with polarizing optical examination
- Biopsy of synovial membrane or SC nodule, processing the specimen anhydrously (urate is water-soluble)

Pathological Findings

- Acute arthritis: Neutrophilic infiltrate throughout synovium
- Chronic arthritis: Intra-articular and periarticular tophi
- Tophi: Macrophages surround MSU crystals, forming a granuloma.
- Gouty nephropathy: MSU crystals deposited in medullary interstitium

DIFFERENTIAL DIAGNOSIS

- Septic arthritis
- Pseudogout (calcium pyrophosphate deposition disease)
- Cellulitis
- Reactive arthritis

- Amyloidosis
- Osteoarthritis
- Hyperparathyroidism
- Spondyloarthropathy
- Rheumatoid arthritis (rarely)

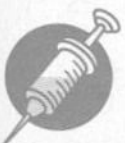

TREATMENT

- Key component is lifestyle adjustment to avoid triggers and reduce risk
- Chronic treatment indicated if >2 attacks per year, tophi present, radiographic evidence of joint damage (2)[C]
- Goal for chronic treatment is serum uric acid less than 6 mg/dL (2)[B]

MEDICATION

First Line

- Acute attack:
  - Nonsteroidal anti-inflammatory drugs (NSAIDs) (e.g., naproxen and indomethacin) at full dosage:
    - Taper a few days after symptoms resolve.
    - Use limited by GI side effects, including GI bleeding (1)[A]
- Chronic treatment:
  - Urate-lowering agents should not be prescribed until 2–3 weeks after acute attack has resolved, but should be continued if patient is taking them prior to attack.
- Xanthine oxidase inhibitors:
  - Allopurinol start at 100 mg daily and adjusted every 2–4 weeks until goal of serum uric acid is <6mg/dL for 3–6 months (2)[B]:
    - Monitor for hypersensitivity reactions: Rash, hepatitis, interstitial nephritis, and toxic epidermal necrolysis.
    - Coprescribe with colchicine 0.5–1 mg/d OR low-dose NSAIDs daily upon initiation of treatment to prevent rebound acute gout attacks (2)[B].
  - Febuxostat:
    - Approved by Food and Drug Administration (FDA) 2/2009 for gout
    - Benefits include more selective xanthine oxidase inhibitor and no renal dose adjustment
    - Starting dose 40 mg daily, titrate to 80 mg daily to goal serum uric acid of <6 mg/dL (3,4)[B]

Second Line

- Acute attack:
  - Colchicine: Should be used within 12–24 hours of attack onset. 1 mg followed by 0.5 mg q2h until absence of symptoms or GI side effects occur (nausea, vomiting, diarrhea) (1)[A].
  - Systemic corticosteroids (5)[B]
  - Intra-articular long-acting corticosteroid is useful if 1 or a few joints involved (2)[B]
  - Adrenocorticotropic hormone (ACTH) 25 USP units SC for acute small-joint monoarticular gout. 40 USP units IM or IV for larger joints or polyarticular gout (2)[B].
- Chronic treatment:
  - Uricosuric agents
  - Use in patients refractory to allopurinol or in whom allopurinol is contraindicated. Ideal for patients <60 years with CrCl >80 mL/min, 24-hour urinary uric acid excretion ≤700 mg on normal diet, and without history of renal calculi:
    - Probenecid: Start at 250 mg p.o. b.i.d. and gradually increase to 500–2,000 mg p.o. (in 2 doses) until desired SUA in those with normal renal function (2)[B].
    - Sulfinpyrazone: Start at 50 mg p.o. b.i.d. and gradually increase to 100–400 mg (in 2 doses) daily until desired SUA in those with normal renal function (2)[B].
    - Initially coprescribe all uricosurics with either colchicine 0.5–1 mg/d for up to 6 months OR low-dose NSAIDs for up to 6 weeks.
  - Fenofibrate and losartan or amlodipine: Consider as alternative therapy for hyperlipidemia and HTN, respectively. Modest uricosuric effect (2,6)[B].
  - Ongoing studies: Puricase (PEG-uricase) for refractory chronic gout (7)[B]

ADDITIONAL TREATMENT

General Measures

Apply ice packs and rest affected joint.

SURGERY/OTHER PROCEDURES

Large tophi that are infected or interfering with joint motion may need to be surgically removed.

ONGOING CARE

FOLLOW-UP RECOMMENDATIONS

Patient Monitoring

Related to medicinal control of the acute attack and suppressing attacks:

- CBC, renal, liver function tests (LFTs), and urinalysis at 1 week, 6 weeks, and every 3 months

DIET

- Reduce ingestion of purine-rich foods of animal origin (meat and shellfish).
- Avoid alcoholic beverages, specifically beer and liquor.
- Increase low-fat dairy foods.
- Maintain adequate hydration.
- Consider additional vitamin C 500 mg daily (8).

PATIENT EDUCATION

Gout and Uric Acid Education Society: http://www.gouteducation.org

PROGNOSIS

- Gout can usually be successfully managed with proper treatment.
- Recurrent attacks may require long-term uric acid-lowering therapy.
- During the 1st 6–12 months of uricosuric or allopurinol therapy, acute gout attacks may occur.

COMPLICATIONS

- Increased susceptibility to infection
- Urate nephropathy
- Renal stones
- Nerve/spinal cord impingement

REFERENCES

1. Schlesinger N, Schumacher R, Catton M, et al. Colchicine for acute gout. *Cochrane Database Syst Rev*. 2006;CD006190.
2. Zhang W, Doherty M, Bardin T, et al. EULAR evidence based recommendations for gout. Part II: Management. Report of a task force of the EULAR Standing Committee for International Clinical Studies Including Therapeutics (ESCISIT). *Ann Rheum Dis*. 2006;65:1312–24.
3. Bruce SP. Febuxostat: a selective xanthine oxidase inhibitor for the treatment of hyperuricemia and gout. *Ann Pharmacother*. 2006;40:2187–94.
4. Schumacher HR, Becker MA, Wortmann RL, et al. Effects of febuxostat versus allopurinol and placebo in reducing serum urate in subjects with hyperuricemia and gout: A 28-week, phase III, randomized, double-blind, parallel-group trial. *Arthritis Rheum*. 2008;59:1540–8.
5. Janssens H, et al. Systemic corticosteroids for acute gout. *Cochrane Database Syst Rev*. 2008;16(2): CD005521.
6. Høieggen A, Alderman MH, Kjeldsen SE, et al. The impact of serum uric acid on cardiovascular outcomes in the LIFE study. *Kidney Int*. 2004;65: 1041–9.
7. Sundy JS, Ganson NJ, Kelly SJ, et al. Pharmacokinetics and pharmacodynamics of intravenous PEGylated recombinant mammalian urate oxidase in patients with refractory gout. *Arthritis Rheum*. 2007;56:1021–8.
8. Huang HY, Appel LJ, Choi MJ, et al. The effects of vitamin C supplementation on serum concentrations of uric acid: results of a randomized controlled trial. *Arthritis Rheum*. 2005;52:1843–7.

ADDITIONAL READING

- Eggebeen AT. Gout: an update. *Am Fam Physician*. 2007;76:801–8.
- Keith MP, Gilliland WR. Updates in the management of gout. *Am J Med*. 2007;120:221–4.
- Liote F, et al. Gout: Update on some pathogenic and clinical aspects. *Rheum Dis Clin N Am*. 2006;32: 295–311.
- Rott KT, Agudelo CA. Gout. *JAMA*. 2003;289: 2857–60.
- Terkeltaub RA. Clinical practice. Gout. *N Engl J Med*. 2003;349:1647–55.

See Also (Topic, Algorithm, Electronic Media Element)

Alcohol Abuse and Dependence; Anemia, Sickle Cell

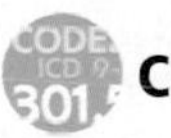

CODES

ICD9

- 274.00 Gouty arthropathy, unspecified
- 274.9 Gout, unspecified
- 274.10 Gouty nephropathy, unspecified

CLINICAL PEARLS

- MSU crystals found in synovial fluid aspirate are pathognomonic for gout.
- Acute gout and sepsis can coexist.
- Asymptomatic hyperuricemia does not require treatment.
- Presentation may vary by age and gender.

GRANULOMA ANNULARE

Ronald Adler, MD

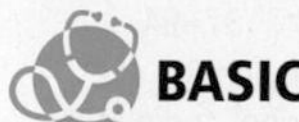

BASICS

DESCRIPTION

A benign skin condition characterized by grouped papules, which typically occur in an annular pattern. 4 variants have been described, the most common of which is localized granuloma annulare (GA). The other types are generalized (or disseminated), subcutaneous, and perforating.

EPIDEMIOLOGY

Incidence

GA is not common, though its occurrence in the general population is unknown. It is seen more often in women, with a ratio of 2:1 over men. The age distribution varies by type, as follows:

- Localized: Children and adults <30 years old
- Generalized: Bimodal: Children <10 and adults 30–60 years old
- Subcutaneous: Children 2–10 years old
- Perforating: Typically children, but also young adults

Prevalence

Among cases of GA, the approximate distribution is as follows:

- Localized: 75%
- Generalized: 10–15%
- Subcutaneous: <5%
- Perforating: <5% (perhaps higher in Hawaii)

RISK FACTORS

No definite risk factors have been identified. There is weak evidence for possible associations with diabetes mellitus, TB, HIV, EBV and other viral infections, trauma, insect bites, and malignancies.

Genetics

There is some evidence for a possible hereditary component.

GENERAL PREVENTION

There are no established strategies for preventing GA.

ETIOLOGY

The cause of GA remains unknown, though it is probably immunologic.

COMMONLY ASSOCIATED CONDITIONS

See Risk Factors. These noted associations are not common.

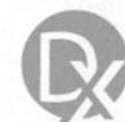

DIAGNOSIS

HISTORY

Cutaneous lesions of GA are generally asymptomatic. They may persist for months or years; longer duration is more often seen in the generalized subtype. They typically resolve spontaneously and they may recur.

PHYSICAL EXAM

- Localized: Small (1–2 mm) papules arranged in a ring, which may enlarge from 5 mm–5 cm. Color may range from flesh tones to red. The most common locations are the dorsal aspects of the distal extremities.
- Generalized: Similar to localized, but a higher number of lesions, which are more widespread, often larger, and typically persist longer.
- Subcutaneous: Firm, nontender, subcutaneous nodule, which tends to grow rapidly. Usually solitary, but may occur in groups. Most common location is lower extremities, especially pretibial; other sites include upper extremities, scalp, buttocks.
- Perforating: Papules may be up to 4 mm and display umbilication, crusting, or scale. Lesions are often generalized and may occur anywhere.

DIAGNOSTIC TESTS & INTERPRETATION

Lab

Initial lab tests

Diagnosis is typically established by the history and physical, so lab investigations are rarely needed. Skin scraping/KOH test may be useful for excluding a fungal process.

Imaging

Initial approach

Rarely indicated, but may occasionally be useful in the workup of suspected subcutaneous subtype

Diagnostic Procedures/Surgery

Occasionally, biopsy is required to confirm the diagnosis. This is most commonly the case for subcutaneous subtype.

DIFFERENTIAL DIAGNOSIS

- Localized: Tinea corporis, annular lichen planus, necrobiosis lipoidica, pityriasis rosea, erythema migrans of Lyme disease, leprosy
- Generalized: Sarcoidosis, lichen planus, cutaneous metastases
- Subcutaneous: Rheumatoid nodule
- Perforating: Molluscum contagiosum

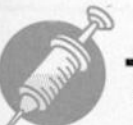

TREATMENT

MEDICATION

- There is no strong evidence supporting any treatment intervention for GA. Multiple therapies have been tried (particularly in generalized cases), and the following medications may be of some use:
  - Corticosteroids, either by intralesional injection or topical application (with or without occlusion)
  - Tacrolimus
  - Pimecrolimus
  - Imiquimod
  - Isotretinoin
  - Dapsone
  - Hydroxychloroquine
  - Cyclosporine
  - Niacinamide
  - Infliximab
  - Doxycycline
  - Allopurinol
- Other therapies:
  - Psoralen ultraviolet A (PUVA)
  - Cryotherapy

ADDITIONAL TREATMENT

General Measures

Given that GA is an asymptomatic condition that is likely to resolve spontaneously, the clinician's primary role after diagnosis is to educate the patient regarding the anticipated natural history and to provide reassurance.

ONGOING CARE

FOLLOW-UP RECOMMENDATIONS

Routine follow-up is not required. However, if treatment is initiated, follow-up may be important to monitor for possible adverse effects associated with treatment.

PATIENT EDUCATION

The patient should be informed that GA is a benign, self-limited condition that may persist a long time, resolve, and recur.

PROGNOSIS

Many cases resolve spontaneously, though recurrence—typically at the original site—is common.

COMPLICATIONS

Complications of treatment are much more likely than complications from GA.

ADDITIONAL READING

- Cyr PR. Diagnosis and Management of Granuloma Annulare. *Amer FP*. 2006;74(10):1729–34.
- Duarte AF, Mota A, et al. Generalized granuloma annulare - response to doxycycline. *J Eur Acad Dermat and Vener*. 2009;23:84–5.
- Mazzatenta C, Ghilardi A, Grazzini M. Treatment of disseminated granuloma annulare with allopurinol: case report. *Dermatologic Therapy*. 2010;23:S24–7.

CODES

ICD9

695.89 Other specified erythematous conditions

CLINICAL PEARLS

This condition is benign. Most proposed treatments are not. *Primum non nocere*.

GRANULOMA INGUINALE

Omar A. Khan, MD, MHS

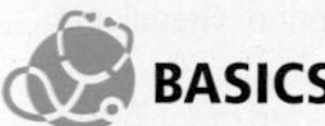

BASICS

DESCRIPTION

Granuloma inguinale is a primarily sexually transmitted, chronic bacterial infection caused by *Calymmatobacterium granulomatis* (which some authorities classify as *Klebsiella granulomatis*), formerly known as *Donovania granulomatis*, an intracellular gram-negative bacillus.

- Also known as *donovanosis*
- Causative organism similar to *Klebsiella* spp., leading to discussions on nomenclature
- Usually manifests as genital or anal lesions
- Sexual/anal intercourse is the main source.
- Also can be acquired via fecal route, passage through an infected birth canal, or contact with laps of infected individuals (children)
- Granuloma inguinale is a risk factor for acquiring HIV infection.
- Four varieties of skin lesions exist: ulcerovegetative, cicatricial, nodular, and verrucous.

EPIDEMIOLOGY

- <100 cases annually in the US (mostly foreign travel)
- Endemic: Tropical and subtropical regions (e.g., New Guinea, Caribbean, West Indies, southern India, sub-Saharan Africa, Southeast Asia, Australia, Brazil)
- Incidence higher in blacks in US
- Predominant sex: Males slightly more susceptible
- Predominant age: 20–40 years; rarely seen in children or elderly; no congenital cases reported

RISK FACTORS

- Residing or traveling in underdeveloped parts of tropical/subtropical countries
- Sexual contact with travelers to endemic area
- Males having unprotected sex with males
- Anal intercourse
- Low socioeconomic background
- HIV positivity

GENERAL PREVENTION

- Safe sex practices
- If infection likely, avoid sexual contact; notify partners.
- Examples of prevention include barrier methods of contraception, avoidance of high-risk sexual activity, and appropriate gynecologic screening (including during the course of pregnancy).
- Sexual contacts within 60 days prior to symptom onset should be evaluated and offered treatment.
- Remaining up to date on HIV care

PATHOPHYSIOLOGY

- Repeated is exposure necessary for clinical infection to occur.
- Communicable as long as the infected person remains untreated and bacteria are present

ETIOLOGY

Bacterial infection caused by caused by the bacillus *Klebsiella/Calymmatobacterium granulomatosis* (previously known as *Donovania granulomatis*)

COMMONLY ASSOCIATED CONDITIONS

Can be associated with other sexually transmitted infections (STIs), including HIV infection

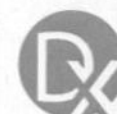

DIAGNOSIS

HISTORY

- Sexual contact ± genital lesions
- Recent travel
- History of HIV infection or other STIs
- Subcutaneous nodules or superficial blisters in the genital area that develop into open sores, usually painless

PHYSICAL EXAM

- Incubation period varies: 1–15 weeks.
- Begins with subcutaneous nodules or superficial blisters in the genital area; may spread to inguinal folds and lead to surrounding depigmentation
- Blister becomes a slowly enlarging open sore; usually painless; may emit a foul odor
- Four types, commonly classified as
  - Ulcerovegetative: This is the most common. The ulcers are fairly large, with raised margins and a prominently erythematous appearance. The base is friable and thus bleeds easily.
  - Cicatricial: This consists of dry ulcers that may coalesce into a plaque.
  - Nodular: Isolated pruritic red nodules are the prominent feature; may develop into the ulcerative type. Owing to their resemblance, these lesions should be distinguished from the buboes of other conditions.
  - Verrucous or hypertrophic: Rare; proliferative reaction; forms large vegetative masses resembling warts
- Genital involvement in 90%, inguinal in 10%
- Males: Lesions usually occur on the genitalia, including the penis and scrotum.
- Association with uncircumcised men if occurring in low-hygiene situations
- Females: Lesions usually occur on the genitalia; about 10% of lesions may be cervical.
- 10–50% infected men and women have lesions in the anal area.
- Extragenital involvement (6%):
  - The most common extragenital sites of infection are the GI tract (including the oral cavity and anus), lymph nodes (may present as pseudobuboes), and hematogenous spread to intraabdominal organs and, rarely, bony structures.

DIAGNOSTIC TESTS & INTERPRETATION

- Mostly a clinical diagnosis; most labs do not have a culture available.
- Consider testing for mimics and common coinfections.
- Staining and biopsy are also appropriate, but results are difficult to assess and not always accurate.

Lab

- Most effective diagnostic method is direct visualization of the organisms within the macrophages, seen as safety pin–shaped intracytoplasmic inclusions (Donovan bodies).
- Tissue crush preparations from ulcer edge may be performed via punch biopsy, curettage, or a thin wedge of skin. Use of Wright-Giemsa or Warthin-Starry stain can help in the visualization of Donovan bodies.
- Polymerase chain reaction (PCR) used for research; may be available clinically in some settings
- Indirect immunofluorescence technique is not accurate for confirming the diagnosis.
- Pap smears may identify Donovan bodies on routine cervical screening.
- Test for other STIs and HIV infection because multiple infections frequently coexist.

Imaging

Consider radiographs if bony involvement is suspected.

DIFFERENTIAL DIAGNOSIS

- Lymphogranuloma venereum
- Condyloma lata of syphilis
- Chancroid
- HIV-associated herpetic ulcers
- Carcinoma of the penis, vulva, or cervix
- Tuberculosis of the cervix

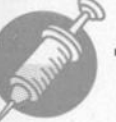

TREATMENT

Usually can be treated in an outpatient setting with appropriate antibiotics and clinical monitoring

MEDICATION

First Line

- All regimens should be administered for 3 weeks or until ulcer resolution.
- Azithromycin: 1 g/d PO 1st day, 500 mg/d after that
- Trimethoprim-sulfamethoxazole DS (Bactrim) PO b.i.d. (avoid in pregnancy)
- Doxycycline: 100 mg PO b.i.d. (avoid in pregnancy)
- HIV-associated granuloma inguinale may take longer to heal; the addition of an aminoglycoside is highly recommended.

Second Line

- Ciprofloxacin: 750 mg PO b.i.d. × 3 weeks (avoid in pediatric and pregnant patients)
- Erythromycin base: 500 mg PO q.i.d. for 3 weeks (use as 1st line in pregnancy)
- Gentamicin: 1 mg/kg IM/IV t.i.d. in pregnancy or if other regimens are ineffective in 1st few days of treatment
- Single-dose regimens of ciprofloxacin, azithromycin, and ceftriaxone have been reported anecdotally.

Pediatric Considerations

Children born to mothers with untreated genital lesions of donovanosis are at risk of infection, and a course of prophylactic antibiotics should be considered.

Pregnancy Considerations

- Use erythromycin, 500 mg PO q.i.d. ± aminoglycoside.
- Doxycycline and ciprofloxacin are contraindicated in pregnancy.
- Sulfonamides are relatively contraindicated.

ADDITIONAL TREATMENT

General Measures

- Empirical treatment should be comprehensive and cover all likely pathogens.
- Antimicrobials given for at least 3 weeks and continued until reepithelialization of the ulcer
- If the ulcer does not respond within the 1st few days of treatment, add an IV aminoglycoside.
- Relapse may occur up to 18 months after treatment.
- Tetracycline is no longer recommended owing to bacterial resistance.
- Care must be taken with pregnant and pediatric patients when choosing antimicrobials.

Issues for Referral

- Surgical referral (e.g., urologic, gynecologic, colorectal), based on complications
- Infectious disease consultation may be helpful if coexisting HIV infection or other STIs are present or suspected.

SURGERY/OTHER PROCEDURES

May need surgical correction for disfiguring genital lesions, abscess drainage, or correction of urethral/lymphatic obstruction

IN-PATIENT CONSIDERATIONS

Initial Stabilization

Usually not a concern unless patient presents with a surgical complication such as lymphatic or urethral obstruction

Admission Criteria

- Extensive, chronic, or necrotizing lesions
- Hematogenous dissemination
- Patient compliance with outpatient regimen a concern

Nursing

- Wound care as needed
- Monitoring for evidence of secondary bacterial infection (i.e., careful review of vital signs)

Discharge Criteria

- Surgical clearance if surgical complications were part of the reason for admission
- Ability to access and tolerate oral antimicrobials if needed
- Clinical improvement

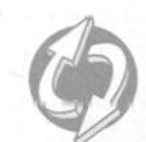

ONGOING CARE

FOLLOW-UP RECOMMENDATIONS

If treated in a timely manner, lesions usually resolve.

Patient Monitoring

- Monitor for hyperkalemia with extended TMP-SMX treatment.
- Other monitoring varies per treatment regimen.
- Monitor patient until resolution of symptoms.

PATIENT EDUCATION

- Patient rapport is critical because many patients may present late secondary to low self-esteem.
- Counseling on safe sex practices should be provided.

PROGNOSIS

- Goal of treatment is to reduce morbidity and prevent complications.
- Relapse may occur up to 18 months after treatment.
- If untreated, lesions may expand for years.

COMPLICATIONS

- Carcinoma (in 0.25%): Squamous cell carcinoma of the penis, vulva, or cervix
- After ulcer healing, fibrosis, stricture formation, phimosis, and scarring can occur, leading to deformity and functional disability.
- Balanitis and secondary infection of ulcers
- Elephantiasis of the genitals may occur secondary to lymphatic obstruction.
- Extragenital involvement with potential fatal spread to the viscera
- Recurrent disease even months to years after treatment (usually associated with HIV infection)

ADDITIONAL READING

- CDC. Sexually transmitted diseases treatment guidelines 2006. *MMWR*. 2006;55:1–118.
- Richens J. Donovanosis (granuloma inguinale). *Sex Transm Inf*. 2006;82(Suppl 4):21–2.
- Velho PE, de Souza EM, Belds Jr. W. Donovanosis. *The Brazilian Journal of Infectious Diseases* 2008;12(6):521–525.

CODES

ICD9

099.2 Granuloma inguinale

CLINICAL PEARLS

- The disease is transmitted usually through sexual activity, including vaginal and anal sex. It can, however, be transmitted through breaks in the skin, such as contact with ulcers of an infected person.
- Antibiotic treatment is available and must be tailored to the patient (e.g., pediatric, pregnant, coexisting conditions).
- It can be transmitted through an infected birth canal from a pregnant woman to her fetus.

GRANULOMA, PYOGENIC

Augustine J. Sohn, MD, MPH

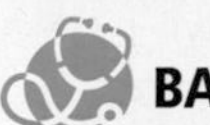

BASICS

DESCRIPTION

- Benign, acquired, solitary vascular proliferation that involves exposed areas such as distal extremities (especially the hands) and face as well as oral cavity (most frequently the gingiva)
- System(s) affected: Gastrointestinal (e.g., colon, small intestine); Skin/Exocrine; External ear canal, eye (e.g., eyelid, lacrimal sac)
- Synonym(s): Pregnancy tumor; Granuloma gravidum; Granuloma telangiectaticum; Lobular capillary hemangioma

EPIDEMIOLOGY

Mean age of patients with pyogenic granuloma is 40.5 years.

Incidence

- In children, accounts for <1% of all skin nodules
- 5% of pregnant women are affected in the US.

Prevalence

Unknown

RISK FACTORS

- Pregnancy
- Trauma
- Intraoral trauma or surgery

GENERAL PREVENTION

Good oral hygiene

ETIOLOGY

- Thought to be an aberrant healing response to minor trauma in many cases
- May be related to hormonal changes in pregnancy
- Not caused by bacterial infection, but associated with capillary proliferation
- Not considered a hemangioma or neoplasm

DIAGNOSIS

HISTORY

- Solitary lesion that develops rapidly from days to weeks after minor trauma and bleeds easily
- Grows early in pregnancy and partially regresses postpartum

PHYSICAL EXAM

- Most commonly located at head and neck lesion and upper extremities (1)[C]
- Among oral lesions, gingiva is the most common location (2)[C]
- Bright red, purple, yellow, or brown with moist and sometimes scaly appearing surface
- Ranges from a few millimeters to 2–3 cm in diameter (usually <1 cm); giant lesions may rarely occur on areas such as the foot
- Soft; sessile or pedunculated
- Granular, smooth, or slightly nodular

DIAGNOSTIC TESTS & INTERPRETATION

Diagnostic Procedures/Surgery

Excisional biopsy

Pathological Findings

Micro:

- Small, endothelial-lined vascular spaces
- Loose or dense connective tissue stroma
- Acute and chronic inflammatory cells
- No true granuloma formation
- Abundant mitotic activity

DIFFERENTIAL DIAGNOSIS

- Peripheral ossifying granuloma
- Giant cell granuloma
- Odontogenic fibroma
- Kaposi sarcoma
- Malignant melanoma
- Angiolymphoid hyperplasia with eosinophilia
- Metastatic carcinoma
- Pilomatricoma
- In AIDS patients: Bacillary angiomatosis, deep mycoses

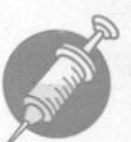

TREATMENT

SURGERY/OTHER PROCEDURES

- Surgical excision with simple closure gives the best result with least recurrence (3)[C].
- Shave excision with cautery may be optimal treatment for a lesion on fingertips (1)[C].
- Topical imiquimod may be useful for children (4)[C].
- Electrosurgery (electrodesiccation and curettage)
- Topical phenol may be used for periungual lesion (5)[C]
- CO_2-laser destruction
- Excision must be adequate to avoid recurrence. Even a small fragment of tissue left behind may lead to recurrence.
- Excisional biopsy should be tried in all situations if possible to ensure a proper diagnosis (i.e., not missing malignancies like amelanotic melanoma or basal cell carcinoma) (1)

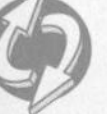

ONGOING CARE

PATIENT EDUCATION

Patient should avoid trauma to area following excision.

PROGNOSIS

- Some lesions spontaneously resolve on their own (usually within 6 months).
- Complete resolution is expected with adequate excision.

COMPLICATIONS

Recurrence: After removal or destruction of solitary lesion, multiple satellite lesions can form around original treatment site.

REFERENCES

1. Giblin AV, Clover AJ, Athanassopoulos A, Budny PG et al. Pyogenic granuloma - the quest for optimum treatment: audit of treatment of 408 cases. *Journal of plastic, reconstructive & aesthetic surgery : JPRAS*. 2007;60:1030–5.
2. Gordón-Nñez MA, Carvalho MD, Benevenuto TG, Lopes MF, Silva LM, Galvão HC et al. Oral Pyogenic Granuloma: A Retrospective Analysis of 293 Cases in a Brazilian Population. *Journal of oral and maxillofacial surgery : official journal of the American Association of Oral and Maxillofacial Surgeons*. 2010;
3. Gilmore A, Kelsberg G, Safranek S et al. Clinical inquiries. What's the best treatment for pyogenic granuloma? *J Fam Pract*. 2010;59:40–2.
4. Tritton SM, Smith S, Wong LC, Zagarella S, Fischer G et al. Pyogenic granuloma in ten children treated with topical imiquimod. *Pediatr Dermatol*. 269–72.
5. Iglesias ME, DE Bengoa Vallejo RB et al. Topical Phenol as a Conservative Treatment for Periungual Pyogenic Granuloma. *Dermatologic surgery : official publication for American Society for Dermatologic Surgery [et al.]*. 2010;

CODES

ICD9

686.1 Pyogenic granuloma of skin and subcutaneous tissue

CLINICAL PEARLS

- Benign, acquired, solitary vascular proliferation that involves exposed areas such as distal extremities and face as well as oral cavity
- Due mainly to aberrant healing response to minor trauma in many cases
- Excision must be adequate to avoid recurrence.
- Excisional biopsy recommended to ensure proper diagnosis (and to not miss a malignant lesion)
- Excision with primary closure or excision with cautery should be the first choice for treatment in most of the lesions.

G

GRAVES DISEASE

Katharine Barnard, MD

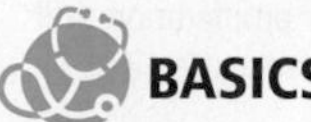

BASICS

DESCRIPTION

Graves disease is an autoimmune disease in which thyroid-stimulating antibodies cause increased thyroid function. In addition to hyperthyroidism, classic findings are goiter and ophthalmopathy.

EPIDEMIOLOGY

Prevalence

- Overall prevalence of hyperthyroidism is estimated to be 2% for women and 0.2% for men.
- Graves disease accounts for 60–80% of all cases of hyperthyroidism.
- Predominant age: 30–40 years

RISK FACTORS

- Female sex (due to sex steroids)
- Postpartum period
- Stressful life events (1)
- Medications: Iodine, amiodarone, lithium, HAART, rarely immune-modulating medications (i.e., interferon)
- Smoking (higher risk of developing ophthalmopathy)

Genetics

Higher risk with personal or family history of any autoimmune disease, especially Hashimoto's thyroiditis

GENERAL PREVENTION

Screening TSH in asymptomatic patients is not recommended. No data conclusively show that treatment of subclinical thyroid dysfunction improves quality of life or clinical outcome measures (2).

PATHOPHYSIOLOGY

- Excessive production of TSH receptor antibodies from B cells primarily within the thyroid, likely due to genetic clonal lack of suppressor T cells
- Binding of these antibodies to TSH receptors in the thyroid causes increased production of thyroid hormone.
- Binding to similar antigen in retro-orbital connective tissue causes ocular symptoms.

COMMONLY ASSOCIATED CONDITIONS

- Mitral valve prolapse
- Hypokalemic periodic paralysis

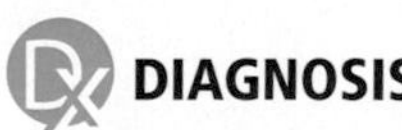

DIAGNOSIS

Thyroid hormone controls metabolic rate and affects many organ systems. Hyperthyroid patients appear hypermetabolic, with increased adrenergic tone.

HISTORY

- Tachycardia, palpitations
- Tremor, restlessness
- Anxiety, emotional lability, insomnia
- Sweating, heat intolerance
- Pruritus, skin changes
- Weight loss
- Fatigue, shortness of breath (due to muscle weakness)
- Oligo-/amenorrhea (women), erectile dysfunction (men), gynecomastia
- Loose, frequent stools
- Blurred vision or diplopia, lacrimation, photophobia, gritty sensation in eyes (ocular dryness), retro-orbital discomfort, painful eye movement, loss of color vision or visual acuity
- Worsening of chronic medical conditions (anxiety or Bipolar disorder, glucose intolerance, heart failure or angina)

Geriatric Considerations

Elderly patients may not display classic symptoms; may present with atrial fibrillation or weight loss

PHYSICAL EXAM

- Thyroid: Enlarged, nontender, and without nodules; possible bruit (increased blood flow)
- Integumentary: Fine hair, warm skin, onycholysis of nails, palmar erythema, possible pretibial myxedema, possible hyperpigmented plaques (dermopathy)
- Cardiac: Resting tachycardia, hyperdynamic circulation, possible atrial fibrillation
- Ophthalmologic (present in 50% of cases): Lid lag, lid retraction, proptosis, corneal irritation, ophthalmoplegia; papilledema and loss of color vision may signify optic neuropathy
- Extremities: Tremor, hyper-reflexia, proximal myopathy; rarely, soft tissue edema of extremities and clubbing of digits (acropachy)

DIAGNOSTIC TESTS & INTERPRETATION

Lab

Initial lab tests

- TSH is initial test. Very low or undetectable TSH confirms hyperthyroidism.
- Next, check T_4 level. T_4 will be high in Graves.

Pregnancy Considerations

Thyroid-stimulating hormone (TSH) level at 36 weeks gestation is most predictive of neonatal hyperthyroidism. This should be checked even in post-treatment pregnant patients taking thyroid hormone replacement.

Imaging

Initial approach

After confirming suppressed TSH and high T_4, next step is radioactive iodine uptake (RAIU) and scan. Graves patients will have diffuse, elevated RAIU (vs focal/nodular elevated uptake in adenoma and multinodular goiter, and decreased uptake in thyroiditis).

DIFFERENTIAL DIAGNOSIS

- Toxic multinodular goiter (multiple hormone-producing nodules)
- Toxic adenoma (single hormone-producing nodule)
- Thyroiditis (hormone leakage):
  - Subacute, usually postviral (thyroid will be tender)
  - Lymphocytic, including postpartum
  - Hashimoto's thyroiditis (anti-TPO antibodies may stimulate TSH receptors)
- Iatrogenic (treatment-induced):
  - Iodine-induced (dietary, radiographic contrast, or medications)
  - Amiodarone
  - Thyroid hormone over-replacement (accidental or intentional)
- Tumor:
  - Pituitary adenoma producing TSH
  - HCG-producing tumors (stimulate TSH receptors)
  - Extraglandular thyroid hormone production (i.e., struma ovarii or metastatic thyroid cancer)

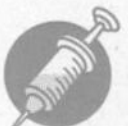

TREATMENT

MEDICATION

Goal of therapy is to correct the hypermetabolic state with the fewest side effects and lowest incidence of post-treatment hypothyroidism.

Pediatric Considerations

- Pediatric cases need treatment, as spontaneous remission occurs in only 30% of cases or less.
- Radioactive iodine is treatment of choice: Fewer side effects, higher cure rate, and no observed increase in future cancer risk or genetic damage. Higher dose radioactive iodine seems to confer even less risk of thyroid cancer than low dose, and so is preferable (3).

First Line

Radioactive iodine:

- Concentrates in the thyroid gland and destroys thyroid tissue
- Treatment of choice in the US for Graves disease
- High cure rate with single treatment, especially with high-dose regimen
- Risks: Side effects (neck soreness, flushing, decreased taste); worsening ophthalmopathy (15% incidence, higher in smokers) (4); post-treatment hypothyroidism (80% incidence, not dosage-dependent); radiation thyroiditis (1% incidence); need to adhere to safety precautions until radiation is eliminated from the body
- Pretreatment with antithyroid medication should be considered in patients with severe disease as symptom control and to reduce risk of post-treatment radiation thyroiditis. Pretreatment may, however, reduce cure rate with radioactive iodine so is not uniformly recommended.
- May be repeated in as soon as 4 months if needed

Pregnancy Considerations

- Radioactive iodine is contraindicated in pregnancy and lactation. There is no effect on future fertility, but it is recommended to avoid pregnancy for 4 months after receiving radioactive iodine.
- Antithyroid drugs: Methimazole (MMI) and propothiouracil (PTU):
  - Compete with the thyroid for iodine, thereby decreasing the synthesis of thyroid hormone; PTU also blocks peripheral conversion of T_4 to T_3
  - Treatment of choice for children and for adults who refuse radioactive iodine
  - May use as pretreatment (symptom control) for older or cardiac patients before radioactive iodine or surgery
  - MMI is usually first choice due to lower cost and once-daily dosing
  - No improvement in remission rates noted with higher-dose MMI; therefore, lowest effective dose should be used (5)
  - Minor side effects (<5% incidence), which may be controlled by switching from one agent to another: Rash, fever, arthralgias, GI side effects
  - Major side effects, which necessitate a change in treatment:
    - Polyarthritis (1–2%)
    - Agranulocytosis (<0.5%)
    - Elevated liver enzymes (30% with PTU) or hepatitis (rare)
    - Cholestasis and jaundice (occurs rarely with MMI)

- Discontinue treatment after 1 year if patient is euthyroid and thyroid-stimulating antibody level is undetectable.
- 60% remission rate with 2 years of treatment (standard regimen); newer studies suggest no increased benefit to treatment beyond 18 months (6)
- Relapse rate of up to 50% in patients who respond initially; higher relapse rate if smoker, large goiter, or positive thyroid-stimulating antibodies at the end of treatment

Pregnancy Considerations

PTU is preferred in pregnancy, as MMI crosses the placenta and may have risks of congenital malformation and for congenital hypothyroidism. Either is safe in breastfeeding (7).

Second Line

Plasmapheresis is under investigation as a treatment option (8).

ADDITIONAL TREATMENT

Issues for Referral

- Endocrinologist:
  - Radioactive iodine therapy
  - Pregnant or breastfeeding patient
  - Graves ophthalmopathy (also should see ophthalmologist)
- Surgeon:
  - Failed drug therapy, or refusing RAI
  - Obstruction
  - Cosmesis

Additional Therapies

- Beta-blockers provide prompt control of adrenergic symptoms. Can be started while workup is in progress. Long-acting propranolol is used most commonly, and titrated to symptom control (40–320 mg daily). Calcium channel blockers are an alternative for heart rate control in patients who cannot take beta-blockers (8).
- Symptom control may be achieved with iodides, which block conversion of T_4 to T_3, and inhibit TSH release. Use for pregnant patients who do not tolerate antithyroid medication, or in conjunction with antithyroid medications. Should not be used long-term (may cause paradoxical increase in TSH release) or in combination with radioactive iodine.
- For corneal protection: Tinted glasses when outdoors, artificial tears, patching or taping the lids at night
- For proptosis: Oral steroid (prednisone 60–80 mg daily for 2–4 weeks, then tapered off)
- For dermopathy, if local discomfort at site of plaques: Topical corticosteroid

SURGERY/OTHER PROCEDURES

- Surgery may be indicated if medication fails, if patient refuses RAI, or in the case of severe disease in second trimester of pregnancy.
- Subtotal thyroidectomy preserves some thyroid function and only holds 25% post-op incidence of hypothyroidism, but has less predictable outcome; therefore, total thyroidectomy is now standard of care. Studies show no increased risk of permanent complications (hypoparathyroidism or laryngeal nerve damage) with total thyroidectomy (9).

IN-PATIENT CONSIDERATIONS

Indications for hospital admission:

- Thyroid storm (rare but life-threatening complication of Graves, with exaggerated symptoms: Tachycardia, hyperpyrexia, neurologic compromise, and GI/liver dysfunction; may be precipitated by trauma, infection, iodine load, or surgery). Admit to ICU for symptom control and antithyroid medications.
- Ophthalmopathy with visual impairment. Admit with ophthalmology consult.
- Severe cardiac symptoms (CHF, rapid atrial fibrillation, angina). Admit for rate control and cardiology consult.

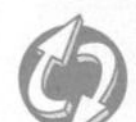

ONGOING CARE

FOLLOW-UP RECOMMENDATIONS

Patient Monitoring

- Monitoring is for resolution of hyperthyroidism and for development of hypothyroidism.
- Check TSH and T_4 levels every 1–2 months for first 6 months after treatment, then every 3 months for a year, then every 6–12 months thereafter. For patients on treatment with PTU and MMI, check anti-TSH receptor antibodies at 12 months of treatment to determine possibility of discontinuing medication.

Pregnancy Considerations

Postpartum exacerbation of hyperthyroidism is common for women not currently under treatment, so TSH and symptoms should be monitored.

DIET

Nutritional supplementation with L-carnitine may diminish hyperthyroid symptoms and may decrease bone demineralization (10).

PATIENT EDUCATION

Adherence to follow-up (surveillance) recommendations and medication regimens are the most important ways to achieve a good outcome and promote lifelong health.

PROGNOSIS

- Generally good with treatment
- May have irreversible ocular, cardiac, and psychiatric consequences
- Increased morbidity and mortality due to osteoporosis, atherosclerotic disease, insulin resistance and obesity, and endothelial cell dysfunction (thromboembolic risk) (8,11)

COMPLICATIONS

Hypothyroidism is most common consequence of treatment (25-80% depending on treatment modality). Patients should be monitored annually, even if asymptomatic.

REFERENCES

1. Matos-Santos A. Relationship between number of and impact of stressful life events and the onset of Graves Disease and toxic multinodular goitre. *Clin Endocrinol*. 2007;55(1).
2. Helfand M, U.S. Preventive Services Task Force. Screening for subclinical thyroid dysfunction in nonpregnant adults: a summary of the evidence for the U.S. Preventive Services Task Force. *Ann Intern Med*. 2004;140:128–41.
3. Rivkees SA, Dinauer C. An optimal treatment for pediatric graves' disease is radioiodine. *J Clin Endocrinol Metab*. 2007;92:797–800.
4. Woeber KA. The year in review: the thyroid. *Ann Intern Med*. 1999;131:959–62.
5. Benker G, Reinwein D. Is there a methimazole dose effect on remission rate in Graves Disease? Results from a longterm prospective study. *Clin Endocrinol*. 2004;49(4).
6. Maugendre D, Gatel A. Antithyroid drugs and Graves Disease - prospective randomized assessment of longterm treatment. *Clin Endocrinol*. 2004;50(1).
7. Streetman DD, Khanderia U. Diagnosis and treatment of Graves disease. *Ann Pharmacother*. 2003;37:1100–9.
8. Reid JR, Wheeler SF. Hyperthyroidism: diagnosis and treatment. *Am Fam Physician*. 2005;72: 623–30.
9. Barakate MS, Agarwal G. Total thyroidectomy is now the preferred option for the surgical management of Graves Disease. *ANZ Journal of Surgery*. 2002;72(5).
10. Benvenga S, Ruggeri RM, Russo A, et al. Usefulness of L-carnitine, a naturally occurring peripheral antagonist of thyroid hormone action, in iatrogenic hyperthyroidism: a randomized, double-blind, placebo-controlled clinical trial. *J Clin Endocrinol Metab*. 2001;86:3579–94.
11. Burggraaf J, Lalezari S, Emeis JJ, et al. Endothelial function in patients with hyperthyroidism before and after treatment with propranolol and thiamazol. *Thyroid*. 2001;11:153–60.

G

ADDITIONAL READING

AACE Thyroid Task Force. American Association of Clinical Endocrinologists medical guidelines for clinical practice for the evaluation and treatment of hyperthyroidism and hypothyroidism. *Endocr Pract*. 2002;8(6).

See Also (Topic, Algorithm, Electronic Media Element)

Algorithms: Weight Loss; Cardiac Arrhythmias; Anxiety

CODES

ICD9

- 242.00 Toxic diffuse goiter without mention of thyrotoxic crisis or storm
- 242.01 Toxic diffuse goiter with mention of thyrotoxic crisis or storm

CLINICAL PEARLS

Thyroid hormone controls metabolic rate and affects many organ systems. Hyperthyroid patients appear hypermetabolic, with symptoms and signs of increased adrenergic tone.

GROWTH HORMONE DEFICIENCY

Lee A. Mancini, MD, CSCS, CSN

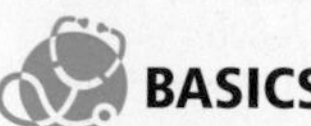

BASICS

DESCRIPTION

- Inadequate production of growth hormone (GH, also called *somatotropin*) in either adults or children
- GH is a polypeptide hormone that stimulates growth and cell reproduction.
- *Hypopituitarism* is often used to describe growth hormone deficiency (GHD). However, hypopituitarism is actually defined as GHD plus a deficiency in at least 1 other anterior pituitary hormone.
- *Panhypopituitarism* is defined as a deficiency in all the hormones produced in the pituitary gland.
- System(s) affected: Endocrine; Musculoskeletal
- Synonym(s): Hypopituitarism

EPIDEMIOLOGY

Incidence

- Most common cause of GHD in children is idiopathic.
- Most common cause of GHD in adults is a pituitary adenoma or treatment of the adenoma with surgery or radiotherapy:
  - 76% of patients with GHD had a pituitary tumor.
  - 13% had an extrapituitary tumor.
  - 8% the cause was unknown
  - 1% had sarcoidosis.
  - 0.5% had Sheehan syndrome.

Prevalence

- In children, isolated GHD has been reported to affect 1 in 4,000.
- Adult-onset idiopathic GHD is extremely rare.

RISK FACTORS

Genetics

A variety of congenital genetic causes of GHD:

- Transcription factor defects (PIT-1, PROP-1, LHX3/4, HESX-1, and PITX-2)
- GHRH receptor gene defects
- GH secretagogue receptor gene defects
- GH gene defects
- GH receptor/postreceptor defects
- Prader-Willi syndrome

PATHOPHYSIOLOGY

- GHD is caused by a complete lack of GH production or a decline in GH production. There are multiple causes.
- Hypothalamus secretes GH-releasing hormone (GHRH), which stimulates the pituitary to secrete GH. Somatostatin is secreted by the hypothalamus to inhibit GH secretion. When GH pulses are secreted into the blood, then insulinlike growth factor (IGF)-1 is released. GHD may result from disruption of the GH axis at numerous places—in the higher brain, the hypothalamus, or the pituitary gland.

ETIOLOGY

- Congenital:
  - Genetic (see Genetics)
  - Structural brain defects:
    - Agenesis of corpus callosum
    - Septo-optic dysplasia
    - Empty sella syndrome
    - Encephalocele
    - Hydrocephalus
    - Arachnoid cyst
  - Associated midline facial defects:
    - Single central incisor
    - Cleft lip/palate
- Acquired:
  - Trauma:
    - Perinatal
    - Postnatal
  - Central nervous system (CNS) infection
  - Tumors of hypothalamus or pituitary:
    - Pituitary adenoma
    - Craniopharyngioma
    - Rathke cleft cyst
    - Glioma/astrocytoma
    - Germinoma
    - Metastatic
  - Cranial irradiation
  - Surgery

COMMONLY ASSOCIATED CONDITIONS

- Macroadenoma
- Sarcoidosis
- Sheehan syndrome

DIAGNOSIS

HISTORY

- Adults:
  - Fatigue
  - Muscle weakness
  - Depression
  - Social withdrawal
  - Poor memory
  - Loss of strength
  - Loss of stamina
- Children:
  - Slower muscular development and delayed gross motor milestones such as standing, walking, and jumping
  - Important questions to ask:
    - Birth weight and length
    - Height of parents
    - Timing of puberty in parents
    - Previous growth points
    - Nutritional history
    - General health of child

PHYSICAL EXAM

- Children with GHD:
  - Most common presentation is short stature
  - Newborns may present with hypoglycemia, jaundice, or micropenis.
  - Severe GHD children have maxillary hypoplasia and forehead prominence; kewpie doll appearance.
  - Accurately measure height and weight.
  - Assess pubertal status using Tanner staging system.
- Adults:
  - Decreased lean body mass
  - Poor bone density

DIAGNOSTIC TESTS & INTERPRETATION

Lab

Initial lab tests

- IGF-1, IGFBP-3
- Multiple GH levels
- Thyroid-stimulating hormone (TSH) (hypothyroidism should be excluded as a cause)
- Serum electrolytes (low bicarbonate levels may indicate renal tubular acidosis)
- Complete blood count (CBC) and erythrocyte sedimentation rate (ESR)
- Karyotype

ollow-Up & Special Considerations
- Testing for GHD by random measurement of GH in a single blood sample is not beneficial, as GH is nearly undetectable for most of the day.
- In children, evaluate those who have significant discrepancy between growth curve.
- Low levels of IGF-1 and IGF binding protein (IGFBP)-3
- Multiple blood-sample testing for GH levels

maging

nitial approach

Radiograph of left hand and wrist to determine skeletal age in children

Follow-Up & Special Considerations

Brain magnetic resonance imaging (MRI) to evaluate for a tumor may be ordered.

Diagnostic Procedures/Surgery

Provocative tests:
- Give a dose of an agent that in a normal person causes a surge in the release of GH: Common agents used include argine, clonidine, glucagons, insulin, levodopa, and propranolol (1)[C]
- After agent is given, GH serum levels are drawn every 15 minutes.
- GH levels are checked for over 60 minutes.

DIFFERENTIAL DIAGNOSIS
- Turner syndrome
- Renal failure
- Small size for gestational age in newborns
- Prader-Willi syndrome
- Idiopathic short stature
- Noonan syndrome
- Russell-Silver syndrome
- Down syndrome

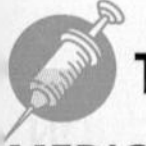

TREATMENT

MEDICATION
- GHD is treated with GH replacement.
- In 1985, GH was synthetically produced from recombinant DNA.
- Several medications are approved for GHD treatment in children:
  - Liquid solutions for SC injection: These are available in multidose pen devices. Daily therapy is more effective than 3-times-a-week therapy. The recommended dose is 0.04 mg/kg/d for children (2)[C].
  - Encapsulated GH in glycolide microspheres for deep SC administration. Either 1.5 mg/kg body weight once a month or 0.75 mg/kg twice a month.
  - Geref (sermorelin) has been removed from the market. It is a synthetic growth hormone-releasing hormone.
- Several growth hormone-releasing peptides (GHRPs) or nonpeptide analogs are to be evaluated in children and adults. It is too early to evaluate their long-term safety and efficacy.

ADDITIONAL TREATMENT

Issues for Referral

Patients with GHD would benefit from a referral to an endocrinologist.

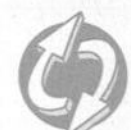

ONGOING CARE

FOLLOW-UP RECOMMENDATIONS
- Children: Regular follow-up with a pediatric endocrinologist
- Adults: Follow-up with an endocrinologist is recommended.

DIET

No restrictions

PROGNOSIS
- In children, the prognosis for GHD is good. GH therapy is effective.
- 5 independent predictors of pubertal growth:
  - Gender
  - Age at onset of puberty
  - Age at end of growth
  - Dose of growth hormone at onset of puberty
  - Deviation of target height from height at onset of puberty

COMPLICATIONS
- In children:
  - Slipped capital femoral epiphysis
  - Scoliosis
- In adults and children:
  - Unmet expectations
  - Metabolic effects
  - Antibodies to growth hormone
  - Cancer: Lymphoma, tumor recurrence
  - Fluid retention: Pseudotumor cerebri, carpal tunnel syndrome, pancreatitis, and edema

REFERENCES

1. Molich ME, et al. Clinical practice guideline: Evaluation and treatment of adult growth hormone deficiency. An endocrine society clinical practice guideline. *J Clin Endocrinol Metabol*. 2006;91: 1621–34.
2. deMuink Keizer-Schrama SM, et al. Dose-response study of biosynthetic human growth hormone in GH-deficient children: Effects on axiological and biochemical parameters. *J Clin Endocrinol Metabol*. 1992;74:898.

ADDITIONAL READING

- Hoffman AR, et al. Efficacy and tolerability of an individualized dosing regimen for adult growth hormone replacement therapy in comparison with fixed body weight-based dosing. *J Clin Endocrinol Metabol*. 2004;87:1974–9.
- Rosenfield RG, et al. Diagnostic controversy: the diagnosis of childhood growth hormone deficiency revisited. *J Clin Endocrinol Metabol*. 1995;80:1532.

See Also (Topic, Algorithm, Electronic Media Element)

Pituitary Tumors

CODES

ICD9
- 253.2 Panhypopituitarism
- 253.3 Pituitary dwarfism

CLINICAL PEARLS

- Most common cause of GHD in children is idiopathic.
- Most common cause of GHD in adults is pituitary adenoma.
- Treatment of pituitary adenoma is either surgery or radiotherapy.
- All patients taking replacement GH therapy need to have their IGF-1 level monitored.

GUILLAIN-BARRÉ SYNDROME

Sheela Swaminatha, MD

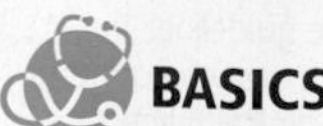

BASICS

DESCRIPTION

- A group of autoimmune diseases targeted at the peripheral nerves and causing acute progressive weakness, usually an ascending paralysis
- Divided into 2 forms:
  - Demyelinating: Acute inflammatory demyelinating polyradiculoneuropathy (AIDP): >90% of cases in Western countries
  - Axonal injury: Uncommon; poor prognosis:
    - Acute motor axonal neuropathy (AMAN): 5% of cases; predominant motor involvement; acute flaccid paralysis with rapid recovery; >50% in northern China; recent *Campylobacter jejuni* gastroenteritis; often summer epidemics in children and adults
    - Acute motor-sensory axonal neuropathy (AMSAN): Hyperacute course: Leads to profound weakness with muscle wasting; poor prognosis
- Occurs mostly in adults
- Synonym(s): Acute inflammatory demyelinating polyradiculopathy; Landry-Guillain-Barré-Strohl syndrome; Acute inflammatory neuropathy; Acute idiopathic polyneuritis; Acute immune-mediated polyneuritis; Landry ascending paralysis

ALERT

30% of the patients have respiratory paralysis requiring mechanical ventilation, but complete or substantial recovery is the natural disease course.

Geriatric Considerations

Worse prognosis >60 years of age

Pediatric Considerations

Disease tends to be milder in children.

Pregnancy Considerations

Uncommon in pregnancy

EPIDEMIOLOGY

Incidence

In the US: 1.8/100,000 (0.8/100,000 in children <18 years of age; 3.2/100,000 in adults >60 years of age)

Prevalence

- In the US: 3–10/100,000
- Predominant age: All ages
- Predominant sex: Male > Female (1.5:1)
- Nonseasonal, nonepidemic

RISK FACTORS

Diabetes mellitus (DM), recent surgery, organ transplantation (i.e., immunosuppression)

PATHOPHYSIOLOGY

Autoimmune disorder targeted against myelin and/or axons of peripheral nerves causing destruction of peripheral nerves in susceptible individuals

ETIOLOGY

Unclear; may be related to viral or bacterial infection

COMMONLY ASSOCIATED CONDITIONS

- Vaccinations: Swine flu (but not other influenza vaccine) and rabies
- Inactivated flu vaccines cause an estimated 1.6 additional cases of Guillain-Barré syndrome per million vaccinations (1)[A].
- 2009 data reveal no increased incidence of Guillain-Barré syndrome (GBS) with the Gardasil vaccine for human papillomavirus (HPV) compared with age-matched controls; incidence was 0.2/100,000 doses (2)[A],(3).
- Malignancies, Hodgkin lymphoma

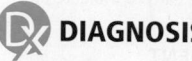

DIAGNOSIS

HISTORY

- Upper respiratory or diarrheal disease within previous 1–3 weeks in 50–70%: *C. jejuni* (~40%), cytomegalovirus (13%), Epstein-Barr virus (10%), *Mycoplasma pneumoniae* (5%), or HIV
- Dysesthesias, paresthesias of feet and hands are usually the earliest symptoms.
- Pain common, especially back pain; can radiate to the legs; no myalgias
- Gait disorder common in all age groups; most common presentation in children
- Neck muscle weakness, dysphagia, and dysarthria are predictors of respiratory failure.
- Most patients reach the plateau phase within 3 weeks of admission, and muscle strength is expected to improve.

PHYSICAL EXAM

- Acute, symmetric, and usually ascending weakness of limbs within days of dysesthesias (4)[A]
- Areflexia or hyporeflexia and muscle weakness, decreased position and vibratory sensation
- Respiratory muscle paralysis 30% if untreated
- Cranial nerve involvement <50%; usually facial weakness, 10–20% ophthalmoparesis
- Dysautonomia (50%): Labile blood pressure, arrhythmias, ileus, urinary retention; more common when seen with severe quadriparesis and respiratory failure
- Miller-Fisher variant: Ophthalmoplegia, ataxia, areflexia

DIAGNOSTIC TESTS & INTERPRETATION

Lab

Initial lab tests

- CSF: Elevated protein and normal white blood cells (WBCs; albuminocytologic dissociation) are characteristic, except that in patients with HIV aseptic meningitis, cell counts may be high. There is a normal opening pressure.
- Blood: Complete blood count (CBC), renal and hepatic function; when appropriate, rheumatoid factor, antineutrophil cytoplasmic antibodies, Sjögren syndrome A&B antibody, angiotensin-converting enzyme (ACE) level, cryoglobulinemia, D-aminolevulinic acid, and Lyme titer
- Urine: 24-hour urine for light chains
- Optional: Drug/toxin, heavy metal screen, HIV; in children, may check arylsulfatase A activity

Follow-Up & Special Considerations

- Special test: Serum anti-GM1 antibody titer in axonal variant (2)[B]; 30% of patients have elevated anti-GM1 antibodies.
- Anti-$GQ1_b$ in ophthalmoplegia form of GBS (Miller-Fisher variant) (5)
- Disorders that may alter lab results: Demyelinating neuropathy of DM may have CSF similar to that of GBS; however, GBS usually has higher CSF protein (>0.4 g/dL).
- Protein normal in 50% patients in 1st week of illness

Imaging

Initial approach

CXR

Follow-Up & Special Considerations

MRI of spinal cord if myelopathy or cord lesion suspected. Diffuse dorsal root enhancement seen on MRI with gadolinium supports GBS.

Diagnostic Procedures/Surgery

- Lumbar puncture for CSF analysis
- Nerve conduction studies (most sensitive test):
  - Initially, may show prolonged F-wave latency
  - Conduction block is common in GBS and characteristic of acquired demyelinating neuropathy.
  - Prolonged distal latency and slowing of conduction velocity in 2 nerves each in arms or legs
  - Formal pulmonary function test (includes negative inspiratory force [NIF] and forced vital capacity [FVC])
  - 12-lead ECG

Pathological Findings

Sural nerve biopsy not indicated unless necessary to rule out vasculitis or amyloidosis: Multifocal inflammatory cell infiltration with segmental demyelination and relative axonal sparing in GBS; axonal degeneration in axonal form of GBS; sensory neuronopathy in so-called Miller-Fisher syndrome

DIFFERENTIAL DIAGNOSIS

- Brain:
  - Acute cerebrovascular strokes (e.g., basilar artery thrombosis)
  - Encephalitis
- Spinal cord syndromes:
  - Transverse myelitis: Can have identical initial presentation
  - Cord compression
  - Carcinomatous meningoradiculitis
- Motor neuron disorder: Poliomyelitis
- Peripheral neuropathy associated with:
  - Vasculitis (e.g., polyarteritis nodosa, Wegner, Churg-Strauss, nonsystemic vasculitis limited to peripheral nerve)
  - Disimmune process (e.g., paraneoplastic syndrome, sensory gangliopathy, angiofollicular lymphoma)
  - Acute ICU neuromyopathy, critical illness neuropathy, ICU myopathy
  - Toxin (e.g., arsenic or thallium poisoning, vitamin B_6 overdose, glue sniffing, chemotherapeutics, organophosphates, neurotoxic fish)
  - Infectious (e.g., tick paralysis, diphtheria, Lyme)
  - Flaring of hereditary/congenital neuropathy (e.g., porphyria, Fabry, mitochondria cytopathy)
- Neuromuscular junction:
  - Myasthenia gravis
  - Eaton-Lambert
  - Botulism
  - Hypermagnesemia
- Muscle:
  - Polymyositis
  - Periodic paralysis (hypokalemia)
  - Toxic myopathy
- Psychiatric: Hysteria

TREATMENT

MEDICATION

Immune globulin IV 2 g/kg over 5 days:
- In severe disease, intravenous immunoglobulin started within 2 weeks from onset hastens recovery as much as plasma exchange (6)[A] *or*

Plasmapheresis on 5 alternate days for a total of 250 mL/kg (7):
- Requires vascular access
- May be difficult in hemodynamically unstable patient given fluid shifts during plasma exchange

Corticosteroids given alone do not significantly hasten recovery from GBS or affect the long-term outcome (8)[A].

ADDITIONAL TREATMENT

General Measures

- Tachyarrhythmias: May not require treatment
- Bradyarrhythmias: If symptomatic, atropine
- Sinus arrest and complete heart block: Temporary pacemaker
- Constipation/ileus from autonomic neuropathy: Laxatives, enemas
- Sucralfate 1 g b.i.d. in mechanically ventilated or nonsteroidal anti-inflammatory drug (NSAID) users
- Urinary retention from autonomic neuropathy: Catheterization
- Depression: Frequent reminders that recovery is the rule; avoid antidepressants.

Additional Therapies

There is no role for high-dose corticosteroids (7).

COMPLEMENTARY AND ALTERNATIVE MEDICINE

Lipoic acid for neuropathic pain control

IN-PATIENT CONSIDERATIONS

Initial Stabilization

- Admitted to ICU; 50% of those need mechanical ventilation; 10–20% of patients have mild disease without need of immune globulin IV or plasmapheresis (9)[A].
- Serial FVC, NIF, and oximetry; intubation for respiratory distress or FVC <20 mL/kg (<1 L in adults), NIF >–20, or difficulty swallowing/aspiration from bulbar palsy; use caution—unfavorable NIF and FVC may precede dyspnea or appreciable rise in pCO_2 on arterial blood gases (ABGs).
- Hypertension (HTN):
  - Often does not need treatment
  - In severe HTN, use morphine bolus to prevent congestive heart failure (CHF).
- Hypotension: Trendelenburg position and volume expansion; pressors if needed
- Pain: Common; can be severe and recalcitrant; analgesics including opioids; carbamazepine; transcutaneous electrical nerve stimulation (TENS)
- Aspiration precautions

Admission Criteria

Any patients suspected of GBS

Nursing

- Prevent complications of immobilization with physical therapy, pneumatic compressor, or subcutaneous heparin.
- Respiratory care and frequent turning; aspiration precaution
- Monitor bowel and bladder function for retention/ileus.

Discharge Criteria

Transfer to rehabilitation facility if patient is able to walk in the plateau phase. Discharge if in the recovery phase.

ONGOING CARE

FOLLOW-UP RECOMMENDATIONS

FVC is the best measurement, as opposed to oximetry/ABGs, which are normal until respiratory failure has occurred.

Patient Monitoring

- Accessory muscle for respiration and spirometry/vital capacity 4×/day at bedside
- Bulbar weakness and airway secretions
- Mechanical ventilation for airway protection or vital capacity <15 mL/kg of body weight or maximum inspiratory pressure ≤25 cm H_2O
- Telemetry monitoring for cardiac condition

DIET

No special diet; enteral feedings if intubated

PATIENT EDUCATION

Important to emphasize expectation of full/significant recovery, regardless of treatment

PROGNOSIS

- If untreated, 3 phases of illness:
  - Initial progression phase 24 hours–3 weeks; >50% reach nadir before 14 days; highest risk of death and complications during this phase (10)[A].
  - Plateau phase same duration as initial phase
  - Recovery phase 1–6 months; in adults, no discernible improvement after 2 years
- Mortality (most often from dysautonomia or complications): 2–5%
- Complete recovery: 50%
- Some residual disability: 45%
- Severe permanent disability: 5%
- Miller-Fisher variant often has more benign prognosis with mean recovery in ~10 weeks.
- Relapses may occur both before and after recovery; acute inflammatory demyelinating polyradiculoneuropathy is the initial presentation of 2% of chronic inflammatory demyelinating polyradiculoneuropathy patients.
- Poor prognostic signs:
  - Rapid progression to severe disease (<7 days)
  - Mechanical ventilation
  - Nerve conduction studies: Compound muscle action potential <10% or mean distal motor amplitude <20%
  - Acute motor axonal neuropathy (see Differential Diagnosis)
  - Preceding *C. jejuni* infection
  - Age >60 years

COMPLICATIONS

- Paralysis, permanent residual weakness
- Respiratory failure, mechanical ventilation
- Hypotension, HTN, labile blood pressure
- Cardiac arrhythmias
- Ileus
- Urinary retention
- Aspiration, pneumonia, sepsis
- Deep vein thrombosis, pulmonary embolism
- Psychiatric problems, including depression

REFERENCES

1. Jefferson T, Di Pietrantonj C, Rivetti A, Bawazeer GA, Al-Ansary LA, Ferroni E et al. Vaccines for preventing influenza in healthy adults. *Cochrane Database Syst Rev*. 2010;7:CD001269.
2. Hiraga A, Mori M, Ogawara K, et al. Recovery patterns and long term prognosis for axonal Guillain-Barré syndrome. *J Neurol Neurosurg Psychiatry*. 2005;76:719–22.
3. Slade BA, Leidel L, Vellozzi C, et al. Postlicensure safety surveillance for quadrivalent human papillomavirus recombinant vaccine. *JAMA*. 2009;302:750–7.
4. Ruts L, van Koningsveld R, van Doorn PA. Distinguishing acute-onset CIDP from Guillain-Barré syndrome with treatment related fluctuations. *Neurology*. 2005;65:138–40.
5. Chiba A, Kusunoki S, Obata H, et al. Serum anti-GQ1b IgG antibody is associated with ophthalmoplegia in Miller Fisher syndrome and Guillain-Barré syndrome: clinical and immunohistochemical studies. *Neurology*. 1993;43:1911–7.
6. Hughes RA, Swan AV, van Doorn PA et al. Intravenous immunoglobulin for Guillain-Barré syndrome. *Cochrane Database Syst Rev*. 2010;6:CD002063.
7. Hughes RA, Wijdicks EF, Barohn R, et al. Practice parameter: immunotherapy for Guillain-Barré syndrome: report of the Quality Standards Subcommittee of the American Academy of Neurology. *Neurology*. 2003;61:736–40.
8. Hughes RA, Swan AV, van Doorn PA et al. Corticosteroids for Guillain-Barré syndrome. *Cochrane Database Syst Rev*. 2010;2:CD001446.
9. Moussouttas M, Chandy D, Dyro F. Fulminant acute inflammatory demyelinating polyradiculoneuropathy: case report and literature review. *Neurocrit Care*. 2004;1:469–73.
10. Green DM, Ropper AH. Mild Guillain-Barré syndrome. *Arch Neurol*. 2001;58:1098–101.

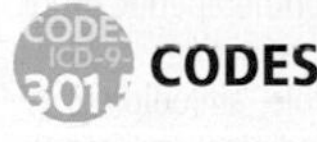

CODES

ICD9

357.0 Acute infective polyneuritis

CLINICAL PEARLS

- GBS is treatable, and if recognized and addressed early, few patients die from this condition.
- The natural history of GBS is to resolve, and treatment with IVIG or plasmapheresis may speed rate of recovery.
- The most useful diagnostic tests are lumbar puncture and a nerve conduction study.
- If GBS is suspected, initial evaluation must include an FVC and NIF to assess for respiratory compromise.

G

GYNECOMASTIA

Timothy L. Black, MD

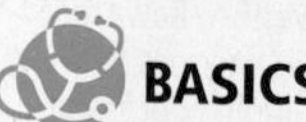

BASICS

DESCRIPTION

- Benign glandular enlargement of male breast that is generally bilateral (may be asymmetric or unilateral):
  - Type 1: Benign adolescent hypertrophy; physiologic discoid subacute mass
  - Type 2: Physiologic gynecomastia; generalized enlargement to greater degree
  - Type 3: Simulated by obesity
  - Type 4: Pectoral muscle hypertrophy
- System(s) affected: Endocrine/Metabolic; Skin/Exocrine
- Synonym(s): Male breast hypertrophy

EPIDEMIOLOGY

- Predominant age: Puberty; >65 years of age (especially with weight gain)
- Predominant sex: Male only

Pediatric Considerations

Transient gynecomastia is seen in neonatal boys.

Geriatric Considerations

Drug-induced form is more common in geriatric patients.

Prevalence

- 38–64% of pubertal males may have mild form. Usual onset is 11–12 years of age, with resolution by age 16–17 years.
- Nonpubertal forms are rare except when drug-induced.

RISK FACTORS

- Obesity
- Liver disease
- Renal disease
- Recovery from prolonged severe illness associated with malnutrition and weight loss (refeeding gynecomastia)
- Multiple therapeutic as well as nontherapeutic drugs (e.g., spironolactone, cimetidine, ranitidine, omeprazole, isoniazid, ketoconazole, amlodipine, captopril, diltiazem, enalapril, nifedipine, verapamil, diazepam, haloperidol, digitalis, statin drugs, anabolic steroids, androgens, estrogens, growth hormone, amphetamines, heroin, methadone, marijuana, and ethanol, among others) (1)
- Family history

Genetics

Some instances of familial gynecomastia may be inherited as male-limited autosomal trait.

GENERAL PREVENTION

In men taking estrogen for prostate cancer: Low-dose radiation prior to institution of diethylstilbestrol

PATHOPHYSIOLOGY

The cause of pubertal gynecomastia is not clear (2)[C].

- May be related to transient imbalance of androgens and estrogens
- May be related to higher leptin levels (may result in altered local estrogen levels)

ETIOLOGY

- Physiologic: Transient in neonatal boys and at puberty:
  - 60–90% of newborn males develop transient breast enlargement related to transplacental estrogen.
  - In pubertal boys, may require 1–3 years to regress or may not regress at all
  - Men age 60–90 years may develop gynecomastia related to declining levels of testosterone.
- Exposure to a high level of estrogen compared with testosterone concentration
- Identifiable syndrome/cause found in 12% of pubertal boys (3)[C]
- Tumors: Estrogen-secreting, gonadotropin-secreting, prolactin-secreting pituitary adenomas, hepatic fibrolamellar carcinoma
- Drugs (10–25% of gynecomastia) (1): Hormones, marijuana, digitalis, spironolactone, cimetidine, ketoconazole, phenytoin, furosemide, verapamil, cytotoxic drugs, antihypertensives, sedatives, antidepressants, amphetamines, heroin, methadone, anabolic steroids (2)[C]
- Systemic disorders: Cirrhosis, thyrotoxicosis, renal failure
- Androgen production deficiency
- Androgen-insensitivity syndromes
- Idiopathic (25% of gynecomastia)

COMMONLY ASSOCIATED CONDITIONS

- Peutz-Jeghers syndrome
- Male pseudohermaphroditism
- Hyperthyroidism
- Hypothyroidism
- Hepatic disease
- Prostate carcinoma
- Adrenal neoplasms (adenoma or carcinoma)
- Renal disease or dialysis
- True hermaphrodism
- Klinefelter syndrome
- Testicular failure (enzymatic defects of testosterone production, androgen insensitivity)
- Testicular neoplasms (germ cell, Leydig cell, Sertoli cell tumors)

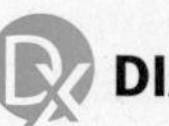

DIAGNOSIS

HISTORY

- Determine onset and duration of symptoms.
- Investigate concurrent drug treatments.

PHYSICAL EXAM

- Careful breast exam to evaluate characteristics of breast:
  - May involve 1 or both breasts
  - Usually asymptomatic but may be tender if it has developed rapidly
  - Usually located concentrically beneath the nipple and areola
- Abdominal exam
- Testicular exam
- Rectal exam

DIAGNOSTIC TESTS & INTERPRETATION

- Most cases in teenage boys are self-limiting and require reassurance alone.
- Full endocrine investigations may be indicated if symptoms of other disease states are indicated.
  - Thyroid function studies, testosterone, estradiol, beta human chorionic gonadotropin, luteinizing hormone (LH), liver functions tests, GGT, prolactin, α-fetoprotein

Lab

Laboratory evaluation rarely indicated in teenage boys

Initial lab tests

If worsening symptoms or clinical suspicion of secondary cause, consider

- Human chorionic gonadotropin (hGC) levels: High levels may indicate choriocarcinoma or other hCG-secreting tumor.
- Plasma testosterone and LH measurements: Help diagnose hypogonadism
- Serum estradiol (E_2)

- Serum prolactin
- Prostate-specific antigen (PSA)
- Liver function tests (LFTs)
- Others if clinically indicated (e.g., thyroid function, chromosomal analysis)

Follow-Up & Special Considerations

Disorders that may alter lab results:

- Cirrhosis
- Thyrotoxicosis
- Renal failure

Imaging

- CT scan of chest and abdomen if adrenal or extragonadal germ cell tumor is suspected
- Testicular ultrasound if there is a palpable mass or abnormality of one or both testicles (rarely indicated)
- MRI of pituitary fossa if prolactin levels are elevated (to exclude a prolactinoma)

Diagnostic Procedures/Surgery

Biopsy, if suspicious

Pathological Findings

- Dense, periductal, hyaline, collagenous connective tissue
- Hyperplastic ductal lining
- Plasma cell infiltrate

DIFFERENTIAL DIAGNOSIS

- Obesity with increase in adipose tissue
- Carcinoma of male breast
- Lipomas
- Neurofibromas
- Cystic hygroma

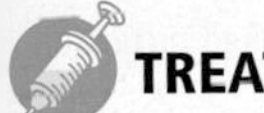

TREATMENT

- In teenage males, only reassurance and follow-up are usually indicated.
  - Spontaneous resolution in majority with the first 1–2 years
  - Persistent idiopathic gynecomastia in 7–8% of teenage boys at 3 years following diagnosis (2)[C]
- There is little evidence to recommend medical treatment of idiopathic gynecomastia in pediatric patients at this time (4).
- Consider medication or illicit drug use in adult males before initiating treatment.

MEDICATION

- Danazol (100 mg b.i.d. × 1 week followed by 100 mg t.i.d. × 2–6 weeks) (5)[B]:
  - Effective in 80% of patients
  - Especially effective in reducing tenderness
  - Dose can be repeated for responders.
  - Drug is licensed for treatment of gynecomastia in the UK.
- Tamoxifen (20–40 mg/d) has been used (5)[B]:
  - May be effective in 78–83% of men with gynecomastia
  - Less effective in breasts with a large amount of fatty tissue
  - May have high relapse rate
  - Short-term tamoxifen treatment also has been used successfully in the treatment of pubertal gynecomastia (6)[C].
- Anastrazole has been studied in pediatric patients with idiopathic gynecomastia and is not effective (4).
- Timing of treatment with medications may influence patient response.
  - Treatment early in the course of developing gynecomastia may be more beneficial (2)[C].
- Testosterone may be of some benefit but has not been well studied and is used infrequently.
- Clomiphene has been used infrequently.

ADDITIONAL TREATMENT

General Measures

- Correct underlying disorder.
- Withdraw causative drug (if feasible).
- Observe with reassurance that the problem is transient.

Issues for Referral

Refer to endocrinologist if abnormally elevated hormone levels are confirmed.

SURGERY/OTHER PROCEDURES

- Biopsy if suspicious for cancer:
  - Needle biopsy or excisional biopsy
  - Gynecomastia is felt to be a risk factor for the development of male breast cancer (7).
- Subcutaneous mastectomy for severe, painful, or persistent cases or for patients with psychologic concerns (8)[C]:
  - Usually performed as outpatient surgery
  - General anesthesia required
  - Liposuction of the subcutaneous tissue may be required as well as skin removal if the breast is pendulous (9).

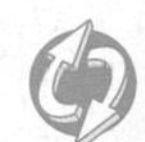

ONGOING CARE

FOLLOW-UP RECOMMENDATIONS

No restrictions

Patient Monitoring

- Every 3–6 months for physiologic gynecomastia
- Until well for nonphysiologic gynecomastia

DIET

- No special diet
- If obesity a problem, weight-loss diet

PATIENT EDUCATION

Surgical procedures for gynecomastia in pubertal boys are rarely covered by insurance because most insurance companies consider these procedures to be cosmetic.

PROGNOSIS

- Type 1: Resolves spontaneously
- Type 2: Clears without treatment (may take up to 2 years)
- Type 3: Little change without substantial weight loss
- Drug-induced: Drug withdrawal should result in resolution of gynecomastia in most cases.
- Other causes: Outcome depends on etiology.
- Good results with subcutaneous mastectomy

COMPLICATIONS

- Nipple inversion may occur following SC mastectomy.
- Asymmetry of breasts
- Postoperative fluid collection
- Withdrawal behavior related to drugs
- Depression
- Weight gain may be associated with danazol treatment.

REFERENCES

1. Eckman A, Dobs A. Drug-induced gynecomastia. *Expert Opin Drug Saf*. 2008;7:691–702.
2. Nordt CA, Divasta AD. Gynecomastia in adolescents. *Curr Opin Pediatr*. 2008;20:375–82.
3. Sher ES, et al. Evaluation of boys with marked breast development at puberty. *Clin Ped*. 1998;37:367–72.
4. Ma NS, Geffner ME. Gynecomastia in prepubertal and pubertal men. *Curr Opin Pediatr*. 2008;20:465–70.
5. Devalia HL, Layer GT et al. Current concepts in gynaecomastia. *Surgeon*. 2009;7:114–9.
6. Derman O, Kanbur NO, Kutluk T. Tamoxifen treatment for pubertal gynecomastia. *Int J Adolesc Med Health*. 2003;15:359–63.
7. Brinton LA, Carreon JD, et al. Etiologic factors for male breast cancer in the U.S. Veterans Affairs medical care system database. *Breast Cancer Res Treat*, epub ahead of print, 2009.
8. Gabra H, et al. Gynaecomastia in the adolescent: A surgically relevant condition. *Eur J Ped Surg* 2004;14:3–6.
9. Cordova A, Moschella F. Algorithm for clinical evaluation and surgical treatment of gynaecomastia. *J Plast Reconstr Aesthet Surg*. 2007.

See Also (Topic, Algorithm, Electronic Media Element)

Algorithm: Gynecomastia

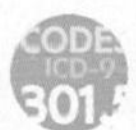

CODES

ICD9

611.1 Hypertrophy of breast

CLINICAL PEARLS

- The initial workup of gynecomastia is history, physical exam, and fasting labs including serum hCG, testosterone, LH, E_2, prolactin, PSA, and LFTs.
- Lab tests do not need to be done in boys with suspected pubertal gynecomastia, but they should be considered if the gynecomastia persists for >1 year.

G

HAMMER TOES

Bryan Beutel, MD
Martin Kerzer, MD

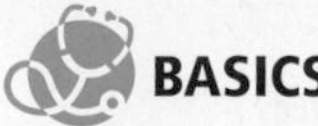

BASICS

Hammer toes are classified as a form of lesser toe (digits 2–5) deformities.

DESCRIPTION

- Plantar flexion deformity of the proximal interphalangeal joint (PIPJ) with varying degrees of hyperextension of the metatarsophalangeal (MTP) and distal interphalangeal (DIP) joints (1). Occurs primarily in sagittal plane.
- Can be flexible, semirigid, or fixed:
  – Flexible: Passively correctable to neutral position
  – Semirigid: Partially correctable to neutral position
  – Fixed: Not passively correctable to neutral position

EPIDEMIOLOGY

Most common deformity of lesser toes, typically affecting only one or two digits; 2nd toe most commonly involved

Incidence

- Undefined with limited data
- Can range from 1–20%
- Increases with age, duration of deformity (from flexible to rigid)

Prevalence

- More common in women than men (2):
  – Female predominance from 2.5:1 to 9:1, depending on age group
- Blacks more affected than whites (2)

RISK FACTORS

- Pes cavus and planus
- Hallux valgus
- Metatarsus adductus
- Ankle equinus
- Neuromuscular disease (rare)
- Trauma
- Improperly fitted shoes (e.g., with narrow toe box) and/or hosiery
- Abnormal metatarsal and/or digit length
- Inflammatory joint disease (e.g., rheumatoid arthritis)
- Connective tissue disease
- Diabetes mellitus

Genetics

- Specific genetic markers not identified
- Seen more frequently in families

GENERAL PREVENTION

- No documented means of prevention
- Modification of shoewear using pressure dispersive devices improves pain (1).
- Foot orthoses modulate biomechanical dysfunction and muscular imbalance, thereby preventing progression (2)
- Control of predisposing factors (e.g., inflammatory joint disease) may slow progression

PATHOPHYSIOLOGY

- Any biomechanical dysfunction that results in loss of function of extensor digitorum longus (EDL) tendon at PIPJ and the flexor digitorum longus (FDL) tendon at the MTP joint. The intrinsic muscles sublux dorsally as the MTP hyperextends. This results in plantar flexion of the PIPJ and hyperextension of the MTP joint (2).
- Specific pathomechanics vary by etiology
  – Toe length discrepancy or narrow toe box induces PIPJ flexion by forcing digit to accommodate shoewear. May also lead to MTP joint synovitis secondary to overuse, with elongation of plantar plate and MTP joint hyperextension.
  – Rheumatoid arthritis causes MTP joint destruction and resultant subluxation

ETIOLOGY

- Congenital
- Acquired:
  – Any condition that compromises intra-articular and periarticular tissues, such as 2nd ray longer than 1st, inflammatory joint disease, improper fitting shoes, and trauma (1)
    ○ Damage to joint capsule, collateral ligaments, or synovia leads to unstable PIPJ or MTP joint.

COMMONLY ASSOCIATED CONDITIONS

- Hallux valgus
- Cavus foot
- Metatarsus adductus
- Dorsal callus

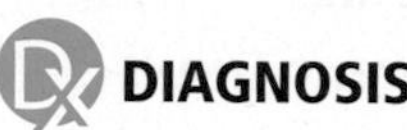

DIAGNOSIS

History and physical exam often sufficient for diagnosis of hammer toes. Additional testing available to exclude other conditions

HISTORY

- Location, duration, severity, and rate of progression of foot deformity (3)[C]
- Type, location, duration of pain
  – Patients often relate sensation of lump on plantar aspect of MTP joint.
- Degree of functional impairment
- Factors that improve and exacerbate the condition
- Type of footwear and hosiery worn
- Peripheral neurological symptoms
- Any prior treatment rendered

PHYSICAL EXAM

- Note MTP joint hyperextension, PIPJ flexion, and DIPJ extension.
- Observe any adjacent toe deformities (e.g., hallux valgus, flexion contractures).
- Assess degree of flexibility and reducibility of deformity in both weightbearing and nonweightbearing positions (2)[C].
- Note any hyperkeratosis over the joint, ulcers, clavi (dorsal PIPJ, metatarsal head), adventitious bursa, erythema, or skin breakdown (2).
- Palpate for pain over dorsal aspect of PIPJ or MTP joint.
- Drawer test of MTP joint
- Palpate webspaces to exclude interdigital neuroma.
- Neurovascular evaluation (e.g., pulses, sensation, muscle bulk)

DIAGNOSTIC TESTS & INTERPRETATION

Lab

Initial lab tests

- Not required unless clinically indicated to rule out suspected metabolic or inflammatory arthropathies (2)[C]
  – Rheumatoid factor, ANA, HLA-B27 serologies for inflammatory disease

Imaging

Initial approach

Weightbearing x-rays of affected foot in anterior-posterior (AP), lateral, and oblique views (2)[C]

- AP view superior for assessing MTP subluxation or dislocation
- Lateral view best for evaluation of gross hammer toe deformity

Follow-Up & Special Considerations

MRI or bone scan if suspect osteomyelitis

Diagnostic Procedures/Surgery

- Nerve conduction studies or EMG if suspect neurologic disorder
- Doppler or plethysmography if impaired circulation and surgery is considered
- Computerized weightbearing pressure testing indicated only in setting of neuromuscular deficiencies of toes

Pathological Findings

Histologic evaluation typically not necessary before treatment

DIFFERENTIAL DIAGNOSIS

Hammer toe: Hyperextension of the MTP and DIP joints and plantar flexion of the PIP joint

- Claw toe: Dorsiflexion of MTP joint and plantar flexion of the DIP joint
- Mallet toe: Fixed or flexible deformity of the distal interphalangeal (DIP) joint of the toe
- Overlapping 5th toe
- Interdigital neuroma
- Plantar plate rupture
- Nonspecific synovitis of MTP joint
- Exostosis
- Arthritis (e.g., rheumatoid, psoriatic)
- Fracture

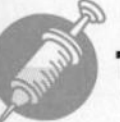

TREATMENT

Goal of treatment is to reduce or relieve symptoms so that patients may return to their normal activity level. Management includes surgical and nonsurgical interventions. Mild cases, however, may not require treatment.

MEDICATION

Indicated if adequate pain relief achievable nonsurgically or patient is poor surgical candidate

First Line

- Nonsteroidal anti-inflammatory drugs (NSAIDs) may be helpful in managing symptoms of pain, as well as soft tissue and joint inflammation.
- Contraindications: Gastrointestinal bleeding or active intracranial bleed; thrombocytopenia; coagulation defects; necrotizing enterocolitis; significant renal dysfunction

Second Line

Anti-inflammatory (cortisone) injectables if local inflammation or bursitis exists (1)[C]

ADDITIONAL TREATMENT

General Measures

Nonsurgical (conservative) treatment includes:

- Shoe modifications, such as wider and/or deeper toe box, may be used to accommodate the deformity and decrease the pressure over osseous prominences. Avoid high-heeled shoes (2)[C].
- Toe sleeve or orthodigital padding of the hammer toe prominence (4)[C]
- Hammer toe straightening orthotics or taping to reduce flexible deformities
- Débridement of hyperkeratotic lesions is effective in reducing symptoms. Topical keratolytics may be helpful (2)[C].
- Shoe orthotics may be used to control abnormal biomechanical influences.
- Physical therapy for stretching and strengthening of the toes may help to preserve flexibility.

Issues for Referral

If nonsurgical (conservative) treatment is unsuccessful and/or impractical or patient has combined deformity of MTP joint, PIPJ, and/or DIPJ, then patient may be referred to an orthopedic surgeon or surgical podiatrist for surgical interventions.

SURGERY/OTHER PROCEDURES

- Surgical procedures for the correction of hammer toes rely on the degree and flexibility of the contracture(s) and the related abnormalities that exist.
- Surgical interventions for <u>flexible</u> hammer toes include (1,4)[C]:
  - PIPJ arthroplasty (most common)
  - Flexor tendon lengthening/flexor tenotomy
  - Extensor tendon lengthening/tenotomy/MTP joint capsulotomy
  - Exostosectomy
  - Implant arthroplasty
- Surgical interventions for semirigid/rigid hammer toes include (1,4)[C]:
  - PIPJ resection arthroplasty or arthrodesis
  - Girdlestone-Taylor flexor-to-extensor transfer
  - Metatarsal shortening (Weil osteotomy)
  - Exostosectomy
  - Diaphysectomy of the proximal phalanx (less common)
  - Middle phalangectomy (less common)
  - Soft tissue releases/lengthening
- Procedures may be performed as isolated operations or in conjunction with other procedures
- Contraindications for surgery: Active infection, inadequate vascular supply, and desire for cosmesis alone

ONGOING CARE

FOLLOW-UP RECOMMENDATIONS

- Radiographs should be taken immediately following surgery or at the first postoperative visit. Subsequent x-rays may be taken as needed.
- Full weightbearing in a postoperative (surgical) shoe or other device is indicated based on the procedure(s) performed and on the individual patient.
- Elevate the foot above nose to minimize swelling, which can lead to pain and delay wound healing.
- Return to regular shoewear depends on the postoperative course.
- Role and efficacy of postoperative physical therapy (3 times per week for 2–3 weeks) unclear

Patient Monitoring

In the absence of complications, the patient should be seen initially within the 1st week following the procedure(s). Frequency of subsequent visits is determined based on the procedure(s) performed and the postoperative course.

PATIENT EDUCATION

- Patients should be aware of mild to moderate swelling and plantar foot discomfort that may persist for many (1–6) months after surgery and may limit footwear options until resolved.
- MTP joint and PIPJ may remain stiff for extended period of time.
- "Molding" of the operative toe (assumes shape of adjacent toes)
- Encourage patients to wear shoes of adequate size with rounded or squared toe box in future.

PROGNOSIS

- Nonoperative (conservative) treatment usually alleviates pain; however, the deformity may progress despite diligent care.
- Surgical treatment of flexible hammer toe deformity reliably corrects the deformity and alleviates pain. Recurrence and progression are common, especially if the patient resumes wearing improperly fitted shoes.
- Surgical treatment of fixed hammer toe deformity provides reliable deformity correction and pain relief. Recurrence is uncommon.

COMPLICATIONS

- Common complications specific to digital surgery include, but are not limited to, the following:
  - Persistent edema
  - Recurrence of deformity
  - Residual pain
  - Excessive stiffness
  - Metatarsalgia
- Less common complications include the following:
  - Numbness (e.g., digital nerve palsy)
  - Flail toe
  - Symptomatic osseous regrowth
  - Malposition of toe
  - Malunion/nonunion
  - Infection
  - Vascular impairment (e.g., toe ischemia, gangrene)

REFERENCES

1. Academy of Ambulatory Foot and Ankle Surgery: Hammertoe Syndrome. National Guideline Clearinghouse. 2003.
2. Clinical Practice Guideline Forefoot Disorders Panel of the American College of Foot and Ankle Surgeons: Diagnosis and Treatment of Forefoot Disorders. Section 1: Digital Deformities. *The Journal of Foot & Ankle Surgery*. 2009;48(2): 230–8.
3. Schrier JC, Verheyen CC, Louwerens JW. Definitions of hammer toe and claw toe: an evaluation of the literature. *J Am Podiatr Med Assoc*. 2009;99: 194–7.
4. Smith BW, Coughlin MJ et al. Disorders of the lesser toes. *Sports Med Arthrosc*. 2009;17:167–74.

ADDITIONAL READING

- Miller JM, Blacklidge DK, Ferdowsian V, Collman DR et al. Chevron arthrodesis of the interphalangeal joint for hammertoe correction. *J Foot Ankle Surg*. 2010;49:194–6.
- O'Kane C, Kilmartin T. Review of proximal interphalangeal joint excisional arthroplasty for the correction of second hammer toe deformity in 100 cases. *Foot Ankle Int*. 2005;26:320–5.
- Pietrzak WS, Lessek TP, Perns SV. A bioabsorbable fixation implant for use in proximal interphalangeal joint (hammer toe) arthrodesis: biomechanical testing in a synthetic bone substrate. *J Foot Ankle Surg*. 2006;45:288–94.

See Also (Topic, Algorithm, Electronic Media Element)

Algorithm: Foot Pain

CODES

ICD9

- 735.4 Other hammer toe (acquired)
- 755.66 Other congenital anomalies of toes

CLINICAL PEARLS

- Hammer toe is plantar flexion deformity of PIPJ.
- Patients may complain of pain at the PIPJ or MTP joint.
- Perform a careful inspection and examination of foot, especially PIPJ and MTP joint.
- Initial management of hammer toe deformity consists of conservative therapy; however, if unsuccessful, surgical interventions are indicated.
- Well-fitting shoewear is vital to minimizing recurrence after treatment.

HEADACHE, CLUSTER

David Cachia, MD
Ann Mitchell, MD

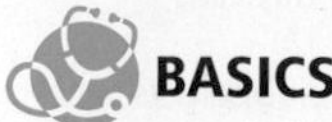

BASICS

DESCRIPTION

- Primary headache disease
- Multiple attacks of short-lived, excruciating, unilateral, sharp, searing, or piercing pain, typically localized in the periorbital area and temple accompanied by signs of ipsilateral autonomic dysfunction. *Severe* pain syndrome.
- Underdiagnosed and suboptimally treated
- Autonomic symptoms: Parasympathetic hyperactivity signs (ipsilateral lacrimation, eye redness, and nasal congestion) and sympathetic hypoactivity (ipsilateral ptosis and miosis)
- Attacks are without prodrome, rapidly escalating in intensity usually within 15 minutes, frequently have a circadian rhythmicity, and often wake patients 60–90 minutes after falling asleep. In contrast to other headache syndromes, the severe pain may cause patients to pace restlessly and occasionally exhibit agitated behavior.
- Individual attacks last 15–180 minutes if untreated and occur from once every other day to 8 times per day. 2 forms exist (ICHD-2 criteria):
  - Episodic: At least 2 cluster periods lasting 7 days–1 year, separated by a pain-free interval of >1 month (80–90% of cases)
  - Chronic: Cluster-free interval of <1 month in a 12-month period or greater

EPIDEMIOLOGY

Incidence

1 year incidence of 53 per 100,000

Prevalence

- Lifetime prevalence 124 per 100,000
- Predominant sex: Male > Female (4.3:1)
- Mean age of onset: Between 29.6 and 35.7 years
- Episodic cluster headaches (CH) > chronic CH

RISK FACTORS

- Male gender
- Age >30 years
- Cigarette smoking
- Family history of CH
- Alcohol induces attacks during a cluster, but not during remission.
- Small amounts of vasodilators (e.g., alcohol, nitroglycerin)
- Strong odors

Genetics

- Usually sporadic inheritance
- Autosomal-dominant inheritance in about 5% of cases, autosomal recessive or multifactorial pattern in other families
- Exact transmission pattern still debated
- 1st-degree relatives carry 5–18-fold; 2nd-degree 1–3-fold increased relative risk of disease.

PATHOPHYSIOLOGY

- Unknown
- Unlikely to arise from a single trigger zone
- Proposed mechanisms include:
  - Pain: Activation of trigeminal nerve
  - Autonomic symptoms: Activation of craniofacial parasympathetic nerve fibers secondary to pathological activation of trigemino-autonomic brainstem reflex. Trigger of trigeminofacial reflex might be in hypothalamus also explaining cyclical nature of cluster headache.

ETIOLOGY

Unknown

COMMONLY ASSOCIATED CONDITIONS

- Increased risk of suicide secondary to the extreme nature of the pain
- Medication-overuse headache
- History of migraine, frequently in female patients
- Sleep apnea
- Increased prevalence of cardiac right-to-left shunt and patent foramen ovale

DIAGNOSIS

- Diagnosis is clinical.
- *International Classification of Headache Disorders* (2nd edition) criteria:
  - At least 5 attacks of severe or very severe unilateral orbital, supraorbital, or temporal pain lasting 15–180 minutes if untreated
- At least 1 of the following:
  - Ipsilateral
    - Conjunctival injection or lacrimation
    - Nasal congestion and/or rhinorrhea
    - Eyelid edema
    - Forehead and facial sweating
    - Miosis and/or ptosis
  - Sense of restlessness or agitation
- Attack frequency: 1 every other day to 8 per day
- Not attributed to another disorder
- Episodic CH: At least 2 cluster periods lasting 7 days–1 year, separated by a pain-free interval of >1 month (80–90% of cases)
- Chronic CH: Cluster-free interval of <1 month in ao12-month period or greater

PHYSICAL EXAM

- Acute distress, crying, screaming, restless, and/or agitated during attacks.
- Ipsilateral lacrimation, injected conjunctivea, ptosis, and miosis
- Nasal stuffiness or rhinorrhea
- Bradycardia or tachycardia
- Nausea

DIAGNOSTIC TESTS & INTERPRETATION

- Diagnosis is primarily clinical; lab tests are not generally indicated.
- Consider neuroimaging (MRI/CT head and vascular imaging of brain):
  - Atypical CH presentation
  - Abnormal neurological exam
  - Suspect secondary CH (see differential diagnosis)

DIFFERENTIAL DIAGNOSIS

- Other trigeminal autonomic cephalgias: Paroxysmal hemicrania, short-lasting unilateral neuralgiform headache attacks with conjunctival injection and tearing (SUNCT)
- Hemicrania continua, hypnic headaches, trigeminal and other facial neuralgias, migraine, temporal arteritis, herpes zoster
- Secondary cluster headache:
  - Vertebral or carotid artery dissection
  - Brain arteriovenous malformations
  - Intracranial artery aneurysms
  - Pituitary adenomas
  - Nasopharyngeal carcinoma
  - Maxillary sinus foreign body/sinusitis
  - Cavernous hemangioma
  - Meningiomas/carcinomas/metastases

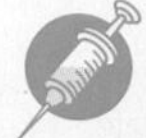

TREATMENT

Many of the medications discussed below are used off-label in the treatment of cluster headache.

MEDICATION

- Avoid pain therapy, especially narcotic analgesics, for acute attacks.
- Goal is abortion of acute attack and prophylaxis for expected duration of the cluster.
- Assess cardiovascular risk before instituting a vasoactive drug such as ergotamine or sumatriptan.

First Line

- For acute attacks:
  - Oxygen: 100% at least 6–12 L/min for 15 minutes via nonrebreathing mask. Relief within 15 minutes. Avoid in severe COPD as might affect hypoxic respiratory drive (1)[A].
  - Sumatriptan (Imitrex): 6 mg SC, maximum 12 mg/24 hours with at least 1 hour between injections (2)[A]. Relief in 10 minutes. Adverse effects: Nonischemic chest pain, distal paresthesias, injection site reactions, nausea and vomiting, fatigue. Triptans contraindicated in ischemic cardiac disease, stroke, uncontrolled hypertension, Prinzmetal angina, basilar migraine, hemiplegic migraine, ischemic bowel disease, and peripheral vascular disease.
  - Sumatriptan nasal spray: 20 mg effective within 30 minutes. Common adverse effect: Bitter taste (3)[B]
  - Zolmitriptan nasal spray: 5 mg and 10 mg dosage both effective to relieve headaches at 30 minutes (4)[A].
  - Zolmitriptan tablet:5 mg and 10 mg tablets shown to be superior to placebo at 30 minutes with episodic CH, but not chronic CH (5)[B]
- Prophylaxis to shorten cluster period and severity and to prevent expected attacks.
  - Verapamil*: Starting dose should be 240 mg to 360 mg daily. (120 mg t.i.d. or in SR formulation). Increase by 80 mg every 2 weeks with ECG control, until 720 mg dose is reached. Recommended clinical dose is 480 mg daily (6). If exceeded, informed consent has to be obtained. Doses up to 1200 mg daily may be required. Has many drug-drug interactions, as it is a CYP3A4 inhibitor. Adverse effects include hypotension, arrhythmias, AV block, bradycardia, pr-prolongation, syncope, gum and ankle swelling, constipation, CHF.
  - Lithium*: One study compared lithium 800 mg daily to placebo in episodic CH. No difference in percentage of patients having cessation of attacks, although those on lithium felt subjectively better. Another study compared verapamil 360 mg daily to lithium 900 mg daily. 50% of verapamil group and 37% in lithium group improved (7)[C]. Seems more effective in chronic CH. Side effects: Confusion, dizziness, diabetes insipidus, polyuria, hypothyroidism, tremor, bradycardia, muscle hyperexcitability, headaches. Monitor levels, liver, renal, and thyroid function. Caution with nephrotoxic drugs, diuretics.

– *Though both verapamil and lithium are given a class C rating based on the trials done, extensive clinical experience as prophylaxis for cluster headaches is available. Verapamil is hence considered 1st-line prophylactic treatment.

Second Line

- Acute attack:
  - Lidocaine/Cocaine: 10% (1 ml) of lidocaine or 40–50 mg of 10% cocaine intranasal. Most common side effects are nasal congestion, unpleasant lidocaine taste.
  - Octreotide: SC 100 μg. Can be considered in patients when triptans are contraindicated. Main side effect is gastrointestinal upset.
- Prophylaxis:
  - Civamide: 100 μL of 0.025% into each nostril daily. Only studied in episodic CH. Most common SE were nasal burning, lacrimation, pharyngitis, rhinorrhea.
  - Melatonin: 10 mg showed reduction in daily headache frequency vs placebo. No SE were reported.
  - Sodium valproate: Did not show any benefit vs placebo. Not advised as preventive treatment.
  - Methylsergide: No studies available to confirm efficacy. Has serious adverse effects including pulmonary and retroperitoneal fibrosis. Cannot be given with triptans and ergots. Avoid use.

ADDITIONAL TREATMENT

Transitional preventive treatment:

- Used until longer-term preventive treatment becomes effective. Longer-term maintenance agents are started concurrently.
  - Steroids: Only 1 study using oral prednisone and it had serious limitations (8). In practice, a commonly used regime is prednisone 60 mg daily for 3 days, then decreased by 10 mg every 3 days for a total of 18 days of treatment. Adverse effects for short-term use: Insomnia, psychosis, hyponatremia, edema, hyperglycemia, peptic ulcer.
  - Suboccipital steroid injection: One class I RCT showed benefit after 72 hours. 12.46 mg betamethasone dipropionate, 5.26 mg betamethasone disodium phosphate, and 0.5 ml 2% Xylocaine used.
  - Dihydroergotamine: 1 mg SC/im b.i.d. for several days
  - Ergotamine tartrate: 1 mg/2 mg daily or in divided doses. Contraindicated with triptans.
- Dihydroergotamine and ergotamine (no trials to prove efficacy)
- See "Acute and preventive pharmacologic treatment of cluster headache" by Francis et al. under Additional Reading

General Measures

- Avoid major changes in sleep habits.
- Stop smoking.
- Avoid use of alcohol during cluster period.
- Avoid prolonged physical exertion.
- Avoid extreme changes in altitude due to changes in oxygen levels.
- Avoid exposure to chemical agents/solvents.

Pregnancy Considerations

Collaboration between headache specialist, obstetrician, and pediatrician strongly encouraged. For abortive treatment, oxygen is most appropriate 1st-line therapy with nasal formulation of sumatriptan (pregnancy category B) or nasal lidocaine (pregnancy category B) as appropriate second line therapies. As preventive therapy, verapamil (pregnancy category C) and steroids (pregnancy category C) remain the preferred options.

Issues for Referral

Consider a neurology or headache center referral for refractory or complicated patients.

SURGERY/OTHER PROCEDURES

- Surgery may be considered for patients who are refractory to or have contraindications to medical therapy.
- The costs and potential benefits of surgery must be carefully weighed. There is a paucity of long-term outcomes data, and available efficacy data are often conflicting.
- Various techniques focused on ablation of segments of trigeminal nerve root and sphenopalatine ganglion
- Occipital nerve:
  - 2 reports of occipital nerve stimulation found that approximately 60% of patients responded to treatment as defined by >50% reduction in headache severity or frequency.
- Deep brain stimulation (DBS):
  - Of the posterior inferior hypothalamus
  - Latest data showing that therapeutic effect of DBS might be related not to direct stimulation of hypothalamus but might modulate a local cluster headache generator in hypothalamus or mesencephalic gray matter or through non-specific anti-nociceptive mechanisms (9).

IN-PATIENT CONSIDERATIONS

Admission Criteria

Suicidal ideation, unwilling to contract for safety

ONGOING CARE

FOLLOW-UP RECOMMENDATIONS

Patient Monitoring

- Anticipate cluster bouts and initiate early prophylaxis.
- Watch for adverse medication response and side effects.
- Watch for unmasking of underlying cardiovascular disorder.
- Educate patient and family.

PROGNOSIS

- Unpredictable course
- With aging attack frequency often decreases
- Poor prognosis associated with older age of onset, male gender, disease duration of >20 years for episodic form.
- Possibility of transformation of episodic cluster to chronic cluster and occasionally chronic cluster to episodic cluster

COMPLICATIONS

- Side effects of medication, including unmasking of coronary heart disease
- Potential for drug abuse
- Problems with high-flow oxygen in patients with COPD or in those who smoke

REFERENCES

1. Cohen AS, Burns B, Goadsby PJ et al. High-flow oxygen for treatment of cluster headache: a randomized trial. *JAMA*. 2009;302:2451–7.
2. Ekbom K, Monstad I, Prusinski A, et al. Subcutaneous sumatriptan in the acute treatment of cluster headache: a dose comparison study. The Sumatriptan Cluster Headache Study Group. *Acta Neurol Scand*. 1993;88:63–9.
3. van Vliet JA, Bahra A, Martin V, Ramadan N, Aurora SK, Mathew NT, Ferrari MD, Goadsby PJ et al. Intranasal sumatriptan in cluster headache: randomized placebo-controlled double-blind study. *Neurology*. 2003;60:630–3.
4. Rapoport AM, Mathew NT, Silberstein SD, Dodick D, Tepper SJ, Sheftell FD, Bigal ME et al. Zolmitriptan nasal spray in the acute treatment of cluster headache: a double-blind study. *Neurology*. 2007;69:821–6.
5. Bahra A, Gawel MJ, Hardebo JE, Millson D, Breen SA, Goadsby PJ et al. Oral zolmitriptan is effective in the acute treatment of cluster headache. *Neurology*. 2000;54:1832–9.
6. Tfelt-Hansen P, Tfelt-Hansen J et al. Verapamil for cluster headache. Clinical pharmacology and possible mode of action. *Headache*. 2009;49: 117–25.
7. Bussone G, Leone M, Peccarisi C, Micieli G, Granella F, Magri M, Manzoni GC, Nappi G et al. Double blind comparison of lithium and verapamil in cluster headache prophylaxis. *Headache*. 1990;30:411–7.
8. Jammes JL et al. The treatment of cluster headaches with prednisone. *Dis Nerv Syst*. 1975;36:375–6.
9. Fontaine D, Lanteri Minet M, Ouchchane L, Lazorthes Y, Mertens P, Blond S, Geraud G, Fabre N, Navez M, Lucas C, Dubois F, Sol JC, Paquis P, Lemaire JJ et al. Anatomical location of effective deep brain stimulation electrodes in chronic cluster headache. *Brain*. 2010;133:1214–23.

ADDITIONAL READING

Francis GJ, Becker WJ, Pringsheim TM et al. Acute and preventive pharmacologic treatment of cluster headache. *Neurology*. 2010;75:463–73.

See Also (Topic, Algorithm, Electronic Media Element)

Algorithm: Headache, Chronic

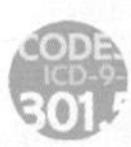

CODES

ICD9

- 339.00 Cluster headache syndrome, unspecified
- 339.01 Episodic cluster headache
- 339.02 Chronic cluster headache

ICD10

G44.0 Cluster headache syndrome

CLINICAL PEARLS

- Patients are often agitated during the headache (vs the quiet and withdrawn appearance of a migraine).
- Alcohol is only a trigger during clusters (not during remission).
- Oxygen and triptans are 1st-line therapy, not narcotics.
- Patients on verapamil should have EKG monitoring, those on lithium should have lithium levels checked.

H

HEADACHE, TENSION

Kaelen C. Dunican, PharmD, RPh
Jill A. Grimes, MD

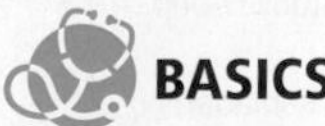

BASICS

DESCRIPTION

- Headache typically characterized by bilateral mild to moderate pain and pressure. May be associated with pericranial tenderness at the base of the occiput.
- 2 types:
  - Episodic tension-type headache (ETTH) divided into:
    - Infrequent: <1 day per month
    - Frequent: ≥1 but <15 days per month
  - Chronic tension-type headache (CTTH): ≥15 days per month for >3 months
- Synonym(s): Muscle contraction headache; Stress headache

EPIDEMIOLOGY

Most common type of primary headache

Prevalence

- Lifetime prevalence is 79%.
- More prevalent in female gender
- Prevalence of CTTH is 3%.
- Prevalence of ETTH decreases with age, whereas the prevalence of CTTH increases with age.

RISK FACTORS

Associated with triggers/precipitating factors:

- Stress
- Change in sleep regimen
- Skipping meals
- Certain foods (caffeine, alcohol, chocolate)
- Physical exertion
- Environmental factors (sun glare, odors, smoke, noise, lighting)
- Poor or sustained posture
- Female hormonal changes
- Medications (e.g., nitrates, selective serotonin reuptake inhibitors [SSRIs], antihypertensives)
- Overuse of abortive headache medication

Genetics

An increased genetic risk has been suggested by studies, particularly for CTTH.

GENERAL PREVENTION

- Identification and avoidance of triggers/precipitating factors
- Minimize emotional stress.
- Encourage relaxation techniques:
  - Biofeedback, relaxation therapy, and physical therapy
  - Consider counseling/psychotherapy.

PATHOPHYSIOLOGY

- Debatable: Peripheral and/or central mechanisms
- Activation of peripheral nociceptors leads to muscle tenderness in ETTH.
- Central sensitization is associated with CTTH:
  - Nitric oxide may play an important role in central sensitization.
  - Debatable: Low platelet serotonin
- Peripheral: May provoke the central mechanism leading from ETTH to CTTH

ETIOLOGY

Stress is the most frequently reported precipitating factor.

COMMONLY ASSOCIATED CONDITIONS

- 83% of patients with migraine headaches also suffer from tension-type headaches.
- Debatable: Increased prevalence of comorbid anxiety and depression

DIAGNOSIS

Diagnosis is based on clinical symptoms:

- Diagnostic criteria provided by the International Headache Society (1):
  - Headache lasting 30 minutes–7 days
  - At least 2 of the following:
    - Bilateral location
    - Pressing/tightening (nonpulsating) quality
    - Mild or moderate intensity
    - Not aggravated by routine physical activity
  - Not associated with nausea or vomiting (chronic type may be associated with nausea)
  - No more than 1 of the following:
    - Photophobia or phonophobia
- Headache not due to another disorder
- Fronto-occipital or generalized pain (dull, pressing, or bandlike)
- Associated symptoms:
  - Fatigue
  - Irritability
  - Difficulty concentrating
  - Muscular tightness, tenderness, or stiffness in neck, occipital, and frontal regions

HISTORY

Obtain a thorough headache history to rule out other headache disorders, including severity, symptoms, onset, location and radiation of pain; quality of pain; concurrent medical conditions and medications; recent trauma or other procedures.

PHYSICAL EXAM

- General physical exam: Vital signs, funduscopic and cardiovascular assessment, and palpation of the head and neck
- Neurologic exam: Mental status, pupillary responses, motor-strength testing, deep tendon reflexes, sensation, cerebellar function, gait testing, and signs of meningeal irritation

Geriatric Considerations

- Onset of new headache in patients >40 years is cause for careful study, including imaging.

DIAGNOSTIC TESTS & INTERPRETATION

Labs and neuroimaging (computed tomography [CT] or magnetic resonance imaging [MRI]) are only necessary when a secondary cause is suspected:

- Atypical pattern of headache (doesn't fit specific category such as migraine, cluster, or tension) (2)[A]
- Focal neurologic findings
- New onset after age 40 years
- Sudden onset or worsening with exertion or Valsalva (2)[A]

Imaging

- CT scan, with and without contrast, is as sensitive as MRI and is the test of choice.
- MRI when lesions of the posterior fossa or aneurysm is the concern

DIFFERENTIAL DIAGNOSIS

- Migraine headache
- Cluster headache
- Head trauma
- Subarachnoid hemorrhage
- Subdural hematoma
- Unruptured vascular malformation
- Ischemic cerebrovascular disease
- Temporal arteritis
- Arterial hypertension (HTN)
- Cerebral venous thrombosis
- Benign intracranial HTN
- Intracranial neoplasm, infection, or meningitis
- Low cerebrospinal fluid pressure
- Medication (nonprescription analgesic dependency, nitrates)
- Caffeine dependency
- Metabolic disorders (hypoxia, hypercapnia, hypoglycemia)
- Toxic effects from drugs or fumes
- Temporomandibular joint syndrome
- Eyes: Glaucoma, refractive errors
- Sinusitis or middle-ear infection
- Cervical spondylosis
- Severe anemia or polycythemia
- Uremia and hepatic disorders
- Paget disease of bone

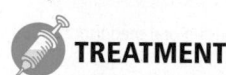

TREATMENT

- Nonsteroidal anti-inflammatory drugs (NSAIDs), acetaminophen (APAP), and aspirin (ASA) are effective for short-term pain relief of ETTH (3)[A].
- NSAIDs are most effective and should be considered 1st line for acute ETTH (3)[A].
- Tricyclic antidepressants (TCAs) are effective prophylaxis of CTTH (3)[A],(4).

MEDICATION

Choice of simple analgesic is based on patient-specific parameters:

- NSAIDs should be considered 1st line in most patients:
  - Ibuprofen and naproxen may be preferred due to better gastrointestinal (GI) tolerability
- APAP should be considered for patients taking warfarin, unable to tolerate NSAIDs, or allergic to ASA or NSAIDs

First Line

- For acute attack (ETTH): NSAIDs, APAP, or ASA:
- NSAIDs:
  - Ibuprofen (Motrin, Advil) 400–800 mg; may repeat q8h PRN (maximum 3.2 g/d)
  - Naproxen (Naprosyn) 375–500 mg or naproxen sodium (Aleve, Anaprox) 440–550 mg; may repeat q8–12h PRN (maximum 1,250 mg naproxen base/d)
  - Ketoprofen (Orudis) 12.5–50 mg; may repeat q6–8h PRN (maximum 300 mg/d)
  - Diclofenac (Voltaren, Cataflam) 50–100 mg; may repeat q8h PRN (maximum 150 mg/d)
- Contraindications:
  - ASA or NSAID allergy or bronchospasm, renal disease, bleeding disorders, increased risk of cardiovascular events (myocardial infarction [MI], stroke, new onset, or worsening of HTN)

- Drug interactions: Antihypertensives, anticoagulants, antiplatelet drugs, ASA, lithium, methotrexate
- Adverse effects:
  - Epigastric distress, peptic ulcer
- APAP (Tylenol) 1,000 mg; may repeat q6h PRN (maximum 4 g/d):
  - Adverse effects (rare): Rash, pancytopenia, liver damage
  - Precaution: Hepatic impairment, consumption of ≥3 alcoholic beverages per day
- Aspirin 500–1,000 mg; may repeat q6h PRN (maximum 4 g/d):
  - Contraindication: ASA or NSAID allergy or bronchospasm, bleeding disorders
  - Drug interactions: Anticoagulants, antiplatelet drugs, angiotensin-converting enzyme inhibitors, β-blockers, corticosteroids, NSAIDs, sulfonylureas
  - Adverse effects: GI irritation/bleeding, thrombocytopenia
- Caffeine combinations: 130 mg caffeine with 500 mg APAP and/or 500 mg ASA q6h PRN
- Isometheptene/dichloralprnhenazone/APAP (Midrin, Duradrin): 1–2 caps q4h PRN (max 8/d)
- Prophylaxis for CTTH: TCAs (amitriptyline, [Elavil]): 10–75 mg/d:
  - Contraindications: Acute recovery phase of MI, use of monamine oxidase inhibitors (MAOIs) within 14 days
  - Drug interactions: Clonidine, MAOIs, quinolone antibiotics, SSRIs, sympathomimetics, azole antifungals, valproic acid
  - Adverse effects: Drowsiness, dry mouth, tachycardia, heart block, blurred vision, urinary retention, seizure

Second Line

- For acute attack (ETTH):
  - Caffeine combinations: 130 mg caffeine with 500 mg APAP and/or 500 mg ASA q6h PRN
  - Isometheptene/dichloralprnhenazone/APAP (Midrin, Duradrin): 1–2 caps q4h PRN (max 8/d)
  - Narcotic analgesics (rarely indicated; consider secondary causes of headache or secondary gain, such as drug-seeking behavior for personal use or diversion/sale)
  - Ketorolac: 60 mg IM single dose
- For CTTH prophylaxis: (although limited evidence of benefit, all are widely used for prophylaxis) (5)
  - Alternative TCAs:
    - Desipramine (Norpramin) 50–100 mg/d
    - Imipramine (Tofranil) 50–100 mg/d
    - Nortriptyline (Pamelor) 25–50 mg/d
    - Protriptyline (Vivactil) 25 mg/d
  - Tizanidine 2 mg/d increase up to 8 mg t.i.d.

ALERT

Use of abortive agents >2 days per week may lead to *medication-overuse headaches*; must withdraw acute treatment to diagnose

Pediatric Considerations

ASA and antidepressants are contraindicated.

ADDITIONAL TREATMENT

The combination of stress management therapy and a TCA (amitriptyline) may be most effective for CTTH.

General Measures

Relief measures: Relaxation routines; rest in quiet, dark room; hot bath or shower; massage of back of neck and temples

Additional Therapies

- Cognitive behavioral interventions such as stress management programs may be helpful.
- Physical therapy, including positioning, ergonomic instruction, massage, transcutaneous electrical nerve simulation, application of heat or cold, and spinal manipulation, may provide limited value.
- Evidence regarding the usefulness of relaxation, biofeedback, and cognitive behavioral therapies is conflicting.

COMPLEMENTARY AND ALTERNATIVE MEDICINE

- Drugs with limited clinical evidence for prevention CTTH:
  - Mirtazapine 15–30 mg/d
  - Topiramate 100 mg/d
  - Venlafaxine XR (Effexor XR): 37.5–300 mg/d
- Drugs with conflicting clinical evidence for CTTH:
  - Tizanidine 2–6 mg t.i.d.
  - Botulinum toxin type A 2–12 U injected into tender cranial muscles
  - Memantine 20–40 mg/day
- Alternative agents:
  - Tiger Balm or peppermint oil applied topically to the forehead may be effective for ETTH.
  - Limited evidence supports use of acupuncture (6)[A].

IN-PATIENT CONSIDERATIONS

Initial Stabilization

Outpatient treatment

ONGOING CARE

FOLLOW-UP RECOMMENDATIONS

- Regulate sleep schedule.
- Regular exercise

DIET

- Identification and avoidance of dietary triggers
- Regulate meal schedule.

PATIENT EDUCATION

For additional information, contact:

- National Headache Foundation (888-643-5552, http://www.headaches.org)
- American Council for Headache Education (800-255-ACHE, http://www.achenet.org)

PROGNOSIS

- Usually follows a chronic course when life stressors are not changed
- Most cases are intermittent.

COMPLICATIONS

- Lost days of work and productivity (>CTTH)
- Cost to health system
- Dependence/addiction to narcotic analgesics
- GI bleeding from NSAID use

REFERENCES

1. Headache Classification Subcommittee of the International Headache Society. The international classification of headache disorders: 2nd edition. *Cephalalgia*. 2004;24:1–151.
2. Detsky ME, McDonald DR, Baerlocher MO, Tomlinson GA, McCrory DC, Booth CM et al. Does this patient with headache have a migraine or need neuroimaging? *JAMA*. 2006;296:1274–83.
3. Lenaerts ME. Pharmacotherapy of tension-type headache (TTH). *Expert Opin Pharmacother*. 2009;10:1261–71.
4. Moja PL, Cusi C, Sterzi RR, et al. Selective serotonin re-uptake inhibitors (SSRIs) for preventing migraine and tension-type headaches. *Cochrane Database Syst Rev*. 2005:CD002919.
5. Verhagen AP, Damen L, Berger MY, Passchier J, Koes BW et al. Lack of benefit for prophylactic drugs of tension-type headache in adults: a systematic review. *Fam Pract*. 2010;27:151–65.
6. Linde K, Allais G, Brinkhaus B, Manheimer E, Vickers A, White AR et al. Acupuncture for tension-type headache. *Cochrane Database Syst Rev*. 2009;CD007587.

See Also (Topic, Algorithm, Electronic Media Element)

Algorithm: Headache, Chronic

Videos: Neck Stretch with Towel; Neck Extension in Prone; Neck Stretches - Chin Tucks; Neck Trigger Point Massage—Trapezius

CODES

ICD9

307.81 Tension headache

CLINICAL PEARLS

- Tension-type headache may be difficult to distinguish from migraine without aura. A tension-type headache is typically described as bilateral, mild to moderate, dull pain, whereas a migraine is typically pulsating; unilateral; and associated with nausea, vomiting, and photophobia or phonophobia.
- Evidence suggests that NSAIDs may be more effective than APAP for episodic tension-type headache. Consider APAP for patients who cannot tolerate or have a contraindication to NSAIDS. APAP 500 mg may not be as effective as 1,000 mg.
- CTTH is difficult to treat, and these patients are more likely to develop medication-overuse headache. Clinical evidence supports the use of amitriptyline plus stress-management therapy for CTTH.
- Medication-overuse headaches must be avoided by limiting use of abortive agents to no more than 2 days per week.

HEARING LOSS

Teresa V. Chan, MD

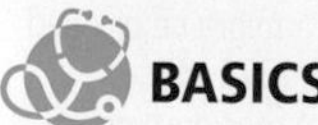

BASICS

DESCRIPTION

- Reduction in hearing manifested as decreased ability to detect or comprehend sound or speech
- May be conductive hearing loss (CHL or air-bone gap), sensorineural hearing loss (SNHL), or both
- System(s) affected: Auditory; External and middle ear (CHL), or inner ear (SNHL)

ALERT

- Any sudden SNHL (usually unilateral) is a medical emergency and should be referred to an otolaryngologist immediately.
- Treatment with high-dose steroids (1 mg/kg/d prednisone for 14 days, followed by taper) should begin ASAP, ideally within 1–2 weeks of onset.
- A simple 512-Hz tuning fork test lateralizes to unaffected ear in sudden SNHL (emergency) and lateralizes to the affected ear in CHL (not an emergency).

EPIDEMIOLOGY

- Predominant age: All ages affected; common in children (CHL) and elderly (SNHL)
- Predominant sex: Male = Female

Incidence

Hearing loss by age group:

- 3 in 10 people >60 years old
- 1 in 6 people ages 41–59 years old
- 1 in 14 people ages 29–40 years old
- At least 1.4 million children (18 or younger)

Prevalence

Hearing loss has doubled in the US during the past 30 years: 13.2 1971 to 28.2 million in 2000

Geriatric Considerations

- Age-related hearing loss is the most common cause in the US.
- ~50% of people >85 years have hearing loss.
- Hearing aids are underutilized.
- Loss of communication is a source of emotional stress and a physical risk for elderly.

Pediatric Considerations

Congenital hearing loss:

- 1–3/1,000 infants have hearing loss.
- Mandatory newborn screening (OAE and ABR testing is ideal)
- NICU screening before discharge
- Audiologic testing after major intracranial infection (meningitis)

Pregnancy Considerations

Otosclerosis (a CHL) can worsen during pregnancy.

RISK FACTORS

- Conductive:
  - Allergy
  - Chronic sinusitis
  - Cigarette smoking, 2nd-hand smoke
  - Sleep apnea with CPAP use
  - Adenoid hypertrophy
  - Nasopharyngeal mass
  - Eustachian tube dysfunction
  - Head trauma
  - Neuromuscular disease
  - Family history/heredity
  - Altered immunity
  - Prematurity and low birth weight
  - Young age
  - Craniofacial abnormalities (e.g., cleft palate, Down syndrome)
  - 3rd mobile window (superior canal dehiscence or large vestibular aqueduct)
- Sensorineural:
  - Aging/older age
  - Loud noise/acoustic trauma
  - Dizziness/vertigo: Especially Ménière disease or history of labyrinthitis
  - Medications (aminoglycosides, loop diuretics, quinine, aspirin, chemotherapeutic agents)
  - Bacterial meningitis
  - Head trauma
  - Atherosclerosis
  - Vestibular schwannoma/skull base neoplasm
  - Previous ear surgery
- Sensorineural, pediatric-specific:
  - Postnatal asphyxia
  - NICU hospitalization
  - Mechanical ventilation lasting ≥5 days
  - In utero infections (TORCH)
  - Toxemia of pregnancy
  - Maternal diabetes
  - Rh incompatibility
  - Prematurity or birth weight <1,500 g
  - Hyperbilirubinemia; exchange transfusions
  - Anomalous temporal bone (Mondini or large vestibular aqueduct)
  - Infectious diseases: Chickenpox, measles, encephalitis, influenza, mumps

Genetics

- Connexin 26 (13q11–12): Most common cause of nonsyndromic genetic hearing loss
- Mitochondrial mutations or disorders:
  - May predispose to aminoglycoside ototoxicity
- Otosclerosis: Familial; no clear genetic cause
- Most common congenital syndromes:
  - Hemifacial microsomia
  - Stickler syndrome
  - Congenital cytomegalovirus
  - Usher syndrome
  - Branchio-oto-renal syndrome
  - Pendred syndrome
  - CHARGE association
  - Neurofibromatosis type II
  - Waardenburg syndrome

GENERAL PREVENTION

- Limit noise exposure; use hearing protection when exposure cannot be avoided.
- Avoid ear canal instrumentation (Q-tips, etc.).
- Limit ototoxic medications.

PATHOPHYSIOLOGY

- CHL:
  - Hearing loss can result from middle ear effusion, obstruction of canal (cerumen/foreign body, osteomas/exostoses, cholesteatoma, tumor), loss of continuity (ossicular discontinuity), stiffening of the components (myringosclerosis, tympanosclerosis, and otosclerosis), and loss of the pressure differential across the TM (perforation).
- SNHL:
  - Damage along the pathway from oval window, cochlea, auditory nerve, and brainstem. Examples include vascular/metabolic insult, mass effect, infection and inflammation, acoustic trauma (see below).
  - Noise-induced hearing loss is caused by acoustic insult that affects outer hair cells in organ of Corti causing them to be less stiff. Over time, severe damage occurs with fusion and loss of stereocilia. Eventually may progress to inner hair cells and auditory nerve as well.
- Large vestibular aqueduct or superior canal dehiscence: 3rd mobile window shunts acoustic energy away from cochlea.

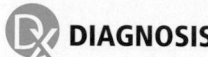

DIAGNOSIS

HISTORY

- Difficulty hearing:
  - Rapid vs gradual decline: Rapid (<2 weeks' duration) is a medical emergency. If suspect sudden SNHL, refer to ENT ASAP.
  - Difficulty with discrimination
  - Difficulty hearing in crowds
  - Frequently having to ask speakers to repeat
  - Friends/family complain of hearing loss
  - TV, phone volume increasing
- Tinnitus, bilateral or unilateral
- Otalgia
- Otorrhea, clear or purulent
- Dizziness or vertigo
- Ear fullness
- Autophony (hearing own voice louder or echoing)
- Facial nerve twitching or asymmetry
- Depression
- Anxiety
- History of ear infections or ear surgeries
- History of trauma or noise exposure
- Family history of hearing loss
- History of recent viral infection
- Nasal obstruction
- Frequent epistaxis

PHYSICAL EXAM

- 512-Hz tuning fork tests:
  - Sensorineural loss:
    - Placed on the forehead: Lateralizes to nonaffected ear (Weber test)
    - Placed on the mastoid and then next to ear; heard louder next to ear (Rinne test)
  - Conductive loss:
    - Placed on the forehead or teeth lateralizes to affected or symptomatic ear
    - Placed on the mastoid and then next to ear; heard louder behind the ear on the side of conductive deficit
- Otoscopy: Assess for deformity, canal patency, and otorrhea, TM integrity/retraction/mobility with insufflation, canal, or middle ear mass.
- Facial symmetry
- Cranial nerve exam
- Nasopharyngoscopy: Adenoid hypertrophy or nasopharyngeal mass (mandatory in adult patient with new unilateral serous effusion)
- Pediatric: Survey for syndromic anomalies

DIAGNOSTIC TESTS & INTERPRETATION

Lab

Often labs are not needed. If indicated:

- Pendred syndrome (goiter, mental retardation + SNHL): Perchlorate test, thyroid function tests
- Alport syndrome (nephritis + SNHL): Urinalysis, renal function tests
- Jervell and Lange-Nielsen syndrome (syncope, family history of sudden death + SNHL): EKG
- Any pediatric patient with SNHL: Genetic testing for connexin 26, mitochondrial studies
- TORCH screening test
- RPR confirmed with FTA-ABS
- Lyme titer in endemic areas
- Antinuclear antibodies and sedimentation rate as a screen for autoimmune disease

Imaging

Often imaging is not required; if indicated:

- Fine-cut CT temporal bones without contrast
- MRI of brain and brainstem with gadolinium

Diagnostic Procedures/Surgery

- Audiometry: Pure tone (air and bone), speech testing, and impedance (middle ear pressure) testing
- Tympanometry: Type B or C tympanograms indicate fluid or retraction, respectively. Negative middle ear peak pressures seen even with normal (Type A) tympanograms.
- Other tests:
  - Auditory brainstem response
  - Otoacoustic emissions: Echo of the cochlea
  - Behavioral (visual reinforcement) audiometry; used in children 6 months–5 years
- Myringotomy for aspiration of middle ear fluid is both diagnostic and therapeutic.

Pathological Findings

Varies depending on etiology

DIFFERENTIAL DIAGNOSIS

- Conductive:
  - Cerumen impaction/foreign body
  - Perforation of tympanic membrane
  - Middle ear fluid (serous otitis media)
  - Acute otitis media
  - Adhesive otitis media
  - Cholesteatoma
  - Ossicular erosion (infection, cholesteatoma)
  - Myringosclerosis/tympanosclerosis
  - Temporal bone fracture
  - Otosclerosis
  - Congenital malleus fixation
  - Glomus tumor
  - Congenital aural atresia
  - Osteogenesis imperfecta
  - Superior canal dehiscence
- Sensorineural:
  - Presbycusis (hearing loss related to aging)
- Noise-induced (recreational, occupational)
  - Ménière disease
  - Ototoxicity (aspirin, quinine, aminoglycosides)
  - Viral labyrinthitis
  - Cerebellopontine angle tumor
  - Large vestibular aqueduct syndrome
  - Syndromic hearing loss
  - Congenital cochlear malformation
  - Labyrinthine artery infarct
  - Idiopathic
  - Syphilis
  - CMV
  - Rubella
  - Temporal bone fracture
  - Metabolic (hyper/hypothyroid)
  - Paget disease
  - Perilymphatic (inner ear) fistula
  - Autoimmune disease

TREATMENT

- Early detection: If sudden single-sided deafness, refer ASAP to otolaryngologist for hearing testing and prompt steroid therapy.
- Hearing rehabilitation: Hearing aids, cochlear implants for patients with bilateral severe to profound hearing loss

MEDICATION

- Depends on cause. Hearing loss is a broad topic with many possible etiologies.
- Sudden SNHL: High-dose oral steroids: 1 mg/kg or 60–100 mg/d prednisone or 12–16 mg/d dexamethasone for 14 days, followed by a taper:
  - Some recent papers suggest simultaneous use of oral and intratympanic steroid use results in better outcomes. There is an ongoing multi-center trial comparing the efficacy of oral steroids and intratympanic steroids (1)[A],(2).
  - Evidence is conflicting regarding use of systemic steroids in sudden SNHL (2)[A].
- Vasodilators and vasoactive substances are being used to treat idiopathic SNHL, but evidence is conflicting (3)[A].

ADDITIONAL TREATMENT

Issues for Referral

- Audiology: If hearing loss is suspected, referral to audiology is warranted. Audiologists also provide hearing aid options and maintenance.
- Genetics: If congenital syndrome or familial hearing loss is suspected
- Speech therapist: If speech delay or speech impediment is present
- Endocrinology: Pendred syndrome, other associated endocrine disorder (hypo-/hyperthyroidism)
- Cardiology: Jervell and Lange-Nielsen syndrome
- Ophthalmology: Usher syndrome
- Neurosurgery: CPA lesion, intracranial complication of middle ear disease

SURGERY/OTHER PROCEDURES

- CHL often has surgical options for repair:
  - Tympanostomy and tube placement
  - Tympanoplasty
  - Mastoidectomy
  - Ossicular chain reconstruction
  - Stapedectomy/stapedotomy
  - Canaloplasty
- Those with profound bilateral SNHL may qualify for cochlear implantation.

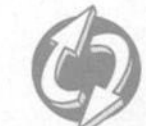

ONGOING CARE

FOLLOW-UP RECOMMENDATIONS

Patient Monitoring

Audiogram and clinical exam are primary means of monitoring patient.

DIET

Salt restriction to 2 g/d is helpful for Ménière disease patients.

PROGNOSIS

SNHL is usually permanent and progressive.

COMPLICATIONS

Acute middle ear problems may become chronic (perforations, cholesteatoma).

REFERENCES

1. Plontke SK, Löwenheim H, Mertens J, et al. Randomized, double blind, placebo controlled trial on the safety and efficacy of continuous intratympanic dexamethasone delivered via a round window catheter for severe to profound sudden idiopathic sensorineural hearing loss after failure of systemic therapy. *Laryngoscope*. 2009;119: 359–69.
2. Wei BP, Mubiru S, O'Leary S et al. Steroids for idiopathic sudden sensorineural hearing loss. *Cochrane Database Syst Rev*. 2006;CD003998.
3. Agarwal L, Pothier DD et al. Vasodilators and vasoactive substances for idiopathic sudden sensorineural hearing loss. *Cochrane Database Syst Rev*. 2009;CD003422.

ADDITIONAL READING

- Chau JK, Lin JR, Atashband S, Irvine RA, Westerberg BD et al. Systematic review of the evidence for the etiology of adult sudden sensorineural hearing loss. *Laryngoscope*. 2010;120:1011–21.
- For information on NIH-funded study. Available at: http://www.suddendeafness.org
- National Institute on Deafness and Other Communication Disorders. At: http://www.nidcd.nih.gov/health/hearing/.
- Ragab A, Shreef E, Behiry E, et al. Randomised, double-blinded, placebo-controlled, clinical trial of ozone therapy as treatment of sudden sensorineural hearing loss. *J Laryngol Otol*. 2008:1–7.

CODES

ICD9

- 389.00 Conductive hearing loss, unspecified
- 389.10 Sensorineural hearing loss, unspecified
- 389.20 Mixed hearing loss, unspecified

CLINICAL PEARLS

- In sudden hearing loss, if a 512-Hz tuning fork test (Weber test) lateralizes to the *unaffected ear*, suspect sensorineural causes (emergent evaluation needed), but if it lateralizes to the *affected* ear, the diagnosis is conductive hearing loss (not an emergency).
- ~50% of people >85 years have hearing loss, so encourage screening and treatment, especially in patients with early dementia (to maximize sensory input and sort out confusion vs lack of hearing).

H

HEAT EXHAUSTION AND HEAT STROKE

Scott A. Fields, MD

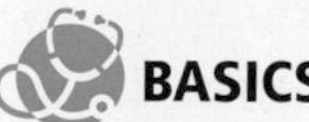

BASICS

DESCRIPTION

- A continuum of increasingly severe heat illnesses caused by dehydration, electrolyte losses, and failure of the body's thermoregulatory mechanisms
  - Heat exhaustion is an acute heat injury with hyperthermia owing to dehydration.
  - Heat stroke is extreme hyperthermia with thermoregulatory failure and profound CNS dysfunction.
- System(s) affected: Endocrine/Metabolic; Nervous
- Synonym(s): Heat illness; Heat injury; Hyperthermia; Heat collapse; Heat prostration

Geriatric Considerations

Elderly persons are more susceptible.

Pediatric Considerations

Children are more susceptible.

Pregnancy Considerations

Pregnant women may be more prone to volume depletion with heat stress.

EPIDEMIOLOGY

- Predominant age: More likely in children or elderly
- Predominant sex: Male = Female

Incidence

Depends on intensity of heat; estimate of 20/100,000 persons per season

Prevalence

- Depends on predisposing conditions in combination with environmental factors
- Roughly 240 deaths per year in the US

RISK FACTORS

- Poor acclimatization to heat or poor physical conditioning
- Salt or water depletion
- Obesity
- Acute febrile or GI illnesses
- Chronic illnesses: Uncontrolled diabetes mellitus or hypertension, cardiac disease
- Alcohol and other substance abuse
- High heat and humidity, poor air circulation in environment
- Heavy, restrictive clothing
- Nutritional supplementation that includes ephedra

GENERAL PREVENTION

- Most important factor in preventing heat stress is adequate fluid replacement.
- Allow acclimatization to hot weather through proper conditioning and activity modification.
- Dress appropriately with loose-fitting, open-weave, light-colored clothing.

PATHOPHYSIOLOGY

Only those associated with major organ system failure

ETIOLOGY

Failure of heat-dissipating mechanisms or an overwhelming heat stress leading to a rise in core temperature, dehydration, and salt depletion

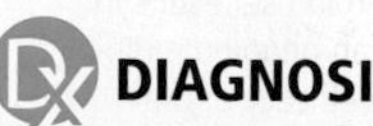

DIAGNOSIS

- Heat exhaustion: Symptoms are milder than in heat stroke, with no severe CNS derangements.
  - Fatigue and lethargy
  - Weakness
  - Dizziness
  - Nausea, vomiting
  - Myalgias
  - Headache
  - Profuse sweating
  - Tachycardia
  - Hypotension
  - Lack of coordination
  - Agitation
  - Intense thirst
  - Hyperventilation
  - Paresthesias
  - Core temperature elevated but $<103^\circ$F ($<39.4^\circ$C)
- Heat stroke: Divided into two categories: Classic and exertional
  - Classic: Caused by environmental exposure, primarily in elderly or chronically ill patients, and may develop gradually over days
  - Exertional: Typically younger, very active patients; rapid onset
    - Exhaustion
    - Confusion, disorientation
    - Delirium
    - Coma
    - Hot, flushed, and dry skin (sweating may continue in exertional heat stroke)
    - Core temperature $>105^\circ$F ($>40.5^\circ$C)

DIAGNOSTIC TESTS & INTERPRETATION

Lab

- Used primarily to detect end-organ damage
- Electrolytes, urinalysis
- Creatinine, blood urea nitrogen
- Liver enzymes, muscle enzymes (creatine phosphokinase)
- Complete blood count
- Increased urine specific gravity
- Results of these studies may indicate hypernatremia, hyperchloremia, and hemoconcentration.
- Drugs that may alter lab results: Diuretics

Diagnostic Procedures/Surgery

Rectal temperature monitoring

DIFFERENTIAL DIAGNOSIS

- Other causes of elevated temperature, dehydration, or circulatory collapse
- Febrile illnesses, sepsis
- Drug-induced fluid loss
- Cardiac arrhythmia or infarction
- Acute cocaine intoxication
- Neuroleptic malignant syndrome
- Malignant hyperthermia (an autosomally inherited disorder of skeletal and cardiac muscle in which patients have abnormal muscle metabolism on exposure to halothane or skeletal muscle reactants)

TREATMENT

MEDICATION

First Line

No medications are required in the initial management. Use isotonic saline solution to rehydrate (1,2)[C].

Second Line

- Consider immunomodulators such as corticosteroids (2)[C].
- Iced gastric, bladder, or peritoneal lavage (1,2)[C]
- Dantrolene 2–4 mg/kg for chemically assisted cooling (2)[C]
- In disseminated intravascular coagulopathy (DIC), consider appropriate replacement therapy.

ADDITIONAL TREATMENT

General Measures

- Fluid and electrolyte replacement with hypotonic oral fluids or IV 0.5–1.0 L normal saline
- Consider central venous pressure (CVP) monitoring.
- Body immersion in ice water (1,2)[C]
- Evaporative cooling: Spraying water over the patient and facilitating evaporation and convection with the use of fans (1,2)[C]
- Immersing the hands and forearms in cold water (1,2)[C]
- Use of ice or cold packs in the neck, groin, and axillae (3)

IN-PATIENT CONSIDERATIONS

Initial Stabilization

- Emergency treatment; best in a hospital setting
- Rapid cooling; remove clothing, wet patient down, apply ice packs.

ONGOING CARE

FOLLOW-UP RECOMMENDATIONS

Rest with legs elevated (1,2)[C]

Patient Monitoring

- Rectal temperature monitoring: Cooling may be discontinued when the core temperature drops to 102°F (38.9°C) and stabilizes.
- Heat stroke patients may require airway management, hemodynamic monitoring, and careful fluid and electrolyte administration and monitoring.
- Consider CVP monitoring.

DIET

- Cool or cold clear liquids only (noncarbonated)
- Avoid caffeine.
- Unrestricted sodium

PATIENT EDUCATION

- The key to prevention is proper hydration.
- Stress the importance of proper conditioning and acclimatization.
- Instruct patients to recognize heat stress signs and symptoms.
- Maintain as much skin exposure as possible in hot, humid conditions while using proper sun block protection.
- Avoid dehydration with proper fluids during activity or exercise: 8 oz fluid intake for every 15 minutes of moderate exercise.
- Never leave children unattended in cars during hot weather.
- Try to gain access to air-conditioned environment during hot weather.

PROGNOSIS

- Good when mental function is not altered and when serum enzymes are not elevated; recovery is within 24–48 h in most cases.
- The mortality rate for heat stroke (10–80%) is directly related to the duration and intensity of hyperthermia, as well as to the speed and effectiveness of diagnosis and treatment.

COMPLICATIONS

- May involve failure of any major organ system
- Cardiac arrhythmias or infarction
- Pulmonary edema, acute respiratory distress syndrome
- Coma, seizures
- Acute renal failure
- Rhabdomyolysis
- DIC
- Hepatocellular necrosis

REFERENCES

1. Cleary M. Predisposing risk factors on susceptibility to exertional heat illness: clinical decision-making considerations. *J Sport Rehabilitation*. 2007;16(3): 204–14.
2. Muldoon S, et al. Identification of risk factors for exertional heat illness: A brief commentary on genetic testing. *J Sport Rehabilitation*. 2007; 16(3):222–26.
3. Gaffin SL, Gardner JW, Flinn SD. Cooling methods for heatstroke victims. *Ann Intern Med*. 2000;132: 678.

ADDITIONAL READING

- American College of Sports Medicine, Armstrong LE, Casa DJ, Millard-Stafford M, Moran DS, Pyne SW, Roberts WO et al. American College of Sports Medicine position stand. Exertional heat illness during training and competition. *Med Sci Sports Exerc*. 2007;39:556–72.
- Bouchama A, Knochel JP. Heat stroke. *N Engl J Med*. 2002;346:1978–88.
- Charaton F. Ephedra supplement may have contributed to sportsman's death. *Br Med J*. 2003;326:464.
- Glazer JL. Management of heatstroke and heat exhaustion. *Am Fam Physician*. 2005;71(11): 2133–40.
- Smith JE. Cooling methods used in the treatment of exertional heat illness. *Br J Sports Med*. 2005;39: 503–7; discussion 507.
- Yeo TP. Heat stroke: a comprehensive review. *AACN Clin Issues*. 2004;15:280–93.

CODES

ICD9

- 992.0 Heat stroke and sunstroke
- 992.5 Heat exhaustion, unspecified

CLINICAL PEARLS

- The diagnosis of heat stroke relies on both hyperthermia and CNS dysfunction (e.g., irritability, ataxia, confusion, seizures, or coma).
- Start the cooling process immediately when heat exhaustion or heat stroke is recognized, beginning with wetting the skin with a cool mist and giving oral rehydration solutions containing saline, if alert and oriented.

HEMATURIA

Tracy O. Middleton, DO

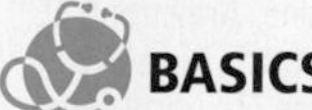

BASICS

DESCRIPTION

- Blood or red blood cells (RBCs) in the urine
- May be:
  - Gross (visible) or microscopic (nonvisible)
  - Symptomatic or asymptomatic

EPIDEMIOLOGY

Prevalence

- Microscopic hematuria in school-aged children: 0.5–2% (1)
- Microscopic hematuria in asymptomatic adults varies from 0.19–21%, depending on population studied (2,3).

RISK FACTORS

- Smoking
- Occupational exposures (dyes, rubber or tire manufacturing) (urothelial cancer)
- Analgesic abuse (e.g., phenacetin)
- Medications (e.g., cyclophosphamide)
- Pelvic irradiation
- Chronic infection, especially with calculi
- Recent upper respiratory tract infection
- Positive family history of renal diseases (stones, glomerulonephritis)
- Underlying primary renal disorder

ETIOLOGY

- Trauma:
  - Exercise-induced (resolves with rest)
  - Abdominal trauma and/or pelvic fracture with renal, bladder, or ureteral injury
  - Iatrogenic from abdominal or pelvic surgery; chronic indwelling catheters
  - Foreign body, physical/sexual abuse
- Neoplasms:
  - Malignancies: 30% of adult patients with gross hematuria and ~10% with microscopic hematuria have a malignancy (2). Urothelial carcinoma of the bladder and renal tumors are of greatest concern in adults.
  - Benign tumors
  - Endometriosis of the urinary tract (suspect in females with cyclic hematuria)
- Inflammatory causes:
  - Urinary tract infection (UTI): The most common cause of hematuria in adults
  - Renal diseases: Radiation nephritis, radiation cystitis, acute and chronic tubulointerstitial nephritis (due to drugs, infections, systemic disease)
  - Glomerular disease:
    - Goodpasture syndrome (antiglomerular basement membrane disease; autoimmune; associated pulmonary hemorrhage)
    - IGA nephropathy
    - Lupus nephritis
    - Henoch-Schönlein purpura
    - Membranoproliferative glomerulonephritis
    - Post-streptococcal glomerulonephritis
    - Rapidly progressive glomerulonephritis
    - Wegener granulomatosis
  - Endocarditis/visceral abscesses
  - Other infections: Schistosomiasis, TB, syphilis
- Metabolic causes:
  - Calculus disease (85% of patients have hematuria):
    - Hypercalciuria: A common cause of both gross and microscopic hematuria in children (1)
    - Hyperuricosuria
- Congenital/familial causes:
  - Cystic disease: Polycystic kidney disease, solitary renal cyst
  - Benign familial hematuria or thin basement membrane nephropathy (autosomal dominant)
  - Alport syndrome (X-linked in 85%; hematuria, proteinuria, hearing loss, corneal abnormalities) (4)
  - Fabry disease (X-linked recessive inborn error of metabolism; vascular kidney disease)
  - Nail-patella syndrome (autosomal dominant; nail and patella hypoplasia; hematuria in 33%)
  - Renal tubular acidosis type 1 (autosomal dominant or autoimmune)
- Hematologic causes:
  - Bleeding dyscrasias (e.g., hemophilia)
  - Sickle cell anemia/trait (renal papillary necrosis)
- Vascular causes:
  - Hemangioma
  - Arteriovenous malformations (rare)
  - Nutcracker syndrome: Compression of left renal vein and subsequent renal parenchymal congestion
  - Renal artery/vein thrombosis
  - Arterial emboli to kidney
- Chemical causes:
  - Nephrotoxins: Aminoglycosides, cyclosporine
  - Other drugs: Analgesics, oral contraceptives, Chinese herbs
- Obstruction:
  - Strictures or posterior urethral valves
  - Hydronephrosis, from any cause
  - Benign prostatic hyperplasia: Rule out other causes of hematuria.
- Other causes: Loin pain hematuria (most often in young women on oral contraceptives)

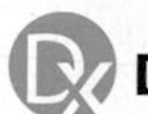

DIAGNOSIS

HISTORY

Considerations:

- Burning, urgency, frequency: UTI
- Dark cola-colored urine: Glomerular origin
- Arthritis/arthralgias/rash: Lupus, vasculitis, Henoch-Schönlein purpura
- Flank pain: Stones, infarction, pyelonephritis
- Recent upper respiratory infection (URI): PSGN, MPGN; concurrent URI: IgA nephropathy
- Excessive vitamin use: Stones
- Marathon runner: Traumatic, rhabdomyolysis
- Travel: Schistosomiasis, tuberculosis
- Painless hematuria and/or weight loss: Malignancy
- Family history: Alport disease (hereditary nephritis), sickle cell, polycystic, IgA nephropathy, thin basement membrane disease

PHYSICAL EXAM

Considerations:

- Elevated BP, edema, and weight gain: Glomerular disease
- Fever: Infection
- Palpable kidney: Neoplasm, polycystic
- Genitalia: Look for meatal erosion, lesions

DIAGNOSTIC TESTS & INTERPRETATION

Pediatric Considerations

- Consider glomerulonephritis, Wilms tumor, child abuse
- Isolated asymptomatic microscopic hematuria may not need full workup, and in fact, these pediatric patients rarely need cystoscopy, but they must be observed for development of HTN, gross hematuria, or proteinuria (1,4)[B].
- Gross, or symptomatic, hematuria needs a full workup.
- If eumorphic RBCs, consider ultrasound (rule out stones, congenital abnormalities) and urinary Ca:Cr ratio (hypercalcemia) (4).
- If dysmorphic RBCs, consider renal consult.
- Renal ultrasound identifies most congenital and malignant conditions; CT reserved for cases of suspected trauma or stones (4)

Geriatric Considerations

- Suspect UTI, sometimes occult
- More likely to have malignant etiology
- Workup includes imaging, cytology, and cystoscopy.

Lab

Initial lab tests

- Urine dipstick:
  - False-negatives are rare, but can be caused by high-dose vitamin C.
  - False-positives: Oxidizers (povidone, bacterial peroxidases, bleach), myoglobin, alkaline urine (>9), semen, food coloring, food (beets, blackberries, rhubarb, paprika) (5)
  - Phenazopyridine may discolor the dipstick, making interpretation difficult.
  - Proteinuria (large) suggests glomerular disease.
- Microscopic urinalysis should always be done to confirm dipstick findings and quantify RBCs (6):
  - American Urological Association (AUA) defines clinically significant microscopic hematuria as ≥3 RBCs/hpf on microscopic evaluation of sediment from 2 of 3 properly collected specimens (2,5)[C]:
    - Criterion is based on a midstream, fresh, clean-catch voided urine sample (7)[C].
  - Exclude factitious or nonurinary causes, such as menstruation, mild trauma, exercise, poor collection technique, chemical/drug causes, through cessation of activity/cause and a repeat urinalysis in 48 hours (1,2)[C].
- Differentiate intrinsic renal disease from other causes. Indicators of renal disease are significant (>500 mg/day) proteinuria, red cell casts (pathognomonic of glomerular disease), dysmorphic RBCs, and increased creatinine (7)[C].
- Urine culture if suspected infection/pyuria (4)
- In patients at high risk for urothelial cancer (e.g., former smokers, age >40, occupational exposures, etc.):
  - Urine cytology; perferably 1st void of morning on 3 consecutive days (AUA recommendation) (2)[C]:
    - Patients with symptoms of bladder cancer should be evaluated with cystoscopy and bladder wash cytology.

- If persistent microscopic hematuria:
  - Renal function tests: BUN and creatinine
  - PT/INR for patients on warfarin or suspected of abusing warfarin
  - CBC:
    - Elevated white blood cells with deeper infections
    - Anemia is unlikely from hematuria, although gross hematuria may produce significant blood loss.
  - Urine Ca:Cr ratio >0.2 mg/mg is suggestive of hypercalcuria in children >6 years (4).

Follow-Up & Special Considerations

Other tests depend on suspected etiology: STD testing, ANCA, C3, C4, ASO titer, hemoglobin electrophoresis (4)

Imaging

Initial approach

- Multidetector CT urography (MDCTU):
  - An exam of the urinary tract by MDCT in the excretory phase, following IV contrast
  - Should be considered as the initial imaging of choice in nonpregnant adults with unexplained hematuria, especially if risk factors are present (5,8)[B]
  - Highly specific (>95%) and relatively sensitive for the diagnosis of urinary tract neoplasms, especially when >1 cm (8)[B]
  - Higher radiation dose; weigh risk of disease vs risk of radiation exposure (9)[B]
  - Does not obviate the need for cystoscopy, particularly in high-risk patients (8)[B]
  - Visualization of ureters is discontinuous.
  - Less cost-efficient
- CT:
  - Perform unenhanced helical CT as 1st test for suspected stone disease (2)[B].
- Intravenous urography (IVU):
  - Limited sensitivity for small renal masses and for differentiating cystic from solid masses (7)[C]
  - Addition of ultrasound or CT often necessary to evaluate renal parenchyma (7)[C]
  - Potential reactions to IV iodine contrast media
- Renal US:
  - Best for differentiating cystic from solid masses
  - Sensitive for hydronephrosis
  - No radiation or iodinated contrast exposure
  - Cost-efficient
  - Poor sensitivity for small renal masses (<3 cm) (7)[C]
  - Main disadvantage is inability to thoroughly evaluate the urothelium for transitional cell cancer
- MRI:
  - Similar to CT in sensitivity for renal masses
  - No radiation exposure
  - Least cost-efficient
  - Limited ability to reliably detect urinary tract calcifications (9)[B]

Pregnancy Considerations

Renal ultrasound is initial imaging choice for pregnant or pediatric patients (5)[C].

Follow-Up & Special Considerations

In the case of glomerulonephritis, consider CXR to rule out cardiac enlargement, effusions, or pulmonary bleeding (5)[C].

Diagnostic Procedures/Surgery

- Renal biopsy:
  - May be necessary to diagnose glomerulonephritis or in the face of increasing renal insufficiency
- Retrograde pyelogram:
  - Used to further evaluate filling defects detected on other modalities (9)[B]
  - Reserved for patients in which findings on MDCTU are equivocal or increased radiation is not justifiable (9)[B]
  - Sensitive for small lesions of supravesicular collecting system
  - Requires cystoscopy
- Cystoscopy:
  - Best for evaluation of bladder pathology, especially small urothelial carcinomas (2)[B]
  - Fluorescence can be used to enhance detection of flat lesions (10)[C].
  - AUA recommends all patients with hematuria who are >40, younger with risk factors for bladder cancer, and/or those with abnormal cytology receive cystoscopy (2,7)[C].
- Ureteroscopy/pyeloscopy:
  - For visualization of suspected supravesical collecting system lesions
  - Biopsy, excision, fulguration, or extraction of lesions/stones possible
  - Requires anesthesia
  - Requires cystoscopy
  - Risk of injury to collecting system

Pathological Findings

Glomerulonephritis

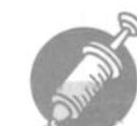

TREATMENT

MEDICATION

None indicated for undiagnosed hematuria

ADDITIONAL TREATMENT

Issues for Referral

Prompt nephrology referral for proteinuria, red cell casts, and elevated serum creatinine (2,7)[C]

SURGERY/OTHER PROCEDURES

Gross hematuria: Clots may require continuous bladder irrigation with a large-bore Foley catheter (2- or 3-way catheter may be helpful) to prevent clot retention.

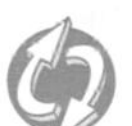

ONGOING CARE

FOLLOW-UP RECOMMENDATIONS

After initial workup, 35% of patients remain without a diagnosis.

Patient Monitoring

Although some experts still recommend periodic urinalysis and cytology, more recent literature suggests after thorough initial negative investigations (imaging, cystoscopy, cytology) no follow-up is indicated unless new symptoms or frank hematuria develops (3)[B].

DIET

Not restricted, except in certain conditions (e.g., increased fluids for stones or clots; restricted animal proteins in stone disease)

PROGNOSIS

- Generally excellent for common causes of hematuria
- Poorer for malignant tumors and certain types of nephritis

REFERENCES

1. Bergstein J, Leiser J, Andreoli S. The clinical significance of asymptomatic gross and microscopic hematuria in children. *Arch Pediatr Adolesc Med*. 2005;159:353–5.
2. McDonald MM, Swagerty D, Wetzel L. Assessment of microscopic hematuria in adults. *Am Fam Physician*. 2006;73:1748–54.
3. Mishriki SF, Nabi G, Cohen NP. Diagnosis of urologic malignancies in patients with asymptomatic dipstick hematuria: prospective study with 13 years' follow-up. *Urology*. 2008;71:13–6.
4. Massengill SF. Hematuria. *Pediatr Rev*. 2008;29:342–8.
5. Choyke PL. Radiologic evaluation of hematuria: guidelines from the American College of Radiology's appropriateness criteria. *Am Fam Physician*. 2008;78:347–52.
6. Rao PK, Gao T, Pohl M, Jones JS et al. Dipstick pseudohematuria: unnecessary consultation and evaluation. *J Urol*. 2010;183:560–4.
7. Grossfeld GD, Wolf JS, Litwan MS, et al. Asymptomatic microscopic hematuria in adults: summary of the AUA best practice policy recommendations. *Am Fam Physician*. 2001;63:1145–54.
8. Sudakoff GS, Dunn DP, Guralnick ML, et al. Multidetector computerized tomography urography as the primary imaging modality for detecting urinary tract neoplasms in patients with asymptomatic hematuria. *J Urol*. 2008;179: 862–7; discussion 867.
9. O'Connor OJ, McSweeney SE, Maher MM. Imaging of hematuria. *Radiol Clin North Am*. 2008;46:113–32, vii.
10. Sharma S, Ksheersagar P, Sharma P et al. Diagnosis and treatment of bladder cancer. *Am Fam Physician*. 2009;80:717–23.

See Also (Topic, Algorithm, Electronic Media Element)

Algorithm: Hematuria

CODES

ICD9

- 599.70 Hematuria, unspecified
- 599.71 Gross hematuria
- 599.72 Microscopic hematuria

CLINICAL PEARLS

- Screening asymptomatic patients for microscopic hematuria is not recommended (2,4,10)[A].
- Asymptomatic hematuria and hematuria persisting after treatment of UTIs must be evaluated (2)[B].
- After initial workup, 35% of patients remain without a diagnosis.
- Routine use of anticoagulants should not cause hematuria unless there is an underlying urologic abnormality (2)[B].

H

HEMOPHILIA

Robyn D. Wing, MD
Patricia McQuilkin, MD

BASICS

DESCRIPTION

- Inherited bleeding disorders caused by a deficiency of coagulant factor VIII (hemophilia A) or factor IX (hemophilia B, also called Christmas Disease). They are clinically indistinguishable but can be differentiated by assays that detect levels of factors VIII and IX.
- Disease severity is determined by the levels of the coagulant factor present:
  - Severe: <1%
  - Moderate: 1–5%
  - Mild: >5%
- Patients with >25% factor activity rarely bleed; however, bleeding after major surgery may occur in patients or carriers with factor VIII levels in the range of 25–35%.
- Synonym(s): Christmas Disease (hemophilia B)

EPIDEMIOLOGY

- Congenital conditions: X-linked–recessive, therefore, they affect males almost exclusively.
- Females are generally asymptomatic carriers unless their factor level is <40%.

Incidence

Incidence of hemophilia A is 1:5,000 live male births; hemophilia B, 1:30,000 live male births.

Prevalence

Affect 500,000 worldwide; 2/3 undiagnosed

RISK FACTORS

Genetics

- Both hemophilia A and B are X-linked–recessive.
- 30% of cases are due to spontaneous mutation.

GENERAL PREVENTION

Consider testing family members for carrier status. 1/3 will have factor levels low enough to cause clinically significant bleeding. Some may wish to use this information in reproductive decision making.

PATHOPHYSIOLOGY

- When blood vessel walls are damaged, exposure of subendothelial tissue initiates the primary hemostatic response, with plasma proteins and platelets interacting with this tissue to generate the platelet plug. Vascular injury also activates the coagulation pathway, which generates thrombin, an element essential to the creation of the fibrin net that stabilizes the platelet plug.
- Deficiencies in factor VIII or factor IX impair the coagulation pathway such that the platelet plug is inadequately stabilized, leading to excessive bleeding.

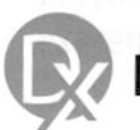

DIAGNOSIS

- Initial presentation:
  - May be known due to family history. All male infants born to known carriers should have factor level testing.
  - Intracranial bleeding, bleeding with circumcision, dental work, surgery, or injury
  - Excessive bruising, hematomas, hemarthroses
- Bleeding:
  - Depends on disease severity:
    - Severe: Spontaneous bleeding
    - Moderate: Bleeding with mild to moderate trauma
    - Mild: Bleeding with major trauma or surgery
  - Joints: Most common sites are ankle (children) and elbows, knees, and ankles (adolescents and adults). May present as irritability or decreased use of limb in an infant. In adults, prodromal stiffness and acute pain and swelling of joint:
    - Progressive arthropathy: Repeated bleeding into a joint damages cartilage and subchondral bone, causing fixed joints and resultant muscle wasting, which may significantly impair mobility.
  - Muscles: Hematoma formation most common in quadriceps, iliopsoas, and forearm
  - Gastrointestinal (GI) tract: Hematomas of bowel wall can cause obstruction or intussuception, as well as pain mimicking appendicitis.
  - Central nervous system (CNS): Intracranial hemorrhage
  - Genitourinary (GU) tract: Hematuria
  - Post-traumatic: Delayed bleeding after injury or surgical procedures
- Compartment syndrome and ischemic nerve damage from large hematomas may occur, for example, femoral nerve neuropathy due to undetected retroperitoneal hemorrhage.
- Pseudotumor syndrome: Untreated hemorrhage causing a hematoma, which calcifies (named because it can be mistaken for cancer)

DIAGNOSTIC TESTS & INTERPRETATION

Lab

Initial lab tests

- Hemophilia A: Diagnostic test is low factor VIII
- Hemophilia B: Diagnostic test is low factor IX
- Activated partial thromboplastin time (PTT): Prolonged
  - Corrected when mixed with normal plasma in absence of inhibitors
- Prothrombin time (PT): Normal
- Platelet count: Normal
- Bleeding time: Prolonged in 15–20% of patients with hemophilia A:
  - Recent aspirin use will increase bleeding time and can lead to confusion with Von Willebrand disease.

Follow-Up & Special Considerations

Inhibitors to factor VIII and IX (see Complications):

- Should be periodically measured with the Bethesda inhibitor assay, which quantifies the antibody titer
- Screen before invasive procedures and at regular intervals.

Diagnostic Procedures/Surgery

Prenatal diagnosis: Genetic testing of a sample of chorionic villus or fluid obtained at amniocentesis

Pathological Findings

In affected joints: Synovial hemosiderosis, articular cartilage degeneration, thickening of periarticular tissues, bony hypertrophy

DIFFERENTIAL DIAGNOSIS

- Von Willebrand disease
- Vitamin K deficiency (factor IX is vitamin K–dependent)
- Other factor deficiencies, afibrinogenemia, dysfibrinogenemia, fibrinolytic defects, platelet disorders
- Child abuse

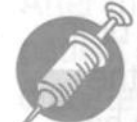

TREATMENT

MEDICATION

First Line

- Primary prophylaxis:
  - Standard of care for patients with severe hemophilia
  - Regular and long-term treatment with deficient factor
  - Goal is to maintain the factor level above 1%, converting patient to moderate or mild hemophilia.
  - 3 times a week factor infusion for hemophilia A and twice weekly infusions for hemophilia B have been demonstrated to reduce bleeding into joints, better prevent joint damage, and decrease frequency of hemorrhages when compared with patients treated on demand (1)[B].
  - Optimal age to start treatment has not been established. Consensus is that it should be initiated before joint bleeds begin in order to most reduce the risk of subsequent arthropathy (usually within the first 2 years of life) (2)[B].
  - Questions remain about what dose of factor should be provided, when to escalate therapy, and how long prophylaxis should be given (1)[B].
  - Barriers include cost and the need for frequent venous access. Stable venous access can be attained by CVLs or AV fistulae.
- On-demand therapy:
  - Hemophilia A:
    - Desmopressin (DDAVP): For mild hemophilia. Raises factor VIII levels by stimulating release of factor VIII from endothelial storage sites.
      - IV or SubQ: 0.3 mcg/kg infused 30 minutes prior to procedure; may repeat if needed
      - Intranasal: >50 kg = 150 mcg to each nostril (total = 300 mcg). <50 kg = 150 mcg to 1 nostril.
      - Adverse effect: Hyponatremic seizures, especially in children. Need to restrict fluids and watch sodium levels and urine output
      - Children may have a lower therapeutic response, which may increase with age (3)[B].
    - Purified factor VIII: Plasma-derived factor replacement is treated to inactivate viruses, an important innovation, because pooled plasma used previously carried high risk of HIV, hepatitis B, and hepatitis C transmission.
    - Recombinant factor VIII: Treatment of choice. Dosing: 1 U of factor VIII (the amount in 1 mL of plasma)/kg body weight will raise the plasma level of the recipient by 2%. Half-life of factor VIII is 8–12 hours. Therefore, b.i.d. or t.i.d. dosing is required with frequent factor-level checks.
  - Hemophilia B:
    - Purified factor IX
    - Recombinant factor IX: Treatment of choice. Dosing: 1 U/kg will raise levels 1%. Half-life of factor IX is 16–17 hours.
  - Amount and duration of factor replacement depends on location and severity of the bleed:
    - A target factor level of >30% is generally sufficient for mild bleeding episodes.
    - Major hemorrhages and large muscle bleeds require correction to levels between 50% and 100%.

- ◦ Life-threatening bleeds require levels between 80–100%, which should be sustained with bolus dosing or continuous infusion.
- – Both hemophilia A and B:
  - ◦ Antifibrinolytic agents: Enhance clot stabilization by inhibiting plasminogen activation. Effective in controlling mucosal bleeding, such as bleeding in oral cavity, epistaxis, and menorrhagia. Can also be used prophylactically, for example, prior to tooth extractions. Tranexamic acid (25 mg/kg p.o. every 6–8 hours or 10 mg/kg IV every 6–8 hours) and aminocaproic acid (Amicar) are also used (4)[B].

Second Line

Patients with inhibitors:

- Low-titer (<5 BU/mL): Transient antibodies, which can be overcome with high amounts or longer duration of factor concentrate
- High-titer: Cannot be treated with deficient factor concentrates; must bypass the deficient factor in the clotting cascade
  - – Prothrombin complex concentrates and activated prothrombin complex concentrates (aPCC) may be used (both contain factors II, VII, IX, and X).
    - ◦ Risk of thrombus formation and disseminated intravascular coagulation (DIC) when used repeatedly or in higher doses.
    - ◦ FEIBA VH dose: 50–100 U/kg every 8–12 hours, but not to exceed 200 U/kg/day (5)[C]
  - – Recombinant activated factor VII (rfVIIa): Avoids the risk associated with pooled donor plasma and does not cause a rise in antibody titer. However, it promotes coagulation only at the local level because it requires tissue factor to be active.
    - ◦ rfVIIa dose: 90–120 mcg/kg every 2 to 3 hours or single dose of 270 mcg/kg for target joint bleeds (5)[B]
- Immune tolerance induction: Protocols to eliminate inhibitors. Regimens include frequent exposure to high-dose factor VIII therapy over 12–18 months, with or without immunosuppressive therapy (corticosteroids, cyclophosphamide, Rituximab), until tolerance develops. Success rate shown to be 60–80% (6)[B].

ADDITIONAL TREATMENT

General Measures

- Avoid aspirin or other nonsteroidal anti-inflammatory drugs.
- Treat early; symptoms may occur before bleeding is clinically apparent.
- For surgical prophylaxis:
  - – If major surgery is undertaken, factor levels should be maintained at >50% for at least 2–3 weeks after the procedure.
  - – Dental extractions: Antifibrinolytics (Amicar, tranexamic acid) may be used.
  - – Small procedures: may use DDAVP
- Hepatitis A and B vaccinations are recommended.
- Encourage physical activity. Patients should avoid high-impact contact sports.
- Female carriers: Majority of females are asymptomatic carriers, although an occasional carrier will bleed at time of surgery.

COMPLEMENTARY AND ALTERNATIVE MEDICINE

Gene therapy:

- Replacement of defective factor gene sequence with a corrected version, which would allow for increased factor production
- Animal studies have demonstrated safe, long-term expression of clotting factors using multiple gene-transfer strategies, but these findings have not been successful in patients (7)[B].
- Dramatic improvements could be seen with even minimal increases in factor levels. For example, a patient may improve from a severe to a mild phenotype by increasing factor from <1% to >5%.

SURGERY/OTHER PROCEDURES

In patients with hemophilic arthropathy from recurrent hemarthrosis:

- Surgical or radionuclide synovectomy
- Total joint replacement

ONGOING CARE

FOLLOW-UP RECOMMENDATIONS

Restrict activities in proportion to the degree of factor deficiency, with efforts to maintain a normal life and adequate physical condition.

Patient Monitoring

Regular evaluations every 6–12 months, including a musculoskeletal evaluation, an inhibitor screen, liver tests, and tests for antibodies to hepatitis viruses and HIV

PATIENT EDUCATION

- National Hemophilia Foundation at: http://www.hemophilia.org
- World Federation of Hemophilia at: http://www.wfh.org

PROGNOSIS

- Survival is normal for those with mild disease; mortality is increased 2–6-fold in those with moderate to severe disease.
- At one time, AIDS surpassed intracranial hemorrhage as the leading cause of death in hemophilia. Risk for HIV infection has declined significantly due to development of recombinant and virus-inactivated factor-replacement products.
- Hemophilic arthropathy is the main cause of morbidity in patients with severe hemophilia, as repeated hemarthroses result in eventual deformity and progressive disability.

COMPLICATIONS

- Hemophilic arthropathy: Symptoms include pain, limitation of motion, and contractures.
- Transmission of bloodborne infections, such as hepatitis A, B, C, D, and HIV. This risk has now been greatly reduced.
  - – Hepatitis B and C increases risk for cirrhosis and hepatocellular cancer.
- Development of inhibitor autoantibodies: IgG antibodies that neutralize the deficient factor
  - – More common in those with hemophilia A (20–30% of patients compared to 5% in hemophilia B) (6)[B]
  - – More common in patients with severe disease requiring multiple transfusions
  - – Risk factors for inhibitor development include:
    - ◦ Specific genetic defect (family history); null mutations have higher inhibitor incidence
    - ◦ Very low or no circulating factor, therefore requiring multiple transfusions
    - ◦ Age of 1st exogenous factor exposure; previous studies report a higher incidence of developing antibodies in those exposed to exogenous factor at <6 months of age, but new studies show this may be due to severity of disease (8)[B].
    - ◦ Concurrent inflammation/infection when administering factor (5)[B] (e.g., surgical prophylaxis).
    - ◦ Duration of factor exposure (5)[B]
  - – No increased risk of bleeding, but when bleeding occurs, it is more difficult to achieve hemostasis due to decreased response to factor replacement

REFERENCES

1. Manco-Johnson MJ, Abshire TC, Shapiro AD, et al. Prophylaxis versus episodic treatment to prevent joint disease in boys with severe hemophilia. *N Engl J Med*. 2007;357:535–44.
2. Carcao M, Chambost H, Ljung R et al. Devising a best practice approach to prophylaxis in boys with severe haemophilia: evaluation of current treatment strategies. *Haemophilia*. 2010;16(Suppl 2):4–9.
3. Castaman G et al. Desmopressin for the treatment of haemophilia. *Haemophilia*. 2008;14(Suppl 1): 15–20.
4. Price VE, Hawes SA, Chan AK. A practical approach to hemophilia care in children. *Paediatr Child Health*. 2007;12:381–3.
5. Kempton CL, White GC et al. How we treat a hemophilia A patient with a factor VIII inhibitor. *Blood*. 2009;113:11–7.
6. Carcao M, Lambert T et al. Prophylaxis in haemophilia with inhibitors: update from international experience. *Haemophilia*. 2010;16(Suppl 2):16–23.
7. Murphy SL, High KA. Gene therapy for haemophilia. *Br J Haematol*. 2008;140:479–87.
8. Gouw SC, van der Bom JG, Marijke van den Berg H et al. Treatment-related risk factors of inhibitor development in previously untreated patients with hemophilia A: the CANAL cohort study. *Blood*. 2007;109:4648–54.

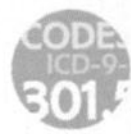

CODES

ICD9

- 286.0 Congenital factor viii disorder
- 286.1 Congenital factor ix disorder
- 286.2 Congenital factor xi deficiency

CLINICAL PEARLS

- Hemophilia A and B are X-linked recessive conditions, affecting males almost exclusively.
- The severity of disease varies based on amount of factor present.
- Standard of care for treatment now includes primary prophylaxis with recombinant factor, as well as on-demand factor replacement with recombinant factor.
- Inhibitor formation should be suspected when treatment with deficient factor fails to correct coagulopathy.

HEMORRHOIDS

Juan Qiu, MD, PhD

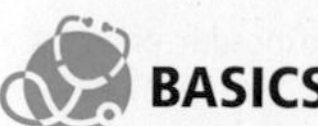

BASICS

DESCRIPTION

- Varicosities of the hemorrhoidal venous plexus
- External hemorrhoids are located below the dentate line and covered by squamous epithelium.
- Internal hemorrhoids are located above the dentate line.
- Both types of hemorrhoids often coexist.
- Classification of internal hemorrhoids:
  - 1st degree: Hemorrhoids do not prolapse.
  - 2nd degree: Prolapse through the anus on straining but reduce spontaneously
  - 3rd degree: Protrude and require digital reduction
  - 4th degree: Cannot be reduced
- Hemorrhoids often progress from itching, bleeding stage to protrusion with easy reduction, then difficult reduction, and finally rectal prolapse. Thrombosis may occur at any protrusion stage.

Geriatric Considerations

Common in elderly along with rectal prolapse

Pediatric Considerations

- Uncommon in infants and children. Look for underlying cause (e.g., venacaval or mesenteric obstruction, cirrhosis, portal HTN).
- Occasionally, as in adults, hemorrhoids may result from chronic constipation, fecal impaction, and straining at stool. Surgery is rarely required in children.

Pregnancy Considerations

- Common in pregnancy
- Usually resolves after pregnancy
- No treatment required, unless extremely painful

EPIDEMIOLOGY

- Predominant age: Adults; peak between 45 and 65 years old
- Predominant sex: Male = Female

Incidence

Common

Prevalence

About 4–5% in general population in US

RISK FACTORS

- Pregnancy
- Pelvic space-occupying lesions
- Liver disease
- Portal HTN
- Constipation
- Occupations that require prolonged sitting
- Loss of muscle tone in old age, rectal surgery, episiotomy, anal intercourse
- Obesity
- Chronic diarrhea

Genetics

No known genetic pattern

GENERAL PREVENTION

- Avoid constipation with high-fiber diet and hydration.
- Lose weight, if overweight.
- Avoid prolonged sitting on the toilet.

ETIOLOGY

- Dilated veins of hemorrhoidal plexus
- Tight internal anal sphincter
- Abnormal distention of the arteriovenous anastomosis
- Prolapse of the cushions and the surrounding connective tissues

COMMONLY ASSOCIATED CONDITIONS

- Liver disease
- Pregnancy
- Portal HTN
- Constipation

DIAGNOSIS

Diagnosis is usually made by history and inspection of the perineum, rectal exam, and anoscopy.

HISTORY

- All cases:
  - Classically, bright red blood per rectum; may be scant blood on toilet paper, or copious in the toilet bowl
  - Constipation or diarrhea
  - Straining with defecation
- Small or minimal external hemorrhoids: Episodic bleeding on stool or toilet paper, pruritus
- More extensive internal hemorrhoids: Feeling of incomplete evacuation

PHYSICAL EXAM

- Anorectal exam including anoscopy
- Inspection following straining at stool
- For protruding hemorrhoids: Mass, more prominent bleeding
- If not reducible, increased risk of strangulation and/or thrombosis with acute pain
- External hemorrhoids cause pain; internal hemorrhoids generally do not.
- Thrombosed hemorrhoids present as acute discomfort and the presence of a painful mass.

DIAGNOSTIC TESTS & INTERPRETATION

Diagnostic Procedures/Surgery

Sigmoidoscopy or colonoscopy depending on coexistent risk factors for malignancy in patients who present with bleeding.

DIFFERENTIAL DIAGNOSIS

- Rectal or anal neoplasia
- Condyloma
- Skin tag
- Inflammatory bowel disease (1)[B]
- Anal fistula, fissure, or abscess (2)[B]

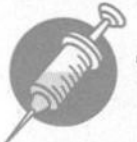

TREATMENT

All these treatments, except surgical, are outpatient with quick recovery time, usually <48 hours.

MEDICATION

- Prevention:
  - Fiber supplements
  - Stool softeners
- Pain:
  - Hydrocortisone ointment (0.5–1.0%)
  - Analgesic sprays or ointments—benzocaine, dibucaine (Nupercainal). Use sprays with caution as they may contain alcohol that can cause burning sensation when applied.
- Pruritus: Hydrocortisone (Anusol-HC, Cortifoam) ointment
- Bleeding:
  - Astringent suppositories (Preparation H)
  - Hydrocortisone (Anusol; Cortifoam) ointment
- Treatment for special cases:
  - Thrombosed external hemorrhoids: Fairly common complication of hemorrhoidal disease. With conservative treatment, the thrombus will be absorbed over the course of weeks and pain improves within 2–3 days (1)[B].
  - With severe acute pain, prompt excision should be performed under local anesthetic and the wound left open without packing. Sitz baths, topical anesthetics, and mild pain relievers for 1st 7–10 days after excision (1)[B].
  - Strangulated hemorrhoid: From irreducible 3rd- or 4th-degree hemorrhoid. If untreated, can progress to ulceration and thrombosis. Treatment requires urgent or emergent hemorrhoidectomy.
  - Acute hemorrhoidal bleeding associated with portal HTN: Bleeding can be life-threatening. Treatment should be suture of the bleeding site with incorporation of the mucosa, submucosa, and internal sphincter. Coagulopathy should be corrected.

ADDITIONAL TREATMENT

General Measures

- Hemorrhoids are a recurrent disease, even after surgical excision; measures for prevention should be taken.
- For mild symptoms or prevention:
  - Avoid prolonged sitting at stool.
  - Avoid straining.
  - Avoid constipation by eating a high-fiber diet or by taking fiber supplements; if necessary, take regular stool softeners.
  - Regular exercise
- For pain, sitz baths warm water or hypertonic Epsom salts (1 cup per 2 quarts of water)
- Mild and minimal hemorrhoids respond to changed diet, relief of constipation, and brief stooling.
- Pruritus or mild discomfort after stooling responds to hydrocortisone ointment, anesthetic ointments or sprays, and warm sitz bath.
- Constipation relief, anal hygiene, local ointments, and sitz baths are effective through the stage of easy reduction, but the more severe stages require rubber band ligation or rectal surgery.

SURGERY/OTHER PROCEDURES

- Indications: Failure of medical and nonoperative therapy, symptomatic 3rd- or 4th-degree (3) symptoms (3) in presence of a concomitant anorectal condition requiring surgery, or patient preference (2)[B],(3)
- Incision of thrombosed hemorrhoid: For severe pain
- Severe protruding hemorrhoids:
  - Rubber band ligation (internal hemorrhoids only)
  - Sclerotherapy: For symptomatic prolapsed stage I or II hemorrhoids; care must be (4) taken injecting near periprostatic parasympathetic nerves. Not for advanced disease or if evidence of infection, inflammation, ulceration is present (1)[B]:
    - Cryotherapy is no longer recommended due to high rate of complications (2)[B].
  - Prolapsed rectum:
    - Requires surgical correction
  - Surgical resection:
    - Gold standard: Conventional hemorrhoidectomy should be considered for grade III hemorrhoids not responding to banding, mixed internal and external, grade IV hemorrhoids, or when complicated by fissures, fistula, or extensive skin tags.
- Newer technique:
  - Stapled hemorrhoidopexy; less painful than traditional surgery, but higher incidence of recurrences (5)[B]
  - Ligasure hemorrhoidectomy; reduces operating time, is superior in patient tolerance, and is equally effective as conventional hemorrhoidectomy in long-term symptom control

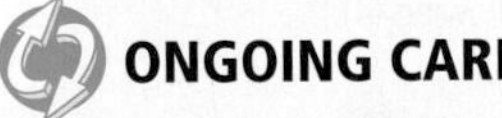

ONGOING CARE

FOLLOW-UP RECOMMENDATIONS

- Encourage physical fitness.
- Avoid prolonged sitting and straining on the toilet.

Patient Monitoring

As needed, depending on treatment

DIET

High-fiber, adequate fluids

PROGNOSIS

- Spontaneous resolution
- Recurrence

COMPLICATIONS

- Thrombosis
- Ulceration
- Anemia (rare)
- Incontinence
- Pelvic sepsis following hemorrhoidectomy (5)[B]

REFERENCES

1. Kaidar-Person O, Person B, Wexner SD. Hemorrhoidal disease: A comprehensive review. *J Am Coll Surg*. 2007;204:102–17.
2. Clinical Practice Committee, American Gastroenterological Association. American Gastroenterological Association medical position statement: Diagnosis and treatment of hemorrhoids. *Gastroenterology*. 2004;126:1461–2.
3. Castellvi J, Sueira A, Espinosa J, Vallet J, Gil V, Pi F. Ligasure versus diathermy hemorrhoidectomy under spinal anesthesia or pudendal block with ropivacaine: a randomized prospective clinical study with 1-year follow-up. *Int J Colorectal Dis*. Published online: 25 April 2009.
4. Nienhuiji S, de Hingh I. Conventional versus LigaSure hemorrhoidectomy for patients with symptomatic hemorrhoids (Review). *The cochrane Library* 2009, Issue 2.
5. Nisar PJ, Acheson AG, Neal KR, et al. Stapled hemorrhoidopexy compared with conventional hemorrhoidectomy: systematic review of randomized, controlled trials. *Dis Colon Rectum*. 2004;47:1837–45.

ADDITIONAL READING

- Giordano P, Gravante G, Sorge R, Ovens L, Nastro P. Long-term Outcomes of stapled hemorrhoidopexy vs conventional hemorrhoidectomy. *Arch Surg*. 2009;144(3):266–72.
- Reese GE, von Roon AC, Tekkis PP et al. Haemorrhoids. *Clin Evid (Online)*. 2009.

See Also (Topic, Algorithm, Electronic Media Element)

Colorectal Malignancy; Portal Hypertension

CODES

ICD9

- 455.0 Internal hemorrhoids without mention of complication
- 455.1 Internal thrombosed hemorrhoids
- 455.2 Internal hemorrhoids with other complication

CLINICAL PEARLS

- Hemorrhoids are uncommon in inflammatory bowel disease, and pain is most related to perianal inflammation, irritation, and swelling. Anal hygiene and symptomatic pain relief are the treatments of choice.
- No pain is associated with internal hemorrhoids. Pain occurs with external hemorrhoids only.

H

HENOCH-SCHÖNLEIN PURPURA

Kimberly A. Pesaturo, PharmD
Evan R. Horton, PharmD
Amy Pelletier, DO

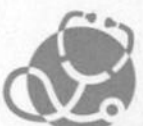

BASICS

DESCRIPTION

- Henoch-Schönlein purpura (HSP) is an immunologically mediated, nonthrombocytopenic, purpuric, systemic vasculitis involving small blood vessels (1).
- HSP is often self-limiting but can result in long-term renal damage (1).

EPIDEMIOLOGY

Incidence

- Up to 20.4/100,000 children <17 years of age per year, but incidence is variable (2)
- Predominant age: Highest incidence between 4 and 6 years of age (2)
- Most common in Caucasians, Japanese, and Native Americans (2)
- Low incidence in Africans and African Americans (2)
- Predominant sex: Male > Female (approximately 1.2:1) (2)

Prevalence

- Year-round occurrence
- More common in late fall to early spring (3)

RISK FACTORS

Genetics

Possible genetic predisposition (1)

PATHOPHYSIOLOGY

- Immune-mediated disorder involving IgA complexes (specifically IgA1) that form and deposit in affected areas, triggering localized inflammation (1)
- Results in leukocytoclastic vasculitis and small blood vessel necrosis
- Proliferative glomerulonephritis with IgA deposit may be seen (4).

ETIOLOGY

- No single etiologic agent has been identified.
- Many cases are associated with preceding infections, usually involving group A β-hemolytic streptococci (3).
- Also reported following infections with (but not limited to): parvovirus B19, adenovirus, hepatitis A and B viruses, Coxsackie virus, Epstein-Barr virus, varicella virus, *B. henselae*, *H. pylori*, and *M. pneumoniae* (3).
- Rare reports after drug ingestion, insect bites, and some vaccines

DIAGNOSIS

Palpable purpura with lower limb predominance with one or more of the following (4):

- Abdominal pain
- Biopsy with predominant IgA
- Arthralgia or arthritis
- Renal involvement (hematuria or proteinuria)

HISTORY

- Previous disease: Infections such as streptococcal infections, upper respiratory infections, and hepatitis (3)
- Rash: Initially may resemble urticaria prior to developing into palpable purpura (1)
- Headache
- Cough
- Vomiting
- Abdominal pain is the most common gastrointestinal symptom (1).
- Transient arthritis of joints, most frequent in lower-limbs (knees and ankles) (1)
- Edema of the periorbital region or ankles
- Hematuria
- Testicular pain or scrotal swelling (1)

PHYSICAL EXAM

- Hypertension may be present.
- Rash is the hallmark of HSP (1). Rash may be petechial or purpuric in a pressure-dependent, symmetric distribution, usually predominating on lower limbs.
  - Rash may be briefly preceded by joint involvement or abdominal pain.
  - Skin lesions may spread to face and trunk; bullous lesions can develop.
- Abdomen often tender to palpation. Some form of bleeding may occur.
  - Abdominal symptoms may precede the rash by up to 2 weeks.
  - Intussusception is a possible complication.
- Orchitis (less common) may occur and can mimic testicular torsion.
  - Swelling and bruising may be noted on the scrotum.
  - Testicular torsion also has been reported.
- Joints (mainly lower limb) should be examined for swelling and limited range of motion.
- CNS involvement may present with headaches, seizures, or behavioral changes (less common).
- Rare pulmonary involvement may be noted.

DIAGNOSTIC TESTS & INTERPRETATION

No definitive tests confirm the diagnosis of HSP.

Lab

The following labs may be useful in diagnosing HSP (1,3):

- CBC:
  - Normal platelet count differentiates from thrombocytopenic purpura.
  - Hemoglobin is usually normal; leukocytosis, eosinophilia especially, may be present.
  - Can detect anemia if there is GI blood loss.
- ESR:
  - Normal or elevated
- Prothrombin (PT) and partial thromboplastin time (PTT):
  - Normal
- IgA:
  - Often elevated in the acute phase of illness, with normal or increased IgG and IgM
- C3/C4:
  - Normal; sometimes decreased
- Antinuclear antibody:
  - Negative
- Throat culture for group A β-hemolytic streptococci:
  - Positive in up to 75% of patients
- Anti-streptolysin O titer:
  - Determines preceding streptococcal infection
- Serum basic/comprehensive chemistries:
  - Elevated BUN and creatinine levels and decreased protein and albumin are seen with renal involvement.
- Urinalysis:
  - Gross hematuria and proteinuria are present in many patients. Microscopic blood, RBCs, WBCs, and casts suggest glomerulonephritis.
- Blood culture:
  - Evaluate for sepsis or bacteremia
- Stool guaiac

Imaging

The following imaging tests may be useful (1):

- Abdominal ultrasound for thickened bowel wall intussusception
- Abdominal radiograph
- Renal tract ultrasound
- CXR

Diagnostic Procedures/Surgery

- Renal biopsy: Severe renal failure
  - Epithelial crescent formation on renal biopsy suggests significant renal damage and inflammation.
- Skin biopsy of purpura: IgA deposition

DIFFERENTIAL DIAGNOSIS

- Petechial and purpuric rashes seen in thrombocytopenia from:
  - Idiopathic thrombocytopenic purpura
  - Sepsis/infection: meningococcemia, Rocky Mountain spotted fever
  - Leukemia
  - Hemolytic-uremic syndrome
  - Coagulopathies
- Vasculitic rashes may result from primary and secondary vasculitides.
  - Polyarteritis nodosa
  - Wegener granulomatosis
  - Infection related
  - Connective tissue diseases (e.g., systemic lupus erythematosus) or Berger disease
  - Infantile acute hemorrhagic edema
  - Rheumatoid arthritis
  - Rheumatic fever
  - Kawasaki disease
- Other: Acute abdomen, bacterial endocarditis, abuse (3)

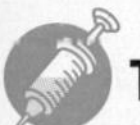

TREATMENT

MEDICATION

- HSP without nephritis usually resolves spontaneously without specific therapy.
- Early oral prednisone (1–2 mg/kg/day of prednisone for two weeks) may reduce intensity of joint and abdominal pain (5)[B].
- Patients with severe renal damage should be considered for aggressive therapy with high-dose steroids and/or immunosuppressants or plasmapheresis; evidence is inconclusive (3)[C].
- Dapsone 1–2 mg/kg/d may be considered for skin rash (6)[C].
- Analgesics and NSAIDs may be used for analgesia, but salicylates and other agents that affect platelet function should be avoided if GI tract bleeding is present.
  - NSAIDs should be avoided in patients with renal disease (3).

ADDITIONAL TREATMENT

General Measures

- Treatment of hypertension may delay or prevent progression of renal disease in patients with glomerulonephritis.
- Rest and elevation of affected areas may limit purpura (3).

Issues for Referral

Pediatric nephrology and/or dermatology

IN-PATIENT CONSIDERATIONS

Hospitalization is often unnecessary. Severe complications may require admission.

Admission Criteria

- Gastrointestinal hemorrhage
- Protein-losing enteropathy requiring total parenteral nutrition
- Renal disease
- Hypertension
- Pulmonary hemorrhage

IV Fluids

Hydration should be maintained.

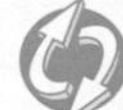

ONGOING CARE

FOLLOW-UP RECOMMENDATIONS

Patient Monitoring

- Patients should be seen weekly during the acute illness. Visits should include history and physical exam, along with BP measurement and urinalysis.
- All patients, even those who did not present with renal involvement, should have urine checked for blood weekly for 6 months and then monthly for 3 years because deterioration of renal function has been observed years after presentation in some patients.
- Women with a history of HSP should be monitored for proteinuria and HTN during pregnancy.

PATIENT EDUCATION

American Family Physician handout on HSP at www.aafp.org/afp/980800ap/980800b.html

PROGNOSIS

- Generally excellent: Most patients are improved within 4 weeks of HSP onset.
- Younger age is associated with better prognosis.
- Recurrence within 1st 6 months in up to 33% (3)
- Extent of renal disease often dictates long-term prognosis (3).

COMPLICATIONS

- Hypertension
- End-stage renal disease
- Intussusception (most common GI tract complication, affecting 1–5% of patients)
- Protein-losing enteropathy
- Hemorrhagic pancreatitis
- Hydrops of the gallbladder
- Intestinal strictures
- Bowel perforations, ischemia, and infarctions, obstructions
- GI hemorrhage
- Pseudomembranous colitis
- Appendicitis
- Skin necrosis
- Subarachnoid, subdural, and cortical hemorrhage and infarction
- Peripheral mononeuropathies and polyneuropathies (Guillain-Barré syndrome)
- Pulmonary hemorrhage (uncommon but may result in death)
- Torsion of the testis and appendix testes and priapism
- Scrotal swelling and pain
- CNS complications
- Myocarditis

REFERENCES

1. McCarthy HJ, Tizard EJ. Diagnosis and management of Henoch-Schönlein purpura. *Eur J Pediatr*. 2010;169:643–650.
2. Gardner-Medwin JM, Dolezalova P, Cummins C, et al. Incidence of Henoch-Schönlein purpura, Kawasaki disease, and rare vasculitides in children of different ethnic origins. *Lancet*. 2002;360: 1197–202.
3. Reamy BV, Williams PM, Lindsay TJ. Henoch-Schönlein purpura. *Am Fam Physician*. 2009;80(7): 697–704.
4. Ozen S, Pistorio A, Iusan SM, et al. EULAR/PRINTO/PRES criteria for Henoch-Schönlein purpura, childhood polyarteritis nodosa, childhood Wegener granulomatosis and childhood Takayasu arteritis: Ankara 2008. Part II: final classification criteria. *Ann Rheum Dis*. 2010;69:798–806.
5. Weiss PF, Feinstein JA, Luan X, et al. Effects of corticosteroid on Henoch-Schönlein purpura: a systematic review. *Pediatrics*. 2007;120:1079–87.
6. Iqbal H, Evans A. Dapsone therapy for Henoch-Schönlein purpura: a case series. *Arch Dis Child*. 2005;90:985–6.

ADDITIONAL READING

- González LM, Janniger CK, Schwartz RA. Pediatric Henoch-Schönlein purpura. *Int J Dermatol*. 2009;48:1157–1165.
- Roberts PF, Waller TA, Brinker TM, et al. Henoch-Schönlein purpura: a review article. *South Med J*. 2007;100:821–4.

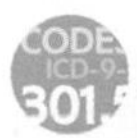

CODES

ICD9

287.0 Allergic purpura

CLINICAL PEARLS

- Rash is the hallmark of HSP.
- HSP without renal involvement is often self-limiting.
- All patients, even those who did not present with renal involvement, should have urine checked for blood weekly for 6 months and then monthly for 3 years because deterioration of renal function has been observed years after presentation in some patients.

H

HEPARIN-INDUCED THROMBOCYTOPENIA

Adam B. Pesaturo, PharmD, BCPS
Patrick Mailloux, DO

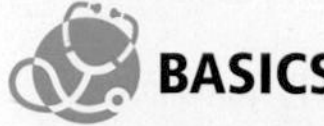

BASICS

DESCRIPTION

- Unexplained decrease in platelet count in a patient treated with heparin:
  - Minimum platelet count fall between 30% and 50% from baseline
- Antibody-mediated prothrombotic disorder initiated by heparin administration
- Idiosyncratic reaction
- 2 types: Nonimmune heparin-associated thrombocytopenia (previously called HIT type I) and HIT (previously called HIT type II):
  - Nonimmune heparin-associated thrombocytopenia: More common, onset 1–4 days after starting heparin, mild thrombocytopenia (>100,000), few complications
  - HIT: Less common, onset 5–14 days after primary exposure to heparin, thrombocytopenia often <100,000 but usually >20,000, high risk of thrombosis:
    - Presentation of thrombocytopenia can be immediate if recent heparin exposure within past 100 days

EPIDEMIOLOGY

Incidence

- 10–15% of heparin-treated patients will experience decrease in platelet count.
- 0.3–3% will develop HIT.

RISK FACTORS

- Postsurgical > medical > obstetric:
  - Postcardiopulmonary bypass being the most significant risk factor
- Bovine unfractionated heparin (UFH) > porcine UFH > low-molecular-weight heparin (LMWH)
- Female > Male
- Heparin duration >4 days

GENERAL PREVENTION

- Inquire about recent heparin exposure and any prior history of HIT
- Proper documentation of past HIT reactions in patient's medical record
- No form of heparin should ever be administered once the diagnosis of HIT is confirmed.

PATHOPHYSIOLOGY

- Nonimmune heparin-associated thrombocytopenia: Potentially a result from direct platelet membrane binding with heparin
- HIT: Heparin can cause an increase in the blood concentration of platelet factor 4 (PF4), a chemokine. PF4 will form a complex with heparin. This heparin/PF4 complex can, in turn, stimulate the production of specific antiheparin/PF4 complex antibodies. These antibodies cause platelet activation and a prothrombotic state. Ultimately, this hypercoagulable state leads to thromboembolic complications in many patients.

COMMONLY ASSOCIATED CONDITIONS

- Venous thrombosis: Deep venous thrombosis (DVT), pulmonary embolism (PE), adrenal vein thrombosis with hemorrhagic infarction
- Arterial thrombosis
- Skin lesions
- Acute systemic reactions

DIAGNOSIS

- Nonimmune heparin-associated thrombocytopenia: Asymptomatic drop in platelet count
- HIT: Thrombocytopenia or thrombosis with the presence of heparin-dependent antibodies:
  - A clinicopathologic syndrome, meaning the foundation for diagnosis is based on both clinical and serologic findings

HISTORY

- Duration of current heparin therapy
- Previous exposure to heparin, including heparin flushes and heparin-coated catheters
- In patients being treated with heparin for thrombosis in which thrombosis recurs during therapy, consider HIT as a potential cause.
- Pretest probability for HIT can be calculated using the "4T's" methodology (1).

PHYSICAL EXAM

- Signs of venous or arterial thrombosis
- Skin necrosis (begins with erythema, progressing to ecchymosis and necrosis)
- Ischemic changes (signs of limb, renal, splenic, mesenteric ischemia)
- Bleeding (less common)

DIAGNOSTIC TESTS & INTERPRETATION

Lab

- Serial platelet counts in patients receiving heparin: Check platelets at baseline, 24 hours, and then every other day for first 14 days (2)[B].
- Confirmatory lab tests needed for a clinical diagnosis can use 1 of 3 serologic assays:
  - Enzyme-linked immunosorbent assay (ELISA) (antigenic assay): Up to 99% sensitive, poor specificity; thus, has an excellent negative predictive value for HIT
  - Heparin-induced platelet activation (platelet activation test): High specificity and low sensitivity
  - Serotonin release assay (platelet activation test): High specificity and moderate sensitivity
- Either a platelet activation assay or an antigenic assay alone may not be adequate for clinical diagnosis; their use in combination is usually recommended.
- The diagnostic interpretation of these laboratory tests must be made in the context of the clinical estimation of the pretest probability of HIT since HIT is a clinicopathologic syndrome. Patients may form heparin-dependent antibodies and still not develop HIT (3).

DIFFERENTIAL DIAGNOSIS

Other potential causes of thrombocytopenia include (list is not all-inclusive):

- Sepsis and other infections
- Drug reactions
- Autoimmune
- Transfusion reactions
- Physical destruction (i.e., during cardiopulmonary bypass)

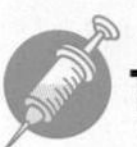

TREATMENT

Treatment is by prompt withdrawal of heparin and replacement with a suitable alternative anticoagulant.

MEDICATION

- Most patients will require anticoagulation either because of:
  - Preexisting thrombosis *OR*
  - Risk of thrombosis during 30 days after HIT diagnosis; consider anticoagulation for 30 days (4)[B]
- Dosing of anticoagulant will depend on indication (prophylaxis vs treatment):
  - In cases where there is clinically a low suspicion/pretest probability of HIT and laboratory confirmation is pending, it may be appropriate to continue antithrombotic prophylaxis using nonheparin anticoagulants.
  - In cases with high suspicion/pretest probability of HIT and laboratory confirmation is pending, it is appropriate to begin anticoagulation treatment with a nonheparin product.
- Direct thrombin inhibitors (DTI) (lepirudin, argatroban, and bivalirudin):
  - They reduce relative risk of thrombosis by 30%, on average (2)[B].
  - DTIs can produce misleading elevation in international normalized ratio (INR) (most likely an in vitro reaction) (5):
    - Argatroban > bivalirudin > lepirudin
  - Lepirudin:
    - Initial dose 0.1 mg/kg/hr, decrease dose with reduced renal function
    - Dose adjustments based on active partial thromboplastin time (aPTT) (goal: 1.5–2 times patient baseline); check aPTT every 4 hours until steady state within goal aPTT range is achieved
  - Argatroban:
    - Initial dose is 2 mcg/kg/min, decrease dose with reduced hepatic function or with critical illness
    - Dose adjustments based on aPTT similar to lepirudin, except aPTT is initially checked every 2 hours
  - Bivalirudin:
    - Favorable pharmacologic profile; however, evidence for use is insufficient compared to lepirudin and argatroban
    - Initial dose is a 0.1 mg/kg bolus, followed by a continuous infusion rate of 0.2 mg/kg/hr, reduced dose with renal insufficiency (CrCl <30 mL/min)
    - Dose adjustments based on aPTT

- Factor Xa inhibitor (fondaparinux):
  - Reports of its use theorized to be useful; however, there is minimal data supporting its efficacy for HIT, and an ideal dose has yet to be determined.
  - Association with the development of HIT has been reported (6)[C]
  - Optional agent for thromboembolic prophylaxis when practitioner wants to avoid heparin
  - Avoid in patients with renal dysfunction (CrCl <30 mL/min).
- Warfarin:
  - Must anticoagulate with an immediate-acting agent before starting warfarin
  - Use of warfarin without other anticoagulants should be avoided, as it can cause thrombosis (2)[A].
  - Begin warfarin after platelet count >150,000 (2)[B]
  - Discontinue other anticoagulant and continue only warfarin after INR is therapeutic (2–3) for at least 5 days (2)[A]. This management differs from the normal heparin-to-warfarin transition in other conditions requiring anticoagulation.
- Low-molecular-weight heparin (LMWH):
  - Although LMWH has a lower risk of initiating a HIT reaction, it should NOT be used when antibodies are already present. These antibodies can cross-react with LMWH and induce thrombosis and thrombocytopenia (2)[A].

ADDITIONAL TREATMENT

General Measures

- Discontinue all heparin products, including flushes and heparin-coated catheters.
- Nonimmune heparin-associated thrombocytopenia generally resolves when heparin is stopped:
  - Consider a nonheparin alternative like fondaparinux if pharmacologic DVT prophylaxis is warranted.
- Avoid platelet transfusions (2)[C].
- Adverse reaction to heparin should be clearly documented in medical record with instruction to avoid all heparin products in the future.
- For patients with a documented history of HIT, under special circumstances only (such as the need for cardiopulmonary bypass), the use of heparin for a short duration may be acceptable if the absence of heparin/PF4 complex antibodies can be documented (7)[C].

IN-PATIENT CONSIDERATIONS

Nursing

- Avoid heparin flushes.
- Avoid platelet transfusion.
- Clearly document reaction in all medical records to avoid the future use of heparin.

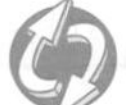

ONGOING CARE

FOLLOW-UP RECOMMENDATIONS

- The transition period of anticoagulation with a DTI and warfarin in patients with HIT can be problematic.
- The INR while administering both a DTI and warfarin should be therapeutic (2–3) for at least 5 days before discontinuing the DTI.
- Warfarin therapy should not be commenced until the platelet count has stabilized within a normal range.
- DTIs can prolong INR; therefore, if INR is >4 while on both warfarin and a DTI, temporarily hold the DTI for 4–6 hours and recheck INR; this second INR will represent only the anticoagulant effect of warfarin.

Patient Monitoring

- Serial platelet counts
- Monitor PTT or INR as determined by the anticoagulation agent

PATIENT EDUCATION

- Patient should inform all health care providers of any previous adverse reaction to heparin.
- HIT information available at: http://medlibrary.org/medwiki/Heparin-induced_thrombocytopenia

PROGNOSIS

- Thrombosis in HIT has 20–30% mortality, with additional morbidity from stroke and limb ischemia
- Platelet counts normalize within weeks after stopping heparin.
- Risk of delayed thrombosis, especially in the first 30 days

REFERENCES

1. Lo GK, Juhl D, Warkentin TE, Sigouin CS, Eichler P, Greinacher A et al. Evaluation of pretest clinical score (4 T's) for the diagnosis of heparin-induced thrombocytopenia in two clinical settings. *J Thromb Haemost*. 2006;4:759–65.
2. Warkentin TE, Greinacher A, Koster A, et al. Treatment and prevention of heparin-induced thrombocytopenia: American College of Chest Physicians Evidence-Based Clinical Practice Guidelines (8th Edition). *Chest*. 2008;133: 340S–380S.
3. Shantsila E, Lip GY, Chong BH. Heparin-induced thrombocytopenia: a contemporary clinical approach to diagnosis and management. *Chest*. 2009;135:1651–64.
4. Dager WE, Dougherty JA, Nguyen PH, et al. Heparin-Induced Thrombocytopenia: Treatment Options and Special Considerations. *Pharmacotherapy*. 2007;27:564–87.
5. Warkentin TE, Greinacher A, Craven S, et al. Differences in the clinically effective molar concentrations of four direct thrombin inhibitors explain their variable prothrombin time prolongation. *Thromb Haemost*. 2005;94:958–64.
6. Warkentin TE, Maurer BT, Aster RH. Heparin-induced thrombocytopenia associated with fondaparinux. *N Engl J Med*. 2007;356:2653–5; discussion 2653–5.
7. Warkentin TE, Kelton JG et al. Temporal aspects of heparin-induced thrombocytopenia. *N Engl J Med*. 2001;344:1286–92.

ADDITIONAL READING

- HIT information. Available at: http://www.heparininducedthrombocytopenia.com/.
- Martel N, Lee J, Wells PS. Risk for heparin-induced thrombocytopenia with unfractionated and low-molecular-weight heparin thromboprophylaxis: a meta-analysis. *Blood*. 2005;106:2710–5.
- Smythe MA, Koerber JM, Mattson JC. The Incidence of Recognized Heparin-Induced Thrombocytopenia in a Large Tertiary Care, Teaching Hospital. *Chest*. 2007.

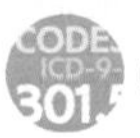

CODES

ICD9

289.84 Heparin induced thrombocytopenia (HIT)

CLINICAL PEARLS

- Heparin exposure through virtually any preparation (including LMWH), any dose, or any route can cause HIT.
- LMWH is contraindicated in HIT; although LMWH is less likely to cause HIT, once HIT is present, the antibodies will cross-react and continue to cause a HIT reaction.
- If a patient is suspected of HIT (with or without confirmatory testing), immediately discontinue of all forms of heparin.
- Patients will require anticoagulation either because of preexisting thrombosis or the risk of thrombosis in first 30 days after HIT.
- A DTI should be used until a patient's INR is therapeutic (2–3) on warfarin for at least 5 days.
- The key to avoiding sequelae from HIT is awareness, vigilance, and a high degree of suspicion.

HEPATITIS A

J. Scott Gaertner, MD

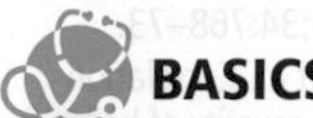

BASICS

DESCRIPTION

Infection with the hepatitis A virus (HAV) primarily involving the liver

EPIDEMIOLOGY

Pediatric Considerations

- Disease is often milder or asymptomatic in pediatric population.
- 70% of infections are asymptomatic in children <6 years of age.
- Hepatitis A infection severity increases with age.

Incidence

- In 2007 there were 2,979 HAV infections reported in the US.
- Prior to release of HAV vaccine, there were 22,000–36,000 cases reported per year in the US (1)[B].
- Estimated cases: 25,000 HAV infections in 2007 (lowest ever recorded in US)
- 1.1/100,000 incidence in US
- Predominant sex: Male = Female

Prevalence

Antibodies in 33% of US population

RISK FACTORS

- Foreign travel to developing countries accounts for over 50% of cases in North America and Europe.
- Employment in health care
- Household exposure
- Intimate exposure, especially men who have sex with men
- Institutionalized individuals
- Clotting factor disorders such as hemophilia
- Blood exposure/transfusion rare

Genetics

Autoimmune hepatitis is associated with human leukocyte antigen class II; DR3 and DR4 after active infection with HAV, although rare

GENERAL PREVENTION

- HAV vaccines: Havrix and Vaqta:
  - 0.5 mL IM for children >1 year. 1 mL IM for adults. 2nd dose at 6–12 months.
  - Separate syringe site from immunoglobulin
  - Used for travelers, day care staff/children, custodial facility employees, sewage workers, military, homosexual men, and food handlers. American Academy of Pediatrics recommends routine administration of HAV vaccine to all children 12–23 months of age in all states according to the Centers for Disease Control-approved immunization schedule.
  - In 2007, self-reporting studies estimated vaccination coverage among adults aged 18–49 years at 12.1% (1)[B].
  - 98% seroprotection at 10 years after primary hepatitis A vaccine
  - HIV infected adults should receive 3 doses at weeks 0, 4, and 24.
  - HAV and hepatitis B virus: Twinrix
- Passive immunization: Immunoglobulin:
  - 0.02–0.06 mL/kg IM given within 2 weeks after exposure prevents illness 80–90%
  - HAV vaccine has similar efficacy to immunoglobulin in postexposure prophylaxis if given within 2 weeks
  - Use immunoglobulin in cases where travelers need immediate protection.
  - Use 0.06 mL/kg q.5 months for long-term travelers if unable to receive vaccine.
  - Do not give immunoglobulin with measles, mumps, rubella, or varicella vaccine.
- Good sanitation
- Good hygiene, including hand washing, especially food handlers, health care, and day care workers
- HAV is NOT killed by freezing.
- HAV is killed by:
  - Heating to 185°F for 60 seconds
  - Chlorine
  - Iodine

Pediatric Considerations

Children <1 year of age

Pregnancy Considerations

Pregnant females who will be traveling

PATHOPHYSIOLOGY

- Hepatitis A vaccine is a single-stranded linear RNA enterovirus and a member of the *Picornaviridae* family.
- Humans are the only natural host.

ETIOLOGY

- Incubation 2–6 weeks (mean of 4 weeks)
- Greatest infectivity is during the 2 weeks before the onset of clinical illness.
- Infection occurs after eating or drinking food or water contaminated with HAV or direct contact with infected person who has poor personal hygiene.
- Food can become contaminated if handled by an infected individual with poor personal hygiene.
- Shellfish, such as clams and oysters, may be contaminated if harvested from waters contaminated with HAV.
- Bloodborne transmission occurs but is rare.
- No chronicity in HAV

COMMONLY ASSOCIATED CONDITIONS

- Arthritis
- Urticaria
- Anemia
- Immune complex nephritis

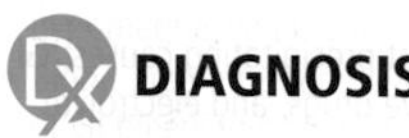

DIAGNOSIS

HISTORY

- Fever: 60%
- Malaise: 67%
- Nausea and vomiting
- Anorexia: 54%
- Dark urine: 84%
- Transient pale stools
- Right upper abdominal pain
- Fatigue
- Myalgias
- Symptom severity has direct correlation to age.
- Pediatric cases frequently asymptomatic

PHYSICAL EXAM

- Hepatomegaly
- Fever
- Jaundice
- Icterus
- Right upper abdominal tenderness

DIAGNOSTIC TESTS & INTERPRETATION

Lab

Initial lab tests

- Aspartate aminotransferase (AST) and alanine aminotransferase (ALT) elevated. May exceed 10,000. ALT usually >AST.
- Anti-HAV immunoglobulin M: Positive at time of onset of symptoms
- Anti-HAV immunoglobulin G: Appears soon after IgM and generally persists for years
- Alkaline phosphatase: Mildly elevated
- Bilirubin: Conjugated and unconjugated fractions usually increased. Usually follows rises in ALT and AST.

- Prothrombin time and partial thromboplastin time: Usually remains normal or near normal range:
  - Significant rises should raise concern
- Complete blood count: Mild leukocytosis. Aplasia and pancytopenia are rare:
  - Initial thrombocytopenia may predict illness severity.
- Albumin, electrolytes, and glucose
- Urinalysis: Bilirubinuria

Follow-Up & Special Considerations

Illness usually resolves within 4 weeks from onset of symptoms.

Imaging

- Usually not needed
- Consider ultrasound to rule out differential diagnosis

Initial approach

Bed rest and appropriate nutrition/hydration

Follow-Up & Special Considerations

Usually can be managed outpatient

Diagnostic Procedures/Surgery

Liver biopsy usually not necessary

Pathological Findings

- Pronounced portal inflammation
- Immunofluorescent stains for HAV-antigen positive
- Positive serum markers in hepatitis A:
  - Acute disease: Anti-HAV IgM and IgG positive
  - Recent disease: Anti-HAV IgM and IgG positive
  - Previous disease: Anti-HAV IgM negative and IgG positive

DIFFERENTIAL DIAGNOSIS

- Other hepatitis virus infections B, C, D, E
- Infectious mononucleosis
- Primary or secondary hepatic malignancy
- Ischemic hepatitis
- Drug-induced hepatitis
- Alcoholic hepatitis
- Autoimmune hepatitis
- Wilson disease

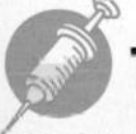

TREATMENT

MEDICATION

Postexposure prophylaxis to persons within 2 weeks of exposure to hepatitis A virus:

- Administer hepatitis A vaccine to persons between the ages of 1 and 40.
- Administer immunoglobulin to persons <1 and >40 years of age.

First Line

- No antiviral medications indicated, as spontaneous resolution occurs in almost all patients.
- Steroids not indicated unless patient with autoimmune hepatitis

Second Line

- Antiemetics: Metoclopramide 5–20 mg IV/IM t.i.d.
- IV fluids

ADDITIONAL TREATMENT

General Measures

- Monitor coagulation defects, fluid and electrolytes, acid-base imbalance, hypoglycemia, and impairment of renal function.
- Report acute cases to local public health department.

Issues for Referral

- Dictated by severity of illness
- Hepatic failure

COMPLEMENTARY AND ALTERNATIVE MEDICINE

Avoid botanicals with hepatotoxicity potential, including:

- Barberry
- Comfrey
- Golden ragwort
- Groundsel
- Huang qin
- Kava kava
- Pennyroyal
- Sassafras
- Senna
- Valerian
- Wall germander
- Wood sage

SURGERY/OTHER PROCEDURES

Liver transplant in fulminant hepatic failure

IN-PATIENT CONSIDERATIONS

Initial Stabilization

Treatment is usually outpatient

Admission Criteria

Dictated by severity of illness

IV Fluids

Treat dehydration and electrolyte imbalances.

Nursing

Routine

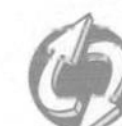

ONGOING CARE

FOLLOW-UP RECOMMENDATIONS

Return to work/school 10–14 days after onset of symptoms with diligence to hygiene

Patient Monitoring

- Monitor coagulation defects, fluid and electrolytes, acid-base imbalance, hypoglycemia, and impairment of renal function.
- Report acute cases to local public health department.
- Usually infectious 4 weeks from initial symptoms

DIET

- Adequate balanced nutrition
- Avoid alcohol.
- Avoid medications that may accumulate in the liver.

PATIENT EDUCATION

- Segregation of food handlers with HAV
- HAV immunity after infection

PROGNOSIS

- Excellent
- Mortality 0.2%

COMPLICATIONS

- Coagulopathy, encephalopathy, and renal failure
- Relapsing HAV: Usually milder than the initial case. Positive anti-HAV IgM. Total duration usually less than 9 months.
- Prolonged cholestasis: Characterized by protracted periods of jaundice and pruritus (>3 mo). Resolves without intervention.
- Autoimmune hepatitis: Good response to steroids
- Hepatic failure: Rare (1–2%)

REFERENCE

1. *Vaccine*. 2009 Feb 25;27(9):1301–5. Epub 2009 Jan 20. Hepatitis A vaccination coverage among adults aged 18–49 years in the United States. Lu PJ, Euler GL, Hennessey KA, Weinbaum CM.

ADDITIONAL READING

- Abreu C. *Acta Med Port*. 2007;20(6):557–66. Epub 2008 Feb 13.
- Bianco E, De Masi S, Mele A, Jefferson T. *Digest Liver Disease*. 2004;36(12):834–42.
- Garner-Spitzer E, Kundi M, Rendi-Wagner P, et al. Correlation between humoral and cellular immune responses and the expression of the hepatitis A receptor HAVcr-1 on T cells after hepatitis A re-vaccination in high and low-responder vaccinees. *Vaccine*. 2008.
- Gilroy, Richard K. eMedicine from WebMD. AAFP. *Hepatitis A*. May 30, 2006.
- Launay O, Grabar S, Gordien E, et al. Immunological efficacy of a three-dose schedule of hepatitis A vaccine in HIV-infected adults: HEPAVAC study. *J Acquir Immune Defic Syndr*. 2008;49:272–5.
- Weiland O. Lakartidningen, 2008;105(19): 1371–2.

See Also (Topic, Algorithm, Electronic Media Element)

Hepatitis B; Hepatitis C

Algorithm: Hyperbilirubinemia

CODES

ICD9

070.1 Viral hepatitis a without mention of hepatic coma

CLINICAL PEARLS

- Hepatitis A vaccine 2 doses 6–12 months apart
- Indicated for travelers, day care staff/children, custodial facility employees, sewage workers, military, homosexual men, and food handlers
- HAV disease severity directly correlates with age; children are often asymptomatic.

HEPATITIS B

Anne M. Walsh, PA-C, MMSc
Jill A. Grimes, MD

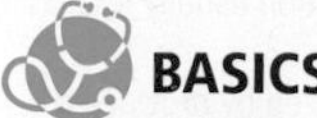

BASICS

DESCRIPTION

Systemic viral infection that may cause acute and chronic liver disease and hepatocellular carcinoma (HCC)

EPIDEMIOLOGY

Incidence

- Predominant age: All ages
- Predominant sex: Fulminant hepatitis B virus (HBV): Male > Female (2:1)
- 60,000 new infections in US in 2008, 70% due to IV drug use

Prevalence

- 2 million people in US with chronic HBV:
  - 5,000 deaths per year
- 350–400 million persons with chronic HBV worldwide:
  - 1,000,000 deaths/year:
    - 10th leading cause of death
    - 2nd most important carcinogen (behind tobacco)
    - 25% of chronic carriers die of cirrhosis or HCC.
    - 75% of chronic carriers are Asian.

RISK FACTORS

- Screen high-risk groups with HBsAg/sAb (1)[A]:
  - Persons born in endemic areas (45% of world)
  - Hemodialysis patients
  - IV drug users (IVDU), past or present
  - Men who have sex with men (MSM)
  - HIV- and HCV-positive patients
  - Household members of HBsAg carriers
  - Sexual contacts of HBsAg carriers
  - Inmates of correctional facilities
  - All patients with chronically elevated aminotransferases (ALT/AST)
- Vaccinate all above groups if negative.
- Additional risk factors:
  - Needle stick/occupational exposure
  - Recipients of blood/products
  - Transplanted organ recipient
  - Intranasal drug users
  - Body piercing/tattoos

Genetics

Family history of HBV and/or HCC to determine exposure and future HCC risk

Pediatric Considerations

- Shorter acute course; fewer complications
- 90% of vertical/perinatal infections become chronic.

Marker	Acute Infection	Chronic Infection	Inactive Carrier	Resolved Infection	
HBsAg	+	+	+	−	
HBsAb	−	−	−	+	
HBcAb	+ IgM	− IgM; + total/IgG	+	+	
HBeAg	+	±	−	−	
HBeAb	−	−/+	+	±	
HBV DNA	Present	Present	Low–negative		
Negative	ALT	Marked elevation	Transient mild elevation	Normal	Normal

Pregnancy Considerations

- Screen all pregnant women for HBsAg (1)[A].
- High viral load at 28 weeks treated with oral meds from 32 weeks on reduces perinatal transmission (2)[B].
- Infant of HBV-infected mother needs HBIg (0.5 mL) plus HBV vaccine within 12 hours of birth and HBV series at 1 and 6 months (1)[A].
- Breastfeeding safe if HBIg and HBV vaccine administered and nipples without fissures
- HIV coinfection significantly increases risk of vertical transmission.
- Continue medications if pregnancy occurs while on oral antiviral therapy to prevent acute flare.

GENERAL PREVENTION

- Most effective: HBV vaccination series (3 doses):
- Vaccinate:
  - All infants at birth
  - All at-risk patients (see Risk Factors)
  - Health care and public safety workers at high risk
  - Sexual contacts of HBsAg carriers
  - Household contacts of HBsAg carriers
- Proper hygiene/sanitation by health care workers, IVDU, tattoo/piercing artists
  - Barrier precautions, safe handling of needles, proper sterilization of equipment
- Do not share personal items exposed to blood (e.g., nail clipper, razor, toothbrush).
- Advocate safe sexual practices, including use of condoms.
- HBsAg carriers cannot donate blood, tissue, or organs.
- Postexposure (e.g., needlestick): HB immune globulin (HBIg) 0.06 mL/kg in <24 hours

ETIOLOGY

HBV is a DNA virus of the family *Hepadnaviridae*.

COMMONLY ASSOCIATED CONDITIONS

Arthritis, polyarteritis nodosa, membranous glomerulopathy, anemia (including aplastic anemia), dermatitis, cardiomyopathy, hepatitis D virus infection, metabolic syndrome

DIAGNOSIS

HISTORY

- Exposure: Detailed family and social history
- Acute HBV:
  - Fever
  - Malaise/fatigue/arthralgias/myalgias
  - Anorexia/nausea/vomiting
  - Jaundice/scleral icterus
  - Dark urine/pale stools
  - Right upper quadrant abdominal pain
  - Headache/meningismus (occasional)
- Chronic HBV: Typically asymptomatic

PHYSICAL EXAM

- Acute: Ill appearing; jaundice/scleral icterus; right upper quadrant tenderness, hepatomegaly
- Typically normal in noncirrhotic chronic HBV

DIAGNOSTIC TESTS & INTERPRETATION

Lab

Initial lab tests

- AST/ALT: Marked elevation in acute HBV, particularly of ALT, 400 to several thousand IU/mL (may be normal or mildly elevated in chronic HBV)
  - Elevate before bilirubin elevates
- Bilirubin: Normal to markedly elevated in acute HBV, conjugated/unconjugated
  - Last test to normalize as acute infection resolves
- Alkaline phosphatase: Mild elevation
- HBcAb IgM may be the only early finding ("window period," when HBsAg/sAb–).
- For acute hepatitis
  - Monitor PT, albumin, electrolytes, glucose, CBC
  - If severe acute HBV, check for superinfection with hepatitis D (HDV).
  - Hepatitis B serologic markers
- Hepatitis B e antigen (HBeAg+) indicates high replication/infectivity; confirmed with high HBV DNA ($\geq 10^5$ copies/mL); these patients benefit from medical therapy.
- HBV precore mutants have undetectable HBeAg despite active viral replication (confirm with HBV DNA level) as well as antibody to e antigen (HBeAb+).
- Screen for HIV, HCV, and immunity to HAV (HAV Ab total/IgG).

Follow-Up & Special Considerations

HBsAg+ persistence >6 months = chronic HBV

- Measure HBV DNA level and ALT every 3–6 months.
- Measure baseline α-fetoprotein (AFP).
- Follow HBeAg for loss (every 6–12 months).
- Lifetime monitoring for progression, need for treatment, and screening for HCC

Imaging

- Ultrasound to demonstrate ascites, exclude obstruction, screen for HCC
- Contrast CT or MRI if abnormal ultrasound or elevated AFP

Diagnostic Procedures/Surgery

Liver biopsy determines extent of injury, excludes other liver disease, guides therapy.

Pathological Findings

Liver biopsy in chronic HBV may show interface hepatitis and variable inflammation, necrosis, cholestasis, fibrosis, cirrhosis, or chronic active hepatitis.

DIFFERENTIAL DIAGNOSIS

- EBV; CMV; hepatitis A,C, or E
- Drug-induced, alcoholic, or autoimmune hepatitis
- Wilson disease or rheumatologic/immunologic disorders

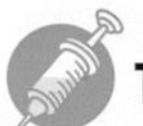

TREATMENT

MEDICATION

First Line

- Acute HBV:
  - Supportive care; antiviral therapy not indicated; spontaneously resolves in 95% of immunocompetent adults

- Chronic HBV: Treatment based on HBeAg status:
  - FDA-approved drugs: Lamivudine 100 mg, adefovir 10 mg, entecavir 0.5–1 mg, telbivudine 600 mg, or tenofovir 300 mg, all given PO every day; pegylated interferon (peg-IFN) α2a SC weekly (1)[A]

- Refer to liver transplant program ASAP if fulminant acute hepatitis, end-stage liver disease, or HCC. Resection/ablation of early or noncirrhotic HCC yields excellent outcomes posttransplant.

COMPLEMENTARY AND ALTERNATIVE MEDICINE

No evidence to support alternative treatments

Table 2 Chronic Hepatitis B Therapy (1)

HBeAg	HBV DNA Viral Load	ALT*	Recommendation
(+)	≥20,000 IU/mL	Elevated	Treat w/mono or combination therapy
(–)	≥2,000 IU/mL	Elevated	(see above)
(+)	≤20,000 IU/mL	Any	Monitor q6–12mo
(–)	≥2,000 IU/mL	Normal	Biopsy; treat if disease
(+)	≥20,000 IU/mL	Normal	(see above)
(–)	≤2,000 IU/mL	Any	Monitor q6–12mo
Cirrhosis	Any	Any	Treat with combination tx (3)
Decomp	Any	Any	Treat + transplant

*ALT elevated if >2 × ULN; ULN for male = 30 IU/mL and for female = 19 IU/mL

- Lamivudine no longer recommended 1st-line due to high rates of resistance
- Entecavir, tenofovir, peg-IFN are preferred 1st-line agents (1,4)[A]
- Oral agents given for extended period:
  - If HBeAg+, treat 6–12 months post loss of eAg/gain of eAb (1)[A]
  - If HBeAg–, treat indefinitely or until HBsAg clearance (1)[A]
- Change/add drug based on development of resistance:
  - Confirm patient compliance with medications before assuming resistance.
  - Combination therapy lowers rate of resistance.
- Dose adjustment made for elevated creatinine
- Standard IFN (Intron A) no longer used in favor of peg-IFN:
  - Peg-IFN (Pegasys) injections given weekly for 48 weeks
  - Best efficacy in genotype A
  - Contraindicated if decompensated cirrhosis
- Goals of therapy: Undetectable HBV DNA, normalization of ALT, loss of HBeAg and appearance of HBeAb; loss of HBsAg (occurs only with IFN therapy)
- Precautions:
  - Oral drugs: Renal insufficiency, acute flare if discontinued, resistance/mutation development
  - Peg-IFN: Coagulopathy, myelosuppression, depression/suicidal ideation
- Interactions: Refer to manufacturer's profile.

Second Line

Emtricitabine effective; pending FDA approval

ADDITIONAL TREATMENT

General Measures

- Monitor coagulation, electrolytes, glucose, renal function, acid/base
- Report all HBsAg+ to public health department
- Providers must be familiar with medication risks/benefits/side effects, monitoring for development of resistance, and HCC screening guidelines.

Issues for Referral

- Refer all HBsAg+ patients to experienced gastroenterologist/hepatologist for consideration of antiviral therapy.

SURGERY/OTHER PROCEDURES

Liver transplantation, operative resection, radiofrequency ablation

IN-PATIENT CONSIDERATIONS

Outpatient treatment usually successful in acute HBV

Admission Criteria

- Worsening course (marked increase in bilirubin, transaminases, or symptoms)
- Hepatic failure (high PT, low albumin)

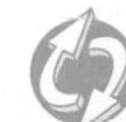

ONGOING CARE

FOLLOW-UP RECOMMENDATIONS

Activity as tolerated; bed rest during acute symptoms (abdominal pain, N/V, jaundice)

Patient Monitoring

- Vaccinate for HAV if seronegative (1)[B].
- Monitor serial ALT and HBV DNA:
  - High ALT + low HBV DNA associated with favorable response to therapy
- Serologic markers: Useful for evaluation of recovery or progression to chronicity (see chart)
- Metabolic complications and renal function
- WBC/platelets with IFN therapy
- Monitor HBV DNA q3–6 months during therapy:
  - Undetectable DNA at week 24 of oral drug therapy associated with low resistance at year 2.
- Monitor for complications (ascites, encephalopathy, variceal bleed) in cirrhosis.

DIET

Adequate calories, balanced nutrition

PATIENT EDUCATION

- Acute HBV:
  - Review transmission precautions (1)[C] and vaccinate seronegative family members and sexual partners (1)[A].
  - Symptoms, especially fatigue, may take several months to resolve.
- Chronic HBV:
  - Alcohol/smoking increase progression of liver disease and should be avoided.
  - If treated, strict compliance with oral medication is critical to prevent flare.
- Patient education materials in English and Spanish available at http://www.cdc.gov/hepatitis/B/PatientEduB.htm.

PROGNOSIS

- 95% of adults recover from acute infection.
- Severity of encephalopathy predicts survival in fulminant hepatic failure.
- Acute HBV: Mortality 1%
- Acute HBV + HDV: Mortality 2–20%
- Chronic HBV:
  - 0.5% per year spontaneously resolve
  - 25% suffer premature death from cirrhosis or HCC.
  - Baseline DNA predictive: Risk of HCC rises with rate of viral replication, even if no cirrhosis
  - US and AFP q 6–12 months for screening (patient-specific guidelines) (1,3)[B]

COMPLICATIONS

- Acute or subacute hepatic necrosis; cirrhosis; hepatic failure
- Hepatocelluar carcinoma (all chronic HBV patients are at risk)
- Severe flare of chronic HBV with corticosteroids:
  - Avoid if able; taper very slowly if used.
- Reactivation of resolved infection if immunosuppressed (e.g., chemotherapy): Prophylactic premedication recommended if HBsAg+ (1,3).

REFERENCES

1. Lok AS, McMahon BJ. Chronic hepatitis B. *Hepatology*. 2007;45:507–39.
2. Tran T, et al. Management of the pregnant hepatitis B patient. *Curr Hep Rep*. 2008;7:12–7.
3. Weinmaum C, et al. Recommendations for identification and public health management of persons with chronic hepatitis B infection. *MMWR*. 2008;57:1–20.
4. Woo G, Tomlinson G, Nishikawa Y, Kowgier M, Sherman M, Wong DK, Pham B, Ungar WJ, Einarson TR, Heathcote EJ, Krahn M et al. Tenofovir and Entecavir are Most Effective Antiviral Agents for Chronic Hepatitis B; A Systematic Review and Bayesian Meta-Analyses. *Gastroenterology*. 2010;

See Also (Topic, Algorithm, Electronic Media Element)

Hepatitis A; Hepatitis C; Cirrhosis of the Liver
Algorithm: Hyperbilirubinemia

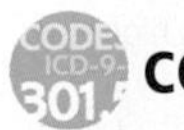

CODES

ICD9

- 070.30 Viral hepatitis b without mention of hepatic coma, acute or unspecified, without mention of hepatitis delta
- 070.32 Chronic viral hepatitis b without mention of hepatic coma without mention of hepatitis delta

CLINICAL PEARLS

- All patients born in endemic countries should be screened with HBsAg.
- Patients with chronic HBV need lifetime monitoring for progressive disease and HCC.

H

HEPATITIS C

Anne M. Walsh, PA-C, MMSc
Frank J. Domino, MD

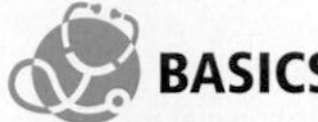 BASICS

DESCRIPTION
Systemic viral infection primarily involving liver; can result in acute and chronic disease

EPIDEMIOLOGY
- Predominant age: All ages; most new diagnoses 40–60 years old
- Predominant sex: Both sexes; Male = Female

Geriatric Considerations
Age >60 less likely to respond; treat earlier if able

Pediatric Considerations
- Prevalence: 0.3%
- Fewer symptoms or abnormal liver tests; more likely to clear spontaneously; slower rate of progression

Pregnancy Considerations
- Vertical transmission 1–5% if HIV negative
- Breastfeeding safe if no fissures (1)
- Ribavirin is teratogenic; contraindicated in pregnancy and in male partners of pregnant or impregnable women without contraception

Incidence
- 40,000 new cases of *chronic* hepatitis C virus (HCV) per year in US:
  - Reports of *acute* infections rare (asymptomatic)
  - 2/3 of people with chronic HCV are undiagnosed.
- Rate of new infections reduced since 1992 when effective donor blood screening began

Prevalence
- ~4 million in US (1.8%) ever infected (HCV Ab+)
- ~3 million have chronic HCV (HCV RNA+)
- ~10,000 deaths annually
- Most common cause of chronic liver disease & liver transplant
- Genotype 1 predominant (75% of cases)

RISK FACTORS
- Screen all patients with persistently elevated alanine aminotransferase (ALT) and all patients with known risk factors (1)[B]:
  - Hemodialysis
  - Blood +/− product transfusion before 1992
  - Hemophilia treatment before 1987
  - IV drug use:
    - 60–70% of new infections
    - *High transmission first use*; "once" is high risk
  - Sexually active homosexual male
  - HIV or hepatitis B infection
  - Household exposure to infected body fluids
  - Organ transplant recipients before 1992
  - Children of HCV+ mothers (test >18 months age)
  - Current sexual partners of HCV+ persons
- Possible risk factors:
  - Inhaled cocaine use; shared works
  - Body piercing and tattoos
  - Unsterile medical equipment
  - Health care worker/occupational risks low unless needlestick
- Universal screening is not recommended.

GENERAL PREVENTION
- No vaccine or postexposure prophylaxis available
- HCV Ab+ does not confer immunity to reinfection.
- Do not share razors/toothbrushes/nail clippers.
- Use and dispose of needles and soiled items properly.
- Sexual transmission rare in long-term partners (1.5%) if monogamous (1)[C].

ETIOLOGY
Single-stranded RNA virus of family *Flaviviridae*

COMMONLY ASSOCIATED CONDITIONS
- Diabetes, metabolic syndrome, iron overload, depression, substance abuse/recovery, autoimmune and hematologic disease
- HIV and hepatitis B coinfections

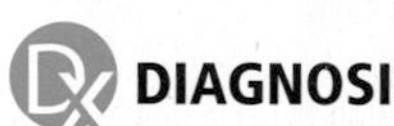 DIAGNOSIS

HISTORY
- Determine exposure: *complete* social history
- Chronic HCV: Vast majority mildly symptomatic (nonspecific fatigue) or asymptomatic elevated ALT/aspartate aminotransferase (AST)
- Acute HCV: *If* symptoms develop (rare):
  - Onset 2+ weeks postexposure
  - Persist 2–12 weeks
  - Spontaneous clearance more likely:
    - Fever
    - Malaise/fatigue, arthralgias/myalgias
    - Nausea/vomiting/anorexia
    - Jaundice/icterus/pruritis
    - Dark urine/ Pale stools
    - Right upper quadrant (RUQ) pain

PHYSICAL EXAM
- Typically normal unless advanced fibrosis/cirrhosis
- May have RUQ tenderness/hepatomegaly

DIAGNOSTIC TESTS & INTERPRETATION
Lab
Initial lab tests
- AST/ALT:
  - Normal or transiently elevated in chronic HCV
  - ALT usually 1–2 × ULN; AST may be normal or elevated but < ALT
  - AST/ALT ratio ≥1 associated with cirrhosis; if ratio >2, rule out alcohol abuse
  - Marked elevation only in acute hepatitis (400 to several thousand U/L)
  - If acute, serial PT to monitor for liver failure
- Alkaline phosphatase and GGT: Usually normal; more likely abnormal if cirrhosis, alcohol/fatty liver, or biliary obstruction
- Bilirubin: Normal in chronic HCV unless end-stage disease; markedly elevated in acute HCV (both direct/indirect); occurs after ALT/AST increase, ≥6 weeks post-exposure
- Albumin and PT normal until liver failure
- Anti-HCV negative until 8–9 weeks postexposure
- HCV RNA is positive 1–3 weeks postexposure
- Persistent HCV RNA >6 months = chronic HCV
- False(+) antibody: Autoimmune disease; false (−): immunosuppressed
- Screen for other liver disease (see Differential Diagnosis):
  - Ferritin (moderately high levels typical in HCV), Ceruloplasmin, ANA, α1-Antitrypsin phenotype, Fasting glucose/lipid panel
- If chronic, baseline α-fetoprotein (AFP) serum markers in Hepatitis C diagnosis

Follow-Up & Special Considerations
Vaccinate if seronegative for hepatitis A/B (1)[C].

Imaging
- US: Hepatomegaly, fatty liver, R/O mass
- MRI with contrast if US or AFP abnormal; Early cirrhosis not detectable by imaging

Diagnostic Procedures/Surgery
Liver biopsy recommended in chronic HCV to determine extent of injury, exclude other disease, guide treatment, and determine prognosis (2)[C]

Pathological Findings
- Periportal lymphocytic inflammation with or without necrosis, steatosis, cholestasis, fibrosis, iron
- Inflammation: Grade 0–4; Fibrosis: Stage 0–4

DIFFERENTIAL DIAGNOSIS
- Hepatitis A or B; EBV, CMV
- Acute/chronic alcoholic hepatitis
- Nonalcoholic steatohepatitis (NASH)
- Hemochromatosis, Wilson disease, α1–Antitrypsin deficiency
- Ischemic, drug induced, or autoimmune hepatitis

Serum Markers in Hepatitis C Diagnosis

Result	Marker (Lab Test)
(+)	Anti-HCV (antibody): • ELISA III • RIBA (distinguishes false-positive HCV Ab from spontaneous clearance)
(+)	HCV RNA (viral load); • Qualitative (TMA) • Quantitative, confirms (+) qualitative (PCR or bDNA)
1, 2, 3, 4, or 6 (rare) (also >50 subtypes)	Genotype: (1)[A] • Indeterminate if RNA too low, spontaneous clearance, or false positive anti-HCV • Best response to therapy: 2a, 2b, 3a • Least responsive: 1a, 1b

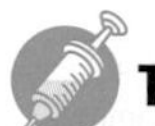 TREATMENT

MEDICATION
- Acute HCV: Antiviral therapy highly effective if given within 12 wks of infection (2)[B]:
  - Pegylated interferon (IFN) alone or in combination with low-dose ribavirin, for 12–24 weeks
- Chronic HCV: Antiviral therapy variably effective
  - Peg-IFN/ribavirin combined therapy (1,3)[A]:
    - Peg-IFN α2b 1.5 μg/kg SC weekly *OR*
    - Peg-IFN α2a 180 mcg SC weekly *WITH*
    - Ribavirin 800–1,400 mg p.o., divided, b.i.d. (weight-based)
  - Duration of therapy: 24–72 weeks based on genotype, presence of cirrhosis, HIV coinfection, and rate/degree viral response (check DNA at 4, 12, 24 wks)

– 32–36 weeks of HCV RNA undetectability optimal duration for genotype 1 (4)
– 24 weeks sufficient for genotype 2/3 if early viral response (EVR):
  ○ Cirrhosis lowers sustained viral response (SVR) by 50% in all genotypes.
  ○ Dose-reduced ribavirin/therapy interruption, especially before RNA negative, reduces SVR (5)[B]

- Contraindications:
  – Mouse IG, egg, or neomycin allergy
  – Pregnancy/breastfeeding
  – Decompensated liver disease or renal failure
  – Untreated psychiatric disease
  – Corticosteroid use or uncontrolled autoimmune disease
  – DDI in HIV patients (substitute comparable agent)
- Precautions:
  – Disorders of coagulation, anemia or myelosuppression
  – Seizures
  – Depression/suicidal ideation; psychiatric clearance and monitoring recommended
  – Retinopathy (diabetic/hypertensive) needs ophthalmology clearance/monitoring

ADDITIONAL TREATMENT

General Measures

- Report acute cases to health department
- Pretreatment patient counseling is critical.
- Control all other conditions prior to treatment (lipids, glucose, gout, mood, etc.).
- Side effects of IFN/ribavirin:
  – Fatigue, weight loss, insomnia, headache, depression/irritability, cognitive changes, nausea, rash, cough, thyroiditis, alopecia (temporary)
  – Premedicate injections with acetaminophen or NSAIDs if not contraindicated; early and prophylactic treatment of somatic and psychiatric side effects is key to adherence (4).
- Growth factors help maintain dose and tolerability (erythropoietin for ribavirin-induced anemia, G-CSF for IFN-induced neutropenia); however, not associated w/ improved SVR (5)[C]
- Team (PCP, GI, counselor, help line/support group, insurance disease management program, family, 12-step sponsor) improves outcomes (4).

Issues for Referral

- Refer all patients to a gastroenterologist or hepatologist experienced with HCV therapy (2)[C]; clinical trial if patient is uninsured.
- Refer to liver transplant program if fulminant acute hepatitis, at 1st complication of end-stage disease, or at diagnosis HCC (2)[A].

Additional Therapies

- Interferon-alfacon-1 (consensus IFN, Infergen) up to 37% cure rate in nonresponders/relapsers (6)[C].
- Addition of third drug (telaprivir, boceprevir) offers improved SVR but increased adverse effects; FDA approval is pending.

COMPLEMENTARY AND ALTERNATIVE MEDICINE

- No medical evidence exists for using herbal or alternative therapy in HCV/cirrhosis/HCC (1)[C].
- Milk thistle (silymarin) generally safe and may reduce ALT but does not eradicate virus nor improve outcomes; avoid while on IFN.
- Rate of HCC tripled in patients on herbal therapy compared to IFN therapy (3).

ONGOING CARE

FOLLOW-UP RECOMMENDATIONS

- If treatment is deferred, annual liver function tests; monitor for complications/associated conditions; and maintain sobriety/recovery.
- No need to monitor serial viral load unless on antiviral therapy; unrelated to disease severity or prognosis, and individual lab assays not well standardized.
- In cirrhosis, lifetime risk HCC 20%; screen with US/AFP every 6–12 months (2)[C].

Patient Monitoring

- Serial ALT/AST; serial fasting glucose
- Serial Hgb/Hct, white blood cells, absolute neutrophil count, platelets
- Follow electrolytes, TSH, renal function, PT
- HCV qualitative RNA negativity at week 4 is rapid viral response (RVR); confers ~90% chance of SVR in all genotypes (1)
- HCV quantitative RNA negativity (or drop of ≥2 log) at week 12 is EVR; confers good chance SVR
- SVR also more likely in patients with (4):
  – Age ≤40; Female gender; Caucasian race
  – Absence of bridging fibrosis/cirrhosis
  – HCV RNA <800,000 IU/mL
  – Genotypes 2 and 3
  – BMI <30 kg/m^2
  – Absence of insulin resistance and steatosis
  – Absence of HIV
  – Recent infection (e.g., needle stick)
- HCV RNA level without 2 log drop at week 24 indicates nonresponse; consider switching to interferon alfacon-1 (Infergen, daily injections) and continue combination therapy ≥6 months.
- HCV RNA positive but ≥2 log drop indicates extending current therapy may be beneficial; continue up to 72 weeks if tolerated (4)[C] or switch to Infergen.
- Monitor for decompensation (low albumin, ascites, encephalopathy, GI bleed) in cirrhotics.
- Goal of therapy is SVR: Eradication of HCV by negative qualitative RNA (TMA) 6 months post-treatment (relapse extremely rare after 6 months)

DIET

- Healthy diet (low-fat, high-fiber) and exercise to prevent/treat obesity/fatty liver
- Extra protein and fluids while on IFN therapy

PATIENT EDUCATION

- Educate patients to avoid alcohol, tobacco, and drugs (including marijuana) at diagnosis; refer to rehab/12-step program and monitor for relapse.
- Caution patients against Internet/alternative medicine claims of false cures.
- Recommend avoidance of herbs (may contain hepatotoxins and contaminants) as well as hepatotoxic medications and vitamins/supplements.

PROGNOSIS

- 70–80% of acute infections become chronic.
- 30% of chronic infections will progress to cirrhosis at a rate of 1–3%/year over 10–30 years.
- 30% of cirrhosis progresses to liver failure and/or cancer (HCC); more rapid if:
  – Older age when infected; Male gender; Alcohol/substance abuse
  – HIV or HBV coinfection; Insulin resistance/diabetes (7)
- IFN therapy, regardless of viral response, slows/improves progressive fibrosis and reduces risk HCC.
- Chronic HCV is *curable* in ~50% of cases; in noncirrhotic genotype 2 or 3, cure rate ~90%

COMPLICATIONS

- Acute/subacute hepatic necrosis, liver failure, transplant and complications, death
- HCC: Risk factors include cirrhosis, age >55, male, obesity/diabetes/fatty liver, and ongoing alcohol/tobacco/marijuana/drug use.

REFERENCES

1. Ghany M, Strader D et al. AASLD Practice Guidelines: Diagnosis, Management, and Treatment of Hepatitis C: An Update. *Hepatology*. 2009;49:1335–74.
2. Chronic Hepatitis C: Current Disease Management, NIH Pub. no. 07-4230 Nov. 2006. Available at: http://digestive.niddk.nih.gov/ddiseases/pubs/chronichepc/ Accessed 5/15/10.
3. Plequezuelo M, et al. Does HCV antiviral therapy decrease the risk of hepatocellular carcinoma? *Curr Hepatitis Rep*. 2008;7:72–9.
4. Agudelo E, et al. Optimizing therapy in treatment-naïve genotype 1 patients. *Curr Hepatitis Rep*. 2008;7:64–71.
5. Shiffman ML. Optimizing the current therapy for chronic hepatitis C virus: peginterferon and ribavirin dosing and the utility of growth factors. *Clin Liver Dis*. 2008;12:487–505, vii.
6. Leevy CB. Consensus interferon and ribavirin in patients with chronic hepatitis C who were nonresponders to pegylated interferon alfa-2b and ribavirin. *Dig Dis Sci*. 2008;53:1961–6.
7. Zein N. Steatosis and metabolic syndrome: An emerging enigma in the natural history of chronic hepatitis C. *Curr Hepatitis Rep*. 2008;7:61–3.

See Also (Topic, Algorithm, Electronic Media Element)

Hepatitis A; Hepatitis B; Cirrhosis of the Liver
Algorithm: Hyperbilirubinemia

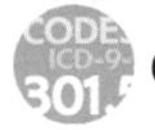

CODES

ICD9

- 070.54 Chronic hepatitis c without mention of hepatic coma
- 070.70 Unspecified viral hepatitis c without hepatic coma

CLINICAL PEARLS

- Hepatitis A&B vaccines if seronegative.
- 1 in 10 patients with hepatitis C have no identifiable risk factors.
- 15–25% of infected persons spontaneously clear their infection without treatment.

H

HEPATOMA

Michael Engels, MD
Nadeem Anwar, MD

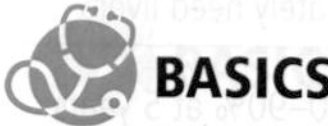

BASICS

DESCRIPTION

Primary malignant tumor of the liver arising from hepatic parenchymal cells (hepatocytes), blood vessels, or cholangioles within the liver, excluding gallbladder and biliary passages; with the exception of the rare fibrolamellar type, 85% are associated with an underlying liver disease, usually cirrhosis.

EPIDEMIOLOGY

Incidence

- 5th most common malignancy worldwide
- 3–4 new cases/100,000 of the US population per year
- Among known cirrhotics, 2–5 cases/100 cirrhotics/year

Prevalence

- Asians > whites > blacks > Hispanics > Native Americans
- Predominant age: Mean age 55–62 years in West, 2–3 decades earlier in Asia and Africa
- Predominant sex: Male > Female (3–4:1)

RISK FACTORS

- For hepatocellular carcinoma (HCC):
  - 80–90% HCC occurs in context of cirrhosis (1)[B]
  - HCC can occur with cirrhosis from any cause: Hepatitis B and C, alcoholism, hemochromatosis, nonalcoholic steatohepatitis, α_1–antitrypsin deficiency, biliary cirrhosis, autoimmune hepatitis, Wilson's disease
  - Fungal aflatoxins (contaminants of grain in Africa and Asia) have a synergistic effect with other causes of liver disease.
  - Choledochal cysts
  - Clonorchiasis
  - Tyrosinemia
  - Nonalcoholic fatty liver disease/nonalcoholic steatohepatitis (2)[C]
- For fibrolamellar type: Risk factors unknown
- For angiosarcoma: Vinyl polymer

Genetics

No known genetic pattern

GENERAL PREVENTION

- The major risk factor for HCC is cirrhosis from any cause. Prevention of cirrhosis and monitoring for tumors in patients with or at risk for cirrhosis are keys to prevention.
- Prevent hepatitis B virus (HBV) and hepatitis C virus (HCV) infection/cirrhosis. Safe sexual practices; avoid shared drug paraphernalia; HBV vaccination in high-risk individuals and all children
- Treat chronic HBV and HCV with lamivudine, adefovir, entecavir, tenofovir, or ribavirin/pegylated interferon according to guidelines to avoid cirrhosis.
- Avoid excessive alcohol use.
- Screening for cancer in at-risk individuals by ultrasonography every 6–12 months
- High risk:
  - HBV
  - HCV
  - Alcoholic cirrhosis
  - Genetic hemochromatosis
  - Primary biliary cirrhosis
  - HCC progresses gradually from dysplastic nodules through eventual vascular invasion (usually occurs after tumor reaches 2 cm diameter). For patients at risk, liver imaging should be done every 6 months (3)[B].
- Patients exposed to 10 years or more of vinyl chloride should have sonography every 6 months. New nodules should be biopsied promptly.

ETIOLOGY

- Cirrhosis accounts for 80–90% HCC. Alcoholic cirrhosis is most important in Western world. Reported risk of hepatoma in alcoholic cirrhosis is 3–10% with micronodular pattern.
- HBV and HCV independent and synergistic risk factors for HCC:
  - Associated with >70% of cases worldwide
  - Most important factor in Africa and Asia
- Chronic alcohol use
- Chronic smoking
- Mycotoxins (aflatoxins): Metabolite of the fungus *Aspergillus flavus* that contaminates foods
- Vinyl polymer, but not the finished product, produces angiosarcoma.

COMMONLY ASSOCIATED CONDITIONS

See Risk Factors.

DIAGNOSIS

- In children:
  - Feminization, precocious puberty
  - Palpable nodule on liver
  - In children aged 2–6 years, abdominal mass in liver, abdominal pain, irregular hepatomegaly
- In adults:
  - Known cirrhosis or prominent clinical signs of cirrhosis: 80%
  - Abdominal pain: 80%; right upper quadrant, dull ache to severe
  - Hepatomegaly: 80–90%; irregular, nodular, firm to hard, tender
  - Weight loss: 30%
  - Hepatic arterial bruit: 20%
  - Friction rub: Rare; more common in metastatic liver disease
  - Nausea, vomiting
  - Paraneoplastic syndrome: Hypertrophic osteoarthropathy, carcinoid syndrome, feminization, polycythemia
  - Hemoperitoneum: Most common tumor cause
  - Unexplained deterioration of stable cirrhosis
  - Budd-Chiari syndrome

DIAGNOSTIC TESTS & INTERPRETATION

Lab

- Liver function test abnormalities
- Rare paraneoplastic syndrome: Erythrocytosis, elevated calcium, low glucose
- Tumor markers:
  - α-Fetoprotein (AFP): Single most important lab test for diagnosis of HCC
  - AFP has low sensitivity for detecting early HCC (25–60% sensitivity, 80% specificity), and it is not recommended as a screening test unless ultrasound (US) is not available (1)[B].
  - Level >400 ng/mL (>400 μg/L) is diagnostic. Level >200 ng/mL highly suspicious for HCC; level does not correlate with prognosis; useful in monitoring for recurrence
  - Fibrolamellar carcinoma usually does not produce AFP.
- Disorders that may alter lab results (all cause a slight elevation in AFP):
  - Acute or chronic hepatitis
  - Germ cell tumors
  - Pregnancy

Imaging

- US (3)[B]:
  - Capable of detecting tumor >1 cm, performance dependent on examiner, technology, cirrhosis (cirrhosis decreases sensitivity)
  - May be positive when AFP is normal
  - Has been useful in serially following cases of cirrhosis to identify hepatocellular cancer when <2 cm and curable
  - If US positive, computed tomography (CT) scan or magnetic resonance imaging (MRI) to confirm (3)[B]
  - Also may be used to guide percutaneous liver biopsy and to guide other percutaneous guided therapy (injection or ablation)
- CT scan:
  - Can detect tumors at 1 cm
  - Valuable in determining extrahepatic spread of the disease
- Positron emission tomography (PET)/PET-CT improves CT detection rates.
- MRI: More sensitive than helical CT scan for early detection of HCC; may help to differentiate benign from malignant tumors; helpful in delineating the details of tumor and invasion of vessels
- Imaging of focal hepatic mass >2 cm with certain characteristic contrast enhancement features can be sufficient for diagnosis (3)[B].
- Hepatic arteriography: Less commonly used as MRI technology improves; used to define vascular anatomy for resection or embolization

Diagnostic Procedures/Surgery

- Tissue diagnosis must be made for mass seen on imaging with atypical findings for HCC or in a noncirrhotic liver. Tissue confirmation is also useful to rule out metastases from other primary sites (3)[B].
- Liver biopsy: Usually US- or CT-guided when nodules are not palpable
- Laparoscopy: Occasionally used to evaluate extent in cirrhosis

Pathological Findings

- Nodular: 75%; usually in cirrhotic liver
- Massive: Common in children and noncirrhotic livers; more prone to rupture
- Diffuse: Rare; a large part of liver is involved
- Hepatocellular origin: Most commonly multicentric, well differentiated; usually superimposed on underlying cirrhosis

DIFFERENTIAL DIAGNOSIS

- Early asymptomatic tumor; underlying liver conditions:
  - Cirrhosis
  - Chronic hepatitis
  - Benign liver nodules
  - Hamartoma
  - Hemangioma
  - Metastatic adenocarcinoma
  - Gallstones
  - Gallbladder polyp
- Late symptomatic tumor with hepatomegaly:
  - Hepatic cyst
  - Adenoma
  - Hemangioma
  - Abscess
  - Metastatic malignancy of liver
  - Cirrhosis
  - Thrombosis of hepatic veins, portal vein, or inferior vena cava
  - Active viral hepatitis or alcoholic hepatitis
- Ruptured tumor: All causes of acute abdomen
- Traumatic hemoperitoneum

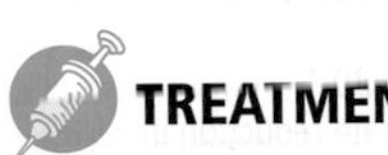

TREATMENT

MEDICATION

- Chemotherapy offers no survival benefit.
- Treatment of hepatoma in patients with HCV with pegylated interferon-α and ribavirin prolongs survival and improves quality of life.

SURGERY/OTHER PROCEDURES

- Surgical resection and liver transplantation offer highest cure rate in HCC (1)[B]:
  - Resection should be considered in children and may include up to 1 lobe of the liver.
  - In noncirrhotic patients with HCC, if preserved liver function, no portal hypertension, resection is preferred treatment. Transplantation is preferred treatment for all others who meet transplantation criteria (1)[B].
  - Advanced liver disease, medical comorbidities, extrahepatic metastases are common and result in only 15–30% of HCC patients being eligible for resection (1)[B].
  - High cure rate for both surgical options when ≤3 or fewer nodules, each <5 cm
- Percutaneous treatments best for unresectable disease, as bridge to surgical resection/transplantation, and for early-stage tumors not eligible for surgery
  - Radiofrequency ablation (RFA) considered superior to alcohol injection for localized therapy (4)[B]
  - Recent trials showed similar survival rates for RFA vs surgical resection in small HCCs, but insufficient evidence to change recommendations favoring surgery at this time (5)[B].
- Embolization of the tumor-supplying artery with chemotherapy, under radiographic guidance, is effective palliation and may make surgery possible (6)[B].
- For patients not appropriate for surgery, 2 approaches:
  - Regional transarterial therapy (which delivers chemotherapy directly to the tumor via its immediate blood supply) for intermediate-stage tumors
  - Local chemical and thermal ablative therapies (which cause tumor necrosis by injecting the agent into the tumor itself) for early-stage tumors
  - The 2 approaches can be used together and may yield a better outcome than either treatment alone (6)[B].
- Fibrolamellar variant should be treated by surgical resection, which yields excellent survival.

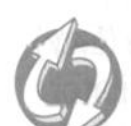

ONGOING CARE

FOLLOW-UP RECOMMENDATIONS

Patient Monitoring

- After successful resection, a high risk for recurrence
- Check AFP every 3 months.
- Ultrasound every 4–6 months

DIET

Attention to nutrition: High-calorie diet

PATIENT EDUCATION

Emphasize preventive measures and HBV vaccine.

PROGNOSIS

- Unresectable symptomatic tumors: Grave; patients seldom live >6 months.
- Resectable asymptomatic tumors:
  - Surgery is curative in >70% of children, 40% of adults
  - Surgery is curative in >80% of tumors <3 cm in cirrhotics.
- Transplantation: Same survival as that for tumor-free patients when hepatoma is incidentally discovered or is <2 cm in diameter; 5-year survival rate of >70% with 1 lesion <5 cm or maximum of 3 lesions <3 cm (UNOS criteria) (3)[B]

COMPLICATIONS

- Rupture
- Hemoperitoneum
- Liver failure
- Cachexia
- Metastases to other organs
- Thrombosis of portal, hepatic, renal veins

REFERENCES

1. Cha CH, Saif MW, Yamane BH, Weber SM et al. Hepatocellular carcinoma: current management. *Curr Probl Surg*. 2010;47:10–67.
2. Siegel AB, Zhu AX et al. Metabolic syndrome and hepatocellular carcinoma: two growing epidemics with a potential link. *Cancer*. 2009;115:5651–61.
3. El-Serag HB, Marrero JA, Rudolph L, Reddy KR et al. Diagnosis and treatment of hepatocellular carcinoma. *Gastroenterology*. 2008;134:1752–63.
4. Cho YK, Kim JK, Kim MY, Rhim H, Han JK et al. Systematic review of randomized trials for hepatocellular carcinoma treated with percutaneous ablation therapies. *Hepatology*. 2009;49:453–9.
5. Delis S, Bakoyiannis A, Papailiou J, Tassopoulos N, Dervenis C et al. Liver resection vs radio-frequency ablation in the treatment of small hepatocellular carcinoma. *Surg Oncol*. 2009;
6. Garrean S, Hering J, Helton WS, et al. A primer on transarterial, chemical, and thermal ablative therapies for hepatic tumors. *Am J Surg*. 2007;194:79–88.

ADDITIONAL READING

- Colli A, Fraquelli M, Casazza G, et al. Accuracy of ultrasonography, spiral CT, magnetic resonance, and alpha-fetoprotein in diagnosing hepatocellular carcinoma: a systematic review. *Am J Gastroenterol*. 2006;101:513–23.
- Stipa F, Yoon SS, Liau KH, et al. Outcome of patients with fibrolamellar hepatocellular carcinoma. *Cancer*. 2006;106:1331–8.

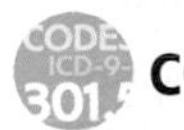

CODES

ICD9

155.0 Malignant neoplasm of liver, primary

CLINICAL PEARLS

- With benign liver tumors, most patients will have normal liver function tests; 97% with HCC will have at least 1 abnormal test.
- Fibrolamellar carcinoma, which occurs at younger age (mean 25 years), is more likely to present with resectable lesions and higher cure rate after resection (6)[B].
- In Africa and Asia, there is a younger onset (3rd and 4th decades); Male:Female ratio is 6–7:1; aflatoxin and HBV are the major factors; more progressive and fulminant; more likely to be unresectable at presentation.

H

HERNIA

Leah A. Burnett, MD

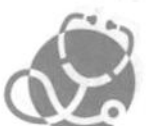

BASICS

DESCRIPTION

This topic pertains to external hernias of the groin and abdominal wall. These are an abnormal protrusion of the contents of the abdominal cavity through a fascial defect in the abdominal wall:

- Definitions:
  - Reducible: Extruded sac and its contents can be returned to its original intra-abdominal position, either spontaneously or with gentle manual manipulation.
  - Irreducible/incarcerated: Extruded sac and its contents cannot be returned to its original intra-abdominal position.
  - Strangulated: Compromise of blood supply to hernia sac contents
  - Richter: Partial circumference of bowel is incarcerated or strangulated. Partial wall damage may occur, increasing potential for bowel rupture and peritonitis.
  - Sliding (wall of a viscus forms part of the wall of the inguinal hernia sac)R-cecum, L-sigmoid colon
- Types:
  - Groin: Inguinal and femoral
  - Inguinal:
    - Direct inguinal: Acquired; herniation through defect in transversalis fascia of abdominal wall medial to inferior epigastric vessels; increased frequency with age as fascia weakens
    - Indirect inguinal: Congenital; herniation lateral to the inferior epigastric vessels, through internal inguinal ring into inguinal canal. A "complete hernia" is one that descends into the scrotum, while an "incomplete hernia" remains within the inguinal canal.
  - Pantaloon: Combination of direct and indirect inguinal hernia with protrusion of abdominal wall on both sides of the epigastric vessels
  - Femoral: Descends through the femoral canal deep to the inguinal ligament. Because of the narrow neck of a femoral hernia, this type of hernia is especially prone to incarceration and strangulation.
  - Other: Obturator, sciatic, perineal
  - Incisional or ventral: Iatrogenic, herniation through a defect in the anterior abdominal wall at the site of a prior surgical incision
  - Umbilical: Defect occurs at umbilical ring tissue
  - Epigastric: Protrudes through the linea alba above the level of the umbilicus. These may develop at exit points of small paramidline nerves and vessels, or through an area of congenital weakness in the linea alba.
- Other:
  - Interparietal (e.g., Spigelian hernia): Hernia sac insinuates itself between layers of the abdominal wall; strangulation common, often mistaken for tumor or abscess

Geriatric Considerations

Abdominal wall hernias increase with advancing age, with significant increase in risk during surgical repair.

Pregnancy Considerations

- Increased intra-abdominal pressure and hormone imbalances may contribute to increased risk of abdominal wall hernias
- Umbilical hernias associated with multiple, prolonged deliveries

EPIDEMIOLOGY

Incidence

- 75–80% groin hernias, including inguinal and femoral
- 2–20% incisional/ventral, depending on whether surgery was associated with infection or contamination
- 3–10% umbilical, considered congenital
- 1–3% other
- Groin:
  - 6–27% lifetime risk in adult men
  - Approximately 50% of children under 2 will have a patent processus vaginalis, decreasing to 40% after age 2. Only between 25% and 50% will become clinically significant.
  - Inguinal hernia found in less than 5% of newborns, but M:F ratio is 10:1
  - Increased incidence in premature infants (1)[B]
  - Increased incidence in patients with abdominal aortic aneurysms
- Incisional/ventral: ~10–23% of abdominal surgeries complicated by an incisional hernia.
- Umbilical: 10–20% of newborns (2)

Prevalence

- Inguinal hernias more prevalent in men; femoral and umbilical hernias are more prevalent in women.
- Incisional/ventral hernias are more prevalent in obese or overweight men, as well as more prevalent among smokers. The opposite may be true for inguinal hernias (3)[C].

RISK FACTORS

Increased abdominal pressure, coughing, heavy lifting, constipation or straining with stool, pregnancy, ascites, prostatism, obesity, advancing age and loss of tissue turgor, smoking, steroid use, low birth weight, prematurity

Genetics

No known genetic pattern

PATHOPHYSIOLOGY

Loss of tissue strength and elasticity, especially with aging or congenital defect in abdominal fascia

ETIOLOGY

In general, a defect in the fascia of the abdominal wall. Most pediatric hernias are congenital defects (e.g., patent processus vaginalis), while most adult hernias are a result of acquired weakness in the tissues of the anterior abdominal wall.

COMMONLY ASSOCIATED CONDITIONS

Obesity, chronic obstructive pulmonary disease, multiple abdominal surgeries, pregnancy, advanced age, Ehlers-Danlos, Marfan, Hurler-Hunter, PKD, osteogenesis imperfecta, Beckwith-Wiedemann syndrome, Down syndrome, abdominal aortic aneurysm

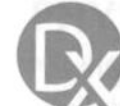

DIAGNOSIS

HISTORY

- While many hernias are asymptomatic, symptoms may include pain, nausea, vomiting, bloating, and relief with reclining.
- Hernia may be directly observed as protrusion through abdominal wall during maneuvers that increase intra-abdominal pressure.

PHYSICAL EXAM

- Examination should initially occur with patient standing and examiner placing finger in inguinal canal via the scrotum. Exam should also be performed with patient in supine position and with cough.
- Inguinal (superior to inguinal ligament):
  - Direct inguinal hernia: Finger in inguinal canal finds defect of the transversalis fascia as a deep (posterior to anterior) bulge palpated by pad of finger with increased intra-abdominal pressure.
  - Indirect inguinal hernia: Finger in inguinal canal finds a persistent process vaginalis as a bulge (lateral to medial) palpated by fingertip, and may extend down into scrotum.
- Femoral (inferior to inguinal ligament): Bulge in upper middle thigh; neck of the sac will protrude lateral to and below a finger placed on the pubic tubercle
- Umbilical: Palpable protrusion at umbilius
- Incisional/ventral: Palpable protrusion at site of prior abdominal incision
- Epigastric: Majority occur just off midline, above umbilicus.

DIAGNOSTIC TESTS & INTERPRETATION

Imaging

Initial approach

Hernia evaluation rarely require imaging; reserve for suspected abdominal hernia or unclear diagnosis. Plain radiographs are often used to look for evidence of obstructive signs including dilated proximal bowel and bowel stacking.

- Ultrasonography can be used to assess inguinal hernias.
- CT or tangential radiography may also be used; best for incisional and abdominal wall hernias.
- Herniography is no longer recommended but may be useful in interpreting obscure hernia symptoms in an atypical presentation (4)[A].
- CT Imaging is frequently used to evaluate post-surgical patients with complaints of abdominal pain and is considered the gold standard there.

Pediatric Considerations

- There is insufficient evidence for contralateral exploration in pediatric patients, except using ultrasonography.

Follow-Up & Special Considerations

For occult hernias not be well appreciated on exam or with imaging, diagnostic laparoscopy may be beneficial.

DIFFERENTIAL DIAGNOSIS

Lymphadenopathy, hydrocele, lipoma, varices, cryptorchidism, abscess, tumor, sports hernia (athletic pubalgia), pelvic fractures, adductor tears, omphalomesenteric duct, urachal cyst.

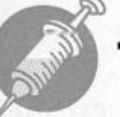

TREATMENT

Acute setting:

- Pain medication recommended for symptomatic hernias.
- Strangulated hernias should be surgically repaired as early as possible to prevent complications such as necrosis and viscus perforation.
- Manual reduction of incarcerated hernia improves outcomes by allowing for elective repair after improvement of acute swelling and inflammation (5).
- Complication rate is near 20 times greater in emergent repair of pediatric inguinal hernias than elective procedures (6)[A].

MEDICATION

- Antibiotics: Antibiotic prophylaxis did not reduce wound infections after groin hernia repairs.
- Pain: Local anesthetic during surgical repair results in significant in reduction of postoperative pain (6)[A]. Tension-free procedures such as Lichtenstein may be performed under local anesthesia.

ADDITIONAL TREATMENT

Geriatric Considerations

Use of a truss (external supportive device) for direct inguinal hernias common; no data exists on their long-term efficacy, and are often considered a temporizing measure

Issues for Referral

Warn patients of symptoms or signs of incarceration or strangulation (acute abdominal pain, fever, bloody bowel movements) mandate immediate self referral to emergency room.

SURGERY/OTHER PROCEDURES

All inguinal hernias should be surgically repaired, but watchful waiting in the asymptomatic patient is a safe option if significant comorbidities may compromise emergent repair (6)[A]:

- Incarceration and strangulation are absolute indications for hernia repair.
- Contraindications: Patients who are not surgical candidates based on cardiovascular risk factors:
  - Elective repair should be avoided in pregnant patients or those with active infections.
- Special considerations:
  - Umbilical hernias < 0.5 cm usually obliterate and can be managed by observation (2).
  - Umbilical hernias in children age 2–4 years may be observed as there is a high rate of spontaneous closure.
  - Semielective surgical repair can be safe during pregnancy if delayed until after 2nd trimester.
  - Women had lower recurrence rates with laparoscopic methods than with Lichtenstein open method.
  - Ascites is not a strict contraindication for surgical repair. There is a greater risk of strangulation and complication without repair than the increased risks associated with repair in the presence of ascites.
  - The more emergent hernia operations can be performed using the same methods for nonacute situations. However, incarceration with strangulation my require laparotomy with partial bowel resection.
- Gold standard:
  - Inguinal hernia:
    - Open: Lichtenstein with mesh (37%) or mesh plug (34%): Decreased recurrence rates (6)[A]
    - Laparoscopic (14%) with mesh: Decreased hospital stay and postoperative pain (6)[A]
      - Requires general anesthesia.
      - Transabdominal preperitoneal (TAPP) versus total extraperitoneal (TEP)
    - Pediatric: Recovery and outcome similar after open and laparoscopic repair. Laparoscopic hernia repair associated with increased operation/anesthesia time and postoperative pain.
  - Incisional/ventral:
    - Laparoscopic repair with mesh for simple, noncomplex hernias
    - Open repair with mesh for complex or recurrent hernias
  - Umbilical:
    - Pediatric: Open excision and closure with suture
    - Adult: Open repair with mesh or plug may reduce hernia recurrence.
- Newer techniques:
  - Prolene hernia system
  - Biologic wound closure system: Reduced recurrence in contaminated procedures
- Complications:
  - Recurrence
  - Postoperative pain, temporary or chronic: Improved in laparoscopic approach versus open
  - Wound infection
  - Injury to cord structures in inguinal herniorrhaphy

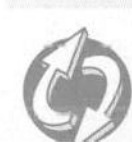

ONGOING CARE

PATIENT EDUCATION

Cleveland Clinic: http://my.clevelandclinic.org/disorders/hernia/hic_hernia.aspx

- Groin hernias: University of Chicago Children's Hospital: http://www.uchicagokidshospital.org/specialties/general-surgery/patient-guides/inguinal-hernia.html
- Incisional/ventral: Society of American Gastrointestinal and Endoscopic Surgeons: http://sages.org/sagespublication.php?doc=PI10
- Umbilical hernias: Boston Children's Hospital: http://www.childrenshospital.org/az/Site1018/mainpageS1018P0.html

PROGNOSIS

- Groin (pediatric): Low recurrence rates (<3%) with surgical treatment; may spontaneously resolve in infants.
- Groin (adult): ≥1%/year risk of bowel strangulation without surgical treatment; 0–10% postoperative recurrence rates, depending on surgeon experience level and method
- Incisional/ventral: 3–5% postoperative occurrence: 2–17% post repair recurrence, increased to 20–46% in larger hernias
- Umbilical (pediatric):
  - High rate of spontaneous resolution
  - Hernia less likely to close further in older children and in children with larger defects
- Umbilical (adult): Up to 11% postoperative recurrence rate
- Epigastric: Most will ultimately become incarcerated and/or strangulated without surgical treatment. Recurrence is high due to frequency of missed defects during repair.

REFERENCES

1. Brandt ML. Pediatric hernias. *Surg Clin North Am*. 2008;88:27–43, vii-viii.
2. Snyder CL. Current management of umbilical abnormalities and related anomalies. *Semin Pediatr Surg*. 2007;16:41–9.
3. Rosemar A, Angerås U, Rosengren A. Body mass index and groin hernia: a 34-year follow-up study in Swedish men. *Ann Surg*. 2008;247:1064–8.
4. Ng TT, Hamlin JA, Kahn AM. Herniography: analysis of its role and limitations. *Hernia*. 2008.
5. Lau ST, Lee YH, Caty MG. Current management of hernias and hydroceles. *Semin Pediatr Surg*. 2007;16:50–7.
6. Matthews RD, Neumayer L. Inguinal hernia in the 21st century: an evidence-based review. *Curr Probl Surg*. 2008;45:261–312.

See Also (Topic, Algorithm, Electronic Media Element)

Algorithms: Lower Abdominal Pain (R, Lt.); Intestinal Obstruction; Pelvic Pain

CODES

ICD9

- 550.10 Unilateral or unspecified inguinal hernia, with obstruction, without mention of gangrene
- 550.90 Unilateral or unspecified inguinal hernia, without mention of obstruction or gangrene
- 552.00 Unilateral or unspecified femoral hernia with obstruction

CLINICAL PEARLS

- Groin: Inguinal and femoral:
- Inguinal:
  - Direct inguinal: Acquired; herniation through defect in transversalis fascia of abdominal wall medial to inferior epigastric vessels; increased frequency with age as fascia weakens
  - Indirect inguinal: Congenital; herniation lateral to the inferior epigastric vessels through internal inguinal ring into inguinal canal. A "complete hernia" is one that descends into the scrotum, while an "incomplete hernia" remains within the inguinal canal.
  - Pantaloon: Combination of direct and indirect inguinal hernia with protrusion of abdominal wall on both sides of the epigastric vessels
  - Femoral: Descends through the femoral canal deep to the inguinal ligament. Because of the narrow neck of a femoral hernia, this type of hernia is especially prone to incarceration and strangulation.
  - Other: Obturator, sciatic, perineal
- Incisional or ventral: Iatrogenic; herniation through a defect in the anterior abdominal wall at the site of a prior surgical incision
- Umbilical: Defect occurs at umbilical ring tissue.
- Epigastric: Protrudes through the linea alba above the level of the umbilicus. These may develop at exit points of small paramidline nerves and vessels, or through an area of congenital weakness in the linea alba.

H

HERPANGINA

Aamir Siddiqi, MD

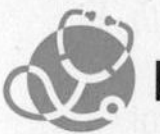

BASICS

DESCRIPTION

- Infectious disease caused by coxsackievirus group A
- Characteristics:
  - Fever of short duration
  - Typical vesicular or ulcerated lesions in the posterior pharynx or on the soft palate
  - Incubation period is 4 days.
- Usual course: Acute and self-limited
- System(s) affected: Endocrine/Metabolic; GI

EPIDEMIOLOGY

Incidence

- Year round in tropical climate; summer and fall in temperate climate (1)[B]
- Predominant age: 3 months–16 years
- Predominant sex: Male = Female.

RISK FACTORS

Contact with infected person

GENERAL PREVENTION

- Avoid contact with infected individual.
- The mode of transfer is fecal-oral, so general hygiene (hand-washing) is suggested.

ETIOLOGY

- Common: Coxsackievirus A, types 1–10, 16, and 22 (2)[B]
- Infrequent:
  - Coxsackievirus B, types 1–5
  - Echovirus, types 6, 9, 11, 17, 22, and 25
  - Other enterovirus (3)[B]

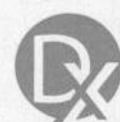

DIAGNOSIS

HISTORY

The patient may have low- or high-grade fever, general malaise, sore throat, and characteristic oropharyngeal lesions.

PHYSICAL EXAM

- Bilateral discrete vesicles, gray base
- Erythematous patches
- Vesicles may rupture to form ulcers.
- Posterior pharynx location: Pharynx, tonsils, soft palate, little involvement of anterior 2/3 of mouth
- Oropharyngeal lesions in the form of vesicles with erythematous edges
- Anorexia
- Drooling
- Sore throat
- Fever
- Malaise
- Irritability
- Listlessness
- Local pain
- Emesis
- Backache
- Headache
- Coryza
- Diarrhea

DIAGNOSTIC TESTS & INTERPRETATION

- This is a clinical diagnosis, so tests are usually not necessary.
- Complement fixation
- Hemagglutinin inhibition tests
- Serum antibodies to coxsackievirus: Titers should show a 4-fold rise in serial samples.

Lab

- Generally no lab work is necessary.
- Slight leukocytosis
- Positive viral culture—mouth washings, stool

DIFFERENTIAL DIAGNOSIS

- Herpes simplex:
  - Multiple ulcers on lips and anterior mouth
  - Diagnose with herpes culture.
- Drug reactions: Cutaneous lesions often present (urticaria, erythema multiforme)
- Recurrent aphthous stomatitis:
  - Buccal, labial, alveolar, mucosal ulcers
  - Recurrent crops
  - Few systemic symptoms
- Lichen planus: Painful ulcer, white lacy pattern on mucosa or may have cutaneous lesions that are purple and pruritic
- Hand, foot, and mouth disease: Classic distribution of vesicular rash on hands, buttocks, feet, and mouth